S0-BHX-649

VASCULAR SURGERY

VASCULAR SURGERY

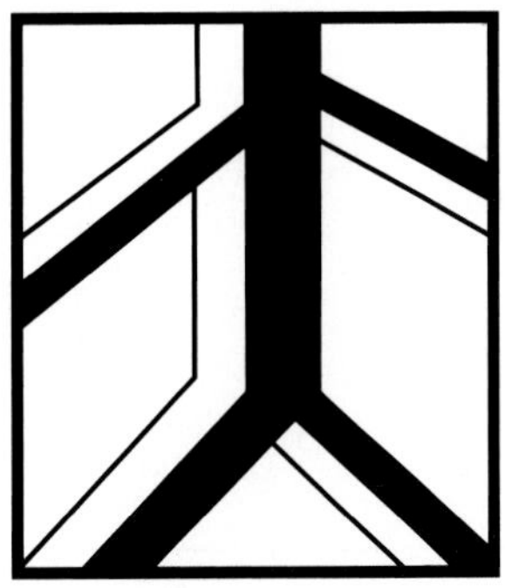

Fourth Edition

Robert B. Rutherford, M.D.
Professor of Surgery
University of Colorado Health Sciences Center
Denver, Colorado

Volume

I

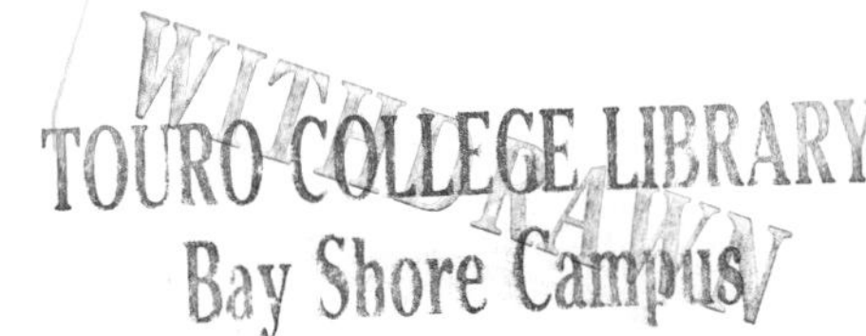

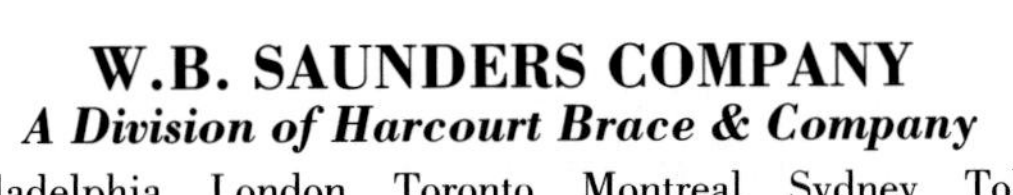
W.B. SAUNDERS COMPANY
A Division of Harcourt Brace & Company
Philadelphia London Toronto Montreal Sydney Tokyo

W.B. SAUNDERS COMPANY
A Division of
Harcourt Brace & Company

The Curtis Center
Independence Square West
Philadelphia, Pennsylvania 19106

Library of Congress Cataloging-in-Publication Data

Vascular surgery / [edited by] Robert B. Rutherford.—4th ed.

p. cm.

Includes bibliographical references.

ISBN 0–7216–3836–8 (set).—
ISBN 0–7216–3837–6 (v. 1).—ISBN 0–7216–3838–4 (v. 2)

1. Blood-vessels—Surgery. I. Rutherford, Robert B.

[DNLM: 1. Vascular Surgery. WG 170 V3311 1995]

RD598.5.V37 1995

617.4′13—dc20
DNLM/DLC 93–40051

VASCULAR SURGERY

ISBN Volume 1 0–7216–3837–6
Volume 2 0–7216–3838–4
Set 0–7216–3836–8

Printed in the United States of America

Last digit is the print number: 9 8 7 6 5 4 3

This book is dedicated to

Richard F. Kempczinski, M.D.

By his contributions to vascular surgery, to this book, and in so many ways, to the profession itself, he has set standards of excellence that are unlikely to be surpassed.

Associate Editors

Assistant Editors

CONTRIBUTORS

M. Samy Abdou, M.D.
Plastic Surgery Research Fellow, UCLA Medical Center; Wadsworth Veterans Administration Medical Center, Los Angeles, California
Excisional Operations for Chronic Lymphedema

Sanford D. Altman, M.D.
Interventional Radiologist, Miami Heart Institute, Department of Radiology, Miami Beach, Florida
Principles of Angiography

Charles M. Anderson, M.D., Ph.D.
Assistant Professor of Radiology, Department of Radiology, University of California, San Francisco; Veterans Administration Medical Center, San Francisco, California
Magnetic Resonance Angiography (Chapter 6)

Enrico Ascer, M.D.
Professor of Surgery, State University of New York Health Science Center at Brooklyn; Chief, Vascular Surgery Services, Maimonides Medical Center, Brooklyn, New York
Secondary Arterial Reconstructions in the Lower Extremity

Eric R. Ashby, M.D.
Research Fellow, Division of Plastic Surgery, UCLA School of Medicine; Resident, General Surgery, Department of Surgery, UCLA School of Medicine, Los Angeles, California
Excisional Operations for Chronic Lymphedema

J. Dennis Baker, M.D.
Professor of Surgery, UCLA School of Medicine, Los Angeles; Chief, Vascular Surgery Section, Veterans Administration Medical Center, Sepulveda, California
The Vascular Laboratory: Diagnosis and Management of Cerebrovascular Disease

William H. Baker, M.D.
Professor of Surgery and Head, Section of Peripheral Vascular Surgery, Stritch School of Medicine, Loyola University, Chicago; Staff, Foster G. McGaw Hospital (LUMC); Attending Staff, Hines Veterans Administration Hospital, Hines, Illinois
Arteriovenous Fistulae of the Aorta and Its Major Branches

Dennis F. Bandyk, M.D.
Professor of Surgery and Director, Division of Vascular Surgery, University of South Florida College of Medicine, Tampa, Florida
Infection in Prosthetic Vascular Grafts

Gary J. Becker, M.D.
Clinical Professor of Radiology, University of Miami School of Medicine; Director of Interventional Radiology, Miami Vascular Institute, Baptist Hospital of Miami, Miami, Florida
Limitations of Peripheral Angioplasty and the Role of New Devices (Chapter 20)

Denis D. Bensard, M.D.
Assistant Professor of Surgery, University of Colorado Health Sciences Center, Denver, Colorado; Pediatric Surgery Fellow, The Children's Hospital and Instructor in Surgery, Ohio State University, Columbus, Ohio
Preoperative Cardiac Evaluation of Patients for Vascular Surgery

Alejandro Berenstein, M.D.
Professor of Radiology and Neurosurgery, New York University School of Medicine; Attending in Radiology and Neurosurgery, New York University Medical Center, New York, New York
Peripheral Arteriovenous Fistulae; Congenital Vascular Malformations

Thomas M. Bergamini, M.D.
Assistant Professor of Surgery, University of Louisville School of Medicine, Louisville, Kentucky
Infection in Prosthetic Vascular Grafts

John J. Bergan, M.D.
Clinical Professor of Surgery, University of California, San Diego, Medical School, San Diego, California, and Uniformed Services University of The Health Sciences, Bethesda, Maryland; Scripps Memorial Hospital, La Jolla, California
Adventitial Cystic Disease of the Popliteal Artery; Sclerotherapy: Technique and Application

Ramon Berguer, M.D., Ph.D.
Professor of Surgery, Wayne State University; Chief, Division of Vascular Surgery, Harper Hospital, Detroit, Michigan
Vertebrobasilar Ischemia: Indications, Techniques, and Results of Surgical Repair

Scott S. Berman, M.D.
Assistant Professor of Clinical Surgery, University of Arizona College of Medicine; Staff Surgeon, University of Arizona Health Sciences Center, Tucson, Arizona
Patient Evaluation and Preparation for Amputation

Victor M. Bernhard, M.D.
Professor and Chief, Vascular Surgery, University of Arizona College of Medicine; Staff, University of Arizona Health Sciences Center and Veterans Administration Center, Tucson, Arizona
Aortoenteric Fistulae; Introduction and General Considerations (Section VIII); Profundaplasty

Fred Bongard, M.D.
Associate Professor of Surgery, UCLA School of Medicine; Chief of Surgical Critical Care and Director of Surgical Education, Harbor–UCLA Medical Center, Los Angeles, California
Thoracic and Abdominal Vascular Trauma

David C. Brewster, M.D.
Associate Clinical Professor of Surgery, Harvard Medical School; Attending Surgeon, Massachusetts General Hospital, Boston, Massachusetts
Prosthetic Grafts; Arterial Thromboembolism; Direct Reconstruction for Aortoiliac Occlusive Disease

T. J. Bunt, M.D., F.A.C.S.
Professor of Surgery, Loma Linda University; Director, Vascular Fellowship, and Chief of Vascular Surgery, Pettit Veterans Administration Medical Center, Loma Linda, California
Revascularization Versus Amputation

Ronald W. Busuttil, M.D., Ph.D.
Professor of Surgery, UCLA School of Medicine, Center for the Health Sciences, Los Angeles, California
Coiling and Kinking of the Carotid Artery

John A. Butler, M.D.
Associate Professor of Surgery and Chief, Surgical Oncology, University of California, Irvine, School of Medicine; UCI Medical Center, Long Beach Veterans Administration Hospital, Orange, California
Long-Term Venous Access

Gary R. Caputo, M.D.
Associate Professor of Radiology and Bioengineering and Associate Director, Magnetic Resonance Science Center, Department of Radiology, University of California, San Francisco, San Francisco, California
Magnetic Resonance Angiography (Chapter 6)

Stephen W. K. Cheng, M.S., F.R.C.S.
Lecturer, Department of Surgery, The University of Hong Kong, Queen Mary Hospital, Hong Kong
Neurogenic Thoracic Outlet Syndrome

Kenneth J. Cherry, Jr., M.D.
Associate Professor, Mayo Graduate School of Medicine; Consultant and Head, Division of Vascular Surgery, Mayo Clinic; Saint Mary's Hospital of Rochester and Rochester Methodist Hospital, Rochester, Minnesota
Arteriosclerotic Occlusive Disease of Brachiocephalic Arteries

Albert K. Chin, M.D.
Vice President of Research, Origin Medsystems, Inc., Menlo Park, California
Arterial Thromboembolism

Richard W. Chitwood, M.D.
Resident, Department of Surgery, St. Joseph Mercy Hospital, Ann Arbor, Michigan
The Natural History, Pathophysiology, and Nonoperative Treatment of Chronic Venous Insufficiency

G. Patrick Clagett, M.D.
Professor of Surgery, The University of Texas Southwestern Medical Center at Dallas; Chief, Vascular Surgery, and Medical Director, Center for Vascular Disease, Zale Lipshy University Hospital and Parkland Memorial Hospital; Attending Staff, Veterans Administration Medical Center, Dallas, Texas
Upper Extremity Aneurysms

Elizabeth T. Clark, M.D.
Vascular Surgery Fellow, University of Chicago School of Medicine and University of Chicago Hospitals and Clinics, Chicago, Illinois
Pseudoaneurysms

Alexander W. Clowes, M.D.
Professor of Surgery, University of Washington School of Medicine; Attending Physician and Vascular Surgeon, Department of Surgery, University of Washington Medical Center, Seattle, Washington
Pathologic Intimal Hyperplasia as a Response to Vascular Injury and Reconstruction

Stanley N. Cohen, M.D.
Professor of Neurology, UCLA School of Medicine; Assistant Chief of Neurology, West Los Angeles Veterans Administration Medical Center, Los Angeles, California
Clinical Manifestations and Evaluation of Patients With Ischemic Cerebrovascular Disease

Anthony J. Comerota, M.D., F.A.C.S.
Professor of Surgery and Vice-Chairman, Department of Surgery, Temple University School of Medicine; Chief of Vascular Surgery, Temple University Hospital, Philadelphia, Pennsylvania
Overview (Chapter 6); Graft Thrombosis and Thromboembolic Complications; Venous Thromboembolism

Timothy P. Connall, M.D.
Surgical Research Fellow, University of California, Irvine, Medical Center; Orange, California
Vascular Access for Hemodialysis

Daniel P. Connelly, M.D.
Associate Professor of Surgery, Uniformed Services University of the Health Sciences; Chairman, Department of Surgery, Malcolm Grow Medical Center, Andrews Air Force Base, Washington, District of Columbia
The Arterial Autograft

Joseph S. Coselli, M.D.
Associate Professor of Surgery, Baylor College of Medicine; Attending Surgeon, The Methodist Hospital, Houston, Texas
Thoracoabdominal Aortic Aneurysm

Earl D. Cottrell, M.D.
Assistant Clinical Professor of Surgery, Loma Linda University School of Medicine, Loma Linda, California; Division Head, Vascular Surgery, Family Health Plan of Utah, Salt Lake City, Utah
Management of Uncommon Lesions Affecting the Extracranial Vessels

Enrique Criado, M.D.
Assistant Professor of Surgery, University of North Carolina School of Medicine, Division of Vascular Surgery; Attending Surgeon, University of North Carolina Hospitals, Chapel Hill, North Carolina
Laboratory Evaluation of the Patient With Chronic Venous Insufficiency

Jack L. Cronenwett, M.D.
Professor of Surgery and Chief, Section of Vascular Surgery, Dartmouth-Hitchcock Medical Center, Lebanon, New Hampshire
Intraoperative Assessment of Technical Adequacy

Bruce S. Cutler, M.D.
Professor of Surgery, University of Massachusetts Medical School; Chairman, Division of Vascular Surgery, University of Massachusetts Medical Center, Worcester, Massachusetts
Cardiac Complications

Michael D. Dake, M.D.
Assistant Professor of Radiology and Medicine, Department of Radiology, Stanford University School of Medicine; Chief, Cardiovascular and Interventional Radiology; Co-Director, Catheterization/Angiography Laboratories, Stanford University Medical Center, Stanford, California
Radiologic Evaluation and Treatment of Renovascular Hypertension

Richard H. Dean, M.D., B.A.
Professor, The Bowman Gray School of Medicine of Wake Forest University; Chief of Surgery, North Carolina Baptist Hospital, Winston-Salem, North Carolina
Renal Complications; Renovascular Hypertension: An Overview; Evaluation and Management of Ischemic Neuropathy; Ex Vivo Renal Artery Reconstructions; Acute Occlusive Events Involving the Renal Vessels

Larry-Stuart Deutsch, M.D., C.M., F.R.C.P.(C.)
Professor and Chief-of-Service: Vascular and Interventional Radiology, University of California, Irvine, Medical Center, Orange, California
Anatomy and Angiographic Diagnosis of Extracranial and Intracranial Vascular Disease

Janette D. Durham, M.D.
Assistant Professor of Radiology, University of Colorado School of Medicine, Denver, Colorado
Endovascular Interventions for Lower Extremity Ischemia

Joseph R. Durham, M.D.
Associate Professor of Surgery, Division of Vascular Surgery, Northwestern University Medical School; Attending Surgeon and Medical Director, Blood Flow Laboratory, Northwestern Memorial Hospital; Chief, Section of Vascular Surgery, and Medical Director, Blood Flow Laboratory, Columbus Hospital, Chicago, Illinois
Lower Extremity Amputation Levels: Indications, Methods of Determining Appropriate Level, Technique, Prognosis

James M. Edwards, M.D.
Assistant Professor of Surgery, Oregon Health Sciences University; Staff Surgeon, Portland Veterans Affairs Hospital, Portland, Oregon
Occlusive and Vasospastic Diseases Involving Distal Upper Extremity Arteries—Raynaud's Syndrome

Errol E. Erlandson, M.D.
Clinical Associate Professor of Surgery, University of Michigan Medical School; Attending Surgeon, St. Joseph Mercy Hospital, Ann Arbor, Michigan
Upper Extremity Revascularization

Calvin B. Ernst, M.D.
Clinical Professor of Surgery, University of Michigan Medical School, Ann Arbor; Head of Vascular Surgery, Henry Ford Hospital, Detroit, Michigan
Infected Aneurysms; Colon Ischemia Following Aortic Reconstruction

Daniel F. Fisher, Jr., M.D.
Associate Professor of Surgery, Chattanooga Unit of the University of Tennessee College of Medicine; Staff Surgeon, Erlanger Medical Center, Chattanooga, Tennessee
Complications of Amputation

Steven Fitzgerald, M.D.
Assistant Professor of Radiology, Northwestern University Medical School; Attending Staff, Northwestern Memorial Hospital, Chicago, Illinois
Computed Tomography and Magnetic Resonance Imaging in Vascular Disease (Chapter 6)

D. Preston Flanigan, M.D.
Clinical Professor of Surgery, University of California, Irvine; Co-Director, Vascular Laboratory, St. Joseph Hospital, Orange, California; Visiting Professor of Surgery, University of Illinois, Chicago, Illinois
Postoperative Sexual Dysfunction Following Aortoiliac Revascularization

Thomas J. Fogarty, M.D.
Professor of Surgery, Stanford University School of Medicine and Stanford University Medical Center, Stanford, California
Fogarty Catheter Thrombectomy (Chapter 21); Arterial Thromboembolism

Richard J. Fowl, M.D.
Associate Professor of Surgery, University of Cincinnati Medical Center, Cincinnati, Ohio
Popliteal Artery Entrapment

John Frazee, M.D.
Associate Professor of Surgery, Division of Neurosurgery, UCLA School of Medicine, Los Angeles, California
Extracranial-Intracranial Bypass: Current Status

Julie A. Freischlag, M.D.
Associate Professor of Surgery, Department of Vascular Surgery, Medical College of Wisconsin; Associate Professor of Surgery, John Doyne Medical Center; Chief, Vascular Surgery, Zablocki Veterans Administration Medical Center, Milwaukee, Wisconsin
Peritoneal Dialysis

James C. A. Fuchs, M.D.
Associate Professor of Surgery, Johns Hopkins University School of Medicine; Chief of Surgery, The Union Memorial Hospital, Baltimore, Maryland
Atherogenesis and the Medical Management of Atherosclerosis

Raju H. Gandhi, M.D.
Lamb Fellow for Vascular Research, Columbia University, and St. Luke's–Roosevelt Hospital Center, New York, New York
Arterial Aneurysms: Etiologic Considerations

Bruce L. Gewertz, M.D.
Dallas B. Phemister Professor of Surgery and Chairman, Department of Surgery, University of Chicago, Pritzker School of Medicine, and University of Chicago Hospitals and Clinics, Chicago, Illinois
Pseudoaneurysms

Joseph M. Giordano, M.D.
Professor and Chairman of the Department of Surgery, George Washington University and George Washington University Medical Center, Washington, District of Columbia
Takayasu's Disease: Nonspecific Aortoarteritis

Seymour Glagov, M.D.
Professor of Pathology, University of Chicago, Pritzker School of Medicine, and University of Chicago Medical Center, Chicago, Illinois
Artery Wall Pathology in Atherosclerosis

Peter Gloviczki, M.D.
Professor of Surgery, Mayo Graduate School of Medicine, Mayo Clinic and Foundation; Staff Surgeon, Saint Mary's Hospital of Rochester and Rochester Methodist Hospital, Rochester, Minnesota
Lymphatic Complications of Vascular Surgery; Ruptured Abdominal Aortic Aneurysms; Lymphedema: Introduction and General Considerations; Clinical Diagnosis and Evaluation of Lymphedema; Nonoperative Management of Chronic Lymphedema; Lymphatic Reconstructions

Michael F. X. Glynn,† M.D., D.Phil.(Oxon.), F.R.C.P.(C.) London
Associate Professor and Assistant Professor of Medicine, University of Toronto School of Medicine; Director of Hemostasis, Toronto General Hospital, Toronto, Ontario, Canada
Perioperative Hemorrhage

Jerry Goldstone, M.D.
Professor and Vice-Chairman, Department of Surgery, University of California, San Francisco; Attending Surgeon, Moffitt-Long Hospitals of UCSF Medical Center and Department of Veterans Affairs Medical Center, San Francisco, California
Aneurysms of the Extracranial Carotid Artery

Michael J. V. Gordon, M.D.
Assistant Professor, University of Colorado; Director, Hand and Microvascular Surgery, University of Colorado Health Sciences Center; University Hospital, Veterans Administration Medical Center, The Children's Hospital, Denver General Hospital, Denver, Colorado
Upper Extremity Amputation

Frank A. Gottschalk, M.D., F.R.C.S.(Ed.), F.C.S.(S.A.) Orth.
Associate Professor, Department of Orthopaedic Surgery, The University of Texas Southwestern Medical Center at Dallas; Attending, Zale Lipshy University Hospital and Parkland Memorial Hospital, Dallas, Texas
Complications of Amputation

†Deceased

Lazar J. Greenfield, M.D.
Frederick A. Coller Professor and Chairman, Department of Surgery, University of Michigan; Surgeon-in-Chief, University of Michigan Hospital, Ann Arbor, Michigan
Caval Interruption Procedures

Sushil K. Gupta, M.D.
Associate Clinical Professor of Surgery, Harvard Medical School, Boston; Chairman, Department of Surgery, MetroWest Medical Center, Framingham, Massachusetts
Secondary Arterial Reconstructions in the Lower Extremity

Vladimir Hachinski, M.D., F.R.C.P.(C.), D.Sc.(Med.)
Professor of Neurology, University of Western Ontario; Chair, Department of Clinical Neurological Sciences, University Hospital, London, Ontario, Canada
Medical Management of Ischemic Cerebrovascular Disease

John W. Hallett, Jr., M.D., F.A.C.S.
Professor of Surgery, Mayo Medical School; Director of Vascular Surgery Fellowship, Mayo Clinic; Staff, Mayo Clinic, Rochester, Minnesota
Iatrogenic Complications of Arterial and Venous Catheterizations

Kimberley J. Hansen, M.D.
Associate Professor of Surgery, Bowman Gray School of Medicine of Wake Forest University; Attending Faculty, North Carolina Baptist Hospital; Courtesy Staff, Forsyth Memorial Hospital and Hoots Memorial Hospital, Winston-Salem, North Carolina
Evaluation and Management of Ischemic Nephropathy

John P. Harris, M.S., F.R.A.C.S., F.R.C.S., F.A.C.S.
Associate Professor of Surgery, University of Sydney, Sydney; Head, Department of Surgery, Royal Prince Alfred Hospital, Camperdown, New South Wales, Australia
Upper Extremity Sympathectomy

Ziv J. Haskal, M.D.
Assistant Professor of Radiology, University of Pennsylvania School of Medicine; Assistant Professor of Radiology and Surgery, Hospital of the University of Pennsylvania, Philadelphia, Pennsylvania
Percutaneous Interventions in Portal Hypertension

George D. Hermann, M.D., B.S.M.E.
Manager, Fogarty Research, Portola Valley, California
Arterial Thromboembolism

Norman R. Hertzer, M.D.
Chairman, Department of Vascular Surgery, The Cleveland Clinic Foundation, Cleveland, Ohio
Postoperative Management and Complications Following Carotid Endarterectomy

Gary S. Hoffman, M.D.
Chairman of Department of Rheumatic and Immunologic Diseases, The Cleveland Clinic Foundation, Cleveland, Ohio
Takayasu's Disease: Nonspecific Aortoarteritis

Martin Holland, M.D.
Resident, Division of Neurosurgery, UCLA School of Medicine, Los Angeles, California
Extracranial-Intracranial Bypass: Current Status

Paul W. Humphrey, M.D.
Resident in Vascular Surgery, University of Missouri–Columbia Hospital and Clinics, Columbia, Missouri
Antithrombotic Therapy

Toshio Inahara, M.D.
Clinical Professor of Surgery, The Oregon Health Sciences University; Director, Peripheral Vascular Fellowship Program, St. Vincent Hospital and Medical Center; Attending Surgeon, St. Vincent Hospital and Medical Center, and Meridian Park Hospital, Portland, Oregon
Femoral and Popliteal Thromboendarterectomy

Bradley A. Jabour, M.D.
Assistant Clinical Professor of Radiology, UCLA School of Medicine, Los Angeles; Director of Radiology, Medical Imaging Center of Southern California; Chief of Neuroradiology, Head and Neck and Neurologic Imaging Associated Medical Group, Inc., Santa Monica, California
Imaging in Cerebrovascular Disease

Kaj H. Johansen, M.D., Ph.D.
Professor of Surgery, University of Washington School of Medicine; Director, Surgical Education, Providence Medical Center, Seattle, Washington
Overview (Section XIV); Operative Therapy for Portal Hypertension

George Johnson, Jr., M.D.
Roscoe B. G. Cowper Distinguished Professor of Surgery and Vice-Chairman, Department of Surgery, University of North Carolina at Chapel Hill; Professor of Surgery, University of North Carolina Hospitals, Chapel Hill, North Carolina
Introduction and General Considerations (Section XVII); Superficial Venous Thrombosis; Varicose Veins: Patient Selection and Treatment

K. Wayne Johnston, M.D., F.R.C.S.(C.)
Professor of Surgery and Chair, Division of Vascular Surgery, University of Toronto, Toronto, Ontario, Canada
Overview (Section VI); Perioperative Hemorrhage; Ischemic Neuropathy; Overview (Section IX)

Darrell N. Jones, Ph.D.
Assistant Professor, Department of Surgery, University of Colorado School of Medicine; Associate Director, Vascular Diagnostic Laboratory, University Hospital, Denver, Colorado
Evaluation of Results, Standard Reporting Practices, and the Computerized Vascular Registry

Sheldon E. Jordan, M.D., F.A.A.N.
Clinical Associate Professor, UCLA School of Medicine, Los Angeles; Staff, UCLA, Department of Neurology, Saint John's Hospital, Santa Monica Hospital, Santa Monica, California
Imaging in Cerebrovascular Disease

John W. Joyce, M.D.
Associate Professor of Medicine, Mayo Medical School, Rochester, Minnesota
Uncommon Arteriopathies

Jeffrey L. Kaufman, M.D.
Associate Professor of Surgery, Tufts University School of Medicine, Boston; Surgeon, Baystate Medical Center, Springfield, Massachusetts
Atheroembolism and Microthromboembolic Syndromes (Blue Toe Syndrome and Disseminated Atheroembolism)

Andris Kazmers, M.D., M.S.P.H.
Director of the Noninvasive Vascular Laboratory, Harper Hospital; Assistant Professor of Surgery, Wayne State University School of Medicine, Detroit, Michigan
Intestinal Ischemia Caused by Venous Thrombosis

Richard F. Kempczinski, M.D.
Professor of Surgery, University of Cincinnati; Chief, Vascular Surgery, and Director, Vascular Diagnostic Laboratory, University Hospital, Cincinnati, Ohio
Overview (Section V); Introduction and General Considerations (Section VIII); Popliteal Artery Entrapment; Vasculogenic Impotence

Lawrence L. Ketch, M.D., F.A.C.S., F.A.A.P.
Associate Professor and Chief, Department of Surgery, University of Colorado; Chief, Division of Plastic and Reconstructive Surgery, University of Colorado Hospital; Chief, Pediatric Plastic Surgery, The Children's Hospital, Denver, Colorado
Microvascular Surgery (Chapter 21); Upper Extremity Amputation

Edouard Kieffer, M.D.
Professor of Surgery, University of Paris; Chief, Department of Vascular Surgery, Pitre-Salptiere University Hospital, Paris, France
Arterial Complications of Thoracic Outlet Compression

Raphael F. Kilcoyne, M.D.
Professor of Radiology, University of Colorado Health Sciences Center; Vice Chairman, Department of Radiology, University Hospital, Denver, Colorado
Principles of Angiography

Young Wook Kim, M.D.
Associate Professor, Department of Surgery, Kyung Pook National University School of Medicine, Taegu, South Korea
Circulation-Enhancing Drugs

William C. Krupski, M.D.
Professor of Surgery, University of Colorado; Chief, Vascular Surgery, University Hospital; Chief, Vascular Surgery, Veterans Administration Hospital, Denver, Colorado
Preoperative Cardiac Evaluation of Patients for Vascular Surgery; Overview (Section X); Infrarenal Aortic Aneurysms; Overview (Section XIX)

David A. Kumpe, M.D.
Professor of Radiology and Surgery, University of Colorado Health Sciences Center; Director, Interventional Radiology, University Hospital; Attending Physician, Denver Veterans Administration Medical Center and Denver General Hospital; Consultant Physician, St. Anthony's Hospital, Rose Medical Center, and Aurora Regional Medical Center, Denver, Colorado
Principles of Angiography; Contrast Arteriography; Percutaneous Transluminal Angioplasty (Chapter 20); Endovascular Interventions for Lower Extremity Ischemia

Stephen G. Lalka, M.D.
Associate Professor of Surgery, Section of Vascular Surgery, Indiana University School of Medicine; Attending Vascular Surgeon, Indiana University Medical Center, Wishard Memorial Hospital, Richard L. Roudebush Veterans Affairs Medical Center, Indianapolis, Indiana
Management of Chronic Obstructive Venous Disease of the Lower Extremity

Robert P. Leather, M.D.
Professor of Surgery, Albany Medical College; Attending Surgeon, Albany Medical Center and St. Peter's Hospital, Albany, New York
Atheroembolism and Microthromboembolic Syndromes (Blue Toe Syndrome and Disseminated Atheroembolism)

Randi Y. Leavitt, M.D., Ph.D.
Assistant Laboratory Chief, Laboratory of Immunoregulation, National Institutes of Allergy and Infectious Diseases, National Institutes of Health, Bethesda, Maryland
Takayasu's Disease: Nonspecific Aortoarteritis

Raymond W. Lee, M.D.
Vascular Surgical Fellow, Oregon Health Sciences University, Portland, Oregon
Diagnosis of Intestinal Ischemia

Robert C. Lowell, M.D.
Fellow in Vascular Surgery, Mayo Graduate School of Medicine, Rochester, Minnesota
Lymphatic Complications of Vascular Surgery

Herbert I. Machleder, M.D.
Professor of Surgery, UCLA Medical School and UCLA Center for Health Sciences, Los Angeles, California
Axillary-Subclavian Vein Thrombosis

John Maher, M.B., B.Ch., B.A.O., M.R.C.P.(I.), F.R.C.P.(C.)
Clinical Fellow, Neurology, University Hospital, London, Ontario, Canada
Medical Management of Ischemic Cerebrovascular Disease

Neil A. Martin, M.D.
Associate Professor, Division of Neurosurgery, UCLA School of Medicine, Los Angeles, California
Extracranial-Intracranial Bypass: Current Status

James May, M.S., F.R.A.C.S., F.A.C.S.
Professor of Surgery, University of Sydney; Chairman, Division of Surgery, Royal Prince Alfred Hospital, Camperdown, New South Wales, Australia
Upper Extremity Sympathectomy

Kenneth E. McIntyre, Jr., M.D.
Professor of Surgery and Chief, Vascular Surgery, University of Texas Medical Branch; Chief, Vascular Surgery, John Sealy Hospital, Galveston, Texas
Patient Evaluation and Preparation for Amputation

Robert H. Meier III, M.D.
Associate Professor and Chairman, Department of Rehabilitation Medicine, University of Colorado Health Sciences Center, Denver, Colorado
Rehabilitation of the Person With an Amputation

Leslie Memsic, M.D.
Assistant Director of Surgery, Department of Surgery, Cedars-Sinai Medical Center, Los Angeles, California
Coiling and Kinking of the Carotid Artery

Louis M. Messina, M.D.
Associate Professor of Surgery, University of Michigan Medical School; Co-Chief, Vascular Surgery Service, Veterans Administration Hospital; Attending Staff, Section of Vascular Surgery, University Hospital, Ann Arbor, Michigan
Respiratory Complications in Vascular Surgery; Renal Artery Fibrodysplasia and Renovascular Hypertension

D. Craig Miller, M.D.
Professor of Cardiovascular and Thoracic Surgery, Stanford University School of Medicine, Stanford, California
Peripheral Vascular Manifestations of Acute Aortic Dissection

Timothy A. Miller, M.D.
Professor of Surgery, Division of Plastic Surgery, UCLA School of Medicine, Los Angeles; Chief, Plastic Surgery Section, Wadsworth Veterans Administration Medical Center, West Los Angeles, California
Excisional Operations for Chronic Lymphedema

Max B. Mitchell, M.D.
Chief Resident, Department of Surgery, University of Colorado Health Sciences Center, Denver, Colorado
Extra-Anatomic Bypass; Infrarenal Aortic Aneurysms

Jerry D. Mohr, M.D.
Clinical Assistant Professor of Surgery, University of Arizona; Chief of General Surgery, Maricopa Medical Center, Phoenix, Arizona
Revascularization Versus Amputation

Gregory L. Moneta, M.D.
Associate Professor of Surgery, Oregon Health Sciences University; Staff Surgeon, Oregon Health Sciences University and Portland Veterans Affairs Hospital, Portland, Oregon
Diagnosis of Intestinal Ischemia; The Natural History, Pathophysiology, and Nonoperative Treatment of Chronic Venous Insufficiency

Wesley S. Moore, M.D.
Professor of Surgery, UCLA School of Medicine; Chief, Section of Vascular Surgery, UCLA Center for the Health Sciences, Los Angeles, California
Anastomotic Aneurysms; Fundamental Considerations in Cerebrovascular Disease; Indications and Surgical Technique for Repair of Extracranial Occlusive Lesions; Results of Medical and Surgical Therapy for Extracranial Arterial Occlusive Disease

Dipankar Mukherjee, M.D., F.A.C.S.
Clinical Assistant Professor of Surgery, Uniformed Services of the Health Sciences F. Edward Hebert School of Medicine, Bethesda, Maryland; Attending Surgeon, Fairfax Hospital, Falls Church; Reston Hospital, Reston; Fair Oaks Hospital, Fair Oaks; and Northern Virginia Doctors Hospital and Arlington Hospital, Arlington, Virginia
Femoral and Popliteal Thromboendarterectomy

Mark R. Nehler, M.D.
Research Resident, Division of Vascular Surgery, Department of Surgery, Oregon Health Sciences University, Portland, Oregon
The Natural History, Pathophysiology, and Nonoperative Treatment of Chronic Venous Insufficiency

Kenneth Ouriel, M.D.
Associate Professor and Director, Noninvasive Vascular Laboratory, University of Rochester School of Medicine and Dentistry, Rochester, New York
Popliteal and Femoral Aneurysms

Thomas F. Panetta, M.D.
Professor of Surgery and Radiology and Chief of Vascular Surgery, State University of New York, Health Science Center at Brooklyn, Brooklyn, New York
Secondary Arterial Reconstructions in the Lower Extremity

William H. Pearce, M.D.
Professor of Surgery, Northwestern University Medical School; Attending Surgeon, Northwestern Memorial Hospital, Chicago, Illinois
Computed Tomography and Magnetic Resonance Imaging in Vascular Disease (Chapter 6)

Malcolm O. Perry, M.D.
Professor of Vascular Surgery, Texas Tech University Health Sciences Center; Chief, Vascular Surgery, University Medical Center, Lubbock, Texas
Acute Limb Ischemia; Injuries of the Brachiocephalic Vessels; Vascular Injuries of the Extremities

John M. Porter, M.D.
Professor of Surgery and Head, Division of Vascular Surgery, Oregon Health Sciences University; Staff Surgeon, Oregon Health Sciences University, and Veterans Affairs Medical Center, Portland, Oregon
Circulation-Enhancing Drugs; Natural History and Nonoperative Treatment of Chronic Lower Extremity Ischemia; Occlusive and Vasospastic Diseases Involving Distal Upper Extremity Arteries—Raynaud's Syndrome; Treatment of Acute Intestinal Ischemia Caused by Arterial Occlusions; Treatment of Chronic Visceral Ischemia; The Natural History, Pathophysiology, and Nonoperative Treatment of Chronic Venous Insufficiency

William J. Quiñones-Baldrich, M.D.
Associate Professor of Surgery, UCLA School of Medicine; Section of Vascular Surgery, UCLA Medical Center, Los Angeles, California
Principles of Thrombolytic Therapy; Results of Medical and Surgical Therapy for Extracranial Arterial Occlusive Disease

Seshadri Raju, M.D.
Professor of Surgery, University of Mississippi Medical Center, Jackson, Mississippi
Operative Management of Chronic Venous Insufficiency

Daniel J. Reddy, M.D.
Clinical Associate Professor of Surgery, University of Michigan Medical School, Ann Arbor; Vascular Surgeon, Henry Ford Hospital, Detroit, Michigan
Infected Aneurysms

Paul L. Redmond, M.B.
Chief of Radiology, Tullamore General Hospital, Offaly, Ireland
Principles of Angiography

Layton F. Rikkers, M.D.
M. M. Musselman Professor of Surgery, Department of Surgery, University of Nebraska Medical Center and University of Nebraska Hospital and Clinics, Omaha, Nebraska
Operative Therapy for Portal Hypertension

Thomas S. Riles, M.D.
Professor of Surgery and Director, Division of Vascular Surgery, New York University Medical Center; Attending Physician, Tisch Hospital and Bellevue Hospital, New York, New York
Overview (Section XI); Peripheral Arteriovenous Fistulae; Congenital Vascular Malformations

Ernest J. Ring, M.D.
Professor of Radiology, University of California, San Francisco; Chief of Vascular and Interventional Radiology, UCSF Mount Zion Campus, San Francisco, California
Percutaneous Interventions in Portal Hypertension; Radiologic Evaluation and Treatment of Renovascular Hypertension

Steven P. Rivers, M.D.
Associate Professor of Surgery, Albert Einstein College of Medicine; Associate Attending Surgeon, Montefiore Medical Center, Bronx, New York
Nonocclusive Mesenteric Ischemia

David L. Robaczewski, M.D., B.S.
Senior Assistant Resident, Department of Surgery, North Carolina Baptist Hospital, Winston-Salem, North Carolina
Renal Complications

Thom W. Rooke, M.D.
Assistant Professor of Medicine, Mayo Medical School; Consultant at Saint Mary's Hospital of Rochester, Rochester Methodist Hospital, and Mayo Medical Center, Rochester, Minnesota
Nonoperative Management of Chronic Lymphedema

Jeffrey S. Rose, M.D.
Chief, Medical Imaging, Colorado Region of Kaiser Permanente, Denver, Colorado
Principles of Angiography

Steven C. Rose, M.D.
Associate Professor of Radiology, University of California at San Diego Medical Center, San Diego, California
Venography

Robert J. Rosen, M.D.

Associate Professor of Radiology, New York University School of Medicine; Director, Vascular and Interventional Radiology, New York University Medical Center, New York, New York

Peripheral Arteriovenous Fistulae; Congenital Vascular Malformations

Carlo Ruotolo, M.D.

Assistant Professor of Surgery, School of Medicine Pitre-Salptiere; Staff Surgeon, Department of Vascular Surgery, Group Hospitalier Pitre-Salptiere, Paris, France

Arterial Complications of Thoracic Outlet Compression

Robert B. Rutherford, M.D.

Professor of Surgery, University of Colorado Health Sciences Center, Denver, Colorado

The Vascular Consultation; Evaluation and Selection of Patients for Vascular Surgery; Contrast Arteriography; Basic Vascular Surgical Techniques (Chapter 21); Evaluation of Results, Standard Reporting Practices, and the Computerized Vascular Registry; Graft Thrombosis and Thromboembolic Complications; Causalgia and Post-Traumatic Pain Syndromes; Extra-Anatomic Bypass; Endovascular Interventions for Lower Extremity Ischemia; Lumbar Sympathectomy: Indications and Technique; Infrarenal Aortic Aneurysms; Diagnostic Evaluation of Arteriovenous Fistulae; Extracranial Fibromuscular Arterial Dysplasia; Varicose Veins: Patient Selection and Treatment

David Saloner, Ph.D.

Associate Professor of Radiology, Department of Radiology, University of California, San Francisco; Veterans Administration Medical Center, San Francisco, California

Magnetic Resonance Angiography (Chapter 6)

Amorn Neil Salyapongse, B.A.

Medical Student, Northwestern University Medical School, Chicago, Illinois

Computed Tomography and Magnetic Resonance Imaging in Vascular Disease (Chapter 6)

George E. Sarris, M.D.

Fellow in Pediatric Cardiac Surgery and Instructor in Cardiothoracic Surgery, Emory University School of Medicine, Atlanta, Georgia

Peripheral Vascular Manifestations of Acute Aortic Dissection

Paul M. Satchell, B.Sc.(Med.), F.R.A.C.P., Ph.D., M.B.A.

Director, Gordon Craig Laboratory, Department of Surgery, University of Sydney, Sydney, New South Wales, Australia

Upper Extremity Sympathectomy

Dhiraj M. Shah, M.D.

Professor of Surgery, Albany Medical College; Attending Physician, Albany Medical Center, Albany Memorial Hospital, St. Peter's Hospital, and Veterans Administration Hospital, Albany, New York

Atheroembolism and Microthromboembolic Syndromes (Blue Toe Syndrome and Disseminated Atheroembolism)

Francis L. Shannon, M.D.

Cardiovascular/Thoracic Surgeon, William Beaumont Hospital and Providence Hospital, Detroit, Michigan

Lumbar Sympathectomy: Indications and Technique

Shigehiko Shionoya, M.D.

Emeritus Professor of Nagoya University, Nagoya, Japan; Sanjay Gandhi Post-Graduate Institute of Medical Sciences, Lucknow, India

Buerger's Disease (Thromboangiitis Obliterans)

Cynthia K. Shortell, M.D.

Clinical Assistant Professor of Surgery and Medicine, University of Rochester School of Medicine and Dentistry; Rochester General Hospital, Rochester, New York

Popliteal and Femoral Aneurysms

Donald Silver, M.D.

Professor and Chairman, Department of Surgery, University of Missouri–Columbia School of Medicine; Surgeon-in-Chief, University of Missouri–Columbia Hospital and Clinics; Consulting Surgeon, Harry S Truman Veterans Administration Hospital; Staff Surgeon, Ellis Fishel Cancer Center, Columbia, Missouri

Antithrombotic Therapy

Louis L. Smith, M.D.

Professor of Surgery, Loma Linda University Medical Center, Loma Linda, California

Management of Uncommon Lesions Affecting the Extracranial Vessels

William H. Snyder III, M.D.

Professor of Surgery, University of Texas Southwestern Medical Center; Active Attending Surgeon, Zale Lipshy University Hospital; Senior Attending Surgeon, Parkland Memorial Hospital; Staff Physician, Veterans Administration Hospital; Visiting Teaching Physician, St. Paul Medical Center; Clinical Consulting Physician, Presbyterian Hospital; Active Staff/Provisional/Courtesy, Medical Arts Hospital; Consulting Physician, Children's Medical Center, Dallas, Texas

Vascular Injuries of the Extremities

James C. Stanley, M.D.

Professor of Surgery, University of Michigan Medical School; Head, Section of Vascular Surgery, University Hospital, Ann Arbor, Michigan

Arterial Fibrodysplasia; Splanchnic Artery Aneurysms; Renal Artery Fibrodysplasia and Renovascular Hypertension

Ronald J. Stoney, M.D.
Professor of Surgery, University of California, San Francisco; Attending Surgeon, Section of Vascular Surgery, University of California Medical Center, San Francisco, California
Endarterectomy (Chapter 21); The Arterial Autograft; Neurogenic Thoracic Outlet Syndrome

Stephen W. Subber, M.D.
Assistant Professor, University of Colorado Health Sciences Center; Chief of Interventional Radiology, Denver Veterans Administration Medical Center, Denver, Colorado
Contrast Arteriography

David S. Sumner, M.D.
Distinguished Professor of Surgery and Chief, Section of Peripheral Vascular Surgery, Southern Illinois University School of Medicine, Springfield, Illinois
Overview (Section II); Essential Hemodynamic Principles; The Vascular Laboratory; Physiologic Assessment of Peripheral Arterial Occlusive Disease; Evaluation of Acute and Chronic Ischemia of the Upper Extremity; Hemodynamics and Pathophysiology of Arteriovenous Fistulae; Diagnostic Evaluation of Arteriovenous Fistulae; Hemodynamics and Pathophysiology of Venous Disease; Diagnosis of Deep Venous Thrombosis

Roy L. Tawes, Jr., M.D.
Associate Clinical Professor of Surgery, University of California, San Francisco; Staff Surgeon, Mills-Peninsula Hospital, Burlingame; Seton Medical Center, Daly City; Sequoia Hospital District, Redwood City, California
Blood Replacement and Autotransfusion in Major Vascular Surgery

Lloyd M. Taylor, Jr., M.D.
Professor of Surgery, Oregon Health Sciences University School of Medicine; Division of Vascular Surgery, Oregon Health Sciences University Medical Center, Portland, Oregon
Circulation-Enhancing Drugs; Natural History and Nonoperative Treatment of Chronic Lower Extremity Ischemia; Treatment of Acute Intestinal Ischemia Caused by Arterial Occlusions; Treatment of Chronic Visceral Ischemia

John Terblanche, Ch.M., F.C.S.(S.A.), F.R.C.S.(Eng.), F.A.C.S.(Hon.), F.A.C.P.(Hon.)
Professor and Chairman, Department of Surgery, Medical School, University of Cape Town; Professor and Chairman, Department and Division of Surgery, Groote Schuur Hospital Teaching Hospital Group, Cape Town, South Africa
Diagnosis and Emergency Management of Variceal Hemorrhage

Erwin R. Thal, M.D.
Professor of Surgery, University of Texas Southwestern Medical Center; Attending Staff, Parkland Memorial Hospital and Zale Lipshy University Hospital; Teaching Staff, St. Paul Medical Center; Consulting Staff, Veterans Administration Medical Center, Children's Medical Center, Baylor University Medical Center, and Presbyterian Hospital, Dallas, Texas
Vascular Injuries of the Extremities

Brian L. Thiele, M.D.
Professor of Surgery and Chief of Vascular Surgery, Pennsylvania State College of Medicine, Hershey, Pennsylvania
The Vascular Laboratory

David S. Thomas, M.D.
Clinical Associate Professor of Surgery, Division of Plastic Surgery, University of Utah, Salt Lake City, Utah
Coiling and Kinking of the Carotid Artery

Robert W. Thompson, M.D.
Assistant Professor of Surgery, Washington University School of Medicine; Attending Surgeon, Section of General Vascular Surgery, Barnes Hospital; Attending Staff, Vascular Surgery, John C. Cochran Veterans Affairs Medical Center, St. Louis, Missouri
Endarterectomy (Chapter 21)

M. David Tilson, M.D.
Ailsa Mellon Bruce Professor of Surgery, Columbia University; Director, Department of Surgery, St. Luke's–Roosevelt Hospital Center, New York, New York
Arterial Aneurysms: Etiologic Considerations

Gail T. Tominaga, M.D.
Assistant Professor of Surgery, University of California, Irvine, College of Medicine; Attending Physician and Surgeon, University of California, Irvine, Medical Center, Orange, California
Long-Term Venous Access

Jonathan B. Towne, M.D.
Professor of Surgery, Medical College of Wisconsin; Chairman, Vascular Surgery, John L. Doyne Hospital, Milwaukee, Wisconsin
The Autogenous Vein; Management of Foot Lesions in the Diabetic Patient

J. Jean E. Turley, M.D., F.R.C.P.(C.)
Assistant Professor of Medicine, University of Toronto; Chief of Neurophysiology, Wellesley Hospital, Toronto, Ontario, Canada
Ischemic Neuropathy

William W. Turner, Jr., M.D.
Director of Surgery, Methodist Hospital of Indiana, Indianapolis, Indiana
Acute Vascular Insufficiency due to Drug Injection

R. James Valentine, M.D.
Associate Professor, Department of Surgery, University of Texas Southwestern Medical Center; Chief, Vascular Surgery Section, Department of Surgery, Veterans Administration Medical Center; Attending Staff, Department of Surgery, Parkland Memorial Hospital and Zale Lipshy University Hospital, Dallas, Texas
Acute Vascular Insufficiency due to Drug Injection

Greg Van Stiegmann, M.D.
Associate Professor of Surgery, University of Colorado School of Medicine; Chief, Surgical Endoscopy, University of Colorado Medical Center and Denver Veterans Administration Hospital, Denver, Colorado
Endoscopic Treatment of Esophageal Varices

Charles W. Van Way III, M.D.
Professor of Surgery and Vice-Chairman, Department of Surgery, University of Missouri–Kansas City; Program Director of Surgery, St. Luke's Hospital, Kansas City, Missouri
Renal Artery Aneurysms and Arteriovenous Fistulae

E. Darracott Vaughan, Jr., M.D.
James J. Colt Professor of Urology, Cornell University Medical College; Urologist-in-Chief and Chairman, Department of Urology, The New York Hospital, New York, New York
Pathophysiology of Renovascular Hypertension

Frank J. Veith, M.D.
Professor of Surgery, Albert Einstein College of Medicine; Chief of Vascular Surgical Services, Montefiore Medical Center and the Jack D. Weiler Hospital of the Albert Einstein College of Medicine, New York, New York
Secondary Arterial Reconstructions in the Lower Extremity; Nonocclusive Mesenteric Ischemia

Heinz W. Wahner, M.D., F.A.C.P
Professor of Radiology and Consultant in Nuclear Medicine, Mayo Clinic, Rochester, Minnesota
Clinical Diagnosis and Evaluation of Lymphedema

Thomas W. Wakefield, M.D.
Associate Professor of Surgery, University of Michigan Medical School; Attending Surgeon, Section of Vascular Surgery, University Hospital; Co-Chief, Vascular Surgery Service, Veterans Administration Hospital, Ann Arbor, Michigan
Arterial Fibrodysplasia

Philip J. Walker, M.D., M.B.B.S., F.R.A.C.S.
Vascular Surgeon, University of Queensland, Royal Brisbane Hospital, Australia
Peripheral Vascular Manifestations of Acute Aortic Dissection

Daniel B. Walsh, M.D.
Associate Professor of Surgery, Dartmouth-Hitchcock Medical School; Staff, Dartmouth-Hitchcock Medical Center; Consulting Surgeon, Veterans Administration Hospital, Lebanon, New Hampshire
Intraoperative Assessment of Technical Adequacy

Kurt R. Wengerter, M.D.
Assistant Professor of Surgery, Albert Einstein College of Medicine; Director of Vascular Diagnostic Laboratory, Montefiore Medical Center, New York, New York
Secondary Arterial Reconstructions in the Lower Extremity

Thomas J. Whelan, Jr., M.D., F.A.C.S.
Professor Emeritus, University of Hawaii John A. Burns School of Medicine, Honolulu, Hawaii
Popliteal Artery Entrapment

Walter M. Whitehouse, Jr., M.D.
Clinical Associate Professor of Surgery, University of Michigan Medical School; Attending Surgeon, St. Joseph Mercy Hospital, Ann Arbor, Michigan
Upper Extremity Revascularization

Anthony D. Whittemore, M.D.
Professor of Surgery, Harvard Medical School; Chief, Division of Vascular Surgery, Brigham and Women's Hospital, Boston, Massachusetts
Infrainguinal Bypass

Samuel E. Wilson, M.D.
Professor, Department of Surgery, College of Medicine, University of California, Irvine; Chair, Department of Surgery, University of California, Irvine, Medical Center, Orange; Attending Staff, Surgical Service, Veterans Affairs Medical Center, Long Beach, California
Vascular Access for Hemodialysis

Charles L. Witte, M.D.
Professor of Surgery, University of Arizona College of Medicine; Attending Surgeon, University Medical Center; Consultant Surgeon, Veterans Administration Hospital, and Kino Community Hospital, Tucson, Arizona
Lymphodynamics and Pathophysiology of Lymphedema

Marlys H. Witte, M.D.
Professor of Surgery and Director of Medical Student Research Program, University of Arizona College of Medicine; Attending Physician in Surgery, University Medical Center, Tucson, Arizona
Lymphodynamics and Pathophysiology of Lymphedema

Creighton B. Wright, M.D.
Clinical Professor, Uniformed Services University of the Health Sciences, Bethesda, Maryland; Director of Surgery, The Jewish Hospital, Cincinnati, Ohio
Acute Vascular Insufficiency due to Drug Injection

James S. T. Yao, M.D., Ph.D.
Magerstadt Professor of Surgery, Northwestern University Medical School; Attending Surgeon and Chief, Division of Vascular Surgery, and Vice-Chairman, Department of Surgery, Northwestern Memorial Hospital, Chicago, Illinois
Occupational Vascular Problems

Christopher K. Zarins, M.D.
Professor of Surgery, Stanford University; Chief, Division of Vascular Surgery, Stanford University Medical Center, Stanford, California
Artery Wall Pathology in Atherosclerosis

Gerald B. Zelenock, M.D.
Professor of Surgery, Section of Vascular Surgery, University of Michigan Medical School; Attending Staff, Section of Vascular Surgery, University Hospital, and Vascular Surgery Service, Veterans Administration Hospital, Ann Arbor, Michigan
Respiratory Complications in Vascular Surgery; Splanchnic Artery Aneurysms

R. Eugene Zierler, M.D.
Associate Professor, Division of Vascular Surgery, Department of Surgery, University of Washington; University of Washington Medical Center, Seattle, Washington
Physiologic Assessment of Peripheral Arterial Occlusive Disease; Arterial Duplex Scanning (Chapter 6)

PREFACE

As another 5 years have passed and yet another, the fourth, edition of *Vascular Surgery* is being published, it is timely to reflect on the many changes that have affected clinical practice in this field during that period. Patient evaluation is being increasingly modified by a burgeoning vascular imaging technology. The "color flow" duplex scan now dominates noninvasive vascular diagnosis, sometimes to the disadvantage of still valuable and less expensive physiologic testing. Spiral computed tomography (CT) is encroaching on conventional CT, while, at the same time, magnetic resonance angiography (MRA) is emerging, with improving software, from standard magnetic resonance imaging (MRI) technology. Both of these improving imaging modalities are increasingly insinuating themselves between duplex scanning and contrast angiography, with the latter as the obvious victim in spite of impressive improvements in digital subtraction techniques. The vascular diagnostic laboratory itself is a changing scene, for this and other reasons, with certified technologists, formal accreditation, demands for quality assurance, and better defined testing indications all favoring the hospital-based laboratory.

At the time of the last edition, endovascular interventions were expected to have the greatest future impact, and they have, but not because of procedures directed at extending the beachhead established by percutaneous transluminal balloon "angioplasty" (PTBA) in the treatment of arterial occlusive disease. In fact, experiences with laser-based interventions and a number of atherectomy devices have generally been disappointing, as has the behavior of many corporations, hospitals, and physicians in association with their use. On the other hand, catheter-directed thrombolytic therapy has had a major impact on our success in dealing with both arterial and venous occlusions, and closely related catheter-directed techniques have allowed embolotherapy to be more effective in managing vascular trauma, gastrointestinal bleeding, and vascular tumors and malformations. Miniaturization has made percutaneous caval filter placement feasible, and for no other good reason, almost doubled its application. Finally, the impact of endovascular stents and their stepchild, vascular endografts, has not yet been fully realized, but it is anticipated that it will steadily increase as inevitable technological advances appear and are applied not only to true and false aneurysms and the acute and chronic sequelae of vascular trauma but also to arterial occlusive disease, after the involved segments are opened with atherectomy or other disobliterating devices.

This may reduce the number of open vascular operations and/or increase their complexity, by operating more often *after* endovascular treatment failure, but it may not significantly reduce the need for qualified vascular surgeons, for this trend may well be offset by a natural attrition of surgeons for whom vascular surgery constitutes a minor portion of their practice, the so-called occasional vascular surgeon. Further, in spite of one intended thrust of anticipated changes in health care delivery in the United States, that is, favoring primary care physicians (with less expensive care perceived to be offered by the less specialized), it will ultimately be recognized that a very significant portion of peripheral vascular disease is best evaluated and treated by committed specialists, in facilities equipped with modern technology, where intervention is actually more selectively and effectively applied.

Although vascular imaging and endovascular procedures have had, and will continue to have, the greatest overall impact on this field, many other lesser changes have nevertheless had significant individual effect—for example, newer cardiac screening methods, preoperative blood banking and increased use of autotransfusion, graft surveillance programs combined with "preventative maintenance" of graft patency, technical improvements in the "in situ" vein bypass for extremity occlusive disease, transjugular intraluminal portasystemic shunting (TIPS), endoscopic sympathectomy, renal revascularization primarily for parenchymal salvage, a more favorable view of carotid endarterectomy after many trials, and a steady refinement in the management of venous disease based on better physiologic evaluation of initial and outcome status.

Because of these and other changes, the fourth edition of *Vascular Surgery* has again undergone major revisions. The previous, third edition, underwent a fundamental basic reorganization, and this has been retained as sound. But, in this edition, a new section on angioaccess has been created, the section on vascular grafts has been completely reorganized, and the section on the general complications of vascular surgery has been greatly expanded. There are also five new section editors, and each of their sections—which deal with vascular diagnosis, aneurysms, amputation, visceral ischemia, portal hypertension, and lymphedema—are essentially all new. In fact, 68 chapters in the book present either completely new topics or topics that have been entirely rewritten by different authors, and an additional 26 chapters have been written by a new coauthor. This means that close to 60 per cent of this edition is new and different, and the remainder has been appropriately updated.

The dedication of this book to Dr. Richard C. Kempczinski, long-time associate editor and heavy contributor to this book since its origin, may have been precipitated by tragedy, but is no less deserved for someone who could have been considered the logical eventual successor to the present editor. To the extent that the other associate and assistant editors of this book have emulated his performance standards, this edition will live on in tribute. To them, and to each of the contributors, I owe my sincere appreciation. In addition, the editors of this book are most grateful for the efforts of the many persons who have assisted our contributors, and us, in the preparation and revision of manuscripts. In particular, I wish to acknowledge the special efforts and talents of Donna Fay, without whom this edition could not have been successfully completed.

ROBERT B. RUTHERFORD, M.D.

CONTENTS

SECTION I

The Surgical Approach to Vascular Problems

Edited by Robert B. Rutherford, M.D.

1

The Vascular Consultation

Robert B. Rutherford, M.D.

• • •

The vascular surgeon is usually consulted to establish a diagnosis and to recommend or carry out appropriate treatment. This involves reaching a presumptive diagnosis on clinical grounds, using noninvasive diagnostic measures to either confirm the diagnosis or grade the functional severity of the condition, weighing the degree of disability and natural course of the underlying disease against the risk and success rate of the various operative and nonoperative therapeutic alternatives, and then, when necessary, confirming the diagnosis and the extent and degree of involvement by angiography (Fig. 1–1). The final decision can be made only by combining the sociologic, pathologic, anatomic, and physiologic findings in the individual patient. Experience and judgment will make this all-important process of patient identification and selection relatively straightforward in most cases, but there will always be some patients in whom the disease process or its management is neither obvious nor definitive.

There are few areas in medicine in which the conditions encountered lend themselves so readily to diagnosis solely on the basis of thoughtful history and careful physical examination as do vascular diseases. The specialist in

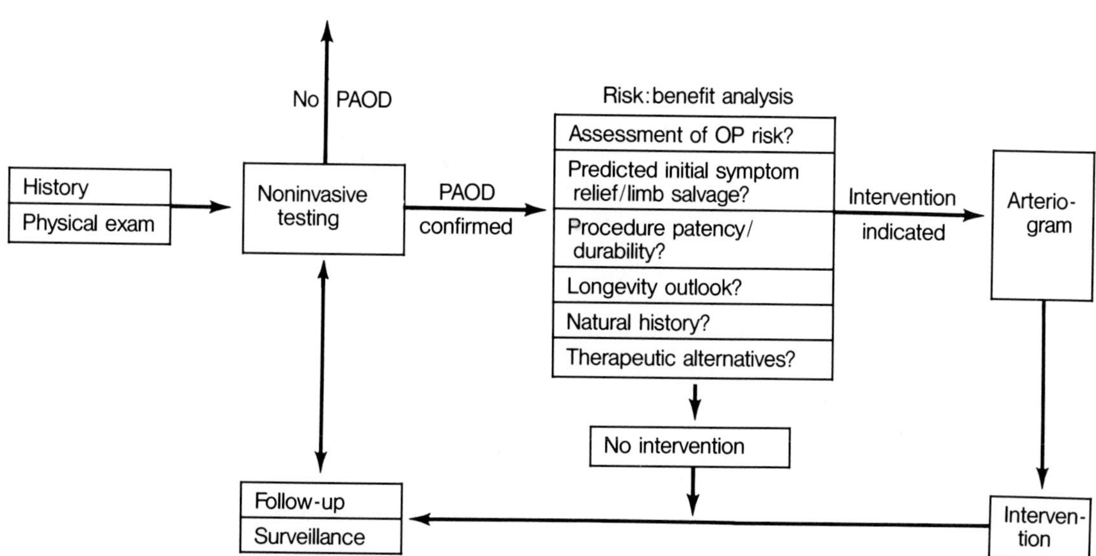

FIGURE 1–1. This algorithm shows the stepwise evaluation and management of patients presenting with peripheral arterial occlusive disease (PAOD). Note the central role played by noninvasive testing and the relegation of arteriography to therapeutic, *not diagnostic*, indications. OP, operative.

this field is often surprised at his or her colleagues' difficulties in assessing peripheral vascular problems. The vast majority of these problems are caused, in the Western world at least, by one of two basic disease processes, arteriosclerosis and thrombophlebitis, which predominantly affect the circulation of the lower rather than of the upper extremity or the viscera; the presenting manifestation is either pain, some form of tissue loss (ulceration or gangrene), or a change in appearance or sensation (swelling, discoloration, or temperature change). By applying a systematic, problem-oriented approach to these complaints, clinicians will soon find that they can often predict the status of the arterial circulation even before examination, recognize the postphlebitic leg at a glance, tell the cause of leg or foot ulcerations by their location and appearance, and predict the cause of leg swelling by its distribution and associated skin changes.

Unfortunately there is a tendency—as the clinician becomes adept at this, and able to turn the anticipated 1-hour consultation with a new patient into a 5-minute interview and spot diagnosis, and handle a clinicful of patients with chronic but familiar vascular problems in an hour or two—to bypass the systematic approach with increasing frequency and to abbreviate consultation notes and clinical records. Eventually the ability to transmit this knowledge to others (colleagues, students, house staff) in an organized fashion is lost or stinted. It may be useful, therefore, for the experienced as well as the inexperienced clinician, to have and maintain some formal framework on which these diagnostic skills can be superimposed. This need can be filled by a diagnostic check list or evaluation form such as the one presented in Figure 1–2. This approach not only avoids embarrassing oversights but also can preserve the details of the initial evaluation for later dictation and can function as a temporary record until the transcribed note reaches the files. It is difficult for the experienced clinician to adhere to this comprehensive approach. He or she will automatically proceed in algorithmic fashion, following the branches of a decision tree out to the area of appropriate focus. Nevertheless, it can still serve as a guideline for students, house staff, and fellows as they first begin evaluating vascular problems, or as a framework for lectures to medical and nursing students. Parts may be filled in by auxiliary personnel, and in larger clinic practices such tabular check lists, particularly if modified for each of the major disease entities or operations encountered, can provide the basis for clinical investigation and computer-based records and registry. The form shown here is intended only as an example. Obviously it will not suit everyone, and physicians should develop their own versions. For most purposes, only the major historical subheadings need to be listed on the form (e.g., location, duration, frequency, course, influencing factors), and instead of using tabular forms for pulses, the location of edema, discoloration, or ulceration, an anatomic silhouette, with or without an outline of the arterial tree, can be used and marked to note the pertinent physical findings. Finally, work forms destined to feed information into a vascular registry must be simpler still, because only essential and unambiguous categorical information should be stored in computers.

HISTORY AND PHYSICAL EXAMINATION

Patients with vascular diseases usually present with key complaints that often can be developed by pointed questioning into a reasonable presumptive diagnosis even before physical examination is carried out. The major diagnostic considerations for the various forms of vascular disease are covered later in appropriate sections of this book. Here, the intention is to demonstrate, mainly by using the lower extremity as an example, the value of knowing which questions to ask and which physical signs to search for. This problem-oriented approach is preferred to the practice of describing an uncorrelated list of vascular signs and symptoms.

The Painful Extremity

The most common presenting symptom in lower extremity vascular disease is pain. Knowing the pain's character, severity, location, frequency and duration, and temporal pattern, and what precipitates or aggravates the pain or makes it subside, often allows one to diagnose or rule out arterial and venous diseases with over 90 per cent certainty *before* the physical examination begins. *Acute arterial occlusion* does not always produce the well-known five Ps—pain, pallor, pulselessness, paresthesias, and paralysis. In fact, if the pain is not severe and sustained, or if patients do not experience motor or sensory loss, they may not even seek immediate medical help, and the absence of pulses may not be detected until later, when patients present with claudication or are examined for other reasons. Nevertheless, the initial pain of acute arterial occlusion usually is fairly characteristic. It begins suddenly and reaches a peak rapidly. Particularly in the case of arterial embolism, patients may describe a sensation of the leg's being "struck" by a severe, shocking pain that renders it weak. If standing at the time, they may be forced to sit down immediately or may even crumple to the ground as the extremity gives way. The pain may quickly subside, and depending on the severity of the ischemia that remains after the initial wave of vasospasm has passed and collateral channels are recruited, it may either resolve completely or settle into one of the typical pain patterns of chronic ischemia. The persistence of pain, particularly if followed by numbness, weakness, or both, indicates that one is dealing with severe, limb-threatening ischemia.

Chronic arterial insufficiency of the lower extremity causes two very characteristic types of pain, intermittent claudication and ischemic rest pain. *Claudication,* although derived from the Latin word for limp, *claudicatio,* has by usage come to mean a discomfort or disability associated with exercise. Depending on the level and extent of the arterial occlusive disease, the patient may present with buttock and thigh claudication, calf claudication, or foot claudication, either singly or in contiguous combination. The most common, *calf claudication,* is easily recognized as a *cramping* pain in the calf that can be consistently reproduced by the same degree of exercise and completely re-

PERIPHERAL VASCULAR WORKSHEET

Name ______ **Date** ______

Past History

Allergies ______ Operations ______
Injuries ______ Major illnesses ______
Pregnancies ______ Phlebitis ______
Pulmonary embolism ______ Serious infections ______
Cardiac: angina ______ CHF ______ MI ______
arrhythmia ______ DOE ______ orthopnea ______
Respiratory ______
Diabetes ______
Hypertension ______
Renal ______
Neurological: cerebrovascular ______
peripheral ______
Venereal disease ______
Arthritis, collagen vascular ______
Other ______

Family History

Same condition ______ Other vascular ______
Diabetes ______ Hypertension ______ CVA ______ Cardiac ______
Clotting abnormalities ______

Personal and Social

Alcohol ______ Tobacco ______
Education ______ Psychological ______
Occupations ______
Travel ______
Drug use: past ______
present ______

PERIPHERAL VASCULAR WORKSHEET

Name ______ **Date** ______

I. Complaints:	**Rank**	**Severity**	**Descriptive Comments**
Pain			
Weakness			
Hot/cold			
Numb/sensitive			
Discoloration			
Swelling			
Ulceration			
Varicose veins			

II. Location: R/L, medial/lateral, dorsal/ventral
Toes ______ Foot ______ Ankle ______ Leg ______ Knee ______
Fingers Hand Wrist Forearm Elbow
Thigh ______ Hip ______ Back ______ Other ______
Arm Shoulder Neck ______

III. Onset: sudden/gradual
IV. Duration: ______ days/weeks/months/years
V. Frequency: ______ times/day/week/month/year
VI. Temporal Pattern: continuous/intermittent/day/night/none
VII. Course: static/better/worse/fluctuates
VIII. Interferes With: sleep/work/exercise/other
IX. Influencing Factors (A-aggravates, R-relieves, O-no effect):
Elevation ______ Dependency ______ Exercise ______ Rest ______ Heat ______
Cold ______ Weather change ______ Menses ______ Emotions ______ Vibration ______
Pressure ______ Position ______
Activity ______
Other (including Rx) ______

FIGURE 1–2. Diagnostic check list for vascular evaluation.

Illustration continued on following page

PERIPHERAL VASCULAR WORKSHEET

Physical Examination

Name ________________ **Date** ________________
Ht.________ Wt. ________ Pulse________ Temperature________ B.P.________
General ________________ Head and neck ________________
Heart________________
Lungs________________ Abdomen ________________

Extremities	**Upper** right	left	**Lower** right	left
Skin Warm/cool				
Atrophied/thickened				
Cyanosis/mottling				
Pallor/rubor				
Capillary filling				
Hair growth				
Nails				
Edema Brawny/pitting/spongy				
Degree				
Extent				
Subcutaneous atrophy				
fibrosis				
Ulceration/tissue loss				
Discoloration/pigmentation				
Erythema/cellulitis				
Lymphangitis				
Musculoskeletal Symmetry/atrophy				
Hypertrophy				
Joint enlargement/swelling				
Range of motion				
Reflexes				
Sensory				
Motor				

PERIPHERAL VASCULAR WORKSHEET

Arterial Survey	**Right** pulse	bruit	aneurysm	**Left** pulse	bruit	aneurysm
Carotid						
Subclavian						
Brachial						
Radial						
Ulnar						
Abdominal aorta						
Iliac						
Femoral						
Popliteal						
Dorsalis pedis						
Posterior tibial						

Venous Survey **Code:** N = normal; P = prominent, tense; V = varicose; T = thrombosed

	Right	**Left**
Greater saphenous		
Lesser saphenous		
Anterolateral thigh		
Posteromedial thigh		
Anterior tibial		
Posterior arch		
Perforators		
Intracutaneous venules		
Tourniquet test		

Demographic Data
Name________________ Date ________ History no. ________
Address________________ Occupation ________________
Age________ Sex ________ Nationality/race________________
Referring physician ________________ Telephone no. ________
Address________________

FIGURE 1–2 *Continued*

lieved by a minute or so of rest. These calf cramps are not to be confused with those that occur at night in older patients, some of whom may even have pulse deficits or other signs of arterial occlusive disease. Nocturnal muscle cramps have no known vascular basis; rather they are thought to result from an exaggerated neuromuscular response to stretch. Experienced clinicians will quickly differentiate between these two unrelated causes of leg cramps. They also realize that it is not unusual for elderly patients to experience no symptoms from superficial femoral artery occlusion because their sedentary existence protects them from claudication, and the occlusive process is gradual enough to allow concomitant development of collateral circulation so there is no ischemia at rest.

Tightness and discomfort in the calf precipitated by exercise may result from a chronic compartment compression syndrome (see Chapter 61). The patients are often athletes (e.g., runners) with large calf muscles. Muscle swelling, increased compartment pressure, and impaired venous outflow constitute a vicious circle. However, this pain usually comes on after considerable exercise and does not quickly subside with rest.

Patients with arterial occlusive disease of more proximal (aortoiliac) distribution usually suffer from buttock and thigh claudication, although a significant number will complain of calf claudication. Buttock and thigh claudication commonly does not produce the severe cramping muscular pain experienced in the calf. The sensation is more of an *aching* discomfort associated with *weakness.* These patients may even deny the existence of pain per se, complaining only that their hip or thigh "gives out" or "tires" after they have walked a certain distance. Patients with osteoarthritis of the hip or knee may complain of similar extremity discomfort that is also brought on by exercise, but important differentiating factors are that the amount of exercise causing their symptoms is variable, the pain does not disappear as promptly with rest, and it varies in severity from day to day, frequently in association with changes in weather conditions or physical activity. Also, neurospinal compression, caused by osteophytic narrowing of the lower (lumbar) neurospinal canal, may simulate claudication secondary to aortoiliac occlusive disease. It is, however, usually more of a numbing weakness that is also produced by standing (or anything increasing lumbar lordosis) rather than just ambulation, and is not relieved by stopping unless the patient sits down, or leans against a lamppost or tree with the upper body bent forward, and straightens out the lumbar spine. Further questioning often reveals that this weakness is associated with either numbness or paresthesias, sometimes involving the perineum. Since older patients not infrequently have diminished femoral pulses and proximal bruits reflecting some degree of aortoiliac occlusive disease, it is not unusual for these other painful conditions to be wrongly ascribed to vascular disease. This is a classic example of the importance of matching symptoms and signs in terms of severity and distribution. It is unusual to have significant hip or buttock pain from iliac artery stenosis without associated thigh claudication. Furthermore, aortic or complete iliac artery occlusion with absence of femoral pulses on at least one side is usually necessary for such proximally distributed symptoms. Finally, bilateral aortoiliac occlusive disease severe enough to produce disabling claudication is nearly always associated with impotence in males. The absence of impotence in a man with bilateral hip or thigh pain should make one suspect that the pain may not be due to aortoiliac occlusive disease, unless the occlusive lesions are limited to the external iliac arteries. Although true claudication is attributable to arterial occlusive disease, thigh claudication can also be experienced because of venous occlusion. This venous "claudication" usually results because recanalization did not occur after ileofemoral venous thrombosis. At rest, collateral vessels allow venous outflow to match arterial inflow without the development of high venous pressures, but they are not able to handle the severalfold increases in arterial inflow associated with exercise. The venous channels in the thigh and/or leg become engorged and tense, and it is this high venous pressure, not ischemia, that is the source of the pain, which is often appropriately described as a "bursting" pain or a tight, heavy sensation. Because this venous engorgement is slow to subside, the pain does not abate as quickly as that of claudication due to arterial occlusive disease.

Foot claudication occurring on an ischemic basis is very rare. It may exist independently of calf claudication if the occlusive lesions are diffuse and involve all the infrapopliteal arteries distally, but it is just as commonly associated with more proximal occlusions and calf pain. It has a greater relative frequency in thromboangiitis obliterans than in arteriosclerosis obliterans because of the typically more distal distribution of occlusive lesions in the former condition. The complaint is usually of a painful ache, a "drawing" pain or cramp in the forefoot, associated only with walking. Patients usually also complain of a "wooden" sensation or numbness in the same distribution, and of a persistently cold foot at night. Frequently they have visited several podiatrists or have tried a variety of arch supports or "orthopedic" shoes. This rarest form of lower extremity claudication usually occurs only with advanced degrees of arterial insufficiency and, therefore, is commonly associated with ischemic rest pain of the foot.

One may encounter cases in which either the clinical diagnosis of arterial claudication is not clear-cut or the symptoms and findings, although compatible with the diagnosis, do not match it in severity. In such cases noninvasive testing can be extremely helpful (see Chapter 5). For example, the ankle pressure after exercise or other forms of induced hyperemia sufficient to reproduce the pain should fall to the vicinity of 50 mmHg or below. If not, the patient may have two causes of leg pain, the lesser of which is related to arterial insufficiency.

Ischemic rest pain is typically a nocturnal pain of disturbing severity that diffusely involves the foot distal to the tarsal bones, although it may be sharply localized to the vicinity of an ischemic ulcer or gangrenous toe. It may be so severe that it is not relieved even by substantial doses of narcotics. Patients who sleep in a horizontal position are typically awakened by this pain and forced to get up and do something about it. They may sit up and rub or hold the painful foot, get up and pace the floor, or walk to the medicine cabinet to take an analgesic. Any of these responses will relieve the pain fairly promptly, but only by the unwitting recruiting of the help of gravity in improving the perfusion pressure to the distal tissues. Although patients may at first wrongly attribute the relief to rubbing the foot, walking, or even an amazingly fast-acting analgesic, eventually they learn to sleep with the foot dependent, either dangling it over the side of the bed and resting it on a chair, or sleeping out the night in a lounge chair. This pain pattern is too characteristic to be missed by the careful interrogator. Occasionally, patients with arthritic changes in the small bones of the feet (metatarsals, usually) can experience "metatarsalgia" that occurs primarily at night and is relieved by standing. This can be seen with either degenerative osteoarthritis or rheumatoid arthritis. Its occurrence is irregular—it may be present or absent for several days to weeks—thus distinguishing it from ischemic rest pain, which occurs whenever the patient lies down for any length of time.

Pain associated with *venous disease* of the lower extremity is not as characteristic as the arterial pain syndromes. Fortunately these conditions usually are easily recognized by their associated physical findings. Severe pain is not a common complaint of patients with primary *varicose veins.* In fact, one must be suspicious when patients with varicose veins present with pain, particularly if the varicosities are of long standing and were not previously painful. Such patients may be suffering from extremity pain of another, more obscure etiology, although blaming it on the visible varicosities. Occasionally varicose veins produce a "pulling," "pricking," "burning," or "tingling" discomfort that is well localized to the varicose veins themselves, unlike the diffuse sensation of fatigue or heaviness that more commonly predominates with deep venous insufficiency. Although, like all venous discomfort, these symptoms are relieved by elevation, the tingling and burning sensation often worsens during the initial period of elevation before it subsides.

Venous thrombosis in the lower extremity may cause little or no acute pain, unless the associated inflammatory reaction is significant, in which case there may also be localized tenderness along the course of the involved vein. Swelling, either early or later in the postphlebitic period, is not uncommonly associated with a moderate aching discomfort and a tight or heavy sensation, but severe, "bursting" pain is rare unless the patient is spending too much time in the upright position or still has significant residual obstruction to venous outflow (venous claudication). It is clear that, although the symptoms associated with venous valvular insufficiency or obstruction (in the absence of associated inflammation) are extremely variable, their aggravation by standing and relief by elevation is consistent, and this relationship should always be explored. The presence of significant discomfort after standing for long periods or walking with chronic venous valvular insufficiency or obstruction (respectively) stands in marked contrast to the lack of discomfort associated with lymphedema (see later discussion).

Patients with other forms of extremity pain are often referred to the vascular surgeon under the false presumption that it is circulatory in origin, and therefore it is important that the surgeon be able to recognize the nonvascular extremity pain syndromes or at least the common ones associated with nerve or musculoskeletal derangements. As previously pointed out, the pain of arthritis or sciatica usually is fairly characteristic and easily distinguishable from that caused by vascular disease. There are, however, two other conditions causing extremity pain that can masquerade as vascular disease because of the associated vascular signs. One is a painful peripheral neuritis commonly seen in diabetics and, because their peripheral pulses may be diminished and they may have rubor and trophic skin changes, the examiner may mistake the problem for arterial insufficiency rather than the early stage of diabetic neuropathy. Later stages of diabetic neuropathy are characteristically painless, and the associated neurologic signs are obvious, but in the early "neuritic" stages, the neurologic signs may be subtle, often no more than a patchy loss of light touch, vibratory sense, and two-point discrimination.

The other misleading type of extremity pain is reflex sympathetic dystrophy, or minor causalgia. Like the neuritis, the pain it produces is usually burning in character. Major causalgia, associated with incomplete nerve injury, usually is easily recognized, but the minor variety, which may follow relatively minimal trauma or acute circulatory problems such as venous or arterial thrombosis, must always be kept in mind by the vascular surgeon. Similarly, there is the patient with residual discomfort following back surgery (disc operations, lumbar fusions), which is often labeled "arachnoiditis" but is really a form of causalgic pain resulting from the "trauma" of long-standing nerve compression. Typically, there are the signs of autonomic imbalance, the "vascular" signs that originally attracted the attention of the referring physician. The causalgic extremity may be warm and dry initially, but later becomes cool, mottled, or cyanotic. Eventually trophic changes develop that are not unlike those of arterial insufficiency. The pain is not always classically superficial, burning, and localized to the distribution of a somatic nerve as originally described. If there are reasonable grounds for suspicion after initial evaluation, relief of the pain by a proximal arterial injection of 10–15 mg of tolazoline hydrochloride, confirmed later by a paravertebral sympathetic block, will establish the diagnosis. This is discussed in more detail in Chapter 49.

Physical examination of the painful extremity is usually carried out by a prejudiced examiner if a careful history has been taken, for the reasons already given, and it is difficult to be systematic when physical findings confirming one's suspicions immediately catch the eye. A complete and thorough initial examination should, however, be carried out. Discovery of a previously undetected diastolic hypertension, carotid bruit, fibrillating heart, or abdominal aortic aneurysm may be the dividend of such thoroughness. Furthermore, documentation of the state of the peripheral pulses may well have future value. Examination of the abdomen should consist of more than a brief palpation for an occult aneurysm. For example, lower abdominal bruits may provide the only physical clue of aortoiliac occlusive disease in a patient with buttock and thigh claudication, since there may be no signs of chronic ischemia and a femoral pulse may be readily palpated because a hemodynamically significant iliac artery stenosis may produce a pressure gradient of as little as 10 mmHg at rest.

If such patients (with "critical" stenoses) exercise to the point of claudication, they usually temporarily "lose" the previously palpable pedal pulses because of the marked decrease in vascular resistance that occurs in exercising muscle distal to an obstruction and the increased distribution of flow to muscle beds proximal to the obstruction. This is the basis for the practice of monitoring ankle pressure following a standard treadmill exercise (see Chapter 5). There is another example of claudication with palpable pulses that should be kept in mind. If one elicits a good history of claudication in a *young* patient with palpable pedal pulses, one should suspect popliteal entrapment (see Chapter 61) and recheck the pulses during active plantar flexion or passive dorsiflexion.

Palpating Pulses. *Femoral pulses* may be difficult to palpate in muscular or obese patients unless the hips are externally rotated and the vessels are palpated over the pubic ramus of the ilium where they lie 1½ to 2 fingerbreadths lateral to the pubic tubercle and are covered by less fat. Even for the experienced examiner, the *popliteal pulses* are often difficult to palpate, so difficult, in fact, that the knowledgeable vascular surgeon who feels them too easily usually suspects at once the possibility of a fusiform popliteal aneurysm. Holding the supine patient's knee partially flexed and allowing it to fall gently back into the examiner's hand, which is positioned so that the proximal interphalangeal joints hook the tendons while the fingertips sink gently into the middle of the popliteal space, is just as effective a means of palpating popliteal pulses as having the patient turn into the prone position with the knee flexed. The location of the *posterior tibial pulse* in the hollow behind the medial malleolus and that of the *dorsalis pedis pulse* along the dorsum of the foot between the first and the second metatarsal bones are well known. It is less well appreciated that one or the other of these pedal pulses is not palpable in almost 10 per cent of normal persons. In such cases the lateral tibial artery, the terminal branch of the peroneal artery, should be sought higher in the foot, just below the ankle and medial to the bony prominence of the fibula. A warm room and a light touch are the best combination for the most accurate detection of pedal pulses. Otherwise it must be hoped that the examiner's and the patient's pulses are distinctly different in rate. Finally, listening for bruits over the course of these major arteries, especially at or above the most proximal pulse that feels weaker than normal, is important. It is surprising how often the telltale bruit of an iliac stenosis is not even auscultated.

Signs of Advanced Ischemia

Severe claudication may be associated with atrophy of the calf muscles, but unless this is unilateral and produces asymmetry it may escape detection. Loss of hair growth over the dorsum of the toes and foot is another relatively common sign of arterial insufficiency, and this may be accompanied by thickening of the toenails secondary to slowness of nail growth. More advanced ischemic changes, however, such as atrophy of the skin and its appendages and the subcutaneous tissue, so that the foot becomes shiny, scaly, and "skeletonized," usually do not appear in the absence of ischemic rest pain. Delayed return of the capillary blush after pressure on the pulp of the digit and slow venous filling after dropping the elevated extremity back into the dependent position are also signs of advanced ischemia. Buerger's sign, i.e., cadaveric pallor on elevation and rubor on dependency, occurs with very restricted arterial inflow and chronic dilatation of the peripheral vascular bed beyond, particularly the postcapillary venules. The dependent toes may appear so red and may refill so rapidly after pressure application that the uninitiated may mistakenly consider this to be evidence of hyperemia rather than an expression of severe ischemia. Localized pallor or cyanosis associated with poor capillary filling is usually a prelude to ischemic gangrene or ulceration. At this advanced stage of ischemia, the foot may be edematous from being continually kept in the dependent position in an attempt to relieve the ischemic pain.

Signs of Venous Insufficiency

As previously stated, lower extremity pain secondary to venous disease is inconstant. In addition, the discomfort caused by venous distention from whatever cause is similar in character, as is its relief by elevation. Therefore, the physical findings associated with these venous problems may be extremely helpful in differentiating between them. For example, *varicose veins* may be the result of primary saphenofemoral incompetence or may be secondary to deep venous and perforator incompetence. In the untreated state, the latter produces brawny edema, stasis dermatitis, and ulceration. By contrast, the edema associated with primary uncomplicated varicose veins is mild and rarely appears early in the day, dermatitis with pigmentation is restricted to the skin immediately overlying prominent varicosities, and ulceration does *not* occur in early cases. Furthermore, primary varicose veins typically involve the main saphenous vein and its major branches rather than scattered tributaries, and they do not refill quickly on standing after a tourniquet has been applied to the upper thigh (positive tourniquet test).

An acutely thrombosed superficial vein feels like a cord, is tender, and may be surrounded by erythema, skin pigmentation, warmth, swelling, induration, and other localized signs of inflammation. Even acute thrombosis of a deep vein, if associated with a sufficient inflammatory reaction, may result in tenderness along its course. Usually, however, it produces a more generalized edema distally. If the deep calf veins are thrombosed, there may be pain on dorsiflexion (Homans' sign), tenderness on anteroposterior but not lateral compression of the calf (Bancroft's sign), and prompt pain in the calf caused by inflating a sphygmomanometer cuff around it to a pressure of 80 mmHg (Löwenberg's sign). These signs, however, are said to be present in fewer than half the patients with acute deep venous thrombosis. The oft-quoted rate of one-third false-positive and one-third false-negative for diagnosis of thrombophlebitis when made on clinical grounds alone applies more to a hospital population of patients at bed rest in whom occult thrombosis is more likely to occur and swelling is more likely to be absent. On the other hand, outpatients with this condition usually present *because of* signs or symptoms, and therefore a higher rate of diagnostic accuracy may be expected in this setting. Nevertheless, it should be remembered that this diagnosis can be made confidently on clinical grounds *only* in cases of extensive, major venous thrombosis (e.g., phlegmasia cerulea dolens or phlegmasia alba dolens) or those associated with a marked inflammatory

Table 1–1. Differential Diagnosis of Chronic Leg Swelling

Clinical Feature	Venous	Lymphatic	Cardiac Orthostatic	"Lipedema"
Consistency of swelling	Brawny	Spongy	Pitting	Noncompressible (fat)
Relief by elevation	Complete	Mild	Complete	Minimal
Distribution of swelling	Maximal in ankles and legs, feet spared	Diffuse, greatest distally	Diffuse, greatest distally	Maximal in ankles and legs, feet spared
Associated skin changes	Atrophic and pigmented, subcutaneous fibrosis	Hypertrophied, lichenified skin	Shiny, mild pigmentation, no trophic changes	None
Pain	Heavy ache, tight or bursting	None or heavy ache	Little or none	Dull ache, cutaneous sensitivity
Bilaterality	Occasionally, but usually unequal	Occasionally, but usually unequal	Always, but may be unequal	Always

reaction. In contrast, the combination of two simple noninvasive tests, plethysmography and venous Doppler examination, and/or examining the veins with a color duplex scanner, is 95 per cent accurate in diagnosing deep venous thrombosis (see Chapter 131).

The Swollen Leg

After the painful leg, the swollen leg is the next most common problem on which the vascular surgeon is called to consult. In examining the swollen leg, the consultant should remember another five Ps: pressure, protein, permeability, paresis, and pendency. Plasma constituents move into the tissues and return to the vascular space normally during circulation according to Starling's law. The balance of factors influencing this process is a delicate one, particularly in the lower extremity, where gravity provides an additional complicating factor. The valved venomotor pump mechanism is presumably an evolutionary adaptation to the assumption of the upright position by humans, for if a normal person were to stand motionless long enough venous pressures at the ankle would stabilize in the range of 80 to 100 mmHg, and swelling and petechial hemorrhages would appear. With a competent venomotor pump mechanism, however, even modest activity of the calf muscles, such as occurs in intermittently shifting one's weight, reduces this pressure to 20 to 30 mmHg, and what little swelling accumulates during the day usually disappears overnight when the body is horizontal. Patients who do not take advantage of this respite, e.g., those who sleep night after night with their feet dependent to relieve ischemic pain, develop chronic swelling, as do patients with peroneal palsy or an arthritic or fused ankle who cannot activate the venomotor pump.

Increased permeability secondary to inflammation results in swelling if the extremity is not kept elevated. Similarly, swelling is seen in secondary aldosteronism. The lymphatics are the route by which extravasated protein is returned to the central circulation. If the clearance capacity of this system is restricted because it is congenitally hypoplastic, because it is obliterated by episodes of lymphangitis, or because its outflow is obstructed or interrupted by surgery or irradiation, protein-rich lymph will accumulate in the tissues. A similar mechanism, in reverse, applies in hypoproteinemia, and this occasional cause of swelling should be considered in obscure cases.

High venous pressure is the most common cause of extremity swelling. The source of this increased peripheral venous pressure may be cardiac in origin, as in right-sided heart failure or tricuspid valvular disease; or it may be due to intrinsic venous obstruction, as in peripheral venous thrombosis, or to extrinsic compression, as of the left iliac vein by the right iliac artery. Most commonly, however, it is due to the unrelenting and unopposed transmission, in the upright position, of gravitational pressure through incompetent valves of the deep and communicating veins of the postphlebitic leg to the superficial tissues. Venous hypertension secondary to arteriovenous fistulae is rarer, and rarely causes swelling in the absence of venous obstruction, but it does cause changes similar to though more localized than those generally ascribed to venous "stasis" (see farther on).

Clinically, the differential diagnosis of swelling may be difficult when it is of brief duration, but in the chronic state, characteristic physical findings appear that greatly simplify matters. When a patient presents with a chronically swollen leg, the experienced examiner may make the correct diagnosis in more than 95 per cent of cases simply by noting the distribution of the swelling, its response to elevation, and the associated discomfort and skin changes. These and other diagnostic considerations pertinent to chronically swollen lower extremities are presented in Table 1–1.

If there are no obvious associated skin changes and the edema "pits" readily on pressure, its cause is usually central or systemic, e.g., heart disease, hypoproteinemia, or secondary aldosteronism. The distribution of this type of swelling, sometimes called orthostatic edema, is diffuse, but the swelling is greatest peripherally and, to some extent, also involves the foot. The edema associated with peripheral venous disease, even in the acute stage, does not "pit" readily. In the chronic stage, it is frankly "brawny" and associated with characteristic skin changes caused by chronic venous hypertension. The breakdown of extravasated red cells causes the characteristic pigmentation and, together with increased fibrin in the interstitial fluid, leads to inflammation and fibrosis in the subcutaneous tissues. Later the skin becomes atrophic and breaks down with minor trauma. These components of so-called stasis dermatitis have a "gaiter" distribution, as shown in Figure 1–3, and even in earlier stages, when edema predominates, the feet often are relatively spared compared with the ankles and lower half of the legs. The reason is that this venous hypertension is transmitted to the superficial veins by in-

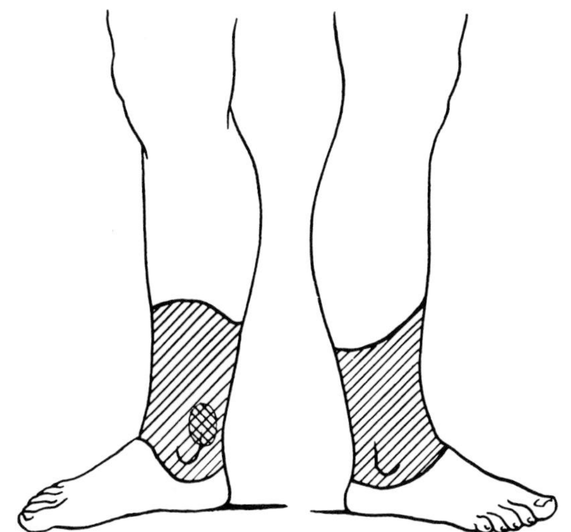

FIGURE 1–3. The "gaiter" distribution of stasis dermatitis and leg ulcers.

competent perforator veins located in this gaiter area. Eventually progression of these chronic changes converts the skin and subcutaneous tissues of the lower leg from a diffusely edematous state to a pigmented, atrophic, tightly scarred zone, which when viewed in contrast to the proximal edema, leads to the descriptive term "inverted-champagne-bottle-leg."

The distribution of *lymphedema* is diffuse, but the swelling is always greater distally, beginning with the toes and moving upward. This swelling is neither pitting nor brawny but firmly "spongy" in character; that is, although it does not significantly resist deformation by pressure, the skin and subcutaneous tissues quickly return to their original position as the pressure is withdrawn. Skin pigmentation and ulceration are rare. If anything, the skin eventually becomes hypertrophic. The end-stage of chronic lymphatic insufficiency, *elephantiasis,* with its folds of thickened, lichenified skin hanging over the ankle, is too characteristic to be missed.

Occasionally, patients with the "postphlebitic syndrome" who progress to stasis dermatitis and ulceration early may not develop typical scarring and contraction of the subcutaneous tissue but have rather more of an elephantiasis appearance. This confusing variant is caused by invasive infection via the chronically ulcerated skin, which obliterates subcutaneous lymphatics and leads to secondary lymphedema.

Not uncommonly, women present with chronically "swollen" legs that have none of the foregoing characteristics. Although often reluctant to admit it, they usually confess that they have always had "thick" ankles. These patients, and often other female members of their family, have maldistribution of fat characterized by excessive peripheral deposition, in the arms as well as the legs. For unknown reasons, these women are prone to superimposed orthostatic edema and complain of a dull ache and sensitivity of the overlying skin. This swelling, sometimes referred to as *lipedema,* never completely subsides with elevation or diuretics. Furthermore, it is symmetric, with a *noticeable* sparing of the feet.

Finally, swelling, which always feels greater to the patient than it appears to the examiner, may represent a form of dysesthesia. If such patients also complain of superficial burning discomfort and show signs of autonomic imbalance, one should suspect a minor form of causalgia or reflex sympathetic dystrophy.

The Ulcerated Leg

The third most common problem for which the vascular specialist is likely to be consulted is leg ulcers. There are only three types of chronic ulceration commonly encountered in the lower extremities—ischemic, stasis, and neurotrophic ulcers—and they are readily distinguished one from the other, as outlined in Table 1–2. *Ischemic ulcers* are usually quite painful, and there is likely to be typical ischemic rest pain in the distal forefoot that occurs nocturnally and is relieved by dependency. These ulcers may have irregular edges at first, but when chronic, they are more likely to be "punched-out." They are commonly located distally over the dorsum of the foot or toes, but may occasionally be pretibial. The ulcer base usually consists of poorly developed, grayish granulation tissue. The surrounding skin may be pale or mottled and the previously described signs of chronic ischemia are invariably present. Probing or débriding the ulcer causes little bleeding.

Table 1–2. Differential Diagnosis of Common Leg Ulcers

Type	Usual Location	Pain	Bleeding With Manipulation	Lesion Characteristics	Associated Findings
Ischemic	Distally, on dorsum of foot or toes	Severe, particularly at night, relieved by dependency	Little or none	Irregular edge, poor granulation tissue	Trophic changes of chronic ischemia, absent pulses
Stasis	Lower third of leg (gaiter area)	Mild, relieved by elevation	Venous ooze	Shallow, irregular shape, granulating base, rounded edges	Stasis dermatitis
Neurotrophic	Under calluses or pressure points (e.g., plantar aspect of first or fifth metatarsophalangeal joint)	None	May be brisk	Punched-out, with deep sinus	Demonstrable neuropathy

Neurotrophic ulcers, on the other hand, are completely painless but bleed with manipulation. They are deep and indolent, and are often surrounded by chronic inflammatory reaction and callus. Their location is typically over pressure points or calluses, e.g., the plantar surface of the first or fifth metatarsophalangeal joint, the base of the distal phalanx of the great toe, the dorsum of the interphalangeal joints of toes with flexion contractures, or the calloused posterior rim of the heel pad. The patient usually has long-standing diabetes with a neuropathy characterized by patchy hypesthesia and diminished positional sense, two-point discrimination, and vibratory perception.

The *stasis ulcer* is located within the gaiter area shown in Figure 1–3, most commonly near the medial malleolus. It is usually larger than the other types of ulcers and irregular in outline, but also shallower and with a moist granulating base. It is always surrounded by a zone of stasis dermatitis, as already described.

More than 95 per cent of all chronic leg or foot ulcers fit into one of these three recognizable types. The remainder are hard to distinguish, except that they are not typical of the other three types. Vasculitis, hypertension, and syphilis all may produce leg ulcers. The first often produces multiple punched-out holes and an inflamed indurated base that, on biopsy, suggests fat necrosis or chronic "panniculitis." Hypertensive ulcers represent focal infarcts and are very painful. They may be located around the malleoli, particularly laterally. Syphilitic ulcers are uncommon today, but in any atypical ulcer this or other systemic causes of ulceration, such as chronic ulcerative colitis with pyoderma gangrenosum or tuberculosis, should be suspected. Long-standing ulcers that are refractory to treatment may represent underlying osteomyelitis or a secondary malignant lesion.

Finally, most patients with ulcers of one of the specific types just described blame trauma as the initiating agent. Occasionally, trauma may actually be the primary etiologic factor, with the chronicity of the ulcer being related either to the slow healing that is characteristic of the lower third of the leg or possibly to a degree of arterial insufficiency that would otherwise be subclinical. Such ulcers often heal with nonspecific therapy such as intermittent elevation and the application of an Unna boot.

In summary, good vascular consultation is exemplified by the problem-oriented approach to the painful, swollen, or ulcerated leg; by careful interrogation; and by thoughtful examination—all guided by experience and an appropriate index of suspicion. Having completed the initial assessment at the bedside or in the office, the vascular surgeon must next consider the need to proceed further diagnostically, either for the sake of diagnosis itself or to provide further objective information on which to base therapeutic decisions. Whether the basic diagnosis is obvious or not, the location and extent of the vascular disease and the degree of circulatory impairment can often be objectively documented by noninvasive diagnostic methods such as those described in the next chapter.

Angiographic confirmation is usually obtained *only* if necessary in order to make major therapeutic decisions, including the feasibility of reconstructive vascular surgery or balloon angioplasty. Since these procedures are not without risk and expense, the choice between operative and nonoperative treatment, as discussed in the next chapter, should usually be made *before* proceeding with angiographic studies (see Fig. 1–1).

2

Evaluation and Selection of Patients for Vascular Surgery

Robert B. Rutherford, M.D.

• • •

KEY CONSIDERATIONS IN THE SELECTION OF PATIENTS

The proper selection of patients for operative treatment is a cornerstone of clinical ability for the vascular surgeon, equal in importance to technical skill. The process can be viewed as a risk : benefit analysis that must always be settled in the patient's favor. The key considerations are outlined in Figure 2–1. One must weigh carefully both the degree of disability and the natural course of the underlying vascular disorder with optimal medical management against the risk and projected benefits of the operation under consideration. The benefits of surgical intervention should be considered in terms of both degree and duration; these will vary from patient to patient for the *same* operation but can

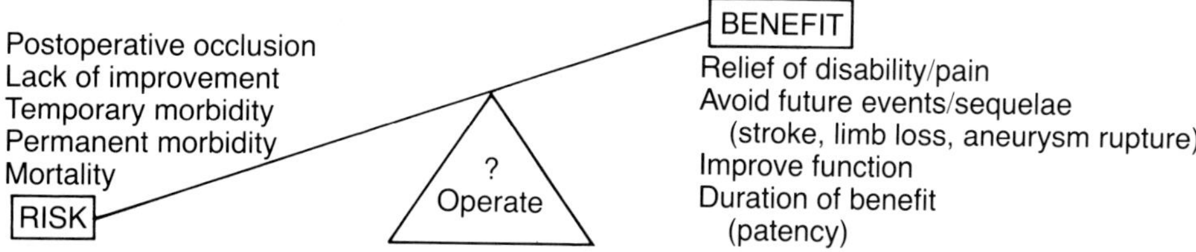

FIGURE 2–1. The risk:benefit analysis that underlies the decision to operate requires accurate assessment of the risks of mortality and morbidity for a given operation, the frequency and consequences of technical and hemodynamic failure (longevity, patency rate), and the likelihood of serious events or sequelae associated with the (medically treated) natural history of the condition.

be estimated by considering specific variables, such as run-off, clinical class, choice of graft, longevity, and known risk factors. The risk of operation also varies with the patient. Therefore, this decision process must be *individualized,* and estimates of longevity, operative risk (morbidity and mortality), hemodynamic benefit, and initial and late patency all must be adjusted to apply to a given procedure being performed on a particular patient by a particular surgeon. Typically this process begins, as depicted in Figure 2–2 (using peripheral *arterial* occlusive disease as an example), with the initial patient interview and examination, complemented by noninvasive testing, when appropriate. This often will establish the nature and severity of the vascular problem and whether the patient is likely to be a candidate for operation. Further studies may be required to evaluate risk, and *only* after these are completed and one is willing to proceed with operation is angiography obtained to assess the morphologic and anatomic characteristics of the involved vascular segment, and thus the most appropriate operation and its technical feasibility. Obtaining an arteriogram at the *end* of the evaluation is like getting a road map. You don't need it unless you are definitely going to make the trip! The relative significance of these factors can best be demonstrated by examples drawn primarily from chronic arterial and venous insufficiency of the lower extremities.

Degree of Disability

Disability constitutes a relative rather than a mandatory indication for operation in that the degree of disability must be considered against the background of the patient's work and other normal activities. Claudication that arises after walking one block may not interfere significantly with the rather sedentary lives of many retired persons, but to

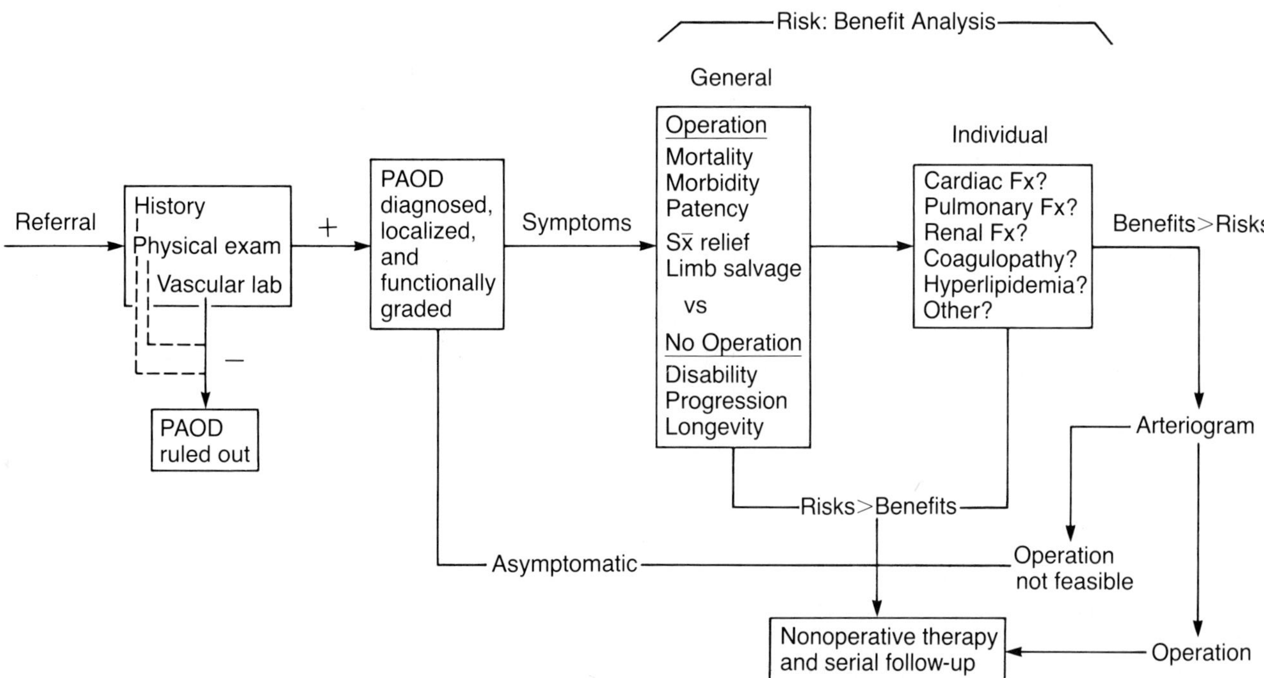

FIGURE 2–2. Stepwise approach to the decision to operate, beginning with initial consultation or outpatient visit and ending, *after* complete evaluation has confirmed the patient to be a surgical candidate with a reasonable operating risk, with arteriography. PAOD, peripheral arterial occlusive disease.

one who has worked long and hard in anticipation of a retirement filled with golf, hiking, or travel, that same degree of claudication constitutes a serious restriction. Claudication usually interferes significantly with the lives of most working persons and is an accepted indication for intervention in those who are not retired when associated risk factors are reasonable. Ischemic rest pain, on the other hand, is an utterly disabling pain that often cannot be controlled even with strong analgesics or narcotics and is, therefore, a universally accepted indication for arterial reconstructive surgery for patients of any age.

However, the absolute concept of claudication as a benign form to be treated conservatively and of chronic critical ischemia as an immediate threat to limb viability that demands arterial reconstruction has been challenged by Taylor and Porter.[9] They have pointed out that, on the one hand, the ultimate risk of limb loss in the claudicator varies directly with the severity of the occlusive disease and can be stratified according to the level of reduction of the ankle-brachial index (ABI). On the other hand, one can succeed in the patient with chronic critical ischemia to preserve limb viability using general supportive measures alone in up to 40 per cent of cases, a perspective gained from control groups in randomized prospective trials of prostanoids and other nonoperative forms of therapy.

A homemaker, however busy, can usually arrange duties so that the postphlebitic leg can be elevated frequently; an automobile assembly line worker, scrub nurse, or shopkeeper may not be able to follow a strict postphlebitic routine and, rather than advising such persons to seek other, less suitable employment, they may be offered one of the procedures designed to combat venous valvular insufficiency or obstruction (see Chapters 139 and 140).

Some disabilities are commonly overlooked by the clinician. Considerable discussion of the impact of claudication from aortoiliac occlusive disease on work or recreation may take place without even broaching the subject of impotence. Similarly, physicians may focus on the ability of drug therapy to control renovascular hypertension without considering the debilitating side effects of multidrug therapy (malaise, asthenia, depression, impotence).

Natural Course of Disease

A further dimension in patient selection is the natural course of the underlying condition, also exemplified by arterial occlusive disease involving the lower extremities. Peabody and associates, in the Framingham study, reported that patients with intermittent claudication ran little more than a 5 per cent risk of major amputation for gangrene within 5 years of the onset of this symptom if treated expectantly, whereas, within the same time frame, 23 per cent developed symptoms of coronary insufficiency, 13 per cent suffered cerebrovascular accidents, and 20 per cent died.[5] From similar experiences, it has been predicted that close to one third of patients operated on for advanced arteriosclerosis obliterans involving the lower extremity will die of heart disease, stroke, or other consequences of atherosclerosis (ruptured aneurysm, mesenteric ischemia) within 5 years. Even though more aggressive surgical treatment of coronary and carotid occlusive disease may invalidate these statistics to some degree in the future, the degree of associated arteriosclerotic coronary disease must still be considered. A patent femoropopliteal bypass can hardly be considered a success if its relief of one-block claudication unmasks two-block angina pectoris. On the other hand, in a reversal of attitudes, many cardiologists are now referring patients with stable angina for peripheral arterial surgery because their claudication prevents participation in a cardiac rehabilitation program that is heavily based on graded ambulatory exercise. Once arteriosclerosis obliterans has progressed to the point of causing ischemic rest pain, however, the likelihood of an eventual major amputation is great if arterial reconstruction is not undertaken. One of the obvious goals of reconstructive surgery is to prevent gangrene, and not long ago established gangrene was treated only by amputation. Since minor (e.g., digital) gangrene due to occlusive disease of major proximal arteries usually requires major proximal (e.g., below-knee) amputation to achieve primary healing, current thinking favors arterial reconstruction in these instances to prevent further tissue loss and to allow healing of tissue subjected to local débridement after a limited (ray, transmetatarsal) amputation. Thus, the surgical attitude changes from conservative to aggressive with increasing severity of peripheral arteriosclerotic occlusive disease, not only because the disability is more severe but also because the eventuality of gangrene and major amputation is increasingly likely. This aggressive attitude toward truly limb-threatening ischemia is reinforced by observations that both the risk and the cost of arterial reconstructions for "limb salvage," using low-risk alternatives when appropriate, are *not* higher than for major amputation. In fact, they are lower in most comparisons (see Chapter 153). Furthermore, older patients are less likely to be rehabilitated or to use a limb prosthesis; they are more likely, in spite of initial support by well-meaning relatives, to end up in nursing homes.

The natural history of untreated deep venous thrombosis of the lower extremity, as summarized in Table 2–1 from Bauer's classic study, is one of increasing frequency of stasis dermatitis and ulceration with the passage of time.[1] Although more recent studies suggest that the frequency of these postphlebitic sequelae may be somewhat less,[4, 7] all recognize that large numbers of potentially productive members of Western society are significantly disabled by chronic venous insufficiency following phlebitis. The indications for operations designed to mitigate these stasis sequelae must not be considered so much in the light of this inevitability, however, as against the established efficacy of nonsurgical treatment, because it has been shown that stasis dermatitis and ulceration can be *completely* controlled in most patients with uncomplicated venous valvular insuffi-

Table 2–1. Natural History of Untreated Deep Venous Thrombosis of the Lower Extremity

Years after phlebitis	5	10	>10
Incidence of stasis dermatitis (%)	45	72	91
Incidence of ulceration (%)	20	52	79

From Bauer GA: A roentgenological and clinical study of the sequels of thrombosis. Acta Chir Scand Suppl 74, p 1, 1942.

ciency who can and will follow a strict postphlebitic routine of intermittent leg elevation and use of proper elastic support. One must consider not only the natural history of the vascular condition under consideration in determining the indications for surgical intervention but also, more specifically, its outlook with appropriate nonoperative therapy. The documented effectiveness of exercise therapy in the claudicator (see Chapter 51) and conservative therapy for chronic venous insufficiency (see Chapter 138) are two obvious examples of this modified perspective.

The natural history of chronic arterial and venous insufficiency of the lower extremities tends to be a continuum, albeit subject to episodic exacerbations. In vascular surgery for other conditions, one may not commonly be faced with patients with few or no symptoms, in whom the outlook for serious, even lethal, symptomatic progression is sufficient to warrant prophylactic intervention. Conditions for which the outlook is serious include abdominal aortic aneurysms, popliteal aneurysms, splenic aneurysms in women of childbearing age, post-stenotic subclavian aneurysms secondary to cervical rib compression, popliteal artery entrapment, "critical" stenosis of the carotid or mesenteric artery, traumatic arteriovenous fistulae involving central vessels, or large "floating tails" of thrombus following deep venous thrombosis. Because of the element of truth in the adage, "it is difficult to make an asymptomatic patient better," the vascular surgeon must be certain of the projections of the threatening natural history of these and similar conditions and of the *relative* safety of the proposed intervention. The latter is particularly pertinent now that the era of endovascular intervention has been ushered in.

Risk and Success Rate of Operative Procedure

The risk of morbidity and death following operation must be weighed. Even though patients with arteriosclerosis are generally at a higher than average risk for their age, they tolerate operations limited to the extremity, neck, or superficial layers of the trunk relatively well, and vascular procedures confined to these areas carry a relatively small risk if one discounts deaths due to ongoing underlying disease rather than due to new problems precipitated by operation. In patients with limb-threatening ischemia, this risk is not greater than that which would attend the major amputation that might be required if arterial reconstruction were not undertaken. In fact, statistics gathered from the major series of amputations for "arterial" gangrene suggest that the risk of major amputation is greater than that of peripheral arterial reconstruction.[2, 3] However, if amputations were taken more seriously, and monitored with the same intensity as arterial reconstructions, one would expect mortality rates to be comparable. Thus, while these risks are not truly comparable, because the patient populations are not comparable, it is clear that the risk of major amputation should not be taken lightly and is significant enough that peripheral arterial reconstruction should not be abandoned in favor of amputation simply because of a presumed lesser risk.

These same patients would, however, be exposed to a considerably greater magnitude of surgical stress if their arterial reconstruction were performed through the abdominal cavity, as in the case of aortoiliac reconstruction. In spite of this, the mortality rates for those undergoing infrainguinal bypass are *not* significantly less than for those undergoing aortic reconstructions. This is because the former population, often heavily loaded with diabetic patients, has proportionately much more visceral atherosclerosis (e.g., coronary, carotid, renal artery involvement). Most patients with chronic limb-threatening ischemia have multilevel occlusive disease and, typically in this situation, one would expect to find superficial femoral artery occlusion in addition to the proximal aortoiliac disease. Parallel experience has also taught us that proximal bypass, performed with a concomitant profundaplasty, thus introducing a full head of systemic arterial pressure into the parallel profunda-geniculate collateral bed, will obviate the need for dealing with the superficial femoral artery occlusion in the vast majority of cases (i.e., 85 to 90 per cent). Although this greatly reduces the time and extent of the operation required, it does not reduce the major risk that is associated with the transabdominal reconstruction. Fortunately, this dilemma has been relieved somewhat by the option now provided by the so-called extra-anatomic bypass procedures, the femorofemoral or axillofemoral bypass. Because of these and other "low-risk" alternatives, such as femoral profundaplasty, it is rare today for the vascular surgeon to have to decline to treat the patient with limb-threatening ischemia (i.e., ischemic rest pain, ulceration, or limited gangrene) because of the risk of reconstructive arterial surgery itself. However, the patency rates of these low-risk alternatives do not compare favorably with those for the direct reconstructive procedures, and thus they are rarely offered for good-risk patients or those with claudication. Furthermore, these low-risk alternatives often carry paradoxically higher mortality rates than those for aortoiliac reconstructions in reported comparisons (see Chapter 54). This is because they are often reserved for patients of prohibitive risk, who, when removed from the ranks of those undergoing direct aortoiliac reconstruction, reciprocally improve the latter's mortality statistics. (See Chapters 52 and 54.)

In predicting the risk and success of a vascular operation, the common practice of quoting the "bottom line" results of some major reported series may be misleading for several reasons. First, the surgeon in question may be more or less experienced than those reporting these experiences, depending on the degree to which the procedures were performed or closely supervised by experienced vascular surgeons. Second, the particular patient to whom this yardstick is being applied is not likely to exactly fit the profile for the average risk of a particular series. The patient's risk with the same operation depends on the coexistence of other significant systemic disorders, such as hypertension, diabetes, and chronic obstructive pulmonary disease, as well as the degree of arteriosclerotic involvement of the coronary and cerebral arteries. The estimation of operative risk clearly must be individualized. Third, the patient is just as unlikely to have the same severity of occlusive disease reflected in the overall data from reported series. These data reflect a mixture of cases with good and poor runoff; the patient in question is likely to have one or the other. For example, the author has reported an overall 5-year patency rate for axillobifemoral bypass performed for occlusive disease of *47 per cent,* but for patients with an open superficial femoral artery this rate was *92 per cent* and for those with poor runoff it was *41 per cent.*[6] Finally, it is not uncommon for large series to extend back over a decade or more and, therefore, to fail to reflect accurately more recent technical advances or the subtle but cumulative benefits of experience.

In the 1960s, in what has been referred to as the golden age of vascular surgery, surgeons were obliged to inform patients of a 5 per cent risk of loss of life and a 10 per cent risk of loss of limb for arterial reconstructive procedures on the lower extremity. Furthermore, in an additional 10 per cent of cases the procedure would fail to either relieve the patient's symptoms or salvage the limb. The overall initial success rate (survival without major morbidity and a patent arterial reconstruction with symptomatic relief) was then 75 per cent. Today, these risks have been greatly reduced and the initial success rate is closer to 95 per cent.

Although series that include data from the 1960s and 1970s may not reflect it, most major vascular surgery services can now point to operative mortality rates for *elective* aortic aneurysmectomy, aortobifemoral bypass, femoropopliteal bypass, and carotid endarterectomy—four of the most commonly performed vascular operations—in the range of 3 to 1 per cent. These figures reflect the development of methods of avoiding recognized complications, more sophisticated monitoring techniques for directing intravenous fluid and drug therapy during the perioperative period, and more careful patient selection (e.g., not operating for acute stroke and using extra-anatomic bypass rather than direct aortoiliac reconstruction in high-risk patients). The risks of permanent neurologic morbidity following carotid endarterectomy and of limb loss following aortoiliac reconstruction are now under 2 per cent. As mentioned earlier, distal arterial reconstructions, which do not invade a major body cavity or cause much blood loss (e.g., femoropopliteal and femorotibial bypasses), and the "low-risk" alternatives, extra-anatomic bypasses and profundaplasty, actually carry a somewhat higher risk of loss of life or limb, in the range of 2 to 5 per cent and 3 to 7 per cent, respectively. This is because the former procedures are performed on patients with more distally distributed atherosclerosis, which is, in turn, associated with a significantly higher incidence of visceral (coronary and carotid) involvement, and the latter procedures are offered *only* to poor-risk patients. Furthermore, both are generally reserved for limb salvage situations, in which multi-segmental disease and poor runoff are invariably present.

The 25 to 50 per cent 5-year failure rate commonly cited in the past for arterial prostheses partly reflected a significant incidence of anastomotic aneurysm and occlusion by sloughing pseudointima or intimal hyperplasia. The abandonment of silk sutures and tightly woven Dacron grafts in favor of polypropylene sutures and knitted velour and polytetrafluoroethylene (PTFE) grafts, respectively, and the avoidance of prosthetic grafts in peripheral, small-caliber (less than 6 mm in diameter) reconstructions in which flexion creases are crossed, runoff is poor, and resting flow rates are slow have contributed to improved results, as have the selective use of antithrombotic drugs and employment of serial graft surveillance protocols. There is no doubt, in the small-caliber, low-flow graft, that saphenous vein grafts (be they in situ, reversed, or translocated in an antegrade orientation after their valves are rendered incompetent) are distinctly superior to any current prosthetic. The rate of failure in "harvesting" a satisfactory saphenous vein graft for femoropopliteal bypass used to be around 20 per cent even for primary operations. Now, with the additional use of lesser saphenous or arm veins, this figure should be closer to 5 per cent for primary infrageniculate bypass (see Chapter 28). Similarly, the frequency of late occlusion of these vein grafts—because of stricture, proliferative or degenerative changes, atheromatous degeneration, intimal fibrosis, or paravalvular stenosis—once noted to be as high as 28 per cent,[8] has decreased now that the causes of damage to the vein during its preparation have been recognized and can be avoided. Finally, technical developments have allowed in situ bypass to be fully utilized in femorodistal bypass. The suitability of the saphenous vein can be established preoperatively by duplex scanning and, because smaller veins can be used and the aforementioned structural changes are rarer, both vein utilization and patency rates have been significantly improved. The improved results with distal bypass using in situ or reversed saphenous veins (now approaching the patency rates achieved with proximal bypass) are in sharp contrast with those achieved with prosthetic or modified biologic grafts when carried below the knee (<40 per cent for below-knee and <20 per cent for tibial/peroneal bypass at 5 years). The lack of a small-caliber graft that can maintain reasonable patency rates when anastomosed to the low-flow, high-resistance arteries of the leg remains the greatest single barrier to successful limb salvage surgery.

The *overall* results in this field do not completely reflect the significant advances that have been made, mainly because more difficult cases are now being subjected to bypass (cases that would have undergone primary amputation in the past) and because of the inability of most patients to refrain from tobacco abuse. Nevertheless, the reconstructive procedures, graft choices, and patency rates have changed significantly since the late 1970s. In recommending appropriate therapy, practicing vascular surgeons need to be as aware of this changing outlook as they are of the technical advances that brought it. Similarly, they must be aware of changes in other modes of therapy, particularly percutaneous transluminal angioplasty. Its low risk and cost compensate for its lesser degree and duration of benefit to make it the initial treatment of choice for discrete stenoses, particularly in the larger, proximal arteries. Now used in close to 25 per cent of patients presenting for treatment, it tends to be complementary and adjunctive rather than a competitive form of therapy (see Chapter 58).

Clearly, it is not possible to predict outcome from past experience; neither should one project outcome on the basis of overall results from others' series. Rather, such reports should serve as a frame of reference on which to project one's own results, for every vascular surgeon should regularly analyze her or his own experiences (see Chapter 25). Furthermore, adjustment should be made not only for the operation and the operator but also for individual considerations such as associated risk factors, runoff, and types of graft.

DIAGNOSTIC STUDIES

The preoperative evaluation of patients for vascular surgery, including angiography, is deliberately dealt with *after* the discussion of case selection, in order to emphasize the sequence of events and priorities that should be observed in clinical practice. This tentative decision is upheld in most cases, although occasionally the unexpected discovery of associated disease or a discouraging angiogram will reverse this judgment. More is required prior to operation than a pertinent history and a physical examination relative to the vascular problem.

The actual assessment of risk is discussed in greater detail in Chapter 22; only the choice of diagnostic studies required to determine operative risk is considered here. Ordinarily, cardiopulmonary and renal function are carefully evaluated. A complete blood count, urinalysis, blood urea nitrogen (BUN) and creatinine level determinations, multiphasic screening or biochemical profile, glucose tolerance test, electrocardiogram (ECG), and chest x-ray films are almost routinely ordered. Special studies for each condition are discussed in detail in the sections and chapters dealing with the individual conditions. Obviously, if the patient's problem is arteriosclerosis, serum cholesterol and triglyceride levels should be determined and serum lipoprotein electrophoresis should be performed; and if the disorder is thromboembolic, a coagulation profile should be obtained. Any intercurrent disease should be investigated on its own merits. More extensive preoperative evaluations may be extended along the lines indicated by history, physical examination, or the results of the previously mentioned routine tests. In patients with known pulmonary problems, an abnormal chest x-ray, or abnormal blood gas values determined with the patient breathing "room air," formal pulmonary function studies are ordered. In patients with an elevated BUN or creatinine level, a creatinine clearance test is obtained, and contrast urography may be performed simultaneously with angiographic study if this is planned. Patients with ECG abnormalities, cardiac symptoms, or evidence of such widespread arteriosclerosis that coronary artery involvement is likely will often undergo radionuclide scanning or Holter's monitoring, or both, to evaluate cardiac perfusion and function; in selected cases, cardiac catheterization and coronary angiography will be performed. Patients with serious cardiac dysfunction with a pressing need for vascular surgery for other problems (e.g., crescendo transient ischemic attacks or a large aortic aneurysm) are best admitted to the intensive care unit for preoperative monitoring and optimization of cardiac function (see Chapter 22).

Noninvasive Studies

Special diagnostic procedures are discussed in detail in the later sections, but the value of selectively employing objective, noninvasive methods of pre- and postoperative monitoring is worthy of emphasis. These studies help avoid misdiagnoses and gauge the extent and severity of the vascular disease prior to angiography; they determine the hemodynamic significance of the lesions visualized by angiography and allow it to be employed more selectively, and when the physiologic data and angiographic anatomy are considered together, the surgeon can not only better choose the most appropriate operation but also better predict the hemodynamic outcome. In some circumstances, noninvasive studies characterize the lesions so well that preoperative arteriography may be obviated (e.g., symptomatic carotid bifurcation disease, infrarenal aortic aneurysms). This will be seen increasingly as newer, improved forms of vascular imaging become generally available (see Chapter 6). Additionally, they provide a readily available means of objectively assessing the initial and continued success of the operation itself.

Furthermore, because they can detect and localize lower extremity occlusive lesions, either singly or in combination, with greater than 95 per cent accuracy, unnecessary "diagnostic" arteriography is eliminated; for all intents and purposes, this study is not obtained until the decision has already been made that the patient should have a particular operation and precise anatomic information is required before embarking on this venture. The availability of endovascular interventions has caused this position to be modified somewhat. However, the cost of routine arteriography in search of short (<5 cm), discrete lesions favorable for this approach cannot be justified. Fortunately, color duplex scanning has filled this screening need. Also fortunately, this and other noninvasive studies can be performed on an outpatient basis.

Radiographic Studies

Equally pertinent to this introductory chapter is a discussion of the use of angiography. Arteriographic and phlebographic studies on selected patients provide invaluable information regarding the location and extent of the disease, and occasionally this anatomic information is supplemented by qualitative impressions regarding the rate of blood flow. Now, however, it is often possible to diagnose the nature and location of the vascular lesion with reasonable certainty by physical examination supplemented by some of the newer noninvasive diagnostic methods so that angiography is selectively rather than routinely employed.

Arteriography. Generally, the vascular surgeon obtains an arteriogram to study the condition of the vessels proximal and distal to the lesion. For example, when confronted with superficial femoral artery occlusion, the vascular surgeon wants to be sure that there is not an occult iliac artery stenosis proximally, that the profunda femoris is widely patent and providing maximal collateral flow, and that the condition of the popliteal and infrapopliteal arteries into which a graft may be placed is suitable. Similarly, if an abdominal aortic aneurysm is large enough to be easily felt, or if its calcific outline on a cross-table lateral film or ultrasound studies indicates it is 5 to 6 cm in diameter, there is little reason for aortography unless there is a suspicion of significant proximal (e.g., renal or mesenteric artery) or distal (e.g., iliac or femoral artery) occlusive disease. In fact, since more abdominal aortic aneurysms are lined by intraluminal clot, their internal diameters often appear misleadingly normal on aortograms. Enhanced com-

Table 2–2. Correlation With Phlebography of Signs and Symptoms in Suspected Leg Deep Venous Thrombosis

	Positive Phlebogram		Negative Phlebogram	
	Per Cent	***No. of Patients Examined***	***Per Cent***	***No. of Patients Examined***
Pain in calf	90	33	97	39
Calf tenderness	84	33	74	39
Decrease of skin temperature	42	26	38	30
Unilateral ankle edema	76	33	76	39
Superficial venous dilatation	33	27	18	34
Homans' sign	33	33	21	37
Löwenberg's sign	20	15	15	15

From Haeger K: Problems of acute deep venous thrombosis. I. The interpretation of signs and symptoms. Angiology, 1969: 20:219. Reprinted with permission of copyright owner: Westminster Publications, Inc., Roslyn, New York, 11576.

puted tomography (CT) scans are better for preoperative screening, because they reveal most of the associated pathology or anomalies that can complicate repair (such as inflammatory aneurysms, horseshoe or ectopic kidney, or caval or renal vein anomalies). Ultrasound is still the most practical method of monitoring for enlargement. Now that segmental limb pressures and plethysmographic studies are readily obtainable, arteriograms are obtained not for diagnostic curiosity but for therapeutic intent. Good quality, multi-plane view arteriograms are absolutely essential in dealing with multi-segmental disease. Particularly important in this regard are oblique views of the iliac and proximal profunda femoris arteries and adequate visualization of "runoff" vessels distally. By the same token, in dealing with carotid occlusive or ulcerative lesions, angiographic demonstration of disease in the arch vessels, contralateral bifurcation, ipsilateral siphon, or vertebral arteries may be as important as what appears to be the primary lesion.

Phlebography. Phlebography also suffers from indiscriminate use. It should never be necessary to use it to rule out deep venous insufficiency in candidates for varicose vein stripping or to localize incompetent perforators in those with more advanced disease. This can nearly always be determined by an adequate history and physical examination, supplemented by venous Doppler examination and plethysmographic measurement of venous reflux and its modification by tourniquet placement. Perforators can be localized by duplex scan (see Chapter 133). The stigmata of the postphlebitic state are readily recognized. On the other hand, the data from Haeger's study, summarized in Table 2–2, indicate that phlebography may be necessary to distinguish initial or recurrent episodes of acute deep venous thrombosis from other causes of leg pain that may mimic it.[3] It is said that at least 30 per cent of patients with a diagnosis of phlebitis carry this stigma unnecessarily, whereas many others suffer deep venous thrombosis without its being recognized either by them or by their physicians. This last is particularly true of patients who have had serious extremity trauma or vascular or orthopedic operations. However, venous Doppler examination and venous plethysmography together, or duplex scan alone, can detect deep venous thrombosis with an accuracy of over 95 per cent. Nevertheless, the consequences of this diagnosis are so far-reaching, in terms of the need for extended anticoagulant therapy and indefinite adherence to a postphlebitic regimen, that if these noninvasive tests are not clearly diagnostic (i.e., disagree with each other or with a strong contrary clinical impression), phlebography should be performed before the patient is committed to long-term therapy. The same rationale applies to the use of pulmonary angiography in cases of suspected pulmonary embolism and particularly in the event of recurrences during anticoagulant therapy.

SUMMARY

It is only after confirming the existence, nature, and extent of the vascular lesion, and balancing the disability it causes, or is likely to cause despite proper nonoperative management, against the feasibility, risk, and anticipated success of alternative surgical, endovascular, and nonsurgical forms of therapy, that the vascular surgeon is in a position to advise the patient or the referring physician regarding the need for surgical intervention. The manner in which this evaluation is carried out and the judgment that is applied to this stepwise process are the foundation for a successful practice in vascular surgery.

References

1. Bauer GA: A roentgenological and clinical study of the sequels of thrombosis. Acta Chir Scand Suppl 74, p 1, 1942.
2. DeWeese JA, Blaisdell FW, Foster JH: Optimal resources for vascular surgery. Arch Surg 105:948, 1972.
3. Haeger K: Problems of acute deep venous thrombosis. I. The interpretation of signs and symptoms. Angiology 20:219, 1969.
4. Lindner DJ, Edwards JM, Phinney ES, et al: Long term hemodynamic and clinical sequelae of lower extremity deep vein thrombosis. J Vasc Surg 4:436, 1986.
5. Peabody CN, Kannel WB, McNamara PM: Intermittent claudication: Surgical significance. Arch Surg 109:693, 1974.
6. Rutherford RB, Patt A, Pearce WH: Extra-anatomic bypass: A closer view. Presented at the Western Vascular Society, Tucson, Arizona, January 23, 1987. J Vasc Surg 6:437, 1987.
7. Strandness DE, Langlois Y, Cramer M, et al: Long term sequelae of acute venous thrombosis. JAMA 250:1289, 1983.
8. Szilagyi DE, Elliot JP, Hageman JH, et al: Biologic fate of autogenous vein implants of arterial substitutes. Surgery 74:731, 1973.
9. Taylor LM Jr, Porter JM: Natural history of chronic lower extremity ischemia. Semin Vasc Surg 4:181, 1991.

SECTION II

Hemodynamics and Diagnosis of Arterial Disease: Basic Techniques and Applications

Edited by David S. Sumner, M.D., and Anthony J. Comerota, M.D.

Overview

David S. Sumner, M.D.

• • •

The sole function of the peripheral circulation can be summarized in one word: transportation. Blood carries oxygen, nutrients, metabolic wastes, hormones, antibodies, leukocytes, medications, and heat to and from all living cells of the body. Energy for this vital function is supplied largely by one source, the heart. Although the muscle pumps of the legs and, to a lesser extent, the respiratory pump do supplement this energy on the venous side, their contribution ordinarily is quite small. Like a roller coaster, blood is given a potential energy boost at the heart, and then must travel in a general downhill direction, periodically accelerating and decelerating as potential energy is transformed back and forth into kinetic energy at each hydraulic hill and valley. All along the way, friction dissipates energy, restricting the velocity of flow. As with the roller coaster, any obstacle or any junction or bend will decrease the total available energy and interfere with the vital function of the bloodstream.

With the exception of some primarily anatomic lesions, such as aortic aneurysms, the pathophysiology of peripheral circulatory disease is largely a study in energy depletion—thus, most vascular surgery is designed to treat a physiologic rather than an anatomic defect. For this reason, precise diagnosis and objective assessment of peripheral vascular disease require recognition of abnormal flow patterns and measurement of energy deficits. The diagnosis, however, is not complete without morphologic information. Planning surgical therapy, assessing the results of therapy, and determining the natural history of the disease all require detailed anatomic knowledge.

With each passing year, vascular diagnostic testing reaches a new level of maturity. Since the last edition of this book appeared, imaging techniques (such as duplex scanning and color duplex imaging) that provide detailed anatomic as well as local physiologic information have become more firmly entrenched as the primary diagnostic modalities. Now that the versatile and sophisticated instruments of these modalities are widely available, there is less emphasis on purely physiologic tests, although the latter continue to play an important role in the hemodynamic assessment of specific problems. Many of the controversies concerning choice of instruments and testing procedures that plagued us during the 2 previous decades have been resolved, but some remain as a challenge for the 1990s. As always, the future promises exciting new developments. Recent advances in three-dimensional imaging provide an inkling of what might be in store.

This section outlines the hemodynamic principles that are basic to our understanding of vascular disease and explores the role of physiologic testing and diagnostic imaging. Although emphasis is placed on diagnostic techniques that have stood the test of time, newer tests whose value remains to be determined are also presented.

3

Essential Hemodynamic Principles

David S. Sumner, M.D.

• • •

Most arterial problems of concern to the surgeon involve obstructive disease, aneurysm formation, or trauma. Less frequently, arteriovenous fistulae and vasospastic phenomena are encountered.

Obstruction or narrowing of the arterial lumen (whether it is the result of atherosclerosis, fibromuscular dysplasia, thrombi, emboli, dissection, trauma, or external compression) interferes with the efficient transport of blood to the peripheral capillary bed. Within the obstructed vessel, the extent of this interference is related to the degree of narrowing and is determined by strict hemodynamic principles. Factors affecting the actual capillary flow deficit are more complex, depending not only on the severity of the local obstructive lesion but also on its location and on the ability of the body to compensate by increasing cardiac work, by developing collateral channels, and by dilating the peripheral arterioles and precapillary sphincters.

The symptoms and signs of obstructive arterial disease reflect the restriction of blood flow to the capillary bed. With mild obstruction, this restriction is evident only when metabolic demands are increased by exercise, trauma, or infection; but with more severe disease, capillary perfusion is compromised even during the basal state. Consequently, the disease may be relatively asymptomatic or symptomatic only during exercise, or may be responsible for continued rest pain and eventual tissue loss.

Except for clot formation and occasional dissection, aneurysms seldom produce symptoms of obstruction. Surgery is indicated to forestall rupture or to reestablish vascular continuity when rupture occurs. The tendency to rupture is determined by both the intraluminal pressure and the diameter of the aneurysm.

This chapter deals with the hemodynamic alterations produced by obstruction, the effects of shear, the rationale for surgery, the elastic properties of the arterial wall, and the stresses that lead to rupture of aneurysms. The pathophysiology of arteriovenous fistulae and other forms of vascular disease is considered in subsequent sections.

BASIC HEMODYNAMIC PRINCIPLES

The flow of blood in the arterial circulation is governed by basic laws of fluid dynamics. Knowledge of these principles permits a better understanding of the physiologic abnormalities associated with arterial obstruction.*

Fluid Energy

We frequently think of pressure as representing the force responsible for the motion of blood. Although it is true that pressure is the most obvious and most important of the forces involved, other forms of energy also play a role. With more precision, we could state that blood moves from one point to another in the vascular system in response to differences in *total fluid energy*.[19]

Total fluid energy (E) consists of potential energy and kinetic energy. In turn, the potential energy component can be broken down into intravascular pressure and gravitational potential energy.

Intravascular pressure (P) is composed of the pressure produced by contraction of the heart, the hydrostatic pressure, and the static filling pressure of the resting circulation.[58] Hydrostatic pressure is caused by the weight of the blood and is given by:

$$P\ (\text{hydrostatic}) = -\rho g h \qquad (3.1)$$

where ρ is the density of blood (about 1.056 $\text{gm} \cdot \text{cm}^{-3}$), g is the acceleration due to gravity (980 $\text{cm} \cdot \text{sec}^{-2}$), and h is the distance in centimeters above a given reference point. In the human body, this reference point is roughly at the level of the right atrium.[18] Obviously, hydrostatic pressure may be quite large in comparison with the dynamic pressure, and cannot be neglected. For example, at ankle level in a man 5 feet 8 inches tall, this pressure is about 89 mmHg.

$$-(1.056\ \text{gm} \cdot \text{cm}^{-3})\ (980\ \text{cm} \cdot \text{sec}^{-2})\ (-114\ \text{cm}) = 117{,}976\ \text{dynes} \cdot \text{cm}^{-2}$$

$$117{,}976\ \text{dynes} \cdot \text{cm}^{-2} \div 1333\ \text{dynes} \cdot \text{cm}^{-2}/\text{mmHg} = 88.5\ \text{mmHg}$$

*It is interesting that three of the early investigators in the fields of fluid dynamics and elasticity, whose names have been applied to classic laws of hemodynamics, were physicians. These include Daniel Bernoulli (1700–1782) of Switzerland, Thomas Young (1773–1829) of England, and Jean-Leonard-Marie Poiseuille (1799–1869) of France.[69]

In contrast, the static filling pressure is quite low, usually about 7 mmHg.[63] This pressure is related to the interaction between the elasticity of the vascular walls and the volume of blood contained within.

Gravitational potential energy ($+\rho gh$) is calculated in the same way as the hydrostatic pressure, but has an opposite sign. It represents the ability of a volume of blood to do work because of its elevation above a given reference point. In many, but not all, circumstances, gravitational potential energy and hydrostatic pressure will cancel each other out.

Finally, kinetic energy represents the ability of blood to do work because of its motion ($\frac{1}{2} \rho v^2$).

Putting these values together, an expression for total fluid energy per unit volume of blood can be obtained:

$$E = P + \rho gh + \tfrac{1}{2} \rho v^2 \quad (3.2)$$

where E is in ergs per cubic centimeter and v refers to the velocity (cm · sec^{-1}) of a particle of blood moving steadily in a straight line.

Bernoulli's Principle

When fluid flows steadily (without acceleration or deceleration) from one point in a system to another further downstream, its total energy content along any given streamline remains constant, provided there are no frictional losses.

$$P_1 + \rho gh_1 + \tfrac{1}{2} \rho {v_1}^2 = P_2 + \rho gh_2 + \rho {v_2}^2 \quad (3.3)$$

This, the *one-dimensional Bernoulli equation*, is derivable from Newton's basic laws of motion and is a fundamental formula in fluid mechanics.[35]

Bernoulli's equation is instructive in that it establishes a relationship among kinetic energy, gravitational potential energy, and pressure in a *frictionless* fluid system. Several apparent paradoxes of fluid flow are readily explained. For example, in Figure 3–1*A*, fluid with the density of blood enters an inclined tube at a pressure of 100 mmHg and flows out at a pressure of 178 mmHg. Thus, fluid moves against the pressure gradient from a point of low pressure to a point where its pressure is high. The total fluid energy remains the same, however, since the gravitational potential energy decreases by an amount exactly equal to the increase in pressure. This situation is analogous to that which exists in the arterial tree of an upright man in which blood pressure in the arteries at ankle level is greater than that in the aortic arch (see Fig. 129–1).

In Figure 3–1*B*, the cross-sectional area of a horizontal tube increases 16 times, resulting in a comparable decrease in fluid velocity. Again, the fluid moves against a pressure gradient, the pressure at the end of the tube being 2.5 mmHg greater than that at the beginning of the tube. The total fluid energy remains the same, however, because of the decrease in kinetic energy. This phenomenon is seldom manifested in the human circulation because associated energy losses effectively mask the slight rise in pressure.

Intravascular pressure measurements made with catheters are subject to error owing to the effect of kinetic energy. If the catheter meets the oncoming blood end-on, the pressure recorded will be too high by a factor of $\frac{1}{2} \rho v^2$. On the other hand, if the catheter faces downstream, the recorded pressure will be too low by the same factor. At a velocity of 50 cm · sec^{-1}, these errors would equal about 1.0 mmHg and would be inconsequential in a high-pressure system such as the aorta. Nevertheless, they could be of importance in low-pressure, high-flow systems such as the vena cava and pulmonary artery.[19]

Energy Losses Associated With Blood Flow

Obviously, the conditions required to fulfill the rigid specifications of Bernoulli's relationship are not met in the human vascular tree. Total fluid energy is always ''lost'' in moving blood from one point to the next in the circulation. Since this energy is almost totally dissipated in the form of heat, Equation 3.3 becomes

$$P_1 + \rho gh_1 + \tfrac{1}{2} \rho {v_1}^2 = P_2 + \rho gh_2 + \tfrac{1}{2} \rho {v_2}^2 + \text{heat} \quad (3.4)$$

There has been interest in using Bernoulli's principle to estimate pressure gradients across cardiac valves and even across peripheral vascular stenoses. With the patient supine, the hydrostatic components (ρgh) on both sides of Equation 3.4 cancel out. If energy losses (heat) are neglected, the following equation is obtained:

$$P_1 - P_2 = \tfrac{1}{2} \rho ({v_2}^2 - {v_1}^2) \quad (3.5)$$

Provided that the upstream velocity (v_1) is quite low, the pressure gradient can be estimated directly from the velocity (v_2) of blood in the orifice of the stenosis—a measurement conveniently made noninvasively with the Doppler technique. Since the density of blood is relatively constant, the $\frac{1}{2} \rho$ term can be replaced by 0.004 when velocity is in

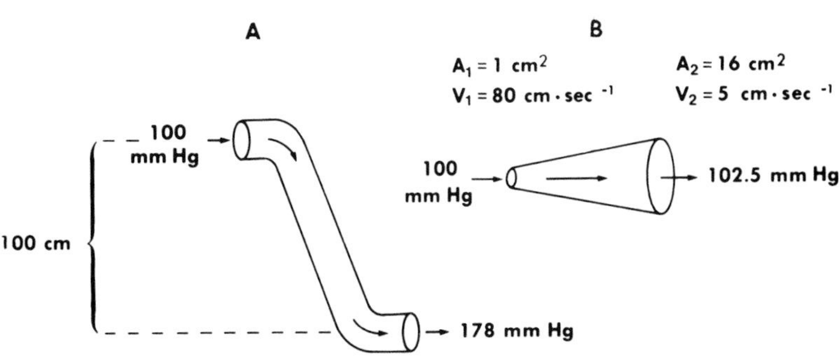

FIGURE 3–1. *A*, Effect of vertical height on pressure in a *frictionless* fluid flowing downhill. *B*, Effect of increasing cross-sectional area on pressure in a *frictionless* fluid system.

cm · sec^{-1} or by 4 when velocity is in m · sec^{-1} to give the pressure gradient in mmHg:

$$\Delta P = 4v_2^2 \qquad (3.6)$$

Although a number of studies have shown reasonably good agreement between pressure drops predicted by this greatly simplified equation and those measured directly across cardiac valves, the agreement, in part, appears to be fortuitous—the underestimation of ΔP due to the neglect of energy losses is balanced by the overestimation of ΔP due to the omission of the upstream velocity (v_1) and the failure to consider the pressure rise that occurs downstream as velocity decreases.[142] As a result, Equation 3.6 tends to overestimate pressure drops across mild to moderate stenoses and to underestimate those across severe stenoses. It seems unlikely, therefore, that Equation 3.6 will predict pressure gradients with sufficient accuracy to be useful when applied to the much longer and more complex lesions found in the peripheral arteries.

Viscosity

Energy losses in the peripheral circulation are related principally to the viscosity of blood and to its inertia. In fluids, viscosity may be defined as the friction existing between contiguous layers of fluid. The friction is due to strong intermolecular attractions; under these conditions, the fluid layers tend to resist deformation. The familiar equation known as Poiseuille's law describes the viscous losses existing in an idealized situation:

$$P_1 - P_2 = \bar{V} \cdot \frac{8L\eta}{r^2} = Q \cdot \frac{8L\eta}{\pi r^4} \qquad (3.7)$$

where $P_1 - P_2$ represents the drop in potential energy (dyne · cm^{-2}) between two points separated by the distance L (cm); Q is the flow (cm^3 · sec^{-1}); and $\bar{V}$ is the mean flow velocity (cm · sec^{-1}) across a tube with an inside radius r (cm). The coefficient of viscosity, η, is expressed in poise (dyne · sec · cm^{-2}).

Under conditions in which Poiseuille's law is operative, the velocities of each concentric layer of fluid describe a *parabolic profile*, with velocity being highest in the center of the stream and becoming progressively lower toward the inner wall. Blood in contact with the wall is stationary. The ratio of the change in velocity (δv) to the change in the radius (δr) between each cylindrical laminar layer is known as the *shear rate* (D); the force required to "shear" the fluid is known as the *shear stress* (τ); and the coefficient of viscosity (η) is the ratio of the shear stress to the shear rate:

$$D = -\frac{\delta v}{\delta r} \quad \text{and} \quad \eta = \frac{\tau}{D} \qquad (3.8)$$

The importance of shear rate and shear stress is discussed later in this chapter.

Because energy losses are inversely proportional to the fourth power of the radius, graphs based on Poiseuille's law are sharply curved (Fig. 3–2). As the diameter of a conduit is reduced, there is little effect on the pressure gradient until a certain degree of narrowing is reached; beyond this point, further reductions in diameter cause the pressure gradient to rise precipitously. Although increasing the rate of flow shifts the curves to the left and linearly increases the pressure gradient at any given radius, these effects are much less marked than those due to changes in radius.

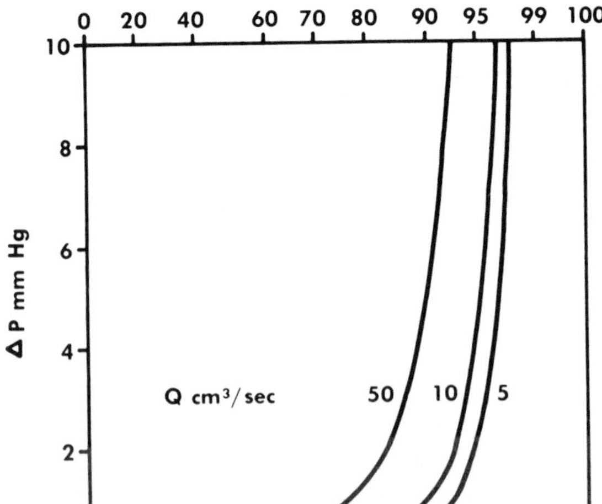

FIGURE 3–2. Curves derived from Poiseuille's law (Eq. 3.7). The stenotic segment is assumed to be 1.0 cm long. Viscosity is 0.035 poise.

Poiseuille's law applies only to steady (nonpulsatile), laminar flow in a straight cylindrical tube with rigid walls. Furthermore, the tube must be long enough to allow a parabolic flow profile to develop.

When fluid passes from a large container into a smaller cylindrical tube, the velocity profile at the entrance is essentially flat (same velocity all across the tube diameter). Just beyond the entrance, friction between the stationary outermost layer and the immediately adjacent concentric layer causes the latter to slow down. This layer in turn exerts a drag force on the next layer and so on down the tube until the "boundary layer," where fluid is sheared, extends to the center of the tube. At this point, flow is said to be fully "developed" and the profile is truly parabolic. The "entrance length" (L_x) in centimeters required to develop a parabolic profile depends on the radius of the tube and the Reynolds number (Re; see later).

$$L_x = k\, r\, Re \qquad (3.9)$$

(The constant, k, varies but approximates 0.16 for Reynolds numbers greater than 50.) All along the entrance length, the velocity profile is "blunt" rather than parabolic. At each branch point in the arterial tree, a certain distance is needed before flow is "developed." Although velocity profiles in smaller arteries, such as the radial or mesenteric arteries, may be essentially parabolic, in larger arteries, such as the iliac or common carotid, the entrance length approaches the length of the artery and flow profiles remain blunt. Many investigators have shown that the flow profile in the human abdominal aorta is blunted.[134, 183]

Entrance effects are, of course, only one of many factors modulating the velocity profile. At branch points or in regions where the vessel curves, the momentum of blood near one wall exceeds that on the other side. As a result, velocity profiles are skewed toward one wall and complicated helical flow patterns develop.[107, 153] Thus, the strict conditions required by Poiseuille's law are seldom, if ever, encountered in the living organism. Furthermore, energy losses almost never are totally viscous; and in many cases, viscous losses are less significant than those related to inertia.

Inertia

Inertial losses depend on the mass or density of the blood, ρ, and on the square of the flow velocity, v:

$$\Delta P = k\ \tfrac{1}{2}\ \rho v^2 \qquad (3.10)$$

Since ρ is a constant, the quantity that changes is v. Changes in velocity occur when blood is accelerated or decelerated as in pulsatile flow, and when blood passes from a vessel of large lumen (where the velocity is low) to one of small lumen (where the velocity is high)—or vice versa. In addition, v is a vector quantity; that is, any change in direction of flow represents an acceleration.

Flow changes direction whenever the blood vessel forms a curve and at all junctions and branch points. There is also a change in direction when the blood vessel gradually narrows, or in pathologic situations in which there is a sudden narrowing and expansion of the flow stream, as in an atherosclerotic stenosis. Moreover, as a result of the expansile nature of the blood vessel wall, velocity vectors must be directed outward during the systolic portion of the pressure wave and inward during the diastolic portion.*

According to the equation of continuity, the product of flow velocity and cross-sectional area is the same at any point along a tube, provided there are no intervening branches to siphon off the fluid.

$$A_1 v_1 = A_2 v_2 \quad \text{or} \quad r_1^2 v_1 = r_2^2 v_2 \qquad (3.11)$$

Because kinetic energy losses depend on the square of the velocity (Eq. 3.10) and because the velocity in a stenotic segment is inversely proportional to the square of its radius (Eq. 3.11), kinetic energy losses—like those attributable to viscosity—are inversely proportional to the fourth power of the radius. As illustrated in Figure 3–3, this creates curves that display little sensitivity to reduction in radius until a certain point is reached, beyond which energy losses increase rapidly. Increasing the velocity of flow has a more marked effect on kinetic energy losses than it does on viscous losses (compare Figs. 3–2 and 3–3). This follows from the fact that the velocity term is squared in Equation 3.10 but enters Equation 3.7 only in the first power.

Turbulence

Turbulence, with its random velocity vectors, also depletes the total fluid energy stores. The point at which flow changes from laminar to turbulent is best defined in terms of a dimensionless quantity known as Reynolds number. Reynolds number is proportional to the ratio of inertial forces acting on the fluid to the viscous forces:

$$Re = \frac{\rho v d}{\eta} = \frac{vd}{\nu} \qquad (3.12)$$

where d is the diameter of the conduit, η is the viscosity, and ν is the kinematic viscosity ($\nu = \eta/\rho$). Above a Reynolds number of 2000, local disturbances in the laminar flow pattern result in fully developed turbulence. Below 2000, local disturbances are damped out by the viscous forces.

Since Reynolds numbers are well below 2000 in most peripheral blood vessels, turbulence is unlikely to occur under normal circumstances.[173] There is evidence, however, that turbulence does develop in the ascending aorta during the peak systolic ejection phase and that it may persist during deceleration.[151] These turbulent flashes are short-lived. Yet, in spite of the absence of fully developed turbulence, the pattern of blood flow in a large portion of the circulation may be characterized as *disturbed.*[5, 202] Energy losses calculated on turbulent friction factors may more closely approximate experimental results than they do when Poiseuille's law is employed.[174]

The Darcy equation is a generalized formula that relates energy losses to flow velocity under conditions of both laminar and turbulent flow.[15, 35]

$$P_1 - P_2 = f\ \frac{L}{4r}\ \rho v^2 \qquad (3.13)$$

where f is a *friction factor* that depends on the shape of the conduit, the roughness of its walls, and the Reynolds number. For laminar flow f = 64/Re, the equation becomes identical to Poiseuille's law. For turbulent flow with Reynolds numbers below 10^5, f can be approximated by $0.316/Re^{1/4}$.

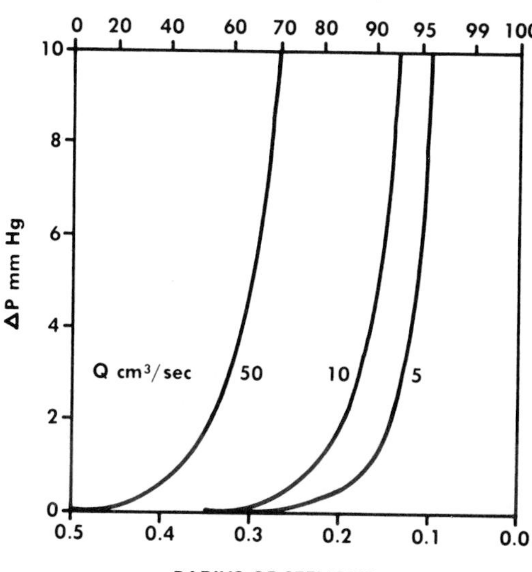

FIGURE 3–3. Effect of increasing stenosis and blood flow on inertial losses at the exit of a stenotic segment that leads into a tube with a radius of 0.5 cm. Curves are based on Equation 3.16. An abrupt exit is assumed.

*Because only flow in the direction of the long axis of the tube is considered in Poiseuille's law, frictional (viscous) energy losses due to molecular interaction involving flow in other directions are neglected in Equation 3.7. Although the magnitude of these losses is difficult to calculate, they are incorporated in a general way in the constant k of Equation 3.10. Thus, *inertial energy loss* is a term of convenience; it should be understood that all these losses are ultimately due to viscous effects.

Pulsatile Flow

Applying any of these equations to pulsatile blood flow is very difficult. For example, in steady flow, kinetic energy can be estimated from the square of the space-averaged velocity of blood flowing past a given point (Eq. 3.10). In pulsatile flow, a more complicated expression must be employed that integrates the instantaneous product of the mass flux and the square of the velocity. This method predicts kinetic energies that sometimes are 10 times as great as would be suspected on the basis of the average velocity of blood flow.[15]

In addition, the shape of the velocity profile must be known before the *spatially averaged velocity* across the lumen of a blood vessel can be used to estimate kinetic energy losses (Fig. 3–4). When the profile is nearly flat, as it is with turbulent flow or when the site of flow measurement is within the entrance length of a blood vessel, the k in Equation 3.10 will be 1.06.[35] But when the profile is parabolic, the k becomes 2.0. With pulsatile flow, a parabolic profile is never really attained (Fig. 3–5).[112] As mentioned previously, in larger blood vessels, such as the aorta, the profile may be quite flat and is often skewed. In smaller arteries, a parabolic profile may be approached, especially during the peak forward phase of the flow pulse.

All these complexities merely add to the energy losses experienced in the circulation. Thus, for a given level of blood flow, the pressure (energy) drop between any two points in the arterial tree may be several times that predicted by Poiseuille's law (Eq. 3.7).[6, 99, 116] Furthermore, the relationship between the pressure gradient and the flow will not be linear, but will define a curve that is concave to the pressure axis (Fig. 3–6). These nonlinearities are all functions of inertial losses and reflect the effect of the v^2 term. Thus, Poiseuille's law cannot be used to predict pressure-flow relationships in the arterial tree, but it can be used to define the *minimal* energy losses that can be expected under any given flow situation.

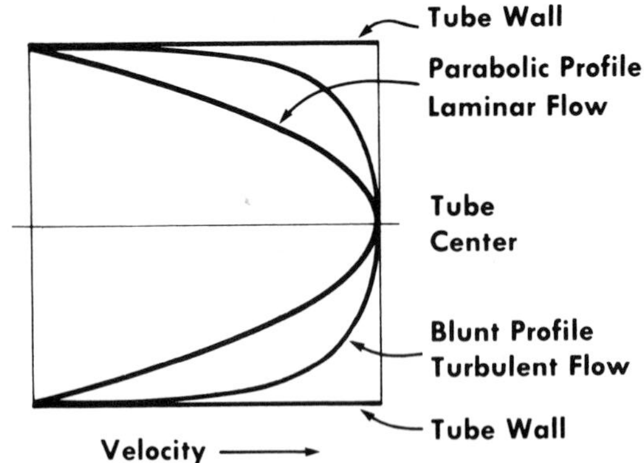

FIGURE 3–4. Velocity profiles of steady laminar and turbulent flow. Velocity is zero at the tube wall and reaches its peak value in the center. A blunt profile is also typical of that seen within the entrance length of a vessel.

Resistance

The concept of hemodynamic resistance is quite useful when one attempts to understand the physiology of arterial disease. Defined simply as the ratio of the energy drop between two points along a blood vessel ($E_1 - E_2$) to the mean blood flow in the vessel (Q), the equation for hemodynamic resistance (R) is analogous to Ohm's law in electric circuits:

$$R = \frac{E_1 - E_2}{Q} = \frac{P_1 - P_2}{Q} \tag{3.14}$$

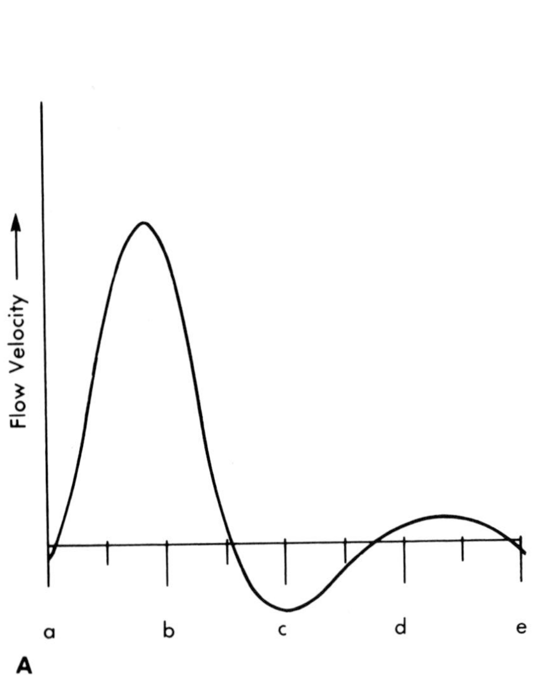

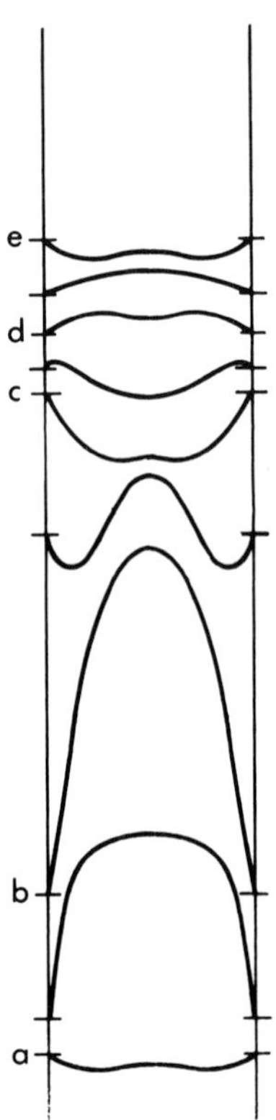

FIGURE 3–5. Velocity profiles *(B)* during various phases of a typical femoral arterial flow pulse *(A)*. Letters indicate corresponding points in the pulse cycle. In all profiles, the velocity at the wall is zero. At point *b*, forward flow is nearly maximal and the profile is almost parabolic. At the next point, flow near the wall is reversed while that in the center continues forward. Note that several profiles, both forward and reverse, are quite blunt. (*A* and *B*, Adapted from McDonald DA: Blood Flow in Arteries. 2nd ed. Baltimore, Williams & Wilkins Co, 1974.)

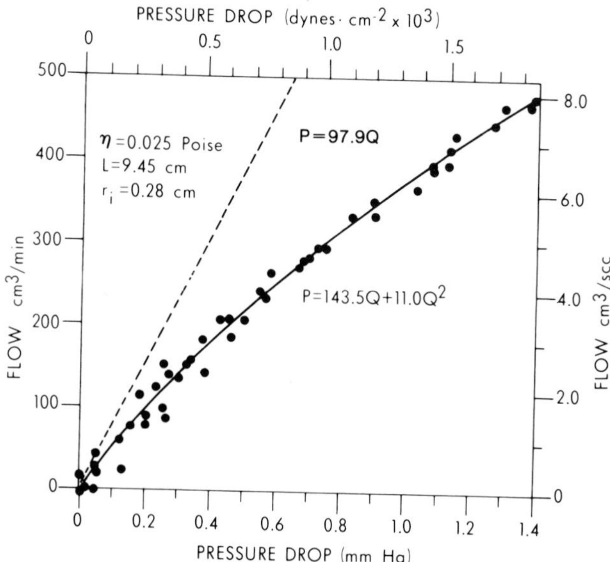

FIGURE 3–6. Pressure drop across a 9.45-cm length of canine femoral artery at varying flow rates. Differential pressure was measured by a specially designed transducer (D. E. Hokanson), and flow, with an electromagnetic flowmeter. Flow rate was varied by constricting a distally located arteriovenous fistula. Note that the line that fits the experimental data best has both a linear and a squared term, corresponding to Poiseuille's law plus kinetic energy losses. Note also that the pressure-flow curve predicted from Poiseuille's law *(dashed line)* depicts much less energy loss than actually is the case.

It is often convenient to drop the kinetic energy term ($\frac{1}{2}\rho v^2$) in Equation 3.2, since it seldom contributes appreciably to the total energy. Also, calculations are simplified if the assumption can be made that the subject is supine. This permits the gravitational terms (ρgh) to cancel. Hence, resistance can be approximated by the ratio of the pressure drop ($P_1 - P_2$) to the flow (Eq. 3.14).

Unlike electric resistance, hemodynamic resistance does not remain constant over a wide range of flows. The minimal possible resistance is given by Poiseuille's law:

$$R_{min} = \frac{8\eta L}{\pi r^4} \tag{3.15}$$

Because of additional energy losses related to acceleration, disturbed flow, and turbulence (all of which are a function of $\frac{1}{2}\rho v^2$), the resistance of a given vascular segment tends to increase as flow velocity increases, provided there is no concomitant change in vascular diameter (Fig. 3–7).

For the purposes of studying arterial and venous flow dynamics in complex hemodynamic circuitry, resistances in series can be added to obtain the total value:

$$R_{total} = R_1 + R_2 + --- R_n \tag{3.16}$$

When resistances are in parallel, the following relationship may be used:

$$\frac{1}{R_{total}} = \frac{1}{R_1} + \frac{1}{R_2} + --- \frac{1}{R_n} \tag{3.17}$$

The dimensions of hemodynamic resistance are dyne $\cdot$ cm^{-5} $\cdot$ sec. It usually is more convenient, however, to use the peripheral resistance unit (PRU), which is millimeters of mercury per milliliter per minute. Thus, one peripheral resistance unit is approximately equal to 8×10^4 dyne $\cdot$ cm^{-5} $\cdot$ sec.

HEMODYNAMICS OF ARTERIAL STENOSIS

Most of the abnormal energy losses in the arterial system result from stenoses or obstruction of the vascular lumen. Since atherosclerosis, the pathologic process in the majority of these lesions, has a predilection for larger arteries, surgical therapy often is possible. Therefore, the study of the hemodynamics of these lesions has a great deal of practical importance.

FIGURE 3–7. Resistance derived from pressure-flow curve in Figure 3–6. The constant resistance predicted by Poiseuille's law is depicted by the *dotted line*. Note that the resistance increases with increasing flow.

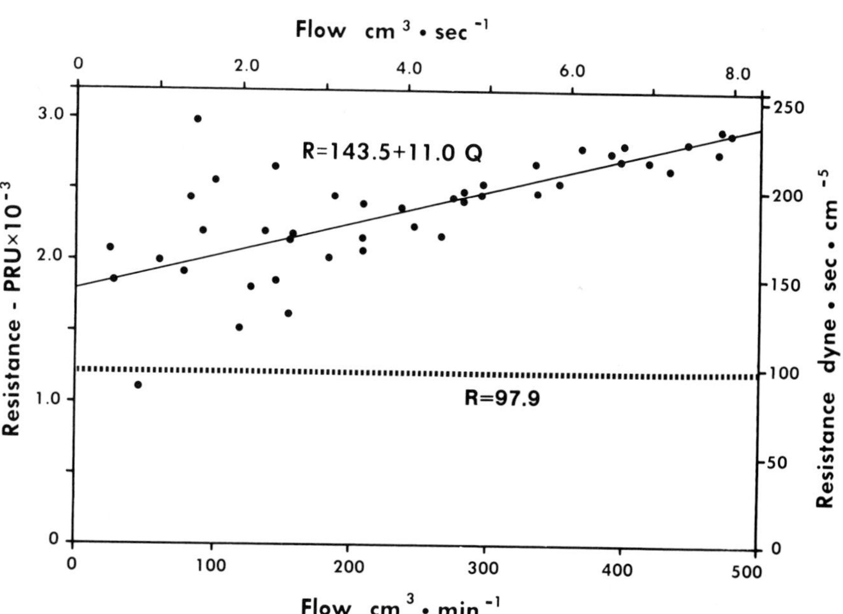

Energy Losses Associated With Stenoses

In accordance with Poiseuille's law (Eqs. 3.7 and 3.15), so-called viscous energy losses within the stenotic segment are inversely proportional to the fourth power of its radius and directly proportional to its length (see Fig. 3–2). Thus, the radius of a stenosis is of much more significance than its length.[22, 52, 83, 110] In addition, *inertial losses*, which are related to the square of the velocity of blood flow, are encountered both at the entrance to the stenosis and at its exit.[15, 110, 173, 204] The magnitude of these losses varies greatly with the shape of the entrance and exit, being much less for a gradual tapering of the lumen than for an abrupt change. Also, energy losses associated with asymmetric stenoses exceed those associated with axisymmetric stenoses even when the lumen is compromised to the same degree.[203] Although energy losses at the entrance can be appreciable, they are usually greater at the exit, where much of the excess kinetic energy resulting from the increased fluid velocity within the stenosis may be dissipated in a turbulent jet (see Fig. 3–3):

$$\Delta P = k \frac{\rho}{2} (v_S - v)^2$$
$$= k \frac{\rho}{2} v^2 \left[\left(\frac{r}{r_S} \right)^2 - 1 \right]^2 \quad (3.18)$$

In this expression, ΔP represents the energy lost in expansion; v_S refers to the mean flow velocity within the stenotic segment; and v to the velocity in the vessel beyond the stenosis. Similarly, r_S and r indicate the radius of the stenotic lumen and that of the uninvolved distal vessel. The constant, k, varies from about 1.0 for an abrupt orifice to less than 0.2 for one that expands gradually at a 6-degree angle.[37]

These concepts are illustrated graphically in Figure 3–8. This figure emphasizes the relatively small contribution of *viscous losses* to the total decrease in available fluid energy produced by the stenosis. Even if the obstruction were diaphragm-like (L in Eq. 3.7 equal to zero), the energy losses would still be 85 per cent of those with the 1.0-cm-long stenosis. In other words, most of the energy losses can be attributed to inertial effects.

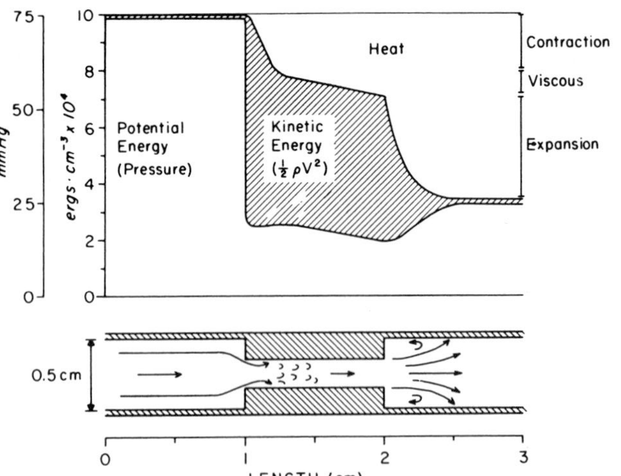

FIGURE 3–8. Diagram illustrating energy losses experienced by blood passing through a stenosis 1 cm long. Flow is assumed to be unidirectional and steady. Note that very little of the total energy loss is attributable to "viscous" losses. Thus, applications of Poiseuille's law greatly underestimate the pressure drop across an arterial stenosis.

Energy losses associated with arterial lesions are inversely proportional to the fourth power of the radius of the stenosis (Eq. 3.7) and to the fourth power of the ratio of the radius of the stenosis to that of the nonstenotic segment (Eq. 3.18). Because these are exponential functions, graphs relating energy losses across a stenosis to the percentage reduction in cross-sectional area are sharply curved, providing theoretical support for the concept of critical stenosis (Fig. 3–9).[15, 22, 110, 119, 204]

Energy losses across stenotic segments also depend on the velocity of blood flow (Eqs. 3.7 and 3.18). In high-flow (low-resistance) systems, significant drops in pressure and flow occur with less severe narrowing than in low-flow systems.[111, 118, 181, 182] Moreover, the curves are less sharply bent when peripheral resistance is low and flow rates are high, as shown in Figure 3–9. Consequently, critical stenosis varies with the resistance of the runoff bed. When peripheral resistances are low, as in the carotid and coronary systems, critical stenosis may be reached with less narrowing of the lumen than in higher resistance systems, such as the resting lower extremity. Even in the leg, lowering the peripheral resistance sufficiently by exercise or reactive hyperemia may cause a stenosis that is noncritical at rest to become critical.[24, 167, 169] This fact is well worth emphasizing. It accounts for the frequent clinical observation that an iliac lesion may severely restrict the patient during exercise, even though it causes no symptoms at rest and may not appear particularly significant on arteriography.[117, 190]

Precise attempts to relate pressure and flow restriction to per cent stenosis are frustrated by the irregular geometry of the vascular lesions and by the nonlinearities introduced by pulsatile blood flow. Empirical formulas have been devised that fit the experimental data.[22] Those formulas that incorporate known viscous and inertial effects are far more instructive, however.[15, 110, 204] Nevertheless, for practical purposes *none of the formulas is very helpful.* Thus, any lesion

Critical Stenosis

How severe does a stenosis have to be to produce a measurable pressure gradient or a decrease in blood flow, or both? This is an important question for the clinician who attempts to assess the severity of an arterial obstruction from its angiographic appearance. Experimentally, appreciable changes in pressure and flow do not occur until the cross-sectional area of a vessel has been reduced by more than 75 per cent (usually 80 to 95 per cent).[111, 118] Assuming that the obstructing lesion is symmetric, this reduction in cross-sectional area corresponds to at least a 50 per cent reduction in diameter. The degree of narrowing at which pressure and flow begin to be affected has been called the *critical stenosis.*

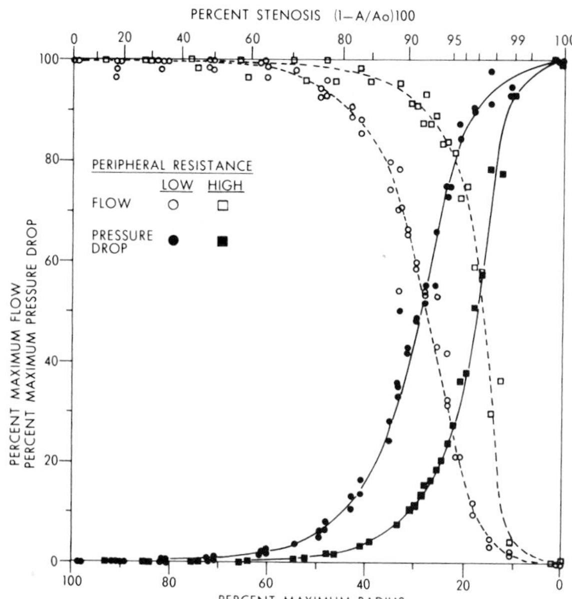

FIGURE 3–9. **Relationship of pressure and flow to degree of stenosis in a canine femoral artery. When peripheral resistance is high, the curves are shifted to the right. Note that percentage change in flow through the stenosis is essentially a mirror image of the percentage of maximal pressure drop across the stenosis.**

that potentially decreases the arterial lumen by about 75 per cent must be suspect, and its hemodynamic significance must be determined by objective physiologic tests.

Length of Stenosis and Stenoses in Series

Not infrequently, the surgeon is faced with a series of lesions involving a single unbranched arterial segment. The question arises whether repair of one of the lesions will benefit the patient significantly. This question is particularly pertinent when one of the lesions is in an inaccessible location. Such a problem is presented by a stenosis at the origin of the internal carotid artery combined with a similar stenosis in the carotid siphon.

The length of a stenosis principally affects energy losses related to viscosity. Since length enters Poiseuille's equation (Eq. 3.7) only in the first power, whereas radius is elevated to the fourth power, the effect of a change of length on viscous losses is far less than that of a change of radius. Doubling the length of a stenosis would merely double the viscous energy losses, but reducing the radius of the vessel lumen by half would increase the losses by a factor of 16. Moreover, the convective acceleration effects at the exit are independent of the length of the stenosis, and are related to the fourth power of the ratio of the diameters of the unstenosed and stenosed portions of the vessel (Eq. 3.18). Therefore, one would predict that the length of a stenosis is far less important than lesion diameter. These predictions are well supported by experimental observations.[17, 22, 52, 110, 184]

Because entrance and exit effects contribute a large portion of the resistance offered by a stenosis, doubling the length of a lesion without changing its diameter would not double its resistance (see Fig. 3–8). In contrast, the total resistance of two separate lesions of equal length and diameter is approximately double that of the individual lesion, since entrance and exit effects occur at each of the stenoses.[53, 80] Thus, separate stenoses of equal diameter are of more significance than a single stenosis of the same diameter whose length equals the sum of the lengths of the shorter lesions.

When two stenoses of unequal diameter are in series, the tighter of the two has by far the greater effect on resistance (Eqs. 3.7 and 3.18). Total resistance is not affected by the sequence of the stenoses; that is, it makes no difference whether the greater occlusion is proximal or distal.[184]

Several practical points emerge from these considerations.

1. The resistances of stenoses in series are roughly additive, although the cumulative effect may be somewhat less than would be anticipated on the basis of the sum of the individual resistances. Therefore, multiple noncritical stenoses may act as a single critical stenosis and result in arterial insufficiency.[53, 80]
2. When two stenotic lesions are of similar caliber, removal of one will provide only a modest improvement in blood flow.
3. If the stenoses are of unequal caliber, removal of the less severe will result in little increase in blood flow; but removal of the more severe will provide significant improvement.

It should be noted that these principles apply only to unbranched arteries. They do not apply to the situation in which the proximal lesion is in an artery feeding a collateral bed that parallels the distal lesion. Thus, endarterectomy of a stenotic iliac artery usually is beneficial even when the superficial femoral artery is completely occluded. In this case, the profunda femoris carries most of the blood to the lower leg, and removal of the proximal iliac obstruction will improve the pressure head at the profunda orifice.[45, 109, 120, 168, 190]

CIRCULATORY PATTERNS IN HUMAN LIMBS

Collateral Circulation and the Peripheral Runoff Bed

Arterial stenoses do not exist in isolation but rather are part of a complex hemodynamic circuit.[173, 177] As shown in Figure 3–10, this circuit includes the diseased major artery, a parallel system of collateral arteries, and a so-called peripheral runoff bed.

Dilatation of the involved artery may compensate for the narrowing caused by small or moderate plaques. This compensatory expansion, which has been demonstrated to occur in human coronary arteries and which may also occur in peripheral arteries, is probably mediated by an endothelium-derived relaxing factor in response to increased shear

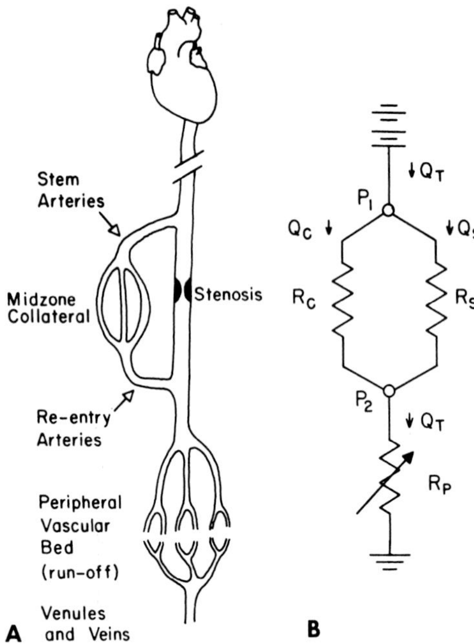

FIGURE 3–10. *A*, The major components of an arterial circuit containing a stenotic major artery. *B*, An electric analogue of this circuit. The battery at the top represents the potential energy source, e.g., the heart; ground potential, at the bottom, indicates the central veins. Q_T is total flow, Q_C is collateral flow, and Q_S is flow through the stenotic artery. Resistances are: R_C, collateral; R_S, stenotic artery; and R_P, peripheral "runoff" bed. R_C and R_S are relatively "fixed"; R_P is "variable."

stress.[59] More severe plaques overwhelm this process and progressively encroach on the residual lumen. To compensate for the increased resistance imposed by a highly stenotic or totally occlusive lesion, two mechanisms are invoked: collateral development and dilatation of the resistance vessels in the peripheral bed.

Collateral vessels consist of distributing branches of large and medium-sized arteries. Anatomically as well as functionally, it is convenient to divide the collateral bed into stem arteries, midzone collaterals, and reentry arteries.[102] For the most part, these vessels are preexisting pathways that enlarge when a stenosis or an occlusion develops in the parallel main arterial supply.[28, 73, 146, 192] Although the mechanism of collateral enlargement is the subject of debate, it appears to be related to an increased pressure gradient across the collateral bed and to an increased velocity of flow (increased shear rate) through the midzone vessels.[28, 68, 73, 81, 192]

In spite of continued expansion of the midzone vessels, the resistance of the collateral bed always exceeds that of the major artery whose function it has replaced.[104, 177] For example, it would take 256 collaterals each with a diameter of 2.5 mm or 10,000 collaterals with a diameter of 1.0 mm to reduce the segmental resistance to that of a major vessel with a diameter of 10 mm (Eqs. 3.15 and 3.17).

Except with gradual dilatation, the resistance of the collateral bed is—for practical purposes—almost fixed. The acute decreases in collateral resistance that occur in response to exercise, sympathectomy, or vasodilator drugs are small and are of relatively little consequence.[10, 26, 44, 104, 177]

In contrast, the peripheral runoff bed has a generally high but quite variable resistance, a large portion of which is concentrated in the terminal arterioles and precapillary sphincters (see Fig. 3–10). Because of their small diameter and heavily muscled walls, these vessels are ideally suited for regulatory function. Their resistance is subject to control by the autonomic nervous system, circulating catecholamines, local metabolic products, and myogenic influences.

Control of Peripheral Vascular Resistance

The cutaneous sympathetic innervation is concerned largely with the regulation of body temperature. Blood vessels within the skin are well supplied with sympathetic vasoconstrictor fibers, especially in the terminal portions such as the fingers, hands, and feet. More proximally (in the forearm, for example), there are vasodilator fibers that act in conjunction with the sudomotor apparatus. Nevertheless, most reflex vasodilatation of cutaneous vessels results from the withdrawal of sympathetic impulses.[157] In contrast, blood vessels within skeletal muscles are innervated by both vasodilator and vasoconstrictor fibers. The former respond to emotional stress and the latter to postural changes.[157] These actions, however, are easily overcome by the powerful vasodilator effect of locally produced metabolites that accumulate during exercise or ischemia.[86, 140] Indeed, exercise is perhaps the best single vasodilator of resistance vessels within skeletal muscle.[25, 92, 135]

Arteriolar constriction also occurs in response to dependency (the venoarterial reflex).[11] By restricting arterial inflow, this reflex serves to limit the increase in venous blood volume that accompanies an elevated hydrostatic pressure.

Finally, we should mention *autoregulation*. This term is used to describe the remarkable ability of most vascular beds to maintain a constant level of blood flow over a wide range of perfusion pressures.[75, 78] In other words, the resistance vessels constrict in response to a rise in blood pressure and dilate in response to a fall. Although the mechanism of autoregulation continues to evoke controversy, it seems to be a myogenic response to stretch that is modified by the local chemical milieu and sympathetic control.[87] Autoregulation is not present when the perfusion pressure drops below a critical level (e.g., about 20 to 30 mmHg for skeletal muscle and about 50 to 60 mmHg for the brain). With pressures below this level, normal blood flow is no longer maintained. Consequently, in these low-pressure situations, flow responds passively to changes in perfusion pressure (Fig. 3–11).

Pressure-Flow Relationships

Normal Limbs

Under resting conditions, blood flow to the normal human leg averages about 300 to 400 ml/min.[25, 54, 97, 139, 185] Calf blood flow hovers around 1.5 to 6.5 ml/min per 100 ml of calf, with an average value of about 3.5 ml/100

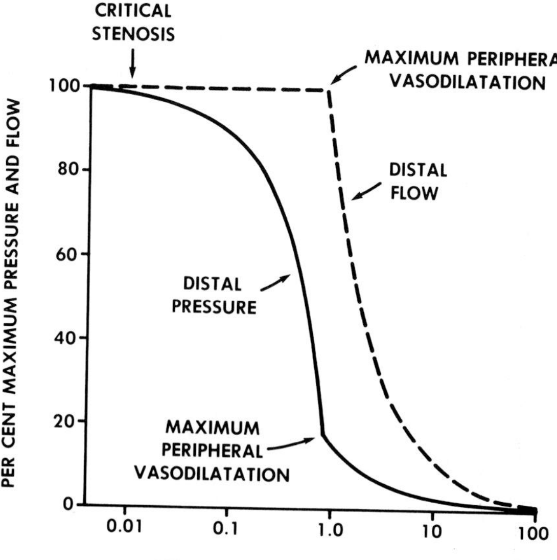

FIGURE 3–11. Although blood pressure distal to a critical stenosis falls progressively with increasing severity of the stenosis, autoregulation maintains normal blood flow to the tissues until maximal peripheral vasodilatation is reached. Beyond this point, pressure and flow are linearly related; increasing stenosis results in a marked decrease in both pressure and flow; and the tissues become ischemic. Compare with Figure 3–9. (From Sumner DS: Correlation of lesion configuration with functional significance. *In* Bond MG, Insull W Jr, Glagov S, et al [eds]: Clinical Diagnosis of Atherosclerosis: Quantitative Methods of Evaluation. New York, Springer-Verlag, 1983.)

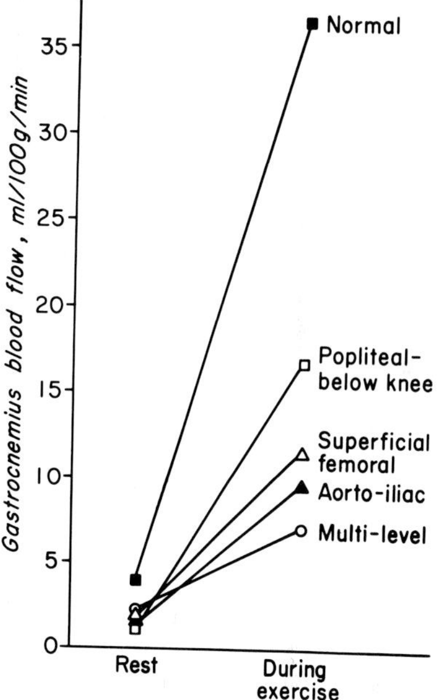

FIGURE 3–12. Mean blood flow at rest and after exercise in normal subjects and in patients with arteriosclerosis obliterans. Location of occlusion is indicated by the labels on the right. Blood flow was measured in the gastrocnemius muscle by the xenon-133 clearance technique. (Data from Wolf EA Jr, Sumner DS, Strandness DE Jr: Correlation between nutritive blood flow and pressure in limbs of patients with intermittent claudication. Surg Forum 23:238, 1972.)

ml/min.[64, 166] Blood flow to the gastrocnemius muscle usually is about 2.0 ml/100 gm/min.[94] This rate of flow is more than adequate to supply all the nutritional needs of the resting limb.

When blood flow is restored to a normal limb that has been rendered ischemic for 5 minutes by means of a proximally placed pneumatic tourniquet, the peripheral arteriolar bed becomes vasodilated. The resulting *reactive hyperemia* reaches peak values of 30 to 40 ml/100 ml/min and then rapidly subsides to resting levels within a minute or two.[163, 166, 209]

Moderate exercise normally increases total leg blood flow from 5 to 10 times.[25, 92, 135] Muscle blood flow rises to 30 ± 14 ml/100 ml/min, reaching 70 ml/100 ml/min during strenous exercise (Fig. 3–12).[92] On cessation of exercise, blood flow decreases rapidly in an exponential fashion, often reaching pre-exercise levels within 1 to 5 minutes.

The mean blood pressure drop across normal arteries from the heart to the ankle is only a few millimeters of mercury.[19] As the pressure wave travels distally, the systolic pressure increases, the diastolic pressure decreases, and the pulse pressure widens (Fig. 3–13).[141] This phenomenon is due to reflection of waves from the high-resistance peripheral arteriolar bed. Under resting conditions, ankle systolic pressures exceed the brachial systolic pressure in normal individuals by about 10 per cent (Fig. 3–14).[199] In normal extremities, moderate exercise produces little or no drop in peripheral pressure at ankle level. With very strenous exercise, the pressure may fall a few millimeters of mercury, but rapidly recovers within a minute or so.[165] These findings contrast sharply with the ankle pressure drop that occurs following exercise in limbs with occlusive arterial disease, as shown in Figure 3–14.

Limbs With Arterial Obstruction

Intermittent Claudication, Ischemic Rest Pain, and Gangrene

Intermittent claudication is the single most important symptom of occlusive arterial disease in the lower extremity. It develops when blood flow to the exercising muscle mass is unable to meet the requirements of the increased

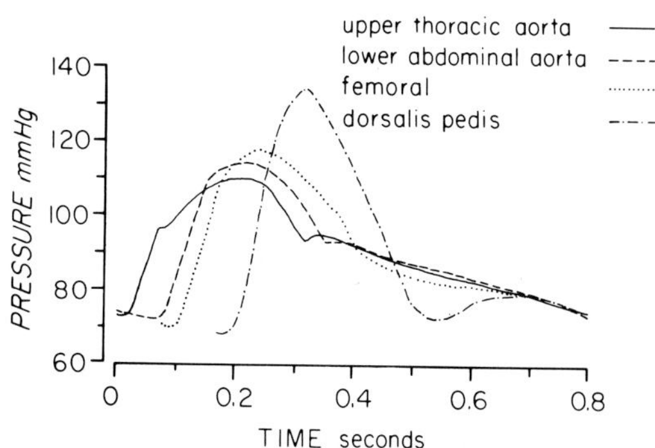

FIGURE 3–13. Pressure pulse contours in a normal subject. (From Strandness DE Jr, Sumner DS: Hemodynamics for Surgeons. New York, Grune & Stratton, 1975; redrawn from Remington JW, Wood EH: Formation of peripheral pulse contour in man. J Appl Physiol 9:433, 1956.)

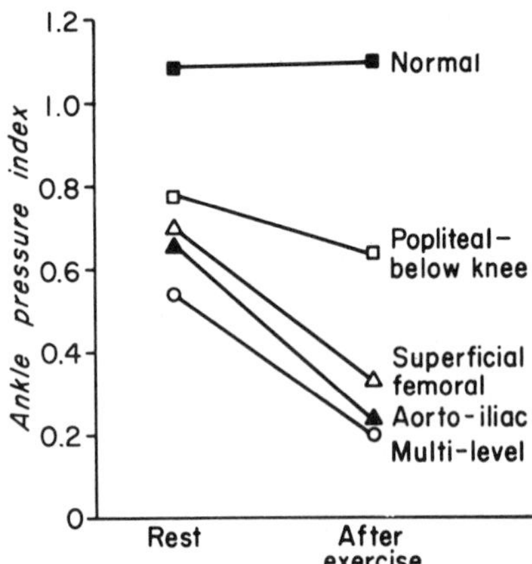

FIGURE 3–14. Mean ankle pressure indices (ankle systolic blood pressure ÷ brachial systolic blood pressure) at rest and after exercise in normal subjects and in patients with arteriosclerosis obliterans. Location of occlusion is indicated by the labels on the right. (Data from Wolf EA Jr, Sumner DS, Strandness DE Jr: Correlation between nutritive blood flow and pressure in limbs of patients with intermittent claudication. Surg Forum 23:238, 1972.)

metabolic activity. Apparently, the pain is related to the abnormal accumulation of metabolic products within the muscle.[98] Pain does not develop in normal extremities during exercise, because these metabolic products are rapidly removed by the copious blood flow.

When intermittent claudication is the sole symptom of arterial obstruction, resting blood flow to the involved limbs will be normal (see Fig. 3–12).[54, 64, 97, 135, 166, 176] With further progression of the disease, however, limb blood flow becomes inadequate even when the patient is at rest (see Fig. 3–11).[90] Ischemic rest pain is experienced in the toes and distal portions of the foot; minor trauma may produce painful nonhealing ulcers; and the toes may become gangrenous.[31]

Effect of Reactive Hyperemia and Exercise on Blood Flow

Reactive hyperemia develops in limbs when the circulation is restored after a 5-minute period of ischemia. In limbs with obstructive arterial disease, this response differs significantly from that observed in normal limbs. Not only is peak blood flow lower in obstructed limbs (averaging about 9 to 20 ml/100 ml/min), but the peak flow may be delayed for from 15 seconds to 2 minutes, and the hyperemia is prolonged for several minutes.[64, 163, 166]

Although blood flow is increased during exercise in limbs with obstructive arterial disease, the increase is far less than that observed in normal limbs undergoing a similar stress (see Fig. 3–12).[55, 92, 135, 194] Flow may even fall below resting levels.[3, 92, 156, 176] After cessation of exercise, the hyperemia is greatly prolonged, subsiding to normal levels in a logarithmic fashion over a 4- to 30-minute period (Fig. 3–15). In some limbs with occlusions at two levels (for example, iliac plus superficial femoral), the peripheral blood flow immediately after exercise may be increased only slightly. Flow then rises for several minutes until a peak level is obtained, before falling gradually to pre-exercise levels (Fig. 3–16). In patients with multi-level occlusions, especially those with rest pain, the flow after exercise may be depressed, peak flow is quite low and very delayed, and the hyperemic state persists for many minutes (Fig. 3–17).[3]

Blood Pressure at Rest and Following Exercise

Under resting conditions, blood pressure distal to an obstructive arterial lesion will be decreased, provided the lesion is hemodynamically significant at the prevailing level of flow.[103, 108, 123] Ordinarily, most lesions of surgical significance will fall into this category (see Fig. 3–14). Measurement of pressures at the ankle by the simple noninvasive techniques described in Chapter 4 provides the clinician with a rapid, accurate, and objective means of assessing the functional severity of the arterial lesion.[23, 57, 171, 176, 193, 194, 199, 201]

When blood flow to the extremity is increased during or following exercise, the blood pressure distal to the arterial lesion falls precipitously, as shown in Figure 3–14. Recovery to pre-exercise levels requires a prolonged period, usually between 10 and 30 minutes (see Figs. 3–15 to 3–17).[96, 169, 176, 194] Even in limbs in which the stenosis is not severe enough to produce a decrease in distal pressure at rest, exercise or reactive hyperemia causes a fall in pressure.[24, 117, 167] The blood pressure begins to recover after peak flows have begun to decline (see Figs. 3–15 to 3–17).[176] These changes account for the disappearance of pedal pulses after exercise in certain patients with stenotic lesions.[38, 39]

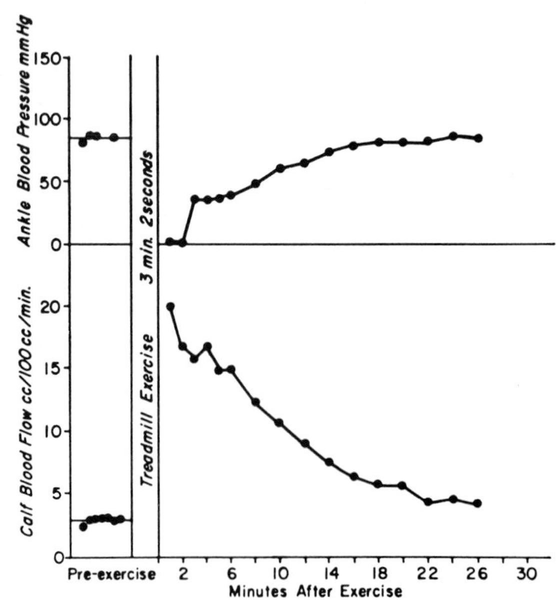

FIGURE 3–15. Ankle blood pressure and calf blood flow before and after exercise in a patient with stenosis of the superficial femoral artery. (From Sumner DS, Strandness DE Jr: The relationship between calf blood flow and ankle blood pressure in patients with intermittent claudication. Surgery 65:763, 1969.)

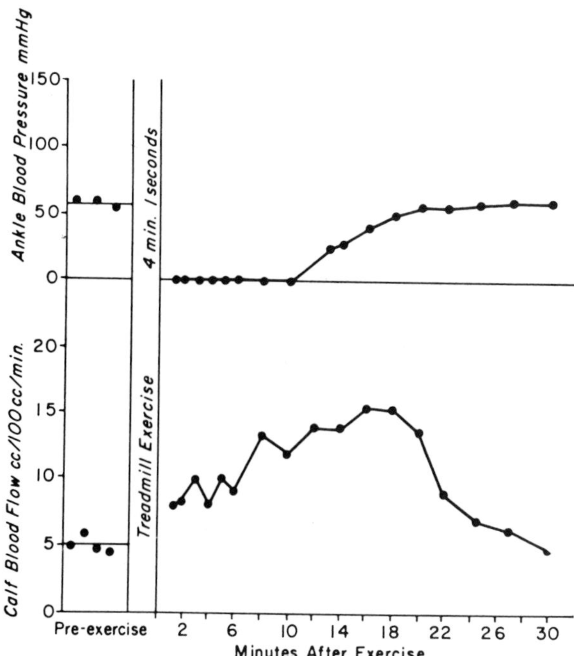

FIGURE 3–16. Ankle blood pressure and calf blood flow before and after exercise in a patient with stenosis of the iliac artery and occlusion of the superficial femoral artery. (From Sumner DS, Strandness DE Jr: The relationship between calf blood flow and ankle blood pressure in patients with intermittent claudication. Surgery 65:763, 1969.)

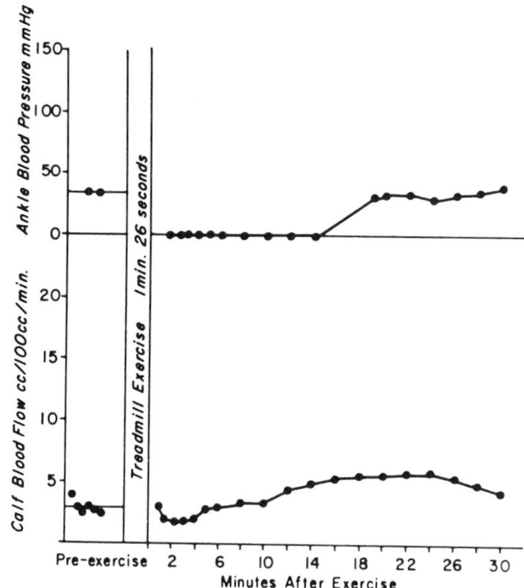

FIGURE 3–17. Ankle blood pressure and calf blood flow before and after exercise in a patient with occlusion of the iliac, common femoral, and superficial femoral arteries. This patient had severe claudication and moderate rest pain. (From Sumner DS, Strandness DE Jr: The relationship between calf blood flow and ankle blood pressure in patients with intermittent claudication. Surgery 65:763, 1969.)

Resistance Changes Accompanying Exercise

Figure 3–18 compares resting and postexercise resistances in normal limbs with those in limbs with occlusive disease of the superficial femoral artery. In normal limbs, *segmental resistance* refers to the resistance of the iliac and femoral arteries. In abnormal limbs, segmental resistance primarily reflects the resistance offered by the collateral arteries bypassing the superficial femoral artery occlusion (parallel resistance; see Eq. 3.17). Calf resistance represents the runoff resistance imposed by intramuscular arterioles, capillaries, and venules, as well as the veins draining the extremity. The major part of this resistance is contributed by the arterioles. In this example, the *total* vascular resistance of the limb can be approximated by adding the segmental and calf resistances (Eq. 3.16).

At rest, values for the total resistance offered by normal and abnormal limbs are essentially equal (for example, in Fig. 3–18, the normal is 37, and the abnormal is 36 peripheral resistance units). Values for distribution of the resistances are markedly different, however.[104, 177] Whereas segmental resistance accounts for less than 3 per cent of the total in normal limbs, it makes up about 38 per cent of the total in abnormal limbs. Resting blood flow rates are equal in both groups of limbs only because peripheral arterioles in the abnormal limbs dilate enough to compensate for the elevated segmental resistance. Thus, calf resistance is much less in the abnormal than in the normal limbs.

During exercise, the intramuscular arterioles become widely dilated, thus markedly reducing calf resistance, as shown in Figure 3–18. After cessation of exercise, calf resistance gradually recovers toward resting values. Recovery is approximately linearly related to time.[177] In normal limbs, there is little change in segmental (collateral) resistance; in abnormal limbs, it may remain unchanged or may drop somewhat.[104, 161, 177] Nevertheless, the total drop in resistance (segmental plus calf) is less in abnormal than in normal limbs. This explains why blood flow during exercise is greater in normal limbs than in limbs with occlusive arterial disease.

Despite the fact that segmental resistance may fall in limbs with arterial obstruction, it actually constitutes a greater percentage of the total resistance than it did at rest. In the example shown in Figure 3–18, segmental resistance

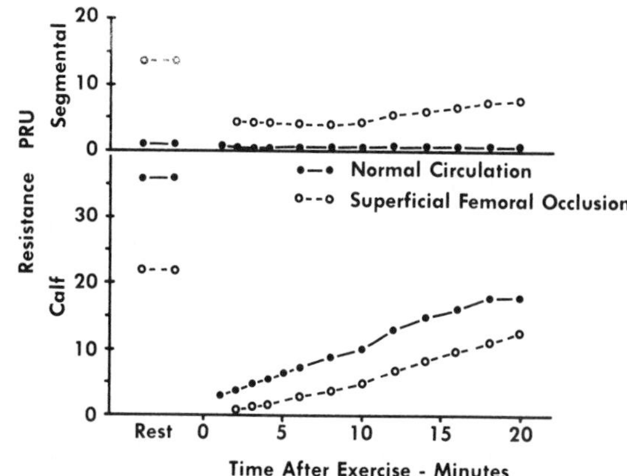

FIGURE 3–18. Segmental (parallel collateral and main channel) resistance and calf (runoff) resistance in normal individuals and in patients with occlusive disease of the superficial femoral artery. Values at rest and after treadmill exercises are shown. PRU, peripheral resistance unit. (Data from Sumner DS, Strandness DE Jr: The effect of exercise on resistance to blood flow in limbs with an occluded superficial femoral artery. Vasc Surg 4:229, 1970.)

makes up 82 per cent of the total resistance immediately following exercise. At that same period, segmental resistance in normal limbs makes up less than 14 per cent of total limb resistance. The relative increase in segmental resistance in abnormal limbs explains the decrease in ankle blood pressure after walking.[104, 176] The following discussion clarifies some of these relationships.

Hemodynamics of Arterial Obstruction

Understanding the hemodynamics of intermittent claudication is facilitated by the use of simple models. Figure 3–10 shows a typical vascular circuit containing a stenotic artery. This circuit consists of a proximal fixed (segmental) resistance made up of the stenotic segment and the bypassing collateral and a runoff bed made up of the distal arteries, arterioles, capillaries, and venules as well as the veins that return blood to the heart. As pointed out earlier, the resistance of the runoff bed largely resides in the arterioles, and consequently is highly variable.

In Figure 3–19, the proximal fixed (segmental) resistance is represented by a compressible tube with a screw-clamp, and the distal runoff resistance by a faucet. The normal situation is depicted in Figure 3–19*A* and *B*. Although, at rest, the resistance of the distal vascular bed is quite high, the proximal resistance is so low that normal flow is maintained (300 ml/min). During exercise, the intramuscular arterioles dilate, reducing the distal runoff resistance to a remarkable degree. In spite of the fact that blood flow (Q_t) is increased five times, there is little pressure drop across the proximal (segmental) resistance:

$$P_2 = P_1 - Q_t R_{seg} \qquad (3.19)$$

(rearranged from 3.14)

Now suppose that an obstruction develops in the proximal vasculature, represented by tightening of the screw-

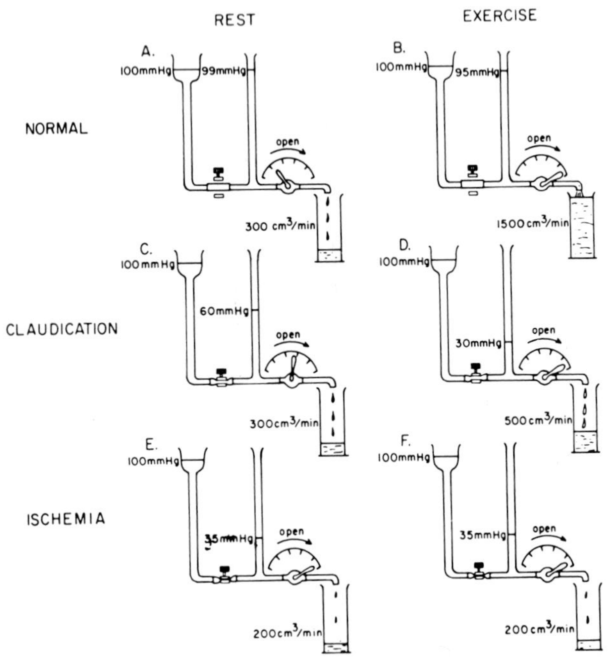

FIGURE 3–19. Hydraulic model of an arterial circuit showing the effect of exercise. See text for explanation.

clamp (Fig. 3–19*C* and *D*). The arterioles within the runoff bed dilate enough to compensate for the increased proximal resistance. Because of this autoregulatory process, resting blood flow remains within normal limits. However, the resting blood pressure distal to the obstructed segment is lower than normal (60 mmHg in this example). This is simply a reflection of the increased energy losses that occur across the increased resistance (Eq. 3.19).

With exercise, the intramuscular arterioles dilate fully (Fig. 3–19*D*). Because of the high proximal resistance, the increase in blood flow is inadequate to meet the metabolic demands of the exercising muscle mass, and claudication ensues. In addition, the blood pressure distal to the obstruction experiences a further fall as a result of the increased rate of flow through the high proximal resistance (see also Fig. 3–15).

Finally, an even worse situation is depicted in Figure 3–19*E* and *F*. Here, the proximal obstruction is so severe that blood flow at rest is only two thirds the normal value (200 ml/min) despite complete peripheral vasodilatation. Consequently, the patient experiences rest pain. Because no further peripheral dilatation is possible, blood flow does not increase with exercise. Blood pressure distal to the obstruction is more profoundly depressed than in the previous examples, because the increase in proximal (segmental) resistance is proportionally greater than the decrease in blood flow (Eq. 3.19; see also Fig. 3–17).

To summarize these points:

1. At rest, peripheral blood flow is normal in claudicators, but is decreased in patients with ischemic rest pain.[54, 64, 90, 135, 166, 176]
2. During exercise, peripheral blood flow increases in claudicators, but the increase is less than that which occurs in normal limbs.[65, 92, 135, 156, 176, 194] In patients with rest pain, exercise may result in no increase in blood flow.[176]
3. At rest, blood pressure levels distal to the arterial lesion will be decreased in claudicators, and even more so in patients with rest pain.[23, 176, 194, 199] Exercise ordinarily results in a further decrease in peripheral pressure.[24, 169, 176, 194]

Multiple Lesions and the Vascular Steal Phenomenon

Obstructing lesions occupying a single arterial segment (such as in the iliac or the superficial femoral artery) commonly cause claudication, but seldom result in ischemia at rest. There are, however, certain exceptions to this rule. When the lesion is located far distally in the foot or toe, the involved vessel may be essentially an endartery with no adequate collateral branches. Blockage of such a vessel will lead to ischemia. In addition, an acute embolic obstruction to the distal aorta, common femoral artery, or popliteal artery also may obstruct stem or reentry collaterals. This, in effect, creates a multi-level occlusion that may be responsible for severe peripheral ischemia.

Multi-level occlusions result when lesions involve two or more major arterial segments. Peripheral blood flow is more severely compromised than in single-level occlusions, because blood must traverse two or more high-resistance collateral beds before reaching the periphery. If the lesions are chronic and confined to two segments (such as the common iliac and the superficial femoral arteries), collateral development usually will be adequate to prevent rest pain or ischemic necrosis. Claudication, however, will be quite severe. Lesions involving three segments (such as the common iliac, femoral, and popliteal) will reduce blood flow markedly and frequently will cause rest pain.

Figure 3–20 illustrates the effect of exercise on pressure-flow relationships in limbs with two levels of obstruction. In this example, the more proximal fixed resistance (R_I) represents a lesion within the iliac artery, and the distal fixed resistance (R_{SF}) is in the superficial femoral artery. The variable resistances imposed by the peripheral vascular beds of the thigh and calf are represented by R_T and R_C, respectively. Normal resting blood flow to the calf and thigh is maintained by nearly complete vasodilatation in the calf (R_C open), and by partial vasodilatation in the thigh (R_T partly open; see Fig. 3–20*A*). Although exercise causes little change in diameter of the calf vessels, which already were nearly maximally dilated (R_C unchanged), the partial dilatation of the thigh vasculature becomes complete, thereby reducing its resistance to a minimal level (R_T open; Fig. 3–20B). Because the total peripheral resistance is reduced, blood flow through the proximal fixed resistance (R_I) increases, leading to a further drop in pressure P_2 (Eq. 3.19). Because the series of resistances leading to the calf have not changed ($R_{SF} + R_C$), and because the pressure head (P_2) perfusing the calf falls, blood flow to the calf decreases. Thus, the effect of exercise is to increase flow to the thigh, to decrease flow to the calf, and to decrease peripheral blood pressure.[3] Stated in another way, the proximal vascular bed *steals* blood from the distal. Calf blood flow will increase only when the thigh blood flow decreases, allowing the distal blood pressure (P_3) to rise (see Fig. 3–16).[3]

In summary, exercise or other causes of peripheral vasodilatation have the following effects in limbs with multiple levels of occlusion.

1. Although blood flow in the more distal tissues may be normal at rest, it may drop to even lower levels during exercise. In fact, the distal tissues may become completely ischemic.[2, 38, 92, 199]

2. Blood pressure below the fixed obstructions will be reduced at rest and will fall to even lower levels during exercise.[169, 176, 199]

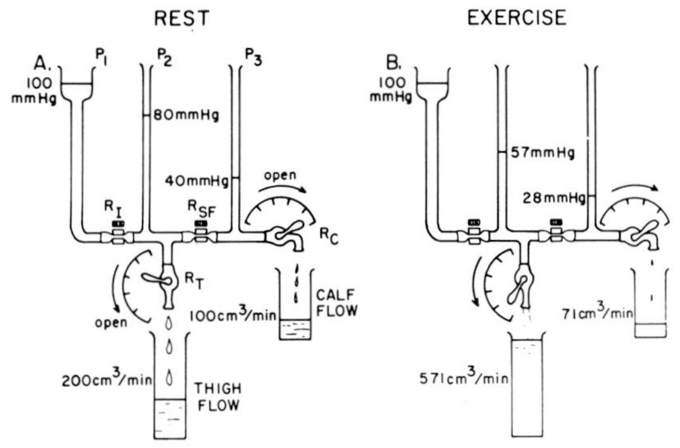

FIGURE 3–20. **Hydraulic model illustrating effect of multiple-level arterial obstructive disease. See text for explanation.**

3. One vascular bed can steal from another only when the artery supplying both beds is functionally obstructed.[48, 173, 178]

Arterial Flow and Pressure Waves

A portion of the left ventricular stroke volume is stored in the compliant aorta during systole and then propelled distally by elastic recoil during diastole. When this surge of blood encounters the high resistance imposed by the arterioles, part is transmitted into the capillaries and part is reflected back up the arterial tree (Fig. 3–21).[173, 191] The magnitude of the reflected wave relative to that of the incident wave is determined by the peripheral resistance, being greatest when the recipient vascular bed is constricted and least when the bed is dilated.[143] As the reflected wave moves up the artery, it subtracts from the forward wave. In normal limbs with a high arteriolar tone, this produces a short period of reversed flow in early diastole. As the reflected wave moves proximally beyond the point of observation, a smaller forward flow wave again appears in late diastole. When the arterioles are dilated (as in exercise) or when the baseline resistance of the recipient bed is low (as in the cerebral circulation), the amplitude of the reflected wave is relatively small and shows up only as a transient downward deflection in the diastolic portion of the flow pulse. In this situation, flow remains antegrade throughout the cardiac cycle; there is no reverse flow component.

Although pressure is also reflected at the periphery, the reflected pressure wave—unlike the flow wave—adds to rather than subtracts from the forward wave, producing a characteristic upward deflection on the downslope of the pressure pulse (Fig. 3–21). As mentioned previously, the additive nature of the reflected pressure wave accounts for the amplification of systolic pressure and the decrease in diastolic pressure that is observed as blood moves from the aorta to the peripheral arteries (see Fig. 3–13).

Although, as a first approximation, it is convenient to think of reflections as arising primarily from the high-resistance microvascular bed, reflections actually occur all along the arterial system where the vessel narrows, gives off branches, or bifurcates. The shape of the pulse is also affected by attenuation of the pressure and flow waves as they move antegrade or retrograde along the artery. Consequently, changes in the waveform attributable to reflections are more clearly seen in peripheral arteries than they are in the proximal aorta, where the amplitude of the reflected wave is greatly diminished.

Fourier analysis permits arterial pressure and flow pulses to be broken down mathematically into a series of harmonics, each having the configuration of a sine wave (see Fig. 4–17).[173] These harmonics are characterized by a modulus (amplitude at peak excursion) and a phase angle, which relates the onset of the sine wave to the beginning of the pulse cycle. The fundamental harmonic has the same frequency as that of the arterial pulse, the second harmonic has twice the frequency, and so on to the *n*th harmonic. Most of the pulsatile information is contained in the lower-frequency harmonics, allowing the raw waveform to be reduplicated fairly accurately by a summation of the first 5 to 10 harmonics. Because the velocity of the various har-

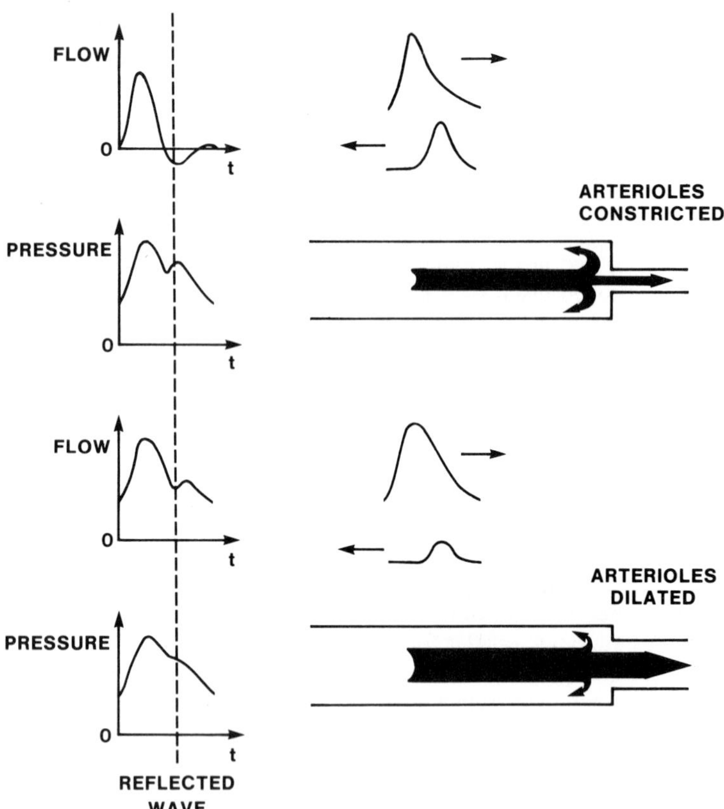

FIGURE 3–21. **Effect of reflected waves on the contour of arterial flow and pressure pulses. Reflected waves subtract from forward flow waves but add to pressure waves. Reflection is accentuated by vasoconstriction and attenuated by vasodilatation. (From Sumner DS: Hemodynamics of abnormal blood flow. *In* Veith FJ, Hobson RW II, Williams RA, Wilson SE [eds]: Vascular Surgery: Principles and Practice. 2nd ed. New York, McGraw-Hill Book Company, 1994. Reproduced with permission of McGraw-Hill.)**

monics depends on their frequency, their relative alignment changes as the pulse wave moves distally along the arterial tree. This is another factor that modifies the overall shape of flow and pressure waves.

Effect of Stenoses on Waveforms

The arterial pulse pressure distal to a stenosis or occlusion is reduced to a greater extent than the mean pressure.[46, 82] This phenomenon is due to energy losses associated with increased velocity flow through high-resistance pathways.[46, 82] Usually, no appreciable decrease in pulse pressure occurs until the stenosis reaches the so-called critical value of 75 to 90 per cent reduction in arterial lumen. Complete absence of pulsation requires a stenosis approaching 99 per cent.[39] The absence of palpable peripheral pulses distal to an arterial occlusion or severe stenosis is due both to reduction in the arterial pressure pulse and to decreased arterial pressure.

In addition to the reduction in pulse pressure, the contour of the pressure pulse is changed radically. The upslope is delayed, the peak becomes more rounded, the wave on the downslope disappears, and the downslope becomes bowed away from the baseline. These changes are reflected in the plethysmographic pulse, thus providing a sensitive indicator of the presence of arterial disease.[29, 36, 171] Further description of abnormal plethysmographic pulses is found in Chapter 5.

Similar changes are also perceived in the flow pulse distal to an obstructed artery (Fig. 3–22). Normal flow pulsations are characterized by a large forward flow component with a steep upslope. After peak flow is reached, the curve falls rapidly toward baseline levels (often actually reversing); typically, it then shows an additional but much smaller forward flow wave in late diastole. Distal to an obstruction, the velocity flow wave rises much more slowly, has a rounded peak, and declines more gradually

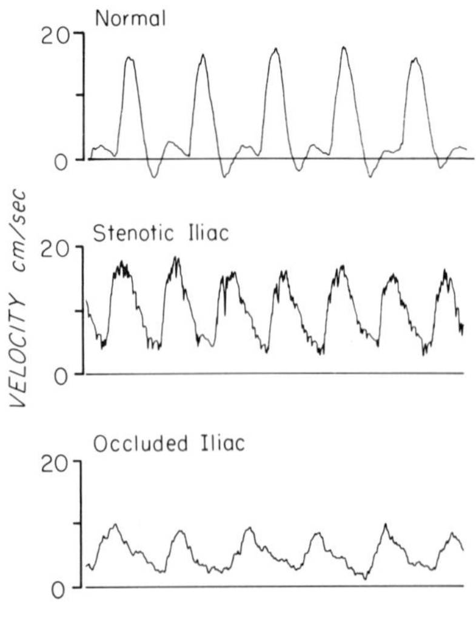

FIGURE 3–22. **Femoral artery flow pulses from a normal subject, a patient with a stenotic external iliac artery, and a patient with an occluded common iliac artery. (From Strandness DE Jr, Sumner DS: Hemodynamics for Surgeons. New York, Grune & Stratton, 1975.)**

toward the baseline during diastole. Almost invariably, the reverse flow components disappear.[57, 60, 172, 199, 200]

A stenosis, even a minor stenosis, disrupts the normal laminar flow pattern, especially in the region of flow separation just beyond the exit (see Fig. 3–8). Because velocity vectors are no longer parallel, multiple frequencies are detected by the Doppler velocimeter, producing a phenomenon known as "spectral broadening." Because the extent of flow disruption is roughly proportional to the degree of stenosis, this finding has proved most useful in detecting and grading the severity of stenoses in both carotid and peripheral arteries.[71, 145] Within the stenosis and in the jet just beyond, velocities are accelerated in accordance with the equation of continuity (Eq. 3.11). If mean flow velocities above and within the stenoses are known with certainty, the relative degree of narrowing can be measured with precision—at least theoretically. In actual practice, however, degrees of narrowing are estimated from peak systolic velocity thresholds.[210] Clinical application of flow signals in the diagnosis of arterial disease is discussed in Chapter 5.

Pulse Wave Analysis

As illustrated in Figure 3–23, the compliance of the arterial wall and that of any collateral channels constitute hydraulic capacitors, which, together with the stenosis, create a situation analogous to a low-pass filter. Passage of a pressure or flow pulse through this circuit attenuates the high-frequency harmonics and alters phase relationships, resulting in a damped waveform. Damping of the flow pulse can be quantitated by an index (PI_F) that relates the sum of the maximal oscillatory energy of the Fourier harmonics (v_r) to the mean flow velocity (v_O).[197]

$$PI_F = \sum_{r=1}^{r=n} v_r^2/v_o^2 \qquad (3.20)$$

Because it is cumbersome to perform Fourier analyses, a simplified definition of pulsatility index (PI_{PP}) was suggested by Gosling and King.[61]

$$PI_{PP} = \frac{\text{Peak-to-peak velocity}}{\text{mean velocity}} \qquad (3.21)$$

This index, which is readily calculated from the flow pulse wave without resorting to elaborate mathematical manipulation, has been shown—both theoretically and experimentally—to be mathematically related to the more complex Fourier index.[61, 77] The pulsatility index has proved to be a good method for detecting disease located proximal to the site at which the flow wave is obtained, provided that the distal vascular bed is unobstructed (see Chapters 4 and 5).[8, 49, 76]

The contour of both flow and pressure pulses above a stenosis is modified by the impedance of the entire outflow tract, which includes the stenotic arteries, the collateral channels, and the peripheral vascular bed, as shown in Figure 3–23. Input impedance is defined as the ratio of the modulus of each pressure wave harmonic to the modulus of the corresponding flow harmonic. The resistance of the outflow tract (mean pressure/mean flow; see Eq. 3.12) is referred to as the impedance at zero frequency.[50, 173] Input impedance is determined by the resistance to outflow, the inertia and viscosity of blood, the stiffness of the arterial wall, the pulse rate, and wave reflections. Arterial stenoses located just distal to the site at which flow and pressure measurements are made reduce the magnitude of the reflected wave, decrease the amplitude of the flow pulse, and increase the amplitude of the pressure pulse.[50, 126] Input

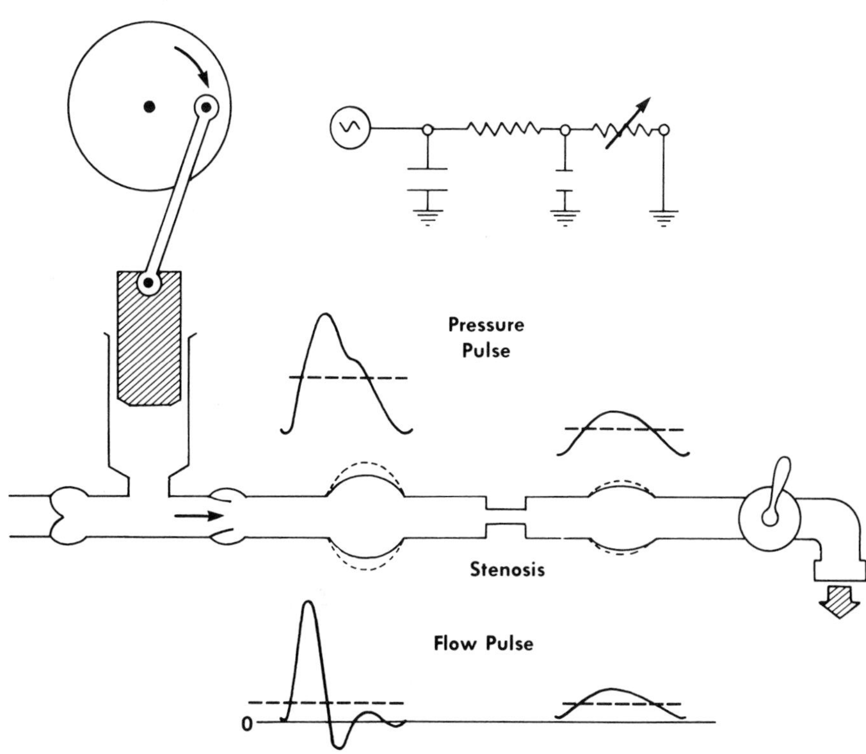

FIGURE 3–23. Effect of a stenosis and compliant vessels on the contour of arterial pressure and flow pulses. Mean pressure *(dashed line)* is reduced, but mean flow *(dashed line)* is unchanged. Faucet represents the variable resistance of the peripheral vascular bed. This, together with the fixed resistance of the stenosis and the compliance of the major arteries, constitutes a model of input impedance. (From Sumner DS: Correlation of lesion configuration with functional significance. *In* Bond MG, Insull W Jr, Glagov S [eds]: Clinical Diagnosis of Atherosclerosis: Quantitative Methods of Evaluation. New York, Springer-Verlag, 1983.)

impedance for the higher harmonics (above the third or fourth) is a function of the resistance of the stenosis and is relatively independent of the state of peripheral vasodilatation.[50]

Because input impedance modifies the contour of the flow pulse (thereby reducing the accuracy of the pulsatility index for detecting proximal disease), Skidmore and Woodcock and their colleagues developed a method for segregating damping caused by proximal stenosis from the effects of arterial wall stiffness and peripheral impedance.[158–160] A computer is used to calculate the Fourier transform of the velocity pulse. From this, the equivalent Laplace transform is evaluated by a curve-fitting procedure. The Laplace transform damping coefficient obtained from the femoral arterial velocity waveform has proved to be a more sensitive method for detecting iliac arterial stenosis than the pulsatility index—particularly in limbs with additional superficial femoral disease.[8] Impedance analysis has also been used as a method of surveillance for identifying infrainguinal bypass grafts that are at risk for failure.[198]

Shear Rate at the Arterial Wall

As mentioned earlier, shear rate (D) is the rate at which the velocity of flow changes between concentric laminae of blood (Eq. 3.8). Although the infinitesimally thin layer of blood in immediate contact with the inner wall of a vessel is static, the contiguous layers are in motion. This creates a shear rate at the wall (D_W) and a corresponding shear stress (τ_W) on the endothelial surface. In terms of mean velocity (V) and mean flow (Q) across a vessel in which the flow profile is parabolic, the shear rate and shear stress at the wall are

$$D_w = 4\frac{V}{r} = 4\frac{Q}{\pi r^3} \quad (3.22)$$

$$\tau_w = 4\eta\frac{V}{r} = 4\eta\frac{Q}{\pi r^3} \quad (3.23)$$

Thus, the shear rate and shear stress at the wall at any instant in the pulse cycle depend on blood viscosity (η) and are directly proportional to the mean velocity of flow and inversely proportional to the inner radius of the vessel. This means that wall shear increases as the mean velocity increases or the radius decreases and that shear decreases as the velocity decreases or the radius increases.

Shear rates at the wall are increased when the velocity profile is blunt, reflecting the decreased radial distance from the wall to the cylindrical plug of maximal velocity flow (see Fig. 3–4). When the profile is skewed (as it is at bifurcations and at areas where the vessel curves), shear is greatest near the wall where the velocity of flow is highest. In these regions, flow may take on a helical pattern, thereby further complicating the pattern of shear.[107] Turbulence not only increases shear stress but also subjects the wall to large oscillatory stresses.[129] At the carotid bulb, shear is greatest near the flow divider and least near the opposite wall, where blood flow may be stagnant or reversed during a large part of the cardiac cycle.[88, 121, 196] In this area of "flow separation," the direction of shear fluctuates during the pulse cycle, corresponding to the direction of the velocity vectors (Fig. 3–24*A*).[88] (Flow is said to be "separated" when the boundary of the main body of flow is no longer attached to the vessel wall but is separated from the wall by a region in which the velocity vectors have a different orientation.) Similarly, in aneurysms, the axial flow stream is separated from flow in the dilated area near the wall, where velocities are low and flow reversal occurs (Fig. 3–24*B*).[196]

Other regions in which flow separation develops include the lateral walls of the common iliac artery at the aortic bifurcation and just beyond stenoses in atherosclerotic vessels (see Fig. 3–8).[144, 155, 196] In stenotic arteries, the longitudinal extent of flow separation depends on the velocity of flow and the degree of narrowing.[127]

The physiologic and pathophysiologic importance of shear rate and shear stress has only recently been recognized. There is good evidence that arteries constrict with decreasing shear[89] and dilate with increasing shear.[70, 79, 115] Teleologically, this may be viewed as an effort to "normalize" shear stress.[207] Apparently, the endothelium in some way senses shear, causing the release of endothelium-derived relaxing factor (EDRF), which in turn relaxes the smooth muscles of the arterial wall, allowing the vessel to expand.[62] The classic example of this phenomenon is the increased diameter of arteries feeding an arteriovenous fistula.[70, 207] As mentioned earlier in this chapter, coronary arteries narrowed by atherosclerotic plaques also tend to dilate, thereby maintaining the lumen at a relatively normal diameter so long as the plaques remain small.[59] This mechanism may be operative in the peripheral circulation as well, where the average diameter of atherosclerotic arteries is usually somewhat larger than that of normal arteries. Post-stenotic dilatation of the axillary artery (frequently observed distal to the site of bony compression in patients with thoracic outlet syndrome) has also been attributed to distorted patterns of shear stress.[129]

Endothelial cells are aligned and are overlapped (like

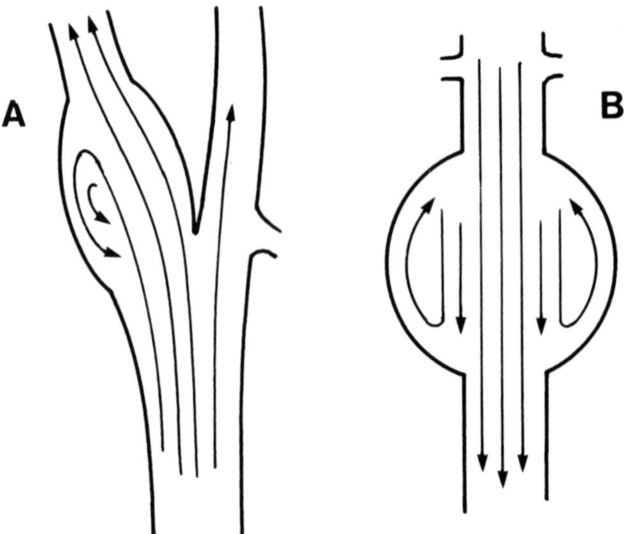

FIGURE 3–24. Diagrammatic representation of flow streamlines in a carotid arterial bifurcation (*A*) and an abdominal aortic aneurysm (*B*). Flow separation and reversal of flow occur in the carotid bulb and in the distended portion of the aneurysm.

shingles) in the direction of the wall shear stress.[164] In areas with reduced shear and where the direction of shear oscillates during the pulse cycle the orientation of these cells is distorted and the pattern of overlap is disrupted. Atherosclerotic plaques tend to form first and develop most rapidly at sites of decreased shear, possibly because the relative stagnation of blood in these regions prolongs the fluid "residence time," modifying mass transport of atherogenic substances from the lumen into the wall and fostering the adherence of platelets and macrophages to the endothelial surface.[88, 121] The endothelial barrier may in turn be more susceptible to penetration owing to the distorted alignment of the cells and the instability of cellular junctions.[88] This explains the preferential location of plaques in the carotid bulb opposite the flow divider and the frequency with which atherosclerotic plaques form at the bifurcations of the terminal aorta, the common femoral artery, and popliteal artery—all areas in which geometry promotes flow separation and decreased shear rates.[88, 155] Once a plaque has formed, further extension may be promoted by the area of stagnant or reversed flow that develops immediately beyond the stenosis (see Fig. 3–8).

Other investigators have observed a positive correlation between shear rate and platelet and fibrin deposition on damaged endothelial surfaces and suggest that increased shear rates may be conducive to arterial thrombosis in certain circumstances.[132]

PHYSIOLOGIC ASPECTS OF TREATING ARTERIAL INSUFFICIENCY

Based on the arguments presented earlier in this chapter, it is evident that the elevated fixed resistance imposed by obstructed major arteries and their associated collaterals is the factor responsible for restricting blood flow to the periphery. It follows that intermittent claudication and other symptoms of peripheral ischemia can be alleviated only by reducing this fixed resistance. Efforts to reduce the resistance of the peripheral vascular bed are seldom beneficial, because this resistance either is automatically adjusted to levels adequate to maintain a normal resting blood flow or already is maximally reduced in limbs with ischemia at rest (see Fig. 3–11). It also is maximally reduced during exercise in patients with intermittent claudication (see Fig. 3–18).[30, 66, 140, 147]

Thus, vasodilators may increase the resting blood flow in limbs when resting blood flow is adequate, but they almost never improve flow in an ischemic limb or during exercise.[27, 188] In fact, they may cause blood to be diverted from areas of relative ischemia to those where the disease is less severe.[93]

Many of these same criticisms can be applied to surgical sympathectomy (Fig. 3–25).[33, 66, 147] Sympathectomy, however, does have the advantage that its effects can be confined to the diseased area. In fact, some relief has been reported in patients with mild rest pain or with superficial ischemic ulcers.[170] Yet even this improvement is difficult to explain, because sympathectomy appears to enhance flow through arteriovenous anastomoses without increasing flow through the nutritive capillary bed.[34]

Because no drugs are available that will produce appreciable collateral dilatation or cause regression of atherosclerotic plaques, satisfactory reduction of the fixed resistance can be accomplished only by direct surgical means. Endarterectomy, replacement grafting, and bypass grafting are all effective surgical measures (Fig. 3–25). Exercise therapy is the only nonoperative treatment that consistently affords any objective relief.[90, 162] Although exercise programs extend maximal walking and claudication distances and appear to decrease the flow debt incurred during muscle activity, there is usually little change in the ankle pressure.[51, 74] This suggests that the benefits are due in large part to metabolic changes rather than to collateral development. Thus, exercise—although helpful in patients with claudication—is applicable only when ischemia is absent at rest and cannot match the hemodynamic improvement provided by reconstructive surgery.

Temporary relief of severe ischemia at rest sometimes can be obtained by rendering the patient hypertensive, thereby increasing the pressure head perfusing the obstructed vascular circuit.[90, 93] Because of the adverse effects of hypertension, this approach is rarely employed. On the other hand, it is well known that hanging the feet over the edge of the bed or walking a few steps often provides complete or partial relief from ischemic rest pain. The temporary improvement in peripheral perfusion that accompanies dependency can be documented objectively by measuring transcutaneous oxygen tensions, which may be increased severalfold compared with levels measured when the patient is supine.[149] According to Equation 3.1, pressure in the dependent arteries, veins, and capillaries is increased

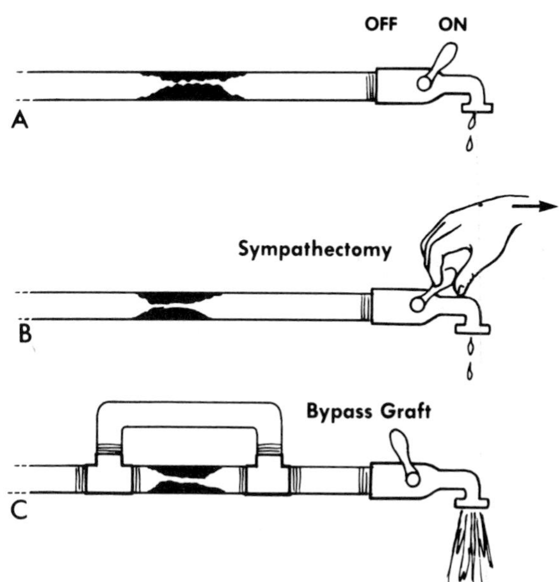

FIGURE 3–25. Hydraulic model contrasting the effects of sympathectomy and bypass grafting on blood flow. *A*, Faucet represents peripheral resistance, which is maximally decreased by exercise. *B*, Resistance cannot be further decreased by sympathectomy. *C*, Bypass graft circumvents the fixed resistance, permitting increased blood flow even with less peripheral vasodilatation. (*A–C*, From Sumner DS: Pathophysiology of arterial occlusive disease. *In* Hershey FB, Barnes RW, Sumner DS [eds]: Noninvasive Diagnosis of Vascular Disease. Pasadena, CA, Appleton Davies, Inc, 1984.)

by gravity commensurate with the vertical distance from the foot to the heart. Although there is no increase in the arteriovenous pressure gradient, the increased hydrostatic pressure dilates capillaries and microvascular vessels, thereby reducing their resistance, which in turn augments blood flow. Augmentation of blood flow does not occur in nonischemic limbs, because the venoarterial reflex that serves to constrict arterioles in the dependent position remains functional.

Because the viscosity of blood increases with hematocrit, it is possible to augment blood flow by hemodilution.[43, 95, 195] The effects, however, are unpredictable, difficult to control, and not applicable on a long-term basis. Pentoxifylline, a drug that increases erythrocyte flexibility, augments walking tolerance somewhat in patients with claudication; but again the results are variable.[138]

Arterial Grafts

When the decision to use a graft has been made, the surgeon often has some latitude in the choice of graft material, diameter, and anastomotic configuration (end-to-end, side-to-end, or end-to-side). Because of the importance of radius in determining both viscous and inertial energy losses, the graft selected should be large enough to carry all the flow required at rest without causing an evident pressure drop. It should also be large enough to accommodate any increased flow that is likely to be required during exercise without an appreciable pressure drop. Any limitation of flow should result from the resistance of the peripheral vascular bed and not from the graft.

Table 3–1 lists the pressure gradients that might be expected through a 40-cm-long femoropopliteal graft at several levels of flow. Since these calculations were made using Poiseuille's equation (Eq. 3.7), they represent minimal values; the actual pressure drops would be several times as great.[148] Clearly a graft with an inside diameter less than 3 mm would be of marginal value at flow rates normally observed at rest (60 to 150 ml/min) and would be completely unsatisfactory during exercise, when rates of 300 to 500 ml/min occur. This coincides with the clinical observation of many surgeons.[21, 47, 128, 189]

Blood flow in the common femoral artery averages about 350 ml/min at rest and may increase by a factor of 5 to 10 during exercise. According to Poiseuille's equation, a 20-cm-long graft with an inside diameter of 7 mm should be capable of carrying flows of 3000 ml/min with a pressure drop of only 4.5 mmHg. Experimentally, the pressure gradient across similar grafts is much higher, approximating 7 to 10 mmHg at a flow rate of 1200 ml/min.[148, 152] At rest, however, a 7-mm graft should result in a pressure gradient of only a few millimeters of mercury. Therefore, under most physiologic conditions, an aortofemoral graft with 7-mm limbs should suffice, restricting flow only during strenuous exercise. Six-millimeter grafts might begin to show some restriction of flow even with mild to moderate exercise.

Table 3–1. Calculated Minimal Pressure Gradients (mmHg) Across a 40-cm Graft (η = 0.035 P)

	Diameter (cm)				
Flow (ml/min)	***0.2***	***0.3***	***0.4***	***0.5***	***0.6***
60	27	5.3	1.7	0.7	0.3
100	45	8.8	2.8	1.1	0.6
150	67	13	4.2	1.7	0.8
300	134	27	8.4	3.4	1.7
500	223	44	14	5.8	2.8

Under ideal flow conditions, prosthetic grafts develop a thin (0.5 to 1.0 mm) layer of pseudointima. Thus, after implantation, a 6-mm prosthetic graft would actually have an internal diameter of 4 to 5 mm, and an 8-mm graft would have a lumen of 6 to 7 mm. For this reason, it seems appropriate, when one performs a femoropopliteal bypass with a prosthetic graft, to select a graft with an original diameter of at least 4 to 5 mm. Similarly, the original diameter of an aortofemoral graft should be at least 6 to 7 mm.

On the other hand, the diameter of the graft must not be too much larger than that of the recipient arteries.[150] It has been shown, both clinically and experimentally, that irregular clots accumulate on the inner walls of grafts of excessive diameter (much as they do in aneurysms) as the flow stream tries to mold itself to the diameter of the recipient vessels. These clots, which are not densely adherent, tend to separate and may be responsible for graft failure. A high flow velocity (high shear) is conducive to the formation of a thin, tightly adherent pseudointima. For a given volume of flow, the wall shear rate (or stress) is inversely proportional to the cube of the radius (Eqs. 3.22 and 3.23). Therefore, the shear rate at the wall in a 7-mm graft would be 1.5 times that in an 8-mm graft and 2.9 times that in a 10-mm graft. In summary, the diameter of a prosthetic graft should be small enough to assure a rapid velocity of flow but large enough to avoid restriction of arterial inflow.

Long-term patency of autogenous vein grafts is compromised by intimal hyperplasia, the development of which has also been shown to be associated with low shear rates.[14, 130] Low shear rates cause smooth muscle cells to become secretory and enhance platelet adherence.[130] On the other hand, a high shear rate fosters continued patency and lessens the tendency for the intima to become hyperplastic. The protective effect of high shear may be due to suppression of the release of endothelin-1, a peptide found in endothelial cells that acts as a vasoconstrictor and a mitogen for smooth muscle cells.[154]

Anastomoses

Because any change in the direction of blood flow increases energy losses due to inertial factors, an end-to-end anastomosis is more hemodynamically efficient than side-to-end or end-to-side anastomoses.[173] The greater the angle subtended by the graft and host vessels, the greater the energy losses become. Even though energy losses may be increased severalfold by an adverse angle, the increase in pressure drop is only a few millimeters of mercury and is ordinarily of no clinical significance. For example, from the point of view of transmitting blood efficiently, it makes little difference whether the donor anastomosis of a femo-

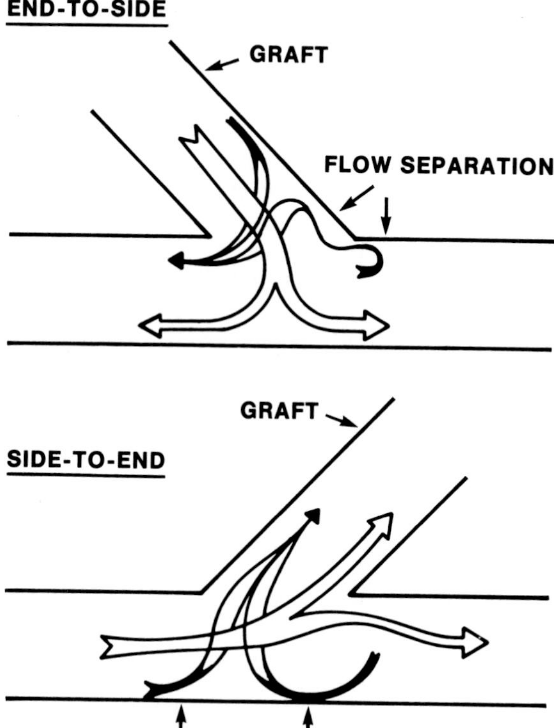

FIGURE 3–26. Flow patterns at end-to-side and side-to-end anastomoses. Near the wall, blood flow may reverse and travel circumferentially to reach the recipient conduit. Areas of flow separation are prone to develop neointimal hyperplasia. (From Sumner DS: Hemodynamics of abnormal blood flow. *In* Veith FJ, Hobson RW, Russell AW, Wilson SE [eds]: Vascular Surgery: Principles and Practice. 2nd ed. New York, McGraw-Hill Book Company, 1994. Reproduced with permission of McGraw-Hill.)

rofemoral graft is made with an angle of 135 degrees (requiring flow to reverse itself) or whether it is made with a more hemodynamically satisfactory angle of 45 degrees.[101, 105]

But energy losses are only part of the story. Any time a graft leaves or enters a host vessel at an angle, flow disturbances are created, resulting in zones of flow separation, stagnation, turbulence, and distorted velocity vectors (Figs. 3–26 and 3–27).[9, 32, 101, 128] The "floor" of an end-to-side anastomosis (in the recipient vessel opposite the anastomosis), the "toe" of the anastomosis (on the near wall just beyond the suture line), and the "heel" (on the near wall proximal to the junction) appear to be prominent sites of flow separation where shear is low and shear stress fluctuates.[9, 128] Low shear and oscillatory shear stresses are conducive to platelet adhesion, intimal hyperplasia, and atherosclerosis, and high shear may result in endothelial damage.[32, 101, 113, 205] The ultimate result will be endothelial thickening or thrombus formation that may lead to graft failure.[100] Therefore, the goal of a long-term graft patency is best achieved by constructing an end-to-end anastomosis or, when this is not feasible, an anastomosis with an acute angle.

VISCOELASTICITY OF THE ARTERIAL WALL

As intraluminal pressure increases during systole, the arterial wall stretches both circumferentially and longitudinally. During diastole, the process is reversed. The magnitude of the stretch is determined by the stiffness of the arterial wall, which in turn is determined by its composition and thickness.

The stiffness of an elastic material can be described by Young's modulus of elasticity (E), which is the ratio of the applied stress (τ) to the resulting strain (ϵ):

$$E = \tau/\epsilon \qquad (3.24)$$

Compliance (C) is the reciprocal of the elastic modulus (1/E). The circumferential stress applied to an arterial wall is a function of the transmural pressure, P (intraluminal pressure minus the extravascular pressure), the inside radius of the artery, r_i, and its wall thickness, δ:[137, 173]

$$\tau = P \cdot \frac{r_i}{\delta} \qquad (3.25)$$

FIGURE 3–27. Flow pattern in a model of an end-to-side anastomosis. Note impingement of high velocity flow on the "floor" of the anastomosis and the helical pattern that develops beyond the anastomosis. Reversal of flow occurs in the proximal segment of the recipient vessel. (*a*, Model tilted toward observer. *b*, Model viewed from above.) From Ojha M, Ethier CR, Johnston KW, Cobbold RSC: Steady and pulsatile flow fields in an end-to-side arterial anastomosis model. J Vasc Surg 12:747–753, 1990.)

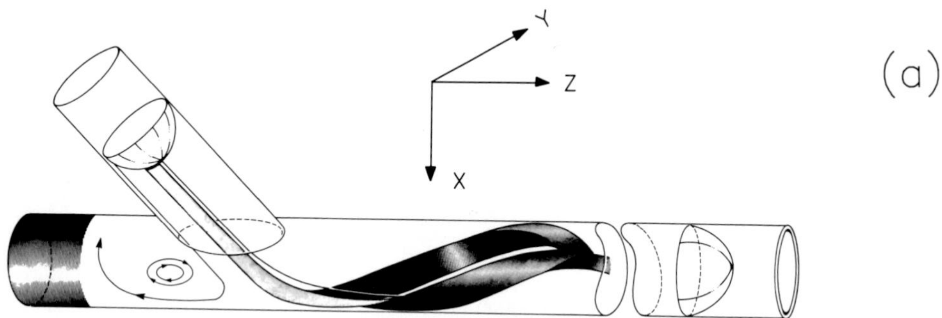

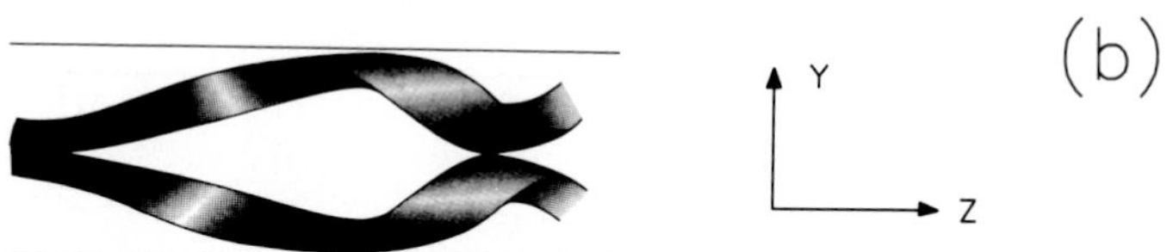

Pressure is in dynes · cm^{-2}, and r_i and δ are in centimeters. Circumferential strain, ε, is proportional to the ratio of the change in outside radius, Δr_o, to the original outside radius, r_o:

$$\epsilon = \Delta r_o/r_o \qquad (3.26)$$

Therefore, an incremental elastic modulus (E_t) can be obtained by substituting Equations 3.25 and 3.26 in 3.24:

$$E_t = \Delta P \frac{r_o}{\Delta r_o} \cdot \frac{r_i}{\delta} \qquad (3.27)$$

Pulse pressure is represented by ΔP. Although this formula allows a first approximation of the stiffness of the materials composing the arterial wall, it fails to take into account the variable stress on the different layers (greatest on the inside and least on the outside) and the tendency of the wall thickness to decrease as the radius increases.[173] A more precise formula that incorporates these variables has been devised by Bergel.[12]

$$E = \Delta P \cdot \frac{r_o}{\Delta r_o} \cdot \frac{(1.5)\, r_i^2}{r_o^2 - r_i^2} \qquad (3.28)$$

Because it is often difficult to obtain precise measurements of arterial wall thickness, several purely descriptive formulas are in common use.[137]

$$E_P = \Delta P \cdot \frac{r_o}{\Delta r_o} \qquad (3.29)$$

Compliance (C) is the reciprocal of E_P.

$$C = \frac{\Delta r_o}{\Delta P \cdot r_o} \qquad (3.30)$$

It should be emphasized that Equations 3.29 and 3.30 relate to the behavior of the entire arterial wall, whereas Equations 3.27 and 3.28 describe the stiffness of the materials composing the wall. In other words, two arteries with the same E value (Eq. 3.28) would have different E_P values if their wall thicknesses were different.

In addition to elasticity, the arterial wall demonstrates viscosity.[13] This property causes the expansion of the artery to lag behind the change in pressure. As a result, the elastic modulus of the arterial wall appears to increase with increasing pulse rate. Wall viscosity may also account for some of the energy losses in pulsatile flow, because the storage of energy during systole and its release during diastole may be incomplete owing to the friction encountered in expansion and contraction of the arterial wall.

Two fibrous proteins, elastin and collagen, determine the mechanical properties of the arterial wall. At low transmural pressures (less than 50 to 75 mmHg), most of the circumferential distending force is sustained by lamellae composed of elastin, which is highly extensible. At higher pressures, the arterial wall stretches and collagen fibers are gradually recruited to bear an increasingly large portion of the load. Because collagen is about 1000 to 2000 times stiffer than elastin, arteries (and veins) become very stiff at high pressures. Therefore, the typical pressure-diameter curve of arteries has two phases: a low-pressure, compliant part, and a high-pressure, stiff part.[40] The elastic modulus of the arterial wall also increases with aging, fibrosis, and calcification—factors that often accompany arteriosclerosis.[122, 173]

Activation of the smooth muscle within the arterial wall has a complex relationship to the elastic modulus, but tends to increase stiffness at a given strain.[42, 173] The effect of muscle contraction becomes evident only in the smaller, muscular arteries of the periphery and is most marked in terminal arterioles. In the absence of muscular contraction, all arteries retain a circular cross section even at zero transmural pressure. Therefore, the phenomenon of "critical closure," in which small arteries appear to collapse (occlude) at low perfusion pressures, can occur only when there is an increase in smooth muscle tone.[7]

Table 3–2 lists some of the stress-strain characteristics of atherosclerotic and normal arteries.

Palpable Pulses

Motion of the arterial wall is responsible for the palpable pulses that are so important in the physical examination of the patient in whom arterial disease is suspected. Yet, it is apparent from the figures in Table 3–2 that a 7.0-mm femoral artery in a young subject would expand only 0.2 mm under the influence of a 50-mmHg pulse pressure. Older, stiffer arteries would expand even less. It seems

Table 3–2. Stress-Strain Characteristics of Human Arteries

Location	Reference	Remarks	Elastic Modulus (E)* (dynes · cm^{-2} · 10^6)	Pressure-Strain Elastic Modulus† (dynes · cm^{-2} · 10^6)	Per Cent Compliance (C)‡ Normalized (ΔP = 50 mmHg)
Infrarenal aorta	173	ASO§	26.0 ± 14.5	9.8 ± 3.5	0.8 ± 0.3
Terminal aorta	173	ASO	37.7 ± 17.2	15.1 ± 4.1	0.5 ± 0.2
Common iliac artery	173	ASO	24.7 ± 21.5	14.8 ± 15.8	0.8 ± 0.4
Common femoral artery	122	Age <35 yr	—	2.6 ± 1.3	3.0 ± 1.0
	122	Age 35–60 yr	—	3.9 ± 2.0	2.1 ± 0.9
	122	Age >60 yr	—	6.3 ± 4.8	1.2 ± 0.9
	186	—	—	2.3 ± 0.2	3.0 ± 0.3

**Equation 3.28.*
†Equation 3.29.
‡Equation 3.30.
§ASO, arteriosclerosis obliterans.

doubtful that the finger could reliably detect this degree of motion. Why, then, are pulses ordinarily so easily felt? When the finger is applied to the skin overlying an artery, the artery is compressed—changing its normally circular cross section into an ellipse. It takes much less energy to bend the wall of an elliptically shaped vessel than it does to stretch the wall of a circular vessel.[122] Therefore, when the artery is partially compressed, its expansion in the direction of the compression is greatly augmented. In addition, as the artery expands longitudinally, the entire vessel moves toward the skin.

As surgeons we are accustomed to grading the peripheral pulses on some arbitrary scale (e.g., from 0 to 4+) and to making some estimate of the degree of proximal obstruction based on the magnitude of the pulse. This is predicated on the assumption that the strength of the pulse is directly related to the pulse pressure, which should be decreased distal to an obstruction. Stiff, calcified vessels may display little or no pulse, however, even though there is no decrease in pulse pressure. On the other hand, relatively good pulses may be palpated despite a proximal arterial obstruction when the arterial wall is compliant, particularly when the systemic pulse pressure is increased.

Although pulse palpation is a valuable tool for the initial evaluation of the patient with suspected arterial disease, both arteriography and noninvasive tests have repeatedly demonstrated its fallibility.

Pulse Wave Velocity

The velocity with which a pulse is propagated in an artery is proportional to the elastic modulus of the arterial wall.[173]

$$\text{Pulse wave velocity} = \left(\frac{E\delta}{\rho(r_o + r_i)}\right)^{1/2}$$

$$\cong \left(0.5\frac{E_P}{\rho}\right)^{1/2} \qquad (3.31)$$

In other words, pulses in older hypertensive patients with stiff arteries should arrive at a given location more rapidly than they would in young, normotensive subjects with compliant arteries. Calcification and an increase in wall thickness (δ) also increase pulse wave velocity. Therefore, one would predict that the pulse arrival time in arteriosclerotic vessels would be decreased.[61] However, in the presence of severe (critical) arterial stenosis, pulse arrival times are often delayed.[197] The delayed arrival in these cases can be attributed to the elongated circuitous collaterals that must be traversed before the pulse reaches the periphery.[61]

Input Impedance and Graft Patency

A comparison of the elastic moduli of grafts listed in Table 3–3 with those of the arteries in Table 3–2 reveals that most synthetic grafts are stiffer than the arteries that they replace. This is especially true for grafts that have been implanted for some time. The ingrowth of fibrous tissue (with its high collagen content) into the interstices of a porous graft and the encapsulation of the graft in an adherent sheath of fibrous tissues are responsible for the increased stiffness.

As discussed earlier in this chapter, input impedance is a function of the stiffness of the arterial conduit. A stiff graft impedes the pulsatile component of blood flow more than a compliant graft, even though their resistances to mean flow may be identical.[131] This raises the level of work required to transmit a given quantity of blood. Although the issue is complex and has not been rigorously tested, it appears that compliant grafts are more likely to remain patent than noncompliant grafts.[1] This may, in part, explain why autogenous vein grafts function better below the inguinal ligament than prosthetic grafts.

Stresses at Graft-Artery Anastomoses and False Aneurysms

Coupling a stiff graft to a compliant artery places additional stresses on the suture line, which may lead to

Table 3–3. Stress-Strain Characteristics of Various Arterial Grafts

Graft Material	Reference	Months Implanted	Pressure-Strain Elastic Modulus* (dynes · cm^{-2} · 10^6)	Per Cent Compliance (C)† Normalized (ΔP = 50 mmHg)
Saphenous vein	186	0	3.0 ± 0.6	2.2 ± 0.4
	106	>36	4.9 ± 2.0	1.7 ± 1.0
Umbilical vein	186	0	3.6 ± 0.5	1.9 ± 0.3
Bovine heterograft	186	0	5.1 ± 0.6	1.3 ± 0.2
	67	12	24.2	0.3
Dacron				
Velour	186	0	7.0 ± 1.1	1.0 ± 0.2
Knitted	67	0	17.8	0.4
	67	12	55.5	0.1
Woven	67	0	166.6	0.04
Teflon woven	67	0	148.1	0.05
PTFE‡	186	0	8.3 ± 1.0	0.8 ± 0.1

**Equation 3.29.*
†Equation 3.30.
‡PTFE, polytetrafluoroethylene.

intimal hyperplasia or the development of a false aneurysm.[9, 114] With the advent of synthetic sutures, most anastomotic disruptions develop in the arterial wall; the sutures themselves remain intact.[84, 125] On the basis of the data in Tables 3–2 and 3–3, the circumference of a young femoral artery measuring 7 mm in diameter would increase 1.32 mm with each 50-mmHg pressure pulse, whereas the circumference of a woven Dacron graft of the same diameter would increase only 0.02 mm, a disparity of 1.30 mm. Repeated 100,000 times per day, this small difference could result in fatigue of the arterial wall.

Paasche and colleagues have analyzed the stresses produced at an end-to-end anastomosis by a compliance mismatch.[133] Three components of the stress system were identified: axial, hoop, and shear. Of these, the last, which is greatest at the suture lines, is the most disruptive. Both theoretically and experimentally, it has been shown that stresses are minimized when the ratio of the diameter of a rigid graft to that of a compliant artery is about 1.4.[85, 133]

Because the impedance of a stiff graft is greater than that of a compliant artery, pulsatile energy is reflected at the proximal suture line. When a Dacron graft with an E_P of 55×10^6 dynes · cm^{-2} is sutured to an infrarenal aorta with an E_P of 9.8×10^6 dynes · cm^{-2}, about 41 per cent of the incident pulsatile energy is reflected.[173] Because this augments the pressure pulsations proximal to the graft, additional stresses are placed on the suture line.[124] This may contribute to disruption of the proximal anastomosis.

Shear stresses produced by vibrations generated at end-to-side anastomoses may also contribute to the formation of false anerurysms.

Arterial Wall Stress and Rupture of Aortic Aneurysms

Aneurysms rupture when the tangential stress within their wall exceeds the tensile strength of the wall at any point.

Tangential stress (τ) within the wall of a cylinder is given by Equation 3.25. This equation explains in part why large aneurysms are more apt to rupture than small aneurysms, and why rupture is more common in hypertensive than in normotensive patients.[16, 56]

Note that Equation 3.25 differs from Laplace's law, which usually is stated as

$$T = Pr \qquad (3.32)$$

where r is commonly taken as the outside radius (though more properly it should be the inside radius), and T is tension in dynes per centimeter of cylindrical length. Laplace's law is truly applicable only to very thin-walled structures, such as soap bubbles, and should not be employed to describe stresses in arterial walls.[136]

Because the wall stress in a sphere is one half that in a cylinder with the same radius and because the typical configuration of an aneurysm is a cross between a sphere and a cylinder, Equation 3.25 may actually overestimate the stress in aneurysm walls.[40] Nonetheless, this does not change the essential argument, namely that wall stress is directly proportional to transmural pressure and to the inner radius of the vessel and is inversely proportional to wall thickness.

Figure 3–28 shows a cylinder with an outside diameter of 2.0 cm and a wall thickness of 0.2 cm. These dimensions are compatible with those found in atherosclerotic terminal aortas.[173, 179] The circumferential wall stress within this structure would be 8.0×10^5 dynes · cm^{-2} when the internal pressure is 150 mmHg. If this tube were distended without increasing the volume of material in the wall, the wall would simultaneously become thinner. In the case illustrated, the tube has been expanded to aneurysmal dimensions, outside diameter 6.0 cm, and the wall thickness has decreased to 0.06 cm (Fig. 3.28, *right-hand panel*). Tripling the radius and decreasing the wall thickness causes the circumferential stress in the wall of the expanded cylinder to increase to 98.0×10^5 dynes · cm^{-2}, provided the pressure remains at 150 mmHg (Eq. 3.25). Thus, the stress per unit area of wall increases by a factor of 12, even though the arterial diameter has increased only three times.

Owing to the sluggish flow and low shear stress on the inner wall of aneurysms, layers of clot develop that tend to maintain the diameter of the lumen near that of the normal artery (see Fig. 3–24). One might think that the thrombus, by increasing the effective thickness of the arterial wall (δ), would reduce wall stress and would therefore afford some protection against rupture (Eq. 3.25). Although this question has not been completely resolved, it is likely that the clot transmits pressure directly to the wall and has little effect on wall stress. Moreover, because the thrombus is so friable and poorly bonded to the inner surface of the residual wall, it exerts little or no retractive force.[40] Therefore, the layers of clot lining the interior of an aneurysm are unlikely to have much influence on the propensity for rupture.

In normal arteries, most of the wall stress imposed by intraluminal pressure is sustained by elastin. It has been suggested that aneurysm formation is related to degeneration of elastic lamellae caused by atherosclerosis or the action of endogenous elastases.[41, 206, 208] Inflammatory cells may also participate in this process, perhaps by serving as a source of elastases.[4] Rupture, however, is prevented by

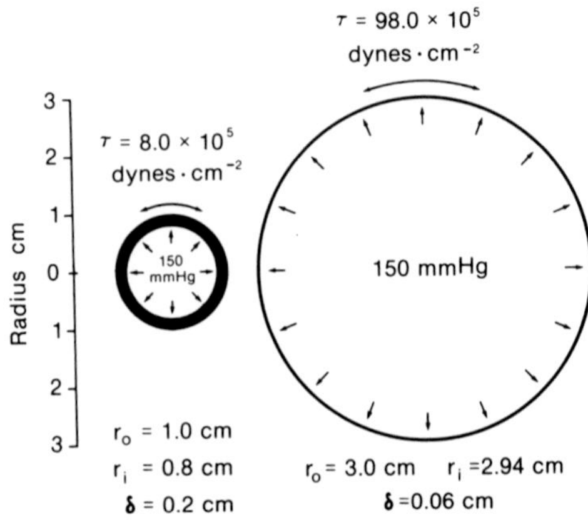

FIGURE 3–28. End-on view of a cylinder 2 cm in diameter before and after expansion to a diameter of 6 cm. Wall area remains the same in the two cases, but wall stress (τ) is greatly increased owing both to the decrease in wall thickness (δ) and to the increase in inside radius (r_i).

collagen fibers, which are principally responsible for the integrity of the arterial wall.[41] Although the tensile strength of collagen (about 5 to 7 $\times$ 10^7 dynes $\cdot$ cm^{-2}) far exceeds the wall stress developed in the dilated tube shown in Figure 3–28, it must be pointed out that collagen fibers make up only about 25 per cent of the atherosclerotic arterial wall, and only 6 to 18 per cent of the aneurysm wall.[175, 180] Therefore, one would predict that each collagen fiber sustains a greater load than would be expected if the entire wall were composed of collagen. In addition, the aneurysm wall is weakened by fragmentation and other degenerative changes within the fibrous network. (Collagenase activity may play an important role in this process.[20]) On the basis of these considerations, it is not hard to imagine how an atherosclerotic artery that has become aneurysmal might rupture. Not only is the wall stress greatly increased, but the collagen fibers are more sparsely distributed, disorganized, and fragmented.

Selected References

Burton AC: Physiology and Biophysics of the Circulation. 2nd ed. Chicago, Year Book Medical Publishers, 1972.

Caro CG, Pedley TJ, Schroter RC, Seed WA: The Mechanics of the Circulation. New York, Oxford University Press, 1978.

Conrad MC: Functional Anatomy of the Circulation to the Lower Extremities. Chicago, Year Book Medical Publishers, 1971.

Dobrin PB: Mechanical properties of arteries. Physiol Rev 58:397, 1978.

Fung YC: Biodynamics: Circulation. New York, Springer-Verlag, 1984.

Milnor WR: Hemodynamics. 2nd ed. Baltimore, Williams & Wilkins, 1989.

Nichols WW, O'Rourke MF: McDonald's Blood Flow in Arteries. Philadelphia, Lea & Febiger, 1990.

Patel DJ, Vaishnav RN: Basic Hemodynamics and Its Role in Disease Processes. Baltimore, University Park Press, 1980.

Shepherd JT: Physiology of the Circulation in Human Limbs in Health and Disease. Philadelphia, WB Saunders Co, 1963.

Strandness DE Jr: Peripheral Arterial Disease, A Physiologic Approach. Boston, Little, Brown & Co, 1969.

Strandness DE Jr: Collateral Circulation in Clinical Surgery. Philadelphia, WB Saunders Co, 1969.

Strandness DE Jr, Sumner DS: Hemodynamics for Surgeons. New York, Grune & Stratton, 1975.

References

1. Abbott WM, Bouchier-Hayes DJ: The role of mechanical properties in graft design. *In* Dardik H (ed): Graft Materials in Vascular Surgery. Miami, Symposia Specialist, 1978, pp 59–78.
2. Allwood MJ: Redistribution of blood flow in limbs with obstruction of a main artery. Clin Sci 22:279, 1962.
3. Angelides NS, Nicolaides AN: Simultaneous isotope clearance from the muscles of the calf and thigh. *In* Puel P, Boccalon H, Enjalbert A (eds): Hemodynamics of the Limbs—1. Toulouse, France, GEPESC, 1979, pp 547–562.
4. Anidjar S, Dobrin PB, Eichorst M, et al: Correlation of inflammatory infiltrate with the enlargement of experimental aortic aneurysms. J Vasc Surg 16:139, 1992.
5. Attinger EO: Flow patterns and vascular geometry. *In* Pulsatile Blood Flow. New York, McGraw-Hill, 1964, pp 179–200.
6. Attinger EO, Sugawara H, Navarro A, et al: Pressure flow relations in dog arteries. Circ Res 19:230, 1966.
7. Azuma T, Oka S: Mechanical equilibrium of blood vessel walls. Jpn J Physiol 21:1310, 1971.
8. Baird RN, Bird DR, Clifford PC, et al: Upstream stenosis, its diagnosis by Doppler signals from the femoral artery. Arch Surg 115:1316, 1980.
9. Bassiouny HS, White S, Glagov S, et al: Anastomotic intimal hyperplasia: Mechanical injury or flow-induced? J Vasc Surg 15:708, 1992.
10. Beaconsfield PA: A. Effect of exercise on muscle blood flow in normal and sympathectomized limbs. B. Collateral circulation before and after sympathectomy. Ann Surg 140:786, 1954.
11. Beiser GD, Zelis R, Epstein SE, et al: The role of skin and muscle resistance vessels in reflexes mediated by the baroreceptor system. J Clin Invest 49:225, 1970.
12. Bergel DH: The static elastic properties of the arterial wall. J Physiol 156:445, 1961.
13. Bergel DH: The dynamic elastic properties of the arterial wall. J Physiol 156:458, 1961.
14. Berguer R, Higgins RF, Reddy DJ: Intimal hyperplasia: An experimental study. Arch Surg 115:332, 1980.
15. Berguer R, Hwang NHC: Critical arterial stenosis. A theoretical and experimental solution. Ann Surg 180:39, 1974.
16. Bernstein EF, Fischer JC, Varco RL: Is excision the optimum treatment for all abdominal aortic aneurysms? Surgery 61:83, 1967.
17. Brice JG, Dowsett DJ, Lowe RD: Hemodynamic effects of carotid artery stenosis. Br Med J 2:1363, 1964.
18. Burch GE, Winsor T: The phlebomanometer. A new apparatus for direct measurement of venous pressure in large and small veins. JAMA 123:91, 1943.
19. Burton AC: Physiology and Biophysics of the Circulation. 2nd ed. Chicago, Year Book Medical Publishers, 1972.
20. Busuttil RW, Abou-Zamzam AM, Machleder HI: Collagenase activity of the human aorta: Comparison of patients with and without abdominal aortic aneurysms. Arch Surg 115:1373, 1980.
21. Buxton B, Lambert RP, Pitt TTE: The significance of vein wall thickness and diameter in relation to the patency of femoropopliteal saphenous vein bypass grafts. Surgery 87:425, 1980.
22. Byar D, Fiddian RV, Quereau M, et al: The fallacy of applying Poiseuille equation to segmented arterial stenosis. Am Heart J 70:216, 1965.
23. Carter SA: Clinical measurement of systolic pressures in limbs with arterial occlusive disease. JAMA 207:1869, 1969.
24. Carter SA: Response of ankle systolic pressure to leg exercise in mild or questionable arterial disease. N Engl J Med 287:578, 1972.
25. Cobb LA, Smith PH, Lwai S, et al: External iliac vein flow: Its response to exercise and relation to lactate production. J Appl Physiol 26:606, 1969.
26. Coffman JD, Mannick JA: A simple objective test for arteriosclerosis obliterans. N Engl J Med 273:1297, 1965.
27. Coffman JD, Mannick JA: Failure of vasodilator drugs in arteriosclerosis obliterans. Ann Intern Med 76:35, 1972.
28. Conrad MC, Anderson JL III, Garrett JB Jr: Chronic collateral growth after femoral artery occlusion in the dog. J Appl Physiol 31:550, 1971.
29. Conrad MC, Green HD: Hemodynamics of large and small vessels in peripheral vascular disease. Circulation 29:847, 1964.
30. Cousins MJ, Wright CJ: Graft, muscle, skin blood flow after epidural block in vascular surgical procedures. Surg Gynecol Obstet 133:59, 1971.
31. Cranley JJ: Ischemic rest pain. Arch Surg 98:187, 1969.
32. Crawshaw HM, Quist WC, Sarrallach E, et al: Flow disturbance at the distal end-to-side anastomosis. Effect of patency of the proximal outflow segment and angle of anastomosis. Arch Surg 115:1280, 1980.
33. Cronenwett JL, Lindenaur SM: Hemodynamic effects of sympathectomy in ischemic canine hind limbs. Surgery 87:417, 1980.
34. Cronenwett JL, Zelenock GB, Whitehouse WM Jr, et al: The effect of sympathetic innervation on canine muscle and skin blood flow. Arch Surg 118:420, 1983.
35. Daily JW, Harleman DRF: Fluid Dynamics. Reading, MA, Addison-Wesley, 1966.
36. Darling RC, Raines JK, Brener BJ, et al: Quantitative segmental pulse and volume recorder: A clinical tool. Surgery 72:873, 1973.
37. Daugherty HI, Franzini JB: Steady flow of incompressible fluids in pipes. *In* Fluid Mechanics With Engineering Applications. 6th ed. New York, McGraw-Hill, 1965, pp 191–245.
38. DeWeese JA: Pedal pulses disappearing with exercise: A test for intermittent claudication. N Engl J Med 262:1214, 1960.
39. DeWeese JA, Van deBerg L, May AG, et al: Stenoses of arteries of the lower extremity. Arch Surg 89:806, 1964.
40. Dobrin PB: Mechanics of normal and diseased blood vessels. Ann Vasc Surg 2:283, 1988.
41. Dobrin PB, Baker WH, Gley WC: Elastolytic and collagenolytic studies of arteries. Implications for the mechanical properties of aneurysms. Arch Surg 119:405, 1984.

42. Dobrin PB, Rovick AA: Influence of vascular smooth muscle on contractile mechanics and elasticity of arteries. Am J Physiol 217:1644, 1969.
43. Dormandy JA: Significance of hemorrheology in the management of the ischemic limb. World J Surg 7:319, 1983.
44. Dornhorst AC, Sharpey-Schafer, EP: Collateral resistance in limbs with arterial obstruction: Spontaneous changes and effects of sympathectomy. Clin Sci 10:371, 1951.
45. Dundas P, Hillestad LK: Profunda revascularization. The early postoperative effect upon calf blood flow. Scand J Thorac Cardiovasc Surg 5:275, 1971.
46. Edholm OG, Howarth S, Sharpey-Schafer EP: Resting blood flow and blood pressure in limbs with arterial obstruction. Clin Sci 10:361, 1951.
47. Edwards WS, Holdefer WF, Mohtashemi M: The importance of proper caliber of lumen in femoral-politeal artery reconstruction. Surg Gynecol Obstet 122:37, 1966.
48. Ehrenfeld WK, Harris JD, Wylie EJ: Vascular ''steal'' phenomenon, an experimental study. Am J Surg 116:192, 1968.
49. Evans DH, Barrie WW, Asher MJ, et al: The relationship between ultrasonic pulsatility index and proximal arterial stenosis in a canine model. Circ Res 46:470, 1980.
50. Farrar DJ, Malindzak GS Jr, Johnson G Jr: Large vessel impedance in peripheral atherosclerosis. Circulation 56(Suppl 2):171, 1977.
51. Feinberg RL, Gregory RT, Wheeler JR, et al: The ischemic window: A method for the objective quantitation of the training effect in exercise therapy for intermittent claudication. J Vasc Surg 16:244, 1992.
52. Fiddian RV, Byar D, Edwards EA: Factors affecting flow through a stenosed vessel. Arch Surg 88:105, 1964.
53. Flanigan DP, Tullis JP, Streeter VL, et al: Multiple subcritical arterial stenoses: Effect on poststenotic pressure and flow. Ann Surg 186:663, 1977.
54. Folse JR: Application of the sudden injection dye dilution principle to the study of the femoral circulation. Surg Gynecol Obstet 120:1194, 1965.
55. Folse R: Alterations in femoral blood flow and resistance during rhythmic exercise and sustained muscular contractions in patients with arteriosclerosis. Surg Gynecol Obstet 121:767, 1965.
56. Foster JH, Bolasny BL, Gobbel WG Jr, et al: Comparative study of elective resection and expectant treatment of abdominal aortic aneurysms. Surg Gynecol Obstet 129:1, 1969.
57. Fronek A, Johansen KH, Dilley RB, et al: Non-invasive physiologic tests in the diagnosis and characterization of peripheral arterial occlusive disease. Am J Surg 126:205, 1973.
58. Gauer OH, Thron HL: Postural changes in the circulation. *In* Hamilton WF, Dow P (eds): Handbook of Physiology. Sect. 2, Circulation. Vol. III. Washington, DC, American Physiological Society, 1965, pp 2409–2439.
59. Glagov S, Weisenberg E, Zarins CK, et al: Compensatory enlargement of human atherosclerotic coronary arteries. N Engl J Med 316:1371, 1987.
60. Gosling RG, Dunbar G, King DH, et al: The quantitative analysis of occlusive peripheral arterial disease by a nonintrusive ultrasonic technique. Angiology 22:52, 1971.
61. Gosling RG, King DH: Continuous wave ultrasound as an alternative and complement to x-rays in vascular examination. *In* Reneman RS (ed): Cardiovascular Applications of Ultrasound. Amsterdam, North-Holland Publishing Co, 1974, pp 266–282.
62. Griffith TM, Lewis MJ, Newby AC, Henderson AH: Endothelium-derived relaxing factor. J Am Coll Cardiol 12:797, 1988.
63. Guyton AC: Venous return. *In* Hamilton WF, Dow P (eds): Handbook of Physiology. Sect. 2, Circulation. Vol. II. Washington, DC, American Physiological Society, 1963, pp 1099–1133.
64. Hillestad LK: The peripheral blood flow in intermittent claudication. V. Plethysmographic studies. The significance of the calf blood flow at rest and in response to timed arrest of the circulation. Acta Med Scand 174:23, 1963.
65. Hillestad LK: The peripheral blood flow in intermittent claudication. VI. Plethysmographic studies. The blood flow response to exercise with arrested and free circulation. Acta Med Scand 174:671, 1963.
66. Hoffman DC, Jepson RP: Muscle blood flow and sympathectomy. Surg Gynecol Obstet 127:12, 1968.
67. Hokanson DE, Strandness DE Jr: Stress-strain characteristics of various arterial grafts. Surg Gynecol Obstet 127:57, 1968.
68. Holman E: Problems in the dynamics of blood flow. I. Conditions controlling collateral circulation in the presence of an arteriovenous fistula and following ligation of an artery. Surgery 26:880, 1949.
69. Hopkins RW: Presidential address: Energy, poise, and resilience—Daniel Bernoulli, Thomas Young, J. L. M. Poiseuille, and F. A. Simeone. J Vasc Surg 13:777, 1991.
70. Ingebrigtsen R, Leraand S: Dilatation of a medium-sized artery immediately after local changes of blood pressure and flow as measured by ultrasonic technique. Acta Physiol Scand 79:552, 1970.
71. Jager KA, Phillips DJ, Martin RL, et al: Noninvasive mapping of lower limb arterial lesions. Ultrasound Med Biol 11:515, 1985.
72. James IM, Millar RA, Purves MY: Observations on the extrinsic neural control of cerebral blood flow in the baboon. Cir Res 25:77, 1969.
73. John HT, Warren R: The stimulus to collateral circulation. Surgery 49:14, 1961.
74. Johnson EC, Voyles WF, Atterbom HA, et al: Effects of exercise training on common femoral artery blood flow in patients with intermittent claudication. Circulation 80:III59, 1989.
75. Johnson PC: Review of previous studies and current theories of autoregulation. Circ Res 14:15, 1964.
76. Johnston KW, Maruzzo BC, Cobbold RSC: Errors and artifacts of Doppler flowmeters and their solution. Arch Surg 112:1335, 1977.
77. Johnston KW, Maruzzo BC, Cobbold RSC: Doppler methods for quantitative measurement and localization of peripheral arterial occlusive disease by analysis of the blood velocity waveform. Ultrasound Med Biol 4:209, 1978.
78. Jones RD, Berne RM: Intrinsic regulation of skeletal muscle blood flow. Circ Res 14:126, 1964.
79. Kamiya A, Tagowa T: Adaptive regulation of wall shear stress to flow change in the canine carotid artery. Am J Physiol 239:H14, 1980.
80. Karayannacos PE, Talukder N, Nerem RM, et al: The role of multiple noncritical arterial stenoses in the pathogenesis of ischemia. J Thorac Cardiovasc Surg 73:458, 1977.
81. Keenan RL, Rodbard S: Competition between collateral vessels. Cardiovasc Res 7:670, 1973.
82. Keitzer WF, Fry WJ, Kraft RO, et al: Hemodynamic mechanism for pulse changes seen in occlusive vascular disease. Surgery 57:163, 1965.
83. Kindt GW, Youmans JR: The effect of stricture length on critical arterial stenosis. Surg Gynecol Obstet 128:729, 1969.
84. Kinley CE, Marble AE: Compliance: A continuing problem with vascular grafts. J Cardiovas Surg 21:163, 1980.
85. Kinley CE, Paasche PE, MacDonald AS, et al: Stress at vascular anastomosis in relation to host artery: Synthetic graft diameter. Surgery 75:28, 1974.
86. Kjellmer I: On the competition between metabolic vasodilatation and neurogenic vasoconstriction in skeletal muscle. Acta Physiol Scand 63:450, 1965.
87. Korner PI: Control of blood flow to special vascular areas: Brain, kidney, muscle, skin, liver and intestine. *In* Guyton AC, Jones CE (eds): MTP International Review of Science, Physiology. Series 1. Vol. 1. Cardiovascular Physiology. London, Butterworths, 1974, pp 123–162.
88. Ku DN, Giddens DP, Zarins CK, Glagov S: Pulsatile flow and atherosclerosis in the human carotid bifurcation. Positive correlation between plaque location and low and oscillating shear stress. Arteriosclerosis 5:293, 1985.
89. Langille BL, O'Donnell F: Reductions in arterial diameter produced by chronic decreases in blood flow are endothelium-dependent. Science 231:405, 1986.
90. Larsen OA, Lassen NA: Medical treatment of occlusive arterial disease of the legs. Walking exercise and medically induced hypertension. Angiologica 6:288, 1969.
91. Lassen NA: Cerebral blood flow and oxygen consumption in man. Physiol Rev 39:183, 1959.
92. Lassen NA, Kampp M: Calf muscle blood flow during walking studied by the Xe^{133} method in normals and in patients with intermittent claudication. Scand J Clin Lab Invest 17:447, 1965.
93. Lassen NA, Larsen OA, Sørensen AWS, et al: Conservative treatment of gangrene using mineral corticoid–induced moderate hypertension. Lancet 1:606, 1968.
94. Lassen NA, Lindberg IF, Dahn I: Validity of the $xenon^{133}$ method for measurement of muscle blood flow evaluated by simultaneous

venous occlusion plethysmography: Observations in the calf of normal man and in patients with occlusive vascular disease. Circ Res 16:287, 1965.

95. LeVeen HH, Moon I, Ahmed N, et al: Lowering blood viscosity to overcome vascular resistance. Surg Gynecol Obstet 150:139, 1980.
96. Lewis JD, Papathanaiou C, Yao ST, et al: Simultaneous flow and pressure measurements in intermittent claudication. Br J Surg 59:418, 1972.
97. Lewis P, Psaila JV, Morgan RH, et al: Common femoral artery volume flow in peripheral vascular disease. Br J Surg 77:183, 1990.
98. Lewis T, Pickering GW, Rothschild P: Observations upon muscular pain in intermittent claudication. Heart 15:359, 1931.
99. Ling SC, Atabek HB, Letzing WG, et al: Non-linear analysis of aortic flow in living dogs. Circ Res 33:198, 1973.
100. LoGerfo FW, Quist WC, Nowak MD, et al: Downstream anastomotic hyperplasia. A mechanism of failure of Dacron arterial grafts. Ann Surg 197:479, 1983.
101. LoGerfo FW, Soncrant T, Teel T, et al: Boundary layer separation in models of side-to-end arterial anastomoses. Arch Surg 114:1369, 1979.
102. Longland CJ: The collateral circulation of the limb. Ann R Coll Surg Engl 13:161, 1953.
103. Lorentsen E, Hoel BL, Hol R: Evaluation of the functional importance of atherosclerotic obliterations in the aorto-iliac artery by pressure/flow measurements. Acta Med Scand 191:399, 1972.
104. Ludbrook J: Collateral artery resistance in the human lower limb. J Surg Res 6:423, 1966.
105. Lye CR, Sumner DS, Strandness DE Jr: Hemodynamics of the retrograde cross-pubic anastomosis. Surg Forum 26:298, 1975.
106. Lye CR, Sumner DS, Strandness DE Jr: The transcutaneous measurement of the elastic properties of the human saphenous vein femoropopliteal bypass graft. Surg Gynecol Obstet 141:891, 1975.
107. Malcome AD, Roach MR: Flow disturbances at the apex and lateral angles of a variety of bifurcation models and their role in the development and manifestations of arterial disease. Stroke 10:335, 1979.
108. Mannick JA, Jackson BT: Hemodynamics of arterial surgery in atherosclerotic limbs. I. Direct measurement of blood flow before and after vein grafts. Surgery 59:713, 1966.
109. Martin P, Frawley JE, Barabas AP, et al: On the surgery of atherosclerosis of the profunda femoris artery. Surgery 71:182, 1972.
110. May AG, DeWeese JA, Rob CA: Hemodynamic effects of arterial stenosis. Surgery 53:513, 1963.
111. May AG, Van deBerg L, DeWeese JA, et al: Critical arterial stenosis. Surgery 54:250, 1963.
112. McDonald DA: Blood Flow in Arteries. 2nd ed. Baltimore, Williams & Wilkins Co, 1974.
113. McMillan DE: Blood flow and the localization of atherosclerotic plaques. Stroke 16:582, 1985.
114. Mehigan DG, Fitzpatrick B, Browne HI, Bouchier-Hayes DJ: Is compliance mismatch the major cause of anastomotic arterial aneurysms? J Cardiovasc Surg 26:147, 1985.
115. Melkumyants AM, Balashov SA, Veselova ES, Khayutin VM: Continuous control of the lumen of feline conduit arteries by blood flow rate. Cardiovasc Res 21:863, 1987.
116. Milnor WR: Pulsatile blood flow. N Engl J Med 287:27, 1972.
117. Moore WS, Hall AD: Unrecognized aortoiliac stenosis. A physiologic approach to the diagnosis. Arch Surg 103:633, 1971.
118. Moore WS, Malone JM: Effect of flow rate and vessel calibre on critical arterial stenosis. J Surg Res 26:1, 1979.
119. Moore WS, Sydorak GR, Newcomb L, et al: Blood pressure gradient to estimate flow changes with progressive arterial stenosis. Surg Forum 24:248, 1973.
120. Morris GC Jr, Edwards W, Cooley DA, et al: Surgical importance of profunda femoris artery. Arch Surg 82:32, 1961.
121. Motomiya M, Karino T: Flow patterns in the human carotid artery bifurcation. Stroke 15:50, 1984.
122. Mozersky DJ, Sumner DS, Hokanson DE, et al: Transcutaneous measurement of the elastic properties of the human femoral artery. Circulation 46:948, 1972.
123. Mundth ED, Darling RC, Moran JM, et al: Quantitative correlation of distal arterial outflow and patency of femoropopliteal reversed saphenous vein grafts with intraoperative flow and pressure measurements. Surgery 65:197, 1969.
124. Newman DL, Gosling RG, Bowden NLR, et al: Pressure amplitude increase on unmatching the aorto-iliac junction of the dog. Cardiovasc Res 7:6, 1973.
125. Nichols WK, Stanton M, Silver D, et al: Anastomotic aneurysms following lower extremity revascularization. Surgery 88:366, 1980.
126. Nicolaides AN, Gordon-Smith DC, Dayandas J, et al: The value of Doppler blood velocity tracings in the detection of aortoiliac disease in patients with intermittent claudication. Surgery 80:774, 1976.
127. Ojha M, Cobbold RSC, Johnston KW, Hummel RL: Pulsatile flow through constricted tubes: An experimental investigation using photochromic tracer methods. J Fluid Mech 203:173, 1989.
128. Ojha M, Ethier CR, Johnston KW, Cobbold RSC: Steady and pulsatile flow fields in an end-to-side arterial anastomosis model. J Vasc Surg 12:747, 1990.
129. Ojha M, Johnston KW, Cobbold RSC: Evidence of a possible link between poststenotic dilation and wall shear stress. J Vasc Surg 11:127, 1990.
130. Okadone K, Yukizane T, Mii S, Sugimachi K: Ultrastructural evidence of the effects of shear stress variation on intimal thickening in dogs with arterially transplanted autologous grafts. J Cardiovasc Surg 31:719, 1990.
131. O'Rourke MF: Steady and pulsatile energy losses in the systemic circulation under normal conditions and in simulated arterial disease. Cardiovasc Res 1:313, 1967.
132. Ouriel K, Donayre C, Shortell CK, et al: The hemodynamics of thrombus formation in arteries. J Vasc Surg 14:757, 1991.
133. Paasche PE, Kinley CE, Dolan FG, et al: Consideration of suture line stresses in the selection of synthetic grafts for implantation. J Biomech 6:253, 1973.
134. Pedersen EM, Hjortdal JØ, Hjortdal VE, et al: Three-dimensional visualization of velocity profiles in the porcine abdominal aortic trifurcation. J Vasc Surg 15:194, 1992.
135. Pentecost BL: The effect of exercise on the external iliac vein blood flow and local oxygen consumption in normal subjects, and in those with occlusive arterial disease. Clin Sci 27:437, 1964.
136. Peterson LH: Physical factors which influence vascular caliber and blood flow. Circ Res 18 and 19(Suppl 1):3, 1966.
137. Peterson LH, Jensen RE, Parnell J: Mechanical properties of arteries in vivo. Circ Res 8:622, 1960.
138. Porter JM, Cutler BS, Lee BY, et al: Pentoxifylline efficacy in the treatment of intermittent claudication. Am Heart J 104:66, 1982.
139. Reagan TR, Miller CW, Strandness DE Jr: Transcutaneous measurement of femoral artery flow. J Surg Res 11:477, 1971.
140. Remensnyder JP, Mitchell JH, Sarnoff SJ: Functional sympatholysis during muscular activity. Circ Res 11:370, 1962.
141. Remington JW, Wood EH: Formation of peripheral pulse contour in man. J Appl Physiol 9:433, 1956.
142. Rijsterborgh H, Roelandt J: Doppler assessment of aortic stenosis: Bernoulli revisited. Ultrasound Med Biol 13:241, 1987.
143. Rittenhouse EA, Maxiner W, Burr JW, et al: Directional arterial flow velocity: A sensitive index of changes in peripheral vascular resistance. Surgery 79:359, 1976.
144. Rittgers SE, Shu MCS: Doppler color-flow images from a stenosed arterial model: Interpretation of flow patterns. J Vasc Surg 12:511, 1990.
145. Roederer GO, Langlois YE, Chan AW, et al: Ultrasonic duplex scanning of extracranial carotid arteries: Improved accuracy using new features from the common carotid artery. J Cardiovasc Ultrasonography 1:373, 1982.
146. Rosenthal SL, Guyton AC: Hemodynamics of collateral vasodilatation following femoral artery occlusion in anesthetized dogs. Circ Res 23:239, 1968.
147. Rutherford RB, Valenta J: Extremity blood flow and distribution: The effects of arterial occlusion, sympathectomy, and exercise. Surgery 69:332, 1971.
148. Sanders RJ, Kempczinski RF, Hammond W, et al: The significance of graft diameter. Surgery 88:856, 1980.
149. Scheffler A, Rieger H: A comparative analysis of transcutaneous oximetry ($tcPo_2$) during oxygen inhalation and leg dependency in severe peripheral arterial occlusive disease. J Vasc Surg 16:218, 1992.
150. Schneider JR, Zwolak RM, Walsh DB, et al: Lack of diameter effect on short-term patency of size-matched Dacron aortofemoral grafts. J Vasc Surg 13:785, 1991.
151. Schultz DL: Pressure and flow in large arteries. *In* Bergel DH (ed): Cardiovascular Fluid Dynamics. Vol. I. New York, Academic Press, 1972, pp 287–314.
152. Schultz RD, Hokanson DE, Strandness DE Jr: Pressure-flow relations of the end-side anastomosis. Surgery 62:319, 1967.

153. Segadal L, Matre K: Blood velocity distribution in the human ascending aorta. Circulation 76:90, 1987.
154. Sharefkin JB, Diamond SL, Eskin SG, et al: Fluid flow decreases preproendothelin mRNA levels and suppresses endothelin-1 peptide release in cultured human endothelial cells. J Vasc Surg 14:1, 1991.
155. Sharp WV, Donovan DL, Teague PC, Mosteller RD: Arterial occlusive disease: A function of vessel bifurcation angle. Surgery 91:680, 1982.
156. Shepherd JT: The blood flow through the calf after exercise in subjects with arteriosclerosis and claudication. Clin Sci 9:49, 1950.
157. Shepherd JT: Physiology of the Circulation in Human Limbs in Health and Disease. Philadelphia, WB Saunders, 1963.
158. Skidmore R, Woodcock JP: Physiological interpretation of Doppler-shift waveforms—I. Theoretical considerations. Ultrasound Med Biol 6:7, 1980.
159. Skidmore R, Woodcock JP: Physiological interpretation of Doppler-shift waveforms—II. Validation of the Laplace transform method for characterization of the common femoral blood-velocity/time waveform. Ultrasound Med Biol 6:219, 1980.
160. Skidmore R, Woodcock JP, Wells PNT, et al: Physiological interpretation of Doppler-shift waveforms—III. Clinical results. Ultrasound Med Biol 6:227, 1980.
161. Skinner JS, Strandness DE Jr: Exercise and intermittent claudication. I. Effect of repetition and intensity of exercise. Circulation 36:15, 1967.
162. Skinner JS, Strandness DE Jr: Exercise and intermittent claudication. II. Effect of physical training. Circulation 36:23, 1967.
163. Snell ES, Eastcott HHG, Hamilton M: Circulation in lower limb before and after reconstruction of obstructed main artery. Lancet 1:242, 1960.
164. Sottiurai VS, Sue SL, Breaux JR, Smith LM: Adaptability of endothelial orientation to blood flow dynamics—A morphologic analysis. Eur J Vasc Surg 3:145, 1989.
165. Stahler C, Strandness DE Jr: Ankle blood pressure response to gradual treadmill exercise. Angiology 18:237, 1967.
166. Strandell T, Wahren J: Circulation in the calf at rest, after arterial occlusion and after exercise in normal subjects and in patients with intermittent claudication. Acta Med Scand 173:99, 1963.
167. Strandness DE Jr: Abnormal exercise response after successful reconstructive arterial surgery. Surgery 59:325, 1966.
168. Strandness DE Jr: Functional results after revascularization of the profunda femoris artery. Am J Surg 119:240, 1970.
169. Strandness DE Jr, Bell JW: An evaluation of the hemodynamic response of the claudicating extremity to exercise. Surg Gynecol Obstet 119:1237, 1964.
170. Strandness DE Jr, Bell JW: Critical evaluation of the results of lumbar sympathectomy. Ann Surg 160:1021, 1964.
171. Strandness DE Jr, Bell JW: Peripheral vascular disease. Diagnosis and objective evaluation using a mercury strain gauge. Ann Surg 161(Suppl):1, 1965.
172. Strandness DE Jr, Schultz RD, Sumner DS, et al: Ultrasonic flow detection—A useful technique in the evaluation of peripheral vascular disease. Am J Surg 113:311, 1967.
173. Strandness DE Jr, Sumner DS: Hemodynamics for Surgeons. New York, Grune & Stratton, 1975.
174. Streeter VC, Keitzer WF, Bohr DF: Pulsatile pressure and flow through distensible vessels. Circ Res 13:3, 1963.
175. Stromberg DD, Weiderhielm CA: Viscoelastic description of a collagenous tissue in simple elongation. J Appl Physiol 26:857, 1969.
176. Sumner DS, Strandness DE Jr: The relationship between calf blood flow and ankle blood pressure in patients with intermittent claudication. Surgery 65:763, 1969.
177. Sumner DS, Strandness DE Jr: The effect of exercise on resistance to blood flow in limbs with an occluded superficial femoral artery. Vasc Surg 4:229, 1970.
178. Sumner DS, Strandness DE Jr: The hemodynamics of the femorofemoral shunt. Surg Gynecol Obstet 134:629, 1972.
179. Sumner DS, Hokanson DE, Strandness DE Jr: Arterial walls before and after endarterectomy, stress-strain characteristics and collagen-elastic content. Arch Surg 99:606, 1969.
180. Sumner DS, Hokanson DE, Strandness DE Jr: Stress-strain characteristics and collagen-elastic content of abdominal aortic aneurysms. Surg Gynecol Obstet 130:459, 1970.
181. Sydorak GR, Moore WS, Newcomb L, et al: Effect of increasing flow rates and arterial caliber on critical arterial stenoses. Surg Forum 23:243, 1972.
182. Van deBerg L, DeWeese JA, Rob CG: The effect of arterial stenosis and sympathectomy on blood flow and the ergogram. Ann Surg 159:623, 1964.
183. Vieli A, Moser U, Maier S, et al: Velocity profiles in the normal human abdominal aorta: A comparison between ultrasound and magnetic resonance data. Ultrasound Biol Med 15:113, 1989.
184. Vonruden WJ, Blaisdell FW, Hall AD et al: Multiple arterial stenosis: Effect on blood flow. Arch Surg 89:307, 1964.
185. Wahren J, Jorfeldt L: Determinations of leg blood flow during exercise in man: An indicator-dilution technique based on femoral venous dye infusion. Clin Sci Mol Med 45:135, 1973.
186. Walden R, L'Italien GJ, Megerman J, et al: Matched elastic properties and successful arterial grafting. Arch Surg 115:1166, 1980.
187. Walker JR, Guyton AC: Influence of blood oxygen saturation on pressure-flow curve of dog hind leg. Am J Physiol 212:506, 1967.
188. Weissenhofer W, Schenk WG Jr: Hemodynamic response to vasodilation and exercise in "critical" arterial stenosis. Arch Surg 108:712, 1974.
189. Wengerter KR, Veith FJ, Gupta SK, et al: Influence of vein size (diameter) on infrapopliteal reversed vein graft patency. J Vasc Surg 11:525, 1990.
190. Wesolowski SA, Martinez A, Domingo RT, et al: Indications for aortofemoral arterial reconstruction: A study of borderline risk patients. Surgery 60:288, 1966.
191. Westerhof N, Sipkema P, Van Den Bos GC, et al: Forward and backward waves in the arterial system. Cardiovasc Res 6:648, 1972.
192. Winblad JN, Reemtsma K, Vernhet JL, et al: Etiologic mechanisms in the development of collateral circulation. Surgery 45:105, 1959.
193. Winsor T: Influence of arterial disease on the systolic blood pressure gradients of the extremity. Am J Med Sci 220:117, 1950.
194. Wolf EA Jr, Sumner DS, Strandness DE Jr: Correlation between nutritive blood flow and pressure in limbs of patients with intermittent claudication. Surg Forum 23:238, 1972.
195. Wolfe JHN, Waller DG, Chapman MB, et al: The effect of hemodilution upon patients with intermittent claudication. Surg Gynecol Obstet 160:347, 1985.
196. Wong PKC, Johnston KW, Ethier CR, Cobbold RSC: Computer simulation of blood flow patterns in arteries of various geometries. J Vasc Surg 14:658, 1991.
197. Woodcock JP, Gosling RG, Fitzgerald DE: A new non-invasive technique for assessment of superficial femoral artery obstruction. Br J Surg 59:226, 1972.
198. Wyatt MG, Muir RM, Tennant WG, et al: Impedance analysis to identify the at risk femorodistal graft. J Vasc Surg 13:284, 1991.
199. Yao ST: Haemodynamic studies in peripheral arterial disease. Br J Surg 57:761, 1970.
200. Yao ST, Hobbs JT, Irvine WT: Pulse examination by an ultrasonic method. Br Med J 4:555, 1968.
201. Yao ST, Hobbs JT, Irvine WT: Ankle systolic pressure measurements in arterial disease affecting the lower extremities. Br J Surg 56:676, 1969.
202. Yellin EL: Laminar-turbulent transition process in pulsation flow. Circ Res 19:791, 1966.
203. Young DF, Tsai FY: Flow characteristics in models of arterial stenoses. I. Steady flow. J Biomech 6:395, 1973.
204. Young DF, Tsai FY: Flow characteristics of models of arterial stenosis. II. Unsteady flow. J Biomech 6:547, 1973.
205. Zarins CK, Giddens DP, Bharadvaj BK, et al: Carotid bifurcation atherosclerosis. Quantitative correlation of plaque localization with flow velocity profiles and wall shear stress. Circ Res 53:502, 1983.
206. Zarins CK, Xu C, Glagov S: Aneurysmal enlargement of the aorta during regression of experimental atherosclerosis. J Vasc Surg 15:90, 1992.
207. Zarins CK, Zatina MA, Giddens DP, et al: Shear stress regulation of artery lumen diameter in experimental atherogenesis. J Vasc Surg 5:413, 1987.
208. Zarins CK, Glagov S, Vesselinovitch D, Wissler RW: Aneurysm formation in experimental atherosclerosis: Relationship to plaque evolution. J Vasc Surg 12:246, 1990.
209. Zellis R, Mason DT, Braunwald E, et al: Effects of hyperlipoproteinemias and their treatment on the peripheral circulation. J Clin Invest 49:1007, 1970.
210. Zwiebel WJ, Zagzebski JA, Crummy AB, et al: Correlation of peak Doppler frequency with lumen narrowing in carotid stenosis. Stroke 13:386, 1982.

4

The Vascular Laboratory

David S. Sumner, M.D., and Brian L. Thiele, M.D.

• • •

OBJECTIVE DIAGNOSTIC TECHNIQUES: ROLE OF THE VASCULAR LABORATORY

The clinical vascular laboratory is largely a phenomenon of the past two decades. Although many of the basic concepts on which peripheral vascular testing is based were formulated before 1960, only sporadic attempts were made to apply these concepts clinically. Technological advances during the 1960s provided, for the first time, simple accurate methods for measuring blood flow and blood pressure noninvasively. It was only natural that investigators in a few scattered laboratories should combine the new technology with the old physiologic principles to evaluate peripheral vascular disease. The 1970s were marked by the proliferation of laboratories, the development of new and improved testing procedures, the expansion into new fields of investigation, and the emergence of an immense body of literature. This process of evolution continued into the 1980s. With the passage of time, some instruments and methods have become entrenched in the armamentarium of the vascular laboratory; others have been discarded, either because they proved to be inaccurate or because better techniques were introduced—these changes are inevitable and will continue.[106]

Ideally, all methods used for physiologic testing of arterial disease should be simple, reliable, and reproducible; capable of intrinsic standardization; easily employed by paramedical personnel; relatively rapid to perform; adaptable to current recording equipment; and applicable to studies during and after exercise.[98] Although a number of well-established physiologic tests that more or less conform to these ideals are available for the objective assessment of arterial disease, some of the modern, more technologically sophisticated methods do not fulfill all of the criteria—especially those related to simplicity. Skilled personnel and careful attention to detail are essential; but because these new modalities either supply unique information or are substantially more accurate than other less demanding methods, the extra effort required for mastering their operation is justified. Most of the techniques and instruments described in this chapter are in widespread use; however, some are employed by only a few laboratories; and others are in the process of being evaluated. All are designed to elucidate those aspects of the pathophysiology of arterial disease that are outlined in Chapter 3. Chapter 5 discusses their application.

Basic Noninvasive Methods

The only parameters that can be measured directly (or almost directly) by noninvasive tests include volume change, blood flow velocity, temperature, and oxygen tension. All others must be derived from these basic measurements.

Plethysmography

Plethysmography was one of the earliest methods devised for measuring blood flow in the extremities, having first been employed for this purpose around the turn of the century.[41] Indeed, much of our basic knowledge of vascular physiology and pathophysiology has been derived from plethysmographic studies. Thanks to the contributions of modern electronics, the simple oscillometers that were popular several decades ago have been replaced by more sophisticated and sensitive instruments, which are now used in clinical vascular laboratories throughout the world.[108]

Although there are a variety of plethysmographs, all perform essentially the same function: the measurement of volume change. With the exception of the lung, transient changes in the volume of most parts of the body are related to their content of blood; and plethysmography is used to measure these changes. Applications vary according to the type of information being sought.

Pulse Plethysmography

With each beat of the left ventricle, the part being examined expands when the arterial inflow exceeds the venous outflow and contracts when the opposite occurs. Because vascular volume is a function of the interaction between intraluminal pressure and the elasticity of the vascular wall, the recorded plethysmographic pulse closely resembles the contour of the arterial pressure pulse (Fig. 4–1). Digital, penile, and segmental limb plethysmography all depend on this technique.[20, 101]

Volume Plethysmography

Pulsatile information is superimposed on less rapid volume changes that result from dilatation or contraction of the arteries and veins.[105] Usually, these volume changes reflect variations in sympathetic activity, venous pressure, and hydrostatic pressure and far exceed those attributed to

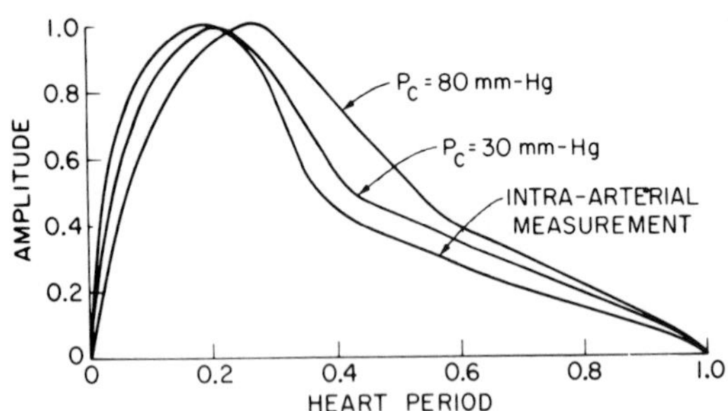

FIGURE 4–1. Comparison of pressure contours obtained with the pulse volume recorder and direct cannulation of the common femoral artery. (From Darling RC, Raines JK, Brener BJ, et al: Quantitative segmental pulse volume recorder: A clinical tool. Surgery 72:873, 1972.)

the arterial pulse (Fig. 4–2). Larger and even more gradual changes in limb volume occur in response to expansion or contraction of the interstitial fluid space, but these changes are seldom measured plethysmographically.

Venous Occlusion Plethysmography

Mean blood flow can be measured in any body part by recording the initial rate at which the volume increases when the venous outflow is suddenly interrupted (Fig. 4–3). In practice, this is usually accomplished by inflating a pneumatic cuff placed around the part proximal to the site of the plethysmographic sensor.[108] (The occluding pressure must exceed venous pressure but be well below arterial pressure in order not to interfere with inflow.) Although this technique is of value to the vascular physiologist, it is too cumbersome to be used in the routine clinical assessment of arterial disease. Moreover, in the resting patient, mean blood flow seldom discriminates between no arterial obstruction and mild or moderate obstruction. The technique, however, has found an important place in the evaluation of venous disease (see Chapters 131 and 133).

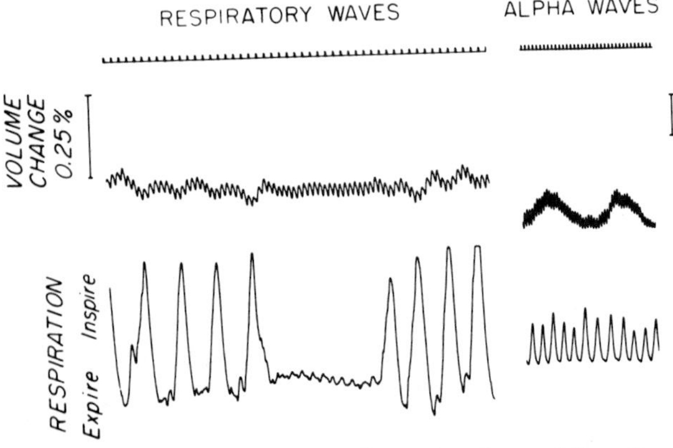

FIGURE 4–2. Plethysmographic tracing of normal fingertip pulse showing relatively large volume changes coinciding with changes in sympathetic activity (respiratory waves and alpha waves). Superimposed are smaller pulses representing the arrival of pressure waves generated by left ventricular contraction. (From Strandness DE Jr, Sumner DS: Hemodynamics for Surgeons. New York, Grune & Stratton, 1975, pp 209–289.)

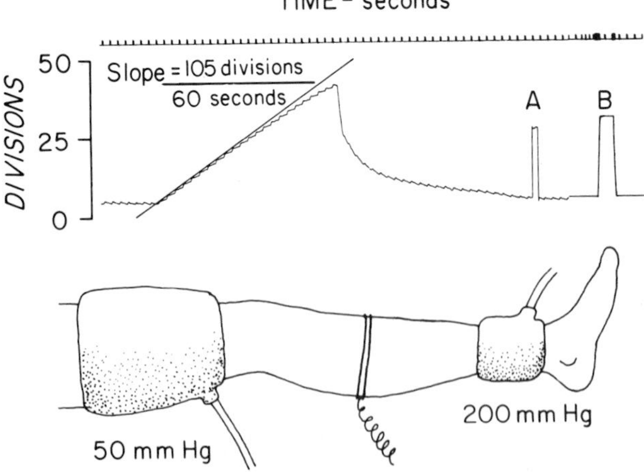

FIGURE 4–3. Technique of measuring blood flow with venous occlusion plethysmography using a mercury strain-gauge. Electrical calibration *(A)* corresponds to a 1.0 per cent increase in resistance. Mechanical calibration *(B)* represents a 0.2-cm stretch of the gauge. Calf circumference is 34.6 cm. On the basis of Equations 4.1 and 4.2, flow is 4.7 ml/100ml/min. (From Strandness DE Jr, Sumner DS: Hemodynamics for Surgeons. New York, Grune & Stratton, 1975, pp 31–46.)

Segmental Plethysmography

The term *segmental plethysmography* is used merely to distinguish between those measurements made on a short segment of a body part and those in which the volume change of the entire part is determined. Either of the two methods can be applied to pulse, volume, or venous occlusion plethysmography; because arterial disease is usually segmental, most clinical plethysmographic measurements are of the segmental variety.[20, 108]

Instrumentation

Because all plethysmographs measure the same thing, volume change, the choice among the many varieties depends on their convenience, simplicity, stability, sensitivity, and ability to be calibrated. Often, it is dictated by personal preference. Although water-displacement plethysmographs measure volume changes directly, none of the varieties commonly used in the vascular laboratory does so.

Air-Filled Plethysmographs. A popular type of air-filled plethysmograph (the pulse volume recorder) employs a pneumatic cuff as a segmental volume sensor.[20] The cuff, which is wrapped around the limb at the site to be tested, is kept in close contact with the skin by inflating it to some relatively low pressure, usually about 65 mmHg. Volume changes in the enclosed limb increase or decrease the pressure of the air entrapped within the cuff (Boyle's law). These pressure changes are readily converted to an analogue recording by means of a pressure transducer. Calibration is accomplished by noting the increase in pressure produced by injecting a known quantity of air into the cuff (Fig. 4–4). Although the frequency response of air-filled plethysmographs is not high, ranging between 8 and 20 Hz, and although some distortion occurs as a result of the re-

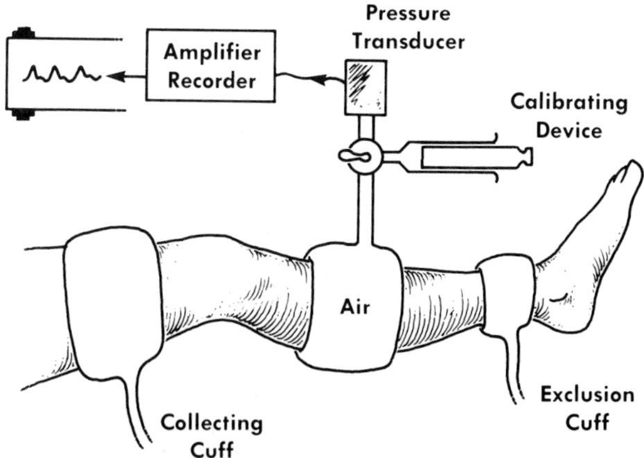

FIGURE 4–4. Segmental air-filled plethysmograph. Collecting and exclusion cuffs are necessary only for venous occlusion plethysmography. (From Sumner DS: Volume plethysmography in vascular disease: An overview. *In* Bernstein EF [ed]: Noninvasive Diagnostic Techniques in Vascular Disease. 3rd ed. St. Louis, CV Mosby Co, 1985, pp 97–118.)

duction in arterial transmural pressure caused by the counterpressure exerted by the cuff, for most practical purposes, these instruments provide a satisfactory rendition of the pulse contour.[22, 80]

Strain-Gauge Plethysmographs. The critical element of the strain-gauge plethysmograph is a fine-bore silicone rubber tube filled with mercury or an indium-gallium alloy.[109, 122] The tube is wrapped around the part being studied with just enough tension to ensure good contact with the skin (Fig. 4–5). As the part expands or contracts, changing its circumference, the length of the gauge changes. If the part has a roughly circular cross-section (as most limbs do), volume changes (ΔV) are related to circumference changes (ΔC) in the following way:

$$\frac{\Delta V}{V} \cong 2\frac{\Delta C}{C} \qquad (4.1)$$

where V and C represent the original volume and circumference, respectively. Because relative changes in the electrical resistance of the gauge (ΔR/R) are proportional to twice the relative change in the length of the gauge (2 ΔL/L), relative changes in resistance and volume are equivalent:

$$\frac{\Delta R}{R} = \frac{\Delta V}{V} \qquad (4.2)$$

This allows for direct calibration of the system in terms of volume change.[43, 93]

Mercury strain-gauges are very sensitive and have a high-frequency response (100 Hz), making them ideally suited for recording pulse volume contours.[76] They are, however, relatively fragile and this, together with their extreme sensitivity, makes them somewhat more difficult to use than other varieties of plethysmographs.

Impedance Plethysmographs. In biologic material, electricity is conducted by the movement of ions in both intracellular and extracellular fluids. Because the concentration of ions in these fluids is relatively constant, the impedance to the passage of an electrical current through any segment of the body is inversely proportional to its fluid content. Although impedance is a vector quantity with resistive, capacitive, and inductive elements, the resistive component predominates. Therefore, by measuring the relative change in resistive impedance (ΔR/R), one can closely approximate the relative change in blood volume (ΔV/V):[108, 120]

$$\frac{\Delta V}{V} = -\frac{\Delta R}{R} \qquad (4.3)$$

In modern impedance plethysmography, four electrodes, consisting of aluminum strips, are applied circumferentially to the limb (Fig. 4–6). A high-frequency oscillator delivers a low-level alternating current (AC) to the two outer electrodes while voltage changes between the two inner electrodes are recorded. Provided the current (I) remains constant, the voltage drop (E) between the two inner

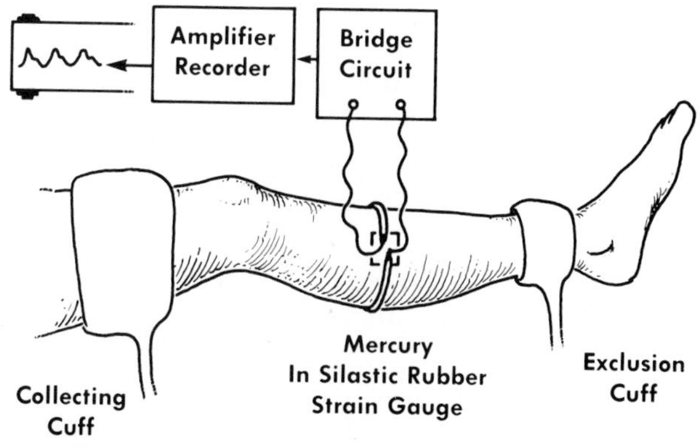

FIGURE 4–5. Mercury strain-gauge plethysmograph. (From Sumner DS: Volume plethysmography in vascular disease: An overview. *In* Bernstein EF [ed]: Noninvasive Diagnostic Techniques in Vascular Disease. 3rd ed. St. Louis, CV Mosby Co, 1985, pp 97–118.)

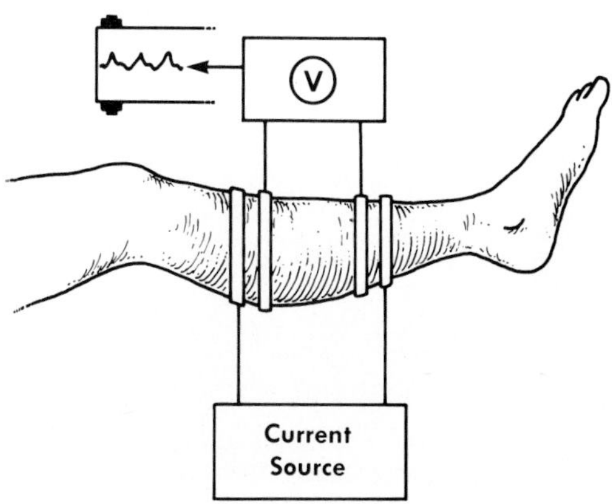

FIGURE 4–6. Impedance plethysmograph. (From Sumner DS: Volume plethysmography in vascular disease: An overview. *In* Bernstein EF [ed]: Noninvasive Diagnostic Techniques in Vascular Disease. 3rd ed. St. Louis, CV Mosby Co, 1985, pp 97–118.)

electrodes is directly proportional to the resistance of the segment:

$$E = IR \tag{4.4}$$

Because the electrical resistance of blood varies with the orientation of red blood cells during the cardiac cycle, pulses recorded with the impedance device have a more rapid upslope and a slower downslope than those obtained with the mercury strain-gauge.[1] Doubts have also been raised about the ability of impedance plethysmography to measure volume changes precisely during venous occlusion plethysmography.[68, 75] As a result, impedance plethysmography is not widely used in the diagnosis of arterial disease. These problems, however, do not affect its utility in the diagnosis of venous disease (see Chapters 107 and 120).

Photoplethysmographs. Photoplethysmographs consist of an infrared light–emitting diode and a photo sensor. Because whole blood is more opaque to red and near-infrared light than the surrounding tissue, the degree to which light is attenuated is proportional to the quantity of blood present.[21, 117] Two basic types of photoplethysmographs are in use. In one, the transilluminated tissue is sandwiched between the light source and the sensor. This type can be used only with thin, relatively transparent organs such as the ear lobe. The more convenient variety depends on reflected light and has the light source and sensor mounted side by side on a small probe, which can be applied easily to the fingers, toes, or virtually any area of the body by means of double-stick transparent tape (Fig. 4–7).

Strictly speaking, the photoplethysmograph is not a true plethysmograph, because it does not actually measure volume change and cannot be reliably calibrated. The recorded output, however, is proportional to the quantity of blood in the cutaneous microvasculature, and the resulting pulse contours closely resemble those obtained with the mercury strain-gauge. When the gauge is coupled to a direct current (DC) amplifier, slower changes in cutaneous blood content can be followed—a feature that permits the instrument to be used for measuring blood pressure and for studying limbs with venous valvular incompetence (see Chapter 133). Because of its simplicity and sensitivity, the photoplethysmograph has become a popular noninvasive instrument.

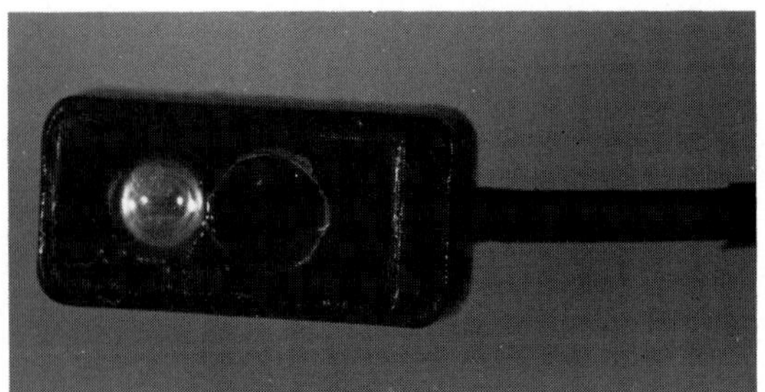

FIGURE 4–7. Photoplethysmograph of the type that depends on light reflected from the superficial tissues. The light-emitting diode and the photoelectric sensor are mounted side by side on the probe. (From Sumner DS: Plethysmography in arterial and venous diagnosis. *In* Zwiebel WJ [ed]: Introduction to Vascular Ultrasonography. New York, Grune & Stratton, 1982, pp 315–346.)

Doppler Ultrasonography

Of all the modalities used in the vascular diagnosis, none has proved more useful than Doppler ultrasonography.[111] Credit for developing the first Doppler flow detector goes to Satomura, whose initial report appeared in 1959.[90] Application of the technique to clinical studies of the peripheral vasculature followed the pioneering work of Rushmer, Strandness, and their coworkers in the mid-1960s.[88, 102, 104] Since then, the instruments have been refined, new applications devised, and much clinical research performed.

The operation of the ultrasonic flow detector depends on a principle formulated by the Austrian physicist Christian Johann Doppler (1803–1853), who demonstrated that the frequency of light or sound emitted by a source moving toward the observer is perceived as higher than the transmitted frequency, whereas that from a source moving away from the observer is perceived as lower than the transmitted frequency.[23] An often cited example is the pitch of a train whistle, which seems higher as the train approaches and lower as the train recedes into the distance.

Ultrasonic flow detectors are classified as continuous-wave (c-w) or pulsed.

Continuous-Wave Instruments

Of the two types of instruments, the continuous-wave or c-w Doppler is the most widely used. In these instruments, two piezoelectric crystals are mounted at the end of a flat or cylindrical probe. One crystal, which serves as the transmitter, emits ultrasonic waves having a frequency ranging from 2 to 10 million cycles per second (2 to 10 MHz). When these waves strike an acoustic interface, part of the energy is backscattered and is detected by the second crystal, which acts as a receiver. If the reflecting object is stationary, the frequency of the backscattered sound is unchanged; but if an object (such as a red blood cell) is moving, the frequency is changed in accordance with the Doppler principle—increasing with motion toward the probe and decreasing with motion away from the probe. The magnitude of the frequency shift (Δf) is inversely proportional to the velocity (C) of sound in tissue (about 1.56×10^5 cm/sec) and directly proportional to the transmitted frequency (f_o), the velocity of the moving object (V), and the cosine of the angle ($\cos \Theta$) at which the incident sound beam intersects the velocity vector.

$$\Delta f = \frac{2\, f_o\, V \cos \Theta}{C} \tag{4.5}$$

This formula can be rearranged to obtain velocity as a function of the frequency shift.

$$V = \frac{C\, \Delta f}{2\, f_o \cos \Theta} \tag{4.6}$$

Because the red blood cells in any cross-section of a blood vessel are traveling at a variety of velocities (ranging from zero at the wall to a peak near the center), the frequency shifts encompass a correspondingly wide range of values (see Chapter 3).

Audible Output. The Doppler signal can be processed in a number of ways. The easiest and most generally useful method is to represent the frequency shift as sound. When the backscattered signal detected by the receiving crystal is mixed with the transmitted signal, a beat frequency identical with the Doppler shift frequency is produced. Because this frequency is in the range of the sensitivity of the human ear (20 Hz to 15 kHz), it can be amplified to drive a loudspeaker or a set of earphones. The pitch of the signal is therefore proportional to the velocity of blood flow in the vessel being examined.

Commercially available instruments have transmitting frequencies ranging from 3 to 10 MHz. Because low frequencies are attenuated less severely than high frequencies by tissue interfaces, they provide better penetration and are necessary when deep vessels, such as the aorta and iliac arteries, are examined.[42] On the other hand, high frequencies are more discriminating and produce a higher-frequency shift for a given velocity. For these reasons, they are preferred when more superficial vessels, such as the smaller arteries of the limbs and digits, are studied.

The audible output has the advantage of containing all of the Doppler-shifted frequencies. A trained observer can easily distinguish between high and low flow velocities, between normal and disturbed flow patterns, and between arterial and venous flow without resorting to more sophisticated methods of analysis.

Audiofrequency Spectral Analysis. The audible output can be more thoroughly examined by means of fast-Fourier analysis of the multiple frequencies contained in the signal.[6, 86] In the resulting display, frequency is on the vertical axis, time is on the horizontal axis, and the amplitude of the backscattered signal at any specific frequency and time is indicated by a continuous gray scale (Fig. 4–8). The intensity of the gray scale is proportional to the number of red cells traveling at a particular velocity at a particular time. By suitable electronic manipulation, the vertical axis may be modified to read velocity rather than frequency—a feature that is of considerable value, because the angle (Θ) of insonation may vary from one study to the next. Some instruments also provide an alternate display with frequency on one axis and amplitude on the other.[39] The operator selects the specific part of the pulse cycle to be depicted in this fashion.

The frequency envelope defines the maximal velocity of the red cells within the lumen at any phase of the pulse cycle. Although this usually represents the velocity of the cells in the center of the flow stream, it may reflect the increased velocity of those cells emerging from a stenosis. Thus, peak velocity has considerable diagnostic significance.

Information concerning the velocity profile can be obtained from analysis of the spectrum. When the velocity profile is parabolic and the entire lumen is completely insonated by the sound beam, the amplitudes at all frequencies should be equal (Fig. 4–9). However, when the velocity profile is blunt (as it frequently is), more cells travel at higher velocities than at lower velocities, the higher amplitude signals parallel the frequency envelope, the spectrum is narrowed, and a ''window'' is produced (Fig. 4–10). Curves, bifurcations, and stenoses change or otherwise disturb the direction of flow relative to the incident sound beam, creating a broad spectrum of amplitudes even among cells traveling at the same speed. This, again, is important diagnostically.

Although visual inspection alone reveals a great deal about the flow pattern, other, more objective, information can be obtained from the spectrum, including measurements of peak, mean, median, and mode frequencies and power at any given frequency—parameters that may prove to be of value for calculating various indices that relate to flow disturbances.[36, 39, 46, 52, 87] Among the many other advantages of spectrum analysis is its ability to segregate noise from the primary signal. Likewise, one can easily separate signals derived simultaneously from adjacent vessels (such as those from an overlapping artery and vein). Because spectrum analysis is free of many of the artifacts that plague other means of processing the Doppler signal, it has become the standard method for depicting flow in the carotid arteries and is replacing other methods in the study of peripheral vascular disease.[48]

Analogue Recordings. Many commercially available Doppler instruments come equipped with a zero-crossing frequency to voltage converter.[6] The output may be displayed on a dial attached to the instrument or recorded on a strip chart. Although under ideal conditions the recordings provide a good rendition of the flow pulse, closely resembling that obtained with an electromagnetic flowmeter, this

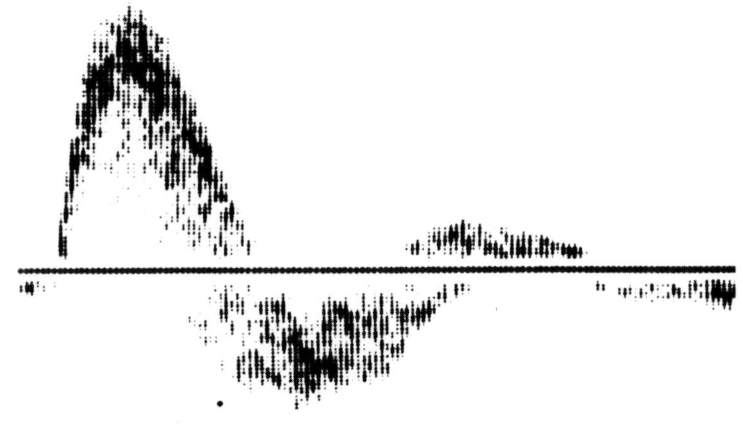

FIGURE 4–8. Spectral analysis of a normal common femoral artery Doppler flow signal. Frequency, corresponding to velocity, is on the vertical axis; and time, on the horizontal. Amplitude of the signal is indicated by the intensity of the gray scale. Note reversed flow in early diastole.

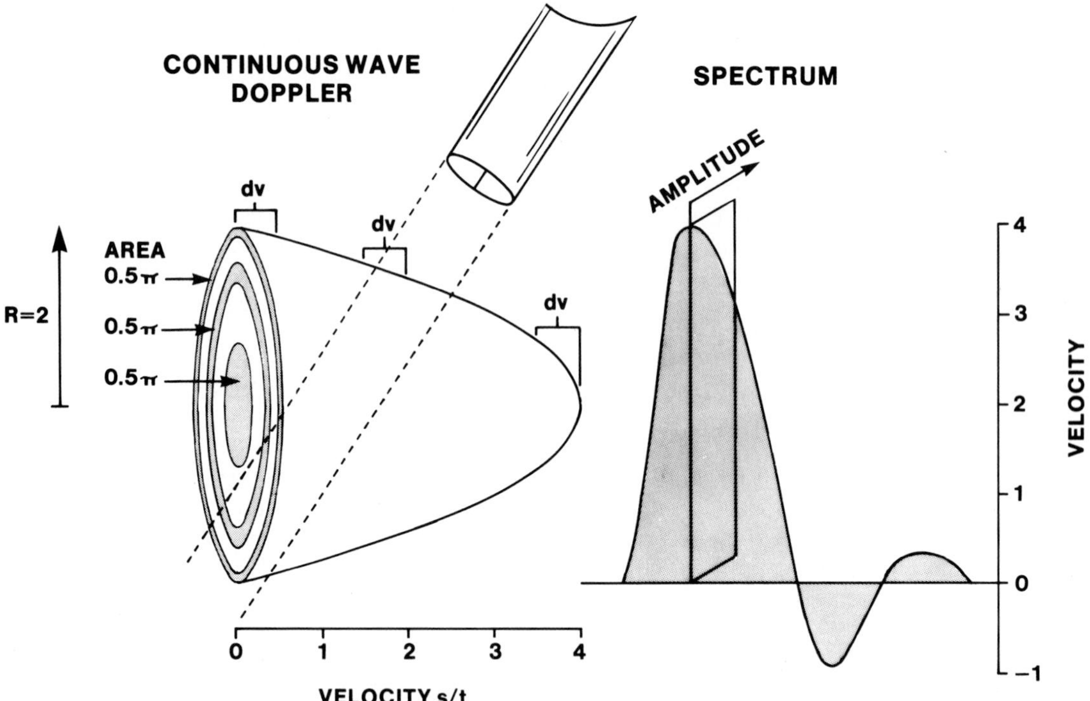

FIGURE 4–9. Instantaneous spectra of constant amplitude occur when a parabolic velocity profile is completely insonated by continuous-wave ultrasound. Since the areas of the annuli corresponding to each velocity increment (dv) are equivalent, the number of red blood cells traveling at any given velocity is identical. (From Sumner DS: Ultrasound. *In* Kempczinski RF, Yao JST [eds]: Practical Noninvasive Vascular Diagnosis. 2nd ed. Copyright © 1987, Year Book Medical Publishers, Chicago, pp 44–79. Reprinted by permission.)

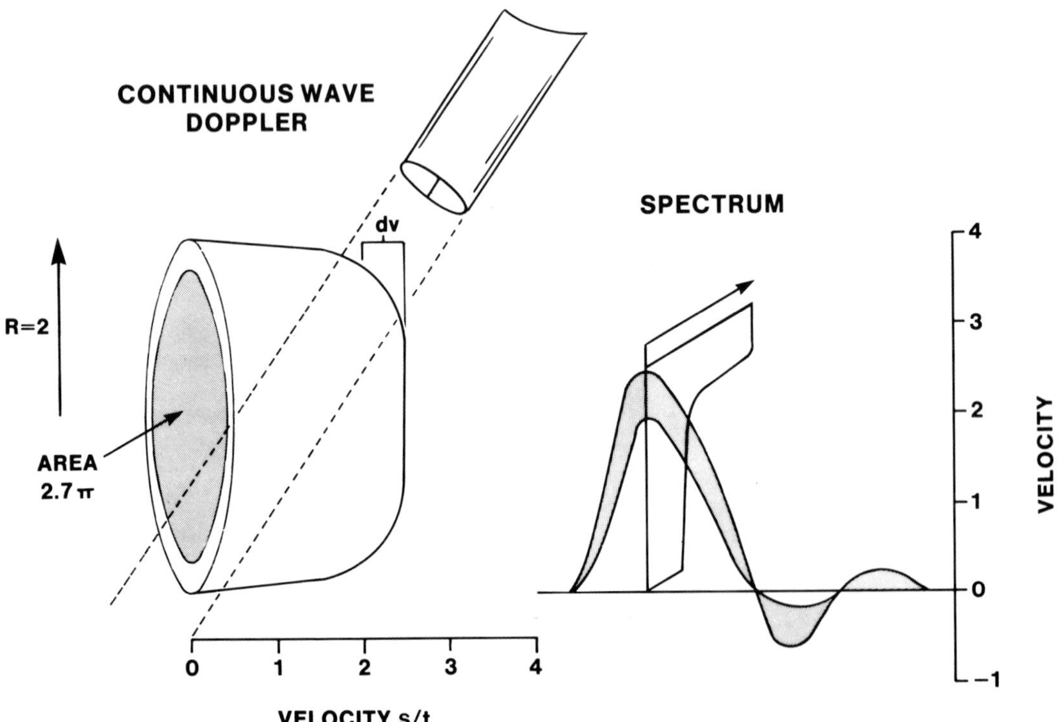

FIGURE 4–10. Complete insonation of a blunt velocity profile with continuous-wave ultrasound yields a spectrum that is skewed toward the peak instantaneous velocity. The area defined by the peak velocity increment (dv) far exceeds that defined by the lower velocities near the vessel wall. (From Sumner DS: Ultrasound. *In* Kempczinski RF, Yao JST [eds]: Practical Noninvasive Vascular Diagnosis. 2nd ed. Copyright © 1987, Year Book Medical Publishers, Chicago, pp 44–79. Reprinted by permission.)

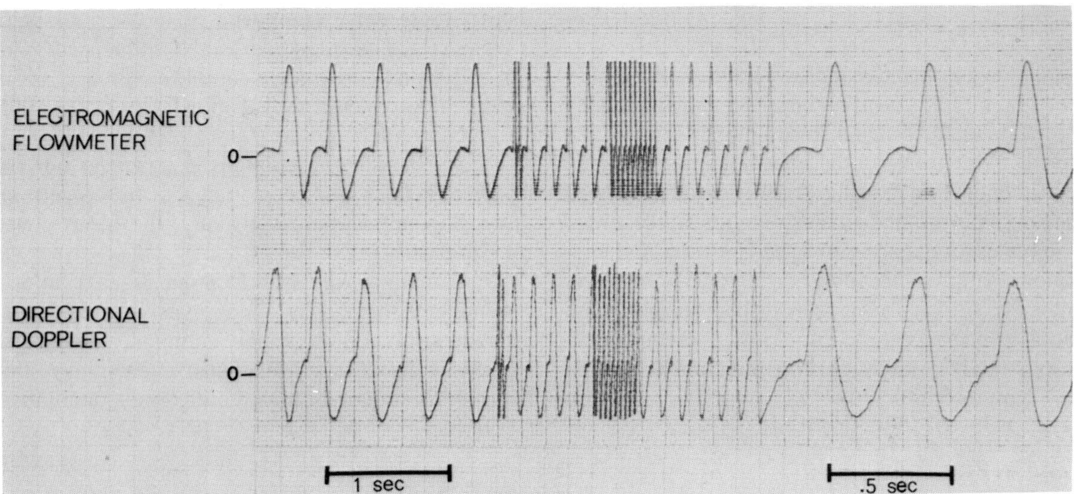

FIGURE 4–11. Flow velocity waveform recorded by a directional Doppler instrument in a normal subject. Note the triphasic pattern with negative flow during diastole. (From Dean RH, Yao JST: Hemodynamic measurements in peripheral vascular disease. Curr Probl Surg 13:1, 1976. Copyright © 1976, Year Book Medical Publishers, Chicago. Reprinted by permission.)

method of processing the Doppler signal is subject to many potentially serious errors (Fig. 4–11). Because the output voltage is proportional to the root mean square frequency rather than the mean Doppler shift frequency, the zero-crosser tends to read velocities that are up to 16 per cent too high.[25] When calibrated in vivo, low velocities tend to be overestimated, whereas high velocities may be underestimated.[26, 82, 92] Incorrect readings due to noise, amplitude and phase distortion, arterial wall movement, and mixing of arterial and venous signals are among the other problems.[48] Nevertheless, the zero-crosser output meets many of the routine needs of the vascular laboratory.

Direction Sensing. Any analysis of blood flow is incomplete without knowledge of its direction. Blood flow, particularly that in normal arteries, often reverses in early diastole; in fact, during the transition phase, antegrade and retrograde flow may coexist (see Chapter 3). Likewise, in areas of flow separation, retrograde flow may be present during most of the cardiac cycle. The direction of blood flow in veins, normally opposite to that in arteries, may reverse when the venous valves are incompetent and may be directed away from the heart in the same direction as it is in the parallel arteries.

A method for separating forward and reverse flow using quadrature phase detection was introduced simultaneously in 1967 by McLeod[65] and Kato and Izumi.[53] Although circuits based on their design have been incorporated in many Doppler flowmeters, there are some important drawbacks. Although the technique provides an accurate differential output, separate recordings of forward and reverse flow yield erroneously low values when blood is moving simultaneously in opposite directions.[6, 18] Moreover, the audio output is not directional.

An "outphasing" circuit, developed by Nippa and colleagues in 1975, overcomes these defects by providing two independent audio channels, one for forward flow and one for reverse.[74] This development not only allows spectral analysis to be performed on flow in both directions but also permits accurate analogue recording of simultaneous forward and reverse flow.

Pulsed-Doppler Instruments

Unlike continuous-wave instruments, which detect blood velocities from the entire cross-section of all vessels in the sound beam, pulsed-Doppler devices are capable of selectively detecting blood flow at a specific distance from the probe.[3] A single crystal acts as both transmitter and receiver. Short bursts of ultrasound, lasting 0.5 to 1.0 μsec, are emitted thousands of times per second. (Pulse repetition frequencies [PRF] of 5 to 16 kHz are commonly employed.) During the quiescent period between bursts, the crystal is activated for a brief period to provide a "gate" for receiving the signal. By adjusting the time between the transmission burst and the activation of the gate, one can select the depth at which the flow signals will be detected. The dimensions of the sample volume are determined by the duration of the sound burst, the width of the crystal, and the dispersion of sound in tissue.[69] Many instruments allow the sample volume to be varied from a minimal length of about 1.0 mm to lengths sufficient to encompass the entire width of the vessel.

Because precise positioning of the sample volume is critical to the interpretation of the Doppler signal, pulsed-Doppler instruments are usually used in conjunction with B-mode ultrasonic imaging devices (duplex scanners). The image also displays the angle (Θ) that the ultrasound beam makes with the long axis of the flow stream and defines the dimensions of the vessel lumen, information that is necessary for the accurate calculation of blood velocity and flow. By adjusting the range gate through a blood vessel from the far to the near wall, one can obtain a rough idea of the velocity profile. Instruments with multiple gates are more useful for this purpose, because they display velocity signals simultaneously at several points across the vessel diameter.[77, 83] Multi-gated pulsed-Dopplers are also used in flow-mapping devices, the newest of which allow real time imaging and are color-coded to indicate velocity (see Chapter 7).[54]

The ability to place the sample volume in the center of the flow stream has greatly enhanced the diagnostic value of the Doppler flow signal. In this location, most of the cells are traveling at nearly the peak velocity. Provided that the flow is undisturbed, spectral analysis of the signal shows a narrow band of frequencies paralleling the envelope of the maximal frequency curve, leaving a large empty space or window (Fig. 4–12). Flow disturbances, however minimal, alter the velocity vectors in respect to the sound beam, producing spectral broadening. Thus, spectral broadening has proved to be a most sensitive indicator of arterial disease (see Chapters 5 and 116).

Laser Doppler Flowmetry

Shifts in the frequency of monochromatic light caused by moving red blood cells can be used to assess skin blood flow. Although the principle is identical to that used in ultrasonic flow measurements, the problems are far more complex.[28] Unlike the relatively well defined geometry of the vessels ordinarily studied with ultrasound, the cutaneous vasculature consists of a complex network of interlacing vessels. Arterioles feed hairpin-like systems of capillaries that rise vertically from the papillae of the corium and return to the subpapillary venous plexus, whereas the larger vessels in the deeper dermis parallel the skin surface. The incident laser beam therefore intersects the flow vectors at multiple angles. Moreover, the light beam is scattered by the tissues both in transmission and again after it is reflected back to the receiving system. As a result, the frequency shifts represent a composite of the various velocities and angles. Because the signal is also influenced by the number of red blood cells in the sample volume, it actually represents the product of the mean velocity of the red blood cells and their concentration.[72, 73]

Depth of penetration is determined not only by the power of the laser beam but also by epidermal thickness and skin pigmentation. Usually, the beam penetrates to a depth of about 1.5 mm.

Although the laser Doppler is easy to use and has stimulated interest as a noninvasive method of assessing cutaneous blood flow, the complexity of the signal precludes calibration. These instruments may, however, be useful in situations that require only qualitative information.[51]

Transcutaneous Measurement of Oxygen Tension

Modified Clark polarographic electrodes are now being evaluated in an increasing number of vascular laboratories as a method for measuring oxygen tension in the cutaneous capillary bed.[16, 17, 27, 121] This technique introduces a potentially important new dimension to noninvasive studies, providing metabolic information to supplement the hemodynamic information supplied by more established testing procedures.

The electrodes are small and can be placed on virtually any area of the body near any lesion of interest. They consist of a circular silver–silver chloride anode surrounding a central platinum cathode. Oxygen diffusing to the surface of the skin is reduced at the cathode to produce a

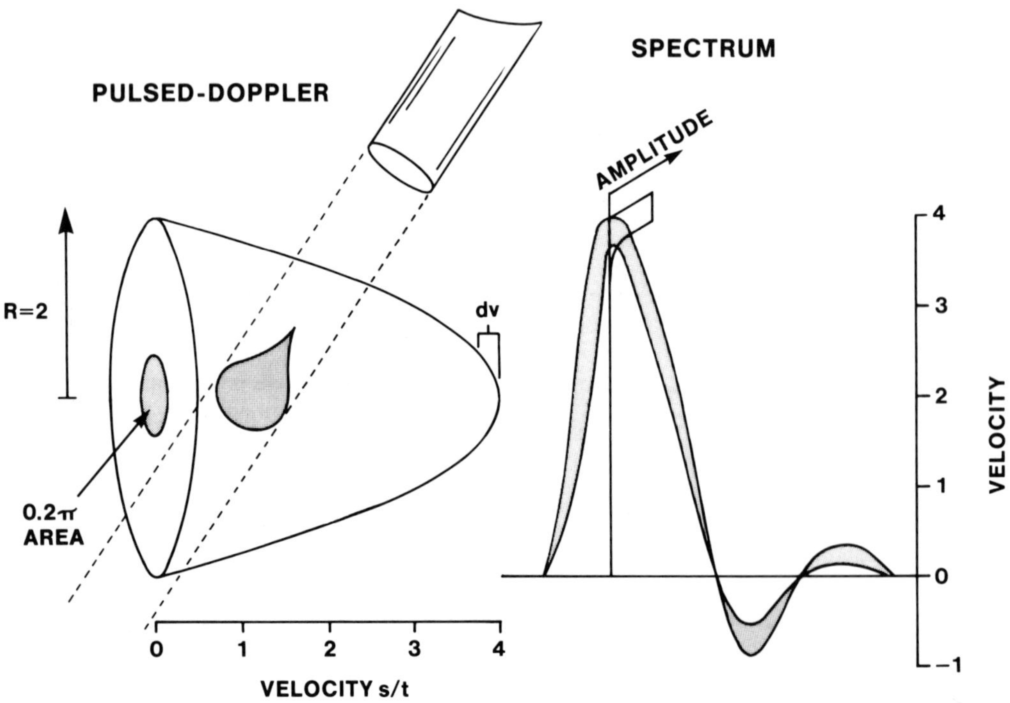

FIGURE 4–12. Sample volume of pulsed-Doppler ultrasound placed in the center of a parabolic velocity profile defines a small area of cells traveling at peak velocity. The resulting spectrum consists of a narrow band of frequencies of high amplitude. (From Sumner DS: Ultrasound. *In* Kempczinski RF, Yao JST [eds]: Practical Noninvasive Vascular Diagnosis. 2nd ed. Copyright © 1987, Year Book Medical Publishers, Chicago, pp 44–79. Reprinted by permission.)

current proportional to the Po_2 within the sensor. Incorporated in the electrode is a servocontrolled heating element, which is set to elevate and maintain the skin temperature at a level conducive to efficient oxygen diffusion and optimal capillary blood flow (about 45°C).

The quantity of oxygen available for diffusion to the skin depends on the difference between the quantity delivered by the influx of blood and that extracted by the tissues to meet local metabolic demands. Provided the arterial Po_2 remains unchanged, transcutaneous oxygen tension measurements reflect the level of tissue perfusion. Because the oxygen-hemoglobin dissociation curve becomes steep below oxygen saturations of about 80 per cent (which is roughly equivalent to a normal venous Po_2 of 40 mmHg), moderate reductions in blood flow have relatively little effect on capillary oxygen tension despite a comparable drop in oxygen saturation. As tissue perfusion becomes marginal, capillary Po_2 begins to drop off rapidly.[66] If inflow is restricted so severely that oxygen delivery is matched or exceeded by the metabolic requirements, no excess oxygen remains for diffusion to the surface of the skin, and transcutaneous oxygen tension measurements approach zero.[116] In other words, even when an arterial lesion becomes hemodynamically significant, no change in transcutaneous oxygen tension would be expected as long as the autoregulatory capacity remains capable of preserving a normal level of peripheral blood flow. Only when the autoregulatory capacity is exhausted will the transcutaneous oxygen tension begin to fall. Thus, transcutaneous oxygen tension measurements are most sensitive at critically low levels of blood flow.

The test is beset by a host of problems, which sometimes make interlaboratory data comparisons difficult.[15] Since skin temperature affects capillary blood flow, oxygen diffusion, and the oxygen-hemoglobin dissociation curve, differences in sensor temperature may account for some of the observed variability. Measurements tend to be unreliable when sympathetic tone is increased, when the body temperature is decreased, when cellulitis is present, and when the area being studied is hyperkeratotic, obese, or edematous. The age of the subject must also be taken into account.[34] Possibly because of changes in the histologic structure of the skin, transcutaneous oxygen tension levels decrease with advancing age. Although these problems make the role of this technique somewhat uncertain, it seems likely that the test will eventually secure a place in the armamentarium of the vascular laboratory.[15, 51]

Temperature Measurement

Because blood conducts heat to (and occasionally away from) the skin, skin temperature is in part determined by the level of cutaneous perfusion.[105] But skin temperature is also a function of environmental factors, including ambient temperature, humidity, and velocity of air circulation. When a body part is immersed in water, heat conduction is markedly enhanced and skin temperature tends to approach that of the surrounding medium. To further complicate matters, cutaneous blood flow increases in response to extrinsic heating and decreases in response to cooling (Fig. 4–13). Sympathetic stimuli lower skin temperature not only by causing cutaneous vasoconstriction but also by increasing

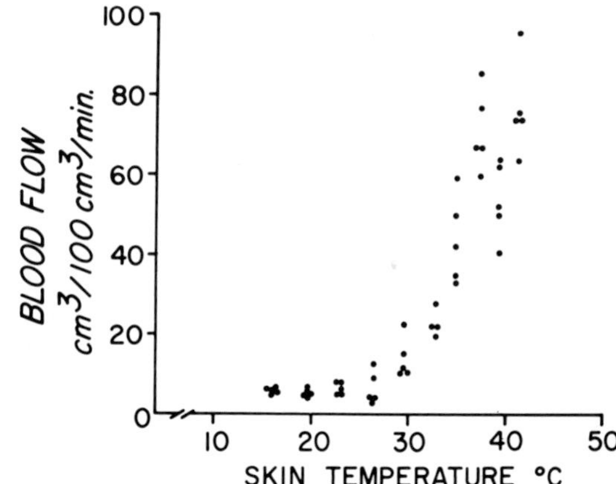

FIGURE 4–13. Relationship between blood flow and skin temperature in a fingertip immersed in a water bath. Skin temperature was varied by adjusting the temperature of the water bath. (From Strandness DE Jr, Sumner DS: Hemodynamics for Surgeons. New York, Grune & Stratton, 1985, pp 582–620.)

the production of sweat, which, by the process of evaporation, dissipates heat. It comes as no surprise, therefore, that the relationship between skin temperature and blood flow is markedly nonlinear. When there is no flow, skin temperature approaches that of the surrounding environment; at high flow rates, it reaches maximal values dictated by the temperature of the inflowing blood; in between, flow rates and skin temperature are mutually responsive.

In the vascular laboratory, thermistors provide the most convenient method for measuring skin temperature and are frequently useful in assessing vasospastic problems.[45, 79]

Liquid crystals are inexpensive; and when applied to the skin, they display specific temperature-related color changes that may be useful in defining the distribution of temperature gradients.[60] Infrared thermography, which requires expensive and sophisticated technology, can hardly be justified from the standpoint of cost-effectiveness.[30]

Other Methods

Radioisotope Techniques. Radioisotope clearance or distribution studies are semi-invasive methods used in some diagnostic vascular laboratories for measuring skin or muscle blood flow. They are described in Chapter 5.

Transcutaneous Electromagnetic Flowmetry. Although the electromagnetic flowmeter has proved to be a reliable invasive method for recording flow, attempts to develop a noninvasive instrument based on similar principles have met with limited success. The Doll system, which permits the recording of pulsatile but not nonpulsatile flow, has been used clinically in Europe, but few laboratories in the United States have any experience with the technique.[10, 59, 89]

Magnetic Resonance (MR) Imaging. Imaging with magnetic resonance is totally noninvasive; nothing is injected and no ionizing radiation is employed. The images are comparable to and, in many cases, better than those obtained with computed x-ray tomography.[67, 84] Because moving blood, unlike the stationary surrounding tissue, produces little or no signal, it appears dark compared with adjacent structures; thus, the MR image can function as an arteriogram or phlebogram. Unfortunately, the expense, high magnetic field, and space required preclude the use of conventional MR imaging in the vascular laboratory. Recently, however, a much smaller and far less expensive instrument that employs permanent magnets rather than giant electromagnets has been introduced specifically for use in the peripheral vascular laboratory. Although this instrument does produce crude cross-sectional images that are color-coded to depict gradations of velocity, it is basically a transcutaneous flow meter, the image serving primarily as a guide to locating a circular cursor, within which flow is assessed. The resulting display includes the contour of the flow wave within the vessel being studied and the mean and peak systolic flow rates. At present, few laboratories have any experience with MR flowmetry; consequently, its role remains uncertain.

MR spectroscopy may be of value in assessing metabolic changes associated with ischemia. Recent studies have shown that impairment of oxidative phosphorylation can be determined both at rest and after exercise.[127] This technique, however, is likely to remain experimental for the foreseeable future.

Derived Measurements

The instruments and methods that have been described furnish the ''raw material'' from which other information can be derived. Basically, the raw material is limited to measurements of volume changes or frequency shifts. Although derived information is necessarily one or more steps removed from the original data and is, therefore, less reliable, it is often equally useful.

Pressure Measurement

As discussed in Chapter 3, the dynamic blood pressure resulting from the contraction of the left ventricle is the major component of the potential energy necessary for moving blood through the vascular tree. No other parameter is more important to the understanding of normal or pathologically altered circulatory dynamics. Although blood pressure can be measured invasively by means of pressure-sensitive transducers, no direct method of noninvasive pressure measurement has been devised. Nonetheless, noninvasive pressure measurements, although inherently subject to error, are among the most valuable—if not *the* most valuable—of the diagnostic studies available in the vascular laboratory.[2]

Pneumatic Cuff Technique

Winsor and colleagues were among the first to employ noninvasive pressure studies in the evaluation of patients with peripheral arterial disease.[123] The method was further popularized by Strandness and his associates, and is now in widespread use in many clinics throughout the world.[100, 101, 103]

The technique is simple, and the equipment is relatively inexpensive. Basically, it consists of a pneumatic cuff and a flow sensor, such as a Doppler ultrasonic velocity detector, a mercury-in-Silastic strain-gauge, a photoplethysmograph, a laser Doppler monitor, or any other suitable device (see Chapter 5).* The cuff is placed around the part being studied, and the Doppler probe is positioned over a peripheral artery, as shown in Figure 4–14, or the strain-

*See references: Doppler ultrasonic velocity detector, 99, 100, 126; mercury-in-Silastic strain-gauge, 64, 103; photoplethysmograph, 11; laser Doppler, 14; other devices, 13, 44, 81, 123.

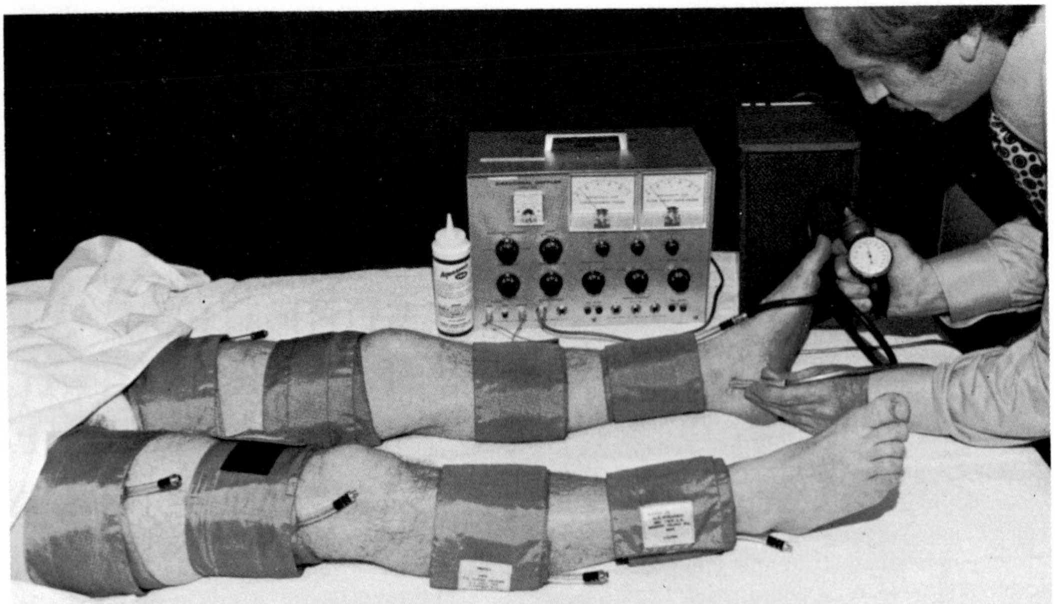

FIGURE 4–14. Technique of measuring segmental arterial systolic blood pressure with a Doppler flow detector and pneumatic cuffs.

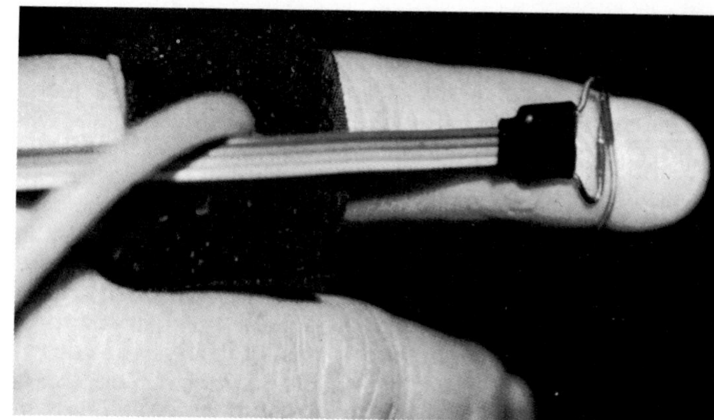

FIGURE 4–15. Technique of measuring digital arterial blood pressure with a mercury-in-Silastic strain-gauge and a pneumatic cuff applied to the proximal phalanx.

gauge is placed around the forearm, calf, finger, or toe (Fig. 4–15). Photoplethysmographs are easily attached to the tip of the toe or finger with double-stick transparent tape.

Measurements are made with the patient in a supine position with the part being studied at the same level as the heart. Owing to gravitational effects, elevating the part would decrease the recorded pressure, whereas lowering the part would cause the pressure to increase (see Chapters 3 and 129).[78]

After the cuff has been inflated to a pressure exceeding systolic, it is gradually deflated. The pressure within the cuff when flow resumes is equal to the systolic pressure in the artery underlying the cuff (Fig. 4–16).

Resumption of flow is most easily recognized by means of the audio output of the Doppler flowmeter (Fig. 4–16). Even when the ultrasonic signals are difficult to obtain, it is almost always possible to record a pressure with the mercury-in-Silastic strain-gauge or a photoplethysmograph. The digit volume changes detected by the plethysmograph are amplified and recorded on a strip chart. As the pneumatic cuff is slowly deflated, the digit volume decreases. When systolic pressure is reached, the volume tracing suddenly begins to rise. Pulses will reappear if they were present before the cuff was inflated, as shown in Figure 4–16. Use of the plethysmograph not only permits pressures to be recorded in fingers and toes but also allows pressures to be measured in the presence of severe obstructive arterial disease when flow velocities are so low that they cannot be detected with the Doppler flowmeter.[37]

Ideally, the width of the pneumatic cuff should be about 1.2 times the diameter of the part around which it is placed.[56] It is also preferable to have a bladder long enough to completely encircle the part.[94] These specifications ensure that even the deepest arteries will be exposed to the full pressure within the cuff. For many purposes, however, the usual clinical blood pressure cuff is adequate. Furthermore, around the upper thigh it may be impractical to use a cuff of ideal width.

In our studies, we employ a cuff with a 40-cm long bladder and a width of 10 cm. This provides an accurate measurement of the blood pressure in the arm and ankle, but results in a distortedly high pressure reading at thigh level. As long as this fact is appreciated, the use of smaller cuffs is not a drawback and, in fact, is necessary if blood pressure is to be measured at multiple levels in the leg.[40]

Estimation of Pressure Gradients: The Modified Bernoulli Equation

A simplification of the Bernoulli equation has been used by cardiologists to estimate pressure gradients across cardiac valves:[85]

$$\Delta P = \tfrac{1}{2}\,\rho(V_S^2 - V_p^2) \qquad (4.7)$$

where V_S and V_p represent the peak velocity measured from the Doppler frequency spectrum in the stenosis and proximal to the stenosis, respectively, and ρ represents the density of blood. As pointed out in Chapter 3, this formula neglects energy losses due to viscosity and assumes that the entire kinetic energy increment is dissipated in the form of heat. Although these assumptions are acceptable in the unique environment of the aortic valve, they introduce significant errors when this formula is applied to peripheral

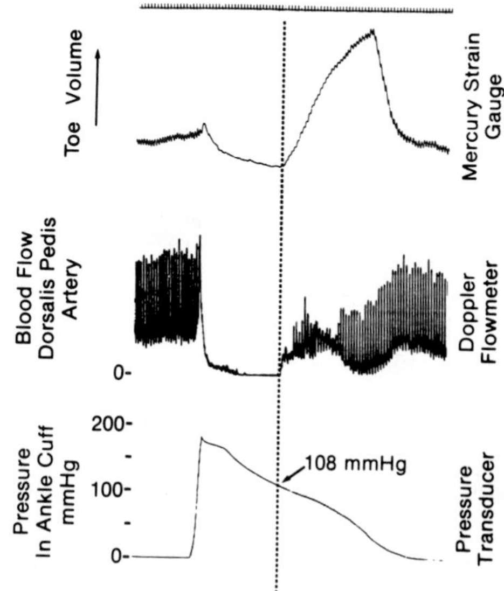

FIGURE 4–16. Systolic blood pressure at ankle level measured simultaneously with the Doppler flow detector and the strain-gauge techniques. The mercury strain-gauge is placed around the distal phalanx of the second toe. Note that the volume of the toe decreases steadily as long as the pressure within the ankle cuff exceeds systolic arterial pressure. When the cuff pressure reaches arterial systolic pressure, blood flow resumes as indicated by the sharp increase in toe volume and the reappearance of the Doppler signal. In this example, digit volume pulses also return.

arterial stenoses, where viscous losses may predominate and where a portion of the velocity increment may be reconstituted as pressure as the velocity returns to prestenotic values further downstream. Experimental data indicate that gradients calculated from the modified Bernoulli equation tend to overestimate gradients across mild stenoses and underestimate those across severe stenoses.[58] Despite some favorable reports, it seems unlikely that this method will ever be sufficiently reliable to be of diagnostic value.

Flow Measurement

As discussed previously, under well-controlled conditions, venous occlusion plethysmography provides reasonably accurate measurements of blood flow to an entire body part (such as a finger, forearm, or calf). Local skin or muscle blood flow can be estimated using radionuclide clearance techniques. Neither, however, can be used to measure flow in a specific vessel. Although MR technology may eventually prove to be a satisfactory method for obtaining noninvasive flow measurements from a single vessel, currently Doppler ultrasound is the only technique widely available for accomplishing this task. Invasive flow measurements can be made using either the electromagnetic flowmeter or the Doppler velocity detector.

Doppler Methods

At first glance, using the Doppler velocity detector to measure blood flow appears quite straightforward.[31] As indicated by Equation 4.6, velocity is directly proportional to the product of the velocity of sound in tissues (usually about 1.56×10^5 cm/sec) and the frequency shift and is inversely proportional to the product of the transmitted frequency and the angle of insonation (Θ). Because the vessel lies hidden under the skin, the first problem is estimating the angle at which the sound beam intersects the flow stream; this problem is relatively easily solved with the duplex scan. Nonetheless, small errors in measuring the angle can be quite significant. For example, if the true angle were 60 degrees, underestimating the angle by 10 degrees would underestimate flow by 22 per cent, and overestimating the angle by 10 degrees would overestimate flow by 46 per cent.

The second problem, that of determining the mean instantaneous velocity across the vascular lumen, presents a far greater challenge. As discussed in Chapter 3, the velocity profile varies with each phase of the pulse cycle, sometimes being almost parabolic and at other times practically flat. Forward flow may even coexist with reversed flow. Curves, bifurcations, and stenoses may skew the profile toward one wall. Whereas the velocity adjacent to the wall is always zero, the peak velocity, although usually found in the center of the flow stream, may be located anywhere in the lumen. Several approaches to determining the mean velocity have been used. If the entire cross-section of the vessel is insonated evenly by the sound beam, the mean Doppler frequency shift derived from frequency spectrum analysis (not from the zero-crosser output) of a continuous-wave Doppler unit or a pulsed-Doppler with an appropriately large sample volume will be proportional to the mean velocity. Obviously, significant errors will be introduced when only a portion of the lumen is insonated.[61] Multi-gated pulsed-Dopplers can be used to measure velocity at several points across the vascular lumen, the velocities being multiplied by the corresponding annular area to obtain a mean velocity. This approach requires small (high resolution) sample volumes and flow symmetry.[31] Instruments are now available that are designed to automatically integrate signals from multiple sampling sites across the entire vessel to produce a spatially averaged velocity. Although initial reports have been encouraging, the accuracy of these instruments in vivo has not been adequately substantiated.[54] Finally, under ideal conditions in which the profile is known to be flat, the peak velocity, which can easily be determined from the frequency envelope of a continuous-wave spectrum or from a single centrally placed gate of a pulsed-Doppler unit, closely approximates the mean velocity. If the profile could be assumed to be parabolic, as it rarely is, the mean velocity would be exactly half the peak velocity, and again a single gate would suffice.

The third problem relates to converting mean velocity to mean flow. This requires multiplying the velocity by the cross-sectional area of the vessel (which, when the lumen is circular, is given by πr^2, where r represents the inside radius). Although B-mode scanning provides the most convenient method for measuring the radius, it is not always accurate.[54] Because the area depends on the square of the radius, a 10 per cent error in measuring the radius translates into a 20 per cent error in the area calculation and a similar error in flow calculation.

Because the spatially meaned velocity varies throughout the pulse cycle (reaching a peak early in systole, often reversing early in diastole, and leveling off in late diastole), it is necessary to average the instantaneous velocities over the entire pulse cycle in order to obtain a mean flow rate. Because flow rates may also vary from cycle to cycle, more representative values may be obtained by averaging flows over several cycles. This problem is relatively easily solved electronically.

Despite all these real and potential problems, flows measured under ideal conditions with well-designed Doppler units are remarkably accurate, agreeing quite well with flows simultaneously measured using timed-collection or the electromagnetic flowmeter. Correlation coefficients of 0.95, slopes ranging from 0.95 to 1.05, and standard errors of 10 to 14 per cent have been reported.[31] It is doubtful, however, that this degree of accuracy can be duplicated in routine clinical studies.

Waveform Analysis

Although a great deal of information can be obtained by simple inspection of the Doppler-derived velocity waveform, a number of waveform indices have been proposed to make the analyses more objective and to facilitate comparison of data between laboratories. Many physiologic and pathophysiologic factors interact to determine the contour of the velocity waveform, including the initial shape of the pulse as it leaves the heart, peripheral reflections, elasticity of the arterial wall, dimensions of the vessels, density and viscosity of blood, and presence and location of branches, bifurcations, and stenoses (see Chapter 3). The problems, therefore, are complex and the solutions only partially successful.

Peak-to-Peak Pulsatility Index

The Doppler-derived velocity pulse wave, like any periodic wave, can be resolved mathematically by Fourier analysis into a series of sine waves that oscillate around a mean velocity. These waves are harmonics of the fundamental frequency (the pulse rate), their frequency being integral multiples of the fundamental. Each harmonic is further characterized by a phase angle and an amplitude (A_n) that is proportional to its peak oscillatory velocity. Because kinetic energy is proportional to velocity squared, Gosling and colleagues reasoned that the sum of the squares of the amplitudes of each harmonic divided by the square of the mean amplitude (A_o) (mean velocity) would provide an index of the maximal oscillatory energy of the wave compared with the energy of mean forward flow:[32]

$$\text{Fourier pulsatility index} = \sum_{n=1}^{\infty} (A_n^2/A_o^2) \quad (4.8)$$

Because stenoses reduce the oscillatory energy of a wave, a reduction in the Fourier pulsatility index is useful for detecting arterial occlusive disease proximal to the site of flow interrogation. The calculation of this index is, however, too time-consuming and cumbersome to be used routinely in the vascular laboratory.

To overcome these difficulties, in 1974, Gosling and King proposed a far less complicated formula that simply relates the maximal excursion of the velocity wave to the mean velocity (Fig. 4–17):[33]

$$PI_{pp} = \text{peak-to-peak velocity/mean velocity} \quad (4.9)$$

This peak-to-peak pulsatility index (PI_{pp}) has been shown to be a function of the Fourier pulsatility index raised to a constant power.[48] Like the Fourier pulsatility index, the PI_{pp} decreases with increasing severity of the stenosis proximal to the Doppler probe site.

Because the relative magnitude of the reverse flow component tends to increase toward the periphery (owing to the increased magnitude of the reflected wave), PI_{pp} tends to increase from the proximal portions of the leg to the distal. In order to quantify these changes and to permit regional localization of arterial occlusions or stenoses, the use of a damping factor (DF) has been proposed.[32]

$$DF = \frac{\text{proximal } PI_{pp}}{\text{distal } PI_{pp}} \quad (4.10)$$

Johnston and coworkers prefer an inverse damping factor (DF^{-1}).[48]

$$DF^{-1} = \frac{\text{distal } PI_{pp}}{\text{proximal } PI_{pp}} \quad (4.11)$$

Thus, a decrease in DF^{-1} between two points indicates an interposed segment of arterial disease.

A major advantage of the pulsatility index is that it is independent of the angle subtended between the sound beam and the axis of flow. A potential and perhaps real disadvantage relates to its sensitivity to changes in peripheral impedance, thereby diminishing its accuracy for detecting proximal disease in the presence of significant distal disease.[115]

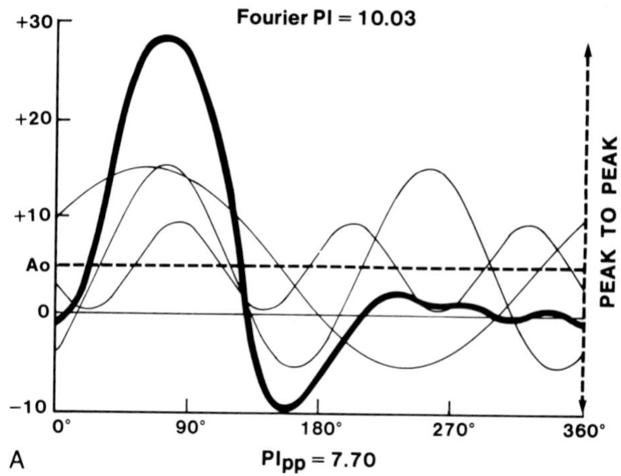

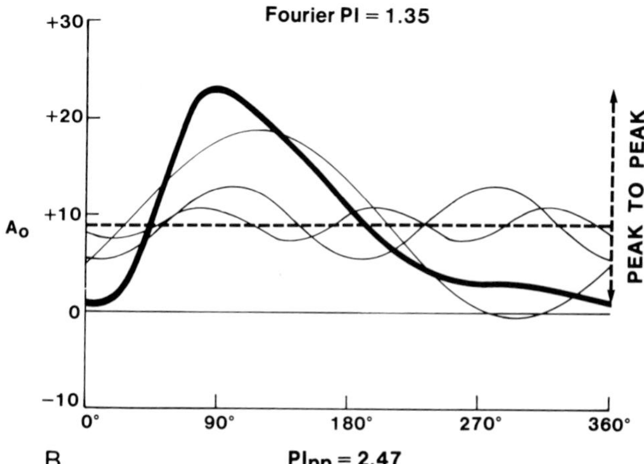

FIGURE 4–17. Waveforms derived from common femoral Doppler signals, showing relationship between Fourier and peak-to-peak pulsatility indices. *A*, Normal iliac artery. *B*, Iliac artery obstruction. The first three harmonics obtained by Fourier analysis are indicated by sine waves. A_o, mean amplitude; vertical arrows, maximal excursion. Note that $PI_{pp} = 1.9$ (Fourier PI)$^{0.57}$.

Laplace Transform Method

Because of the perceived problems with the pulsatility index (a time-domain processing technique), Skidmore and Woodcock and their colleagues investigated frequency domain processing of the Doppler velocity signal.[95–97] The calculations are complex and are best accomplished by an on-line computer. Initially the waveform is digitized and the Fourier transform calculated, from which the equivalent Laplace transform is obtained using a curve-fitting procedure. The roots of the resulting equation are plotted on an Argand diagram, from which parameters that are functions of arterial stiffness (ω_o), peripheral impedance (γ), and proximal lumen diameter (δ) are obtained. Segregation of the various factors that determine the contour of the velocity pulse has been shown by some investigators to improve the accuracy with which proximal disease is diagnosed in the presence of distal occlusions (e.g., aortoiliac stenoses in the presence of superficial femoral artery occlusions), but others have not confirmed these observations.[5, 47, 50, 97] Although the technique is theoretically appealing, its value to the vascular diagnostician remains to be established.

Other Methods

From time to time, many other methods have been proposed for evaluating the velocity pulse. Some are simple, being merely measurements of readily apparent features of the pulse; others, such as principal component analysis, are more complex.[35, 36, 43, 62, 63, 71] All may suffer because the velocity waveform is studied at some distance from the lesion. With the advent of Duplex scanning, direct investigation of the artery at the site of stenosis has become feasible. Simple pattern recognition applied to the velocity spectrum combined with equally simple velocity measurements have proved to be at least as accurate, if not more so, than the more complicated methods of waveform analysis.[57, 70]

Pulse Wave Velocity and Transit Time

The velocity (c) with which the pulse is transmitted in the arterial system is given by the Moens-Korteweg equation (see Chapter 3):

$$c = (E\delta/\rho d)^{1/2} \qquad (4.12)$$

where E is the elastic modulus of the arterial wall; δ, its thickness; d, the mean diameter of the artery; and ρ, the density of blood. Velocity is therefore proportional to the "stiffness" of the arterial wall (E) and the relative wall thickness (δ/d), both of which are increased in diseased arteries. Consequently, one would expect an increased pulse wave velocity in atherosclerotic vessels.[38]

In practice, pulse transit times (TT) between two sites in the arterial system are usually measured rather than pulse wave velocities:

$$TT = \frac{S}{c} \qquad (4.13)$$

where S represents the distance between the two sites. One method measures the time between the electrocardiographic R wave to a specified point on the Doppler velocity waveform (often the peak or foot of the wave); another, the time delay between the arrival of the Doppler signal at proximal and distal sites of the arterial tree.[19, 24] Simultaneous recordings of the Doppler signal are made, for example, from the common femoral and popliteal arteries or from the popliteal and posterior tibial arteries. Because transit time is a function of the distance the pulse must travel, any delay in pulse arrival implies an elongation of the arterial pathway—an elongation that can usually be attributed to the presence of interposed collateral channels. Thus, although pulse wave velocity may increase in diseased arteries, transit times are usually increased. Even in the presence of a totally occluded artery, transit times can vary depending on the length of the collateral arteries.

Although transit time determinations may have some value as ancillary studies, they do not provide the discrimination required for most diagnostic purposes and are rarely used in most laboratories.

Invasive Methods

Although this chapter is primarily concerned with noninvasive measurements, cannulation of vessels to measure blood pressure and the use of the electromagnetic flowmeter are two invasive methods that are often used by surgeons in the evaluation of vascular problems.

Direct Intravascular Pressure Measurement

The ready availability of pressure transducers and the simplification of recording techniques have increased the use of invasive methods, not only in the diagnostic laboratory but also in the radiologic suite and the operating room.[2] Monitoring radial artery pressure during extensive vascular procedures is now commonplace; measurement of carotid back pressure is used by many surgeons; pull-through pressures are employed by radiologists in conjunction with Grüntzig dilatations; and direct femoral artery pressures are used by a growing number of surgeons to assess the hemodynamic status of the inflow to the leg (see Chapter 7).

Theoretically, invasive techniques should be more accurate than the more indirect noninvasive methods. This is particularly true in areas such as the femoral artery, where noninvasive methods are quite fallible. Moreover, they permit the measurement of diastolic as well as systolic pressure and allow visualization of the pressure waveform. Many of the newer commercial devices display a continuous image of the pressure wave and provide convenient digital readings of the systolic, diastolic, and mean pressures.

Although direct intra-arterial pressure measurements are often considered to be the "gold standard," they are subject to many technical errors that all too frequently affect the results. In most communications, the possible existence of such errors is ignored. Hydrostatic problems related to the height of the transducer in relation to the heart are usually given the appropriate amount of attention, and the proper zero is determined. Seldom, however, is more than cursory attention given to the hydraulic system that leads to the transducer. Most needle, catheter, and transducer systems are underdamped and frequently have a low resonant frequency.[12] This is particularly true when bubbles are present in the system. Consequently, the pulse pressure tends to be amplified, leading to spuriously high systolic pressure readings.[12, 105] In fact, it is not unusual to hear the nurse complain that the radial artery systolic pressure is 20 to 40 mmHg higher than the pressure measured at the brachial level with the conventional Riva-Rocci sphygmomanometer.

To obtain truly accurate pressure recordings, the resonant frequency and the damping factor of the hydraulic system must be known.[29, 105] In working with an underdamped system, every effort should be made to achieve a high resonant frequency. Because even small air bubbles interfere, it has been recommended that only boiled distilled water be used and that all hydraulic parts be flushed for up to 24 hours.[29] Unfortunately, in clinical practice, analysis of the properties of the system and extensive preparations are seldom practical; but one can strive to use stiff tubing, eliminate leaks, use a minimal number of stopcocks, and free the apparatus of air bubbles. When small differences in pressure are critical—as in measuring the gradient across an arterial segment—it is important to make sure that the same equipment is used at both levels or, if two sets are used, that they are equally matched. This is especially important when systolic gradients are being measured. Mean pressures are less likely to be distorted. Finally, because there is no convenient way of eliminating errors, the surgeon must be aware that they may exist and use this knowledge in interpreting results.

Electromagnetic Flowmeter

The electromagnetic flowmeter is useful not only during reconstructive surgery but also during experimental studies in animal models. In addition, the technique is often regarded as the "gold standard" for evaluating newer flow measuring devices. Therefore, knowledge of the principles governing its function and the errors to which it is subject is essential for those interested in using the electromagnetic flowmeter either clinically or in the research laboratory.

Principles of Operation[113, 119, 124]

When a fluid conductor moves at right angles through a magnetic field, an electrical potential is induced in the fluid perpendicular to both the magnetic field and the direction of flow. The magnitude of this voltage (E) depends on the spatially averaged velocity flow (v in cm/sec), the strength of the magnetic field (B in gauss), and the diameter of the blood vessel (d in cm):

$$E = dBv \cdot 10^{-8} \qquad (4.14)$$

In practice, the standard noncannulating electromagnetic flow probe consists of an electromagnet and two electrodes embedded in a C-shaped plastic device for easy application to the vessel (Fig. 4–18). The electrodes are located opposite each other and at right angles to the poles of the electromagnets. A voltage proportional to the velocity of flow appears at the interface between the fluid and the vessel wall. In turn, this voltage is conducted across the vessel wall, where it is picked up by the electrodes and amplified to drive a recording system. Volume flow Q in cubic centimeters per second can be measured, provided that the cross-sectional area of the vessel is known:

$$E = \frac{4BQ}{\pi d} \cdot 10^{-8} \qquad (4.15)$$

Although the principle of operation is quite simple, many technological problems needed to be solved before a reliable instrument could be constructed. Currently, systems employing gated sine waves, square waves, and pulsed waves are in use. The last-named systems have the advantage of providing an interval between pulses when the magnetic field is zero, thereby permitting a more reliable determination of electronic (nonocclusive) zero.

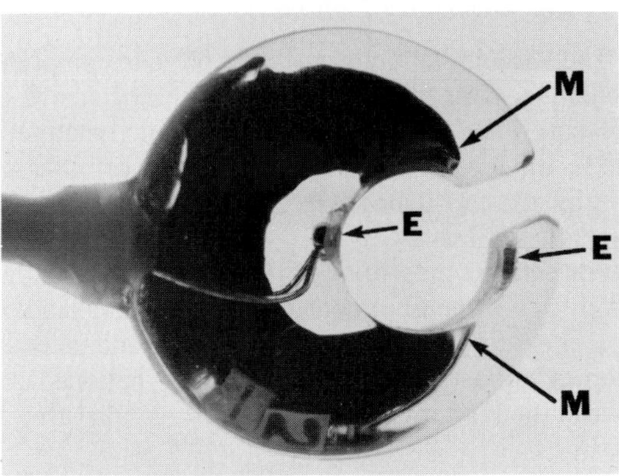

FIGURE 4–18. Electromagnetic flow probe. E, electrodes; M, poles of electromagnet.

Sources of Error

The shape of the velocity profile does not affect the output of the electromagnetic flowmeter as long as the profile is axisymmetric, but readings may be distorted when these conditions are not met.[91] Errors of 23 per cent have been recorded at sites within six diameters of a 30-degree curve, and errors of 83 per cent have been recorded just downstream from a 25 per cent diameter stenosis.[112] These inaccuracies can be minimized by placing the probe on a straight, uniform section of the vessel some distance from a junction, sharp bend, or atherosclerotic plaque. Every effort should be made to ensure good electrical contact with the vessel wall by selecting a probe with a diameter 5 to 20 per cent less than that of the vessel to which it is applied and by making sure that the space between the probe and the vessel is completely filled with conducting fluid. Flows measured with a "dry" probe may be 50 per cent higher than the actual value.[118]

Although flow signals increase with a decreasing hematocrit and decrease with an increasing hematocrit, for hematocrits between 30 and 50 per cent, the sensitivity will be within 10 per cent of that at a hematocrit of 40 per cent.[114] Outside this range, errors may be appreciable. The output of the flowmeter is also affected by the relative impedance of the flowing blood and that of the surrounding vessel wall. Thus, flow values may be altered when the arterial wall is excessively thickened by atherosclerotic plaque. Likewise, measurements obtained when the probe is applied to synthetic grafts may not be reliable.[124]

Calibration

Most clinical flow measurements will be made with precalibrated probes. To minimize errors, those situations (discussed previously) that are known to distort the output of the flowmeter should be avoided. Because this is not always possible, the surgeon must realize that the recorded flow measurements may not be accurate and should not attach undue significance to measurements made under less than ideal circumstances. If possible, the probe should be calibrated in vivo by the timed collection of blood or by the use of an infusion pump. Although this is seldom feasible during a vascular operation, it should always be done as an integral part of all experimental work in which accuracy is critical.[125]

THE ROLE OF THE VASCULAR LABORATORY

In 1976, the Inter-Society Commission for Heart Disease Resources issued a report on medical instrumentation in peripheral vascular disease that stated their belief that "a clinical vascular laboratory is desirable in any institution that is doing angiography of the distal aorta, iliac, femoropopliteal circulation or of the coronary and cerebral vessels."[8] They also emphasized the importance of a vascular laboratory in institutions that treat trauma patients, that perform arterial reconstructive surgery, and that care for patients suffering from venous thromboembolism. Clearly, to comply with this recommendation, vascular laboratories would be required in most of the largest hospitals and in large numbers of smaller facilities. (More than 1000 are in existence today.)

The vascular laboratory has undergone a transition from being a facility primarily involved with clinical research studies to one that has become an essential component of the comprehensive practice of vascular surgery. Not only has the profile of activity changed but also the individuals involved in performing these studies are no longer exclusively vascular surgeons, but represent a wide variety of medical disciplines. It is perhaps this latter feature more than any other that clearly establishes that the diagnostic capabilities of the laboratory are now part of accepted medical practice.

The Function of the Laboratory

The vascular laboratory has provided those involved with the diagnosis and treatment of vascular diseases objective and often quantitative information to both identify and stratify the severity of disease, as well as to evaluate the effects of intervention. As with most new technologies, the procedures usually performed are complementary to other diagnostic procedures and have tended to provide functional rather than morphologic data.

The diagnostic procedures supplied by vascular laboratories have gradually decreased in number but, as one would expect, increased in complexity. Today, the majority of clinical evaluations are performed with duplex ultrasonography, which is discussed in detail in Chapter 6, although in the assessment of patients with lower extremity occlusive disease, for example, a variety of techniques are still effectively utilized. The specific applications of the technologies available are best considered by reviewing their use in individual clinical circumstances.

Cerebrovascular Disease

Duplex ultrasonography is the primary method for diagnosing extracranial vascular disease.[4] This technique should provide detailed information regarding the degree of stenosis of the carotid bifurcation, as well as the presence of disease in the other extracranial vessels. Information about plaque morphology should be supplied in simple terms.[7] The categories of degree of stenosis should be such that critical lesions are clearly identified and disease progression can also be detected.

Appropriate indications for examination of the extracranial arteries include the evaluation of cervical bruits, of patients with symptomatic cerebral ischemia, and of patients following carotid endarterectomy. Serial evaluation at 6-month intervals is appropriate in patients with asymptomatic carotid disease and those in whom endarterectomy has been performed.

Venous Disease

Acute Venous Thrombosis

Duplex ultrasonography is also becoming the preferred method for evaluating patients with suspected acute venous thrombosis.[9] Recent studies have documented the poor performance of plethysmography as a technique for examining patients at high risk who do not have any symptoms.[49] Duplex ultrasonography has clearly established its place in evaluating these patients, as well as those in the symptomatic group. Plethysmography, particularly impedance plethysmography, does, however, still have a useful role in the evaluation of the symptomatic patient.[107]

Chronic Venous Disease

Patients with chronic venous disease can now be evaluated with duplex ultrasonography, which has proved to be a useful method of detecting residual obstruction and valvular reflux in the thigh and knee areas.[110] Unfortunately, it cannot assess quantitatively the overall functional effect of obstruction or reflux. These issues are best evaluated plethysmographically with either air or photoplethysmographic techniques.[128, 129]

Peripheral Occlusive Disease

Vascular laboratories should be capable of evaluating patients who present for the first time with symptoms suggestive of lower extremity ischemia or upper extremity ischemia, as well as being able to monitor the efficacy of all forms of lower extremity revascularization.

Lower Extremity Ischemia

The vascular laboratory should provide comprehensive techniques to determine whether vascular occlusive disease is present, what the severity of the hemodynamic disturbance is, the location of the abnormality (aortoiliac or femoropopliteal), and if possible, to provide some idea of the therapeutic options available.

For patients presenting with critical ischemia, these are recommended: measurement of ankle-brachial index, segmental pressure, or waveform evaluation and selective use of duplex ultrasonography. In diabetic patients or those with calcified arteries, toe pressures should also be included.

In patients with claudication, the ankle-brachial index and segmental pressure or waveform studies should be supplemented with an exercise treadmill examination to deter-

Table 4–1. Cerebrovascular Disease

Indication	Technique
Hemispheric symptoms	Duplex carotids
Nonlocalizing	Extracranial duplex, brachial pressures
After endarterectomy	Duplex carotids (6-mo intervals)

mine the true claudication distance and also to confirm the presence of abnormal hemodynamics consistent with claudication.[130]

Duplex ultrasonography should be used selectively in patients with symptoms of lower extremity ischemia to identify focal areas of stenosis or short-segment occlusion.[131] These types of lesions may be amenable to balloon dilatation. Suitable patients include those with mild claudication or those with bruits in the iliac fossa or groin regions, as well as those with bruits along the course of the superficial femoral artery.

An important application of duplex ultrasonography in the lower extremities is in the area of graft surveillance where studies should be performed at 3-month intervals for the first 12 months, and thereafter at 6-month intervals. This technique provides a mechanism not only for measuring graft velocities but also for identifying areas of focal stenosis.[132]

Upper Extremity Ischemia

The evaluation of upper extremity symptoms revolves primarily around the diagnosis of hemodynamically significant proximal vessel disease and the evaluation of Raynaud's phenomenon. In the former patients, simple brachial blood pressure measurement is generally adequate, but this may be supplemented with duplex ultrasonography to evaluate the subclavian arteries. For the vasospastic group of patients, plethysmographic techniques are usually required to evaluate the individual digital artery pressure and waveform features as well as the response to cold stimuli.[133]

Extended Applications

Technical advances in instrumentation have been responsible for the application of duplex ultrasonography to evaluate the splanchnic[134] and renal circulation,[135] as well as the status of transplanted kidneys.[136] These studies involve the measurement of blood flow velocities in the appropriate arteries with the subjective evaluation of waveform patterns, particularly in the case of renal transplant evaluation.

Table 4–3. Lower Extremity Ischemia

Indication	Technique
Ischemic rest pain	Ankle-brachial index Segmental pressures *or* segmental waveforms Duplex ultrasonography
Claudication	Ankle-brachial index Segmental pressures or waveforms Exercise treadmill Duplex ultrasonography
Graft surveillance	Ankle-brachial index Duplex ultrasonography (every 3 mo 1st year, then every 6 mo)

Quality Controls

Quality control has become increasingly important in the activities of vascular laboratories to ensure that diagnostic studies of appropriate accuracy are performed. The quality assurance activity should be comprehensive and include, but not be limited to, such issues as training and continuing education of both physicians and technologists, the use of examination protocols for studies, the application of appropriate diagnostic criteria, and the review of incorrect studies in comparison with other studies for the purpose of maintaining acceptable accuracies. As instrumentation becomes more sophisticated, careful maintenance checks also become essential. Other important issues include those of the patient's safety, as well as measures used to ensure that reporting of results is achieved in a timely fashion.

Summary

The preceding section outlines the broad scope of vascular laboratory activities as it has evolved since the early 1970s. What was once primarily a small research facility has now matured to a well-recognized and essential clinical service. The general uses of this technology and the indications are presented in Tables 4–1 through 4–5.

To summarize this discussion of the vascular laboratory, one cannot improve on the definition provided by Dr. Richard Kempczinski: ". . . the term 'vascular diagnostic laboratory' does not imply a specific battery of tests or instruments, but rather reflects a commitment to study vascular occlusive disease with whatever objective, noninvasive techniques are most applicable to each institution and to the training and requirements of the personnel establishing the laboratory."[55]

Table 4–2. Venous Disease

Indication	Technique
Acute venous thrombosis	Duplex ultrasonography Impedance plethysmography
Chronic venous disease	Duplex ultrasonography Air plethysmography Photoplethysmography

Table 4–4. Upper Extremity Ischemia

Indication	Technique
Arm claudication	Brachial blood pressure
Peripheral embolization	Subclavian duplex ultrasonography
Raynaud's phenomenon	Brachial blood pressure Subclavian duplex ultrasonography Digital plethysmography

Table 4–5. Abdominal Vascular Diseases

Indication	Technique
Renovascular hypertension Renal insufficiency	Renal duplex ultrasonography
Mesenteric insufficiency	Mesenteric duplex ultrasonography
Aneurysmal disease	Abdominal duplex ultrasonography

Selected References

Atkinson P, Woodcock JP: Doppler Ultrasound and Its Use in Clinical Measurements. London, Academic Press, 1982.

Bernstein EF (ed): Noninvasive Diagnostic Techniques in Vascular Disease. 3rd ed. St. Louis, CV Mosby Co, 1985.

Kempczinski RF, Yao JST (eds): Practical Noninvasive Vascular Diagnosis. 2nd ed. Chicago, Year Book Medical Publishers, 1987.

References

1. Anderson FA Jr, Penny BC, Patwardhan NA, et al: Impedance plethysmography: The origin of electrical impedance changes measured in the human calf. Med Biol Eng Comput 18:234, 1980.
2. Baker AR, Macpherson DS, Evans DH, et al: Pressure studies in arterial surgery. Eur J Vasc Surg 1:273, 1987.
3. Baker DW: Pulsed ultrasonic Doppler blood-flow sensing. IEEE Trans Sonics Ultrasonics 17:170, 1970.
4. Langlois YE, Roederer GO, Strandness DE Jr: Ultrasonic evaluation of the carotid bifurcation. Echocardiography 4:141, 1987.
5. Baker JD, Machleder HI, Skidmore R: Analysis of femoral artery Doppler signals by Laplace transform damping method. J Vasc Surg 1:520, 1984.
6. Beach KW, Phillips DJ: Doppler intrumentation for the evaluation of arterial and venous disease. *In* Jaffe CC (ed): Vascular and Doppler Ultrasound. New York, Churchill Livingstone, 1984, pp 11–49.
7. Bluth EI, Kay D, Merritt CRB, et al: Sonographic characterization of carotid plaque: Detection of hemorrhage. AJR 146:1061, 1986.
8. Bergan JJ, Darling RC, DeWolfe VG, et al: Report of the Inter-Society Commission for Heart Disease Resources. Medical instrumentation in peripheral vascular disease. Circulation 54:A-1, 1976.
9. Killewich LA, Bedford GR, Black KW, Strandness DE Jr: Diagnosis of deep venous thrombosis: A prospective study comparing duplex scanning to contrast venography. Circulation 79:810, 1989.
10. Boccalon H, Candelon B, Doll HG, et al: Noninvasive electromagnetic measurement of the peripheral pulsatile blood flow: Experimental study and clinical applications. Cardiovasc Res 12:66, 1978.
11. Bone GE, Pomajzl MJ: Toe blood pressure by photoplethysmography: An index of healing in forefoot amputation. Surgery 89:569, 1981.
12. Bruner JMR, Krenis LJ, Kunsman JM, et al: Comparison of direct and indirect methods of measuring arterial blood pressure. Med Instrum 15:11, 1981.
13. Carter SA: Clinical measurement of systolic pressure in limbs with arterial occlusive disease. JAMA 207:1869, 1969.
14. Castronuovo JJ, Pabst TS, Flanigan DP, et al: Noninvasive determination of skin perfusion pressure using a laser Doppler. J Cardiovasc Surg 28:253, 1987.
15. Cina C, Katsamouris A, Megerman J, et al: Utility of transcutaneous oxygen tension measurements in peripheral arterial occlusive disease. J Vasc Surg 1:362, 1984.
16. Clark LC Jr: Monitor and control of tissue oxygen tensions. Trans Am Soc Artif Intern Organs 2:41, 1956.
17. Clyne CAC, Ryan J, Webster JHH, et al: Oxygen tension on the skin of ischemic legs. Am J Surg 143:315, 1982.
18. Coughlan BA, Taylor MG: Directional Doppler techniques for detection of blood velocities. Ultrasound Med Biol 2:181, 1976.
19. Craxford AD, Chamberlain J: Pulse wave form transit ratios in the assessment of peripheral vascular disease. Br J Surg 64:449, 1977.
20. Darling RE, Raines JK, Brener BJ, et al: Quantitative segmental pulse volume recorder: A clinical tool. Surgery 72:873, 1972.
21. DePater L, VandenBerg JW, Bueno AA: A very sensitive photoplethysmograph using scattered light and a photosensitive resistance. Acta Physiol Pharmacol Neerl 10:378, 1962.
22. Dohn K: Three plethysmographs usable during functional states recording volume changes in ml per 100 ml of extremity. Rep Steno Mem Hosp 6:147, 1956.
23. Doppler C: Uber das Farbige Licht der Dopplesterne und einiger anderer Gestirne des Himmels. Abh K Boh Ges Wiss (Prague) 2:465, 1842.
24. Fitzgerald DE, Gosling RG, Woodcock JP: Grading dynamic capability of arterial collateral circulation. Lancet 1:66, 1971.
25. Flax SW, Webster JG, Updike SJ: Statistical evaluation of the Doppler ultrasonic flowmeter. Biomed Sci Instrum 7:201, 1970.
26. Flax SW, Webster JG, Updike SJ: Pitfalls using Doppler ultrasound to transduce blood flow. IEEE Trans Biomed Eng 20:309, 1973.
27. Franzeck VK, Talke P, Bernstein EF, et al: Transcutaneous Po_2 measurements in health and peripheral arterial disease. Surgery 91:156, 1982.
28. Fronek A: Noninvasive evaluation of the cutaneous circulation. *In* Bernstein EF (ed): Noninvasive Diagnostic Techniques in Vascular Disease. 3rd ed. St. Louis, CV Mosby Co, 1985, pp 694–707.
29. Gabe IT: Pressure measurement in experimental physiology. *In* Bergel DH (ed): Cardiovascular Fluid Dynamics. London, Academic Press, 1972, vol. 1, pp 11–50.
30. Gershon-Cohen J, Haberman-Brueschke JD, Brueschke EE: Medical thermography. Radiol Clin 3:403, 1965.
31. Gill RW: Measurement of blood flow by ultrasound: Accuracy and sources of error. Ultrasound Biol Med 11:625, 1985.
32. Gosling RG, Dunbar G, King DH, et al: The quantitative analysis of occlusive peripheral arterial disease by a nonintrusive ultrasonic technique. Angiology 22:52, 1971.
33. Gosling RG, King DH: Continuous wave ultrasound as an alternative and complement to x-rays in vascular examination. *In* Reneman RS (ed): Cardiovascular Applications of Ultrasound. New York, Elsevier North-Holland, 1974, pp 266–282.
34. Gothgen I, Jacobsen E: Transcutaneous oxygen tension measurement. I. Age variation and reproducibility. Acta Anaesthesiol Scand 67 (Suppl): 66, 1978.
35. Green IL, Taylor AD, Greenhalgh RM: Femoral artery pulse rise time: An objective test for aortoiliac disease. Eur J Vasc Surg 1:121, 1987.
36. Greene FM Jr, Beach K, Strandness DE Jr: Computer-based pattern recognition of carotid arterial disease using pulsed Doppler ultrasound. Ultrasound Biol Med 8:161, 1982.
37. Gundersen J: Segmental measurement of systolic blood pressure in the extremities including the thumb and great toe. Acta Chir Scand Suppl 426:1, 1972.
38. Harris PL, Taylor LA, Cave FD, et al: The relationship between Doppler ultrasound assessment and angiography in occlusive arterial disease of the lower limbs. Surg Gynecol Obstet 138:911, 1974.
39. Harward TRS, Bernstein EF, Fronek A: The value of power frequency spectrum analysis in the identification of aortoiliac disease. J Vasc Surg 5:803, 1987
40. Heintz SE, Bone GE, Slaymaker EE, et al: Value of arterial pressure measurements in the proximal and distal part of the thigh in arterial occlusive disease. Surg Gynecol Obstet 146:337, 1978.
41. Hewlett AW, van Zwaluwenburg JG: The rate of blood flow in the arm. Heart 1:87, 1909.
42. Hill CR: Ultrasonic attenuation and scattering by tissues. *In* deVlieger M, Holmes JH, Kazner E, et al (eds): Handbook of Clinical Ultrasound. New York, John Wiley & Sons, 1978, pp 91–98.
43. Hokanson DE, Sumner DS, Strandness DE Jr: An electrically calibrated plethysmograph for direct measurement of limb blood flow. IEEE Trans Biomed Eng 22:25, 1975.
44. Holstein P, Sager P, Lassen NA: Wound healing in below-knee amputations in relation to skin perfusion pressure. Acta Orthop Scand 50:49, 1979.
45. Jansson IG, Thomsen MB, Elfstrom JL: Bilateral ankle skin temperature as a predictor of early graft patency. Br J Surg 74:795, 1987.
46. Johnston KW, Baker WH, Burnham SJ, et al: Quantitative analysis of continuous-wave Doppler spectral broadening for the diagnosis of carotid disease: Results of a multicenter study. J Vasc Surg 4:493, 1986.
47. Johnston KW, Kassam M, Cobbold RSC: Relationship between Doppler pulsatility index and direct femoral pressure measurements in the diagnosis of aortoiliac occlusive disease. Ultrasound Med Biol 9:271, 1983.

48. Johnston KW, Marruzzo BC, Cobbold RSC: Doppler methods for quantitative measurement and localization of peripheral arterial occlusive disease. Ultrasound Med Biol 4:209, 1978.
49. Comerota AJ, Katz ML, Greenwald AA, et al: Venous duplex imaging: Should it replace hemodynamic tests for deep venous thrombosis? J Vasc Surg 14:780, 1991.
50. Junger M, Chapman BLW, Underwood CJ, et al: A comparison between two types of waveform analysis in patients with multisegmental arterial disease. Br J Surg 71:345, 1984.
51. Karanfilian RG, Lynch TG, Zirul VT, et al: The value of laser Doppler velocimetry and transcutaneous oxygen tension determination in predicting healing of ischemic forefoot ulcerations and amputations in diabetic and nondiabetic patients. J Vasc Surg 4:511, 1986.
52. Kassam MS, Cobbold RSC, Johnston KW, et al: Method for estimating the Doppler mean velocity waveform. Ultrasound Biol Med 8:537, 1982.
53. Kato K, Izumi T: A new ultrasonic Doppler flowmeter that can detect flow direction. Med Ultrasonics 5:28, 1967.
54. Keagy BA, Palmer GJ, Crouch JD, et al: The use of angiodynography to quantify blood flow in the canine aorta. J Vasc Surg 6:269, 1987.
55. Kempczinski RF: Vascular diagnostic laboratory: Organization and operation. *In* Kempczinski RF, Yao JST (eds): Practical Noninvasive Vascular Diagnosis. 2nd ed. Chicago, Year Book Medical Publishers, 1987, pp 2–15.
56. Kirkendall WM, Burton AC, Epstein FH, et al: Recommendations for human blood pressure determination by sphygmomanometers. Circulation 36:980, 1967.
57. Kohler TR, Nance DR, Cramer MM, et al: Duplex scanning for diagnosis of aortoiliac and femoropopliteal disease: A prospective study. Circulation 76:1074, 1987.
58. Kohler TR, Nicholls SC, Zierler RE, et al: Assessment of pressure gradient by Doppler ultrasound: Experimental and clinical observations. J Vasc Surg 6:460, 1987.
59. Lee B, Trainor F, Kavner D, et al: A clinical evaluation of a noninvasive electromagnetic flowmeter. Angiology 26:317, 1975.
60. Lee BY, Trainor FS, Madden JL: Liquid crystal tape: Its use in the evaluation of vascular diseases. Arch Phys Med Rehab 54:96, 1973.
61. Long JW Jr, Stevens R, Lichti E, et al: Reliability of continuous-wave Doppler probes. J Vasc Surg 5:558, 1987.
62. MacPherson DS, Evans DH: Pulsatility index, transfer function analysis, and principal component analysis. A comparison of their value in detecting the severity of implanted stenoses in an animal model. *In* Puel P, Boccalon H, Enjalbert A (eds): Hemodynamics of the limbs—2. Toulouse, France, GEPESC, 1981, pp 35–42.
63. MacPherson DS, Evans DH, Bell PRF: Common femoral artery Doppler waveforms: A comparison of three methods of objective analysis with direct pressure measurements. Br J Surg 71:46, 1984.
64. Mason DT, Braunwald E: A simplified plethysmographic system for the measurement of systemic arterial pressure and peripheral blood flow. Am Heart J 64:796, 1962.
65. McLeod FD: Directional Doppler demodulation. Proc Ann Conf Eng Med Biol 9:27, 1967.
66. Megerman J, Abbott WM: Transcutaneous oxygen tension determination. *In* Kempczinski RF, Yao JST (eds): Practical Noninvasive Vascular Diagnosis. 2nd ed. Chicago, Year Book Medical Publishers, 1987, pp 210–228.
67. Mills CM, Brant-Zawadzki M, Crooks LE, et al: Nuclear magnetic resonance: Principles of blood flow imaging. AJR 142:165, 1984.
68. Mohapatra SN, Arenson HM: The measurement of peripheral blood flow by the electrical impedance technique. J Med Eng Technol 3:132, 1979.
69. Morris RL, Histand MB, Miller CW: The resolution of the ultrasound pulsed Doppler for velocity measurements. J Biomech 6:701, 1973.
70. Nicholls SC, Kohler TR, Martin RL, et al: Diastolic flow as a predictor of arterial stenosis. J Vasc Surg 3:498, 1986.
71. Nicolaides AN, Gordon-Smith IC, Dayandas J, et al: The value of Doppler blood velocity tracings in the detection of aortoiliac disease in patients with intermittent claudication. Surgery 80:774, 1976.
72. Nilsson GE, Tenland T, Oberg PA: A new instrument for continuous measurement of tissue blood flow by light beating spectroscopy. IEEE Trans Biomed Eng 27:12, 1980.
73. Nilsson GE, Tenland T, Oberg PA: Evaluation of a laser Doppler flowmeter for measurement of tissue blood flow. IEEE Trans Biomed Eng 27:12, 1980.
74. Nippa JH, Hokanson DE, Lee DR, et al: Phase rotation for separating forward and reverse blood velocity signals. IEEE Trans Sonics Ultrasonics 22:340, 1975.
75. O'Donnell JA, Hobson RW II: Comparison of electrical impedance and mechanical plethysmography. J Surg Res 25:459, 1978.
76. Parrish D, Strandness DE Jr, Bell JW: Dynamic response characteristics of a mercury-in-Silastic strain-gauge. J Appl Physiol 10:363, 1964.
77. Peronneau PA, Hinglais JR, Xhaard J, et al: The effects of curvature and stenosis on pulsatile blood flow in vivo and in vitro. *In* Reneman RS (ed): Cardiovascular Applications of Ultrasound. New York, Elsevier North-Holland, 1974, pp 203–215.
78. Pollak EW, Chavis P, Wolfman EF Jr: The effect of postural changes upon the ankle arterial perfusion pressure. Vasc Surg 10:219, 1976.
79. Porter JM, Snider RL, Bardana EJ, et al: The diagnosis and treatment of Raynaud's phenomenon. Surgery 77:11, 1975.
80. Raines JK: Diagnosis and analysis of arteriosclerosis in the lower limbs from the arterial pressure pulse. PhD dissertation, Massachusetts Institute of Technology, Cambridge, 1972.
81. Raines JK, Darling RG, Buth J, et al: Vascular laboratory criteria for the management of peripheral vascular disease of the lower extremities. Surgery 79:21, 1976.
82. Reneman RS, Clarke HF, Simmons N, et al: In vivo comparison of electromagnetic and Doppler flowmeters: With special attention to the processing of the analogue Doppler flow signal. Cardiovasc Res 7:557, 1973.
83. Reneman RS, van Merode T, Hick P, et al: Flow velocity patterns in and distensibility of the carotid artery bulb in subjects of various ages. Circulation 71:500, 1985.
84. Rhodes RS, Cohen AM: Magnetic resonance imaging and spectroscopy in the study of cardiovascular disease. J Vasc Surg 2:354, 1985.
85. Rijsterborgh H, Roelandt J: Doppler assessment of aortic stenosis: Bernoulli revisited. Ultrasound Med Biol 13:241, 1987.
86. Rittgers SE, Putney WW, Barnes RW: Real-time spectrum analysis and display of directional Doppler ultrasound blood velocity signals. IEEE Trans Biomed Eng 27:723, 1980.
87. Rittgers SE, Thornhill BM, Barnes RW: Quantitative analysis of carotid Doppler spectral waveforms. Ultrasound Med Biol 9:255, 1983.
88. Rushmer RF, Baker DW, Stegall HF: Transcutaneous Doppler flow detection as a nondestructive technique. J Appl Physiol 21:554, 1968.
89. Salles-Cunha SX, Battocletti JH, Towne JB, et al: Transcutaneous electromagnetic flowmetry. *In* Puel P, Boccalon H, Enjalbert A (eds): Hemodynamics of the Limbs—2. Toulouse, France, GEPESC, 1981, pp 25–34.
90. Satomura S: Study of flow patterns in peripheral arteries by ultrasonics. J Acoust Soc Jpn 15:151, 1959.
91. Shercliffe JA: The Theory of Electromagnetic Flow Measurement. Cambridge, MA, Cambridge University Press, 1962.
92. Shoor PM, Fronek A, Bernstein EF: Quantitative transcutaneous arterial velocity measurements with Doppler flowmeters. Arch Surg 114:922, 1979.
93. Sigdell JE: A critical review of the theory of the mercury strain-gauge plethysmograph. Med Biol Eng 7:365, 1969.
94. Simpson J, Jamieson G, Dickhaus D, et al: Effect of cuff bladder on accuracy of measurements of indirect blood pressure. Am Heart J 70:208, 1965.
95. Skidmore R, Woodcock JP: Physiologic interpretation of Doppler-shift waveforms. I. Theoretical considerations. Ultrasound Biol Med 6:7, 1980.
96. Skidmore R, Woodcock JP: Physiologic interpretation of Doppler-shift waveforms. II. Validation of the Laplace transform method for characterization of the common femoral blood-velocity waveform. Ultrasound Biol Med 6:219, 1980.
97. Skidmore R, Woodcock JP, Wells PNT, et al: Physiologic interpretation of Doppler-shift waveforms. III. Clinical Results. Ultrasound Biol Med 6:227, 1980.
98. Spittell JA Jr, DeWolfe V, Hume M, et al: Prevention and early detection of peripheral vascular disease. Circulation 42:A-43, 1970.
99. Stegall HF, Kardon MB, Kemmerer WT: Indirect measurement of blood pressure by Doppler ultrasonic sphygmomanometry. J Appl Physiol 25:793, 1968.

100. Strandness DE Jr: Peripheral Arterial Disease: A Physiologic Approach. Boston, Little, Brown & Co, 1969.
101. Strandness DE Jr, Bell JE: Peripheral vascular disease. Diagnosis and objective evaluation using a mercury strain-gauge. Ann Surg 161(Suppl 1):1, 1965.
102. Strandness DE Jr, McCutcheon EP, Rushmer RF: Application of a transcutaneous Doppler flowmeter in evaluation of occlusive arterial disease. Surg Gynecol Obstet 122:1039, 1966.
103. Strandness DE Jr, Radke HM, Bell JW: Use of a new simplified plethysmograph in the clinical evaluation of patients with arteriosclerosis obliterans. Surg Gynecol Obstet 112:751, 1961.
104. Strandness DE Jr, Schultz RD, Sumner DS, et al: Ultrasonic flow detection: A useful technique in the evaluation of peripheral vascular disease. Am J Surg 113:320, 1967.
105. Strandness DE Jr, Sumner DS: Hemodynamics for Surgeons. Orlando, FL, Grune & Stratton, 1975.
106. Sumner DS: Presidential address: Noninvasive testing of vascular disease—Fact, fancy, and future. Surgery 93:664, 1983.
107. Hull R, Van Aken WG, Hirsh J, et al: Impedance plethysmography using the occlusive cuff technique in the diagnosis of venous thrombosis. Circulation 53:696, 1976.
108. Sumner DS: Volume plethysmography in vascular disease: An overview. *In* Bernstein EF (ed): Noninvasive Diagnostic Techniques in Vascular Disease. 3rd ed. St. Louis, CV Mosby Co, 1985, pp 97–118.
109. Sumner DS: Mercury strain-gauge plethysmography. *In* Bernstein EF (ed): Noninvasive Diagnostic Techniques in Vascular Disease. 3rd ed. St. Louis, CV Mosby Co, 1985, pp 133–150.
110. Van Bemmelen PJ, Bedford G, Strandness DE Jr: Quantitative segmental evaluation of venous valvular reflux with ultrasonic duplex scanning. J Vasc Surg 10:425, 1989.
111. Sumner DS: Ultrasound. *In* Kempczinski RF, Yao JST (eds): Practical Noninvasive Vascular Diagnosis. 2nd ed. Chicago, Year Book Medical Publishers, 1987, pp 44–79.
112. Terry HJ: The electromagnetic measurement of blood flow during arterial surgery. Biomed Eng 7:466, 1972.
113. Terry HJ: The electromagnetic flowmeter. *In* Verstraete M (ed): Methods in Angiology. The Hague, Martinus Nijhoff Publishers, 1980, pp 21–37.
114. Terry HJ, Taylor GW: Quantitation of blood flow in femoropopliteal grafts. Surg Clin North Am 54:85, 1974.
115. Thiele BL, Bandyk DF, Zierler RE, et al: A systematic approach to the assessment of aortoiliac disease. Arch Surg 118:477, 1983.
116. Tonnesen KH: Transcutaneous oxygen tension in imminent foot gangrene. Acta Anaesthesiol Scand 68:107, 1978.
117. Uretzky G, Palti Y: A method for comparing transmitted and reflected light plethysmography. J Appl Physiol 31:132, 1971.
118. Weissenhofer W, Schmidt R, Schenk WG Jr: Technique of electromagnetic blood flow measurements: Notes regarding a potential source of error. Surgery 73:474, 1973.
119. Wetterer E: Flowmeters: Their theory, construction, and operation methods based on the electromagnetic-induction principle. *In* Hamilton WF, Dow P (eds): Handbook of Physiology. Sec 2. Circulation. Baltimore, Williams & Wilkins, 1963, vol. II, pp 1311–1324.
120. Wheeler HB, Penny BC: Impedance plethysmography: Theoretic, experimental, and clinical considerations. *In* Bernstein EF (ed): Noninvasive Diagnostic Techniques in Vascular Disease. 3rd ed. St. Louis, CV Mosby Co, 1985, pp 119–132.
121. White RA, Nolan L, Harley D, et al: Noninvasive evaluation of peripheral vascular disease using transcutaneous oxygen tension. Am J Surg 144:68, 1982.
122. Whitney RJ: The measurement of volume changes in human limbs. J Physiol (Lond) 121:1, 1953.
123. Winsor T: Influence of arterial disease on the systolic blood pressure gradients of the extremity. Am J Med Sci 220:117, 1950.
124. Woodcock JP: Theory and Practice of Blood Flow Measurement. London, Butterworth & Co, 1975.
125. Yao JST, Graham LM, Ricco J-B, et al: Application of the electromagnetic flowmeter in reconstructive vascular surgery. *In* Rutherford RB (ed): Vascular Surgery. 2nd ed. Philadelphia, WB Saunders, 1984, pp 136–147.
126. Yao JST, Hobbs JT, Irvine WT: Ankle systolic pressure measurements in arterial diseases affecting the lower extremities. Br J Surg 56:676, 1969.
127. Zatina MA, Berkowitz HD, Gross GM, et al: ^{31}P nuclear magnetic resonance spectroscopy: Noninvasive biochemical analysis of the ischemic extremity. J Vasc Surg 3:411, 1986.
128. Abramowitz HB, Queral LA, Flinn WR, et al: The use of photoplethysmography in the assessment of venous insufficiency: A comparison to venous pressure measurements. Surgery 86:434, 1979.
129. Christepouldos DV, Nicholaides AN, Szendro G, et al: Air plethysmography and effect of elastic compression on leg vein hemodynamics. J Vasc Surg 5:148, 1987.
130. Carter SA: Response of ankle systolic pressure to leg exercise in mild or questionable arterial disease. N Engl J Med 287:578, 1972.
131. Kohler TR, Nance DR, Cramer MM, et al: Duplex scanning for diagnosis of aortoiliac and femoropopliteal disease: A prospective study. Circulation 76:1074, 1987.
132. Bandyk DF, Schmitt DD, Seabrook GR, et al: Monitoring functional patency of in-situ saphenous vein bypasses. J Vasc Surg 9:286, 1989.
133. Porter JM, Rivers SP, Anderson OJ, et al: Evaluation and management of patients with Raynaud's syndrome. Am J Surg 142:183, 1981.
134. Nichols SC, Kohler TR, Martin BS, Strandness DE Jr: Use of hemodynamic parameters in the diagnosis of mesenteric insufficiency. J Vasc Surg 3:507, 1986.
135. Kohler TR, Zierler RE, Martin RL, et al: Non-invasive diagnosis of renal artery stenosis by ultrasonic duplex scanning. J Vasc Surg 4:450, 1986.
136. Fleischer AC, Hinton AA, Glick AD, Johnson K: Duplex Doppler sonography of renal transplants. Correlation with histopathology. J Ultrasound Med 8:89, 1989.

5

Physiologic Assessment of Peripheral Arterial Occlusive Disease

R. Eugene Zierler, M.D., and David S. Sumner, M.D.

• • •

As pointed out in the introduction to this section, peripheral arterial surgery should be designed to treat a physiologic rather than an anatomic defect. It makes little difference how aesthetically unappealing the arteriosclerotic plaque becomes if it does not restrict blood flow. The mere presence of disease, however widespread, rarely causes any problems. Aneurysms, with their potential for rupture, are, of course, an exception.

For these reasons, the surgeon who evaluates peripheral arterial disease must concentrate on the physiologic defects that the lesions produce. From the history, the surgeon gains an appreciation of how these defects limit the patient's activities. Unfortunately, the interpretation of symptoms is highly subjective, from both the patient's and the surgeon's point of view. Beyond a gross estimate of the physiologic limitations imposed by claudication or the suffering due to rest pain, the history yields nothing measurable. The physical examination affords more objectivity, in that pulses can be graded, ischemic ulcers measured, gangrenous areas delineated, and pallor, dependent rubor, and skin temperature noted. But even the most skilled surgical diagnostician will make some errors; and the nonspecialist physician will make many more.[10, 155, 174] Quite frequently, the physical examination fails to provide an accurate assessment of the severity of the disease.

Arteriography serves to define the anatomic lesion. Although good x-ray films are indispensable for most vascular surgery, they provide little objective data regarding physiologic disability. From clinical experience, the surgeon may have a fairly good idea of the type of limitations to be expected when the patient presents with an iliac occlusion, a superficial femoral occlusion, or multi-level disease. He or she may also be able to estimate the efficacy of the collateral circulation. Nevertheless, the experienced surgeon will recall many cases in which lesions shown on radiographs produced considerably more or less disability than expected.

Thus, a comprehensive assessment of atherosclerotic occlusive disease requires the integration of physiologic, anatomic, and clinical information. This chapter reviews the diagnostic information that can be derived from the noninvasive instruments and methods introduced in Chapter 4 and then discusses the application of this information to specific clinical situations.

PRESSURE MEASUREMENT

Measurement of pressure has distinct advantages over the measurement of flow for identifying the presence of arterial disease and for assessing its severity. Even though resting flow levels remain normal, there is almost always a pressure drop across an increased arterial resistance—even at rest.[42, 240, 253, 268, 272] Pressure measurements can be made more sensitive by augmenting blood flow through a stenotic segment. This can be accomplished by exercise, by reactive hyperemia, or by the intra-arterial administration of vasodilating drugs. With increased blood flow, pressure drops are greater, and even those that were not noticeable under baseline conditions become evident (see Figs. 3–14 to 3–17).[14, 32, 43, 231, 272]

Ankle Pressure

Of all the noninvasive tests available for evaluating the functional severity of peripheral arterial disease, none is more useful than measurement of systolic blood pressure at the ankle. Not only does it provide a simple, reliable means of diagnosing obstructive arterial disease but it is also readily applicable to follow-up studies.

The method has been described in Chapter 4. A pneumatic cuff is wrapped around the ankle and a Doppler probe is placed over the posterior tibial or dorsalis pedis artery. Ordinarily, the pressure measured at these two sites should differ by no more than 10 mmHg. A pressure difference greater than 15 mmHg suggests that there is a proximal occlusion or stenosis in the artery with the lower pressure.[42] The pressure at the site giving the highest value is taken as the ankle pressure.

At times, no audible Doppler signal can be obtained over either the posterior tibial or the dorsalis pedis artery. In these cases, a careful search will often reveal a peroneal collateral signal anteriorly, near the lateral malleolus. When no Doppler signal can be found, the ankle pressure can be measured with a plethysmograph placed around the foot or applied to one of the toes.

Normally, the systolic pressure at the ankle exceeds that in the arm by 12 ± 8 to 24 ± 9 mmHg.[27, 43, 151] This reflects the augmentation of the systolic pressure that occurs

Table 5–1. Segmental Pressure Indices in Normal Subjects (mean ± SD)*

Author and Year	Thigh	Above Knee	Below Knee	Ankle
Carter (1968)[41]	—	1.16 ± 0.05§	—	1.15 ± 0.08‡
Yao (1970, 1973)[272, 273]	—	—	—	1.11 ± 0.10
Wolf et al (1972)[268]	—	—	—	1.09 ± 0.08†
Fronek et al (1973)[80]	1.34 ± 0.27‖	1.32 ± 0.23‖	1.26 ± 0.24‖	1.08 ± 0.10‡
Cutajar et al (1973)[61]	1.53 ± 0.17†	—	1.17 ± 0.13‡	1.08 ± 0.09‡
Hajjar and Sumner (1976)[94]	1.37 ± 0.20†	1.26 ± 0.11†	1.16 ± 0.10†	1.08 ± 0.08†
Rutherford et al (1979)[207]	1.28 ± 0.17†	1.24 ± 0.17†	1.16 ± 0.17†	1.08 ± 0.17†

**Pressure index equals systolic pressure at site of measurement divided by brachial systolic pressure.*
†Cuff 10 × 40 cm.
‡Cuff 12.5 × 30 cm (standard).
§Cuff 15 × 45 cm.
‖Cuff 17 × 50 cm.

as the pressure wave travels peripherally. Distal to a hemodynamically significant lesion, the ankle pressure is almost invariably decreased.[27, 236, 240, 241] A single stenosis of 50 per cent or more or multiple mild irregularities of the arterial lumen will reduce the ankle pressure by at least 10 mmHg.[210] Typical ankle-arm pressure gradients are: isolated superficial femoral obstruction, 53 ± 10 mmHg; isolated aortoiliac obstruction, 61 ± 15 mmHg; and multilevel obstruction, 91 ± 23 mmHg.[240]

Ankle-Brachial Index

Because the ankle systolic blood pressure varies with the central aortic pressure, it is convenient to normalize the values by dividing the ankle pressure by the brachial blood pressure.[41, 42, 266, 276] This ratio, which is commonly referred to as the ankle pressure index or ankle-brachial index (ABI), normally averages about 1.1 when the well-rested subject is lying supine (Table 5–1). Although an occasional patient with functionally significant arterial stenosis will have an ABI that exceeds 1.0,[1, 41, 79, 184, 276] in the vast majority of patients with arterial disease, the resting index will be much lower.[1, 61, 268, 273, 276] In fact, an ABI less than 1.0 is highly suggestive of functional arterial obstruction;[41, 42, 61, 272, 273] only rarely does a normal limb have an index less than 0.92.[94, 184]

As shown in Figure 5–1 and Table 5–2, the ABI varies somewhat with the location of the arterial obstruction.[240, 268, 273] Values tend to be highest when the lesion is confined to the popliteal or below-knee arteries and lowest in limbs with multi-level disease.[42, 207, 268, 276] Carter found that the ABI exceeded 0.50 in 85 per cent of patients with a single block but was below 0.50 in 91 per cent of those with two or more blocks.[42] In addition, the ABI decreases as the functional severity of the disease increases, the lowest values being obtained in limbs with impending gangrene and the highest in limbs with mild claudication (Fig. 5–2).[61, 185, 194, 197, 272, 273] The ABI also correlates with arteriographic findings.[210, 276] Values are lowest when there is complete occlusion and highest when there is minimal atheromatous change (Fig. 5–3).[41, 61, 250, 276] As one would predict, based on the hemodynamic principles outlined in Chapter 3, the length of the occlusive process and the length of the bypassing collaterals are less important than their diameters.[66]

Since the ABI is reasonably stable from one examination to the next in the same individual (provided there is not change in the obstructive process), it constitutes an effective means of following the patient's course. A consistent decrease indicates advancing disease or a failure of arterial reconstruction.[23, 167, 168, 183, 244] A spontaneous rise in the ABI is usually attributable to the development of collateral circulation.[218, 219] After successful reconstructive surgery, there will be an increase in the ABI.[61, 233, 243, 244, 276] If all obstructions have been totally removed or bypassed, the index will exceed 1.0; however, if there are residual sites of obstruction, the ABI will increase, although not to normal levels (Fig. 5–4).[243]

Table 5–2. Segmental Pressure Indices in Patients With Occlusive Arterial Disease of the Legs (mean ± SD)*

Location of Obstruction	Author and Year	Upper Thigh	Above Knee	Below Knee	Ankle
Aortoiliac	Fronek et al (1973)[80]	0.72 ± 0.25	0.70 ± 0.24	0.62 ± 0.21	0.57 ± 0.18
	Rutherford et al (1979)[207]	0.81 ± 0.25	0.76 ± 0.25	0.71 ± 0.25	0.68 ± 0.32
	Ramsey et al (1979)[196]	0.81 ± 0.27	0.72 ± 0.25	0.59 ± 0.22	0.54 ± 0.22
Femoropopliteal	Fronek et al (1973)[80]	1.26 ± 0.39	0.92 ± 0.39	0.73 ± 0.30	0.51 ± 0.28
	Rutherford et al (1979)[207]	1.25 ± 0.27	0.86 ± 0.22	0.75 ± 0.18	0.65 ± 0.18
	Ramsey et al (1979)[196]	1.19 ± 0.21	0.87 ± 0.23	0.70 ± 0.18	0.60 ± 0.19
Combined aortoliac and femoropopliteal	Fronek et al (1973)[80]	0.97 ± 0.34	0.79 ± 0.32	0.61 ± 0.28	0.48 ± 0.31
	Rutherford et al (1979)[207]	0.89 ± 0.17	0.72 ± 0.17	0.58 ± 0.17	0.53 ± 0.28
	Ramsey et al (1979)[196]	0.79 ± 0.21	0.62 ± 0.17	0.49 ± 0.15	0.39 ± 0.15

**Pressure index equals systolic pressure at site of measurement divided by brachial systolic pressure.*

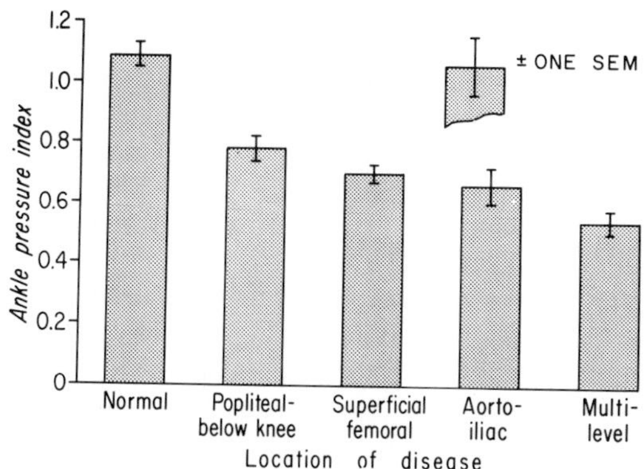

FIGURE 5–1. Resting ankle blood pressure indices (ankle systolic/arm systolic) measured in normal limbs and in limbs with arterial obstruction localized to different anatomic levels. (From Strandness DE Jr, Sumner DS: Hemodynamics for Surgeons. New York, Grune & Stratton, 1975; data from Wolf EA Jr, Sumner DS, Strandness DE Jr: Correlation between nutritive blood flow and pressure in limbs of patients with intermittent claudication. Surg Forum 23:238, 1972.)

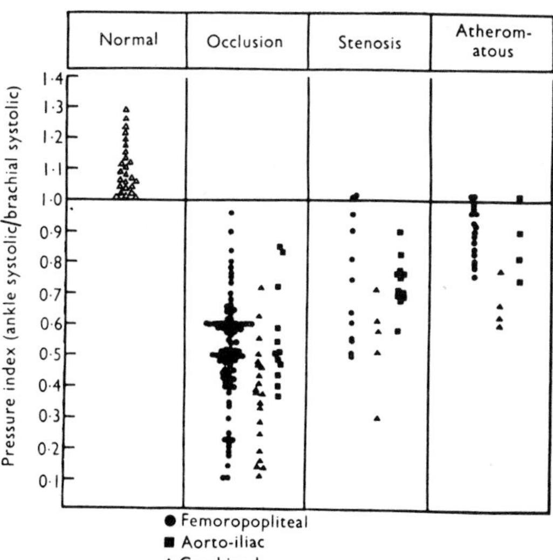

FIGURE 5–3. Relationship of ankle pressure index to the severity of the occlusive process. Note that the index exceeds 1.0 in all normal limbs in this series. (From Yao JST, Hobbs JT, Irvine WT: Ankle systolic pressure measurements in arterial diseases affecting the lower extremities. Br J Surg 56:676, 1969.)

Technical Errors

Ankle pressure measurements are easily made and are remarkably free of error. The standard deviation between two measurements repeated within a few minutes is about 5 mmHg, and only 8 to 9 mmHg when the measurements are repeated from one day to the next.[176] These figures do not take into account variations in central arterial pressure. When the ABI rather than the absolute value is considered, the day-to-day results are even more consistent. This test is also subject to interobserver and intraobserver variability, as well as to nonpathologic biologic variability. A change in the ABI of 0.15 or more almost certainly lies beyond the 95 per cent confidence limits of "normal" variation and therefore usually implies a significant physiologic change.[7, 120]

Medial calcification, which renders the underlying arteries incompressible, is responsible for most of the errors made in measuring ankle pressure.[79, 107, 194, 232, 245] Since pa-

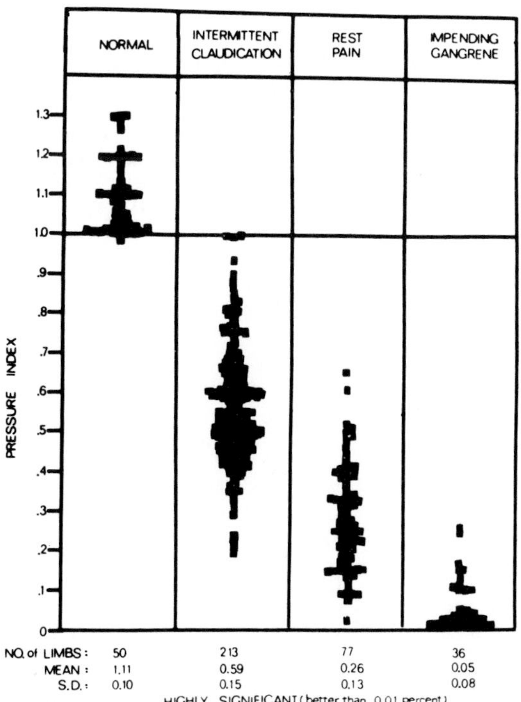

FIGURE 5–2. Relationship of ankle pressure index to functional impairment produced by the occlusive process. (From Yao JST: Hemodynamic studies in peripheral arterial disease. Br J Surg 57:761, 1970.)

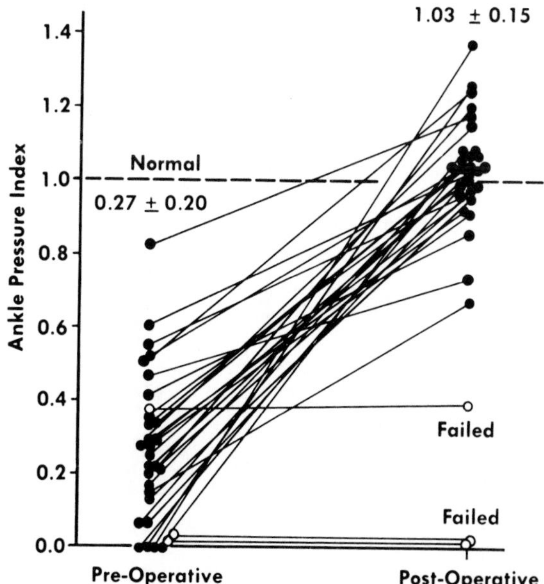

FIGURE 5–4. Results of femorotibial and femoroperoneal grafts. Ankle pressure indices before and after 31 bypass grafts from femoral to tibial, peroneal, or dorsalis pedis arteries. *Open circles* indicate grafts that failed within 30 days. Mean and standard deviations of the patent grafts are indicated. (From Sumner DS, Strandness DE Jr: Hemodynamic studies before and after extended bypass grafts to the tibial and peroneal arteries. Surgery 86:442, 1979.)

tients with diabetes are particularly prone to this problem, one can anticipate that ankle pressure measurements in diabetics may be 5 or 10 per cent too high.[194] In these cases, it is sometimes possible to estimate the pressure by elevating the foot and noting the vertical distance from the bed at the point at which the Doppler signal disappears.[86] Multiplying this distance (in centimeters) by 0.735 will give the pressure in mmHg.

Confusion between arterial and venous flow can also occur when the arterial flow velocity is decreased and the signal becomes less pulsatile.[1] Venous signals can, however, be distinguished from arterial signals with the directional Doppler flowmeter. Moreover, venous signals can be augmented by foot compression (see Chapter 131), but arterial signals either are not affected or will diminish. If doubt still remains, a plethysmograph can be substituted to sense the return of flow as the cuff is deflated.

Segmental Pressure

Further diagnostic information can be obtained by measuring the pressure gradient down the leg.[105, 128, 232, 266] Only rarely do these measurements need to be made when the ankle pressure is normal.[79]

The following is but one of a number of techniques that have been advocated. Pneumatic cuffs (width 10 cm) are placed around the thigh at groin level, around the thigh just above the knee, around the calf below the knee, and at ankle level. Blood pressure is measured at each level by the method described in Chapter 4 (see Fig. 4–14).

Upper Thigh Pressure

In most normal individuals, blood pressures measured with the cuff technique at the upper thigh exceed those measured at the brachial level by 30 to 40 mmHg.[1, 61, 105, 266] Indices, obtained by dividing the thigh pressure by the brachial pressure, are comparably elevated, averaging around 1.30 to 1.50 (see Table 5–1).

It must be remembered that these values do not accurately reflect the femoral artery pressure, which, when measured by invasive techniques, is almost identical to the brachial pressure.[187] Moreover, as indicated by the standard deviations in Table 5–1, upper thigh pressures are highly variable even in normal subjects. Owing to the disparity between cuff width and thigh diameter, higher pressures are obtained in patients with large thighs and lower, more accurate pressures are obtained in patients with small thighs.[232]

A thigh pressure equal to or lower than the arm pressure usually indicates hemodynamically significant aortoiliac disease.[61] When the thigh pressure exceeds arm pressure but exceeds it by less than 15 to 30 mmHg, iliac disease may be suspected but could be absent if the diameter of the thigh is small.[105, 207] Comparison of the pressures obtained from the two thighs is of some value in these cases.[80] A 20-mmHg difference is said to be significant; however, some authors have not found this difference to be a reliable indicator.[196]

Thigh pressure indices associated with aortoiliac obstructive disease are shown in Table 5–2 and Figure 5–5. It is apparent from Figure 5–5 that the thigh index may be lower than 1.0 in limbs with superficial femoral obstructions even when there is no hemodynamically significant

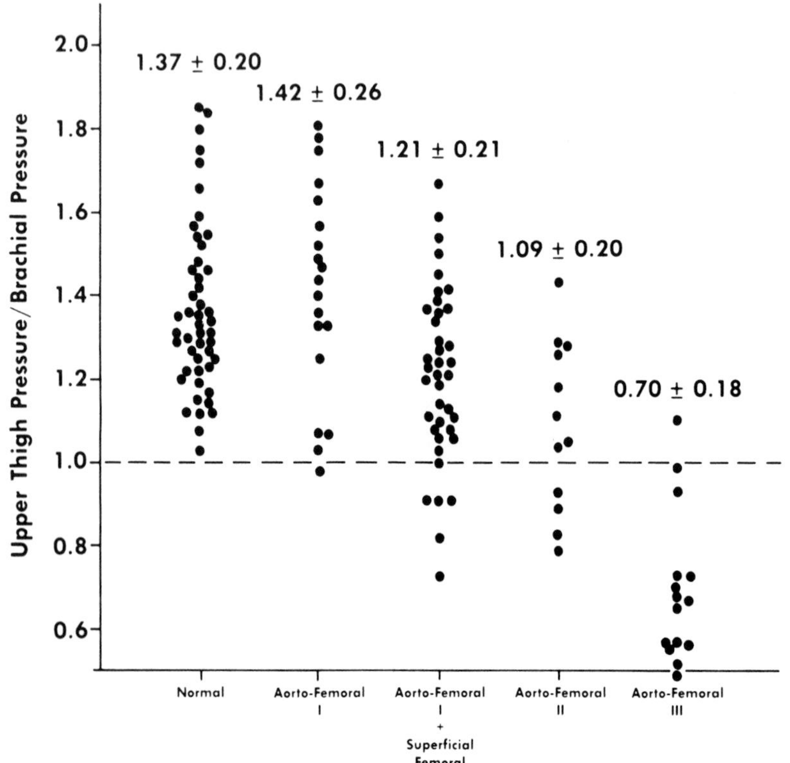

FIGURE 5–5. Identification of aortofemoral obstruction. Upper thigh index in normal limbs and in limbs with arteriosclerotic disease of the aortofemoral segment. Grading of aortofemoral disease is: I, less than 50 per cent diameter stenosis; II, more than 50 per cent diameter stenosis; and III, occlusion. Grades II and III are hemodynamically significant.

Table 5–3. Pressure Gradients in Normal Subjects (mean ± SD)

Author and Year	Arm–Upper Thigh	Upper Thigh–Above Knee	Above Knee–Below Knee	Below Knee–Ankle
Winsor (1950)[266]*	−22	13	11	8
Bell (1973)[19]†	−6 ± 12	2 ± 8	—	—
Hajjar and Sumner (1976)[94]‡	−46 ± 24	13 ± 19	12 ± 4	10 ± 9
Rutherford et al (1979)[207]‡	−35 ± 18	5 ± 12	10 ± 15	11 ± 15

Cuff 13 cm width.
†Cuff 18 × 60 cm.
‡Cuff 10 × 40 cm.

disease in the aortoiliac segment.[26] This is somewhat more likely to occur in the presence of concomitant stenosis of the profunda femoris artery. Although the thigh index seldom exceeds 1.0 in limbs with occlusion of the iliac artery, it is not uncommon to find normal indices in limbs with hemodynamically significant stenoses of the iliac arteries.[26] This is most likely to occur when the thighs are large. There is, however, another possible explanation. Because compression of the upper thigh by the cuff temporarily restricts arterial inflow, the pressure gradient across the external iliac artery is reduced. Consequently, when a stenosis is confined to this artery, the upper thigh reading may be spuriously high.[79]

If an upper thigh index of 1.0 is taken as the lower limit of normal, the data in Figure 5–5 indicate that there would be no mistakes in the normal control group; but in the patient groups, the sensitivity for detecting hemodynamically significant disease would be only 67 per cent, whereas the specificity for identifying the absence of disease would be 90 per cent.[207] Cutajar and coworkers reported that values over 1.20 are normal, those below 0.80 suggest occlusion, and those in between usually indicate the presence of aortoiliac occlusive disease.[61] According to these criteria, the data in Figure 5–5 show that only 10 per cent of the studies with indices exceeding 1.20 would be falsely classified as negative and that only 7 per cent of limbs with indices less than 0.80 would have no hemodynamically significant disease. Between these limits, however, significant disease was found in only 33 per cent. Moreover, 19 per cent of normal control limbs had indices below 1.20.

Pressure Gradients

Between any two adjacent levels in the normal leg, the pressure gradient usually does not exceed 20 to 30 mmHg (Table 5–3).[1, 232] Gradients greater than 30 mmHg strongly suggest that a significant degree of arterial obstruction is present in the intervening artery.[1, 84, 105] When the arterial segment is occluded, the gradient generally exceeds 40 mmHg.[80, 232] Rutherford and associates found that an upper thigh to above-knee gradient of 15 mmHg best distinguished limbs with superficial femoral occlusion from those without.[207] Similar gradients between the above-knee and the below-knee levels and between the below-knee and the ankle levels were found to have some predictive value related to disease in the popliteal and below-knee segments, respectively; but there was a great deal of overlap.

In addition to measuring "longitudinal" gradients along the leg, it is frequently helpful to compare pressures in one leg with those at the same level in the other leg. A "horizontal" difference of 20 mmHg in normotensive patients may be significant, implying greater disease at or above this level in the leg with the lower pressure.[80]

The ratio of the pressures at all levels in the leg to that in the arm should exceed 1.0 (see Tables 5–1 and 5–2). Values lower than this at any level imply significant obstructive disease in the proximal arteries. This is fairly reliable. Theoretically, by making both "longitudinal" and "horizontal" comparisons of the segmental pressures or indices, the examiner should be able to locate the site or sites of arterial obstruction and obtain some idea of their functional significance. Idealized values illustrating this point are shown in Table 5–4. Isolated disease in the aortoiliac or superficial femoral segments can usually be identified; but in limbs with multi-level disease, identification is frequently suboptimal. For example, superficial femoral obstructions may not produce an abnormal gradient in limbs with aortoiliac disease, iliac stenoses may not be recognized in limbs with superficial femoral disease, and below-knee disease is commonly misdiagnosed or overlooked when there is concomitant superficial femoral obstruction (Table 5–5).[105, 207]

Table 5–4. Typical Segmental Systolic Arterial Pressures (mmHg)

		Arterial Disease			
	Normal	*Iliac*	*Superficial Femoral*	*Iliac and Superficial Femoral*	*Below Knee*
Arm	120	120	120	120	120
Upper thigh	160	110	160	110	160
Above knee	250	100	100	70	150
Below knee	140	90	90	60	140
Ankle	130	80	80	50	90

Table 5–5. Accuracy of Segmental Pressures for Locating Arterial Obstructive Disease*

	Diagnosis Based on Segmental Pressure Data (%)					
Arteriographic Diagnosis	*Normal*	*Aortoiliac*	*Aortoiliac and Superficial Femoral*	*Superficial Femoral*	*Superficial Femoral and Popliteal*	*Popliteal*
Normal	97.2	1.4	—	—	1.4	—
Disease						
Aortoiliac	12.5	75.0	12.5	—	—	—
Aortoiliac and superficial femoral	6.3	6.3	78.0	3.1	6.3	—
Superficial femoral	15.0	—	10.0	55.0	15.0	5.0
Superficial femoral and popliteal	8.0	—	4.0	24.0	60.0	4.0
Popliteal	57.0	—	7.0	—	—	36.0

**Modified from Rutherford RB, Lowenstein DH, Klein MF: Combining segmental systolic pressures and plethysmography to diagnose arterial occlusive disease of the legs. Am J Surg 138:211, 1979.*

Note: *Popliteal includes popliteal artery or two or more of the peroneal-tibial arteries.*

The location and severity of lower extremity arterial lesions can be directly assessed by duplex scanning, as discussed later in this chapter.

Technical Errors

In an effort to achieve a more accurate assessment of the thigh pressure, some investigators have advocated using a single wide cuff (19 cm) rather than two 10-cm cuffs, one at the upper thigh and the other above the knee.[106] Gray and colleagues compared thigh pressures obtained with a wide cuff and direct measurements of the femoral arterial blood pressure in an effort to see how accurately the noninvasive pressure predicted aortoiliac disease.[91] A normal thigh-brachial index (exceeding 0.90) was generally reliable in ruling out inflow disease (only 13 per cent false-negative results). The thigh pressure, however, was spuriously low in 59 per cent of the studies, implying the presence of aortoiliac disease when in fact there was none. All of these false-positive errors occurred in limbs with occlusions of the superficial femoral artery. Thus, it would appear that the wide cuff is less accurate than the narrow cuff for diagnosing aortoiliac stenoses. Moreover, Heintz and associates have shown that detection of superficial femoral disease by means of the "wide cuff to below-knee pressure gradient" is considerably less accurate than it is with the narrow cuff technique, which allows gradients across both the thigh and the knee to be analyzed.[105] Others have reached similar conclusions.[75, 206]

Not infrequently, the pressure gradient between two adjacent segments of the leg may appear to be reversed. For example, the above-knee pressure may exceed that recorded at the upper thigh or the below-knee pressure may be greater than that recorded at the above-knee level. This reversal of the normal pattern of progression is usually due to local arterial incompressibility or to varying relationships between the size of the cuff and the limb.[1, 79] In hypertensive patients, the gradient between any two adjacent levels may be increased. On the other hand, when the cardiac output is low, the pressure drop may be diminished.[266]

Normal blood pressure gradients may be obtained in limbs with arterial obstructions when collateral channels are quite large. These findings do not really constitute errors, since the measurements are designed to reveal *functional* rather than *anatomic* obstruction.[232] For example, the pressure gradient from the below-knee level to the ankle is typically normal in limbs in which either the anterior tibial or the posterior tibial artery is patent.[1, 110, 152, 216, 232]

Obstructions of arteries such as the internal iliac or the profunda femoris, which are not directly responsible for perfusion of the distal leg and ankle, may be missed.[1, 41] As pointed out earlier in this chapter, occlusions of the profunda femoris artery will become evident when the superficial femoral artery is also occluded. In these cases, the profunda femoris constitutes the major collateral channel supplying the lower leg and foot. Therefore, if both of these arteries are obstructed, the upper thigh pressure will be abnormally low even though the aortoiliac segment is completely patent.

Because of the errors inherent in noninvasive assessment of the upper thigh pressure, direct femoral arterial pressure measurements, as discussed later in this chapter, are being used more frequently.[14, 32, 73, 165, 255] It should be noted, however, that direct pressure measurements are also subject to errors that are easily overlooked; most systems, for example, are underdamped, giving spuriously high systolic pressures.[36] Many laboratories also use segmental plethysmography or Doppler flow signal analysis to supplement segmental pressure studies.[194, 207]

Toe Pressure

Toe pressures are measured as described in Chapter 4.[54, 92, 147, 175] A pneumatic cuff of appropriate width (about 1.2 times the diameter of the digit) is wrapped around the proximal phalanx, and a flow sensor is applied distally. Although mercury strain-gauges work well for this purpose, photoplethysmographs, which are more stable and occupy less space on the tip of the digit, are generally more convenient to use.

At toe level, the systolic blood pressure is usually somewhat lower than the brachial pressure. According to Nielsen and associates, in the supine position, toe pressures of young normal individuals averaged 4.8 ± 6.6 mmHg

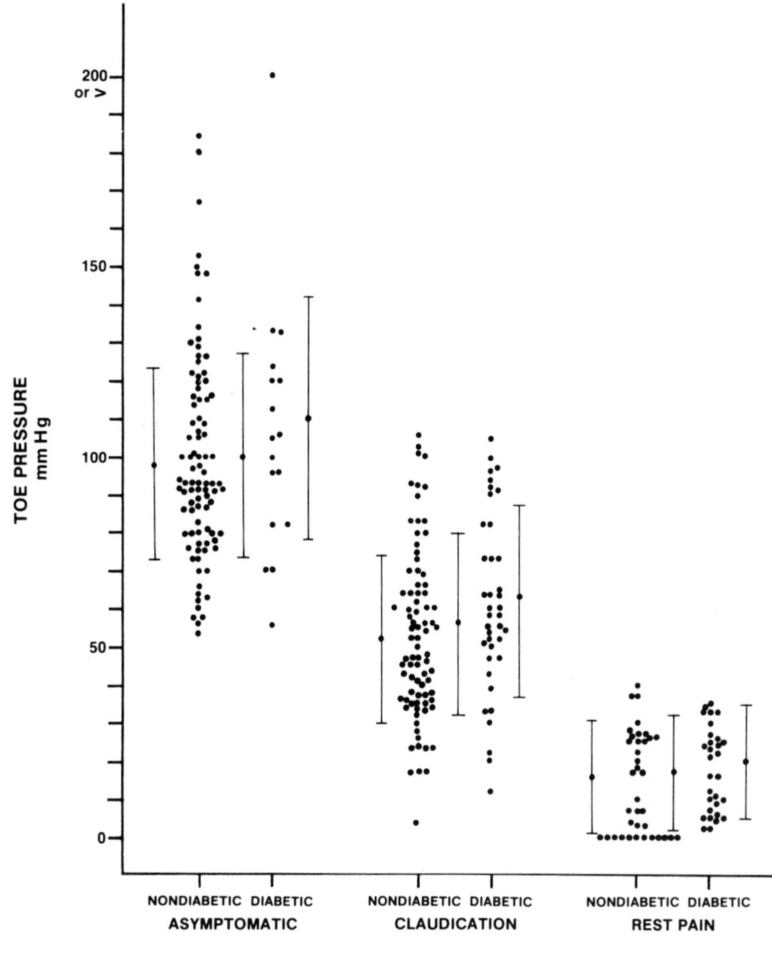

FIGURE 5–6. Toe blood pressures grouped according to symptoms and presence of diabetes in patients with arterial disease. Mean and standard deviations for the nondiabetic and diabetic subgroups and for the two groups combined are indicated by *vertical bars.* (From Ramsey DE, Manke DA, Sumner DS: Toe blood pressure—A valuable adjunct to ankle pressure measurement for assessing peripheral arterial disease. J Cardiovasc Surg 24:43, 1983.)

below those in the arm.[175] In older subjects, toe pressures were 9.8 ± 10.7 mmHg less than those in the arm.

Figure 5–6 shows the distribution of toe pressures in 296 limbs with arteriosclerosis obliterans.[197] No asymptomatic patient had a toe pressure less than 50 mmHg, and only 11 per cent of those whose complaints were limited to claudication had toe pressures less than 30 mmHg. In contrast, 81 per cent of the limbs with ischemic rest pain had toe pressures less than 30 mmHg, and none had pressures above 40 mmHg. Eighty-one per cent of the limbs with toe pressures less than 30 mmHg and almost all of those with pressures less than 15 mmHg had ischemic symptoms at rest. Patients with rest pain usually have toe pressures below 20 to 30 mmHg, but those with ischemic ulcers often have somewhat higher pressures.[45, 112, 197, 254]

Toe indices (toe pressure divided by brachial pressure) of patients with arteriosclerosis obliterans are listed in Table 5–6 according to the severity of their symptoms. Interestingly, there is little difference between the mean values of diabetic and nondiabetic patients. Spuriously high pressures due to arterial calcification (which is common in diabetics) seldom occur at toe level. For this reason, toe indices are a reliable indicator of the physiologic severity of arterial occlusive disease and should be used when there is any doubt about the validity of the ankle pressure.[260]

Toe pressures are particularly valuable for recognizing

Table 5–6. Toe Indices in Patients With Arterial Disease (mean ± SD)

		Claudication		Ischemia*	
Author and Year	**No Symptoms**	***Nondiabetic***	***Diabetic***	***Nondiabetic***	***Diabetic***
Carter and Lezack (1971)[45]	0.91 ± 0.13†	0.43 ± 0.17	0.42 ± 0.16	0.24 ± 0.14	0.19 ± 0.10
Vollrath et al (1980)[260]	0.89 ± 0.16	0.47 ± 0.24	0.60 ± 0.17	0.19 ± 0.15	0.16 ± 0.13‡
Ramsey et al (1983)[197]	0.72 ± 0.19	0.35 ± 0.15	0.38 ± 0.15	0.11 ± 0.10	0.12 ± 0.09

**Ischemic rest pain, ulcers, or gangrene.*
†Normal subjects, 52 ± 6 years old; 21 ± 4 years old: 0.86 ± 0.12.
‡Diet-controlled; insulin-dependent: 0.23 ± 0.15.

arterial disease confined to the pedal or digital arteries.[80] In limbs with ischemic ulcers or gangrene, normal ankle pressures and normal ankle pressure indices are often associated with toe pressures that lie in the ischemic range (Fig. 5–7).[110, 197]

Normally, toe pressures average 24 ± 7 to 41 ± 17 mmHg less than ankle pressures.[19, 45, 175] Ankle to toe gradients that exceed 44 mmHg in young patients or 64 mmHg in older patients are abnormal.[175] In our experience, the toe-ankle index (obtained by dividing the toe pressure by the ipsilateral ankle pressure) averaged 0.64 ± 0.20 in asymptomatic limbs, 0.52 ± 0.20 in claudicating limbs, and 0.23 ± 0.19 in limbs with ischemic rest pain or ulcers.[197] This suggests that obstruction of the pedal or digital arteries plays a major role in causing gangrene or ischemic rest pain.[260]

The use of toe pressures for predicting healing of foot lesions or amputations is discussed later in this chapter.

Penile Pressure

The penis is supplied by three paired arteries: the dorsal penile, the cavernosal (deep corporal), and the urethral (spongiosal) arteries. These vessels are terminal branches of the internal pudendal artery, which originates from the internal iliac, or hypogastric, artery. The cavernosal artery is most important for erectile function. Obstruction of any of the arteries leading to the corpora cavernosa—including the common iliac artery or terminal aorta—can be responsible for vasculogenic impotence.

A pneumatic cuff measuring 2.5 cm in width is applied to the base of the penis. Return of blood flow when the cuff is deflated can be detected by a mercury strain-gauge plethysmograph, a photoplethysmograph applied to the anterolateral aspect of the shaft, or a Doppler flow probe.* Although some investigators have positioned the probe over the dorsal penile arteries, others have emphasized the importance of detecting flow in the cavernosal artery.† Because the penile blood supply is paired and obstruction may occasionally be limited to only one side, it has been recommended that pressures be measured on both sides of the penis.[195]

In normal men under 40 years of age, the penile-brachial index (penile pressure divided by brachial systolic pressure) was found by Kempczinski to be 0.99 ± 0.15.[132] In other words, in the absence of any arterial disease, the penile and brachial pressures are roughly equivalent. Older men without symptoms of impotence tend to have lower indices.[132] Penile-brachial indices greater than 0.75 to 0.80 are considered compatible with normal erectile function; an index less than 0.60 is diagnostic of vasculogenic impotence, especially in patients with peripheral vascular disease.[48, 83, 132, 146, 171, 192] A brachial to penile pressure gradient less than 20 to 40 mmHg suggests adequate penile blood flow.[35, 132, 146] Gradients in excess of 60 mmHg suggest arterial insufficiency.[132]

Knowledge of the penile pressure can be used to guide the vascular surgeon in planning the operative approach to aneurysmal or obstructive lesions of the aorta and iliac arteries.[171] Maintenance of blood flow to the internal iliac artery will preserve potency, and restoration of flow to this

*See references: mercury strain-gauge plethysmograph, 35; photo plethysmograph, 146; Doppler flow probe, 132.

†See references: dorsal arteries, 192; cavernosal artery, 171.

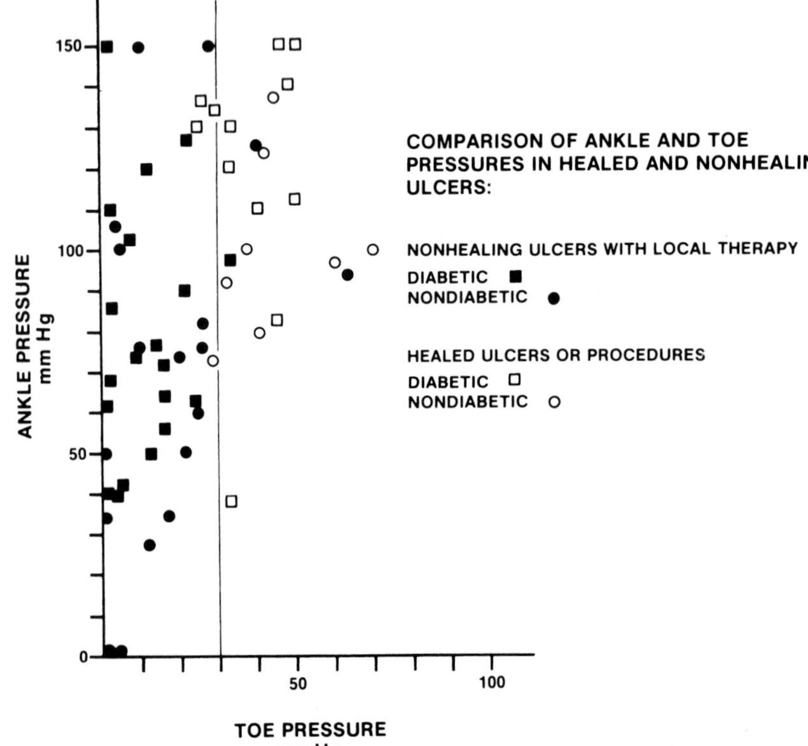

FIGURE 5–7. Comparison of ankle and toe pressures in 58 limbs with healed or nonhealing ischemic ulcers or toe amputations. Note that a toe pressure of 30 mmHg provides good separation between those limbs that healed and those that did not. *Solid symbols* indicate nonhealing ulcers: ■ diabetic, ● nondiabetic; *open symbols* indicate healed ulcers or procedures: □ diabetic, ○ nondiabetic. (From Ramsey DE, Manke DA, Sumner DS: Toe blood pressure—A valuable adjunct to ankle pressure measurement for assessing peripheral arterial disease. J Cardiovasc Surg 24:43, 1983.)

artery will often improve penile pressure and erectile function.[192]

Stress Testing

Exercise

Reducing the resistance of the peripheral vascular bed by having the patient exercise is an effective physiologic method for stressing the peripheral circulation (see Chapter 3). Under such stress, lesions that may not appear particularly significant at rest can be evaluated.[43] In addition, exercise testing allows the surgeon to better appreciate the functional disability that the arterial obstruction produces.[194] It also permits the surgeon to judge the relative magnitude of the disability produced by arterial obstruction in relation to the restrictions imposed by orthopedic, neurologic, or cardiopulmonary disease.

It should be emphasized that exercise testing (or other stress testing) is not required for the evaluation of patients with ischemia at rest. Patients with ischemic rest pain, ulcers, or gangrene will always have decreased digital artery pressures and will usually have low ankle pressures. Their disease is seldom subtle. Moreover, the vast majority of patients with claudication will have a decreased ankle pressure at rest; consequently, supplementary stress testing is only occasionally necessary to establish the diagnosis.[185] Nevertheless, exercise testing is indicated in certain selected patients for the reasons mentioned in the preceding paragraph. Therefore, it has a restricted but important role in the diagnostic armamentarium.

Although many different programs are possible, the following has proved reliable in the authors' hands. After the patient has rested supine for about 20 minutes, a baseline ankle pressure is obtained. The patient then walks on a treadmill at 2 mph up a 10 per cent grade for 5 minutes or until forced to stop because of claudication (or because of other restrictions). The time at which symptoms appear in the leg is noted as well as which muscle group is first affected. In addition, the final walking time is recorded.[240, 268]

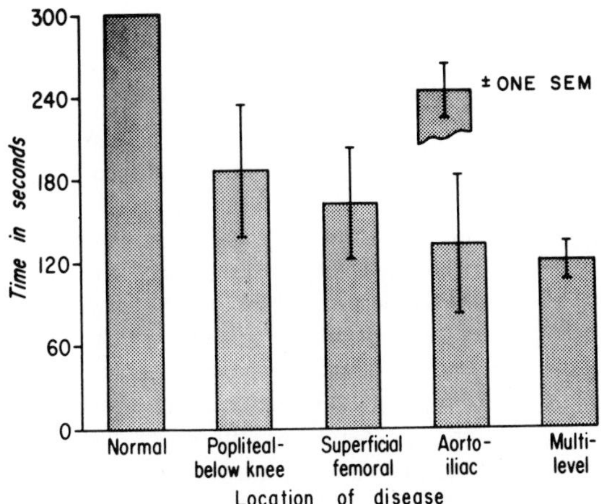

FIGURE 5–8. Treadmill walking times in patients with occlusive arterial disease. Normal subjects almost always will be able to exceed 5 minutes (300 seconds). Treadmill set at 2 mph, 12 per cent grade. (From Strandness DE Jr, Sumner DS: Hemodynamics for Surgeons. New York, Grune & Stratton, 1975.)

The patient then promptly assumes a supine position on the examining table. Ankle and arm pressures are obtained immediately and every 2 minutes until pre-examination levels are reached or until 20 minutes have elapsed. A normal individual, regardless of age, usually will be able to walk for 5 minutes and will experience little or no drop in ankle pressure.[136, 223, 226, 231, 268] Patients with obstructive arterial disease seldom will be able to walk for 5 minutes and will always experience an immediate drop in ankle pressure (Fig. 5–8; see also Figs. 3–14 to 3–17).[231, 240, 268] The magnitude of this drop reflects the extent of the functional disability. Patients with multi-level arterial disease usually will walk for a shorter distance and will experience a much more profound drop in ankle pressure.[268, 273] Often, the ankle pressure will be unobtainable for several minutes (see Figs. 3–16 and 3–17).

Brachial systolic pressure increases after exercise. The increase in pressure is usually much more pronounced in patients with arterial disease than it is in normal subjects. Although an occasional patient with minimal or no symptoms may not demonstrate a distinct decrease in ankle pressure following exercise, the arm to ankle gradient will be increased.[249] Arterial disease may be diagnosed when the postexercise arm pressure exceeds the ankle pressure by more than 20 mmHg. It is rare for such patients to require arterial reconstruction for claudication.

Location of the disease also has an effect on the magnitude of the pressure drop and the time required for the pressure to return to baseline levels (see Fig. 3–14). Pressure drops following exercise indicate that the obstruction involves arteries supplying the gastrocnemius and soleus muscles. Because a large portion of the blood supply to these muscles is derived from the sural arteries, which have their origin from the popliteal, a drop in ankle pressure following exercise signifies an obstruction of the upper popliteal, superficial femoral, or more proximal vessels. When the obstruction is confined to below-knee vessels, exercise seldom causes claudication or a significant drop in ankle pressure—in fact, the pressure may even rise.[231, 232]

In general, the more proximal the occlusive disease is, the more effect it has on the ankle pressure response to exercise. For example, an isolated aortoiliac lesion usually has more functional significance than a lesion confined to the superficial femoral artery.[240, 273] This phenomenon occurs because the more proximal arteries supply a greater muscle mass than the distally located arteries do. Consequently, there is a more severe and prolonged diversion of blood away from the ankle to the proximal muscle masses (see Chapter 3).[236, 240]

Walking time itself is not a particularly important indicator because it is not very reproducible.[185] Motivation, pain tolerance, and ancillary symptoms dictate its duration. It correlates poorly with estimated walking tolerance and with objective hemodynamic measurements.

Reactive Hyperemia

Reactive hyperemia, by increasing the rate of blood flow through stenotic arteries or high-resistance collateral vessels, causes a drop in the ankle pressure similar to that observed after exercise (see Chapter 3).[6, 113, 118, 257] A pneumatic cuff, placed around the thigh, is inflated well above systolic pressure for 3 to 7 minutes. After release of the compression, ankle pressures are monitored at 15-, 20-, or 30-second intervals for 3 to 6 minutes or until measurements return to preocclusion levels. In normal limbs, ankle pressures immediately decrease to about 80 per cent of preocclusion levels but rapidly rise, reaching 90 per cent levels within about 30 to 60 seconds. In limbs with obstructive arterial disease, the decrease in pressure coincides well with that seen following exercise, but recovery to resting levels is much faster.[6, 113] The magnitude of the pressure drop depends on the anatomic extent of the disease process and on the degree of functional impairment.[118, 257] Although recovery times are also correlated with the severity of the disease (from less than 1 minute to more than 3 minutes), the correlation is not as good as that given by the maximal depression of the ankle pressure.[185]

In some laboratories, reactive hyperemia has supplanted treadmill exercise for stress testing.[113] Compared with treadmill exercise, the test is less time-consuming, can be done in the patient's room, and uses simple inexpensive equipment. Since the duration of cuff occlusion can be prescribed and walking time cannot, the stress may be more standardized than that afforded by exercise testing. It is less dependent on patient motivation. Another frequently cited reason for preferring reactive hyperemia is that it can be used on patients who cannot walk on the treadmill because of neurologic, cardiac, pulmonary, or orthopedic problems or because of general disability, prior amputation, rest pain, or ischemic ulceration.

To the authors, these last arguments are not very convincing. Stress testing is not required to diagnose arterial disease in limbs with rest pain, ulcers, or gangrene. Disease of that severity is easily detected and evaluated with ankle or toe pressures.[185] There is no need to seek out occult disease. In those who cannot walk because of other problems, disease of sufficient severity to jeopardize the limb is readily detected without stress testing; and in such patients, arterial reconstruction for low-grade disease would not be justified. Finally, exercise duplicates the stress responsible for claudication (reactive hyperemia does not) and permits neurologic, cardiopulmonary, and orthopedic problems to be evaluated vis-à-vis the arterial disease.[113]

Some disadvantages of using the reactive hyperemia response can be listed. The test causes mild to moderate discomfort, thigh compression may be hazardous in limbs with femoropopliteal grafts, and rapid pressure measurements are required to get reproducible results.[6, 113, 185] Ouriel and coworkers found that reactive hyperemia was a less sensitive and less specific indicator than resting ankle pressures or exercise tests.[185] Still, the method has some good points, and its use may occasionally be justified.

Direct Measurement of Arterial Pressure

As noted in Chapter 3, the relationship between arterial pressure, flow, and resistance can be expressed by Poiseuille's law. The degree of narrowing at which pressure and flow begin to decline is called the critical stenosis. However, in the intact arterial circulation, autoregulation can maintain normal flow rates distal to a critical stenosis, even when a significant pressure drop is present. Therefore, pressure measurements are more likely than flow measurements to indicate the presence of arterial disease. Furthermore, measurements of flow rates or peripheral resistance are extremely difficult to perform in the clinical setting.

The direct measurement of arterial pressure avoids the cuff artifacts and other potential errors associated with noninvasive pressure measurements. Direct pressure measurements have been applied primarily to the assessment of lower extremity arterial disease. Specific approaches include pull-through aortoiliac artery pressures during arteriography, percutaneous measurement of common femoral artery pressures, and intraoperative pressure measurements during arterial reconstructions. As with the noninvasive methods, direct pressure measurements can be made both in the resting state and following some form of hemodynamic stress. Although a pedal ergometer exercise test has been described for use with percutaneous common femoral artery pressure measurements, a large proportion of patients are unable to adequately perform this test, and it has not been widely used.[222] A simpler technique that does not require strict patient cooperation or any specialized equipment is intra-arterial injection of papaverine to produce peripheral vasodilatation.

Although direct arterial pressure measurements are generally regarded as the reference standard for the physiologic evaluation of peripheral arterial disease, this approach is subject to certain errors that must be recognized. The proper zero level for a particular measurement must be selected, taking into account the relative height of the patient's heart, the transducer, and the site of measurement. Underdamping of the needle, transducer, and catheter system is common, especially when air bubbles are present.[36] This tends to augment the pulse pressure and result in excessively high systolic pressure values, although the mean pressure component is less likely to be affected. These problems can be minimized during clinical measurements by using stiff tubing with few stopcocks and eliminating fluid leaks and air bubbles.

Percutaneous Pressure Measurement

The direct measurement of arterial pressure is indicated to assess the physiologic severity of aortoiliac disease found on either arteriography or noninvasive testing. Although arteriography is usually adequate to evaluate the significance of infrainguinal arterial disease, the same is not true for more proximal arterial lesions.[165] Even biplane arteriography may not allow an accurate assessment of the aortoiliac system.[74]

Since arteriographic procedures are most commonly performed using a femoral puncture site, direct measurements of arterial pressure during arteriography generally include the aortic, iliac, and femoral segments. Pull-through pressures taken with the arteriogram catheter indicate the hemodynamic significance of any lesions present in the aortoiliac system. Intra-arterial injection of papaverine can be used as a pharmacologic stress test to assess the pressure gradients during high flow conditions. Studies of hemodynamically normal patients suggest that a hemodynamically significant lesion in the aortoiliac segment is present when the systolic pressure gradient is more than 10 mmHg at rest or 20 mmHg following injection of papaverine hydrochloride (30 mg) into the arteriogram catheter.[248]

Direct measurement of femoral artery pressure is performed by percutaneous puncture of the common femoral artery with a 19-gauge needle attached by rigid fluid-filled tubing to a calibrated pressure transducer. The femoral artery systolic pressure is compared with the brachial artery systolic pressure, and the femoral-brachial index (FBI) is calculated. As with the ABI, the brachial artery pressure, as measured by Doppler ultrasound, is presumed to represent systemic arterial pressure. A resting FBI of greater than or equal to 0.9 is considered normal.[74] Values less than 0.9 indicate the presence of a hemodynamically significant lesion proximal to the common femoral artery. If the resting FBI is normal, the injection of papaverine can be used to look for less severe lesions that are apparent only at increased flow rates. This is accomplished by injecting 30 mg of papaverine hydrochloride directly through the needle in the common femoral artery and monitoring both the common femoral and the brachial artery pressures. It is particularly important to measure the brachial artery pressure during this test, because papaverine often causes a slight decrease in systemic arterial pressure. The mean decrease in FBI following papaverine injection is 6 per cent for normal subjects, and a decrease of 15 per cent or more is indicative of a hemodynamically significant lesion.[74] A peak flow increase of 50 per cent or greater is sufficient for a valid test; reasons for an invalid test include fixed outflow resistance and extravascular injection of papaverine.

Intraoperative Pressure Measurement

The basic principles and techniques for intraoperative pressure measurements are identical to those described for the percutaneous approach. Common femoral artery pressures, both before and after papaverine injection, can be used to assess the aortoiliac segment when it is not feasible to obtain these measurements preoperatively. Sequential pressure measurements along a native artery or bypass graft can localize areas of hemodynamic abnormality. In this manner, the inflow, graft segment, and distal runoff of an arterial reconstruction can be evaluated and specific problems corrected.

Intraoperative pressure measurements are performed by puncturing the exposed vessel with a hypodermic needle attached to rigid fluid-filled tubing. A 19-gauge or larger needle provides optimal pressure waveforms, smaller needles are satisfactory for measurement of pressure gradients. The same pressure transducer setup used by the anesthesiologist for monitoring radial artery pressure can be used for these measurements. In addition to looking for significant pressure gradients along an arterial reconstruction, the intraoperative pressures can be compared with the systemic pressure, which is typically based on the reading from a radial artery pressure line.

DOPPLER ULTRASONOGRAPHY

Although the absolute magnitude of blood flow measured at rest is of little help in the diagnosis or objective assessment of peripheral arterial obstructive disease, the contour of the velocity pulse wave and disturbances of the flow pattern in individual arteries provide a great deal of important information. Before the development of transcutaneous Doppler ultrasonography, this information was essentially unavailable. The presence of a bruit signifies a flow disturbance of some type; however, bruits are difficult to quantify, do not appear until the arterial lumen is significantly narrowed, disappear when the stenosis is very severe, and are absent when the artery is totally occluded. Moreover, bruits may arise from arteries adjacent to the vessel of interest, causing additional confusion. Although the electromagnetic flowmeter is capable of displaying the contour of the velocity pulse, it can only be used on exposed vessels, and even then it does not furnish much information regarding subtle flow disturbances. As discussed in Chapter 4, the transcutaneous electromagnetic flowmeter has not filled this void. The noninvasive assessment of arterial blood flow with magnetic resonance is being evaluated (see Chapter 6), but for many reasons it is unlikely that this modality will soon assume an important role. Laser Doppler flowmetry is applicable only to the cutaneous tissues and cannot be quantified.

Doppler ultrasonography has, therefore, become an essential part of the noninvasive evaluation of peripheral arterial disease. The instruments are not only rugged and easy to use but also provide instantaneous information. Many levels of data analysis are available, ranging from the simple to the extremely complex.

Examination Technique

For most purposes, a pencil-type probe is preferred. Optimal signals are obtained by placing the probe directly over the vessel to be examined at an angle of 45 to 60 degrees. In the lower limb, the common femoral artery is examined at the groin at or slightly above the inguinal skinfold to avoid confusion with signals arising from the profunda femoris or the proximal superficial femoral artery. Persson and coworkers have emphasized the importance of accurately locating the common femoral artery, using the line drawn between the anterior-superior iliac spine and the pubic tubercle to determine the site of the inguinal ligament.[188] The inguinal skin crease, especially in obese patients, is often well below the inguinal ligament.

Signals from the superficial femoral artery are best detected with the probe positioned medially on the thigh in the groove between the quadriceps and the adductor muscle bellies. When the patient is supine, flexion of the knee and mild external rotation of the leg provide access to the popliteal artery. Alternatively, the popliteal artery can be examined with the patient prone, the feet being supported by a pillow to flex the knee. At the ankle level, the posterior tibial arterial signal is obtained just behind the medial malleolus. The dorsalis pedis is consistently located slightly lateral to the extensor hallucis longus tendon a centimeter or so distal to the ankle joint. Finally, the lateral tarsal artery (representing the termination of the peroneal artery) can usually be studied by placing the probe anterior and medial to the lateral malleolus over the navicular bone.

Although these represent the sites incorporated in the routine diagnostic evaluation, virtually the entire length of the arteries of the leg can be examined, provided the patient's limb is not too large. For example, the posterior tibial and anterior tibial arteries are usually readily detected in mid-calf in their respective anatomic positions, medial and posterior to the tibia and toward the middle of the anterior compartment. The peroneal artery is more difficult to study but can sometimes be located by placing the probe posterior and medial to the fibula. Examination of these more deeply situated arteries is greatly facilitated by the use of a duplex scanner, which allows accurate identification of the vessel and permits precise evaluation of flow.

Although simple nondirectional devices suffice for many clinical applications, direction-sensing instruments supply more information and are necessary for any detailed analysis of the Doppler signal. Even in routine surveys of the peripheral arteries, direction sensing is often a valuable adjunct. The choice of frequency depends on the depth of the vessel being examined. Whereas superficial vessels are best studied with a high-frequency probe (10 MHz), the deeper vessels of the leg require the use of lower frequencies (5 MHz). A 3-MHz probe may be necessary to adequately evaluate flow in the aorta, iliac arteries, and mesenteric vessels.

Audible Interpretation

The ear serves as the simplest and most readily available means of interpreting the output of the Doppler flowmeter. Skilled observers can derive a great deal of information from the audible signal without resorting to recordings or complex methods of analysis. Since good quality, continuous-wave (c-w), nondirectional devices meet most of the requirements for audible interpretation, there is no need for bulky, expensive instrumentation. For many purposes, a hand-held Doppler flowmeter suffices.

Normal arterial signals are biphasic or triphasic.[234] The first sound corresponds to the large, high-velocity, forward-flow systolic component of the pulse wave; the second, to the smaller reversed-flow component in early diastole; and the third, to the even smaller, low-velocity, forward-flow component that usually appears in late diastole. The pitch of the signal rises rapidly to a peak during systole and then falls abruptly in early diastole. The pitch of the two subsequent signals is always much lower. Finding a clear, crisp, multi-phasic signal with a high systolic velocity implies patency of the proximal arteries and almost invariably rules out hemodynamically significant disease.

The characteristics of abnormal Doppler flow signals vary depending on whether the probe is positioned above, at, or well below the site of the occlusive process. Distal to a stenosis or an occlusion, flow signals are typically low-pitched and monophasic, the high-frequency components of the pulse wave having been filtered out by passage through the stenosis or high-resistance collateral channels. As long as the velocity of flow exceeds a certain minimal level (determined by the ultrasound transmission frequency and the cutoff frequency of the high-pass filter used to eliminate extraneous signals arising from wall motion), arterial signals will be obtained despite the absence of palpable pulses. Absence of a signal implies either a flow velocity below the threshold level or occlusion of the arterial segment being evaluated. In cases of severe arterial obstruction, the Doppler signal may lose much of its characteristic pulsatility and be difficult to distinguish from an adjacent venous signal. A directional Doppler will usually resolve this issue.

Signals detected over a stenosis or from an artery immediately below a stenosis are high-pitched, noisy, and monophasic. These characteristics reflect the increased velocity of flow within the narrowed lumen and the development of disturbed or turbulent flow patterns in the jet of blood emerging from the stenosis.

Signals obtained from a pulsating artery a few centimeters proximal to an occlusion have a characteristic "to-and-fro" or "thumping" quality. This sound is composed of a low-frequency forward-flow wave followed by a relatively large flow wave reflected from the obstruction. In questionable cases, a directional instrument equipped with frequency meters may aid in the interpretation of the audible signal. When the artery is obstructed distal to the probe and there are no intervening branches to provide outflow, the meters will indicate no mean forward flow or low-velocity flow of equal magnitude in both the forward and the reversed channels.

Waveform Analysis

The main drawback to the audible interpretation of the Doppler signal is its inherent subjectivity. Waveform analysis is not only objective but also permits more information to be extracted from the Doppler shifted signal. As discussed in Chapter 4, several methods are available for processing and recording the velocity signal. Although the zero-crossing output is simple to use, it is often inaccurate and, consequently, is seldom suitable for quantitative work. It does, however, provide a quick method of examining the contour of the waveform, especially in conjunction with segmental pressure measurements. For all serious work, spectral analysis of the Doppler signal is the method of choice.

Qualitative Analysis

Contour

Simply inspecting the contour of the waveform obtained from the zero-crosser or audiofrequency spectrum often is of considerable diagnostic value. As illustrated in Figure 5–9, the normal velocity waveform is triphasic. Velocity increases rapidly in early systole, reaches a peak, and then drops almost equally as rapidly, reversing in early diastole.[126] In late diastole, the velocity tracing again becomes positive before returning to the zero-flow baseline. With increasing peripheral vasoconstriction, the reversed flow component becomes more exaggerated.[203, 236] When peripheral resistance is reduced following exercise, artifi-

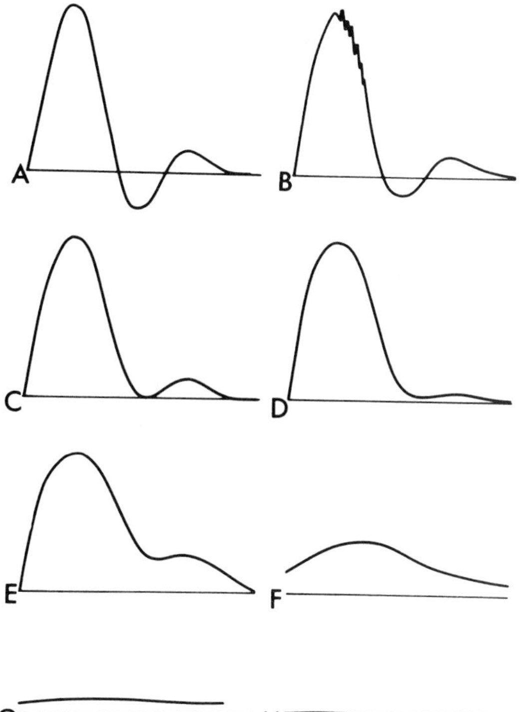

FIGURE 5–9. Different patterns of flow velocity waveforms. *A*, Normal. *B*, Atherosclerotic changes of artery causing turbulence during systolic phase (high frequency). *C* and *D*, Loss of reverse flow due to progression of degree of stenosis. *E–H*, With increasing arterial stenosis, the flow velocity waveform becomes progressively damped. (*A–H*, From Johnston KW, Maruzzo BC, Kassam M, et al: Methods for obtaining, processing and quantifying Doppler blood velocity waveforms. *In* Nicolaides AN, Yao JST [eds]: Investigation of Vascular Disorders. Churchill Livingstone, New York, 1981, p 543.)

cially induced reactive hyperemia, or infusion of vasodilating drugs, the reverse-flow component disappears, the baseline rises above the zero-flow level, and the wave assumes a biphasic rather than a triphasic contour. To maintain the characteristics of the normal waveform, recordings should be made in a warm room with the patient resting comfortably in a supine position.

Atherosclerotic changes in arteries proximal to the site of the probe initially produce a disturbance of the contour of the systolic forward-flow wave at the peak or in the early deceleration phase. With increasing stenosis, the reversed-flow component is damped and then disappears entirely. As the stenosis becomes more severe, progressing to total occlusion, the rate of acceleration of the forward flow decreases, the peak becomes rounded, and the wave becomes continuous and less pulsatile.[236]

Above a stenosis or occlusion, the wave may have a nearly normal contour, especially when the disease process is located well below the site being evaluated and when there are large outflow branches that serve to reduce the peripheral resistance. It is not uncommon, however, to find that the contour is modified perceptively by increased input impedance and that the resulting wave takes on some of the characteristics commonly associated with proximal stenosis.[281] For example, recordings made from common femoral arteries proximal to superficial femoral occlusions often resemble the waves in Figure 5–9*C* and *D*, even in the absence of any significant iliac stenosis. This must always be kept in mind when one attempts to use the contour of the common femoral waveform to rule in or out inflow disease.

By comparing the contours of the Doppler waveforms obtained from the common femoral, popliteal, and pedal arteries, one can usually identify the presence of hemodynamically significant disease and can often localize the disease to the aortoiliac, superficial femoral, or below-knee segment. The presence of multilevel disease is implied when severely dampened waveforms, such as those shown in Figure 5–9*F*, *G*, and *H*, are recorded from the pedal arteries. Absence of a recordable signal from any of the pedal arteries is indicative of severe arterial disease.

Quantitative Analysis

As discussed in Chapter 4, several methods have been proposed for quantitating the Doppler flow signal.

Peak-to-Peak Pulsatility Index

In normal legs, the peak-to-peak pulsatility index (PI_{pp}; see Eq. 4.9) increases as the recording site moves from the proximal to distal portions of the limb, being greatest in the dorsalis pedis and posterior tibial arteries and least in the common femoral artery.[123, 124] When, however, there is an intervening arterial stenosis or occlusion, the PI_{pp} value obtained below the involved segment tends to decrease (Table 5–7). Damping factors (DF; see Eq. 4.10) increase

Table 5–7. Typical Pulsatility Indices (PI) and Inverse Damping Factors (DF^{-1})*

	Location of Arterial Obstruction							
	None		*Aortoiliac*		*Superficial Femoral*		*Aortoiliac and Superficial Femoral*	
Recording Site	PI	DF^{-1}	PI	DF^{-1}	PI	DF^{-1}	PI	DF^{-1}
Common femoral	13.0		2.4		6.1		3.1	
Popliteal	16.7	1.3	2.7	1.1	4.4	0.7	2.4	0.8
Dorsalis pedis	17.7	1.1	5.6	2.1	5.6	1.3	3.7	1.5
Posterior tibial	18.0		4.6		4.6		3.1	

Data from Johnston KW, Maruzzo BC, Cobbold RSC: Doppler methods for quantitative measurement and localization of peripheral arterial occlusive disease by analysis of the blood velocity waveform. Ultrasound Med Biol 4:209, 1978.

Table 5–8. Common Femoral Pulsatility Indices (PI) in Limbs With Aortoiliac Occlusive Disease (mean ± SD)

	Severity of Diameter Stenosis				
Author and Year	**Normal**	**Minimal**	**Less Than 50%**	**Greater Than or Equal to 50%**	**Occluded**
Johnston et al (1978)[123]	9.6 ± 2.8	8.1 ± 2.8	4.9 ± 1.3	2.3 ± 1.2	1.6 ± 0.7
Baker et al (1984)[8]	8.3 ± 7.9	7.6 ± 5.0	3.9 ± 1.2	2.4 ± 0.8	1.8 ± 1.1
Harris et al (1974)[97]	7.1 ± 1.8	5.7 ± 3.2		2.8 ± 1.1	1.6 ± 0.9
Ward and Martin (1980)[262]	11.1 ± 5.4	4.1 ± 1.8		3.0 ± 1.0	1.9 ± 0.7
Baird et al (1980)[3]	11.8 ± 5.3	7.4 ± 1.6		3.6 ± 1.6	
Aukland and Hurlow (1982)[2]		6.1 ± 2.3		4.3 ± 2.0	1.3 ± 0.6
Hirai and Schoop (1984)[106]	8.0 ± 2.3	6.1 ± 3.0		3.7 ± 1.6	2.0 ± 0.4

and inverse damping factors (DF^{-1}; see Eq. 4.11) decrease across segments with significant arterial disease (Table 5–7).

The PI_{pp} has been advocated as a method for determining the presence or absence of iliac artery disease. As shown in Table 5–8, mean values obtained by several investigators from the common femoral artery agree reasonably well for the various categories of disease severity; however, the standard deviations are large, and data from adjacent categories frequently overlap. When arteriography is used as the gold standard, the sensitivity of the PI_{pp} for identifying diameter reductions of the iliac artery greater than 50 per cent (hemodynamically significant stenoses) varies widely from 41 to 100 per cent, depending on the laboratory making the measurements and the value of the index chosen as the dividing point between positive and negative studies (Table 5–9). Specificities are equally variable. Similar data are reported when the pressure drop across the aortoiliac segment, a physiologic gold standard, is substituted for the arteriographic image (Table 5–10).

In general, assessment of the hemodynamic status of the iliac artery seems to be more accurate in the absence of concomitant disease in the superficial femoral artery.[69, 199] Distal arterial obstruction tends to lower the femoral pulsatility index in limbs with no stenosis or low-grade stenoses of the iliac arteries, thereby increasing the number of false-positive study results and reducing specificity (Table 5–10).[8, 69, 122, 199, 248, 262] Some investigators, however, maintain that distal arterial obstruction has little effect on accuracy.[2, 28, 121, 122, 125]

In theory, simple, objective measurements, such as the PI_{pp}, should be relatively consistent from one laboratory to the next. Since pulsatility indices are independent of heart rate and probe angle, there is no obvious explanation for the observed differences other than biologic variability. It is difficult, therefore, to reconcile the disparate opinions expressed in the literature concerning the value of the PI_{pp} for detecting iliac stenosis.[3, 92, 122, 125, 199] Nonetheless, the assumption that a normal femoral pulsatility index (e.g., greater than 4.0) probably rules out significant iliac stenosis is consistent with many reports.[248] An abnormal index, on the other hand, must be interpreted cautiously, particularly in the presence of infrainguinal obstructive disease.[248]

The mean popliteal pulsatility index in normal limbs was found by Harris and associates to be 9.3 ± 3.6, with a range of 4 to 20.[97] In limbs with femoropopliteal disease, mean indices for stenoses less than 50 per cent are reported to be 5.9 ± 3.2 and 7.7 ± 1.1; for hemodynamically significant stenoses, they are 4.7 ± 4.0 and 5.9 ± 1.2; and for occlusion, they are reduced to 1.6 ± 0.9 and 2.3 ± 0.2.[2, 97] Obviously, there is a great deal of overlap between values for different grades of disease, but it is usually possible to distinguish between occlusion and no stenosis. Calculation of DFs provides somewhat better discrimination.

Table 5–9. Accuracy of Femoral Pulsatility Indices (PI) for Detecting ≥50% Diameter Stenoses of the Aortoiliac Arterial Segment

Author and Year	**Superficial Femoral Artery**	**PI Criterion***	**Sensitivity (%)**	**Specificity (%)**
Flanigan et al (1982)[72]	—	2.5	70	81
Baird et al (1980)[3]	—	3.0	41	55
Baker et al (1984)[8]	—	3.0	76	81
Johnston et al (1984)[122]	—	3.0	95	97
Baird et al (1980)[3]	—	4.0	55	71
Baker et al (1984)[8]	—	4.0	94	66
Campbell et al (1984)[40]	—	4.0	92	75
Junger et al (1984)[125]	Occluded	5.0	90	95
Baker et al (1984)[8]	—	5.5	100	53
Junger et al (1984)[125]	Patent	7.6	78	89

**PI below which ≥50 per cent stenosis is predicted.*

Table 5–10. Accuracy of Femoral Pulsatility Indices (PI) for Detecting Hemodynamically Significant Pressure Drops Across the Aortoiliac Segment

Author and Year	Critical Pressure Drop (mmHg)	Distal Arteries	PI Criterion*	Sensitivity (%)	Specificity (%)
Flanigan et al (1982)[72]	5	—	2.5	62	69
Johnston et al (1983)[121]	10	Patent	5.5	95	100
	10	Occluded	5.3	92	92
Thiele et al (1983)[248]	10	Patent	4.0	95	82
	10	Occluded	4.0	96	45
	20†	Patent	4.0	92	92
	20†	Occluded	4.0	92	51
Bone (1982)[28]	10%‡	—	4.5	94	100

**PI below which pressure drop exceeding the critical value is predicted.*
†Critical pressure drop during papaverine-induced hyperemia.
‡Critical drop in femoral/brachial index after reactive hyperemia.

Johnston and coworkers state that a DF^{-1} less than 0.9 suggests superficial femoral occlusion.[123] Aukland and Hurlow report DFs of 0.8 ± 0.1, 1.3 ± 0.2, and 2.1 ± 0.2 for minimal disease, hemodynamically significant stenosis, and occlusion of the superficial femoral artery, respectively.[2] A DF exceeding 1.0 identifies most superficial femoral occlusions; whereas a DF less than 1.9 is highly specific (95 per cent) for the absence of significant disease.[5]

Pulsatility indices obtained from the dorsalis pedis or posterior tibial arteries at the ankle are probably of little practical value in the assessment of below-knee disease. According to Aukland and Hurlow, the mean index in limbs with patent popliteal-tibial segments (6.5 ± 1.4) did not differ significantly from that in limbs in which these arteries were occluded (4.1 ± 0.8).[2] Although Harris and associates found a significant difference between the pedal indices in normal limbs (8.3 ± 3.1) and in limbs with below-knee disease, there was no statistically significant difference between any of the angiographic grades (less than 50 per cent stenosis, 3.1 ± 2.9; greater than 50 per cent stenosis, 1.9 ± 2.4; occlusion, 1.1 ± 0.6).[97] On the other hand, the data of Johnston and coworkers suggest that a DF^{-1} less than 1.0 is indicative of severe popliteal-tibial occlusive disease and that a value greater than 1.0 is consistent with normal arteries or arteries with minimal stenosis.[123]

Laplace Transform

The Laplace transform method of waveform analysis was developed to circumvent some of the problems inherent in the interpretation of pulsatility indices (see Chapter 4). It has evoked the most interest as a method for identifying stenoses of the aortoiliac segment, especially in limbs with multilevel disease. Analysis of the femoral waveform yields three parameters, ω_o, γ, and δ, that theoretically relate to arterial wall stiffness, peripheral impedance, and proximal stenosis, respectively.[217] Typical values for δ are given in Table 5–11. These values, which may range from 0.0 to 1.0, tend to increase with increasing severity of stenosis. Statistically significant differences were noted between the means of all adjacent stenosis categories by the first three investigative teams listed in Table 5–11;[3, 122, 217] and Baker and associates, the last team in the list, reported statistically significant differences between the means for stenoses less than 50 per cent and for those greater than 50 per cent.[8] All studies, however, have demonstrated appreciable overlapping of individual values from the various categories of stenosis.

The reported accuracy of Laplace δ values for detecting hemodynamically significant stenoses of the aortoiliac segment (greater than or equal to 50 per cent diameter reduction) has generally been quite acceptable, most studies indicating sensitivities and specificities well over 85 per cent (Table 5–12). Although some proponents of the Laplace transform method maintain that the δ value is not influenced by distal impedance,[3, 8, 217] others have noted that, like PI_{pp}, the δ value is also sensitive to the presence of superficial femoral arterial occlusive disease.[122, 125] For example, Junger and coworkers found that clamping surgically exposed superficial femoral arteries increased the δ value by 8 to 38 per cent.[125] As pointed out by Johnston and associates, δ is most affected by superficial femoral

Table 5–11. Laplace Transform Damping Values (δ) in Limbs With Aortoiliac Occlusive Disease (mean ± SD)

	Severity of Diameter Stenosis			
Author and Year	*Normal*	*<50%*	*>50%*	*Occluded*
Skidmore et al (1980)[217]	0.38	0.50	––––––– 0.70 –––––––	
Baird et al (1980)[3]	0.33 ± 0.06	0.50 ± 0.15	––––– 0.78 + 0.16 –––––	
Johnston et al (1984)[122]	0.41 ± 0.15	0.53 ± 0.18	0.73 ± 0.21	0.89 ± 0.10
Baker et al (1984)[8]	0.39	0.62	0.82	0.88

Table 5–12. Accuracy of Laplace Transform for Detecting ≥50% Diameter Stenosis of the Aortoiliac Arterial Segment

Author and Year	Superficial Femoral Artery	δ Criterion*	Sensitivity (%)	Specificity (%)
Baird et al (1980)[3]	—	0.60	85	84
Baker et al (1984)[8]	—	0.60	100	93
Campbell et al (1984)[40]	—	0.55	86	69
Junger et al (1984)[125]	Patent	0.44	88	92
	Occluded	0.52	75	96
	Occluded	0.70	90	88
Johnston et al (1984)[122]	Patent	0.66	99	90

*δ *above which* ≥*50 per cent stenosis is predicted.*

arterial occlusion when the aortoiliac segment is normal or minimally stenotic.[122] In limbs without inflow disease but with occluded superficial femoral arteries, δ averaged 0.50 ± 0.18, a figure considerably larger than the normal value of 0.35 ± 0.10. The detrimental effect of distal disease on accuracy is most apparent when the δ value is used to distinguish between normal or minimally diseased aortoiliac arteries and those with less than 50 per cent stenosis, greater than 50 per cent stenosis, or total occlusion—superficial femoral arterial occlusion dropping the sensitivity from 94 to 75 per cent and the specificity from 97 to 86 per cent.[122]

Conclusions regarding the relative accuracy of PI_{pp} and δ values differ. Although some authors feel strongly that δ is the better test,[3, 8] others have found both to be equally good.[122, 125, 153] In fact, receiver operator characteristic (ROC) curves of both tests were identical in the study reported by Junger and coworkers.[125] The data of Campbell and coworkers suggest that PI_{pp} is the better method for detecting iliac stenosis greater than 50 per cent but that δ is better for identifying stenosis of less than 50 per cent.[40] On the other hand, Junger and coworkers found that PI_{pp} was slightly more accurate than δ for identifying low-grade stenoses.[125] If the results of the two tests eventually prove to be comparable, PI_{pp}, which has the advantage of simplicity and ease of calculation, would be the method of choice.

In contrast to δ, the other parameters, ω_o and γ, have received much less attention. Skidmore and associates found that ω_o was related to the stiffness of the arterial wall, increasing as systemic blood pressure increased;[217] however, Junger and coworkers observed no change in wall stiffness with advancing age, although age would be expected to be associated with increasing wall stiffness.[125] Similarly, Junger's group could not confirm Skidmore and associates' observations concerning the correlation of γ and peripheral impedance, finding that γ did not discriminate between normal limbs and those with superficial femoral arterial occlusions.

A ratio of the ω_o calculated from the femoral waveform and that calculated from the posterior tibial or dorsalis pedis artery has been investigated by Campbell and associates as a method for identifying femoropopliteal occlusive disease.[39] In their study, almost all limbs with ratios exceeding 1.0 had occlusions in this arterial segment, and the results seemed to be independent of the presence or absence of concomitant aortoiliac disease. Although almost all limbs with normal femoropopliteal segments had ratios less than 1.0, an appreciable number of limbs with occlusions did also. These researchers attributed the false-negative studies to the presence of well-developed collaterals. The overall sensitivity and specificity for identifying superficial femoral arterial occlusion was 75 per cent and 92 per cent, respectively—an accuracy considerably greater than that achieved by calculating damping factors from PI_{pp}.

Velocity Measurements

Fronek and colleagues have advocated quantitative measurement of flow velocities in the common femoral, posterior tibial, and dorsalis pedis arteries as an adjunctive method for assessing peripheral arterial occlusive disease.[77] By making the recordings with the Doppler probe oriented to obtain the maximal output, they minimize the problem posed by the angle of insonation. Measurements include peak forward and reverse velocity, mean velocity, acceleration, and deceleration. From these, peak velocity/mean velocity and acceleration/deceleration indices are calculated. Selected values are listed in Table 5–13. Although the mean values of most of the measurements in diseased limbs are significantly different from those obtained from normal limbs, and mean values from limbs with multisegmental disease differ significantly from many of those from limbs with localized obstructions, the standard deviations are quite large, suggesting that individual measurements are not sufficiently reliable to have much predictive value.[106] When combined with other tests, however, they may be helpful.

Power Frequency Spectrum Analysis

The Doppler frequency spectrum is usually recorded with time on the horizontal axis and frequency on the vertical axis (see Chapter 4). The power (amplitude) at any given frequency is depicted by a gray scale. An alternative format plots frequency at any selected time during the pulse cycle on the horizontal axis and power at the various frequencies on the vertical axis (see Fig. 4–10). Harward and colleagues used this format to study the power frequency spectrum of the common femoral Doppler signal at peak systole.[98] After examining several parameters that could be derived from the power frequency spectrum, they concluded that the frequency bandwidth at 50 per cent of the

Table 5–13. Arterial Flow Velocity Measurements (mean ± SD)*

Parameter	Velocity			
	Normal	*Aortoiliac*	*Popliteal*	*Femoral-Popliteal*
PEAK FORWARD VELOCITY (cm/sec)				
Femoral artery	41 ± 11	26 ± 9†	30 ± 15†	21 ± 11†
Posterior tibial artery	16 ± 10	13 ± 12	17 ± 7	12 ± 8†
Dorsalis pedis artery	17 ± 6	15 ± 6‡	11 ± 9†‡	7 ± 7†
DECELERATION (cm/sec^2)				
Femoral artery	251 ± 60	123 ± 76†	181 ± 117†‡	91 ± 71†
Posterior tibial artery	130 ± 76	79 ± 62‡	77 ± 90†‡	43 ± 40†
Dorsalis pedis artery	138 ± 54	80 ± 51†‡	72 ± 56†‡	29 ± 21†
PEAK VELOCITY/MEAN VELOCITY				
Femoral artery	4.8 ± 1.6	3.1 ± 1.1†	3.6 ± 0.8†‡	2.7 ± 0.8†
Posterior tibial artery	4.8 ± 2.5	3.0 ± 0.8†‡	2.8 ± 1.1†‡	2.1 ± 0.8†
Dorsalis pedis artery	6.0 ± 4.1	3.4 ± 1.5†‡	2.6 ± 0.9†‡	2.0 ± 0.7†

**From Fronek A, Coel M, Bernstein EF: Quantitative ultrasonographic studies of lower extremity flow velocities in health and disease. Circulation 53:957, 1976. By permission of the American Heart Association, Inc.*
†$p < .01$ compared with normal.
‡$p < .01$ localized versus combined disease.

maximal amplitude ($f_{50\%}$) provided the most diagnostic information. This parameter is essentially a measure of "spectral broadening" (see Chapter 4). To obtain maximal $f_{50\%}$ values, recordings were made during postocclusive reactive hyperemia, which augments flow through the femoral artery, enhances flow disturbances, and increases spectral broadening.

Analysis of their data demonstrated that a maximal postocclusion $f_{50\%}$ of 2000 Hz proved to be the best discriminator between a positive and a negative test for inflow disease. Values less than 2000 Hz were characteristic of limbs with hemodynamically significant aortoiliac stenosis; whereas values above this level were found in normal limbs and in limbs with less severe aortoiliac stenoses. The presence or absence of superficial femoral artery stenosis had no effect on the results—a most important observation. Retrospectively applied, the test had a 93 per cent sensitivity and specificity for detecting isolated aortoiliac disease and a 93 per cent sensitivity and 88 per cent specificity for identifying the presence or absence of hemodynamically significant aortoiliac stenoses in limbs with multi-level disease.

Although these data are encouraging, prospective studies are required before the utility of the test can be determined.

Reactive Hyperemia

Although resting blood flow in limbs with arterial occlusive disease is ordinarily normal and has no diagnostic value, the capacity to increase blood flow in response to peripheral vasodilation is limited (see Chapter 3). This constitutes the rationale for using reactive hyperemia as a test for the presence of arterial disease. Fronek and associates induce reactive hyperemia by inflating a pneumatic cuff placed below the knee to suprasystolic pressures for 4 minutes.[81] Mean flow velocities in the common femoral artery are recorded with a Doppler probe before cuff inflation and then continuously after cuff deflation until velocities return to baseline values. Two parameters are monitored: the percentage increase in velocity, representing the maximal hyperemic response, and the time required for the velocity to return to 50 per cent of its peak value ($T_{1/2}$). In normal limbs, the maximal velocity increase averages about 210 ± 96 per cent of the resting value, and the $T_{1/2}$ averages about 26 ± 9 seconds.[24] Percentage velocity increases are significantly lower in limbs with localized aortoiliac disease, femoropopliteal obstruction, and multi-level disease, averaging 137 ± 112 per cent, 48 ± 54 per cent, and 43 ± 60 per cent, respectively.[24] Similarly, the $T_{1/2}$ is prolonged to 47 ± 22 seconds, 64 ± 51 seconds, and 41 ± 21 seconds in the same disease categories.[24] In the study reported by Ward and Martin, T proved to be a good method for discriminating between normal iliac segments and those with less than 50 per cent stenosis, more than 50 per cent stenosis, and total occlusion, the corresponding mean values being 15 ± 5, 49 ± 14, 68 ± 33, and 91 ± 22 seconds.[262] Hirai and Schoop, however, found that neither the maximal velocity increase nor the $T_{1/2}$ reliably distinguished between less than 50 per cent and greater than 50 per cent diameter stenosis or occlusion of the iliac artery.[106] Because variances are large, this test is largely of supplementary value.

Pulse Transit Time

As discussed in Chapters 3 and 4, the increased wall thickness and decreased wall compliance associated with advancing age and plaque formation tend to accelerate the velocity with which the arterial pulse wave is transmitted in atherosclerotic vessels. Pulse transit times (TTs), however, are often prolonged, owing to the extended length of the pathway provided by the more compliant collateral vessels. TTs are, therefore, most sensitive to the presence of total occlusions, which are always associated with the development of collateral vessels.[2, 114, 262] Most investigators report little difference between the TTs in normal limbs and those in limbs with patent but severely stenosed arteries. For example, Aukland and Hurlow found that the TT from the common femoral to the popliteal artery averaged 35 ± 9 msec over femoropopliteal segments with less than 50 per cent stenosis, 43 ± 7 msec over segments with more than 50 per cent stenosis, and 68 ± 16 seconds over occluded segments.[2] Ward and Martin, who measured TTs from the R wave of the electrocardiogram to the foot of the common femoral pulse, reported mean values of about 150 msec for normal limbs and limbs with both low-grade and severe iliac arterial stenoses.[262] However, in limbs with occluded iliac arteries, the mean TT was significantly increased to 230 msec.

In an effort to enhance the accuracy of Doppler studies for detecting disease of the femoropopliteal segment, a number of investigators, following the lead of Gosling, plot damping factors obtained from the PI_{pp}s of the common femoral and popliteal arteries (see Eq. 4.11) against the TTs measured across the same segment.[88] To reduce the possible effects of blood pressure variation and age on TTs, the observed TTs are divided by the average "normal" TT across the same segment in limbs of comparable blood pressure and age. (Gosling has provided tables of normal values for this purpose.[88]) Similarly, the observed DF is divided by the mean DF found in normal subjects across the same segment (DF equals 0.7 for the normal femoropopliteal segment).[88] When a scattergram was constructed by plotting the normalized values of the two parameters (DF_N, TT_N) against one another, Gosling and King observed that values obtained from limbs with patent femoropopliteal arteries fell in a box whose upper limits were defined by a DF_N equal to 1.5 and a TT_N equal to 1.5.[89] Occluded arteries had DF_N and TT_N values over 1.2. Severely stenotic arteries also had TT_N values in excess of 1.2 but DF_N values less than 1.2. When the superficial femoral arteries were occluded and the collaterals were short, the values for TT_N were less than 2.5; when collaterals were long, values for TT_N exceeded this. The results of Humphries and coworkers' study were similar but did not achieve the 90 per cent accuracy reported by Gosling.[114] Using a cut-off point of 1.9 for both parameters, Baker and associates reported an excellent specificity of 95 per cent but a sensitivity of only 70 per cent.[5]

Although TTs are reasonably successful as a method for identifying total occlusions, this diagnosis can usually be made clinically. Consequently, the applicability of TT measurements is limited.

Rise Time

Rise time (RT) is defined as the duration of the systolic upswing of the flow velocity waveform and is measured from the foot of the wave to the point at which peak velocity is reached. Below an arterial obstruction, RT is delayed, reflecting the decreased acceleration of the velocity tracing. Obstructions distal to the recording site have little effect on this parameter. In a small series, Hamilton and associates found that RT measured at the common femoral artery discriminated well between limbs with and without significant iliac stenosis.[95] Humphries and coworkers reported good results in detecting severe stenosis or occlusion of the superficial femoral artery when the ratio of the RT at the popliteal and common femoral arteries was plotted against the transit time between these two sites.[114] RT proved to be as good as DF for this purpose and was much easier to calculate.

Comment on Waveform Analysis

The large number of methods that have been devised in an effort to provide meaningful quantitation of the Doppler signal suggests that none has proved to be sufficiently accurate. All initially have evoked enthusiasm, but with further experience, their inadequacies have become apparent. The interplay of the multiple factors that dictate the contour and power content of the flow or velocity pulse is indeed complex—so much so that it may be impossible to devise any simple measurement that will afford diagnostic information applicable to all the pathophysiologic situations encountered in clinical practice. Many, despite the aura of accuracy that numbers convey, are little better than simple pattern recognition—and perhaps not as good. A major problem is that most derive their information from sites remote from that of the principal lesion where flow patterns have reverted toward a more normal configuration. For this reason, the direct investigation of the artery at the site of the lesion, as accomplished by duplex scanning, is becoming the preferred noninvasive method for evaluating peripheral arterial disease.[137]

Duplex Scanning

More precise information on the location and severity of arterial disease can be obtained by surveying the arteries of the abdomen and lower extremities with the duplex scanner.[108, 115, 116, 137, 138, 164, 173, 247, 278] The B-mode image permits the sample volume of the pulsed Doppler to be placed in the vicinity of suspected arterial lesions. Certain features of the pulsed Doppler signal can then be used to characterize the flow disturbances and classify the severity of disease at a specific site. The technique and interpretation of duplex scanning for abdominal and lower extremity arterial disease are discussed in Chapter 6.

Spectral Waveform Analysis

Spectral waveform analysis is a signal processing technique that displays the complete frequency and amplitude content of the Doppler signal. Pulsed Doppler signals are most suitable for spectral analysis because they permit evaluation of flow patterns at discrete sites. As discussed in Chapter 4, Doppler shift frequency is directly proportional to blood cell velocity, whereas amplitude depends on the number of blood cells moving through the Doppler sample volume. Spectral waveform information is presented graphically with frequency or velocity on the vertical axis, time on the horizontal axis, and amplitude indicated by shades of gray. Although several methods have been developed for performing real-time spectral analysis, the digital fast-Fourier transform is most commonly used in duplex scanning.

The flow pattern in a normal artery is uniform or laminar, and the center stream pulsed Doppler spectral waveform shows a relatively narrow band of frequencies. As shown in Figure 5–10, stenoses and other arterial wall abnormalities disrupt this normal pattern and produce flow

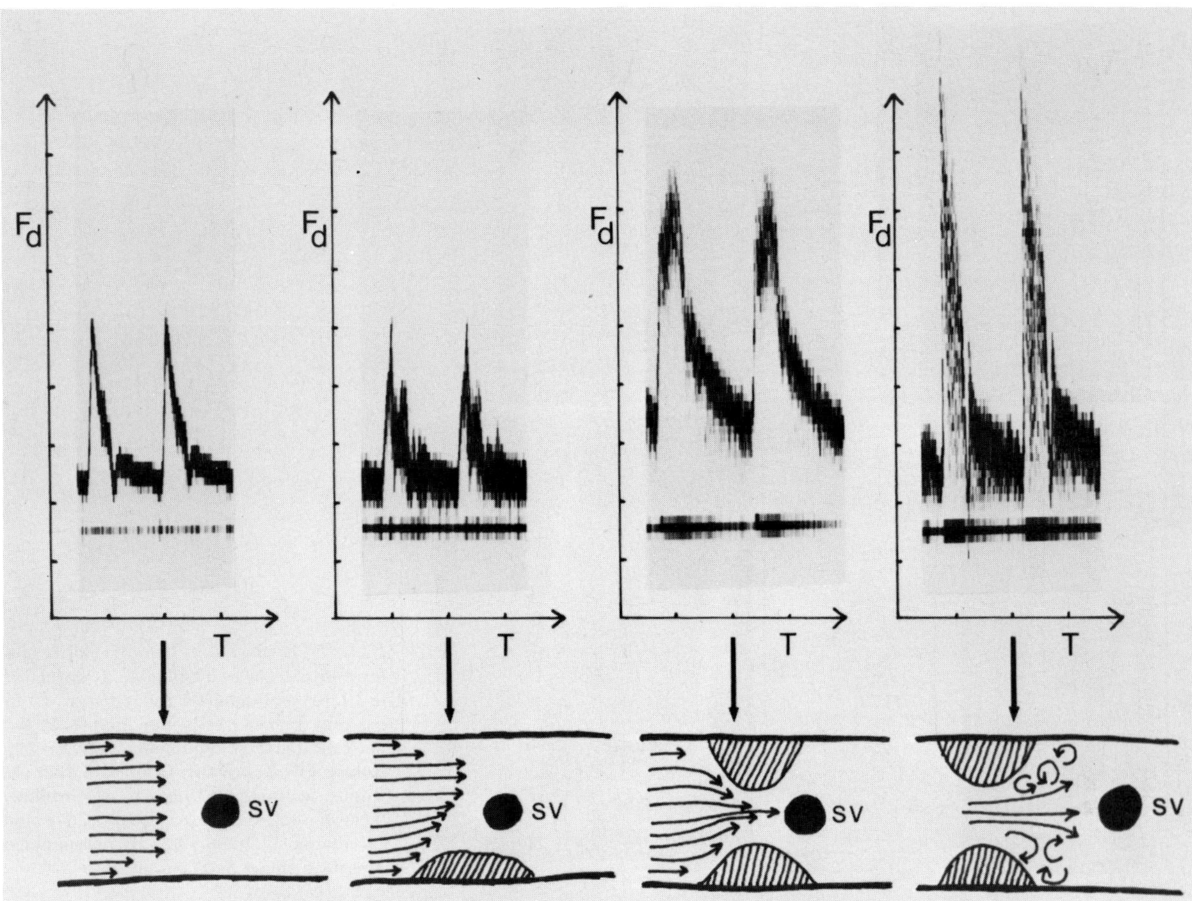

FIGURE 5–10. Spectral waveform characteristics of normal and abnormal flow patterns. *Left panel* represents laminar center stream flow with a narrow band of frequencies, particularly in systole; the *second panel* depicts a minor lesion that results in disturbed flow with spectral broadening in late systole and diastole but no increase in peak frequency. The *third panel* shows a severe stenosis that produces a high-velocity jet at the site of the lesion, and the *last panel* shows the high peak frequencies and spectral broadening that are present distal to a severe stenosis. F_d, Doppler shift frequency (proportional to velocity); T, time; SV, site of pulsed Doppler sample volume. (Courtesy of David L. Phillips, M.D.)

disturbances that are apparent in the Doppler spectrum as a wider range of frequencies and amplitudes. This increase in the width of the frequency band is referred to as spectral broadening. An abnormal increase in the peak systolic frequency or velocity is associated with severe stenoses that produce high-velocity jets. End-diastolic frequency is also increased in very high-grade stenoses (Fig. 5–10). These spectral features have been used to define sets of criteria for classifying the severity of arterial lesions (see Chapter 6). Table 6–2 summarizes the spectral waveform criteria for classification of lower extremity arterial lesions; Table 6–3 gives the criteria for classification of renal artery disease by duplex scanning. Representative spectral waveforms for the various degrees of lower extremity arterial disease are shown in Figure 5–11.

It is important to recognize that some changes in Doppler shift frequency and spectral width can result from artifacts or errors in examination technique. For example, if the pulsed Doppler sample volume is placed near the arterial wall instead of in the center stream, the severity of disease may be overestimated owing to spectral broadening from the velocity gradients that are normally present at that site. A sample volume that is large in relation to the vessel being examined will also detect velocity gradients near the arterial wall even when it is positioned in the center of the lumen. Therefore, in the majority of applications, a small sample volume size provides the most reliable information. In duplex scanning, the beam-to-vessel angle can be monitored and adjusted using the B-mode image and the superimposed Doppler cursor. Whether the Doppler scale is set to units of frequency or velocity, a constant angle should be maintained throughout the examination, preferably 60 degrees or less. Variations in this angle between measurements, or use of angles approaching 90 degrees, can produce significant errors in the calculation of velocity using the Doppler equation.[189] Finally, in order to accurately display the Doppler shift, a pulsed Doppler system must have an adequate pulse-repetition frequency (PRF). The highest Doppler frequency shift that can be displayed is one half of the PRF and is called the Nyquist limit. For example, if a pulsed Doppler has a PRF of 10 kHz, the highest Doppler shift that can be correctly displayed is 5 kHz. When the Nyquist limit is exceeded, the phenomenon of "aliasing" is observed. A spectral waveform with aliasing is "cut off"

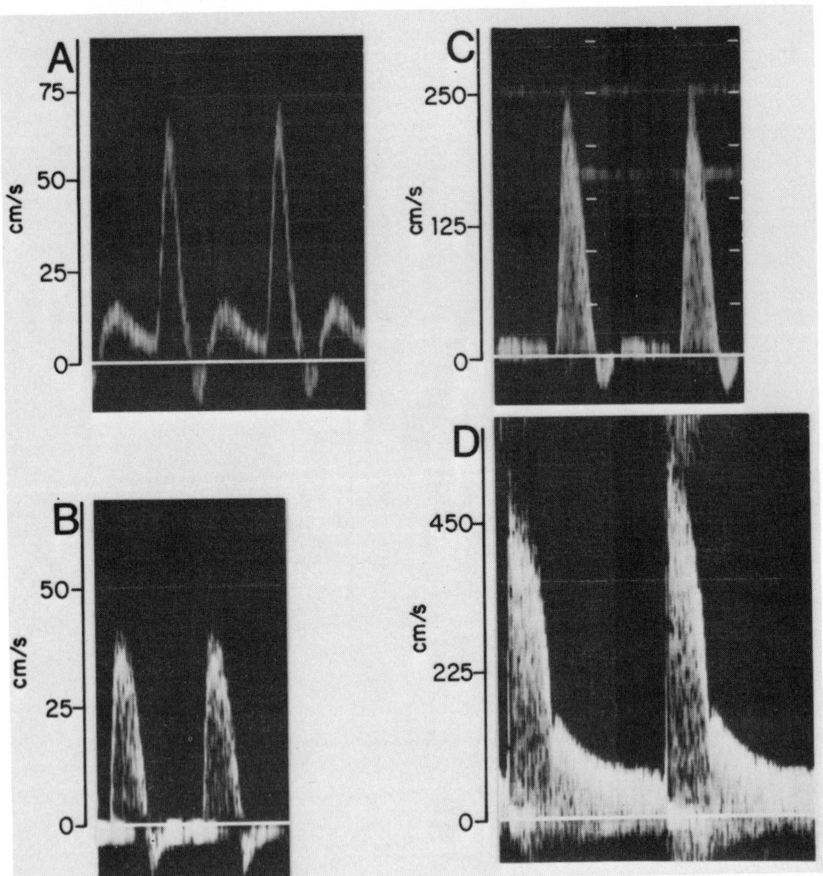

FIGURE 5–11. Typical velocity spectra for four categories of stenosis: *A*, normal; *B*, 1 to 19 per cent diameter reduction; *C*, 20 to 49 per cent diameter reduction; and *D*, 50 to 99 per cent diameter reduction. (*A–D*, From Kohler TR, Nance DR, Cramer MM, et al: Duplex scanning for diagnosis of aortoiliac and femoropopliteal disease: A prospective study. Circulation 76:1074, 1987. By permission of the American Heart Association, Inc.)

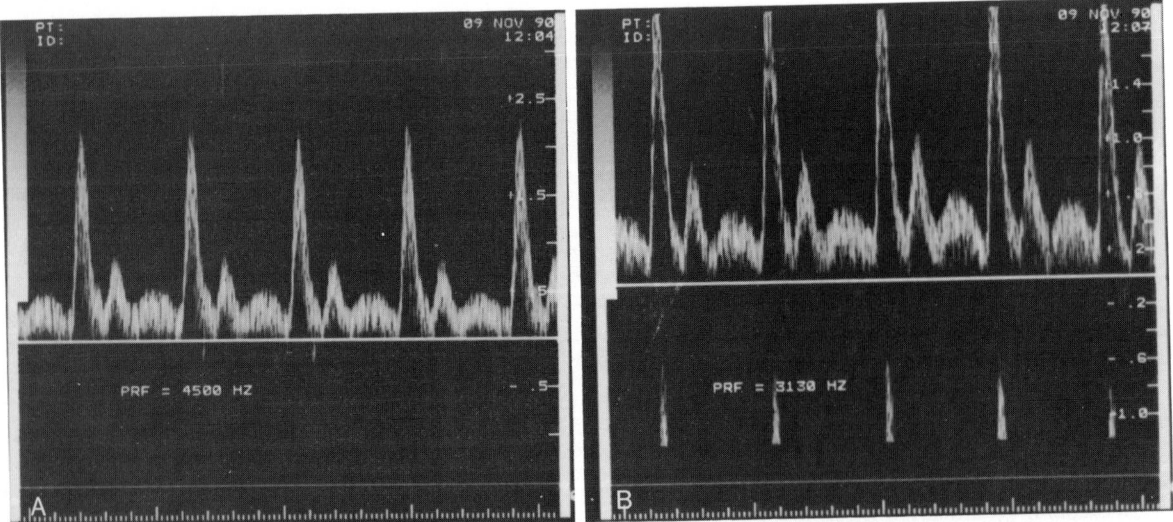

FIGURE 5–12. *A*, Normal triphasic peripheral artery spectral waveforms without aliasing; PRF is set at 4500 Hz. *B*, Spectral waveforms from the same vessel taken with a PRF of 3130 Hz; peaks of the aliased waveforms are cut off and appear below the zero baseline. (*A* and *B*, From Zierler RE, Zierler BK: Duplex sonography of lower extremity arteries. *In* Zwiebel WJ [ed]: Introduction to Vascular Ultrasonography. 3rd ed. Philadelphia, WB Saunders, 1992, p 240.)

at the Nyquist limit, and the missing portion of the waveform appears below the baseline as flow in the opposite direction (Fig. 5–12).

Color Flow Imaging

The real-time color flow image is an alternative to spectral waveforms for displaying pulsed Doppler information. Whereas spectral waveform analysis evaluates the entire frequency and amplitude content of the pulsed Doppler signal at a selected arterial site, color flow imaging provides a single estimate of the Doppler shift frequency or flow velocity for each site within the B-mode image. Thus, spectral waveforms actually give more information on flow at each individual site than color flow imaging does. The main advantage of the color flow display is that it presents flow information on the entire image, even though the absolute amount of data for each site is reduced. Because of these differences, it is often difficult to compare the Doppler information obtained by spectral waveform analysis and color flow imaging. Spectral waveforms contain a range of frequencies and amplitudes, allowing determination of flow direction and parameters such as mean, mode, peak, and bandwidth. In contrast, color assignments are based on flow direction and a single mean or average frequency estimate. Consequently, the peak or maximal Doppler frequency shifts seen with spectral waveforms are generally higher than the frequencies indicated by color flow imaging.

Because color flow imaging is based on pulsed Doppler ultrasound, it is subject to the same physical limitations as spectral waveform analysis. For example, because the Doppler frequency shift depends on the beam-to-vessel angle, color assignments will be accurate only if this angle is properly set and remains constant along the length of a vessel. Unfortunately, blood vessels are seldom straight, so color differences may represent either true velocity changes or variations in the frequency shift resulting from changes in the Doppler angle. This potential source of error should always be considered when interpreting color flow images.

Another problem that can occur with both spectral waveform analysis and color flow imaging is aliasing. As previously noted, aliasing in spectral analysis produces an abrupt loss of the waveform above the Nyquist limit, with the missing portion appearing below the baseline as flow in the reverse direction. When aliasing is present in a color flow image, high velocities, such as those associated with severe stenoses, are assigned colors that indicate flow in the direction opposite to normal arterial flow. The frequency at which aliasing occurs will vary according to the PRF of the Doppler system. Lower PRF values are required to obtain Doppler signals from deeply located vessels like those in the abdomen. Theoretically, aliasing should be more common with color flow systems than with spectral waveform analysis, since lower PRF values are generally required to generate the color flow images.

Because of the extremely large amount of Doppler and B-mode information that they require, color flow images are acquired at relatively slow frame rates. Consequently, some of the rapid variations in flow velocity that occur during the cardiac cycle may be missed. For example, if it takes 33 msec to generate each frame of the color image (about 30 frames/sec), flow transients with time constants near 20 msec, such as those occurring at the onset of systole, will not be reliably detected. This can result in temporal and spacial distortion of the color flow image. Correct interpretation of color flow images requires an understanding of the errors and artifacts that can occur. Color flow images provide an estimate of the flow velocities within the image plane; they should not be considered equivalent to the anatomic images obtained by arteriography.

Comment on Duplex Scanning

Duplex scanning with spectral waveform analysis has several distinct advantages over the indirect noninvasive tests for peripheral arterial disease: Lesions can be accurately localized; lesions can be detected at multiple levels in the same limb; stenoses can be classified according to the degree of severity; minor lesions can be recognized; and severe stenoses can be distinguished from total occlusions.[137, 164, 278] In addition, it is possible to study virtually all the major arteries of the abdomen and lower extremities, including the aortoiliac segment, the renal and mesenteric vessels, and the common femoral, profunda femoris, superficial femoral, and popliteal arteries. It is also feasible to examine the anterior tibial, posterior tibial, and peroneal arteries when clinically necessary. Kohler and associates compared the results of duplex scanning with spectral waveform analysis to arteriography in 383 lower extremity arterial segments.[137] In this study, duplex scanning had a sensitivity of 82 per cent, a specificity of 92 per cent, a positive predictive value of 80 per cent, and a negative predictive value of 93 per cent for identifying hemodynamically significant stenoses (greater than or equal to 50 per cent diameter reduction). A similar study by Moneta and coworkers reported sensitivities for detecting hemodynamically significant stenoses that ranged from 89 per cent in the iliac arteries to 67 per cent in the popliteal arteries; stenosis was correctly distinguished from occlusion in 98 per cent of patients.[164]

The addition of color flow imaging can facilitate certain aspects of the arterial duplex examination. Color flow imaging is extremely helpful for identifying vascular structures, especially when they are deeply located, such as the abdominal vessels, or small, like the arteries below the knee.[100, 101, 164] When Cossman and associates used color flow duplex scanning to examine 84 lower extremities in 61 patients, the sensitivity and specificity for differentiating between normal and diseased arteries were 83 per cent and 96 per cent, respectively.[56] For identifying stenoses of greater than 50 per cent diameter reduction the sensitivity was 87 per cent and the specificity was 99 per cent; occluded arterial segments were detected with a sensitivity of 81 per cent and a specificity of 99 per cent. Color flow imaging correctly determined the location and length of occlusion in 48 of 51 extremities (94 per cent). In spite of these favorable results, it is often difficult to assess the severity of arterial lesions based on the color flow image alone, and spectral waveforms are still necessary for the most accurate classification of arterial disease.[101]

PLETHYSMOGRAPHY

Although direct noninvasive testing has assumed a more prominent role in recent years; plethysmography remains one of the most valuable noninvasive diagnostic modalities available in the vascular laboratory. As outlined in Chapter 4, a variety of instruments are in use, any one of which can be employed in most situations. All measure the same physiologic parameter: volume change. Although the division may be somewhat arbitrary, it is convenient to discuss segmental and digital plethysmography separately.

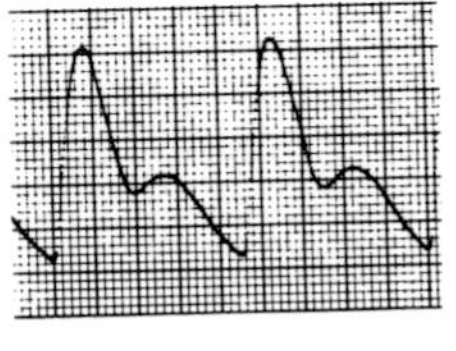

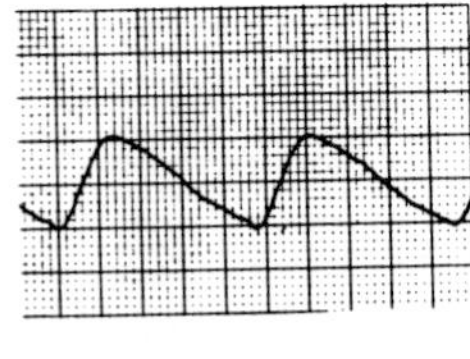

FIGURE 5–13. Normal and abnormal pulse volume contours recorded at ankle level. Normal form shows a prominent dicrotic wave on the downslope. (Cuff pressure, 65 mmHg; cuff volume, 75 ml).

Segmental Plethysmography

Although mercury or indium-gallium strain-gauges are quite sensitive and provide excellent recordings of limb volume change, the air plethysmograph, owing to its rugged construction and the ease with which it is used, has become the standard device employed in segmental plethysmography. The impedance plethysmograph, although useful for diagnosing deep venous thrombosis, has not proved to be a reliable tool for studying peripheral arterial disease.

Much of the original work with the air plethysmograph was done by Raines and colleagues, who called their specific instrument the pulse-volume recorder, or PVR.[63, 193] This term has now become almost synonymous with segmental plethysmography. Their approach has been to apply pneumatic cuffs to the upper thigh, calf, and ankle. Larger cuffs are used around the thigh (bladder = 18 × 36 cm) and smaller cuffs around the other two sites (bladder = 12 × 23 cm). The cuffs are inflated to 65 mmHg, a pressure that should require about 400 ± 75 ml of air for the thigh cuff and 75 ± 10 ml of air for each of the other two. Recordings are then made successively from each site. Measurements may be repeated after the patient has exercised on a treadmill.

Pulse Contour

The normal segmental pulse contour is characterized by a steep upstroke, a sharp systolic peak, a downslope that bows toward the baseline, and a prominent dicrotic wave (Fig. 5–13).[63] Significant occlusive disease in arterial segments proximal to the recording cuff is virtually excluded by the presence of a dicrotic wave. Its absence, however, is of less diagnostic significance. For example, during the hyperemic period following exercise, the dicrotic wave, which represents reversed flow, may disappear.[134]

Below an arterial obstruction, the upslope is less steep, the peak becomes rounded and is delayed, the downslope bows away from the baseline, and the dicrotic wave disappears (Fig. 5–13).[63] As the proximal obstruction becomes more severe, the rise and fall times become more nearly equal and the amplitude decreases. A ''mildly abnormal'' form has been identified, the contour of which lies between normal and distinctly abnormal.[134] This pulse retains the rapid upslope and sharp systolic peak characteristic of the normal form but loses the dicrotic wave. The downslope tends to bow away from the baseline. Arterial occlusions distal to the recording cuff may produce a ''mildly abnormal'' waveform in limbs with no proximal disease. Deterioration toward a distinctly abnormal wave following exercise indicates the presence of significant proximal obstruction.

Pulse Amplitude

According to Darling, Raines, and their associates, the amplitude of the plethysmographic pulse remains highly reproducible in the individual patient provided constant cuff pressures and volumes are used.[63] Amplitudes, however, vary from patient to patient and are influenced by cardiac stroke volume, blood pressure, blood volume, vasomotor tone, and the size and position of the limb. With progressively severe proximal disease, the pulse amplitude decreases. Pulses may be classified into five categories that combine amplitude and specific features of the wave contour (Table 5–14).[194] Category 1 designates a normal pulse wave, and categories 2 through 5 represent waves associated with increasingly severe obstructive disease. Although the actual volume change with each pulse (DV) is greater in the thigh than it is in the calf, the chart deflection at calf level normally exceeds that at the thigh by 25 per cent or more (Table 5–14).[133, 207] This so-called augmentation has proved to be an important diagnostic criterion, its absence signifying the presence of superficial femoral stenosis.

In normal limbs, pulse amplitude increases following treadmill exercise, reflecting the increased blood flow. On the other hand, pulse amplitude at the ankle uniformly diminishes after exercise in limbs with arterial disease, owing to the diversion of blood to the proximal musculature.[193]

Analysis of Pulses

Pulse volume recordings are generally reported to be reasonably accurate for detecting and locating arterial obstructions in the lower extremity. Typical tracings from normal limbs and from those with various combinations of peripheral arterial disease are shown in Figure 5–14.[207] When disease is confined to the aortoiliac segment, pulse contours at all levels are abnormal, but the amplitude of the calf pulse exceeds that of the thigh (a manifestation of the augmentation phenomenon). Although pulse contours are also abnormal at all levels when there is combined aortoiliac and superficial femoral arterial disease, the amplitude of the calf pulse is less than that of the thigh pulse. In limbs with isolated superficial femoral arterial obstruction, the thigh pulse is normal but the calf and ankle pulses are abnormal.

Table 5–14. Definition of Pulse Volume Recorder Categories

Pulse Volume Recorder Category	Chart Deflection (mm)		DV* (mm³)		
	Thigh and Ankle	*Calf*	*Ankle*	*Calf*	*Thigh*
1	>15†	>20†	>160	>213	>715
2	>15‡	>20‡	>160	>213	>715
3	5–15	5–20	54–160	54–213	240–715
4	<5	<5	<54	<54	<240
5	Flat	Flat	0	0	0

**DV, maximal segmental volume change per heartbeat.*
†With reflected wave.
‡No reflected wave.

The thigh pulse, according to Kempczinski, tends to underestimate the severity of aortoiliac disease.[133] If, however, moderately abnormal waves were considered to be positive, the PVR correctly identified 95 per cent of the significant stenoses in this segment. There were no false-negative results in his series. All false-positive results occurred in limbs with stenosis of the profunda femoris artery and occlusions of the superficial femoral segment. Limbs with mildly abnormal thigh pulses were subjected to treadmill exercise at 2 mph up a 10 per cent incline. If the contour of the ankle pulse became more abnormal and if its amplitude decreased, significant aortoiliac obstruction was present; but if there was no change in the pulse, the abnormal thigh pulse was attributed to superficial femoral disease.[133]

The PVR correctly assessed patency of the superficial femoral artery in 97 per cent of the limbs studied by Kempczinski, but pulse changes did not become evident unless the stenosis exceeded 90 per cent diameter reduction.[133] Isolated mid-popliteal occlusions were associated with normal augmentation of the calf pulse. All false-positive results for superficial femoral disease occurred in limbs with aortoiliac disease, and all false-negative results occurred in limbs with well-developed collaterals bypassing short segmental occlusions of the superficial femoral artery.

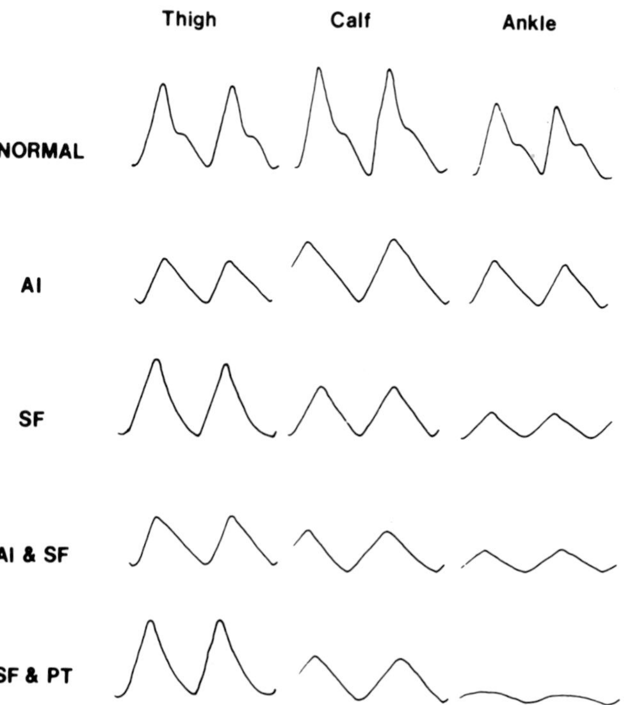

FIGURE 5–14. Pulse volume recorder (PVR) tracings from normal limbs and from limbs with various combinations of peripheral vascular disease. AI, aortoiliac; SF, superficial femoral; PT, popliteal-tibial. (From Rutherford RB, Lowenstein DH, Klein MF: Combining segmental systolic pressures and plethysmography to diagnose arterial occlusive disease of the legs. Am J Surg 138:216, 1979.)

Reidy and colleagues reported that the PVR was 100 per cent sensitive to the presence of stenoses of more than 50 per cent of the diameter of the aortoiliac arteries when disease was isolated to that segment; however, the sensitivity fell to 83 per cent in limbs with concomitant superficial femoral arterial occlusions.[200] Although negative predictive values were good for aortoiliac stenoses (87 per cent), positive predictive values were low (64 per cent). Therefore, they considered a positive study to be of little diagnostic value. On the other hand, negative and positive predictive values were quite acceptable (85 and 91 per cent, respectively) when the PVR was used to detect femoropopliteal disease.[133] On the basis of a similar study, Francfort and coworkers concluded that the PVR was inaccurate for detecting aortoiliac disease but that it was highly sensitive to superficial femoral lesions, even in limbs with proximal disease.[75]

Rutherford and associates found that the PVR correctly identified 97 per cent of normal limbs, about 70 per cent of limbs with isolated or combined disease of the aortoiliac and superficial femoral segments, and 100 per cent of limbs with disease confined to the below-knee arteries.[207] When PVR results were considered in conjunction with segmental limb pressures, the accuracy of the combined tests was distinctly better than that of either test alone, ranging between 86 and 100 per cent for all categories of disease. Other investigators have confirmed the complementary roles of the two tests.[75, 133] Therefore, the simultaneous use of PVR and segmental limb pressure measurement is generally advocated. Indeed, this approach was originally recommended by Raines and associates.[194] PVR findings are especially important in subjects with calcified arteries, in whom the segmental systolic pressures are often unreliable.[184]

Digital Plethysmography

Although digital plethysmography may be considered a form of segmental plethysmography, pulses obtained

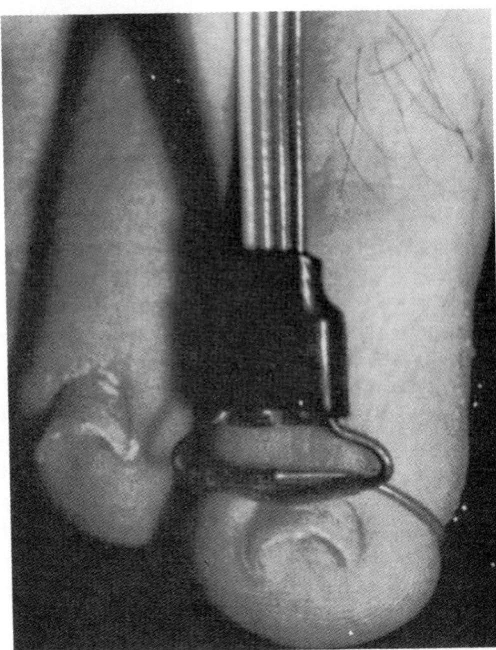

FIGURE 5–15. A mercury strain-gauge applied to the second toe.

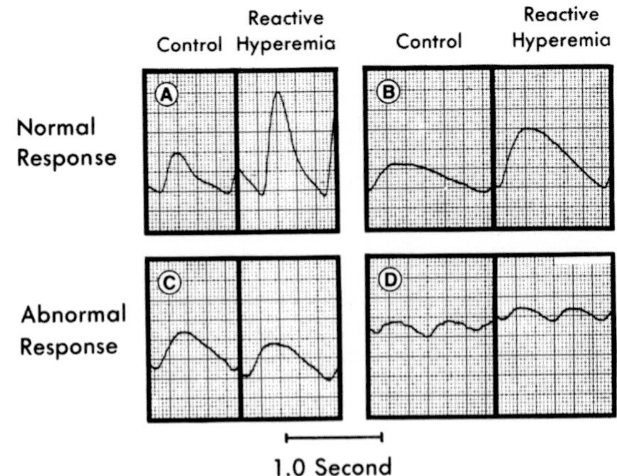

FIGURE 5–16. Reactive hyperemia test; digit pulse, second toe. Digit pulse volume more than doubles in the normal response *(upper panels)*. Little change in pulse volume is evident in abnormal response *(lower panels)*. *A*, Normal circulation (pressure: arm 130, ankle 140). *B*, Superficial femoral occlusion (pressure: arm 100, ankle 80). *C*, Diabetic for 20 years (pressure: arm 135, ankle 135). *D*, Iliac and superficial femoral arterial disease (pressure: arm 118, ankle 46). Attenuation of recorder: *A*, ×10; *B–D*, ×20.

from the tips of the toes or fingers (see Chapter 65) have special diagnostic significance. Because the recordings are made from the most distal portion of the extremities, they reflect the physiologic status of all proximal arteries, from the arterioles to the aorta. They are sensitive, therefore, not only to mechanical obstruction but also to vasospasm.

Digit pulses may be recorded with specially designed air plethysmographs that use cuffs with bladders measuring 7 × 2 cm or 9 × 3 cm; however, mercury strain-gauges or photoplethysmographs (PPG) are usually employed because of their greater sensitivity (Fig. 5–15). Although the PPG does not provide quantitative data, it is the most easily used of the three devices and consequently is preferred by many laboratories.

To obtain optimal recordings, studies should be conducted in a warm room (about 72 to 75°F) in which relative humidity is maintained at about 40 per cent. In order to avoid vasospasm, the feet and toes must be warm. This may require immersing the foot in warm water or placing the patient under an electric blanket. At times, it may be necessary to induce postischemic reactive hyperemia, as discussed later.[232] Although interpretation of good volume pulses is relatively easy, it is futile and misleading to attempt to assess those of inferior quality.

Pulse Contour

The contour of the digit pulse resembles that of the segmental pulses obtained more proximally in the limb (Fig. 5–16).[54, 227, 232, 267, 277] Normally, there is a rapid upslope, a sharp peak, and a downslope that bows toward the baseline. A dicrotic wave or notch is usually present on the downslope. Distal to an obstruction, the pulse is considerably more rounded, having a slower upslope, a downslope that bows away from the baseline, and no dicrotic wave. In severe cases of arterial obstruction, no pulse may be perceptible.

Finding a normal toe pulse contour is good evidence that all arteries from the digital arteries to the heart are free of functionally significant arterial disease. Similarly, finding an obstructive pulse contour indicates that there are one or more functionally significant areas of obstruction lying somewhere between the heart and the digital arteries. Thus, digital pulses are especially important in the investigation of ischemia of the toes or forefoot.[239] Pedal or digital artery disease, which may contribute greatly to the ischemic process, may escape detection if the investigation is carried no further than the ankle level. Such errors are easily made in diabetic patients, because the ankle arteries are often incompressible and the disease is more likely to involve pedal vessels. As shown in Figure 5–17, perfusion of the toes may be inadequate even in the presence of a good ankle pressure.

Although more complex methods for describing digital pulse contours have been proposed (including measurements of slope, pulse width at half maximal excursion, and relative amplitudes at various parts of the curve), these measurements have little physiologic meaning and are unnecessary in clinical work.[20, 23]

Pulse Amplitude

The volume of the toe pulse is not in itself a very reliable indicator of the severity of arterial disease.[54, 227, 277] Although the digital pulse volume corresponds quite closely with digital blood flow (provided that the same gauge is used on the same toe of the same subject during the same examination), it is impossible to compare toe pulses from day to day in the same subject or between subjects as an index of relative blood flow.[279] Moreover, digital blood flow is highly variable, depending more on sympathetic activity than on the presence of anatomic arterial disease.

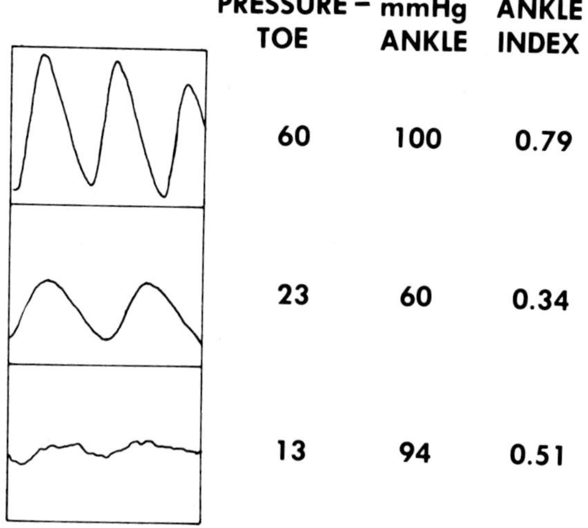

FIGURE 5–17. The configuration of the toe plethysmogram is closely correlated with the toe pressure but is poorly correlated with the ankle pressure or ankle index. *Upper tracing* implies good digital artery perfusion; *middle tracing*, borderline perfusion; *lower tracing*, ischemia. (From Sumner DS: Rational use of noninvasive tests in designing a therapeutic approach to severe arterial disease of the legs. *In* Puel P, Boccalon H, Enjalbert A [eds]: Hemodynamics of the Limbs—2. Toulouse, France, GEPESC, 1981, pp 369–376.)

Reactive Hyperemia

The reactive hyperemia test is valuable as an indicator of the extent of peripheral vascular disease and as a predictor of the efficacy of surgical sympathectomy.[225, 232] A pneumatic cuff is placed around the ankle, calf, or thigh; inflated to above systolic pressure; kept at that level for 3 to 5 minutes; and rapidly deflated. The volume of the toe pulse is then followed over the next several minutes. In normal limbs, the pulse returns almost immediately, attains half its preocclusive amplitude within a few seconds, and then rapidly reaches a peak volume (Table 5–15).[78, 93, 239] Maximal excursion is usually more than twice that recorded during the control period (see Fig. 5–16).

The reappearance time of the toe pulse is frequently delayed in legs with arterial occlusive disease, often exceeding 120 seconds in severely impaired extremities.[78, 93] Because it is difficult to define precisely the time at which the first pulse returns, the time required for the pulse to reach half the preocclusive volume seems to be a more practical measurement. This value is closely related to the severity of the disease and to the extent of arterial occlusion (Table 5–15). Bernstein and colleagues found that the functional results of aortofemoral bypass procedures can be predicted quite well by determining the time required for the pulse to reach half the control volume.[25] When the time was less than 10 seconds, 63 per cent of the limbs became asymptomatic and another 37 per cent were improved. However, when the time exceeded 90 seconds, only 10 per cent of the limbs became asymptomatic and only 50 per cent improved.

Table 5–15. Pulse-Reappearance Time After Release of Arterial Occlusion (sec)*

Location of Occlusive Disease	Pulse-Reappearance Time	Time Required to Reach Half Control Volume
No occlusions	0.2 ± 0.1	3.4 ± 0.8
Aortoiliac	7.2 ± 4.0	23.9 ± 6.7
Femoropopliteal	3.7 ± 3.7	26.5 ± 12.7
Popliteal trifurcation	15.2 ± 9.3	23.9 ± 9.4
Multi-level	45.3 ± 5.5	71.2 ± 5.5

**Modified from Fronek A, Coel M, Bernstein EF: The pulse-reappearance time: An index of over-all blood flow impairment in the ischemic extremity. Surgery 81:376, 1977.*

The relative increase in pulse volume during reactive hyperemia is an excellent indicator of the functional severity of the arterial obstruction. As discussed in Chapter 3, the peripheral vascular bed is nearly maximally dilated in limbs with severe ischemia; consequently, little further vasodilatation is possible (see Fig. 5–16). Approximately 85 per cent of limbs with obstruction confined to a single segment (e.g., aortoiliac, femoropopliteal, or popliteal trifurcation) display at least a 25 per cent increase in the volume of the toe pulse.[78] In contrast, only about half of the limbs with multi-level disease show a response of this magnitude. Because of proximal steal phenomena, the pulse volume in such limbs may remain decreased for a long period and may never exceed that recorded during the control period.[239]

Experience has shown that surgical sympathectomy is most likely to provide a satisfactory result if the peak reactive hyperemia pulse is twice the size of the control pulse. If less dilatation is seen, it is much less likely that sympathectomy will increase peripheral blood flow. Since reactive hyperemia can occur in a fully sympathectomized extremity, the reactive hyperemia test reveals nothing about the integrity of the sympathetic innervation; what the test does is to substantiate the ability of the peripheral vessels to dilate in response to a release of vascular tone. The ''deep breath test'' or one of its modifications is necessary to demonstrate continued function of the sympathetic nervous system.[67] In response to a deep breath, the pulse volume will temporarily decrease, provided sympathetic innervation is intact. Absence of this response implies impaired sympathetic activity and should be considered a contraindication to sympathectomy.

TRANSCUTANEOUS OXYGEN TENSION

Unlike the methods previously discussed in this chapter, which are sensitive to hemodynamic changes, transcutaneous oxygen tension ($tcPo_2$) measurements reflect the metabolic state of the target tissues. Although the technique is susceptible to a host of confounding variables, the potential importance of the information derived is so great that the method deserves close attention.

Although measurements may be obtained from almost any area of interest, common locations include the dorsum of the foot, the anteromedial calf about 10 cm below the patella, the thigh about 10 cm above the patella, and the chest in the subclavicular region. In normal limbs, most—but not all—investigators have observed a modest decrease (5 to 6 mmHg) in $tcPo_2$ from the more proximal parts of the leg to the foot.[38, 49, 156] With increasing age, $tcPo_2$ tends to decrease, paralleling a similar decline in arterial Po_2.[49, 90, 104, 169, 182] For this reason, Hauser and Shoemaker have advocated dividing the limb $tcPo_2$ by that measured at the subclavicular region to obtain a regional perfusion index (RPI) that is independent of age, cardiac output, and arterial Po_2.[104] Others maintain that this calculation does not significantly enhance the predictive value of the test.[38, 49, 169] Values for $tcPo_2$ also depend on the vertical distance between the measurement site and the heart, decreasing when the limb is elevated and increasing when the limb is dependent.[38, 76, 103, 104, 156] In addition, there may be some increase in $tcPo_2$ with an elevation of venous pressure.[76]

As discussed in Chapter 4, $tcPo_2$ values represent a complex function of cutaneous blood flow, metabolic activity, oxyhemoglobin dissociation, and oxygen diffusion though the tissues. Changes are not ordinarily perceptible in limbs with mild degrees of arterial disease, because the oxygen supply far exceeds that required to meet metabolic demands. Under conditions of stress, however, the metabolic demands may utilize a larger portion of the available oxygen supply, thereby reducing the $tcPo_2$. Likewise, in cases of severe arterial obstruction, oxygen delivery is often marginal: The quantity of free O_2 reaching the sensor is reduced and the $tcPo_2$ falls. Thus, $tcPo_2$ is most sensitive to the higher grades of arterial obstruction. Even at low levels of perfusion, $tcPo_2$ values are not linearly related to blood flow.[157] In fact, $tcPo_2$ may fall to zero in areas where cutaneous blood flow is still detectable by other methods.[157] This does not mean that no oxygen is reaching the tissue but does imply that all available oxygen is being consumed and that none remains for diffusion to the sensor.[36, 49, 76]

Because the arterial pressure at any given site represents the potential energy available for transporting blood through the tissues, it is not surprising that statistically significant correlations between segmental pressures and $tcPo_2$ values are reported.[50, 156, 182, 270] The correlation coefficients, however, are quite poor, especially in diabetic extremities.

Resting Values

Representative $tcPo_2$ values obtained from resting supine subjects are given in Table 5–16. The tendency for the values to decrease from the more proximal to the more distal parts of the leg is minimal in normal limbs but becomes more pronounced with increasing severity of disease. Irrespective of the site of measurement, normal $tcPo_2$ hovers around 60 mmHg. Measurements in normal younger subjects are usually about 10 mmHg higher than those given in the table, which correspond to values observed in patients in the age groups most susceptible to atherosclerosis.[49, 104, 169] In general, a $tcPo_2$ greater than 55 mmHg may be considered normal at any measurement site regardless of age.[49] The average normal RPI is about 90 per cent.[104]

Peripheral measurements reflect the deleterious effect of increasing obstructive disease more dramatically than the more proximal measurements do. For example, there is little difference among the thigh $tcPo_2$ values of any of the disease groups listed in Table 5–16. Although statistically significant differences are often demonstrated between the values of normal and claudicating extremities and between claudicating extremities and those with rest pain, there is enough overlap to prevent individual tests from discriminating accurately among the various disease categories.[49] Many claudicants have resting $tcPo_2$ values that fall in the normal range, even at foot level.[38] Values in limb-threatening ischemia are, however, significantly reduced. At foot level, $tcPo_2$ values are usually less than 20 mmHg in legs with severe rest pain, ischemic ulcers, or gangrene.[38, 49, 181] In the series reported by Wyss and coworkers, 46 per cent of nondiabetic limbs with $tcPo_2$ values less than 20 mmHg required amputation.[270]

Enhancement Procedures

Recordings may be made after exercise, following a period of ischemia, during oxygen inhalation, and with the legs in a dependent position. These are among the various modifications of the basic measurement procedure that have been advocated to enhance the discriminatory ability of the $tcPo_2$ values.

Dependent Position

Franzeck and colleagues observed an average increase of 15 ± 7 mmHg in the $tcPo_2$ on the dorsum of the foot in normal subjects when they moved from a supine to a sitting position.[76] In this position, the sensor was 54 cm below the heart. With standing, which extended the distance to 84 cm, the $tcPo_2$ rose by an average of 28 ± 14 mmHg. The increase in $tcPo_2$ that accompanies standing occurs at all

Table 5–16. Representative $tcPo_2$ Values at Rest, Supine Position (mmHg, mean ± SD)

	Normal*			Claudication			Rest Pain		
Author and Year	*Foot*	*Calf*	*Thigh*	*Foot*	*Calf*	*Thigh*	*Foot*	*Calf*	*Thigh*
Clyne et al (1982)[50]	59 ± 4	63 ± 5	64 ± 6	51 ± 10	64 ± 9	67 ± 9	36 ± 16	50 ± 16	55 ± 18
Hauser and Shoemaker (1983)[104]	59 ± 10	56 ± 10	64 ± 7	46 ± 12	49 ± 9	57 ± 9	—	—	—
Cina et al (1984)[49]†	64 ± 4	64 ± 4	—	46 ± 5	55 ± 4	—	17 ± 4	42 ± 6	—
Byrne et al (1984)[38]	60 ± 7	63 ± 8	66 ± 8	56 ± 4	59 ± 5	66 ± 7	4 ± 4	29 ± 20	50 ± 14
				37 ± 12	48 ± 10	54 ± 7‡			
Kram et al (1985)[143]	47 ± 12	53 ± 15	—	33 ± 14	37 ± 13	—	20 ± 16	29 ± 20	—

**Older subjects.*
†Values estimated from published graphs.
‡More severe claudication.

levels of the leg but is most evident at foot level, where the hydrostatic pressure is greatest.

As a rule, the augmentation in $tcPo_2$ increases commensurate with the severity of limb ischemia. Byrne and associates, for example, noted an average increase of 20 mmHg in limbs with rest pain compared with an average increase of 10 mmHg in normal limbs.[38] Based on their data, it appears that $tcPo_2$ rises by about 18 per cent in normal limbs, 22 per cent in claudicating limbs with normal resting $tcPo_2$ values, 58 per cent in claudicating limbs with abnormal resting values, and 88 per cent in limbs with rest pain. Oh and colleagues, working in the same laboratory, retrospectively separated severely ischemic extremities into two groups based on the change in $tcPo_2$ that occurred with standing.[181] Group I was defined by a $tcPo_2$ increase of less than 15 mmHg (average 4 ± 5 mmHg), and group II, by an increase of more than 15 mmHg (average 36 ± 11 mmHg). Despite the fact that both groups had similar supine $tcPo_2$ values (4 ± 5 mmHg and 6 ± 5 mmHg, respectively), the manifestations of disease were more severe in group I limbs (61 per cent ulcers or gangrene, 48 per cent rest pain, and 39 per cent claudication) than in group II limbs (29 per cent ulcers or gangrene, 46 per cent rest pain, and 68 per cent claudication).

The increase in oxygen tension that occurs when a patient with an ischemic limb sits or stands may explain how dependency relieves rest pain. As discussed in Chapter 3, elevation of the hydrostatic pressure dilates capillaries and other resistive vessels, thereby permitting more blood to flow at the same arteriovenous pressure gradient. In addition, any muscular activity with the leg dependent may decrease venous pressure and increase the arteriovenous pressure gradient (see Chapter 129). With the increase in capillary blood flow, more oxygen is delivered to the tissues. In the most severely ischemic extremities, these physiologic buffers are nearly exhausted, and the increase in blood flow is inadequate to provide relief.

Exercise

In limbs with restricted arterial inflow, dilatation of intramuscular vessels induced by exercise diverts blood away from cutaneous vascular beds, causing $tcPo_2$ to fall. In normal limbs, this "steal" is not evident, because the arterial blood supply is adequate to supply both vascular beds. It is not surprising, therefore, to find that postexercise/pre-exercise ratios of ankle pressures and ankle $tcPo_2$ values are highly correlated ($r = 0.918$), as demonstrated by the treadmill studies of Matsen and associates.[158]

Byrne and associates observed that $tcPo_2$ values measured on the dorsum of the foot during treadmill exercise remained at about the same level as those obtained during quiet standing (which is somewhat difficult to explain); however, during the period following exercise, after the subjects had resumed a supine position, the $tcPo_2$ values fell in all patients with significant arterial obstruction, even in those with normal resting values (Table 5–17).[38] No fall was evident in normal subjects. Similar, but less marked, changes occurred at calf level. They concluded that postexercise $tcPo_2$ measurements accurately distinguished all subjects with vascular claudication from those who were normal.

Hauser and Shoemaker found that the chest $tcPo_2$ increased in claudicators during exercise, perhaps explaining the failure of limb values to decrease.[104] However, the RPI (limb $tcPo_2$/chest $tcPo_2$) at foot level did decrease during exercise, even in normal extremities. When RPIs obtained during exercise were compared with values obtained when the patient was standing, a decrease of more than 10 per cent at the thigh or more than 15 per cent at the calf was found to be highly specific for intermittent claudication. Normal limbs measured at these levels demonstrated no fall in RPI. After exercise, the RPI at the foot in normal limbs always returned to pre-exercise values within 1 minute. In claudicating limbs, the average time to recover one half of the exercise drop was about 4 minutes.

Reactive Hyperemia

Inflation of a pneumatic cuff to suprasystolic pressure is followed by a rapid decline in the $tcPo_2$ measured further down the leg. When the cuff is deflated after a period of ischemia (usually about 4 minutes), the $tcPo_2$ rapidly returns to preocclusion levels in normal extremities. In limbs with occlusive arterial disease, the rate of recovery is much slower. Recovery rates are usually expressed as the time required for the $tcPo_2$ to return to one half of the preocclusive value ($T_{1/2}$).

Representative results are shown in Table 5–18. Cina and coworkers reported a range of 43 to 60 seconds in normal limbs and 75 to 150 seconds in claudicating limbs; there were no overlapping values.[49] Kram and associates found that postischemic recovery times based on the RPI (limb $tcPo_2$/chest $tcPo_2$) were more diagnostic of arterial

Table 5–17. Effect of Exercise on Foot $tcPo_2$ (mmHg, mean ± SD)*

Type of Obstruction	$tcPo_2$ Values			
	Supine	*Standing*	*Exercise*	*Postexercise*†
Normal	60 ± 7	71 ± 7	75 ± 9	69 ± 7
Claudication‡	56 ± 4	58 ± 8	53 ± 10	33 ± 16
Claudication	37 ± 12	58 ± 12	49 ± 18	23 ± 20
Rest Pain	4 ± 4	25 ± 20	26 ± 26	5 ± 7

Data from Byrne P, Provan JL, Ameli FM, et al: The use of transcutaneous oxygen tension measurements in the diagnosis of peripheral vascular insufficiency. Ann Surg 200:159, 1984.

†Postexercise measurements made with patient supine.

‡Claudicators with normal resting $tcPo_2$ values.

Table 5–18. Postischemic Transcutaneous Oxygen Recovery Rate $T_{1/2}$ (sec)

	Normal		Claudication		Rest Pain	
Author and Year	*Foot*	*Calf*	*Foot*	*Calf*	*Foot*	*Calf*
Franzeck et al (1982)[76]	87 ± 27	60 ± 15	136 ± 73	131 ± 69	—	—
Cina et al (1984)[49]	49 ± 6	—	114 ± 2	—	—	—
Kram et al (1985)[143]	66 ± 18	48 ± 18	156 ± 60	126 ± 42	204 ± 78	126 ± 66

**Based on limb/chest $tcPo_2$ ratio.*

disease than toe-pulse recovery times.[141] Values for $T_{1/2}$ in excess of 84 seconds at the calf and 102 seconds at the foot were considered pathologic.[141, 143]

Oxygen Inhalation

Inhalation of pure oxygen markedly augments the $tcPo_2$ in normal limbs but has less effect in limbs with severe arterial occlusion. Ohgi and associates reported that pretibial values increased from 70 ± 9 to 365 ± 87 mmHg in normal legs, from 34 ± 33 to 115 ± 109 mmHg in legs with chronic occlusions, and from 23 ± 30 to 96 ± 57 mmHg in legs with acute occlusions.[182] According to Harward and colleagues, the prediction of amputation healing by means of $tcPo_2$ determinations may be enhanced by oxygen inhalation.[99]

Comment on $tcPo_2$ Measurements

Although $tcPo_2$ measurements made after exercise or a period of ischemia can be used to distinguish between normal and claudicating limbs, other less demanding tests are equally efficacious. It would seem that a more appropriate role for $tcPo_2$ measurement is to assist in the assessment of severe ischemia.[252] Because the results are not affected by arterial calcification, this test is particularly valuable for evaluating diabetic vascular disease.[49, 76, 103, 127]

LASER DOPPLER

A relative index of cutaneous blood flow can be obtained with the laser Doppler (see Chapter 4). The output, which is expressed in millivolts (mv), is roughly proportional to the average blood flow in a 1.5 mm^3 volume of skin, lying 0.8 to 1.5 mm below the skin surface. According to Karanfilian and associates, tracings from normal skin exhibit three major characteristics: (1) pulse waves that coincide with the cardiac cycle, (2) vasomotor waves that occur four to six times per minute, and (3) a mean blood flow velocity that is represented by the elevation of the tracing above a zero baseline.[126] In the leg, the highest velocities are obtained from the skin of the big toe, followed, in descending order, by velocities from the skin of the plantar surface of the foot, dorsal foot, distal leg, thigh, and proximal leg.

In limbs with peripheral vascular disease, pulse waves are attenuated, mean velocities are decreased, and vasomotor waves may disappear (Table 5–19).[127] The reactive hyperemic response to a period of cuff-induced ischemia is diminished, and the time to reach maximal hyperemia is markedly delayed (Table 5–19).[127] Karanfilian and coworkers investigated the ability of laser Doppler studies to predict healing of ulcers or forefoot amputations in a series of ischemic limbs.[127] When the mean velocity recorded from the plantar aspect of the foot or big toe exceeded 40 mv and the pulse wave amplitude exceeded 4 mv, 96 per cent of the lesions or amputations healed. On the other hand, when these criteria were not met, 79 per cent of the feet failed to heal. These results were not quite as good as those obtained on the same extremities using $tcPo_2$.

The laser Doppler can also be used in conjunction with a pneumatic cuff to estimate skin blood pressure at almost any level of the upper or lower extremities. These measurements are made with the probe (which merely serves as a flow sensor) placed under the pneumatic cuff. Castronuovo and associates obtained cutaneous pressure averaging 47 ± 28 mmHg in normal forearms and thighs and 73 ± 28 mmHg in the plantar skin of the big toe.[47] These pressures are similar to those in precapillary vessels. Much lower values were found in the plantar skin of the toe (17 ± 15 mmHg) and in the dorsal skin of the foot (10 ± 10 mmHg) in limbs with rest pain, ulceration, or gangrene.

Although the laser Doppler is a valid physiologic test, it has not been widely used in vascular laboratories. It

Table 5–19. Laser Doppler Measurements From the Big Toe (mean ± SD)*

	Baseline Values		Reactive Hyperemia Test	
	Velocity (mv)	*Pulse Amplitude (mv)*	*Peak/Baseline† Ratio*	*Time (sec) to Maximal Velocity*
Normal	197 ± 174	77 ± 63	3.1 ± 0.9	18 ± 7
Ischemic	67 ± 42	5 ± 4	1.7 ± 1.6	150 ± 48

**Data from Karanfilian RG, Lynch TG, Lee BC, et al: The assessment of skin blood flow in peripheral vascular disease by laser Doppler velocimetry. Am Surg 50:641, 1984.*

†Ratio of peak postischemic velocity to preischemic velocity.

cannot be calibrated in terms of actual blood flow, and much of the information that it provides is already supplied by more established techniques.

CLINICAL APPLICATIONS

After the history and physical examination have been completed, the next logical step in the evaluation of a patient for arterial disease is physiologic testing.[20] These tests are designed to answer the following questions:

1. Is significant arterial occlusive disease present?
2. If so, how severe is the physiologic impairment?
3. What is the approximate location of the disease?
4. In multi-level disease, which arterial segments are most severely affected?
5. In limbs with tissue loss, what is the potential for healing?

Armed with this information, the surgeon is better able to decide whether the deficit is severe enough to warrant diagnostic arteriography as a prelude to possible intervention.

Some surgeons protest that physiologic testing is unnecessary, provided a careful history and physical examination have been carried out. This argument fails to take into account a number of clinical problems that are not easily resolved even with the help of arteriography. For example, patients with pseudoclaudication may be identified and spared further vascular work-up.[46, 87, 130, 246] Patients with demonstrable arterial disease may have concomitant orthopedic or neurologic problems. With the help of physiologic testing, the physician can determine the relative magnitude of the deficit caused by each of the diseases and advise the patient accordingly. In limbs with multi-level disease, it is usually possible to identify which of the lesions is most significant, allowing the surgeon to focus on the more critical lesion.[3, 25, 32, 173, 188, 243, 262] Stenoses that appear mild on arteriograms frequently cause significant physiologic deficits; others that appear severe may be relatively inconsequential.

Physiologic tests are helpful in determining whether an ulcer is due to neuropathy, stasis, infection, or ischemia and in deciding whether foot pain is primarily neuropathic or ischemic.[112, 197] They may also enhance the ability of the surgeon to assess the healing potential of a foot lesion or amputation and thus help in selecting the appropriate site for amputation.[17, 29, 109, 166, 259] In cases of suspected vascular trauma, physiologic findings, if negative, may avert an unnecessary vascular exploration or, if positive, may alert the surgeon to the need for immediate operation.[117] Similarly, the recognition and evaluation of suspected iatrogenic vascular injuries, such as those that follow cardiac catheterization or interventional radiology, are facilitated by physiologic testing.[16] Physiologic tests are uniquely applicable to the diagnosis of intermittent arterial obstructions, such as those arising from entrapment syndromes, and for distinguishing between fixed arterial obstructions and those due to vasospasm. These are but a few of the many areas in which physiologic tests complement the information gleaned from the routine history, physical examination, and arteriogram.

Once all the data have been analyzed, the surgeon must decide among various therapeutic options. No matter what course is elected, physiologic testing continues to offer valuable supplementary information (Fig. 5–18). If the choice is made to defer operation, a baseline physiologic study should be performed and the patient should be carefully followed to detect disease progression. If an interventional approach, such as arterial reconstruction, balloon angioplasty, laser disobliteration, or sympathectomy, is selected, a preoperative evaluation is of value to establish a baseline against which the therapeutic outcome can be measured. During the operation and at the completion of the reconstruction, physiologic testing may alert the surgeon to the presence of a mechanical defect that might adversely affect the result of the surgery (see Chapter 24).[237] Repeat studies in the recovery room and during the first few days after interventional therapy will permit early recognition of failure. Follow-up monitoring helps identify early failure, deteriorating physiologic parameters that herald impending failure, and the lack of significant improvement despite continued patency of the reconstruction—any of which may signify the need for arteriographic evaluation and possible repeat surgery.[23, 183, 244] Objective assessment of the physiologic improvement resulting from arterial reconstruction or other interventional measures supplies valuable data that can be used by the surgeon to perfect the therapeutic approach to specific vascular problems.[243, 244]

Although many different methods for studying the arterial circulation have been discussed in this chapter, not all are indicated in the evaluation or follow-up of each patient.[20] Some tests are not as accurate as others, some are more difficult to perform, and many provide overlapping information or information that is not pertinent to the questions being asked. The best policy is to select those modalities that supply the most information, have been shown to be reliable by critical prospective evaluation, and are known to be economical in terms of time and money. The remainder of this chapter is devoted to the application of these tests to specific arterial problems.

Intermittent Claudication

When the presenting complaint is limited to exercise-induced pain or fatigue in the muscles of the leg or buttocks, the two most important questions are: (1) Is arterial disease present? and (2) If so, is it severe enough to account for the discomfort? If the ankle pressures are clearly normal, further investigation is seldom required.[185, 238] If, however, the symptoms are highly suggestive of intermittent claudication, or if the ankle pressure is equivocal, the patient should undergo a treadmill exercise evaluation at 2 mph up a 10 per cent grade (Fig. 5–19).[43] A drop in ankle pressure indicates that blood flow is inadequate to sustain normal metabolism during walking, confirming the diagnosis of claudication. If, on the other hand, the resting ankle pressure is clearly abnormal, exercise testing is required only to substantiate the diagnosis, to evaluate the extent of the disability, and to provide a baseline for follow-up studies. When, despite a drop in ankle pressure, the patient stops walking because of angina, dyspnea, or pain in the hip or knee, the limiting cardiac, pulmonary, or orthopedic

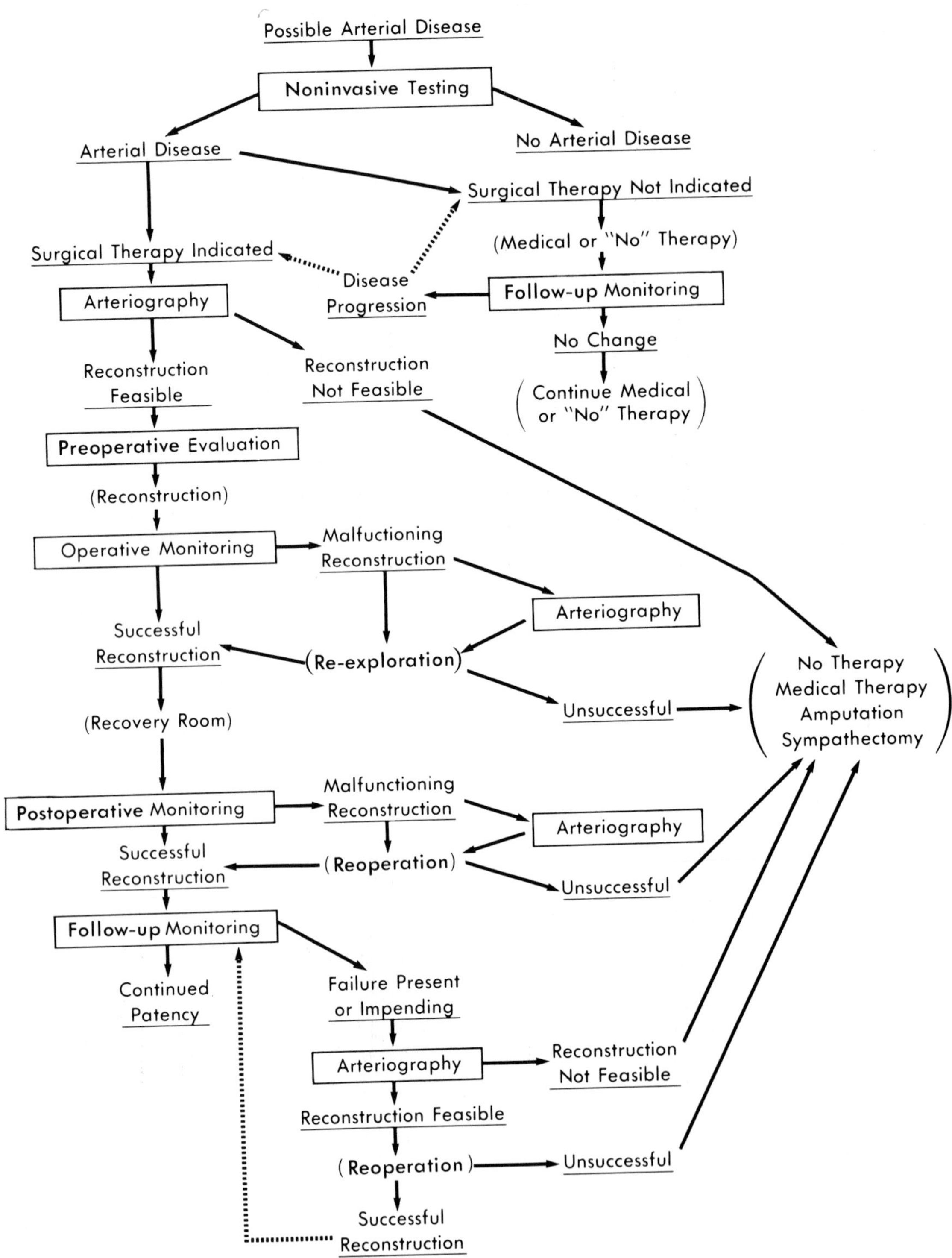

FIGURE 5–18. Physiologic approach to the diagnosis and management of peripheral arterial disease. In this diagram, diagnostic procedures are enclosed in *boxes*; conclusions, interpretations, and results are *underlined*; therapeutic procedures are enclosed in *parentheses*. Feedback loops are indicated by *broken lines*.

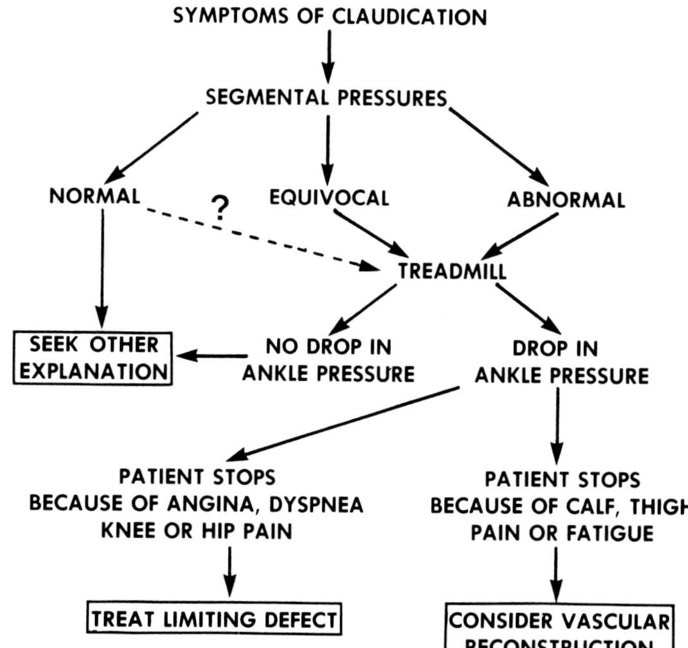

FIGURE 5–19. Algorithm illustrating diagnostic approach to patients with claudication. (Modified from Sumner DS: Algorithms using noninvasive diagnostic data as a guide to therapy of arterial insufficiency. *In* Puel P, Boccalon H, Enjalbert A [eds]: Hemodynamics of the Limbs—1. Toulouse, France, GEPESC, 1979, pp 543–566.)

defect should be treated before arterial reconstruction is considered. Cessation of walking with little or no drop in ankle pressure suggests neurogenic claudication (pseudoclaudication).[46, 87, 130, 246] Rarely, the ankle pressure may not drop even though the resting ankle pressure is decreased. This may occur when the arterial obstruction is limited to the distal vessels of the leg below the origin of the major blood supply to the calf muscles (sural arteries). In this event, the more proximal segmental pressures, plethysmographic tracings, and Doppler velocity signals will usually be normal. These patients may complain of foot claudication. Foot claudication in conjunction with normal ankle pressures is also seen in some patients with thromboangiitis obliterans in whom the obstruction is limited to the pedal arteries.[227]

A more common cause of a "normal" resting ankle pressure in limbs with symptoms suggestive of claudication is medial calcification in patients with diabetes. In such cases, abnormal Doppler signals, abnormal segmental or digital plethysmographic waveforms, or duplex scanning can be used to substantiate the diagnosis. Cutaneous oxygen tension measurements, however, are often normal at rest, even in limbs with significant proximal arterial disease and definite claudication.[38] A drop in the $tcPo_2$ after treadmill exercise and a delayed recovery are quite specific for intermittent claudication, even in patients with diabetic extremities (see Table 5–17).[38, 104] Raines and associates concluded that limiting claudication was unlikely if the postexercise ankle pulse volume recordings fell into categories 2 or 3; but that claudication was probable when the recordings fell into categories 4 or 5 (see Table 5–14).[194]

As discussed previously in this chapter, reactive hyperemia tests can be substituted for treadmill exercise to evaluate the severity of the obstructive process. Unfortunately, reactive hyperemia testing does not provide information regarding nonvascular conditions that limit walking and is rarely useful. If the patient cannot walk on the treadmill, treatment for claudication is not indicated and the information supplied by reactive hyperemia is superfluous. Nonetheless, the half-time required for recovery to preischemic pulse volumes or $tcPo_2$ values has been shown to discriminate well between normal and claudicating extremities; therefore, these tests may have a role in the evaluation of diabetic patients with incompressible arteries.[49, 78, 143]

It should be noted that the absolute level of the ankle blood pressure is of less importance than the ABI in assessing the severity of claudication. For example, a patient with a brachial systolic pressure of 100 mmHg and an ankle pressure of 110 mmHg will have no claudication, but a patient with an arm pressure of 150 mmHg and an ankle pressure of 110 mmHg will be significantly limited by claudication. Although both will have normal resting blood flows, the muscle blood flow during exercise in the patient with an ankle index of 0.73 will be restricted (see Chapter 3).

Rest Pain

Absence of pedal pulses, dependent rubor, trophic skin changes, and decreased skin temperature—all hallmarks of severe ischemia—are generally present in patients with rest pain, even when there is no evident tissue loss. When the ischemia has been present for only a short time, the skin may appear relatively normal. Other causes of pain, such as orthopedic problems and infections, are usually easily recognized, but neuropathic pain associated with diabetes mellitus may present a diagnostic challenge, particularly in limbs with concomitant arterial obstruction. The function of noninvasive testing is not only to identify the presence of arterial obstruction but also to ascertain whether the blood flow at rest is sufficiently compromised to be responsible for the symptoms.

Again, the first step is to measure the ankle systolic

pressure (Fig. 5–20).[238, 239] Stress testing is not necessary; subtle degrees of arterial obstruction are of no concern. If the ankle pressure is clearly within the ischemic range, vascular reconstruction should be strongly considered. When the ankle pressure is normal or when it is abnormal (below arm pressure) but above ischemic levels, digital plethysmography should be employed and toe pressures obtained. If the toe pressures and plethysmographic tracings are normal or are abnormal but above the ischemic range, it is most unlikely that the patient has an ischemic foot (see Fig. 5–6).[197] In the absence of a skin lesion, other explanations for the pain must be sought. If, on the other hand, toe pressures and plethysmographic tracings are compatible with severe ischemia, arterial reconstruction should be considered in any limb with a decreased ankle pressure, because even a moderate elevation of the perfusion pressure may relieve pain. In limbs with ischemic feet but normal ankle pressures, therapeutic options are limited to amputation or possibly to sympathectomy.

Measurements of $tcPO_2$ levels from the skin of the dorsum of the foot may be diagnostic of rest pain and may also provide an objective assessment of the degree of ischemia (see Table 5–16).[38, 49, 270] Such measurements are likely to be of most value in patients with diabetic extremities, in which pressure data are frequently unreliable.[49, 271] In the same situation, the diagnosis of rest pain is probable when the ankle pulse volume recordings are in the range of categories 3 to 4 and is likely when the categories are in the range of 4 to 5 (see Table 5–14).[194]

There is no absolute definition of what constitutes an ischemic ankle pressure. Certainly, pressures less than 35 mmHg in nondiabetic patients and less than 55 mmHg in diabetic patients must be regarded as ischemic or nearly so.[194] The use of the ABI is inappropriate, since the critical concern is not the severity of the obstructive process but rather the head of pressure available to pump blood through the pedal arteries and the vascular bed of the foot. A patient with a high systemic blood pressure may have an adequate ankle pressure despite a markedly reduced ABI.

Ischemic Ulcers and Gangrene

Foot ulcers may be neuropathic or ischemic, or they may have a combined neuropathic-ischemic etiology. Although purely neuropathic ulcers are usually easily distinguished from those due to ischemia by their characteristic location and the normal appearance of the surrounding skin, many foot ulcers are not so readily categorized. Gangrene, on the other hand, always implies ischemia; however, its presence does not define the location or extent of the occlusive process responsible for the impaired blood flow. The role of noninvasive testing, therefore, is to ascertain whether ischemia is present, to determine its severity, and to assess the potential for healing.

The basic approach is similar to that employed in the evaluation of rest pain (Fig. 5–21).[238] Ankle pressures are used to identify obstructions in arteries above the foot, and toe pressures and digital plethysmography are used to determine the degree of ischemia in the feet of limbs with normal ankle pressures or in limbs with abnormal but "not ischemic" ankle pressures.[197] Determination of $tcPO_2$ values or pulse volume recordings may be used instead of, or in conjunction with, the digital studies.[252] When the ankle pressure is ischemic (less than 40 to 50 mmHg in nondiabetics or less than 80 mmHg in diabetics) or when the ankle plethysmogram is markedly abnormal or absent (pulse volume categories 4 or 5), there is little hope that ulcers will respond to local treatment or that forefoot amputations will be successful.[194] In this event, arterial reconstruction—if technically feasible, safe, and otherwise not contraindicated—should be performed in order to avoid a major amputation.[178]

Arterial reconstruction should also be considered in limbs with abnormal but not ischemic ankle pressures when the digital pressures, toe plethysmograms, or $tcPO_2$ values are indicative of severe pedal ischemia (Fig. 5–21). Despite the presence of significant pedal arterial disease, the increase in pressure resulting from a successful arterial reconstruction is often sufficient to ensure the success of local

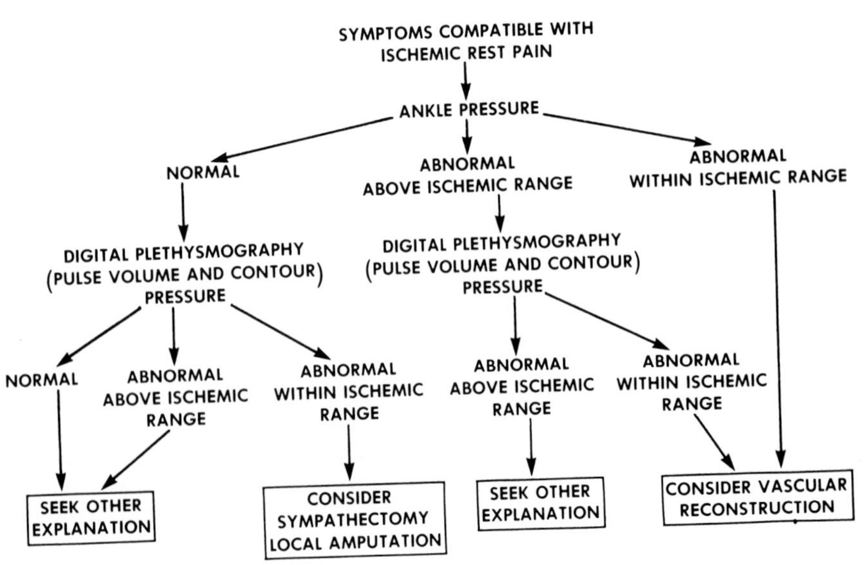

FIGURE 5–20. Algorithm illustrating diagnostic approach to patients with rest pain of the feet.

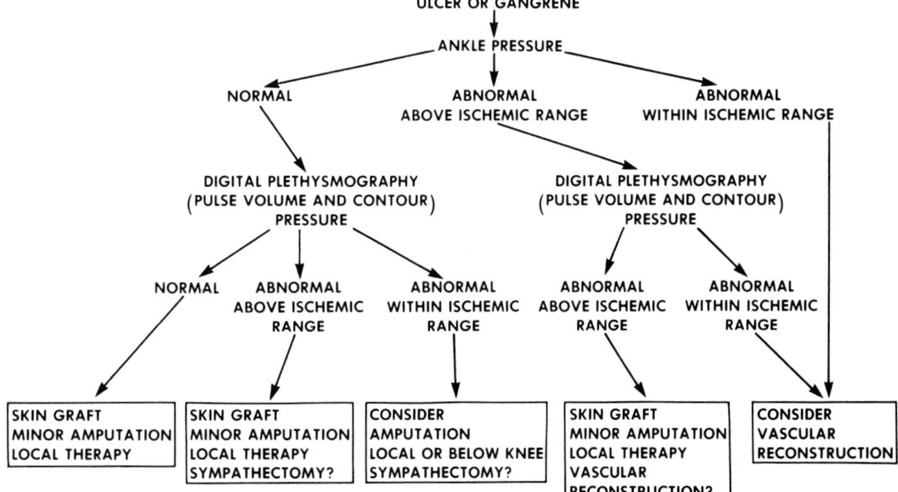

FIGURE 5–21. Algorithm illustrating diagnostic approach to patients with ulcers or gangrene of the feet. (From Sumner DS: Algorithms using noninvasive diagnostic data as a guide to therapy of arterial insufficiency. *In* Puel P, Boccalon H, Enjalbert A [eds]: Hemodynamics of the Limbs—1. Toulouse, France, GEPESC, 1979, pp 543–566.)

therapy. Even when healing can be expected on the basis of pedal hemodynamic parameters, arterial reconstruction may accelerate the healing process.

In limbs with normal ankle pressures or normal ankle plethysmograms, arterial reconstruction will not increase blood flow to the foot. If the toe or $tcPo_2$ studies are normal or, if abnormal, are not indicative of ischemia, there should be no problem with healing. Ischemic values, however, present a different problem. In this situation, ischemia is attributable solely to digital or pedal arterial obstruction; reconstruction at this level is not feasible and a Syme's or below-knee amputation is usually required. Sympathectomy is seldom if ever beneficial.

Criteria for Predicting Healing of Foot Lesions or Forefoot Amputations

A blood supply adequate to ensure healing under ideal circumstances may be insufficient when complicating factors, such as infection, diabetes, poor nutrition, or local trauma, are present. Owing to localized end-artery obstruction, some areas of the foot may be ischemic while others remain adequately perfused. For example, a heel ulcer can exist and be recalcitrant to treatment in a foot with viable toes. The skill of the surgeon and compliance of the patient are also immensely important. It is not surprising, therefore, that noninvasive criteria for predicting healing vary from laboratory to laboratory. In view of the multiple factors determining healing potential, this should not be considered an indictment of the tests; rather, it emphasizes that the results of noninvasive tests should be used only as guidelines in predicting the outcome of foot lesions and amputations. Nevertheless, when used in conjunction with clinical observations, noninvasive test results are frequently quite helpful to the surgeon who is faced with the perplexing decision of whether to revascularize the extremity, amputate immediately, or persist with nonoperative therapy.

Table 5–20 lists criteria that have been used by various investigators to discriminate between lesions or amputations that are likely to heal and those that are not. Predictive values obtained from the raw data are normalized to a 65 per cent healing rate and a 35 per cent failure rate. These figures represent the average distribution of healing and failure based on clinical assessment alone, as reported by the investigators whose data are included in the table. (The healing rate varied from 35 to 84 per cent.)

As indicated in Table 5–20, ankle pressures tend to be less predictive than tests that are designed to assess perfusion of the foot itself. This is particularly true in diabetic limbs for two reasons: (1) The arteries at ankle level are often incompressible, giving spuriously high values, and (2) pedal arterial obstruction, which is frequently present, may be responsible for severe ischemia even in the absence of disease above the ankle. Moreover, there is little or no correlation between ankle pressures and pedal skin blood flow.[263] Even when the ankle pressure exceeds 80 mmHg, a distal healing failure rate of about 20 per cent can be expected. Although ankle pressures less than 60 to 80 mmHg accurately predict failure in only about 60 per cent of cases, the potential for healing is markedly reduced at lower levels. For example, Carter reported that all limbs with ischemic lesions required amputation when the ankle pressure was less than 55 mmHg, and Holstein and coworkers found that only 11 per cent of skin lesions healed when the pressure fell below 50 mmHg.[44, 112] It is very unlikely that healing will occur at foot level in any limb with an ankle pressure less than 30 or 40 mmHg (see Fig. 5–7).[197, 259]

With tests of more peripheral vessels, it is generally possible to define a limit above which healing is to be expected, but the converse is somewhat less likely to be true. In other words, healing may occur when the noninvasive parameters are below the "critical" level (see Table 5–20). There are at least three possible explanations for these observations: (1) The test results are inaccurate, (2) the test does not measure the proper parameter, and (3) the minimal value required for healing may be very low under ideal circumstances. For these reasons, most surgeons are reluctant—and rightly so—to base their decision to proceed to a major amputation exclusively on noninvasive test findings.

Table 5–20. Predicting Healing of Foot Lesions and Forefoot Amputations in Diabetic and Nondiabetic Patients

			Correctly Predicted (%)		Normalized Predictive Value (%)‡	
Modality	**Author and Year***	**Criterion†**	*(Sensitivity) Nonhealing*	*(Specificity) Nonhealing*	*(Positive) Healing*	*(Negative) Nonhealing*
Ankle pressure	Cumulative[a]	80 mmHg	79	63	80	62
	Cumulative[b]	70 mmHg	68	40	68	40
	Cumulative[c]	60 mmHg	87	46	75	66
Toe pressure	Cumulative[d]	40 mmHg	97	81	91	94
	Cumulative[e]	30 mmHg	73	87	91	64
	Schwartz et al (1982)[213]	20 mmHg	96	80	90	92
$tcPo_2$	Karanfilian et al (1986)[127]	10 mmHg	100	88	94	100
	Harward et al (1985)[99]	10 mmHg	71	57	75	51
Skin pressure	Faris and Duncan (1985)[70]	40 mmHg	97	80	90	94
Elevation	Gilfillan et al (1985)[86]	35 cm	96	85	92	92
Laser Dopplers	Karanfilian et al (1986)[127]	40 mv	79	96	97	71
Peripheral vascular resistance	Gibbons et al (1979)[85]	Moderate	46	94	93	48

**References: a = 29, 70, 112, 197, 213, 259; b = 85, 172; c = 9, 18, 44, 86; d = 29, 70; e = 18, 44, 112, 197.*
†Level above which healing is expected.
‡Assumes 65% healing rate.

Raines and associates suggest that healing of foot lesions is likely with PVR categories 1 and 2, probable with category 3, and unlikely with categories 4 and 5 when tracings are obtained at ankle level (see Table 5–14).[194] Although strong or moderate forefoot pulse volumes were found to be highly predictive of successful healing by Gibbons and associates, absent or low-volume waveforms predicted failure in only 48 per cent of the diabetic limbs included in their study (see Table 5–20).[85] In our experience, toe plethysmographic tracings are equally predictive (see Fig. 5–17).[239]

Carter found that foot lesions usually heal if toe pressures exceed 30 mmHg in nondiabetic patients or 55 mmHg in diabetics.[44] On the other hand, Holstein and coworkers noted no appreciable difference between the two groups.[112] In their study, healing occurred in 91 per cent of the limbs when toe pressures were greater than 30 mmHg, in 50 per cent when pressures were between 20 and 29 mmHg, and in only 29 per cent when pressures were less than 20 mmHg. Bone and Pomajzl noted failure of toe amputations in all patients in whom the toe pressures were less than 45 mmHg and in 25 per cent of patients with pressures between 45 and 55 mmHg; healing occurred in all patients with toe pressures greater than 55 mmHg.[29] Other investigators have reported uniform healing when toe pressures exceeded 10 to 25 mmHg.[18, 213] Several successful toe amputations have been reported in toes with undetectable pressures.[18] Because the pressure in any gangrenous digit will almost certainly be zero, it is wise to use the pressure from nongangrenous adjacent digits to predict healing.[29, 213]

In a study by Ramsey and coworkers, toe pressures proved to be of more prognostic value than ankle pressures (see Fig. 5–7).[197] Lesions and toe amputations failed to heal in 92 per cent of limbs with an ankle pressure less than 80 mmHg, but they also failed to heal in 45 per cent of limbs with higher pressures. There were three failures in limbs with ankle pressures of 150 mmHg; in all three cases, the toe pressures were less than 30 mmHg. When toe pressures were less than 30 mmHg, the failure rate was 95 per cent, but when the pressures were above 30 mmHg, only 14 per cent of the lesions or amputations did not heal. This experience suggests that toe pressures below 20 mmHg almost uniformly predict an unsuccessful result.

Although $tcPo_2$ measured at foot level is a promising method for ascertaining healing potential, the minimal value consistent with a successful result remains uncertain. For example, the discrimination provided by a $tcPo_2$ of 10 mmHg was excellent in the study by Karanfilian and coworkers,[127] but was less so in the study by Harward and colleagues (see Table 5–20).[99] Other investigators have suggested that healing is unlikely if the $tcPo_2$ is less than 20, 40, or 50 mmHg.[49, 76, 129] Hauser reported uniform failure of amputations when the RPI was less than 0.40 and nearly complete success when the index exceeded 0.60.[102] Laser Doppler, another technique for assessing skin blood flow, was found by Karanfilian and coworkers to be somewhat less accurate than $tcPo_2$ in a comparative study of the two modalities.[127]

An interesting and apparently highly predictive method of measuring foot perfusion pressure has been advocated by Gilfillan and associates (see Table 5–20).[86] With the patient supine, the foot is elevated 65 cm above the level of the right atrium, kept in this position until the foot blanches, and then lowered gradually until the color returns. At the point at which color returns, the perfusion pressure in centimeters of blood is equivalent to the height of the foot above the atrium. Listening for the return of blood flow in the pedal arteries with the Doppler flowmeter is a variation of this technique that we have occasionally employed in diabetic limbs with incompressible vessels. Isotope clearance methods for measuring skin blood pressure, as reported by Faris and Duncan, have also proved efficacious (see Table 5–20).[70] These techniques are further discussed in Chapter 149.

Because rigid guidelines cannot be established, it is best to think of the results of the various noninvasive tests as being indicative of the probability that a foot lesion or forefoot amputation will heal. When the probability is low, vascular reconstruction should be performed if at all possible (see Fig. 5–21). Even a small increase in perfusion may tip the balance in favor of healing. Noer and associates, for example, found that foot ulcers gradually healed when, as a result of vascular reconstruction, the toe pressure rose 15 to 20 per cent of the arm pressure, an increase of only 20 to 30 mmHg.[178]

Criteria for Predicting Healing of Major Amputations

Major amputations become necessary in limbs with severe ischemia or gangrene when arterial reconstruction is not feasible or when the extent of infection or tissue loss precludes salvage by localized amputation. Since the chance of rehabilitation is better the more distal the amputation site, Syme's amputations are preferred over below-knee, and below-knee over above-knee amputations. Unfortunately, the potential for healing is just the opposite, diminishing as the site of amputation moves from proximal to distal levels of the leg. Keagy and coworkers, reporting on a large series from a major university hospital, found that the failure rate for above-knee amputations (AKAs) was 9 per cent compared with 19 per cent for below-knee amputations (BKAs).[131] These findings are in basic agreement with those of other investigators, who, like Keagy and coworkers, selected the amputation site exclusively on the basis of clinical judgment. Although many factors determine the success or failure of an amputation, it is obvious that healing will not occur without an adequate blood supply. Various noninvasive methods of assessing perfusion at the intended site of amputation have, therefore, been proposed in an effort to decrease the number of failures.

Almost all limbs with a Doppler-derived calf systolic pressure in excess of 65 to 70 mmHg will heal a BKA.[17, 18, 85, 172, 194] It is, however, difficult to define a calf pressure below which BKAs consistently fail. Although Raines and associates[194] stated that healing is unlikely when the calf pressure is less than 65 mmHg, Gibbons and associates[85] noted no failures in 11 limbs with pressures less than this. Nicholas and colleagues found that 68 per cent of the BKAs with calf pressures less than 70 mmHg in their series healed.[172] Barnes and coworkers reported a 75 per cent healing rate when the below-knee pressure was less than 70 mmHg and a 44 per cent healing rate when the pressure was less than 50 mmHg.[17] In a subsequent study, Barnes and colleagues found no significant difference between the mean below-knee pressures of those limbs that healed a BKA and those that did not.[18] In fact, eight limbs with no recordable calf pressure healed. This, of course, does not mean that there was no blood pressure at the site of the amputations; it implies that the velocity of flow below the cuff was insufficient to obtain a Doppler signal.

As one would expect, a low (or zero) ankle pressure does not necessarily predict an unsuccessful BKA, since the pressure at the more proximal amputation site may be entirely satisfactory.[18, 65, 85, 172, 191] On the other hand, a reliable ankle pressure (i.e., one that is not artificially elevated because of arterial calcification) that exceeds 30 mmHg is a favorable prognostic sign, because the pressure at all proximal levels will exceed this value.[172, 194]

If the data obtained from skin blood pressure measurements can be assumed to be representative of the actual perfusion pressure, the circulatory support necessary to heal BKAs is quite low indeed. For example, Holstein and associates found that healing of BKAs occurred in 25 per cent of limbs with skin pressures less than 20 mmHg, in 67 per cent with pressures between 20 and 30 mmHg, and in 90 per cent with pressures greater than 30 mmHg.[111] They used the clearance rate of a radionuclide injected intradermally 10 cm below the knee joint to monitor the cessation of cutaneous blood flow as pressure on the skin was increased with a pneumatic cuff. Similar results were reported by Stockel and associates, who used a photodetector to sense the return of blood flow as the counterpressure was reduced.[224] Because the critical below-knee pressure seems to be less than 20 mmHg, it may be impossible to measure it accurately with the usual noninvasive methods.

Raines and associates have stated that healing of BKAs is unlikely if the pulse volume tracing obtained at calf level is flat or shows a minimal pulse and the below-knee pressure is less than 65 mmHg.[194] Others, however, have found pulse volume recordings to have little predictive value.[85, 172]

Transcutaneous oxygen tension measurements are plagued with much the same problems that beset pressure measurements. Although most investigators agree that over 90 per cent of BKAs will heal when the $tcPo_2$ obtained from the skin of the calf about 10 cm below the knee is greater than 35 to 40 mmHg, a minimal level below which failure is to be expected has proved more difficult to define.[49, 102, 129, 169, 198] The level most often cited is 30 to 35 mmHg. However, Ratliff and associates[198] observed that 67 per cent of the BKAs in limbs with $tcPo_2$ values less than 35 mmHg healed, and Harward and colleagues[99] reported that 82 per cent with values less than 10 mmHg healed. In fact, Harward's group found that 98 per cent of the BKAs with $tcPo_2$ values greater than 10 mmHg were successful. Of those that healed, 55 per cent had midcalf $tcPo_2$ values below 30 mmHg and 4 per cent had values of zero, even after oxygen inhalation. Malone and associates, in a study of AKAs, BKAs, and transmetatarsal amputations, found that $tcPo_2$ values of 20 mmHg provided perfect separation between those limbs that healed and those that did not.[154] The clearance rate of xenon-133, a technique previously advocated by their group, was not reliable as a prospective test for selecting the level of amputation (see Chapter 148). Kram and coworkers advocated using a critical Po_2 index, defined as the calf-brachial $tcPo_2$ ratio, to predict healing of BKAs.[140] They measured calf and brachial $tcPo_2$ in 40 patients prior to BKA. Successful healing occurred in 50 per cent of limbs with calf $tcPo_2$ less than 20 mmHg and in

96 per cent of limbs with calf $tcPo_2$ greater than 20 mmHg. The critical Po_2 index provided better predictive accuracy: All patients with an index of 0.20 or less failed to heal, and 97 per cent of patients with an index greater than 0.20 healed successfully.

In summary, a calf pressure greater than 40 mmHg, an ankle pressure greater than 30 mmHg, or a mid-calf $tcPo_2$ greater than 35 mmHg provides reasonable assurance that a BKA will heal; however, lower values should not deter the surgeon from attempting an amputation at this level if other signs are favorable and the patient is expected to benefit from preservation of the knee joint.

Acute Arterial Obstructions

The clinical diagnosis of acute arterial obstruction is seldom difficult and is usually easily made on the basis of the history and physical examination. Simple noninvasive tests, however, are frequently useful in an adjunctive role.

Embolism and Thrombosis

It is sometimes difficult to distinguish between an embolic obstruction and one caused by thrombosis of a previously stenotic artery. Finding normal pulses, Doppler signals, and ankle pressures in the opposite extremity suggests that the process is likely to be embolic. Abnormal findings in the opposite extremity suggest thrombosis, because chronic occlusive arterial disease is often bilateral. This distinction is important because the therapeutic approaches to the two conditions differ. Although preoperative arteriography is seldom necessary if the obstruction is embolic, angiography is very helpful in cases of thrombotic obstruction, which often require arterial reconstruction.

A quick survey of the involved limb with the Doppler flowmeter will usually identify the site of obstruction. This information can influence the choice of incision. Although a palpable pulse may be present (e.g., in the femoral artery), no flow may be detected, indicating that the underlying artery is occluded. An abrupt, ''thumping'' signal strongly suggests that all or nearly all of the outflow is occluded. This finding is typical in cases of embolic obstruction of the distal common femoral artery in which both the superficial femoral and the profunda femoris arteries are occluded.

Although unrelenting pain, loss of sensation, and reduced motor function indicate severe ischemia and demand immediate surgical intervention, there are situations in which ischemia is present but is not immediately limb-threatening.[230] In these cases, there may be some subjective numbness and coldness of the foot but no objective loss of sensation, limitation of movement, or pain. When velocity signals are present in the pedal arteries and when the ankle pressure exceeds 30 or 40 mmHg, it is possible to delay intervention because collateral circulation is adequate to sustain viability—at least for a brief period. The time gained may be used to improve the patient's condition. Such patients may also be candidates for thrombolytic therapy. An ABI greater than 0.50 indicates excellent collateral circulation.[230] In this situation, flow will often improve even if nothing is done, although the patient may subsequently experience claudication. If, on the other hand, no velocity signals are obtained from the pedal arteries or if the systolic pressure is less than 30 mmHg, implying marginal collateral input, the surgeon should move expeditiously to restore circulation.

Occasionally, patients with a low cardiac output present with symptoms and signs suggestive of an acute occlusion when in fact there has been no anatomic change in the status of the limb circulation. In this situation, there is almost invariably a degree of preexisting chronic arterial disease. Although one leg may be worse than the other, both are usually involved. Doppler signals are usually present in the pedal arteries and a Doppler survey of the common femoral, superficial femoral, and popliteal arteries will reveal no site of acute occlusion, although the signals in these areas are often abnormal. Because of preexisting arterial disease, the ABI is usually low and the absolute ankle systolic pressure may fall in the ischemic range. With correction of the cardiac failure, the ankle pressure will improve even though the index does not change. Diagnosis in these patients can be difficult, and frequent careful monitoring during the period of resuscitative therapy is required to avoid missing an acute occlusion.

Trauma

Finding reduced or absent velocity signals in arteries distal to the site of penetrating or blunt limb trauma indicates the need for arteriography or surgical exploration. The mere presence of a Doppler signal never rules out an arterial injury. Even when peripheral pulses are palpable, a decreased systolic blood pressure in the limb below the area of injury is also highly suggestive of arterial damage. It must be remembered, however, that the Doppler survey is useful mainly when it is positive; a negative study does not exclude arterial trauma when there is major hemorrhage, hematoma formation, penetrating wounds, fractures in the vicinity of major arteries, or other indications for surgical exploration.[15]

In patients in whom only one of the three below-knee arteries has been injured, noninvasive tests can be helpful in evaluating the adequacy of the residual perfusion to the foot; a normal or near-normal study provides reassurance to the surgeon, who may then elect to ligate rather than reconstruct the injured vessel. A Doppler study can also identify which of the vessels is damaged. It must be emphasized that the presence of Doppler signals does not eliminate the possibility of a developing compartment syndrome.[15]

During the Vietnam war, the ultrasonic flow detector proved to be a valuable method for ascertaining the viability of limbs in which palpable pulses did not return or were lost after arterial repair. In the experience reported by Lavenson and associates, all extremities with audible signals remained viable, whereas all extremities with absent signals required further reconstruction or amputation.[148] Thus, noninvasive examination identified those limbs in which it was safe to defer definitive arterial repair long enough to permit control of infection.

Kram and Shoemaker have advocated the use of $tcPo_2$ measurements as an adjunctive diagnostic method in patients with trauma of the limbs.[142] They found that the mean

$tcPo_2$ in limbs with arterial injury (34 ± 21 mmHg) was significantly lower than that in traumatized limbs without arterial injury (58 ± 14 mmHg). A ratio of 0.90, obtained by dividing the $tcPo_2$ in the injured limb by that in the opposite uninjured extremity, identified major arterial injury with a sensitivity and specificity of 80 per cent and 91 per cent, respectively. It would seem, however, that $tcPo_2$ measurements would be more appropriately used to assess the viability of a traumatized limb rather than to detect arterial injury.

Diagnostic Arterial Catheterization

Ankle pressures and brief Doppler surveys help identify unsuspected arterial obstruction that could make catheterization difficult or hazardous, in which case, another limb can be used.[16] After the procedure, pressure data can be used to determine whether an accident has occurred and to help formulate a therapeutic approach. With arterial spasm, the blood pressure drops only moderately and recovers rapidly. When peripheral pressures are above 40 mmHg, one can afford to wait an hour or two to see whether clot lysis will take place. If there is no response or if the initial pressures are quite low, immediate repair is indicated. When the ABI is greater than 0.50, surgical intervention is not required for limb preservation and can be delayed if there are significant medical contraindications.

Not infrequently, it is difficult to distinguish between a hematoma at the groin and an early false aneurysm. In these cases, duplex scanning, particularly with instruments that provide color flow images, has proved to be extremely valuable. Although a hematoma may appear to pulsate and may have a configuration similar to that of a false aneurysm, no flow will be detected; flow within the mass identifies it as a false aneurysm.

Popliteal Entrapment and Adventitial Cystic Disease

Popliteal artery entrapment should be considered when young men present with intermittent claudication (see Chapter 61). The claudication may be atypical, occurring with walking but not with running, and peripheral pulses may be normal.[160] In these cases, noninvasive tests can be used to demonstrate compression of the popliteal artery by the medial head of the gastrocnemius muscle. Hyperextension of the knee, passive dorsiflexion of the ankle, and active plantar flexion of the foot with the knee moderately flexed are three maneuvers that have little effect on the distal circulation of normal limbs but decrease the ankle systolic blood pressure, diminish the amplitude of the pedal arterial Doppler signals, and reduce the volume of pulses recorded at the ankle in limbs with popliteal entrapment (Fig. 5–22).[52, 62, 162] Unfortunately, these maneuvers, if conducted very vigorously, may produce positive results even in normal extremities, leading some investigators to question their reliability.[160] As an alternative, exercise testing has been recommended. A drop in the ABI after treadmill exercise at 3 mph with a zero grade or at 4 mph with a 10 per cent grade documents the presence of intermittent or

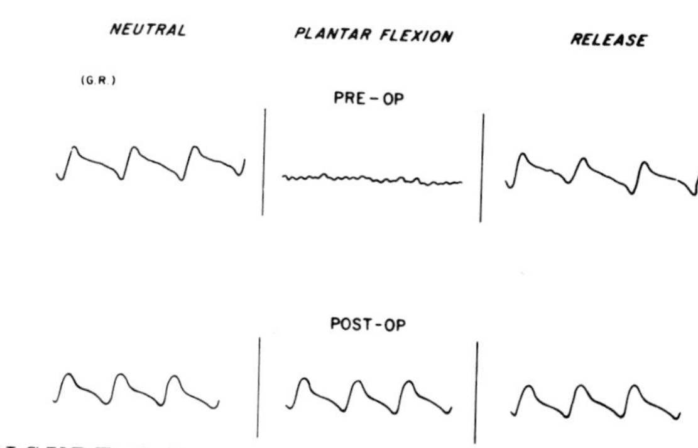

FIGURE 5–22. Pulse volume recordings at ankle level before and after surgery for popliteal artery entrapment. Prior to operation, pulses disappear during plantar flexion. After surgical correction, plantar flexion has no effect on pulse volume.

fixed arterial obstruction.[160] A negative response, on the other hand, provides reasonable assurance that the patient does not have the popliteal entrapment syndrome.

Cystic adventitial disease of the popliteal artery is another cause of intermittent claudication that characteristically affects young athletic males (see Chapter 60). Unlike popliteal entrapment, circulatory changes are typically absent when the leg is extended but develop when the knee is sharply flexed.[21] Segmental pressures, Doppler-derived waveforms, and plethysmographic pulses are normal above the knee and abnormal below. Treadmill exercise testing will establish the presence of partial arterial obstruction.

Preoperative Evaluation

Once the decision to operate has been made based on the history, physical examination, and noninvasive findings, arteriography is usually the next logical step. An anatomic assessment of the distribution of disease is necessary to determine the feasibility of reconstruction and to plan the operative approach. Unfortunately, the preoperative arteriogram may provide insufficient information in two commonly encountered situations: (1) severe peripheral ischemia with below-knee obstructive disease, and (2) multilevel disease involving both the aortoiliac and the femoropopliteal segments.

Identification of Recipient Arteries for Femoral-Distal Bypass

Despite the best efforts of the angiographer to enhance blood flow pharmacologically or by reactive hyperemia, arteriographic visualization of the distal crural vessels may be inadequate in limbs with gangrene, ischemic ulcers, or rest pain. Ricco and coworkers reported complete nonvisualization of calf vessels in 20 per cent of preoperative arteriograms and limited visualization in another 20 per cent.[201] In the majority of such limbs, a velocity signal can be obtained with the Doppler probe from one or more of the pedal arteries, indicating the presence of a residual channel that is at least partially patent. The presence of a signal does not, however, always identify a vessel suitable for accepting a graft. The lumen may be too small or the communications with the remainder of the pedal vessels too poor to ensure patency of the graft or to provide adequate perfusion for the foot. Occasionally, the signal may arise from a neighboring collateral artery. Nonetheless, the correlation between the results of carefully conducted Doppler surveys and the findings obtained with intraoperative arteriography or surgical exploration are gratifyingly high.[201, 215] In the series reported by Ricco and coworkers, Doppler examination correctly identified arteries suitable for bypass in 71 per cent of the limbs with nonvisualization of distal vessels and in 83 per cent of the limbs in which preoperative angiographic visualization was inadequate (Fig. 5–23).[201] A simple scoring system developed by Shearman and colleagues, based on a combination of clinical data, Doppler signals from the pedal arteries, and the ABI, was found in a prospective study to be highly predictive of the need for a bypass to the popliteal trunk, to the popliteal trifurcation, or to a distal calf artery.[215] Encouraged by these results, they have curtailed their use of preoperative arteriography in patients requiring distal bypass grafts and have relied instead on intraoperative arteriography.

Doppler surveys are initiated by examining the dorsalis pedis and posterior tibial arteries at ankle level. To get some idea of the length of vessel available for bypass and to exclude the possibility that the signal is arising from a collateral channel, one can attempt to follow the signal up the leg or down into the foot. It is often possible to trace the medial plantar artery for a short distance beyond its origin from the posterior tibial and to follow the dorsalis pedis distally in the first metatarsal space to the origin of the deep plantar artery. The patency of the peroneal artery, which cannot be examined directly, can be determined by placing the probe over the anterior lateral malleolar artery. Although the ankle pressure obtained from these arteries may provide some insight into the status of their inflow, medial calcification often renders this assessment unreliable. If manual compression of the anterior tibial or posterior tibial arteries in the proximal leg just below the popliteal trifurcation has little or no effect on the signal obtained from the dorsalis pedis or posterior tibial arteries at ankle level, it can be assumed that the proximal portion of the artery being compressed is occluded or severely stenotic.[202] On the other hand, augmentation of the velocity signal in one artery during proximal compression of the other indicates that the proximal portion of the artery being evaluated is patent. Not infrequently, the signal from the dorsalis pedis artery will disappear when the posterior tibial artery is compressed at ankle level (or vice versa), establishing the fact that the compressed artery is serving as the source of inflow for both vessels. In such cases, reversed flow may be detected in one of the two arteries.[202]

Patency of the pedal arch has an important influence on graft function and graft survival. Patency of the pedal arch signifies a low-resistance vascular bed and usually implies that the potential for revascularizing the distal foot is good. Yet, even when the preoperative arteriogram opacifies the arteries at ankle level, the pedal arch is seldom adequately visualized. A technique, analogous to Allen's test in the hand, has been proposed by Roedersheimer and associates for assessing the patency of the pedal arch noninvasively.[204] With the Doppler probe applied to the first metatarsal space over the deep plantar artery, the tibial arteries are alternately compressed. If the pedal arch is patent, compression of one of the vessels may attenuate but will not abolish the signal. Disappearance of the signal

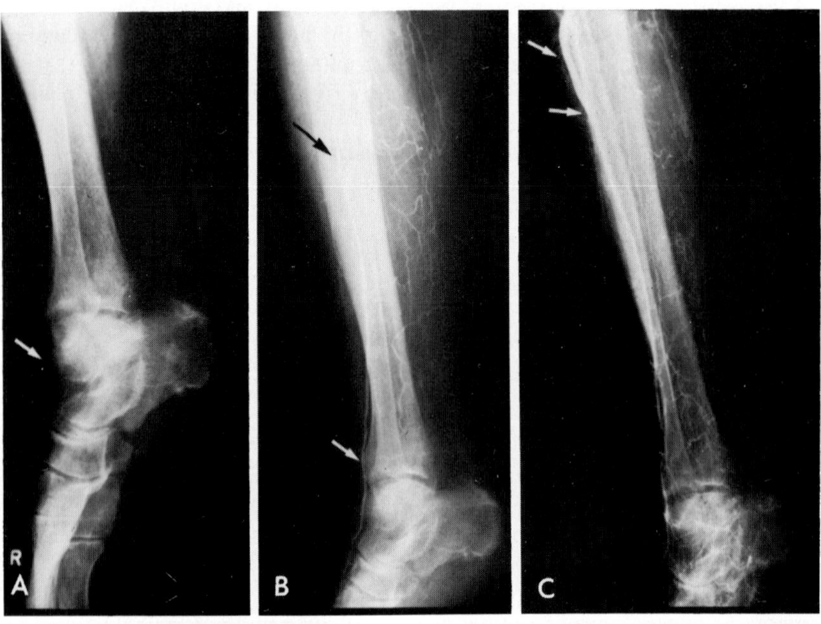

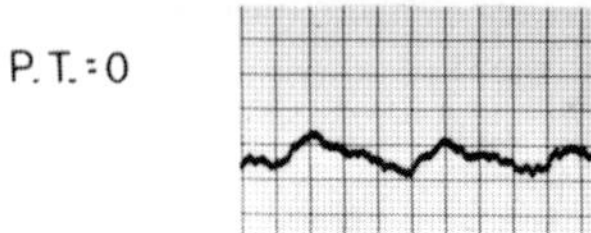

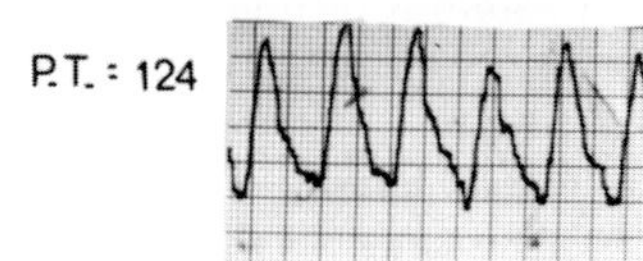

FIGURE 5–23. Doppler flow detection in femorodistal bypass. *A*, Although the tibial vessels did not fill on arteriography, the Doppler instrument detected pulsatile flow over the dorsalis pedis artery *(arrow)*. *B*, The intraoperative, prebypass arteriogram confirmed the presence of a patent anterior tibial artery *(arrows)*. *C*, Note the change in pulsatile flow patterns after a successful femoral–anterior tibial bypass *(arrows)*.

indicates an incomplete arch supplied by the artery being compressed. They observed a 96 per cent correlation between the results of this test and findings obtained with intraoperative arteriography.

Duplex scanning with color flow imaging is becoming established as a rapid and accurate method for determining the patency of the below-knee arteries in limbs with distal occlusive disease. In a study of 150 patients undergoing both color flow imaging and arteriography, Moneta and coworkers reported overall sensitivities for predicting distal arterial obstruction of 90 per cent for the anterior tibial, 90 per cent for the posterior tibial, and 82 per cent for the peroneal arteries.[164] Although duplex scanning can provide useful clinical information on the status of the tibial vessels, it appears to be somewhat more accurate for classifying the severity of arterial disease proximal to the level of the knee.[101, 164] When Hatsukami and coworkers used color flow imaging to distinguish between patent and occluded arteries, sensitivities were 97 per cent for the superficial femoral and 100 per cent for the popliteal, but only 83 per cent for the anterior and posterior tibial arteries.[101] It appears that the ability of duplex scanning to detect distal arterial lesions is not affected by the presence of more proximal occlusive disease.

Multi-Level Disease

Failure to recognize a significant inflow lesion adversely affects the chances for patency of a femoropopliteal or femorotibial bypass graft. On the other hand, aortoiliac reconstruction in limbs with hemodynamically significant lesions of the femoropopliteal segment may fail to alleviate symptoms. In 9 to 57 per cent of patients with multi-level disease, reconstructions limited to lesions above the inguinal ligament do not relieve claudication or rest pain and may not allow ischemic ulcers to heal.[42, 67, 82, 114, 137, 139, 206, 212, 243]

Difficulties encountered in interpreting arteriograms of the aortoiliac segment are directly or indirectly responsible for many of the unsatisfactory results.[165] Although the surgeon, swayed by the presence of large atheromatous plaques, may overestimate the extent of the disease, it is more likely that he or she will underestimate the degree of iliac arterial stenosis. Asymmetric plaques, which typically lie on the posterior wall, are often not perceptible on the routine anteroposterior projection, their severity becoming apparent only on lateral or oblique views.[33, 214, 255] Although the interpretation of arteriograms of the femoropopliteal segment is more straightforward, the degree of physiologic impairment is greatly influenced by collateral development, which cannot always be reliably estimated. Likewise, palpation of femoral pulses and auscultation of bruits are apt to be unreliable, especially when the examiner is inexperienced.[10, 34, 119, 170, 221]

These problems have spawned a great body of literature concerned with the development of noninvasive methods for ascertaining the relative physiologic significance of concomitant disease in the aortoiliac and femoropopliteal segments. Although it would appear that noninvasive tests are ideally suited for this type of investigation, the results have not been particularly encouraging. In fact, Campbell and coworkers concluded that conventional clinical assessment was more accurate than most noninvasive methods for detecting severe aortoiliac disease; however, laboratory tests were more helpful for lesser degrees of stenosis.[40]

Measurement of ankle pressure immediately following completion of an inflow procedure has been recommended as a method for identifying those limbs that require additional distal bypass.[82] Unfortunately, this simple test has not proved to be as discriminating as originally hoped. Although an immediate rise of 0.10 in the ABI has consistently been a favorable prognostic sign, no change or even a fall does not necessarily portend a poor result.[4, 82, 139, 243] In fact, an index that is initially decreased may rise to preoperative levels within 1 or 2 hours and may exceed preoperative values within 3 to 24 hours.[139, 179] If, however, the ABI has not risen by 0.10 in 5 to 7 days, the results of aortofemoral reconstruction are likely to be unsatisfactory.[212] In a series of patients undergoing proximal reconstructions for multi-level arterial disease, the ABI in 56 per cent of limbs attained maximal values within 10 days following aortofemoral reconstruction; in another 22 per cent, maximal values were reached in 3 months; and in the remainder, the levels continued to increase for 3 to 26 months.[243]

Theoretically, patients with low upper thigh pressures should have more severe disease in the iliac segment and should benefit more from an inflow procedure than those with high upper thigh pressures. Bone and associates reported that all limbs with an upper thigh pressure index of 0.85 or less were improved after aortofemoral bypass.[30] All unimproved limbs had preoperative thigh indices greater than 0.85, but 65 per cent of those limbs within this range also improved. Others have noted no appreciable difference between the thigh pressure indices in limbs with multi-level disease that improved following aortofemoral reconstruction and those that did not.[180, 243]

It seems logical that poor results would be expected to accompany a large pressure gradient between the upper thigh and the ankle, because this situation implies a high resistance in the arterial segments that lie distal to the aortofemoral reconstruction. In the study reported by Bone and associates, 24 per cent of the limbs with one abnormal pressure gradient (greater than 30 mmHg across the thigh, the knee, or below the knee) failed to improve.[30] When there were two abnormal gradients, 71 per cent showed no improvement. All proximal reconstructions were successful in limbs with isolated aortoiliac disease (no abnormal gradients). In a separate study, however, the pressure gradient proved to be of no prognostic value in limbs with multi-level disease.[243]

The problem with these observations lies not with the theory but with the inaccuracies inherent in the noninvasive measurement of thigh pressure. When the femoral artery pressure is measured accurately by means of direct arterial puncture and a pressure transducer, the rise in ankle pressure (or toe pressure) following a successful aortofemoral reconstruction is directly proportional to the rise in femoral arterial pressure.[177, 264] Therefore, preoperative knowledge of the arm-to–femoral arterial pressure gradient and the noninvasively determined ankle pressure can be used to predict the likelihood of a successful result after proximal reconstruction in limbs with multi-level disease.

Because of the fallibility of noninvasive thigh pressure measurements, attention has shifted to the interpretation of

Doppler-derived common femoral velocity waveforms as a method for determining the hemodynamic significance of lesions within the aortofemoral segment. Simple inspection of the pulse contour is the most direct method (see Fig. 5–9).[71] Persson and coworkers reported that the presence of a triphasic flow pattern with reversed flow in early diastole correctly identified 94 per cent of iliac arteries with either no disease or with stenoses that reduced the diameter by less than 50 per cent.[188] Absence of reversed flow detected stenoses greater than 50 per cent with a sensitivity of 96 per cent. Reverse flow may be absent, however, in limbs with concomitant superficial femoral arterial obstruction despite a normal aortoiliac segment; but in these cases, the systolic portion of the wave is usually normal, displaying a rapid rise, sharp peak, and rapid fall to baseline, and the diastolic portion is usually flat and is not elevated above the zero baseline. A triphasic waveform, on the other hand, does not reliably exclude low-grade iliac stenoses of the type that permit normal flow during resting conditions but restrict flow during exercise.[33, 71, 96]

As discussed earlier in this chapter, more sophisticated methods for analyzing the common femoral waveform have been developed. These include pulsatility indices and Laplace transform methods. Their accuracies for detecting hemodynamically significant stenoses of the aortoiliac segment are summarized in Tables 5–9, 5–10, and 5–12. Although sensitivities and specificities are generally acceptable, the reported results are quite variable, and it is by no means certain that they are significantly more reliable than simple inspection of the pulse contour. All have been reported to be affected by the presence of superficial femoral arterial occlusions. Thiele and associates found that 92 per cent of limbs with normal femoral pulsatility indices (PI ≥ 4) had hemodynamically normal aortoiliac segments as determined by direct measurement of femoral artery pressure after papaverine injection.[248] The presence or absence of concomitant superficial femoral artery occlusion made little difference. Although 88 per cent of limbs with abnormal femoral pulsatility indices (PI < 4) and patent superficial femoral arteries had hemodynamically significant aortoiliac disease, when the superficial femoral artery was occluded only 45 per cent of the limbs with abnormal pulsatility indices were found to have significant inflow disease. From these data, they devised an algorithm that should afford correct localization of the disease process in almost all cases (Fig. 5–24).

Duplex scanning, which allows direct investigation of the aortoiliac segment, is the most valuable noninvasive technique for assessing inflow disease (see Chapter 6).[56, 100, 101, 116, 137, 164] The ability to evaluate flow disturbances at the site where they are produced rather than at a considerable distance downstream is a major advantage of this technique. Moreover, infrainguinal disease has little or no effect on local flow disturbances. The reported sensitivity of duplex scanning for identifying iliac artery stenoses associated with a significant pressure gradient or more than 50 per cent diameter reduction is 89 per cent.[137] The main disadvantage of lower extremity duplex scanning is that it is time-consuming and requires relatively expensive equipment and highly trained personnel. At present direct arterial pressure measurement remains the gold standard for assessing aortoiliac disease.[14, 32, 73, 74, 135] Because pressure measurements are no more invasive than arteriography and can be made intraoperatively, they should be obtained whenever there is any question regarding the validity of the noninvasive assessment.[33]

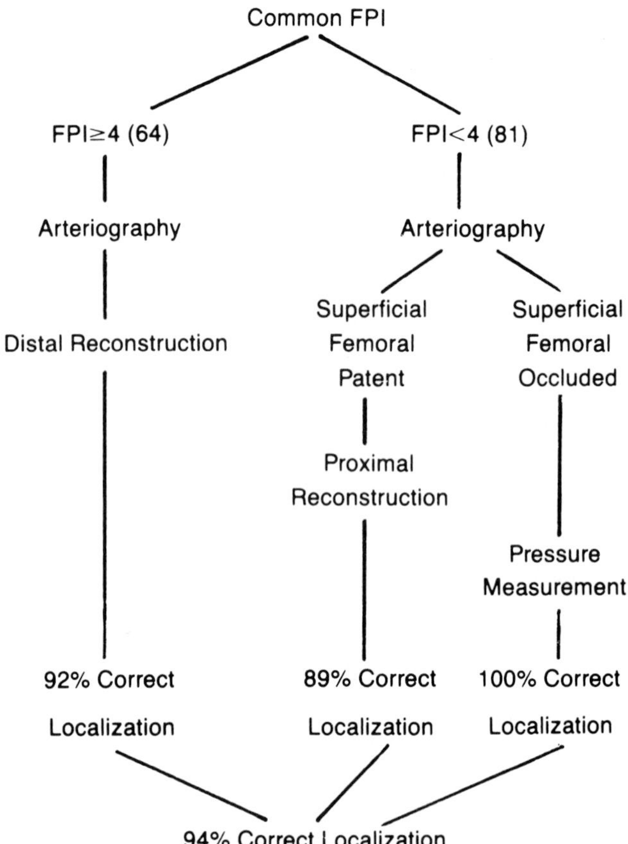

FIGURE 5–24. Algorithm for localizing hemodynamically significant disease in lower limb arterial segments in claudicants with palpable femoral pulses (n = 145). FPI indicates femoral pulsatility index. (From Thiele BL, Bandyk DF, Zierler RE, et al: A systematic approach to the assessment of aortoiliac disease. Arch Surg 118:477, 1983. Copyright 1983, American Medical Association.)

Femorofemoral Bypass

Candidates for femorofemoral bypass present problems analogous to those encountered in patients with multilevel disease. The success or failure of the operation is determined by the functional capacity of the donor iliac artery, which must carry roughly twice the blood flow that it normally does without a significant increase in the pressure gradient from the aorta to the femoral artery.[242] When the donor iliac artery is free of disease, there is no problem, the increased gradient being too small to be recognized. If, however, the donor artery contains atherosclerotic plaques, which it usually does, a minor pressure drop that is tolerable preoperatively may become a major pressure drop postoperatively. Although a modest drop in the resting ankle pressure in the donor limb may be a small price to pay for a significant rise in the ankle pressure of an ischemic recipient limb, a large drop in the postexercise ankle pressure in the donor limb is likely to be unacceptable when the operation has been performed for disabling claudication.[96] Figure 5–25 illustrates this situation in a man with a stenotic donor iliac artery, an occluded recipient artery, and no infrainguinal arterial obstruction.[242] Following construction of a femorofemoral graft, the ankle pressure response to exercise improved in the recipient limb but deteriorated in the donor limb, becoming essentially identical, and the patient's treadmill walking time decreased from 3 minutes to 2 minutes, indicating a worsening of his claudication.

Harris and associates, reporting on a series of femorofemoral bypasses performed for claudication, found that the ankle pressure responses to exercise deteriorated in 45 per cent of the donor limbs, despite the fact that none of the donor iliac arteries appeared significantly stenotic on arteriography.[96] Of the donor limbs with impaired exercise responses, 90 per cent had normal triphasic femoral arterial velocity waveforms, indicating that this test is not sufficiently sensitive to detect the low-grade lesions responsible for the postexercise pressure drops. In two thirds of the hemodynamically impaired donor limbs, direct femoral artery pressure measurements obtained after injection of papaverine also failed to detect an abnormality. It is probable that papaverine, which usually results in a doubling of the blood flow, does not duplicate the stresses imposed by exercise, which may increase blood flow by a factor of five to ten. Nonetheless, direct pressure measurement remains the best physiologic test available for assessing donor limb hemodynamics. In the future, however, it may be supplanted by duplex scanning, which is more sensitive to low-grade lesions.

Comment on Preoperative Studies

Regardless of whether noninvasive testing has been used to make the diagnosis of arterial occlusive disease, preoperative studies are of value as a baseline for follow-up evaluation. At a minimum, these should consist of ankle pressure determinations. In patients with severe ischemia (especially diabetic patients with incompressible ankle vessels), toe pressures and tcPO_2 measurements are also valuable. In patients being treated for claudication, treadmill exercise testing provides an objective method for ascertaining the benefits of the procedure.

Saphenous vein mapping with the duplex scanner is a new and potentially important adjunctive use of preoperative noninvasive testing (see Chapter 6).[205]

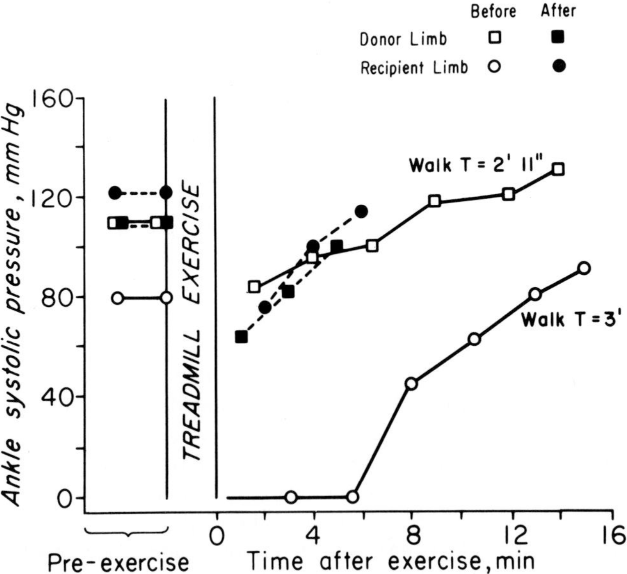

FIGURE 5–25. Ankle pressure response to exercise before and after femorofemoral grafting in a patient with a severely narrowed donor iliac artery. (From Sumner DS, Strandness DE Jr: The hemodynamics of the femorofemoral shunt. Surg Gyencol Obstet 134:629, 1972. By permission of Surgery Gynecology & Obstetrics.)

Predicting Success of Operations

Bernstein and associates have stated, ". . . the area in which the noninvasive laboratory has the greatest opportunity to influence patient care lies in its potential as a predictive tool."[25] Although some may take issue with this statement, the ability to accurately estimate the likelihood of success or failure of a specific management plan is certainly of great importance.

Sympathectomy

With the advent of reconstructive surgery, there are few indications for lumbar sympathectomy. Treating claudication by means of sympathetic denervation has no physiologic basis (see Chapter 3). Some surgeons feel that it may be beneficial in patients with mild rest pain or superficial ulcers; however, this too is open to question. It certainly has no role in the management of the severely ischemic leg. Sympathetic dystrophy and hyperhidrosis remain the only compelling indications for the procedure.

The use of digital plethysmography to identify the presence of sympathetic activity and the ability of the peripheral arterioles to dilate in response to sympathetic denervation has been discussed earlier in this chapter.

As one might expect, the success of sympathectomy in elevating cutaneous blood flow is related to the local perfusion pressure. With pressures below a certain level, the arterioles are completely dilated and therefore do not respond further to sympathetic denervation. Uhrenholdt demonstrated that pedal blood flow increased in response to a sympathetic block when the skin pressure exceeded 40 mmHg but decreased when the pressure was less than 20 mmHg.[256] Similarly, Thulesius and colleagues, in a series of patients with rest pain or ischemic ulcers, found that the toe temperature increased following a sympathectomy when the ankle pressure was more than 60 mmHg but fell when the pressure was less than 60 mmHg.[251] These results suggest that sympathectomy may result in a steal in limbs with low pedal blood pressures and, therefore, might actually be harmful. In the series reported by Yao and Bergan, 96 per cent of limbs with severe ischemia and ABIs below 0.21 required amputation following a sympathectomy.[275] When the indices exceeded 0.35, the results were satisfactory. More recently, Walker and Johnston observed that sympathectomy was unlikely to be beneficial in any ischemic limb with an associated neuropathy.[261] In the absence of neuropathy, a successful outcome was likely in limbs with rest pain or digital gangrene, provided the ankle pressure exceeded 30 mmHg. About 50 per cent of limbs with more severe ischemia (forefoot or heel gangrene) were predicted to respond favorably when the ankle pressure was greater than 60 mmHg.

Plecha and associates observed that a distal thigh-arm index greater than 0.7 was associated with 78 per cent good results from sympathectomy and that an index below this level uniformly predicted a poor outcome.[190] Neither the presence or the absence of diabetes nor the level of ankle pressure had any discernible effect. In fact, five of six limbs with zero ankle pressures and favorable thigh indices (greater than 0.7) responded well. Neuropathy was not considered in their study, and no limbs with extensive tissue necrosis, forefoot gangrene, or uncontrolled infection were included. Again, their findings confirm the importance of adequate inflow to the success of surgical sympathectomy.

In summary, it appears that sympathectomy is likely to be successful only in limbs with ankle pressures greater than 30 to 60 mmHg—in other words, in limbs with low-grade ischemia that would probably respond quite well to judicious medical management. There is little likelihood of success in limbs with low ankle pressures and even some chance that the procedure might be detrimental.

Profundaplasty

When performed for limb salvage, profundaplasty as an isolated procedure is effective in 33 to 86 per cent of cases.[31] To be successful, the operation must be performed on a severely stenotic profunda femoris artery, and the profundopopliteal collateral bed must be well developed. If collateral resistance is too high, the reduction in total limb resistance following profundaplasty will be insufficient to alleviate ischemia. In order to better predict the outcome of profundaplasty, Boren and associates developed an index of popliteal collateral arterial resistance.[31] This index is calculated by dividing the gradient across the knee (above-knee pressure minus below-knee pressure) by the above-knee pressure. When the index was less than 0.25, 67 per cent of the operations were successful; when the index was greater than 0.50, there were no successful results.

Femoropopliteal and Femorotibial Reconstruction

Because one of the major factors determining the potential for graft survival is the resistance of the recipient vascular bed, it seems logical that the preoperative ABI should correlate inversely with the incidence of femoropopliteal graft failure.[64]

Dean and colleagues found that 90 per cent of autogenous saphenous vein femoropopliteal grafts inserted in limbs with ABIs less than 0.20 failed in the early postoperative period.[64] Based on this observation, they suggested that attempting femoropopliteal reconstruction in such limbs may be unwarranted. Others, having had a less dismal experience, are not as pessimistic.[55, 68, 208, 211] The combined early and late failure rates of femoropopliteal bypasses in legs with ABIs less than 0.2 were 47 per cent in the series reported by Corson and associates[55] and 33 per cent in that of Samson and coworkers.[208] Even when no preoperative ankle pressure can be measured owing to the absence of pedal Doppler signals, many femoropopliteal grafts survive.[68, 211, 264]

Although there appears to be a general trend toward better graft survival as the preoperative ABI increases, the data overlap so extensively that statistical significance is not reached.[55, 64, 68] Thus, the individual ABI has little prognostic value. In fact, Samson and coworkers[208] found no difference between the preoperative ABIs in limbs with grafts that failed and those that remained patent and almost identical failure rates in those with indices below and above 0.2. Although Corson and associates observed no statistically significant correlation between failure rate and ABIs, they did note that an index greater than 0.5 appeared to be a favorable prognostic indicator because only 3 per cent of the grafts placed under these circumstances failed in the early postoperative period and only 15 per cent failed later.[55] Preoperative pulse volume recordings are also of no value in predicting femoropopliteal graft survival.[208]

Because grafts to the distal peroneal, posterior tibial, anterior tibial, and dorsalis pedis arteries bypass the below-knee obstructive disease that may be responsible for the failure of grafts terminating at the popliteal area, ABIs would not be expected to correlate well with graft survival. In one report, only 2 of 11 distal bypass grafts in limbs with preoperative ABIs less than 0.2 failed within 30 days (see Fig. 5–4).[244] Moreover, the average preoperative ABI of limbs in which grafts failed within 6 months (0.28 ± 0.22) was not significantly different from that of limbs whose grafts remained patent for more than 12 months (0.32 ± 0.26). Although Samson and coworkers found that the mean preoperative ABI associated with graft survival (0.37 ± 0.30) was significantly greater than that associated with graft failure (0.27 ± 0.27), there was so much variability that individual values were meaningless.[208] Early failure occurred in 37 per cent of legs with ABIs less than 0.2 and in 31 per cent of legs with pulse volume recordings less than 5 mm; but about 50 per cent of the grafts in legs with no detectable ankle pressure or pulse volume recorded pulses survived.

In summary, preoperative ABIs and pulse volume recordings are only roughly correlated with infrainguinal graft survival: Indices of 0.2 or pulse volume recordings of 5 mm are poor discriminators, and many grafts survive in limbs in which no ankle pressures or pulses are detected preoperatively. Therefore, the decision to perform a bypass graft should not be influenced by noninvasive test results.[55, 68, 208, 211, 244]

Aortofemoral Reconstruction

Aortofemoral reconstructions are functionally successful only when hemodynamically significant disease is present in the aorta or iliac arteries.[206] Accurate assessment of the severity of arteriographically demonstrated lesions may be difficult, especially when there is concomitant involvement of the infrainguinal arteries. Physiologic methods for diagnosing and evaluating the relative importance of disease in these two locations have been discussed earlier in this chapter.

Bernstein and colleagues followed 80 patients who had undergone aortofemoral bypass grafting to determine the predictive value of a battery of noninvasive tests performed preoperatively.[25] When the ABI was greater than 0.80, 94 per cent of the limbs became asymptomatic or improved. An index less than 0.40 was associated with a 64 per cent improvement rate. The time required for the toe pulse to regain half its baseline amplitude after a 4-minute period of cuff-induced ischemia (TPRT/2) proved to be the best discriminator. All limbs with a TPRT/2 less than 10 seconds either became asymptomatic or improved, but only 60 per cent of those with a TPRT/2 of 90 seconds were similarly benefitted. Combining these two studies enhanced the predictive value somewhat, particularly in patients with two levels of disease.

The ability to predict minimal increases in the ABI may be helpful to the surgeon who is debating whether to bypass one segment or two in patients with multi-level disease. Williams and colleagues, using a method originally devised by Noer and associates, predicted postoperative ABIs in limbs undergoing aortofemoral bypasses by increasing the preoperative ABI by the same percentage that the directly measured FBI would be expected to increase if it attained a normal value of 1.0 after bypass.[177, 178, 264] Mathematically, this equates to the ratio obtained by dividing the preoperative ABI by the preoperative femoral artery pressure index. When the actual postoperative ABIs were compared with those predicted, a surprisingly high correlation coefficient was obtained ($r = 0.874$). Only 4 per cent of the actual values failed to increase to within 10 per cent of the predicted value, and most were higher than predicted.

These calculations, of course, are not applicable when the ABI is zero or extremely low. Although the "additive transmission" method described by Rutherford and colleagues[206] could be used in this situation, it proved to be only 77 per cent accurate for predicting postoperative ABIs to within ± 0.10. In this method, the estimated increase in the thigh/brachial index is simply added to the preoperative ABI. Inaccuracies inherent in estimating femoral pressure by the cuff technique were undoubtedly partially responsible for the relatively poor results obtained by these investigators.

Postoperative Monitoring

Monitoring the patency of an arterial reconstruction once the patient reaches the recovery room is of obvious importance to the successful outcome of the surgical procedure. Assuming that the intraoperative assessment (discussed in Chapter 24) revealed no abnormalities, the surgeon is obligated to detect early signs of graft failure in order to correct the responsible defect as expeditiously as possible. The problem is likely to be technical but may be a thrombosis for which there is no apparent explanation. Early correction of a minor problem often ensures long-term patency.

The reappearance of peripheral pulses in limbs in which the pulse was not palpable preoperatively is good evidence of graft patency, and the disappearance of pulses palpable in the operating room at the termination of the procedure is highly suggestive of occlusion. But pedal pulses may be weak immediately after operation and may be absent in limbs with residual distal disease even when a graft is patent. Although the presence of a palpable pulse in a graft is reassuring, it does not necessarily imply patency. Despite the absence of blood flow, a graft can continue to pulsate when its terminal end is occluded as long as the column of blood remains liquid or is incompletely thrombosed. Furthermore, it is seldom possible to palpate graft pulsations when the graft is placed deeply within the leg.

The Doppler flowmeter is the most versatile noninvasive instrument for assessing graft patency in the immediate postoperative period (Fig. 5–26). The presence of pulsatile, often hyperemic flow clearly establishes patency. Absence of a velocity signal or the presence of an abrupt signal with a thumping quality indicates occlusion even when the graft may continue to pulsate. Unfortunately, it is frequently impossible to detect a flow signal through a polytetrafluoroethylene (PTFE) graft soon after it has been placed, owing to the severe damping of ultrasound by air trapped in the interstices of the graft material. Later, as these areas are infiltrated by body fluids, the signal is readily detected. There is no problem in investigating grafts of autogenous vein, umbilical vein, or Dacron. It is, however, difficult to examine aortofemoral grafts at groin level because of the fresh incision, the depth of the graft, and the disruption of tissue planes, all of which interfere with the transmission of ultrasound.

Signals from the dorsalis pedis, posterior tibial, and anterior medial tarsal arteries should be assessed in all patients. It must be emphasized that the mere presence of an audible signal does not connote graft patency. In the hands of an experienced observer, the quality of the Doppler signal can, nevertheless, be quite informative. For example, hyperemic flow or a normal triphasic signal is excellent evidence of graft patency. On the other hand, a barely audible, nonpulsatile signal or the absence of a signal in a pedal artery that was patent preoperatively and is known to be in continuity with the reconstruction must be viewed with concern. Immediately after proximal (aortoiliac, femorofemoral, or axillary femoral) reconstruction in limbs with associated severe femoropopliteal/tibial occlusion, flow signals may not be detected at the ankle.[274] In this event, an audible signal in the popliteal area usually signifies patency of the proximal reconstruction. If the pedal

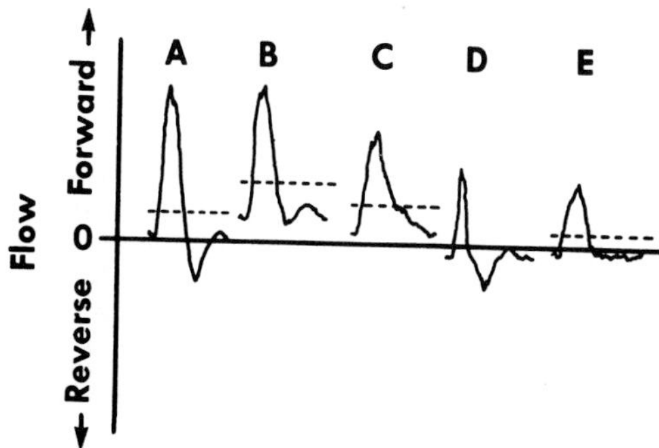

FIGURE 5–26. Contour of flow pulse in a vein graft. *Dotted line* indicates mean flow. *A*, Unobstructed graft with peripheral vasoconstriction. *B*, Unobstructed graft with peripheral vasodilation. *C*, Stenosis proximal to the site of the flow probe. *D*, Complete obstruction several centimeters distal to site of flow probe. Note that the pulse contour is nearly normal but mean flow is zero. *E*, Stenosis just below site of flow probe.

flow signals remain inaudible 4 to 6 hours after the operation, the possibility of thrombosis must be entertained.

Measurement of ankle pressure can be accomplished in all cases with an audible pedal Doppler signal except those in which the terminal anastomosis is at foot level or those in which peripheral incisions make the examination too painful. An increase in the ABI of more than 0.15 compared with the preoperative value is indicative of graft patency.[209] Ordinarily, the increase will be appreciably greater than this. Failure to demonstrate an increase in the ABI suggests, but does not conclusively establish, the existence of a problem. If other evidence is compatible with continued graft function, it is usually safe to delay arteriography or re-exploration for a variable period of time (depending on the type of operation) while the ankle pressure is carefully monitored.[274] The limit should be no more than 4 hours following a femoropopliteal bypass. If, after that time, the ankle pressure does not improve, the patient should be returned to the operating room for correction of the problem. In limbs with chronic obstructions below the site of the distal anastomosis, it may take much longer for the ABI to rise. For example, improvement may not be apparent for 4 to 6 hours following a bypass to a blind popliteal segment, for 6 to 12 hours after an aortofemoral bypass in a limb with multi-level disease, and for 24 hours after a profundaplasty.[274]

Pulse volume recordings may be useful in limbs in which ankle pressures cannot be obtained either because of arterial calcification or because of painful incisions.[63, 209] An increase of more than 5 mm in the amplitude of the ankle PVR tracing compared with that obtained preoperatively is indicative of graft patency. A decrease in the amplitude is strongly suggestive of obstruction.

Follow-Up Studies

After the immediate postoperative period, noninvasive studies continue to be important, affording an objective assessment of improvement and permitting failure or impending failure of the reconstruction to be detected.

Assessing Results of Surgery

Ankle pressure measurements provide the most convenient method of evaluating the results of reconstructive arterial surgery. An increase of 0.15 or more in the resting ABI can be taken as definite evidence of improvement. If all involved segments have been bypassed, the result should be an ankle index of 1.0 or higher, provided the diameter of the graft is sufficiently large to carry the required flow with a minimal pressure gradient. During the hyperemic phase following revascularization of a severely ischemic extremity, ABIs, although improved, may remain low when the graft diameter is less than 3.5 mm.[12] This situation is most likely to be encountered when in situ grafts terminate far distally in the leg, but it may also occur in association with femoropopliteal bypasses. As the hyperemia decreases, the ankle pressure gradually rises, perhaps requiring a month before reaching a maximal level. If, however, all diseased arterial segments have not been bypassed or otherwise reconstructed, the ABI will rise commensurate with the reduction in total resistance but will not attain normal levels.[177, 206, 264] Many examples of this, including aortofemoral bypasses in limbs with superficial femoral obstruction and bypasses to a blind popliteal segment, occur.

Unfortunately, as repeatedly emphasized in this chapter, ankle pressure measurements may be unreliable in 5 to 10 per cent of revascularized limbs, owing to medial calcification of the peripheral arteries. In addition, the presence of pedal arterial disease may continue to restrict perfusion of the foot despite adequate inflow pressures. Pulse volume recordings at ankle or foot level, digital plethysmography, measurement of toe pressures, and $tcPo_2$ determinations are often quite helpful for assessing functional results in such cases.[141, 145]

When surgery has been performed to alleviate claudication, exercise testing affords a sensitive means of judging physiologic improvement. In the ideal case, the patient will be able to walk for 5 minutes without experiencing a drop in ankle pressure (Fig. 5–27).[228] When residual disease is present or when the diameter of the graft restricts flow, there will be a postexercise pressure drop even though the resting ABI is normal and the patient walks for 5 minutes without developing claudication (Fig. 5–28).[232] Other patients may be symptomatically improved, walking for a longer time on the treadmill with a less severe drop in ankle pressure, but will be far from normal. This result is commonly seen when arterial reconstruction is limited to the aortofemoral segment in patients with multi-level disease (Fig. 5–29).[229]

Obtaining a baseline study early after reconstruction is important for further follow-up. Patient testimony and the physical examination may be unreliable.[228] Often, the ankle pressure and exercise tolerance continue to increase for several days to several months, possibly in response to the increased head of pressure made available by a proximal reconstruction.[276] Although the explanation is not readily

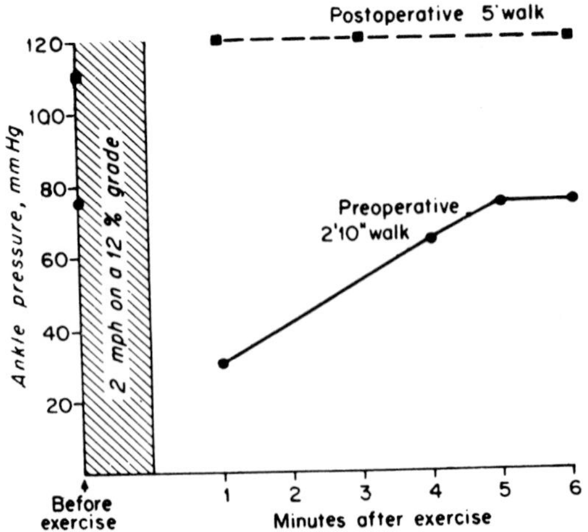

FIGURE 5–27. Resting ankle pressure and ankle pressure response to exercise in a 50-year-old man with calf and thigh claudication due to occlusion of left common iliac artery. After bypass grafting, ankle pressure and ankle pressure response to exercise returned to normal. The patient was relieved of symptoms. (From Strandness DE Jr: Exercise testing in the evaluation of patients undergoing direct arterial surgery. J Cardiovasc Surg 11:192, 1970.)

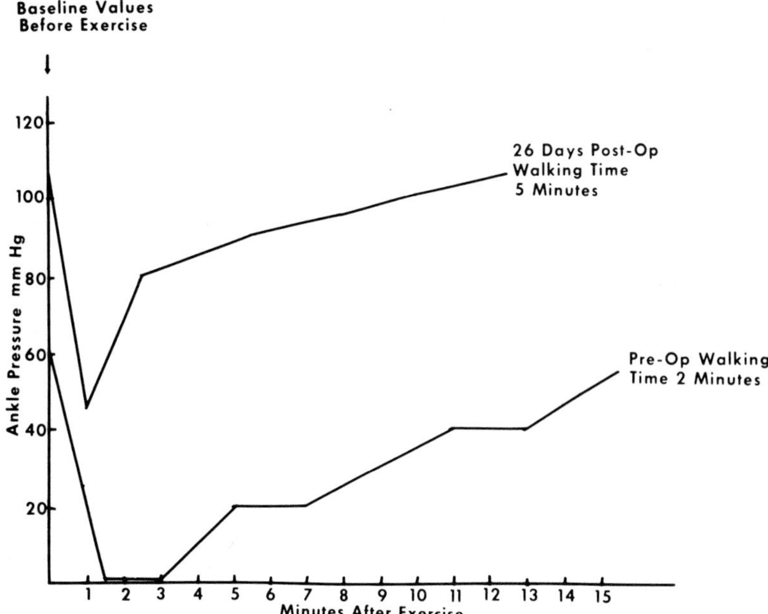

FIGURE 5–28. Effect of exercise on ankle pressure response before and after a "successful" femoropopliteal bypass graft. Following the operation, the patient regained his popliteal and pedal pulses and became asymptomatic. His resting ankle pressure returned to normal levels. Although he could walk 5 minutes on the treadmill without experiencing claudication, his ankle pressure response to exercise remained abnormal. (From Strandness DE Jr: Abnormal exercise responses after successful reconstructive arterial surgery. Surgery 59:325, 1966.)

apparent, many patients with femoropopliteal bypasses also improve.[233, 276]

Predicting Early Failure of Bypass Grafts

Corson and associates observed that 88 per cent of vein bypass grafts to the popliteal, tibial, or peroneal arteries failed in the early (less than 30 days) postoperative period when the postoperative ABI was less than 0.50 and that 91 per cent of early failures had postoperative indices below 0.70.[55] When the increase in the postoperative index compared with that obtained preoperatively was less than 0.10, 88 per cent of the grafts failed early. All early failures were in limbs in which the increase in the index was less than 0.40. Samson and coworkers, on the other hand, found that neither the absolute value of the postoperative ABI, the pulse volume recording amplitude, nor the increase in these two measurements had any predictive value.[208] Other investigators have reached similar conclusions.[68, 244]

Bandyk and colleagues, who used pulsed Doppler ultrasound to examine blood flow in in situ vein bypass grafts, found that a peak systolic velocity less than 40 cm/sec was associated with technical errors.[12] Even in the absence of an identifiable problem, low velocities predicted early failure. Owing to the hyperemia that follows successful arterial reconstruction, diastolic forward flow is typically present and is a good prognostic sign. Absence of diastolic forward flow indicates a high peripheral resistance, an observation that correlates with early failure.[11, 12]

Recognition of Impending Graft Failure

Stenoses or other problems that jeopardize graft survival are best corrected prior to the development of thrombosis.[13, 22, 23, 51, 144, 150, 258] Once a graft has thrombosed, suc-

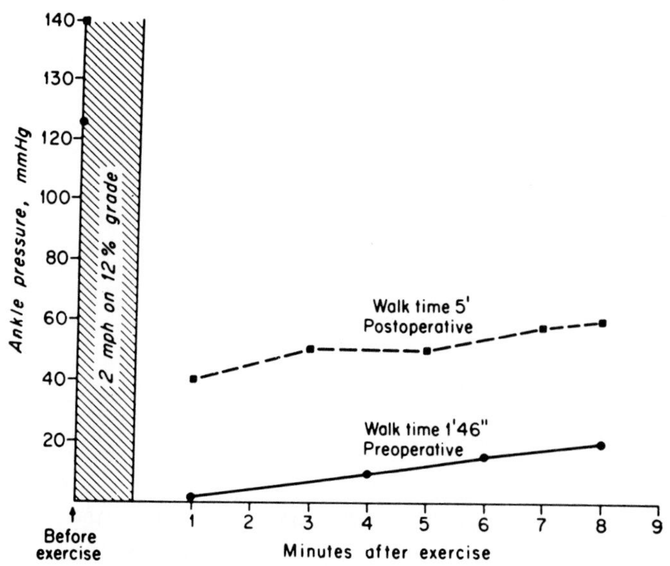

FIGURE 5–29. Effect of aortofemoral grafting on exercise response in a patient with combined iliac stenosis and superficial femoral occlusion. Walking time increased greatly, but ankle pressure response to exercise, although improved, remained abnormal. (From Strandness DE Jr: Physiologic evaluation of peripheral arterial occlusion. *In* Dale WA [ed]: Management of Arterial Occlusive Disease. Chicago, Year Book Medical Publishers, 1971, pp 13–29.)

cessful thrombectomy does not ensure long-term patency, even when appropriate measures have been taken to rectify the responsible defect.

Stenoses may develop in femoropopliteal or femorotibial grafts without producing any symptoms or any alteration of the pulses in the grafts or at the periphery.[22, 23] Many of these "silent" stenoses can be detected if the ankle pressure is followed closely in the months and years after operation.[23, 51, 183, 244, 254, 258] Close surveillance is particularly important during the first year, since about three quarters of the problems arise within this early period. A previously stable ABI that drops by 0.15 or more (or a decrease in the pulse volume recording amplitude of 5 mm or more) suggests the need for arteriographic investigation.[7, 22, 23, 120, 254] As a rule, operative correction is easily accomplished, after which the ankle pressure should return to the original postoperative level.

Unfortunately, in an appreciable number of limbs, no drop in ankle pressure will be evident prior to graft failure.[11, 144, 163, 269] For this reason, Bandyk and coworkers recommend following the velocity of blood flow in recently implanted grafts as a supplement to ankle pressure measurements.[11–13] A decrease in systolic flow velocity below 40 cm/sec has, in their experience, proved to be an ominous sign. Diastolic flow velocity, on the other hand, has little predictive value. It normally decreases in the weeks following graft insertion—essentially disappearing by 3 months—at which time, a typical triphasic flow pattern is established (see Fig. 5–26*A*).[12]

The function of a graft and its longevity may also be compromised by the progression of atherosclerotic or fibrodysplastic disease at the anastomoses or in the inflow or outflow arteries.[244, 254] Again, these changes, which may not be clinically apparent, can often be detected by a fall in the ABI (Fig. 5–30). Segmental pressures may help to distinguish stenoses developing in a bypass graft or endarterectomized segment from disease progression in arteries above or below the reconstruction.[167, 168]

Duplex scanning with color flow imaging is a powerful method for following bypass grafts.[11, 13, 37, 60, 144, 149, 150, 161, 163, 220] Not only can the presence of a graft-threatening defect be detected but the problem can also be localized to the inflow or outflow arteries, the anastomoses, or the graft itself. Moreover, stenoses can be identified before they become hemodynamically significant, that is, before the ABI begins to fall or before exercise test results become abnormal.[11, 144, 161, 163] Although the natural history of these early lesions has not been established, it seems logical to predict that many, if not most, will progress.[161, 269] Duplex scanning also facilitates the recognition of residual arteriovenous fistulae and valve leaflets, problems unique to in situ bypass grafting.[13, 60, 149, 220] In addition, aneurysms involving the graft, anastomotic false aneurysms, and perigraft seromas are easily evaluated (see Chapter 6).

Laborde and associates performed routine postoperative surveillance on 124 in situ saphenous vein bypass grafts using both ABIs and color flow duplex scanning.[144] Of 38 graft and native artery stenoses demonstrated by arteriography, only 16 (42 per cent) were identified by a fall in ABI of more than 0.15, whereas duplex scanning detected 37 (97 per cent). The duplex criteria used to indicate a significant stenosis were a localized threefold increase in peak systolic velocity or a peak velocity throughout the graft of less than 45 cm/sec. It appears that a localized velocity increase correlates with the presence of a significant stenosis at that site; however, the defect responsible for an abnormally low graft velocity may lie proximal or distal to the graft. The finding of a low graft velocity without any intrinsic graft lesions suggests either inflow obstruction or severely limited outflow. Whatever the underlying cause, a low graft velocity is highly suggestive of some problem that threatens graft patency.

Among 379 infrainguinal reversed vein bypass grafts followed with duplex scanning by Mills and coworkers, only 2 per cent of 280 grafts with peak systolic velocities over 45 cm/sec occluded within 6 months of examination.[163] Arteriography was performed on 75 of the 99 grafts with peak velocities less than 45 cm/sec, with identification of stenotic lesions involving 48 grafts, occlusion of 19 grafts, limited outflow in 4 grafts, and dilatation alone in 4 grafts. Only 29 per cent of the grafts that were abnormal by duplex scanning were associated with a reduction in ABI of 0.15 or greater.

Long-term patency of grafts in which significant steno-

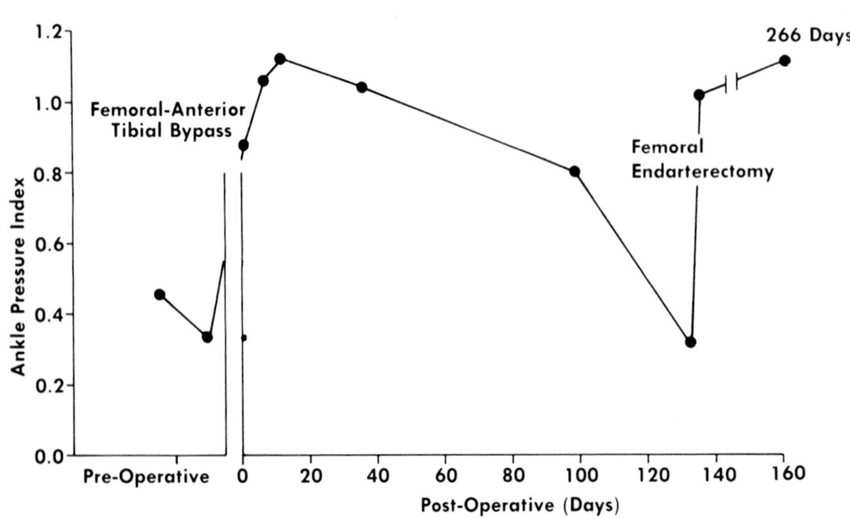

FIGURE 5–30. Salvage of femoral anterior tibial graft prior to failure. The drop in ankle pressure following a femoral anterior tibial bypass called attention to the development of a stenosis in the common femoral artery above the proximal anastomosis. An endarterectomy restored normal function. (From Sumner DS, Strandness DE Jr: Hemodynamic studies before and after extended bypass grafts to the tibial and peroneal arteries. Surgery 86:442, 1979.)

ses have been detected by duplex scanning is poor, unless the lesions are corrected before thrombosis occurs. Mattos and colleagues, in a study of 170 infrainguinal autogenous vein bypass grafts, found that the cumulative 2-year assisted primary patency rate of grafts with a localized twofold increase in velocity was only 33 per cent, a rate significantly lower than that in grafts in which stenoses identified by this criterion had been revised (90 per cent).[280] In studies based on a routine protocol of postoperative graft surveillance, the prevalence of lesions that could lead to graft failure is in the range of 10 to 30 per cent.[13, 144, 150, 163, 220] Therefore, it is important to follow all bypass grafts with serial noninvasive tests, preferably by duplex scanning. One recommended follow-up protocol includes examinations at 3-month intervals during the first postoperative year and every 6 to 12 months thereafter.[163]

Hemodynamic Failure

Continued patency of a bypass graft or endarterectomy has been the traditional standard for success of reconstructive surgery. The reconstruction may remain patent, however, without providing functional improvement or relief of symptoms.[183, 206, 243] If patent but hemodynamically failed grafts are recognized, the condition responsible for the lack of physiologic improvement may be susceptible to correction. Any lesion within the graft or inflow or outflow arteries can be responsible.[167, 168, 183] Of particular interest is the occurrence of hemodynamic failure in the absence of any new or residual lesion. For example, the diameter of the graft may merely be too small to permit a flow rate adequate to relieve symptoms.[183] Segmental pressure studies, Doppler surveys, exercise testing, and duplex scanning are all valuable methods for identifying and evaluating the severity of hemodynamic failure (Fig. 5–31).

Directional Doppler flow studies are especially helpful in the evaluation of the functional results of femorofemoral bypass grafting (see Fig. 5–25).[242] Of 51 such grafts examined by O'Mara and coworkers, 2 were found to have flow going in the opposite direction to that originally intended.[183]

Natural History and Prognosis

Symptoms and physical signs are too unreliable and arteriography is too invasive to be used to study the prevalence, incidence, and natural history of peripheral arteriosclerotic occlusive disease.[58, 155] Because of their objectivity and ability to be repeated frequently without subjecting the patient to undue discomfort or risks, noninvasive tests are ideally suited for population surveys and longitudinal studies of disease progression.

Criqui and coworkers reported that only 1.9 per cent of a geographically defined population ranging in age from 38 to 82 years (mean, 66 years) complained of intermittent claudication, but noninvasive testing of this same population revealed an 11.7 per cent prevalence of large vessel peripheral arterial disease.[57] The prevalence ranged from less than 3 per cent in subjects under the age of 60 years to more than 20 per cent in subjects older than 75 years. Identification of any symptom that could possibly be called claudication or the recognition of any pulse abnormality had a positive predictive value of only 37 per cent. Similarly, Marinelli and colleagues found that 165 (36 per cent) of 458 diabetic patients had positive noninvasive test results, indicating the presence of hemodynamically significant peripheral arterial disease.[155] Nearly one third of the patients with no history of intermittent claudication and one fifth of those with normal physical examinations had abnormal test results. Using noninvasive methods, Strandness and Stahler detected disease progression in 52 per cent of patients with lower extremity arterial disease who were followed for an average of 3 years.[235] Almost 40 per cent of patients with disease progression experienced no increase in symptoms. Clearly, clinical evaluation alone underestimates both the prevalence of arteriosclerosis obliterans and its rate of progression.

Based on a 5-year follow-up study of nondiabetic patients with intermittent claudication due to occlusion of the superficial femoral artery, Wilson and associates concluded that symptoms are likely to improve or remain unchanged when the ABI exceeds 0.60 but are likely to progress when

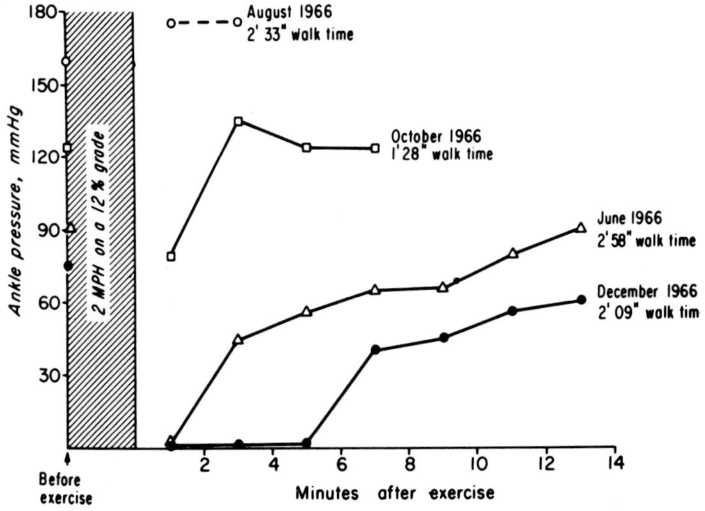

FIGURE 5–31. Changes in ankle pressure and postexercise response in a 65-year-old man who underwent an aortic bifurcation graft in June 1966. In August 1966, ankle pressure was normal and there was no drop in pressure following exercise. By October 1966, however, the exercise response was abnormal, and by December 1966, the objective tests were worse than they were prior to operation. Although the graft remained patent, the patient developed an occlusion in the superficial femoral artery. (From Strandness DE Jr: Techniques in the evaluation of vascular disease. *In* Cooper P, Nyhus LM [eds]: Surgery Annual. Norwalk, CT, Appleton-Century-Crofts, 1971, pp 181–197.)

the index is less.[265] Of those patients whose symptoms improved, only 46 per cent demonstrated any objective increase in the ABI. With more severe disease, the outcome may become evident over a much shorter period of time. Mazza and coworkers found that 57 per cent of limbs with an ABI between 0.30 and 0.50 could be managed nonoperatively, whereas 92 per cent of limbs with ABIs less than 0.30 required reconstruction or amputation within 2 years.[159] Paaske and Tønnesen found that 82 per cent of patients with a toe/brachial pressure index less than 0.07 underwent a major amputation within 2 years, and 27 per cent died.[186] The amputation and death rates were 38 and 33 per cent, respectively, in those with toe indices of 0.08 to 0.13 and were 27 and 18 per cent, respectively, in patients with toe indices of 0.14 to 0.25. An ABI less than 0.30 is associated with a 32 per cent amputation rate and a 60 per cent death rate over a 6-year period.[53] This contrasts with a 13 per cent amputation rate and 33 per cent death rate in patients of similar age (72 ± 11 years) with ankle indices between 0.30 and 0.50 ($p < .05$).

Not all investigators have been able to confirm a strong association between the initial ABI and symptom progression in limbs with intermittent claudication. For example, Cronenwett and colleagues found that the values overlapped too extensively to establish valid criteria for predicting outcome.[59] Most studies, however, do suggest that noninvasive tests have prognostic value and confirm the association between disease progression, limb loss, early death, and the severity of the atherosclerotic process.

References

1. Allan JS, Terry HJ: The evaluation of an ultrasonic flow detector for the assessment of peripheral vascular disease. Cardiovasc Res 3:503, 1969.
2. Aukland A, Hurlow RA: Spectral analysis of Doppler ultrasound: Its clinical application in lower limb ischemia. Br J Surg 69:539, 1982.
3. Baird RN, Bird DR, Clifford PC, et al: Upstream stenosis. Its diagnosis by Doppler signals from the femoral artery. Arch Surg 115:1316, 1980.
4. Baird RJ, Feldman P, Miles JT, et al: Subsequent downstream repair after aorta-iliac and aorta-femoral bypass operations. Surgery 82:785, 1977.
5. Baker AR, Evans DH, Prytherch DR, et al: Haemodynamic assessment of the femoropopliteal segment: Comparison of pressure and Doppler methods using ROC curve analysis. Br J Surg 73:559, 1986.
6. Baker JD: Poststress Doppler ankle pressures. A comparison of treadmill exercise with two other methods of induced hyperemia. Arch Surg, 113:1171, 1978.
7. Baker JD, Dix D: Variability of Doppler ankle pressures with arterial occlusive disease: An evaluation of ankle index and brachial-ankle gradient. Surgery 89:134, 1981.
8. Baker JD, Machleder HI, Skidmore R: Analysis of femoral artery Doppler signals by Laplace transform damping method. J Vasc Surg 1:520, 1984.
9. Baker WH, Barnes RW: Minor forefoot amputations in patients with low ankle pressure. Am J Surg 133:331, 1977.
10. Baker WH, String ST, Hayes AC, et al: Diagnosis of peripheral occlusive disease: Comparison of clinical evaluation and noninvasive laboratory. Arch Surg 113:1308, 1978.
11. Bandyk DF, Cato RF, Towne JB: A low flow velocity predicts failure of femoropopliteal and femorotibial bypass grafts. Surgery 98:799, 1985.
12. Bandyk DF, Kaebnick HW, Bergamini TM, et al: Hemodynamics of in situ saphenous vein arterial bypass. Arch Surg 123:477, 1988.
13. Bandyk DF, Schmitt DD, Seabrook GR, et al: Monitoring functional patency of in situ saphenous vein bypasses: The impact of a surveillance protocol and elective revision. J Vasc Surg 9:286, 1989.
14. Barber GG, Fong H, McPhail NV, et al: Hemodynamic assessment of the aortoiliac segment: A prospective study. Can J Surg 23:542, 1980.
15. Barnes RW: Noninvasive methods to evaluate acute vascular problems. *In* Haimovici H (ed): Vascular Emergencies. New York, Appleton-Century-Crofts, 1982, pp 7–26.
16. Barnes RW, Hafermann MD, Petersen J, et al: Noninvasive assessment of altered limb hemodynamics and complications of arterial catheterization. Radiology 107:505, 1973.
17. Barnes RW, Shanik GD, Slaymaker EF: An index of healing in below-knee amputation: Leg blood pressure by Doppler ultrasound. Surgery 79:13, 1976.
18. Barnes RW, Thornhill B, Nix L, et al: Prediction of amputation wound healing. Roles of Doppler ultrasound and digit photoplethysmography. Arch Surg 116:80, 1981.
19. Bell G: Systolic pressure measurements in occlusive vascular disease to assess run-off preoperatively. Scand J Clin Lab Invest 31(Suppl 128):173, 1973.
20. Bergan JJ, Yao JST: Invited overview: Role of the vascular laboratory. Surgery 88:9, 1980.
21. Bergan JJ, Yao JST, Flinn WR: Surgical management of young claudicants: Adventitial cysts. *In* Bergan JJ, Yao JST (eds): Evaluation and Treatment of Upper and Lower Extremity Circulatory Disorders. Orlando, FL, Grune & Stratton, 1984, pp 457–464.
22. Berkowitz HD, Greenstein SM: Improved patency in reversed femoral-infrapopliteal autogenous vein grafts by early detection and treatment of the failing graft. J Vasc Surg 5:755, 1987.
23. Berkowitz HD, Hobbs CL, Roberts B, et al: Value of routine vascular laboratory studies to identify vein graft stenosis. Surgery 90:971, 1981.
24. Bernstein EF: How does a vascular laboratory influence management of arterial disease? *In* Greenhalgh RH, Jamieson CW, Nicolaides AN (eds): Vascular Surgery, Issues in Current Practice. London, Grune & Stratton, 1986, pp 101–117.
25. Bernstein EF, Rhodes GA, Stuart SH, et al: Toe pulse-reappearance time in prediction of aortofemoral bypass success. Ann Surg 193:201, 1981.
26. Bernstein EF, Witzel TH, Stotts JS, et al: Thigh pressure artifacts with noninvasive techniques in an experimental model. Surgery 89:319, 1981.
27. Bollinger A, Mahler F, Zehender O: Kombinierte Druck- und Durchflussmessungen in der Beurteilung arterieller Durchblutungsstörungen. Dtsch Med Wochenschr 95:1039, 1970.
28. Bone GE: The relationship between aorto-iliac hemodynamics and femoral pulsatility index. J Surg Res 32:228, 1982.
29. Bone GE, Pomajzl MJ: Toe blood pressure by photoplethysmography: An index of healing in forefoot amputation. Surgery 89:569, 1981.
30. Bone GE, Hayes AC, Slaymaker EE, et al: Value of segmental limb blood pressures in predicting results of aortofemoral bypass. Am J Surg 132:733, 1976.
31. Boren CH, Towne JB, Bernhard VM, et al: Profunda-popliteal collateral index. A guide to successful profundaplasty. Surgery 115:1366, 1980.
32. Brener BJ, Raines JK, Darling RC, et al: Measurement of systolic femoral arterial pressure during reactive hyperemia. Circulation 49–50(Suppl II):259, 1974.
33. Breslau PJ, Jorning PJG, Greep JM: Assessment of aorto-iliac disease using hemodynamic measures. Arch Surg 120:1050, 1985.
34. Brewster DC, Waltman AC, O'Hara PJ, et al: Femoral artery pressure measurements during arteriography. Circulation 60(Suppl I):120, 1979.
35. Britt DB, Kemmerer WT, Robison JR: Penile blood flow determination by mercury strain gauge plethysmography. Invest Urol 8:673, 1971.
36. Bruner JMR, Krenis LJ, Kunsman JM, et al: Comparison of direct and indirect methods of measuring arterial blood pressure. Med Instrum 15:11, 1981.
37. Buth J, Disselhoff B, Sommeling C, et al: Color flow duplex criteria for grading stenoses in infrainguinal vein grafts. J Vasc Surg 14:716, 1991.
38. Byrne P, Provan JL, Ameli FM, et al: The use of transcutaneous

oxygen tension measurements in the diagnosis of peripheral vascular insufficiency. Ann Surg 200:159, 1984.
39. Campbell WB, Baird RN, Cole SEA, et al: Physiological interpretation of Doppler shift waveforms: The femorodistal segment in combined disease. Ultrasound Med Biol 9:265, 1983.
40. Campbell WB, Cole SEA, Skidmore R, et al: The clinician and the vascular laboratory in the diagnosis of aorto-iliac stenosis. Br J Surg 71:302, 1984.
41. Carter SA: Indirect systolic pressure and pulse waves in arterial occlusive disease of the lower extremities. Circulation 37:624, 1968.
42. Carter SA: Clinical measurement of systolic pressures in limbs with arterial oclusive disease. JAMA 207:1869, 1969.
43. Carter SA: Response of ankle systolic pressure to leg exercise in mild or questionable arterial disease. N Engl J Med 287:578, 1972.
44. Carter SA: The relationship of distal systolic pressures to healing of skin lesions in limbs with arterial occlusive disease, with special reference to diabetes mellitus. Scand J Clin Lab Invest 31(Suppl 128):239, 1973.
45. Carter SA, Lezack JD: Digital systolic pressures in the lower limb in arterial disease. Circulation 43:905, 1971.
46. Castronuovo JJ, Flanigan DP: Pseudoclaudication of neurospinal origin. Vasc Diagn Ther 5:21, 1984.
47. Castronuovo JJ Jr, Pabst TS, Flanigan DP, et al: Noninvasive determination of skin perfusion pressure using a laser Doppler. J Cardiovasc Surg 28:253, 1987.
48. Chiu RC-J, Lidstone D, Blundell PE: Predictive power of penile/brachial index in diagnosing male sexual impotence. J Vasc Surg 4:251, 1986.
49. Cina C, Katsamouris A, Megerman J, et al: Utility of transcutaneous oxygen tension measurements in peripheral arterial occlusive disease. J Vasc Surg 1:362, 1984.
50. Clyne CAC, Ryan J, Webster JHH, et al: Oxygen tension on the skin of ischemic legs. Am J Surg 143:315, 1982.
51. Cohen JR, Mannick JA, Covek NP, et al: Recognition and management of impending vein-graft failure. Arch Surg 121:758, 1986.
52. Cohrs P, Seller K, Brantigan CO: Popliteal artery entrapment syndrome: Noninvasive diagnosis. Bruit 7:20, 1983.
53. Colgan MP, Howell MA, Seeger RW, et al: Relationship of severity of lower limb peripheral vascular disease to mortality and morbidity—A six-year follow-up study. Unpublished observations, 1988.
54. Conrad MC, Green HD: Hemodynamics of large and small vessels in peripheral vascular disease. Circulation 29:847, 1964.
55. Corson JD, Johnson WC, LoGerfo FW, et al: Doppler ankle systolic blood pressure. Prognostic value in vein bypass grafts of the lower extremity. Arch Surg 113:932, 1978.
56. Cossman DV, Ellison JE, Wagner WW, et al: Comparison of dye arteriography to arterial mapping with color-flow duplex imaging in the lower extremities. J Vasc Surg 10:522, 1989.
57. Criqui MH, Fronek A, Barrett-Connor E, et al: The prevalence of peripheral arterial diseae in a defined population. Circulation 71:510, 1985.
58. Criqui MH, Fronek A, Klauber MR, et al: The sensitivity, specificity, and predictive value of traditional clinical evaluation of peripheral arterial disease: Results from noninvasive testing in a defined population. Circulation 71:516, 1985.
59. Cronenwett JL, Warner KG, Zelenock GB, et al: Intermittent claudication. Current results of nonoperative management. Arch Surg 119:430, 1984.
60. Cullen PJ, Lehay AL, Ryan SB, et al: The influence of duplex scanning on early patency rates of in situ bypass to the tibial vessels. Ann Vasc Surg 1:340, 1986.
61. Cutajar CL, Marston A, Newcombe JF: Value of cuff occlusion pressures in assessment of peripheral vascular disease. Br Med J 2:392, 1973.
62. Darling RC, Buckley CJ, Abbott WM, et al: Intermittent claudication in young athletes: Popliteal artery entrapment syndrome. J Trauma 14:543, 1974.
63. Darling RC, Raines JK, Brener BJ, et al: Quantitative segmental pulse volume recorder: A clinical tool. Surgery 72:873, 1972.
64. Dean RH, Yao JST, Stanton PE, et al: Prognostic indicators in femoropopliteal reconstructions. Arch Surg 110:1287, 1975.
65. Dean RH, Yao JST, Thompson RG, et al: Predictive value of ultrasonically derived arterial pressure in determination of amputation level. Am Surg 41:731, 1975.
66. Delius W, Erikson U: Correlation between angiographic and hemodynamic findings in occlusions of arteries of the extremities. Vasc Surg 3:201, 1969.
67. Delius W, Kellerova E: Reactions of arterial and venous vessels in the human forearm and hand to deep breath or mental strain. Clin Sci 40:271, 1971.
68. Dolgin C, Collins R, Martin E, et al: The prognostic value of the noninvasive vascular laboratory in autologous vein bypass of the lower extremity. J Cardiovasc Surg 24:231, 1983.
69. Evans DH, Barrie WW, Asher MJ, et al: The relationship between ultrasonic pulsatility index and proximal arterial stenosis in a canine model. Circ Res 46:470, 1980.
70. Faris I, Duncan HP: Skin perfusion pressure in the prediction of healing in diabetic patients with ulcers or gangrene of the foot. J Vasc Surg 2:536, 1985.
71. Faris IB, Jamieson CW: The diagnosis of aorto-iliac stenosis: A comparison of thigh pressure measurements and femoral artery flow velocity profile. J Cardiovasc Surg 16:597, 1975.
72. Flanigan DP, Collins JT, Schwartz JA, et al: Hemodynamic and arteriographic evaluation of femoral pulsatility index. J Surg Res 32:234, 1982.
73. Flanigan DP, Ryan TJ, Williams LR, et al: Aortofemoral or femoropopliteal revascularization? A prospective evaluation of the papaverine test. J Vasc Surg 1:215, 1984.
74. Flanigan DP, Williams LR, Schwartz JA, et al: Hemodynamic evaluation of the aortoiliac system based on pharmacologic vasodilatation. Surgery 93:709, 1983.
75. Francfort JW, Bigelow PS, Davis JT, et al: Noninvasive techniques in the assessment of lower extremity arterial occlusive disease. The advantages of proximal and distal thigh cuffs. Arch Surg 119:1145, 1984.
76. Franzeck UK, Talke P, Bernstein EF, et al: Transcutaneous Po_2 measurements in health and peripheral arterial occlusive disease. Surgery 91:156, 1982.
77. Fronek A, Coel M, Bernstein EF: Quantitative ultrasonographic studies of lower extremity flow velocities in health and disease. Circulation 53:957, 1976.
78. Fronek A, Coel M, Bernstein EF: The pulse-reappearance time: An index of over-all blood flow impairment in the ischemic extremity. Surgery 81:376, 1977.
79. Fronek A, Coel M, Bernstein EF: The importance of combined multisegmental pressure and Doppler flow velocity studies in the diagnosis of peripheral arterial occlusive disease. Surgery 84:840, 1978.
80. Fronek A, Johansen KH, Dilley RB, et al: Noninvasive physiologic tests in the diagnosis and characterization of peripheral arterial occlusive disease. Am J Surg 126:205, 1973.
81. Fronek A, Johansen K, Dilley RB, et al: Ultrasonographically monitored postocclusive reactive hyperemia in the diagnosis of peripheral arterial occlusive disease. Circulation 48:149, 1973.
82. Garrett WV, Slaymaker EE, Heinz SE, et al: Intraoperative prediction of symptomatic result of aortofemoral bypass from changes in ankle pressure index. Surgery 82:504, 1977.
83. Gaylis H: The assessment of impotence in aorto-iliac disease using penile blood pressure measurements. S Afr J Surg 16:39, 1978.
84. Gibbons GE, Strandness DE Jr, Bell JW: Improvements in design of the mercury strain gauge plethysmograph. Surg Gynecol Obstet 116:679, 1963.
85. Gibbons GW, Wheelock FC, Siembieda C, et al: Noninvasive prediction of amputation level in diabetic patients. Arch Surg 114:1253, 1979.
86. Gilfillan RS, Leeds FH, Spotts RR: The prediction of healing in ischemic lesions of the foot. A comparison of Doppler ultrasound and elevation reactive hyperemia. J Cardiovasc Surg 26:15, 1985.
87. Goodreau JJ, Creasy JK, Flanigan DP, et al: Rational approach to the differentiation of vascular and neurogenic claudication. Surgery 84:749, 1978.
88. Gosling RG: Extraction of physiologic information from spectrum analyzed Doppler-shifted continuous wave ultrasound signals obtained noninvasively from the arterial system. IEE Med Electr 4:73, 1976.
89. Gosling RG, King DH: Processing arterial Doppler signals for clinical data. *In* deVlieger M, Holmes JH, Kazner E, et al (eds): Handbook of Clinical Ultrasound. New York, John Wiley & Sons, 1978, pp 613–646.
90. Gothgen I, Jacobsen E: Transcutaneous oxygen tension measure-

ment. I. Age variation and reproducibility. Acta Anaesthesiol Scand Suppl 67:66, 1978.
91. Gray B, Kmiecik JC, Spigos DD, et al: Evaluation of Doppler-derived upper thigh pressure in the assessment of aorto-iliac occlusive disease. Bruit 4:29, 1980.
92. Gundersen J: Segmental measurement of systolic blood pressure in the extremities including the thumb and great toe. Acta Chir Scand Suppl 426:1, 1972.
93. Gutierrez IZ, Gage AA, Makuta PA: Toe pulse study in ischemic arterial disease of the legs. Surg Gynecol Obstet 153:889, 1981.
94. Hajjar W, Sumner DS: Segmental pressures in normal subjects 16 to 32 years of age. Unpublished observations, 1976.
95. Hamilton WAP, Fulton TJ, Gay P, et al: Locating aortofemoral disease by measuring flow velocity in the femoral artery with Doppler ultrasound. Vasc Diag Ther 3:37, 1982.
96. Harris JP, Flinn WR, Rudo ND, et al: Assessment of donor limb hemodynamics in femorofemoral bypass for claudication. Surgery 90:764, 1981.
97. Harris PL, Taylor LA, Cave FD, et al: The relationship between Doppler ultrasound assessment and angiography in occlusive arterial disease of the lower limbs. Surg Gynecol Obstet 138:911, 1974.
98. Harward TRS, Bernstein EF, Fronek A: The value of power frequency spectrum analysis in the identification of aortoiliac artery disease. J Vasc Surg 5:803, 1987.
99. Harward TRS, Volny J, Golbranson F, et al: Oxygen inhalation–induced transcutaneous Po_2 changes as a predictor of amputation level. J Vasc Surg 2:220, 1985.
100. Hatsukami TS, Primozich J, Zierler RE, et al: Color Doppler characteristics in normal lower extremity arteries. Ultrasound Med Biol 18:167, 1992.
101. Hatsukami TS, Primozich J, Zierler RE, et al: Color Doppler imaging of infrainguinal arterial occlusive disease. J Vasc Surg 16:527, 1992.
102. Hauser CJ: Tissue salvage by mapping of skin surface transcutaneous oxygen tension index. Arch Surg 122:1128, 1985.
103. Hauser CJ, Klein SR, Mehringer CM, et al: Superiority of transcutaneous oximetry in noninvasive vascular diagnosis in patients with diabetes. Arch Surg 119:690, 1984.
104. Hauser CJ, Shoemaker WC: Use of a transcutaneous Po_2 regional perfusion index to quantify tissue perfusion in peripheral vascular disease. Ann Surg 197:337, 1983.
105. Heintz SE, Bone GE, Slaymaker EE, et al: Value of arterial pressure measurements in the proximal and distal part of the thigh in arterial occlusive disease. Surg Gynecol Obstet 146:337, 1978.
106. Hirai M, Schoop W: Hemodynamic assessment of the iliac disease by proximal thigh pressure and Doppler femoral flow velocity. J Cardiovasc Surg 25:365, 1984.
107. Hobbs JT, Yao ST, Lewis JD, et al: A limitation of the Doppler ultrasound method of measuring ankle systolic pressure. Vasa 3:160, 1974.
108. Hoffmann U, Edwards JM, Carter S, et al: Role of duplex scanning for the detection of atherosclerotic renal artery disease. Kidney Int 39:1232, 1991.
109. Holstein P, Dovey H, Lassen NA: Wound healing in above-knee amputations in relation to skin perfusion pressure. Acta Orthop Scand 50:59, 1979.
110. Holstein P, Sager P: Toe blood pressure in peripheral arterial disease. Acta Orthop Scand 44:564, 1973.
111. Holstein P, Sager P, Lassen NA: Wound healing in below-knee amputations in relation to skin perfusion pressure. Acta Orthop Scand 50:49, 1979.
112. Holstein P, Noer I, Tønnesen KH, et al: Distal blood pressure in severe arterial insufficiency. Strain-gauge, radioisotopes, and other methods. *In* Bergan JJ, Yao JST (eds): Gangrene and Severe Ischemia of the Lower Extremities. New York, Grune & Stratton, 1978, pp 95–114.
113. Hummel BW, Hummel BA, Mowbry A, et al: Reactive hyperemia vs. treadmill exercise testing in arterial disease. Arch Surg 113:95, 1978.
114. Humphries KN, Hames TK, Smith SWJ, et al: Quantitative assessment to the common femoral to popliteal arterial segment using continuous wave Doppler ultrasound. Ultrasound Med Biol 6:99, 1980.
115. Jager K, Bollinger A, Valli C, et al: Measurement of mesenteric blood flow by duplex scanning. J Vasc Surg 3:462, 1986.
116. Jager KA, Phillips DJ, Martin RL, et al: Noninvasive mapping of lower limb arterial lesions. Ultrasound Med Biol 11:515, 1985.
117. Johansen K, Lynch K, Paun M, et al: Noninvasive vascular tests reliably exclude occult arterial trauma in injured extremities. J Trauma 31:515, 1991.
118. Johnson WC: Doppler ankle pressure and reactive hyperemia in the diagnosis of arterial insufficiency. J Surg Res 18:177, 1975.
119. Johnston KW, Demorais D, Colapinto RI: Difficulty in assessing the sensitivity of aortoiliac disease by clinical and arteriographic method. Angiology 32:609, 1981.
120. Johnston KW, Hosang MY, Andrews DF: Reproducibility of noninvasive vascular laboratory measurements of the peripheral circulation. J Vasc Surg 6:147, 1987.
121. Johnston DW, Kassam M, Cobbold RSC: Relationship between Doppler pulsatility index and direct femoral pressure measurements in the diagnosis of aortoiliac occlusive disease. Ultrasound Med Biol 9:271, 1983.
122. Johnston KW, Kassam M, Koers J, et al: Comparative study of four methods for quantifying Doppler ultrasound waveforms from the femoral artery. Ultrasound Med Biol 10:1, 1984.
123. Johnston KW, Maruzzo BC, Cobbold RSC: Doppler methods for quantitative measurement and localization of peripheral arterial occlusive disease by analysis of the blood velocity waveform. Ultrasound Med Biol 4:209, 1978.
124. Johnston KW, Maruzzo BC, Kassam M, et al: Methods for obtaining, processing and quantifying Doppler blood velocity waveforms. *In* Nicolaides AN, Yao JST (eds): Investigation of Vascular Disorders. London, Churchill-Livingstone, 1981, pp 532–558.
125. Junger M, Chapman BLW, Underwood CJ, Charlesworth D: A comparison between two types of waveform analysis in patients with multisegmental arterial disease. Br J Surg 71:345, 1984.
126. Karanfilian RG, Lynch TG, Lee BC, et al: The assessment of skin blood flow in peripheral vascular disease by laser Doppler velocimetry. Am Surg 50:641, 1984.
127. Karanfilian RG, Lynch TG, Zirul VT, et al: The value of laser Doppler velocimetry and transcutaneous oxygen tension determination in predicting healing of ischemic forefoot ulcerations and amputations in diabetic and nondiabetic patients. J Vasc Surg 4:511, 1986.
128. Karpman HL, Winsor T: The plethysmographic peripheral vascular study. J Int Coll Surg 30:425, 1958.
129. Katsamouris A, Brewster DC, Megerman J, et al: Transcutaneous oxygen tension in selection of amputation level. Am J Surg 147:510, 1984.
130. Kavanaugh GJ, Svien HJ, Holman CB, et al: "Pseudoclaudication" syndrome produced by compression of the cauda equina. JAMA 206:2477, 1968.
131. Keagy BA, Schwartz JA, Kotb M, et al: Lower extremity amputation: The control series. J Vasc Surg 4:321, 1986.
132. Kempczinski RF: Role of the vascular diagnostic laboratory in the evaluation of male impotence. Am J Surg 138:278, 1979.
133. Kempczinski RF: Segmental volume plethysmography in the diagnosis of lower extremity arterial occlusive disease. J Cardiovasc Surg 23:125, 1982.
134. Kempczinski RF: Segmental volume plethysmography: The pulse volume recorder. *In* Kempczinski RF, Yao JST (eds): Practical Noninvasive Vascular Diagnosis. 2nd ed. Chicago, Year Book Medical, 1987, pp 140–153.
135. Kikta MJ, Flanigan DP, Biskhara RA, et al: Long-term follow-up of patients having infrainguinal bypass performed below stenotic but hemodynamically normal aortoiliac vessels. J Vasc Surg 5:319, 1987.
136. King LT, Strandness DE Jr, Bell JW: The hemodynamic response of the lower extremity to exercise. J Surg Res 5:167, 1965.
137. Kohler TR, Nance DR, Cramer MM, et al: Duplex scanning for diagnosis of aortoiliac and femoropopliteal disease: A prospective study. Circulation 76:1074, 1987.
138. Kohler TR, Zierler RE, Martin RL, et al: Noninvasive diagnosis of renal artery stenosis by ultrasonic duplex scanning. J Vasc Surg 4:450, 1986.
139. Kozloff L, Collins GJ Jr, Rich NM, et al: Fallibility of postoperative Doppler ankle pressures in determining the adequacy of proximal arterial revascularization. Am J Surg 139:326, 1980.
140. Kram HB, Appel PL, Shoemaker WC: Multisensor transcutaneous

oximetric mapping to predict below-knee amputation wound healing: Use of a critical Po_2 index. J Vasc Surg 9:796, 1989.
141. Kram HB, Appel PL, White RA, et al: Assessment of peripheral vascular disease by postocclusive transcutaneous oxygen recovery time. J Vasc Surg 1:628, 1984.
142. Kram HB, Shoemaker WC: Diagnosis of major peripheral arterial trauma by transcutaneous oxygen monitoring. Am J Surg 147:776, 1984.
143. Kram HB, White RA, Tabrisky J, et al: Transcutaneous oxygen recovery and toe pulse-reappearance time in the assessment of peripheral vascular disease. Circulation 72:1022, 1985.
144. Laborde AL, Synn AY, Worsey MJ, et al: A prospective comparison of ankle/brachial indices and color duplex imaging in surveillance of the in situ saphenous vein bypass. J Cardiovasc Surg 33:420, 1992.
145. Lalka SG, Malone JM, Anderson GG, et al: Transcutaneous oxygen and carbon dioxide pressure monitoring to determine severity of limb ischemia and to predict surgical outcome. J Vasc Surg 7:507, 1988.
146. Lane RJ, Appleberg M, Williams WA: A comparison of two techniques for the detection of the vasculogenic component of impotence. Surg Gynecol Obstet 155:230, 1982.
147. Lassen NA, Tuedegaard E, Jeppesen FI, et al: Distal blood pressure measurement in occlusive arterial disease strain gauge compared to xenon-133. Angiology 23:211, 1972.
148. Lavenson GS Jr, Rich NM, Strandness DE Jr: Ultrasonic flow detector value in the management of combat-incurred vascular injuries. Arch Surg 103:644, 1971.
149. Leopold PW, Shandall AA, Kay C, et al: Duplex ultrasound: Its role in the noninvasive follow-up of the in situ saphenous vein bypass. J Vasc Technol 11:183, 1987.
150. Londrey GL, Hodgson KJ, Spadone DP, et al: Initial experience with color-flow duplex scanning of infrainguinal bypass grafts. J Vasc Surg 12:284, 1990.
151. Lorentsen E: Calf blood pressure measurements. The applicability of a plethysmographic method and the result of measurements during reactive hyperemia. Scand J Clin Lab Invest 31:69, 1973.
152. Lorentsen E: The vascular resistance in the arteries of the lower leg in normal subjects and in patients with different degrees of atherosclerotic disease. Scand J Clin Lab Invest 31:147, 1973.
153. Macpherson DS, Evans DH, Bell PRF: Common femoral artery Doppler wave-forms: A comparison of three methods of objective analysis with direct pressure measurements. Br J Surg 71:46, 1984.
154. Malone JM, Anderson GG, Lalka SG, et al: Prospective comparison of noninvasive techniques for amputation level selection. Am J Surg 154:179, 1987.
155. Marinelli MR, Beach NW, Glass MJ, et al: Noninvasive testing vs clinical evaluation of arterial disease. A prospective study. JAMA 241:2031, 1979.
156. Matsen FA III, Wyss CR, Pedegana LR, et al: Transcutaneous oxygen tension measurement in peripheral vascular disease. Surg Gynecol Obstet 150:525, 1980.
157. Matsen FA III, Wyss CR, Robertson CC, et al: The relationship of transcutaneous Po_2 and laser Doppler measurements in a human model of local arterial insufficiency. Surg Gynecol Obstet 159:418, 1984.
158. Matsen FA III, Wyss CR, Simmons CW, et al: The effect of exercise upon cutaneous oxygen delivery in the extremities of patients with claudication and in a human laboratory model of claudication. Surg Gynecol Obstet 158:522, 1984.
159. Mazza G, Henry M, Betts RK, et al: Correlation of noninvasive testing with the natural history of lower extremity arterial disease. Bruit 7:23, 1983.
160. McDonald PT, Easterbrook JA, Rich NM, et al: Popliteal artery entrapment syndrome. Clinical, noninvasive, and angiographic diagnosis. Am J Surg 139:318, 1980.
161. McShane MD, Gazzard VM, Clifford PC, et al: Duplex ultrasound monitoring of arterial grafts: Prospective evaluation in conjunction with ankle pressure indices after femorodistal bypass. Eur J Vasc Surg 1:385, 1987.
162. Miles S, Roediger W, Cooke P, et al: Doppler ultrasound in the diagnosis of the popliteal artery entrapment syndrome. Br J Surg 64:883, 1977.
163. Mills JL, Harris EJ, Taylor LM, et al: The importance of routine surveillance of distal bypass grafts with duplex scanning: A study of 379 reversed vein grafts. J Vasc Surg 12:379, 1990.
164. Moneta GL, Yeager RA, Antonovic R, et al: Accuracy of lower extremity arterial duplex mapping. J Vasc Surg 15:275, 1992.
165. Moore WS, Hall AD: Unrecognized aortoiliac stenosis. Arch Surg 103:633, 1971.
166. Moore WS, Henry RE, Malone JM, et al: Prospective use of xenon-133 clearance for amputation level selection. Arch Surg 116:86, 1981.
167. Mozersky DJ, Sumner DS, Strandness DE Jr: Long-term result of reconstructive aortoiliac surgery. Am J Surg 123:503, 1972.
168. Mozersky DJ, Sumner DS, Strandness DE Jr: Disease progression after femoropopliteal surgical procedures. Surg Gynecol Obstet 135:700, 1972.
169. Mustapha NM, Redhead RG, Jain SK, et al: Transcutaneous partial oxygen pressure assessment of the ischemic lower limb. Surg Gynecol Obstet 156:582, 1983.
170. Myers KA, Scott DF, Devine TJ, et al: Palpation of the femoral and popliteal pulses: A study of the accuracy as assessed by agreement between multiple observers. Eur J Vasc Surg 1:245, 1987.
171. Nath RL, Menzoian JO, Kaplan KH, et al: The multidisciplinary approach to vasculogenic impotence. Surgery 89:124, 1981.
172. Nicholas GG, Myers JL, DeMuth WE Jr: The role of vascular laboratory criteria in the selection of patients for lower extremity amputation. Ann Surg 195:469, 1982.
173. Nicholls SC, Kohler TR, Martin RL, et al: Use of hemodynamic parameters in the diagnosis of mesenteric insufficiency. J Vasc Surg 3:507, 1985.
174. Nicolaides AN. Value of noninvasive tests in the investigation of lower limb ischemia. Ann R Coll Surg Engl 60:249, 1978.
175. Nielsen PE, Bell G, Lassen NA: The measurement of digital systolic blood pressure by strain gauge technique. Scand J Clin Lab Invest 29:371, 1972.
176. Nielsen PE, Bell G, Lassen NA: Strain gauge studies of distal blood pressure in normal subjects and in patients with peripheral arterial diseases. Analysis of normal variation and reproducibility and comparison to intraarterial measurements. Scand J Clin Lab Invest 31(Suppl 128):103, 1973.
177. Noer I, Tønnesen KH, Sager P: Preoperative estimation of runoff in patients with multiple level arterial obstructions as a guide to partial reconstructive surgery. Ann Surg 188:663, 1978.
178. Noer I, Tønnesen KH, Sager P: Minimal distal pressure rise after reconstructive arterial surgery in patients with multiple obstructive arteriosclerosis. Acta Chir Scand 146:105, 1980.
179. O'Donnell TF, Cossman D, Callow AD: Noninvasive intraoperative monitoring: A prospective study comparing Doppler systolic occlusion pressure and segmental plethysmography. Am J Surg 135:539, 1978.
180. O'Donnell TF Jr, Lahey SJ, Kelly JJ, et al: A prospective study of Doppler pressures and segmental plethysmography before and following aortofemoral bypass. Surgery 86:120, 1979.
181. Oh PIT, Provan JL, Amelie FM: The predictability of the success of arterial reconstruction by means of transcutaneous oxygen tension measurements. J Vasc Surg 5:356, 1987.
182. Ohgi S, Ito K, Mori T: Quantitative evaluation of the skin circulation in ischemic legs by transcutaneous measurement of oxygen tension. Angiology 32:833, 1981.
183. O'Mara CS, Flinn WR, Johnson ND, et al: Recognition and surgical management of patent but hemodynamically failed arterial grafts. Ann Surg 193:467, 1981.
184. Osmundson PJ, Chesebro JH, O'Fallon WM, et al: A prospective study of peripheral occlusive arterial disease in diabetes. II. Vascular laboratory assessment. Mayo Clin Proc 56:223, 1981.
185. Ouriel K, McDonnell AE, Metz CE, et al: A critical evaluation of stress testing in the diagnosis of peripheral vascular disease. Surgery 91:686, 1982.
186. Paaske WP, Tønnesen KH: Prognostic significance of distal blood pressure measurements in patients with severe ischemia. Scand J Thorac Cardiovasc Surg 14:105, 1980.
187. Pascarelli EF, Bertrand CA: Comparison of blood pressures in the arms and legs. N Engl J Med 270:693, 1964.
188. Persson AV, Gibbons G, Griffey S: Noninvasive evaluation of the aorto-iliac segment. J Cardiovasc Surg 22:539, 1981.
189. Phillips DJ, Beach KW, Primozich J, et al: Should the results of ultrasound Doppler studies be reported in units of frequency or velocity? Ultrasound Med Biol 15:205, 1989.
190. Plecha FR, Bomberger RA, Hoffman M, et al: A new criterion for predicting response to lumbar sympathectomy in patients with severe arteriosclerotic occlusive disease. Surgery 88:375, 1980.
191. Pollack SB Jr, Ernst CB: Use of Doppler pressure measurements in

predicting success in amputation of the leg. Am J Surg 139:303, 1980.
192. Queral LA, Whitehouse WM Jr, Flinn WR, et al: Pelvic hemodynamics after aorto-iliac reconstruction. Surgery 86:799, 1979.
193. Raines JK: Diagnosis and analysis of arteriosclerosis in the lower limbs from the arterial pressure pulse. Doctoral thesis, Massachusetts Institute of Technology, 1972.
194. Raines JK, Darling RG, Buth J, et al: Vascular laboratory criteria for the management of peripheral vascular disease of the lower extremities. Surgery 79:21, 1976.
195. Ramirez C, Box M, Gottesman L: Noninvasive vascular evaluation in male impotence: Technique. Bruit 4:14, 1980.
196. Ramsey DE, Johnson F, Sumner DS: Anatomic validity of segmental pressure measurement. Unpublished observations, 1979.
197. Ramsey DE, Manke DA, Sumner DS: Toe blood pressure—A valuable adjunct to ankle pressure measurement for assessing peripheral arterial disease. J Cardiovasc Surg 24:43, 1983.
198. Ratliff DA, Clyne CAC, Chant ADB, et al: Prediction of amputation wound healing: The role of transcutaneous Po_2 assessment. Br J Surg 71:219, 1984.
199. Reddy DJ, Vincent GS, McPharlin M, et al: Limitations of the femoral pulsatility index with aortoiliac stenosis: An experimental study. J Vasc Surg 4:327, 1986.
200. Reidy NC, Walden R, Abbott WA, et al: Anatomic localization of atherosclerotic lesions by hemodynamic tests. Arch Surg 116:1041, 1981.
201. Ricco J-B, Pearce WH, Yao JST, et al: The use of operative prebypass arteriography and Doppler ultrasound recordings to select patients for extended femoro-distal bypass. Ann Surg 198:646, 1983.
202. Rittenhouse EA, Brockenbrough EC: A method for assessing the circulation distal to a femoral artery obstruction. Surg Gynecol Obstet 129:538, 1969.
203. Rittenhouse EA, Maixner W, Burr JW, et al: Directional arterial flow velocity: A sensitive index of changes in peripheral vascular resistance. Surgery 79:350, 1976.
204. Roedersheimer LR, Feins R, Green RM: Doppler evaluation of the pedal arch. Am J Surg 142:601, 1981.
205. Ruoff BA, Cranley JJ, Hannon LA, et al: Real-time duplex ultrasound mapping of the greater saphenous vein before in situ infrainguinal revascularization. J Vasc Surg 6:107, 1987.
206. Rutherford RB, Jones DN, Martin MS, et al: Serial hemodynamic assessment of aortofemoral bypass. J Vasc Surg 4:428, 1986.
207. Rutherford RB, Lowenstein DH, Klein MF: Combining segmental systolic pressures and plethysmography to diagnose arterial occlusive disease of the legs. Am J Surg 138:211, 1979.
208. Samson RH, Gupta SK, Veith FJ, et al: Perioperative noninvasive hemodynamic ankle indices as predictors of infrainguinal graft patency. J Vasc Surg 2:307, 1985.
209. Samson RH, Gupta SK, Veith FJ, et al: Evaluation of graft patency utilizing the ankle-brachial pressure index and ankle pulse volume recording amplitude. Am J Surg 147:786, 1984.
210. Sanchez SA, Best EB: Correlation of plethysmographic and arteriographic findings in patients with obstructive arterial disease. Angiology 20:684, 1969.
211. Satiani B, Biggers K, Burns R, et al: Are noninvasive Doppler arterial studies useful in predicting success of infrainguinal bypass grafts? J Vasc Surg 21:237, 1987.
212. Satiani B, Hayes JP, Evans WE: Prediction of distal reconstruction following aortofemoral bypass for limb salvage. Surg Gynecol Obstet 151:500, 1980.
213. Schwartz JA, Schuler JJ, O'Connor RJA, et al: Predictive value of distal perfusion pressure in the healing of amputations of the digit and the forefoot. Surg Gynecol Obstet 154:865, 1982.
214. Sethi GK, Scott SM, Takaro T: Multiple-plane angiography for more precise evaluation of aortoiliac disease. Surgery 78:154, 1975.
215. Shearman CP, Gwynn BR, Curran F, et al: Noninvasive femoropopliteal assessment: Is that angiogram really necessary? Br Med J 293:1086, 1986.
216. Siggard-Anderson J, Ulrich J, Engell HC, et al: Blood pressure measurements of the lower limb. Arterial occlusions in the calf determined by plethysmographic blood pressure measurements in the thigh and at the ankle. Angiology 23:350, 1972.
217. Skidmore R, Woodcock JP, Wells PNT, et al: Physiological interpretation of Doppler-shift waveforms. III. Clinical results. Ultrasound Med Biol 6:227, 1980.
218. Skinner JS, Strandness DE Jr: Exercise and intermittent claudication. I. Effect of repetition and intensity of exercise. Circulation 36:15, 1967.
219. Skinner JS, Strandness DE Jr: Exercise and intermittent claudication. II. Effect of physical training. Circulation 36:23, 1967.
220. Sladen JG, Reid JDS, Cooperberg PL, et al: Color flow duplex scanning of infrainguinal grafts combining low- and high-velocity criteria. Am J Surg 158:107, 1989.
221. Sobinsky KR, Borozan PG, Gray B, et al: Is femoral pulse palpation accurate in assessing the hemodynamic significance of aortoiliac disease? Am J Surg 148:214, 1984.
222. Sobinsky KR, Williams LR, Gray G, et al: Supine exercise testing in the selection of suprainguinal versus infrainguinal bypass in patients with multisegmental arterial occlusive disease. Am J Surg 152:185, 1986.
223. Stahler C, Strandness DE Jr: Ankle blood pressure response to graded treadmill exercise. Angiology 18:237, 1967.
224. Stockel M, Ovesen J, Brochner-Mortensen J, et al: Standardized photoelectric technique as routine method for selection of amputation level. Acta Orthop Scand 53:875, 1982.
225. Strandness DE Jr: Long-term value of lumbar sympathectomy. Geriatrics 21:144, 1966.
226. Strandness DE Jr: Abnormal exercise responses after successful reconstructive arterial surgery. Surgery 59:325, 1966.
227. Strandness DE Jr: Peripheral Arterial Disease: A Physiologic Approach. Boston, Little, Brown & Co., 1969.
228. Strandness DE Jr: Exercise testing in the evaluation of patients undergoing direct arterial surgery. J Cardiovasc Surg 11:192, 1970.
229. Strandness DE Jr: Physiologic evaluation of peripheral arterial occlusion. *In* Dale WA (ed): Management of Arterial Occlusive Disease. Chicago, Year Book Medical, 1971, pp 13–29.
230. Strandness DE Jr: Noninvasive tests in vascular emergencies. *In* Bergan JJ, Yao JST (eds): Vascular Surgical Emergencies. Orlando, FL, Grune & Stratton, 1987, pp 103–111.
231. Strandness DE Jr, Bell JW: An evaluation of the hemodynamic response of the claudicating extremity to exercise. Surg Gynecol Obstet 119:1237, 1964.
232. Strandness DE Jr, Bell JW: Peripheral vascular disease, diagnosis and objective evaluation using a mercury strain gauge. Ann Surg 161(Suppl 4):1, 1965.
233. Strandness DE Jr, Bell JW: Ankle pressure responses after reconstructive arterial surgery. Surgery 59:514, 1966.
234. Strandness DE Jr, Schultz RD, Sumner DS, et al: Ultrasonic flow detection: A useful technic in the evaluation of peripheral vascular disease. Am J Surg 113:311, 1967.
235. Strandness DE Jr, Stahler C: Arteriosclerosis obliterans. Manner and rate of progression. JAMA 196:1, 1966.
236. Strandness DE Jr, Sumner DS: Hemodynamics for Surgeons. New York, Grune & Stratton, 1975.
237. Sumner DS: Perioperative assessment of patient revascularization: Intraoperative assessment by Doppler ultrasound. *In* Bergan JJ, Yao JST (eds): Gangrene and Severe Ischemia of the Lower Extremities. New York, Grune & Stratton, 1978, pp 349–372.
238. Sumner DS: Algorithms using noninvasive diagnostic data as a guide to therapy of arterial insufficiency. *In* Puel P, Boccalon H, Enjalbert A (eds): Hemodynamics of the Limbs—1. Toulouse, France, GEPESC, 1979, pp 543–546.
239. Sumner DS: Rational use of noninvasive tests in designing a therapeutic approach to severe arterial disease of the legs. *In* Puel P, Boccalon H, Enjalbert A (eds): Hemodynamics of the Limbs—2. Toulouse, France, GEPESC, 1981, pp 369–376.
240. Sumner DS, Strandness DE Jr: The relationship between calf blood flow and ankle blood pressure in patients with intermittent claudication. Surgery 65:763, 1969.
241. Sumner DS, Strandness DE Jr: The effect of exercise on resistance to blood flow in limbs with an occluded superficial femoral artery. J Vasc Surg 4:229, 1970.
242. Sumner DS, Strandness DE Jr: The hemodynamics of the femorofemoral shunt. Surg Gynecol Obstet 134:629, 1972.
243. Sumner DS, Strandness DE Jr: Aortoiliac reconstruction in patients with combined iliac and superficial femoral arterial occlusion. Surgery 84:348, 1978.
244. Sumner DS, Strandness DE Jr: Hemodynamic studies before and after extended bypass grafts to the tibial and peroneal arteries. Surgery 86:442, 1979.
245. Taguchi JT, Suwangool P: Pipe-stem brachial arteries: A cause of pseudohypertension. JAMA 228:733, 1974.

246. Tait WF, Charlesworth D, Lemon JG: Atypical claudication. Br J Surg 72:315, 1985.
247. Taylor DC, Kettler MD, Moneta GL, et al: Duplex ultrasound in the diagnosis of renal artery stenosis—A prospective evaluation. J Vasc Surg 7:363, 1988.
248. Thiele BL, Bandyk DF, Zierler RE, et al: A systematic approach to the assessment of aortoiliac disease. Arch Surg 118:477, 1983.
249. Thulesius O: Systemic and ankle blood pressure before and after exercise in patients with arterial insufficiency. Angiology 29:374, 1978.
250. Thulesius O, Gjöres JE: Use of Doppler shift detection for determining peripheral arterial blood pressure. Angiology 22:594, 1971.
251. Thulesius O, Gjöres JE, Mandaus L: Distal blood flow and blood pressure in vascular occlusion; influence of sympathetic nerves on collateral blood flow. Scand J Clin Lab Invest 31(Suppl 128):53, 1973.
252. Tønneson KH: Transcutaneous oxygen tension in imminent foot gangrene. Acta Anaesthesiol Scand 68:107, 1978.
253. Tønneson KH, Noer I, Paaske W, et al: Classification of peripheral occlusive arterial diseases based on symptoms, signs, and distal blood pressure measurements. Acta Chir Scand 146:101, 1980.
254. Turnipseed WD, Acker CW: Postoperative surveillance. An effective means of detecting correctable lesions that threaten graft patency. Arch Surg 120:324, 1985.
255. Udoff EJ, Barth KH, Harrington DP, et al: Hemodynamic significance of iliac artery stenosis: Pressure measurements during angiography. Radiology 132:289, 1979.
256. Uhrenholdt A: Relationship between distal blood flow and blood pressure after abolition of the sympathetic vasomotor tone. Scand J Clin Invest 31(Suppl 128):63, 1973.
257. Van De Water JM, Indech CDV, Indech RB, et al: Hyperemic response for diagnosis of arterial insufficiency. Arch Surg 115:851, 1980.
258. Veith FJ, Weiser RK, Gupta SK, et al: Diagnosis and management of failing lower extremity arterial obstructions prior to graft occlusion. J Cardiovasc Surg 25:381, 1984.
259. Verta MJ Jr, Gross WS, vanBellen B, et al: Forefoot perfusion pressure and minor amputation for gangrene. Surgery 80:729, 1976.
260. Vollrath KD, Salles-Cunha SX, Vincent D, et al: Noninvasive measurement of toe systolic pressures. Bruit 4:27, 1980.
261. Walker PM, Johnston KW: Predicting the success of a sympathectomy: A prospective study using discriminant function and multiple regression analysis. Surgery 87:216, 1980.
262. Ward AS, Martin TP: Some aspects of ultrasound in the diagnosis and assessment of aortoiliac disease. Am J Surg 140:260, 1980.
263. Welch GH, Leiberman DP, Pollack JG, et al: Failure of Doppler ankle pressure to predict healing of conservative forefoot amputations. Br J Surg 72:888, 1984.
264. Williams LR, Flanigan DP, Schuler JJ, et al: Prediction of improvement in ankle blood pressure following arterial bypass. J Surg Res 37:175, 1984.
265. Wilson SE, Schwartz I, Williams RA, et al: Occlusion of the superficial femoral artery. What happens without operation. Am J Surg 140:112, 1980.
266. Winsor T: Influence of arterial disease on the systolic blood pressure gradients of the extremity. Am J Med Sci 220:117, 1950.
267. Winsor T, Sibley AE, Fisher EK, et al: Peripheral pulse contours in arterial occlusive disease. Vasc Dis 5:61, 1968.
268. Wolf EA Jr, Sumner DS, Strandness DE Jr: Correlation between nutritive blood flow and pressure in limbs of patients with intermittent claudication. Surg Forum 23:238, 1972.
269. Wolfe JHN, Thomas ML, Jamieson CW, et al: Early diagnosis of femorodistal graft stenoses. Br J Surg 74:268, 1987.
270. Wyss CR, Matsen FA III, Simmons CW, et al: Transcutaneous oxygen tension measurements on limbs of diabetic and nondiabetic patients with peripheral vascular disease. Surgery 95:339, 1984.
271. Wyss CR, Robertson C, Love SJ, et al: Relationship between transcutaneous oxygen tension, ankle blood pressure, and clinical outcome of vascular surgery in diabetic and nondiabetic patients. Surgery 101:56, 1987.
272. Yao JST: Hemodynamic studies in peripheral arterial disease. Br J Surg 57:761, 1970.
273. Yao JST: New techniques in objective arterial evaluation. Arch Surg 106:600, 1973.
274. Yao JST: Postoperative evaluation of graft failure. *In* Bernhard VM, Towne JB (eds): Complications in Vascular Surgery. Orlando, FL, Grune & Stratton, 1985, pp 1–24.
275. Yao JST, Bergan JJ: Predictability of vascular reactivity relative to sympathetic ablation. Arch Surg 107:676, 1973.
276. Yao JST, Hobbs JT, Irvine WT: Ankle systolic pressure measurements in arterial diseases affecting the lower extremities. Br J Surg 56:676, 1969.
277. Zetterquist S, Bergvall V, Linde B, et al: The validity of some conventional methods for the diagnosis of obliterative arterial disease in the lower limb as evaluated by arteriography. Scand J Clin Lab Invest 28:409, 1971.
278. Zierler RE, Strandness DE Jr: Duplex scanning for the diagnosis of aortoiliac and lower extremity disease. J Vasc Technol 11:99, 1987.
279. Zweifler AJ, Cushing G, Conway J: The relationship between pulse volume and blood flow in the fingers. Angiology 18:591, 1967.
280. Mattos MM, van Bemmelen PS, Hodgson KJ, et al: Does correction of stenoses identified with color duplex scanning improve infrainguinal graft patency? J Vasc Surg (In press).
281. Nicolaides AN, Gordon-Smith IC, Dayandas J, et al: The value of Doppler blood velocity tracings in the detection of aortoiliac disease in patients with intermittent claudication. Surgery 80:774, 1976.

6

Vascular Imaging Techniques

Overview

Anthony J. Comerota, M.D., F.A.C.S.

• • •

The evolution of technology for the evaluation of vascular disease has made remarkable progress. Its application to clinical practice has improved our understanding of disease and modified patient care. The needs of physicians are to make an appropriate diagnosis, to grade disease severity, and to follow patients after intervention. Diagnostic requirements vary depending on the specific vascular problem and treatment options. Occlusive disease of the lower extremity can be accurately diagnosed by history and physical examination over 90 per cent of the time. On the other hand, patients with suspected renovascular disease, mesenteric occlusive disease, pelvic venous thrombosis, or aortic dissection can challenge our most advanced interventional diagnostic techniques.

Proper use of diagnostic studies mandates an understanding of the underlying pathology and a familiarity with the fundamentals of each of the diagnostic procedures. Having this background, physicians can "fine-tune" the diagnostic work-up, taking advantage of the strengths of individual diagnostic tests and minimizing the shortcomings of others by avoiding them. As an example, what information is important to properly evaluate the patient with suspected aortic dissection? Of course, identification of the entry point is critical. In the patient whose entry point is distal to the left subclavian and whose blood pressure can be controlled, what additional information is necessary? The size of the dissected aorta and perfusion of the viscera, kidneys, and lower extremities are the most important data. Whether perfusion is through a true or a false lumen is less important than establishing that perfusion exists, especially when the decision is being made about the appropriate treatment option.

Another illustration of the utility of an understanding of the patient's disease assisting proper use of diagnostic studies is the evaluation of pelvic venous thrombosis. This assumes much greater importance in patients with suspected pulmonary emboli and a non–high-probability ventilation-perfusion (V/Q) scan following a pelvic operation for cancer than it does in a similar patient scenario following a total knee replacement.

The diagnosis of critical lower extremity ischemia is not difficult; however, the key information for the surgeon is the levels at which there is unobstructed inflow and unimpeded outflow, respectively. Since either of these may not be completely present (i.e., varying degrees of obstruction may exist), judgments must be made as to what is acceptable based on the available information about the disease. Diagnostic studies not offering these important details will compromise outcome. Although, in contrast, the diagnostic evaluation of patients with intermittent claudication may be somewhat easier, we cannot relax our diagnostic standards, since any intervention carries potential complications not imminent as a result of the disease itself.

The development of duplex scanning, computed tomography, and magnetic resonance angiography offers the opportunity for comprehensive evaluation of vascular disease (in centers appropriately equipped and experienced) without requiring contrast arteriography. Most clinicians treating patients with vascular disease have come to rely on contrast arteriography, and its risks have diminished. However, in many instances, its findings are not definitive and potential complications are still an unattractive feature. Because the risk of the diagnostic procedure is part of the therapeutic morbidity/mortality equation, there is a continuing search to obtain the required information noninvasively. With improved preoperative, anesthetic, and postoperative critical care, patients have been beneficiaries of reduced operative complications and mortality. In certain areas, such as extracranial cerebrovascular disease, complications of invasive angiography approach 25 to 50 per cent of the operative neurologic complication rate in some centers, thereby challenging the need for routine arteriography and justifying the search for alternative methods offering the same information at reduced or no risk.

Duplex ultrasonography has witnessed rapid advances in probe technology and softwear data processing. This technique can be both an anatomic and a physiologic evaluation of the vascular tree (Table 6–1). In certain areas, one can evaluate the vessel wall as well as the pathophysiologic consequences of luminal compromise on vascular hemody-

Table 6–1. Duplex Ultrasound

Advantages	Disadvantages
Noninvasive/no risk	Operator-dependent
Repeatable	Probe angle of 90 degrees to axis of blood flow shows little or no Doppler information
Good availability	Color information represents mean or mode velocities; therefore, spectral waveform still required to assess severity of stenosis
Portable	Obesity and bowel gas interfere with abdominal vascular evaluation
Anatomic and physiologic information	All instruments are not comparable; therefore, data from one center cannot be extrapolated to another
Vessel wall and lumen evaluation (selected sites)	Most estimates of stenosis are based on velocity
Good image resolution for superficial vessels	

namics. Classification of occlusive disease is based on the principle that as plaque develops, hemodynamics evolve in sequence from disordered, turbulent flow to increased systolic velocity, to increased diastolic velocity, and finally, to the reduced velocities associated with preocclusive lesions. Although interpretation criteria vary with the specific arterial bed (proximity to the heart and outflow resistance), the principles remain the same. The addition of the color flow feature has gained increasing popularity with duplex users; however, although, color can speed and facilitate a study, it cannot substitute for the technologist's ability, perseverance, and attention to detail. Color information represents mean or mode velocities; therefore, the severity of the disease cannot be accurately assessed with color alone, and spectral waveform analysis is still required.

Duplex imaging is the least invasive, least expensive, most repeatable, and most operator-dependent of the newer diagnostic techniques. The clinical utility of duplex scanning is clearly and concisely elucidated here by Eugene Zieler. His algorithms place arterial duplex scanning into good clinical perspective. Surveillance of lower extremity bypass grafts has become our responsibility following lower extremity revascularization and is a routine part of patient care. Although briefly mentioned in this section, it is covered in more detail in Chapter 35.

Since the late 1970s, surgeons have increasingly used *computed tomography* (CT) for the diagnosis and treatment of patients with vascular disease, especially aneurysmal disease. This technique evaluates multiple slices of x-ray images that are stacked and subsequently computer-analyzed. The best images are viewed in cross section (transverse planes) but coronal and sagittal slice images also can be obtained (Table 6–2). William Pearce has presented the underlying principles of CT imaging in understandable detail. CT is particularly useful for the evaluation of large arteries and veins, permits evaluation of surrounding tissues, and is more readily available than magnetic resonance angiography. Claustrophobia may be a problem with CT scans; however, not to the degree experienced with MRA.

Table 6–2. Computed Tomography (CT)

Advantages	Disadvantages
Good visualization of central vessels (thorax and abdomen)	Claustrophobia may be a problem
Evaluates surrounding tissue	Radiation exposure
More readily available than magnetic resonance angiography	Overestimates vessel/aneurysm diameter with tortuosity
	Contrast required for vascular studies can be toxic
	Cannot assess stenosis
	Cannot assess patency of medium and small-sized vessels (unless rapid infusion CT technique is used)
	CT slices may be too thick to identify important details

There is the small risk of radiation exposure as well as the associated risk of contrast, if it is required for imaging of vascular structures. Vessel and aneurysm diameters may be overestimated if they are tortuous. Unfortunately, CT scans cannot accurately assess degrees of stenosis, and unless one uses rapid sequential imaging with contrast, the patency of medium or small-sized vessels cannot be reliably evaluated either. Specific areas of importance to the surgeon should be brought to the attention of the radiologist, so that ''thinner'' slices can be made where appropriate and important detail not be missed (e.g., the origin of mesenteric and renal arteries relative to aortic aneurysms, the presence of a retroaortic renal vein).

Magnetic resonance angiography (MRA) is potentially the ideal vascular imaging technique. It can offer broad views of the vascular system and show surrounding tissues and has no inherent risk (Table 6–3). Gary Caputo and his associates from the University of California, San Francisco, offer a current view of the changing field of MRA. MRA is based on blood flow relative to surrounding tissues, and therefore MRA should be regarded as a ''hemodynamic'' as well as an anatomic study. Intraluminal signals can occur with blood flowing out of an imaging slice or field, while blood flowing into an imaging slice provides signals of greater intensity than adjacent stationary tissue and results in flow-related enhancement. This effect varies with blood velocity, slice thickness, and the imaging parameters used by the radiologist. Additionally, data acquisition that coincides with diastole, when blood flow is

Table 6–3. Magnetic Resonance Angiography

Advantages	Disadvantages
Potentially the ideal imaging technique	Limited availability; may have to move patient to another building
Noninvasive	Limited validation
No risk	Claustrophobia a problem
Shows vessels and surrounding tissue	Overestimates stenosis
Anatomic and physiologic information available	Image is based on blood flow
	Patients with metallic attachments/implants cannot be studied

minimal or absent, generates a high-intensity signal that fails to image the artery. There can also be loss of magnetic resonance signal at the vessel wall owing to boundary layer separation, thereby giving the appearance of a partially recanalized thrombus.

Imaging parameters can be manipulated to maximize intravascular signal and to minimize the signal from the stationary tissue. To the nonexpert observer, this gives the appearance of ''dialing in'' the arteriogram and maximizing or minimizing the disease. At which point one decides to accept that the manipulated image is arbitrary and can be problematic.

Claustrophobia is a problem with some patients, and the limited availability and cost of the MRA will restrict its use in the immediate future.

The degree of stenosis is frequently overestimated and high-grade stenoses are commonly identified as segmental occlusions. Improved image quality and detail will parallel the rapid development of coils for vascular imaging.

With the growth in the newer diagnostic studies, there is a tendency to minimize the clinical evaluation of our patients. Even as diagnostic vistas widen, a careful history and physical examination remains a necessity for good patient care. Although newer imaging techniques may offer an improved understanding of the natural history of vascular disease, this new information must be put into proper perspective. We must avoid treating ''diseased blood vessels'' simply because the diagnosis is confirmed. Incidental diagnosis of occlusive disease that does not cause unacceptable limitations on the patient's life or increased morbidity/mortality (based on its natural history) should not be dilated, atherectomized, stented, endarterectomized, or bypassed.

As one understands the advantages and disadvantages of each of the new techniques as well as the details important for good patient management, the concept of sequential data acquisition emerges for selected patients. Although, in the future, sequential diagnostic studies will be limited by the payors of medical care, they may be justified in certain patient scenarios.

Validation of the findings of these newer techniques is critical, and physicians must take advantage of every opportunity to confirm their own results in an ongoing quality assurance effort.

It is always tempting to predict future applications of new technology. It is evident that increasing numbers of patients will have their diagnoses established and therapy completed without standard contrast angiography, as we know it today. Ongoing advances in technology will permit evaluations not yet conceived by most clinicians and will challenge clinical investigators to design accurate validation studies. Above all, physicians must meet their responsibilities to their patients while at the same time showing sound fiscal judgment in selecting diagnostic studies from the tempting array offered by this new technology.

Arterial Duplex Scanning

R. Eugene Zierler, M.D.

The evolution of duplex scanning as a diagnostic tool is a prime example of how advances in technology can be exploited for clinical purposes. In the early 1970s, efforts to use B-mode imaging to evaluate arterial walls and atherosclerotic plaques were just beginning. At the same time, continuous-wave and pulsed Doppler techniques were being used to characterize flow patterns within blood vessels. While these two diagnostic approaches were being applied separately, a fortuitous clinical observation suggested that a combination of imaging and flow detection might be superior to either method used alone.[1] The carotid artery bifurcation was the initial site of interest because of the high prevalence of disease and easy accessibility to ultrasound. One of the first patients evaluated with a prototype real-time B-mode imaging system at the University of Washington appeared to have widely patent carotid vessels; however, when an arteriogram was done, the internal carotid artery was found to be occluded. It was immediately apparent that the occluding material had acoustic properties that were similar to those of flowing blood and, therefore, could not be detected solely on the basis of the image.

The proposed solution to this problem was to incorporate a Doppler system into the instrument to directly assess the patency of vessels seen on the B-mode image.[2, 3] This concept of combining ultrasound techniques for anatomic imaging and flow detection became known as duplex scanning. Although the capabilities of the prototype instrument were limited, it was clear from the initial clinical experience that duplex scanning would be a valuable diagnostic technique. However, in contrast to the emphasis on B-mode image interpretation that characterized the early work, it was found that the degree of arterial narrowing could be determined most accurately by analysis of pulsed Doppler flow signals. Thus, the important components of a duplex scanner are a B-mode imaging system, a pulsed Doppler flow detector, and some method for analyzing the Doppler signals. The signal processing methods that have been most successful in the clinical setting are real-time spectral waveform analysis and color flow imaging (Chapter 5).

Although the applications of duplex scanning were initially limited to superficial vessels by technical considerations such as ultrasound transmitting frequency and scanhead design, advances in technology have expanded the applications of modern duplex scanning to include the deeply located vessels in the abdomen and extremities. Improvements in signal processing techniques have provided detailed information on flow patterns in both normal and diseased arteries. The more recent development of high-resolution B-mode imaging systems has renewed interest in the use of ultrasound imaging for the assessment of the arterial wall and atherosclerotic plaques. This chapter reviews basic principles of arterial duplex scanning and discusses current clinical applications.

GENERAL PRINCIPLES OF DUPLEX SCANNING

Although contrast arteriography has always been used to validate the results of duplex scanning, it should be emphasized that arteriography and duplex scanning are fundamentally different. Arteriography is strictly an anatomic investigation of the vascular lumen; duplex scanning is both an anatomic and a physiologic test that evaluates the vessel wall and the hemodynamic effects of arterial lesions. An arteriogram report typically specifies whether an artery is patent or occluded and gives the maximal degree of stenosis expressed as a percentage of the normal lumen diameter. Duplex scanning assesses the physiologic significance of a vascular lesion and classifies the severity of disease according to relatively broad categories. Although the details of disease classification by duplex scanning differ for the various arterial segments, the underlying principles relating the severity of arterial disease to localized flow disturbances remain the same.

Interpretation of Duplex Scan Results

In conventional arterial duplex scanning, vessels are visualized with the B-mode image and a single sample volume pulsed Doppler device is placed within the arterial lumen at a site of interest. The local flow pattern is then assessed by spectral waveform analysis. An important aspect of duplex scanning is the use of a pulsed Doppler device, which permits evaluation of the arterial flow pattern at a discrete site. The sample volume of a pulsed Doppler device is the region in which flow is actually detected. By adjusting the size and position of the sample volume, center stream flow patterns can be assessed without interference from flow disturbances near the arterial wall or flow in adjacent vessels. The spectral waveform features that are used to classify arterial lesions include a widening of the frequency band or spectral broadening, which represents turbulent flow, and increased peak systolic frequency, which results from the high-velocity jet within a stenosis. It is especially important to sample flow at closely spaced intervals along the vessel because the flow disturbances associated with arterial lesions are quite localized.

Color flow imaging is an alternative to spectral waveform analysis for displaying the Doppler information obtained by duplex scanning. Within certain technical limitations, the color flow image permits visualization of moving blood in the plane of the B-mode image (Chapter 5). The principal advantage of the color flow display is that it presents flow information on the entire image, even though the amount of information on each site is reduced. Color flow imaging can be helpful for identifying vessels, particularly when they are small, deeply located, or anatomically complex.[4] However, because the color assignments in the flow image represent mean (or mode) rather than peak velocities, it is difficult to determine disease severity based on the color flow image alone. Therefore, even when color flow imaging is used, spectral waveforms are still necessary for accurate disease classification.

B-mode imaging has been used to evaluate the histologic and surface features of arterial lesions with varying degrees of success.[5, 6] Although the sonographic characteristics of atherosclerotic plaque may correlate qualitatively with histologic composition, the clinical value of this information is uncertain. In general, lipid is the least echogenic component of a plaque, and as the collagen content increases relative to lipid content, the echogenicity also increases. Fibrous plaque is usually homogeneous, but focal deposits of thrombus or lipid can produce a more heterogeneous appearance. Calcification, which typically occurs at sites of hemorrhage or necrosis, is extremely echogenic and results in bright echoes with acoustic shadows. In spite of these sonographic features, it is difficult to accurately measure the size of the arterial lumen on a B-mode image because the acoustic properties of noncalcified plaque, thrombus, and flowing blood are often similar. Furthermore, acoustic shadows from calcified plaques may prevent complete visualization of the arterial wall. These limitations are largely overcome by duplex scanning.

CLINICAL ROLE OF DUPLEX SCANNING

In the clinical setting, duplex scanning can be used to perform three distinct functions: screening, definitive diagnosis, and follow-up. The purpose of screening is to detect the presence of disease, particularly severe disease, in a relatively large and diverse patient population. Although the patients being screened may have risk factors or other characteristics that raise the suspicion of disease, it is to be expected that most of the patients in the population will not have the disease in question. Therefore, in order to be effective as a screening tool, a diagnostic test must have a high sensitivity and be capable of detecting disease whenever it is present. This requires a very low rate of false-negative tests. Other requirements for a useful screening test are a high degree of safety and relatively low cost. These features are clearly necessary if the test is to be performed on a large number of patients or repeated at frequent intervals. Because contrast arteriography is not a suitable screening test, duplex scanning plays an important role in screening for arterial disease.

Definitive diagnosis is necessary for planning specific approaches to treatment. In a patient with arterial disease, the essential information includes the precise location and severity of occlusive lesions. Such information helps determine whether endarterectomy, bypass grafting, or balloon angioplasty is most appropriate. Although invasive contrast studies have traditionally served this purpose, the need for routine use of arteriography has been questioned in order to reduce the overall costs and risks of treatment.

The goal of follow-up testing is to detect progressive or recurrent disease after treatment has been carried out. Specific examples of follow-up testing are the detection of recurrent stenosis after carotid endarterectomy and surveillance of lower extremity bypass grafts for lesions that could threaten long-term patency. The general requirements for an optimal follow-up test are similar to those for screening, because most patients who require follow-up studies will be doing well clinically. Thus, invasive tests are not appropriate for routine follow-up testing, and duplex scanning plays a major role as well.

Table 6–4. Criteria for Classification of Internal Carotid Artery Disease by Duplex Scanning With Spectral Waveform Analysis of Pulsed Doppler Signals*

Arteriographic Lesion	Spectral Criteria
A. 0% diameter reduction	Peak systolic frequency less than 4 KHz; no spectral broadening
B. 1–15% diameter reduction	Peak systolic frequency less than 4 KHz; spectral broadening in deceleration phase of systole only
C. 16–49% diameter reduction	Peak systolic frequency less than 4 KHz; spectral broadening throughout systole
D. 50–79% diameter reduction	Peak systolic frequency greater than or equal to 4 KHz; end-diastolic frequency less than 4.5 KHz
D+. 80–90% diameter reduction	End-diastolic frequency greater than or equal to 4.5 KHz
E. Occlusion (100% diameter reduction)	No internal carotid flow signal; flow to zero in common carotid artery

**Criteria are based on a pulsed Doppler with a 5-MHz transmitting frequency, a sample volume that is small relative to the internal carotid artery, and a 60-degree beam-to-vessel angle of insonation. Approximate angle-adjusted velocity equivalents are: 4 KHz = 125 cm/sec and 4.5 KHz = 140 cm/sec.*

EXTRACRANIAL CAROTID ARTERY DISEASE

Technique and Interpretation

A carotid duplex scan usually begins with visualization of the common carotid artery low in the neck. This vessel is then followed distally to the area of the bifurcation, where the carotid bulb may be apparent as a localized dilatation of the lumen. The internal and external carotid arteries are identified by their typical location with the internal branch posterolaterally and the external branch anteromedially. When anatomic variations alter these relationships, the branches can usually be identified by their characteristic Doppler flow signals. The internal carotid flow pattern is characteristic of an artery supplying a low-resistance vascular bed with forward flow throughout the cardiac cycle; the triphasic external carotid waveform is typical of peripheral arteries that supply high-resistance vascular beds. Sites routinely evaluated with the pulsed Doppler sample volume include the low and high common carotid, the carotid bulb, the proximal, middle, and distal internal carotid, and the external carotid arteries. Any sites with abnormal flow patterns are carefully examined. Flow patterns in the subclavian and vertebral arteries can also be assessed during the carotid duplex examination.

The spectral waveform criteria for classification of internal carotid artery stenoses have been validated by comparisons with contrast arteriograms.[7–9] A set of currently used criteria is given in Table 6–4 and illustrated in Figure 6–1. These criteria distinguish between normal and diseased internal carotid arteries with a specificity of 84 per cent and a sensitivity of 99 per cent. The accuracy for detecting 50 to 99 per cent diameter stenosis or occlusion is 93 per cent.

Some degree of variability is unavoidable with any physiologic or anatomic test. In carotid duplex scanning, the greatest variability has been noted for the normal to moderate stenosis categories, which are designated A, B, and C lesions in Table 6–4. Agreement is much better for classification of lesions that reduce the carotid artery diameter by 50 per cent or more.[10] Similarly, carotid arteriography is subject to the most variability when the arteries are normal or minimally diseased.[11] In general, the agreement between duplex scanning and arteriography is equivalent to the agreement between two radiologists interpreting the same arteriograms.

Clinical Applications

The main goal in the noninvasive evaluation of carotid artery disease is to identify patients who are at risk for stroke. Once this is accomplished, decisions can be made regarding the need for arteriography and the potential benefits of carotid endarterectomy. Although attempts have been made to predict clinical outcome based on the sonographic features of carotid plaques, the degree of stenosis at the carotid bifurcation has been the most consistently reliable feature for assessing neurologic risk. The major indications for carotid duplex scanning are (1) an asymptomatic carotid bruit; (2) hemispheric cerebral or ocular transient ischemic attacks; (3) prior stroke with good neurologic recovery; (4) screening prior to major cardiac or peripheral vascular surgery; and (5) follow-up after carotid endarterectomy.[12]

The auscultation of a bruit in the neck is one of the most common reasons for requesting a noninvasive evaluation of the carotid arteries. Among 100 patients with 165 asymptomatic bruits, duplex scanning showed a normal internal carotid in 12 (7 per cent), less than 50 per cent diameter stenosis in 83 (50 per cent), a 50 per cent or greater stenosis in 61 (37 per cent), and internal carotid occlusion in 9 (6 per cent).[13] Thus, although most neck bruits are associated with disease of the carotid artery, only about one third are related to severe internal carotid stenoses.

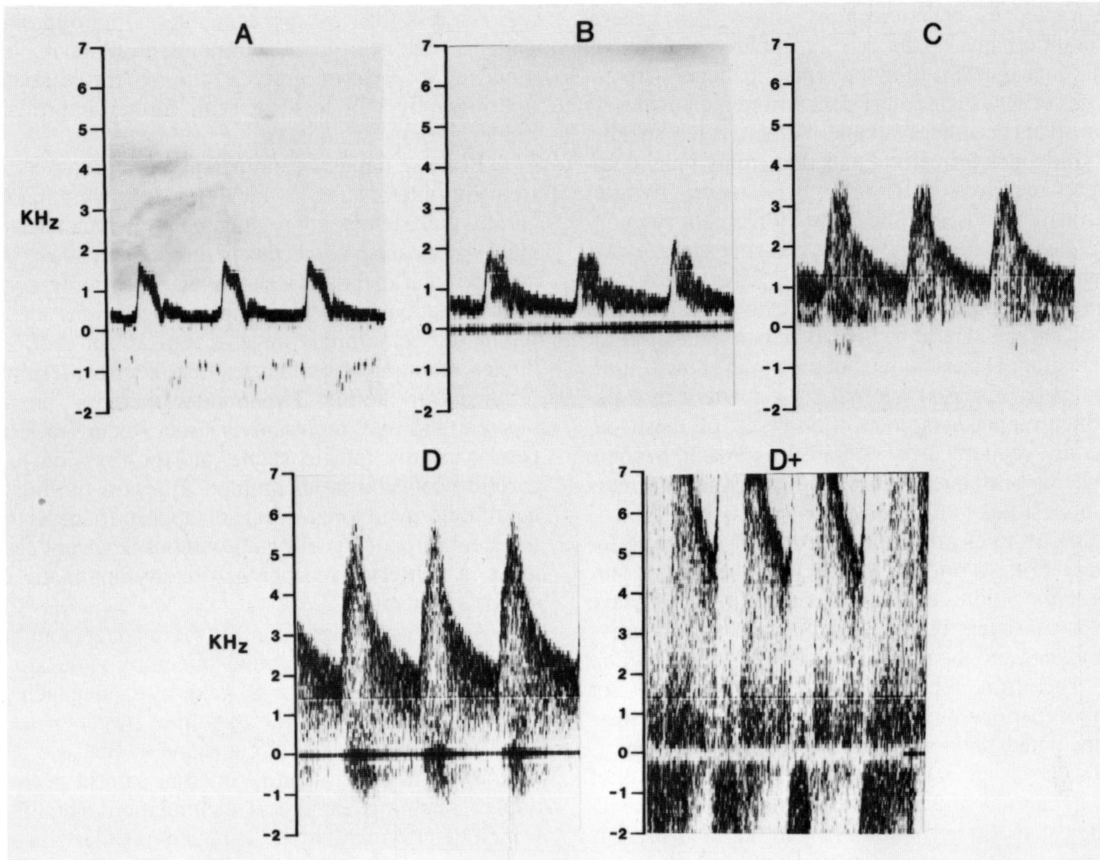

FIGURE 6–1. Internal carotid spectral waveforms classified according to the criteria given in Table 6–4. *A*, Normal; *B*, 1–15 per cent diameter reduction; *C*, 16–49 per cent diameter reduction; *D*, 50–79 per cent diameter reduction; and *D+*, 80–99 per cent diameter reduction. (*A–D+*, From Zierler RE, Strandness DE Jr: Noninvasive dynamic and real-time assessment of extracranial cerebrovasculature. *In* Wood JH [ed]: Cerebral Blood Flow: Physiologic and Clinical Aspects. New York, McGraw-Hill, 1987, p 317. Reproduced with permission of McGraw-Hill.)

Therapeutic decisions for patients with asymptomatic carotid disease must take into account not only the severity of stenosis but also the natural history of the lesions. In a serial follow-up study of 167 patients with asymptomatic neck bruits, duplex scanning showed progression of disease in 60 per cent of the internal carotid arteries.[14] The mean annual rate for development of ipsilateral neurologic symptoms (transient ischemic attack or stroke) was 4 per cent. There was a strong correlation between the presence of an 80 to 99 per cent internal carotid stenosis and the occurrence of neurologic symptoms or internal carotid occlusion. Patients with lesions of this severity had a 46 per cent incidence of one or more of these events, whereas those with less severe stenoses had only a 1.5 per cent incidence. Thus, duplex scanning can be used as a screening test to identify patients with especially severe carotid stenoses who are at increased risk for neurologic events.

Although the finding of an asymptomatic 80 to 99 per cent internal carotid stenosis by duplex scanning identifies a high-risk group of patients, the clinically important question is whether this risk can be reduced by carotid endarterectomy. Although this question will ultimately be answered by randomized clinical trials, follow-up data are available on 129 asymptomatic 80 to 99 per cent internal carotid stenoses, of which 56 were treated by carotid endarterectomy and 73 were followed without surgery.[15] The operated and nonoperated patients were similar with regard to characteristics such as age and prevalence of diabetes mellitus, hypertension, ischemic heart disease, and aspirin use. During a 24-month follow-up period, neurologic symptoms and internal carotid occlusion were significantly more frequent in the nonoperated patients (48 per cent) than in the operated patients (9 per cent). These results strongly suggest that endarterectomy improves the natural history of *high-grade* asymptomatic internal carotid stenoses. Asymptomatic patients with less than 80 per cent internal carotid stenoses by duplex scanning can be safely followed at approximately 6-month intervals. If neurologic symptoms or progression to an 80 to 99 per cent stenosis are observed, then the patient should be considered for carotid endarterectomy.

The purpose of carotid screening in patients with hemispheric neurologic symptoms is to identify lesions that could reduce hemispheric blood flow or be the source of cerebral emboli. In the North American Symptomatic Carotid Endarterectomy Trial (NASCET), surgery was highly beneficial for patients with recent hemispheric transient ischemic attacks or mild strokes and 70 to 99 per cent stenosis of the ipsilateral internal carotid artery.[16] Based on these results, symptomatic patients with severe carotid stenoses should be treated by endarterectomy unless their general medical condition makes the risk of surgery prohibitive. The optimal management of symptomatic patients with carotid stenoses of less than 70 per cent will remain uncertain until further data become available. Although the specific NASCET guidelines for carotid endarterectomy in symptomatic patients require a 70 to 99 per cent stenosis by arteriography, many stenoses in the 50 to 79 per cent category and all the stenoses in the 80 to 99 per cent category by duplex scanning will fall into this group. Thus, the duplex scan finding of a 50 to 99 per cent carotid lesion in a symptomatic patient should be considered an indication for further evaluation. Occasionally a duplex scan shows a normal or minimally diseased internal carotid artery in a patient with neurologic symptoms. Follow-up of these patients generally supports a nonoperative approach, because the incidence of subsequent neurologic events is extremely low and a noncarotid cause for symptoms may exist.[17]

It is difficult to clearly define the role of screening for carotid artery disease prior to cardiac or other major surgical procedures. Studies that have reviewed this issue have not shown a consistent relationship between perioperative neurologic events and the presence of asymptomatic carotid stenoses.[18] Therefore, routine carotid endarterectomy for prevention of perioperative stroke is difficult to justify. However, as noted previously, severe asymptomatic internal carotid stenoses are associated with an increased risk of neurologic symptoms and carotid occlusion. If endarterectomy is indicated for asymptomatic carotid stenosis, this may take precedence over other elective surgical procedures.

Although conventional contrast arteriography is still considered to be the definitive diagnostic test for carotid artery disease, there has been increasing interest in performing carotid endarterectomy based on the clinical evaluation and duplex scan findings alone. This trend has been stimulated by improvements in the accuracy and reliability of carotid duplex scanning, along with increasing demands to minimize both the costs and the risks of medical care. Carotid bifurcation lesions that are suitable for endarterectomy include high-grade stenoses in asymptomatic patients and moderate to severe stenoses in patients with hemispheric neurologic symptoms. These categories of lesions can be accurately detected by duplex scanning. Although duplex scanning does not provide any direct information on lesions involving the proximal aortic arch branches or the intracranial circulation, significant lesions proximal or distal to the carotid bifurcation are uncommon and rarely have an adverse effect on the outcome of carotid endarterectomy.[19] In addition, most stenoses in the proximal brachiocephalic vessels can be suspected on the basis of common carotid flow abnormalities or unequal arm blood pressures.

Although the specific indications for carotid surgery without arteriography remain controversial, the results of arteriography rarely alter the clinical treatment plan when a technically adequate duplex scan shows an 80 to 99 per cent stenosis in an asymptomatic patient or an ipsilateral 50 to 99 per cent stenosis in a patient with hemispheric neurologic symptoms.[20] Arteriography is most likely to be of value when the duplex scan is nondiagnostic, for atypical lesions that appear to extend beyond the carotid bifurcation, and for less than 50 per cent internal carotid stenoses in patients with neurologic symptoms. It is inevitable that the tendency to perform more carotid surgery without contrast arteriography will increase with further improvements in the technology of noninvasive testing.

Because duplex scanning can be repeated at relatively frequent intervals, it is ideal for follow-up testing after carotid endarterectomy to document the incidence and clinical significance of recurrent carotid stenosis. Although symptomatic recurrent stenosis occurs in only about 5 per cent of patients, when asymptomatic lesions are included the incidence is in the range of 9 to 21 per cent.[21, 22] Serial duplex scanning also indicates that recurrent lesions tend to occur during the first 2 years after operation, are smoothly tapered, and may regress over time. Recurrent lesions that persist usually remain stable, and progression to internal carotid occlusion is uncommon. Because the incidence of neurologic symptoms does not appear to be significantly different in patients with and without recurrent carotid stenosis, a conservative approach to asymptomatic recurrent stenosis is justified.

A suggested algorithm for the management of carotid artery disease based on initial screening with duplex scanning is given in Figure 6–2. Like most management algorithms, it provides general guidelines but does not account for all possible clinical circumstances. Because it is occasionally difficult to identify internal carotid occlusions by duplex scanning, equivocal examinations should be confirmed by arteriography if the patient is otherwise a surgical candidate.

LOWER EXTREMITY ARTERIAL DISEASE

Technique and Interpretation

The detection of arterial lesions in the abdomen and lower extremities by duplex scanning is based on the same general principles that apply to the carotid duplex evaluation. However, certain details of the examination technique and interpretation of spectral waveforms differ according to the specific segment being evaluated. In average-sized adults, the abdominal vessels can be studied with a 3- or 5-MHz transducer. Scanheads with transducer operating frequencies as low as 2.25 MHz are necessary for obese patients. Examination of the arteries in the legs can be performed with 5-, 7.5-, or 10-MHz transducers. When the abdominal vessels need to be scanned, patients should be examined after an overnight fast to reduce interference from bowel gas. A complete lower extremity duplex study begins with the upper abdominal aorta and proceeds distally. B-mode images and pulsed Doppler spectral waveforms are recorded from any areas where increased velocities or other flow disturbances are noted. Recordings are generally made from the proximal and distal abdominal aorta, the common and external iliac arteries, the common and deep femoral arteries, the proximal, middle, and distal superficial femoral arteries, and the popliteal arteries. If the status of the tibial and peroneal arteries is of clinical interest, recordings can

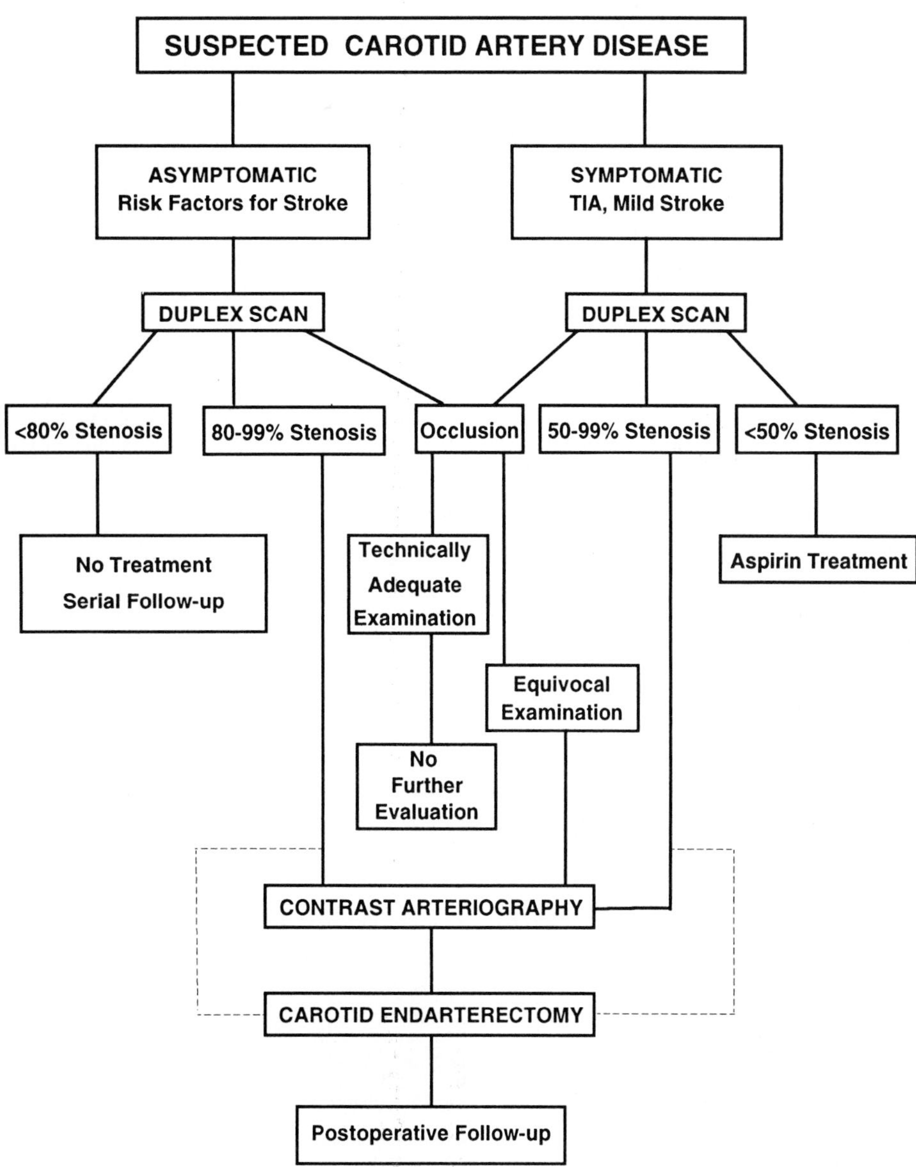

FIGURE 6–2. Clinical management algorithm for symptomatic and asymptomatic carotid artery disease based on screening with duplex scanning. The option of proceeding directly to carotid endarterectomy based on the duplex scan results alone is indicated by the *dotted lines*. TIA, transient ischemic attack.

also be obtained from the proximal and distal segments of these vessels. A complete examination of the aortoiliac and lower extremity arteries may require as much as 2 hours to perform.

The spectral waveform criteria for classification of lower extremity arterial stenoses are summarized in Table 6–5. As with carotid duplex scanning, the distinction between normal and minimally diseased peripheral arteries is relatively subjective, and diagnostic accuracy is better for severe stenoses.[23] For identifying stenoses that produce a significant pressure gradient or are greater than 50 per cent diameter reducing at the time of arteriography, the lower extremity duplex scan has a sensitivity of 82 per cent, a specificity of 92 per cent, a positive predictive value of 80 per cent, and a negative predictive value of 93 per cent. The correlation is especially good for the iliac artery segment where significant stenoses are detected with a sensitivity of 89 per cent and a specificity of 90 per cent.[24]

Clinical Applications

The major clinical application of aortoiliac and lower extremity duplex scanning is in screening patients who may be candidates for intervention. Duplex scanning is particularly helpful for examining the aortoiliac arterial segment, which is difficult to evaluate by any other noninvasive method (Fig. 6–3). The same duplex techniques can also be used for intraoperative assessment and follow-up after treatment. Duplex scanning has been especially valuable in monitoring the function of bypass grafts in the leg. Transformation of the normal triphasic graft flow waveform to a biphasic or monophasic configuration, combined with a peak systolic graft velocity of less than 45 cm/sec, correlates with a high risk of graft failure.[26] Early detection of grafts at risk for occlusion facilitates revision and maintenance of graft patency.[25, 26]

The results of duplex scanning often indicate which

Table 6–5. Criteria for Classification of Lower Extremity Arterial Lesions Based on Duplex Scanning With Spectral Waveform Analysis of Pulsed Doppler Signals

Normal
Triphasic waveform; no spectral broadening

1–19% Diameter Reduction
Triphasic waveform with minimal spectral broadening only; peak systolic velocities increased <30% relative to the adjacent proximal segment; proximal and distal waveforms remain normal

20–49% Diameter Reduction
Triphasic waveform usually maintained, although reverse-flow component may be diminished; spectral broadening is prominent with filling-in of the clear area under the systolic peak; peak systolic velocity is increased from 30 to 100% relative to the adjacent proximal segment; proximal and distal waveforms remain normal

50–99% Diameter Reduction
Monophasic waveform with loss of the reverse-flow component and forward flow throughout the cardiac cycle; extensive spectral broadening; peak systolic velocity is increased >100% relative to the adjacent proximal segment; distal waveform is monophasic with reduced systolic velocity

Occlusion
No flow detected within the imaged arterial segment; preocclusive "thump" may be heard just proximal to the site of occlusion; distal waveforms are monophasic with reduced systolic velocities

type of intervention would be most appropriate. Whether a particular arterial segment is suitable for an endovascular procedure or direct surgical reconstruction depends on the specific features of the lesion. For example, focal stenoses or short occlusions in the iliac or superficial femoral arteries are usually quite amenable to percutaneous transluminal angioplasty (PTA), whereas arterial segments with long, irregular stenotic lesions or extensive occlusions are better treated by a surgical approach. The anatomic features that are particularly important in making this determination are the site, severity, and length of the lesion. In addition, it is essential to assess the status of the inflow and the quality of the distal runoff. Duplex scanning provides a practical and cost-effective method for obtaining this information without resorting to arteriography.

Among 110 patients who underwent lower extremity duplex scanning prior to arteriography, 50 lesions were considered suitable for balloon angioplasty on the basis of the duplex scan findings.[27] Of these, the procedure was actually carried out in 47 (94 per cent). In the remaining 3 cases, lesions were present as predicted by the duplex scan, but angioplasty was not done for various technical reasons. No angioplasties were performed in patients who were found not to be candidates by duplex scanning.

In a study designed to ascertain whether duplex scanning could replace arteriography in planning intervention for lower extremity arterial occlusive disease, six vascular surgeons were asked to select a treatment plan based on a brief clinical description and information from either the duplex scans or the arteriograms.[28] For the 29 patients reviewed, the clinical decisions made using the duplex scan results were very similar to those based on arteriography.

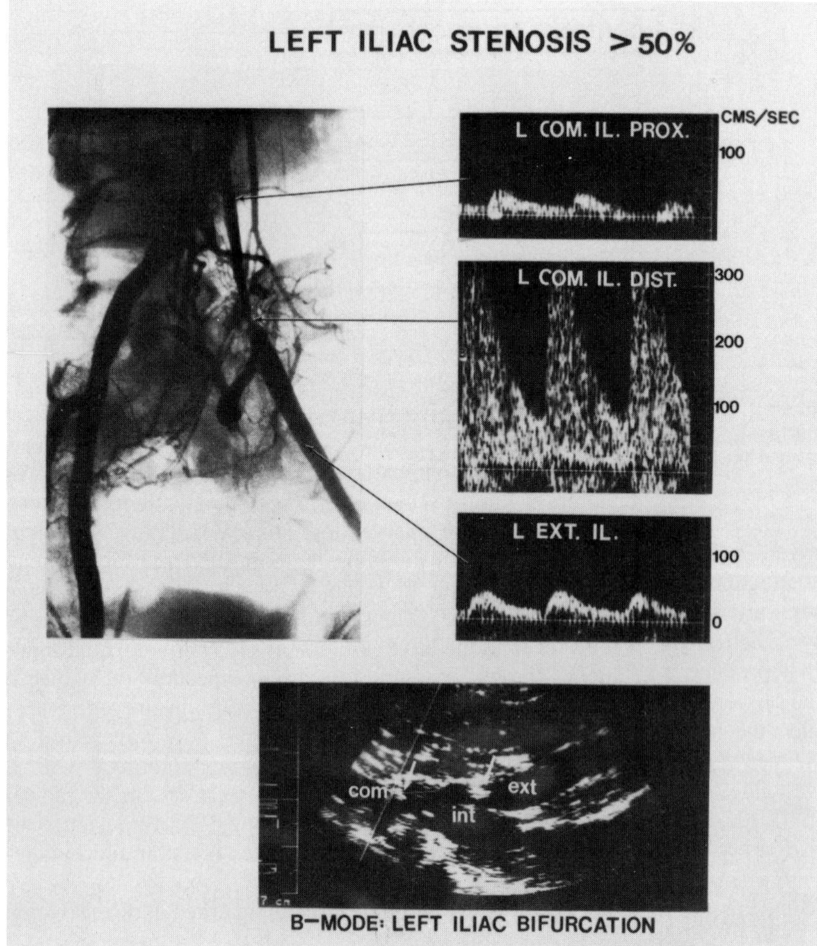

FIGURE 6–3. Duplex scan and arteriogram of a tight (>50 per cent diameter reducing) left iliac artery stenosis. The severity and focal nature of the stenosis are indicated by the localized high-velocity jet in the distal common iliac artery. The external iliac waveform beyond the stenosis is monophasic and damped. (From Zierler RE, Zierler BK: Duplex sonography of lower extremity arteries. *In* Zwiebel WJ [ed]: Introduction to Vascular Ultrasonography. 3rd ed. Philadelphia, WB Saunders, 1992, p 248.)

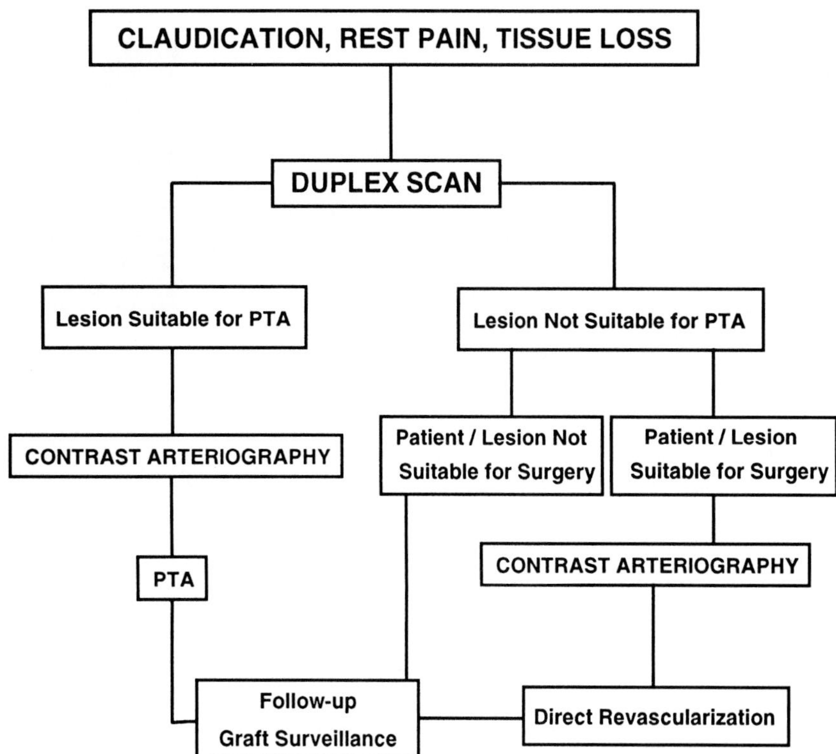

FIGURE 6–4. Clinical management algorithm for lower extremity arterial disease based on duplex scanning prior to arteriography. PTA, percutaneous transluminal angioplasty.

However, significant differences were noted in the treatment plans chosen by the various surgeons, suggesting that much of the disparity resulted from diverse approaches to common patterns of disease.

An algorithm for the management of lower extremity arterial disease based on initial screening with duplex scanning is given in Figure 6–4.

RENAL AND MESENTERIC ARTERIAL DISEASE

Technique and Interpretation

Duplex scanning is the only method available for noninvasive evaluation of the renal and mesenteric vessels. The general technique is similar to that described previously for the aortoiliac arteries. Classification of renal artery disease is based on spectral waveforms from the renal artery and abdominal aorta. The normal triphasic flow pattern of the aortoiliac and lower extremity arteries is a result of the relatively high vascular resistance of the peripheral circulation. In contrast, the normal kidney offers a low vascular resistance, and the renal artery spectral waveform is monophasic with a rounded systolic peak and forward flow throughout the cardiac cycle (Fig. 6–5). This low-resistance waveform is also characteristic of the normal internal carotid artery and celiac axis.

Because the peak velocity associated with a significant renal artery stenosis increases relative to aortic peak velocity, the ratio of peak systolic velocities (or frequencies) in the renal artery and adjacent aorta can be used as an index of renal artery stenosis. This is referred to as the renal-aortic ratio or RAR. Renal artery occlusion is diagnosed when the artery is visualized but no flow signal can be detected in the proximal segment. A retrospective review of 43 renal arteries evaluated by both duplex scanning and arteriography found that an RAR of 3.5 or greater was highly predictive of a renal artery stenosis of 60 per cent diameter reduction or more.[29] In a subsequent prospective study of 58 renal arteries in 29 patients, an RAR of 3.5 or greater had a sensitivity of 84 per cent and a specificity of 97 per cent for detection of severe renal artery stenoses.[30] The duplex scan classification of renal artery disease has been refined by noting that a renal artery velocity above 180 cm/sec is an accurate predictor of an abnormal renal artery, and an RAR of 3.5 or more characterizes a high-grade renal artery stenosis.[31] The criteria for classification of renal artery disease by duplex scanning are summarized in Table 6–6.

Duplex scanning can also detect stenotic lesions of the celiac and superior mesenteric arteries.[32–34] Atherosclerotic lesions usually involve the origins and proximal segments of the mesenteric vessels. Because these lesions are relatively uncommon, the results of mesenteric duplex scanning have not been compared with arteriography in a large number of patients; however, the spectral waveform features associated with severe stenoses include localized high-velocity jets and spectral broadening.

Clinical Applications

Duplex scanning is becoming established as a noninvasive screening test for renal artery stenosis in patients who may have renovascular hypertension or renal failure secondary to chronic renal ischemia. The diagnostic tests

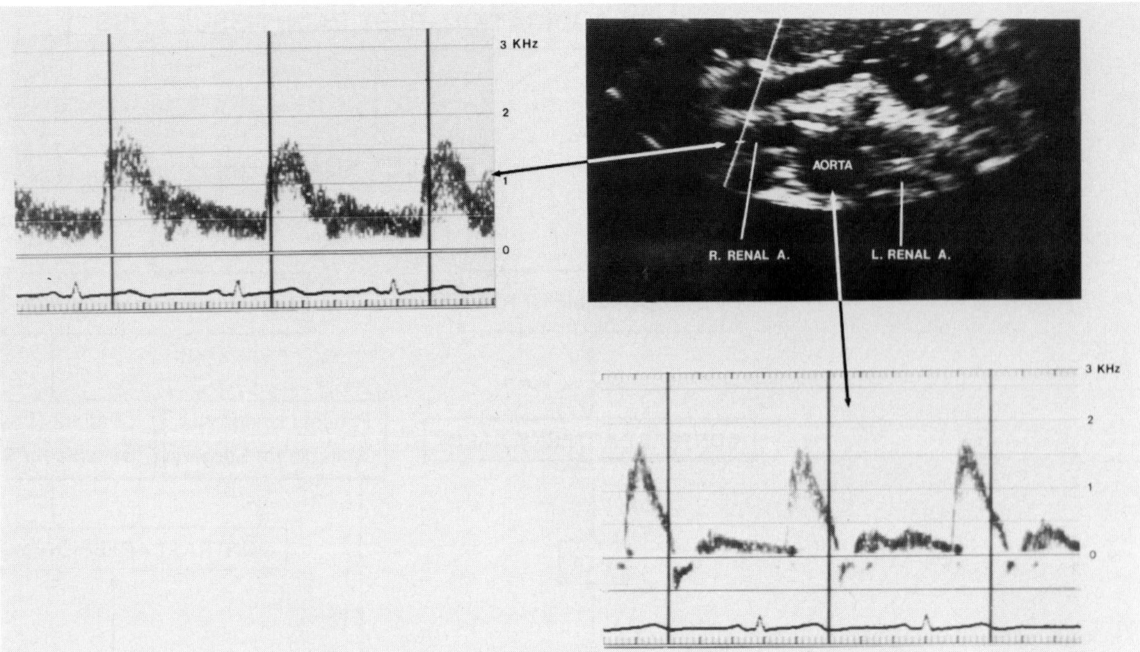

FIGURE 6–5. Normal renal and aortic spectral waveforms. Aortic waveform *(lower right)* is triphasic with reversed flow in late systole. The renal artery waveform *(upper left)* is monophasic with forward flow throughout the cardiac cycle. (From Kohler TR, Zierler RE, Martin RL, et al: Noninvasive diagnosis of renal artery stenosis by ultrasonic duplex scanning. J Vasc Surg 4:450, 1986.)

that have been used to screen for the presence of renal artery stenosis and renovascular hypertension include peripheral plasma renin assays, the rapid-sequence intravenous pyelogram, isotope renography, and renal arteriography. Experience has shown that, with the exception of arteriography, none of these methods is sufficiently sensitive to serve as a reliable screening test.[35] However, because of the costs and risks involved, arteriography is not suitable for screening purposes, particularly for patients with impaired renal function. Although duplex scanning is reliable for detecting lesions in the main renal arteries, accessory renal arteries are difficult to identify. Furthermore, the duplex scan findings do not predict the clinical response to renal revascularization. Once a renal artery stenosis has been identified, its functional significance must still be assessed. This is usually accomplished by either renal vein renin determinations or split renal function studies.

The symptoms of chronic mesenteric ischemia occur when there is insufficient blood flow to support the normal intestinal functions of motility, secretion, and absorption.[36]

Table 6–6. Criteria for Classification of Renal Artery Disease by Duplex Scanning

Renal Artery Diameter Reduction	Renal Artery PSV	RAR
Normal	<180 cm/sec	<3.5
<60%	≥ 180 cm/sec	<3.5
≥60%	< or ≥ 180 cm/sec	≥3.5
Occlusion	No signal	No signal

Key: *PSV, peak systolic velocity; RAR, renal aortic ratio (ratio of the peak systolic velocity in the renal artery to the peak systolic velocity in the aorta).*

Although stenosis or occlusion of the celiac, superior mesenteric, or inferior mesenteric arteries is relatively common in patients with widespread atherosclerosis, the collateral blood supply to the splanchnic circulation is remarkably efficient, and relatively few patients develop the clinical syndrome. Most patients who develop the typical signs and symptoms are found to have significant occlusive lesions in at least two of the major mesenteric arteries. Duplex scanning can be used as a screening test for mesenteric arterial disease in patients with suspected mesenteric ischemia.[34]

An algorithm for the management of renal and mesenteric arterial disease based on screening with duplex scanning is given in Figure 6–6.

CONCLUSIONS

The development of duplex scanning has made it possible to document the presence and severity of vascular lesions in the carotid, abdominal, and peripheral arteries without resorting to invasive contrast studies. Initial clinical decisions regarding the need for specific intervention or further diagnostic tests can usually be based on the duplex scan results alone. Thus, the screening role of duplex scanning is firmly supported and established. Because duplex scanning provides definitive diagnostic information in most arterial applications, arteriography should rarely be necessary solely for diagnosis. Therefore, the clinical role of arteriography is primarily that of an adjunct to intervention, either as a final investigation prior to direct arterial surgery or as a component of a percutaneous procedure. There is a growing trend to regard duplex scanning as a definitive diagnostic test for carotid disease and perform carotid end-

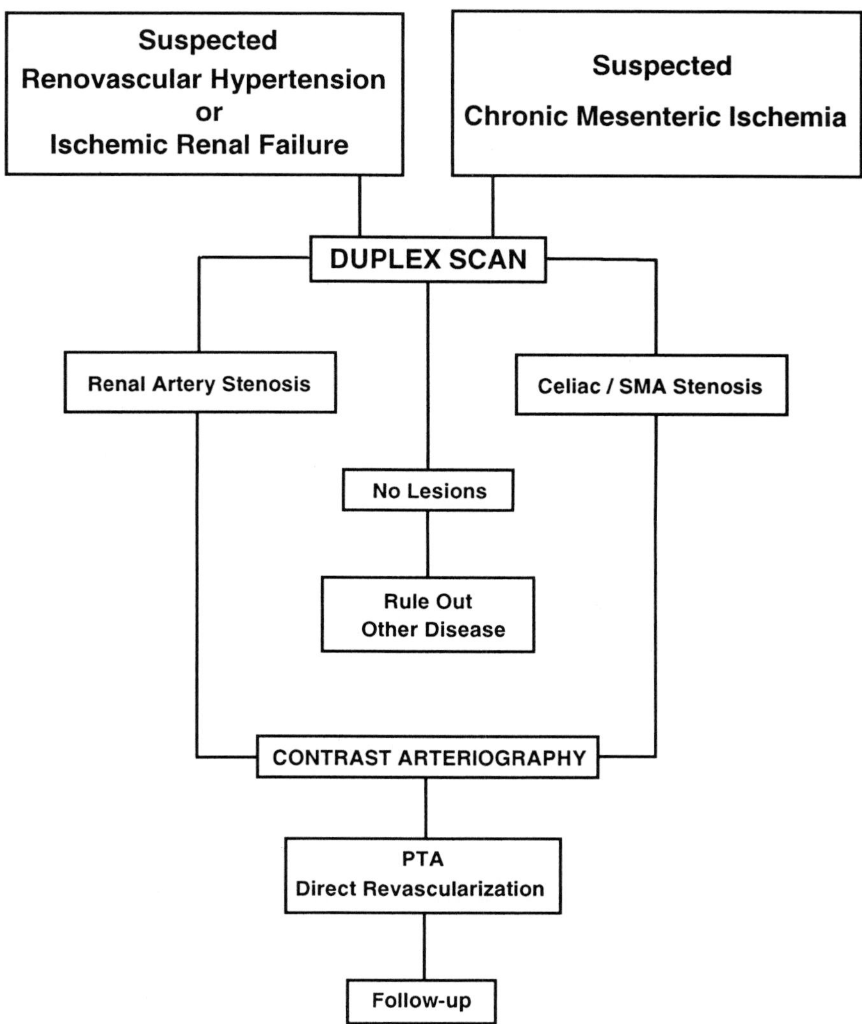

FIGURE 6–6. Clinical management algorithm for renal and mesenteric arterial disease based on duplex scanning prior to arteriography. SMA, superior mesenteric artery; PTA, percutaneous transluminal angioplasty.

arterectomy without preliminary arteriography. In contrast to carotid duplex scanning, duplex techniques for evaluating abdominal and peripheral arteries are still being actively developed and refined, so arteriography is still necessary for planning intervention. Duplex scanning is the method of choice for follow-up testing of patients with arterial disease. This allows early detection of disease progression and surveillance of bypass grafts for lesions that might threaten long-term patency.

References

1. Strandness DE Jr: Historical aspects. *In* Duplex Scanning in Vascular Disorders. New York, Raven Press, 1990.
2. Barber FE, Baker DW, Nation AWC, et al: Ultrasonic duplex echo Doppler scanner. IEEE Trans Biomed Eng 21:109, 1974.
3. Barber FE, Baker DW, Strandness DE Jr, et al: Duplex scanner II for simultaneous imaging of artery tissues and flow. Ultrasonics Symposium Proc IEEE 74CH0896–ISU, 1974.
4. Zierler RE, Phillips DJ, Beach KW, et al: Noninvasive assessment of normal carotid bifurcation hemodynamics with color-flow ultrasound imaging. Ultrasound Med Biol 13:471, 1987.
5. Comerota AJ, Cranley JJ, Katz AK, et al: Real-time B-mode carotid imaging: A three-year multicenter experience. J Vasc Surg 1:84, 1984.
6. Hennerici M, Reifschneider G, Trockel U, et al: Detection of early atherosclerotic lesions by duplex scanning of the carotid artery. J Clin Ultrasound 12:455, 1984.
7. Fell G, Phillips DJ, Chikos PM, et al: Ultrasonic duplex scanning for disease of the carotid artery. Circulation 64:1191, 1981.
8. Langlois YE, Roederer GO, Chan AW, et al: Evaluating carotid artery disease—The concordance between pulsed Doppler/spectrum analysis and angiography. Ultrasound Med Biol 9:51, 1983.
9. Roederer GO, Langlois YE, Chan AW, et al: Ultrasonic duplex scanning of extracranial carotid arteries: Improved accuracy using new features from the common carotid artery. J Cardiovasc Ultrasonog 1:373, 1982.
10. Kohler T, Langlois Y, Roederer GO, et al: Sources of variability in carotid duplex examination: A prospective study. Ultrasound Med Biol 4:571, 1985.
11. Chikos PM, Fisher LD, Hirsh JA, et al: Observer variability in evaluating extracranial carotid artery stenosis. Stroke 14:885, 1983.
12. Strandness DE Jr, Andros G, Baker JD, et al: Vascular laboratory utilization and payment: Report of the Ad Hoc Committee of the Western Vascular Society. J Vasc Surg 16:163, 1992.
13. Fell G, Breslau P, Knox RA, et al: Importance of noninvasive ultrasonic Doppler testing in the evaluation of patients with asymptomatic carotid bruits. Am Heart J 102:221, 1981.
14. Roederer GO, Langlois YE, Jager KA, et al: The natural history of carotid arterial disease in asymptomatic patients with cervical bruits. Stroke 15:605, 1984.
15. Moneta GL, Taylor DC, Nicholls SC, et al: Operative versus nonoperative management of asymptomatic high-grade internal carotid ar-

tery stenosis: Improved results with endarterectomy. Stroke 18:1005, 1987.

16. North American Symptomatic Carotid Endarterectomy Trial Collaborators: Beneficial effect of carotid endarterectomy in symptomatic patients with high-grade carotid stenosis. N Engl J Med 325:445, 1991.
17. Zierler RE, Kohler TR, Strandness DE Jr: Duplex scanning of normal or minimally diseased carotid arteries: Correlation with arteriography and clinical outcome. J Vasc Surg 12:447, 1990.
18. Barnes RW, Liebman PR, Marszalek PB, et al: The natural history of asymptomatic carotid disease in patients undergoing cardiovascular surgery. Surgery 90:1075, 1981.
19. Roederer GO, Langlois YE, Chan ARW, et al: Is siphon disease important in predicting outcome of carotid endarterectomy? Arch Surg 118:1177, 1983.
20. Dawson DL, Zierler RE, Kohler TR: Role of arteriography in the preoperative evaluation of carotid artery disease. Am J Surg 161:619, 1991.
21. Healy DA, Zierler RE, Nicholls SC, et al: Long-term follow-up and clinical outcome of carotid restenosis. J Vasc Surg 10:662, 1989.
22. Bernstein EF, Torem S, Dilley RB: Does carotid restenosis predict an increased risk of late symptoms, stroke, or death? Ann Surg 212:629, 1990.
23. Jager KA, Phillips DJ, Martin RRL, et al: Noninvasive mapping of lower limb arterial lesions. Ultrasound Med Biol 11:515, 1985.
24. Kohler TR, Nance DR, Cramer MM, et al: Duplex scanning for diagnosis of aortoiliac and femoropopliteal disease: A prospective study. Circulation 76:1074, 1987.
25. Londrey GL, Hodgson KJ, Spadone, DP, et al: Initial experience with color-flow duplex scanning of infrainguinal bypass grafts. J Vasc Surg 12:284, 1990.
26. Bandyk DF, Schmitt DD, Seabrook GR, et al: Monitoring functional patency of in situ saphenous vein bypasses: The impact of a surveillance protocol and elective revision. J Vasc Surg 9:286, 1989.
27. Edwards JM, Coldwell DM, Goldman ML, et al: The role of duplex scanning in the selection of patients for transluminal angioplasty. J Vasc Surg 13:69, 1991.
28. Kohler T, Andros G, Porter J, et al: Can duplex scanning replace arteriography for lower extremity arterial disease? Ann Vasc Surg 4:28, 1990.
29. Kohler TR, Zierler RE, Martin RL, et al: Noninvasive diagnosis of renal artery stenosis by ultrasonic duplex scanning. J Vasc Surg 4:450, 1986.
30. Taylor DC, Kettler MD, Moneta GL, et al: Duplex ultrasound in the diagnosis of renal artery stenosis—A prospective evaluation. J Vasc Surg 7:363, 1988.
31. Hoffmann U, Edwards JM, Carter S, et al: Role of duplex scanning for the detection of atherosclerotic renal artery disease. Kidney Int 39:1232, 1991.
32. Nicholls SC, Kohler TR, Martin RL, et al: Use of hemodynamic parameters in the diagnosis of mesenteric insufficiency. J Vasc Surg 3:507, 1985.
33. Jager K, Bollinger A, Valli C, et al: Measurement of mesenteric blood flow by duplex scanning. J Vasc Surg 3:462, 1986.
34. Jager KA, Fortner GS, Thiele BL, et al: Noninvasive diagnosis of intestinal angina. J Clin Ultrasound 12:588, 1984.
35. Grim CE, Luft FC, Weinberger MH, et al: Sensitivity and specificity of screening tests for renal vascular hypertension. Ann Intern Med 91:617, 1979.
36. Zelenock GB, Graham LM, Whitehouse WM, et al: Splanchnic atherosclerotic disease and intestinal angina. Arch Surg 115:497, 1980.

Computed Tomography and Magnetic Resonance Imaging in Vascular Disease

William H. Pearce, M.D., Amorn Neil Salyapongse, B.A., and Steven Fitzgerald, M.D.

• • •

Advances in imaging technology have given a unique view of the pathology of many vascular diseases. Until recently, the diagnosis and treatment of these diseases were based on arteriography and venography in combination with noninvasive blood flow testing. Contrast arteriography and venography supply the anatomic information needed to plan surgical procedures or percutaneous intervention. Although these studies provide the anatomic detail, noninvasive testing is necessary to determine the physiologic importance of the anatomic lesion. In some cases, ultrasound imaging provides both anatomic and hemodynamic information, but there is limited application. In the abdomen, the ultrasound is limited by bowel gas and does not give the anatomic detail of other intra-abdominal organs as does computed tomography (CT) or magnetic resonance imaging (MRI). In the chest, the ultrasound is limited to intracardiac pathology and, more recently, the thoracic aorta using an esophageal probe. With the development of CT in the late 1960s and MRI in the early 1970s, these modalities have provided more complete anatomic detail important in planning many vascular surgical procedures.

The CT scan was first developed in 1963 for intracranial imaging by Godfried Hounsfield of EMI Limited.[1] Early generations of the CT scan quickly proved their clinical usefulness in intracranial disease. Continued evolution of CT from second- to third-, and now fourth-generation scanners has provided better images with improved spatial resolution and faster scanning times. During the 1980s, the role of CT in the diagnosis of vascular disease has become more clearly defined. The CT scan can detect a variety of arterial and venous disorders, including the intraluminal pathology of atherosclerotic embolic disease, the nature of cerebral infarctions, arterial aneurysms, venous malformations, and postoperative complications.

MRI was introduced in 1973 into clinical practice by Paul Lauterbur.[2] Like the CT scan, the MRI was used initially to image intracranial disease. With improvements in software and surface coils, other portions of the body may now be imaged. The role of MRI in the management of patients with vascular disease is evolving, much like that of the CT scan in the early 1980s.

The advantages of MRI over the CT scan have become evident in evaluating cerebral and spinal diseases. The MRI is able to reconstruct the image not only in a transaxial plane but also in coronal and sagittal planes. This multiplanar reconstruction capability is valuable in straight vessels lying within a single plane and in vascular malformations. Further, the MRI provides anatomic detail and blood information without contrast. However, CT scan remains superior in pelvic pathology. In this chapter the role of the CT scan and MRI in a variety of vascular diseases is reviewed. In many instances, both modalities provide identical information and the selection of the test is based on local factors. At the authors' institution, the CT scan is readily available, whereas the MRI exists in a separate facility. As a result, the majority of the authors' experience has been with the CT scan as opposed to the MRI. This may not be true in other institutions, where the MRI is more readily available. In each clinical application, the relative merits of each technique as well as its drawbacks will be discussed.

BASIC PRINCIPLES

Interpreting images generated by CT and MRI requires an understanding of the physical principles on which they are based. In addition, such knowledge allows the physician to recognize the strengths and limitations of each modality. Rather than attempt an exhaustive explanation of the complexities of each modality, this section presents a conceptual approach to the physics and terminology relevant for the clinician.

Computed Tomography (CT)

The most commonly encountered form of CT is transmission CT. Using a finely collimated x-ray beam, extremely sensitive detectors, and powerful computer workstations, scanners translate measurements of x-ray transmission through a body into an image representing the structure the beam has traversed.[3]

In essence, CT uses the same physical principles as the standard x-ray. An x-ray tube directs a beam of photons of a given energy level (usually 40 to 150 kV) at a body. As the photons pass through the body, some interact with the atoms composing the tissues, leading to a reduction in the strength of the beam (Fig. 6–7). This process of attenuation arises primarily from two types of x-ray interaction with matter, the photoelectric and the Compton effects.

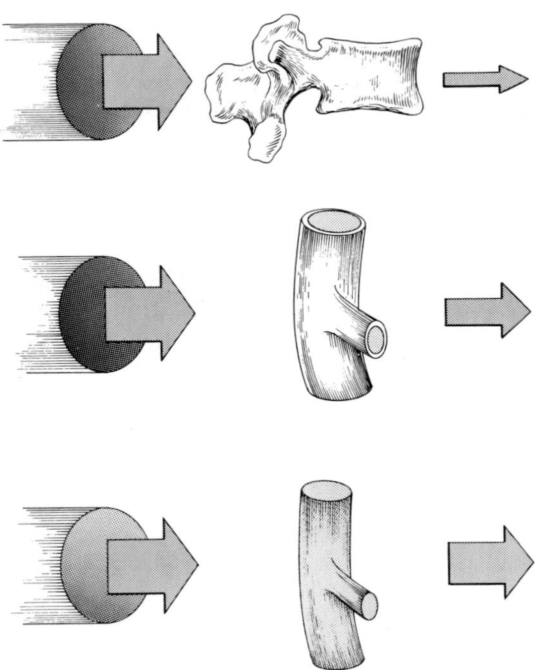

FIGURE 6–7. Attenuation of the photon beam depends on the molecular structure of the tissue traversed. Greater attenuation occurs with dense, mineralized tissue, such as bone.

The photoelectric effect consists of three stages. First, a photon collides with and transfers its energy to an electron in one of the deeper shells of an atom. This added energy allows the electron to escape from its orbit, leaving a vacant spot in that shell. Following this, an electron belonging to an outer shell falls into the void left by the previous electron, thus moving from a higher to a lower energy state and releasing energy in the form of radiation. The probability of a photoelectric interaction occurring depends on the number of protons in the nucleus of an atom. As a result, variations in the type and number of atoms in each tissue yield variations in the degree to which the x-ray beam is attenuated.

The Compton effect occurs when a photon strikes an electron of significantly lower energy, knocking it out of the atom. Instead of being absorbed, the photon imparts a small portion of its energy to the displaced electron and scatters in a direction ranging from 0 to 180 degrees from its initial course. As a result, the photon no longer contributes to the strength of the transmitted beam. The Compton effect varies according to electron density, and because electron density does not vary greatly between tissues, this effect contributes less to attenuation than does the photoelectric effect.

The final step in x-ray imaging involves measuring the degree of attenuation of the original beam. Because the transmitted beam represents the result of the attenuation caused by each tissue through which the beam has passed, a variety of shades are produced. Whereas x-ray relies on a wide beam, CT employs a pencil-thin, collimated beam. The x-ray film gives way to a reusable, extremely sensitive, high-pressure xenon detector, which receives the transmitted beam and converts it to an electrical signal. The electrical signals constitute the raw data from which the computer will reconstruct the CT image.

The ultimate goal of reconstructing an image involves generating a matrix, a rectangular array of elements consisting of rows and columns. To this end, the many contiguous scans through volumes of the same size as the beam are obtained by rotating the x-ray tube and detector around the body. Thus, each image is derived from readings obtained through the same volume at different angles. Each intersection between two readings represents a small volume whose specific attenuation may be derived by analyzing all intersections via a complex algorithm and whose physical position determines its position in the matrix. Having obtained a value for each intersection, or volume element (''voxel''), the computer may assign a gray-scale intensity from black to white to each value and display this image on a monitor. This final image is composed of picture elements (''pixels''), which are a two-dimensional representation of the three-dimensional information from each voxel.

The traditional CT scanner employs an x-ray tube rotating with a series of detectors to generate the data sets. This technology limits the CT scan to individual slices that are not related to the slice immediately above. Two new technologies are available that allow acquisition of a volume data set in which the slices are linked to one another. The spiral CT scan uses a continuous gantry rotation while the patient is advanced through the x-ray beam. This volume data set is obtained rapidly, avoiding motion artifacts such as respiration. By having the data sets linked, it is possible to reconstruct the image in three dimensions. Since this technique is rapid (less than 30 seconds) intravenous contrast injection will produce a CT angiogram (CTA). The ultrafast scanner is another method to obtain volume data sets in a rapid fashion. Instead of using a mechanical device to rotate around the patient, the ultrafast scanner magnetically guides the electron beams circumferentially as the patient passes through the scanner. The ultrafast scanner dramatically reduces scan time and can obtain 32 1-cm slices in 1 second. Each of these technologies allow the generation of data either as a CT angiogram or in three dimensions (Fig. 6–8). The spiral CT and ultrafast CT scanners hold great promise for diagnosing and treating patients with vascular disease. In preliminary studies, these techniques have been valuable in diagnosing abdominal aortic aneurysms, renal artery stenosis, and carotid artery stenosis.[4]

Magnetic Resonance Imaging

MRI resembles CT in that both attempt to characterize the types of tissue contained within small, carefully proscribed volumes. Whereas CT generates data by measuring the attenuation of an x-ray beam, MRI obtains data by measuring the behavior of atoms when subjected to a strong magnetic field. MRI scanners consist of a powerful magnet (typically, 0.5 to 1.5 Tesla), superconducting or permanent, an array of sensors, and a computer workstation for analyzing the received signal and transforming it into the final image.

A magnetic field will affect any atom placed therein; however, only those atoms possessing an odd number of protons or neutrons are capable of generating an MRI signal. Because hydrogen has the highest natural abundance and sensitivity to the MRI signal[5] of all the suitable atoms, MRI scanners use hydrogen nuclei to generate the signal that will form the image.

Each hydrogen atom has a spinning, charged nucleus; as a result, a magnetic dipole moment (MDM) is formed, and the hydrogen nucleus can be considered a tiny bar magnet. When this MDM, or "spin," is placed in a strong magnetic field, it will tend to align itself with the field (Fig. 6–9). The MRI scanner generates a signal by bombarding these aligned spins sequentially with two radiofrequency (RF) pulses whose vectors are perpendicular to one another

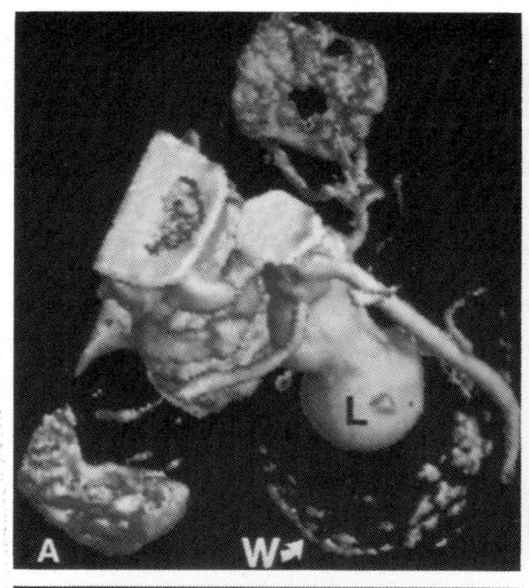

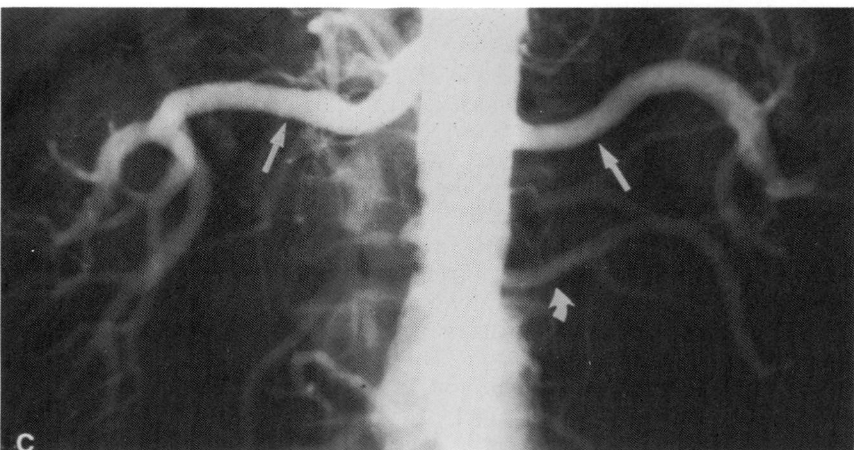

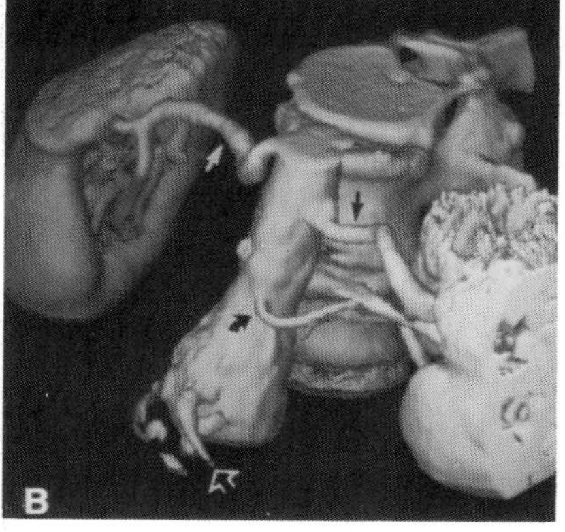

FIGURE 6–8. *A*, Shaded surface display (SSD) image of abdominal aortic aneurysm demonstrates both contrast-filled lumen (L) and mural calcifications (W). *B*, SSD image in another patient with abdominal aortic aneurysm. Although main renal arteries *(straight arrows)* arise above neck of aneurysm, small left accessory artery *(curved arrow)* and patent inferior mesenteric artery arise from posterior aspect of aneurysm. *C*, Conventional aortogram in same patient as in *B*. (From Rubin GD, Napel S, Dake MD, et al: Spiral CT creates 3-D neuro, body angiograms. Diagn Imaging, August, pp 66–69, 72–74, 1992.)

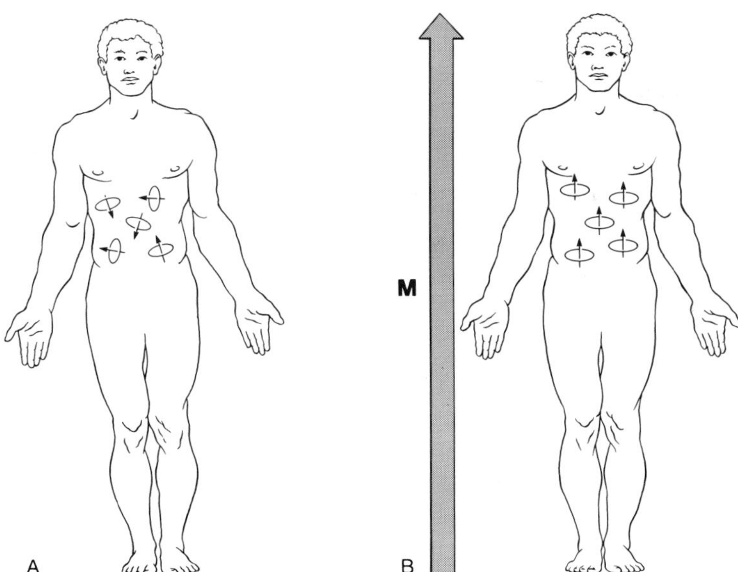

FIGURE 6–9. *A* and *B*, Realignment of the body's hydrogen nuclei when placed in a strong magnetic field (M).

and to the vector of the initial magnetic field. This causes the spins to absorb energy and ''tip'' out of the initial field. As the MDMs begin to realign with the magnetic field, they release the acquired energy in the form of radio signals, which can be received by coils surrounding the portion of the body to be imaged. The strength of this signal depends primarily on two factors, termed T1 and T2 relaxation, which vary across tissues.

T1, or ''spin-lattice,'' relaxation represents the time required for the MDM to lose its excess energy to the surrounding molecules, or lattice, and realign with the magnetic field. Tissues with shorter T1 relaxation times will realign more completely and thus have a greater magnitude when ''tipped'' during the next excitation than those tissues having longer T1 relaxation times (Fig. 6–10). Because the released radio signal depends on the magnitude of the tipped MDM, a shorter T1 implies a stronger or brighter signal.

Absence of irregularities that each spin experiences in the magnetic field results in a more rapid loss of magnetization, T2 relaxation. Immediately following the first 90-degree RF pulse, all MDM vectors spin at the same rate about their origins. Because the pulse aligns them in the same direction, these vectors are ''in phase.'' Variation in the magnetic field an MDM experiences will cause a change in the frequency at which it spins, its rate of precession. Thus, nonuniformities in the magnetic field caused by changes in local chemical environment or irregularities in the macroscopic field strength will vary the rates of precession of the vectors, resulting in a ''dephasing'' of the spins. Overall, this yields a reduction in the net magnetization in the direction of the 90-degree pulse and a consequent reduction in signal. Because this form of relaxation occurs through the interaction of neighboring molecules, it has acquired the name spin-spin relaxation.

Although variation in relaxation times provides the basis for tissue differentiation, the imaging parameters employed for the scan strongly affect the role each relaxation time plays in generating an image. The most important controlled parameters are repetition time (TR) and echo time (TE) of the RF pulse. These parameters, together with other factors such as additional magnetic fields, compose a pulse sequence.

TR represents the time allowed for the tipped spins to relax between two successive RF pulses. Values for TR can range from a few hundred to a few thousand milliseconds. Since a shorter TR will allow less time for relaxation to occur, a tissue with a shorter T1 will repolarize more completely between RF pulses than a tissue with a longer T1 and therefore yield a stronger signal. Such scan sequences are referred to as T1-weighted. A long TR will allow the spins of most atoms to realign, placing the role of tissue contrast on TE.

The time lag between the initial RF pulse and the reading of the radio signal generated by the excited tissue

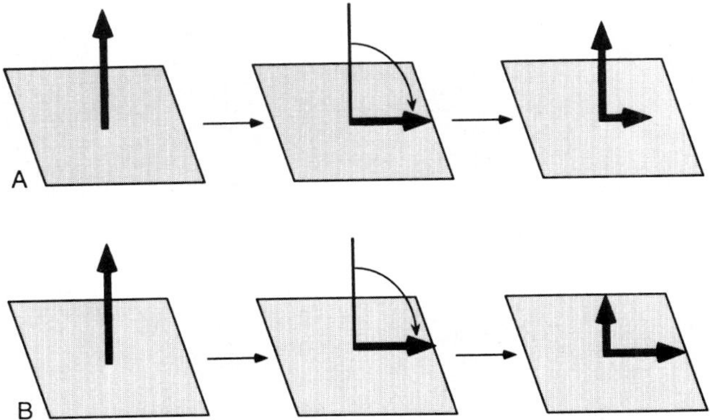

FIGURE 6–10. The ''tipping'' and relaxation of two spins with different T1 values. Initially as well as immediately after being tipped, both spins have equal magnitude. As the spins relax, however, spin *A* regains its magnitude in the z-axis, the original direction of the external magnetic field, more rapidly than spin *B*. Spin *A* represents a tissue with a shorter T1.

constitutes TE. TE has standard values between 15 and 150 msec, significantly less than TR. Given a long TE, tissues possessing a short T2, those consisting of more proteinaceous material, will have lost their energy and appear dark, whereas tissues with a longer T2, such as water, will appear bright. A sequence employing both long TR and long TE results in a heavily T2-weighted image. Using a long TR and short TE yields an image that depends mostly on the proton density of the tissue.[6]

Multiple excitations of each slice yield measurements in the form of radio signals. Receiving coils record this information and pass it to the computer workstation where a complex algorithm involving either two or three Fourier transformations converts information in the form of a wave into a matrix. This matrix receives gray-scale values in a similar manner to the CT matrices, thus providing the recognizable video image.

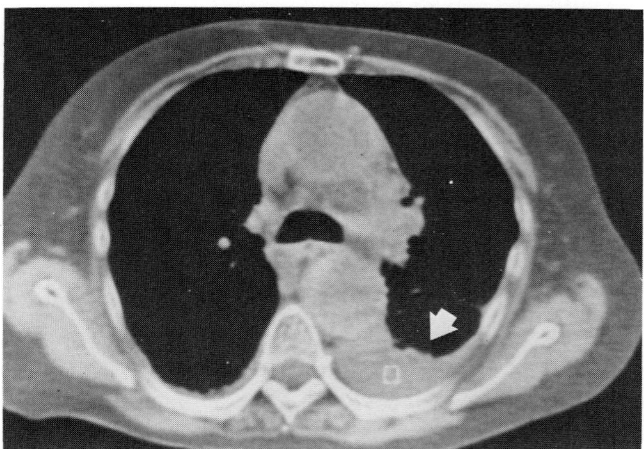

FIGURE 6–12. Aortic dissection with left pleural effusion *(arrow)*.

CLINICAL APPLICATIONS

Thoracic Aorta

The thoracic aorta and brachiocephalic vessels are imaged with either CT or MRI. Until recent years, ultrasound imaging of the thoracic aorta was limited to the ascending aorta because of intrathoracic air. With the introduction of transesophageal echo, the intrathoracic aorta may now be visualized.[7] However, since transesophageal echo is not always available, CT and MRI are more commonly used to diagnose aortic dissection and atherosclerotic thoracic aneurysms. CT appears to be as accurate as aortography in diagnosing aortic dissection.[8,9] CT findings in aortic dissection include two contrast-filled lumens representing the patent true and adjacent false lumen (Fig. 6–11). The channels are separated by a thin band and may appear to rotate as the dissection spirals down the aorta. When the false lumen has thrombosed, enlargement of long aortic segments with crescent soft tissue density may be suggestive of an aortic dissection. Another CT clue may be displacement of calcified plaques between the true and the false lumens. As the dissection occurs, mural calcification is displaced to the center of the aorta. With rupture, a left pleural effusion or atelectasis may be present (Fig. 6–12).

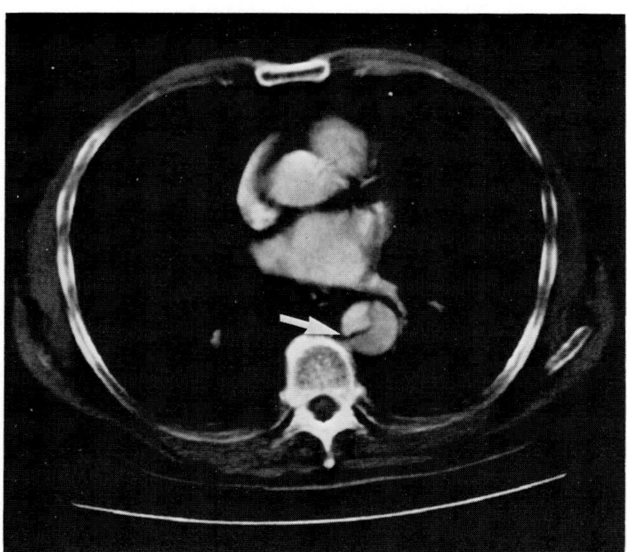

FIGURE 6–11. Aortic dissection with contrast-filled tissue showing true and false lumens separated by displaced intima and media *(arrow)*.

The CT diagnosis of aortic dissection may be difficult when there is insufficient contrast to clearly delineate both lumens or when motion artifacts created by the movement of the heart produce a linear streak that may be interpreted as an intimal flap. Also, calcified plaques appear to be displaced with partial volume averaging. With 10-mm thick slices or with dilating and tortuous vessel, the smaller calcified ring is averaged with a larger calcified ring, producing a calcified artifact within a larger calcified ring. Thinner CT slices resolve this problem.

Like CT, MRI has a similarly high sensitivity and specificity for the diagnosis of aortic dissection.[10–12] When both lumens are patent, flowing blood will produce a double flow void.[11] When there is differential flow, phase shift can be used to display the differences in flow (Fig. 6–13). However, when the false lumen is thrombosed, it may be difficult to diagnose aortic dissection. With the CT scan, displacement of a calcified plaque is seen; however, because calcium is not visualized with MRI, this sign is not useful.

Thoracic atherosclerotic aneurysms appear as a focal or diffuse enlargement of the aorta on CT scanning (Fig. 6–14). The wall is readily identified by intramural calcium. The contrast-filled lumen is surrounded by less dense thrombus. Other findings of aortic aneurysms include erosion of the vertebral body, extravasation of contrast, and pleural effusion. On the other hand, acute traumatic aortic disruptions are not well visualized with either CT or MRI. In these patients, aortography remains essential because aortic diameter may be normal and the intimal flap missed with either CT or MRI. Chronic traumatic aneurysms, such as atherosclerotic aneurysms, are, however, easily identified.

Overall, for thoracic vascular disease, CT is rapidly

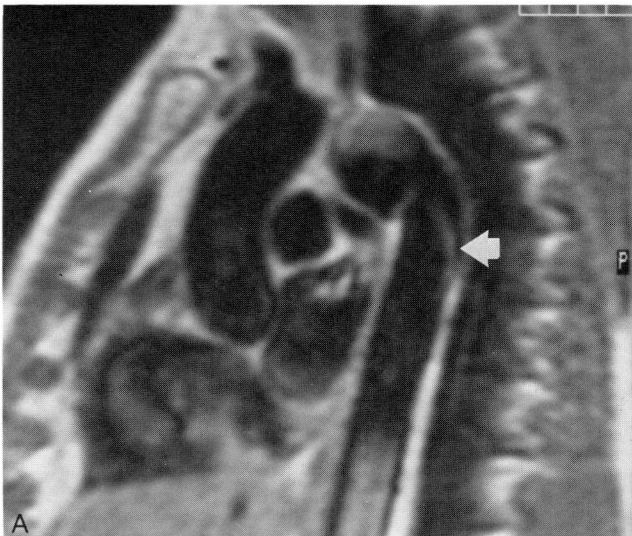

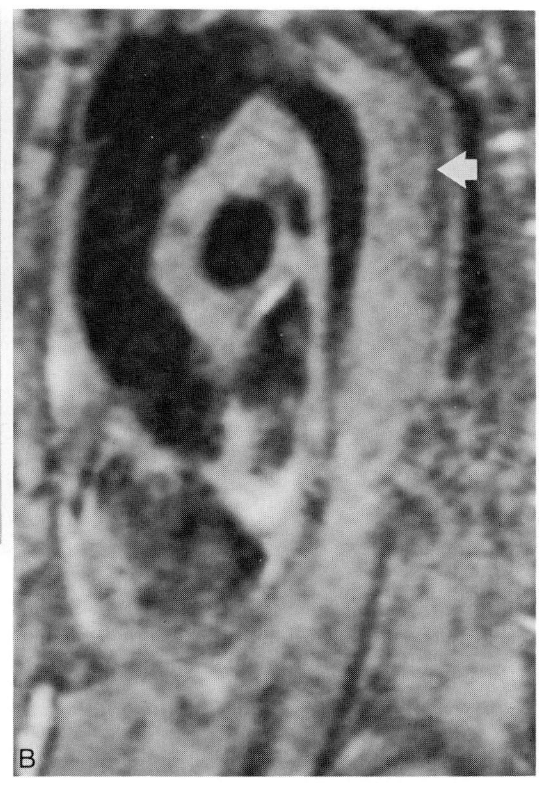

FIGURE 6–13. *A*, Sagittal reconstruction of an aortic dissection originating at the left subclavian *(arrow)* intimal flap. *B*, With phase shift, differential blood flow is demonstrated *(arrow)*.

performed, but requires contrast infusion. Aortic dissections, aneurysms, and intraluminal thrombi are clearly visualized. MRI does not require contrast, accurately depicts flow, and may be reconstructed in many planes. However, long imaging times are required for MRI in potentially unstable patients. CT scanning is rapid with short interscan delay and motion artifact, which may be problematic with MRI, is avoided.

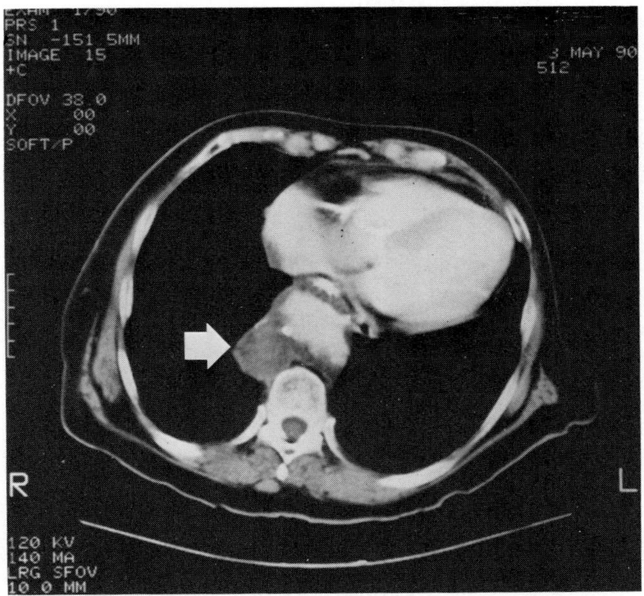

FIGURE 6–14. Thoracic aortic aneurysm appears as a thrombus-filled aortic dilatation *(arrow)*.

Abdominal Aorta and Iliac Vessels

The abdominal aorta from the diaphragm to the iliac bifurcation is also well visualized with either CT or MRI. An abdominal ultrasound is useful to screen patients for abdominal aortic aneurysm (AAA), but for follow-up, further imaging techniques are required prior to surgery (either aortography or CT/MRI). In uncomplicated AAA, CT/MRI are performed on all patients in our practice and aortography is performed selectively. In patients with uncontrolled hypertension, renal failure, complex aneurysms, juxtarenal, supraceliac, and iliac aneurysms, and horseshoe kidneys, aortography is essential (Fig. 6–15).

The characteristic CT findings of AAA are dilatation of the calcified arterial wall. The contrast-filled lumen is surrounded by varying degrees of thrombus that may be irregular in nature.[13–15] Disruption of the calcium with obliteration of adjacent soft tissue may represent rupture. The identification of a chronic contained rupture is particularly helpful in planning a surgical repair (Fig. 6–16).[16] Calcification of the thrombus may occur but must be differentiated from rupture or dissection. Erosion of the vertebral bodies adjacent to the AAA is rare. With CT, associated aortic aneurysms and aneurysms of peripheral vessels are detected. In addition, aneurysms complicated by inflammation or infection may be identified. Inflammatory aortic aneurysms are characterized by thickening of the aortic wall, which enhances with contrast and is adhered to bowel, vena cava, or left renal vein.[17, 18] Mycotic aneurysms appear as eccentric thick aortic walls with intramural air.

Because the treatment of AAA is dependent on size, the normal diameter for a variety of different locations is

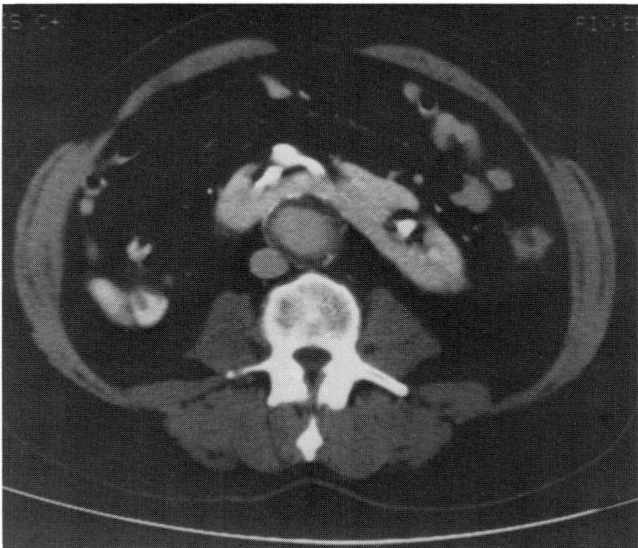

FIGURE 6–15. Congenital anomalies of the kidneys are readily demonstrated with computed tomography (CT). In this patient, the horseshoe kidney and collecting system are positioned directly over the aortic aneurysm.

not known. Few studies have reported normal aortic diameters for selected location. The greatest infrarenal aortic diameter is frequently compared with the diameter of the aorta at the level of the left renal vein. Aortic diameter, though, is dependent on age, gender, and body size.[19–21] Also, the aorta tapers from the thoracic aortic to the bifurcation. Therefore, the absolute measurement of the diameter of the aorta may be of little relevance in a given patient. In practice, the greatest diameter of the aortic aneurysm is compared with the aorta at the level of the left renal vein. A 50 per cent enlargement is considered significant.

CT images of the abdominal aorta also demonstrate major arterial branches including celiac, superior mesenteric, and occasionally renal arteries. Because these vessels are often tortuous, only short segments are seen. However, visceral artery aneurysms are easily detected with CT. Visceral aneurysms, like other aneurysms, are seen as calcified masses that enhance with contrast infusion (Fig. 6–17). For treatment, visceral artery aneurysms still require selective visceral angiography.

The images MRI provides are similar to those of CT.[22–24] However, MRI offers the advantage of sagittal reconstruction to demonstrate the longitudinal extent of the aneurysm. The length of the neck of the aneurysm is often difficult to determine with CT scanning, and aortography is, therefore, necessary. However, with sagittal MRI reconstruction, the relationship of the aneurysm to the renal arteries is better seen. MRI, similar to CT, is able to differentiate inflammatory aneurysms. On T1 images, the thick wall demonstrates an intermediate signal that is slightly higher on T2.

In surgical patients, it is valuable to define associated venous and renal abnormalities. Retroaortic left renal veins, circumaortic renal veins, duplication of the vena cava, and left inferior vena cava are readily seen with both CT and MRI.[25–28] MRI multi-planar reconstruction is not advantageous because these vessels are tortuous. Transaxial views are necessary to image such vessels. CT is also important in diagnosing postoperative complications. Arterial graft infections and anastomotic aneurysms are readily identified with CT scanning. Initially, loculated air is found surrounding aortic graft for up to 4 weeks.[29, 30] Beyond this time, perigraft air may represent infection (Fig. 6–18). Intra-abdominal and groin anastomotic aneurysms appear as other aneurysms with dilatation and laminated thrombus. The presence of subcutaneous air in the groin is suspicious for infection. There is limited experience with MRI in postoperative complication.

Peripheral Arteries

Pathology of the popliteal and femoral arteries is accurately defined by MRI and CT. Arterial diameter, intra-

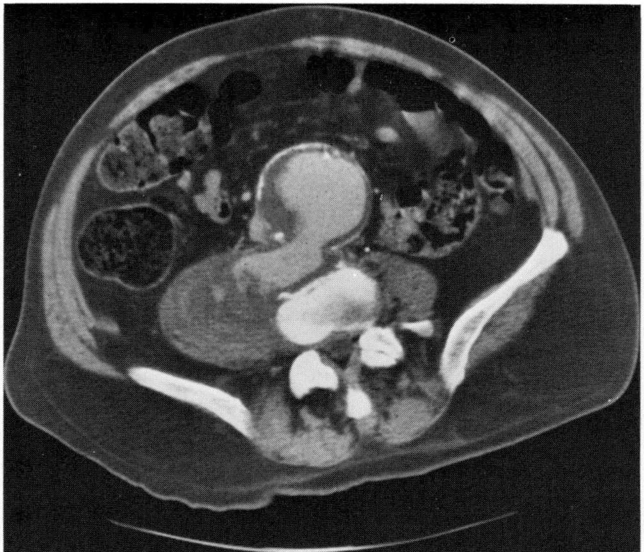

FIGURE 6–16. Large contained rupture of an abdominal aortic aneurysm.

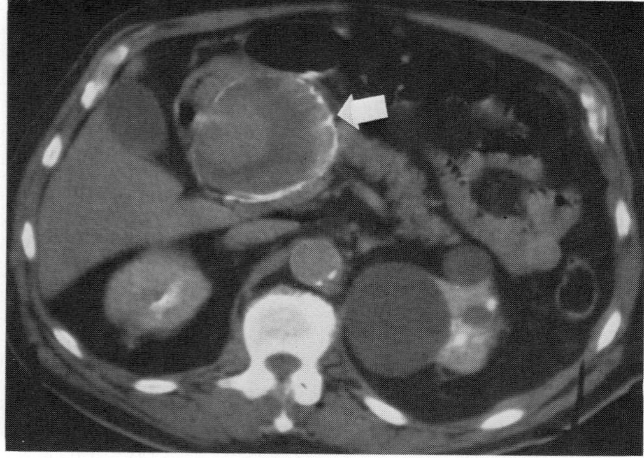

FIGURE 6–17. A pulsatile mass of the upper abdomen is a large hepatic artery aneurysm *(arrow)*.

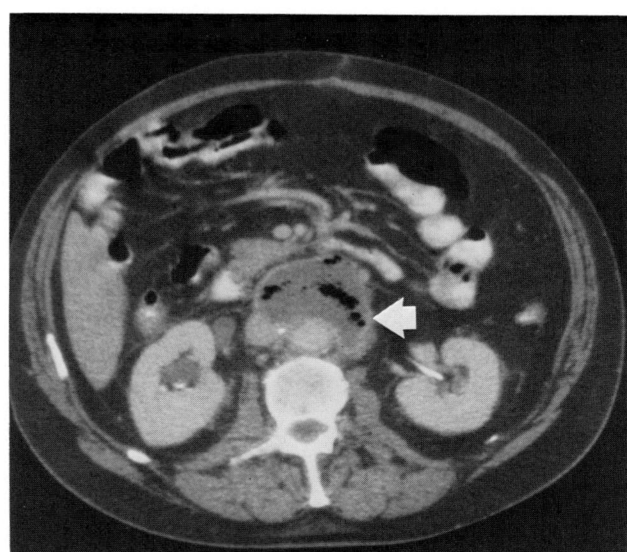

FIGURE 6–18. Loculated air adjunct to a previously placed aortic graft (24-month) *(arrow)*. Enterococcus was cultured at the surgery.

luminal thrombus, and extent can be determined with both techniques. Furthermore, it is important to define adjacent muscle abnormalities in young patients with claudication. When compared with arteriography, CT accurately diagnosed popliteal artery pathology in 98 per cent of 45 popliteal disorders versus 70 per cent diagnosed with arteriography.[31] CT was found to be particularly useful in detecting asymptomatic disease in the contralateral leg in patients with popliteal artery aneurysms or entrapment. Bilateral popliteal aneurysms were identified in 75 per cent of patients as opposed to 37 per cent by arteriography. Associated aneurysmal disease of either the aorta or the femoral artery was found in 60 per cent of all patients. CT findings of entrapment depend on the anatomic variant.[32–34] In the most common variant, the artery and vein are separated by an identifiable muscle band or medial displacement of the lateral head of the gastrocnemius muscle (Fig. 6–19). In type 1 entrapments, there is also medial displacement of the popliteal artery. With MRI, the abnormal musculature is seen passing between the flow voids created by the popliteal artery and vein on the transaxial reconstruction. Adventitial cystic disease appears as fluid-filled eccentric localized dilatation that does not enhance with contrast.[35, 36] It may be difficult to exclude aneurysm formation, but patient age and the discrete abnormality establish the diagnosis. The septa of multi-loculated adventitial cysts may be seen on CT (Fig. 6–20). Interestingly, since MR is preferred in detecting joint pathology, asymptomatic popliteal artery entrapment is identified in the occasional patient.

Vena Cava

Accurate imaging of the inferior vena cava and collateral pathways often require multiple modalities.[37] Both intrinsic and extrinsic diseases produce occlusions of the inferior vena cava. Therefore, vena cavography is combined with either CT or MRI to exclude adjacent malignancy. The CT scan is sensitive for thrombosis and tumor; however, the intrahepatic vena cava is poorly seen. Here vena cavography and MRI are more useful. Because the location of the vena cava is constant, the MRI with multi-planar reconstruction provides more information than CT. However, other venous branches are tortuous and do not lie in a single plane; therefore, MRI offers no advantage over CT.

Using any technique, it is difficult to differentiate vena caval occlusion from thrombosis or tumor invasion from either renal cell carcinoma or primary leiomyosarcomas. In general, a bland thrombosis will not expand the diameter of the vena cava, whereas a thrombus will enlarge the vena cava. MRI may be helpful in differentiating tumor thrombus from bland, but MRI findings are not consistent enough to be sufficiently diagnostic. Hence, cavography remains essential in planning the surgical procedure. Congenital abnormalities of the inferior vena cava and renal veins, although rare, present technical problems that may be recognized preoperatively. Duplication of the cava, circumaortic renal veins, retroaortic left renal veins (Fig. 6–21), and left-sided inferior vena cava are seen on transaxial views and variability on sagittal and coronal reconstructions.

The mesenteric venous system may be visualized by ultrasound, CT, and MRI. The portal, splenic, and superior

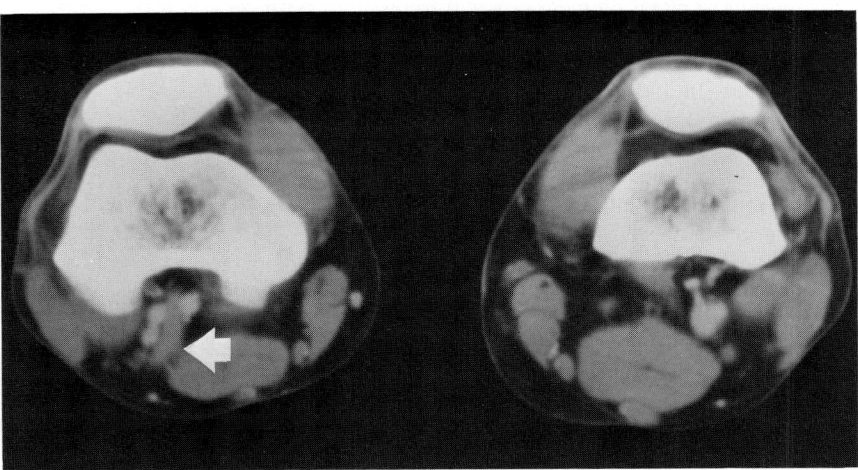

FIGURE 6–19. CT of right popliteal fossa. The peripheral artery and vein are separated by a thick muscular band *(arrow)*.

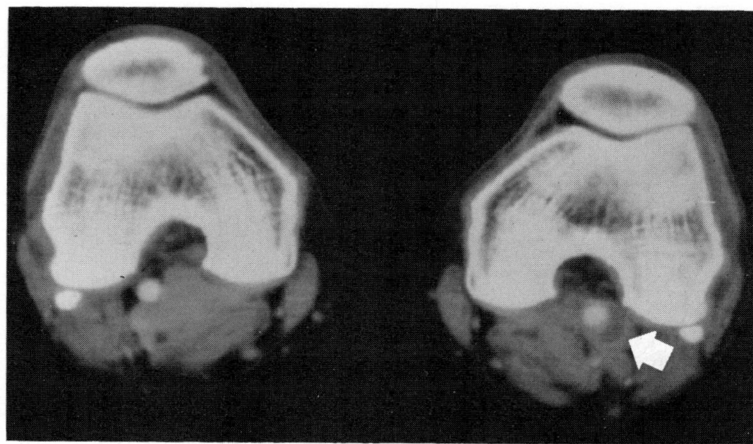

FIGURE 6–20. CT of left popliteal fossa. A small cystic structure surrounds the popliteal artery, which appears to be loculated *(arrow)*.

mesenteric veins may be imaged in the absence of excessive bowel gas. With an acute abdomen and an adynamic ileus, ultrasound imaging of the portal venous system is impossible. Both MRI and CT are sensitive in detecting mesenteric venous thrombosis. The transaxial reconstruction of MRI is most useful and as such does not offer a significant advantage over CT. Since CT is more readily available and is as sensitive, CT remains our diagnostic test of choice in mesenteric venous thrombosis. With mesenteric venous thrombosis, the mesenteric vein is enlarged with a low-density center surrounded by an enhancing wall. In addition, there is marked edema of the mesentery with bowel wall thickening and, rarely, portal air.

Peripheral Veins

Imaging of the deep vein of the legs is best performed using color flow duplex ultrasound or venography. Although CT and MRI will define deep venous thrombosis, these techniques are not cost-effective. However, complex arteriovenous malformations require many different imaging modalities to clearly define the anatomic location and feeding vessels. Arteriography is necessary to delineate the feeding vessels. Arteriography also crudely estimates the degree of arteriovenous shunting. However, arteriography does not define the fascial planes or involvement of adjacent musculoskeletal elements. Not infrequently, with angiography the entire limb segment is filled with contrast, making it difficult to determine accurately the location of these masses. In addition, angiography is particularly difficult to perform in infants. Ascending phlebography and closed-space phlebography are valuable in accurately defining the postcapillary venous dilatation, sinusoids, and isolated venous abnormalities. However, both of these techniques tend to underestimate the full extent of the lesion.

CT scanning with contrast enhancement will identify the location and often demonstrate the specific muscle groups involved. Deep intramuscular lesions give a mottled appearance, and with administration of contrast, there is enhancement that depends on the rate of arteriovenous shunting and the degree of cellularity of the lesions.[38, 39] Congenital vascular malformations that are highly cellular with very little vascular space may not enhance. Here, the CT scan will underestimate the extent of the lesion. Unfortunately, without more sophisticated hardware, CT scanning is performed only in transverse sections. To create sagittal sections, multiple axial images are required. Finally, the optimal technique for administration of the contrast medium by either bolus or constant infusion has yet to be determined.

MRI provides a noninvasive method for assessing the anatomic extent, flow patterns, and cellularity of congenital vascular malformations.[40–42] Of greatest interest to the vascular surgeon is the ability of MRI to image and quantify blood flow. If the signal from the area of interest is received after the pulsed protons in blood have moved out of the field and been replaced by nonpulsed, oriented protons flowing in, no signal will be seen and a black "flow" void will appear in the image. These "black holes" identify high-flow feeding arteries and draining veins in cross-sectional images (Fig. 6–22*A* and *B*). Further, another more sophisticated form of MRI, called even-echo rephasing, allows identification of vessels with slow laminar flow, such as seen in some venous channels. Intravascular thrombus is seen in some cases based on its signal intensity. Venous thrombosis is very different from either rapid flow or slow laminar flow. In addition, highly cellular tumors will produce more signal intensity because of increased water density than will spongy tumors that may be very vascular but

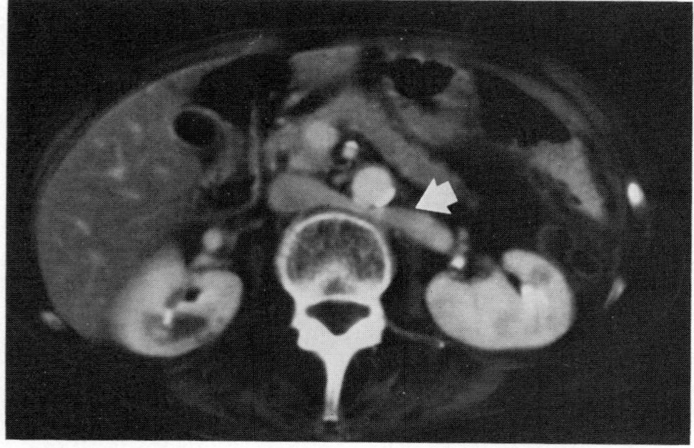

FIGURE 6–21. Retroaortic left renal vein *(arrow)*.

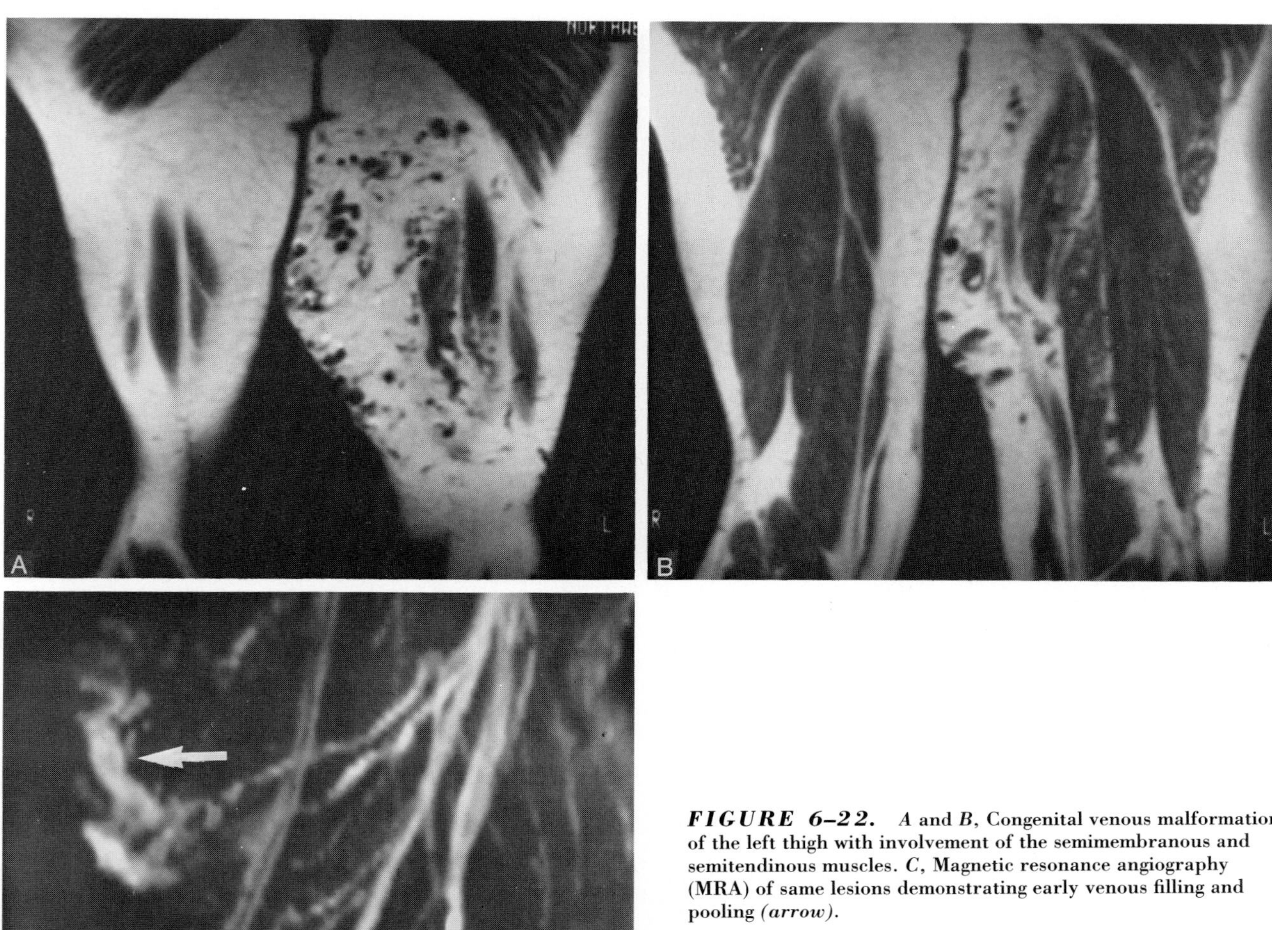

FIGURE 6–22. *A* and *B*, Congenital venous malformation of the left thigh with involvement of the semimembranous and semitendinous muscles. *C*, Magnetic resonance angiography (MRA) of same lesions demonstrating early venous filling and pooling *(arrow)*.

that give less intense signals because of the "flow-void" phenomenon. With magnetic resonance angiography (MRA), both the anatomy and the arterial hemodynamics can be determined (Fig. 6–22*C*). Overall, MRI is highly sensitive in detecting and determining noninvasively the anatomic extent of a CT congenital vascular malformation.

Cerebrovascular Disease

The diagnosis of stroke is made on the basis of history and physical examination. However, the information provided by CT and MRI directs subsequent diagnostic and therapeutic interventions. In symptomatic patients, it is important to distinguish intracranial hemorrhage, ischemic infarcts, and other inflammatory and vascular diseases of the brain. The diagnosis of an ischemic stroke by the CT within the first 24 hours is limited. After 24 hours, the CT scan is positive in the majority of patients who sustain an ischemic infarction.[43–45] During this early period, the MRI is significantly more sensitive than CT in detecting ischemic infarction.[46] MRI is more sensitive than CT for detecting brain stem or cerebellar infarctions. However, CT is more sensitive than MRI in detecting acute intracerebral hemorrhages.[47–49] The characteristic increased intensity seen on T1-weighted MRI requires several days to develop.[50, 51] Although the presence of a mass effect and location of the lesion is helpful, early intracranial hemorrhages are rarely detected with MRI. In later phases, the MRI is better able than CT to distinguish intracranial hemorrhages from infarctions. The MRI remains abnormal for many months as the hematoma reabsorbs, in contrast to the CT scan, which may rapidly return to normal.

In sequential follow-ups of patients with either subarachnoid hemorrhages or ischemic stroke, the MRI appears to be more sensitive and to provide more data involving size and progression of infarct than is CT.

In conclusion, MRI appears to be superior to CT in the detection of early ischemic infarctions. However, the diagnosis of stroke is made on the basis of the history and physical examination. In patients with acute neurologic symptoms, the use of anticoagulants is determined by the presence of an intracranial hemorrhage. Therefore, CT is an essential early study. For natural history studies of stroke and intracranial hemorrhages, MRI is more appropriate. Furthermore, the lack of artifact produced by the skull makes MRI more useful in diagnosing any disease of the brain stem or cerebellum.

COMMENTS

MRI and CT provide anatomic detail important in diagnosing and treating many vascular diseases. Both techniques provide similar information, even though the technology is vastly different. In Table 6–7, the relative merits of each technology are summarized. Depending on the specific equipment, the relative merits of each modality may vary. Accelerating technology is transforming how vascular surgeons diagnose many vascular diseases. New developments in software and hardware will provide three-dimensional images and flow characteristics using both technologies. Currently, MRI is the technique of choice for multiplanar reconstruction. However, with ultrafast CT and spiral CT, three-dimensional reconstruction is possible. With dynamic CT, CT angiography (CTA) is also possible. Therefore, both MRI and CT will provide nearly identical information. Then the choice of using either CT or MRI will depend on other factors related to the institution, patient, and cost.

Local institutional factors play an important role in the decision to use either MRI or CT. CT and MRI development has not been parallel. As such, CT scanners of different generations may be present with advanced, high-quality MRI scans. In this situation, it may be preferable to use MRI. In addition, certain patient factors may determine which technology is to be used. CT continues to require contrast, which may present problems to patients with renal failure and allergic reaction. Although metallic objects produce significant artifacts with CT, the artifacts may be greater with MRI. Patients with large metallic objects or pacemakers are ineligible for MRI. MRI also requires a long imaging time, which in certain patients is uncomfortable and not well tolerated. A final consideration is the cost of each examination. If there is no clear advantage of one technique over the other, CT is less expensive than MRI. Therefore, in deciding which modality to use, it is first necessary to determine whether the information provided by MRI or CT is significantly different from the other. If the data are comparable, other factors such as locale, patient tolerance, and cost become important considerations.

Table 6–7. CT Versus MRI

Feature	Advantage
Resolution	CT*
Reconstruction	MRI/spiral CT
Directional flow	MRI/CTA
Noncontrast	MRI
Low cost	CT
Patient factors	CT
Variation in tissue density	MRI
Calcification	CT
Intracranial	
Intracranial hemorrhage (early)	CT
Ischemic stroke (early)	MRI
Brain stem/cerebellum	MRI

**Conventional CT (512 × 512 matrix) versus conventional MRI (256 × 256 matrix)*

Key: *CTA, CT angiography.*

References

1. Hounsfield GN: Computerized transverse axial scanning (tomography). Part I. Description of system. Br J Radiol 46:1016, 1973.
2. Lauterbur PC: Image formation by induced local interactions: Examples employing nuclear magnetic resonance. Nature 247:190, 1973.
3. Morgan CL: Basic Principles of Computed Tomography. Baltimore, University Park Press, 1983.
4. Kalender WA, Seissler W, Klotz E, Vock P: Spiral volumetric CT with single-breath-hold technique, continuous transport, and continuous scanner rotation. Radiology 176:181, 1990.
5. Edelman RR, Hesselink JR: Clinical Magnetic Resonance Imaging. Philadelphia, WB Saunders, 1990.
6. Riles TS, Litt AW: Magnetic resonance angiography. *In* Yao JST, Pearce WH (eds): Technologies in Vascular Surgery. Philadelphia, WB Saunders, 1992.
7. Erbel R, Engberding R, Daniel W, et al: Echocardiography in the diagnosis of aortic dissection. Lancet 1:P457, 1984.
8. Farmer DW, Moore E, Amparo E, et al: Calcific fibrosing mediastinitis: Demonstration of pulmonary vascular obstruction by magnetic resonance imaging. AJR 143:1189, 1984.
9. Thorsen MK, San Dretto MA, Lawson TL, et al: Dissecting aortic aneurysm: Accuracy of computed tomographic diagnosis. Radiology 148:773, 1983.
10. Amparo EG, Higgins CB, Hricak H, Sollitto R: Aortic dissection: Magnetic resonance imaging. Radiology 155:399, 1985.
11. Dinsmore RE, Wedeen VJ, Miller SW, et al: MRI of dissection of the aorta: Recognition of the intimal tear and differential flow velocities. AJR 147:1286, 1986.
12. Geisinger MA, Risius B, O'Donnel JA, et al: Thoracic aortic dissections: Magnetic resonance imaging. Radiology 155:407, 1985.
13. Mark AS, McCarthy SM, Moss AA, et al: Detection of abdominal aortic graft infection: Comparison of CT and In-labeled white blood cell scans. AJR 144:315, 1985.
14. Gomes NM, Hufnagel CA: CT scanning: A new method for the diagnosis of abdominal aortic aneurysms. J Cardiovasc Surg 20:511, 1979.
15. Papanicolaou N, Wittenberg J, Ferrucci JT Jr, et al: Preoperative evaluation of abdominal aortic aneurysms by computed tomography. AJR 146:711, 1986.
16. Flinn WR, Courtney DF, Yao JST, et al: Contained rupture of aortic aneurysm. *In* Bergan JJ, Yao JST (eds): Aortic Surgery. Philadelphia, WB Saunders, 1989, pp 341–350.
17. Ramirez AA, Rioles TS, Imparato AM, et al: CAT scans of inflammatory aneurysms: A new technique for preoperative diagnosis. Surgery 91:390, 1982.
18. Wadlington VR, Nemcek AA, Vogelang RL, et al: CT and MR imaging of inflammatory abdominal aortic aneurysms. RNSA 185(P):258, 1992.
19. Liddington MI, Heather BP: The relationship between aortic diameter and body habitus. Eur J Vasc Surg 6:89, 1992.
20. Mohiaddin RH, Schoser K, Amanuma M, et al: MR imaging of age-related dimensional changes of thoracic aorta. J Comput Assist Tomogr 14:748, 1990.
21. Horejs D, Gilbert PM, Burstein S, et al: Normal aortoiliac diameters by CT. J Comput Assist Tomogr 12:602, 1988.
22. Evancho AM, Osbakken M, Weidner W: Comparison of NMR imaging and aortography for preoperative evaluation of abdominal aortic aneurysm. Magn Reson Med 2:41, 1985.
23. Flak B, Li DKB, Ho BYB, et al: Magnetic resonance imaging of aneurysms of the abdominal aorta. AJR 144:991, 1985.
24. Lee JKT, Ling D, Heiken JP, et al: Magnetic resonance imaging of abdominal aortic aneurysms. AJR 143:1197, 1984.

25. Reed MD, Friedman AC, Nealey P: Anomalies of the left renal vein: Analysis of 433 CT scans. J Comput Assist Tomogr 6:1124, 1982.
26. Royal SA, Callen PW. CT evaluation of anomalies of the inferior vena cava and left renal vein. AJR 132:750, 1979.
27. Hricak H, Amparo E, Fisher MR, et al: Abdominal venous system: Assessment using MRI. Radiology 156:415, 1985.
28. Bartle EJ, Pearce WH, Sun JH, et al: Infrarenal venous anomalies and aortic surgery: Avoiding vascular injury. J Vasc Surg 6:590, 1987.
29. O'Hara PJ, Borkowski GP, Hertzer NR, et al: Natural history of periprosthetic air on computerized axial tomographic examination of the abdomen following abdominal aortic aneurysm repair. J Vasc Surg 1:429, 1984.
30. Qvarfordt PG, Reilly LM, Mark AS, et al: Computerized tomographic assessment of graft incorporation after aortic reconstruction. Am J Surg 150:227, 1985.
31. Rizzo RJ, Flinn WR, Yao JST, et al: Computed tomography for evaluation of arterial disease in the popliteal fossa. J Vasc Surg 11:112, 1990.
32. Williams LR, Flinn WR, Yao JST, et al: Extended use of computed tomography in the management of complex aortic problems: A learning experience. J Vasc Surg 4:264, 1986.
33. Muller N, Morris DC, Nichols DM: Popliteal artery entrapment demonstrated by CT. Radiology 151:157, 1984.
34. Williams LR, Flinn WR, McCarthy WJ, et al: Popliteal artery entrapment: Diagnosis by computed tomography. J Vasc Surg 3:360, 1986.
35. Wilbur AC, Spigos DG: Adventitial cyst of the popliteal artery: CT-guided percutaneous aspiration. J Comput Assist Tomogr 10:161, 1986.
36. Fitzjohn TP, White FE, Loose HW, et al: Computed tomography and sonography of cystic adventitial disease. Br J Radiol 59:933, 1986.
37. Sonin AH, Mazer MJ, Powers TA: Obstruction of the inferior vena cava: A multiple-modality demonstration of causes, manifestations, and collateral pathways. Radiographics 12:309, 1992.
38. Rauch RF, Silverman PM, Korobkin M, et al: Computed tomography of benign angiomatous lesions of the extremities. J Comput Assist Tomogr 8:1143, 1984.
39. Bernardino ME, Jing BS, Thomas JL, et al: The extremity soft-tissue lesion: A comparative study of ultrasound, computed tomography and xeroradiography. Radiology 189:53, 1981.
40. Pearce WH, Rutherford RB, Whitehill TA, et al: Nuclear magnetic resonance imaging: Its diagnostic value in patients with congenital vascular malformations. J Vasc Surg 8:64, 1988.
41. Cohen JM, Weinreb JC, Redman HC: Arteriovenous malformations of the extremities: MR imaging. Radiology 158:475, 1986.
42. Amparo EG, Higgins CB, Hricak H: Primary diagnosis of abdominal arteriovenous fistula by MR imaging. J Comput Assist Tomogr 8:1140, 1984.
43. Wall S, Brant-Zawadski M, Jeffrey R, et al: High-frequency CT findings within 24 hours after cerebral infarction. AJR 138:307, 1982.
44. Tatemichi TK, Mohr JP, Rubinstein LV, et al: CT findings and clinical course in acute stroke: The NINCDS Pilot Stroke Data Bank. Stroke 16:138, 1985.
45. Wall SK, Brant-Zawadzki M, Jeffrey RB, et al: High frequency CT findings within 24 hours after cerebral infarction. AJNR 2:553, 1981.
46. Black SE, Helpern JA, Kertesz AS, et al: Nuclear magnetic resonance imaging and spectroscopy in stroke. *In* Moore WS (ed): Surgery for Cerebrovascular Disease. New York, Churchill Livingstone, 1987, pp 217–253.
47. Dolinskas C, Bilaniuk L, Zimmerman R, et al: Computed tomography of intracerebral hematomas. I. Transmission CT observations on hematoma resolution. AJR 129:681, 1977.
48. Dolinskas C, Bilaniuk L, Zimmerman R, et al: Computed tomography of intracerebral hematomas. II. Radionuclide and transmission CT studies of the perihematoma region. AJR 129:689, 1977.
49. Bentson JR: Computed tomography of stroke. *In* Moore WS (ed): Surgery for Cerebrovascular disease. New York, Churchill Livingstone, 1987, pp 201–216.
50. DeLaPaz RL, New PFJ, Buonanno FS, et al: NMR imaging of intracranial hemorrhage. J Comput Assist Tomogr 8:599, 1984.
51. Swensen SJ, Keller PL, Berquist TH, et al: Magnetic resonance imaging of hemorrhage. AJR 145:921, 1985.

Magnetic Resonance Angiography

Gary R. Caputo, M.D., Charles M. Anderson, M.D., Ph.D., and David Saloner, Ph.D.

• • •

The term magnetic resonance angiography (MRA) does not describe a specific technique but rather a wide variety of methods for studying blood vessels and blood flow in the body using magnetic resonance imaging (MRI). These techniques range from standard cardiac gated spin-echo images of the heart and aorta to three-dimensional time-of-flight angiograms of the carotid arteries to phase mapping blood velocity measurements of the portal vein. Magnetic resonance has proved to be a very flexible method for the investigation of vascular disorders, particularly since the vascular space, the vessel wall, the end-organ, as well as the blood motion itself may be visualized using proper sequences.[1–28]

It is important to recognize that MRA can be dissimilar to conventional contrast x-ray angiography (XRA). The degree of similarity depends on blood flow conditions and well-chosen acquisition parameters. Although MRA and XRA might be strikingly similar in carotid arteries with moderate to severe disease, they may appear different in more slowly flowing vessels, such as the internal carotid in the vicinity of a critical lesion, or in a distal extremity vessel.

It is important to understand the strengths and limitations of MRA viewed as a unique modality rather than as a substitution for conventional angiography methods.

Comparison With Doppler Ultrasound and Conventional Angiography

The first question the surgeon must ask is: How does MRA compare with the traditional modalities of Doppler ultrasound and XRA in the detection and staging of vascular diseases?

Ultrasound is readily available and inexpensive. Its two chief limitations are that it does not provide a three-dimensional image of a blood vessel nor can one find suitable acoustic access to many vessels of interest in the body.

For example, the carotid bifurcation is usually well seen by ultrasound, yet one cannot directly visualize the origins of the carotid arteries, the distal internal carotid arteries, or the circle of Willis. Therefore a screening examination based on ultrasound alone might be incomplete for surgical purposes. Ultrasound is also highly operator-dependent, with skilled technologists providing more reliable information than the novice.

The weaknesses of ultrasound as a noninvasive screening examination are complemented by MRA. MRA can access virtually any vessel in the body, such as the carotid artery from the arch to the circle of Willis, and is not obscured by overlying bone, bowel gas, adipose tissue, or dense vascular calcifications. It displays vessel anatomy as a rotatable three-dimensional angiogram that can be readily interpreted by those who did not perform the study.[29, 30] Like ultrasound, it can be used to measure blood flow volumes and blood velocity, although it lacks the temporal resolution of Doppler devices.

MRA has other attributes that also complement XRA. Unlike XRA, it is noninvasive and may be safely applied to patients with compromised renal function or severe contrast allergies. There is no danger of emboli as might occur with catheter manipulation during XRA. Unlike XRA, in MRA one must choose between fine detail and coverage over a large area. That is, in MRA one may do a coarse survey over a large field of view or a fine-resolution study of a small field of view. In comparison, XRA can provide high detail of the aorta and the lower extremity vessels in a run-off arteriogram.

A weakness of XRA has been abdominal venography. Large volumes of contrast must be injected in visceral arteries in order to opacify the splenic and portal veins. With MRA, these vessels may be quickly examined with high-image contrast.

Vascular Problems Amenable to MRA

Based on preliminary clinical evaluation, and keeping in mind the relative strengths of the imaging modalities, we can identify several areas in which MRA plays a contributory role. These include:

- Heart disease, especially congenital heart disease, cardiac function studies, and coronary artery occlusion.
- The aorta, including intravascular anatomy as well as the detection of dissection, leak, and rupture, and graft infection.
- Detection and grading of carotid artery stenosis.
- Detection of proximal intracranial aneurysms, vascular malformations, and detection of intracranial hemorrhage.
- Abdominal and thigh venography including studies of deep venous thrombosis, portal vein velocities and thrombosis, and imaging of collateral vessels.
- Screening of proximal renal arteries for stenosis.
- Examination of lower extremity trifurcation vessels and grafts for patency and measurements of blood flow (e.g., runoff visualization beyond a proximal obstruction).

This list encompasses a wide variety of applications that are of interest to the vascular surgeon.

Contraindications to MRA

There are several situations in which MRA is likely to be unsuccessful.

Patients who require intensive monitoring or mechanical respiration are difficult to study by MRA because of poor access to the patient and because of the need to use specialized monitoring and respiratory equipment that does not generate RF frequency noise and is not attracted by the magnet. It is generally more convenient to study these patients by other modalities.

Patients who are claustrophobic will require sedation before the study. Again, these patients might be more conveniently studied by a different modality.

Patients must be able to hold still for approximately 4 to 8 minutes at a time, otherwise the images will be considerably degraded. Images are also degraded by the presence of small pieces of metal in the body near the vessel of interest. This includes surgical clips and small fragments from surgical instruments. Hemostatic clips placed around a carotid endarterectomy graft or near a portocaval shunt will distort the appearance of those structures and render an interpretation impossible.

Patients with intracranial aneurysm clips or cardiac pacemakers are excluded from having MR studies.

TECHNIQUES FOR MRA

MRI is a flexible modality in that new software is constantly being created to image different physical properties of vessels and tissues. Several techniques are well established and are certain to be in use for many years. These include the traditional spin-echo method, which is usually associated with the term MRI, as well as the gradient recalled echo (GRE) method and new angiographic methods including time-of-flight (TOF) and phase-contrast (PC).

Spin-Echo

Spin-echo, although it does not produce an angiogram per se, is often used to answer vascular questions.[31] It is the method most frequently used to study the heart and aorta and to evaluate hemorrhage and trauma in the extremities. It can be acquired as either a so-called T1-weighted or a T2-weighted image. These two weightings have different image appearance. On a T1-weighted image, intravascular blood usually appears dark, and hemorrhage greater than a few days old appears bright. T1-weighted images of the heart and aorta can unveil complex anatomy. Unlike conventional angiography, one sees the surrounding tissues as well as the vascular space. For example, it can visualize the true size of an aneurysm, even if it is mostly thrombosed. A T1-weighted spin-echo image is most similar to CT in its information content.

As a T2-weighted image, MRI is most often applied to study perigraft fluid and graft infection.

Cine Gradient Recalled Echo Imaging

Cardiac-triggered acquisition of the heart and aorta is best performed with the so-called gradient recalled echo (GRE) method. Eight to 16 images are acquired through the cardiac cycle; then played as a cine loop to show cardiac wall or blood motion.[13, 32–37] These studies provide not only functional information but may also be the best method for detecting moving structures such as atrial myxomas and pedunculated thrombus that may not be conspicuous on nontriggered studies.

Time-of-Flight

TOF is the most commonly applied method for angiography in most parts of the body. It is relatively simple to understand. The common artifacts and limitations of TOF derive directly from its mechanism. Therefore, it is useful to consider the basics of how this sequence works.

The Mechanism of TOF

TOF can be acquired as a series of two-dimensional, or as one or several three-dimensional acquisitions.[2, 6] We will consider the two-dimensional case first. Protons, including those in blood, which are pulsed rapidly and repeatedly by radio waves, lose their magnetization and therefore lose their signal on MRI. This process of suppressing the signal of tissues is called saturation. Tissues that have not been pulsed for several seconds recover their magnetization and again appear bright on MRI. This process is called relaxation. The strategy of TOF is to pulse radio waves into a slice so that it becomes dark. Blood outside of the slice is bright, and as it is carried into the slice it remains bright for several pulses before it too becomes suppressed. The process of carrying bright vascular signals into a dark slice is called in-flow phenomena. Vessels appear as bright disks where they traverse the slice. After one thin slice has been acquired, a second adjacent slice is obtained. This process is repeated sequentially until the region of interest has been covered. After the slices are all acquired, the bright disks that represent the blood vessels are then stacked up and projected to provide an angiogram-like image. The brightness of the vessels is directly dependent on the rate at which blood enters the slice. That is to say that contrast is velocity-dependent.

In its three-dimensional form, blood flow plays an even more important role. Relaxed blood must enter not a single thin slice, but rather a slab several centimeters thick. Three-dimensional TOF is best suited for relatively rapid velocity vessels such as the carotid and intracranial arteries. The choice of two-dimensional or three-dimensional TOF is important because each has different advantages. Generally speaking, two-dimensional TOF is more sensitive to slow flow and can better be used to differentiate very slow flow from complete thrombosis. The three-dimensional method provides finer resolution and better sensitivity to flow in multiple directions, such as occurs in a tortuous vessel, and better contrast in turbulent flow situations. The flip angle in the acquired slice should be adjusted so as to minimize pulsatility artifact while achieving the greatest background suppression possible. Usually this is between 15 and 45 degrees. However, it will vary from instrument to instrument. The repetition time should be at least 35 msec and could be as high as 50 msec in slow-flow situations.[38]

Phase-Contrast

The weakness of the TOF method is that the radio wave pulses used to suppress background also suppress blood signal. The PC method was devised to eliminate this problem.[8] In PC, the background is eliminated without substantially saturating blood. Two or more images are obtained at each position. In one, the direction (or phase) of the magnetization is altered in a certain sense according to the velocity of blood flow. In the second image, the direction is altered in the opposite sense. In stationary tissues, there is no change in the direction of magnetization. When the magnetization of the two acquisitions is subtracted as vectors, stationary tissue disappears and moving tissue has a brightness dependent on its velocity. As one might imagine, the PC method has shown good results in slow-flowing situations such as the dural venous sinuses and small collateral vessels. It has three disadvantages with respect to TOF. First, the time of the study is more prolonged; second, one must have an idea of the blood velocity before the acquisition begins; and third, the sequence is more prone to artifact from turbulent blood flow. PC also requires an MRA instrument with good eddy current compensation.

INSTRUMENT CONSIDERATIONS

A number of instrument-specific factors affect image appearance in an MRA study. For this reason, the most favorable protocol for obtaining an MRA of a specific vascular territory will vary from one system to another.

Field Strength

The signal:noise ratio in an MRA study improves with increasing field strength. Whereas high-field MRA systems operate at 1.5 Tesla, acceptable MRA has been shown on 1 and 0.5 Tesla systems. MRA on mid-field systems might require signal averaging and increased scan time.

MRA techniques generally work by producing images with high signal strength from flowing blood and low signal strength from the surrounding stationary tissue. Protons attached to lipids and protons attached to free water have slightly different resonant conditions, and the signal strength from stationary tissue containing a mixture of both will depend on the echo time of the sequence. The desired echo time, namely that at which the background signal is at a minimum, will in turn depend on the field strength of the machine.

Gradient Strength

Spatial localization is achieved using magnetic field gradients. In order to properly encode the position and account for the motion of flowing spins, the gradients must be rapidly varied. Gradients that can be adjusted rapidly, that can be applied with strong spatial variation, that have well-defined spatial variations, and that do not generate secondary magnetic field disturbances (eddy currents) are important for high-quality MRAs. These gradient features can be used to produce short echo time sequences that generate images unaffected by flow disturbances.[39]

Radiofrequency Coils

Transmission and reception of RF excitation is provided by RF coils. The most suitable design of these coils depends on the anatomy of interest. Each manufacturer provides a variety of coils so that all body parts can be imaged. Although MRA and MRI both demand sensitive coils, the coil requirements for MRA differ somewhat from those of routine clinical MRI. For example, in studies of the carotid bifurcation, it is desirable to have a coil that provides both RF transmission and reception and in which the sensitive volume of the coil can be placed over the bifurcation. Transmit/receive coils provided by manufacturers for imaging of the head and neck typically image the bifurcation at the edge of the sensitive volume. Coil placement by the technologist can significantly affect the quality of the MRA. Dedicated coil designs for MRA studies are currently under development and these should further contribute to an improvement in the quality of MRA studies.[40–42]

THE HEART

MRA is a completely noninvasive technique using no ionizing radiation or contrast media for imaging the heart. Various MRI techniques are utilized, depending on whether demonstration of anatomic or functional abnormalities is the primary goal. Anatomic abnormalities are best demonstrated with electrocardiogram (ECG) gated spin-echo techniques, which provide static images with high signal:noise ratios. Gradient refocused techniques using shallow flip angles (less than 90 degrees) can achieve temporal resolutions of 30 frames per cardiac cycle and are therefore most effective for demonstrating ventricular contractile function.[43]

Orthogonal imaging planes (transverse, sagittal, and coronal) are used to show cardiac anatomy, and images along the cardiac axes are acquired for measurement of cardiac dimensions and derivation of functional parameters. The plane most often used for cardiac quantitation is referred to as the short-axis plane, which is perpendicular to a plane transecting the mid-point of the aortic valve and apex of the left ventricle (long-axis plane) (Fig. 6–23). Short-axis imaging requires a two-step angulation of the slice-selective gradient relative to the orthogonal axes[44] and, consequently, increases total imaging time.

Natural high contrast between the blood pool and the myocardium is obtained by both spin-echo and GRE techniques. Spin-echo techniques represent flowing blood as a signal void, and the continual entry of saturated spins into the imaging planes results in the bright signal seen with GRE techniques. Flow abnormalities within the blood pool cause increased signal intensity when spin-echo techniques

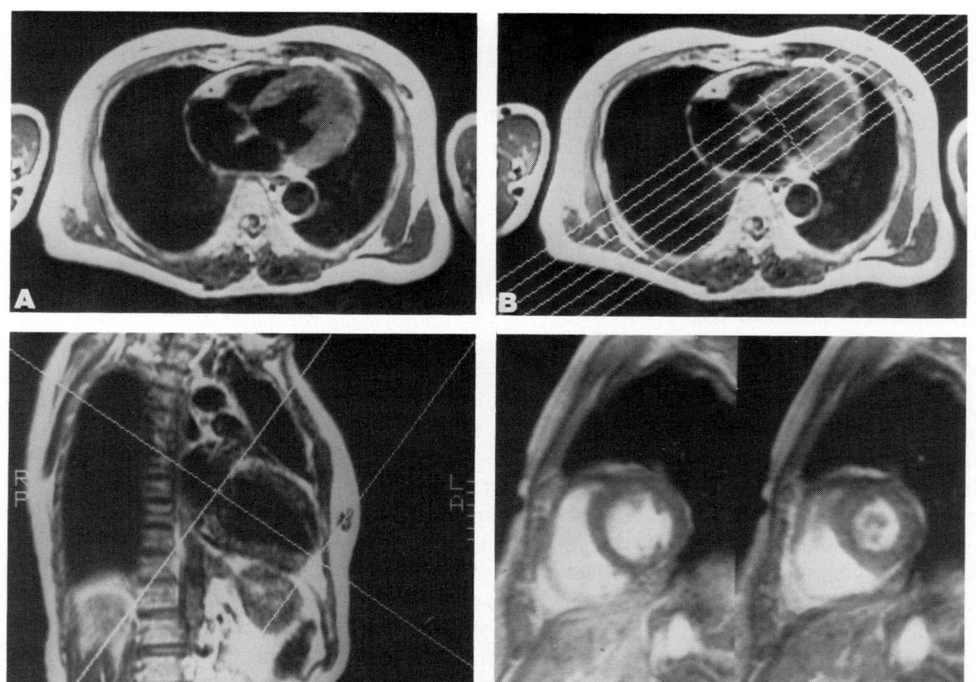

FIGURE 6–23. *A*, Transaxial electrocardiogram (ECG)–gated magnetic resonance imaging (MRI) of the heart at mid-ventricular level. *B*, Slice-selective gradient reorientation *(lines)* superimposed on *A* (long-axis image through left atrium and left ventricle). *C*, Long-axis image used to reorient slice-selective gradient to short-axis plane. Parallel lines passing through atrioventricular valve plane and apex are perpendicular to third line coinciding with long axis of left ventricle. *D*, *Left*, Short-axis cine MRI at end-diastole. *Right*, Short-axis cine MRI at end-systole. Note the increase in wall thickness and the decrease in chamber size that occur between end-diastole and end-systole. LA, left anterior; RP, right posterior. (*A–D*, From Caputo GR, Higgins CB: Advances in cardiac imaging modalities: Magnetic resonance, fast computed tomography, and positron emission tomography. Invest Radiol 25:838–854, 1990.)

are used[45] and a focal signal void within the high-intensity blood pool on GRE techniques.[46, 47]

Evaluation of Pathoanatomy With MRI

Many cardiac abnormalities have been effectively evaluated with MRI.[48–72] These include intracardiac thrombus,[48, 49] intracardiac and paracardiac tumors,[48–52] ischemic heart disease,[53–55] cardiomyopathy,[56, 57] pericardial disease,[58–60] congenital heart disease,[61–64] and thoracic aortic disease.[65–69]

The primary diagnostic imaging technique for the evaluation of ischemic heart disease has been cardiac scintigraphy. However, MRI has demonstrated complications of myocardial infarction, such as intraventricular thrombus, as well as true and false aneurysms of the left ventricle.[54] In the future, MRI may demonstrate residual myocardium in a region of previous infarct; coronary artery bypass graft patency; and regional myocardial perfusion using MRI contrast agents.[73]

Two-dimensional echocardiography is the diagnostic technique most frequently used to evaluate cardiomyopathies. MRI is capable of showing the distribution and extent of hypertrophied muscle in patients with hypertrophic cardiomyopathy and has been particularly useful in the evaluation of variant forms.[74]

MRI may be considered the primary diagnostic modality for the evaluation of pericardial disease, especially constrictive pericarditis, paracardiac and intracardiac masses, thoracic aortic disease, and certain forms of congenital heart disease. MRI has effectively characterized various pericardial diseases.[58–60] Direct visualization of the pericardium is possible,[59] enabling the diagnosis of constrictive pericarditis to be made on the basis of pericardial thickness (greater than 4 mm).[58] The major differential diagnostic consideration is restrictive cardiomyopathy, which has characteristic atrial chamber signal intensity and enlargement, out of proportion to ventricular size.[57] Although echocardiography remains the technique of choice for evaluating pericardial effusions, pericardial hematoma can be specifically identified by MRI by its characteristic signal intensity (Fig. 6–24).

Intracardiac thrombi[48] and tumors[50–52] are effectively demonstrated using MRI. Both primary and metastatic tumors to the heart, as well as mediastinal tumors invading cardiovascular structures, have been effectively demonstrated by MRI.[75] An MRI examination is most often requested when an intracardiac hyperechoic area is demonstrated by echocardiography, raising the question of the presence of a mass. One study[48] found that in every instance when an intracardiac mass was suspected on echocardiography, MRI confirmed the presence of a mass or demonstrated an anatomic abnormality that mimicked an intracardiac mass on echocardiography. In some cases, MRI showed a normal study that was confirmed by clinical follow-up. Several patients diagnosed as having tumor by echocardiography were ultimately found not to have tumor on follow-up MRI examination, demonstrating MRI's role in excluding false-positive echocardiographic examinations.

In many congenital heart lesions, MRI remains a secondary diagnostic technique to echocardiography. However, it may obviate the need for invasive angiography because of its ability to precisely demonstrate cardiac anatomy. In many instances, when MRI follows echocardiography in place of angiography in the evaluation of congenital heart disease, it is less expensive and less invasive and at least as effective. MRI can be considered the technique of choice in the preoperative and postoperative evaluation of aortic arch[68, 69] and pulmonary arterial anomalies (Fig. 6–25).[71]

MRI has become the primary diagnostic technique for the evaluation of thoracic aortic disease.[66, 67] In the presence of aortic dissection, MRI clearly demonstrates the intimal flap and the extent of dissection within the aorta (Fig. 6–25). True and false lumen, the presence of thrombus, and the involvement of arch and visceral arterial branches are easily demonstrated. Although in the past, contrast angiography has been used in this setting, it requires ionizing radiation and potentially nephrotoxic quantities of contrast media. Patients with aortic disease often have reduced renal

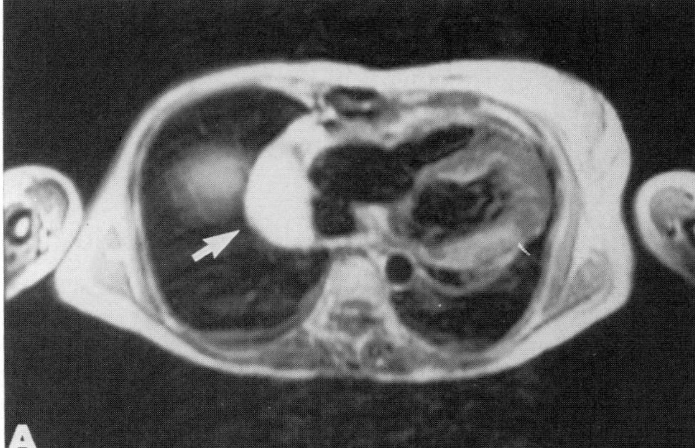

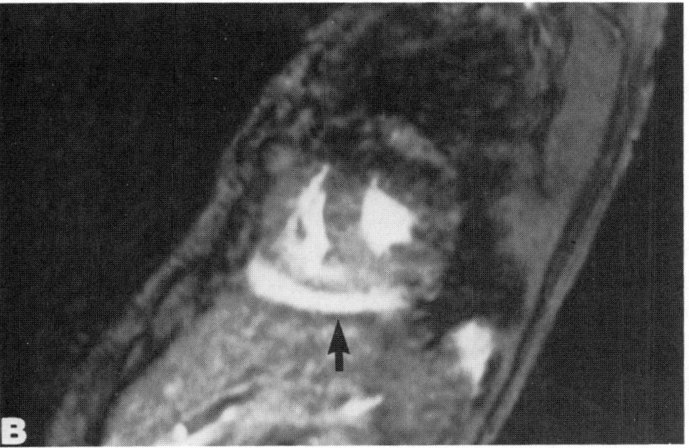

FIGURE 6–24. *A*, Transaxial ECG-gated spin-echo image through the heart at mid-ventricular level. A pericardial hematoma can be seen as an area of bright signal intensity overlying the right atrium *(arrow)*. *B*, Short-axis cine MRI in the same patient as in *A* with the hematoma again appearing bright along the undersurface of the heart *(arrow)*. (From Caputo GR, Higgins CB: Advances in cardiac imaging modalities: Magnetic resonance, fast computed tomography, and positron emission tomography. Invest Radiol 25:838–854, 1990.)

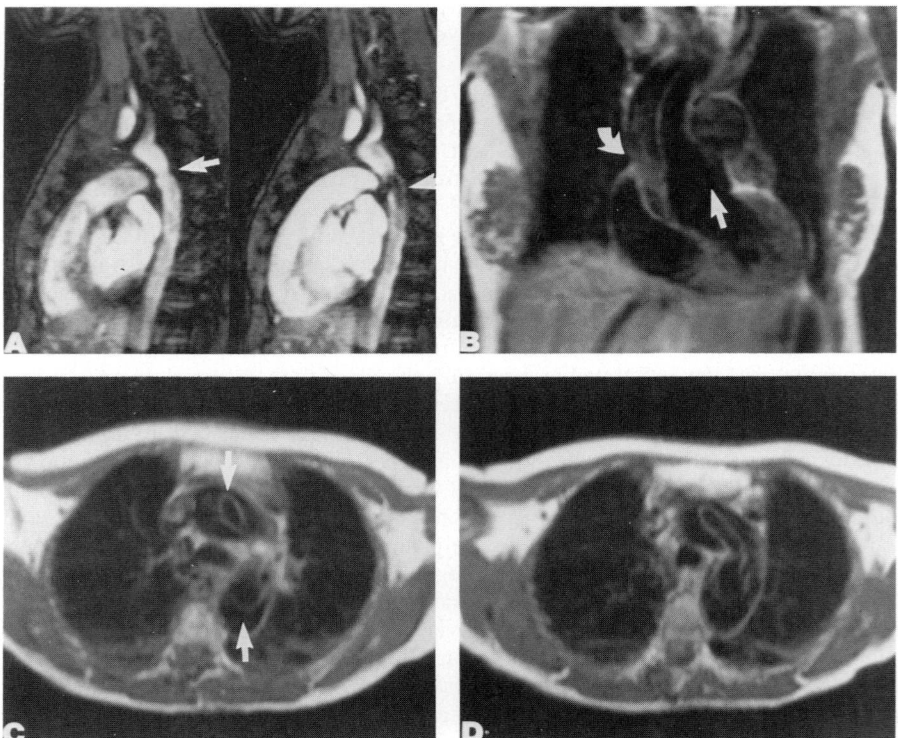

FIGURE 6–25. *A, Left,* Sagittal cine MRI through the heart at end-diastole demonstrating a coarctation of the aorta *(arrow)*. *Right,* Same sagittal imaging plane at end-systole. Note the area of disordered flow across the area of coarctation resulting in the signal void *(arrow)*. *B,* Coronal spin-echo image through the heart in a patient with Marfan's syndrome and a type I aortic dissection. The dissection flap separates the false lumen *(small arrow)* from the true lumen *(curved arrow)*. *C,* Axial spin-echo image through the ascending and descending thoracic aorta demonstrating the dissection flap encircling the true lumen *(small arrows)*. *D,* Axial spin-echo image through the aortic arch shows findings similar to those in *C*. (*A–D,* From Caputo GR, Higgins CB: Advances in cardiac imaging modalities: Magnetic resonance, fast computed tomography, and positron emission tomography. Invest Radiol 25:838–854, 1990.)

reserves secondary to hypertensive renal disease, and emergent vascular surgery can cause further renal embarrassment. Although angiography provides luminal information, a further limitation is its inability to provide information regarding the aortic wall and periaortic abnormalities, which is provided by MRI. In a recent study,[67] MRI had a sensitivity and specificity in excess of 90 per cent in the evaluation of suspected thoracic aortic disease.

Evaluation of Pathophysiology With MRI

GRE techniques have now made it possible to evaluate cardiac function with MRI. Evaluation of abnormal blood flow patterns,[45, 47] left ventricular and right ventricular dimensions and stroke volumes,[46, 76] left ventricular mass,[77, 78] and regional myocardial function[79, 80] can be accomplished using cine MRI. Cine MRI provides sufficient temporal resolution to capture end-diastole and end-systole, permitting accurate calculation of stroke volumes and ejection fraction,[46, 81, 82] which correlate well with echocardiographic measurements.[46] MRI offers the advantage of providing truly three-dimensional tomographic volumetric information, because it encompasses the entire heart and is unencumbered by the geometric assumptions made by angiography, which are erroneous in the presence of conformational or significant wall motion abnormalities.

Recent studies have been performed in the authors' laboratory in normal volunteers and in patients with dilated cardiomyopathy or left ventricular hypertrophy. In these examinations separated by a short time interval, the interstudy variability for left ventricular mass (less than 5 per cent), ejection fraction and end-diastolic volume (less than 6 per cent), and end-systolic volume (less than 10 per cent) were small. Similarly, interobserver variability for left ventricular mass, ejection fraction, and end-diastolic volume (less than 5 per cent) and end-systolic volume (less than 14 per cent) were also small. These results suggest that cine MRI may be useful in the serial monitoring of therapeutic responses in various disease states.

MRI accurately measures left ventricular mass in canine studies[77, 78] and closely correlates with human angiographic estimates.[83] This may prove to be important clinically, because serial monitoring of progression or regression of left ventricular hypertrophy may reflect therapeutic response to such interventions as aortic valve replacement for aortic stenosis or the pharmacologic treatment of hypertension. In the presence of ischemic heart disease, MRI can evaluate systolic performance of the left ventricle by quantitating wall thickening. Regions of prior myocardial infarction demonstrate a reduction in, or absence of, wall thickening during systole.[84]

Assessment of Valvular Regurgitation With Cine MRI

The homogeneous high signal intensity of the blood pool seen with cine MRI persists throughout most of the cardiac cycle, with the exception of the signal loss caused by the opening and rapid closure of the atrioventricular valves. The high-velocity jet associated with either atrioventricular or semi-lunar valve regurgitation generates a signal void in the otherwise high signal intensity blood pool. This signal void emanating from the closed incompe-

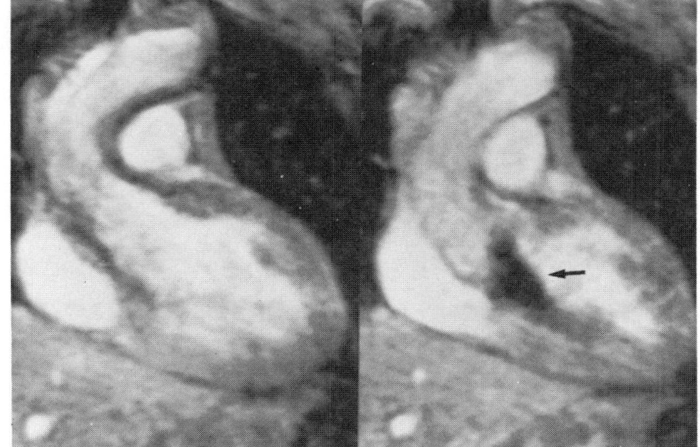

FIGURE 6–26. Coronal cine MRI through the heart of a patient with severe aortic regurgitation. Systolic image is shown on the *left*. The diastolic image on the *right* demonstrates the turbulent regurgitant flow through the leaking aortic valve resulting in the signal void *(arrow)*. (*Left* and *right*, From Caputo GR, Higgins CB: Advances in cardiac imaging modalities: Magnetic resonance, fast computed tomography, and positron emission tomography. Invest Radiol 25:838–854, 1990.)

tent valve is a marker for regurgitation. Because the stroke volumes of both ventricles of normal subjects are equal, the severity of valvular regurgitation can be determined by comparison of right and left ventricular stroke volumes used to calculate regurgitant fraction, volumes, or stroke volume ratios.[47] This technique correlates well with independent imaging techniques in differentiating patients with moderate or severe regurgitation from normals and patients with mild regurgitation.[84] Quantitation of regurgitation has been accomplished by measuring the entire volume of the signal void as it appears on multiple tomographic images encompassing the recipient chamber. Preliminary results with this technique demonstrate that the signal void increases significantly with increasing severity of aortic and mitral regurgitation (Fig. 6–26).[85]

Cine MRI can precisely define left ventricular myocardial function by correlating changes in blood pressure during the cardiac cycle with ventricular dimensions at these times, yielding measurements of left ventricular wall stress. As expected, these measurements are markedly elevated in patients with dilated cardiomyopathy compared with normal controls.[86] Serial determinations may prove clinically useful in assessing the efficacy of therapeutic regimens used in patients with dilated cardiomyopathy and other forms of dilated cardiac diseases.

MRI Phase-Velocity Mapping

Blood flow imaging has been accomplished and shown to be practical clinically using PC MRA.[87–90] Flow-encoding gradient pulses are used to assign phase shifts to moving spins that are proportional to velocity while leaving stationary spins unaffected. In this manner, images are produced that contain information from moving spins, while signals from stationary tissue are suppressed (Fig. 6–27).

Velocity mapping provides a quantitative two-dimensional method of measuring blood velocities in the vascular system. The instantaneous flow in the ascending aorta at different points in the cardiac cycle can be integrated over time providing left ventricular stroke volume, which, when multiplied by the heart rate, yields cardiac output. These stroke volumes correlate well with those stroke volumes obtained in the same patients using conventional MRI techniques. This method of measuring flow should be accurate provided that the flowing blood generates sufficient signal to calculate phase, the velocity phase-encoding gradients are accurately calibrated, and the correct range of flows in the vessels being interrogated have been selected. MRI velocity mapping should prove to be of value in the study of diseases throughout the cardiovascular system.

Clinical MRI flow quantification is still in an inchoate stage; however, it has enormous potential. Most clinical noninvasive flow applications have involved the use of Doppler ultrasound. Preliminary studies[91–93] have demonstrated the clinical capabilities of MRI flow quantification. Because MRI phase-velocity mapping is not limited by patient body habitus, it may be possible to accurately measure flow in medium or relatively small-sized vessels deep within the body that are difficult to approach with Doppler ultrasound.

Phase-velocity mapping has been used successfully for measuring intracardiac shunts and coarctation of the aorta.[91] Phase-velocity mapping shows the velocity profile in a cross section of a vessel. Because phase-velocity mapping is bipolar, flow in one direction is encoded with high signal intensity and flow in the opposite direction is encoded with low signal intensity. This allows separation and quantification of antegrade and retrograde flow in the same vessel. Excess mid- to late-systolic retrograde flow has been recognized in patients with pulmonary hypertension,[92] and retrograde flow in the aorta was significantly reduced in coronary artery disease compared with normal subjects.[93] Further studies will be required to determine whether these findings are related to the severity of the disease process and to elucidate the significance of these findings.

A potential advantage of velocity flow mapping over Doppler echocardiography is its ability to acquire images in oblique imaging planes, thereby minimizing the error introduced by the angle between the flow-encoding direction and the direction of true flow. Studies in the authors' laboratory[94] have employed this approach to measure both right and left pulmonary arterial flow. The sum of the flows in the right and left pulmonary arteries correlated closely with the flow in the main pulmonary artery. The relative flows measured using oblique angle phase-velocity map-

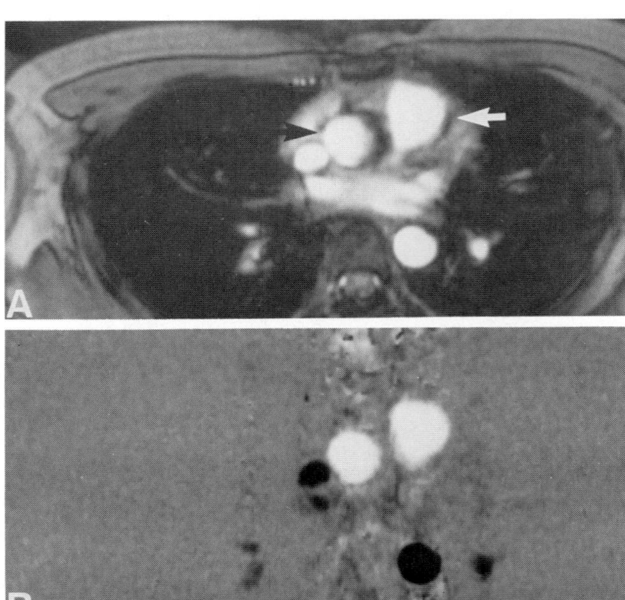

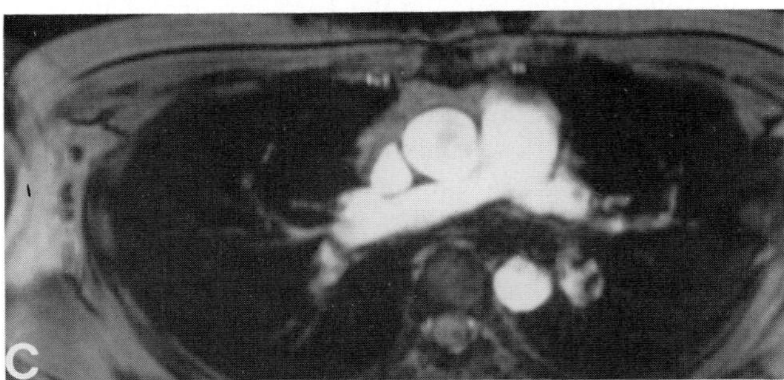

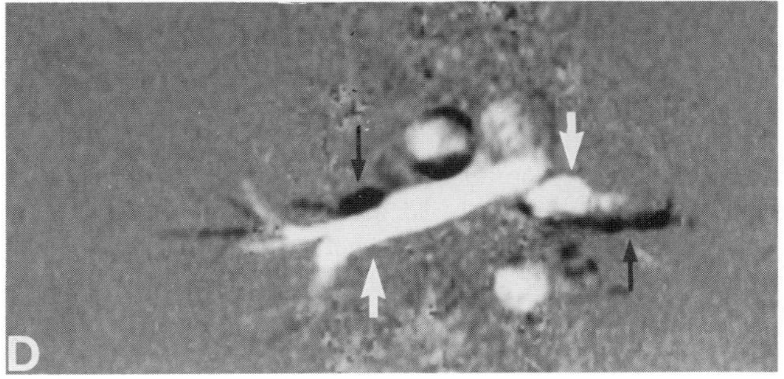

FIGURE 6–27. *A*, Transaxial cine MRI at the level of the aortic root *(black arrow)* and right ventricular outflow tract *(white arrow)*. *B*, Phase-contrast image at same level with velocity encoded in slice-select direction. Flow in the cranial direction (aorta and right ventricular outflow tract) is white, and flow in the caudal direction (superior vena cava and descending aorta) is black. Right ventricular outflow tract velocity and stroke volume were calculated as 67 cm/sec and 64 cc, which closely correlate with the left ventricular values of 69 cm/sec and 69 cc, respectively. *C*, Transaxial cine MRI at the level of the ascending aorta and bifurcation of the main pulmonary artery. *D*, Phase-contrast image at the same level with velocity encoded in the frequency direction (right to left). Flow toward the right side of the body is white (right pulmonary artery and left pulmonary vein *[white arrows]*), and flow toward the left side of the body is black (left pulmonary artery and right pulmonary vein *[black arrows]*). (*A–D*, From Caputo GR, Higgins CB: Advances in cardiac imaging modalities: Magnetic resonance, fast computed tomography, and positron emission tomography. Invest Radiol 25:838–854, 1990.)

ping correlated well with values measured using nuclear techniques.[95] Left-to-right shunts in patients with congenital heart disease have been successfully quantitated in our laboratory using this oblique flow-encoding approach. The stroke volumes measured in the main pulmonary artery and ascending aorta have correlated closely with values measured directly from the cardiac chamber using biphasic spin-echo MRI.[96, 97] Pulmonary to systemic flow ratios have correlated well with values measured in the cardiac catheterization laboratory.

Preliminary studies in the authors' laboratory have demonstrated the efficacy of phase-velocity mapping in quantifying aortic regurgitation.[98] Time-integrated flow throughout the cardiac cycle provides both total antegrade flow during systole and retrograde flow during diastole through the incompetent aortic valve. Left ventricular stroke volume in the ascending aorta was significantly larger than right ventricular stroke volume measured in the main pulmonary artery and correlated well with left ventricular stroke volume measured directly from the cardiac chamber using biphasic MRI. Subtraction of aortic retrograde flow from total antegrade flow yielded a similar value to main pulmonary artery antegrade flow. The magnitude of the regurgitant volume may be utilized to grade the severity of aortic regurgitation.

MRI is effective for both the anatomical and the functional evaluation of cardiac disease. Because imaging planes and positions can be reliably reproduced and volume quantitation can be done accurately, it is an ideal technique for monitoring the response of the heart to therapy. The eventual role of MRI for cardiovascular diagnosis will be modified by the traditional reliance on two-dimensional echocardiography and nuclear cardiac imaging as well as referral patterns previously established.

THE AORTA

MRI studies of the aorta have concentrated on four disease states, each of surgical interest. These include screening and evaluation of aortic dissection, evaluation of aortic aneurysm, measurement of the degree of coarctation, and evaluation of aortic grafts for infection or pseudoaneurysm. One disease missing from this list is suspicion of aortic transection or rupture following trauma. If these patients become unstable, they are difficult to resuscitate in the magnet room. Anatomic studies of the aorta are generally performed with cardiac-triggered spin-echo sequences and with the application of saturation bands on the aorta above and below the acquired slices so that blood appears black.

Aortic Dissection

Intimal flaps are easily recognized as bright lines extending across the dark lumen of the aorta on a spin-echo sequence.[99–101] Sensitivity for detection of these flaps is approximately equivalent to CT but is superior to conventional angiography. Conventional angiography is less sensitive because one does not see the flap directly but rather infers its presence when, for example, the aortic wall appears too thick.

Although detection of a flap is straightforward, it is more difficult to discern if the false lumen is patent or thrombosed. Often very slow flowing blood cannot be distinguished from thrombus on a spin-echo sequence.[102–104] Other MRI techniques are available to make this differentiation. For example, velocity measurements may be undertaken to demonstrate the motion of blood in the false lumen.[105] A more sensitive technique is to inject gadolinium contrast and perform very fast gradient-echo acquisitions. Any portion of the vessel that is not thrombosed will appear bright on this sequence.[106]

Aortic Aneurysm

MRI provides information on aortic aneurysm that is not available from conventional angiography. Specifically one sees both the intervascular volume and the mural plaque and the vessel wall.[102, 107–110] Coronal acquisitions are very effective in determining the precise relationship of the aneurysm to the origins of the renal arteries. Unlike ultrasound, one may study the entire aorta from the aortic valve to the iliac arteries. A potential disadvantage with respect to conventional angiography is difficulty visualizing the visceral arteries. Generally only the first several centimeters of celiac, superior mesenteric, and renal arteries can be evaluated, and then only following lengthy examinations. Fortunately this information is generally not necessary in the routine work-up and surveillance of aortic aneurysms.

It has not been possible to characterize mural plaque as to its fat or blood content. Calcifications are difficult to see with MRI and are better examined by CT.

Aortic Grafts

The salient features of an aortic graft are perigraft fluid, which is bright on a T2-weighted spin-echo sequence, as well as bright signal in surrounding structures, especially the psoas muscle.[111] Following surgery, perigraft fluid can be expected for approximately 4 weeks. Fluid that persists beyond that point is a sign of nonincorporation and fluid that develops or increases after the postsurgical period usually indicates infection. Hemorrhage also has identifiable signal characteristics.[1, 112, 113] A blood collection that is more than 1 week old appears bright on a T1-weighted sequence. Blood that is several months old is usually surrounded by a dark rim of hemosiderin. A graft that leaks intermittently will generate concentric rings of thrombus.

CAROTID AND VERTEBRAL ARTERIES

Blood flow in the carotid arteries is generally rapid and laminar, permitting high-quality angiograms by the TOF technique. Clinical trials comparing MRA with conventional angiography or Doppler ultrasound in assessment of carotid stenosis, although still preliminary, have already shown considerable success.[19, 26, 114]

There is some debate as to whether carotid angiography should be performed with two- or three-dimensional TOF methods, or if, in fact, both methods should be used on every patient. Two-dimensional TOF is simple to perform. It provides a high-contrast angiogram with good sensitivity even to slow flow. Because the slices are collected sequentially, only a limited number of slices are degraded if a patient moves midway through the study. One of the major limitations to the TOF is in-plane saturation. This means that blood vessels that change their direction (e.g., tortuous carotids) will be poorly visualized by two-dimensional TOF. Additionally, an internal carotid artery that originates at right angles to the common carotid may be poorly seen, and a redundant cervical loop will not be appreciated.

Three-dimensional TOF provides superior resolution (Fig. 6–28) and is not compromised by tortuous vessels. It is more degraded by patient motion and is less able to differentiate very slow flow from total occlusion.

A strategy to combine the advantages of both two- and three-dimensional TOF is to first run a two-dimensional localizer consisting of approximately 10 slices spaced through the neck. Then the area of suspicion, generally the bifurcation, is acquired with a high-resolution three-dimensional TOF sequence. Another strategy that partially combines the advantages of two-dimensional and three-dimensional TOF is to acquire sequential thin three-dimensional slabs. Because the slabs are thin, there is less difficulty with saturation than with the typical thick three-dimensional slab.

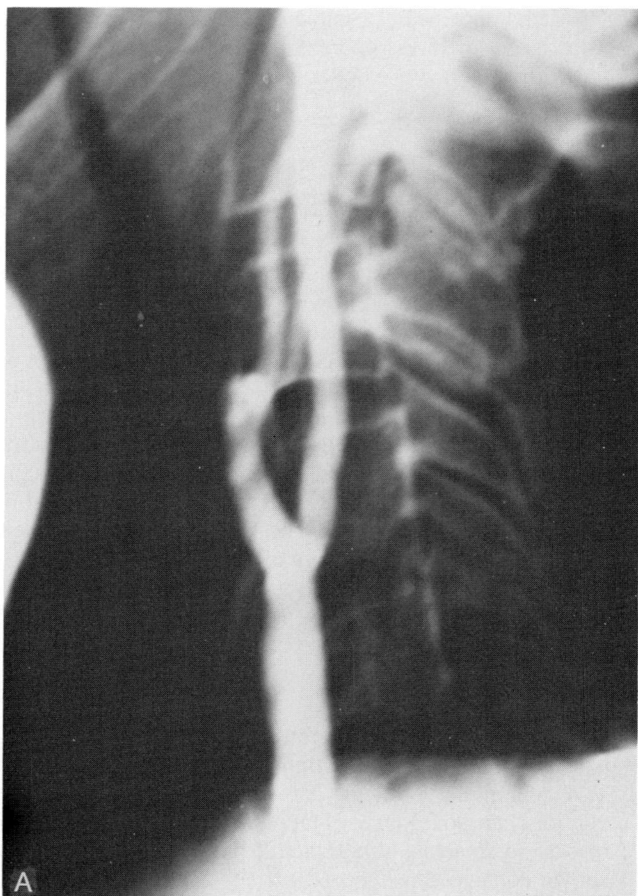

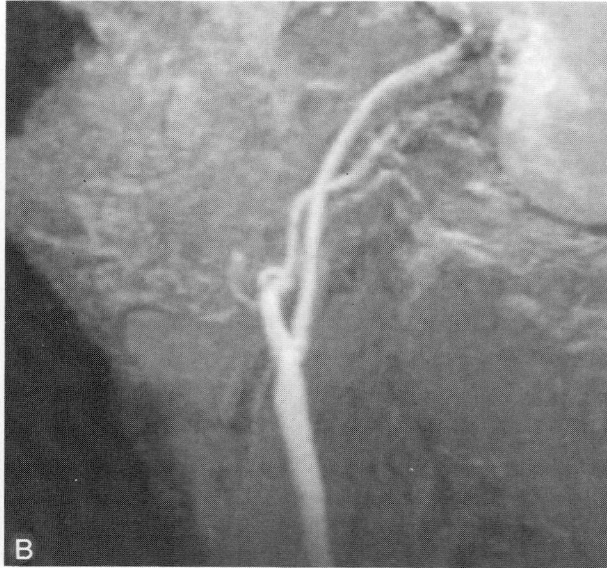

FIGURE 6–28. Comparison of conventional and three-dimensional time-of-flight (TOF) magnetic resonance angiography (MRA) of carotid bifurcation. *A*, Conventional x-ray angiogram of carotid bifurcation shows minimal narrowing of distal common carotid artery. *B*, MRA in same projection, again showing slight stenosis.

Grading of Stenosis

MRI is extremely sensitive to the presence of vascular stenosis (Fig. 6–29). Where there is a difficulty, it is usually in specificity. That is to say, a stenosis may be overestimated but rarely missed or underestimated. This overestimation results from turbulence. Wherever there is chaotic or mixing flow, or blood flow that is accelerating and decelerating rapidly, the vascular signal may be lost, and this loss of signal may be misinterpreted as a stenosis. What makes this problem especially troublesome is that turbulent flow is likely to occur in the jet within and following a tight stenosis (Fig. 6–30).

Considerable effort has been made to reduce the artifacts of turbulence. Very short echo-time sequences and very high resolution as well as superior motion compensation are all technical factors that have been used to minimize this artifact.[39, 115] With sequences currently available, there is little turbulence artifact below about 85 per cent stenosis. Above this level, and especially in long, very narrow stenoses, the vascular signal may be completely lost, as if the vessel were interrupted.

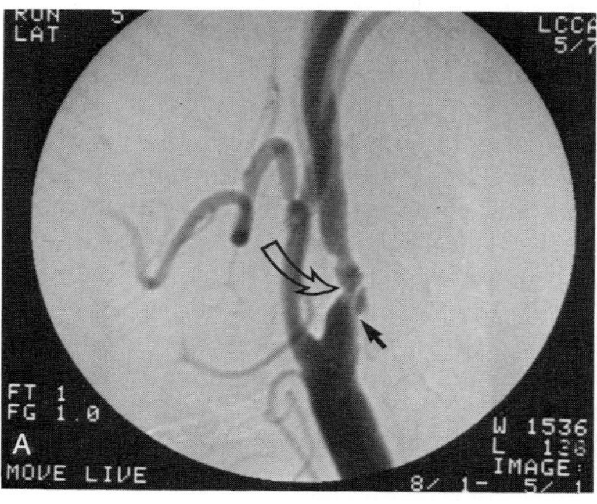

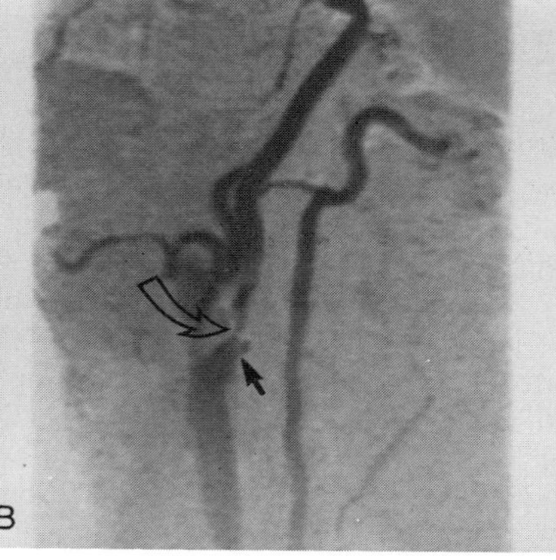

FIGURE 6–29. Carotid ulcer and stenosis detection by MRA. *A*, Conventional angiogram of carotid bifurcation. *B*, Three-dimensional TOF angiogram in same projection. Both studies reveal severe stenosis *(open arrows)* of proximal internal carotid artery, as well as ulceration *(small arrows)* of carotid bulb. Both stenoses and ulcerations have been implicated in the generation of emboli leading to stroke.

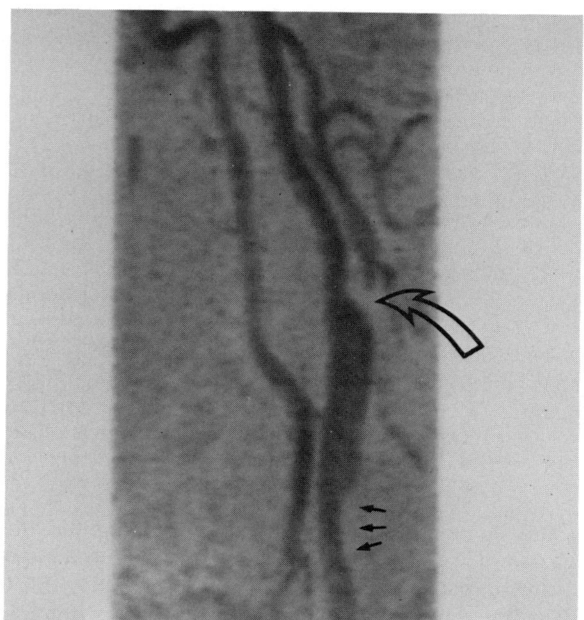

FIGURE 6–30. Carotid stenosis detection by MRA showing effect of turbulence. Three-dimensional TOF angiogram of carotid bifurcation shows approximately 2-cm-long plaque in proximal common carotid artery *(small arrows)* as well as critical stenosis at origin of external carotid artery *(open arrow)*. Blood signal is lost in the immediate vicinity of the critical stenosis because of turbulence effects.

A second problem in interpretation that was encountered initially was the differentiation between slow flow and occlusion of the distal internal carotid artery. This differentiation can be easily made if one uses the proper protocol. If occlusion is suspected, it should be confirmed either by two-dimensional TOF slices extending as high as the carotid canal in the base of skull. by PC images, or by the injection of gadolinium and repetition of three-dimensional acquisition.

Caution should be used when interpreting MRAs, because these angiograms are sensitive to blood flow in one direction only. Unless reverse flow is suspected—for example, in the case of retrograde flow of the left vertebral artery in left subclavian steal phenomena—it will not be visualized on the MRA.

Carotid Origins

The aortic arch and proximal neck vessels are best studied with overlapping sets of transverse three-dimensional TOF acquisitions (Fig. 6–31). If one does not have a neck coil that extends as low as the aortic arch, this study can be successfully acquired in the body coil. Although the carotid origins are usually reliably seen, vertebral origins may be too small in comparison with pixel size for accurate grading of origin stenosis.

Carotid Siphon

Although the carotid siphons are not generally surgically accessible, the presence of severe disease in the siphons might change the surgical approach (Fig. 6–32). When interpreting angiograms of the siphons, one should keep in mind the irregular blood flow that results from the tortuous course of the vessel. This may lead to flow artifacts and differences in flow velocity across the vessel diameter. These artifacts are best eliminated by a very short echo time sequence. Another technical factor that has improved siphon imaging is the reduction in time between the so-called phase and frequency encoding gradients. With the use of short echo time sequences, examination of the siphons is nearly always successful.

Comparison of MRA, XRA, and Doppler Ultrasound

Doppler ultrasound is likely to remain the initial screening method of the carotid bifurcation in most cases. MRA may be used as a screening method in two situations. First, if one plans to obtain an MRI of the brain to assess prior ischemic events, one can easily include screening images of the bifurcation with very little additional expense. Second, MRA may be used for patients whose findings are equivocal by ultrasound. This includes patients with unfa-

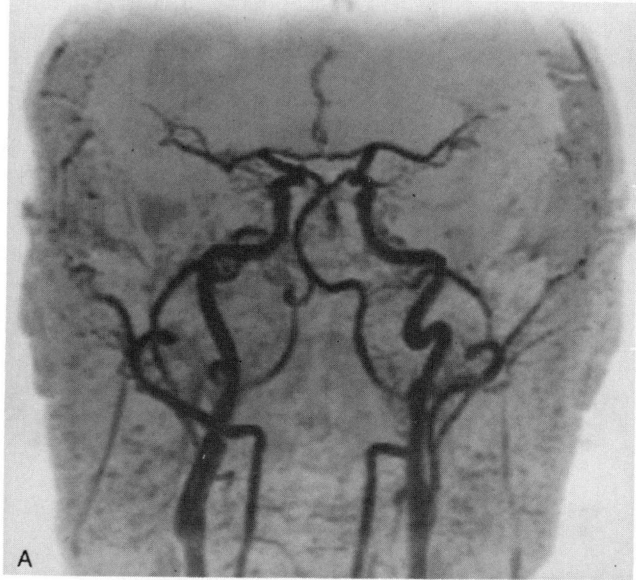

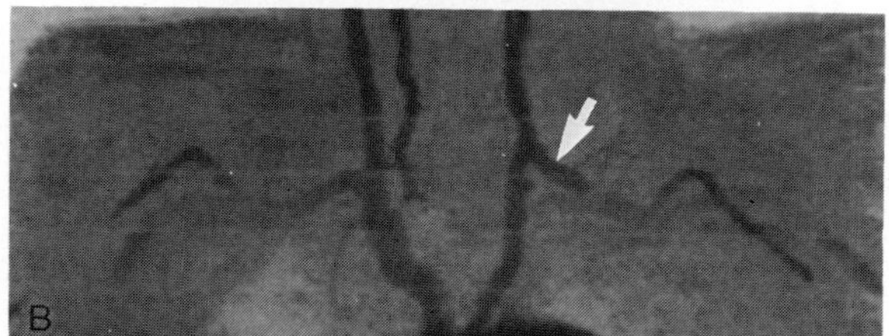

FIGURE 6–31. MRA may image vessels inaccessible to ultrasound. *A*, Three three-dimensional TOF angiograms have been stacked to provide a high-resolution angiogram from the carotid bifurcation to the circle of Willis. *B*, Angiogram of the aortic arch, again using stacked three-dimensional technique, reveals occlusion of left subclavian artery. A bypass has been constructed *(arrow)* between the left common carotid artery and the left subclavian artery beyond the occlusion.

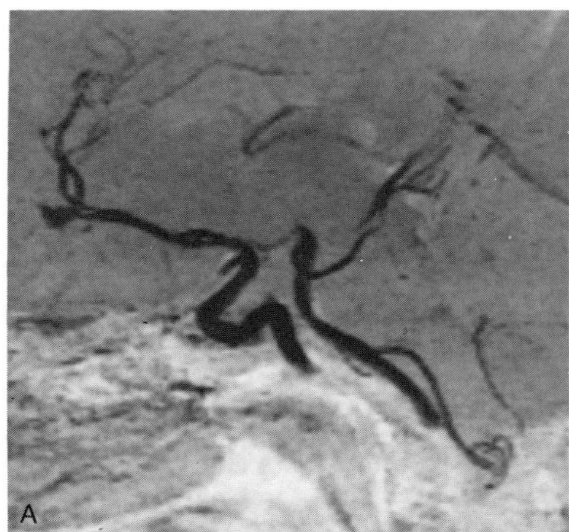

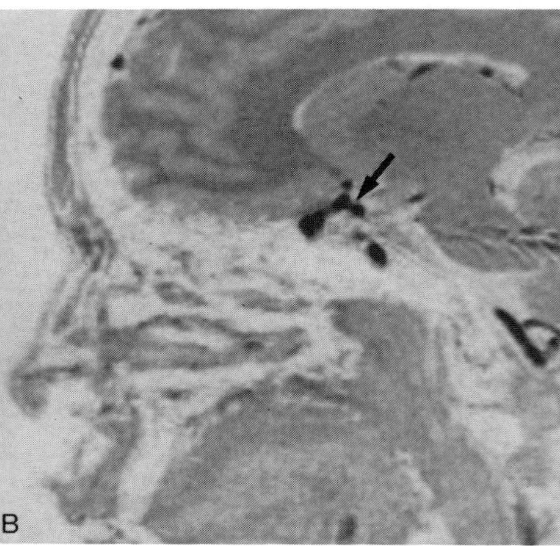

FIGURE 6–32. Stenosis of carotid siphon. *A*, Three-dimensional TOF angiogram of normal siphon in lateral projection. *B*, Single sagittal slice of three-dimensional TOF set in a different patient with focal stenosis of the siphon *(arrow)*.

vorable anatomy, such as a high bifurcation, tortuous vessels that are difficult to identify, considerable overlying adipose tissue that may obscure the vessel, or dense vascular calcifications that cause acoustic shadowing. If the ultrasound procedure shows a dampened waveform consistent with the presence of a tandem lesion, MRA can provide a noninvasive assessment of those portions of the carotid not accessible to the ultrasound transducer. One might also consider MRA on patients in whom the ultrasound findings are discrepant with clinical presentation. Another advantage of MRA is for the study of patients with neck wounds where one would prefer not to apply the transducer.

Often XRA of the carotid arteries is performed prior to surgery in order to visualize carotid origins, to confirm patency of vertebral arteries, to obtain higher-resolution views of the anatomy, or to identify ulcerations that may be a nidus for embolic thrombus formation and that are often missed by ultrasound. Here MRA may be chosen as an alternative procedure. Although the resolution of MRA is slightly inferior to that of XRA, it is usually more than adequate for operative decision making. The entire length of the carotid artery may be examined. A variety of methods exist to determine which parts of the brain are perfused by each of the neck vessels. For example, one can acquire an intracranial angiogram while presaturating the inflow from one of the vessels and see which part of the intracranial anatomy becomes dark.[22, 116] Alternatively, one can measure the direction and velocity of blood flow in intracranial vessels. This capability may be of use when determining the risk of carotid procedures. The incidence of angiographically induced stroke is approximately 1 per cent. The overall complication rate for carotid surgical procedures should include the diagnostic work-up as well. Therefore, substitution of MRA for XRA when applicable will reduce procedure-related complications.

Intracranial Vessels

Because of the small size of intracranial arteries, three-dimensional TOF or PC sequences are most often used. Structures that are most readily seen are the basilar and distal vertebral arteries, proximal pica and superior cerebellar arteries (Fig. 6–33), the circle of Willis (Fig. 6–34), and the proximal 5 cm of the cerebral arteries.

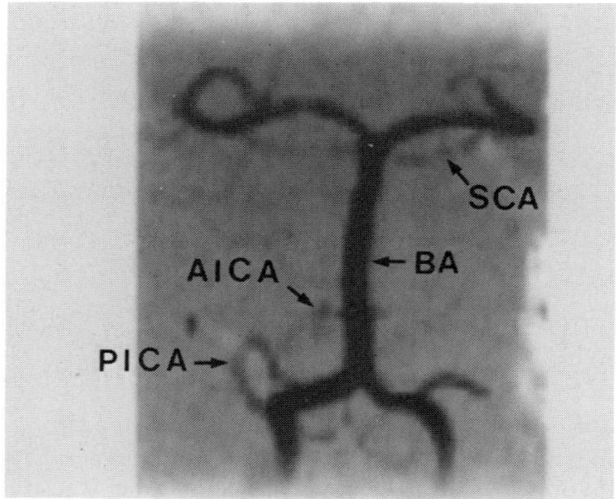

FIGURE 6–33. Posterior circulation by MRA. Three-dimensional TOF angiogram of distal vertebral arteries, basilar artery (BA), and proximal posterior cerebral arteries. Posterior inferior cerebellar arteries (PICA), anterior inferior cerebellar arteries (AICA), and superior cerebellar arteries (SCA) are visible.

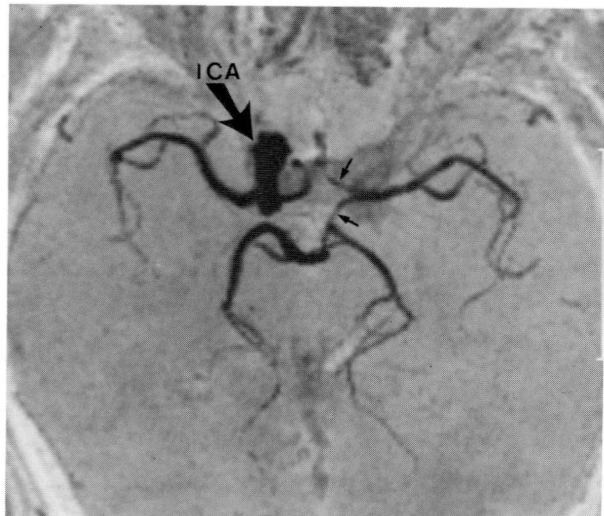

FIGURE 6–34. Collateral intracranial circulation. Three-dimensional TOF angiogram of the circle of Willis. Left internal carotid artery (ICA) occluded. Perfusion of left middle cerebral circulation through prominent left posterior and anterior communicating arteries *(small arrows)*.

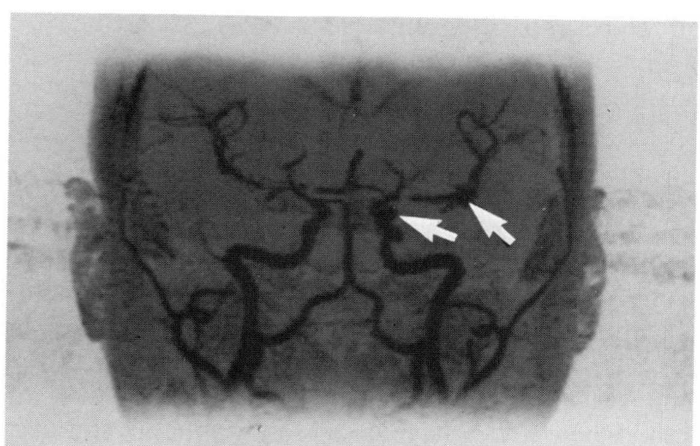

FIGURE 6–35. Intracranial aneurysm. Three-dimensional TOF angiogram in frontal projection shows intracranial aneurysms at the origin and at the trifurcation of the left middle cerebral artery *(arrows)*.

Aneurysm Detection

Aneurysms as small as 3 mm are routinely detected by MRA so long as these aneurysms are near the circle of Willis and not in the most distal branches of the cerebral arteries (Fig. 6–35).[1, 10, 11, 117–120] Paradoxically, large aneurysms are more difficult to see than small ones by MRA. This is because the rate of blood exchange within a small aneurysm may be very slow, particularly if it has a narrow neck. It is sometimes difficult to determine what portion of an aneurysm is thrombosed and what portion is dark simply because of slow flow. In that case, injection of gadolinium contrast may provide an answer. By viewing individual slices or by rotating the projected calculation, one can often see the neck and determine its point of communication with the cerebral vessels. At the same time that an MRA is performed, one can acquire additional GRE or spin-echo slices to detect hemorrhage.

Vascular Malformations

Vascular malformations are most easily seen with sequential two-dimensional TOF (Fig. 6–36) or with PC. Small arteriovenous malformations and venous angiomas are often visualized.[121–123] One may use MRA to assess the results of radiation therapy.

Tumor Perfusion. It is sometimes possible to determine the vessels perfusing a tumor; however, this is far from routine because a tumor may recruit small vessels from a variety of sources both intracranial and extracranial. One practical application of MRA in preparation for tumor resection is to acquire an angiogram of cortical veins and superimpose this on a gadolinium-enhanced acquisition of the tumor. The surgeon may then confirm the location of a deep tumor from the pattern of cortical veins seen through the craniotomy.

Dural Sinus Thrombosis. Angiograms of the sagittal sinus and other dural sinuses may be acquired with two-dimensional TOF or PC acquisition. This confirms the presence of sinus thrombosis or invasion of the dural sinus by adjacent tumor.[124, 125]

ABDOMEN

When the abdomen is studied, three-dimensional acquisition is usually not practical because of respiratory motion. Instead, rapid two-dimensional slices are acquired sequentially, one with each breath-hold. For vessels that are relatively fixed, such as the proximal renal arteries, three-dimensional PC or TOF acquisition is often successful.[20, 126, 127]

Abdominal Veins

Abdominal venography by MRA is particularly rewarding because high-contrast studies may be quickly acquired without exposing the patient to the typically high contrast loads involved in portacaval studies by conventional angiography. Often a small number of two-dimensional slices strategically placed along the portal (Fig. 6–37) or splenic vein or perpendicular to the inferior vena cava will answer the clinical question.

For example, in screening for a thrombosis of iliac veins or inferior vena cava, one can acquire transverse two-dimensional slices with a slight gap and cover the abdomen in approximately 30 slices. Venous thrombosis is seen as a dark filling defect within the vascular space (Fig. 6–38). Screening by this method is advantageous in comparison with ultrasound because ultrasonography is usually obscured by overlying bowel gas. X-ray venography is also difficult to perform in the inferior vena cava because of dilution of contrast medium unless a catheter is placed

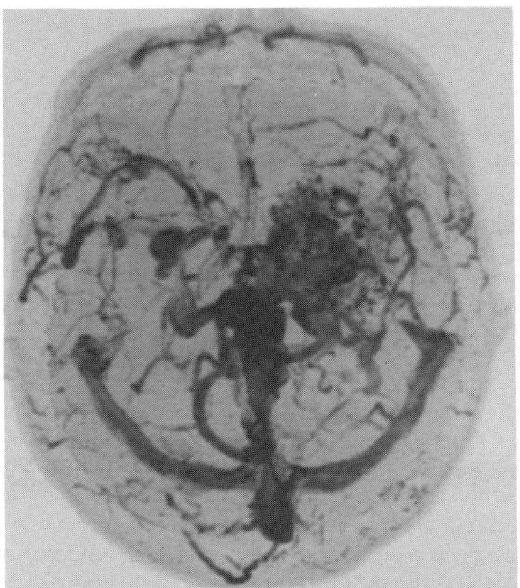

FIGURE 6–36. Arteriovenous malformation of the brain. Set of transverse two-dimensional TOF angiograms through nidus of malformation projected in submental-vertex direction. Nidus and draining veins are apparent.

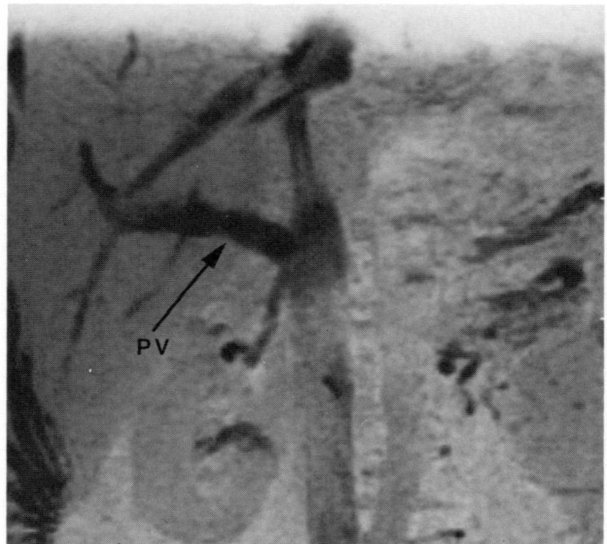

FIGURE 6–37. Portal vein angiogram. Several coronal two-dimensional TOF slices, each obtained in a breath-hold to eliminate respiratory motion, are combined to demonstrate the portal vein (PV).

directly into the caval system. The portal and splenic veins are also readily studied with two-dimensional methods acquired in either a coronal or a transverse plane. Coronal acquisition has the advantage of providing a frontal view that is familiar to those who do conventional abdominal studies. Once patency has been established, MRA can then be used to measure the direction and velocity of blood flow. Deep Doppler imaging can often be used to make similar determinations; however, for vessels that pass retroperitoneally or when collateral vessels are present, MRA is advantageous because an adequate acoustic window is usually not possible. Furthermore, MRA provides a three-dimensional depiction.

A common problem in abdominal venous studies, particularly in surgically introduced shunts, is the presence of hemostatic clips. These may eliminate all local vascular signal so that it is impossible to rule out stricture or thrombus in the area of a clip.

Arterial Studies

There is considerable interest in the use of MRA to detect renal artery stenosis because these patients cannot tolerate the large osmotic loads of intravascular contrast. MRA of the renal arteries has been performed either with angled coronal two-dimensional slices placed precisely at the renal ostium or with three-dimensional PC acquisition. Using either of these methods, it is possible to differentiate normal from stenosed proximal arteries.[8, 15, 20, 127, 128] If a renal vessel is significantly stenosed, the velocity might be substantially reduced and the stenosis difficult to grade. In very-slow-flowing arteries, PC appears to have some advantages. So far, MRA has not been sufficiently specific to replace contrast angiography but it is sensitive enough to be used as a screening examination. Also, small secondary renal arteries are often missed by MRA. Therefore, it does not appear to be adequate for planning renal transplant procedures.

LOWER EXTREMITIES

The term angiography connotes the demonstration of vascular anatomy using ionizing radiation and iodinated contrast media. The contrast media used with MRA is flowing blood and as such results in a projected three-dimensional ''flow map'' of the vasculature. This flow map image incorporates both pathoanatomic and pathophysiologic information. Two general approaches have been applied to provide projection images of blood vessels coursing through a large thickness of the body. TOF flow effects are related to the increase in amplitude of the signal returning from flowing blood entering the area imaged (flow-related enhancement). Phase effects relate to the increase in phase angle of this returning signal, which is proportional to the velocity of flowing blood.[129]

With MRA, undesirable flow phenomena such as turbulence cause signal loss and visual overestimation of the severity of a stenosis.[130] Therefore, taken alone, the MRA can be misleading in terms of the hemodynamic significance of a stenosis (not unlike the findings from conventional angiography when compared with those from duplex sonographic findings).[131–134] Previous duplex sonographic studies[135] have demonstrated that the systolic, early diastolic, and late diastolic phases of the cardiac cycle produce distinct segments of the velocity waveform in a peripheral artery. As blood is accelerated into and distends peripheral arteries during systole, a positive waveform occurs, terminating at peak systole. As the blood decelerates with filling of the arterial high-pressure reservoirs, the positive waveform decreases and finally terminates as a negative wave-

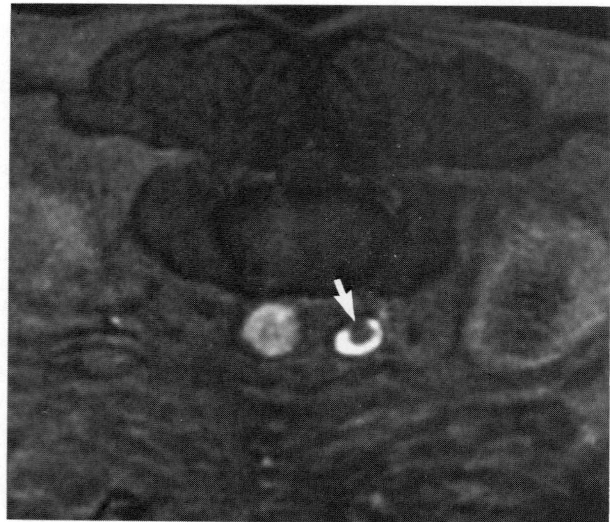

FIGURE 6–38. Deep venous thrombosis. An image from a set of transverse two-dimensional TOF slices through the lower inferior vena cava. Thrombus is seen against the posterior wall of cava *(arrow)*. A series of such slices may be acquired from the knee to the heart in less than 15 min.

form as the distended arterial reservoirs undergo recoil contraction, forcing blood flow in a reversed direction toward the heart. Finally, in late diastole, a positive waveform smaller than that occuring during systole is produced as the distended arterial reservoirs force blood antegrade if the peripheral resistance allows perfusion in late diastole.

When a hemodynamically significant arterial obstruction (greater than 50 per cent reduction in diameter) occurs, the triphasic waveform dampens in the artery, resulting in amplitude reduction and broadening of the systolic segment with absence of diastolic segments (monophasic waveform). In the presence of a more severe obstruction, the pulsatility of the velocity waveform is completely absent. This flow profile has been clearly demonstrated using duplex sonography.

One approach to deal with the problem of overestimation of the severity of a stenosis by MRA is to employ a TOF technique to demonstrate a stenosis, followed by phase-velocity mapping[136, 137] perpendicular to the vessel above and below the diseased segment to measure the velocity along the direction of flow throughout systole and diastole. The curve created would demonstrate a triphasic or monophasic pattern indicating the hemodynamic severity of a stenosis in a manner analogous to duplex sonographic evaluations, extracting conventional waveform parameters such as the pulsatility index,[138, 139] which are insensitive to angular correction and vessel size.

Arterial Morphology and Flow in Normal Subjects

Studies performed in the authors' laboratory[140] have demonstrated the morphology of the popliteal and tibioperoneal arteries in healthy subjects using two-dimensional TOF MRA (Fig. 6–39) and have compared their MRI phase-velocity mapping waveform patterns with those acquired by means of color-coded ultrasound (Fig. 6–40).

There was no significant difference between velocity-encoded cine MRI and color-coded sonographic velocity

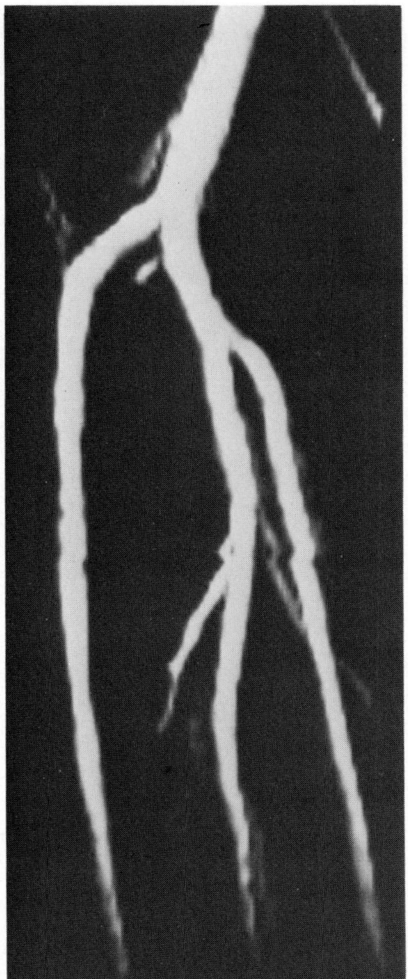

FIGURE 6–39. Two-dimensional TOF MRA of the popliteal and tibioperoneal arteries in a normal volunteer. (From Caputo G, Kondo C, Higgins CB: Quantification of blood flow using magnetic resonance imaging. *In* Higgins C, Hricak H, Helms C (eds): Magnetic Resonance Imaging of the Body. New York, Raven Press, 1992, pp 339–352.)

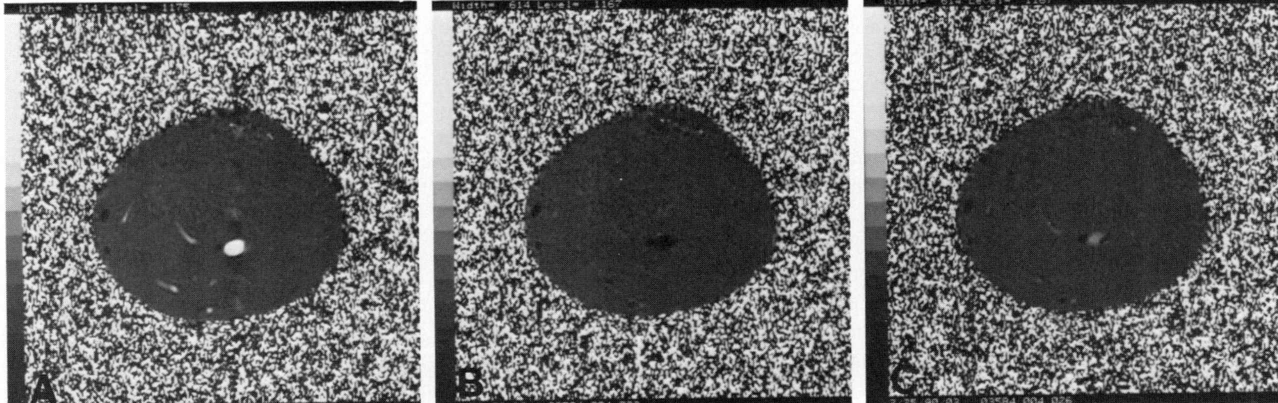

FIGURE 6–40. Transaxial velocity-encoded cine MRI through the popliteal artery of a normal volunteer. *A*, At peak systole, maximal antegrade velocity is indicated by high signal intensity. *B*, In early diastole, retrograde flow is indicated by low signal intensity *C*, In late diastole, flow once again is antegrade (high signal intensity), although at a much lower velocity than in *A*. (*A–C*, From Caputo G, Kondo C, Higgins CB: Quantification of blood flow using magnetic resonance imaging. *In* Higgins C, Hricak H, Helms C (eds): Magnetic Resonance Imaging of the Body. New York, Raven Press, 1992, pp 339–352.)

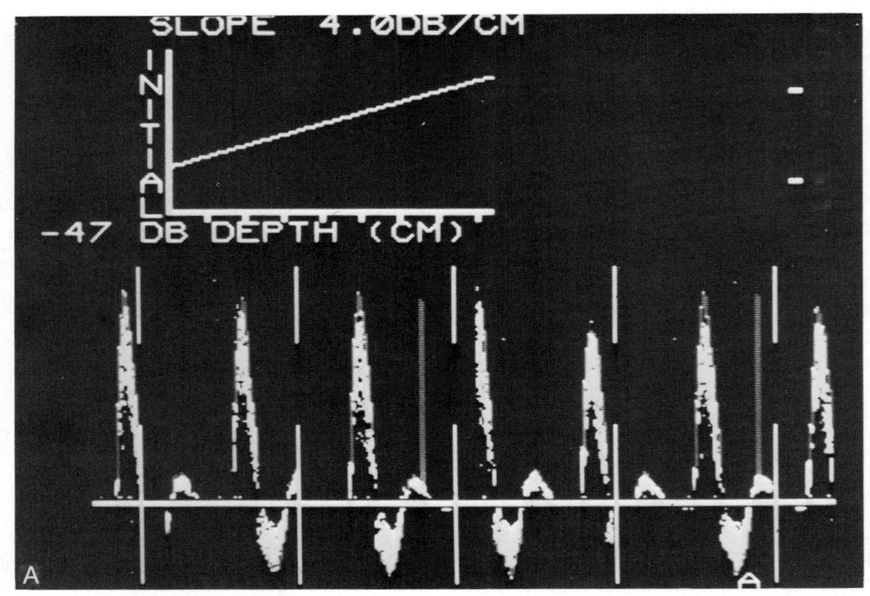

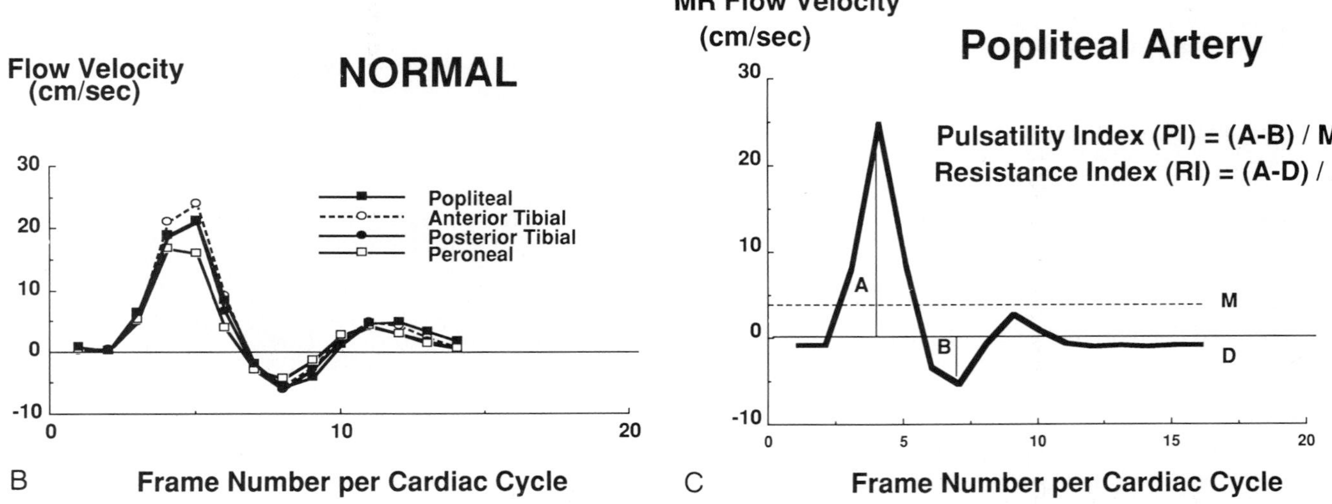

FIGURE 6–41. *A*, Duplex sonogram of the popliteal artery in a normal volunteer demonstrating the normal triphasic waveform pattern. *B*, Popliteal and trifurcation arteries' MRI velocity waveform. Note the triphasic waveform pattern similar to the normal triphasic waveform obtained with duplex sonography. *C*, Diagram depicting the normal MRI triphasic waveform and the parameters used for calculating pulsatility index. (*A–C*, From Caputo G, Kondo C, Higgins CB: Quantification of blood flow using magnetic resonance imaging. *In* Higgins C, Hricak H, Helms C (eds): Magnetic Resonance Imaging of the Body. New York, Raven Press, 1992, pp 339–352.)

measurements in the popliteal, anterior tibial, and peroneal arteries. Velocity measurements were significantly different for the posterior tibial artery ($p < .05$). As expected, the spatial mean velocities were significantly lower than the spatial maximal velocity. Interobserver variability was small for the spatial mean velocities measured with velocity-encoded cine MRI in the popliteal, anterior, and posterior tibial arteries and slightly larger for the peroneal artery.[140]

The normal triphasic waveform was observed for the popliteal and tibioperoneal arteries using color-coded sonography. The waveforms obtained using velocity-encoded cine MRI correlated well with the waveforms obtained with color-coded sonography. There was no significant difference between pulsatility indices calculated for the popliteal artery using velocity-encoded cine MRI and color-coded sonography (Fig. 6–41).

Morphology and Flow in Obstructive Disease

Preliminary studies in the authors' laboratory,[141] using the same velocity-encoded cine MRI techniques, demonstrated monophasic waveforms above and below hemodynamically significant popliteal artery stenoses (Fig. 6–42). Furthermore, excellent quality two-dimensional TOF MRAs were obtained in the same patients as long as the presaturation band was kept far enough away from the imaging slice to avoid the dark, horizontal, stripe artifacts described in prior studies (Fig. 6–43).[140] Further studies are

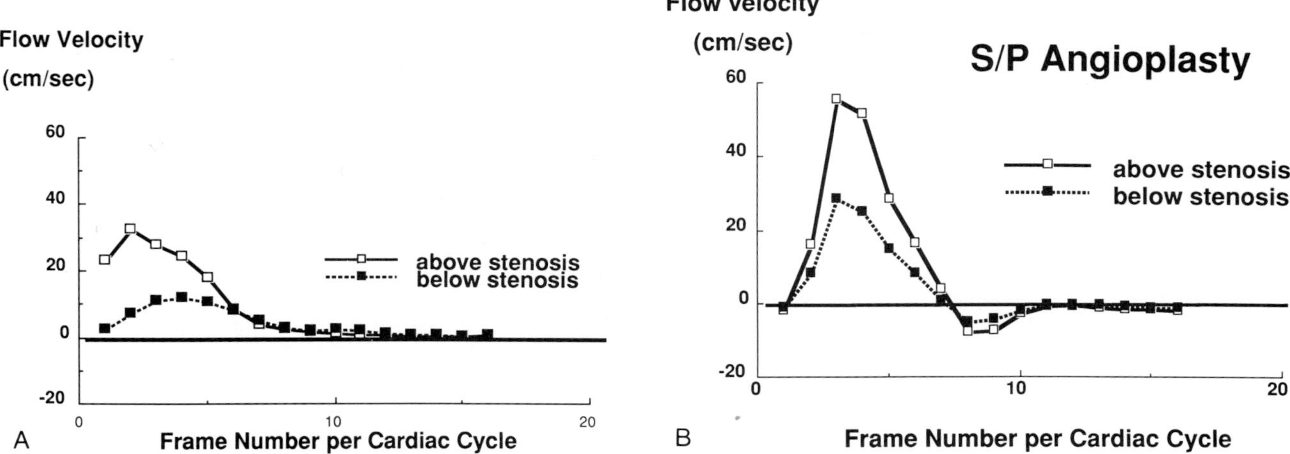

FIGURE 6–42. *A*, Abnormal monophasic MRA waveform obtained above and below a significant popliteal stenosis prior to angioplasty. This is the typical pattern obtained with duplex sonography. *B*, Return of the normal triphasic waveform above and below the same popliteal stenosis status post (S/P) angioplasty. This is the pattern typically seen using duplex sonography. (From Caputo G, Kondo C, Higgins CB: Quantification of blood flow using magnetic resonance imaging. *In* Higgins C, Hricak H, Helms C (eds): Magnetic Resonance Imaging of the Body. New York, Raven Press, 1992, pp 339–352.)

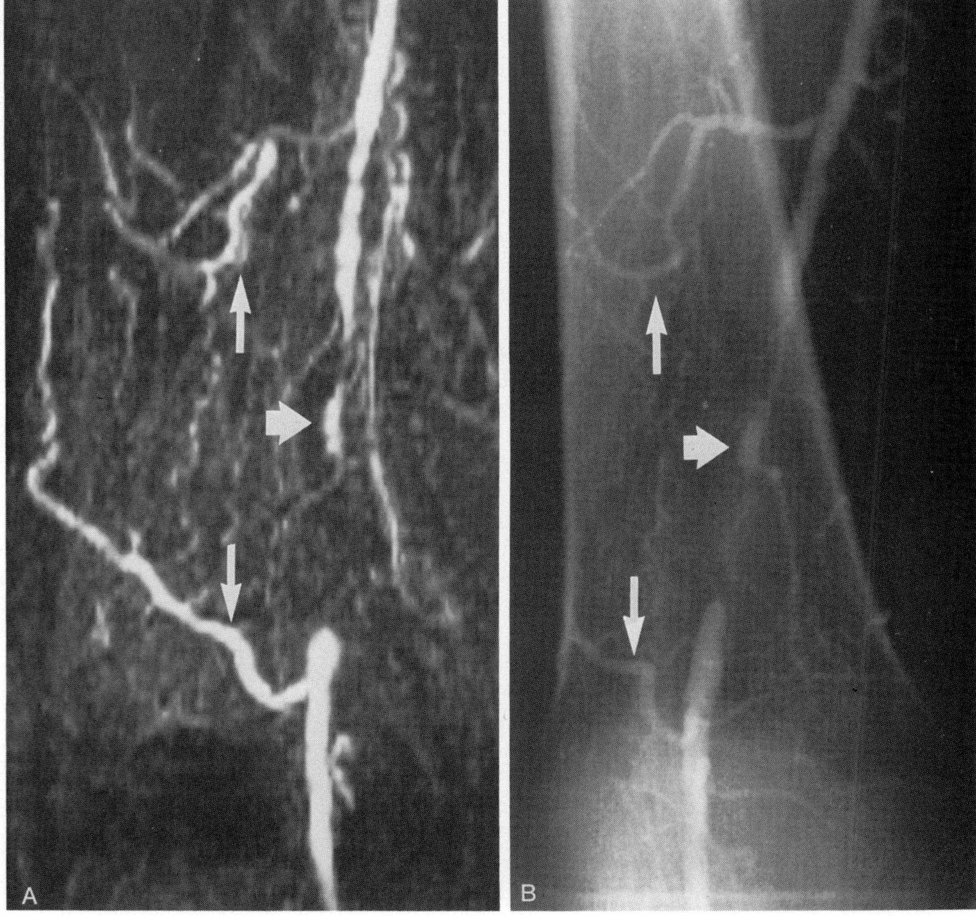

FIGURE 6–43. MRA *(A)* and conventional angiogram *(B)* of the popliteal artery with arterial occlusive disease. Obstruction of the popliteal artery *(thick arrow)* and serpiginous collateral circulation *(thin arrows)* are identically observed on both MRA and conventional angiograms.

required to define the role of combining MRA and velocity-encoded cine MRI in a complementary manner to evaluate the pathoanatomy and pathophysiology of the wide spectrum of peripheral vascular disease. Velocity-encoded cine MRI may be useful in assessing the hemodynamic significance of a peripheral vascular stenosis whose severity might be overestimated using MRA alone. When two-dimensional TOF MRA is combined effectively with velocity-encoded cine MRI, the anatomic information from contrast angiography and the physiologic information from duplex sonography[142] can be obtained during the course of one magnetic resonance examination. In the popliteal and tibioperoneal arteries, velocities determined by velocity-encoded cine MRI showed excellent interobserver reproducibility and correlated well with those obtained by color-coded sonographic studies.

Color-coded sonographic velocities in the popliteal and tibioperoneal arteries correlated well with uncorrected MR velocities. The assumption was made that an angle less than 20 degrees ($\cos \theta \geq .94$) existed between the MRI flow-encoding direction (transaxial slice selection direction, parallel to the long axis of the extremity coil) and the true direction of flow. An angle of 20 degrees would result in a 6 per cent underestimation of flow velocity; however, it would have minimal if any effect on the pulsatility index, which is calculated as a ratio of velocities equally affected by the angle between the flow-encoding direction and the true direction of flow. For vessels running at steeper angles to the flow-encoding gradients, either cosine correction[143] or the use of oblique flow-encoding gradients would be required. The triphasic waveforms and pulsatility indices obtained using velocity-encoded cine MRI correlated well with the color-coded sonographic findings in normal volunteers.

Other investigators have examined peripheral vessels using MRA without concurrent phase-velocity mapping.[144–152] Yucel and associates[144] found that MRA had a 94 per cent accuracy in showing the status of runoff vessels when correlated with conventional angiography or surgery. Owen and coworkers[145] studied 23 patients with peripheral arteriosclerosis and arterial insufficiency with MRA. MRA detected all vessels identified by conventional angiography, whereas conventional arteriography failed to detect 22 per cent of runoff vessels identified by MRA. Overall, these authors found MRA to be more sensitive for detecting distal runoff vessels in patients with peripheral arterial occlusive disease. Lossef and associates[146] concluded that gadolinium enhancement combined with a magnitude contrast technique appreciably improved MRA of lower extremity arteries.

Nakatsuka and colleagues[147] performed PC MRA of veins in the lower extremities of normal volunteers and of patients with deep venous thrombosis of the lower extremities. In all normal volunteers, MRA demonstrated bilateral large popliteal veins. In patients with deep venous thrombosis, obstruction of the femoral veins and development of collateral veins were clearly visualized. They concluded that MRA may be a valuable technique for the evaluation of the patency of veins in the lower extremities.

Internal dialysis shunts have been evaluated using MRA techniques.[148, 149] In patients with chronic renal failure, dialysis grafts were clearly visualized, and the graft stenoses later confirmed by digital subtraction angiography were also well defined.[148] However, MRA of dialysis shunts may be limited by the patient positioning required, resulting in pain in the shoulder of the extremity imaged.[149]

The signal:noise available in MRA is an important limitation in its application to the peripheral vascular system and can result in relatively long acquisition times. Either a large field of view at poor resolution or several smaller fields of view (perhaps 16 cm) at high resolution can be imaged. However, at present, it is not feasible to obtain a high-resolution study covering the infrarenal aorta to the dorsalis pedis. MRA appears to be suited best for surveillance of known lesions or follow-up of an arterial segment suspected of having new disease.

MRA may have its earliest application in screening a specific site for the presence of disease. Grafts can be evaluated to rule out thrombosis. MRA might be used for periodic surveillance of patients with known disease at a site. Following angioplasty, a baseline study and serial examinations could be made of the angioplasty site to detect recurrence of the stenosis.[152]

SUMMARY

MRA should become a useful adjunct to conventional contrast angiography in the detection or serial evaluation of specific arterial segments without the incumbent morbidity and discomfort of injection of iodinated contrast media. The recent proliferation of investigative work in this area will define MRA's clinical role within the near future.

References

1. Atlas SW, Mark AS, Fram EK, Grossman RI: Vascular intracranial lesions: Applications of gradient-echo MR imaging. Radiology 169:455, 1988.
2. Laub GA, Kaiser WA: MR angiography with gradient motion refocusing. J Comput Assist Tomogr 12:377, 1988.
3. Bogren HG, Klipstein RH, Firmin DN, et al: Quantitation of antegrade and retrograde blood flow in the human aorta by magnetic resonance velocity mapping. Am Heart J 117:1214, 1989.
4. Edelman RR, Zhao B, Liu C, et al: MR angiography and dynamic flow evaluation of the portal venous system. AJR 153:755, 1989.
5. Haacke EM, Masaryk TJ: The salient features of MR angiography. Radiology 173:611, 1989.
6. Keller PJ, Drayer BP, Fram EK, et al: MR angiography with two-dimensional acquisition and three-dimensional display. Work in progress. Radiology 173:527, 1989.
7. Atkinson D, Burstein D, Edelman R: First-pass cardiac perfusion: Evaluation with ultrafast MR imaging. Radiology 174:757, 1990.
8. Dumoulin CL, Yucel EK, Vock P, et al: Two- and three-dimensional phase contrast MR angiography of the abdomen. J Comput Assist Tomogr 14:779, 1990.
9. Edelman RR, Mattle HP, Wallner B, et al: Extracranial carotid arteries: Evaluation with "black blood" MR angiography. Radiology 177:45, 1990.
10. Masaryk TJ, Laub GA, Modic MT, et al: Carotid-CNS MR flow imaging. Magn Reson Med 14:308, 1990.
11. Ross JS, Masaryk TJ, Modic MT, et al: Intracranial aneurysms: Evaluation by MR angiography. AJR 155:159, 1990.
12. Spritzer CE, Blinder RA: Practical aspects of vascular imaging using MRI. Crit Rev Diagn Imaging 31:145, 1990.
13. Atkinson D, Edelman R: Cineangiography of the heart in a single breath hold with a segmented turboFLASH sequence. Radiology 178:357, 1991.
14. Blatter DD, Parker DL, Robison RO: Cerebral MR-angiography with

multiple overlapping thin slab acquisition. 1. Quantitative analysis of vessel visibility. Radiology 179:805, 1991.
15. Debatin JF, Spritzer CE, Grist TM, et al: Imaging of the renal arteries: Value of MR angiography. AJR 157:981, 1991.
16. Finn JP, Edelman RR, Jenkins RL, et al: Liver transplantation: MR angiography with surgical validation. Radiology 179:265, 1991.
17. Haacke EM, Lin WL: Technologic advances in magnetic resonance angiography. Curr Opin Radiol 3:240, 1991.
18. Haacke E, Lidskog E, Lin W: A fast, partial-Fourier technique capable of local phase recovery. J Magn Reson Imaging 92:126, 1991.
19. Kido DK, Barsotti JB, Rice LZ, et al: Evaluation of the carotid artery bifurcation—Comparison of magnetic resonance angiography and digital subtraction arch aortography. Neuroradiology 33:48, 1991.
20. Lewin JS, Laub G, Hausmann R: Three-dimensional time-of-flight MR angiography: Applications in the abdomen and thorax. Radiology 179:261, 1991.
21. Link KM, Elster AD, Margosian P, Sattin B: Clinical utility of three-dimensional magnetic resonance angiographic imaging. Clin Neurosurg 37:275, 1991.
22. Mattle H, Edelman RR, Wentz KU, et al: Middle cerebral artery: Determination of flow velocities with MR angiography. Radiology 181:527, 1991.
23. Mohiaddin RH, Paz R, Theodoropoulos S, et al: Magnetic resonance characterization of pulmonary arterial blood flow after single lung transplantation. J Thorac Cardiovasc Surg 101:1016, 1991.
24. Mohiaddin RH, Amanuma M, Kilner PJ, et al: MR phase-shift velocity mapping of mitral and pulmonary venous flow. J Comput Assist Tomogr 15:237, 1991.
25. Parker DL, Yuan C, Blatter DD: MR angiography by multiple thin slab 3D acquisition. Magn Reson Med 17:434, 1991.
26. Anderson CM, Saloner D, Lee RE, et al: Assessment of carotid artery stenosis by MR angiography: Comparison with x-ray angiography and color-coded Doppler ultrasound. AJNR 13:989, 1992.
27. Boesiger P, Maier SE, Liu KC, et al: Visualization and quantification of the human blood flow by magnetic resonance imaging. J Biomech 25:55, 1992.
28. Haltom J, Harms S, Glastad K, et al: MR angiographic evaluation of peripheral vascular disease with poor visualization at conventional angiography. J Magn Reson Imaging 2(P):75, 1992.
29. Laub G: Displays for MR angiography. Magn Reson Med 14:222, 1990.
30. Cline HE, Dumoulin CL, Lorensen WE, et al: Volume rendering and connectivity algorithms for MR angiography. Magn Reson Med 18:384, 1991.
31. Higgins C: The vascular system. *In* Higgins C, Hricak H, Helms C (eds): Magnetic Resonance Imaging of the Body. New York, Raven Press, 1992, pp 629–678.
32. Futatsuya R, Seto H, Kakishita M, Kurimoto M: Cine MR angiography—Application to cerebrovascular disease [in Japanese]. Nippon Rinsho 49:1610, 1991.
33. Gefter WB, Hatabu H, Dinsmore BJ, et al: Pulmonary vascular cine MR imaging—A noninvasive approach to dynamic imaging of the pulmonary circulation. Radiology 176:761, 1990.
34. Iwai F, Sostman HD, Evans AJ, et al: Cine phase-contrast magnetic resonance imaging for analysis of flow phenomena in experimental aortic dissection. Invest Radiol 26:1071, 1991.
35. Mohiaddin RH, Wann SL, Underwood R, et al: Vena caval flow: Assessment with cine MR velocity mapping. Radiology 177:537, 1990.
36. Nayler GL, Firmin DN, Longmore DB: Blood flow imaging by cine magnetic resonance. J Comput Assist Tomogr 10:715, 1986.
37. Underwood SR: Cine magnetic resonance imaging and flow measurements in the cardiovascular system. Br Med Bull 45:948, 1989.
38. Ruggieri PM, Laub GA, Masaryk TJ, Modic MT: Intracranial circulation: Pulse-sequence considerations in three-dimensional (volume) MR angiography. Radiology 171:785, 1989.
39. Schmalbrock P, Yuan C, Chakeres DW, et al: Volume MR angiography: Methods to achieve very short echo times. Radiology 175:861, 1990.
40. Anderson CM, Saloner D, Lee RE, Fortner A: Dedicated coil for carotid MR angiography. Radiology 176:868, 1990.
41. Rajan SS, Patt RH, Jarso S, et al: An extended-length coil design for peripheral MR angiography. Magn Reson Imaging 9:493, 1991.
42. Masaryk TJ, Tkach J, Glicklich M: Flow, radiofrequency pulse sequences, and gradient magnetic fields: Basic interactions and adaptations to angiographic imaging. Top Magn Reson Imaging 3:1, 1991.
43. Sechtem U, Pflugfelder PW, White RD, et al: Cine MRI: Potential for the evaluation of cardiovascular function. AJR 148:239, 1987.
44. Dinsmore RF, Wismer GL, Levine RA, et al: Magnetic resonance imaging of the heart: Positioning and gradient angle selection for optimal imaging planes. AJR 143:1135, 1984.
45. von Schulthess GK, Fisher MR, Crooks LE, Higgins CB: Gated MR imaging of the heart: Intracardiac signal in patients and healthy subjects. Radiology 156:125, 1985.
46. Sechtem U, Pflugfelder PW, Gould RG, et al: Measurement of right and left ventricular volumes in healthy individuals with cine MR imaging. Radiology 163:697, 1987.
47. Sechtem U, Pflugfelder PW, Cassidy MM, et al: Mitral or aortic regurgitation: Quantification of regurgitant volumes in patients with cine MR imaging. Radiology 167:425, 1988.
48. Dooms GC, Higgins CB: MR imaging of cardiac thrombi. J Comput Assist Tomogr 10:415, 1986.
49. Sechtem U, Hugenbeg K, Smoley J, et al: Detection of left ventricular thrombi: Comparison of MRI, computed tomography, echocardiography, angiography, and surgery. J Am Coll Cardiol 11(Suppl A):158, 1988.
50. Amparo EG, Higgins CB, Farmer D, et al: Gated MRI of cardiac and paracardiac masses. AJR 143:1151, 1984.
51. Go RT, O'Donnell JK, Underwood DA, et al: Comparison of gated cardiac MRI and 2D echocardiography of intracardiac neoplasms. AJR 145:21, 1985.
52. Winkler M, Higgins CB: Suspected intracardiac masses: Evaluation with MR imaging. Radiology 165:117, 1987.
53. Higgins CB, Lanzer P, Stark D, et al: Imaging by nuclear magnetic resonance in patients with chronic ischemic heart disease. Circulation 69:523, 1984.
54. McNamara MT, Higgins CB, Schechtmann N, et al: Detection and characterization of acute myocardial infarctions in man with the use of gated magnetic resonance imaging. Circulation 71:717, 1985.
55. Fisher MR, McNamara MT, Higgins CB: Acute myocardial infarction: MR evaluation in 29 patients. AJR 148:247, 1987.
56. Higgins CB: MR of the heart: Anatomy, physiology, and metabolism. AJR 151:239, 1988.
57. Sechtem U, Higgins CB, Sommerhoff BA, et al: Magnetic resonance imaging of restrictive cardiomyopathy. Am J Cardiol 59:480, 1987.
58. Soulen RL, Stark DD, Higgins CB: Magnetic resonance imaging of constrictive pericardial heart disease. Am J Cardiol 55:480, 1985.
59. Sechtem U, Tscholakoff D, Higgins CB: MRI of the normal pericardium. AJR 147:239, 1986.
60. Sechtem U, Tscholakoff D, Higgins CB: MRI of the abnormal pericardium. AJR 147:245, 1986.
61. Higgins CB, Byrd BF III, Farmer D, et al: Magnetic resonance imaging in patients with congenital heart disease. Circulation 70:851, 1984.
62. Diethelm L, Dery R, Lipton MJ, Higgins CB: Atrial level shunts: Sensitivity and specificity of MR in diagnosis. Radiology 162:185, 1987.
63. Didier D, Higgins CB, Fisher M, et al: Congenital heart disease: Gated MR imaging in 72 patients. Radiology 158:227, 1986.
64. Didier D, Higgins CB: Identification and localization of ventricular septal defects by gated magnetic resonance imaging. Am J Cardiol 57:1363, 1986.
65. Amparo EG, Higgins CB, Hricak H, Sollitto R: Aortic dissection: Magnetic resonance imaging. Radiology 15:399, 1985.
66. White RD, Dooms GC, Higgins CB: Advances in imaging thoracic aortic disease. Invest Radiol 21:761, 1986.
67. Sommerhoff BK, Higgins CB, White RD, et al: Aortic dissection: Sensitivity and specificity of MR imaging. Radiology 3:651, 1988.
68. Sommerhoff BK, Sechtem UP, Fisher MR, Higgins CB: MR imaging of congenital anomalies of the aortic arch. AJR 149:9, 1987.
69. von Schulthess GK, Higashino SM, Higgins SS, et al: Coarctation of the aorta: MR imaging. Radiology 158:469, 1986.
70. Bissett GS III, Strife JL, Kirks DR, Bailey WW: Vascular ring: MR imaging. AJR 149:251, 1987.
71. Sommerhoff BK, Sechtem UP, Higgins CB: Evaluation of pulmonary blood supply by magnetic resonance imaging in patients with pulmonary atresia. J Am Coll Cardiol 11:166, 1988.

72. Higgins CB, Byrd BF III, McNamara MT, et al: Magnetic resonance imaging of the heart: A review of the experience in 172 subjects. Radiology 155:671, 1985.
73. Brown JJ, Higgins CB: Myocardial contrast agents for magnetic resonance imaging. AJR 151:239, 1988.
74. Higgins CB, Byrd BF III, Stark D, et al: Magnetic resonance imaging in hypertrophic cardiomyopathy. Am J Cardiol 55:1121, 1985.
75. Brown JJ, Barakos J, Higgins CB: MRI of paracardiac and intracardiac masses. J Thorac Imaging 4:58, 1989.
76. Markiewicz W, Sechtem U, Kirby R, et al: Measurement of ventricular volumes in the dog by nuclear magnetic resonance imaging. J Am Coll Cardiol 10:170, 1987.
77. Caputo GR, Sechtem U, Tscholakoff D, Higgins CB: Measurement of myocardial infarct size at early and late time intervals using MR imaging: An experimental study in dogs. AJR 149:237, 1987.
78. Maddahi J, Crues J, Berman DS, et al: Noninvasive quantitation of left ventricular mass by gated proton magnetic resonance imaging. J Am Coll Cardiol 10:682, 1987.
79. Sechtem U, Sommerhoff BK, Markiewicz W, et al: Assessment of regional left ventricular wall thickening by magnetic resonance imaging: Evaluation in normal persons and patients with global and regional dysfunction. Am J Cardiol 59:145, 1987.
80. Pflugfelder PW, Sechtem UP, White RD, Higgins CB: Quantitation of regional myocardial function by rapid (cine) magnetic resonance imaging. AJR 150:523, 1988.
81. Utz JA, Herfkens RJ, Heinsimer JA, et al: Cine MR determination of left ventricular ejection fraction. AJR 148:839, 1987.
82. Pflugfelder PW, Sechtem UP, White RD, et al: Noninvasive evaluation of mitral regurgitation by analysis of left atrial signal loss in cine magnetic resonance imaging. Am Heart J 117:1113, 1989.
83. Mogelvang J, Thomson C, Horn T, et al: Determination of left ventricular volume (mass) by magnetic resonance imaging. Am J Noninvasive Cardiol 1:231, 1977.
84. Higgins CB, Holt W, Pflugfelder P, Sechtem U: Functional evaluation of the heart with MRI. Magn Reson Med 6:121, 1988.
85. Wagner S, Aufferman W, Buser P, et al: Diagnostic accuracy and estimation of the severity of valvular regurgitation from signal void on cine MRI. Am Heart J 118:760, 1989.
86. Holt WW, Pflugfelder P, Auffermann W, et al: Noninvasive measurement of left ventricular systolic wall stress by cine MRI [Abstract]. *In* Book of Abstracts. Berkeley, CA, Society of Magnetic Resonance in Medicine, 1987, p 727.
87. Nayler GL, Firmin DN, Longmore DB: Blood flow imaging by cine magnetic resonance. J Comput Assist Tomogr 10:715, 1986.
88. Firmin DN, Nayler GL, Klipstein RH, et al: In vivo validation of MR velocity imaging. J Comput Assist Tomogr 11:751, 1987.
89. Pettigrew RI, Dannels W, Galloway JR, et al: Quantitative phase-flow MR imaging in dogs by using standard sequences: Comparison with in vivo flow-meter measurements. AJR 148:411, 1987.
90. Bendel P, Buonocare E, Bockisch A, Besozzi MC: Blood flow in the carotid arteries: Quantification by using phase-sensitive MR imaging. AJR 152:1307, 1989.
91. Underwood SR, Firmin DN, Klipstein RH, et al: Magnetic resonance velocity mapping: Clinical application of a new technique. Br Heart J 57:404, 1987.
92. Bogren HG, Klipstein RH, Mohiaddin RH, et al: Pulmonary artery distensibility and blood flow patterns: A magnetic resonance study of normal subjects and of patients with pulmonary arterial hypertension. Am Heart J 118:990, 1989.
93. Bogren HG, Mohiaddin RH, Klipstein RH, et al: The function of the aorta in ischemic heart disease: A magnetic resonance and angiographic study of aortic compliance and blood flow patterns. Am Heart J 118:234, 1989.
94. Caputo GR, Kondo C, Masui T, et al: Pulmonary branch arterial flow can be measured by cine MR velocity mapping. Radiology 177:144, 1990.
95. Karvonen J, Ahowen A, Kari-Koskinen O, et al: Determination of reference values for regional lung ventilation and perfusion. *In* Hutas I, Debreczeni LA (eds): Respiration. Advances in Physiological Sciences, vol. 10. Elmsford, NY, Pergamon Press, 1981.
96. Brenner LD, Steiman D, Caputo GR, et al: Velocity-encoded cine MR measurement of left-to-right shunts and pulmonary blood flow in patients with congenital heart disease. Circulation 84(Suppl):II-352, 1991.
97. Caputo GR, Suzuki JI, Kondo C, et al: Determination of left ventricular volumes and mass using efficient biphasic spin-echo magnetic resonance imaging: Comparison with cine MRI. Radiology 177:773, 1990.
98. Caputo GR, Steiman D, Funari M, et al: Quantification of aortic regurgitation by velocity-encoded cine MR. Circulation 84(Suppl):II-203, 1991.
99. Fishman MC, Naidich JB, Stein HL: Vascular magnetic resonance imaging. Radiol Clin North Am 24:485, 1986.
100. Mendelson DS, Apter S, Mitty HA, et al: Residual dissection of the thoracic aorta after repair—MRI-angiographic correlation. Comput Med Imaging Graph 15:31, 1991.
101. Chang JM, Friese K, Caputo GR, et al: MR measurement of blood flow in the true and false channel in chronic aortic dissection. J Comput Assist Tomogr 15:418, 1991.
102. Dinsmore RE, Wedeen V, Rosen B, et al: Phase-offset technique to distinguish slow blood flow and thrombus on MR images. AJR 148:634, 1987.
103. Gehl HB, Bohndorf K, Klose KC, Gunther RW: Two-dimensional MR angiography in the evaluation of abdominal veins with gradient refocused sequences. J Comput Assist Tomogr 14:619, 1990.
104. Pan X, Rapp J, Harris H, et al: Identification of aortic thrombus by magnetic resonance imaging. J Vasc Surg 9:801, 1989.
105. Caputo G, Kondo C, Higgins CB: Quantification of blood flow using magnetic resonance imaging. *In* Higgins C, Hricak H, Helms C (eds): Magnetic Resonance Imaging of the Body. New York, Raven Press, 1992, pp 339–352.
106. Anderson CM, Saloner D, Lee RE: Gadolinium turbo-FLASH screening of the aorta in forty seconds. Proceedings of the 9th Annual Meeting of the Society for Magnetic Resonance Imaging, 1991, p 417.
107. Bandyk DF: Preoperative imaging of aortic aneurysms—Conventional and digital subtraction angiography, computed tomography scanning, and magnetic resonance imaging. Surg Clin North Am 69:721, 1989.
108. Rapp JH, Pan XM, Hale J, et al: ''Angiography'' by magnetic resonance imaging: Detailed vascular anatomy without ionizing radiation or contrast media. Surgery 105:662, 1989.
109. Edelman RR, Mattle HP, Atkinson DJ, Hoogewoud HM: MR angiography. AJR 154:937, 1990.
110. Zeitler E: Magnetic resonance angiography—The body and extremities [in German]. Vasa Suppl 27:394, 1989.
111. Lim TH, Saloner D, Anderson CM: Current applications of magnetic resonance vascular imaging. Cardiol Clin 7:661, 1989.
112. Gomori J, Grossman R, Goldberg H: Intracranial hematomas, imaging by high-field MR. Radiology 157:87, 1985.
113. Sevick RJ, Tsuruda JS: Magnetic resonance imaging and computed tomography of cerebral vascular disease. Curr Opin Radiol 3:31, 1991.
114. Litt AW, Eidelman EM, Pinto RS, et al: Diagnosis of carotid artery stenosis: Comparison of 2DFT time-of-flight MR angiography with contrast angiography in 50 patients. AJR 156:611, 1991.
115. Nishimura DG, Macovski A, Jackson JI, et al: Magnetic resonance angiography by selective inversion recovery using a compact gradient echo sequence. Magn Reson Med 8:96, 1988.
116. Edelman RR, Mattle HP, Oreilly GV, et al: Magnetic resonance imaging of flow dynamics in the circle of willis. Stroke 21:56, 1990.
117. Huston J, Rufenacht DA, Ehman RL, Wiebers DO: Intracranial aneurysms and vascular malformations: Comparison of time-of-flight and phase-contrast MR angiography. Radiology 181:721, 1991.
118. Masaryk TJ, Modic MT, Ross JS, et al: Intracranial circulation: Preliminary clinical results with three-dimensional (volume) MR angiography. Radiology 171:793, 1989.
119. Ruggieri PM, Masaryk TJ, Ross JS, Modic MT: Magnetic resonance angiography of the intracranial vasculature. Top Magn Reson Imaging 3:23, 1991.
120. Sevick RJ, Tsuruda JS, Schmalbrock P: Three-dimensional time-of-flight MR angiography in the evaluation of cerebral aneurysms. J Comput Assist Tomogr 14:874, 1990.
121. Edelman RR, Wentz KU, Mattle HP, et al: Intracerebral arteriovenous malformations: Evaluation with selective MR angiography and venography. Radiology 173:831, 1989.
122. Marchal G, Bosmans H, Van Fraeyenhoven L, et al: Intracranial vascular lesions: Optimization and clinical evaluation of three-dimensional time-of-flight MR angiography. Radiology 175:443, 1990.
123. Pernicone JR, Siebert JE, Potchen EJ: Demonstration of an early

draining vein by MR angiography. J Comput Assist Tomogr 15:829, 1991.
124. Padayachee TS, Bingham JB, Graves MJ, et al: Dural sinus thrombosis. Diagnosis and follow-up by magnetic resonance angiography and imaging. Neuroradiology 33:165, 1991.
125. Rippe DJ, Boyko OB, Spritzer CE, et al: Demonstration of dural sinus occlusion by the use of MR angiography. AJNR 11:199, 1990.
126. Koch M, Von Schulthess GK: Magnetic resonance angiography in the abdomen and pelvis. Curr Opin Radiol 3:463, 1991.
127. Kim D, Edelman RR, Kent KC, et al: Abdominal aorta and renal artery stenosis: Evaluation with MR angiography. Radiology 174:727, 1990.
128. Mitchell DG, Tobin M, LeVeen R, et al: Induced renal artery stenosis in rabbits: Magnetic resonance imaging, angiography, and radionuclide determination of blood volume and blood flow. Magn Reson Imaging 6:113, 1988.
129. Caputo GR, Higgins CB: Advances in cardiac imaging modalities: Magnetic resonance, fast computed tomography, and positron emission tomography. Invest Radiol 25:838–854, 1990.
130. Masaryk TJ, Modic MT, Ruggieri PM, et al: Three-dimensional (volume) gradient-echo imaging of the carotid bifurcation: Preliminary clinical experience. Radiology 171:801, 1989.
131. Sacks D, Robinson JL, Marinelli DL, Perlmutter GS: Evaluation of the peripheral arteries with duplex ultrasound after angioplasty. Radiology 176:39, 1990.
132. Fronek A, Loel M, Bernstein EF: Quantitative ultrasonographic studies of lower extremity flow velocities in health and disease. Circulation 53:957, 1976.
133. Kohler TR, Nance DR, Carner MM, et al: Duplex scanning for diagnosis of aortoiliac and femoropopliteal disease: A prospective study. Circulation 76:1074, 1987.
134. de Morais D, Johnston KW: Assessment of aortoiliac disease by noninvasive quantitative Doppler waveform analysis. Br J Surg 68:789, 1981.
135. Gerlock AJ, Giyanani VL, Krebs C: Applications of Noninvasive Vascular Techniques. Philadelphia, WB Saunders, 1988, pp 296–298.
136. Kondo C, Caputo GR, Semelka R, Higgins CB: Right and left ventricular stroke volume measurements with velocity encoded cine NMR imaging: In vitro and in vivo validation. AJR 157:9, 1991.
137. Pelc NJ, Shimakawa A, Glover GH: Phase contrast cine MRI. Book of Abstracts of the Eighth Annual Meeting of the Society of Magnetic Resonance in Medicine, 1989, p 101.
138. Nelson TR, Pretorius DH: The Doppler signal: Where does it come from and what does it mean? AJR 151:439, 1988.
139. Johnston KW, Taraschuk I: Validation of the role of pulsatility index in quantitation of the severity of peripheral arterial occlusive disease. Am J Surg 131:295, 1976.
140. Caputo GR, Masui T, Gooding GAW, et al: Popliteal and tibioperoneal arteries: Feasibility of two-dimensional time-of-flight MR angiography and phase velocity mapping. Radiology 182:387, 1992.
141. Masui T, Caputo GR, Bowersox JC, Higgins CB: Assessment of femoropopliteal occlusive disease with two-dimensional MR angiography and velocity encoded cine MR imaging: In vivo validation. J Comput Assist Tomogr (In press).
142. Maier SE, Meir D, Boesiger P, et al: Human abdominal aorta: Comparative measurements of blood flow with MR imaging and multigated Doppler ultrasound. Radiology 171:487, 1989.
143. Caputo GR, Kondo C, Masui T, et al: Right and left lung perfusion: In vitro and in vivo validation with oblique-angle, velocity-encoded cine MR imaging. Radiology 180:693, 1991.
144. Yucel EK, Dumoulin CL, Waltman AC: MR angiography of lower extremity arterial disease: Preliminary experience. J Magn Reson Imaging 2:303, 1992.
145. Owen RS, Carpenter JP, Baum RA, et al: Magnetic resonance imaging of angiographically occult runoff vessels in peripheral arterial occlusive disease. N Engl J Med 326:1577, 1992.
146. Lossef SV, Rajan SS, Patt RH, et al: Gadolinium-enhanced magnitude contrast MR angiography of popliteal and tibial arteries. Radiology 184:349, 1992.
147. Nakatsuka H, Hashimoto H, Tsubakimoto M, et al: MR-angiography of veins in the lower extremities [in Japanese, English Abstract]. Nippon Igaku Hoshasen Gakkai Zasshi 51:1498, 1991.
148. Nakatsuka H, Tsubakimoto M, Hashimoto H, et al: MR angiography of the forearm—Visualization of the internal dialysis shunt [in Japanese, English Abstract]. Nippon Igaku Hoshasen Gakkai Zasshi 51:1105, 1991.
149. Gehl HB, Bohndorf K, Gladziwa U, et al: Imaging of hemodialysis fistulas: Limitations of MR angiography. J Comput Assist Tomogr 15:271, 1991.
150. Mulligan SA, Matsuda T, Lanzer P, et al: Peripheral arterial occlusive disease: Prospective comparison of MR angiography and color duplex US with conventional angiography. Radiology 178:695, 1991.
151. Wendt RE III, Nitz W, Morrisett JD, Hedrick TD: A technique for flow-enhanced magnetic resonance angiography of the lower extremities. Magn Reson Imaging 8:723, 1990.
152. Lim TH, Saloner D, Anderson CM: Current applications of magnetic resonance vascular imaging. *In* Wolfe CL (ed): Cardiac Imaging: Diagnosis and Assessment of Cardiac Disorders. Philadelphia, WB Saunders, 1989, pp 661–683.

7

Principles of Angiography

Sanford D. Altman, M.D., David A. Kumpe, M.D., Paul L. Redmond, M.B., Raphael F. Kilcoyne, M.D., and Jeffrey S. Rose, M.D.

• • •

HISTORY OF ANGIOGRAPHY

Only 2 months after Roentgen discovered x-rays in 1895, investigators had begun to study the circulation by injecting opaque substances into the blood vessels of cadavers. In both Europe and America, scientists were extolling the marvels of the new rays, which were able to delineate the fine vascular structures of the body.[60, 103] The pulmonary vessels, as well as the peripheral vessels, were displayed. Hickey, in Detroit, injected a suspension of bismuth in glycerin into the blood vessels of the chest in a cadaver.[63] Although some in vivo injections were made, investigations with cadavers remained the mainstay of angiographic studies until the development of nontoxic contrast materials. In 1910, Franck and Alwens successfully injected bismuth in oil intravenously into rabbits and dogs and studied the blood flow in the veins, heart, and lungs fluoroscopically.[50] Heuser performed the first contrast study of blood vessels in a living human being in 1919 by injecting potassium iodide into a dorsal vein on the hand of a child with congenital syphilis. He followed the flow of the substance from the arm to the heart.[62] By 1923 and 1924, investigators in three countries had performed angiograms in living humans. In Germany, Berbereich and Hirsch used an aqueous solution of strontium bromide;[17] in France, Sicard and Forestier used iodized poppyseed oil;[136] and in the United States, Brooks used sodium iodide.[26]

The search for safe contrast media led to the development of the predecessor of the modern water-soluble organic iodides by Binz and colleagues in 1929; the agent was marketed as Selectan Neutral.[22] At the same time that contrast media were being improved, other investigators focused on methods of injecting these media into appropriate vessels. Direct arterial injection had been used to deliver Salvarsan into the internal carotid arteries for syphilis therapy.[16] Moniz* and associates used this direct method to introduce sodium iodide, and later thorium dioxide (Thorotrast), into the carotid arteries (Fig. 7–1).[98, 99] He was the first to perform direct arterial injections in humans.

A number of different approaches were developed for studying the heart and thoracic aorta. Nuvoli (who died at age 36 years) inserted a needle through the anterior chest wall into the ascending aorta.[105] A similar approach was used from the posterior direction to the aorta and left ventricle. Because of the hazards of these direct approaches, Castellanos and associates, and later Robb and Steinberg, described an indirect method that remained popular for many years.[30, 123] They injected contrast media into arm veins and filmed the heart and great vessels. Dilution of the contrast agent by blood in the heart and pulmonary vessels caused the aorta to be seen successfully in only 75 per cent of cases.

Moniz and colleagues also pioneered in cardiac and pulmonary angiography. They called the study angiopneumography, and employed a catheter from an arm vein into the heart.[100] This approach had been devised earlier by a young resident, Werner Forssmann, who was looking for a safer method of injecting epinephrine into the heart in cases of anesthetic-induced cardiac arrest than the direct insertion of a needle into the cardiac chamber through the anterior chest wall. Forssmann practiced on cadavers and then performed the catheter procedure on himself. He injected sodium iodide into the right atrium and studied the flow in his own heart and lungs by having an assistant hold a mirror in front of the fluoroscope.[49] His work went unrecognized for some time because his superiors could not see the utility of the method. Ultimately, in 1956, along with Cournand and Richards, he received the Nobel Prize (for bravery?).[2] The circulation to the right side of the heart was studied by this approach in 1936.[7]

Selective catheterization of the pulmonary vessels was reported by Bolt and Rink in 1951.[24] The term angiocardiography was coined by Rousthoi, who used retrograde passage of a catheter into the left ventricle in 1933.[126] Thoracic aortography was performed by Castellanos and Pereiras by a retrograde injection into the brachial artery.[31] Radner modified this method by threading a catheter from the radial artery into the thoracic aorta for better visualization.[115] Jonsson used retrograde passage of a catheter down

*This great Portuguese neurologist received the Nobel Prize in Medicine in 1949, not for his important contributions in angiography of the brain and chest, but rather for developing the controversial prefrontal lobotomy for treatment of mental illness.[57]

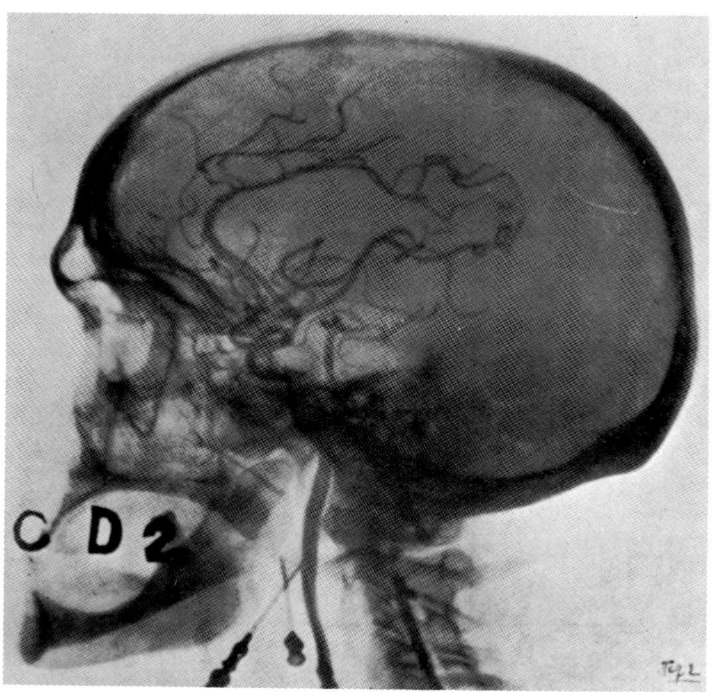

FIGURE 7–1. **Internal carotid arteriogram from Moniz' original article. A 30 per cent solution of sodium iodide was injected into a cadaver. (From Moniz E: Rev Neurol [Paris] 34:72, 1927.)**

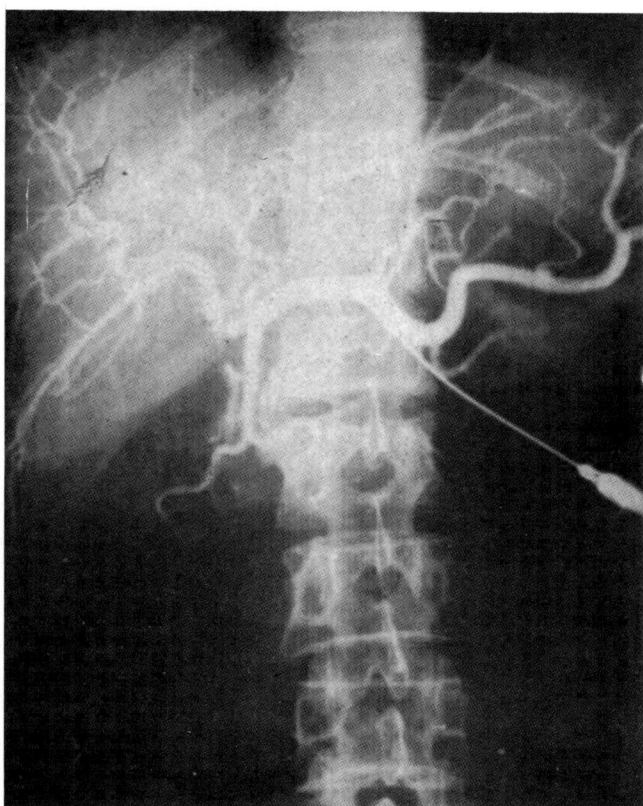

FIGURE 7–2. Dos Santos and coworkers' example of a translumbar injection directly into the celiac axis. (Sodium iodide, 10 ml of a 100 per cent solution.) (From dos Santos R, Lamas A, Caldas J: L'arteriographie des membres, de l'aorta et de ses branches abdominales. Bull Mem Soc Natl Chir 55:589, 1929.)

the common carotid artery.[75] An interesting route to the thoracic aorta was Euler's transesophageal puncture of the descending aorta.[44] Early coronary angiography included some novel techniques, such as cardiac arrest on occlusion of the aorta by a balloon catheter.[11, 40]

In 1929, dos Santos and coworkers used a translumbar needle to inject contrast medium directly into the abdominal aorta (Fig. 7–2).[39] This method gave way only gradually to the approach by way of a catheter inserted percutaneously from a femoral or axillary artery. Farinas pioneered the catheter approach from the femoral artery in 1941, a method perfected by Seldinger in 1953.[45, 131] Good results in peripheral angiography were obtained as early as 1931 (Fig. 7–3).[113] Venography was introduced by some of the same investigators in the 1920s and 1930s.[17, 128, 136]

NEEDLES, CATHETERS, AND GUIDEWIRES

Inserting a needle or cannula directly into a blood vessel is the simplest method of injecting contrast material. Because some blood vessels are inaccessible to direct injection, methods were devised for either remote injection of contrast media or remote insertion of a catheter. Dos Santos and coworkers' translumbar approach to aortography and Moniz's needle insertions into the carotid artery are two examples of the direct method.[39, 98] Catheter techniques did not become popular until Seldinger showed how to introduce the catheter percutaneously into the femoral artery over a guidewire.[131] Odman perfected this approach and made selective injections into aortic branches with specially shaped catheters.[108] This method has become the one used for most selective angiography. More recent developments include the mass production by many manufacturers of specifically shaped catheters for various arterial branches. Tip deflecting systems and external magnetic fields have been used to direct catheters into vessels;[67] however, they have not become clinically significant because of the wide variety of specialized catheter and guidewire systems available enabling fluoroscopic superselective catheterization of essentially every named vessel for diagnostic and therapeutic purposes.

CONTRAST MEDIA

History

Radiographic contrast media are substances whose primary purpose is to enhance diagnostic information of med-

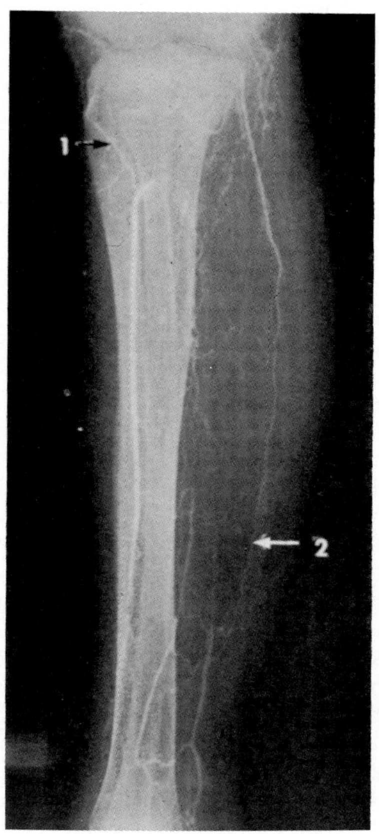

FIGURE 7–3. An early femoral arteriogram showing popliteal artery occlusion with filling of the anterior and posterior tibial arteries by collateral arteries (1,2). Skiodan in a 40 per cent solution was used as contrast medium. (From Pearse H, Warren S: The roentgenographic visualization of the arteries of the extremities in peripheral vascular disease. Ann Surg 94:1094, 1931.)

ical systems.[139] Opaque contrast media were not used successfully in living humans until the development of nontoxic substances. Investigators searched for a material sufficiently radiodense, soluble in water, and relatively harmless to the patient. Strontium and bismuth held early promise, but proved to be too toxic. In 1896, Sehrwald had conducted experiments that showed that iodine and other halogens were opaque to the new roentgen rays.[130] The soluble ionic solutions sodium and potassium iodide were less toxic than strontium when injected intravenously, yet sometimes they too produced convulsions, paralysis, or death. Oil-soluble compounds also were less toxic chemically, but they did not remain as an intact bolus long enough and also produced dangerous emboli, especially in the lung capillaries. In 1923, Osborne realized that sodium iodide, injected into the blood, was excreted in urine.[110] Thorium dioxide (Thorotrast) held promise when introduced by Moniz and coworkers in 1931, but unfortunately this material is radioactive and has a very long half-life.[99] Once deposited in the body, it can lead to the development of a variety of malignant tumors.[14]

In 1926, Binz and Rath discovered that a heterocyclic pyridine ring had a detoxifying effect on arsenic and iodine.[22, 54] In the following year, a real breakthrough in the search for intravascular contrast occurred when Binz and colleagues synthesized an organic iodine preparation of pyridine called Selectan Neutral. This compound was initially used as a therapeutic agent in the treatment of staphylococcal infections of the gallbladder.[1] Swick successfully used Selectan Neutral and a less toxic derivative, Uroselectan, in the first intravenous urograms.[147] Two years after the introduction of Uroselectan, two improved pyridine products, Diodrast and NeoIopax, were developed. Each carried two iodine atoms instead of one, as with Uroselectan, and therefore increased diagnostic efficacy while decreasing toxicity.[54] Owing to the greater opacity of these agents, investigators were able to study the heart and great vessels in the early 1930s. These contrast agents were used for the next 20 years.

In 1933, Swick and Wallingford proposed a 6-carbon (benzene) ring as a carrier of iodine; however, it took 20 years to produce this concept.[55, 80] Their benzene ring was the precursor to modern-day water-soluble contrast media. Adding a carboxyl group at C-1 made this ring an acid (benzoic acid). An amino group at C-3 allowed the addition of 3 iodine atoms at the C-2, C-4, and C-6 positions, which increased absorption of x-rays further and therefore improved diagnostic efficacy. Acetylation of the amino group at C-3 resulted in decreased toxicity. This compound, introduced in the early 1950s, was known as Urokon. The addition of a second acetylated amino group (acetamide chain) at C-5 decreased toxicity even further.[112] This compound, diatrizoic acid, which was introduced in 1954, is the main building block for all standard high-osmolarity contrast agents in use today (e.g., Hypaque and Renografin). These agents are salts and are completely dissociated/ionized in solution as contrast media. For every three iodine atoms in solution, there are two particles (1 anion [$RCOO^-$] and 1 cation [sodium or meglumine]). In 1962, further modifications of the basic tri-iodinated molecule produced iothalamate meglumine (Conray) and metrizoate sodium (Isopaque). The tri-iodinated compounds produce excellent radiodensity, and the high iodine content counteracts dilution of the medium by blood. Since the introduction of diatrizoate, the incidences of transverse myelitis and kidney damage after abdominal aortography have decreased markedly.[93] The slight modification of the diatrizoate formula into iothalamate created a compound less viscous and, therefore, easier to inject under pressure.

The pioneering work of Torsten Almen, a radiologist from Malmo, Sweden, led to the synthesis of the nonionic contrast medium metrizamide (Amipaque).[5] Substituting a nondissociating amide group for the ionic carboxyl group reduced the molar concentration by half without reducing the iodine content. With a large number of hydrophilic hydroxyl groups on the side chains, these compounds remained water-soluble. Metrizamide, however, is not sufficiently stable in solution to allow sterilization by autoclaving; a freeze-dried lyophilized form that must be reconstituted prior to use is available. Substitution of different side chains of metrizamide has led to the introduction of the more soluble compounds iopamidol (Niopam, Isovue), iohexol (Omnipaque), iopentol (Nycomed), ioversol (Optiray), iopromide (Ultravist), and ioxilan (Biophysica),[144] which are available in solution like conventional contrast media.[6, 114]

An alternative approach to reduce osmolarity has been to link two tri-iodinated benzene rings together, with only one of the rings having an ionizing carboxyl group. The result is a monoacid dimer, providing six atoms of iodine for two particles in solution.[36] Using this approach, Guerbet (Paris) introduced ioxaglate (Hexabrix). Nonionic dimers, iotrol (Iotrolan) and iodixanol (Nycomed), are currently under development. Their osmolarity is close to that of plasma; however, they are highly viscous. These may find particular application in myelography where their larger molecular size and higher viscosity offer an advantage.[141] The lower osmolarity of these newer agents offers significant theoretical advantages; however, they are much more expensive than the conventional contrast media, and, if used for all contrast studies, could add over $1 billion per year to current health care costs. Current research on new contrast media should yield compounds that are easier (and cheaper) to manufacture and even less toxic than currently available agents.

Chemical and Physical Characteristics

The surgeon dealing with vascular disease often relies on contrast-enhanced roentgenologic methods to plan, execute, and follow therapeutic regimens. Although many of the technical aspects of angiography are properly the responsibility of the vascular radiologist, it is essential that the referring physician possess some knowledge of the nature and incidence of complications inherent in a requested examination. Only in light of such knowledge can diagnostic procedures with intrinsic morbidity be requested in the best interests of the patient. The pathophysiologic effects of contrast media and the general hazards of vascular catheterization, as well as the risks incurred by the patient during specific procedures, are discussed later in this chapter. Several suggestions are made regarding preparation of the patient for angiography. More detailed information regarding these issues may be found in other sources.[74, 125, 129, 156]

The roentgenographic demonstration of vascular structures requires a contrast material that absorbs x-rays prodigiously. Iodine, with its high atomic number, has a K shell binding energy close to the mean energy of most diagnostic x-rays. Iodine therefore absorbs x-rays through photoelectric interactions that provide excellent contrast with minimal scatter.[32] There are four different groups of contrast media with different chemical structures in use today. They are all tri-iodinated derivatives of benzoic acid and exist as either ionic monomers, ionic dimers, nonionic monomers, or nonionic dimers. The triiodobenzoic acid molecules contain iodine covalently bonded at the 2, 4, and 6 positions on the benzene ring (Fig. 7–4). The ionic monomers have organic side chains of different kinds attached to the 3 and 5 positions of the ring to maximize solubility, but two major side chain types have proved least toxic, and they define the diatrizoate family and the iothalamate family of contrast media (Fig. 7–5). The carboxyl group at the number 1 carbon of the ring dissociates in solution to form an acid and, therefore, must be combined with a cation to form a stable soluble salt; the major media use either sodium or methylglucamine (meglumine), or a mixture of the two as cations (Fig. 7–6). Monomeric ionic contrast agents have three iodine molecules for every two particles (cation and anion) in solution. These are referred to as ratio 1.5 contrast media (i.e., 1.5 iodine atoms per particle in solution).

The osmolarity of the conventional monomeric ionic contrast agents is five to eight times that of plasma (280 mOsm/kg), and the concentration cannot be reduced significantly without compromising roentgen opacity. Much of the toxicity of these agents is caused by their hypertonicity. In recent years, two types of low-osmolarity contrast media have become available. Nonionic monomeric contrast media are the more widely used low-osmolarity contrast agents, and iopamidol and iohexol constitute the second generation of these compounds, based on the parent substance metrizamide (Fig. 7–7). They were designed to provide a high iodine content per number of particles in solution, and to be without charge, and therefore without electrical effects. They contain three iodine atoms for every particle in solution (i.e., ratio 3.0 contrast media). Ioxaglate (Hexabrix), which represents the second type of low-osmolarity contrast medium, is a monoacid dimer (Fig. 7–7). Two tri-iodinated benzene rings are linked by a short chain, with only one of the rings containing an ionizing carboxyl group. Each molecule has six iodine atoms per two particles in solution (i.e., ration 3.0 contrast media). By reducing the number of osmotically active particles by half, one would expect a reduction of 50 per cent in the osmolarity of these agents. However, the osmolarity of the new media is, in fact, one third that of the conventional high-osmolarity agents at the same iodine concentration, and this is due to the aggregation of some of the molecules of the new media when in solution, further reducing the number of osmotically active particles.[54] The commonly used angiographic agents are listed in Table 7–1.

The other contrast agent commonly applied in vascular roentgenology is ethiodized oil (Ethiodol), a poppy seed oil–based medium with a 37 per cent iodine content. It is used in small amounts for lymphography, and, more recently, it has been mixed with chemotherapeutic agents for chemoembolization of liver tumors.[23] This agent has its own unique set of composition-related ill effects, which are reviewed later in the chapter.

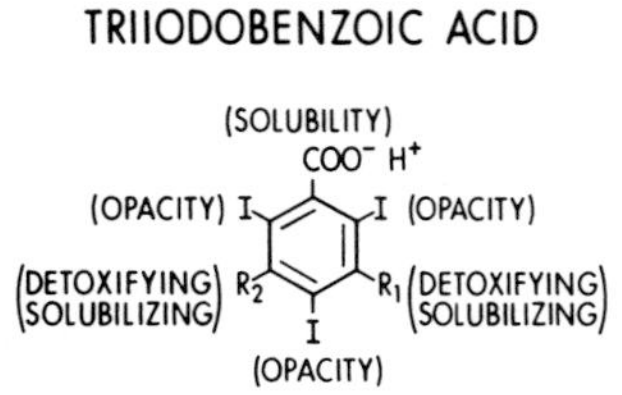

TRIIODOBENZOIC ACID

(SOLUBILITY) COO⁻ H⁺ — (OPACITY) I, I (OPACITY) — (DETOXIFYING, SOLUBILIZING) R_2, R_1 (DETOXIFYING, SOLUBILIZING) — I (OPACITY)

FIGURE 7–4. Triiodobenzoic acid. This is the parent compound of all modern angiographic contrast agents.

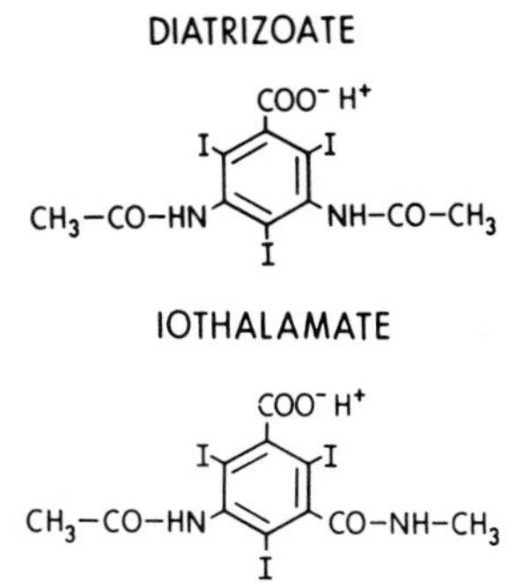

DIATRIZOATE

COO⁻ H⁺, I, I, CH_3–CO–HN, NH–CO–CH_3, I

IOTHALAMATE

COO⁻ H⁺, I, I, CH_3–CO–HN, CO–NH–CH_3, I

FIGURE 7–5. The anions of the two major ionic agents in current use, shown as the acids.

Pathophysiologic Characteristics

Sovak states that contrast media are drugs by default. The ideal contrast agent should be biologically inert, pharmacologically inactive, and efficiently and innocuously excreted.[139] A substantial number of toxic effects are induced in tissues perfused with contrast media. These appear to be related to the dose administered, the ionic composition of the contrast media, the osmolarity of the agent (Table 7–2), the intrinsic chemotoxicity of the agent, the duration of exposure, and the sensitivity of the specific tissue.

Intravascular Consequences

Contrast media exert a direct toxic effect on endothelium. Cellular metabolism is altered, and there is disruption of the normal intercellular junctions.[74] These effects are partly due to hyperosmolarity and partly due to the intrinsic chemotoxicity of the contrast medium. Vasodilatation, which is correlated with hyperosmolarity, may result in

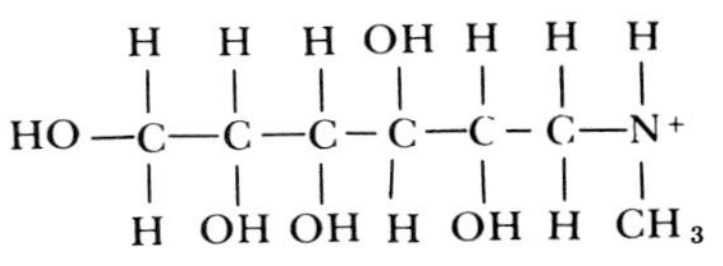

```
 H   H   H  OH  H   H   H
 |   |   |   |   |   |   |
HO—C—C—C—C—C—C—N+
 |   |   |   |   |   |   |
 H  OH  OH  H  OH  H  CH3
```

FIGURE 7–6. Structural formula for methylglucamine.

Table 7–1. Trade Names and Formulations of Commonly Used Angiographic Contrast Agents in the United States

Trade Name (Manufacturer)	Iodine (mg/ml)	Concentration (per cent)	Anion	Cation(s) (per cent)	Viscosity (centipoise at 37°C)	Osmolality (mOsm/kg)
Conray 43 (Mallinckrodt)	202	43	Iothalamate	Methylglucamine (43)	2.0	1000
Omnipaque 240 (Winthrop)	240	51.8	Iohexol*	—	3.1	504
Conray	282	60	Iothalamate	Methylglucamine (60)	4.0	1400
Hypaque 60% (Winthrop)	282	60	Diatrizoate	Methylglucamine (60)	4.1	1415
Reno-M-60 (Squibb)	282	60	Diatrizoate	Methylglucamine (60)	4.0	1500
Renografin-60 (Squibb)	288	60	Diatrizoate	Methylglucamine (52) and sodium (8)	4.0	1420
Hypaque sodium 50% (Winthrop)	300	50	Diatrizoate	Sodium (50)	2.4	1550
Isovue 300 (Squibb)	300	61	Iopamidol*	—	4.7	616
Omnipaque 300 (Winthrop)	300	64.7	Iohexol*	—	6.8	709
Renovist II (Squibb)	310	69	Diatrizoate	Methylglucamine (28.5) and sodium (29.1)	3.8	1517
Hexabrix (Mallinckrodt)	320	58.9	Iothalamate	Methylglucamine (39.3) and sodium (19.6)	7.5	600
Omnipaque 350 (Winthrop)	350	75.5	Iohexol*	—	11.2	862
Diatrizoate meglumine USP 76% (Squibb)	358	76	Diatrizoate	Methylglucamine (76)	9.2	1980
Renografin-76 (Squibb)	370	76	Diatrizoate	Methylglucamine (76) and sodium (10)	8.4	1940
Isovue 370 (Squibb)	370	76	Iopamidol*	—	9.6	796
Renovist (Squibb)	372	69	Diatrizoate	Methylglucamine (34.3) and sodium (35.0)	5.7	1900
Hypaque-M 75% (Winthrop)	385	75	Diatrizoate	Methylglucamine (50) and sodium (25)	8.0	2108
Conray 400 (Mallinckrodt)	400	66.8	Iothalamate	Sodium (66.8)	4.5	2300
Vascoray 400 (Mallinckrodt)	400	78	Iothalamate	Methylglucamine (52) and sodium (26)	9.0	2400
Hypaque-M 90% (Winthrop)	462	90	Diatrizoate	Methylglucamine (60) and sodium (30)	19.5	2938
Angio-Conray (Mallinckrodt)	480	80	Iothalamate	Sodium (80)	9.0	2400
Angiovist 282 (Berlex)	282	60	Diatrizoate	Methylglucamine (60)	4.1	1000
Angiovist 292 (Berlex)	292	60	Diatrizoate	Methylglucamine (52) and sodium (8)	4.0	1090
Angiovist 370 (Berlex)	370	76	Diatrizoate	Methylglucamine (66) and sodium (10)	9.0	1380
Optiray 160 (Mallinckrodt)	160	34	Ioversol		1.9	355
Optiray 240 (Mallinckrodt)	240	51	Ioversol	—	3.0	502
Optiray 320 (Mallinckrodt)	320	68	Ioversol	—	5.8	702
Optiray 350 (Mallinckrodt)	350	74	Ioversol	—	9.0	792

**Nonionic; no anion or cation.*

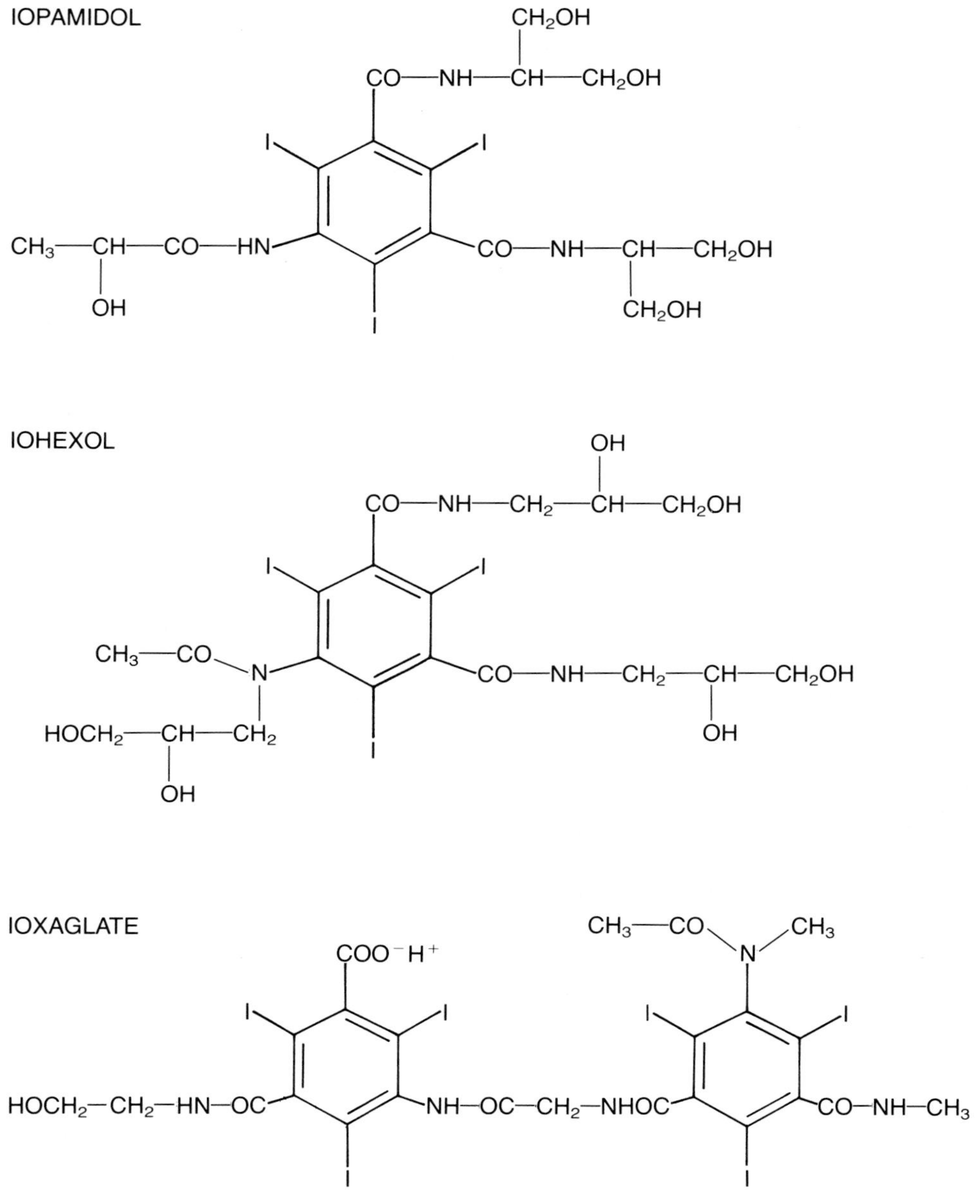

IOPAMIDOL

IOHEXOL

IOXAGLATE

FIGURE 7–7. **Structural formulas for the currently used low-osmolar contrast agents.**

Table 7–2. Adverse Effects of High-Osmolarity Contrast Agents

Hemodynamic Effects
Vasodilatation (local and general)
Hemodilution
Hypervolemia
Changes in pulmonary artery pressure, cardiac output and pulmonary and systemic resistance
Adverse Effects Upon Erythrocytes
Crenation, rigidity
Mobility resulting in tissue anoxia and increased peripheral resistance in microcirculation
Adverse Effects Upon Capillary Endothelium Resulting in
Tissue anoxia
Increased capillary permeability
Vasodilatation
Systemic hypotension
Osmotic hypervolemia

From Stolberg HO, McClennan BL: Ionic versus nonionic contrast use. Curr Probl Diagn Radiol 20:47, 1991.

systemic hypotension with pooling of blood in capillaries and veins and resultant decrease in systemic venous return to the heart.[56] These vasodilatory changes are greatly decreased with nonionic media.[102]

Contrast media cause increased rigidity of red blood cells, an effect that is less marked with the use of low-osmolarity agents. The reduced ability of stiffened erythrocytes to pass through capillaries may lead to regional increases in peripheral vascular resistance with resultant tissue anoxia.[47, 54] These changes may result in serious complications in patients with pulmonary hypertension undergoing pulmonary arteriography.[55] Damage to capillary endothelial cells may result in the release of substances that cause intravascular coagulation, platelet aggregation, and possibly anaphylactoid reactions.[56, 84] Ratio 3 nonionic monomers cause less capillary endothelial damage.

Contrast has an inhibitory effect on the thrombin fibrinogen reaction as well as platelet aggregation. Most authors agree that contrast agents have some anticoagulant effect on blood due chiefly to the inhibition of the final step of coagulation. These inhibitory effects are greater with ionic media than with nonionic media.[145, 146] In vitro experiments have shown an increase in clot formation with nonionic media.[29] Ioxaglate (Hexabrix) is the one low-osmolarity contrast medium that demonstrates more inhibition of coagulation than currently used high-osmolarity contrast.[12, 83, 117] To reduce the frequency of thromboembolic complications while using nonionic contrast media, catheter manipulations should be performed carefully, catheters should be flushed continually, and blood–contrast media contact should be avoided.[120, 124] Vascular pain that occurs during the arterial or venous passage of injected contrast media is attributable to the osmolarity of the contrast solution.[143] Low-osmolarity contrast media produce much less pain when injected intravascularly than do high-osmolarity contrast media. The subsequent sensation of heat is thought to be secondary to vasodilatation, and is also lessened with the use of low-osmolarity contrast media.[143]

Cardiopulmonary Consequences

The adverse effects of intravascular contrast agents on the heart are accentuated in patients with reduced myocardial reserve and severe coronary artery stenosis.[144] Intravascular contrast has deleterious electrophysiologic, inotropic, and volumetric effects on the heart. Electrophysiologic changes related to contrast agents include decrease in impulse generation and conductivity delay, which may result in bradycardia, asystole, ventricular tachycardia, and ventricular fibrillation. Osmolarity is felt to play a major role in these reactions, which are seen less frequently with low-osmolarity contrast agents.[65]

Contrast media are vasodilators and can lower blood pressure during left ventriculography or peripheral arteriography.[156] Hypotension can have serious consequences in patients with ischemic myocardial or cerebrovascular disease. There is less vasodilatation with the low-osmolarity agents.[106, 121]

Intracoronary injection of a conventional ionic contrast medium has a direct depressant effect on the myocardium, an effect that is not shared by the low-osmolarity media, and the conventional media have a greater propensity to cause electrocardiographic changes and arrhythmias.[66] Binding of calcium by chelating agents in ionic media is felt to be one of the reasons for myocardial depression and arrhythmia. This is avoided with the use of nonionic contrast media.[144] Patients in congestive heart failure should be imaged with low-osmolarity contrast media (if contrast is needed) because of possible severe changes that may be induced by the increased osmotic load of high-osmolarity contrast media. An intravenous or direct pulmonary artery injection can cause a transient increase in pulmonary artery pressure. This may be detrimental in patients with pulmonary artery hypertension. This effect is greatly reduced with the use of low-osmolarity contrast media.[133]

Other substantial ill effects of contrast media may be manifested by the cardiopulmonary system. Patients with a pheochromocytoma may experience hypertensive crisis with contrast injection, especially following adrenal arteriography and venography. If patients need to be studied with contrast agents, premedication with an alpha blocker such as phenoxybenzamine is indicated.[106, 112, 156]

Renal Consequences

Greater than 99 per cent of contrast excretion occurs through the kidneys, making them the target organ for contrast toxicity.[37, 52]

Contrast media are excreted by glomerular filtration without significant secretion or resorption.[52, 142, 148] The glomerular filtration rate (GFR) in a normal 70-kg adult is 180 L/day. GFR, however, varies with age, sex, body size, circulatory dynamics, and underlying renal disease. The filtered load of contrast agent is highly dependent on the amount and rate of contrast administration.[144] High-osmolarity contrast media induce an osmotic diuresis. This causes an initial increase followed by a decrease in renal blood flow. Although the exact mechanism of contrast-induced nephropathy is not known, this decrease in renal blood flow seen with high-osmolarity contrast agent superimposed on abnormal baseline renal macrovasculature and microvasculature could incite local tissue ischemia and serve as a major contributing factor to contrast-induced nephropathy.[13, 28, 37, 52, 149] Direct toxicity on renal tubular cells is another proposed cause of contrast-induced nephrotoxicity. This too is lessened with the use of low-osmolarity contrast media.[35, 37]

Contrast nephropathy is an acute impairment of renal function following exposure to radiographic contrast. Alterations in serum creatinine are thought to be logarithmically related to alterations in GFR (i.e., a change in serum creatinine from 0.7 to 1.4 = 50% decrease in GFR).[21] Measurements of serum creatinine in the first 5 days after exposure to contrast media is the most practical method of identifying contrast-induced nephropathy. Authors have defined various degrees of rise of serum creatinine to indicate contrast-induced nephropathy. A good definition appears to be a rise of 1.0 mg/dl within 48 hours of contrast administration.[64] Contrast-induced acute renal failure may occur with or without oliguria (less than 400 ml urine/24 hr).

Many studies have been performed to determine risk factors for contrast-induced nephropathy. To date, the most important risk factors appear to be

1. Chronic renal insufficiency:[59, 64, 150] Patients with baseline serum creatinine greater than 1.5 should be viewed with caution.[101]

2. Diabetes: Diabetic patients, especially insulin-dependent diabetics with impaired renal function, are at increased risk. Diabetics with normal renal function are no longer felt to be at increased risk for contrast-induced nephrotoxicity.[18, 33, 58, 59, 64]

3. Dehydration: Dehydrated patients are at greater risk for contrast-induced nephropathy; all patients, therefore, should be well hydrated prior to administration of intravascular contrast.[37] The practice of ordering "NPO [nothing by mouth] after midnight" for patients who are to have an arteriogram the following day is to be avoided.

4. Dose and administration: Large, repeated doses of contrast media produce increased risk.[18, 104]

5. Advanced age: Patients greater than 60 years of age are at increased risk. This most likely is secondary to the

greater incidence of vascular disease with concurrent decrease in GFR.[37]

6. Recent surgery or vascular interventional procedures.[144]

These risk factors may be additive.[21] Myeloma, once felt to be a risk factor, is now felt to be of no greater risk than patients with similar creatinine levels who are well hydrated.[38, 64, 153]

Although contrast-induced renal failure usually reverts back to baseline preprocedure creatinine levels within 1 to 2 weeks, more serious complications such as oliguria and anuria lasting several days, permanent renal damage requiring chronic dialysis, and uremia resulting in death have been described.[18, 77, 104] Since nonionic low-osmolarity contrast media appear to have a less toxic effect on the kidneys, it may be prudent to use these agents on patients in the high-risk groups.[87]

Neurologic Consequences

The endothelium of cerebral capillaries has a continuous basement membrane that acts as a selective filter controlling the free passage of serum contents between blood and brain.[25, 82, 92, 109, 118, 127, 140, 154] Water-soluble contrast media should not cross a normal intact blood-brain barrier. Damage to the blood-brain barrier is a specific example of contrast-induced endothelial damage and hyperosmolarity is generally regarded as the inciting factor.[118, 119, 127] Hyperosmolarity and a direct chemotoxic effect of contrast are two major etiologic factors in contrast-induced neurotoxicity. Specific complications related to contrast may include convulsions, paresis, cortical blindness, and frank stroke.[82, 156] The effects of contrast media on the central nervous system may be responsible for many of the systemic adverse effects of these agents, from nausea (stimulation of the chemoreceptor trigger zone) to temperature variations (hypothalamic effect) to pulmonary edema and ventricular fibrillation (abnormal sympathetic neural discharge).[82]

Conventional ionic sodium-containing agents are more neurotoxic than the meglumine media, and diatrizoate products are slightly more dangerous than iothalamates.[95] When conventional ionic media are used, a weight-volume concentration not exceeding 60 per cent should be employed if neurologic complications are to be minimized.[89–91]

Low-osmolarity nonionic contrast media cause less damage to the blood-brain barrier than conventional media and are significantly better tolerated by the central nervous system during contrast examinations.[41]

Idiosyncratic Reactions to Contrast Agents

In addition to the nonidiosyncratic dose-dependent pathophysiologic effects of contrast media just described, there are a number of unusual, "idiosyncratic" responses that are not dose-related. These idiosyncratic reactions are termed anaphylactoid or anaphylactic-like. Unlike true allergic or anaphylactic reactions, there are no identifiable circulating antibodies found after an anaphylactoid reaction. Also, not all patients with a history of prior anaphylactoid reactions have repeat reaction when reexposed to contrast media, as would be expected with true anaphylactic reactions.[112] These "allergic" clinical symptoms constitute the familiar "contrast reactions," and they are generally categorized as follows (Table 7–3): *Minor reactions* are self-limited discomforts of short duration that are not life-threatening and do not require treatment; they include nausea, vomiting, headache, chills, dizziness, itching, sweating, transient hives, and edema. *Intermediate reactions* are transient but more serious. They require treatment but are not life-threatening. Vasovagal hypotension, refractory skin conditions, edema, urticaria, and mild bronchospasm are examples. *Major reactions* are life-threatening responses, such as severe hypotension, convulsions, pulmonary edema, severe bronchospasm, laryngeal edema, and cardiac arrhythmia.

Table 7–3. Classification of Severity of Reactions to Contrast Media

Minor	Intermediate	Major
Nausea	Faintness	Hypotensive shock
Vomiting (limited)	Vomiting (severe)	Pulmonary edema
Urticaria (limited)	Urticaria (profound)	Respiratory arrest
Pruritus	Facial edema	Cardiac arrest
Diaphoresis	Laryngeal edema	Convulsions
	Bronchospasm (mild)	

From Bush WH, Swanson DP: Acute reactions to intravascular contrast media: Types, risk factors, recognition, and specific treatment. AJR 157:1153, 1991.

The basis of these adverse reactions to contrast media is very poorly understood, and the demarcation between chemotoxic and idiosyncratic responses is not entirely clear. Suspected mechanisms for the etiology of these anaphylactoid reactions are: (1) cellular-released mediators such as histamine from mast cells and basophils;[144] (2) antigen-antibody reactions;[84, 122] (3) psychogenic factors;[144] and (4) acute activation or release of vasoactive substances including the complement and coagulation systems, kinins, and fibrinolysins. This last mechanism is felt to play a major role in idiosyncratic reactions.[7, 26, 84, 85] The incidence of allergic reactions occurring following a variety of studies is given in Table 7–4. The following list includes some important features of these reactions.

1. Idiosyncratic reactions are probably caused by the medium rather than by free iodine. A history of allergy to iodine is significant in predicting a reaction to water-soluble media, but no more so than a history of any other kind of allergy.[1]

2. Patients with a history of any allergy are twice as likely to have a mild idiosyncratic reaction to contrast me-

Table 7–4. Incidence of Allergic Reactions to 36 Contrast Media

Type of Study	Incidence of Reaction (per cent)
Urography	4.8
Intravenous cholangiography	8.0
Arteriography	
Aortography	2.7
Cerebral arteriography	2.0
Other	3.6
All types	5.0

dia as nonallergic individuals,[134] and are four times as likely to have a severe reaction.[9] Patients with a history of asthma have up to five times the risk of idiosyncratic reaction as the general population.[26, 27, 91]

3. An individual with a history of a previous reaction is three to six times as likely to have a reaction again as an individual without this history.[9, 135]

4. Most fatal reactions occur in patients over the age of 50 years.[2] There is a significant increase in the risk of death if the patient has cardiopulmonary disease or is an alcoholic.[1, 9]

5. Most of the less serious reactions occur in patients between 30 and 50 years of age.[134, 157]

6. Patients in all age groups may suffer major reactions.[131]

7. The absence of a history of reaction to contrast medium administration does not ensure that no reaction to its readministration will occur.[9, 135]

8. There is no reliable sensitivity test to predict the idiosyncratic response, and a patient may suffer a severe reaction to small amounts of contrast media in "test doses."[9, 159]

9. Anxiety and apprehension may play a role in all grades of reaction.[82]

The prevalence of idiosyncratic reactions is less with intra-arterial injections than with intravenous injections; however, intra-arterial injections have a higher percentage of severe reactions.[151] Intravenous bolus injections are associated with a lower reaction rate than is intravenous drip infusion.[8]

Because patients with previous mild reactions are at an increased risk of similar adverse responses with reexposure, and because many of the clinical manifestations of such reactions appear to be "allergic," prophylactic premedication of such patients with steroids and antihistamines has been tried. There is no conclusive evidence to support the efficacy of this practice. The reactions are not often "immune-mediated," and the major benefit of antihistamine administration may result from mild sedation and a decrease in the patient's (and the physician's) anxiety. Wolf claims that it is safer to be a high-risk patient given low-osmolarity nonionic contrast than it is to be a low-risk patient pretreated with steroids and given high-osmolarity ionic contrast.[21, 27, 86, 158]

There is a reduced incidence of minor reactions with low-osmolarity contrast media.[34] Ioxaglate, however, causes a higher incidence of nausea and vomiting than the nonionic media.[88] The risk of a fatal reaction following intravascular administration of a conventional contrast medium is between 1 in 16,000 and 1 in 117,000. Comprehensive statistics on the incidence of major reactions caused by the newer media suggest that the likelihood of a severe reaction may be somewhat lower with the low-osmolarity media.[93, 159] Katayama has shown an overall decrease in all adverse drug reactions from 12.6 per cent in those patients receiving intravenous ionic high-osmolarity contrast media to 3.1 per cent for those receiving intravenous nonionic low-osmolarity contrast agents.[76] He has also shown a decrease in severe reactions from 0.22 per cent in those receiving ionic high-osmolarity contrast agents to 0.04 per cent for those receiving nonionic low-osmolarity contrast media.[76] It is thought, therefore, that acute, potentially life-threatening systemic reactions to contrast media are less frequent with nonionic low-osmolarity contrast agents; however, such reactions are still not eliminated.[27]

Although the likelihood of recurrence may be less for a major reaction than for a less severe reaction, the magnitude of such an event mandates careful evaluation of the reasons for readministration of contrast medium. Despite the questionable efficacy of prophylactic premedication, the use of prednisone and antihistamines in these patients prior to the procedure has been recommended.[78] Low-osmolarity media have been used safely in patients with a history of previous reaction, both with and without premedication, and their use has also been recommended.[69, 116] The vascular surgeon and the radiologist must be prepared to institute basic life-support measures and to treat major reactions with facility.

Which Contrast Agent—Low-Osmolarity or High-Osmolarity?

Low-osmolarity contrast media clearly cause less patient discomfort than the conventional media. In addition, there is less cardiotoxicity, less neurotoxicity, less nephrotoxicity, and less endothelial toxicity with a newer media.

The major problem with the newer agents is their cost, which in the United States is as much as 20 times that of conventional high-osmolarity media. To change completely to the use of low-osmolarity agents would have major financial implications for the health budget of both the individual health care institution and the nation as a whole. It has been estimated that to make the transition from ionic high-osmolarity agents to nonionic low-osmolarity contrast media would increase health care expenditure by $1.1 billion per year.[13]

The use of low-osmolarity agents in selected high-risk groups has therefore been recommended. Replacement of contrast-enhanced procedures with alternative imaging techniques that are less expensive and not associated with the use of ionizing radiation offers an opportunity for substantial cost reduction. This includes replacing significant numbers of intravenous urograms with ultrasonographic evaluations, using duplex sonography instead of venography as the initial examination for suspected deep venous thrombosis, and using duplex sonography or magnetic resonance angiography, or both, instead of contrast arteriography in the evaluation of extracranial carotid and vertebral artery disease. Although clinicians requesting contrast examinations should confer with their colleagues in radiology regarding the type of contrast media to be used, a list of high-risk factors for contrast reactions might include the following:

1. Previous reaction to contrast medium.
2. History of asthma or allergy.
3. Cardiovascular disease.
4. Renal failure.
5. Diabetes mellitus.
6. Pulmonary arteriography.
7. Poorly hydrated patients.
8. Sickle cell disease.[111]

Table 7–5. Guide for Treatment of Acute Reactions to Contrast Media

Signs and Symptoms	Treatment	Treatment Dose/Route of Administration: Adults	Treatment Dose/Route of Administration: Children	Treatment Interval	Treatment Precautions
Nausea/vomiting					
Transient	Supportive				Observe patient
Severe, protracted	Prochlorperazine injectable (Compazine)	5–10 mg/intramuscular, IV	>2 years old: 0.13 mg/kg/intramuscular <2 years old: not recommended	Every 3–4 hr	IV–administer slowly; drowsiness
Urticaria					
Scattered, transient	Supportive				Observe patient
Scattered, protracted	Diphenhydramine injectable (Benadryl)	25–50 mg/IV, intramuscular	1.25 mg/kg/IV, intramuscular	Every 2–3 hr	Drowsiness
Profound	Cimetidine injectable (Tagamet)	300 mg (diluted—10 ml)/IV	5–10 mg/kg (diluted)/IV	Every 6–8 hr	Administer slowly; drowsiness
	or				
	Ranitidine injectable (Zantac)	50 mg (diluted—10 ml)/IV	Use not established	Every 6–8 hr	Administer slowly
Bronchospasm	Oxygen	3 L/min	3 L/min		
Mild-moderate	Subcutaneous epinephrine 1:1000	0.1–0.2 mg (0.1–0.2 ml)/subcutaneous	0.01–0.02 mg/kg to 0.2 mg maximum/subcutaneously	Every 10–15 min	Noncardioselective beta-blockers
Accelerating, severe	IV epinephrine 1:10,000	0.1 mg (1 ml)/IV	0.01 mg/kg to 0.1 mg maximum/IV	Every 2–3 min	Administer slowly; beta-blockers (especially noncardioselect)
Wheezing-protracted, isolated	Metaproterenol (Alupent) *or* Terbutaline (Brethaire) *or* Albuterol (Proventil)	Two deep inhalations (all)/metered-dose inhaler	If possible: one to two deep inhalations (all)/metered-dose inhaler	Every 4–6 hr	Proper inhalation technique (use of insert)
Hypotension					
Normal sinus rhythm, tachycardia	IV fluids (e.g., normal saline, Ringer's solution)	1–2 L/IV (rapid)	10–20 ml/kg/IV (rapid)	As per blood pressure, urine output	Fluid overload
Bradycardia	IV fluids (e.g., normal saline, Ringer's solution)	1–2 L/IV (rapid)	10–20 ml/kg/IV (rapid)	As per blood pressure, urine output	Fluid overload
	plus Atropine injectable	1 mg/IV (push)	0.02 mg/kg to 0.60 mg maximum/IV	Every 3–5 min to total 3 mg for adults or 2 mg for children	Monitor pulse rate
Seizures/convulsions					
Isolated	See Hypotension				
Multiple, continuous	Diazepam injectable (Valium)	5–10 mg/IV	0.2–0.5 mg/kg/IV	Every 20 min	Respiratory depression

From Bush WH, Swanson DP: Acute reactions to intravascular contrast media: Types, risk factors, recognition, and specific treatment. AJR 157:1153, 1991.

As long as there remains such a large price differential between ionic and nonionic contrast media, the decision to use nonionic agents poses a financial and ethical dilemma. The use of nonionic contrast in high-risk patients, however, is recommended (Table 7–5).

INDICATIONS FOR ANGIOGRAPHY

In determining basic criteria for any diagnostic test, certain variables must be considered. Geographic variation in disease may make a particular study commonplace in one community and rare in another. Subspecialists with skewed patient populations may convert rare procedures into routinely performed examinations. Furthermore, depending on the strengths or weaknesses of particular radiology departments, vascular abnormalities may be initially evaluated with noninvasive techniques in one and invasive techniques in another department.

Based on the underlying premise that the angiographer who is to perform the requested study, in consultation with the patient's referring clinician, is the person who is in the best position to determine the appropriateness of any diagnostic arteriogram, the Society of Cardiovascular and Interventional Radiology (SCVIR) has created detailed guidelines for ordering invasive intravascular procedures.[129] The SCVIR also recommends that, in all cases, the indications for any given procedure should be documented in the patient's medical record.

COMPLICATIONS OF ANGIOGRAPHY

Complications in diagnostic angiography occur with variable incidence, depending on the procedure being performed and the patient's condition at the time of the study. In most cases, the complications are related to the contrast medium, as reviewed previously, and in the remainder of cases, they are due to mechanical damage to the vascular system during catheter insertion and manipulation. The effects of instrumentation depend on the approach route selected for the study, the total time of catheterization, the size of the catheter utilized, the degree of vessel selectivity necessary to achieve the examination, and the expertise of the angiographer.[61, 89–91, 156] Complications for interventional radiologic procedures (e.g., angioplasty, intra-arterial infusion of fibrinolytic agents, embolization) are higher than those for diagnostic arteriography. The risks inherent in vascular studies commonly requested by vascular surgeons are reviewed. Clinical factors that may influence the basic risks are outlined in the hope that awareness of these problems will reduce the overall incidence of angiography-related morbidity.

Thoracic, Visceral, and Peripheral Arteriography

The incidence of idiosyncratic contrast reactions in general arteriography varies slightly depending on the specific study performed (see Table 7–4), but generally is less than 4 per cent.[134] The incidence of reactions requiring additional hospitalization is less than 0.1 per cent, and death occurs in fewer than 1 in 20,000 patients.[134]

The development of abnormal central nervous system function during angiography or shortly thereafter may be thought of as separate from catheter-related complications because it may occur even when the catheter is nowhere near the cerebral vessels.[61] Whether such neurologic events are related to contrast media or embolic debris or whether they simply represent spontaneous unrelated events is not clear. The incidence of neurologic complications has been observed to be roughly equivalent in patients who were scheduled for but did not undergo angiography and in those who have had an examination.[15] In thoracic, visceral, and peripheral arteriography, the neurologic complications range from seizures and transient ischemic attacks (less than 0.1 per cent) to completed strokes (less than 0.02 per cent).[61] These neurologic complications occur with an overall incidence of 0.3 per cent with a transfemoral route, 0.02 per cent with a translumbar route, and 0.6 per cent with a transaxillary route. The reason for the differences among approach routes is incompletely understood but may relate in part to the different proximity of the catheter to the intracranial circulation in each method.

Local catheter complications at the puncture site include hemorrhage, thrombosis, pseudoaneurysm creation, and arteriovenous fistula formation, with the first two being more frequent.[61] Bleeding is the most common overall complication of arterial catheterization and, although it may occur during the procedure, is most often a problem after the study. Traumatic arterial punctures, use of a large catheter, decreased arterial wall elasticity due to calcification or sclerosis, excessive manipulation of the catheter, coagulopathy, high blood pressure, and suboptimal postprocedure hemostasis all influence the occurrence of this complication. Although the incidence of minor bleeding (hematoma) is variable and may be as high as 10 per cent,[61, 155] major hematomas (i.e., those requiring transfusion, surgical evacuation, or delay in discharge) should occur in only 0.5 to 2 per cent of the population.[129] The use of smaller catheters has reduced the incidence of bleeding, and outpatient angiography is now widely practiced. These outpatient procedures are usually performed via the femoral route with 4 to 5 Fr catheters or via the brachial route with 4 Fr catheters.

Thrombosis is the other major local catheter-related complication. The incidence of this is less than 1 per cent. The primary factor influencing this hazard appears to be the catheter size relative to the artery being cannulated.[51] This factor explains the more frequent occurrence of thrombosis in the brachial artery and after catheterization in children.[61, 156] The degree of intimal damage, coagulation status, duration of cannulation, and presence of vascular spasm will also affect thrombosis, and intraprocedure anticoagulation may be helpful when such a problem is anticipated.[73, 156] The increasing use of smaller catheters should help to reduce the incidence of thrombosis.

Pseudoaneurysms and arteriovenous fistulae are rare puncture site complications, occurring in less than 1 per cent of patients undergoing diagnostic arteriography. Duplex sonographic evaluation may aid in the diagnosis of both as well as in the treatment[46] of the former. Clinically significant infection at the puncture site is very rare, and, therefore, antibiotic prophylaxis is not recommended for routine diagnostic arteriography.[132]

The distal complications of catheterization—embolization, catheter breakage, and vascular mural disruption—are independent of the approach route. These represent the least frequent group of complications. Intramural injection of contrast medium occurs more frequently in translumbar aortography and should probably be considered a puncture site complication.[61] Subintimal contrast injections elsewhere may occur as a result of wire or catheter manipulation; this happens more frequently when small vessels are selectively cannulated, when stiff catheters or wires are used, and when venous studies are performed.[61] Overall, these complications have decreased in recent years, in part owing to advances in guidewire and catheter technology.

Whether thromboembolism is induced by the catheter depends on the patient's coagulation status, the material of which the catheter is made, the duration of cannulation, and the condition of the vascular system.[42] Clinically significant thromboembolic events are most common in cerebral angiography, in which the incidence of neurologic complications approximates 2.6 per cent among patients being evaluated for vascular symptoms. The majority of these complications are transient, with the incidence of permanent neurologic damage approximating 0.33 per cent.[43] Atheromatous plaques may be displaced from diseased intima, and patients with medial necrosis are at a greater risk of vascular dissection and perforation. Thromboembolic consequences of catheterization should be treated as conservatively as possible, but clear-cut ischemic changes should alert the surgeon to the potential need for embolectomy or intra-arterial thrombolytic administration.

Cerebral Arteriography

The incidence of idiosyncratic contrast reactions in patients undergoing cerebral arteriography is lower than in those undergoing thoracic, visceral, and peripheral angiography, for unknown reasons (see Table 7–4).

The overall incidence of neurologic effects of cerebral angiography is around 1 per cent if a transfemoral approach is used and would be expected to be higher with a transaxillary route.[61, 89–91] Most neurologic abnormalities are transient, with permanent neurologic deficit occurring in less than 0.33 per cent of patients.[79, 89–91] Most of these events are presumed to be caused by emboli or the neurotoxic effects of contrast media, and they depend, to a large extent, on the condition of the patient at the time of the study. Those individuals with clinically suspected vascular occlusive disease, subarachnoid hemorrhage, and post-traumatic brain conditions have an overall complication rate up to four times that of patients being evaluated for seizure, headache, or suspected tumor.[79, 125]

The reported incidence of catheter-related complications at the puncture site (0.2 per cent) is slightly less than that for thoracic, visceral, and peripheral arteriography, probably because smaller catheters have been used in cerebral studies.[61, 79] Mortality figures for cerebral arteriography are in the same range (0.02 per cent) as those for general angiography.[89–91]

Pediatric Arteriography

The incidence of contrast-related reactions in children is similar to that in adults, although severe reactions may occur less often.[134] The major problem in pediatric angiography is overdose of the contrast agent with resultant renal damage.[156]

There is evidence that patients under the age of 40 years have fewer cerebral complications during selective catheterization of the head vessels,[89–91] although extensive data on neurologic complications during arteriography in children are not available. Whether healthier blood vessels or increased brain resilience accounts for this phenomenon and whether the data can be extrapolated to infants and children are not established.

The major difference between adult and pediatric arterial catheterizations is the tendency for younger patients to develop arterial spasm and thrombosis at the puncture site, which can occur in up to 30 per cent of children.[73] The use of small catheters combined with systemic heparinization during the procedure and careful postprocedure care may greatly reduce the incidence of this complication.[152] Other complications in children occur as described for thoracic, visceral, and peripheral arteriography in adults.

Comprehensive data on the mortality rate for noncardiac angiography in children are not available, but a rate of around 0.03 per cent is probably reasonable.

Axillary Hematoma and Brachial Plexus Palsy

The sequelae of hematoma formation depend on the site of the puncture and the amount of blood lost. The axillary artery may bleed more substantially than the femoral artery, not only because it is more difficult to compress after cannulation but also because there is a relative lack of surrounding firm tissue for tamponade. Injury to the brachial plexus may occur following axillary artery puncture, most commonly due to a hematoma within the medial brachial fascial compartment, which is a tough fascial tunnel that surrounds the axillary sheath.[137] With the increasing use of the axillary approach for arterial access, the use of large angioplasty catheters and the more aggressive administration of anticoagulants and thrombolytic agents, this complication is likely to occur more frequently. In the majority of reported cases of nerve injury, the hand is affected with both sensory and motor dysfunction. The forearm is involved to a lesser extent, whereas the arm (shoulder to elbow) is usually spared. In most cases, the hematoma at the puncture site first compresses the median and ulnar nerves; proximal extension of the hematoma is required to compress the radial, musculocutaneous, axillary, and suprascapular nerves. Distal pulses are typically normal even in the presence of severe neurologic symptoms. Patients who have brachial plexus compression complain of severe pain and sensory disturbance in the hand and arm. Motor weakness subsequently develops—initially in the median nerve distribution, and subsequently in the ulnar and radial nerve territories (i.e., affecting the forearm and hand). The musculocutaneous and axillary nerve territories (shoulder and upper arm) are infrequently affected. The overall size, or presence, of a visible hematoma does not correlate well with the development of neuropathy, and, if neurologic changes are present following an axillary puncture, the absence of a visible hematoma should not alter therapy. Symptoms usually begin within 24 hours, but have been reported as late as 15 days.[97] When only minor sensory symptoms are present, careful observation without surgery may suffice; however, with severe sensory symptoms or the smallest of motor dysfunction, immediate surgical decompression is imperative. The prognosis for recovery of motor function worsens with time, and is poor if surgery is delayed for 24 hours or more after the onset of motor dysfunction.[107] Patients having an axillary artery puncture must be advised of the symptoms of brachial plexus compression, and warned to return to their physician immediately for urgent surgical decompression should they notice any of these symptoms.

Taken together, local adverse effects of catheterization in thoracic, visceral, and peripheral arteriography occur with an incidence of 0.5 per cent with a transfemoral route, 0.6 per cent with a translumbar route, and 2.0 per cent with a transaxillary route.[61]

The rate of mortality directly related to arteriography is difficult to assess because many patients studied are extremely ill and at considerable risk of death irrespective of the procedure. In fact, the mortality rate has been noted to be twice as high in a group of potential cardiac catheterization patients who did not undergo the invasive study as in the patients who did.[68] There is, nevertheless, a small but definite risk of death in arteriography, and a mortality rate of 0.03 per cent is probably reasonable.[61]

Pulmonary Angiography

Allergic reactions to contrast media during pulmonary angiography occur in approximately 1 per cent of patients when ionic contrast are used, and presumably with decreased frequency when nonionic contrast are used.[96] Catheter-related complications occur during venous catheterization and passage of the catheter through the heart. The risks of hemorrhage and thromboembolism are less significant in venous catheterization than in arterial catheterization. Venous thrombosis is the major concern in venous cannulation. Myocardial perforation can occur when a straight catheter is used for pulmonary arteriography but is rare now that catheters with pigtail configuration are employed.[96] Cardiac conduction abnormalities, which may result from irritation of the myocardium by the catheter, may lead to asystole, especially in the patient with a preexisting left bundle branch block. A temporary transvenous pacing wire should be inserted prior to pulmonary arteriography when left bundle branch block is present, and a physician who is experienced in managing cardiac arrhythmias should be present during the procedure.

The death rate in pulmonary angiography approaches 0.2 per cent, which is considerably higher than in other angiographic procedures. Poor condition of the patient at the time of the study and the intrinsic morbidity of right heart catheterization may account partially for this higher mortality rate; patients with pulmonary arterial hypertension are at still greater risk of dying during pulmonary angiography, particularly if the right ventricular end diastolic pressure exceeds 20 mmHg.[96] Low-osmolarity contrast agents may be safer in these patients, and have become the preferred agents in pulmonary arteriography because they induce less coughing and therefore provide an examination of superior quality with more diagnostic detail.

Central Venous Angiography

Allergic reactions with central venous contrast injections occur in less than 3 per cent of patients, and the mortality rate reported in such studies is accounted for almost entirely by adverse reactions to contrast media.[134]

The puncture of the femoral or basilic veins is rarely associated with hemorrhage and is infrequently complicated by significant thrombosis.[156] Because patients with preexisting venous thrombosis may be at an increased risk of pulmonary thromboembolism if the catheter is passed through the clot, preliminary venous injections of contrast agent through the introducing needle are performed with fluoroscopic guidance.

Patients undergoing adrenal venography have an additional risk of prolonged back pain and even of adrenal ablation if overly vigorous contrast injections produce venous rupture. If both adrenal glands are affected, adrenal insufficiency may result.[61]

Peripheral Venous Angiography

Lower extremity phlebography remains the definitive test for the diagnosis of deep venous thrombosis, but the procedure is not without risk. Systemic reactions to contrast agents are the same as with any other intravenous injection.[134, 144]

Postvenography thrombophlebitis may be documented in as many as 26 per cent of patients undergoing the examination with a conventional contrast medium, although the incidence is usually lower.[125] Diluting the contrast medium and infusing heparinized saline solution on completing the venogram help reduce the incidence of thrombophlebitis.[10, 19] Sequelae of thrombophlebitis induced by contrast media have not been documented, but Doppler ultrasonography and plethysmographic studies represent reasonably accurate alternative means of diagnosing venous thrombosis, particularly in patients at increased risk of adverse reactions.[72] Contrast-induced thrombophlebitis occurs less frequently with low-osmolarity media.[3] One investigator states that, ''The only contrast suitable for IV phlebography are non-ionic low osmolar agents.''[4]

Extravasation of contrast media in the foot may lead to a chemical ''burn,'' cellulitis that may ulcerate and result in tissue necrosis and skin sloughing. This is more common in patients who have arterial or venous insufficiency, or both, or when the deep venous system is occluded. This complication has thus far not been described with nonionic low osmolarity contrast agents.[53, 70, 81]

Lymphography

Lymphography involves the slow infusion of an ethiodized oil–based contrast medium (Ethiodol) into a cannulated lymphatic vessel after a cutdown on the dorsum of the foot. Allergic reactions to Ethiodol are rare (less than 0.1 per cent), but a history of allergy to iodine may have more significance in patients who have reactions, because free iodine is liberated as the oil-based agent decomposes.[1, 138] A few patients may react to the aniline dye that is injected subcutaneously to opacify the lymph vessels prior to cannulation.

The other untoward effects of lymphography involve the pulmonary reactions to the oily contrast media that embolize to the lungs. Embolization occurs if excessive amounts of media are used, if inadvertent venous cannulation occurs, or if postoperative lymphovenous fistulae are present. The oil in the embolized droplets reduces pulmonary diffusion capacity and stimulates a chemical pneumonitis, either of which may be deleterious to patients with abnormal cardiopulmonary status.[1, 74] Patients with right-to-left circulatory shunts should not undergo lymphography because of the possibility of oil embolism through the shunt to the brain.[1, 138]

Local infection at the cutdown site occasionally occurs but is usually without significant sequelae. Death resulting directly from lymphography is extremely rare.[61, 138]

Preparation of the Patient

The basic principles of proper patient preparation for angiography should be evident in light of the complications already reviewed. The cardinal rule in this regard should be avoidance of an invasive study if the results of such an investigation are not likely to alter the treatment plan. When the benefits of a study are judged to outweigh the risks, and the patient's condition and the morbidity of the specific examination to be obtained are taken into account, the following guidelines will help to ensure safe angiography. The consulting surgeon should:

1. Keep the patient well hydrated before and after the administration of intravascular contrast media. A clear liquid diet for 8 hours prior to the study is usually sufficient to prevent intraprocedure vomiting and aspiration. Orders for no oral intake should be made *only* if an intravenous line is in place to maintain fluid status.

2. Review aspects of the medical history that may be pertinent to adverse contrast reactions (e.g., diabetes mellitus, renal failure, previous allergy) or to complications of catheterization (e.g., recent myocardial infarction, hypertension, coagulopathy). Obtain careful baseline documentation of the patient's vascular and neurologic status prior to angiography so that accurate postprocedure care can be rendered and complications can be quickly identified.

3. Assess carefully medications the patient is currently taking, especially to ascertain whether narcotic or barbiturate preprocedure sedation has been ordered, so as to avoid adverse drug interactions and to identify conditions that might be aggravated by such premedication (e.g., porphyria, ischemia, allergy). Most angiographers do not currently premedicate patients on call to the angiographic suite, preferring instead to medicate patients immediately prior to or during the procedure with short-acting neuroleptics (e.g., midazolam hydrochloride [Versed] and fentanyl citrate [Sublimaze]).

4. Obtain baseline laboratory data on renal function for all patients who are to receive intravascular contrast media, and order appropriate coagulation studies if a bleeding diathesis is suggested by the medical history.

5. Search by means of physical examination and relevant laboratory and noninvasive diagnostic studies for risk factors specific to the desired examination; for example, exclude left bundle branch block prior to pulmonary angiography and right-to-left circulatory shunts prior to lymphography.

6. Consult the vascular radiologist when requesting the examination to determine the safest, most productive study available for each diagnostic problem. Discuss specific risk factors and arrange for the examination to be done so that it will not follow soon after other studies involving contrast media, such as intravenous urography, computed tomography, and barium gastrointestinal studies.

SUMMARY

The safe performance of a diagnostically complete vascular radiologic study requires knowledge about the adverse effects of contrast media and awareness of potential catheter-related complications in a number of different settings.

The best studies are obtained when the vascular radiologist is aware of clinical and vascular laboratory findings, so that he or she can anticipate the degree of vascular compromise in each region to be studied and is aware of what specific information is required from each study. A close and continuing contact between consulting surgeon and vascular radiologist, including a prolonged effort of mutual education so that each is thoroughly aware of the techniques and limitations of the other's discipline, not only proves personally rewarding but also produces optimal angiograms with minimal risk to patients.

References

1. American College of Radiology, Committee on Drugs, Commission on Public Health and Radiation Protection: Prevention and management of adverse reactions to intravascular contrast media. July, 1977.
2. Abrams H: Angiocardiography and thoracic aortography. *In* Brewer A (ed): Classic Descriptions in Diagnostic Roentgenology. Springfield, IL, Charles C Thomas, 1964, pp 492–501.
3. Albrechtsson U, Fagher B, Lagerstedt C, et al: Double-blind comparison between iohexol and metrizoate in phlebography of the lower limb. Acta Radiol Suppl 366:58, 1983.
4. Albrechtsson U: Contrast media in phlebography. *In* Felix R, Fischer HW, Kormano M, et al (eds): Contrast Media from the Past to the Future. Stuttgart, Georg Thieme, 1987, pp 63–73.
5. Almén T: Contrast agent design. Some aspects on the synthesis of water-soluble contrast agents of low osmolality. J Theor Biol 24:216, 1969.
6. Almén T: Experience from 10 years of development of water-soluble nonionic contrast media. Invest Radiol 15:S283, 1980.
7. Ameuille P: Remarques sur quelques cas d'arteriographie pulmonarie chez l'homme vivant. Bull Mem Soc Med Hop Paris 52:749, 1936.
8. Ansell G: Adverse reactions to contrast agents: Scope of the problem. Invest Radiol 5:374, 1970.
9. Ansell G, Tweedie M, West C, et al: The current status of reactions to intravenous contrast media. Invest Radiol 15:S32, 1980.
10. Arndt R, Grollman J, Gomes A, et al: The heparin flush: An aid in preventing post phlebography thrombophlebitis. Radiology 130:249, 1979.
11. Arnulf G, Buffard P: Arteriographie der Koronarien mittels Azetylcholin. Fortschr Roentgenstr 92:115, 1960.
12. Arroyave CM: In vitro assay for radiographic contrast media idiosyncrasy. Invest Radiol 15(Suppl):S21, 1980.
13. Barrett BJ, Parfrey PS, McDonald JR, et al: Nonionic low-osmolality versus ionic high-osmolality contrast material for intravenous use in patients perceived to be at high risk: Randomized trial. Radiology 183:105, 1992.
14. Baserga R, Hidejiro Y, Henegar G: Thorotrast-induced cancer in men. Cancer 13:1021, 1960.
15. Baum S, Stein G, Kuroda K: Complications of "no arteriography." Radiology 86:835, 1966.
16. Benedek L, Thurzo E: Zur Technick der interkarotidealen Injectionen von untersichtigen Kolloidlosungen. Dtsch Z Nervenheilkd 78:243, 1923.
17. Berbereich J, Hirsch S: Die röntgenographische Darstellung der Arterien und Venen am lebenden Menschen. Klin Wochenschr 2:2226, 1923.
18. Berg KJ, Jacobsen JA: Nephrotoxicity related to contrast media. *In* Enge I, Edgren J (eds): Patient Safety and Adverse Events in Contrast Medium Examinations. International Congress Series, vol. 816. Amsterdam: Excerpta Medica, 1989.
19. Bettmann M, Paulin S: Leg phlebography: The incidence, nature and modification of undesirable side effects. Radiology 122:101, 1977.
20. Bettmann MA: Ionic versus nonionic contrast agents for intravenous use: Are all the answers in? Radiology 175:616, 1990.
21. Bettmann MA: The evaluation of contrast-related renal failure. AJR 157:66, 1991.
22. Binz A, Rath C, von Lichtenberg A: Die Wiedergabe von Nieren und Harnwegen ina Rontgenbildedurch. Jodpyridon-deprivate Angew Chem 43:452, 1929.
23. Bismuth H, Morino M, Sherlock D, et al: Primary treatment of hepatocellular carcinoma by arterial chemoembolization. Am J Surg 163:387, 1992.
24. Bolt W, Rink H: Selektive Angiographie der Lungengefasse bei Lungenturberkulose. Schweiz Z Tuberk 8:380, 1951.
25. Bradbury M: The Concept of the Blood-Brain Barrier. New York, John Wiley & Sons, 1979.
26. Brooks B: Intra-arterial injection of sodium iodide. JAMA 82:1016, 1924.
27. Bush WH, Swanson DP: Acute reactions to intravascular contrast media: Types, risk factors, recognition, and specific treatment. AJR 157:1153, 1991.
28. Caldicott WJH, Hollenberg NK, Abrams HL: Characteristics of response of renal vascular bed to contrast media: Evidence for vaso-

constriction induced by renin angiotensin system. Invest Radiol 5:539, 1970.
29. Casalini E: Role of low-osmolality contrast media in thromboembolic complications: Scanning electron microscopy study. Radiology 183:741, 1992.
30. Castellanos A, Pereiras RAG: La angiocardiografia radioopaca. Arch Soc Estud Clin 31:523, 1937.
31. Castellanos A, Pereiras R: Counter-current aortography. Rev Cuba Cardiol 2:187, 1939.
32. Curry TS III, Dowdey JE, Murry RC Jr: Christensen's Introduction to the Physics of Diagnostic Radiology. Philadelphia, Lea & Febiger, 1984.
33. D'Elia JA, Gleason RE, Alday M, et al: Nephrotoxicity from angiographic contrast material: A prospective study. Am J Med 72:719, 1982.
34. Dahlstrom K, Shaw D, Clauss W, et al: Summary of U.S. and European intravascular experience with iohexol based on the clinical trial program. Invest Radiol 20:S117, 1985.
35. Dawson P: Some aspects of contrast agent nephrotoxicity. Acta Radiol (Suppl) 366:174, 1983.
36. Dawson P, Grainger R, Pitfield J: The new low-osmolar contrast agents: A simple guide. Clin Radiol 34:221, 1983.
37. Dawson P: Aspects of contrast agent nephrotoxicity. *In* Felix R, Fischer HW, Kormano M, et al (eds): Contrast Media From the Past to the Future. Stuttgart, Georg Thieme, 1987, pp 137–148.
38. Defronzo R, Humphrey RL, Wright JR: Acute renal failure in multiple myeloma. Medicine 54:209, 1975.
39. dos Santos R, Lamas A, Caldas J: L'arteriographie des membres, de l'aorta et de ses branches abdominales. Bull Mem Soc Natl Chir 55:587, 1929.
40. Dotter C, Friscke L: Visualization of coronary circulation by occlusion aortography: A practical method. Radiology 71:502, 1958.
41. Drayer B, Velaj R, Bird R, et al: Comparative safety or intracarotid iopamidol, iothalamate meglumine and diatrizoate meglumine for cerebral angiography. Invest Radiol 19:S212, 1986.
42. Durst S, Leslie J, Moore R, et al: A comparison of the thrombogenicity of commercially available catheters. Radiology 122:101, 1977.
43. Earnest F, Forbes G, Sandok BA, et al: Complications of cerebral angiography: Prospective assessment of risk. AJR 142:247, 1984.
44. Euler H: Die perioesophegeale Aortenpunktien: Ihre diagnostischen und therapeutischen Möglichkeiten. Arch Klin Exp Ohren Nasen Kehlokopfheilkd 155:536, 1949.
45. Farinas P: A new technique for the examination of the abdominal aorta and its branches. AJR 46:641, 1941.
46. Fellmeth BD, Roberts AC, Bookstein JJ, et al: Postangiographic femoral artery injuries: Nonsurgical repair with US-guided compression. Radiology 178:671, 1991.
47. Fischer HW: Hemodynamic reactions to angiographic media. Radiology 91:66, 1968.
48. Fitzer PM, Ammann AM: Pretreatment with corticosteroids to prevent reactions to IV contrast material. AJR 150:1443, 1988.
49. Forssmann N: Ueber Kontrastdarstellung der Hohlen des lebenden rechten Herzen und der Lungenschlagader. Munch Med Wochenschr 78:489, 1931.
50. Franck O, Alwens W: Kreislaufstudien am Rontgenschirm. Munch Med Wochenschr 57:1950, 1910.
51. Franken E, Girod A, Sequciro F: Femoral artery spasm in children: Catheter size is the principal cause. AJR 138:295, 1982.
52. Golman K, Almén T: Urographic contrast media and methods of investigative uroradiology. *In* Sovak M (ed): Radiocontrast Agents. Handbook of Experimental Pharmacology, vol. 73. Heidelberg, Springer-Verlag, 1984.
53. Gordon I: Evaluation of suspected deep venous thrombosis in the arteriosclerotic patient. AJR 131:531, 1978.
54. Grainger RG: Osmolality of intravascular radiological contrast media. Br J Radiol 53:739, 1980.
55. Grainger RG: Intravascular contrast media—The past, the present, and the future. MacKinzie Davidson Memorial Lecture, April 1981. Br J Radiol 55:1, 1982.
56. Grainger RG: Osmolality and osmolality-related side effects. *In* Felix R, Fischer HW, Kormano M, et al (eds): Contrast Media From the Past to the Future. Stuttgart, Georg Thieme, 1987, pp 25–32.
57. Guerra M: An elegy to Egas Moniz. *In* Veiga-Pires J, Grainger R (eds): Pioneers in Angiography. Lancaster, UK, MTP Press, 1982.
58. Haerkoenen S, Kjellstrand C: Exacerbation of diabetic renal failure following intravenous pyelography. Am J Med 63:939, 1977.
59. Haerkoenen S, Kjellstrand C: Contrast nephropathy. Am J Nephrol 1:69, 1981.
60. Haschek E, Lindenthal O: A contribution to the practical use of photography according to Rontgen. Wien Chir Wochenschr 9:63, 1896.
61. Hessel SJ, Adams DF, Abrams HL: Complications of angiography. Radiology 138:273, 1981.
62. Heuser C: Pieloradiografia con ioduro potasico y las injecciones intravenosas de ioduro potasico en radiografia. Sem Med 26:424, 1919.
63. Hickey P: The interpretation of radiographs of the chest. Trans Am Roentg Ray Soc 5:136, 1905.
64. Hietala S, Almén T: Patient risk factors of importance in nephrotoxicity of contrast media. *In* Enge I, Edgren J (eds): Patient Safety and Adverse Events in Contrast Medium Examinations. International Congress Series, vol. 816. Amsterdam, Excerpta Medica, 1989.
65. Higgins CB: Contrast media in the cardiovascular system. *In* Sovak M (ed): Radiocontrast Agents. Handbook of Experimental Pharmacology, vol. 73. Heidelberg, Springer-Verlag, 1984.
66. Higgins C: The cardiotolerance of iohexol. Survey of experimental evidence. Invest Radiol 20:S65, 1985.
67. Hilal S, Michelsen J, Driller J, et al: Magnetically guided devices for vascular exploration and treatment. Radiology 113:529, 1974.
68. Hildner F, Javier R, Ramaswany K, et al: Pseudocomplications of cardiac catheterization. Chest 63:15, 1973.
69. Holtas S: Iohexol in patients with previous adverse reactions to contrast agents. Invest Radiol 19:563, 1984.
70. Homans J: Thrombosis as complication of venography. JAMA 119:136, 1942.
71. Hou S, Bushinsky DA, Wish JB, et al: Hospital-acquired renal insufficiency: A prospective study. Am J Med 74:243, 1983.
72. Hull R, Hirsch J, Sackett D, et al: Replacement of venography in suspected venous thrombosis by impedance plethysmography and ^{125}I-fibrinogen leg scanning: A less invasive approach. Ann Intern Med 94:12, 1981.
73. Jacobsson B, Curlgren L, Hedvall G, et al: A review of children after arterial catheterization of the leg. Pediatr Radiol 1:96, 1973.
74. Johnsrude I, Jackson D: A Practical Approach to Angiography. Boston, Little, Brown, 1979.
75. Jonsson G: Thoracic aortography by means of a cannula inserted percutaneously into the common carotid artery. Acta Radiol 31:376, 1949.
76. Katayama H: Report of the Japanese committee on the safety of contrast media. Radiological Society of North America. RSNA, 1988.
77. Katzberg RW: Contrast media and renal effects. *In* Stolberg HO (ed): Proceedings of the Radiology Speakers Program, Hong Kong. Montreal, Medicopea International, 1989, pp 29–33.
78. Kelly J, Patterson R, Lieberman P, et al: Radiographic contrast media studies in high-risk patients. J Allergy Clin Immunol 62:181, 1978.
79. Kerber C, Cromwell L, Drayer B, et al: Cerebral ischemia. I. Current angiographic techniques, complications and safety. AJR 130:1097, 1975.
80. King BF: Low-osmolality contrast media: A current perspective. Mayo Clinic Proc 64:946, 1989.
81. Kinnunen J, Rainikainen M, Laasonen EM: Hautnekrose nach aszendierender Beinphlebographie. ROFO 136:104, 1982.
82. Lalli AF: Contrast media reactions: Data analysis and hypothesis. Radiology 134:1, 1980.
83. Lasser EC, Lang JH: Contrast protein interactions. Invest Radiol 5:446, 1970.
84. Lasser EC, Lang JH, Hamblin AE, et al: Activation systems in contrast idiosyncrasy. Invest Radiol 15(6 Suppl):S2, 1980.
85. Lasser EC: Adverse systemic reactions to contrast media. *In* Sovak M (ed): Radiocontrast Agents. Handbook of Experimental Pharmacology, vol. 73. Heidelberg, Springer-Verlag, 1984.
86. Lautin EM, Freeman NJ, Schoenfeld AH, et al: Radiocontrast-associated renal dysfunction: Incidence and risk factors. AJR 157:49, 1991.
87. Lautin EM, Freeman NJ, Schoenfeld AH, et al: Radiocontrast-asso-

ciated renal dysfunction: A comparison of lower-osmolality and conventional high-osmolality contrast media. AJR 157:59, 1991.
88. Manhire A, Dawson P, Dennet R: Contrast agent–induced emesis. Clin Radiol 35:369, 1984.
89. Mani RL, Eisenberg RL: Complications of catheter cerebral arteriography. Analysis of 5000 procedures. I. Criteria and incidence. AJR 131:861, 1978.
90. Mani RL, Eisenberg RL: Complications of catheter cerebral arteriography. Analysis of 5000 procedures. II. Relation of complication rates to clinical and arteriographic diagnosis. AJR 131:867, 1978.
91. Mani RL, Eisenberg RL: Complications of catheter cerebral arteriography. Analysis of 5000 procedures. I. Criteria and incidence. AJR 131:861, 1978.
92. Martin JB, Reichlin S, Brown GM: Clinical Neuroendocrinology. Philadelphia, FA Davis, 1977, pp 240–243.
93. McAfee J: A survey of complications of abdominal aortography. Radiology 68:825, 1957.
94. McClennan B: Low-osmolarity contrast media: Premises and promises. Radiology 162:1, 1987.
95. Melartin E, Tuohimaa P, Dabb R: Neurotoxicity of iothalamates and diatrizoates. I. Significance of concentration and cation. Invest Radiol 5:13, 1970.
96. Mills S, Jackson D, Older R, et al: The incidence, etiologies, and avoidance of complications in pulmonary angiography in a large series. Radiology 136:295, 1980.
97. Molnar W, Paul DJ: Complications of axillary arteriotomies. An analysis of 1,762 consecutive studies. Radiology 104:269, 1972.
98. Moniz E: L'encephalographie arterielle, son importance dans la localization des tumeurs cerebrales. Rev Neurol 2:272, 1927.
99. Moniz E, Pinto A, Lima A: Le thorotrast dans l'encephalographie arterielle. Rev Neurol 2:646, 1931.
100. Moniz E, de Carvaldo L, Lima A: Angiopneumographie. Presse Med 53:996, 1931.
101. Moore RD, Steinberg EP, Powe NR, et al: Nephrotoxicity of high-osmolality versus low-osmolality contrast media: Randomized clinical trial. Radiology 182:649, 1992.
102. Morris TW: General effects of intravascular contrast media. *In* Skulcas J (ed): Radiographic Contrast Agents. Rockville, MD: Aspen Publishers, 1989, vol. 2, 129–138.
103. Morton W, Hammer E: The X-ray or Photography of the Invisible and Its Value in Surgery. American Technical Book Co, 1896.
104. Mudge GH: Nephrotoxicity of urographic radiocontrast drugs. Kidney Int 18:540, 1980.
105. Nuvoli L: Arteriografia dell'aorta toracica mediante punture dell'aorta ascendente o del ventriculos. Policlinico (Prat) 43:227, 1936.
106. Nyman U, Almén T, Landtman M: Effect of contrast media on femoral blood flow: Comparison between the nonionic and ionic monomeric and monoacidic dimeric contrast media in the dog. Acta Radiol 362(Suppl):43, 1980.
107. O'Keefe D: Brachial plexus injury following axillary arteriography. Case report and review of the literature. J Neurosurg 53:853, 1980.
108. Odman P: Percutaneous selective angiography of the main branches of the aorta. Acta Radiol 45:1, 1956.
109. Oldendorf WH: The blood-brain barrier and its relevance to modern nuclear medicine. *In* Magistretti PL (ed): Functional Radionuclide Imaging of the Brain. 5th ed. New York, Raven Press, 1983, pp 1–10.
110. Osborne ED, Sutherland CG, Scholl AJ Jr, et al: Roentgenography of the urinary tract during excretion of sodium iodide. JAMA 80:368, 1923.
111. Palmer FJ: The RACR survey of intravenous contrast media reactions—Final report. Australas Radiol 32:426, 1988.
112. Parker JE, Bettmann MA: Angiographic contrast media. Cardiac Vascular Radiology 2(135A):1, 1992.
113. Pearse H, Warren S: The roentgenographic visualization of the arteries of the extremities in peripheral vascular disease. Ann Surg 94:1094, 1931.
114. Pitre D, Felder E: Development, chemistry and physical properties of iopamidol and its analogues. Invest Radiol 15:S301, 1980.
115. Radner S: Thoracic aortography by catheterization from the radial artery. Acta Radiol 29:178, 1948.
116. Rapoport S, Bookstein J, Higgins C, et al: Experience with metrizamide in patients with previous severe anaphylactoid reactions to contrast agents. Radiology 142:321, 1982.
117. Rapoport SI, Levitan H: Neurotoxicity of x-ray contrast media: Relationship to lipid solubility and blood-brain barrier permeability. AJR 122:186, 1974.
118. Rapoport SI, Thompson HK, Bidinger JM: Equi-osmolar opening of the blood-brain barrier in the rabbit by different contrast media. Acta Radiol (Diagn) 15:21, 1974.
119. Rapoport SI, Fredericks WR, Ohno K, et al: Quantitative aspects of reversible osmotic opening of the blood-brain barrier. Am J Physiol 238:R421, 1980.
120. Rasuli P: Blood clot formation in angiographic syringes containing nonionic contrast media [Letter]. Radiology 165:582, 1987.
121. Reidy J: Iopamidol in peripheral angiography. Invest Radiol 19:S206, 1984.
122. Ring J, Sovak M: Release of serotonin from human platelets in vitro by radiographic contrast media. Invest Radiol 16:245, 1981.
123. Robb G, Steinberg I: A practical method of visualization of the chambers of the heart, the pulmonary circulation, and the great blood vessels in man. J Clin Invest 17:507, 1936.
124. Robertson HJF: Blood clot formation in angiographic syringes containing nonionic contrast media. Radiology 162:621, 1987.
125. Rose J: Risk and patient care. Chicago, Year Book Medical, 1982.
126. Rousthoi P: Uber Angiokardiographic. Acta Radiol 14:419, 1933.
127. Sage MR: Neuroangiography. *In* Skucas J (ed): Radiographic Contrast Agents. 2nd ed. Rockville, MD, Aspen Publishers, 1989, pp 170–188.
128. Saito M, Kanikawa K, Yanagizawa H: A new method of blood vessel visualization (arteriography: veinography, angiography) in vivo. Am J Surg 10:225, 1930.
129. Society of Cardiovascular and Interventional Radiology (SCVIR): SOP Committee Draft 5/13/92—Standard of practice for diagnostic angiography. *In* Standards of Practice Committee. James B, Spies M (Chairmen) (eds): Fairfax, VA, SCVIR, 1992, pp 1–18.
130. Sehrwald E: Das Verhalten der Halogene gegen Rontgenstrahlen. Dtsch Med Wochenschr 30:477, 1896.
131. Seldinger S: Catheter replacement of the needle in percutaneous arteriography. Acta Radiol 39:368, 1953.
132. Shawker TH, Kluge RM, Ayella RJ: Bacteremia associated with angiography. JAMA 229:1090, 1974.
133. Shehadi WH: Contrast media adverse reactions: Occurrence, recurrence and distribution patterns. Radiology 143:11, 1975.
134. Shehadi W, Toniolo G: Adverse reactions to contrast media. Radiology 137:299, 1980.
135. Shehadi W: Contrast media adverse reactions: Occurrence, recurrence, and distribution patterns. Radiology 143:11, 1982.
136. Sicard J, Forestier G: Injections intravascularies d'huile iodee sous controle radiogique. CR Soc Biol 88:1200, 1923.
137. Smith DC, Mitchell DA, Peterson GW, et al: Medial brachial fascial compartment syndrome: Anatomic basis of neuropathy after transaxillary arteriography. Radiology 173:149, 1989.
138. Sokol G, Clouse M, Kotner L, et al: Complications of lymphangiography in patients of advanced age. AJR 128:43, 1977.
139. Sovak M: Introduction: State of the art and design principles of contrast media. *In* Sovak M (ed): Radiocontrast Agents. Handbook of Experimental Pharmacology, vol. 73. Heidelberg, Springer-Verlag, 1984.
140. Sovak M: Contrast media for imaging of the central nervous system. *In* Sovak M (ed): Radiocontrast Agents. Handbook of Experimental Pharmacology, vol. 73. Heidelberg: Springer-Verlag, 1984.
141. Spataro RF, Fischer HW, Boylan L: Urography with low-osmolality contrast media. Comparative urinary excretion of iopamidol, hexabrix and diatrizoate. Invest Radiol 17:494, 1982.
142. Spataro RF. Urography. *In* Skucas J (ed): Radiographic Contrast Agents. Rockville, MD, Aspen Publishers, 1989, pp 245–269.
143. Speck U, Siefert HM, Klinik G: Contrast media and pain in peripheral arteriography. Invest Radiol 15:335, 1980.
144. Stolberg HO, McClennan BL: Ionic versus nonionic contrast use. Curr Probl Diagn Radiol 20:47, 1991.
145. Stormorken H, Skalpe IW, Testart MC: Effects of various contrast media on coagulation, fibrinolysis and platelet function. An in vitro and in vivo study. Invest Radiol 21:348, 1986.
146. Stormorken H: Effects of contrast media on the hemostatic and thrombotic mechanisms. Invest Radiol 23(2 Suppl):S318, 1988.
147. Swick M: Intravenous urography by means of Uroselectan. Am J Surg 8:405, 1930.

148. Taenzer V: Optimum dosage in urography. *In* Felix R, Fischer HW, Kormano M (ed): Contrast Media From the Past to the Future. Stuttgart: Georg Thieme, 1987, pp 123–135.
149. Talner L, Davidson A: Renal hemodynamic effects of contrast media. Invest Radiol 3:310, 1968.
150. Tervel JL, Marcen R, Onaindia JM, et al: Renal function impairment caused by intravenous urography. Arch Intern Med 141:1271, 1981.
151. Thrall JH: Adverse reactions to contrast media. *In* Swanson DP, Chilton HM, Thrall JH (eds): Pharmaceuticals in Medical Imaging. New York, Macmillan, 1990, pp 253–277.
152. Totty N, Gilula L, McClennan B, et al: Low-dose intravascular fibrinolytic therapy. Radiology 143:56, 1982.
153. Vix V: Intravenous pyelography in multiple myeloma. Radiology 87:896, 1966.
154. Walton JN: Brain's Diseases of the Nervous System. 8th ed. Oxford: Oxford University Press, 1977, p 317.
155. Waugh JR, Sacharias N: Arteriographic complications in the DSA era. Radiology 182:243, 1992.
156. White R Jr: Fundamentals of Vascular Radiology. Philadelphia, Lea & Febiger, 1976.
157. Witten D. Reactions to urographic contrast media. JAMA 231:974, 1975.
158. Wolf GL: Adult peripheral angiography: Results from four North American randomized clinical trials of ionic media versus iohexol. Acta Radiol 366:166, 1983.
159. Wolf G: Safer, more expensive iodinated contrast agents. How do we decide? Radiology 159:557, 1986.

8

Contrast Arteriography

Stephen W. Subber, M.D., David A. Kumpe, M.D., and Robert B. Rutherford, M.D.

• • •

Although alternative means of vascular imaging, such as duplex sonography, computerized tomography, and magnetic resonance angiography, have become increasingly useful, the workhorse and gold standard for the accurate evaluation of blood vessels remains contrast angiography. This entails the percutaneous passage of a catheter into a vessel using needles, guidewires, and fluoroscopic guidance, with subsequent contrast injection and serial filming over the anatomic distribution of the vessel injected. Image recording may be done using conventional film-screen technique with 14-inch films or by digital imaging.

The angiographer must select the best roentgenographic projection; decide how many images are to be obtained over what time period; determine the proper contrast agent, injection rate, and volume; and position the catheter appropriately. Although techniques will vary from one angiographer to another, the following descriptions and recommendations are fairly representative.

With the exception of intraoperative studies, arteriography should optimally be performed by a physician with a minimum of 4 to 6 months training in catheter angiography. The physician should preferably be a radiologist, because training in radiology equips the physician to handle problems of exposure factors, projectional geometry, and radiation safety. Complex angiography and most interventional procedures should be performed only by formally trained and experienced angiographers, owing to the greater technical skills required and the greater risks of these procedures.

EQUIPMENT

Optimal evaluation of the cardiovascular system requires rapid acquisition of multiple images in multiple projections, as well as an accurate means of delivering contrast medium to a specific area of interest. Fluoroscopic monitoring of an intravascular catheter is essential for all but the simplest direct needle injection, and a specialized angiography room is usually necessary to achieve satisfactory images.

Angiography Room and Imaging System

Basic Angiographic Equipment

One typical room configuration (Fig. 8–1) includes two or more x-ray tubes supplied by high-capacity generators. For fluoroscopy, radiation from a fixed, floor-mounted under-table tube penetrates the tabletop and the patient, and is sensed by an image intensifier located immediately over the table; the live fluoroscopic image is displayed on a television monitor. A high-resolution imaging system is necessary for accurate manipulation of small, thin-walled catheters and the demonstration of vascular luminal anatomy and pathology. Standard (film-screen) x-ray images are made using a separate overhead tube and under-table film-holding/changing device; an additional tube and film

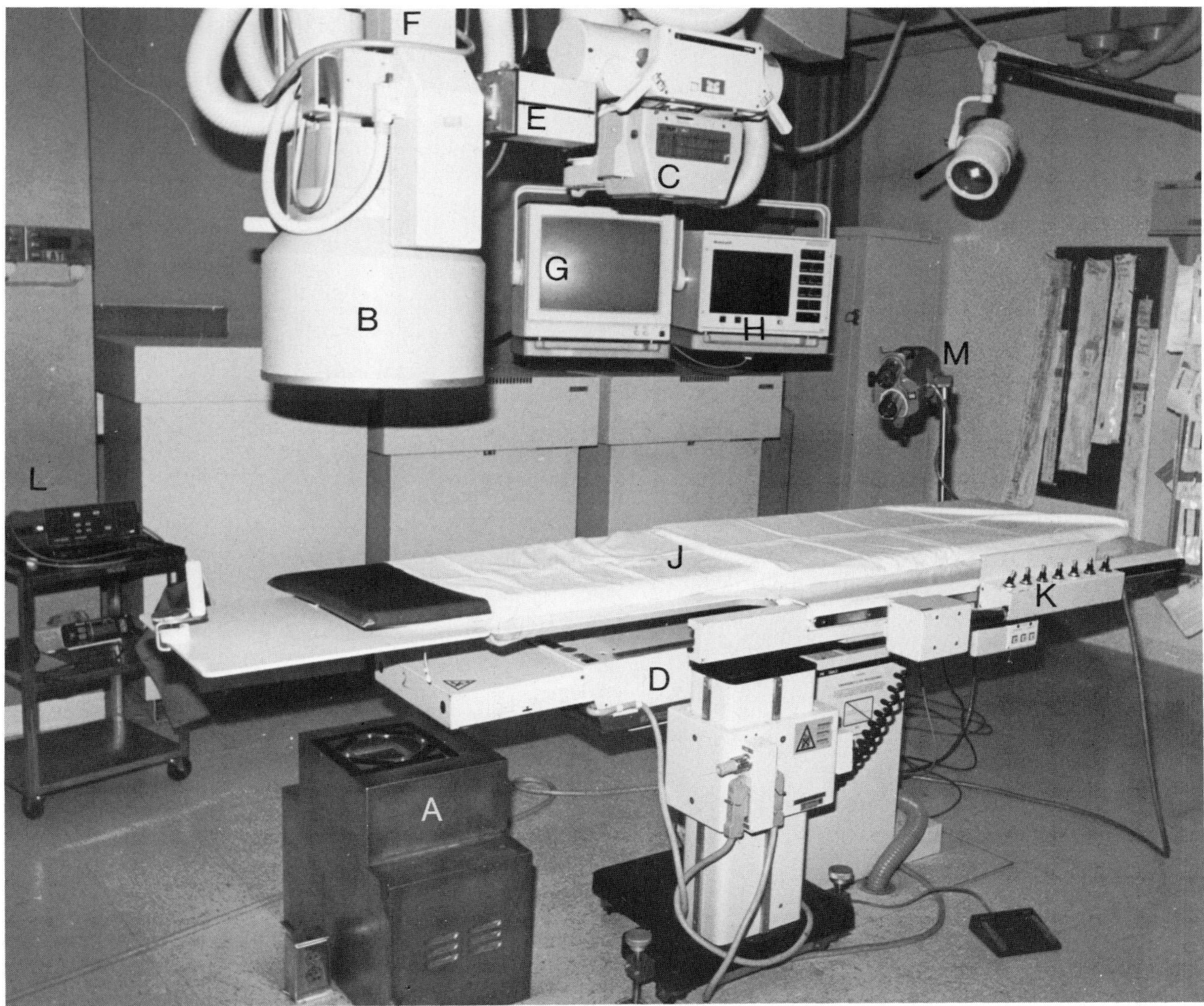

FIGURE 8–1. Examining room for general and peripheral angiography. *A*, Floor-mounted tube for fluoroscopy; *B*, ceiling-mounted image intensifier (moved aside during conventional filming); *C*, ceiling-mounted tube for film-screen roentgenography; *D*, PUCK film changer; *E*, camera for digital imaging; *F*, 105-mm spot-film camera; *G*, television monitor; *H*, ECG and pressure monitor; *J*, angiographic table; *K*, table and fluoroscopy controls; *L*, vital signs monitor and pulse oximeter; *M*, injector.

changer may be available to perform exposures in a lateral (or other) projection during the same contrast injection (''biplane filming'').

Another configuration (Figs. 8–2 and 8–3) uses a single x-ray tube fixed to one limb of a movable C- or U-arm, with an interchangeable image intensifier and film changer on the opposing limb of the arm. Rotation or angling of the C-arm around the patient permits fluoroscopy or filming in virtually any desired projection. A supplemental tube and film changer may be used to perform biplane filming. This configuration has become increasingly common during the 1980s because it permits optimal visualization of vascular anatomy, which may be poorly seen in standard anteroposterior (AP) and lateral projections, and because it adapts better to the increasingly wide variety of vascular and nonvascular procedures performed by an interventional radiologist.

The table on which the patient is positioned is specifically designed for angiography and interventional radiologic procedures. It has a free-floating top and can be elevated for the angiographer's convenience or to perform magnification filming studies. Newer tables can be tilted and are of value for nonvascular interventional procedures. Lateral pivoting of the table is particularly useful in evaluating the upper extremities. The angiographic table usually incorporates a stepping device that changes the longitudinal position of the table during filming so that the arteries of the lower extremities can be radiographed with a single injection of contrast medium.[1] In the past, ordinary tilting tables, designed for gastrointestinal radiology and general roentgenography, have been used for diagnostic angiographic procedures if a film changer was available, with the tabletop extended beyond either end of the table over the film changer. This arrangement can be used to produce

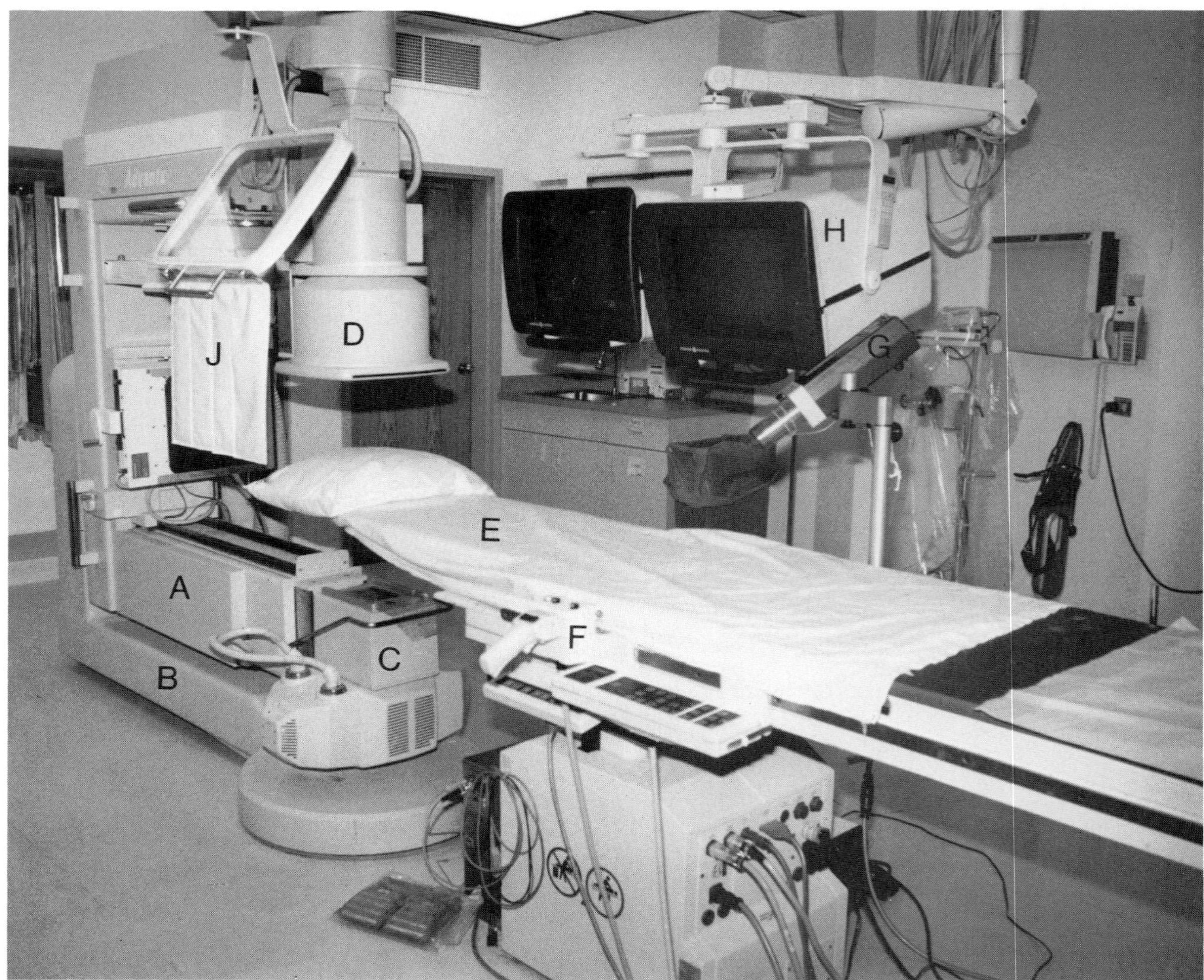

FIGURE 8–2. Examing room for general and peripheral angiography, U-arm configuration (arranged for fluoroscopy or digital imaging). *A*, U-arm, mounted within *B*, floor-mounted L-arm; *C*, tube mounted on one limb of U-arm; *D*, image intensifier (interchangeable with film changer) mounted on opposing limb of U-arm; *E*, table; *F*, table and fluoroscopy controls; *G*, injector; *H*, monitors; *J*, radiation protection shield for operator and medical personnel.

satisfactory diagnostic angiographic films and is still used in hospitals where the angiographic case load does not justify installation of specialized equipment. However, such arrangements are inappropriate for performing complex angiographic or interventional procedures.

Image Recording Techniques and Equipment

Conventional (film-screen) angiography is performed using a rapid-sequence film changer. Cut film changers are the most commonly used, transporting up to 30 individual films, 14 inches square, and changing them at rates up to 6 films per second. The most popular model is the PUCK unit, which can deliver up to 30 films at up to 4 films per second. It is reliable and lightweight enough to use on a C-arm stand. Other basic types of changers include cassette changers, which move individual cassettes containing single films, and roll-film changers, which use a continuous roll of film; these represent older designs that are seldom used today.

Aside from the standard 14 × 14-inch (35.5 × 35.5 cm) angiographic films, usually performed with a PUCK changer, permanent images can be acquired by other recording devices. The fluoroscopic image from the image intensifier can be rapidly recorded by camera on videotape (video fluoroscopy) or on ''spot films'' with relatively low radiation exposure to the patient. The 105-mm spot films[10] can be obtained at up to 12 films per second, with good resolution. If a movie camera is added to the imaging system, rapid-sequence filming can be performed (cineradiography). This technique has been the mainstay of cardiac and coronary angiography in the past but has more recently been replaced by digital recording techniques for coronary

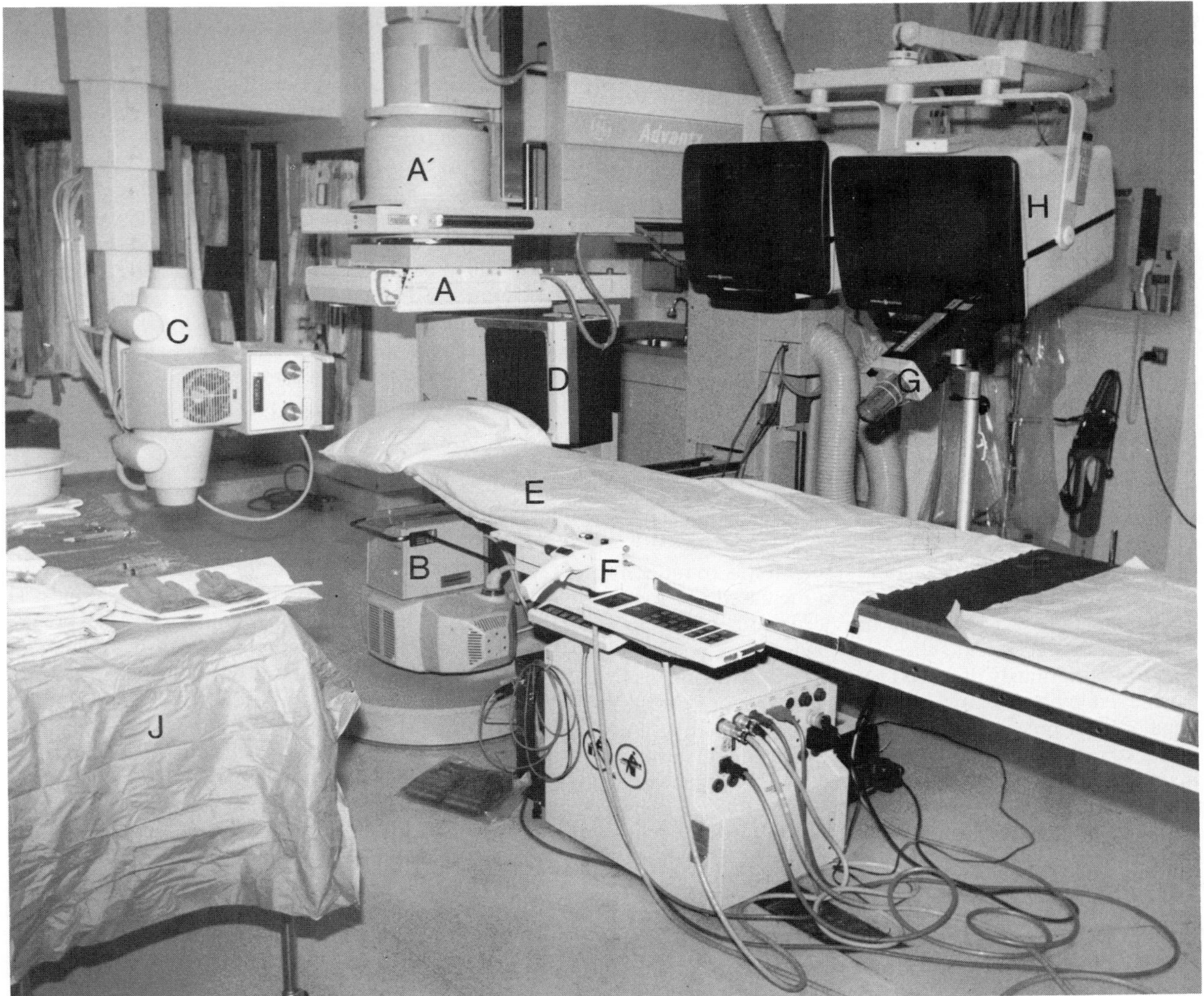

FIGURE 8–3. Examining room for general and peripheral angiography, U-arm configuration (arranged for conventional biplane filming). *A*, U-arm–mounted film changer in place below image intensifier *(A′)*; *B*, opposing U-arm–mounted tube; *C*, ceiling-mounted tube in place for lateral filming; *D*, film changer for lateral filming; *E*, table; *F*, table and fluoroscopy controls; *G*, power injector; *H*, monitors; *J*, table for angiographic instruments.

arteriography. Inferior image resolution makes the sole use of cineradiography or video fluoroscopy inadequate for routine arteriography.[6]

Digital imaging, with or without subtraction, is rapidly replacing direct film acquisition. This involves the electronic conversion of the fluoroscopic image into digital form, without the use of film as a recording medium. An angiographic run can be obtained at any time during the procedure, without needing to move the patient so that the area to be examined lies over a film changer. Current fluoroscopes are 14 to 16 inches in diameter, so that the area normally covered by conventional 14 × 14-inch angiographic film can be encompassed in a digital angiographic run. The sequence of images in an angiographic run is obtained with the fluoroscope, processed by a computer, stored on a hard disc, and displayed on a screen using a matrix of either 512 × 512 or 1024 × 1024 pixels. The angiographic images are then displayed on the fluoroscopy monitor and can be reviewed immediately after they are acquired, so that there is no delay while waiting for films to be developed. Hard-copy images are later selected for printing on a laser printer, which records 1 to 12 images on a single 14 × 17-inch film. In digital subtraction angiography (DSA), a preliminary or ''mask'' image is obtained immediately prior to contrast injection and automatically subtracted from subsequent images, eliminating background information and ideally demonstrating only the contrast-filled vessels of interest. Logarithmic amplification of an initially high x-ray signal combined with such digital subtraction processing permits the detection and enhancement of small density differences. Contrast sensitivity is consequently very high, and smaller volumes or lower concentrations of contrast material can be used for any single angiographic run, with improved patient comfort and reduced risk of nephrotoxicity. There is still a problem acquiring subtracted images with a moving table technique; hence, several injections of contrast medium are usually required to study an extremity, although a variety of new techniques under development by manufacturers of digital equipment may soon eliminate this problem.

The advantages of DSA include rapid acquisition (at up to 30 frames per second) and processing, with images available for immediate review. These features facilitate the performance of more complex, multi-step interventional procedures such as transcatheter embolization of arteriovenous malformations and vascular tumors with multiple arterial feeders, during which 30 or more angiographic runs may be needed. Conventional filming and development, along with contrast requirements, would simply not be practical in such procedures. Film costs are dramatically reduced as well because only the selected best images are photographically reproduced on film, with more than one image per film.

Disadvantages of DSA include susceptibility to motion artifacts, inferior spatial resolution, and increased radiation dose. In situations where motion has occurred between acquisition of the mask and subsequent images, the resulting image can be seriously degraded. An acceptable image may be achieved by using an unsubtracted image or through computer post-processing, whereby multiple images are "averaged" together or the mask is changed or shifted. Although several variables are involved, a 1024 digital image has a theoretical spatial resolution of 3 to 4 line pairs per mm, and conventional film-screen angiography may permit resolution of 5 line pairs per mm. This difference is generally acceptable, as fine detail is not always required in diagnostic or therapeutic studies. The superior contrast resolution of DSA is of particular advantage in demonstrating the small arteries of the ankle and foot, which are notoriously difficult to visualize using film-screen techniques in patients who have critical ischemia and multiple levels of occlusion. This same superior sensitivity to contrast, however, may obscure intraluminal abnormalities in larger arteries, such as intimal flaps and localized atheromata. Although subject to several variables, radiation dose for DSA examinations is significantly higher (by at least several times) than for conventional filming.

Parenthetical note might be made here of the use of carbon dioxide gas as a "negative" contrast agent. Using techniques developed and advocated by Hawkins,[7] the high-contrast sensitivity of DSA permits the obtaining of images of diagnostic quality in selected areas[21] with intra-arterial injection of carbon dioxide. Carbon dioxide is highly soluble in serum, nonallergenic, nontoxic, of low viscosity (permitting high-volume injections via very small catheters), and very inexpensive and causes little discomfort. Despite favorable results, clinical acceptance has been exceedingly slow. Layering of the gas over blood can occur in larger vessels and high compressibility can make delivery difficult, although automated injection devices are currently being developed. The use of this contrast medium can expand the use of arteriography in patients with hypersensitivity reactions or renal insufficiency.

Needles, Guidewires, and Catheters

A wide variety of specialized angiographic catheters and guidewires are currently in use. Nomenclature and sizes are confusing and arcane, but general principles are straightforward.

Units of measurement include inches, millimeters, French scale, and gauge. In the United States, needle sizes are generally stated in Stubs needle gauge, guidewire diameters in thousandths of an inch, catheter diameters in French units (1 French unit = ⅓ mm); catheter and guidewire lengths are given in centimeters. Metric units can be used as a conversion between the others and are used (mm) for guidewire diameters in Europe.

Needles

A variety of needle assemblies are available for vascular access. They are typically of thin-walled construction relative to standard hypodermic needles, resulting in a larger lumen for a given outer diameter, so that they may accommodate angiographic guidewires. The simplest arterial needle is 2 or 3 inches long, with a sharp bevel and no stylet. This single-wall needle is designed to puncture a vessel through its most superficial wall. The standard arterial needle is a double-wall needle, of similar length but with a beveled stylet. This needle is passed through both walls of a vessel; the stylet is then removed and lumen access is achieved during withdrawal of the cannula.

An 18-gauge thin-walled needle will accept a 0.038-inch wire, and 19-gauge needles will accept 0.035-inch wires. Micropuncture sets permit vessel puncture with a 21-gauge needle, through which a heavy-duty 0.018-inch wire can be placed, permitting conversion via a coaxial dilator assembly to a standard (i.e., 0.035 or 0.038-inch) guidewire. These devices are useful in difficult punctures (e.g., for puncture of clotted extra-anatomic grafts) or when risk of bleeding from unsuccessful needle passes is high (e.g., when a fibrinolytic infusion is anticipated).

Guidewires

Guidewires are used to guide the catheter percutaneously into an artery or vein and to advance it safely to its final position within the targeted vessel. Made of stainless steel, the standard guidewire consists of an outer, tightly coiled spring—or spring guide—surrounding a tapered inner core—or mandrel—that runs the length of the wire for added strength. The mandrel is tapered at its tip and terminates before the end of the spring guide, providing for a smooth transition from a stiffer wire shaft to a flexible tip. Multiple wire configurations are available. Tips are commonly straight or precurved into a J shape, with a typical radius of curvature of 1.5 mm or 3 mm (up to 15 mm).

The outer surface of the guidewire is usually Teflon-coated, reducing friction between the spring guide and catheter lumen. The usual guidewire length is 145 cm in adults. Exchange guidewires measure 260 to 300 cm and permit catheter exchange while leaving the wire tip in a desired position. Guidewire diameters are sized in thousandths of an inch, range from 0.012 to 0.052 inch, and must be matched to both needle and catheter in a particular case. The most commonly used sizes are 0.035 and 0.038 inch.

Many special-application guidewires are available. Movable-core guidewires permit movement of the mandrel to adjust the length of the terminal flexible section of the wire. At least 3 cm of flexible tip should be used to prevent damage to the vessel wall. In infusion wires, the mandrel can be completely removed and the hollow spring guide used for pressure measurements, limited contrast injections for superselective studies, or infusion of pharmacologic agents, often with simultaneous coaxial infusion via the more proximal catheter tip through which the wire passes.

The glidewire or Terumo wire is of fundamentally different construction from conventional guidewires. This wire consists of a nickel-titanium (nitinol) tapered core, surrounded with polyurethane. A thin layer of a hydrophilic polymer coats the wire, resulting in an extremely slippery surface when wet. This low-friction wire can be difficult to handle but is steerable with excellent torque control, owing to its single-piece construction, and can traverse complex curves. It has proved to be a near-revolutionary development, making superselective catheterization a routine procedure.

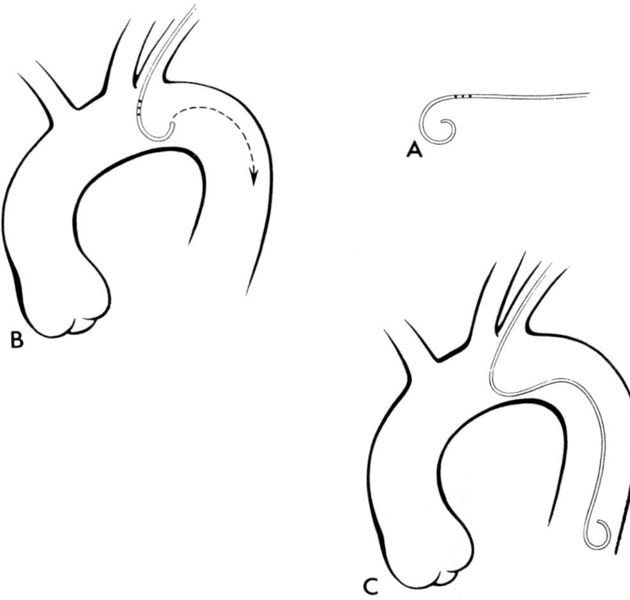

FIGURE 8–4. Technique of abdominal aortic catheterization from a left axillary approach. *A*, The pigtail catheter. *B*, The catheter is positioned at the top of the aortic arch with its tip oriented toward the descending aorta. A guidewire, inserted through the catheter, is directed into the descending aorta, as indicated by the *dotted line*. *C*, Final catheter position. A catheter inserted in this manner may be advanced as far as the aortic bifurcation if the aortic lumen will accommodate the curled catheter tip. Catheterization from the right axillary artery is analogous.

Catheters

Catheters provide the means by which contrast or other agents (e.g., pharmacologic, embolic) may be safely and selectively delivered within the vascular system. Direct-needle injections have been used in the past, prior to widespread use of catheters, but this approach has limited application at present. Sheath needles are sometimes used; after the needle is inserted into the vessel, the integral overlying plastic sheath is advanced until its hub reaches the skin and the needle is removed. This is essentially a very short catheter and is suitable for nonselective injections of easily accessible vessels; however, the risk of vascular injury is lower when a guidewire is used to lead a catheter.

The French or Charriere scale is used to size catheters. One French unit is ⅓ mm, so a 6 Fr catheter has an *outside* diameter of 2 mm; the lumen diameter is obviously smaller and depends on the thickness of the catheter wall. Three to 6 Fr catheters are routinely used in pediatric angiography, and 4 to 7 Fr catheters are commonly used in adults. The trend is toward smaller-sized, thin-walled catheters and the use of smaller volume injections of more dilute contrast to obtain DSA images. Generally, thin-walled catheters with relatively larger lumens, multiple side holes, and curved "pigtail" configurations at the tips (Fig. 8–4) are used for larger-dose, rapid, nonselective aortic injections, and catheters with thicker walls and relatively smaller lumens are used for the lower-dose, slower delivery needed for selective studies. Selective catheterization is easier with the better torque control provided by thicker catheter walls.

Standard catheters are constructed of thermoplastic (may be shaped when heated) material with or without reinforcement, such as stainless steel mesh, in the catheter wall, and are usually impregnated with a radiopaque substance, such as a barium, lead, or bismuth salt, to provide better fluoroscopic visibility. The ideal catheter is nonthrombogenic and has good memory, torque control (to facilitate rotational positioning), and sufficient bursting strength to accommodate the high injection pressures needed during a high flow rate of contrast.

Polyethylene, Teflon, polyurethane, and nylon or nylon composites are used to make catheter tubing, which is formed by extruding the molten plastic through a die to create a long tube that is then cut into the desired lengths. Polyethylene is the most commonly used catheter material. It is easy to shape with steam heat and has reasonable torque control, but is soft and flexible enough not to damage vessel intima. Most selective catheters are made of polyethylene. Teflon is very strong and can tolerate high flow rates. It has a very low coefficient of friction but is very stiff and requires very high heat to shape. Teflon catheters can damage vessels if used for selective catheterization. Polyurethane, although softer than Teflon, is stiffer than polyethylene and more difficult to shape. It is rubbery, and generally is reinforced with wire mesh, compromising lumen size. A higher coefficient of friction in polyurethane requires the use of Teflon-coated guidewires. Nylon is stiffer than polyethylene but has a lower coefficient of friction and can withstand higher injection pressures; it is used for high-flow, nonselective (e.g., aortogram) pigtail catheters. Copolymer catheters made of polyurethane with an inner nylon wall are strong, have thin walls, will accommodate high flow rates, and can be used for selective studies.

Coaxial systems have been developed for precision superselective catheterization in which small, 2 to 3 Fr catheters with very soft, flexible tips and relatively stiffer shafts can be introduced through conventional preshaped diagnostic catheters. The diagnostic catheter is positioned selectively in the proximal portion of the vessel being superselectively catheterized and acts as a guiding catheter, providing proximal support. The inner microcatheters, with correspondingly small steerable guidewires, can access very small or tortuous vessels for diagnostic or therapeutic purposes. These tiny catheters and wires have gold or platinum markers at their tips to make them visible. A high-resolution imaging system is necessary to perform superselective catheterization safely.

CATHETER TECHNIQUES

Puncture Sites

Prior to the 1950s, arteriography was performed via either direct-needle puncture or surgically placed catheters. In 1953, Seldinger[20] described the technique for percutaneous catheter placement that remains the mainstay of vascular access today (Fig. 8–5). Following percutaneous needle puncture, a guidewire is passed into the vessel, the needle is withdrawn, and a tapered catheter is threaded over the wire. Manual compression at the puncture site prevents excessive bleeding around and dislodgment of the wire. The catheter is gently advanced over the guidewire through the skin and subcutaneous tissues into the artery. Fluoroscopic monitoring then allows exact positioning of the catheter. When the catheter has been correctly placed, the guidewire is removed. The wire must not be removed prematurely, because advancing a sharp-tipped, straight catheter without a guidewire may injure the vessel wall. Backflow of blood from the catheter should be present, and a test injection of contrast material should always be observed fluoroscopically prior to filming to ensure satisfactory positioning of the catheter.

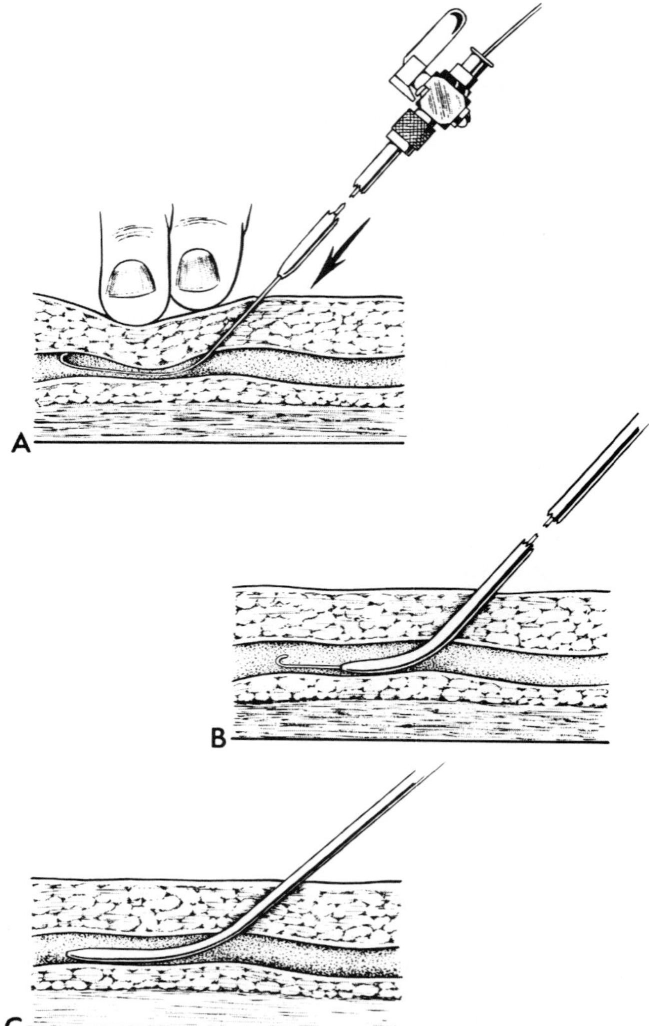

FIGURE 8–5. Technique of percutaneous catheterization. *A*, After a guidewire has been inserted into the vessel and the needle removed, a tapered-tip catheter is threaded over the guide. *B*, With the guidewire fixed, the catheter is slid over the wire into the vessel. *C*, After the catheter has been advanced to the desired location, the guidewire is removed.

The common femoral artery is the preferred site for vascular access, owing to its relatively large size, superficial location, and ease of manual compression against the femoral head for achieving hemostasis after removal of the catheter. If both femoral pulses are absent or if selective catheterization cannot be achieved from a femoral approach, an axillary arterial puncture can be utilized, again using the Seldinger technique.[17, 19] Disadvantages of the axillary approach compared with the femoral approach include increased patient discomfort, more difficult access due to smaller vessel size and greater vessel mobility, and the risk of brachial plexus injury from an axillary hematoma following catheter removal.[8, 15] A left axillary approach provides straightforward access to the descending aorta and its branches; a curved or pigtail catheter is frequently needed to direct the wire down the aorta (see Fig. 8–4).[5] A right transaxillary approach can also be used, although the course is less direct and the catheter traverses all of the brachiocephalic artery origins; there is consequently a slightly increased risk of neurologic complications.

The brachial artery may be utilized for antegrade access to the forearm or hand, but is inadvisable for retrograde puncture owing to its small size, with increased risk of spasm or thrombotic occlusion. Only catheters of 4 Fr or smaller should be placed in the brachial artery.

In the absence of femoral or axillary access, a translumbar approach, described by dos Santos and coworkers in 1929,[23] can be used for aortography and even selective brachiocephalic arteriography if no other access route is available. With the patient prone, a long needle is positioned in the aorta using external landmarks (Fig. 8–6). In the "high" translumbar approach used when visualizing the major visceral branches as well as the pelvic vessels, the needle is introduced just below the 12th rib and enters the aorta above the celiac trunk. In the "low" translumbar approach, used for arteriography of the pelvic and femoral vessels, the needle is inserted halfway between the 12th rib and the iliac crest and penetrates the aorta distal to the

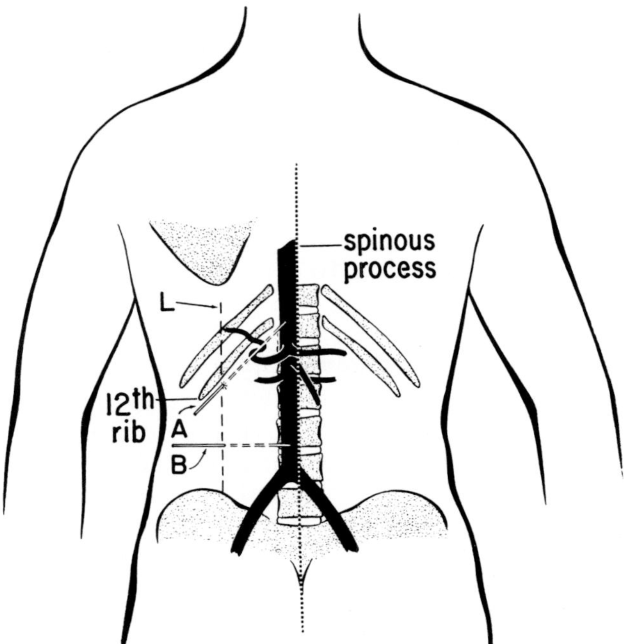

FIGURE 8–6. Landmarks for translumbar cannulation of the aorta. The patient is prone. Puncture is from the left side. Needle A (high translumbar puncture) is directed toward the right shoulder. Needle B (low translumbar puncture) is directed transversely. Both needles enter the skin along line L, halfway between the midline and the flank, and are inclined at about a 45-degree angle from the tabletop.

origins of the renal arteries. Using an intermediate approach is not recommended owing to the risk of injury to the visceral branches. A plastic-sheath needle or closed-tip steel needle with side holes should be used to reduce the risk of subintimal or extravascular injection. The former is preferable, and if used with a low translumbar approach, the sheath may be advanced with the aid of a guidewire, either upstream or downstream, thus correcting a possibly suboptimal puncture level.

Retroperitoneal hemorrhage occurs in nearly all cases of translumbar catheterization,[2] since no direct compression for hemostasis can be applied, but is usually of no clinical consequence; in fact, hemorrhagic complications requiring treatment are more frequent in transaxillary than in either transfemoral or translumbar approaches.[8] Patients with uncontrolled hypertension or a coagulopathy should not be considered for translumbar access, nor should aortic grafts be punctured from a translumbar approach. Direct translumbar aortic puncture precludes the use of anticoagulation and, consequently, the performance of angioplasty or fibrinolysis by this route. For this reason, translumbar aortography has been used with decreasing frequency during the past decade as such interventional procedures more commonly accompany a diagnostic extremity arteriogram.

Use of other puncture sites, including the superficial femoral artery, profunda femoris, and even the popliteal artery, may be necessary for therapeutic and occasionally diagnostic access in highly selected cases.

Aortography

Abdominal aortography typically involves placement of a high-flow catheter in the lower thoracic aorta, with biplane filming during rapid injection of a large volume of contrast. A pigtail catheter is usually utilized. This has a tightly curled tip with multiple side holes proximal to the resulting terminal loop (see Fig. 8–4). A large lumen size and the side holes permit rapid injection of contrast, and the pigtail tip reduces the force of the jet of contrast through the end hole of the catheter.

Lower Extremities

Arteriography of the lower extremities—a ''runoff'' angiogram—is usually performed via a pigtail catheter in the infrarenal abdominal aorta. During a single prolonged contrast injection, a motorized, or ''stepping,'' table moves the patient in a preset sequence so that first the pelvis, then the thighs, then the knees, and so on, are positioned over the film changer. Films are obtained while the table is stationary in each position. If the sequence is properly programmed, the contrast agent may be followed all the way to the foot. Fluoroscopic timing of the interval between injection of a test dose of contrast material and its appearance at the level of the knees is helpful in planning the timing of the film program for the arteriogram.

Single-extremity runoff examinations can be performed in the same way, via either the same aortic catheter (thereby using more than the needed volume of contrast) or a catheter selectively placed at the common or external iliac level from a contralateral or ipsilateral puncture.

DSA can be utilized for evaluation of the lower extremities. Standard DSA images can be obtained while separate contrast injections are performed at each station. Alternatively, the table can be moved through sequential positions during a single injection of contrast medium; these images are not subtracted, but the high contrast can often provide adequate vascular detail. Even with conventional filming, DSA is excellent for supplemental images or projections in regions not well visualized with conventional filming, particularly distal to the popliteal artery.

Selective Catheterization

An experienced angiographer can cannulate any aortic branch using standard catheters and maneuvers. An appropriately shaped catheter may be inserted into the desired arterial branch after the catheter tip has been positioned at the branch orifice. Because the exact location and orientation of each patient's arterial branch orifice usually is not known in advance, the angiographer may need to try a variety of catheters and maneuvers. The catheter is positioned with a combination of axial and rotary movement. Because the fluoroscopic image provides only a two-dimensional image, hand-eye coordination is essential to sense the third dimension. Using steerable guidewires and small flexible catheters, superselective catheterization of vessels can be achieved, permitting embolization or perfusion with thrombolytic or other pharmacologic agents. These selective and superselective catheterization techniques require a considerable amount of experience and should be employed only by physicians specifically trained in their use.

INJECTION TECHNIQUES

Injections of contrast agent may be made by a hand-held syringe or an automatic injector. Injecting by hand into either a catheter or an intra-arterial needle is less reliable and requires the angiographer to be in the examining room, with consequent exposure to scattered radiation. Most automatic injectors initiate the filming sequence at a preset time, thus improving the reliability of the entire examination.

In selective arteriography, the contrast agent should be injected at a rate the same as or slightly above the blood flow rate in the targeted vessel. If the injection rate is too slow, the contrast agent will become diluted with blood, and the vessels will be poorly visualized on film. If the rate is too fast, contrast agent will overflow into the parent vessel. The unwanted opacification of the parent vessel and its branches may obscure details of the vascular bed being studied selectively. When the injection rate is correct, all filled branches are clearly seen until the injection is completed. Thereafter, progressive dilution gradually diminishes the degree of opacification.

For aortic injections, the contrast agent does not displace flowing blood but mixes with blood already there. Accordingly, a more concentrated solution of contrast agent is used in an attempt to compensate for dilution. If the injection is too slow, the contrast agent may actually layer dependently beneath the flowing blood, not filling branches that arise on the nondependent side of the aorta. If injection is too fast, there will be mixing with blood upstream from the point of injection. Clearly, there are correct injection rates for all arteriograms. The selected flow rate is based on previous experience and observation under fluoroscopy of the flow rate in the individual patient. DSA permits the use of a smaller contrast volume or the same volume of more dilute contrast.

INTERPRETIVE PITFALLS IN ARTERIOGRAPHY

Time and effort in mutual education are required to ensure that the vascular surgeon and angiographer are aware of each other's capabilities and limitations. The vascular surgeon must educate the vascular radiologist as to the types of operations in his or her repertoire and the diagnostic information desired from the angiogram in order to perform these operations. Likewise, the experienced vascular and interventional radiologist must make the surgeon aware of what can be accomplished with various combinations of angioplasty, intra-arterial fibrinolytic infusion, and selective embolization in order to provide optimal care to the widest spectrum of patients with vascular disease.

Appropriate treatment planning depends on an accurate understanding of the patient's pathologic anatomy. Most experienced angiographers have achieved an almost automatic awareness of the many potential pitfalls in interpretation of angiograms performed to evaluate vascular disease. The vascular surgeon should at least be familiar with those that occur frequently, particularly since some of the more common ones are quite simple.

Problems Relating to Roentgenography

High-Contrast Roentgenographic Techniques

X-rays will not efficiently penetrate a radiodense structure. Accordingly, a vessel outline may be obscured by an overlying dense bone or another opacified vessel. The penetration of the x-rays may be increased by raising the kilovoltage, producing an image with less contrast in which the relative opacity of the overlapping structure is decreased without unacceptably compromising the opacity of the contrast medium in the vessel. Thus, low-contrast (high-kilovoltage) film angiography should be used to assess diseases of the vessels, whereas high-contrast (low-kilovoltage) angiography should be reserved for assessment of organ disease (Fig. 8–7). Even with appropriate high-contrast filming techniques, web-like narrowings may be difficult to detect when contrast material is injected at a distance from the lesion. Injection of contrast medium selectively at the site of the lesion is necessary to provide the necessary detail (Fig. 8–8).

DSA is inherently a high-contrast imaging technique; despite its many favorable characteristics, DSA remains subject to serious motion and density artifacts. Its high-contrast detection is extremely useful for delineating small arteries distal to the popliteal fossa, but the same high contrast often obscures mural abnormalities—plaques, intimal flaps, mural thrombi—in larger arteries.

Superimposed Vessels

Because atherosclerotic plaques frequently form at arterial bifurcations, demonstrating the luminal configuration at these junctional segments is particularly important. An atherosclerotic narrowing in one branch may be obscured by the superimposed image of the other and may not be appreciated unless the roentgenographic projection shows the bifurcation in profile. This problem occurs most frequently at the carotid, iliac, and femoral bifurcations and at the left vertebral artery orifice as seen in the oblique arch projection (Figs. 8–9 and 8–10). Stenoses of the origins of the external iliac and profunda femoris arteries are concealed with notorious frequency by the adjacent overlapping internal iliac and superficial femoral arteries, respectively. In each instance, an additional projection can show the bifurcation in profile. The iliac bifurcation is best evaluated in the ipsilateral posterior oblique projection, whereas the opposite obliquity (i.e., anterior oblique) is best for the ipsilateral femoral bifurcation. Using low-contrast techniques already described, the luminal contour of both vessels may be seen in spite of superimposition (Fig. 8–11*A*).

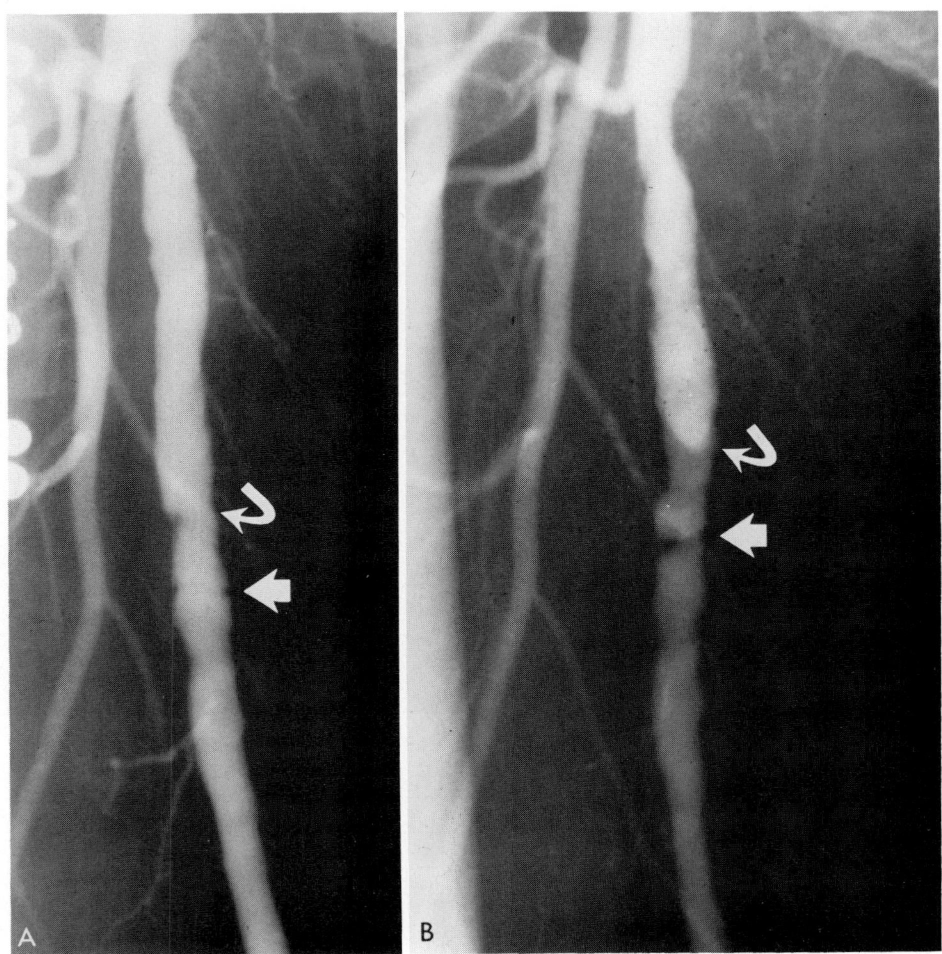

FIGURE 8–7. Femoral arteriograms (separate studies, same patient). Web-like narrowing *(straight arrow)* and thick posterior plaque *(curved arrow)* are present. *A*, High-contrast study. The lesions are poorly defined. *B*, Low-contrast study. The lesions are clearly seen.

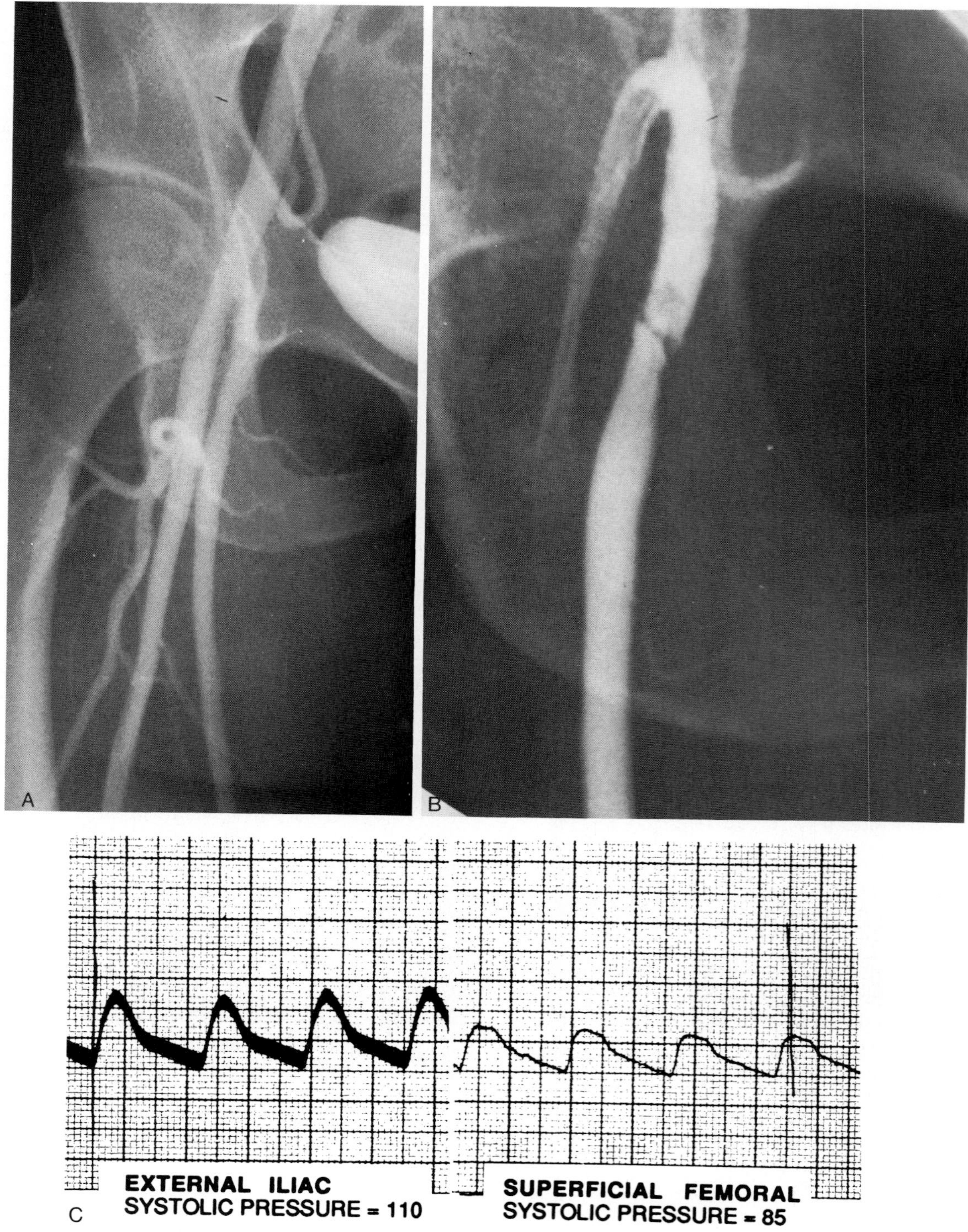

FIGURE 8–8. *A*, Contrast injected in the common iliac artery. Web-like narrowing of common femoral artery is poorly seen. *B*, Contrast injected in the common femoral artery. There is an obvious web-like narrowing causing a pressure gradient, which is documented by intra-arterial pressure measurement *(C)*.

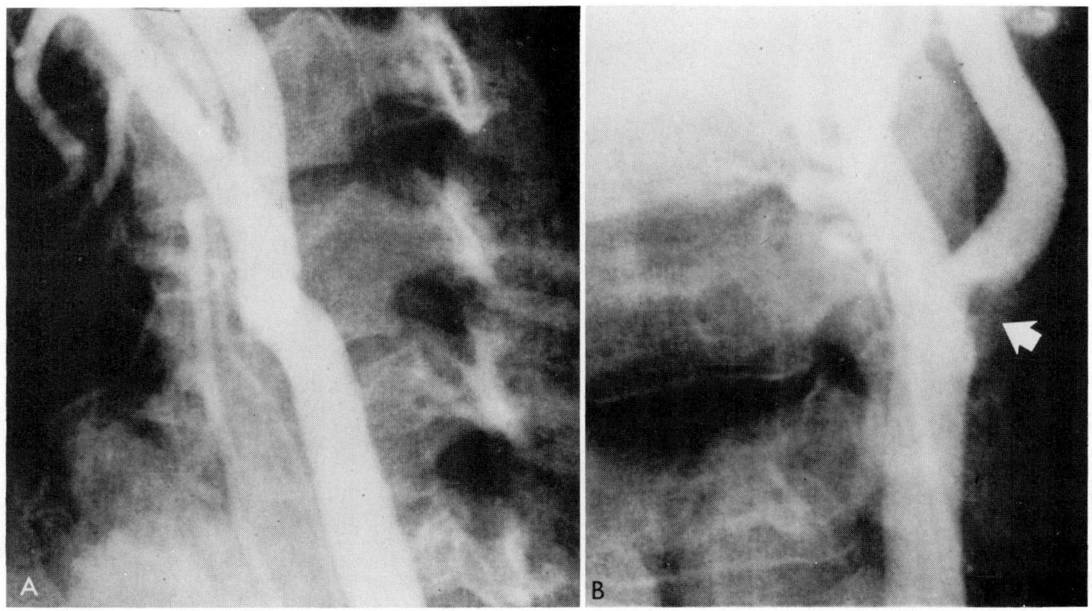

FIGURE 8–9. Left carotid arteriograms. *A*, Oblique projection. The branches are superimposed. *B*, Frontal projection. The bifurcation is seen in profile. A stenosis is present *(arrow)*.

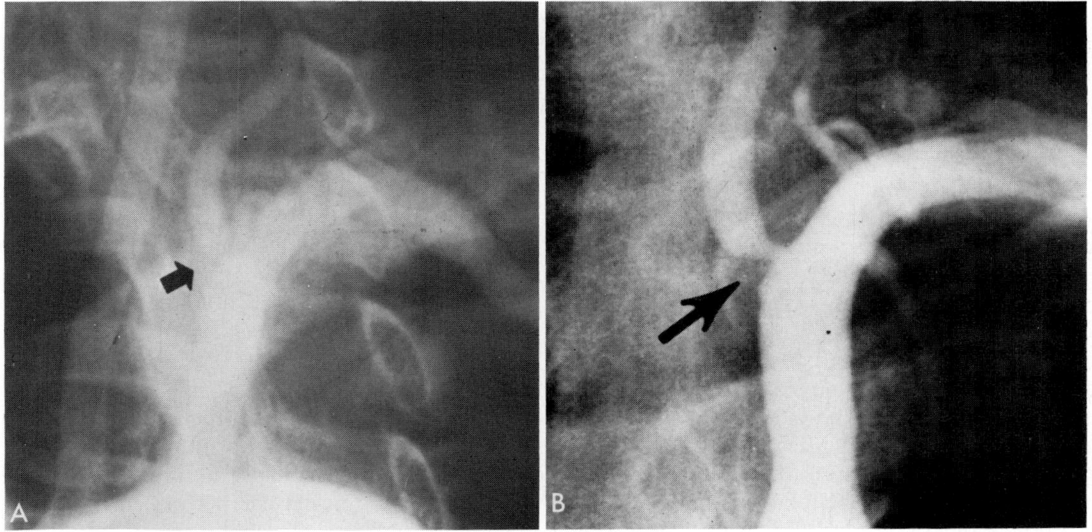

FIGURE 8–10. Left vertebral artery stenosis *(arrows)*. *A*, Arch injection, oblique projection. The stenosis is hidden. *B*, Subclavian injection, frontal projection. The stenosis is well shown.

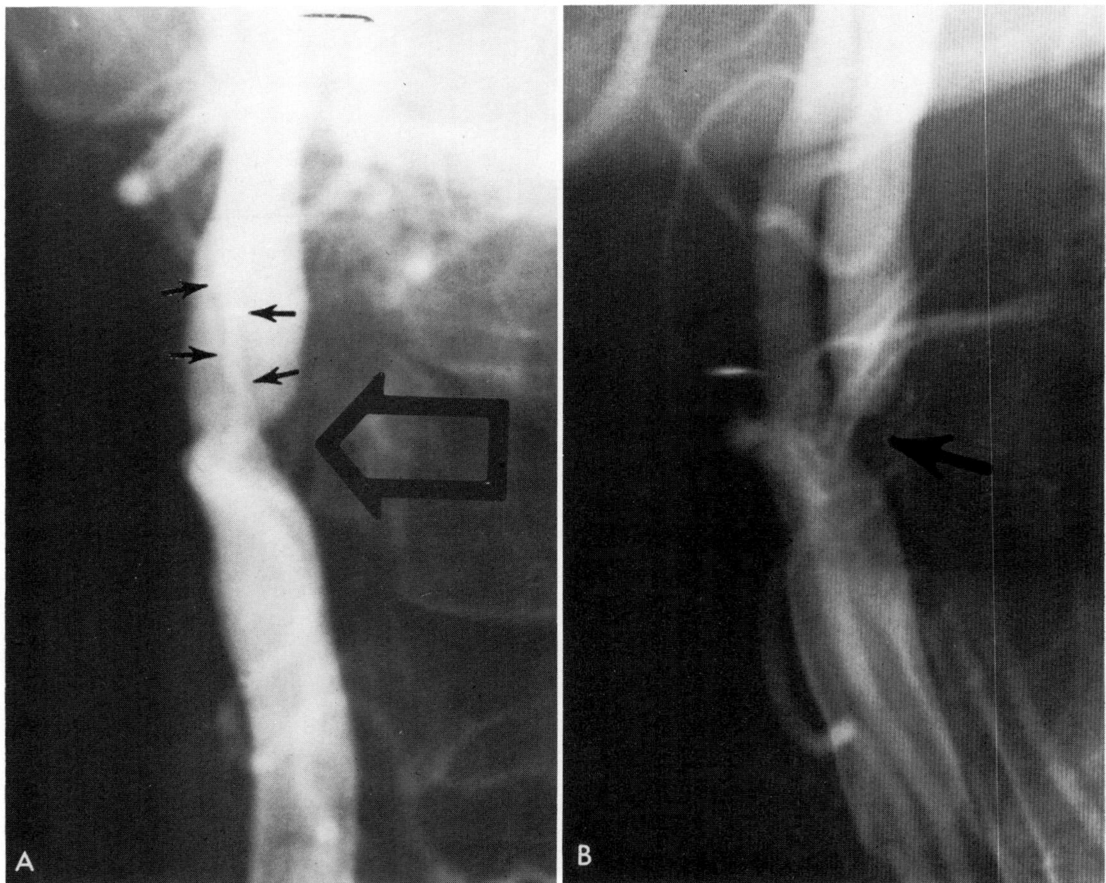

FIGURE 8–11. Right carotid arteriograms. Internal carotid branch stenosis *(large arrows)*. *A*, Frontal projection. The branches are superimposed, but their separate contours can be identified *(solid arrows)*. *B*, Oblique projection. The bifurcation is seen in profile.

If either vessel appears to be abnormal, additional filming in another projection should be obtained for confirmation (Fig. 8–11*B*); DSA can quickly provide these supplemental projections.

Moore and Hall have pointed out that aortoiliac stenoses are frequently unrecognized on aortograms because the atherosclerotic plaques develop primarily on the posterior surface of that segment and are consequently not seen in profile if only single-plane anterior-posterior projection films are obtained.[16] Simultaneous biplane filming of the abdominal aorta, iliac vessels, and common femoral artery bifurcations usually demonstrates any significant abnormalities in this segment and should be performed routinely if the angiographic equipment has this capability. Supplementary oblique views of these vessels may be necessary if biplane filming is not available. Biplane filming distal to the femoral bifurcation is technically difficult and seldom useful clinically. Intra-arterial pressure measurements obtained proximal and distal to a stenosis also provide valuable data about the hemodynamic significance of an angiographically demonstrated lesion.

Physical findings and noninvasive vascular diagnostic laboratory data are of great value in planning the arteriogram and should be known by the arteriographer before the puncture is performed. For example, if the arteriographer knows that the physical findings and vascular laboratory tests suggest the presence of a right iliac lesion, extra views of this region can be obtained if the standard projections are unrevealing. If the infrapopliteal vessels on one side are not visualized because of incorrect timing of the films, but the vascular laboratory data indicate that no infrapopliteal lesion is present, an extra run is probably not necessary.

Superimposed Bones

The tibial arteries are frequently obscured by overlying bone cortex. This may be minimized by the use of low-contrast (high-kilovoltage) filming techniques (Fig. 8–12). An additional run may be performed using a different projection. Subtraction techniques cannot be performed on conventional films from a stepping-table run, since no film of this area without contrast is available to use as a mask. Another run using DSA (automatically subtracting bone) or limited to one station using conventional films (providing a mask prior to contrast injection) can provide the desired information.

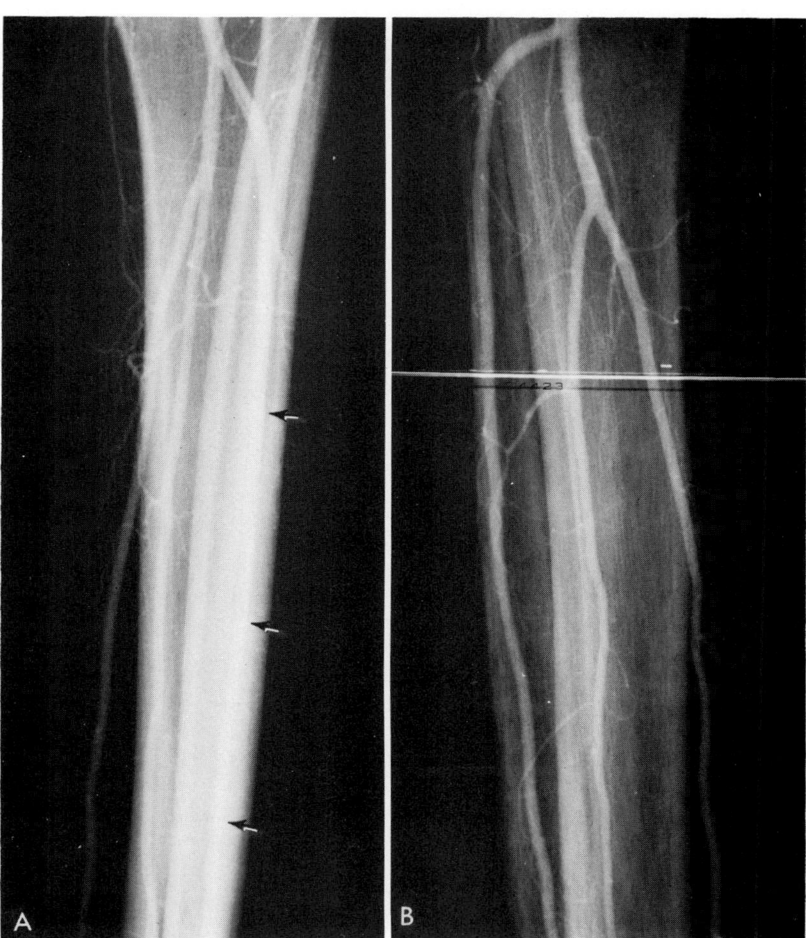

FIGURE 8–12. Femoral arteriograms (different patients). *A*, High-contrast technique. The anterior tibial artery *(arrows)* is obscured by bone. *B*, Low-contrast technique. All vessels are seen, even where they are projected over bone.

Problems Related to Blood Flow

Nonfilled Vessels

Proximal origin of either the radial or the ulnar artery is not unusual,[12] and a brachial arteriogram performed on a patient with such an anomaly will fail to show the anomalous branch if the injection is made distal to its origin. Similarly, a selective left subclavian arteriogram will not demonstrate a left vertebral artery that arises from the aortic arch. In both instances, the unwary observer may conclude that the anomalous artery is occluded. More frequently, patent distal arteries are not visualized because the arteriographic technique is at fault—either the volume of contrast is too small or the film is exposed too soon after injection (Fig. 8–13). At least one of two criteria must be met if occlusion is to be verified: branches that arise from the occluded vessels are well filled while the parent vessel remains unopacified; or a distal, patent portion of the occluded artery is filled (Figs. 8–14 and 8–15). The length of an occlusion can be overestimated by arteriography if films are obtained too soon. What appears to be a sharply circumscribed proximal point of occlusion may merely be the head of the slowly advancing column of contrast material (Fig. 8–16). Such an appearance is found only when blood flow is markedly reduced. Similarly, the distal extent of an occlusion may be overestimated when collateral vessels reenter at several different levels and there is greater flow through the more distally entering collaterals. In this situation, opacification of the proximal patent vessel will be seen only on later films. If knowing the exact extent of occlusion is critical in planning the most appropriate revascularization procedure, another angiographic run with prolonged serial filming centered over the critical area may be necessary.

Owing to its superior contrast resolution, DSA may demonstrate patent distal vessels that are not evident on conventional studies. DSA is especially helpful in the hand and for assessing patency of the distal tibial arteries and the plantar arch of the foot, so long as motion artifact can be controlled.

In acute occlusions, the distal arteries may be poorly seen because of markedly reduced flow. Rather than use repeated injections of large volumes of contrast material, intra-arterial fibrinolytic therapy can be instituted. Fibrinolysis will often clear out the acute thrombus and allow diagnostic visualization of the distal arterial tree so that appropriate arterial reconstruction can be planned.

Prolonged filming is often necessary in evaluating a graft anastomosis for the presence of a false aneurysm, since opacification of the aneurysm lumen occurs slowly when the point of communication with the lumen is small. In most instances, color Duplex scanning is the preferred

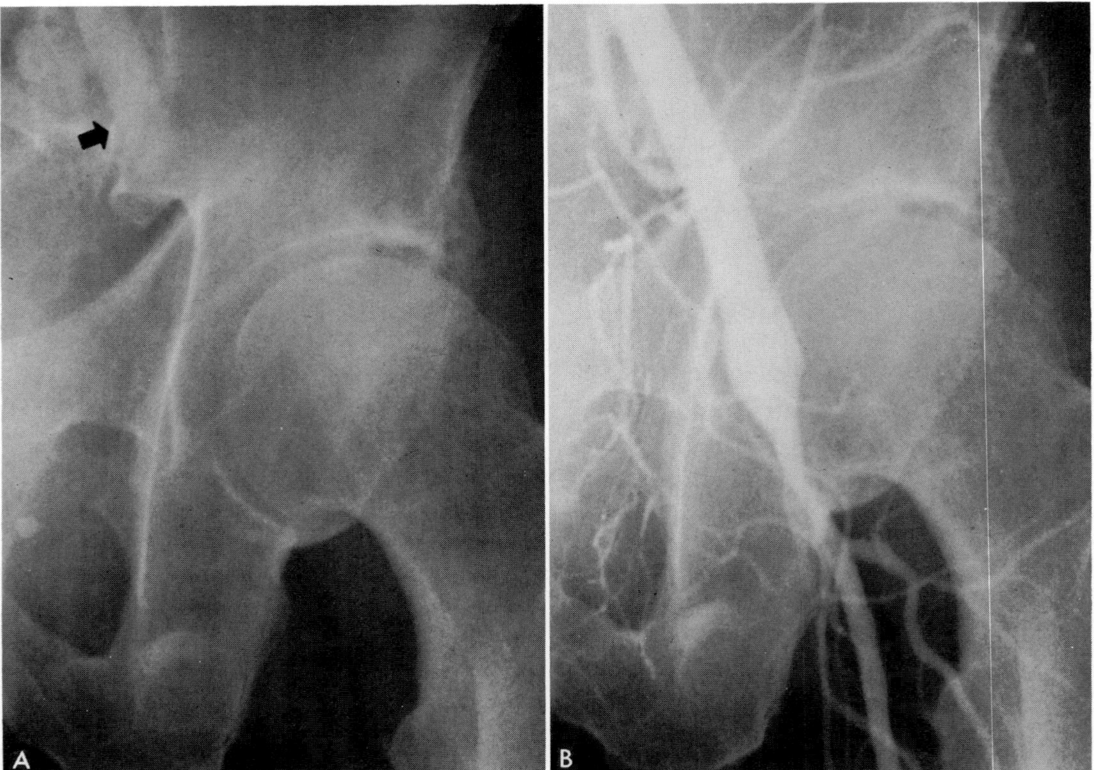

FIGURE 8–13. Iliac arteriogram following aortofemoral bypass. *A*, Early film. Only the upper part of the bypass is seen *(arrow)*. *B*, Later film. Good filling of all vessels.

technique for diagnosis of an anastomotic aneurysm or a false aneurysm at an accessible site of arterial trauma.

Embolism Versus Thrombosis

When an acute arterial occlusion occurs, it is important to differentiate, if possible, between embolism and thrombosis of a previously stenosed artery. The only absolute arteriographic sign of embolism is the demonstration of the embolus itself as an intraluminal filling defect surrounded by contrast agent (Fig. 8–17). Unfortunately, the embolus is frequently not demonstrated because the stagnant column of blood proximal to the point of occlusion will form adjacent thrombus within a few hours, and the angiographic differentiation from primary thrombosis may not be possible. When collateral vessels are small and little atherosclerosis is present in the visualized vessels, embolism should be suspected (Fig. 8–18). Thrombosis of a preexisting stenosis may produce a similar focal arteriographic appearance, but collateral vessels are larger, and atherosclerosis is usually present in the adjacent segments (Fig. 8–19).

Anatomic Obstruction Versus Spasm

Mechanical stimulation of the internal arterial wall by an angiographic or embolectomy catheter can induce arterial spasm, which can simulate the arteriographic appearance of a stenosis or even occlusion. Spasm should be suspected when a narrowing or an apparent occlusion is present in a vessel through which a catheter passes (particularly the external iliac artery) or when the catheter tip or guidewire has just been advanced into the artery.[9] The proximal internal and external carotid arteries are particularly prone to catheter-induced spasm. Spasm in the iliofemoral vessels occurs most commonly in children. Following balloon catheter embolectomy in either the upper or the lower extremity, lesions that appear on an intraoperative arteriogram to be organic narrowings or even occlusions often turn out to be spasm artifacts. Unless residual intraluminal thrombus or a sharp arterial cutoff is seen, an apparent obstruction on an intraoperative arteriogram may be due to spasm. A larger-volume contrast injection with a later film may be necessary either to demonstrate the point of obstruction or to establish that no obstruction exists. The intra-arterial administration of tolazoline (25 mg) or a bolus of nitroglycerin (100 to 300 μg) may be helpful in this circumstance, just as it is during diagnostic and interventional arteriography.

Other than awareness of the clinical situations in which it occurs, the differentiation of arterial spasm from a fixed anatomic lesion may be difficult. Failure of a second arteriogram performed minutes later to demonstrate the same finding may be the only way to confirm the diagnosis of spasm.

Early Venous Filling

The veins draining an extremity are usually seen on delayed films following arterial injection. Occasionally, they may fill earlier than anticipated, particularly when ar-

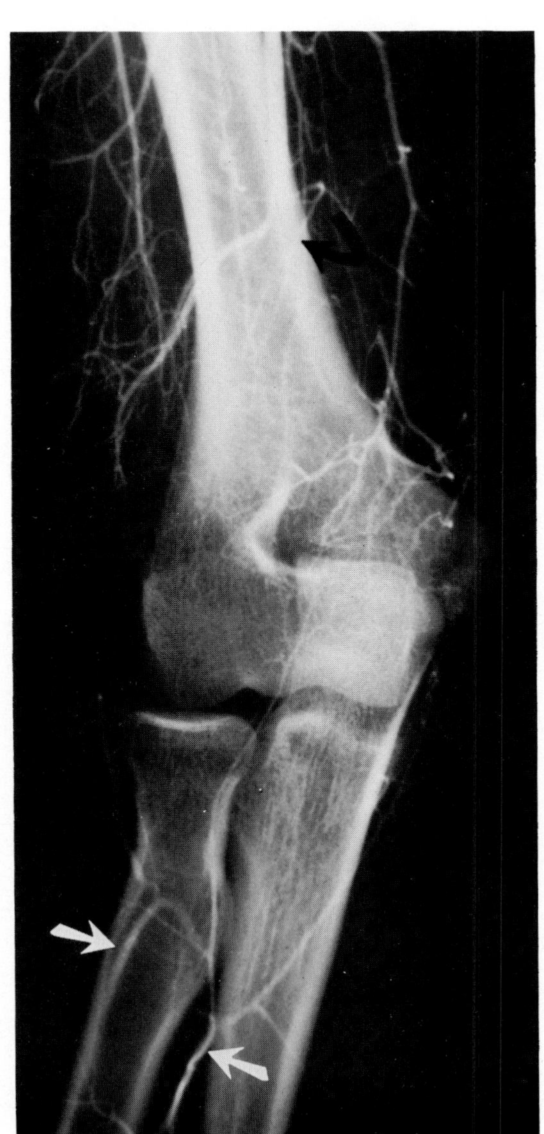

FIGURE 8–14. Brachial arteriogram. Point of brachial artery occlusion *(curved arrow)* is not well defined, but peripheral branch filling *(straight arrows)* proves that occlusion is present.

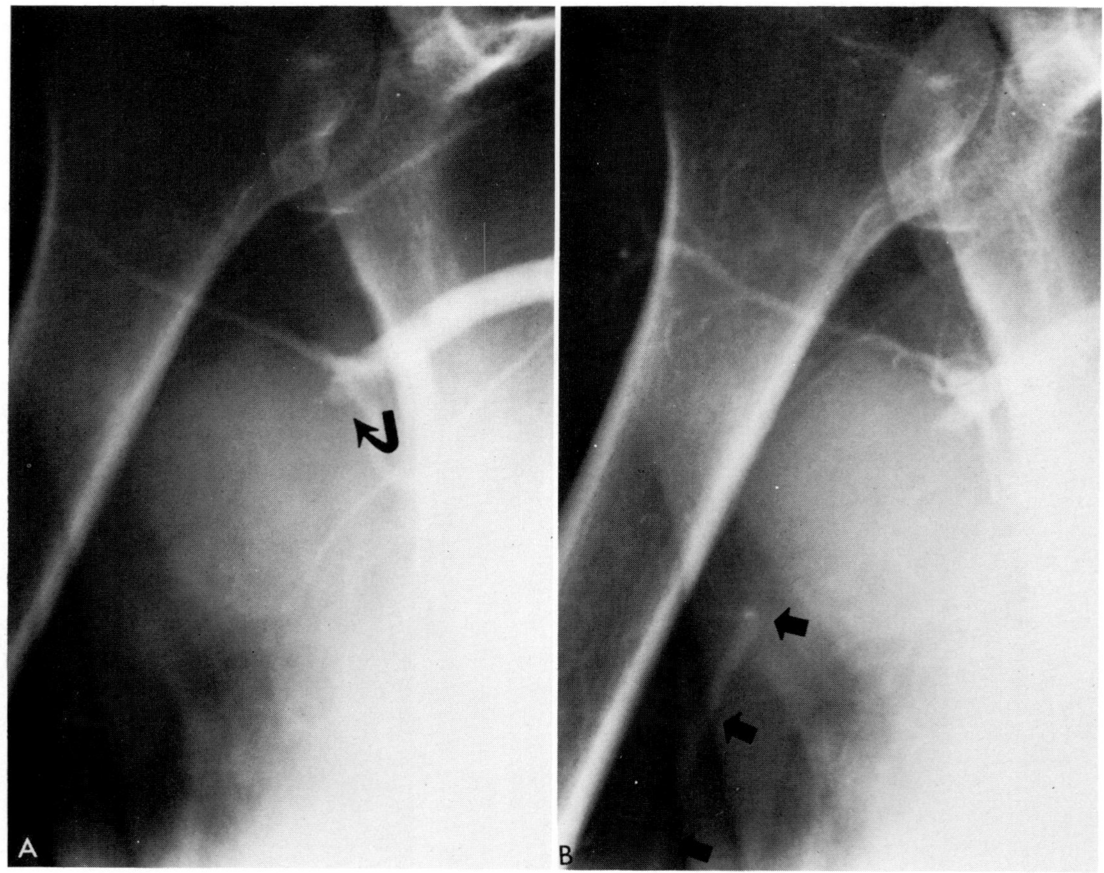

FIGURE 8–15. Arteriogram of occluded axillary artery. *A*, Early film. Axillary artery terminates abruptly *(curved arrow)*. *B*, Delayed film. Filling of distal artery *(straight arrows)* proves the presence of occlusion.

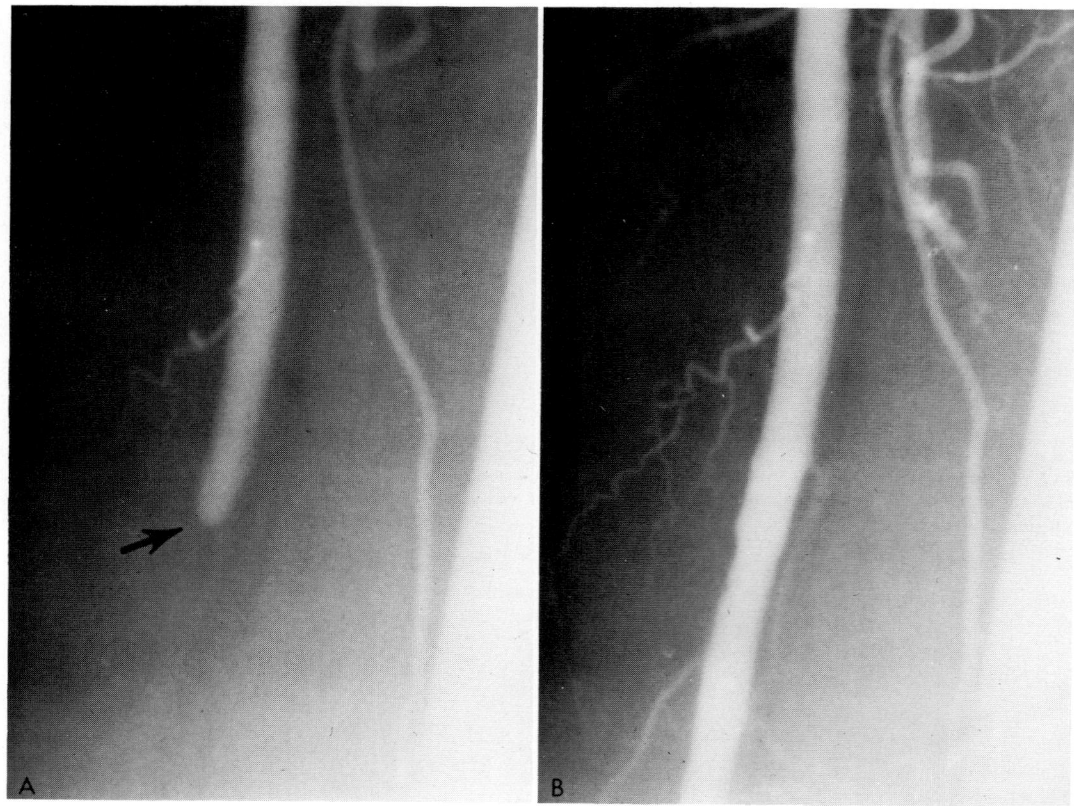

FIGURE 8–16. Femoral arteriogram. Flow in the superficial femoral artery was slow. *A*, Early film. Superficial femoral artery appears to terminate abruptly *(arrow)*. *B*, Late film. The entire vessel is filled.

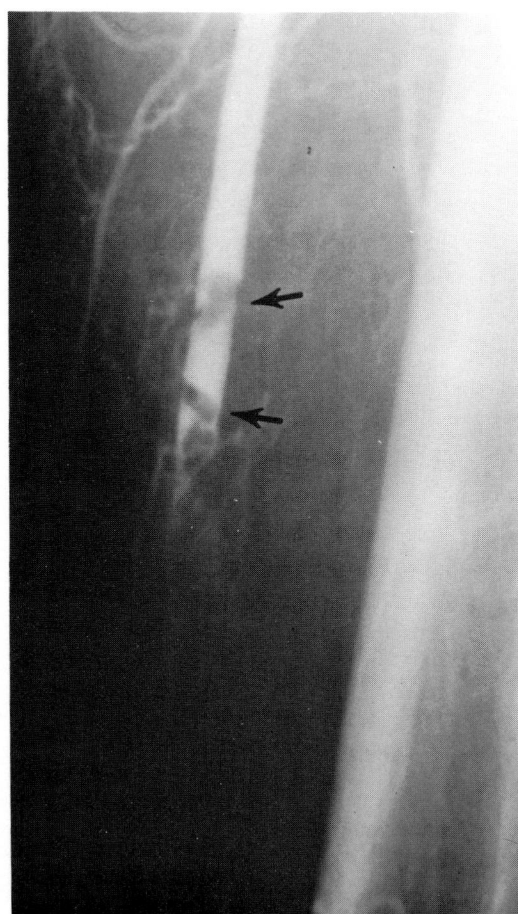

FIGURE 8–17. Femoral arteriogram. Embolus *(arrows)* is outlined.

terial occlusion is present. Although the significance of this finding has been debated, the entity should not be confused with an arteriovenous fistula.[4, 13] When a fistula is present, only the affected vein and its proximal drainage will be filled with contrast (Fig. 8–20*A*). Additionally, the fistula itself is usually visualized. When a fistula is not present, all the muscular tributary veins will be filled, and a contrast agent will be diluted (Fig. 8–20*B*).

Intraoperative Arteriography

Intraoperative arteriography requires several modifications of conventional arteriographic technique, because all the information must be obtained on a single exposure in one projection. Despite the suboptimal conditions, surprisingly good and consistent results can be obtained if the surgeon who carries out the procedure follows certain principles. First, the surgeon should be in charge of all stages of the procedure, except setting the x-ray exposure, and should have some practical knowledge of performing arteriography. If unskilled at angiography, she or he should consult with an angiographer about proper injection rates and timing of x-ray exposures. Second, an adequate x-ray machine is essential. In most hospitals, a portable x-ray unit is used to expose a single appropriately sized film in a screen cassette. If available, a C-arm image intensifier, with a video disc recorder to record a fluoroscopic sequence and ''freeze-frame'' the best image, can be very helpful and is faster than intraoperative arteriographic filming, because no film development is required. There are two types of image acquisition available on portable fluoroscopy units: (1) recording of an individual fluoroscopic frame; or (2) a single electronic spot film that is exposed with a higher dose and that contains more detail. Hard copies of these images can then be made with a number of devices. The image can be printed on film using a multi-format camera. Printing can

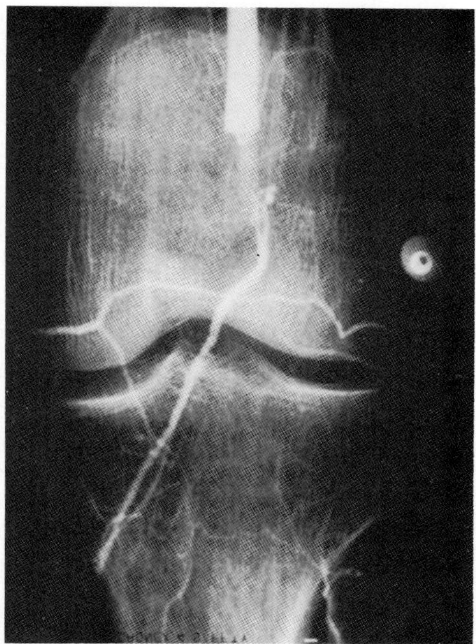

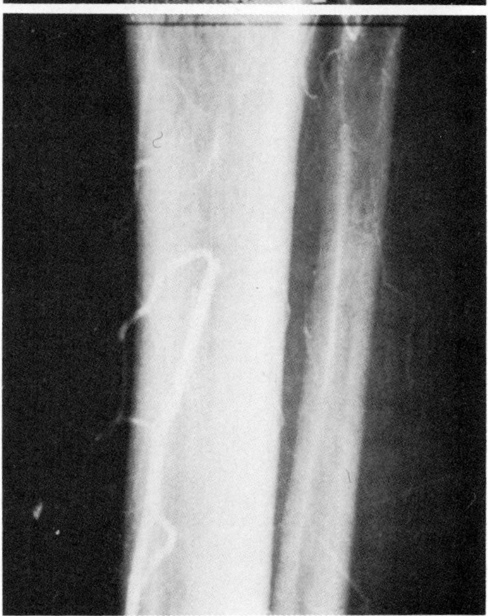

FIGURE 8–18. Femoral arteriogram. Embolic occlusion of popliteal artery. Embolus is not outlined. Collateral vessels are small. Distal vessels do not show atherosclerosis.

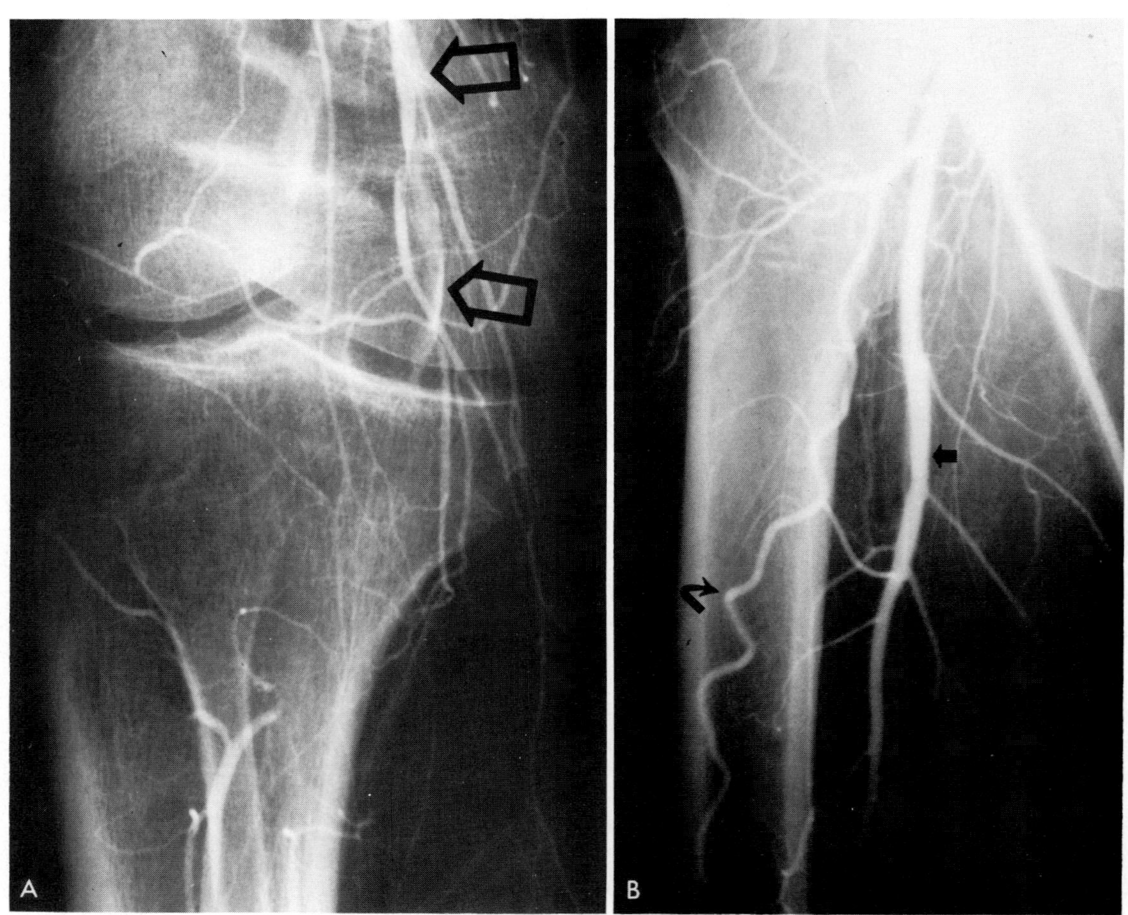

FIGURE 8–19. Femoral arteriogram. Acute thrombosis of popliteal artery. *A*, Popliteal area. Filling defects *(open arrows)* look like emboli. *B*, Upper thigh. Deep femoral artery *(straight arrow)* and collateral branch *(curved arrow)* are enlarged.

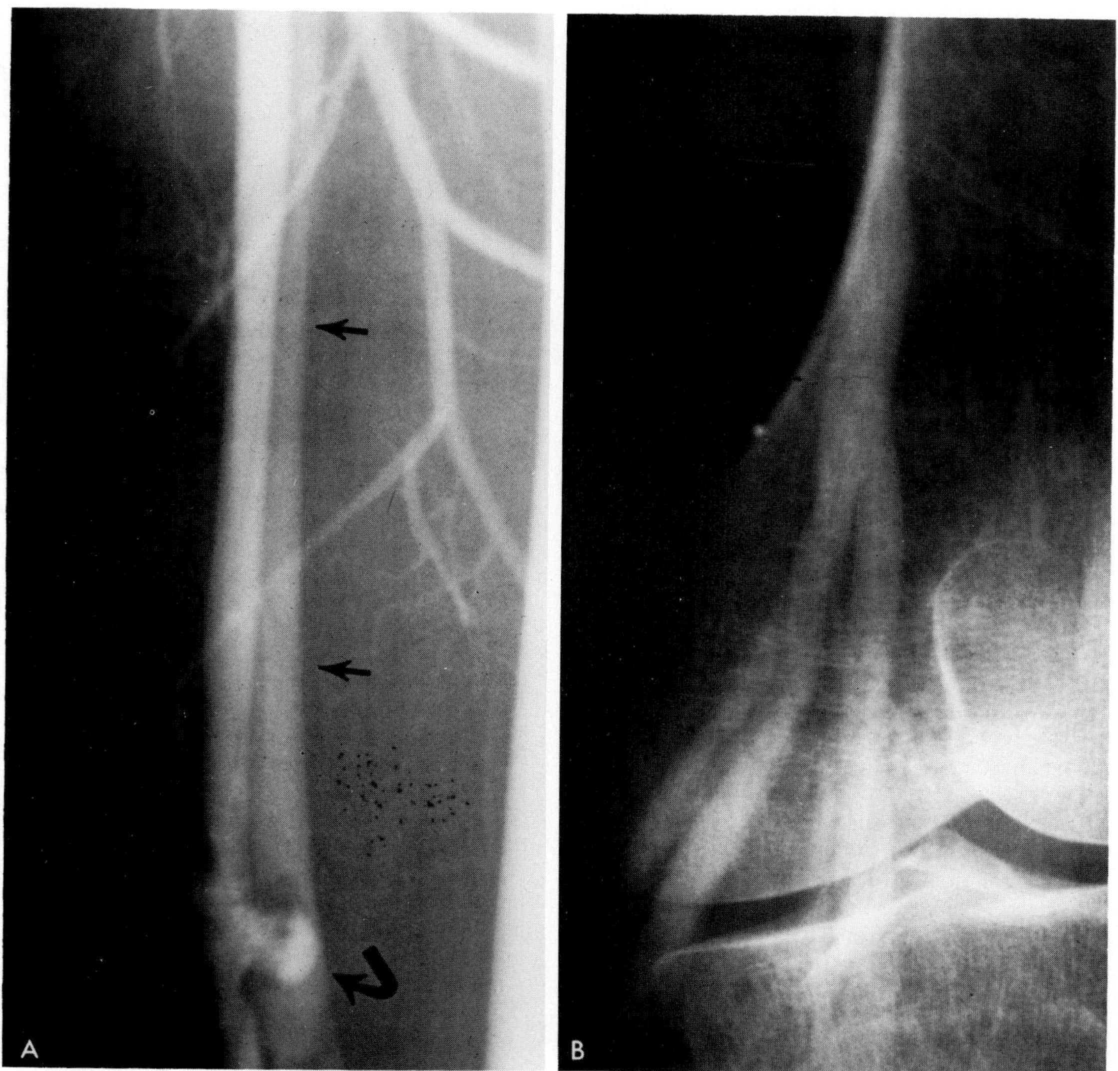

FIGURE 8–20. Femoral arteriograms (different patients). *A*, Arteriovenous fistula *(curved arrow)* fills adjacent vein *(straight arrows)*. *B*, Early venous filling (5-sec film). Several branches are filled.

also be done on Polaroid film using a specifically designed multi-format camera, or on special paper using a multi-scan video printer. The latter two resemble photographs of the angiographic image and can be incorporated in the patient's clinical record. More than one type of hard copy can be made of the same recorded image. The image can thus be printed on x-ray film for the hospital archives and on paper for the clinical chart. The detail of these images is not as good as that of cassette films, but is usually sufficient for documentation of the anatomy. The convenience of speed, that the image is immediately available in the operating suite where changes are assessed by the minute, and being able to make hard copies in several formats usually outweigh the lack of detail. Third, an experienced x-ray technologist must be present and must be familiar with intraoperative arteriography because exposure factors for arteriography are not the same as for skeletal roentgenography.

Technique

The cassette and the patient should be positioned by the surgeon. To optimize film detail, positioning should be accomplished so that the part to be studied is as close to the film as possible (minimizing object-to-film distance) and the distance between the x-ray tube and the film should be as great as practical (maximizing x-ray source-to-film distance). The latter is accomplished by lowering the operating table and placing the x-ray tube as high as possible above the table.

The cassette may be placed in the cassette rack under the operating table. For examination of extremities, however, it is often more convenient and accurate to wrap the screen cassette in a sterile plastic sheet and position it directly under the limb. The area of interest should be centered on the film so that vessels proximal and distal to this site are visualized.

The surgeon needs shielding from unnecessary irradiation, but wearing a lead apron during the entire procedure or changing in and out of one is unnecessary. She or he can stand behind an apron draped over an IV stand and covered with a sterile plastic drape. Use of extension tubing keeps the hands and contrast-filled syringe away from the field of exposure. A typical setup for operative arteriography during lower extremity revascularization is seen in Figure 8–21.

The patient should be positioned so that vessels will not project over each other or over a heavy bone. For the arteries of the thigh and popliteal space, straight anteroposterior projection is appropriate. In the calf, slight internal rotation of the foot gives the least overlay of the three tibial arteries. Visualization of the distal tibial arteries just above the ankle and of the dorsalis pedis and plantar arch of the foot is best with the foot in external rotation and plantar flexion. Vessels of the antecubital space, forearm, and hand are best demonstrated with the hand in anatomic position (palm up in a supine patient), so that there is no overlap of the radial, ulnar, and interosseous arteries.

Injection of the contrast medium should be made into the vessel as close to the level of interest as practical, although the technique of temporary inflow occlusion usually yields satisfactory arterial delineation even at some

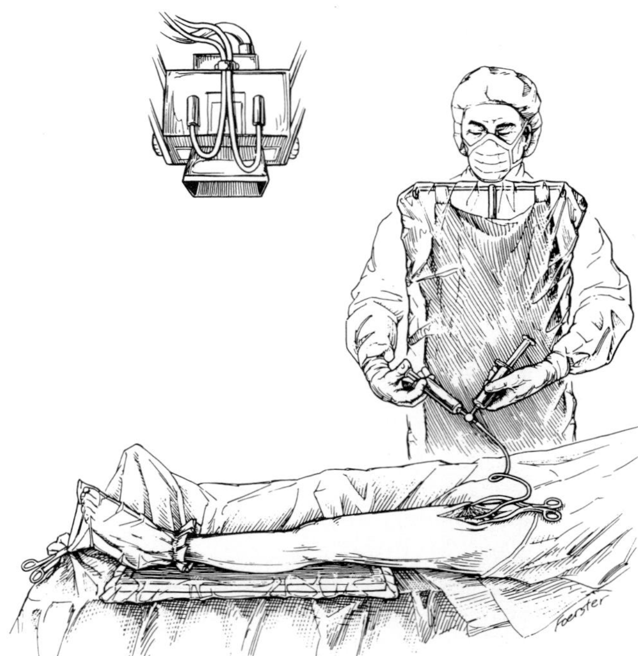

FIGURE 8–21. The major features of intraoperative arteriography are demonstrated, including draping and exposure of the leg, placement of the x-ray cassette, positioning of the cathode tube, positioning of the operator behind a sterile lead apron shield, and using extension tubing to keep the operator's hands away from the field of exposure. (From Rutherford RB: *Atlas of Vascular Surgery: Basic Techniques and Exposures.* Philadelphia, WB Saunders, 1993.)

distance from the injection site. Temporary inflow occlusion with a vascular clamp or even digital pressure greatly slows the distal arterial circulation so that the single exposure is more likely to capture a moment when there is adequate opacification of the lumen. Alternative methods of injecting during inflow occlusion are shown in Figure 8–22.

The volume of contrast agent must be sufficient to fill the arterial bed being studied. If it is excessive, however, venous filling may obscure the arteries. The flowing volumes are usually appropriate: 5 ml for the renal artery, 10 ml for the brachial artery, 20 ml in the axillary artery for visualization of the brachial artery or for the distal popliteal artery when injection is near the area of interest, 30 ml in the proximal femoral artery for visualization of the popliteal and tibial vessels, and 40 ml for the distal aorta and proximal iliac arteries. After exposure, a similar volume of heparinized saline solution is injected to flush out the contrast agent.

Lower Extremity

Most commonly, the femoral artery is the site of injection. With temporary inflow occlusion, a volume of 20 to 30 ml of 60 per cent contrast agent (e.g., Renografin-60, Conray 60, or Hypaque meglumine 60 per cent; see Chapter 7) will give very satisfactory visualization of the femoropopliteal segment and the proximal tibial arteries. The injections should be made with only moderate force, and the exposure is made just as the injection is completed. The

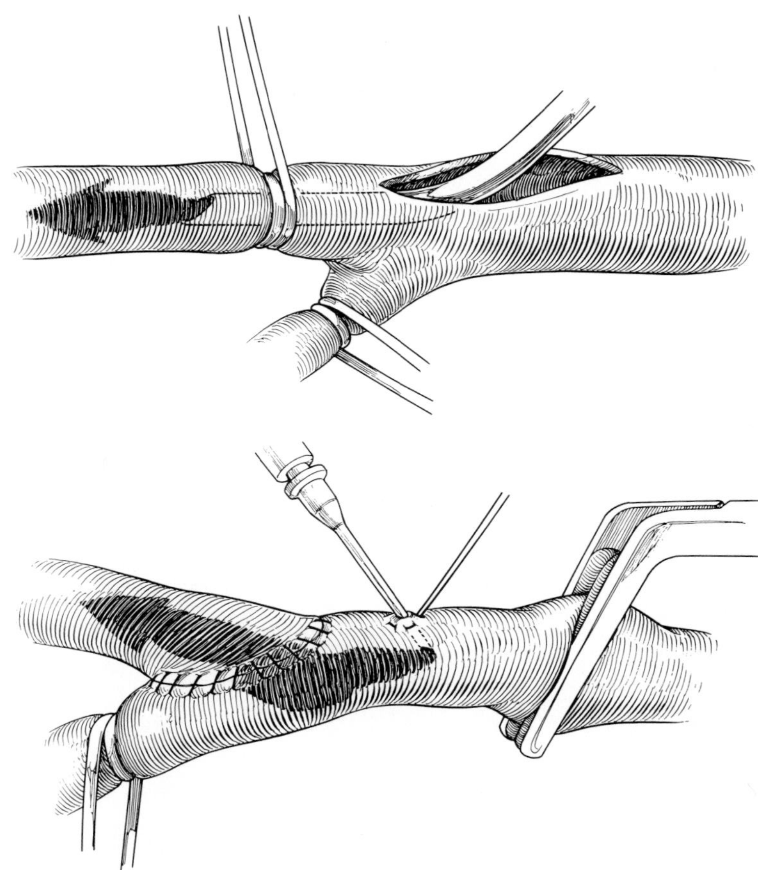

FIGURE 8–22. Alternative techniques for intraoperative arteriography. *A*, After thromboembolectomy, catheter is placed through open arteriotomy. *B*, After completion of a bypass, contrast media is injected through a needle or short catheter inserted through pursestring suture. (From Rutherford RB: *Atlas of Vascular Surgery: Basic Techniques and Exposures*. Philadelphia, WB Saunders, 1993).

more distal the visualization site, the larger the volume of contrast required. Injection must be made through a larger bore catheter because of resistance to flow offered by contrast medium. A 5 to 10 Fr catheter, a 16-gauge ''intracath,'' or an 18-gauge or larger needle, connected through a length of extension tubing and a three-way stopcock to a 30-ml syringe is usually sufficient.

Although this technique is generally used to evaluate an operative result, it is also valuable when critical ischemia due to acute arterial thromboembolic or traumatic occlusion necessitates an operation before conventional arteriography can be obtained. If the location and nature of the occlusion are obvious, intraoperative arteriography can be performed after thromboembolectomy or repair of the vessel (Figs. 8–23 and 8–24). Following embolectomy, a large-bore plastic or rubber catheter is inserted into the superficial femoral artery through the common femoral arteriotomy. Backbleeding is controlled by double-looped Silastic tape, and arteriography is obtained prior to closure in case further embolectomy is required. In such operative arteriograms, balloon catheter–induced spasm is extremely common and must be considered when there is apparent residual occlusion, as outlined in the previous discussion.

During femoropopliteal bypass grafting using autogenous saphenous vein, arteriography can be performed through the same catheter that was used to irrigate the vein and test for leaks. Arteriography is performed after the distal anastomosis and passage of the graft through the tunnel to the upper incision are complete, thus allowing the distal anastomosis and the course of the graft through its new anatomic pathway to be checked before performance of the proximal anastomosis. During exploration for distal bypass, when dealing with either an isolated popliteal segment or infrapopliteal occlusive disease not well delineated by conventional arteriography, injection of a smaller volume (10 to 15 ml) of contrast agent directly into the popliteal artery may demonstrate the tibial vessels, collaterals, and plantar arch. This information is essential to choosing the most appropriate bypass procedure.

It is more difficult to visualize the arterial tree proximal to the point of exploration. A Fogarty aortic occluding balloon catheter can be passed upward through a femoral arteriotomy to provide inflow occlusion. A second catheter (e.g., embolectomy irrigating type) is then passed up from below, and 40 ml of contrast agent is injected in the distal abdominal aorta. An alternative method is possible when the abdomen is already open. The aorta is cross-clamped and contrast agent is injected distal to the clamp in the fashion described by Minken and Rob for evaluating the location of accessory renal arteries when a horseshoe kidney is unexpectedly encountered.[14]

Other Sites

Intraoperative arteriography is used primarily to evaluate the adequacy of a vascular procedure in the extremities, such as embolectomy or a bypass graft, but it has been used following carotid endarterectomy, renal artery reconstruction, and other intra-abdominal procedures.[3, 18]

Intraoperative arteriography to delineate an area of

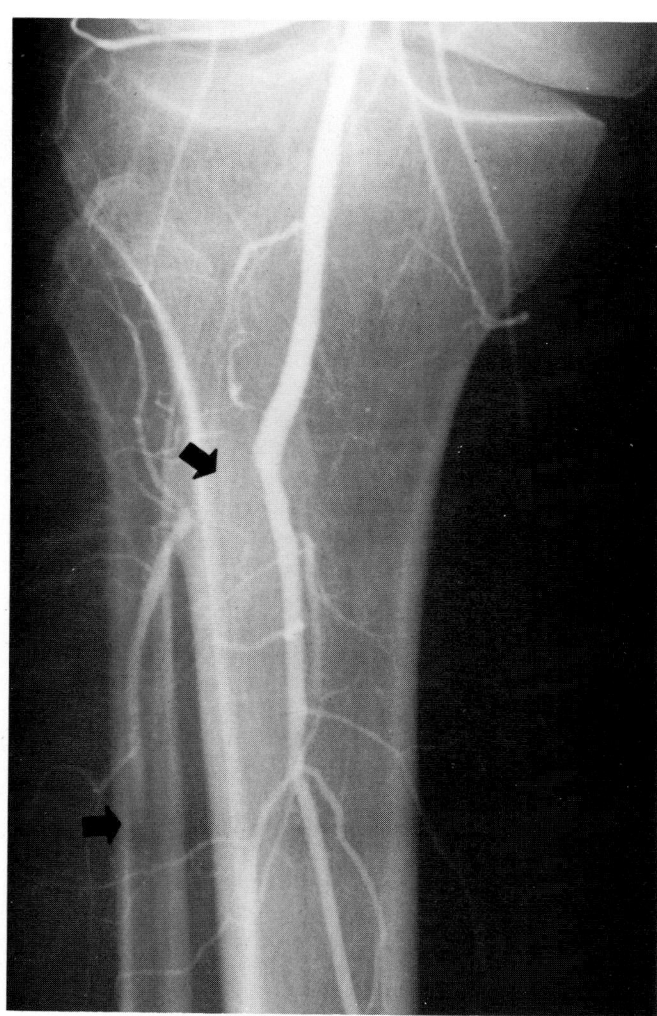

FIGURE 8–23. Operative right popliteal arteriogram following embolectomy. Although the posterior tibial artery is patent, certain segments of the anterior tibial artery *(arrows)* are still occluded. Further instrumentation was required to reopen this vessel.

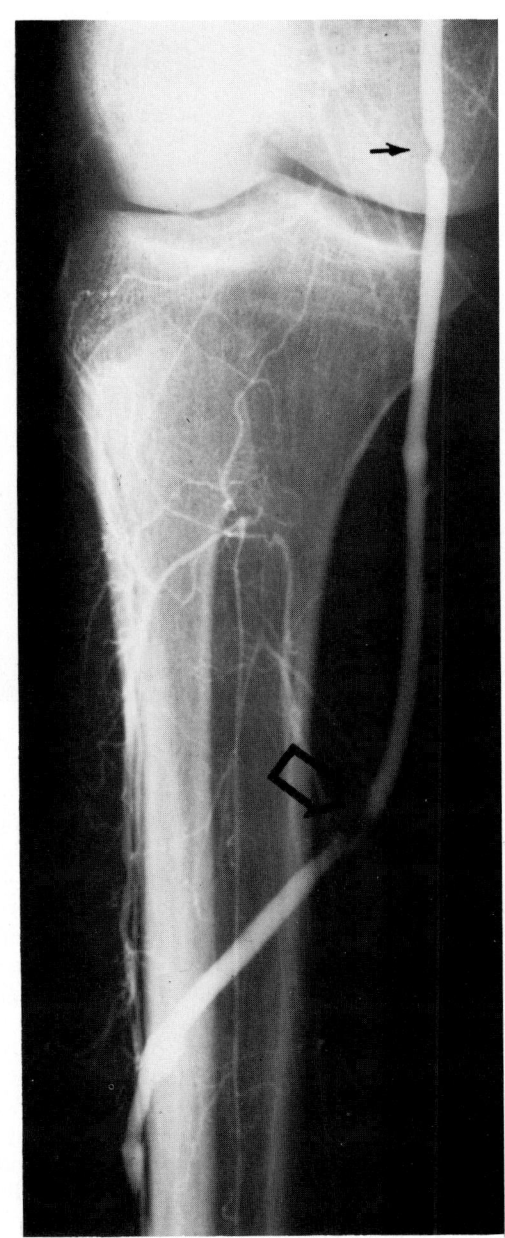

FIGURE 8–24. Operative arteriogram following insertion of a femorotibial bypass. Poor pulse at the distal end of the bypass suggested a partially obstructing thrombus *(open arrow)*. The additional localized narrowing *(straight arrow)* was not anticipated. After this arteriogram was obtained, both of the abnormalities were corrected.

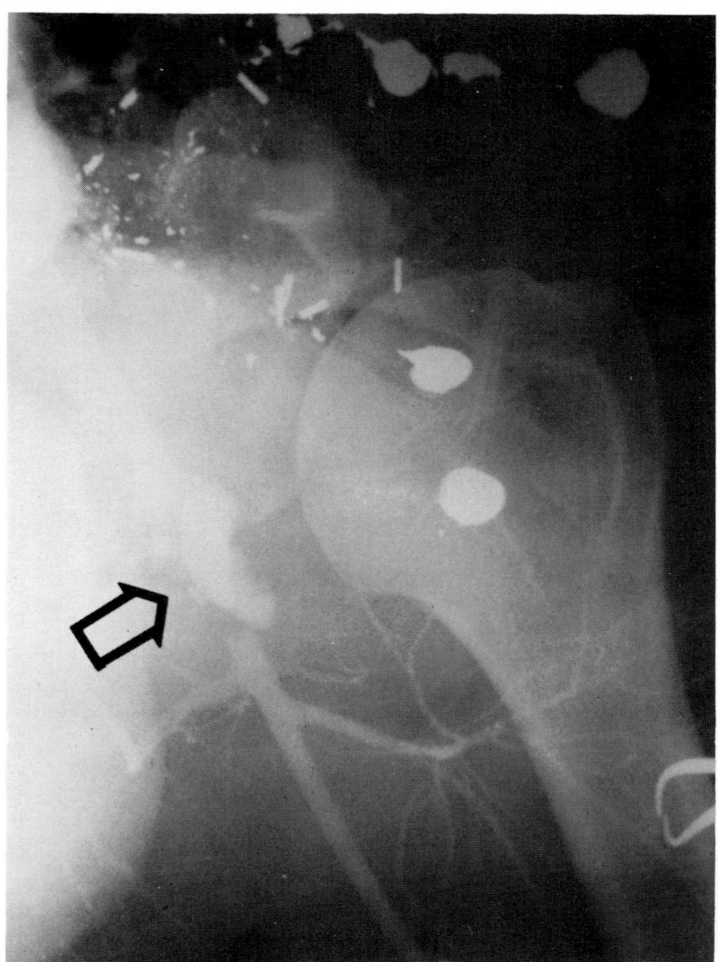

FIGURE 8–25. Operative arteriogram demonstrating disruption *(arrow)* of the left axillary artery. The patient had been shot in the shoulder and was bleeding profusely. Contrast medium was injected into the subclavian artery via the supraclavicular needle approach. The film was obtained at a second attempt because the first film was too dark and the contrast volume too small. The film was available to the surgeon approximately 45 min after his decision to perform arteriography. A better film could have been obtained within 30 min in the angiographic room, and immediate temporary control of bleeding could then have been provided with a balloon catheter.

vascular injury is occasionally done in the course of an emergency operation. If, however, an angiogram can be done *pre*operatively, it should be obtained in an angiographic facility, where better films can be obtained more quickly. Indeed, if bleeding from an undetermined site is the problem, it may be more quickly diagnosed and may be temporarily treated by balloon catheter occlusion or embolization techniques rather than by surgical exploration (Fig. 8–25).[11, 22]

Other technical variations of intraoperative arteriography are too numerous to describe here, and the vascular surgeon must often improvise when dealing with the situation at hand. The volume of the injection may vary from 5 to 50 ml, depending on the site of interest and its distance from the point of injection. Satisfactory studies almost always result, however, when the basic principles are observed: use of temporary inflow occlusion, nonforceful injection of contrast material, immediate exposure of the roentgenogram at the end of the injection, and flushing with an equal volume of heparin-containing saline solution immediately after the exposure.

References

1. Agee O, Kaude J: Arteriography of the pelvis and lower extremities with moving table technique. AJR 107:860, 1969.
2. Amendola MA, Tisnado J, Fields WR, et al: Evaluation of retroperitoneal hemorrhage by computed tomography before and after translumbar aortography. Radiology 133:401, 1979.
3. Dardik I, Ibrahim I, Sprayregen S, et al: Routine intraoperative angiography. An essential adjunct in vascular surgery. Arch Surg 110:184, 1975.
4. Giargiana F, White R, Greyson N, et al: Absence of arteriovenous shunting in peripheral arterial disease. Invest Radiol 9:222, 1976.
5. Glenn J: Abdominal aorta catheterization via the left axillary artery. Radiology 115:227, 1975.
6. Gyepes M, Abrams H: Peripheral cinearteriography. Radiology 88:736, 1967.
7. Hawkins IF: Carbon dioxide digital subtraction arteriography. AJR 139:19, 1982.
8. Hessel SJ, Adams DF, Abrams HL: Complications of angiography. Radiology 138:273, 1981.
9. Lindbom A: Arterial spasm caused by puncture and catheterization: An arteriographic study of patients not suffering from arterial disease. Acta Radiol Diagn 47:449, 1957.
10. Maddison F, Handel S: A rapid-sequence 105 mm photospot device. Appl Radiol 3:41, 1974.
11. Margolies M, Ring E, Waltman A, et al: Arteriography in the management of hemorrhage from pelvic fractures. N Engl J Med 287:317, 1972.
12. McCormack L, Cauldwell E, Anson B: Brachial and antebrachial arterial patterns. A study of 750 extremities. Surg Gynecol Obstet 96:43, 1953.
13. Milne E: The significance of early venous filling during femoral arteriography. Radiology 88:513, 1967.
14. Minken S, Rob C: Abdominal aneurysms and horseshoe kidney: A case report and collective review. Surgery 61:719, 1967.

15. Molnar W, Paul DJ: Complications of axillary arteriotomies. Radiology 104:269, 1972.
16. Moore W, Hall A: Unrecognized aortoiliac stenosis. Arch Surg 103:633, 1971.
17. Newton HT: Axillary artery approach to arteriography of aorta and its branches. AJR 89:275, 1963.
18. Rosental J, Gaspar M, Movius H: Intraoperative arteriography in carotid thromboendarterectomy. Arch Surg 106:806, 1973.
19. Roy P: Percutaneous catheterization via the axillary artery. AJR 94:1, 1965.
20. Seldinger S: Catheter replacement of the needle in percutaneous arteriography. Acta Radiol 39:368, 1953.
21. Weaver FA, Pentecost MJ, Yellin AE, et al: Clinical applications of carbon dioxide/digital subtraction arteriography. J Vasc Surg 13:266, 1991.
22. Wholey M, Stockdale R, Hung T: A percutaneous balloon technique for the immediate control of hemorrhage. Radiology 95:65, 1970.
23. dos Santos R, Lamas A, Pereira-Caldas J: Arteriografia da aorta e dos vasos adominais. Med Contemp 47:93, 1929.

SECTION III

Arterial Diseases

Edited by Robert B. Rutherford, M.D.

9

Artery Wall Pathology in Atherosclerosis

Christopher K. Zarins, M.D., and Seymour Glagov, M.D.

• • •

Atherosclerosis is the principal pathologic process affecting the large arteries. Atherosclerosis is a degenerative disease characterized by the accumulation of cells, matrix fibers, lipids, and tissue debris in the intima, which may result in narrowing of the lumen and obstruction of blood flow or ulceration, embolization, and thrombosis. Intimal plaque deposition may be accompanied by arterial enlargement and thinning of the underlying artery wall. Such enlargement may compensate for the enlarging intimal plaque and prevent lumen stenosis. It may also, under certain circumstances, lead to aneurysm formation with eventual artery wall rupture. Dissection, arteritis, and other degenerative conditions may also result in similar clinical complications, but these are rare compared with the prevalence of atherosclerosis and are dealt with elsewhere. This chapter discusses the problem of atherosclerosis as it relates to the functional biomechanical properties of the artery wall. Both normal and pathologic responses of the artery wall are considered, as are differences in the evolution of atherosclerotic lesions. Local differences that may account for the propensity of certain areas to form extensive and complex plaques or aneurysms are also discussed.

STRUCTURE AND FUNCTION OF THE ARTERY WALL

Arteries are not simply a passive system of tubes of uniform and fixed composition that distribute blood to organs. Investigation revealed that the major arteries are intricate biomechanical structures well suited to carry out their metabolic and mechanical functions under a wide range of conditions.[1] Arteries respond to acute hemodynamic alterations by changing caliber, either by constriction or dilatation.[2] Several mechanisms operate to limit hemorrhage in the event of disruptive injury and to restore wall integrity without long-term sequelae.[3] Arteries also adapt to gradual changes in local hemodynamic stresses and to systemic environmental conditions in order to maintain optimal diameter and mechanical characteristics and to ensure continued adequate blood flow.[4] A brief review of the functional microanatomy of the artery wall will indicate the range and limits of artery wall adaptability.

Intima

The intima is the innermost layer of the artery wall and extends from the lumen surface to the internal elastic lamina. The luminal surface is lined by the endothelium, a continuous monolayer of flat, polygonal cells. Between the endothelium and the internal elastic lamina, the intima is normally very narrow, with the endothelium lying directly on the internal elastic lamina and containing only a few scattered leukocytes, smooth muscle cells, and connective tissue fibers. It is in this region that atherosclerotic lesions develop.

Endothelium. The endothelium rests on a basal lamina that provides a continuous, pliable, and compliant substrate. Changes in cell shape and in the extent of junctional overlap among adjacent endothelial cells occur in relation to changes in artery diameter associated with pulsatile wall motion, in relation to changes in configuration associated with bending or stretching, and in relation to the intimal accumulation of cells and matrix fibers during the development of intimal atherosclerotic plaques.[5] These changes act to prevent the development of discontinuities in the endothelial lining.

The endothelium also has numerous focal attachments to the underlying internal elastic lamina.[6] These relatively tight and rigid junctions contribute to stability by preventing slippage, telescoping, or detachment of endothelial cells and disruption or denudation by elevations in shear stress or by other mechanical forces. The endothelium presents a thromboresistant surface as well as a selective interface for diffusion, convection, and active transport of circulating substances into the underlying artery wall.[7] The endothelium plays a critical role in regulating the ingress, egress, and metabolism of lipoproteins and other agents that may participate in intimal plaque initiation and progression.[3, 5]

Endothelial Injury. The endothelial surface can be injured or disrupted by various means but regenerates rapidly after focal denudation. The healing response, if extensive, may be accompanied by smooth muscle cell proliferation and migration and intimal thickening.[8, 9] A series of reactions set into motion by focal endothelial denudation has been proposed as the initiating event in the pathogenesis of atherosclerosis. According to the *original endothelial injury hypothesis,* mechanical forces such as elevated wall shear stress and hypertension, metabolic intermediates such as those that characterize hyperlipidemia, immunologic reactions, and increased exposure to vasoactive agents cause endothelial injury and desquamation. Endothelial desquamation would expose subendothelial tissues to the circulation and stimulate platelet deposition, the release of a platelet-derived growth factor, cellular proliferation, and eventual lipid deposition and plaque formation.[10] Focal, repeated disruptive endothelial injuries and responses to those injuries would account for the localized nature of plaque deposition. However, there is little evidence to support the belief that endothelial injury or disruption in the form of desquamation, with or without platelet adhesion, occurs in regions of the vascular tree at highest risk for future lesion development.[11] In addition, there is no direct evidence that experimentally induced endothelial damage or removal results in eventual sustained lesion formation,[12] even in the presence of hyperlipidemia. On the contrary, evidence has been advanced that the formation of experimental intimal plaques may require the presence of an endothelial covering.[13, 14] Although platelets may play a role in the transition of early plaques to more complex and advanced forms,[15] their effect on plaque initiation remains questionable. Platelet-derived growth factor has now been isolated from other cellular elements that participate in plaque formation,[16] and smooth muscle cell proliferation may be an aspect of an overall healing reaction of arteries rather than the underlying primary event in atherosclerosis. More recent studies have attempted to define injury in terms of functional alterations that may predispose to the formation of atherosclerotic lesions.[17, 18]

Under normal circumstances, the vascular endothelium functions as an antithrombotic surface and contributes to the regulation of vascular tone and artery lumen diameter through the secretion of vasoconstrictors (e.g., angiotensin II) and vasodilators and inhibitors of platelet aggregation (e.g., prostacyclin and endothelium-derived relaxing factor).[19] Such factors maintain the smooth muscle cells of the media in a contractile, nonproliferative phenotype with low cholesterol ester content. In response to endothelial cell activation or injury, endothelial cells become increasingly permeable to low-density lipoprotein, have higher replicative rates, develop prothrombotic properties, and express surface glycoproteins that promote the adhesion and ingress of neutrophils, monocytes, and platelets.[20] Endothelial cells and monocytes release cytokines, growth factors, and leukotrienes in preference to prostacyclin production, which further promotes monocyte adhesion and diapedesis. The net effect of cytokine and growth factor production is the stimulation of smooth muscle cell proliferation and migration. As a result of these changes, extracellular lipid as well as foam cells containing cholesterol esters accumulate in the intima.

These observations suggest that humoral mediators, growth factors, and cytokines from altered endothelial cells and from inflammatory cells interacting with other arterial cells are important mediators of macrophage infiltration, smooth muscle cell proliferation, and lipid deposition. Although physical and mechanical endothelial disruption and denudation may not be reactions initiating or precipitating events in atherosclerotic plaque formation, biologic reactions of the endothelium and artery wall during injury and repair may play important roles in the proliferative and lipid deposition stage of plaque formation.

Media

The media extends from the internal elastic lamina to the adventitia. Although an external elastic lamina demarcates the boundary between the media and adventitia in many vessels, a distinct external elastic lamina may not be present, particularly in vessels with a thick and fibrous adventitial layer. The outer limit of the media can nevertheless be distinguished in nearly all intact arteries because, in contrast to the adventitia, the media consists of closely packed layers of smooth muscle cells in close association with elastin and collagen fibers. The *smooth muscle cell* layers are composed of groups of similarly oriented cells, each surrounded by a common basal lamina and a closely associated interlacing basket-work of type III collagen fibrils arranged so as to tighten about the cell groups as the media is brought under tension; this configuration tends to hold the groups of cells together and prevent excessive stretching or slippage. In addition, each cellular subgroup or fascicle is encompassed by a system of similarly oriented *elastic fibers* such that the effective unit of structure is a musculoelastic fascicle. In relation to the curvature of the artery wall, each fascicle is oriented in the direction of the imposed tensile stress. Focal tight attachment sites between smooth muscle cells and elastic fibers are normally abundant.[21]

The aorta and its immediately proximal, larger branches are called *elastic arteries* because of the prominence of their elastic fibers. In such vessels, the elastin fiber systems of the musculoelastic fascicles are thick and closely packed, resulting in an appearance on transverse cross section of elastin lamellae alternating with smooth muscle layers. Thicker, crimped, type I collagen bundles are woven between adjacent large elastic lamellae.[22] The elastin fibers are relatively extensible and allow for compliance and recoil of the artery wall in relation to pulse propagation during the cardiac cycle. The extensive interconnected transmural arrangement of the elastic fibers of the musculoelastic fascicles tends to ensure uniform distribution of tensile mural stresses and prevent the propagation of flaws that develop in the media with age. The thick, crimped collagen fiber bundles provide much of the tensile strength

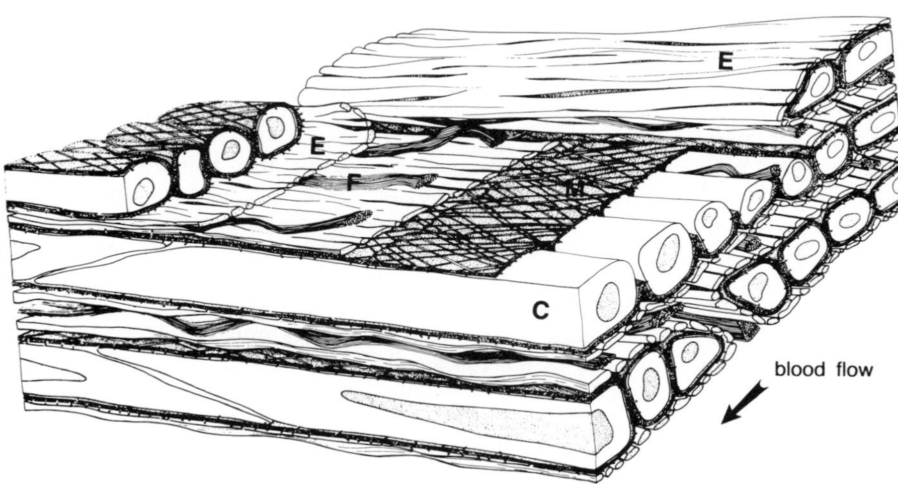

FIGURE 9–1. Transmural organization of the media of large elastic arteries such as the aorta. Groups of smooth muscle cells (C), oriented with their long axes perpendicular to the longitudinal axis of the artery (axis of blood flow), are surrounded by a network of fine type III collagen fibrils within a matrix of basal lamina (M). They are surrounded by a closely associated system of elastic fibers (E) oriented in the same direction as the smooth muscle cells. Wavy bundles or fibers (F) of type I collagen are woven between the adjacent large elastic lamellae and provide much of the tensile strength of the media. Elastin fibers allow for compliance and recoil of the artery during the cardiac cycle. (From Clark JM, Glagov S: Transmural organization of the arterial wall: The lamellar unit revisited. Arteriosclerosis 5:19, 1985.)

of the media and because of their high elastic modulus limit distension and prevent disruption even at very high blood pressures (Fig. 9–1).[23]

The smaller-caliber *muscular arteries* contain relatively less collagen and elastin and more smooth muscle cells than elastic arteries and can therefore alter their diameter rapidly by constricting or dilating. The musculoelastic fascicles, which are most clearly evident in elastic arteries, are also the structural unit of muscular arteries and, as in elastic arteries, are generally aligned in the direction of the tensile forces. However, because of the preponderance of smooth muscle cells relative to elastin and collagen fibers, they are less prominent and the layering of the media is therefore less distinct (Fig. 9–2).[23]

Medial thickness and the number of musculoelastic layers, or *lamellar units,* are closely related to the lumen radius and to mural tangential tension. Tangential tension on the artery wall is, in general, proportional to the product of pressure and radius (Laplace's law), whereas the actual tensile stress per unit of cross-sectional area is inversely proportional to the wall thickness. The average tension per lamellar unit tends to be constant for homologous vessels in mammals. With increasing species size, mammalian adult aortic radius increases with a corresponding increase in medial thickness and in the number of musculoelastic layers, or lamellar units.[24] Because aortic pressure is similar for most adult mammals and individual medial layers tend to be of similar thickness regardless of species, there is a

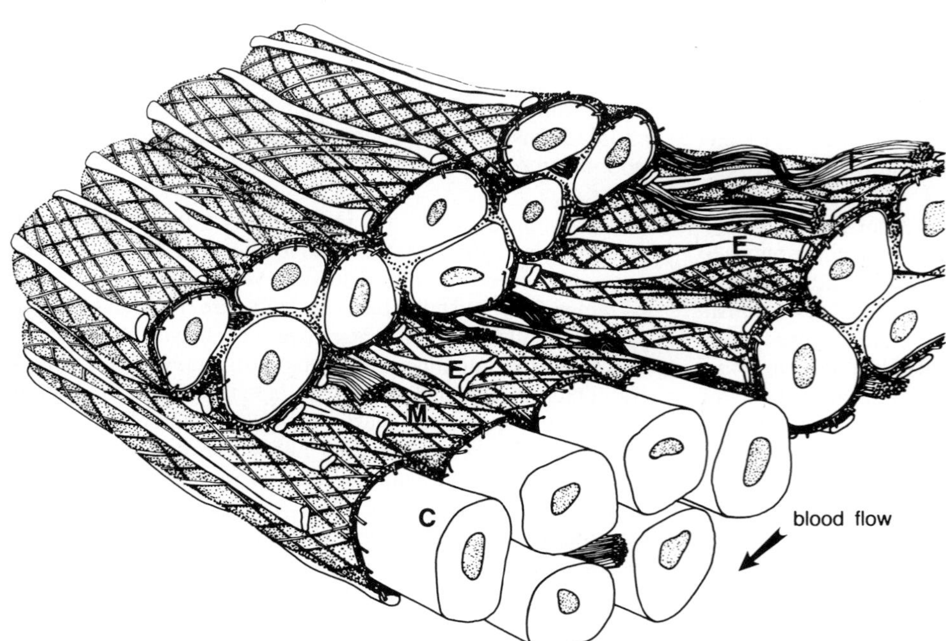

FIGURE 9–2. Transmural organization of a muscular artery. Smooth muscle cells (C) are more numerous and prominent and are organized in groups oriented with their long axes perpendicular to the long axis of the artery. Contraction or relaxation of smooth muscle cells allows for rapid alterations in lumen diameter. Smooth muscle cells are surrounded by a basal lamina matrix containing a meshwork of type III collagen fibrils (M). Elastin fibers (E) and type I collagen fibers (F) are present but are less prominent than in elastic arteries. (From Clark JM, Glagov S: Transmural organization of the arterial wall: The lamellar unit revisted. Arteriosclerosis 5:19, 1985.)

very nearly linear relationship between adult aortic radius and the number of medial fibrocellular lamellar units. On the average, the tangential tension per aortic lamellar unit is close to 2000 dynes/cm. For the pulmonary trunk, wall tension is about 1000 dynes/cm. For muscular arteries, such as the coronary and renal vessels, total tangential tension and the number of transmural layers are also linearly related.[24] In addition, the relative proportions of collagen and elastin differ between muscular and elastic arteries. The media of the proximal aorta and that of the major brachiocephalic elastic arteries contain a larger proportion of elastin and a lower proportion of collagen than the abdominal aorta or the distal peripheral vessels.[25] The proximal major vessels are therefore more compliant than the abdominal aorta but are also more fragile and prone to tear when sutured.

Medial smooth muscle cells, in addition to synthesizing the collagen and elastin fibers, which determine the mechanical properties of the aortic wall, are actively engaged in metabolic processes that contribute to wall tone and may be related to susceptibility to plaque formation.[26] Under conditions of increased pulse pressure, increased wall motion, and increased wall tension, such as exist proximal to an aortic coarctation, medial smooth muscle cell metabolism is increased, as is plaque formation.[27] Conversely, when wall motion, pulse pressure, and smooth muscle cell metabolism are decreased, as in areas distal to a severe arterial stenosis, intimal plaque formation is inhibited, despite the continued presence of strong atherogenic stimuli such as marked hyperlipidemia.[28] In vitro studies have revealed that cyclic stretching of smooth muscle cells grown on elastin membranes results in increased biosynthetic activity,[29] and acute arterial injury experiments have revealed that an intact, metabolically active media may be required for intimal plaque formation.[30] The composition and microarchitecture of the media are designed to ensure stability, whereas the metabolic state of the media appears to be an important factor in the pathogenesis of atherosclerotic lesions.

Adventitia

The adventitia is composed of fibrocellular connective tissue and contains a network of vasa vasorum composed of small arteries, arterioles, capillaries, and venous channels, as well as nerves that mediate smooth muscle tone and contraction. The adventitia varies in thickness and organization. In some arteries, such as the proximal renal and mesenteric trunks, the adventitia is a layered structure composed of both collagen and elastic fibers and may be thicker than the associated media. In the normal aorta, removal of the adventitia has little effect on static pressure-volume relationships.[31] In atherosclerotic arteries, on the other hand, increasing intimal plaque thickness may be associated with atrophy of the underlying media.[32] Under these circumstances, a thickened adventitia may contribute to tensile support. The tensile strength and adequacy of the adventitia to provide such support are well demonstrated following carotid or aortoiliac endarterectomy. In these procedures, the entire intima and most or all of the media are usually removed, leaving only the adventitia to provide support, and aneurysmal degeneration after endarterectomy is very rare.

Vasa Vasorum. The inner layers of the aortic media are nourished by diffusion from the lumen. Diffusion of nutrients is apparently sufficient to nourish the inner 0.5 mm of the adult mammalian aortic media, which corresponds to approximately 30 medial fibrocellular lamellar units.[33] When the aorta is thicker than 30 medial lamellar layers, the outer layers of the media are nourished by vasa vasorum that penetrate into the media. Vasa vasorum usually arise from the parent artery at branch junctions and arborize in the adventitia. In thick-walled arteries, mural stresses and deformations may affect vasa vasorum blood flow, and hypertension may impair vasal flow.[34] Intimal plaque formation increases intimal thickness and may thereby increase the diffusion barrier from the lumen to the smooth muscle cells of the media. This increase in wall thickness may be accompanied by an ingrowth of vasa vasorum, and vasa vasorum have been identified in atherosclerotic lesions. Both intraplaque hemorrhage and plaque breakdown or disruption may be potentiated by changes in the vascular supply of the artery wall and plaque.

ADAPTIVE RESPONSES OF THE ARTERY WALL

Adaptive responses of arteries and the healing response to arterial injuries serve to maintain the structural and functional integrity of the arterial tree. Normal responses to altered biomechanical and hemodynamic conditions result in compensatory alterations in artery wall thickness, lumen diameter, or both, whereas abnormal or pathologic conditions may engender alterations in wall thickness and lumen diameter that proceed to lumen stenosis, aneurysm formation, or obstructive intimal hyperplasia.[1]

Wall Thickness

Artery wall thickness and composition are closely related to *tangential tension* in the wall. During normal growth and development, arteries adapt to increases in tangential tension by increasing the number of medial lamellar units and by the accumulation of matrix fibers to increase wall thickness.[35] For example, at birth the ascending aorta and pulmonary trunk are equal in diameter, in wall thickness, and in the concentration of elastin and collagen. However, in the immediate postnatal period, with expansion of the lungs, pressure in the pulmonary artery falls while pressure in the aorta rises. Volume flow and diameter remain equivalent in the two vessels, but a marked difference in blood pressure develops, resulting in profound alterations in medial growth and development. The high-pressure aortic media becomes thicker with an increased number of medial lamellae. The differences can be attributed to different rates of collagen and elastin accumulation, which correspond closely to the differences in total tangential tension for the two vessels.[36] At any given interval during early postnatal growth, however, the number of cells is the same for the two vessel segments. Thus, smooth muscle cells of the media are apparently capable of a remarkable range of biosynthetic activity in response to imposed tensile stress.

In adult life, arterial wall thickening also occurs in response to increases in tangential tension, but this thickening occurs not by increases in the number of medial lamellar units but by intimal thickening and changes in matrix volume and composition. In patients with hypertension, arterial and arteriolar intimal thickening develops as an adaptive response to the increase in wall tension and the relative proportion of matrix fiber changes in favor of collagen.[37] Similarly, the performance of a distal arterial bypass increases wall tension by increasing pressure as well as by producing a large increase in lumen radius at the anastomotic site. The resulting increase in tangential wall tension would be expected to stimulate intimal thickening as an adaptive response to the increase in tension. The factors that differentiate a normal adaptive intimal thickening from an inappropriate intimal hyperplastic response resulting in lumen stenosis at a vascular anastomosis are unclear and deserve further study.

Lumen Diameter

Under normal conditions, adaptive alterations in lumen diameter are determined by *blood flow* in the artery. During embryologic development, arteries with high-volume flow enlarge, and those with low flow become smaller.[38] When parallel flow channels exist, the one with higher flow enlarges and persists, whereas the one with lesser flow atrophies and disappears. During extrauterine growth, increases in artery lumen diameter also keep pace with changes in flow.[39] Arteries exposed to abnormal increases in flow, such as those feeding an arteriovenous fistula, may also increase in size, whereas arteries exposed to abnormal decreases in flow, such as vessels supplying an amputated limb, will adapt with a decrease in size.[40]

The mechanism for adjustment of lumen diameter appears to be mediated by wall *shear stress,* which is the effective velocity gradient at the endothelial-blood interface.[4] Because shear stress is inversely related to the cube of the radius, small alterations in radius will have a major effect on wall shear stress. In mammals, wall shear stress normally ranges between 10 and 20 dynes/cm^2 at all levels of the arterial tree.[41] In experimentally produced arteriovenous fistulae, the afferent artery has been shown to enlarge just enough to restore shear stress to baseline levels.[42] Wall shear stress thus appears to act as a regulating signal to determine artery size, and this response seems to be dependent on the presence of an intact endothelial surface.[43] The response may be mediated by the release of endothelial-derived relaxing factor or other vasoactive agents.[44] Atherosclerotic arteries are also capable of enlarging in response to increases in wall shear stress, but this process may be limited because such vessels may eventually become occluded.[45] This is further discussed later in this chapter. The nature and mechanisms of the adaptive processes allowing living arteries to adjust lumen diameter require further study. Definition of the limits of the process and identification of the consequences for the vessel wall of shear stress that is persistently higher or lower than normal are important and should have clinical relevance.

FUNCTIONAL PATHOLOGY OF ATHEROSCLEROSIS

The features that distinguish normal arterial adaptation to changing hemodynamic and mechanical conditions from pathologic processes affecting the artery wall are not well defined. Intimal thickening and changes in wall thickness and lumen diameter occur both as a function of age and as a function of atherosclerosis. A prominent feature distinguishing atherosclerotic plaques is the presence of lipid in intimal lesions. However, it is unclear whether all lesions containing lipids are necessarily precursors of clinically significant atherosclerotic plaques.

Intimal Thickening

As noted earlier, intimal thickening can reflect an adaptive response to diminish lumen caliber under conditions of reduced flow or can be a response designed to augment wall thickness when tensile stress increases. Focal intimal thickenings have been observed in infants and fetuses at or near branch points and probably represent local remodeling of vessel wall organization related to growth and the associated redistribution of tensile stress.[46] Diffuse fibrocellular intimal thickening can occur as a more generalized phenomenon without a clear relationship to branches or curves and may result in a diffusely thickened intima that is considerably thicker than the media. Lipid accumulation is not a prominent feature in such intimal thickening, and the lumen remains regular and normal or slightly larger than normal in diameter.[47] Although there is little direct evidence that diffuse intimal thickening is a precursor of lipid-containing atherosclerotic plaques, both intimal thickening and plaques tend to occur in similar locations, and intimal thickening is most evident in vessels that are especially susceptible to atherosclerosis.[48] Evidence has also been presented that diffuse forms of intimal thickening do not develop uniformly and that foci of relatively rapid thickening undergo dystrophic changes, which give rise to necrosis and other features characteristic of plaques.[49] The relationship of these findings to usual atherosclerosis remains to be defined.

Fatty Streaks

Fatty streaks are flat yellow focal patches or linear streaks seen on the lumen surface of arteries. They correspond to the accumulation of lipid-laden foam cells in the intima. Fatty streaks are evident in most individuals over the age of 3 years. They are found with increasing frequency between the ages of 8 and 18, after which many apparently resolve despite the frequent presence of matrix materials among the characteristic cells. Fatty streaks may be seen at any age and may be noted adjacent to or even superimposed on advanced atherosclerotic plaques. Fatty streaks and atheromata, however, do not have identical patterns of localization, and fatty streaks usually do not compromise the lumen or ulcerate.[50] In experimental animals, diet-induced lesions resembling fatty streaks occur early, before characteristic atherosclerotic lesions prevail. These lesions are characterized by foam cells under a preserved and intact endothelial surface with no evidence of disruption.[51] Some evidence has been presented that endothelial cells covering experimental fatty streak–type lesions are attenuated and fragile and may predispose to endothelial disruption, platelet adhesion, and possible transformation into a fibrous plaque.[52] On the other hand, attachment of endothelial projections to underlying basal lamina and elastin remains prominent in early fatty streak lesions. Although morphologic studies have identified transitional features, a firm line of evidence linking fatty streaks to fibrous plaque formation has not yet been established.

Fibrous Plaques

Fibrous plaque is the term used to identify the characteristic and unequivocal atherosclerotic lesion. These intimal deposits appear in the 2nd decade of life but usually do not become predominant or clinically significant until the 4th decade. Fibrous plaques are usually eccentric, and most are covered by an intact endothelial surface.

Although there is considerable variation in plaque composition and configuration, a characteristic architecture prevails for manifest advanced plaques. The immediate subendothelial region usually consists of a compact and well-organized stratified layer of smooth muscle cells and connective tissue fibers known as the *fibrous cap* (Fig. 9–3). This structure may be quite thick and may present architectural features resembling the media, including the formation of a subendothelial elastic lamina. The fibrous cap may provide structural support or function as a barrier to sequester thrombogenic debris in the underlying necrotic core of the plaque from the lumen. Its lumen surface is regular and maintains a concave contour corresponding to the circular or oval cross-sectional lumen contour of the uninvolved vessel wall segment. The *necrotic core* usually occupies the deeper central regions of the plaque and contains amorphous as well as crystalline and droplet forms of lipid. Cells with morphologic and functional characteristics of smooth muscle cells or macrophages are noted about the necrotic core and at the edges or shoulders of the plaques.[53] Both cell types may contain lipid vacuoles. In addition, calcium salts and myxoid deposits, as well as matrix fibers, including collagen, elastin, fine fibrillar material, structures resembling basal lamina, and amorphous ground substance, are evident. Atherosclerotic plaques show evidence of uneven or episodic growth, including dense fibrocellular regions adjacent to organizing thrombus and foci of atheromatous debris. Intermittent ulceration and healing may occur, and there is evidence that thrombi formed on lesions are incorporated into them and resurfaced with a fibrocellular cap and an intact endothelial layer.

Vasa vasorum penetrate from the adventitia or possibly from the lumen to supply the plaque and fibrous cap and serve to organize thrombotic deposits.[54] The *media* underlying an atherosclerotic plaque may become thin and

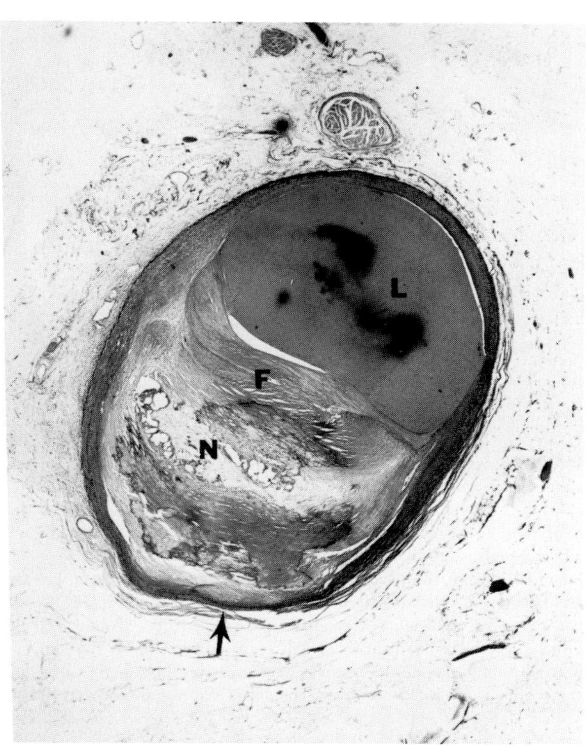

FIGURE 9–3. Cross section of a human artery with an advanced atherosclerotic plaque. The fibrous cap (F) is a well-organized layer of smooth muscle cells and fibrous tissue that separates the necrotic core (N) of the plaque from the lumen (L). The media beneath the plaque may become thin and atrophic (*arrow*). The lumen contains a gelatin cast used to redistend and maintain lumen contour.

attenuated, with bulging of the plaque toward the adventitia (see Fig. 9–3), but the tissue between the necrotic core and the media is usually densely fibrotic. Support of the artery wall may also be taken up by the fibrous cap or a thickened adventitial layer. Some *advanced lesions,* particularly those associated with aneurysms, may appear to be atrophic and relatively acellular, consisting of dense fibrous tissue, prominent calcific deposits, and only minimal evidence of a necrotic center. *Calcification* is a prominent feature of advanced plaques and may be quite extensive, involving both the superficial and deeper reaches of the plaques. Although there is no consistent relationship between plaque size or complexity and the degree of calcification, calcific deposits are most prominent in plaques in older individuals and in areas such as the abdominal aortic segment and coronary arteries, where plaques form earliest.[55] Advanced lesions are called fibrocalcific, lipid-rich, fibrocellular, necrotic, myxomatous, and so forth, depending on their morphologic features. The presence of large quantities of lipid, necrotic material and cells tends to make a lesion *soft* and friable, in contrast to the *hard,* rubbery, or brittle consistency of a mainly fibrocalcific lesion.

Plaque Morphology

The common perception that atherosclerotic plaques bulge into the lumen of arteries reflects the fact that most

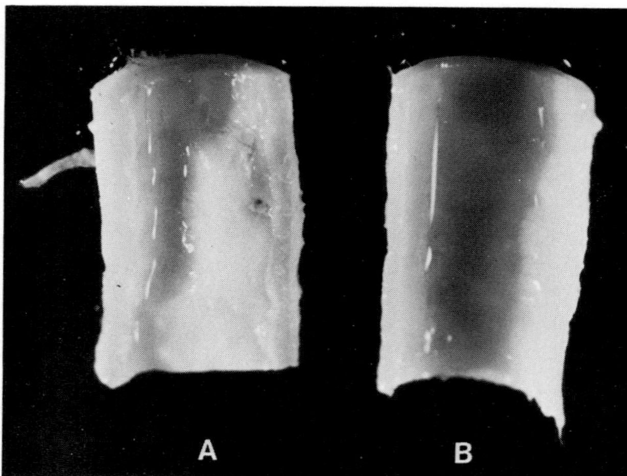

FIGURE 9–4. Effect of vessel collapse on the luminal surface appearance of atherosclerotic plaques. *A*, The artery was fixed while collapsed with no distending intraluminal pressure. Note the apparent bulge of the plaque into the lumen. *B*, The vessel was fixed while distended with an intraluminal pressure of 100 mmHg. Note that there is no visible protrusion of plaque into the lumen and that the lumen contour is rounded. Both segments are from the same human superficial femoral artery, and multiple histologic sections confirm that both segments have the same volume of intimal plaque.

often, plaques are evaluated by angiography, which reveals the lumen contour in a longitudinal or axial projection. A narrowing of the lumen thus is usually perceived as a protrusion of plaque into the lumen (Fig. 9–4). This perception is supported by gross observations by vascular surgeons and pathologists, who usually examine the luminal surface of atherosclerotic arteries en face or on cross section with the arteries collapsed. Without distending intraluminal pressure, the relatively uninvolved sector of the artery wall recoils and the eccentric plaque is usually thrown up as a protrusion or bulge. Viewed en face in vessels laid open by longitudinal section, the fibrous or complex plaque is seen as an elevation, with either smooth or irregular surface contours (see Fig. 9–4). The purely descriptive term *raised plaque* has been used to contrast this appearance with that of the fatty streak, which usually does not appear to be elevated in such preparations. Restoration of in vivo configuration can be achieved by redistending the artery during fixation at controlled levels of intraluminal pressure.[56] Under these circumstances, the cross-sectional lumen contour is usually regular and round or oval, even in the presence of very large and extensive atherosclerotic lesions.[57] The usual eccentric atherosclerotic plaque therefore presents a concave luminal contour on transverse section, does not protrude into the lumen, and instead tends to bulge outward from the lumen. Thus, the external cross-sectional contour of an atherosclerotic artery tends to become oval, whereas the lumen tends to remain circular. Although plaques may appear as focal or segmental projections into the lumen on longitudinal angiographic or ultrasonic images, cross-sectional views reveal rounded lumen contours. Cross-sectional lumen contours in pressure perfusion–fixed arteries that are irregular or slit-like, with protrusions of the plaque or its contents into the lumen, usually signify that a complication of plaque evolution such as ulceration, hemorrhage, dissection, or thrombosis has occurred. On the other hand, circumferential, rigid fibrocalcific plaques may retain an in vivo circular lumen configuration, even when dilating pressure is absent.

Atherosclerotic Arterial Enlargement

As intimal plaques enlarge, a closely associated enlargement of the affected artery segment tends to limit the stenosing effect of the enlarging intimal plaque (Fig. 9–5). Such enlargement of atherosclerotic arteries has been demonstrated in experimental atherosclerosis,[58–60] as well as in human coronary,[45, 61] carotid,[62] and superficial femoral arteries[63] and the abdominal aorta. Enlargement may proceed by mechanisms suggested by the demonstrated adaptive

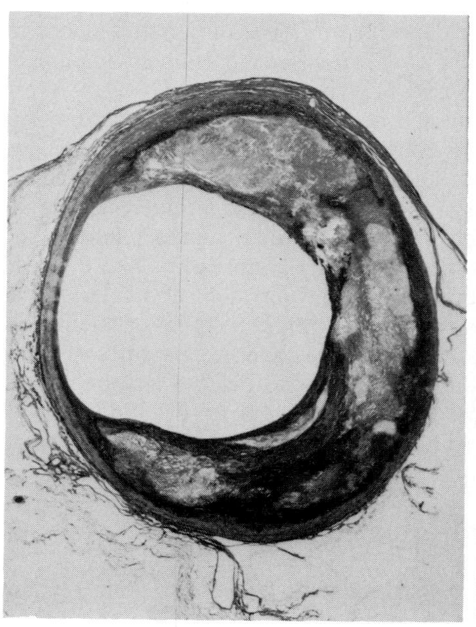

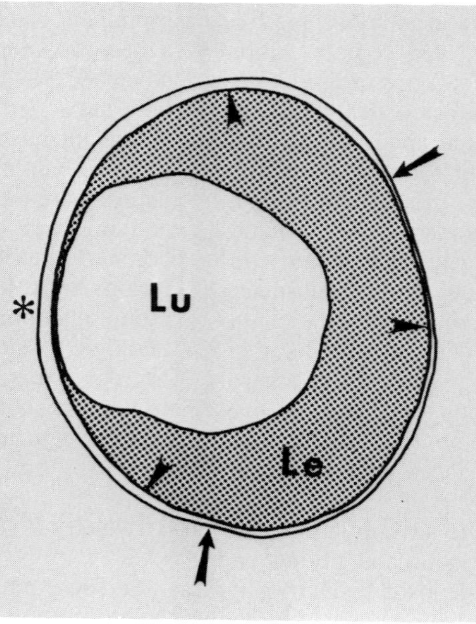

FIGURE 9–5. Cross section of a human left main coronary artery demonstrating atherosclerotic arterial enlargement. Despite an enlarging lesion (Le) area, the lumen (Lu) area is preserved owing to artery enlargement. The lumen contour remains rounded, but the external artery contour becomes oval because of the eccentric nature of the plaque. When intimal plaque area exceeds 40 per cent of internal elastic lumina area (*arrowheads*), compensatory enlargement apparently fails and stenosis develops. Enlargement may occur by dilatation of the uninvolved artery wall segment (*asterisk*) or atrophy of the media underlying the plaque (*arrows*). (From Glagov S, Weisenberg E, Zarins CK, et al: Compensatory enlargement of human atherosclerotic coronary arteries. Reprinted by permission of The New England Journal of Medicine, 316:1371, 1987.)

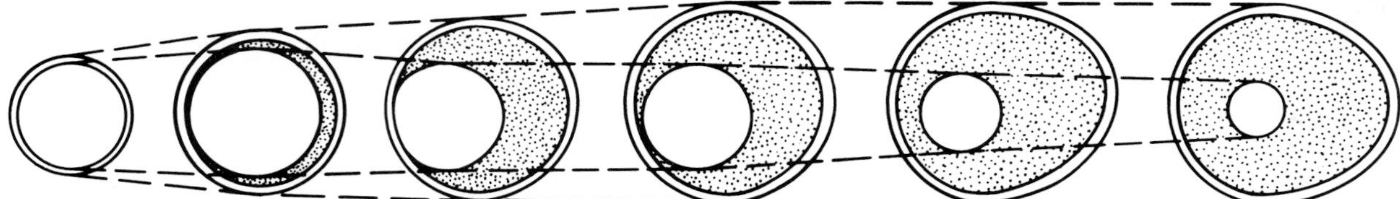

FIGURE 9–6. Possible sequence of changes in atherosclerotic arteries in response to enlarging atherosclerotic plaques. In the early stages of intimal plaque deposition, the lumen remains normal or enlarges slightly (*left*). When intimal plaque enlarges to involve the entire circumference of the vessel and produces more than 40 per cent stenosis, the artery is no longer able to enlarge at a rate sufficient to prevent narrowing of the lumen. (From Glagov S, Weisenberg E, Zarins CK, et al: Compensatory enlargement of human atherosclerotic coronary arteries. Reprinted by permission of The New England Journal of Medicine, 316:1371, 1987.)

response to altered flow or by direct effects of the plaque on the artery wall.[64] Focal intimal plaque deposition would tend to decrease lumen diameter, thereby increasing local blood flow velocity and wall shear stress and inducing dilatation of the artery to restore baseline shear stress levels. Atrophy of the media underlying the plaque could also result in outward bulging of the artery in the region of the plaque in order to maintain an adequate lumen caliber. Thus, an increase in intimal plaque volume appears to induce an increase in artery size. In the human left main coronary artery, such enlargement keeps pace with increases in intimal plaque and is effective in preventing lumen stenosis until plaque area occupies, on the average, approximately 40 per cent of the cross-sectional area encompassed by the internal elastic lamina area (i.e., the potential lumen area if a plaque were not present) (Fig. 9–6). Continued plaque enlargement or complication apparently exceeds the ability of the artery to enlarge, and lumen stenosis may then develop.[45]

However, different segments of the coronary tree respond differently to increasing intimal plaque. In the distal left anterior descending coronary artery, arterial enlargement occurs more rapidly than intimal plaque deposition. This may result in a net increase in lumen area rather than lumen stenosis in the most severely diseased arteries.[61] Thus, it appears that the development of lumen stenosis, the maintenance of a normal lumen cross-sectional area, or the development of an increase in lumen diameter is determined by the relative rates of plaque growth and artery enlargement. Further study of this phenomenon of artery enlargement, particularly in regions associated with great morbidity related to plaque deposition, is needed in order to fully understand the processes involved in the development of atherosclerotic stenoses and aneurysms.

ATHEROSCLEROTIC PLAQUE LOCALIZATION

Atherosclerosis is a generalized disorder of the arterial tree, and epidemiologic studies have identified a number of clinical risk factors that are associated with the development and complication of plaques. These include cigarette smoking, elevated serum lipid levels, hypertension, obesity, diabetes mellitus, physical inactivity, emotional stress, and genetic predisposition.[65] Certain of these factors appear to be more closely associated with atherosclerosis in some arterial beds than in others. For example, serum cholesterol and low-density lipoprotein levels are strongly related to coronary heart disease but only moderately related to cerebrovascular or peripheral occlusive disease. Cerebrovascular disease is closely related to hypertension,[66] whereas cigarette smoking is the principal risk factor for peripheral occlusive disease.[67] In addition to differences in systemic risk factor associations, differences in local hemodynamic and artery wall properties appear to exert major selective effects on plaque formation.[68, 69] Certain regions of each vascular bed are especially prone to plaque formation, whereas others are usually spared.[70] For example, the coronary arteries, carotid bifurcation, infrarenal abdominal aorta, and iliofemoral arteries are particularly susceptible to plaque formation, whereas the thoracic aorta and the common carotid, distal internal carotid, renal, mesenteric, and upper extremity arteries are particularly resistant. Such differences have been associated with variations in the distribution of shear and tensile stresses produced by variations in geometry and flow in differing segments of the arterial tree.[1] Although plaques may occur in straight vessels away from branch points, they are usually located at bifurcations or bends, where variations in hemodynamic conditions are especially likely to occur.

Hemodynamic Considerations in Plaque Localization

A number of hemodynamic variables have been proposed to account for the selective distribution of plaques. These include shear stress, flow separation and stasis, oscillation of shear stress vectors, turbulence, and hypertension. Several texts have provided detailed, in-depth consideration of the relevant fluid dynamic principles.[1, 4]

Wall Shear Stress

Wall shear stress is the tangential drag force produced by blood moving across the endothelial surface. It is a function of the velocity gradient of blood near the endothelial surface. Its magnitude is directly proportional to blood flow and blood viscosity and inversely proportional to the

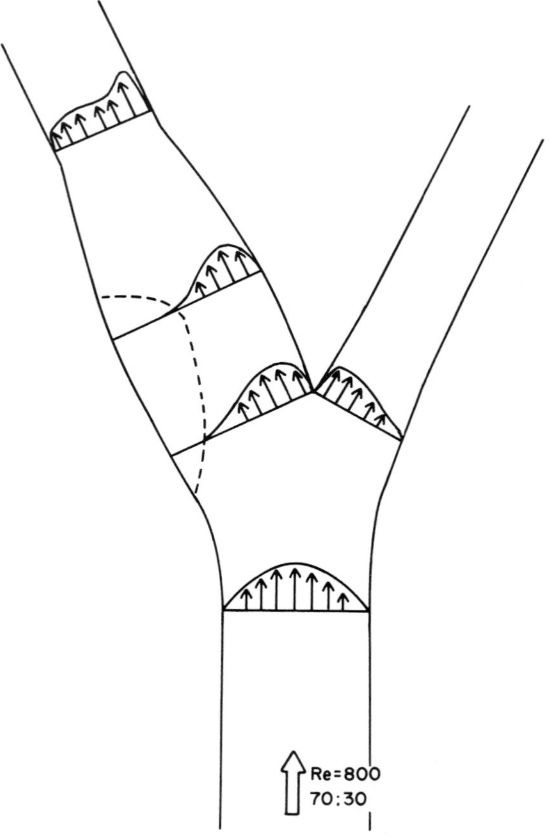

FIGURE 9–7. Axial velocity profiles measured with laser Doppler anemometry in a glass model carotid bifurcation under conditions of steady flow (Reynolds number, 800; flow division ratio of internal carotid : external carotid, 70 : 30). The velocity profile is skewed toward the inner wall of the carotid bifurcation, resulting in a steep velocity gradient and high wall shear stress. Along the outer wall of the internal carotid sinus, the velocity profile is flat and there is an area of flow separation with very low flow velocities (*dotted line*) and very low wall shear stress. It is in this region of the human carotid bifurcation that intimal plaques form. (From Zarins CK, Giddens DP, Bharadvaj BK, et al: Carotid bifurcation atherosclerosis: Quantitative correlation of plaque localization with flow velocity profiles and wall shear stress. Circ Res 53:502, 1983.)

cube of the radius. Thus, a small change in the radius of a vessel will have a large effect on wall shear stress. High shear stress was implicated in atherogenesis when endothelial desquamation and smooth muscle proliferation were considered to be prime factors in plaque initiation,[10] and experimental studies showed that acute experimental elevations of shear stress could cause endothelial disruption.[71] Chronic elevations of shear stress were, however, not associated with endothelial injury, and regions of relatively high shear stress appeared to be selectively spared from plaque formation.[72]

It is now evident that atherosclerotic plaques localize preferentially in regions of *low shear stress* and not in regions of high shear stress. This has been demonstrated in quantitative studies correlating early plaque formation in pressure perfusion–fixed human carotid bifurcations with wall shear stress determinations in analogous geometrically precise flow models (Fig. 9–7).[73] Plaques form where shear stress values are near zero (i.e., at the lateral wall opposite the flow divider), and it has been suggested that a threshold value may exist below which plaque deposition tends to occur.[74] Similar quantitative studies of the human aortic bifurcation have also shown that plaques localize in regions of low rather than high shear stress.[75] Low shear rates may retard the transport of atherogenic substances away from the wall, resulting in an increased accumulation of lipids.[76] In addition, low shear stress may interfere with endothelial surface turnover of substances essential both to artery wall metabolism and to the maintenance of optimal endothelial metabolic function.[77]

Flow Separation and Stasis

In especially susceptible areas, such as the outer wall of the carotid bifurcation, where flow velocity is reduced and where flow separation occurs, fluid and particles are cleared slowly (Fig. 9–8) and have an *increased residence time.*[4, 74, 78] The vessel wall would therefore have a prolonged exposure to atherogenic particles. Time-dependent lipid particle–vessel wall interactions would thus be facilitated and favor plaque formation. In addition, blood-borne

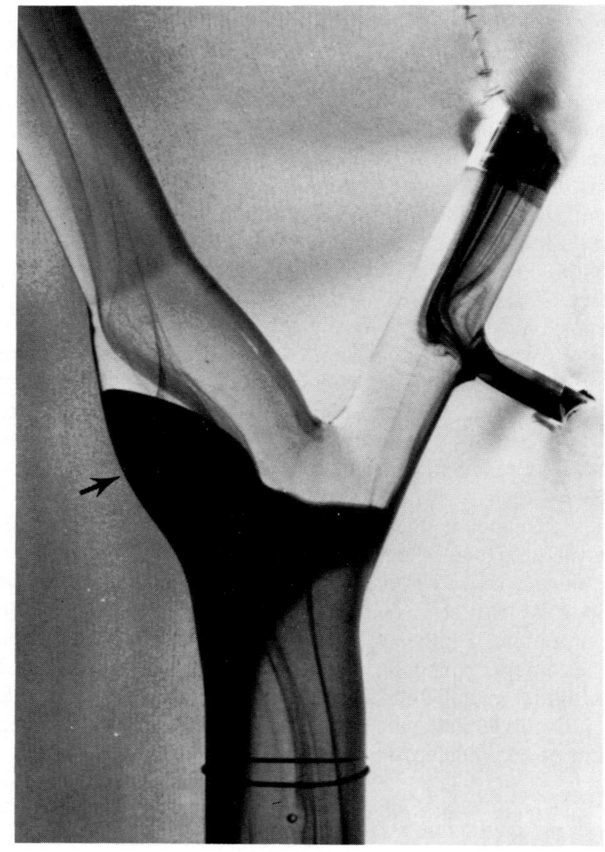

FIGURE 9–8. Flow visualization with dye injection in a glass model carotid bifurcation illustrating slow clearance from the separated flow region along the outer wall of the internal carotid sinus (*arrow*). Dye remains along the outer wall and within the separation zone long after it has been convected away from the region of the flow divider and distal internal carotid artery. (From Zarins CK, Giddens DP, Bharadvaj BK, et al: Carotid bifurcation atherosclerosis: Quantitative correlation of plaque localization with flow velocity profiles and wall shear stress. Circ Res 53:502, 1983.)

cellular elements that may play a role in atherogenesis would have an increased probability of deposition, adhesion, or diapedesis into the vessel wall in such regions.[79] Flow separation has, for example, been shown to favor deposition of platelets in vitro,[80] which may contribute to plaque induction and complication. Radiographic and ultrasound studies confirm the presence of flow separation and stasis in this outer wall region of the carotid bifurcation.[81] Not only do early intimal thickenings and plaques localize in this region, but complications, stenoses, and ulcerations also predominate in this same location.

Oscillation of Flow

Blood velocity varies markedly during the course of the cardiac cycle, resulting in a fluctuation in the magnitude of wall shear stress, which is a normal feature at the blood-artery interface. Along the inner wall of the carotid bifurcation on the side of the flow divider, blood flow and shear stress vary but the vector is always in the forward direction. Along the outer wall of the carotid bifurcation, opposite the flow divider where intimal plaques form, there is a reversal of axial flow direction during systole and phasic retrograde flow along the wall (Fig. 9–9). This results in a directional oscillation of the shear stress vector during the cardiac cycle.[74] Variations in shear stress direction associated with pulsatile flow may favor increased endothelial permeability by direct mechanical effects on cell junctions, whereas relatively high unidirectional shear stresses may not be injurious[82] and may even favor endothelial mechanical integrity. Endothelial cells are normally aligned in the direction of flow[83] in an overlapping arrangement.[84] Cyclic shifts in the relationship between shear stress direction and the orientation of intercellular overlapping borders may disturb the relationships between ingress and egress of particles through junctions. This hypothesis agrees well with reports of increased permeability of cultured, confluent endothelial cells subjected to changes in shear stress[85] as well as increased permeability to Evans blue dye in relation to differences in endothelial cell orientation,[86] which may be associated with different flow patterns.

Because oscillation of shear stress direction at susceptible sites occurs during systole, the number of such oscillations over time is directly related to the number of systoles (i.e., to heart rate). Heart rate has been implicated as an independent risk factor in coronary atherosclerosis and is discussed further in the section dealing with the coronary arteries.

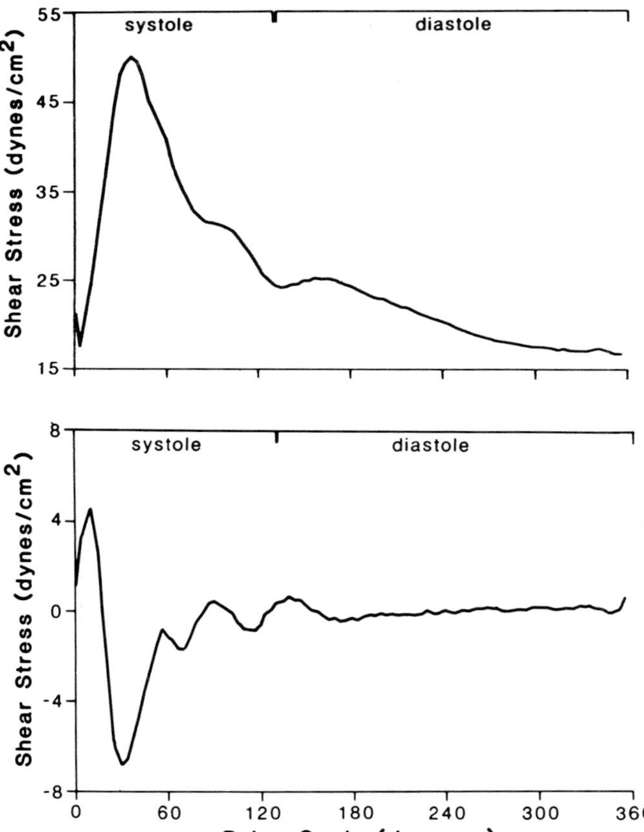

FIGURE 9–9. Shear stress alterations in the carotid bifurcation during the cardiac cycle. *Top*, Along the inner wall of the internal carotid sinus, shear stress is high and always in the forward direction (18–50 dynes/cm^2). Plaque does not form in this area. *Bottom*, Along the outer wall of the sinus, shear stress is low (+5 to −6 dynes/cm^2) and changes direction during the cardiac cycle from a forward to a reverse vector with multiple oscillations. This oscillation in the shear stress vector is highly correlated with early plaque formation. (From Ku DN, Giddens DP, Zarins CK, et al: Pulsatile flow and atherosclerosis in the human carotid bifurcation: Positive correlation between plaque location and low and oscillating shear stress. Arteriosclerosis 3:293, 1985.)

Turbulence

Turbulence is defined as random, disordered flow and is rarely seen in the normal vascular tree. Turbulent flow has often been implicated as a factor in plaque pathogenesis.[87, 88] However, in vitro observations and experimental atherosclerosis studies fail to support this concept. In model studies of the carotid bifurcation, a zone of complex secondary and tertiary flow patterns including counterrotating helical trajectories is demonstrable in regions of plaque formation, but turbulence does not occur (Fig. 9–10).[89] In vivo pulsed Doppler ultrasound studies of carotid arteries have confirmed this finding in normal human subjects.[90] Turbulence may, however, develop in association with stenoses and irregularities of the flow surface caused by atherosclerotic plaques, but turbulence is located distal to the lesion, not at the lesion. Experimentally produced stenoses reveal that turbulence is greatest two to four vessel diameters distal to the stenosis in an area that frequently develops post-stenotic dilatation but does not readily develop diet-induced plaques.[91–93] Thus, turbulence per se has not been shown to be an initiating factor in atherogenesis. Nevertheless, turbulence may play a role in plaque disruption or thrombogenesis. Further investigation is needed to establish these relationships.

Hypertension

Hypertension has been identified as an important risk factor in the development of clinical complications of atherosclerosis, such as myocardial infarction and stroke.[94] Postmortem studies have revealed that hypertension is associated with an increase in both the extent and the severity of atherosclerosis.[70] Elevated blood pressure alone does not

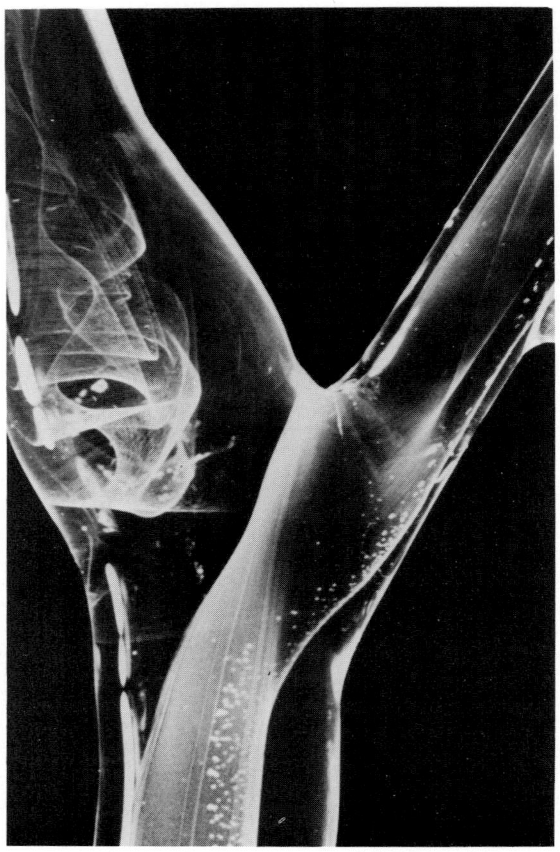

FIGURE 9–10. Hydrogen bubble flow visualization in a glass model carotid bifurcation. Streamlines are skewed toward the apex of the carotid flow divider, and in the outer wall of the carotid sinus, there is a zone of complex secondary and tertiary flow patterns, including flow reversal and counterrotating helical trajectories. However, no random, disordered flow or turbulence is present.

induce atherosclerosis in experimental animals. In the presence of hyperlipidemia, however, hypertension enhances plaque formation.[95–97] Yet atherosclerotic plaque will not form despite the presence of hypertension and severe hyperlipidemia when pulse pressure, wall motion, or both are decreased.[98, 99] Although hypertension has been shown to enhance experimental plaque formation, it has been noted to inhibit plaque regression when cholesterol levels are reduced.[100] Hypertension has further been shown to enhance coronary artery plaque progression despite the reduction of hypercholesterolemia.[101] These observations suggest that factors other than blood pressure per se may be of primary importance in plaque pathogenesis. However, hypertension may play an important role in atherosclerotic plaque evolution and the clinical complications of atherosclerotic plaques.

Susceptible Regions of the Vascular Tree

Carotid Arteries

The carotid bifurcation is particularly prone to plaque formation, with focal plaque deposition occurring principally at the origin of the internal carotid artery, whereas the proximal common carotid artery and the distal internal carotid artery are relatively spared. The geometry of the carotid bifurcation is an important determinant of the hemodynamic conditions that favor plaque formation. The internal carotid sinus has a cross-sectional area twice that of the immediately distal internal carotid segment. This configuration, in combination with the branching angle, results in a large area of flow separation and low and oscillating shear stress along the outer wall of the sinus and a region of laminar flow and high unidirectional shear stress along the inner wall of the sinus.[73, 74] The manner in which these differences may determine plaque localization at the outer wall of the sinus has been discussed. As plaques enlarge at the outer wall, however, the geometric configuration of the lumen is modified so that other flow patterns may develop that favor plaque formation on the side and inner walls. In its most advanced and stenotic form, carotid bifurcation atherosclerotic disease may therefore involve the entire circumference of the sinus, including the region of the flow divider, but the plaques are nevertheless largest and most complicated at the outer and side walls of the proximal internal carotid bifurcation.[102] The modified hemodynamic conditions that exist at the carotid bifurcation, including the turbulence that may underlie the characteristic bruit, may also compromise integrity of existing carotid plaques and contribute to their tendency to fissure, ulcerate, and form thromboemboli.

Coronary Arteries

Velocity profile and wall shear stress measurements in model human coronary arteries reveal that low wall shear stress, flow separation, and oscillation occur at susceptible sites for plaque localization.[103] These near-wall flow field characteristics are similar to those found in susceptible regions of the carotid bifurcation.

Several special hemodynamic features of the coronary arteries may explain their particular propensity to develop clinically significant plaques. The epicardial coronary tree has a complex geometric configuration of branchings and curves. Mechanical torsions and flexions of the vessels are evident during the cardiac cycle as the configuration of the cardiac chambers changes. In addition, there are marked variations in flow rate during the cardiac cycle.[104] The coronary arteries experience two different systolic pulses of flow during each cardiac cycle.[105] If oscillation in the direction of the shear stress vector during systole is indeed a major factor in plaque localization,[106] the coronary arteries would be expected to have increased vulnerability to plaque formation compared with other systemic arteries in which only a single systolic pulse is present. In experimental atherosclerosis, a 20 per cent reduction in mean heart rate resulted in a 50 per cent reduction in diet-induced coronary artery atherosclerotic plaques.[107] Similarly, there was a significant reduction in carotid bifurcation atherosclerosis with reduction in heart rate.[59, 108] In humans, a number of major prospective clinical studies have found high heart rates in men at rest to be predictors of future clinical coronary heart disease, whereas low heart rates had a protective effect.[109, 110] The beneficial effects of exercise on limiting coronary atherosclerosis may result from a reduction in resting heart rate, an intermittent increase in coronary flow and wall shear stress, or a combination of the two.

Abdominal Aorta

Atherosclerotic plaques in humans are found throughout the length of the aorta but are rarely clinically significant in the thoracic segment. In contrast, the infrarenal abdominal aorta is particularly prone to the development of clinically significant lesions, with the formation of obstructive plaques, ulcerations, thrombi, and aneurysmal degeneration. The differences in susceptibility between the thoracic and abdominal aortas may be related to differences in flow conditions, mural architecture, or vasa vasorum blood supply.[110] The thoracic aorta is the main conduit carrying blood flow to the viscera and extremities. Much of the cardiac output is delivered to the cerebral and upper extremity vessels as well as to the visceral organs; the renal arteries alone take up to 25 per cent of the cardiac output.[112] Levels of flow in the infrarenal aorta, in contrast, are largely dependent on the muscular activity of the lower extremities. With mechanized transportation and an increasingly sedentary lifestyle, reduced physical activity may result in an overall reduction in flow velocity in the abdominal aortic segment. The long-term effect of reduced flow velocity may be further accentuated by the tendency of the aorta to enlarge with age. Although the human thoracic aortic media is furnished with intramural vasa vasorum, the abdominal aorta is relatively avascular.[68] Thus, reduced and marked variations in luminal flow rate as well as discrepancies between medial thickness and medial nutrition may combine to enhance the accumulation of atherogenic substances in the abdominal aortic intima.

Superficial Femoral Artery

The arteries of the lower extremities are frequently affected by atherosclerotic plaques, whereas vessels of similar size in the upper extremities are usually spared. In addition to differences in hydrostatic pressure, the arteries of the lower extremities are subjected to more marked variations in flow rate depending on the level of physical activity. As in the abdominal aorta, a sedentary lifestyle would tend to favor low flow rates and lead to increased plaque deposition in vessels of the lower extremities. Cigarette smoking and diabetes mellitus are the risk factors most closely associated with atherosclerotic disease of the lower extremities.[113] The manner in which these factors and the special hemodynamic conditions are mutually enhancing in the vessels of the lower extremities remains to be elucidated. The arterial media in the lower extremities may be rendered more dense by increased smooth muscle tone induced by nicotine.[114] Such a change could interfere with transmural transfer of materials entering the intima and favor accumulation of atherogenic materials, as has been suggested by recent pharmacologic experiments.[115] Of the arteries of the lower extremity, the superficial femoral artery is the most common site of multiple stenotic lesions, and the profunda femoris tends to be spared. Plaques in the superficial femoral artery have not been shown to occur preferentially at branching sites, but stenotic lesions tend to appear earliest at the adductor hiatus, where the vessel is straight and branches are few. Increased susceptibility to plaque formation because of mechanical trauma caused by the closely associated adductor magnus tendon has been proposed to explain the selective localization of occlusive disease in this area.[116] However, studies have suggested that the adductor canal segment of the superficial femoral artery is not more prone to plaque formation but rather is limited in its ability to dilate or enlarge in response to increasing intimal plaque. Thus, an equivalent volume of intimal plaque results in more stenosis at the adductor canal.[63]

EVOLUTION OF ATHEROSCLEROTIC LESIONS

Atherosclerosis is not necessarily a continuous process leading inexorably to artery stenosis or other clinically significant complications. Plaque formation involves an interaction among systemic risk factors and local conditions in the lumen and artery wall in the context of a living tissue capable of healing and remodeling. The evolution of atherosclerotic lesions therefore involves initiating and sustaining processes, as well as adaptive responses and involutional changes. The natural history of atherosclerotic lesions in humans is poorly understood despite the available experimental data concerning plaque progression and regression.

Plaque Initiation

Plaque initiation refers to the earliest detectable biochemical and cellular events leading to or preceding the formation of atherosclerotic lesions. Possible mechanisms of plaque initiation have received a great deal of attention. Research has centered principally on several possibilities, including altered endothelial function or turnover resulting in increased permeability, oxidative alteration of insudated lipids by endothelium, and subsequent ingress of macrophages.[117] Other possibilities include various stimuli to smooth muscle proliferation, including circulating mitogens,[118] and limitations of transmural transfer or egress related to the composition and organization of subendothelial tissues and media.[119] High levels of specific lipoprotein cholesterol fractions have also been implicated.[120] Although each of these can be related to early lesion development in experimental models and may be related to one or another of the epidemiologically identified risk factors, none has as yet been demonstrated to underlie the mural disturbance that leads to plaque formation. Some or several of these changes may well prove to be significant.

On the other hand, it is not clear that inhibiting the possible initiating injury to the artery wall will be of primary importance in the clinical control of atherosclerosis. More recent research has centered principally on several possibilities. These include altered endothelial function linked to an inflammatory response to injury with leukocyte adhesion, diapedesis, and cell proliferation, as well as smooth muscle cell migration and macrophage foam cell formation with lipid accumulation in both cell types. These lipids include cholesterol, cholesterol esters, and triglycerides. Increased lipoprotein infiltration coupled with disregulation of the cholesterol ester cycle activity and cholesterol efflux processes has been proposed to explain the pathobiology of this lipid accumulation process. Moreover, T-cells, macrophages, and smooth muscle cells may release specific biologic response modifiers that may participate in the disregulation of lipid metabolism, thereby enhancing lipid accumulation.[20, 26] It is well recognized that very old people with no clinically manifest atherosclerotic disease during life have substantial and advanced atherosclerotic plaques at autopsy. Longevity and good health in these people were associated not with the prevention of plaque initiation or formation but with the stable nature of the plaque, control of progression, adequate artery adaptation, and prevention of lesion complications.

Plaque Progression

Plaque progression refers to the continuing increase in intimal plaque volume, which may result in narrowing of the lumen and obstruction of blood flow. Progression may be rapid or slow, continuous or episodic. Rates of accretion may also vary with the stage of plaque development, plaque composition, and cell population of the lesion. Some of these may be modulated by clinical risk factors, whereas others are related to the changes in circulation and wall composition associated with lesion growth. At the tissue level, progression involves cellular migration, proliferation, and differentiation; intracellular and extracellular accumulation of lipids; extracellular matrix accumulation; and degeneration and cell necrosis. Progression also implies evolution and differentiation of plaque organization and stratification. In general, these features are designed to maintain an adequate lumen channel for as long as possible. The formation of a fibrous cap, the sequestration of necrotic and degenerative debris, and the persistence of a regular and round lumen cross section, as well as adaptive enlargement of the artery, reflect an overall healing process. In the long term, these reactive processes may prove inadequate, but they may also retard or arrest the atherogenic process. If plaque enlargement occurs under these conditions, plaque progression is well tolerated. Lumen diameter and blood flow are maintained even in the face of advanced and extensive lesions. Plaque modeling also includes incorporation and organization of mural thrombi and healing and reendothelialization of ulcerations, suggesting further means of restoring and preserving optimal conditions for adequate laminar flow. Plaque disruptions that undergo remodeling may leave defects corresponding to healed or restructured walls without the development of clinical symptoms.

The processes that regulate plaque development, differentiation, and healing must be understood in order to understand why one plaque progresses unfavorably with stenosis, ulceration, or thrombosis and another progresses without obstruction or complication. It is likely that rates of cell proliferation, lipid deposition, fibrous cap formation, necrosis and healing, calcification, and inflammation vary over time and may differ with location at the same point in time. Such differences probably account for the spectrum of morphologic changes in plaques in a given patient at the same time. Changes in local hemodynamics that occur during plaque progression may also alter plaque composition and the rate of progression. Increases in shear stress in a developing stenosis may inhibit further plaque formation but may also favor erosion of the fibrous cap and ulceration. Developing stenoses may also alter hemodynamic conditions to enhance lesion formation and complication distally.[121] Severe, hemodynamically significant stenoses, on the other hand, enhance plaque formation in the proximal arterial segments[122] while inhibiting it distally[99] because of changes in pulse pressure, wall motion, and medial smooth muscle metabolism.[123]

Plaque Regression

Plaque regression refers to a discernible decrease in intimal plaque volume; this may occur by resorption of lipids or extracellular matrix or by cell death or cell migration out of the plaque. Significant reduction in lesion volume has been demonstrated in a number of animal models in which experimentally elevated serum lipid levels have been markedly reduced by diet alteration or by lipid-lowering drugs.[124–126] Lesions previously induced by an atherogenic diet respond readily, although not uniformly. Coronary and aortic lesions in monkeys tend to regress, but carotid lesions appear to be resistant.[127] Severe, long-standing lesions in swine are much more resistant to regression than early foam cell lesions.[128] Animal studies usually involve induction and regression periods of several months. Whether human lesions, which may have accumulated over decades, also decrease significantly in volume is as yet unclear.

Just as local hemodynamic conditions exert a profound influence on plaque progression, so they are important in regression. Severe proximal stenosis inhibits plaque formation[122] but also inhibits plaque regression in the distal arterial tree.[100] Hypertension promotes continued experimental plaque progression in the coronary arteries despite the reduction of hypercholesterolemia.[101] Despite plaque regression elsewhere and despite the reversal of hypercholesterolemia, experimental plaque formation and complication can continue in the arteries distal to a stenosis, indicating again that local hemodynamic factors and metabolic conditions in the artery wall may greatly modify systemic influences on plaque function during both progression and regression.[100]

Human Regression Studies. Apparent regression of atherosclerosis has been documented by serial contrast arteriography in humans. Angiographic regression of atherosclerotic lesions has been demonstrated in humans in coronary[129–131] and peripheral[59] arteries. Each of these trials has demonstrated luminal changes on angiography rather than by direct evidence of plaque regression. It should be noted that each trial to date has demonstrated simultaneous angiographic lesion progression *and* regression of different lesions during the treatment, indicating the complexity of the process.

Although regression is usually thought of as simply a resorption of plaque material, it may proceed by different mechanisms. A decrease in intimal plaque volume may occur owing to a change in plaque metabolism, resulting in dissolution of the fibrous cap, ulceration and erosion, and embolization of the necrotic core.

Apparent regression may also take place when the rate of artery wall enlargement exceeds the rate of plaque deposition. Most human regression studies performed to date have used angiography to document lesion regression.[132] However, angiography provides information only on lumen diameter and contour, not on the volume and composition of the atherosclerotic lesion itself. Thus, if intimal plaque deposition and artery wall dilatation keep pace, no change will be noted on arteriography despite continued plaque progression. Conversely, if dilatation exceeds plaque deposition, this will be taken as evidence of regression even if plaque deposition continues.[133] Such a phenomenon occurs at the outset of plaque formation in some vessels and is quite prominent in some locations. Certainty with regard to reduction in lesion volume or regression of atherosclerosis in humans must be based on a direct assessment of the plaque and artery wall as well as of lumen caliber.

Although plaque regression may a priori seem desirable, regression regimens could alter plaque composition and organization, especially for plaques with soft, semifluid, or pultaceous contents, and lead to plaque ulceration or disruption, release of plaque ulceration or disruption, release of plaque debris, and thrombosis and embolism. In certain circumstances, particularly with well-organized sclerotic plaques, the plaque may provide mechanical support to the artery wall. This may be especially significant in situations in which there has been medial atrophy underneath the plaque. Plaque dissolution under these circumstances could leave a weakened artery wall and potentiate aneurysm formation. Experimental studies have revealed aneurysm formation in monkeys undergoing cholesterol-lowering regression regimens.[134, 135] Further studies of the direct effects of regression regimens on plaques and the artery wall are needed, and regression must be defined in terms of its specific effects on well-established atherosclerotic plaques. An alternate therapeutic goal may be arrest or control of progression, plaque stabilization, and enhancement of artery wall adaptation.

Plaque Complications and Stability

Clinical sequelae of atherosclerotic lesions are usually caused by plaque complications. Complications such as plaque disruption or ulceration may result in embolization of plaque materials or the exposure of plaque components to the circulation, thereby causing occlusive or embolizing thrombi. Critical lumen narrowing or the presence of plaque complications at a few critical locations in the vascular tree is the predominant determinant of clinical symptoms rather than plaque size per se.

Susceptibility of plaques to disruption, fracture, or fissuring is likely to be associated with plaque structure, composition, and consistency. Thus, plaques may be relatively soft and pliable, friable or cohesive, densely sclerotic, or calcific and brittle. Some have well-formed fibrous caps, similar in architecture and thickness to a normal artery wall, thereby effectively sequestering the plaque and its contents from the lumen, whereas the necrotic interior of other plaques is separated from the lumen only by a narrow zone of connective tissue or by endothelium alone.[136] Advanced plaques with intact, well-organized fibrous caps would be expected to present smooth and regular lumen surfaces to the bloodstream, but abnormal levels of wall shear stress and departures from laminar, unidirectional flow may favor local accumulation, adhesion, and deposition of thrombocytes, monocytes, and fibrin. These are likely to occur distal to stenoses, at foci of endothelial surface irregularity or extrinsic mechanical trauma, and in regions of softened plaque consistency. Local mechanical stresses resulting from sudden changes in pressure, flow, or pulse rate, or from torsion and bending in relation to organ movements, may precipitate disruption of friable or brittle plaques. Conversely, changes in vessel configuration associated with plaque progression and stenosis may create conditions favoring the development of complex flow instabilities and vibrations. Although vessel segments distal to tight stenoses tend to be spared, degrees of stenosis not tight enough to prevent distal plaque formation may nevertheless engender unstable flow conditions that could modify plaque composition and configuration. In experimental animals, plaques located immediately distal to a region of moderate narrowing have been shown to be more complex in structure and composition than those that occur in the same region in the absence of a proximal stenosis.[121] The likelihood of turbulence is also enhanced as vessels enlarge and become tortuous with age or when multiple plaques occur in the same vessel in close axial proximity. Because regions of high flow velocity tend to be spared, increasing flow velocity at progressive narrowings could also conceivably be associated with local slowing of the atherogenic process. Decreased flow velocity due to distal obstruction, decreased pressure, or increased peripheral resistance would have the opposite effect. Further information is needed concerning the factors that determine plaque complication or stability in human atherosclerosis.

ANEURYSM FORMATION

The association between atherosclerosis and aneurysm formation has long been recognized in humans. The demonstration of increased proteolytic enzyme activity[137–139] and the demonstration of a familial tendency for abdominal aortic aneurysm formation[140] have led some investigators to suggest that aneurysm formation is primarily a genetically controlled connective tissue dysfunction with little or no relation to atherosclerosis. However, experimental evidence reveals that aneurysms can be induced in animals by feeding them high-cholesterol atherogenic diets for prolonged periods and that aneurysm formation is associated with destruction of the medial lamellar architecture of the aortic wall.[141, 142] Furthermore, aneurysm formation was noted to be related to plaque regression in both controlled[135] (Fig. 9–11) and uncontrolled[134, 143] trials.

Increasing intimal plaque is associated with arterial enlargement and atrophy of the underlying arterial media, as described earlier in this chapter. Under these circumstances, the atherosclerotic plaque may contribute to the structural support of the artery wall. Significant plaque regression by resorption of lipid and extracellular matrix can reduce plaque volume. Further reduction in plaque vol-

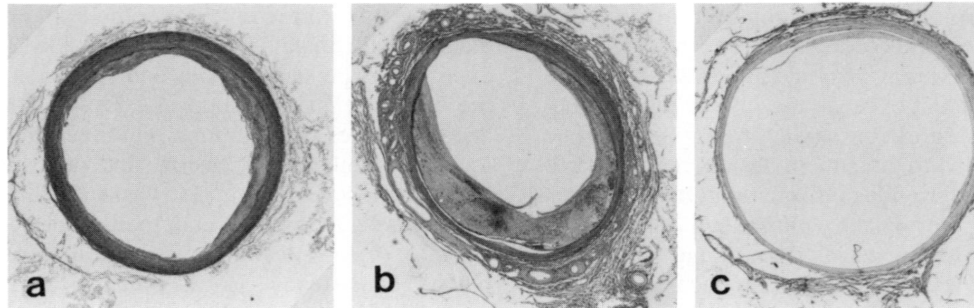

FIGURE 9–11. Aneurysmal enlargement of the abdominal aorta in a controlled trial of regression of experimental atherosclerosis. Transverse sections of the abdominal aorta from three groups of monkeys are shown. In group I, there was moderate plaque formation after a 6-month diet containing 2% cholesterol and 25% peanut oil *(a)*. In group II, plaques were much larger and the media was slightly thinner after 12 months of the atherogenic diet, but the artery size (internal elastic lumina area) did not change significantly *(b)*. After 6 months of the atherogenic diet, followed by a low-cholesterol regression diet (group III), plaques were significantly smaller and were absent in some regions. The media was thin, and the artery size (internal elastic lumina area) was increased twofold *(c)*. (Weigert–van Gieson, original magnification ×10.) (*a–c*, From Zarins CK, Xu C-P, Glagov S: Aneurysmal enlargement of the aorta during regression of experimental atherosclerosis. J Vasc Surg 15:90, 1992.)

ume can occur by erosion of the fibrous cap, elution of the necrotic core, and plaque ulceration. The net effect may be a thinned artery wall incapable of supporting the increased mural tension brought about by earlier atherosclerotic arterial enlargement. This increase in wall stress, together with the biologic interaction between metabolic plaque resorption and proteolytic enzyme activity on the arterial wall, can result in progressive arterial dilatation and aneurysm formation. Histologic examination of the aorta in animals with experimentally induced aneurysms and in humans with aneurysms reveals similar atrophic characteristics of atherosclerotic plaque, with loss of the elastin lamellar architecture of the artery wall (Fig. 9–12). Loss of elastin is a prominent feature along with the loss of collagen and thinning of the aortic wall. In humans, a strong association exists between atherosclerosis and aneurysm formation. They have risk factors in common. Aneurysms form in the same distributions as atherosclerotic plaques, but the greatest vulnerability to aneurysm formation is in the abdominal aorta. The abdominal aorta is particularly susceptible to plaque formation and may be particularly vulnerable because of its medial lamellar architecture and limited aortic wall nutrition, as discussed earlier. These considerations suggest that abdominal aortic aneurysm formation may complicate the atherosclerotic process under special experimental and human clinical conditions. It appears at a relatively late phase of plaque evolution, when plaque regression and media atrophy predominate, rather than in earlier phases, when cell proliferation, fibrogenesis, and lipid accumulation characterize plaque progression.

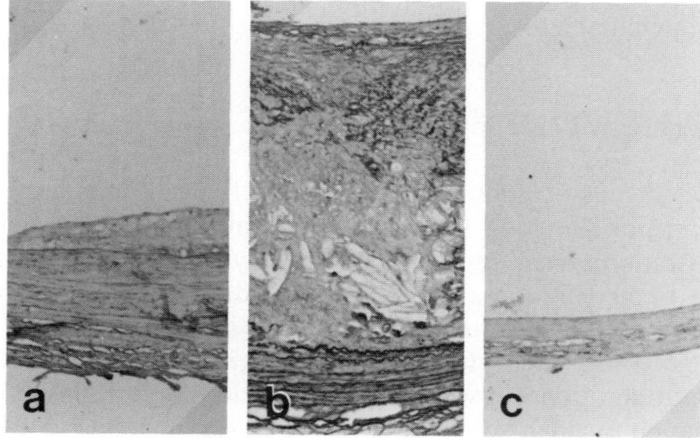

FIGURE 9–12. Histologic changes in the abdominal aorta of the sections shown in Figure 9–11. After 6 months of the atherogenic diet (group I; *a*), a moderate amount of plaque formed, with characteristic foamy cell prevalence and little change in the media. After 12-months of the atherogenic diet (group II; *b*), plaques were complex, with the formation of fibrous caps and evidence of necrosis and cholesterol accumulation. The media appeared normal, with clearly stained elastic lamellae and smooth muscle cells. After 6 months of the atherogenic diet and 6 months of the regression diet (group III; *c*), plaques were much smaller and largely fibrotic. The media was thinned, and elastic lamellae were largely inapparent. These histologic changes are similar to those seen in human aneurysms. (Weigert–van Gieson, original magnification ×75.) (*a–c*, From Zarins CK, Xu C-P, Glagov S: Aneurysmal enlargement of the aorta during regression of experimental atherosclerosis. J Vasc Surg 15:90, 1992.)

SUMMARY

Atherosclerosis is a systemic disorder with localized plaque deposition in selected sites on the arterial tree. Low or oscillatory wall shear stress, or both, and increased particle residence time due to flow stasis are the hemodynamic conditions associated with plaque formation. Alterations in local hemodynamic conditions also result in adaptive changes in the artery wall to maintain an adequate lumen caliber for blood flow. The primary adaptive response to enlarging intimal plaque is compensatory artery enlargement. Other responses, such as sequestering the plaque to one side and walling it off with a fibrous cap, can permit long-term clinical stability despite extensive atherosclerotic plaque formation. Clinical complications of atherosclerosis occur when the normal adaptive and compensatory mechanisms fail and complications such as stenosis, ulceration, embolization, and thrombosis develop. A better understanding is needed of the normal adaptive responses of arteries, the processes and evolution of atherosclerotic lesions, and the means by which plaques can be stabilized to prevent local plaque complications and subsequent clinical consequences.

Acknowledgments: *This work was supported by NHLBI grant HL-15062 and NSF grant CME 7921551.*

References

1. Glagov S, Zarins CK, Giddens DP, Ku DN: Hemodynamics and atherosclerosis. Arch Pathol Lab Med 112:1018, 1988.
2. Zarins CK: Adaptive responses of arteries. J Vasc Surg 9:382, 1989.
3. Schwartz S, Heimark R, Majesky M: Developmental mechanisms underlying pathology of arteries. Physiol Rev 70:1177, 1990.
4. Giddens DP, Zarins CK, Glagov S: Response of arteries to near-wall fluid dynamic behavior. Appl Mech Rev 43(5):S96, 1990.
5. Taylor KE, Glagov S, Zarins CK: Preservation and structural adaptation of endothelium over experimental foam cell lesions. Arteriosclerosis 9:881, 1989.
6. Ts'ao CH, Glagov S: Basal endothelial attachment: Tenacity at cytoplasmic dense zone in the rabbit aorta. Lab Invest 23:520, 1970.
7. Jaffe EA: Biology of Endothelial Cells. Boston, Martinus Nijhoff, 1984.
8. Clowes AW, Clowes MM, Reidy MA: Kinetics of cellular proliferation after arterial injury. III. Endothelial and smooth muscle growth in chronically denuded vessels. Lab Invest 54:295, 1986.
9. Clowes AW, Reidy MA: Prevention of stenosis after vascular reconstruction: Pharmacological control of intimal hyperplasia—A review. J Vasc Surg 13:885, 1991.
10. Ross R, Glomset JA: The pathogenesis of atherosclerosis. N Engl J Med 295:369, 1976.
11. Zarins CK, Taylor KE, Bomberger RA, et al: Endothelial integrity at aortic ostial flow dividers. Scanning Electron Micros 3:249, 1980.
12. Reidy MA: Biology of disease: A reassessment of endothelial injury and arterial lesion formation. Lab Invest 53(5):513, 1985.
13. Chidi CC, Klein L, DePalma R: Effect of regenerated endothelium on collagen content in the injured artery. Surg Gynecol Obstet 148:839, 1979.
14. Falcone DJ, Hajjar DP, Minick CR: Lipoprotein and albumin accumulation in reendothelialized and deendothelialized aorta. Am J Pathol 114:112, 1984.
15. Faggiotto A, Ross R: Studies of hypercholesterolemia in the nonhuman primate. II. Fatty streak conversion to fibrous plaque. Arteriosclerosis 4:341, 1984.
16. DiCorleto PE, Bowen-Pope DF: Cultured endothelial cells produce a platelet-derived growth factor–like protein. Proc Natl Acad Sci USA 80:1919, 1983.
17. Bevilacqua MP, Pober JS, Majeau GR, et al: Interleukin 1 (IL-1) induces biosynthesis and cell surface expression of procoagulant activity in human vascular endothelial cells. J Exp Med 160:618, 1984.
18. Einhorn S, Eldor A, Vladavsky I, et al: Production and characterization of interferon from endothelial cells. J Cell Physiol 122:200, 1985.
19. Whatley R, Zimmerman G, McIntyre T, Prescott S: Lipid metabolism and signal transduction in endothelial cells. Prog Lipid Res 29:45, 1990.
20. Hajjar DP, Pomerantz KB: Signal transduction in atherosclerosis: Integration of cytokines and the eicosanoid network. FASEB J 6:2933, 1992.
21. Clark JM, Glagov S: Structural integration of the arterial wall. I. Relationships and attachments of medial smooth muscle cells in normally distended and hyperdistended aortas. Lab Invest 40:587, 1979.
22. Gay S, Miller EJ: Collagen in the Physiology and Pathology of Connective Tissue. Stuttgart, New York, Gustav Fischer, 1978.
23. Clark JM, Glagov S: Transmural organization of the arterial wall: The lamellar unit revisited. Arteriosclerosis 5:19, 1985.
24. Wolinsky H, Glagov S: A lamellar unit of aortic medial structure and function in mammals. Circ Res 20:99, 1967.
25. Fischer GM, Llaurado JG: Collagen and elastin content in canine arteries from functionally different vascular beds. Circ Res 19:3984, 1966.
26. Pomerantz K, Hajjar D: Eicosanoids in regulation of arterial smooth muscle cell phenotype, proliferative capacity, and cholesterol metabolism. Arteriosclerosis 9:413, 1989.
27. Davis HR, Runyon-Hass A, Zarins CK, et al: Interactive arterial effects of hypertension and hyperlipidemia. Fed Proc 43(3):711, 1984.
28. Lyon RT, Zarins CK, Glagov S: Artery wall motion proximal and distal to stenoses. Fed Proc 44:1136, 1985.
29. Leung DYM, Glagov S, Mathews MB: Cyclic stretching stimulates synthesis of matrix components by arterial smooth muscle cells in vitro. Science 191:475, 1976.
30. Bomberger RA, Zarins CK, Glagov S: Medial injury and hyperlipidemia in development of aneurysms or atherosclerotic plaques. Surg Forum 31:338, 1980.
31. Wolinski H, Glagov S: Structural basis for the static mechanical properties of the aortic media. Circ Res 14:400, 1964.
32. Crawford T, Levene CI: Medial thinning in atheroma. J Pathol 66:19, 1953.
33. Wolinsky H, Glagov S: Nature of species differences in the medial distribution of aortic vasa vasorum in mammals. Circ Res 20:409, 1967.
34. Heistad DD, Marcus ML, Law EG, et al: Regulation of blood flow to the aortic media in dogs. J Clin Invest 62:133, 1978.
35. Wolinsky H, Glagov S: Zonal differences in modeling of the mammalian aortic media during growth. Fed Proc 26:357, 1967.
36. Leung DYM, Glagov S, Mathews MB: Elastin and collagen accumulation in rabbit ascending aorta and pulmonary trunk during postnatal growth: Correlation of cellular synthetic response with medial tension. Circ Res 41:316, 1977.
37. Wolinsky H: Long-term effects of hypertension on the rat aortic wall and their relation to concurrent aging changes. Circ Res 30:301, 1972.
38. Thoma R: Untersuchungen über die Histogenase and Histomechanik des Gefass Systems. Stuttgart, F Enke, 1893.
39. Mulvihill DA, Harvey SC: The mechanism of the development of collateral circulation. N Engl J Med 104:1032, 1931.
40. Holman E: Problems in the dynamics of blood flow. I. Condition controlling collateral circulation in the presence of an arteriovenous fistula, following the ligation of an artery. Surgery 26:889, 1949.
41. Kamiya A, Togawa T: Adaptive regulation of wall shear stress to flow change in the canine carotid artery. Am J Physiol 239:H14, 1980.
42. Masuda H, Bassiouny HS, Glagov S, Zarins CK: Artery wall restructuring in response to increased flow. Surg Forum 40:285, 1989.
43. Langille BL, O'Donnell F: Reductions in arterial diameter produced by chronic decreases in blood flow are endothelium-dependent. Science 231:405, 1986.
44. Furchgott RF: Role of endothelium in responses of vascular smooth muscle. Circ Res 53:557, 1983.
45. Glagov S, Weisenberg E, Zarins CK, et al: Compensatory enlargement of human atherosclerotic coronary arteries. N Engl J Med 316:1371, 1987.
46. Wilens SL: The nature of diffuse intimal thickening of arteries. Am J Pathol 27:825, 1951.
47. Movat HZ, More TH, Haust MD: The diffuse intimal thickening of the human aorta with aging. Am J Pathol 34:1023, 1958.
48. Tejada C, Strong JP, Montenegro MR, et al: Distribution of coronary and aortic atherosclerosis by geographic location, race and sex. Lab Invest 18:5009, 1968.
49. Tracy RE, Kissling GE: Age and fibroplasia as preconditions for atheronecrosis in human coronary arteries. Arch Pathol Lab Med 111:957, 1987.
50. McGill HC Jr: Atherosclerosis: Problems in pathogenesis. *In* Paoletti R, Gotto AM (eds): Atherosclerosis Reviews. New York, Raven Press, 1977, pp 27–65.
51. Taylor KE, Glagov S, Zarins CK: Preservation and structural adaptation of endothelium over experimental foam cell lesions. Arteriosclerosis 9:881, 1989.
52. Faggiotto A, Ross R: Studies of hypercholesterolemia in the nonhuman primate. II. Fatty streak conversion to fibrous plaque. Arteriosclerosis 4:341, 1984.
53. Stary HO: The intimal macrophage in atherosclerosis. Artery 8:205, 1980.
54. Paterson JC: Vascularization and haemorrhage of the intima of arteriosclerotic coronary arteries. Arch Pathol 22:312, 1936.

55. Rifkin RD, Parisi HF, Follard E: Coronary calcification in the diagnosis of coronary artery disease. Am J Cardiol 44:141, 1979.
56. Glagov S, Eckner FAO, Lev M: Controlled pressure fixation apparatus for hearts. AMA Arch Pathol 76:640, 1963.
57. Zarins CK, Zatina MA, Glagov S: Correlation of postmortem angiography with pathologic anatomy: Quantitation of atherosclerotic lesions. *In* Bond MG, Insull W Jr, Glagov S, et al (eds): Clinical Diagnosis of Atherosclerosis. New York, Springer-Verlag, 1983, pp 283–303.
58. Bond MG, Adams MR, Bullock BC: Complicating factors in evaluating coronary artery atherosclerosis. Artery 9:21, 1981.
59. Beere PA, Glagov S, Zarins CK: Experimental atherosclerosis at the carotid bifurcation of the cynomolgus monkey. Atherosclerosis Thromb 12:1245, 1992.
60. Armstrong ML, Heistad DD, Marcus MI, et al: Structural and hemodynamic responses of peripheral arteries of macaque monkeys to atherogenic diet. Arteriosclerosis 5:336, 1985.
61. Zarins CK, Weisenberg E, Kolettis G, et al: Differential enlargement of artery segments in response to enlarging atherosclerotic plaques. J Vasc Surg 7:386, 1988.
62. Masawa N, Glagov S, Bassiouny H, Zarins CK: Intimal thickness normalizes mural tensile stress in regions of increased intimal area and artery size. Arteriosclerosis 8:621a, 1988.
63. Blair JM, Glagov S, Zarins CK: Mechanism of superficial femoral artery adductor canal stenosis. Surg Forum 41:359, 1990.
64. Zarins CK, Zatina MA, Giddens DP, et al: Shear stress regulation of artery lumen diameter in experimental atherogenesis. J Vasc Surg 5:413, 1987.
65. Strong JP, Eggen DA: Risk factors and atherosclerotic lesions. *In* Jones RJ (ed): Atherosclerosis II. New York, Springer-Verlag, 1970, pp 355–364.
66. Wolfe PA, Kannel WB, Verter J: Epidemiologic appraisal of hypertension and stroke risk. *In* Guthrie GP Jr, Kotchen TA (eds): Hypertension and the Brain. Mount Kisco, NY, Futura Publishing, 1984.
67. Greenhalgh RM: Biochemical abnormalities and smoking in arterial ischaemia. *In* Bergan JJ, Yao JST (eds): Gangrene and Severe Ischemia of the Lower Extremities. New York, Grune & Stratton, 1978, pp 39–60.
68. Glagov S: Hemodynamic risk factors: Mechanical stress, mural architecture, medial nutrition and the vulnerability of arteries to atherosclerosis. *In* Wissler RW, Geer JC (eds): The Pathogenesis of Atherosclerosis. Baltimore, Williams & Wilkins, 1972, pp 164–199.
69. Texon M: The hemodynamic concept of atherosclerosis. Bull NY Acad Med 36:263, 1960.
70. Glagov S, Rowley DA, Kohut R: Atherosclerosis of human aorta and its coronary and renal arteries. Arch Pathol Lab Med 72:558, 1961.
71. Fry DL: Acute vascular endothelial changes associated with increased blood velocity gradients. Circ Res 22:165, 1968.
72. Bassiouny HS, Lieber BB, Giddens DP, et al: Quantitative inverse correlation of wall shear stress with experimental intimal thickening. Surg Forum 39:328, 1988.
73. Zarins CK, Giddens DP, Bharadvaj BK, et al: Carotid bifurcation atherosclerosis: Quantitative correlation of plaque localization with flow velocity profiles and wall shear stress. Circ Res 53:502, 1983.
74. Ku DN, Giddens DP, Zarins CK, et al: Pulsatile flow and atherosclerosis in the human carotid bifurcation: Positive correlation between plaque location and low and oscillating shear stress. Arteriosclerosis 5(3):293, 1985.
75. Friedman MH, Hutchins GM, Bargeron CB, et al: Correlation between intimal thickness and fluid shear in human arteries. Atherosclerosis 39:425, 1981.
76. Caro CG, Fitz-Gerald JM, Schroter RC: Atheroma and arterial wall shear: Observation, correlation and proposal of a shear dependent mass transfer mechanism for atherogenesis. Proc R Soc Lond [Biol] 117:109, 1971.
77. Robertson AJ Jr: Oxygen requirements of the human arterial intima in atherogenesis. Prog Biochem Pharmacol 4:305, 1968.
78. Talukder N, Giddens DP, Vito RP: Quantitative flow visualization studies in a carotid artery bifurcation model. *In* 1983 Biomechanics Symposium, AMD, vol. 56; FED, vol. 1. New York, American Society of Mechanical Engineers, 1983, pp 165–168.
79. Gerrity RG, Goss JA, Soby L: Control of monocyte recruitment by chemotactic factor(s) in lesion-prone areas of swine aorta. Arteriosclerosis 5:55, 1985.
80. Parmentier EM, Morton WA, Petschek HE: Platelet aggregate formation in a region of separated blood flow. Phys Fluids 20:2012, 1981.
81. Fox JA, Hugh AE: Static zones in the internal carotid artery: Correlation with boundary layer separation and stasis in model flows. Br J Radiol 43:370, 1976.
82. Fry DL: Hemodynamic forces in atherogenesis. *In* Scheinberg P (ed): Cerebrovascular Disease. New York, Raven Press, 1976, pp 77–95.
83. Nerem RM, Levesque MJ, Cornhill JF: Vascular endothelial morphology as an indicator of the pattern of blood flow. J Biomech Eng 103:171, 1981.
84. Clark JM, Glagov S: Luminal surface of distended arteries by scanning electron microscopy. Eliminating configurational artifacts. Br J Exp Pathol 57:129, 1976.
85. Dewey CF, Bussolari SR, Gimbrone MA, et al: The dynamic response of vascular endothelial cells to fluid shear stress. J Biomech Eng 103:177, 1981.
86. Fry DL: Responses of the arterial wall to certain physical factors. Ciba Found Symp 12:93, 1973.
87. Davies PF, Remuzzi A, Gordon EJ, et al: Turbulent fluid shear stress induces vascular endothelial cell turnover in vitro. Proc Natl Acad Sci USA 83:2114, 1986.
88. Gutstein WH, Farrell GA, Armellini C: Blood flow disturbance and endothelial cell injury in pre-atherosclerotic swine. Lab Invest 29:134, 1973.
89. Bharadvaj BK, Mabon RF, Giddens DP: Steady flow in a model of the human carotid bifurcation. Part II. Laser Doppler anemometer measurements. J Biomech Eng 15:363, 1982.
90. Ku DN, Giddens DP: Pulsatile flow in a model carotid bifurcation. Arteriosclerosis 3:31, 1983.
91. Ku DN, Zarins CK, Giddens DP, et al: Reduced atherogenesis distal to stenosis despite turbulence and hypertension [Abstract]. Circulation 74(Suppl II):457, 1986.
92. Khalifa AMA, Giddens DP: Characterization and evolution of post-stenotic flow disturbances. J Biomech 14:279, 1981.
93. Coutard M, Osborne-Pellegrin MJ: Decreased dietary lipid deposition in spontaneous lesions distal to a stenosis in the rat caudal artery. Artery 12:82, 1983.
94. Kannel WB, Schwartz MJ, McNamara PM: Blood pressure and risk of coronary heart disease: The Framingham study. Dis Chest 56:43, 1969.
95. Hollander W, Madoff I, Paddock J, et al: Aggravation of atherosclerosis by hypertension in a subhuman primate model with coarctation of the aorta. Circ Res 38(Suppl 2):63, 1976.
96. McGill HC Jr, Carey KD, McMahan CA, et al: Effects of two forms of hypertension on atherosclerosis in the hyperlipidemic baboon. Arteriosclerosis 5:481, 1985.
97. Folkow BL: Physiological aspects of primary hypertension. Physiol Rev 62:347, 1982.
98. Lyon RT, Runyon-Hass A, Davis HR, et al: Protection from atherosclerotic lesion formation by inhibition of artery wall motion. J Vasc Surg 5(1):59, 1987.
99. Bomberger RA, Zarins CK, Taylor KE, et al: Effect of hypotension on atherogenesis and aortic wall composition. J Surg Res 28:402, 1980.
100. Zarins CK, Bomberger RA, Taylor KE, et al: Artery stenosis inhibits regression of diet-induced atherosclerosis. Surgery 88(1):86, 1980.
101. Xu C-P, Glagov S, Zatina MA, Zarins CK: Hypertension sustains plaque progression despite reduction of hypercholesterolemia. Hypertension 18(2):123, 1991.
102. Bassiouny HS, Davis H, Masawa N, et al: Critical carotid stenoses: Morphologic and biochemical similarity of symptomatic and asymptomatic plaques. J Vasc Surg 9(2):202, 1989.
103. Tang TD, Giddens DP, Zarins CK, Glagov S: Velocity profile and wall shear measurements in a model human coronary artery. ACME 17:261, 1990.
104. Klocke FJ, Mates RE, Canty JM, et al: Coronary pressure-flow relationships. Controversial issues and probable implications. Circ Res 56:310, 1985.
105. Granata L, Olsson RA, Huvos A, et al: Coronary inflow and oxygen usage following cardiac sympathetic nerve stimulation in unanesthetized dogs. Circ Res 16:114, 1965.
106. Ku DN, Giddens DP: Pulsatile flow in a model carotid bifurcation. Arteriosclerosis 3:31, 1983.
107. Beere PA, Glagov S, Zarins CK: Retarding effect of lowered heart rate on coronary atherosclerosis. Science 226:180, 1984.

108. Bassiouny HS, Zarins CK, Hovanessian A, Glagov S: Heart rate and experimental carotid atherosclerosis. Surg Forum 48:373, 1992.
109. Dyer AR, Persky V, Stamler J, et al: Heart rate as a prognostic factor for coronary heart disease and mortality: Findings in three Chicago epidemiologic studies. Am J Epidemiol 112:736, 1980.
110. Williams PT, Wood PD, Haskell WL, et al: The effects of running mileage and duration on plasma lipoprotein levels. JAMA 247:2674, 1982.
111. Wolinsky H, Glagov S: Comparison of abdominal and thoracic aortic medial structure in mammals: Deviation from the usual pattern in man. Circ Res 25:677, 1969.
112. Guyton AC: Textbook of Medical Physiology. 2nd ed. Philadelphia, WB Saunders, 1961, p 356.
113. Gordon T, Kannel WB: Predisposition to atherosclerosis in the head, heart and legs. The Framingham Study. JAMA 221:661, 1972.
114. Winniford MD, Wheelan KR, Kremers MS, et al: Smoking-induced coronary vasoconstriction in patients with atherosclerotic coronary artery disease: Evidence for adrenergically mediated alterations in coronary artery tone. Circulation 73:662, 1986.
115. Caro CG, Fish PJ, Jay M, et al: Influence of vasoactive agents on arterial hemodynamics: Possible relevance to atherogenesis. Abstr Biorheol 23:197, 1986.
116. Balaji MR, DeWeese JA: Adductor canal outlet syndrome. JAMA 245:167, 1981.
117. Ross R: The pathogenesis of atherosclerosis—An update. N Engl J Med 314:488, 1986.
118. Benditt EP, Barrett T, McDougall JK: Viruses in the etiology of atherosclerosis. Proc Natl Acad Sci 80:6388, 1983.
119. Caro CG: Transport of material between blood and wall in arteries. *In* Atherogenesis: Initiating Factors. Ciba Found Symp 12:127, 1973.
120. Ross R, Harker L: Hyperlipidemia and atherosclerosis. Science 193:1094, 1976.
121. Bomberger RA, Zarins CK, Glagov S: Subcritical arterial stenosis enhances distal atherosclerosis. Resident Research Award. J Surg Res 30:205, 1981.
122. Davis HR, Runyon-Hass A, Zarins CK, et al: Interactive arterial effects of hypertension and hyperlipidemia. Fed Proc 43(3):711, 1984.
123. Cozzi PJ, Lyon RT, Davis HR, et al: Aortic wall metabolism in relation to susceptibility and resistance to experimental atherosclerosis. J Vasc Surg 7:706, 1988.
124. Malinow MR: Experimental models of atherosclerosis regression. Atherosclerosis 48(2):105, 1983.
125. Wissler RW, Vesselinovitch D: Combined effects of cholestyramine and probucol on regression of atherosclerosis in rhesus monkey aortas. Appl Pathol 1(2):89, 1983.
126. Stary HC: Regression of atherosclerosis in primates. Virchows Arch [A] 383:117, 1979.
127. Clarkson TB, Bond MG, Bullock BC, et al: A study of atherosclerosis regression in Macaca mulatta. V. Changes in abdominal aorta and carotid and coronary arteries from animals with atherosclerosis induced for 38 months and then regressed for 24 or 48 months at plasma cholesterol concentrations of 300 or 200 mg/dl. Exp Mol Pathol 41(1):96, 1984.
128. Daoud AS, Jarmolych J, Augustyn JM, et al: Sequential morphologic studies of regression of advanced atherosclerosis. Arch Pathol Lab Med 105(5):233, 1981.
129. Blankenhorn DH, Nessim SA, Johnson BL, et al: Beneficial effects of combined colestipol-niacin therapy on coronary atherosclerosis and coronary venous bypass grafts. JAMA 257:3233, 1987.
130. Brown G, Albert JJ, Fisher LD, et al: Regression of coronary artery disease as a result of intensive lipid-lowering therapy in men with high levels of apolipoprotein B. N Engl J Med 323:1290, 1990.
131. Buchwald H, Varco RL, Matts PJ, et al: Effect of partial ileal bypass surgery on mortality and morbidity from coronary heart disease in patients with hypercholesterolemia: Report of the Program on the Surgical Control of the Hyperlipidemias (POSCH). N Engl J Med 323:946, 1990.
132. Barndt R, Blankenhorn DH, Crawford DW, et al: Regression and progression of early femoral atherosclerosis in treated hyperlipoproteinemic patients. Ann Intern Med 86:139, 1977.
133. Zarins CK, Zatina MA, Glagov S: Correlation of postmortem angiography with pathologic anatomy: Quantitation of atherosclerotic lesions. *In* Bond MG, Insull W Jr, Glagov S, et al (eds): Clinical Diagnosis of Atherosclerosis: Quantitative Methods of Evaluation. New York, Springer-Verlag, 1983, pp 283–306.
134. Zarins CK, Glagov S, Wissler, RW, Vesselinovitch D: Aneurysm formation in experimental atherosclerosis: Relationship to plaque evolution. J Vasc Surg 12(3):246, 1990.
135. Zarins CK, Xu C-P, Glagov S: Aneurysmal enlargement of the aorta during regression of experimental atherosclerosis. J Vasc Surg 15:90, 1992.
136. Glagov S, Zarins CK, Giddens DP, et al: Atherosclerosis: What is the nature of the plaque? *In* Strandness DE Jr, Didisheim P, Clowes AW, et al (eds): Vascular Diseases: Current Research and Clinical Applications. Orlando, FL, Grune & Stratton, 1987, pp 15–33.
137. Campa JS, Greenhalgh RM, Powell JT: Elastin degradation in abdominal aortic aneurysms. Atherosclerosis 65:13, 1987.
138. Dobrin PB, Baker WH, Gley WC: Elastolytic and collagenolytic studies of arteries: Implications for the mechanical properties of aneurysms. Arch Surg 119:405, 1984.
139. Menashi S, Campa JS, Greenhalgh RM, Powell JT: Collagen in abdominal aortic aneurysm: Typing, content and degradation. J Vasc Surg 6:578, 1987.
140. Johansen K, Koepsell T: Familial tendency for abdominal aortic aneurysm. JAMA 256:1934, 1986.
141. Bomberger RA, Zarins CK, Glagov S: Medial injury and hyperlipidemia in development of aneurysms or atherosclerotic plaques. Surg Forum 31:338, 1980.
142. Zatina MA, Zarins CK, Gewertz BL, Glagov S: Role of medial lamellar architecture in the pathogenesis of aortic aneurysms. J Vasc Surg 1:442, 1984.
143. DePalma RG, Koletsky S, Bellon EM, Insull W Jr: Failure of regression of atherosclerosis in dogs with moderated cholesterolemia. Atherosclerosis 27:297, 1977.

10

Atherogenesis and the Medical Management of Atherosclerosis

James C. A. Fuchs, M.D.

• • •

Atherosclerosis is the vascular disease responsible for most of the surgical procedures described in this text. Despite the large number of sophisticated operations available to surgeons, progression of the basic disease is commonly unaltered. Evidence suggests that atherosclerosis evolves over a long period before patients become candidates for surgery and that it tends to progress even after surgical intervention.[17, 46, 53, 58] This concept is reinforced by follow-up of patients with arterial bypass grafts and by repeated angiographic or noninvasive assessment of patients with vascular disease. Any patient with atherosclerosis has the potential for enlargement of present lesions or for development of the disease in a previously normal site. For this reason, it is important that surgeons be fully aware of information about the origin, development, and nonoperative treatment of atherosclerotic vascular disease. The data necessary to clarify the underlying principles and indications for the long-term medical management of these patients are summarized here.

Extremely important to this issue are whether atherosclerosis can be arrested and whether regression of established lesions can occur. The pathologic changes of atherosclerosis can be reduced or even cleared in experimental animals by the use of diet and drugs.[8, 52, 70, 71] Evidence is accumulating that such changes may also occur in humans.[13, 14, 84, 103, 105] Although it appears that certain lesion patterns are resistant to regression, the fact that the course of this disease is not necessarily inexorable underscores the importance of factors involved in its development and treatment.[32] It is hoped that the application of such therapy to patients with atherosclerosis will continue the encouraging trend of decreasing the mortality rate of ischemic disease.[61, 67, 97]

PATHOGENESIS OF ATHEROSCLEROSIS

In order to design any rational treatment program, it is first necessary to understand clearly the pathogenesis of the underlying disease. In the case of atherosclerosis, no single etiologic factor is known. As a result, much of our knowledge has been achieved through inductive examination of data from patients with the disease. This has stimulated worldwide epidemiologic studies to determine the features associated with atherosclerotic vascular disease.[62, 102] Considerable information has come from retrospective and ongoing prospective analyses. In the first place, there is a universal difference in the incidence of atherosclerosis. For example, a 10-fold difference in the incidence of coronary disease exists between middle-aged men in parts of Northern Europe and men of the same age group in the Mediterranean area.

When specific high-risk populations are examined, certain features appear to be related to vascular atherogenesis. A prime example of such a study is that in which six leading centers combined their data to form the Pooling Project of the American Heart Association Council on Epidemiology. Prospective studies following 12,381 men, free of coronary disease at entry into the study, have been done for 98,741 person-years with the goal of determining the factors, both major and minor, that will predict the risk of developing atherosclerosis or the future course of established disease.[83] Three major risk factors have emerged as significant contributors to this disease in North America (Table 10–1).

Epidemiologic Factors

Hypertension has been found to be associated with a greater incidence of coronary atherosclerosis in most popu-

Table 10–1. Risk Factors for Atherosclerosis*

Major Factors
Hypertension
Hypercholesterolemia
Cigarette smoking
Minor Factors
Obesity
Diabetes mellitus
Hypertriglyceridemia
Sedentary living
Stress
Family history

From Fuchs JCA: Dietary and pharmacologic management of atherosclerosis. In Sabiston DC Jr, Spencer FC (eds): Gibbon's Surgery of the Chest. 4th ed. Philadelphia, WB Saunders, 1983.

**Epidemiologic surveys have defined major factors that have a strong correlation with vascular disease and minor ones that are associated less positively. This particular set of features applies to the population surveyed in the United States.*

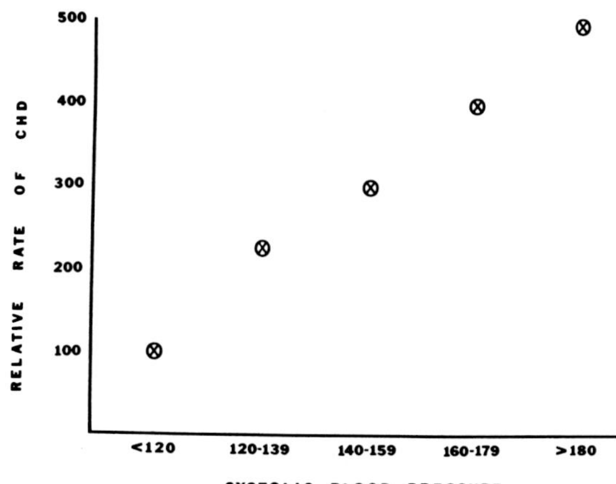

FIGURE 10–1. Relative risk of developing coronary heart disease (CHD) in the Framingham, Massachusetts, population compared with the systolic blood pressure on entry into the study. (Data from Stamler J: The coronary risk factors. *In* Preventive Cardiology. New York, Grune & Stratton, 1967.) This linear relationship has been found to apply to the diastolic pressure as well. (From Fuchs JCA: Dietary and pharmacologic management of atherosclerosis. *In* Sabiston DC Jr, Spencer FC [eds]: Gibbon's Surgery of the Chest. 4th ed. Philadelphia, WB Saunders, 1983.)

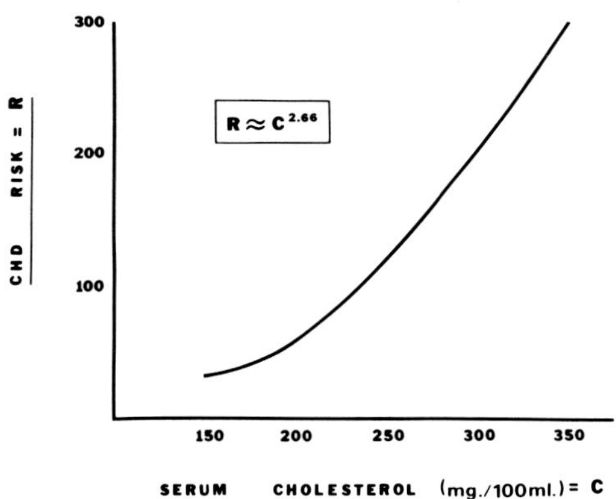

FIGURE 10–2. Risk of developing CHD compared with the serum level of total cholesterol. Biostatistical analysis has revealed an exponential relationship between these entities. (Data from Cornfield J: Joint dependence of risk of coronary heart disease on serum cholesterol and systolic blood pressure: A discriminant function analysis. Fed Proc 21(Suppl 2):58, 1962. From Fuchs JCA: Dietary and pharmacologic management of atherosclerosis. *In* Sabiston DC Jr, Spencer FC [eds]: Gibbon's Surgery of the Chest. 4th ed. Philadelphia, WB Saunders, 1983.)

lations surveyed. In addition, high blood pressure is associated with heightened susceptibility to peripheral and cerebral vascular involvement.[60] The relationship between hypertension and coronary artery disease is continuous, and each increment of pressure increases the risk (Fig. 10–1).

Hypercholesterolemia is a frequent single factor correlated with atherosclerosis. Appreciation of this concept started with clinical observations that certain diseases such as hypothyroidism, nephrotic syndrome, diabetes mellitus, and familial xanthomatosis were associated with persistent hypercholesterolemia. In these situations, premature atherosclerosis is a significant problem. The argument that elevated serum lipid concentrations contribute to the development of atherosclerosis has gained considerable support from prospective population surveys.[62] In fact, a patient's risk of developing the disease increases exponentially at high levels of serum cholesterol (Fig. 10–2).[26] The incidence of coronary atherosclerosis in a specific population has been found to vary directly with the mean serum cholesterol level (Fig. 10–3). In addition, cardiovascular mortality varies with the serum cholesterol level, particularly in younger patients.[6] This is one risk feature that holds true regardless of the population examined. Greater specificity for the predictive value of serum cholesterol is obtained when the lipid is expressed in terms of lipoprotein fractions. In particular, low-density lipoprotein cholesterol has been found to be an important risk factor positively related to coronary disease in both men and women well into the 7th or 8th decade of life.[45] Two serum factors appear to increase the risk of coronary artery disease: elevated low-density lipoprotein and decreased high-density lipoprotein cholesterol.[108]

It has also been established that lowering of elevated blood cholesterol levels will reduce the risk of myocardial infarction from coronary heart disease.[68] Such results have lent support to the rationale of programs of diet and drug therapy for large groups of the population for whom elevated blood cholesterol offers a potential threat.[24]

Cigarette smoking is remarkably constant in its positive relationship to death from atherosclerosis. Studies confirm a strong relationship between cigarette consumption and the extent and character of aortic atherosclerosis and cerebral vascular involvement.[50] The risk of coronary events is more than three-fold greater in men smoking more than one pack per day than in nonsmokers.[83] Particularly relevant to this concept is the fact that before the Surgeon General's Report on Smoking and Health in 1964, there was a steady increase in mortality in coronary heart disease. Since the report appeared, there has been a decrease in the proportion of both male and female smokers and a corresponding decline in coronary artery disease and death rates.[61]

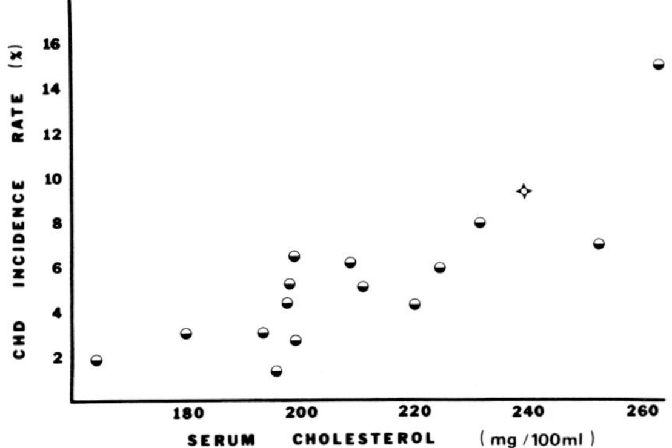

FIGURE 10–3. The incidence of CHD in national populations compared with the mean level of serum cholesterol. The relationship is a linear one. The incidence in the United States (*star*) is exceeded only by that in Finland. (Data from Keys A [ed]: Coronary heart disease in seven countries. Circulation 41 [Suppl 1]:1, 1970. From Fuchs JCA: Dietary and pharmacologic management of atherosclerosis. *In* Sabiston DC Jr, Spencer FC [eds]: Gibbon's Surgery of the Chest. 4th ed. Philadelphia, WB Saunders, 1983.)

The remaining "minor" risk factors have a more variable correlation with atherosclerotic disease. Categorized as such are diabetes mellitus, obesity, hypertriglyceridemia, hyperuricemia, sedentary lifestyle, psychosocial tensions, and a family history of the disease (see Table 10–1). Although these are common features in patients with atherosclerosis, they are classified as minor because they cannot be separated as *independent* predictors of the disease.

Pathologic Changes

In addition to the epidemiologic data, the second major source of information concerning the course of atherosclerotic disease has been the observations of pathologists. The appearance and distribution of arterial lesions was well known by 18th and 19th century anatomic pathologists. Although gross vascular lesions were thought to be related to aging, significant discrepancies have been found in the age-related incidence of this disease. Comprehensive examinations have revealed the presence of early lesions in a young, otherwise healthy population, and the disease may be minimal in some elderly individuals.[98] Rather than being an inevitable consequence of aging, the disease may, as suggested by its early appearance and variable course, have a prolonged pathogenesis in selected individuals. Such information has encouraged the search for the underlying etiologic factors, as just delineated.

The gross appearance of raised yellow plaques, often with ulcerated or thrombosed surfaces, is familiar to the cardiovascular surgeon. The lesions are limited primarily to the tunica intima of the artery and to the adjacent portion of the tunica media. Histologic study of such tissue provides the following information that is pertinent to the probable evolution of this disease process (Fig. 10–4).

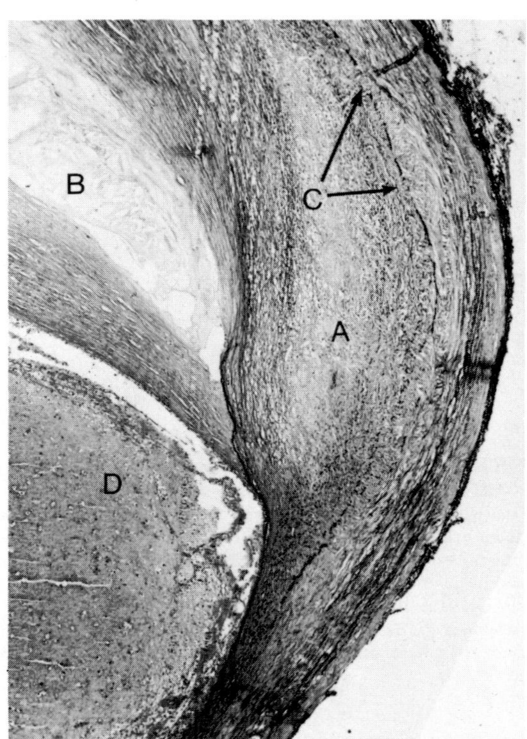

FIGURE 10–4. Atherosclerosis involving the right coronary artery of a 41-year-old man with type II hyperlipidemia. Tissue proliferation within the intimal region (A) intrudes into the lumen, and the cholesterol clefts of lipid deposition are present (B). The intrinsic structures of elastic fibers are disrupted (C), and thrombosis has occurred within the lumen (D). (From Fuchs JCA: Dietary and pharmacologic management of atherosclerosis. *In* Sabiston DC Jr, Spencer FC [eds]: Gibbon's Surgery of the Chest. 4th ed. Philadelphia, WB Saunders, 1983.)

Tissue proliferation is characteristic of all lesions. Basic investigation suggests that this response involves migration and duplication of intrinsic smooth muscle cells.[86, 101] In addition to cellular proliferation, increased amounts of collagen and ground substance are produced. The resulting tissue build-up is largely responsible for the encroachment of the atherosclerotic plaque on the vascular lumen. *Tissue disruption* of medial elastic fibers occurs as the disease extends deeper into the wall. The resulting structural disintegration leads to a loss of tensile strength and elasticity that may contribute to the vascular dilatation seen in degenerating atherosclerotic vessels.

Lipid infiltration, both intracellular and extracellular, is a histopathologic hallmark of atherosclerosis. The cholesterol clefts of the plaques were among the earliest identified components of this disease. Biochemical assays show free and esterified cholesterol to be the major lipid constituents of the plaque. The observations of an increased lipid content with severe disease and the presence of immunologically intact lipoproteins in early lesions implicate these compounds in the possible etiology of atherosclerosis.[3]

Tissue reaction adjacent to areas of atherosclerosis is characterized by platelet build-up and thrombosis on the luminal surface and by infiltration of inflammatory cells in the periplaque region. The thrombus may be secondary to intimal ulceration and it can, in turn, induce damage to the endothelial surface. Injected lipids will incite an inflammatory response, and accumulation of these agents may be responsible for the cellular inflammation seen with this disease.[2]

Theories of Pathogenesis

The pathologic changes and epidemiologic factors listed here have been used to construct hypotheses for the etiology and course of atherosclerosis. Any theory of atherosclerosis must account for such diverse factors as hypertensive pressure, hemodynamic shear stress, vascular permeability, platelet and thrombus encrustation, alterations in lipid content, changes in biochemical metabolism, protein accumulations within diseased arterial tissue, endothelial and smooth muscle cell replication, mutagenic agents, growth factors, hypoxia, and inflammation. The need to explain so many complicated factors has engendered numerous hypotheses of pathogenesis. Although each explanation of the etiology and progression of arterial lesions is usually presented as a self-contained concept, there is considerable overlap in the elements of these theories. For practical purposes, these hypotheses can be classified into three groups: response to injury, reaction to serum lipids, and mutagenic cellular transformation.

There are similarities in these three approaches in the

detailed explanations for atherogenesis. This arises because certain features of atherosclerosis are so consistent that they must be part of any comprehensive hypothesis. Such recurrent concepts provide the most solid rationale for the treatment or prevention of atherosclerotic arterial disease. Although the features of atherogenesis are hypothetical and the risk factors delineated by epidemiologic surveys may be more circumstantial than causal, they nonetheless suggest means for the medical management of this complicated problem.

Injury Hypothesis

The practical approach of explaining atherosclerosis by an injury hypothesis began as early as 1852 with Rokitansky. Modified over the years by increasingly sophisticated concepts of injury and of tissue response, this hypothesis continues to be the subject of investigation.[15, 40, 86, 91] Atherogenesis is seen to begin with an endothelial injury—in the form of hypertensive pressure, hemodynamic shearing forces, thrombosis, humoral stimuli, chemical irritation, immunologic trauma, hypoxia, or lipid build-up. Such an injury disrupts or stimulates the endothelium and brings about a multi-phasic response that ultimately produces the mature atherosclerotic lesion or plaque. An important proliferative response occurs in the medial and subintimal smooth muscle cells, possibly related to growth factors released by adherent platelets and monocytes or from the endothelium itself.[87, 90, 91] Initially, the smooth muscle cell replication produces the histologic picture of intimal hyperplasia, similar to that seen postoperatively in grafted vascular tissues.[72, 88] This cell proliferation may regress if its initiating factors are reversed, or it may evolve into the mature lesions of occlusive arterial disease under the influence of repeated injury (Fig. 10–5).

With disease maturation, there is a fibrous transformation of the vascular wall brought about by increased collagen synthesis and glycopeptide accumulation.[73] The resulting thickened and scarred arterial wall can induce local hypoxia by interrupting normal periluminal diffusion or by decreasing the transport of oxygen through the vasa vasorum.[4] Hypoxic changes in cellular metabolism that have been demonstrated in plaques may be responsible for the necrosis and inflammation of mature lesions.[41]

Lipid Hypothesis

The pivotal role of lipids or lipoproteins in the initiation and development of atherosclerosis is the basis for the lipid hypothesis. Such substances are seen to begin and maintain the early stages of the process.[89] Basic investigations have revealed that certain lipoproteins stimulate replication of smooth muscle cells before being metabolized into component lipids by intracellular enzymes. The validity of this hypothesis is strengthened by the demonstration of serum lipids and lipoproteins in the regions of developing plaques in amounts corresponding to the severity of the disease. In advanced lesions, the lipid accumulation is predominantly cholesterol, particularly in its esterified form. Distinct changes in arterial wall metabolism that may favor the production of certain cholesteryl esters have been documented in atherosclerosis. Although the quantity of these products of altered metabolism is small when compared with that of imbibed serum lipids and lipoproteins, these products are known to elicit the cellular responses seen in fibrous plaques.[2] The lipid theory thus considers that serum lipids—in particular, cholesterol and low-density lipoproteins—can both initiate and mature the lesions of arterial atherosclerosis.

Monoclonal Hypothesis

A different explanation for atherogenesis is offered by the monoclonal hypothesis. This theory views each arterial

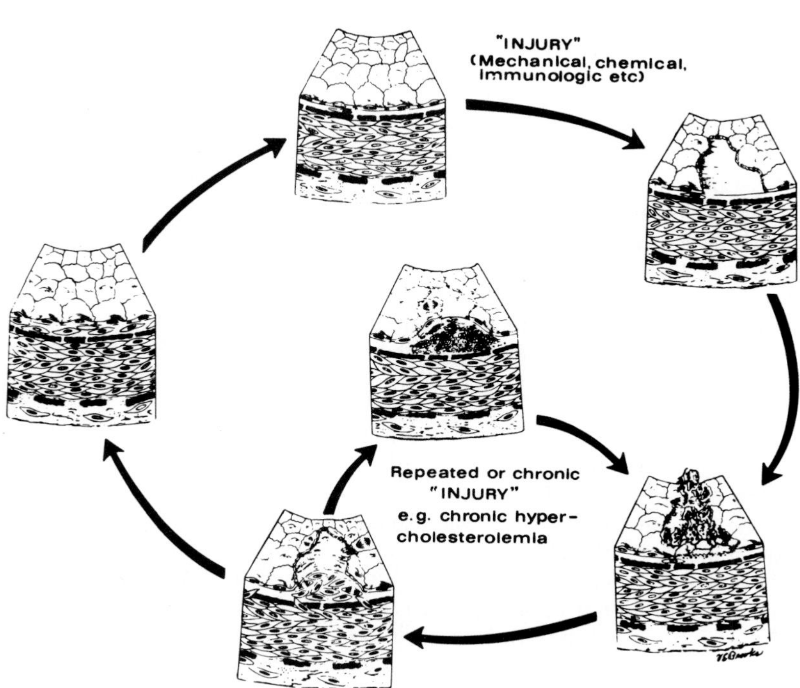

FIGURE 10–5. **Proposed description of the vascular cellular response to injury. Injury from any noxious stimulus leads to desquamation of endothelial cells. Platelets adhere to the denuded surface and release substances that stimulate proliferation of myointimal and medial smooth muscle cells. With no further injury, this process can resolve, leaving a slightly thickened intima lined with endothelium. On repeated injury, the proliferating smooth muscle cells undergo further degeneration and accumulate the intracellular and extracellular lipids and ground substance associated with mature atherosclerotic lesions. (From Ross R, Glomset JA: Pathogenesis of atherosclerosis. Reprinted with permission from The New England Journal of Medicine, 295:369, 420, 1976.)**

plaque as a benign tumor arising from a single smooth muscle cell. Proof for this concept is found in the monotypic enzyme pattern of plaque tissue from heterozygous individuals, as compared with the bimorphic values seen in undiseased artery wall.[11, 81] Factors that bring about smooth muscle cell transformation are considered mutagens, and progression of the replication occurs under conditions that stimulate cell proliferation. The maturing process—of fibrosis, necrosis, calcification, and thrombosis—is the same as that in other hypotheses.

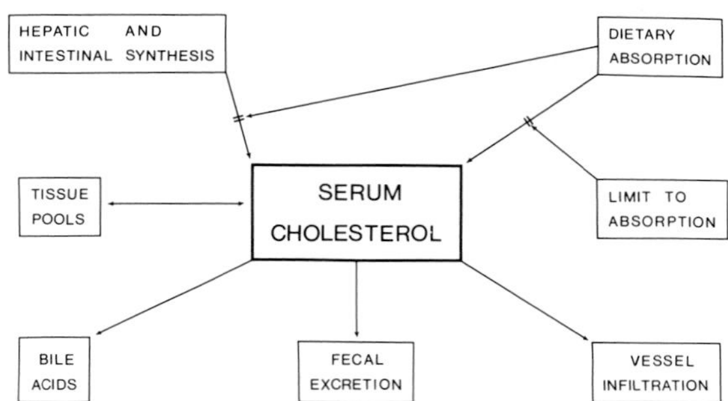

FIGURE 10–6. Features contributing to the level of serum cholesterol. The sources are endogenous synthesis in the liver and intestine, dietary absorption, and mobilization from the body stores. There is a limit to absorption, and elevated serum levels will inhibit hepatic synthesis. The circulating cholesterol can be excreted in the stool in a free or bile acid form, or it can be shunted into the tissue pools. As a low-density lipoprotein, serum cholesterol is found within normal arterial tissue. (From Fuchs JCA: Dietary and pharmacologic management of atherosclerosis. *In* Sabiston DC Jr, Spencer FC [eds]: Gibbon's Surgery of the Chest. 4th ed. Philadelphia, WB Saunders, 1983.)

THERAPY

The basis for nonoperative therapy for atherosclerosis lies in the risk factors found to be strongly associated with the disease. Many of the measures employed embody principles of good general medical care. Treatment programs involving cessation of cigarette smoking, control of hypertension, changes in patterns of activity and stress, weight loss, and the regulation of diabetes mellitus have been practiced for years. They produce major changes in lifestyle and require extensive follow-up periods for successful application. These approaches offer patients an improved sense of well-being and have been found to be beneficial by both epidemiologic surveys and prospective trials. Such basic medical treatment programs are beyond the scope of this chapter, and some are covered elsewhere in this text.

Three particular issues—lipids, platelets, and cigarette smoking—are pertinent to the course of atherosclerosis, and most treatment programs involve manipulation of these entities. Each of these topics is discussed in terms of background data, involvement in atherogenesis, indications for treatment, and therapeutic programs available for use. It is hoped this information will help surgeons to design practical treatment programs that will give patients the greatest chance to receive continued benefit from their vascular operations.

Lipids

Lipid Metabolism

Lipids are organic substances that are soluble only in certain nonaqueous solvents. Within tissue, they form the basic structure of membranes, act as storage or carrier agents of metabolic fuel, or convey biologic activity in the form of hormones or vitamins. The following brief description of the structure and metabolism of lipids is essential in order to understand the means available for antilipid therapy for atherosclerosis.

Cholesterol. A sterol-structured neutral lipid, cholesterol was first found to be a constituent of human tissue when it was extracted from gallstones. It was then identified in the circulating blood and was isolated from atherosclerotic plaques by Vogel in 1835. Because of this distribution, cholesterol has long been implicated in the process of atherosclerosis. Serum cholesterol has three possible origins (Fig. 10–6). It can be synthesized in the liver or intestine from acetate fragments. One of the enzymes essential for this reaction, 3-hydroxy-3-methylglutaryl coenzyme A (HMG CoA) reductase, is a rate-limiting factor influenced by serum constituents or drugs (Fig. 10–7). Cholesterol is readily absorbed from the diet, depending on levels of bile acids, dietary fat, and intestinal enzyme activity. In addition, cholesterol can be mobilized from tissue pools. Measured serum cholesterol thus depends on several interrelated and balanced metabolic pathways. In the serum, cholesterol usually exists as esters of fatty acids. The esterification reaction is mediated by the lecithin-cholesterol acyltransferase enzyme system (Fig. 10–8).[43] Although a similar pathway may be involved in tissues, direct acylation through fatty acyl coenzyme A is more likely.[1] This system favors the production of monounsaturated fatty acids, which have been found to be plentiful in atherosclerotic plaques.

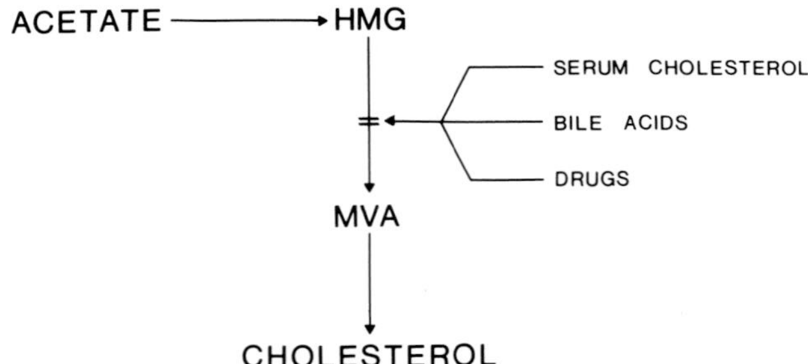

FIGURE 10–7. Pathway of endogenous cholesterol synthesis. Acetate is used to form beta-hydroxymethylglutarate (HMG). The enzyme system (hydroxymethylglutaryl coenzyme A reductase) involved in its conversion to mevalonate (MVA) is inhibited by elevated serum cholesterol levels and by certain pharmacologic agents. Inhibition at this early stage of synthesis avoids the build-up of toxic metabolites because other pathways are available to the HMG. Mevalonate fragments combine to form long-chain structures that are converted to sterols. (From Fuchs JCA: Dietary and pharmacologic management of atherosclerosis. *In* Sabiston DC Jr, Spencer FC [eds]: Gibbon's Surgery of the Chest. 4th ed. Philadelphia, WB Saunders, 1983.)

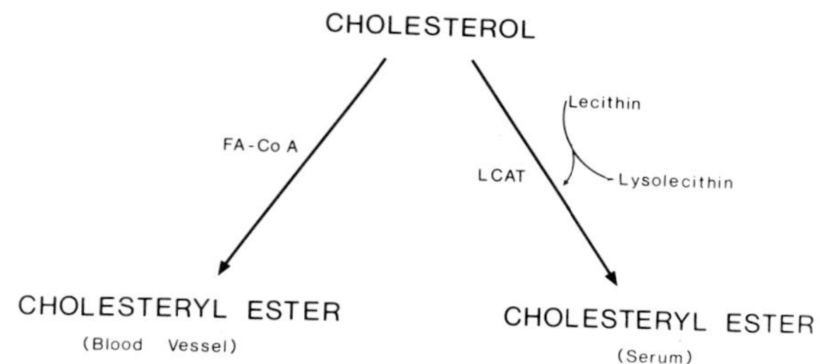

FIGURE 10–8. Cholesterol esterification. In the serum, the lecithin-cholesterol acyltransferase system (LCAT) mediates the transfer of the more unsaturated fatty acid chain from the position of lecithin to the hydroxy position of cholesterol. This system favors the production of cholesteryl linoleate, the major component of low-density lipoproteins. In tissues, another enzyme system utilizing coenzyme A (FA-CoA) mediate the acylation of cholesterol with the production of more saturated cholesteryl esters such as cholesteryl oleate. (From Fuchs JCA: Dietary and pharmacologic management of atherosclerosis. *In* Sabiston DC Jr, Spencer FC [eds]: Gibbon's Surgery of the Chest. 4th ed. Philadelphia, WB Saunders, 1983.)

Triglycerides. Triacyl esters of glycerol, triglycerides are basic units of energy storage in fat deposits that are synthesized by the liver, intestine, or adipose tissue. The free fatty acids for this reaction can be either created de novo in the liver, absorbed from the breakdown of dietary triglycerides, or arise from mobilization of storage pools of triglycerides.

Phospholipids. Phospholipids constitute another important group of lipids. The glycerophospholipids have a basic structure of glycerol with fatty acids esterified in positions 1 and 2 and a phosphoric acid at position 3. The latter is linked to various compounds such as choline, ethanolamine, or an alcohol to form components that are major constituents of organic membranes. Phosphatidylcholine, or lecithin, also plays an important part in the esterification of serum cholesterol, as shown in Figure 10–8. A very significant function of these polar substances is to facilitate the dispersion of insoluble lipids in the intestinal lumen or in the serum.

Because of their insolubility, the lipids just described do not exist as free entities in the serum. Instead, they are combined with polypeptides or apoproteins to form lipoproteins.[59] In human serum, these large lipoprotein complexes are categorized in four distinct groups (Fig. 10–9).

Chylomicrons. Triglyceride-rich conglomerates, chylomicrons are formed by the lipids absorbed following a meal. Their constituents are derived from exogenous diet and are transported to liver, blood vessels, or adipose tissue, where they are metabolized. This clearing process is mediated through lipoprotein lipases and can be accelerated by heparin. Such lipolytic enzyme activity exists in vascular endothelium and in the apoprotein components of some of the lipoproteins. Fragments of metabolized chylomicrons are taken up by the liver, where they may be combined with apoproteins to form triglyceride-rich very-low-density lipoprotein (VLDL) (Fig. 10–10).

Very-Low-Density Lipoproteins. Because the half-life of VLDLs far exceeds that of chylomicrons, an increase in these lipoproteins will produce prolonged hypertriglyceridemia. Carbohydrate ingestion, especially in the form of sucrose, stimulates this production, possibly through elevated levels of insulin.[37, 64] Fatty acid mobilization brought on by starvation or by stress-induced elevations of catecholamines will also increase their hepatic synthesis. In addition, ethanol ingestion brings about hypertriglyceridemia through a mechanism different from that of carbohydrate induction. Regulation of hepatic synthesis of VLDL

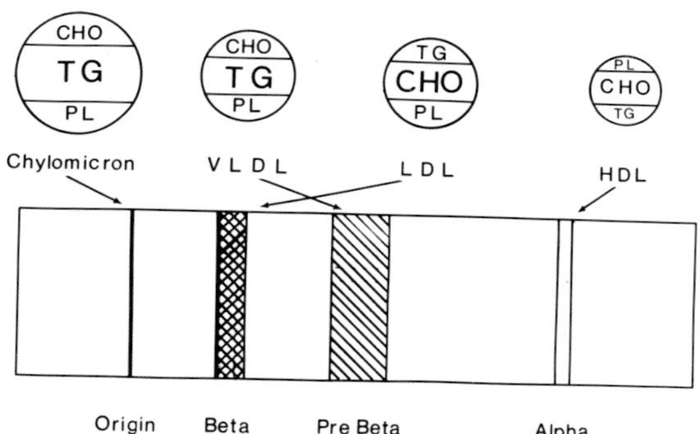

FIGURE 10–9. Lipoproteins. These entities are arranged in order of increasing density from left to right: chyomicrons, very-low-density lipoproteins (VLDL), low-density lipoproteins (LDL), and high-density lipoproteins (HDL). The lipid content (the predominant fraction is represented by larger letters) is made up of triglycerides (TG), cholesterol (CHO), and phospholipids (PL). When placed in an electromagnetic field, the chylomicrons remain at the origin. The low-density lipoproteins migrate in the area of beta-globulins and are called beta-lipoproteins. The very-low-density lipoproteins precede the beta and are named pre-beta lipoproteins. The high-density lipoproteins migrate in the zone of alpha-globulins and are called alpha-lipoproteins. (From Fuchs JCA: Dietary and pharmacologic management of atherosclerosis. *In* Sabiston DC Jr, Spencer FC [eds]: Gibbon's Surgery of the Chest. 4th ed. Philadelphia, WB Saunders, 1983.)

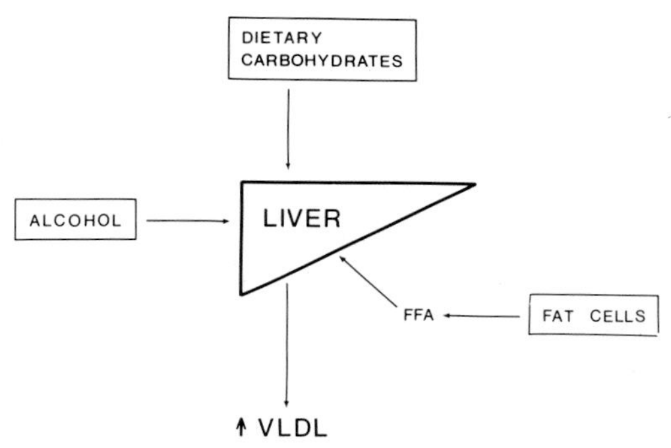

FIGURE 10–10. Lipoprotein metabolism. Very-low-density lipoprotein (VLDL) synthesized by the liver undergoes lipolysis by tissue lipases. The intermediate-density lipoprotein formed is predominantly transformed to low-density lipoprotein by further degradation of triglycerides. (A small portion of intermediate-density lipoprotein is cleared by the liver.) Cholesterol-rich low-density lipoprotein transports cholesterol into cells. Excess tissue cholesterol cannot be catabolized and is cleared by high-density lipoprotein and returned to the liver for further metabolism. (From Fuchs JCA: Dietary and pharmacologic management of atherosclerosis. *In* Sabiston DC Jr, Spencer FC [eds]: Gibbon's Surgery of the Chest. 4th ed. Philadelphia, WB Saunders, 1983.)

is thus a process subject to both endogenous and exogenous influences.

Intermediate-Density and Low-Density Lipoproteins. As they circulate, molecules of VLDL are hydrolyzed by lipases to form smaller, intermediate-density lipoproteins, as shown in Figure 10–10. A small portion of IDL is cleared by the liver, but most is further degraded to low-density lipoprotein (LDL).[93] Consisting largely of cholesteryl esters, LDL carries half to two thirds of the plasma cholesterol and has the important function of transporting this substance to peripheral tissues. Because of its small size, it appears to travel easily across the endothelium through microvascular pores. In addition, there are receptors on cell membranes to facilitate cellular entry. Absence of these receptors may lead to failure of inhibition of intracellular cholesterol synthesis or may decrease LDL catabolism, thus resulting in hyperlipidemia characterized by elevated levels of LDL and of intracellular cholesterol.[44]

High-Density Lipoproteins. Peripheral cells cannot catobolize cholesterol. Instead, this substance must be transported back to the liver for further metabolism through a mechanism that involves high-density lipoproteins (HDLs). These small complexes are half protein by weight. Originally found as discs, they enlarge and become spherical as they accumulate cholesteryl esters. Esterification of tissue cholesterol may be mediated by the apoprotein moiety of HDL, which has lecithin-cholesterol acyltransferase enzyme activity, as shown in Figure 10–8. This process of mobilization and accumulation of tissue cholesterol is thought to account for the inverse relation between the HDL cholesterol level and atherosclerosis.[49] Another possibility is that HDL may block uptake of LDL at tissue receptor sites.[21] Whatever the case, there is a strong negative association between HDL levels and the extent of atherosclerosis, and future therapy will probably involve agents or regimens that can increase this plasma lipoprotein.

Apoproteins. With increasing knowledge of apoprotein constituents, this topic appears more complicated than the simple scheme just presented. Each classification of lipoproteins can have up to several different apoproteins or protein moieties and is therefore a heterogenous collection rather than a distinct molecular entity. Epidemiologic review of the serum content of apolipoproteins shows that apolipoprotein B-100 is associated with an increased incidence of myocardial infarction, whereas apolipoproteins A-I and A-II are associated with a decreased risk of this event. Although these observations raise interesting concepts of the role of the protein content of lipoproteins, they really add little to the prognostic value of the simpler determinations of total and HDL cholesterol.[111]

Apoproteins have enzymatic activities, which may explain variable lipoprotein activity and metabolism. In addition, the apoproteins are not peculiar to particular lipoprotein groups but can be exchanged during stages of lipoprotein interconversion. Because of the importance of apoproteins in lipid metabolism, lipoproteins may someday be classified in terms of dominant apoprotein rather than of density or separation characteristics. Lipoprotein (a) is an example of such an entity. This subfraction of LDL appears structurally similar to standard LDL particles except for the presence of apoprotein (a) in addition to the apolipoprotein B-100 of LDL. Lipoprotein (a) in the serum has been linked to coronary artery disease, premature atherosclerosis, and degree of stenosis in autologous vein arterial bypass grafts.[113] The peculiar enzymatic or immunologic features of lipoprotein (a) may implicate this entity in the processes of thrombosis, cholesterol transport, or atherogenesis.

Currently, there are no ways known to regulate the levels of individual apoprotein fractions. For this reason, most antilipid therapy for atherosclerosis is designed to alter the distribution and balance of major lipoprotein fractions–VLDLs, LDLs, and HDLs. This approach can apply to normolipidemic individuals as well as to those with clinically recognized hyperlipidemia.

Appreciation of the role of lipoproteins in specific clinical situations has been a major advance in medical care. A significant contribution was made by Frederickson and coworkers, who classified abnormal lipoprotein patterns into types I to V on the basis of specific clinical presentations.[38] It is of particular interest that some types of lipoproteinemia are characterized by virulent atherosclerosis. With background knowledge of lipids and lipoproteins, a rational means of therapy can be designed to correct derangement in lipoprotein homeostasis and thereby possibly alter the progress of vascular disease.[65] Serum lipoprotein patterns can definitely be altered, and beneficial effects have been seen in established atherosclerotic lesions and in the prognosis of some patients with atherosclerosis.[14, 69]

A high incidence of atherosclerotic vascular disease is found in hyperlipoproteinemia types II, III, and IV.[18] A common denominator of these entities is high levels of LDL and high total cholesterol:HDL cholesterol ratios. Ordinarily, only types II and IV hyperlipoproteinemia are seen with frequency in routine vascular surgical patients. A discussion of the methods of correcting these metabolic defects and the results of therapeutic trials follows. As this therapy proves to be of value for hyperlipidemic populations, it may be applicable to patients without fully developed hyperlipidemias who are nevertheless at high risk for atherosclerosis.

Antilipid Diet Therapy

Dietary treatment requires a commitment of instructional time that may be unavailable to active surgeons. Still, basic advice can be given to each patient and provisions made for follow-up analysis after intensive instruction by a dietitian. If a program can be begun while a patient is hospitalized, the simultaneous presentation of dietary instructions with palatable, modified meals will enhance acceptance of these principles. Practical instructions and literature are available to help design and carry out a program of this nature.[34, 39]

Five features must be considered in selecting a diet to alter the factors associated with arterial atherosclerosis.

Calorie content is important, especially if obesity is present. This situation is common in patients who show high serum levels of VLDL, as in types III and IV hyperlipidemia. Increased serum levels of free fatty acids, from either excessive mobilization or decreased clearing, stimulate hepatic synthesis of VLDL. Loss of adipose tissue through caloric restriction and weight reduction will reverse these abnormal features and often results in a marked reduction of both adipose tissue and serum triglycerides.

Carbohydrate restriction, particularly of sucrose-rich sweet concentrates, will also reduce serum levels of VLDL.[57] Oral carbohydrates enhance the endogenous synthesis and transport of triglycerides through a mechanism related to glucose-insulin balance.[64] The fact that weight reduction usually accompanies carbohydrate restriction makes the independent value of this principle difficult to establish. Nonetheless, low carbohydrate intake is a basis of the diet therapy for types III and IV hyperlipidemia.

The contribution of dietary *cholesterol* to atherosclerosis is still an unsettled issue. However, serum cholesterol levels in humans can be changed by altering the oral intake of this substance, and values of serum cholesterol do indeed correlate with the harmful consequences of atherosclerosis.[6, 92] The complicating features of variable dietary absorption and feedback control of cholesterol synthesis enter into this relationship, however (see Fig. 10–6).[48] Whatever the degree of intestinal absorption in humans, dietary cholesterol above 300 mg/day appears to elevate the serum levels. Because the average American diet contains between 600 mg and 1 gm, restriction of cholesterol intake to 300 mg/day is usually recommended.

The ubiquitous correlation of dietary cholesterol and vascular disease is supported by the animal models of atherosclerosis, which usually rely on a large oral dose of cholesterol. Particularly convincing is the work in nonhuman primates in which a cholesterol-rich diet will produce atherosclerotic lesions that are reversible on return to a diet low in that substance.[8, 70] In humans, epidemiologic studies reaffirm that it is possible to control serum cholesterol with diet and that these values are definitely related to the course of atherosclerotic vascular disease.[74, 92]

Fat restriction was one of the earliest dietary maneuvers for the control of hyperlipidemia. The degree of saturation of the fatty acid chains of ingested triglycerides is as important as the amount of fat consumed. The average American diet has 40 per cent of its caloric content as fat, with a ratio of polyunsaturated:saturated fats of 1:2. Decrease of serum lipids and lipoproteins can be produced by both increasing the ratio of unsaturated:saturated fats and reducing the total intake of dietary fats.[12, 33, 100] It is generally agreed that the entire population over the age of 2 should reduce total fat consumption to 30 per cent of total daily caloric intake and should increase the polyunsaturated fat component of these lipids.[24] The mechanism whereby saturated fats elevate and unsaturated fats lower the serum cholesterol level may be related to the control of fecal excretion of sterols or to the balance between tissue and serum cholesterol levels.[23]

Alcohol ingestion can lead to elevated serum triglyceride levels. This may be the result of a direct stimulatory effect of ethanol on hepatic fatty acid synthesis and can occur with consumption within the range of social drinking. In this situation, alcohol may add extra unneeded calories that lead to obesity and hyperlipidemia. A new and interesting development is an appreciation of the positive correlation between ethanol consumption and serum HDL levels.[56] Studies have revealed this to be a dose-related phenomenon that occurs within the low and moderate ranges of daily alcohol consumption. This response may account for the beneficial or inverse relationship between daily moderate alcohol consumption and complications of atherosclerotic disease.[54]

Because these dietary alterations have potential for influencing the course of atherosclerosis, multiple prospective intervention trials and retrospective epidemiologic surveys have been undertaken to test the relation between diet and arterial disease.[95] The first major one, the National Diet Heart Study, was administered to a controlled, free-living population. This plan proved feasible, and the diet produced a 14 per cent reduction in serum cholesterol by lowering intake of saturated fats and cholesterol.[77] These principles have been applied on a large scale to groups of patients with existing atherosclerotic disease. Modifications of fat and cholesterol intake have succeeded in lowering the serum cholesterol and LDL values, usually in the range of 14 to 17 per cent.[66] Favorable results are also beginning to appear in the form of reduction of atherosclerotic events such as myocardial infarction and peripheral vascular complications.[31, 66, 75] More stringent dietary programs coupled with angiographic evaluation of atherosclerotic lesions have shown a beneficial effect in plaque evolution when serum lipoproteins have been favorably altered by diet.[9] Twenty-year follow-up of epidemiologic surveys strongly underscores the importance of dietary constituents and the value of modification in terms of coronary heart disease.[92, 99]

A safety question has arisen in that some epidemiologic surveys have found low serum cholesterol levels to be associated with increased noncoronary deaths, especially from bowel cancer.[79, 82] This association is considered tentative by experienced investigators.[47] The American Heart Association, however, feels secure in recommending a diet to lower serum cholesterol. Their "prudent" diet can be recommended to normolipidemic patients with atherosclerosis and is applicable to the population in general (Table 10–2).[5]

Patients with specific lipoprotein abnormalities require more intensive control of diet. Those with an elevated level of LDL, or *type II hyperlipidemia,* should practice a diet reduced in cholesterol and in which unsaturated fats are used to replace saturated animal fats. With this plan, the total serum cholesterol and LDL content can be reduced as much as 15 per cent.[33] The other common lipid disorder, that of elevated VLDL levels, or *type IV hyperlipidemia,* requires a basic treatment program consisting of weight loss and a reduction of the oral intake of carbohydrates and alcohol. As the weight returns to normal, calories can be supplied by the addition of polyunsaturated fats. With good patient compliance, this dietary regimen is very successful and is often the only therapy required.

Antilipid Drug Therapy

Diet therapy alone has consistently been found to have a limit in terms of lipid reduction. Maximal lowering of serum cholesterol and LDL levels has been in the range of 12 to 15 per cent.[33] The decision to begin drug therapy is made only after diet has failed to control serious, docu-

Table 10–2. Diet Factors in Atherosclerosis Therapy*

	Average	American Heart Association Recommendations
Cholesterol (mg/day)	>500	<300
Fats (per cent daily caloric intake)	40	30
Saturated fats (per cent daily caloric intake)	15	<10
Polyunsaturated fats (per cent daily caloric intake)	5	15
Polyunsaturated:saturated ratio	0.3	>1.5

From Fuchs JCA: Dietary and pharmacologic management of atherosclerosis. In *Sabiston DC Jr, Spencer FC (eds): Gibbon's Surgery of the Chest. 4th ed. Philadelphia, WB Saunders, 1983.*

**The composition of an average American diet as compared with the "prudent" diet of the American Heart Association.*

mented hyperlipidemia. Antilipidemic drugs should be limited to these situations, as serious toxic sequelae can occur with any pharmacologic agent.

For patients with high levels of LDL, or *type II hyperlipidemia,* the type of drug therapy depends on the degree of hypercholesterolemia. In severe cases, usually familial in origin, in which the serum cholesterol level is well above 300 mg/100 ml, a *bile acid–binding resin* is selected. These agents, either cholestyramine or colestipol, are nonabsorbable resins to which quaternary amine groups are attached. When these agents are taken orally, their charged sites are bound to chloride. Internally, the chloride exchanges with bile acids, which remain bound to the resin and are excreted in the stool. Interruption of the enterohepatic pathway stimulates bile acid synthesis from body cholesterol. Most patients experience a lowering of LDL levels to 20 to 25 per cent below the values achieved by diet alone.[96] Administered in a total daily dose of 16 to 20 gm, this drug is not absorbed from the gut and consequently has few systemic side effects. It is, however, unpalatable and can produce severe constipation and problems with adsorption of concurrently administered drugs.

Large-scale trials have evaluated the effect of bile acid–binding resins on the progression of disease and mortality of patients with coronary heart disease, hyperlipidemia, or both.[14, 63, 68, 69] In all situations, the drug was effective in lowering total serum cholesterol by 25 to 30 per cent. A more dramatic decrease of greater than 40 per cent was seen in LDL cholesterol, with a similar elevation in HDL cholesterol values. The latter changes corresponded dramatically with decreased incidence of nonfatal myocardial infarction and reduced progression of atherosclerotic lesions in these patients. The Lipid Research Clinics data confirmed these benefits in 3800 hypercholesterolemic patients randomly assigned to receive either resins or placebos over a 7-year period. When the drug trial was completed and the patients were followed up for another 6 years, the two groups became similar in profile, and no lasting benefits were seen in the drug-treated patients. Even though no statistically significant adverse effects of the resin therapy were detected, there was a modest increase in colorectal neoplasia and cholelithiasis in the resin-treated group.[110]

With lower levels of hypercholesterolemia, other drugs can be selected. *Niacin,* or *nicotinic acid,* is effective in lowering both VLDL and LDL levels, with serum reduction in the range of 20 per cent.[22] It appears to limit the mobilization of free fatty acids from adipose tissue, thereby reducing hepatic synthesis of VLDL. Lowering of serum cholesterol occurs through interference of the conversion of VLDL to LDL and decreased endogenous synthesis by inhibition of HMG CoA reductase (see Fig. 10–7). The side effects of this drug can be impressive. It produces sufficient gastrointestinal irritation to preclude its use in patients with peptic ulcer. Abnormalities in liver function are frequent, and prolonged use can result in histologic liver damage and cholangitis. Probably the most limiting feature of nicotinic acid is that, in the usual dosage of 3 to 6 gm/day, it causes unpleasant sensations of cutaneous flushing and itching that are so intense that patients are unwilling to continue its use. These responses can be minimized by gradual increase of daily doses to the therapeutic range. This agent is often given as a second drug with other agents to intensify the hypolipedemic response.[14]

Dextrothyroxine, the D-isomer of the naturally occurring hormone L-thyroxine, will lower the serum LDL level as much as 20 per cent in euthyroid patients. This drug may produce mild hyperthyroid symptoms that can be reduced with the use of beta-blocking agents. Because of the increased mortality rate in patients with previous myocardial infarction, this drug is contraindicated in patients with coronary artery disease and thereby has limited application in adult patients with diffuse atherosclerosis.[27] Dextrothyroxine appears to augment the catabolism and excretion of endogenous cholesterol.[94] The starting doses are 1 to 2 mg/day, with a gradual increase of 1 mg every 2 to 4 weeks until reduction of serum cholesterol is seen. The usual daily dosage selected is 4 to 8 mg.

A newer drug, *probucol,* appears to lower serum LDL levels through a mechanism that is not fully understood. It appears to have the undesirable side effect of reducing HDL cholesterol as well. This may contribute to the animal toxicity described below. Given in doses of 1 gm/day, this agent may inhibit the initial steps of cholesterol synthesis or enhance fecal sterol excretion. The significant cardiac toxicity seen in animals on markedly atherogenic diets suggests that this is not an innocuous drug. Its use is at present indicated in cases of mild hypercholesterolemia that are not responsive to diet or as an additional drug for more severe cholesterolemia.

A number of HMG CoA reductase inhibitors (see Fig. 10–7) have been approved for use as LDL cholesterol–lowering agents. The longest experience in humans is with the drug lovastatin, which has been found effective in lowering the LDL cholesterol almost 40 per cent while increasing the HDL cholesterol volume up to 13 per cent. This agent has been used in trials involving patients with very significant hypercholesterolemia, usually familial in origin, and in patients with moderate hypercholesterolemia.[104] The early studies are too small to evaluate the effects on coronary disease incidence and mortality; however, the lipoprotein changes would probably bring about favorable results. Because it interferes with cholesterol synthesis at an early stage, this drug is contraindicated in pregnancy. Potential complications of lenticular opacities and derangement of hepatic enzymes necessitate regular slit-lamp examinations and liver function studies. It is presently recommended only in patients with significant hypercholesterolemia that is unresponsive to diet therapy.

The other common lipid abnormality associated with atherosclerosis is *type IV hyperlipidemia,* with elevation of the serum level of VLDL. Although this disorder is often quite responsive to weight loss and diet, many situations remain in which drug therapy is useful. The agents most commonly selected are clofibrate and gemfibrozil. These drugs are markedly successful in reducing serum lipids, with triglyceride reduction of 50 per cent and cholesterol reduction of 20 per cent being reported. After oral ingestion, such drugs are well absorbed and are strongly bound to serum albumin. Serum free fatty acids decrease with clofibrate, possibly owing to inhibition of albumin anionic binding sites, and this can diminish synthesis of VLDL in the liver.[10] Release of albumin-bound thyroxine has also been suggested as the basis of the action of this drug. The cholesterol reduction is thought to be due to inhibition of the HMG CoA reductase in endogenous synthesis or to reduction of very-low-density to low-density transformation of lipoprotein. The final result of clofibrate therapy is a reduction of total body cholesterol. Some of this is produced through biliary excretion, and this may be responsible for the increased gallstone formation seen with its use.[29]

Given in a daily adult dose of 2 gm for clofibrate or 1.2 gm for gemfibrozil, these drugs have documented complications of gastrointestinal distress, skin rashes, muscle soreness, leukopenia, and genitourinary dysfunction. Coumarin-type anticoagulants are potentiated by these drugs and must usually be reduced in dosage when they are administered. Animal studies have found hepatic tumorogenicity with clofibrate, although this has not been a documented risk in human subjects. The large-scale population studies using clofibrate have raised sufficient problems to limit its use to patients with unresponsive and persistent hyperlipidemia. The chemical and pharmacologic similarity of gemfibrozil has raised concern about the use of this agent.

Clofibrate has been the study drug in two of the largest multi-center cooperative trials designed to assess the use of pharmacologic agents in long-term prevention of coronary heart disease.[25, 28] The Coronary Drug Project compared 3000 myocardial infarction patients receiving placebos with 1000 similar patients who were given clofibrate. No significant improvement in the number of subsequent myocardial infarction events was seen with this drug, even though there was a 10 per cent decrease in serum cholesterol and a 22 per cent reduction of triglycerides.[28] Drug-treated patients did show a higher incidence of cholelithiasis and biliary tract disease with its associated complications.[29]

The World Health Organization coordinated trial in three cities compared 5000 drug-treated healthy volunteers with 5000 volunteers receiving placebos. Both groups consisted of individuals whose serum cholesterol values were in the upper third of those who volunteered. Another 5000 individuals whose serum cholesterol values were in the lower third were given placebo and used as a second set of control subjects. After 5 years, the drug-treated subjects had a 9 per cent decrease in serum cholesterol and a 25 per cent decrease in nonfatal myocardial infarctions. The incidence of fatal infarctions was unchanged by clofibrate. The rate of ischemic heart disease remained low in the control group composed of those with initially lower serum cholesterol values. An alarming finding in the clofibrate-treated subjects was an increased death rate from noncardiovascular disease, half of which were malignant. This stimulated the Food and Drug Administration to recommend that such agents not be used for community-wide prevention of ischemic heart disease but rather be limited to patients with documented lipid disorders.

Platelets

Platelet Function

Platelets appear to play a role in the course of atherosclerotic vascular disease. The possible involvement of platelets in the initiation and progression of early atherosclerotic lesions has already been mentioned.[86] In addition, they are associated with accumulation of particulate material on the surface of arterial lesions. Such deposits can embolize, lead to subsequent thrombosis, or contribute to vasoconstriction. These blood particles thus appear to be important in the development of intra-arterial plaques as well as contributing to thromboembolic complications of mature lesions.

Normally platelets circulate as flat discs with a mean survival time of 9 or 10 days. When they encounter a thrombogenic surface, such as denuded endothelium, these particles adhere, release factors that stimulate further platelet aggregation, and lead to coagulation. Through the arachidonate pathways, platelets form thromboxane A_2, a substance that stimulates platelets adherence and intense vasospam. From the same metabolic precursors, endothelium synthesizes prostacyclin, which acts as a potent vasodilator and inhibits platelet aggregation. This substance may account for the antithrombotic qualities of endothelial cells.[76] Manipulation of platelet function offers the potential for control of atherogenesis as well as prevention of some of the acute complications arising in the course of clinical atherosclerosis. A discussion of the means to accomplish these goals and the results of preliminary trials follows. The actions and other therapeutic applications of these drugs are discussed in Chapter 17.

Antiplatelet Drug Therapy

Antiplatelet agents are used primarily to prevent thromboembolic complications from existing arterial lesions.[78] They may be of some benefit in terms of altering the process of atherogenesis if the mechanisms already discussed are operable.[86] Although there is epidemiologic support for the prophylactic value of these drugs, there are insufficient data to recommend them for routine prevention of atherosclerosis.[16] On the other hand, multiple clinical trials have produced information concerning their value in the secondary prevention of cardiovascular events, and one study has suggested that antiplatelet agents will decrease the progression of atherosclerotic lesions in patients with demonstrated lower extremity occlusive disease.[55]

Platelet function can be altered through several means. Primary among these is the inhibition of arachidonate metabolism in order to limit thromboxane A_2 synthesis by platelets. *Aspirin* will irreversibly acetylate platelet cyclooxygenase and thereby decrease the endoperoxides available for conversion to thromboxane A_2.[19] Because endoperoxides are also necessary for endothelial production of the potent antiaggregant prostacycline, an appropriate dose of aspirin must be selected so as not to inhibit endothelial cyclooxygenase. A total dose of 600 to 1200 mg/day is generally given, and this drug can be administered once or twice a day.

Sulfinpyrazone at a total daily dose of 800 mg appears to produce *reversible* inhibition of cyclooxygenase and therefore requires a more frequent dosing schedule. Despite the inconvenience of the multiple daily doses, this agent lacks some of the undesirable side effects of aspirin and does appear to have more favorable effects on platelet survival and endothelial stability.[20, 51]

Dipyridamole inhibits phosphodiesterase and may thereby tend to increase platelet content of cyclic adenosine monophosphate. Increased cyclic adenosine monophosphate appears to stabilize platelets and will decrease their adhesion, aggregation, and release of granules. Such changes in platelet composition have not been conclusively demonstrated, but theoretically this drug could limit the induction of smooth muscle cell replication during atherogenesis, as well as prevent thromboembolic complications from intravascular lesions.[36] The total daily dose is usually 75 to 300 mg (administered three to four times a day). Because its activity differs from that of aspirin, dipyridamole is frequently given in conjunction with that drug to achieve greater interference with platelet function.

Numerous clinical trials have been performed on patients with coronary artery and cerebrovascular disease, in whom antiplatelet agents offer the possibility of relief from severe thromboembolic complications. Among aspirin-treated patients with previous myocardial infarctions, there is a trend toward a reduced mortality rate and a slightly significant reduction of recurrent nonfatal infarctions.[42] The small benefit seen with the drug and the incidence of complications have discouraged its routine use in patients surviving myocardial infarction.[7] Concomitant administration of dipyridamole did not significantly change the results achieved with aspirin alone. Sulfinpyrazone was used as a single drug and appeared to be related to a significant reduction of the risk of sudden death during the initial 6 months following myocardial infarction.[8] The time course of these benefits suggests that these properties may arise from a mechanism of action other than antiplatelet activity.

Studies of patients with transient ischemic attacks and carotid artery disease have shown the use of aspirin to be beneficial.[35] In one trial, there appeared to be preferential protection from further stroke in the men using this drug.[20] These data are consistent, and they suggest that the use of aspirin will reduce the risk of further ischemic attacks and the incidence of subsequent stroke.[80] These benefits are found whether aspirin is used as primary medical therapy or as a postendarterectomy adjuvant.

Large-scale studies have examined the role of low-dose aspirin as prophylaxis for coronary and peripheral artery atherosclerosis.[106, 107, 112] These protocols have involved ostensibly normal subjects as well as patients with atherosclerosis or diabetes. The initial results support the benefit of such regimens in terms of a decreased incidence of myocardial infarction and peripheral arterial surgery, but not in terms of a reduction in total cardiovascular death or in the development of new peripheral arterial symptoms. It seems, therefore, that this drug influences the thromboembolic complications of atherosclerosis, rather than the actual progression of the arterial disease. For the present, low-dose aspirin seems a reasonable prophylaxis in those at risk for cardiovascular disease.

Cigarette Smoking

Reference has been made to the strong incrimination of cigarette smoking in the development of atherosclerosis.[30, 83] Smoking appears to be the greatest single risk factor for the development of atherosclerotic peripheral vascular disease. It also augments the progression of disease with the other risk factors. Symptoms from peripheral vascular occlusive disease and death from abdominal aortic aneurysm are both increased dramatically by cigarette smoking.[109] Although the exact mechanism of the detrimental effects of cigarette smoking is unknown, it probably involves features of the effects of carbon monoxide or nicotine on vessel walls, alterations in blood components, or changes in serum lipids. There are equally cogent data to support the value of discontinuing tobacco consumption by patients with arterial occlusive disease.[61] Perhaps even more relevant are the studies showing that the long-term benefits of peripheral vascular reconstructive procedures vary with the ability of the patient to stop smoking. Patency of arterial prostheses is definitely enhanced when patients can control this habit.[85]

The evidence is clear—every patient with atherosclerotic arterial disease should stop smoking! Success in breaking this addiction often requires a team approach involving patient, family, and psychological counseling. Individual determination to stop smoking is probably most critical for success in this effort. This can be supported by behavior modification programs, nicotine replacement therapy, group efforts toward smoking cessation, or multiple-intervention trials. Although relapse rates may be high, this risk factor is so critical that it must be attacked over and over again until success is achieved.

SUMMARY

Many of the major issues in the medical management of atherosclerosis have yet to be firmly settled. Certainly, the management of possible contributors such as hypertension, diabetes, and cigarette smoking is to be recommended.

Some of the more controversial points, however, still await the results of ongoing and future clinical trials. In the meantime, the results from past studies allow the safe recommendation of diet modification to the general population and suggest the use of drugs in specific cases of lipidemia or in patients at risk from the thromboembolic complications of vascular disease. If more physicians follow this lead and advise appropriate treatment, the value of this therapeutic rationale will become obvious. The importance of such information is so great as to justify the time and effort required for the total care of patients with atherosclerotic vascular disease.

References

1. Abdulla YH, Adams CWM, Bayliss OB: The location of lecithin: Cholesterol transacylase activity in the atherosclerotic arterial wall. J Atheroscler Res 10:229, 1969.
2. Abdulla YH, Adams CWM, Morgan RS: Connective-tissue reactions to implantation of purified sterol, sterol esters, phosphoglycerides, glycerides and free fatty acids. J Pathol Bacteriol 94:63, 1967.
3. Adams CWM: Tissue changes and lipid entry in developing atheroma. *In* Atherogenesis: Initiating Factors. New York, Association of Scientific Publishers, 1973.
4. Adams CWM, Bayliss OB: The relationship between diffuse intimal thickening, medial enzyme failure, and intimal lipid deposition in various human arteries. J Atheroscler Res 10:327, 1969.
5. American Heart Association Committee Report: Diet and coronary heart disease. Circulation 58:762A, 1978.
6. Anderson KM, Castelli WP, Levy D: Cholesterol and mortality. JAMA 257:2176, 1987.
7. Anturane Reinfarction Trial Research Group: Sulfinpyrazone in the prevention of sudden death after myocardial infarction. N Engl J Med 302:250, 1980.
8. Armstrong ML, Warner ED, Conner WE: Regression of coronary atherosclerosis in rhesus monkeys. Circ Res 27:59, 1970.
9. Arntzenius AC, Kromhont D, Barth JD, et al: Diet, lipoproteins, and the progression of coronary atherosclerosis—The Leiden Intervention Trial. N Engl J Med 312:805, 1985.
10. Barrett AM, Thorp JM: Studies on the mode of action of clofibrate. Br J Pharmacol Chemother 32:381, 1968.
11. Benditt EP: Implications of the monoclonal character of human atherosclerotic plaques. Am J Pathol 86:693, 1977.
12. Bierenbaum MI, Fleischman AI, Raichelson RI, et al: Ten-year experience of modified-fat diets on younger men with coronary heart disease. Lancet 1:1404, 1973.
13. Blankenhorn DH: Will atheroma regress with diet and exercise? Am J Surg 141:644, 1981.
14. Blankenhorn DH, Nessim SA, Johnson RL, et al: Beneficial effects of combined colestipol-niacin therapy on coronary atherosclerosis and coronary venous bypass grafts. JAMA 257:3222, 1987.
15. Bomberger RA, Zarins CK, Glagov S: Subarterial stenosis enhances distal atherosclerosis. J Surg Res 30:205, 1981.
16. Boston Collaborative Drug Surveillance Group: Regular aspirin intake and acute myocardial infarction. Br Med J 1:440, 1974.
17. Bourassal MG, Goulet C, Lesperance J: Progression of coronary arterial disease after aortocoronary bypass grafts. Circulation 47/48(Suppl 3):127, 1973.
18. Brown DF, Daudiss K: Hyperlipoproteinemia prevalance in a free-living population in Albany, New York. Circulation 47:558, 1973.
19. Burch JW, Stanford N, Majeruo PW: Inhibition of platelet prostaglandin synthetase by oral aspirin. J Clin Invest 61:314, 1978.
20. Canadian Cooperative Study Groups: A randomized trial of aspirin and sulfinpyrazone in threatened stroke. N Engl J Med 299:53, 1978.
21. Carew TE, Koschinsky T, Hayes SB, et al: A mechanism by which high-density lipoproteins may slow the atherogenic process. Lancet 1:1315, 1976.
22. Committee on Nutrition: Childhood diet and coronary heart disease. Pediatrics 49:305, 1972.
23. Connor WE, Connor SL: Dietary factors in the treatment of hyperlipidemic disorders. *In* Casdorph H (ed): Treatment of Hyperlipidemic States. Springfield, IL, Charles C Thomas, 1971.
24. Consensus Conference—Lowering Blood Cholesterol to Prevent Heart Disease. JAMA 253:2080, 1985.
25. Cooperative trial in the primary prevention of ischemic heart disease using clofibrate. Br Heart J 40:1069, 1978.
26. Cornfield J: Joint dependence of risk of coronary heart disease on serum cholesterol and systolic blood pressure: A discriminant function analysis. Fed Proc 21(Suppl 2):58, 1962.
27. Coronary Drug Project: Findings leading to further modification of its protocol with respect to dextrothyroxine. JAMA 220:996, 1972.
28. Coronary Drug Project: Clofibrate and niacin in coronary heart disease. JAMA 231:306, 1975.
29. Coronary Drug Project Research Group: Gallbladder disease or a side effect of drugs influencing lipid metabolism. N Engl J Med 296:1185, 1977.
30. Couch N: On the arterial consequences of smoking. J Vasc Surg 3:807, 1986.
31. Dayton S, Pearce ML: Prevention of coronary heart disease and other complications of atherosclerosis by modified diet. Am J Med 46:751, 1969.
32. DePalma RG, Koletsky S, Bellon EM, et al: Failure of regression of atherosclerosis in dogs with moderate cholesterolemia. Atherosclerosis 27:297, 1977.
33. Ernst N, Fisher M, Bowen P, et al: Changes in plasma lipids and lipoproteins after a modified fat diet. Lancet 2:111, 1980.
34. Eshleman R, Soderquist K (eds): The American Heart Association Cookbook. New York, David McKay, 1973.
35. Fields WS, Lemak NA, Frankowski RF, et al: Controlled trial of aspirin in cerebral ischemia. Circulation 62(V):90, 1980.
36. Fitzgerald GA: Dipyridamole. N Engl J Med 316:1247, 1987.
37. Ford S Jr, Bozian RC, Knowles HC Jr: Interaction of obesity, insulin and glucose levels in hypertriglyceridemia. Clin Res 15:428, 1967.
38. Frederickson DS, Levy RI, Lees RS: Fat transport in lipoproteins—An integrated approach to mechanisms and disorders. N Engl J Med 276:34, 94, 148, 215, 273, 1967.
39. Frederickson DS, Levy RI, Jones E, et al: The Dietary Management of Hyperlipoproteinemia: A Handbook for Physicians. Washington, DC, US Government Printing Office, 1970.
40. Fry DL: Hemodynamic forces in atherosclerosis. *In* Steinberg P (ed): Cerebrovascular Disease, Tenth Princeton Conference. New York, Raven Press, 1976.
41. Gainer JL, Chisholm GM III: Oxygen diffusion and atherosclerosis. Atherosclerosis 19:135, 1974.
42. Genton E: A perspective on platelet-suppressant drug treatment in coronary artery and cerebrovascular disease. Circulation 62(Suppl VIII):21, 1980.
43. Glomset JA: The plasma lecithin: Cholesterol acyltransferase reaction. J Lipid Res 9:155, 1968.
44. Goldstein JL, Brown MS: The low density lipoprotein pathway and its relation to atherosclerosis. Annu Rev Biochem 46:897, 1977.
45. Gordon T, Castelli WP, Hjortland MC, et al: Predicting coronary heart disease in middle-aged and older persons. JAMA 238:497, 1977.
46. Griffith LSC, Achuff SC, Conti CR, et al: Changes in intrinsic coronary circulation and segmental ventricular motion after saphenous-vein coronary bypass graft surgery. N Engl J Med 288:589, 1973.
47. Grundy SM: The relationship between low cholesterol levels and cancer symptoms: Nutrition and heart disease. The 1981 Perspective, New York City, 6/17/81.
48. Grundy SM, Ahrens EH Jr, Davignon J: The interaction of cholesterol absorption and cholesterol synthesis in man. J Lipid Res 10:304, 1969.
49. Hamel RJ: High density lipoproteins, cholesterol transport and coronary heart disease. Circulation 60:1, 1979.
50. Hammond EC, Garfinkel L: Coronary heart disease, stroke and aortic aneurysm—Factors in the etiology. Arch Environ Health 19:167, 1969.
51. Harker L, Wall RT, Harlan JM, et al: Sulfinpyrazone prevention of homocysteine-induced endothelial cell injury and arteriosclerosis. Clin Res 26:554A, 1978.
52. Henahan J: Regression of atherosclerosis: Preliminary but encouraging news. JAMA 246:2309, 1981.
53. Henderson RR, Rowe GG: The progression of coronary atherosclerotic disease as assessed by cinecoronary arteriography. Am Heart J 86:165, 1973.
54. Hennekens CH, Willett W, Rosner B, et al: Effects of beer, wine, and liquor in coronary deaths. JAMA 242:1973, 1979.

55. Hess H, Mietaschik A, Deischel G: Drug-induced inhibition of platelet function delays progression of peripheral occlusive arterial disease. Lancet 1:415, 1985.
56. Hulley SB, Gordon S: Alcohol and high-density lipoprotein cholesterol: Causal inference from diverse study designs. Circulation 64(Suppl III):57, 1981.
57. Hulley SB, Wilson WS, Burrows MI, et al: Lipid and lipoprotein response of hypertriglyceridemic out-patients to a low carbohydrate modification of the AHA fat controlled diet. Lancet 2:551, 1972.
58. Imparato AM, Bracco A, Kim GE, et al: Intimal and neointimal fibrous proliferation causing failure of arterial reconstructions. Surgery 72:1007, 1972.
59. Jackson RL, Morrisett JD, Gotto AM Jr: Lipoprotein structure and metabolism. Physiol Rev 56:259, 1976.
60. Kannel WB, Dawber TR, Skinner JJ, et al: Epidemiological aspects of intermittent claudication—The Framingham study. Circulation 32(Suppl 2):21, 1965.
61. Kannel WB, Thom TJ: Declining cardiovascular mortality. Circulation 70:331, 1984.
62. Keys A: Seven Countries, a Multivariate Analysis of Death and Coronary Heart Disease. Cambridge, MA, Harvard University Press, 1980.
63. Kuo PT, Hayase K, Kosis JB, et al: Use of combined diet and colestipol in long-term (7–7½ years) treatment of patients with type II hyperlipidemia. Circulation 59:199, 1979.
64. Lees RS, Frederickson DS: Carbohydrate induction of hyperlipidemia in normal man. Circ Res 13:327, 1965.
65. Lees RS, Wilson DE: The treatment of hyperlipidemia. N Engl J Med 284:186, 1971.
66. Leren P: The Oslo diet-heart study. Circulation 42:935, 1970.
67. Levy RI: Declining mortality in coronary heart disease. Arteriosclerosis 1:312, 1981.
68. Levy RI, Brenskie JF, Epstein SE, et al: The influence of changes in lipid values induced by cholestyramine and diet on progression of coronary artery disease: Results of the NHL BI Type II Coronary Intervention Study. Circulation 69:325, 1984.
69. Lipid Research Clinics Program: The Lipid Research Clinics coronary primary prevention trial results. I. Reduction in the incidence of coronary heart disease. JAMA 251:351, 1984.
70. Malinow MR: Atherosclerosis: Regression in nonhuman primates. Circ Res 46:311, 1980.
71. Malinow MR, McLaughlin P, McNulty WP, et al: Treatment of established atherosclerosis during cholesterol feeding in monkeys. Atherosclerosis 31:185, 1978.
72. McCann RL, Larson RM, Mitchener JS, et al: Intimal thickening and hyperlipidemia in experimental primate vascular autografts. Ann Surg 189:62, 1979.
73. McCullagh KG, Ehrhart LA: Increased arterial collagen synthesis in experimental canine atherosclerosis. Atherosclerosis 19:13, 1974.
74. McGill HC Jr: The relationship of dietary cholesterol to serum cholesterol concentration and to atherosclerosis in man. Am J Clin Nutr 32:2664, 1979.
75. Miettinen M, Turpeinen O, Karvonen MJ, et al: Effect of cholesterol-lowering diet on mortality from coronary heart disease and other causes—a twelve year clinical trial in men and women. Lancet 2:835, 1972.
76. Moncada S, Gryglewski R, Bunting S, et al: An enzyme isolated from arteries transforms prostaglandin endoperoxides to an unstable substance that inhibits platelet aggregation. Nature 263:663, 1976.
77. National Diet Heart Study Research Group: The National Diet Heart Study final report. Circulation 37(Suppl 1):26, 1968.
78. Packham MA, Mustard JF: Pharmacology of platelet-affecting drugs. Circulation 62(Suppl V):26, 1980.
79. Pearce ML, Dayton S: Incidence of cancer in men on a diet high in polyunsaturated fat. Lancet 1:464, 1971.
80. Persantine Aspirin Trial in Cerebral Ischemia. Part II. End-point results. Stroke 16:406, 1985.
81. Person TA, Kramer EC, Solez K, et al: The human atherosclerotic plaque. Am J Pathol 86:657, 1977.
82. Peterson B, Trell E, Sternby NH: Low cholesterol level as risk factor for noncoronary death in middle-aged men. JAMA 245:2056, 1981.
83. Pooling Project Research Group: Relationship of blood pressure, serum cholesterol, smoking habit, relative weight and EKG abnormalities to incidence of major coronary events. J Chronic Dis 31:201, 1978.
84. Rafflenbeul W, Smith LR, Rogers WJ, et al: Quantitative coronary arteriography: Coronary anatomy of patients with unstable angina pectoris reexamined 1 year after optimal medical therapy. Am J Cardiol 43:699, 1979.
85. Robicsek F, Daugherty HK, Mullen DC, et al: The effect of continued cigarette smoking on the patency of synthetic vascular grafts in Leriche syndrome. J Thorac Cardiovasc Surg 70:107, 1975.
86. Ross R: Arteriosclerosis: A problem of the biology of arterial wall cells and their interactions with blood components. Arteriosclerosis 1:293, 1981.
87. Ross R: Pathogenesis of atherosclerosis—An update. N Engl J Med 314:488, 1986.
88. Ross R, Glomset JA: Pathogenesis of atherosclerosis. N Engl J Med 295:369, 420, 1976.
89. Ross R, Harker L: Hyperlipidemia and atherosclerosis. Science 193:1094, 1976.
90. Ross R, Vogel A: The platelet derived growth factor. Cell 14:203, 1978.
91. Schwartz SM, Gajdusek CM, Selden SC III: Vascular wall growth control: The role of endothelium. Arteriosclerosis 1:107, 1981.
92. Shebelle RB, Shyrock AM, Paul O, et al: Diet serum cholesterol and death from coronary heart disease. N Engl J Med 304:65, 1981.
93. Sigurdsson G, Nicole A, Lewis B: Conversion of very low density lipoprotein to low density lipoprotein. J Clin Invest 56:1481, 1975.
94. Simons LA, Myant NB: The effect of D-thyroxine on the metabolism of cholesterol in familial hyperbetalipoproteinemia. Atherosclerosis 19:103, 1974.
95. Stamler J: Population studies. *In* Levy R, Rifkind B, Dennis B, et al (eds): Nutrition, Lipids and Coronary Heart Disease. New York, Raven Press, 1979.
96. Steinbert D, Grundy SM: Management of hyperlipidemia—Diet and drugs. Arch Surg 113:55, 1978.
97. Stern MP: Ischemic heart disease: An epidemic on the wane? Am J Surg 141:646, 1981.
98. Strong JP, Guzman MA: Decrease in coronary atherosclerosis in New Orleans. Lab Invest 43:297, 1980.
99. Turpeinen O: Effects of cholesterol-lowering diet on mortality from coronary heart disease and other causes. Circulation 59:1, 1979.
100. Wilson WS, Hulley SB, Burrows MI, Nichaman MZ: Several lipid and lipoprotein responses to the American Heart Association fat controlled diet. Am J Med 51:491, 1971.
101. Wissler RW: The arterial medial cell smooth muscle or multifunctional mesenchyme. J Atheroscler Res 8:201, 1968.
102. Wright IS, Frederickson DT: Atherosclerosis and epidemiology study groups: Primary prevention of atherosclerotic disease. *In* Cardiovascular Diseases: Guidelines for Prevention and Care. Washington, DC, US Government Printing Office, 1973.
103. Blankenhorn DH, Kramsch DM: Reversal of atherosis and sclerosis. Circulation 79:1, 1989.
104. Bradford RH, Shear CL, Dujovne C, et al: Expanded clinical evaluation of lovastatin (EXCEL) study results. I. Efficacy in modifying plasma lipoproteins and adverse event profile in 8,245 patients with moderate hypercholesterolemia. Arch Intern Med 151:43, 1991.
105. Brown G, Albers JJ, Fisher LD, et al: Regression of coronary artery disease as a result of intensive lipid-lowering therapy in men with high levels of apolipoprotein B. N Engl J Med 323:1289, 1990.
106. ETDRS Investigators: Aspirin effects on mortality and morbidity in patients with diabetes mellitus. JAMA 268:1292, 1992.
107. Goldhaber SZ, Manson JE, Stampfer MJ, et al: Low-dose aspirin and subsequent peripheral arterial surgery in the Physicians' Health Study. Lancet 340:143, 1992.
108. Gotto AM Jr, LaRosa JC, Hunninglake D, et al: The cholesterol facts. A summary of the evidence relating dietary fats, serum cholesterol and coronary heart disease. Circulation 81:1721, 1990.
109. Krupski WC, Rapp JH: Smoking and atherosclerosis. Perspect Vasc Surg 1:103, 1988.
110. The Lipid Research Clinics coronary primary prevention trial: Results of 6 years of post trial follow-up. Arch Intern Med 152:1399, 1992.
111. Stampfer MJ, Sacks FM, Simonetta S, et al: A prospective study of cholesterol, apolipoproteins and the risk of myocardial infarction. N Engl J Med 325:373, 1991.
112. Steering Committee of the Physicians' Health Study Research Group: Final report on the aspirin component of the ongoing physicians' health study. N Engl J Med 321:129, 1989.
113. Valentine RJ: Lipoprotein (a): A new risk factor for vascular disease. Perspect Vasc Surg 5(2):84, 1992.

11

Buerger's Disease (Thromboangiitis Obliterans)

Shigehiko Shionoya, M.D.

• • •

Buerger's disease (thromboangiitis obliterans) is a disease of misconceptions. When he called it "endarteritis obliterans" in 1878, Winiwarter indicated his belief that the essential nature of the vascular lesions leading to what was characterized as "presenile spontaneous gangrene" was a proliferation of intimal cells.[40] In 1908, Buerger reported that the disease was an inflammation of the artery resulting in a cellular type of thrombosis. He concluded, "Taking the true nature of the lesion into consideration, I would suggest that the names 'endarteritis obliterans' and 'arteriosclerotic gangrene' be discarded . . . and that we adopt the term 'obliterating thromboangiitis' of the lower extremities when we wish to speak of the disease under discussion."[6] However, the crucial words "of the disease under discussion" came to be ignored. Buerger's advice that the term "arteriosclerotic gangrene" be abandoned was followed, but out of its intended context, with the result that *all* cases of lower extremity gangrene at any age came to be diagnosed as thromboangiitis obliterans.[11]

Even worse, the disease became defined primarily by pathohistologic criteria and its characteristic clinical profiles were disregarded. Furthermore, clinicians and pathologists tended to stretch the concept of the disease so that "thromboangiitis obliterans" soon bore little resemblance to the original "presenile spontaneous gangrene." After World War II, skepticism about this overdiagnosed and ill-defined disease entity arose. For example, Wessler and associates claimed that the disease described by Buerger was indistinguishable from atherosclerosis, systemic embolization, or idiopathic peripheral arterial thrombosis.[39] However, controversy regarding the existence of the disease has dwindled, and there is abundant proof of the existence of this peculiar form of occlusive disease afflicting the peripheral arteries of young smokers. As the specificity of the disease is derived from its clinical characteristics, "Buerger's disease" is a better name than "thromboangiitis obliterans," which tends to be associated with impractical histopathologic criteria.

EPIDEMIOLOGY

Although Buerger's disease affects all races, it is more prevalent in the Middle and Far East than in Europe and the United States. At the Mayo Clinic, the annual patient registration almost doubled, from 119,337 in 1949 to 204,000 in 1978. However, the rate of patients with the diagnosis of Buerger's disease steadily declined, from 104 per 100,000 patients registered in 1949 to 10 per 100,000 patients registered in 1978.[20] At the International Symposium on Buerger's disease in Bad Gastein, Austria, in 1986, Cachovan reported the rate of Buerger's disease in patients with chronic arterial occlusive disease in Europe and other countries: 1 to 3 per cent in Switzerland, 0.5 to 5 per cent in West Germany, 1.2 to 5.6 per cent in France, 4 per cent in Belgium, 0.5 per cent in Italy, 0.25 per cent in the United Kingdom, 3.3 per cent in Poland, 6.7 per cent in East Germany, 11.5 per cent in Czechoslovakia, 39 per cent in Yugoslavia, 80 per cent in Israel (Ashkenazim), 45 to 63 per cent in India, and 16 to 66 per cent in Korea and Japan.[8]

These rates are derived from patients presenting for care at specialized institutions rather than from the population as a whole. In this regard, in 1976, the Buerger's Disease Research Committee of the Ministry of Health and Welfare of Japan studied 3034 patients with the disease from all over Japan (2930 men; 104 women) and estimated its incidence to be about 5 per 100,000 population.[17] In 1986, the Epidemiology of Intractable Diseases Research Committee of the Ministry of Health and Welfare of Japan estimated the number of patients with the disease in Japan during the previous year to be 8858, or about 5 per 100,000 population.[24] Although frequent clinical reports on Buerger's disease come from India, Indonesia, and Israel, its incidence in these countries is as yet unknown because no nationwide epidemiologic studies have been carried out. Finally, the number of new patients with Buerger's disease in Japan seems to be decreasing, but the number of patients under the care of a physician remains almost unchanged because of recurrence. At the author's institution, the current ratio of new patients with Buerger's disease:new patients with arteriosclerosis obliterans is about 1:3, so that Buerger's disease is still quite prevalent.

ETIOLOGY

Although the cause of Buerger's disease is not yet known, smoking is very closely related to exacerbations and remissions of the disease. In general, if the patient absolutely abandons smoking, the natural history will invariably be benign, but if smoking continues, any treatment will ultimately prove futile and the course will progressively worsen. Essentially all patients with Buerger's disease are smokers, and *true nonsmokers* should never develop the disease, although the influence of passive smoking on the cardiovascular system should be taken seriously.[9] Cotinine, the major metabolite of nicotine, is a sensitive marker for measuring levels of active smoking and the exposure of nonsmokers to tobacco smoke because it has a relatively long half-life, and cotinine levels can be determined by noninvasive means in urine.[12] In a study by Matsushita and colleagues, those with urinary cotinine levels above 50 ng/mg creatinine were considered to be active smokers; those with levels between 10 and 50 ng/mg creatinine, passive smokers; and those with levels below 10 ng/mg creatinine, nonsmokers who experienced no noticeable passive smoking.[22] A cooperative epidemiologic and clinical study that is based on the long-term and timely evaluation of the effect on health of involuntary exposure to tobacco smoke may provide the evidence to support the hypothesis that passive smoking can influence the occurrence of Buerger's disease and the worsening of the disease process. Because the incidence is very low, even among heavy smokers, an immunopathogenesis for the disease has been considered probable. Evidence of this includes increases in complement factor C4, antielastin,[5] and anticollagen antibody; cellular sensitivity to human type I or type III collagen;[1] and organ-specific autoantibodies (IgM, IgG, and IgA) and C3 component in the diseased vessels[13] in patients with Buerger's disease. HLA analysis in patients with Buerger's disease shows significantly high frequencies of Aw24, Bw40, Bw54, Cw1, and DR2 antigens and a low frequency of DR9 and DRw52 as compared with those in normal Japanese individuals.[26] It has been speculated that there may be a gene in Japanese controlling susceptibility to the disease, linked to the presence or absence of some HLA antigens. However, the significance of these immunologic findings remains to be resolved.

In the Far East, the majority of patients have been outdoor workers, suggesting a relation to socioeconomic conditions, work environment, or both. Although a hypercoagulable state has been observed in association with exacerbations of ischemic symptoms in patients with the disease, its causal significance is unknown. Similarly, hepatitis B virus[28] or a rickettsiosis[3] may contribute to the pathogenesis of the disease, but their role is obscure.

Whether or not other etiologic factors contribute to Buerger's disease, one thing is clear. Tobacco smoking, whether it is a direct etiologic factor or only a strongly contributory one, plays a pivotal role in disease development and progression.

PATHOLOGIC FINDINGS

Buerger's disease is an inflammatory occlusive disease primarily involving the medium-sized muscular and smaller arteries of the extremity. Arguments concerning the status of Buerger's disease as a distinct entity center on the specificity of the acute lesion. Understanding of the pathologic arterial changes in Buerger's disease has been handicapped by the relative paucity of anatomic material available for study, particularly from early stages. However, in superficial arteries, such as the radial or the posterior tibial artery, an acute lesion is not uncommonly recognized, for the skin over the artery reddens and subsequently darkens or blackens. This interesting appearance implies a marked periarterial inflammation. Whether the initial vascular lesion of Buerger's disease is primarily thrombotic or primarily inflammatory has never been satisfactorily settled and probably never will be, in the strict sense of the word.[21] Removed at a time when the area is painful and tender and the pulse is reduced or absent, the specimen shows the characteristics of the acute lesion, as described in the following sections.[34]

Early Stage. Macroscopically, the occluded artery appears to be tense or swollen, and the periarterial tissue edematous. The lumen is obstructed with a fresh thrombus in which a focal inflammation, consisting of multi-nucleated giant cells, epithelioid cells, and leukocytes, in the form of microabscesses, is frequently observed. Careful examination of serial sections not infrequently reveals phagocytic giant cells in the cellular thrombus. Inflammatory cells, mainly lymphocytes and fibroblasts, infiltrate throughout the media and adventitia, but no necrotizing lesions are found in the media. Intimal cells proliferate slightly, but the internal elastic membrane remains essentially intact. The granulomatous reaction with giant cells lends a characteristic appearance to the thrombotic lesion of Buerger's disease at this early stage; it is characteristic in that this picture is *never* seen in thrombi associated with arteriosclerosis obliterans or simple arterial thrombosis. Two conditions are necessary for the presence of phagocytic giant cells in a thrombus: (1) the existence of slightly soluble materials, such as fibrin, and (2) local mesenchymal cell activation.[37] Detailed study of biopsy specimens results in a higher rate of detection of characteristic acute lesions in Buerger's disease.

Late Stage. Macroscopically, the occluded artery appears to be contracted and indurated. The artery and veins may be bound into a rather firm cord so that they can be separated only with difficulty. The advanced lesion is characterized by some recanalization of the thrombus, a fibrous thickening of the intima, and increased fibrous tissue in the media and adventitia. Although the internal elastic membrane is partially destroyed or fragmented, the general architecture of the vessel wall is well preserved.[21] The histopathologic features in involved superficial veins bear a close resemblance to those in the affected artery.

PATHOPHYSIOLOGY AND CORRELATIVE HEMODYNAMIC FINDINGS

The most characteristic pathophysiologic change in Buerger's disease is the breakdown of microvascular regulating and defense systems due to multiple arterial occlusions from the beginning of the disease, and the majority of the patients develop critical limb ischemia.[25] Ischemic symptoms are manifested mainly in the distal parts of the extremity, and trophic lesions occur exclusively in the fingers and toes. Arterial flow velocity in the foot during reactive hyperemia has been noninvasively measured by means of a tracer technique with technetium ^{99m}-pertechnetate.[35] The mean velocity in the foot in healthy persons was 6.8 ± 1.9 cm/sec; the velocity was less than 2.0 cm/sec in 52 of 57 limbs with Buerger's disease and was usually less than 1.0 cm/sec in 30 of 31 limbs with ischemic ulceration due to the disease. Because the initial occlusive lesions of Buerger's disease are found in the arteries below the ankle, ankle pressure determinations are not always a good indicator of ischemia. Toe systolic pressure measurements are more appropriate to evaluate the degree of ischemia in the foot,[15] and finger pressure measurements are useful for diagnosis of arterial involvement in the hand.

When the pedal arterial velocity is less than 1.0 cm/sec and the toe pressure index is less than 0.3, ischemic ulceration is either imminent or present. When toe pressure is less than 30 mmHg, the likelihood of spontaneous healing of toe lesions is poor. *Foot claudication* is characteristic of exercise-induced muscle ischemia in Buerger's disease, when arterial occlusion involves the lower leg and foot. Because the pain occurs more frequently in the sole than in the instep, the term *foot claudication* is appropriate. With crural artery occlusion, xenon-133 clearance curves from the flexor hallucis brevis in patients with foot claudication were found to be significantly different from those in patients without foot claudication. It has been concluded that foot claudication is caused by ischemia of the *plantar* muscles during walking in patients with involvement of the posterior tibial artery, the plantar artery, or both.[14]

Although *calf claudication* usually occurs in cases of suprapopliteal occlusion, it is sometimes seen in patients with infrapopliteal occlusion due to Buerger's disease. In such cases, calf claudication pain might be attributed to obstruction of muscular nutritive arteries.[18] Here, the xenon-133 clearance method can be used for separate measurement of muscle blood flow in the anterior tibial, soleus, and gastrocnemius muscles. Finally, the majority of patients with Buerger's disease perspire freely and suffer from coldness of the fingers or toes. However, typical Raynaud's vasospastic phenomena are not frequently seen because the chronically dilated and atonic digital arteries do not respond to cold or mental stimuli.

CLINICAL PRESENTATION

Based on the observation that obstructive lesions have been demonstrated angiographically in the arteries of the finger, hand, toe, or foot in *asymptomatic* patients with Buerger's disease, the disease seems to commence peripherally and extend proximally. As the disease may pass unnoticed until the occlusive lesions involve the forearm or crural arteries, it is not surprising that the first clinical manifestations are multifarious: coldness, paresthesias, skin color changes, skin lesions, rest pain, and intermittent claudication. Therefore, Fontaine's stepwise classification, which is useful for the clinical staging of arterial insufficiency due to arteriosclerosis obliterans, is not valuable in gauging the degree of ischemia in Buerger's disease. Gangrene or ulceration does not always follow claudication and may precede it.[34]

Characteristically, the fingers or toes are cold and damp to the touch. The patient often complains of paresthesia of the finger or the foot after manual labor or walking, respectively. The skin color changes are characteristic of the disease: the affected fingers and toes are purplish-red, particularly with pendency. Venous filling time in the foot usually requires more than 20 seconds. Differences in the delay in the return of skin color or in the degree of reactive hyperemia reflect regional differences in the degree of ischemia. These skin color changes often persist after sympathectomy.

Although foot claudication is a characteristic symptom associated with ischemia of the foot due to infrapopliteal arterial occlusion, calf claudication may be experienced if the disease progresses to the suprapopliteal segment. Gangrene and ulceration may occur spontaneously (particularly gangrene), but in the majority of cases, such trophic lesions follow various forms of trauma, including iatrogenic. Necrotic lesions develop most commonly on the tip of a digit, particularly the big toe. As a result of secondary infection, such lesions spread proximally and are associated with intractable pain. Rest pain is characteristically localized to the digits or immediately adjacent areas and often precedes gangrene or ulceration. Skin color is usually purplish-red but is occasionally pale, as in acute arterial occlusion.

Recurrent superficial thrombophlebitis develops on the arm, the lower leg, or the foot. Redness of the skin over the affected vein and tenderness usually disappear in 2 to 3 weeks, leaving a blackish-brown pigmentation. *Phlebitis migrans* is a pathognomonic episode characteristic of Buerger's disease (as an angiitis), but its occurrence often escapes the patient's attention.

CLINICAL CORRELATIONS

From 1977 through 1988, 255 new patients with Buerger's disease were treated at the author's institution: 249 were men (98 per cent) and 6 were women (2 per cent). Despite changing smoking habits, the incidence in women is still low. The age at onset of symptoms ranged from 19 to 49 years (average, 35.8 ± 7.7 years). The major presenting symptoms were paresthesia, coldness, or cyanosis in 94 patients (36.9 per cent), gangrene or ulcer in 47 (18.4 per cent), foot claudication in 38 (14.9 per cent), calf claudication in 42 (16.5 per cent), rest pain in 26 (10.2 per cent), and thrombophlebitis in 8 (3.1 per cent). From the onset of symptoms to the end of follow-up, gangrene or ulceration occurred in 184 (72.2 per cent) of the 255 patients, phlebitis migrans in 109 (42.7 per cent) and involvement of the upper extremity in 230 (90.2 per cent). These findings are summarized in Table 11–1. Although the upper limb was involved in the majority of the patients, ischemic symptoms of the fingers were recognized in only 41 per cent. Two limbs were affected in 17 per cent of the 255 patients, three in 43 per cent, and four in 40 per cent. Thus, 83 per cent of all the cases had involvement of three or four limbs, and none had single-limb involvement. The accompanying veins of the main crural arteries are often involved in Buerger's disease, but as a rule, no disturbance of venous return in the deep system is seen.

DIAGNOSIS

The author's clinical criteria for the diagnosis of Buerger's disease are (1) smoking history, (2) onset before the age of 50 years, (3) infrapopliteal arterial occlusive lesions,

Table 11–1. Clinical Presentation and Progression of Buerger's Disease in 255 Patients*

	Primary Presenting Problem	Eventual Incidence
Paresthesia, coldness, or cyanosis	94 (36.9%)	—
Gangrene or ulcer	47 (18.4%)	184 (72.2%)
Foot claudication	38 (14.9%)	—
Calf claudication	42 (16.5%)	—
Rest pain	26 (10.2%)	
Phlebitis	8 (3.1%)	109 (42.7%)
Upper extremity involvement	—	230 (90.2%)

**Occurrence in patients followed up from 1 to 12 years at the author's institution.*[34]

(4) either upper limb involvement or phlebitis migrans, and (5) absence of atherosclerotic risk factors other than smoking.[34] The clinical diagnosis of Buerger's disease is made when all five requirements are met. Arteriographic findings serve as supporting evidence, and characteristic pathohistologic findings corroborate the existence of the disease.

Migrating phlebitis and upper extremity involvement are considered to be systemic manifestations of Buerger's disease. In the author's series, involvement of the upper extremity occurred in 90.2 per cent and phlebitis migrans developed in 42.7 per cent; both upper limb involvement *and* phlebitis migrans occurred in 33 per cent. Patients with *both* involvements were compared to those with *either,* and no significant difference in clinical course was found between the two groups.[34] Therefore, either upper limb involvement *or* phlebitis migrans seems sufficient to support the clinical diagnosis of Buerger's disease.

Differential Diagnosis

Buerger's disease may affect men in their 50s, but they might be expected to respond in a different manner to etiologic factors than younger men because their aged vessels may show arteriosclerotic degenerative changes. When the onset of ischemic symptoms occurs after 50 years of age, patients should be studied carefully with arteriosclerosis obliterans in mind. In female patients with extremity ischemia, Buerger's disease must be distinguished from collagen diseases, such as scleroderma or systemic lupus erythematosus, because not only the digital arteries but also the infrabrachial and infrapopliteal arteries may be occluded in collagen vascular diseases. It should be kept in mind, in this regard, that the natural course of Buerger's disease is uneventful unless smoking continues, whereas the natural history of collagen diseases is progressive irrespective of smoking.

Diagnostic Studies

History taking and physical examination are usually sufficient to make the diagnosis of Buerger's disease, but additional diagnostic procedures are required to evaluate the degree of ischemia objectively and to select the most appropriate therapy.

Noninvasive Diagnostic Techniques. As local impairment of distal arterial blood flow is the essential characteristic of Buerger's disease, the monitoring of ankle and toe pressures and plethysmography, digital artery flow velocity,[35] or both have practical clinical value. Typical findings were described earlier, and the techniques are discussed in detail in Chapter 5. In addition, thallium-201 perfusion scans are helpful in determining the healing potential of ulcers.[27] Such tests are also useful in predicting the response to sympathectomy and in documenting the response to any therapeutic intervention.

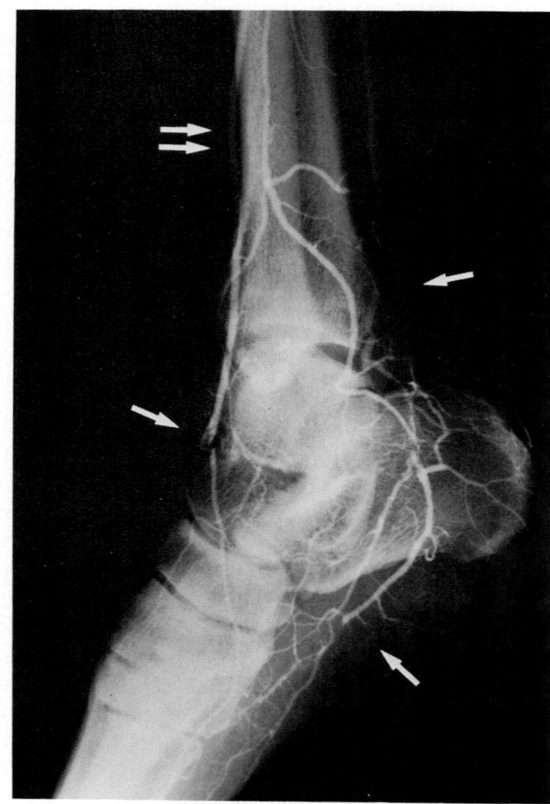

FIGURE 11–1. Right femoral arteriogram of a 42-year-old man with Buerger's disease (onset at the age of 40 years). Multiple segmental occlusive lesions seen around the ankle show an abrupt obstruction *(single arrows).* The anterior tibial artery has a corrugated appearance *(double arrow).* The right foot was asymptomatic, although the patient experienced rest pain in the left foot.

Arteriography. Multiple segmental occlusions of distal extremity arteries are characteristic of Buerger's disease, with each occlusion being either tapered or abrupt. The arterial wall proximal to the occlusion is usually smooth. A corrugated or accordion-like appearance is sometimes seen, mostly in the femoral or crural arteries, but this is not a characteristic of the Buerger lesion itself. Rather, it represents an associated arterial spasm (Figs. 11–1 to 11–3). Generally, there is an extensive reticular network of collateral vessels around each occlusion, so that arterial circulation in the extremity is somehow maintained by collaterals in spite of occlusion of almost all the main arteries (Fig. 11–3). These collateral vessels characteristically have a corkscrew or root-like appearance (Figs. 11–3 and 11–4). The arteriographic appearance with upper extremity involvement is the same as that in the lower extremity (Fig. 11–5). Unlike in arteriosclerosis obliterans, neither calcification of the vessel wall nor a motheaten defect of the arterial silhouette is seen. Although in clinically obvious cases it is possible to diagnose and treat Buerger's disease without arteriography, it may be indicated for diagnosis in obscure cases and of course is essential whenever arterial reconstruction is being contemplated. Arteriography is frequently employed in the author's practice.

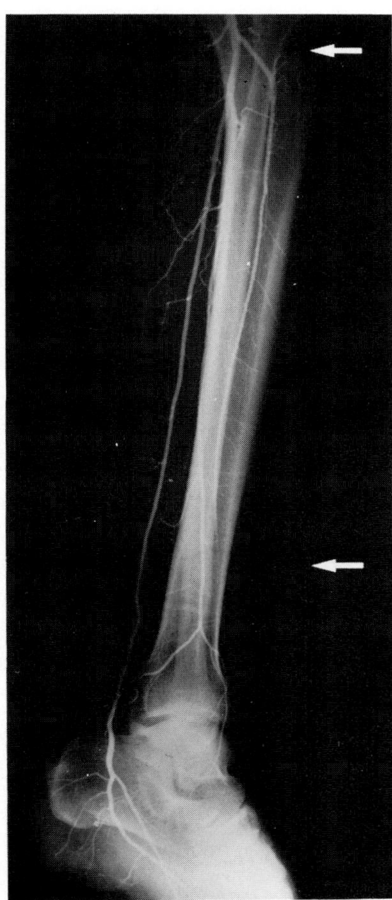

FIGURE 11–2. Left femoral arteriogram of a 34-year-old man with Buerger's disease (onset at the age of 32 years). The anterior tibial artery shows a tapering occlusion with a corrugated appearance (*arrows*). The left foot suffered from coldness.

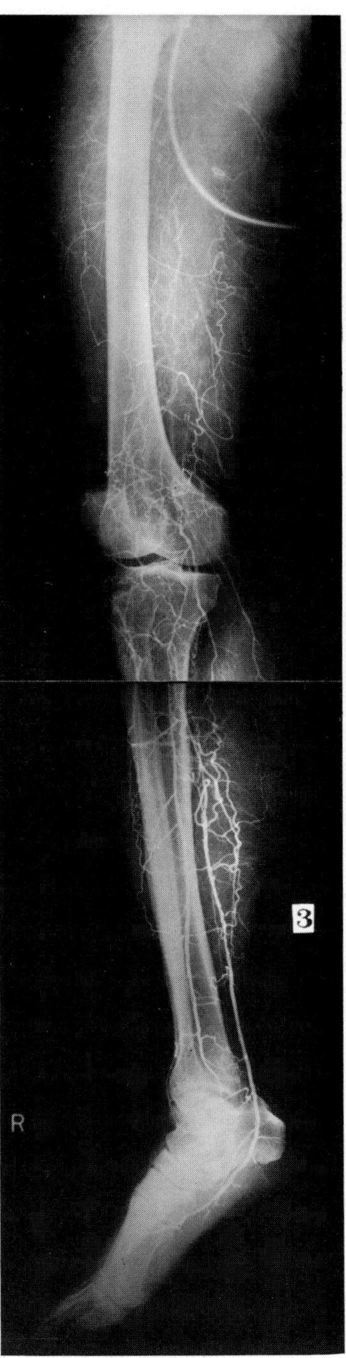

FIGURE 11–3. Right femoral arteriogram of a 45-year-old man with Buerger's disease (onset at the age of 35 years). The femoropopliteal segment is occluded, and the posterior tibial artery and the peroneal artery are visualized by collateral vessels that show a corkscrew appearance. The right foot had ischemic ulceration.

CLINICAL COURSE

In the lower extremity, the disease commences in the digital arteries and the small arteries in the foot and then proceeds to involve the crural arteries. After the crural arteries are affected, the pattern of infrapopliteal arterial occlusive disease is set, up to a certain point, although there

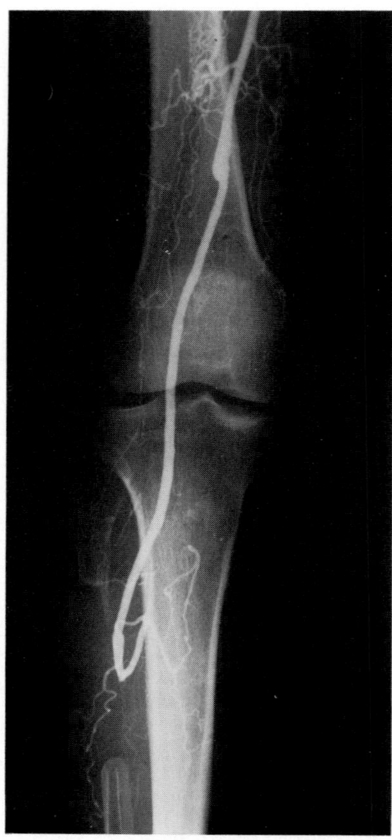

FIGURE 11–4. Right femoral arteriogram of a 52-year-old man with Buerger's disease (onset at the age of 40 years). At the age of 47, a right femoroperoneal bypass with an autologous vein was performed. The graft remains patent even though the distal vessels have become occluded for the most part. The collateral vessels around the site of proximal occlusion show a root-like appearance. Although there was digital gangrene in the right foot at the time of the bypass, the foot is now asymptomatic.

is often further deterioration in the distal vessels. Because of the proximal lesions, the distal vessels are not well visualized by conventional arteriography. Further progression of the disease takes one of two forms: (1) continuous progression or (2) skip progression. Characteristically, in the arteriograms of patients with Buerger's disease, an apparently normal, smooth-walled artery tapers toward or abruptly ends in the occlusion. However, stenosis, dilatation, or irregularity of the proximal artery, principally of the popliteal segment, is sometimes seen.[19] This so-called skip lesion is considered an early stage in the proximal progression of the disease. Such preexisting lesions in the popliteal artery favor the eventual occurrence of thrombotic occlusion, as a form of *skip progression,* in contrast to contiguous segmental involvement with progressive thrombosis, or *continuous progression.*

In the clinical course of Buerger's disease, there appears to be an interval, often from 1 to 2 years, between the initial onset of symptoms and the eventual involvement of the suprapopliteal segment, which is usually signaled by the development of calf claudication. The disease may involve segments as far proximal as the external iliac artery. More proximal occlusion is caused by secondary thrombosis or an iatrogenic event, such as failure of an aortofemoral bypass. In the author's series, arterial occlusion was limited to the infrapopliteal segment in 60 per cent of patients at the time of initial evaluation.[34] Arterial occlusion had already progressed to the femoropopliteal segment in 32 per cent and to the aortoiliac region in 8 per cent. In the upper extremity, the process begins in the digital arteries and small arteries in the hand and then proceeds to involve the forearm arteries. In contrast to the situation in the lower extremity, involvement of the brachial artery rarely follows involvement of the forearm arteries.

Although there are a number of reports of *generalized* Buerger's disease,[4, 7, 30] occlusive lesions typical of Buerger's disease at nonextremity sites should be viewed with skepticism. The majority of reported cases lacked symptoms of peripheral arterial occlusion, and diagnosis was based on the histologic similarity of the arterial lesions with those seen in Buerger's disease. As the specificity of Buerger's disease depends on its clinical characteristics, histologic resemblance alone is an insufficient basis for diagnosis; in other words, not all inflammatory arteritides are Buerger's disease. According to the annual reports of autopsy cases in Japan from 1966 to 1971, only 3 of 129,113 patients had been diagnosed as having Buerger's disease during their lifetime: their causes of death were peritonitis, pneumonia, and sepsis. Although the aorta and the coro-

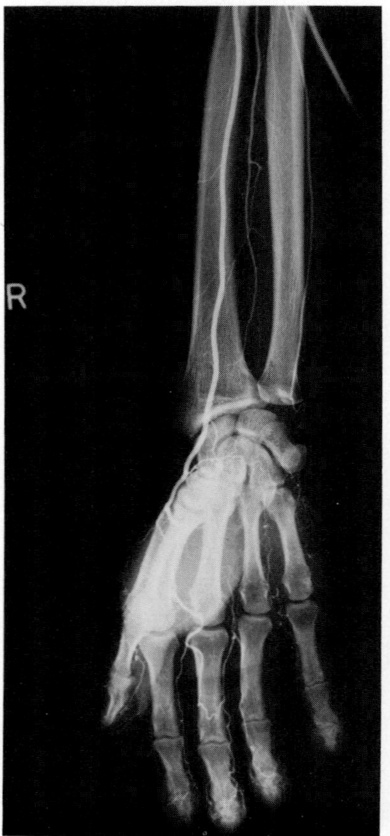

FIGURE 11–5. Right brachial arteriogram of a 51-year-old man with Buerger's disease (onset at the age of 46 years). The ulnar artery narrows and is occluded at the wrist. The digital and metacarpal arteries are extensively obstructed. The only symptom is cyanosis of the fifth finger.

nary, renal, celiac, and superior mesenteric arteries were thrombosed in one case, *no* histologic features typical of thromboangiitis obliterans were seen in the visceral arteries.[17] Of 255 patients with Buerger's disease treated and followed from 1 to 12 years at the author's institution, 5 died. The causes of death were mesenteric thrombosis in 3 patients and myocardial infarction in 2. The 3 patients with thrombosis had juxtarenal aortic occlusion due to proximal propagation of thrombus, and 2 of them had previously undergone aortofemoral bypass grafting that later occluded. Their ages at death were 33, 47, and 60 years, respectively. No characteristic pathohistologic features of Buerger's disease were found in the mesenteric vessels in 2 autopsied cases. The 2 patients who had myocardial infarction died at the ages of 48 and 51 years, respectively; one patient had previously undergone brachioulnar bypass; the other, femoropopliteal bypass. Visceral vessel involvement is rare in Buerger's disease, which explains the fact that these patients have normal survival rates.[23] Although there is no evidence that patients with Buerger's disease are more susceptible to arteriosclerosis, aging is inevitable for them as for everyone, and the development of arteriosclerotic lesions later in life in these patients should not be unexpected.

Finally, the clinical course is primarily influenced by whether or not the patient completely stops smoking. The disease is marked by the episodic appearance of new lesions, but exacerbations producing rapidly increased arterial insufficiency of the affected limbs do *not* occur if the patient stops smoking completely. On the other hand, if the patient continues to smoke, sudden progression in arterial occlusion, gradual worsening of the peripheral ischemia, or both, ultimately render any surgical or medical treatment ineffective. If the patient with Buerger's disease *completely* abstains from smoking, the clinical course will be uneventful, and a good prognosis can be assured.

MEDICAL TREATMENT

The only way to arrest the disease is abstinence from smoking. Any therapeutic procedure not accompanied by a cessation of smoking will be unsuccessful in treating the arterial insufficiency. Initially, a number of extremity arteries are spared from obstructive lesions. The goal of medical treatment is to protect and develop flow through the remaining patent vessels and the compensatory collateral network. Because there are no vasodilating drugs that can act selectively on these collateral vessels, the value of systemically administered vasodilators is very much in question (see Chapter 18). Although antithrombotic therapy consisting of a fibrolytic agent and heparin may restrain fulminant thrombotic progression of arterial lesions, the effectiveness of long-term anticoagulant therapy remains unproven.

Selection of Patients for Interventional Therapy

As efforts are concentrated on the healing of *trophic* lesions, it is essential to determine which lesions will heal with conservative management and which will require a surgical procedure or an amputation. An objective, reliable method of predicting the healing potential of ischemic ulceration is needed to prevent either unnecessarily prolonged hospitalization or premature surgery. The ability to develop an inflammatory response with local hyperemia is necessary for spontaneous healing.[38] Gauged by means of a post-stress imaging study following a single intravenous injection of thallium-201, ulcers with a *hot spot* in the initial distribution of this radionuclide can be predicted to respond well to conservative treatment, whereas lesions with a hot spot only in the redistribution phase will require a surgical procedure to prevent protracted hospitalization, with only a slim chance of spontaneous ulcer healing. Healing of ulcerations without a hot spot throughout all phases of thallium-201 distributions cannot be expected, even with optimal conservative treatment, and if arterial reconstruction is not feasible, the necrotic tissue must be removed after the line of demarcation becomes apparent.[27] As a hot spot is seen to some degree in the majority of the trophic lesions, most have some spontaneous healing potential. Medical treatment must be designed to facilitate the spontaneous healing process.

Prostaglandin Therapy. The discovery of prostaglandins has opened new vistas in medical treatment of extremity arterial insufficiency. When administered by the intra-arterial route, prostaglandin E_1 (PGE_1) is able to produce maximal vasodilation and inhibition of platelet aggregation at such a low concentration that its pharmacologic effects are restricted to the target area. Adverse systemic effects are avoided because of the extensive degradation of PGE_1 during passage through the pulmonary circulation.[33] Controversy continues regarding the degree of efficacy of PGE_1 in the treatment of ischemic ulceration.[32] However, variances in the reported beneficial effects of the drug might be related to differences in patients admitted into the clinical trials.

In the Nagoya experience, 29 patients with intractable ulceration, in whom neither arterial reconstruction nor sympathectomy was feasible, underwent continuous intra-arterial infusion of PGE_1 in a dose of 0.05 to 0.06 ng/kg/min. With a 13- to 79-day infusion (average, 43 days), ulcers healed in 9 (31 per cent) of 29 patients, improved in 14 (48 per cent) and were unchanged in 6 (21 per cent). In view of the practical advantages of the intravenous over the intra-arterial route and because of a perception of beneficial effects in the contralateral limb during intra-arterial infusion of the drug, the efficacy of intravenous injection of PGE_1 for ischemic ulceration was compared with that of intra-arterial administration. However, although an intravenous drip infusion of PGE_1, in a dose of 5 to 10 ng/kg/min, brought about a certain measure of improvement, the intravenous route was clearly inferior to intra-arterial administration in regard to the healing of trophic lesions.[33] The lesser efficacy of the intravenous infusion of PGE_1 might be attributed to an underdose in the target area. Nevertheless, the intravenous route is preferred to the intra-arterial route in cases with involvement of the iliofemoral segment because of difficulties caused by the intra-arterial insertion of the perfusing catheter. In addition, long-term intravascular insertion of the catheter into the *deep* femoral artery carries the risk of damaging collateral circulation and is less effective than insertion into a patent superficial femoral artery. The discovery and recent availability in stable form of prostacyclin (prostaglandin I_2), a powerful inhibitor of platelet aggregation as well as a vasodilator, offers promise for the treatment of peripheral vascular diseases with prostaglandins. In this regard, it is important to determine *at the outset* which patients will respond well to prostaglandins by objectively evaluating the drug-induced hemodynamic change in the affected limb. For example, this has been done by means of thermography: if the temperature decreases in the target area during infusion of the drug, no therapeutic benefit can be expected because of a steal phenomenon.[16]

Other Measures. There is no evidence that prostaglandins alter the clinical course of Buerger's disease. No panacea for the disease exists, but it is essential that something be done to try to help the patient through the difficult time between the onset of acute symptoms and eventual clinical improvement.[10] The most difficult aspect is the war against intractable pain. Epidural anesthesia gives quick relief, and a 1- to 2-week administration via an indwelling catheter provides relief for the patient, who otherwise must keep his or her leg dependent around the clock. In addition, alleviation of dependent edema speeds healing. Although epidural anesthesia produces sympathectomy-like vasodilation, it will subsequently need to be supplemented by surgical sympathectomy in the more serious cases. Hyperbaric oxygen therapy may also relieve pain and accelerate healing of ischemic ulcers.[31] *Bridging therapy* is the term used for the appropriate use of epidural anesthesia, prostaglandin infusion, antithrombotic agents, or hyperbaric oxygen to help the patient through periods of acute exacerbation.

Epidural spinal electrical stimulation has been introduced into clinical practice for the treatment of intractable ischemic pain.[2] In the author's recent experience, the procedure was effective for relieving pain and promoting skin healing of trophic lesions in some patients with Buerger's disease.

SURGICAL TREATMENT (Table 11–2)

As surgical treatment does not constitute direct, specific therapy for underlying Buerger's disease, good initial results will give way to recurrence unless the patient abstains from smoking.

Arterial Reconstruction. Although direct arterial reconstruction is not often feasible because of the multiple occluded distal arteries, when successful it provides the most effective healing of ischemic lesions. Some cases of suprapopliteal involvement permit arterial reconstruction. Thromboendarterectomy is usually not feasible, and only bypass procedures are considered. Although synthetic grafts are employed for aorto- or iliofemoral bypasses, autologous vein is the graft of choice for infrainguinal and infra-axillary bypasses. The greater saphenous vein is frequently occluded or of inadequate diameter because of inflammatory changes; the lesser saphenous, the cephalic, or the basilic vein should be used in such circumstances, if at all possible, because autologous vein is superior for bypasses crossing a joint and will remain patent in spite of poor runoff (see Figure 11–4).

Bypass procedures were performed in only 44 (17.3 per cent) of 255 patients in the author's series: aorto- or iliofemoral bypass in 10, femorofemoral in 2, femoropoplit-

Table 11–2. Surgical Treatment of Buerger's Disease in 255 Patients*

Indication	Bypass		Sympathectomy
Coldness or paresthesia	—		26 (19.4%)
Claudication	11 (21.5%)		—
Rest pain	10 (19.6%)		24 (17.9%)
Gangrene or ulcer	28 (54.9%)		84 (62.7%)
Graft infection	2 (4.0%)		—
Procedure	**Bypass**	**Procedure**	**Sympathectomy**
Aorto- or iliofemoral	10 (19.6%)	Lumbar	108 (80.6%)
Femorofemoral	2 (4.0%)	Thoracic	26 (19.4%)
Femoropopliteal	8 (15.6%)	Both	4 (3.0%)
Femorocrural	21 (41.0%)		
Popliteocrural	4 (7.8%)		
Tibiotibial	2 (4.0%)		
Axilloradial	1 (2.0%)		
Brachioradial	1 (2.0%)		
Brachioulnar	2 (4.0%)		
Bypass	44/255 (17.3%)	Sympathectomy (134 limbs)	130/255 (51.0%)
Concomitant lumbar sympathectomy	24/44 (54.5%)	Concomitant bypass	24/130 (18.5%)
Amputation			
Below-knee	6 (2.4%)		
Above-knee	1 (0.4%)		

**From 1977 to 1988 at the author's institution. Seven patients underwent two separate bypasses: both lumbar and thoracic sympathectomy were performed in four patients.*[34]

eal in 8, femorocrural in 21, popliteocrural in 4, tibiotibial in 2, axilloradial in 1, brachioradial in 1, and brachioulnar in 2 (7 patients underwent two separate operations).[34] The indications for arterial reconstruction were gangrene or ulceration in 28 cases (54.9 per cent), rest pain in 10 (19.6 per cent), claudication in 11 (21.5 per cent), and graft infection in 2 (4.0 per cent). Concomitant lumbar sympathectomy was performed in 24 (see Table 11–2). The rationale for concomitant sympathectomy was increased flow through the revascularized segment as a result of reduced peripheral resistance. The effect of postoperative anticoagulant or antiplatelet therapy on patency of the revascularized segment is still controversial, and this type of therapy was not used consistently. Follow-up ranged from 1 to 12 years. The cumulative life table patency of 12 suprainguinal grafts was 90 per cent at 1 year, 70 per cent at 2 years, and 70 per cent at 10 years; that of 34 infrainguinal grafts was 56 per cent, 48 per cent and 32 per cent, respectively. Unsatisfactory long-term results might be attributable to impaired runoff, disease recurrence, poor quality of the vein graft, or a combination of factors.

Preoperative measurement of distal blood pressure and blood flow were not predictive of early graft failure. In an effort to determine whether resistance offered by the arteries of the foot (below the ankle) influenced the results of arterial reconstruction, a *distal runoff resistance index* was calculated by dividing the difference in blood pressure between the ankle and the toe by the brachial systolic pressure (A-T gradient). No correlation between the preoperative A-T gradient and graft patency could be demonstrated.[36] Although the increase in toe pressure was significantly smaller than that in ankle pressure after the arterial reconstruction, the postoperative toe pressure was of value in predicting healing of ischemic ulcerations: a toe pressure of more than 30 mmHg correlated with healing of the lesion.[15] Patency of the graft for even a few months allowed time for the healing of trophic lesions, and if the graft failed after the lesions healed, they did not recur unless the patient resumed smoking.

Sympathectomy. Surgical sympathetic denervation has a long history and is still the most valuable of the standard methods of treatment in Buerger's disease. It provides permanent freedom from vasoconstrictor activity in the distal part of the limb, which is the part usually affected by the disease. Worsening of ischemia after sympathectomy is rare, so the operation tends to be freely employed. Sympathectomy was performed in 130 (51.0 per cent) of the 255 patients with Buerger's disease in the author's series: lumbar in 108 (concomitant with arterial reconstruction in 24) and thoracic in 26 (both lumbar and thoracic in 4).[34] The indications for sympathectomy were gangrene or ulceration in 84 (62.7 per cent), rest pain in 24 (17.9 per cent), and coldness or paresthesia in 26 (19.4 per cent) (see Table 11–2).

The purpose of sympathetic denervation is to remove vasoconstrictor tone in the peripheral region of the extremity; it cannot be expected to benefit ischemic limbs with chronically dilated arteries lacking vasospastic reactivity. Postoperative clinical course correlated better with flow velocity in the foot than with distal blood pressure, as there was a reduction in toe blood pressure in some instances.[35] Ulceration healed more frequently and rapidly in the limbs with postoperative normalization of the flow velocity in the foot.

Sympathectomy is indicated for superficial trophic lesions of the skin or vasospastic symptoms, such as coldness or cold sensitivity. Because no significant improvement in muscle circulation occurs after sympathetic denervation, it is not indicated for intermittent claudication. The technique and extent of sympathectomy are as recommended in Chapters 59 and 72 (i.e., L2, 3 for the lower extremity and T2, 3 and the lower one third of the stellate ganglion for upper extremity sympathectomy). These are sufficient for maximal effect and avoid loss of ejaculation and Horner's syndrome, respectively.

Local Treatment. Local management of necrotic lesions in Buerger's disease is the same as in other chronic arterial occlusive diseases: that is, it is not influenced by underlying etiology but by the ischemic nature of the lesions. Although local infection plays an important role in the development of an intractable lesion and contributes to the difficulty in healing, systemic administration of antibiotics alone is insufficient because of the lack of adequate blood supply to the target areas. Furthermore, local application of the drugs and antiseptics frequently damages the ischemic skin and granulation tissue.

Débridement. Débridement of the necrotic tissue is accomplished either by the use of an enzymatic débriding agent or by gentle surgical technique. The necrotic lesion should be soaked daily for 5 to 10 minutes, using saline warmed to body temperature. The lesion may be treated conservatively with the hope of self-amputation, with the necrotic tissue being removed after the boundary between living and gangrenous tissue is well demarcated.

Amputation. Digital gangrene or ulceration occurs in the majority of patients with Buerger's disease, and excising the dry gangrene at a line of demarcation or amputation of a finger or toe is frequently required. However, no major amputation should be necessary if the disease is detected early enough and is appropriately managed. In the 255 patients in the Nagoya series, below-knee amputation was performed in 6 and above-knee amputation in 1, for a 2.7 per cent major amputation rate.[34] As long as the patient strictly abstains from tobacco use, the long-term outlook for limb salvage is favorable because of the excellent healing potential of ischemic ulcerations.

THERAPEUTIC APPROACH

After the diagnosis is made, the first step is to warn the patient about the effects of smoking. Protection against cold and safeguards against trauma are enough for patients with coldness or cold sensitivity. The patient should also pay attention to asymptomatic limbs because of the possibility of latent occlusive lesions. Sympathectomy is indicated only in advanced cases. There is no remedy except walking training for foot claudication due to infrapopliteal arterial occlusions. Arterial reconstruction is sometimes indicated for calf claudication due to suprapopliteal arterial occlusion when the patient's work and quality of life are significantly compromised by the claudication. Synthetic graft is used for arterial reconstruction of the aortoiliac segment, but autologous vein is the graft of choice for infrainguinal revascularization. In cases in which there is no suitable autologous vein, walking training is preferred over synthetic bypass grafting for calf claudication due to occlusion of the leg arteries. Bridging therapy is necessary for patients with acute intractable pain due to severe ischemia.

Employment of the medical or surgical treatment of choice is based on clinical diagnostic techniques for predicting ischemic ulcer healing. Because of the good natural healing potential of most trophic lesions in Buerger's disease, the digital necrotic lesion should be conservatively managed at first. Continuous intra-arterial infusion with PGE_1 is indicated for intractable ulceration in patients for whom no surgical procedure is feasible. In cases of poor spontaneous healing potential, sympathectomy or arterial reconstruction should be considered. Because of occlusion of the infrapopliteal and foot arteries, lumbar sympathectomy is preferably performed at the same time as arterial reconstruction if the latter is feasible; otherwise, it is done alone. All efforts should be concentrated on the healing of ulceration or successful auto- or surgical amputation of gangrene. Although minor amputation, such as digital or transmetatarsal, is frequently necessary, *foot salvage* is easily accomplished. By definition, this means retention of a functional foot that allows standing and walking without a prosthesis.[29] Because of the natural history of the disease and the treatment modalities available, major amputation is almost always avoidable.

SUMMARY

Buerger's disease is characterized by peripheral arterial occlusion of the extremities in young smokers, and true Buerger's lesions outside the extremities are questionable. Although the incidence of this disease is low in Europe and the United States, the treatment of patients with the disease is still one of the most important aspects of vascular surgery in the Middle and Far East. The etiology remains unknown, but there is an extremely close relationship between the use of tobacco and the occurrence or recurrence of the disease. If the patient absolutely and permanently abandons smoking, the natural history is uneventful. In spite of a high incidence of digital gangrene and ulceration, a functional foot can almost always be preserved because of the good spontaneous healing potential of the trophic lesions. An understanding of the natural course of the disease not only has prognostic value but also places the role of surgical or conservative treatment in the proper perspective. Surgeons treating patients with Buerger's disease should take note of this and avoid premature and possibly unnecessary surgery.

References

1. Adar R, Papa MZ, Halpern Z, et al: Cellular sensitivity to collagen in thromboangiitis obliterans. N Engl J Med 308:1113, 1983.
2. Augustinsson LE, Carlsson CA, Holm J, et al: Epidural electrical stimulation in severe limb ischemia. Ann Surg 202:104, 1985.
3. Bartolo M, Rulli F, Raffi S: Buerger's disease: Is it a rickettsiosis? Angiology 31:660, 1980.
4. Birnbaum W, Prinzmetal M, Connor CL: Generalized thromboangiitis obliterans. Report of a case with involvement of retinal vessels and suprarenal infarction. Arch Intern Med 53:410, 1934.
5. Bollinger A, Hollmann B, Schneider E, et al: Thromboangiitis obliterans: Diagnose und Therapie im Licht neuer immunologischer Befunde. Schweiz Med Wochenschr 109:537, 1979.
6. Buerger L: Thrombo-angiitis obliterans: A study of the vascular lesions leading to presenile spontaneous gangrene. Am J Med Sci 136:567, 1908.
7. Buerger L: The Circulatory Disturbances of the Extremities: Including Gangrene, Vasomotor and Trophic Disorders. Philadelphia, WB Saunders, 1924, pp 307–320, 368–374.
8. Cachovan M: Epidemiologie und geographisches Verteilungsmuster der Thromboangiitis obliterans. *In* Heidrich H (ed): Thromboangiitis obliterans Morbus Winiwarter-Buerger. Stuttgart, Georg Thieme, 1988, pp 31–38.
9. Davis JW, Shelton L, Watanabe IS, et al: Passive smoking affects endothelium and platelets. Arch Intern Med 149:386, 1989.
10. Eastcott HHG: Buerger's disease. *In* Arterial Surgery. London, Pitman Medical Publishing, 1969, pp 94–110.
11. Eastcott HHG: Buerger's disease. *In* Bergan JJ, Yao JST (eds): Evaluation and Treatment of Upper and Lower Extremity Circulation Disorders. Orlando, FL, Grune & Stratton, 1984, pp 483–497.
12. Fielding JE, Phenow KJ: Health effects of involuntary smoking. N Engl J Med 319:1452, 1988.
13. Gulati SM, Madhra K, Thusoo TK, et al: Autoantibodies in thromboangiitis obliterans (Buerger's disease). Angiology 33:642, 1982.
14. Hirai M: Intermittent claudication of the foot in view of foot muscle blood flow measured by 133-Xe clearance technique and arteriographic findings. Jpn Circ J 40:313, 1976.
15. Hirai M, Kawai S, Ohta T, et al: The value of toe blood pressure measurement in arterial reconstructive surgery. Vasc Surg 15:380, 1981.
16. Hirai M, Nakayama R: Haemodynamic effects of intra-arterial and intravenous administration of prostaglandin E1 in patients with peripheral arterial disease. Br J Surg 73:20, 1986.
17. Ishikawa K (ed): Annual Report on Buerger's disease. Tokyo, Japanese Ministry of Health and Welfare, 1970, pp 3–17, 18–19.
18. Kinmonth JB: Thromboangiitis obliterans. Results of sympathectomy and prognosis. Lancet 255:717, 1948.
19. Lambeth JT, Yong NK: Arteriographic findings in thromboangiitis obliterans. With emphasis on femoropopliteal involvement. Am J Roentgenol Rad Ther Nucl Med 109:553, 1970.
20. Lie JT: Thromboangiitis obliterans (Buerger's disease) in women. Medicine 64:65, 1987.
21. Lie JT: Thromboangiitis obliterans (Buerger's disease) revisited. Pathol Ann 23:257, 1988.
22. Matsushita M, Shionoya S, Matsumoto T: Urinary cotinine measurement in patients with Buerger's disease—Effects of active and passive smoking on the disease process. J Vasc Surg 14:53, 1991.
23. McPherson JR, Jergens JL, Gifford RW Jr: Thromboangiitis obliterans and arteriosclerosis obliterans. Clinical and prognostic differences. Ann Intern Med 59:288, 1963.
24. Nishikimi N, Shionoya S, Mizuno S, et al: Result of national epidemiological study of Buerger's disease. J Jpn Coll Angiol 27:1125, 1987.
25. Nishikimi N, Sakurai T, Shionoya S, et al: Microcirculatory characteristics in patients with Buerger's disease. Angiology 43:312, 1992.
26. Numano F, Sasazuki T, Koyama T, et al: HLA in Buerger's disease. Exp Clin Immunogenet 3:195, 1986.
27. Ohta T: Noninvasive technique using thallium-201 for predicting ischaemic ulcer healing of the foot. Br J Surg 72:892, 1985.
28. Roncon A: Endarterie obliterante do jovem. Estudo clinico e histopatologico. Doctoral dissertation, University of Porto, 1982.
29. Rutherford RB, Flanigan DP, Gupta SK, et al: Suggested standards for reports dealing with lower extremity ischemia. J Vasc Surg 4:80, 1986.
30. Sachs IL, Klima T, Frankel NB: Thromboangiitis obliterans of the transverse colon. JAMA 238:336, 1977.
31. Sakakibara K, Takahashi H, Kobayashi S: Clinical experience of hyperbaric oxygen therapy (OHP) for chronic peripheral vascular disorders. *In* Shiraki D, Matsuoka S (eds): Hyperbaric Medicine and Underwater Physiology. Bethesda, MD, Undersea Medical Society, 1983, pp 337–344.

32. Schuler JJ, Flanigan DP, Holcroft JW, et al: Efficacy of prostaglandin E1 in the treatment of lower extremity ischemic ulcers secondary to peripheral vascular occlusive disease. Results of a prospective randomized, double-blind, multicenter clinical trial. J Vasc Surg 1:160, 1984.
33. Shionoya S: Clinical experience with prostaglandin E1 in occlusive arterial disease. Int Angiol 3:99, 1984.
34. Shionoya S: Buerger's disease. Pathology, diagnosis and treatment. Nagoya, The University of Nagoya Press, 1990, pp 57–77, 101–116, 189–197, 199–233.
35. Shionoya S, Hirai M, Kawai S, et al: Hemodynamic study of ischemic limb by velocity measurement in foot. Surgery 90:10, 1981.
36. Shionoya S, Matsubara J, Hirai M, et al: Measurement of blood pressure, blood flow and flow velocity in arterial reconstruction of the lower extremity. Angiology 34:244, 1983.
37. Shionoya S, Tsunekawa S, Kamiya K: Elastolysis and giant cell reaction against disintegrated elastic fibres. Nature 207:311, 1965.
38. Siegel ME, Giarhiana FA Jr, Rhodes BA, et al: Perfusion of ischemic ulcers of the extremity. A prognostic indicator of healing. Arch Surg 110:265, 1975.
39. Wessler S, Ming SC, Gurewich V, et al: A critical evaluation of thromboangiitis obliterans. The case against Buerger's disease. N Engl J Med 262:1149, 1960.
40. Winiwarter FV: Ueber eine eigentümliche Form von Endarteritis und Endophlebitis mit Gangrän des Fusses. Arch Klin Chir 23:202, 1878.

12

Takayasu's Disease: Nonspecific Aortoarteritis

Joseph M. Giordano, M.D., Gary S. Hoffman, M.D., and Randi Y. Leavitt, M.D., Ph.D.

• • •

Takayasu's disease is an arteritis of unknown etiology affecting primarily the aorta and its main branches, resulting in segmental stenosis, occlusion, dilatation, and aneurysm formation in vessels. The stenotic and occlusive lesions, in the absence of adequate collateral flow, may cause regional ischemia. Although the majority of reported cases are from the Far East, the disease occurs worldwide.[1–11] In addition, Takayasu's arteritis predominantly affects females but has been described in males.[1–8, 10, 11] Patients who have the disease can present with a systemic illness with acute or chronic ischemia, the asymptomatic absence of pulses, or a combination of these findings. Takayasu's arteritis is a rare disease that requires both long-term medical and surgical follow-up to achieve improved survival and quality of life. This chapter reviews the current literature on Takayasu's arteritis but focuses primarily on clinical features of the disease, diagnostic modalities, and the treatment of this complex disorder.

INCIDENCE AND ETIOLOGY

Takayasu's arteritis is a rare disease that appears to occur most frequently in the Far East.[1] A postmortem series in Japan demonstrated evidence of Takayasu's arteritis in approximately 1 of every 3000 autopsy cases.[12] A population study of Olmsted County, Minnesota, revealed a yearly incidence rate of 2.6 cases per 1 million inhabitants, and a hospital-based study in a defined area of Sweden estimated the yearly incidence of this disease to be 6.4 cases per 1 million inhabitants.[8, 13] It has been observed that the last figure might be high because the series included several elderly patients who may actually have had giant cell (temporal) arteritis.[10]

The cause of Takayasu's arteritis remains unclear, and no consistent immunologic findings have been reported. Because of the known association of microorganisms and aortitis, infectious etiologies have been considered.[14] There have been reports of a relationship between tuberculosis and Takayasu's arteritis, with one series reporting active tuberculous infection in 60 per cent of autopsy cases of nonspecific aortitis and other series noting a high incidence of tuberculin-positive skin hypersensitivity.[6, 10, 11, 15] However, other analyses of similar groups of patients have not borne out this association.[8–11] Several studies have proposed various HLA associations with Takayasu's arteritis, suggesting a genetic predisposition for the disease.[16–22] The strong predilection for women, geographic incidence, and occasional familial occurrence also intimate the role of genetic factors. However, investigators have not consistently found the same associations, and further studies need to be performed. Using the technique of restriction fragment length polymorphism, investigators have demonstrated an association between Takayasu's arteritis and the HLA-D gene at the genomic level.[21] Furthermore, another report proposed a negative association between this disease and HLA-DR1, implying a protective effect of this antigen.[22] The tendency for the disease to affect women of reproductive age has suggested to some investigators a potential role for hormonal influences in the pathogenesis of the disorder.[7]

CLINICAL FEATURES

Takayasu's arteritis occurs in females seven to eight times more frequently than in males.[1–13] It generally occurs in patients younger than 40 years of age, but older patients may be affected.[2, 5, 11, 23, 24] It has been called a "great imitator" in medicine because of its nonspecific and varied clinical presentations.[25, 26]

The disease has been subdivided into an early, systemic inflammatory, "prepulseless" phase and a late, occlusive, "pulseless" phase.[6, 8, 9, 11, 14, 26, 27] Although in many patients these phases are not distinct and may overlap, awareness of the varied presentations of Takayasu's arteritis may enable the diagnosis to be established early in the course of the illness. Some patients present with nonspecific signs and symptoms of a systemic inflammatory illness such as fever, myalgias, arthralgias, and weight loss. Other patients complain of pain over a presumably inflamed vessel, such as carotodynia. Clues to the diagnosis during this phase include hypertension, vascular bruits, asymmetric arm blood pressures, and early ischemic symptoms. The disease can be very difficult to diagnose during this stage. Some patients present with both systemic inflammatory disease and ischemic manifestations simultaneously. Many patients present in the late, occlusive stage of disease and never manifest a recognized systemic inflammatory component.[14]

Most patients present with symptoms of vascular insufficiency.[6–11, 14] Takayasu's arteritis is a diffuse aortitis that may affect the entire aorta and its branches, as well as the pulmonary arteries.[6–10, 25, 28] The disease has been divided into types based on sites of involvement: type I is localized to the aortic arch and its branches; type II involves the descending and abdominal aorta and is also called atypical coarctation of the aorta; type III manifests features of types I and II; and type IV combines features of types I through III with pulmonary artery disease.[6] Most reported cases fall into the category of type III disease, emphasizing the diffuse nature of the aortitis.[6, 11] The most commonly affected vessels are the subclavian artery, descending aorta, renal artery, carotid artery, mesenteric arteries, ascending aorta, and abdominal aorta.[6–11] However, the vertebral, splenic, pulmonary, coronary, iliac, femoral, brachial, and tibial arteries have also been affected with Takayasu's arteritis.[6–10] Symptoms referable to vascular disease may include syncope, dizziness, claudication, and angina; stroke or myocardial infarction may occur.

This disease was first described by an ophthalmologist, and ocular signs such as blurred vision, amaurosis fugax, and diplopia have been reported. Hypertension due to renal artery stenosis or coarctation of the aorta may occur. Dilatation of the proximal aorta may lead to aortic insufficiency. Congestive heart failure may result from hypertension, aortic insufficiency, and coronary ischemia.[10, 29] Coronary artery involvement may cause angina; the coronary ostia are more frequently affected than distal sites.[10, 29, 30] Although pulmonary artery disease is often asymptomatic, it is found in approximately 50 per cent of patients; occasionally patients may present with severe pulmonary hypertension.[10, 29, 31, 32] Perfusion lung scans may be useful in screening and following up these patients.[33] Although obstructive lesions are commonly seen in the visceral arteries, they are rarely symptomatic because of the development of collateral vessels.[34, 35] However, mesenteric infarction secondary to these lesions has been reported in several patients.[34, 35]

Physical findings generally associated with this disorder include vascular bruits, absent or diminished pulses, hypertension, and asymmetry of the blood pressure between the right and the left sides and between the upper and the lower extremities. The retinopathy noted in early reports but not in the more recent series is believed to be secondary to ischemia leading to neovascularization.[2, 6–10]

Cutaneous disease such as erythema nodosum and pyoderma gangrenosum occurs in up to 16 per cent of patients.[10, 36, 37] Various forms of glomerulonephritis have been noted but are uncommon.[10, 38, 39] Takayasu's arteritis has been reported in association with juvenile rheumatoid arthritis, sarcoidosis, and inflammatory bowel disease.[10, 40–42]

There are no specific laboratory markers associated with Takayasu's arteritis. During the systemic inflammatory phase, patients commonly present with an elevated erythrocyte sedimentation rate, anemia of chronic disease, and leukocytosis.[3, 8–10]

ANGIOGRAPHY

Several distinctive angiographic findings have been described, including (1) narrowing of the aorta and other arteries, which may be short and segmental, long and diffuse, or progress to complete occlusion of the vessel; (2) arterial dilatation and aneurysm formation, both fusiform and saccular; and (3) any combination of these findings.[5, 43] The majority of patients have both dilatative and stenotic lesions. These radiographic features are usually diagnostic, especially when other supportive clinical data are present. However, occasionally a single lesion is identified in an asymptomatic patient or angiographic findings suggest atherosclerotic changes, and the diagnosis can be established only by careful observation of the patient. The authors believe that serial angiography should be part of the initial evaluation of all patients with suspected Takayasu's arteritis, regardless of the clinical assessment of disease activity. Angiograms obtained at 3- to 6-month intervals, correlated with clinical features of disease, provide a good assessment of disease activity.[44] New vascular lesions suggest active arteritis, whereas progressive vessel stenosis in a previously diseased area may be a result of either scarring or active disease. The potential complications associated with angiography, such as bleeding, anaphylaxis, radiation exposure, and infection, require that each procedure be carefully considered. Because of the diffuse nature of this disease, the angiographer should attempt to visualize as much of the arterial tree as possible. It is particularly important to visualize the brachiocephalic vessels; the entire aorta; and the renal, celiac, and mesenteric arteries. In the absence of symptoms, the authors do not routinely perform coronary or pulmonary angiography. Studies have indicated that noninvasive imaging techniques such as ultrasonography and magnetic resonance imaging may play an increasing role in the diagnosis and management of patients with this disease in the future, but at present, angiography remains the principal means of establishing a diagnosis of Takayasu's arteritis.[45–49]

At the time of angiography, blood pressure should be measured directly in the ascending aorta, and this value should be compared with measurements obtained in the extremities.[50] Subclavian and axillary artery disease can interfere with accurate peripheral measurements and make the assessment of systemic hypertension difficult in these patients. This is important because hypertension leads to significant long-term morbidity associated with Takayasu's arteritis.[51]

PATHOLOGY

Histologically, the formation of stenotic lesions is secondary to intimal proliferation and fibrotic contraction of the media and adventitia, whereas aneurysms may form in areas where there is inflammation of the media and disruption of the elastic lamina.[4, 25, 34, 52] Active lesions are characterized by granulomatous vasculitis leading to disruption of the media; a lymphocytoplasmic infiltrate is seen in the media, as are Langhans' and foreign body giant cells. Adventitial fibrosis and intimal proliferation may be noted. Chronic lesions are characterized by transmural sclerosis with little or no inflammatory infiltrate. Adventitial fibrosis tends to be seen in the older chronic or "healed-stage" lesions.[25, 34] Thrombosis may occur, and lesions can be mistaken for atherosclerosis.[25] The diagnosis of Takayasu's arteritis is usually based on the combination of clinical features and compatible angiographic findings. Pathology specimens are usually obtained secondarily at surgery or from autopsy examinations. The authors believe that it is important to obtain specimens from affected vessels at the time of revascularization procedures. It is increasingly realized that histologic proof of inflammation may be found in normal-appearing vessels serving as the origin or insertion of bypass grafts.[34, 50] However, the treatment of patients with clinically and angiographically quiescent disease who have an inflammatory lesion on biopsy remains controversial. Although symptoms of acute inflammation often abate with glucocorticosteroid therapy, it is not clear that therapy inhibits the inflammatory process in the aorta.[3, 6] Because therapy is associated with many untoward side effects, the authors believe that more data on the correlation between histopathologic findings and surgical outcome must be accrued before firm recommendations can be made.

MEDICAL THERAPY

The medical management of Takayasu's arteritis is directed at (1) relieving the systemic manifestations of the disease and decreasing the inflammation in affected vessels and (2) identifying and treating the complications of the vascular disease both medically and surgically.[44] Glucocorticosteroid therapy, prednisone given at 1 mg/kg/day, is generally effective in controlling clinical manifestations and disease progression in patients with active disease.[8–10, 44, 53] The authors maintain patients on this initial dose of daily prednisone for 3 months. After this, in the absence of any evidence of active disease, they attempt to taper the prednisone over a year.[44] However, some patients fail to respond to prednisone therapy and either have signs of active disease while they are receiving high doses of daily prednisone or are unable to have the drug tapered.[3, 9, 44] The authors believe that the side effects of high-dose prednisone over long periods are significant and are rarely justified in treating this disease. Cyclophosphamide has been effective in treating some patients with Takayasu's arteritis who have had progressive disease while receiving daily glucocorticosteroids.[9] However, cyclophosphamide is associated with a number of toxic effects, including infertility, cystitis, and bladder carcinoma.[54] Several groups have successfully treated these patients with low-dose weekly oral methotrexate at a dose of 0.15 to 0.35 mg/kg/wk.[55, 56] Patients who manifest convincing features of active disease, such as systemic complaints, progressive new angiographic lesions, and an elevated erythrocyte sedimentation rate despite aggressive therapy, may need to be maintained on daily prednisone at the lowest effective dose. The authors do not think that long-term glucocorticosteroid therapy is warranted in a patient with the isolated finding of an elevated erythrocyte sedimentation rate. The value of antiplatelet drugs, such as aspirin and dipyridamole, has not been established in Takayasu's arteritis and deserves further study.

The cause of death in Takayasu's arteritis is usually related to the vascular complications of the disease, including hypertension, aortic insufficiency, and stroke.[10, 51] Patients should be followed up expectantly for secondary complications and treated aggressively, both medically and surgically.

More recent studies have indicated improved survival rates compared with those of older studies; one series reported an overall 5-year survival rate of 94 per cent.[7–10, 51, 53] This result is probably due to earlier recognition of the disease, anti-inflammatory therapy, and recognition and treatment of disease complications that have been associated with poor outcomes.[7–10, 44, 51, 53] However, many questions about the treatment of Takayasu's disease remain unanswered and should be addressed in future clinical studies.

PERCUTANEOUS TRANSLUMINAL ANGIOPLASTY

Percutaneous transluminal angioplasty (PTA) is an accepted modality for the treatment of patients with peripheral vascular disease due to atherosclerosis. Excellent results have been obtained in arteries involved with short-segment stenoses, particularly in the iliac and renal arteries, with less impressive results reported for longer or occluded lesions in the more distal arterial segments. Because Takayasu's arteritis affects arteries that would be treated with PTA if they had atherosclerotic occlusive disease involvement, it is not surprising that angioplasty is advocated as a primary form of treatment in arterial segments affected with Takayasu's arteritis.[57–60]

Takayasu's arteritis presents the angiographer with unique technical problems not found in atherosclerosis. The disease is a panarteritis with active and chronic phases that may involve all three arterial wall layers. It is unclear whether the trauma of balloon dilatation in the active phase of the disease exacerbates inflammation and restenosis. Although this theory is unproved, some angiographers recommend PTA *only* if the disease is in an inactive phase, as determined in part by a normal sedimentation rate.[57, 58] In the chronic phase, extensive periarterial wall fibrosis, intimal thickening, and widespread transmural chronic changes produce a stenotic artery that is rigid and noncompliant. Dilatation may not be possible, or three to five attempts at balloon dilatation may be necessary before the "waist" of the stenosis is eliminated. Restenosis in these noncompliant vessels can quickly recur. The introduction of arterial stents may reduce the incidence of restenosis. Distal embolization resulting from PTA in an artery involved with Takayasu's arteritis is unusual because the intima is thickened, and unlike in atherosclerosis, it is smooth and not calcified or ulcerated.

Hypertension due to renal artery stenosis from Takayasu's arteritis is commonly treated with PTA. A short-segment narrowing just beyond the orifice is technically advantageous for PTA. If the adjacent aortic wall is not involved, the stenosis can be traversed with a catheter. Multiple attempts at dilatation may be necessary before the stenosis is eliminated. Statistically, 85 per cent of patients with renal artery stenoses from Takayasu's arteritis have successful dilatation, with 82 per cent of this group achieving initial clinical improvement in the control of their hypertension.[59] Provided overdistention of the artery with the balloon is not attempted, complications, including dissection and occlusion, are unusual. Restenosis is most likely to occur in renal arteries that have a residual stenosis of 20 to 30 per cent after the initial dilatation.[59]

Isolated reports of successful balloon dilatation of the abdominal aorta, subclavian artery, and mesenteric vessels have been published.[57, 58, 60] The common carotid and the iliac arteries often have long-segment stenoses that preclude PTA.

Although these reports suggest that short-segment stenoses of arteries affected with Takayasu's arteritis can be dilated, the follow-up of these patients has been short. The good long-term results of PTA on arteries affected with arteriosclerotic occlusive disease should not be extrapolated to arteries with Takayasu's disease. Even after only 6 months of follow-up, restenosis of dilated arteries has been reported in the majority of cases.[61] This is not surprising, given the nature of the arterial pathology, the effects of trauma from balloon dilatation, and the poor compliance of arteries with Takayasu's disease. Nevertheless, because of the low complication rate and good initial results, it appears reasonable to attempt balloon dilatation on renal and other arteries with short-segment stenoses.

GENERAL PRINCIPLES OF SURGICAL TREATMENT

1. Patients with Takayasu's arteritis present the surgeon with problems that are different from the clinical problems of atherosclerosis. Treatment for patients with Takayasu's arteritis must be individualized. There must be careful coordination between medical and surgical treatment and provision for long-term follow-up.

2. The surgeon should not assume that, because most patients with Takayasu's arteritis are young, complications from systemic medical problems are uncommon. These patients may have significant cardiac problems, including a low but definite incidence of coronary artery involvement.[20, 29, 30, 62] In 54 patients studied in India, 35 had hypertension, 24 had congestive heart failure, and 27 had ejection fractions under 45 per cent.[29] Of 32 North American patients, 5 had ischemic heart disease and 18 eventually developed significant hypertension.[8] Systemic hypertension is frequently unrecognized and untreated because of subclavian involvement leading to left ventricular hypertrophy and congestive heart failure.

3. Most patients do not need urgent or emergency surgery but can undergo elective surgical procedures, allowing time for a complete evaluation.

4. Although it is not always possible, avoiding surgical procedures during the acute phase of the disease is preferred. Reports have suggested but not proved that fewer surgical complications occur if medical treatment has initially controlled the acute phase of the illness.[61] Surgical procedures can be performed once the erythrocyte sedimentation rate returns to normal.

5. Bypass of obstructive lesions is the preferred surgical approach. To minimize anastomotic complications, the proximal and distal anastomoses are performed in arteries free of disease on arteriography. It is advisable not to use arteries for anastomotic sites that have a high incidence of involvement.[34, 63] These arteries may later become involved, causing stenoses of the anastomotic site. Again, it should be emphasized that even arteries that appear normal on arteriography may have microscopic evidence of disease.[34, 50] Endarterectomy with patch grafting is technically difficult because involvement of all three arterial layers may be present. Even if endarterectomy is possible, suturing arteries affected with disease may cause anastomotic problems later.

CEREBROVASCULAR SYSTEM

Cerebrovascular symptoms in this young patient population are common because of the high incidence of involvement of the major branches of the aortic arch. The lateralizing cerebrovascular symptoms of stroke, transient ischemic attacks, and amaurosis fugax occur in 8 to 35 per cent of patients.[8, 34, 61, 63] The incidence of stroke alone was 14 per cent.[63] A high incidence of nonlateralizing symptoms, such as dizziness and syncope, has also been reported.[8, 34, 61, 63] Although it is easy to postulate that these symptoms are consistent with extensive involvement of the aortic arch arteries that limits cerebral blood flow, documentation of this is lacking. Not all patients with dizziness allegedly due to cerebrovascular involvement have a reduction in ocular pressures, indicating that hemodynamically significant carotid arterial disease may not always be present.[8] Nonlateralizing symptoms could be due to causes other than stenoses of aortic arch arteries, such as accelerated hypertension, arrhythmias, and congestive heart failure.

Arteriograms of the aortic arch and its branches usu-

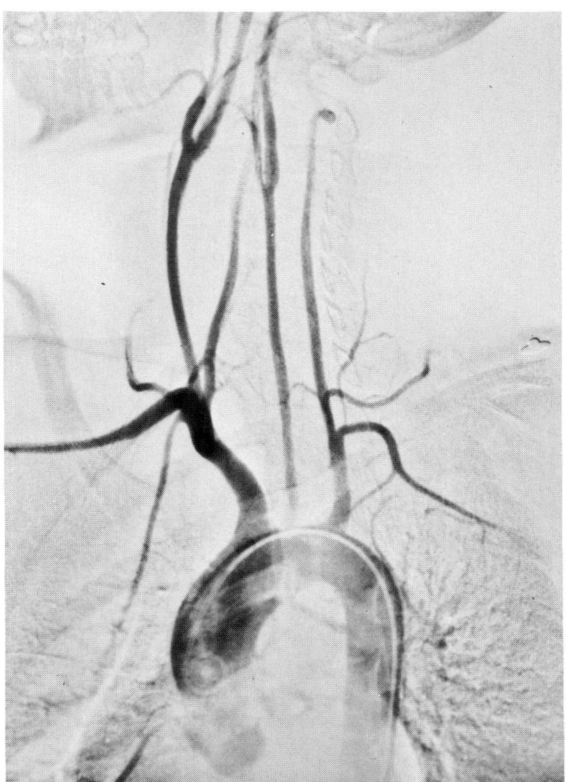

FIGURE 12–1. Characteristic long tapered stenosis of the left common carotid artery, with sparing of the carotid bifurcation.

ally show a long area of stenosis involving the common carotid artery and usually sparing the carotid bifurcation and the internal carotid artery (Fig. 12–1). The intima of the involved artery appears smooth, without evidence of ulcerations or segmental narrowing that could cause local turbulence. Therefore, it is unlikely to be a source of major emboli. Stroke more likely occurs from total occlusion of one or more aortic arch arteries. Because the common carotid and subclavian arteries are so frequently involved, blood flow is restricted to not only the internal carotid but also the external and vertebral arteries, reducing blood flow to the circle of Willis. The innominate artery itself is at times occluded. If one or all of these involved vessels suddenly occlude, the patient could sustain a stroke from the marked reduction in cerebral blood flow. In the authors' series, all four patients who sustained a major stroke had occlusion of one or more thoracic aortic arch arteries, suggesting that the stroke occurred from a reduction in cerebrovascular blood flow.[63]

Bypass is recommended to prevent stroke in patients who have hemodynamically significant stenoses of either the innominate or carotid arteries. These bypasses should originate from the ascending aorta, not the more commonly involved subclavian artery. The ascending aorta has only a 5 per cent incidence of involvement, reducing the potential for proximal anastomotic stenosis. The authors observed that strokes did not occur in the seven patients who underwent bypass.[63]

RENOVASCULAR HYPERTENSION

The incidence of hypertension in patients with Takayasu's arteritis is high, ranging from 20 to 72 per cent.[6, 8, 9, 34] This diagnosis is important because the major morbidity and mortality from the disease (i.e., that caused by congestive heart failure, cardiomyopathy, hemorrhagic stroke, hypertensive encephalopathy, and myocardial infarction) are due to the effects of uncontrolled hypertension. However, the frequent involvement of both subclavian arteries may mask the diagnosis of hypertension, leaving patients with significantly elevated blood pressure that is both undiagnosed and untreated. Most cases of hypertension are due to renal artery stenosis. Some reviews report a high incidence of mid-abdominal aortic coarctation that can cause renovascular hypertension.[6, 34] It is not clear from these reports whether this mid-abdominal aortic coarctation is due to developmental abnormalities or Takayasu's disease.

Bypass of renal artery stenosis is recommended for renovascular hypertension and kidney salvage. The role of PTA has already been discussed. The authors recommend an aggressive approach with this young patient population rather than prolonged periods of antihypertensive medication.

Renal artery disease is usually confined to the proximal segment, leaving an uninvolved segment available for the distal anastomosis (Fig. 12–2). The frequent involvement of the infrarenal aorta may preclude the use of this artery for the proximal anastomosis. Therefore, it may be necessary to use the hepatic or supraceliac abdominal aorta as the inflow site, provided there is no evidence of disease in these arteries. Vein is the preferred conduit for the bypass. Stenotic involvement of the descending thoracic or mid-abdominal aorta has been reported in European studies to be a common cause of renovascular hypertension.[34, 64] This requires a more extensive procedure: revascularization of the distal abdominal aorta combined with bypass to both renal arteries. Surgical treatment for renovascular hypertension due to Takayasu's arteritis has been reported in only a small number of cases, but follow-up has been extensive.[8, 34, 61] In general, the results are comparable to those of the larger series of surgical treatment for renovascular hypertension due to atherosclerosis.

VISCERAL ARTERY INVOLVEMENT

The incidence of celiac and superior mesenteric artery involvement varies from 5 to 66 per cent.[8, 9, 34] Arterial blood flow to the visceral circulation could also be compromised by stenoses of the thoracic or suprarenal aorta. Despite this high incidence of disease, clinical problems are unusual, with few indications for surgical correction.[34, 35] An aggressive approach to visceral artery involvement was reported from Russia.[64] In a large series of 300 patients, 25 per cent had visceral artery involvement. Nine patients developed chronic visceral ischemia. Forty-one patients underwent visceral artery reconstruction, which included 13 graft bypasses and 28 transaortic endarterectomies. The rec-

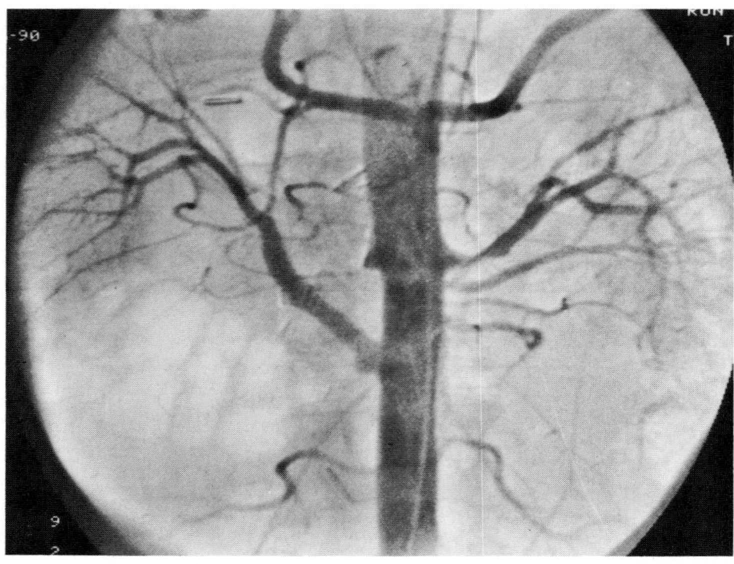

FIGURE 12–2. Classic involvement of the left renal artery with Takayasu's arteritis. Note the bypass of the right renal artery.

ommendation is made that involvement of the visceral circulation should be corrected even if patients are asymptomatic. This experience is not consistent with that reported in series from North America.[8, 61, 63] In addition, endarterectomy of these lesions can be difficult because of inflammatory disease and severe fibrosis in the arterial wall. The authors recommend observation of asymptomatic patients with visceral artery involvement. A bypass originating from the uninvolved abdominal aorta is recommended only for the rare patients with symptoms of chronic intestinal ischemia.

UPPER AND LOWER EXTREMITY ARTERIAL DISEASE

Symptoms of upper extremity ischemia are common because of the frequent involvement of the subclavian and axillary arteries. Unlike atherosclerosis, which is characterized by short-segment proximal stenosis or occlusion, Takayasu's arteritis involves much longer segments of these arteries (Fig. 12–3). Because the subclavian artery is usually involved both proximal and distal to the origin of the vertebral artery, the subclavian steal syndrome is rare. With long-segment arterial involvement, symptoms of upper extremity ischemia tend to be more severe in patients with Takayasu's arteritis than in those with atherosclerosis. Because these patients are young and active, bypass for upper arm ischemia is sometimes necessary. Measurement of blood pressure in the upper arm may be inaccurate because of involvement of both subclavian arteries. In view of the potentially devastating morbidity of uncontrolled hypertension, it is appropriate in some cases to consider upper extremity revascularization to provide access for accurate determination of systemic blood pressure.

Bypass with grafts originating from the ascending aorta is the preferred method for revascularization of the upper extremity. The use of the common carotid artery as the inflow vessel, even if it is uninvolved, should be discouraged. The high incidence of disease in the common carotid arteries places the patient at increased risk for graft occlusion at a later date. Revascularization of the subclavian artery is frequently done concomitantly with a bypass of one or both common carotid arteries with hemodynamically significant stenosis. The use of a bifurcation graft from the ascending aorta with limbs to both subclavian arteries and the use of a bifurcation graft with one limb to the subclavian artery and one to the carotid artery are two common clinical approaches.

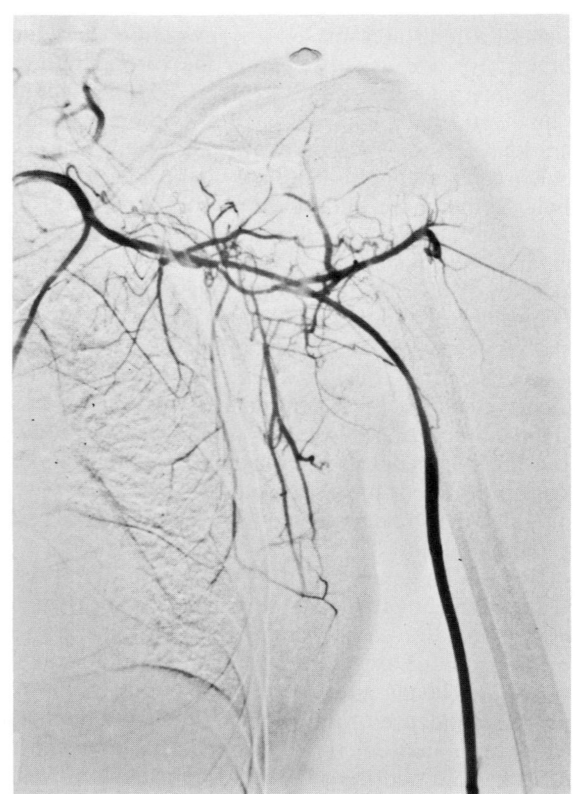

FIGURE 12–3. Long-segment involvement of the subclavian and axillary arteries classic for Takayasu's disease.

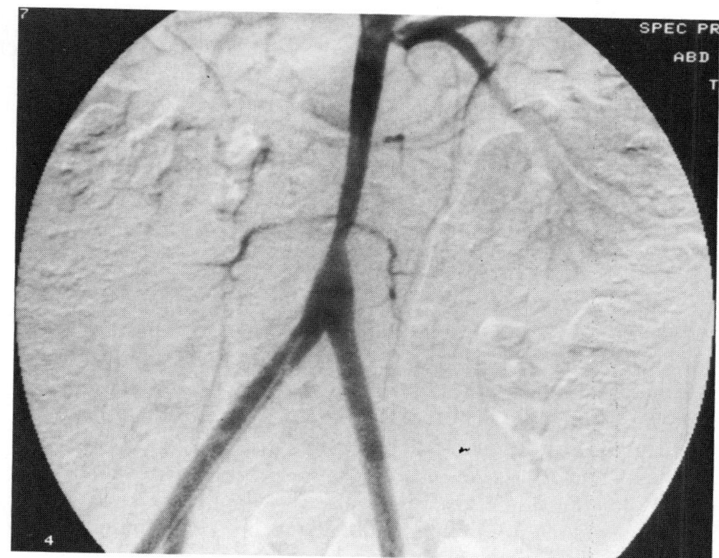

FIGURE 12–4. Involvement of the infrarenal abdominal aorta. Note the sparing of the distal aorta. Bypass from the thoracic aorta to the left iliac artery perfuses both legs.

Claudication of the lower extremity is considerably less common than upper extremity ischemic symptoms.[8, 61] This is due to less frequent involvement of the iliac arteries and the low incidence of the disease in the femoral and distal arterial circulation. Most cases of lower extremity claudication result from abdominal aortic involvement, particularly in the infrarenal abdominal aorta. It is peculiar that the disease may cause marked narrowing of the aorta below the renal arteries but spare the distal aorta (Fig. 12–4). Rest pain, gangrene, and nonhealing ulcerations occur but are unusual.

Claudication symptoms can be severe, and it is not clear whether conservative measures, such as a walking program, increase exercise tolerance. Because these patients are young and have severe symptoms, a more aggressive approach is at times warranted. Most cases involve bypass of the stenotic abdominal aorta. Because the disease usually affects the aorta below the renal arteries, the proximal anastomosis of a bifurcation graft is placed in the supraceliac aorta. Another approach is bypass with a 10-mm tube graft from the lower thoracic aorta retroperitoneally to the left external iliac artery. Both legs are then perfused through the spared lower distal abdominal aorta.[65]

ANEURYSMS

The incidence of aneurysm formation from Takayasu's arteritis varies in different parts of the world. The largest series of aneurysms were from studies in Japan[66] and India,[67] where aneurysms occurred in 31.9 per cent (36 of 113) and 22.2 per cent (30 of 135) of cases, respectively. Both studies reported that the aneurysms were multiple, saccular and fusiform, associated with stenotic lesions, and most commonly found in the ascending, thoracic, and abdominal aorta. Other arteries such as the subclavian and brachiocephalic were less commonly involved. These studies reported a low incidence of aneurysm resection and rupture, with each study noting only one ruptured aneurysm. Aneurysms were more common in Japanese patients older than 40 years of age, but this finding was not confirmed in the report from India. Other studies reported a lower incidence of aneurysms, with a 10 per cent occurrence in a large series from Russia and an even lower incidence from North America (Fig. 12–5).[8, 63, 64]

The incidence of aneurysm rupture is low, and most series report that only a small percentage of patients with aneurysms undergo resection. Nevertheless, localized fusi-

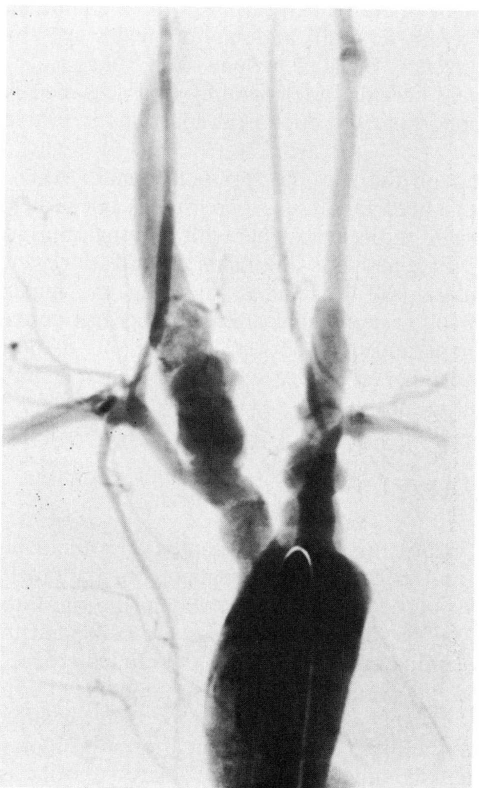

FIGURE 12–5. Extensive aneurysmal involvement of the ascending aorta and its main branches in a 17-year-old patient.

form or saccular aneurysms in a medically stable patient should be resected. These patients are young and can anticipate a long life. The risk of aneurysm resection is probably lower than the risk of rupture in patients followed up for a long period. Resection and aortic valve replacement are also recommended for aneurysms of the ascending aorta causing clinically significant aortic insufficiency.

SURGICAL RESULTS

Reports of surgical series have emphasized that patients with Takayasu's arteritis can undergo revascularization with minimal morbidity and mortality.[34, 61, 63] These excellent results are due to careful preoperative evaluation, avoidance of procedures in patients with active disease, careful patient selection, and the use of maximal medical therapy to control the disease process. None of these series are large, and the follow-up on all patients has been limited. Because these patients have a much longer life expectancy than the older patient population surgically treated for atherosclerosis, 20- to 30-year follow-up may yield less gratifying results.

The available evidence suggests that these patients have an acceptable incidence of anastomotic problems. Although one series reported the development of 5 false aneurysms in 90 patients undergoing procedures over a 35-year period, other series reported that false aneurysms did not occur.[61, 63, 68] Anastomotic stenoses have been reported, but the incidence is acceptable, and their occurrence is not necessarily related to the activity of disease at the time of surgery.[61, 63] The anastomotic stenoses may be related to the development of intimal hyperplasia from compliance mismatch of synthetic grafts and may not necessarily be due to local recurrence. Because patients with Takayasu's arteritis should have periodic arteriography to assess disease activity, the opportunity to document anastomotic problems exists.

Although the surgical series are small, good clinical results have been reported. Aggressive surgical therapy can be performed in these patients with minimal morbidity and mortality. Patients with significant carotid lesions have had successful bypass procedures, reducing the incidence of stroke in follow-up. Renal artery bypass has cured or decreased hypertension. The long-term results of procedures to relieve upper or lower extremity ischemia have been successful in most cases.

SUMMARY

Takayasu's disease is a complex arteritis of unknown etiology that affects a young patient population. Stenoses and occlusion of the major arteries are the life-threatening sequelae of this disease. Surgeons are consulted to assess and to recommend treatment for the clinical consequences of arterial involvement, but few surgeons have experience with this unusual disease. It is important for surgeons to appreciate the differences between arterial problems due to atherosclerosis and those due to Takayasu's disease. It is equally important for the treating physicians to coordinate medical and surgical therapy carefully. Follow-up must be intense and long term. Thoughtful medical and surgical therapy should produce excellent long-term results.

References

1. McKusick VA: A form of vascular disease relatively frequent in the Orient. Am Heart J 63:57, 1962.
2. Judge RD, Currier RD, Gracie WA, et al: Takayasu's arteritis and the aortic arch syndrome. Am J Med 32:379, 1962.
3. Nakao K, Ikeda M, Kimata S-I, et al: Takayasu's arteritis. Clinical report of eighty-four cases and immunological studies of seven cases. Circulation 35:1141, 1967.
4. Vinijchaikul K: Primary arteritis of the aorta and its main branches (Takayasu's arteriopathy). A clinicopathologic autopsy study of eight cases. Am J Med 43:15, 1967.
5. Hachiya J: Current concepts of Takayasu's arteritis. Semin Roentgenol 5:245, 1970.
6. Lupi-Herrera E, Sanchez-Torres G, Marcushamer J, et al: Takayasu's arteritis. Clinical study of 107 cases. Am Heart J 93:94, 1977.
7. Ishikawa K: Natural history and classification of occlusive thromboaortopathy (Takayasu's disease). Circulation 57:27, 1978.
8. Hall S, Barr W, Lie JT, et al: Takayasu arteritis. A study of 32 North American patients. Medicine 64:89, 1985.
9. Shelhamer JH, Volkman DJ, Parrillo JE, et al: Takayasu's arteritis and its therapy. Ann Intern Med 103:121, 1985.
10. Hall S, Buchbinder R: Takayasu's arteritis. Rheum Dis Clin North Am 16:411, 1990.
11. Procter CD, Hollier LH: Takayasu's arteritis and temporal arteritis. Ann Vasc Surg 6:195, 1992.
12. Nasu T: Takayasu's truncoarteritis in Japan. A statistical observation of 76 autopsy cases. Pathol Microbiol 43:140, 1975.
13. Waern AU, Andersson P, Hemmingsson A: Takayasu's arteritis: A hospital-region based study on occurrence, treatment and prognosis. Angiology 34:311, 1983.
14. Lande A, Berkmen YM: Aortitis. Pathologic, clinical and arteriographic review. Radiol Clin North Am 14:219, 1976.
15. Kinare SG: Aortitis in early life in India and its association with tuberculosis. J Pathol 100:69, 1970.
16. Isohisa I, Numano F, Maezawa H, et al: Takayasu disease. Tissue Antigens 12:246, 1978.
17. Naito S, Arakawa K, Saito S, et al: Takayasu's disease: Association with HLA-B5. Tissue Antigens 12:143, 1978.
18. Sasazuki T, Ohta N, Isoshisa I, et al: Association between Takayasu disease and HLA-DHO. Tissue Antigens 14:177, 1979.
19. Volkman DJ, Mann DL, Fauci AS: Association between Takayasu's arteritis and a B-cell alloantigen in North Americans. N Engl J Med 306:464, 1982.
20. Numano F, Isohisa I, Maezawa H, et al: HL-A antigens in Takayasu's disease. Am Heart J 98:153, 1979.
21. Takeuchi Y, Matsuki K, Saito Y, et al: HLA-D region genomic polymorphism associated with Takayasu's arteritis. Angiology 41:421, 1990.
22. Khraisis MM, Gladman DD, Dagenais P, et al: HLA antigens in North American patients with Takayasu arteritis. Arthritis Rheum 35:573, 1992.
23. Kerr G, et al: Personal communication.
24. Morales E, Pineda C, Martinez-Lavin M: Takayasu's arteritis in children. J Rheumatol 18:1081, 1991.
25. Lie JT: The classification and diagnosis of vasculitis in large and medium-sized blood vessels. Pathol Annu 22(Pt 1):125, 1987.
26. Strachan RW: The natural history of Takayasu's arteriopathy. Q J Med 33:57, 1964.
27. Volkman DJ, Fauci AS: Takayasu's arteritis. *In* Lichtenstein L, Fauci AS (eds): Current Therapy in Allergy and Immunology 1983–1984. Philadelphia, BC Decker, 1983, p 143.
28. Lande A, Gross A: Total aortography in the diagnosis of Takayasu's arteritis. Am J Roentgenol 116:165, 1972.
29. Panja M, Kar AK, Dutta AL, et al: Cardiac involvement in nonspecific aorto-arteritis. Int J Cardiol 34:289, 1992.
30. Amano J, Suzuki A: Coronary artery involvement in Takayasu's arteritis. J Thorac Cardiovasc Surg 102:554, 1991.
31. Lupi E, Sanchez G, Horwitz S, et al: Pulmonary artery involvement in Takayasu's arteritis. Chest 67:69, 1975.
32. Haas A, Stiehm ER: Takayasu's arteritis presenting as pulmonary hypertension. Am J Dis Child 140:372, 1986.

33. Umehara I, Shibuya H, Nakagawa T, et al: Comprehensive analysis of perfusion scintigraphy in Takayasu's arteritis. Clin Nucl Med 16:352, 1991.
34. Lagneau P, Michel JB, Vuong PN: Surgical treatment of Takayasu's disease. Ann Surg 205:157, 1987.
35. Nussaume O, Bouttier S, Duchatelle J-P, et al: Mesenteric infarction in Takayasu's disease. Ann Vasc Surg 4:117, 1990.
36. Perniciaro CV, Winkelmann RK, Hunder GG: Cutaneous manifestations of Takayasu's arteritis. J Am Acad Dermatol 17:998, 1987.
37. Frances C, Boisnic S, Bletry O, et al: Cutaneous manifestations of Takayasu arteritis. Dermatologica 181:266, 1990.
38. Hellmann DB, Hardy K, Lindenfeld S, et al: Takayasu's arteritis associated with crescentic glomerulonephritis. Arthritis Rheum 30:451, 1987.
39. Koumi S-I, Endo T, Okumura H, et al: A case of Takayasu's arteritis associated with membranoproliferative glomerulonephritis and nephrotic syndrome. Nephron 54:344, 1990.
40. Hall S, Nelson AM: Takayasu's arteritis and juvenile rheumatoid arthritis. J Rheumatol 13:431, 1986.
41. Rose CD, Eichenfield AH, Goldsmith DP, et al: Early onset sarcoidosis with aortitis—"Juvenile systemic granulomatosis?" J Rheumatol 17:102, 1990.
42. Achar KN, Al-Nakib B: Takayasu's arteritis and ulcerative colitis. Am J Gastroenterol 81:1215, 1986.
43. Lande A, Rossi P: The value of total aortography in the diagnosis of Takayasu's arteritis. Radiology 114:287, 1975.
44. Leavitt RY, Fauci AS: Takayasu's arteritis. *In* Lichtenstein LM, Fauci AS (eds): Current Therapy in Allergy, Immunology and Rheumatology. 4th ed. Philadelphia, BC Decker, 1992, p 218.
45. Buckley A, Southwood T, Culham G, et al: The role of ultrasound in evaluation of Takayasu's arteritis. J Rheumatol 18:1073, 1991.
46. Maeda H, Handa N, Matsumoto M, et al: Carotid lesions detected by B-mode ultrasonography in Takayasu's arteritis: "Macaroni sign" as an indicator of the disease. Ultrasound Med Biol 17:695, 1991.
47. Dashefsky SM, Cooperberg PL, Harrison PB, et al: Total occlusion of the common carotid artery with patent internal carotid artery: Identification with color flow doppler imaging. J Ultrasound Med 10:417, 1991.
48. Oneson SR, Lewin JS, Smith AS: MR angiography of Takayasu arteritis. J Comput Assist Tomogr 16:478, 1992.
49. Tanigawa K, Eguchi K, Kitamura Y, et al: Magnetic resonance imaging detection of aortic and pulmonary artery wall thickening in the acute stage of Takayasu's arteritis. Arthritis Rheum 35:476, 1992.
50. Kieffer E, Piquois AL, Bertal A, et al: Reconstructive surgery of the renal arteries in Takayasu's disease. Ann Vasc Surg 4:156, 1990.
51. Ishikawa K: Survival and morbidity after diagnosis of occlusive thromboaortopathy (Takayasu's disease). Am J Cardiol 47:1026, 1981.
52. Nasu T: Pathology of pulseless disease. Angiology 14:225, 1963.
53. Fraga A, Mintz G, Valle L, et al: Takayasu's arteritis: Frequency of systemic manifestations (study of 22 patients) and favorable response to maintenance steroid therapy with adrenocorticosteroids (12 patients). Arthritis Rheum 15:617, 1972.
54. Hoffman GS, Kerr GS, Leavitt RY, et al: Wegener's granulomatosis: A prospective analysis of 158 patients. Ann Intern Med 116:488, 1992.
55. Hoffman GS, Leavitt RY, Kerr GS, et al: Treatment of Takayasu's arteritis with methotrexate. Arthritis Rheum 34(9)(Suppl):74, 1991.
56. Liang GC, Nemickas R, Madayag M: Multiple percutaneous transluminal angioplasties and low-dose pulse methotrexate for Takayasu's arteritis. Rheumatology 16:1370, 1989.
57. Sharma S, Rajani M, Kaul U, et al: Initial experience with percutaneous transluminal angioplasty in the management of Takayasu's arteritis. Br J Radiol 63:517, 1990.
58. Park JH, Han MC, Kim SH, et al: Takayasu's arteritis: Angiographic findings and results of angioplasty. Am J Radiol 153:1069, 1989.
59. Sharma S, Saxena A, Talwar KK, et al: Renal artery stenosis caused by non-specific arteritis (Takayasu's disease). Results of treatment with percutaneous transluminal angioplasty. Am J Radiol 158:417, 1992.
60. Kumar S, Mandalam R, Rao VRK, et al: Percutaneous transluminal angioplasty in non-specific aortoarteritis (Takayasu's disease): Experience in 16 cases. Cardiovasc Intervent Radiol 12:321, 1990.
61. Weaver FA, Yellin AE, Campen DH, et al: Surgical procedures in the management of Takayasu's arteritis. J Vasc Surg 12:429, 1990.
62. Talwar KD, Kumar K, Chopra P, et al: Cardiac involvement in nonspecific aortoarteritis (Takayasu's arteritis). Am Heart J 122(6):1666, 1991.
63. Giordano J, Leavitt RY, Hoffman G, et al: Experience with surgical treatment of Takayasu's disease. Surgery 109:252, 1991.
64. Prokrovsky AV: Nonspecific aortoarteritis. *In* Rutherford RB (ed): Vascular Surgery. 3rd ed. Philadelphia, WB Saunders, 1989, p 217.
65. Giordano J: Surgical treatment of Takayasu's disease. *In* Ernst CB, Stanley JC (eds): Current Therapy in Vascular Surgery. 2nd ed. Philadelphia, BC Decker, 1991, p 169.
66. Matsumura K, Hirano T, Takeda K, et al: Incidence of aneurysms in Takayasu's arteritis. Angiology 42(4):308, 1991.
67. Kumar S, Subramanyan R, Ravi Mandalam K, et al: Aneurysmal form of aortoarteritis (Takayasu's disease). Analysis of thirty cases. Clin Radiol 42:342, 1990.
68. Takagi A, Tada J, Sato O: Surgical treatment for Takayasu's arteritis. J Cardiovasc Surg 30(4):553, 1989.

13

Arterial Aneurysms: Etiologic Considerations

M. David Tilson, M.D., and Raju H. Gandhi, M.D.

• • •

An arterial aneurysm may be defined as a permanent localized arterial dilatation with a 50 per cent or greater increase over the normal diameter of the affected artery. Since the mid-1980s, numerous investigations into the etiology of aneurysms have led to significant changes in concepts of aneurysm pathogenesis. Classification systems have emerged based on etiology, site, morphology, and size. In this chapter, the classification based on etiologic factors as suggested by the Society of Vascular Surgery/International Society of Cardiovascular Surgery (SVS/ISCVS) Subcommittee on Reporting Standards for Arterial Aneurysms is used, with minor modifications (Table 13–1).[1] All classification schemes have imperfections. Should post-stenotic dilatations be considered congenital in the

Table 13–1. Etiologic Classification of Arterial Aneurysms

Congenital
Primary connective tissue disorders
Marfan's syndrome
Ehlers-Danlos syndrome
Other
Focal medial agenesis
Tuberous sclerosis
Turner's syndrome
Menkes' syndrome
Mechanical (hemodynamic)
Post-stenotic
Arteriovenous fistula and postamputation related
Traumatic (pseudoaneurysms)
Penetrating arterial injuries
Blunt arterial injuries
Pseudoaneurysms
Inflammatory (noninfectious)
Associated with arteritis
Takayasu's disease
Giant cell arteritis
Systemic lupus erythematosus
Behçet's syndrome
Kawasaki's disease
Periarterial (i.e., pancreatitis)
Infectious (mycotic)
Bacterial
Fungal
Spirochetal
Pregnancy related
Degenerative
Nonspecific
Inflammatory variant
Anastomotic (postarteriotomy) and graft aneurysms
Infection
Arterial wall failure
Suture failure
Graft failure

sense that there may be a predisposing developmental anatomic variant such as a cervical rib, or should they be in the hemodynamic group? The authors decided on hemodynamic because it is the cervical rib that is congenital, whereas the aneurysm is acquired. Should the inflammatory aneurysm be discussed as a variant of the nonspecific group or as a variant of the inflammatory (noninfectious) group? Some day, the inflammatory aneurysm might be reclassified as infectious if some microbial agent is discovered (analogous to the situation with Lyme disease). Should not the degenerative, nonspecific aneurysm (atherosclerotic) now be considered congenital because many, if not most, investigators believe that there is a strong probability of genetic predisposition in many patients? These are some of the questions that are presently unanswerable.

A form of aortic disease not dealt with in detail in this chapter is the aortic dissection, which poses another entymologic problem. Dissections are frequently referred to imprecisely as "dissecting aneurysms" when the media has separated after an intimal tear. Many dissections begin in vessels of relatively normal diameter, and some occur in aneurysmal thoracic aortae. Approximately 10 per cent of acute dissections heal, at which point the term *aneurysm* may become appropriate if the false channel is conspicuously dilated. Perhaps these should be classified as false aneurysms because the dilatated portion does not contain all layers of the normal vessel.

Structural weakness and mechanical and hemodynamic forces are the basic etiologic factors responsible for the development of aneurysmal disease. Some combination of the two is necessary for the initiation and progression of most aneurysms. The relative contribution of each varies according to the type of aneurysm. For example, hemodynamic stresses, mechanical stresses, or both appear to be the major etiologic contributors in the development of post-stenotic dilatations; however, increased levels of enzyme activity that may lead to mural weakness have been detected in the arterial tissue adjacent to the stenotic segment.[2] In most other true aneurysms, mural weakness is thought to be the primary developmental abnormality; again, however, other mechanical or hemodynamic factors such as hypertension may play a role.

Before each type of aneurysm is discussed, a brief review of arterial wall architecture is important for understanding the processes that cause structural failure in aneurysm development. Collagen and elastin are the major structural proteins of the arterial wall. Collagen imparts tensile strength to the vessels, whereas elastin is responsible for its recoil capacity. Arteries have three distinct layers: the intima, the media, and the adventitia. The intima consists of a layer of endothelial cells that adhere to a basement membrane to form the lumen flow surface. In the media, elastic fibers are disposed in layers between smooth muscle cells to form lamellar units. The number of units is a function of arterial wall tension; this relationship is well preserved throughout mammalian species, with the exception of the human abdominal aorta, which contains fewer units than expected from the load it bears.[3] This interesting fact may be one of the reasons that the abdominal aortic aneurysm is common in humans. The adventitia is a layer of investing connective tissue that also contains elastin, along with most of the load-bearing collagen. Studies have suggested that failure of the collagen in this important zone is a pivotal event in aneurysm development.[4]

CONGENITAL

By definition, congenital disease is present at the time of birth, although the majority of aneurysms that have been labeled as congenital develop or are clinically detected later in childhood or even in adulthood. These aneurysms are associated with the primary inherited connective tissue disorders (Marfan's syndrome or Ehlers-Danlos syndrome) or other inherited disease associated with vessel wall weakness. As mentioned earlier, congenital anomalies that cause hemodynamic changes predisposing to aneurysm formation are classified under the mechanical group. Cases of truly idiopathic congenital aneurysms are rare and may be considered secondary to undiagnosed underlying disease.

Primary Disorders

Marfan's Syndrome

Marfan described features of the syndrome that bears his name nearly a century ago, but not until about 1950 did skeptics become convinced that the disease was due to a single mutant gene.[5] The identification of this gene has resulted from a combination of classic and reverse genetics. The classic approach is to begin with a candidate protein and pursue it to the gene level, whereas the reverse approach is to start with genomic DNA of members of affected families and to study the segregation of different chromosomes (or their fragments) with the phenotype by analysis of marker restriction fragment length polymorphisms within the family. The reverse approach initially led to the exclusion of most chromosomes other than 15 and eventually led to the assignment of the Marfan gene to the long arm of chromosome 15 in several Finnish families.[6] Along the classic line, McKusick is credited with suggesting that an understanding of the biochemical feature that the aorta and the suspensory ligament of the lens have in common might lead to characterization of the underlying defect.[7] Fibrillin, a microfibrillar protein of connective tissue discovered by Sakai and coworkers in 1986, was such a candidate.[8] In 1990, Hollister and coworkers described abnormalities of fibrillin in both skin and cultured fibroblasts from patients with Marfan's syndrome.[9] Other investigators mapped genes for the fibrillins to chromosomes 5 and 15, and it has now been shown that the gene on chromosome 15 is linked to the Marfan phenotype.[10] Closing the loop, Dietz and colleagues demonstrated identical point mutations in the fibrillin gene in two patients with Marfan's syndrome; this mutation changed the codon for arginine at residue 239 to a glycine.[11] This story is a paradigm for the power of the new biology in uncovering the molecular basis of vascular diseases.

Ehlers-Danlos Syndrome

A prototype of the classic form of Ehlers-Danlos syndrome (ED) was described by vanMeekeren in the 17th century.[12] A young Spanish man could stretch the skin from his right chest to his left ear. Barabas noted that the heterogeneity of the syndrome is implied even by its name,[13] and at present multiple phenotypic variations of the syndrome are recognized. Ehlers described a case with excess bruising, and Danlos described a case with excess scarring. Both patients had hyperextensibility of the skin and hypermobility of the joints. The eponym *Ehlers-Danlos* was coined by Weber in 1936.[14]

Ten clinical types of this syndrome have been assigned roman numerals I through X. ED-I and -IV are the types associated with vascular catastrophies. ED-I (gravis) is an autosomal dominant disorder with severe joint hypermobility and hyperextensibility of skin. Arterial ruptures may occur in type I disease, but they are not common.

In 1967, Barabas described two patients with severe arterial complications who had soft, thin skin with an extreme tendency to bruise.[15] This ecchymotic variant was subsequently classified as type IV. Spontaneous perforations of the colon also occur in type IV disease. Tears of peripheral arteries occur spontaneously or after trivial trauma, and visceral branches are also prone to disruptions. Gentle application of vascular clamps may result in uncontrollable hemorrhage, and surgery under such conditions has been described by Wesley and associates as a ''surrealistic'' experience.[16]

The first abnormalities of collagen in ED-IV were discovered in 1975, when Pope and coworkers reported deficiency of type III collagen in tissue and cultured fibroblast.[17] This group subsequently suggested that there were both clinical and molecular heterogeneities among the ED-IV patients.[18] Both Pope and coworkers and Barabas have taken the position that disease should not be classified as ED-IV, even with proven abnormalities in type III collagen, unless the classic skin changes are present.[13, 19] This has led Barabas to argue that the presence of true aneurysms in ED-IV is a misconception.[13]

A family has been described in which several members have had abdominal aortic aneurysms associated with a point mutation in the type III procollagen gene, but members of this family do not have the classic skin changes of ED-IV.[20] The question now is whether to adhere to earlier rigid criteria whereby skin changes are a requirement for the ED-IV phenotype or to classify the disease in such a family as a new subtype. One of the authors of this chapter believes that considering the established relationship of type III collagen to the occurrence of arterial disease and its central role in the original formulation of ED-IV, the most sensible approach is to define a new subset within the ED-IV category.[21]

According to this proposal, ED-IVA would be the classic type, referred to as acrogeria, with characteristic skin, facies, and arterial ruptures. ED-IVB would be the Sack-Barabas type, with severe ecchymoses along with ruptures of arteries and bowel. ED-IVC would be the aneurysmal type, and it is also likely to have several subsets, depending on the mutations in type III collagen detected and the site of the associated aneurysmal lesions.

Other Congenital Forms

Other congenital systemic disorders associated with aneurysm development include focal medial agenesis, tuberous sclerosis, gonadal dysgenesis (Turner's syndrome), Menkes' kinky-hair syndrome, and neurofibromatosis. *Focal medial agenesis* has been mainly responsible for intracranial berry aneurysms, with rare reports of peripheral aneurysms.[22] *Tuberous sclerosis,* an autosomal dominant developmental abnormality of the central nervous system associated with seizures, mental retardation, and adenoma sebaceum in infants and children, has been associated with thoracic and abdominal aneurysms. Possible etiologic contributors to these disorders include aortic medial defects (i.e., elastin fragmentation and fibromuscular dysplasia) and hypertension.[23] Patients with gonadal dysgenesis (*Turner's syndrome*; 45, XO karyotype) can manifest skeletal and connective tissue abnormalities.[24, 25] The aneurysms are often associated with stenotic aortic segments (coarctations); however, infrarenal aneurysms have been reported.

Menkes' kinky-hair syndrome, a rare X-linked syndrome manifested by rapid central nervous system and arterial degeneration, is caused by an abnormality in copper transport.[26] The blotchy mouse is believed to represent a counterpart of this disease.[27–29] The lack of available copper prevents the normal cross-linking of collagen and elastin required for a stable connective tissue matrix because the formation of the desmosines, along with that of other cross-links such as pyridinoline, is dependent on the activity of the copper-dependent metalloenzyme lysyl oxidase.

MECHANICAL (HEMODYNAMIC)

Post-stenotic aneurysms begin as post-stenotic dilatations but become true aneurysms when the diameter criterion is met and the ectasia becomes permanent and fixed. These aneurysms have historically been thought to occur in a normal arterial wall purely as a result of mechanical factors. Coarctation of the aorta is a classic example. Other disease entities included in this category are pulmonary and aortic valvular disease, cervical rib, and impingement on peripheral arteries caused by any abnormally situated anatomic structures (e.g., popliteal entrapment secondary to an abnormal insertion of the medial head of the gastrocnemius). Mechanical factors postulated as initiators of post-stenotic dilatation include elevated lateral wall pressures, turbulence, abnormal shear stress, and vibratory forces. Application of Bernoulli's principle predicts, in rigid-walled cylinders with laminar flow, an increase in the post-stenotic lateral pressures created by the acceleration of flow past the stenosis. Attempts to demonstrate this phenomenon in human and animal experiments have failed. In vitro and in vivo studies have documented significant turbulence in the flow exiting a stenotic segment. Trauma secondary to arterial wall vibration generated by the turbulence may be responsible for the post-stenotic dilatation.[30] The development of elevated shear stress has also been reported in the post-stenotic segment. The abnormal shear stress has been suggested to produce a cyclic pulling on the arterial wall, causing local weakening and dilatation. In addition, endothelial cells exposed to abnormal shear stress can secrete vasoactive substances and other factors that could lead to remodeling and dilatation of the vessel. An increase in the collagenase activity of aortic tissue distal to a stenosis has been shown in the cynomolgus monkey.[2] This finding suggests that factors other than purely mechanical forces may be associated with the initiation and progression of post-stenotic aneurysm development. In addition, once dilatation has developed, increased resultant tension (lateral pressure) may accelerate the process, as predicted by Laplace's law (tension varies directly with radius when pressure is constant). Again, critics point out that this law properly applies only to thin-walled structures such as soap bubbles, so its relevance in this situation is unclear.

TRAUMATIC

Full-thickness traumatic disruption of the normal arterial wall is the leading cause of pseudoaneurysms. They are false aneurysms because the wall lacks all three layers of a normal artery. The capsule is composed of the surrounding compacted periadventitial tissue. False aneurysms are basically pulsatile hematomas. Both penetrating and blunt trauma can be responsible for the formation of this type of aneurysm. Penetrating injuries are most commonly related to gunshot and stab wounds. Other etiologic factors in this category that have been noted with increasing frequency include iatrogenic injuries from invasive techniques and repeated arterial punctures in drug addicts. After the injury, a hematoma forms within the surrounding tissues, and a fibrous wall subsequently develops. If a communication persists between the artery and the hematoma sac, a pseudoaneurysm develops. Common examples of blunt trauma resulting in the formation of pseudoaneurysms include deceleration injuries of the descending thoracic aorta and compression injuries of the abdominal aorta from seat belts. Of note, blunt injuries generally produce linear transverse tears in the artery similar to those seen with aortic dissections, but the tear tends to be full thickness in the intrinsically normal vessel when it sustains this kind of injury.

INFLAMMATORY

Associated With Arteritis

Multiple specific forms of arteritis have been associated with arterial aneurysms. *Takayasu's disease* (pulseless disease) is the most common of these disorders. It was first described in 1908 as an ophthalmic disease with "peculiar ocular lesions."[31] Only recently has the full spectrum of vascular disease encompassed in this syndrome been identified. Occlusive or stenotic changes in the aorta and its major branches are the most frequently identified lesions, but aneurysms have been reported in up to 31 per cent of patients.[32] These patients are more commonly female and tend to be younger than patients with nonspecific aneurysms. Aneurysms are found at almost any level of the aorta and in many visceral arteries. Aneurysmal degeneration has traditionally been attributed to post-stenotic changes, but evidence now suggests that primary arterial wall abnormalities may also be present.

Giant cell or *temporal arteritis* is characterized by panarteritis with mononuclear and giant cell infiltration, similar to the lesion of Takayasu's disease.[33] Occurring in elderly patients, aneurysms associated with this disorder can involve any portion of the aorta and its branches, with a particular propensity for the ascending aorta and the axillary-brachial segment. There are rare reports of aneurysms associated with *systemic lupus erythematosus,* and along with the aneurysms associated with *periarteritis nodosa,* these tend to be visceral. *Behçet's disease* variably includes oral and genital ulcerations, posterior uveitis, arthritis, and a hypercoagulable state that may result in episodes of venous thrombosis.[34]

Kawasaki's disease, or mucocutaneous lymph node syndrome, is a multi-system disease of children. Common manifestations include skin rash, conjunctivitis, lymphadenopathy, myocarditis, and aneurysms. Aneurysms most commonly occur in the coronary arteries but have been reported throughout the arterial tree.[35]

Periarterial

Periarterial inflammatory etiologies of a noninfectious nature imply digestion of the arterial wall from an extrinsic source. The prototypical example is digestion of the splenic artery from pancreatitis or the contents of a pseudocyst, resulting in marked thinning of the arterial wall with the potential for rupture.

INFECTIOUS (MYCOTIC)

Although the association between bacterial endocarditis and distal arterial disruptions had already been noted by Koch, Osler was the first to use the term *mycotic aneurysm* in his Gulstonian lectures of 1884. Osler used the term to describe multiple aortic aneurysms laden with fungal vegetations in a patient with bacterial endocarditis. Since then, the term *mycotic* has been applied to any aneurysm that is believed to have developed secondary to any infectious process, although this term is a misnomer in the sense that a true fungal etiology is rare. Historically, bacterial endocarditis and syphilis were the most common causes of mycotic aneurysms. The advent of antibiotics has reduced the incidence of these entities, so that at present an initial traumatic event is the leading cause.

There are several mechanisms of infection. *Direct extension* from a contiguous septic focus causing arterial disruption with aneurysm formation is the rarest mode of development, demonstrating the exceptional resistance of the normal arterial wall to extravascular infection. *Embolomycotic* aneurysms are thought to result from septic emboli lodging within vessel orifices or their vasa vasorum. Bacterial endocarditis remains the most common etiologic factor in this category. *Cryptogenic* mycotic aneurysms form when microbes from an unknown primary site infect a segment of vessel wall. The syphilitic (luetic) aneurysm, which is the classic type, was responsible for more than 50 per cent of all aneurysms in the preantibiotic era and usually affected the ascending aorta. The abdominal aorta is now the most common location for cryptogenic mycotic aneurysms. Older series reported predominantly gram-positive organisms, including *Streptococcus* species and *Staphylococcus* species, with *Salmonella* species being the most common gram-negative organisms. *Salmonella* species seem to have a special affinity for normal arterial walls. More recent series have reported *Staphylococcus aureus* to be the predominant isolate from mycotic aneurysms.[36] In addition, gram-negative and anaerobic infections are now more commonly encountered, with unusual species such as fungi, yeasts, and mycobacteria found in immunocompromised patients.

Penetrating arterial trauma is the most common cause of mycotic aneurysms; the aneurysm results from the introduction of an inoculum at the site of arterial injury or adjacent hematoma. The large increase in the incidence of this type of aneurysm can be attributed to an increase in the use of invasive techniques and the current epidemic of substance abuse with intra-arterial injections of illicit drugs. This kind of infected aneurysm was one of the earliest forms of aneurysmal disease clearly recognized, during the preantiseptic era when bloodletting was commonplace.

A special case of an aneurysm infected from extravascular sources is the *infected anastomotic aneurysm.* Usually presumed to originate from contamination at the time of surgery, in the aortic location it may result from erosion of an anastomotic aneurysm into the duodenum.

Infection of a preexisting aneurysm is also known to occur occasionally. Although it is not proper to consider such aneurysms mycotic in origin, infection may occur from bacteremia, resulting in sepsis, fever, and rapid expansion of the aneurysm. Interestingly, organisms can be cultured from approximately 10 per cent of routine abdominal aortic aneurysms,[37] suggesting that simple colonization is much more common and less virulent than a true invasive infection.

PREGNANCY ASSOCIATED

Arterial rupture is a leading cause of maternal death. Vessels that have been reported to be the site of aneurysmal rupture during pregnancy most commonly include the splenic, cerebral, and aortic, followed by the renal, iliac, coronary, and ovarian. More than 50 per cent of ruptured aneurysms suffered by women under the age of 40 years are pregnancy-related.[38, 39] Etiologic factors that may contribute to aneurysm development or rupture during pregnancy can be divided into hemodynamic changes and arterial wall changes. Manalo-Estrella and Barker described decreased levels of acid mucopolysaccharides and fragmentation of reticular fibers in the aortic walls of 16 patients dying of other causes during pregnancy.[40] Twelve age-adjusted nonpregnant control subjects did not manifest these changes. Thus, in addition to obvious connective tissue changes during pregnancy, such as the relaxation of pelvic ligaments before parturition, the effects of hormonal changes on other connective tissue structures (e.g., vascular) may be a generalized phenomenon.

Hemodynamic changes associated with pregnancy include increased cardiac output and circulating blood volume, with a concomitant reduction in peripheral resistance. This generally results in a decrease in systemic blood pressure until the third trimester, when prepregnancy levels or higher return. This factor would theoretically add to the stress on an already susceptible vascular wall. Thus, both hemodynamic and arterial wall changes are potentially important in aneurysm development and rupture during pregnancy, but the exact role of each and why only a small subset of pregnant women is affected remain obscure.

DEGENERATIVE

Nonspecific

The most common form of aneurysmal disease, which usually affects the infrarenal abdominal aorta as well as the popliteal, femoral, and iliac arteries, has historically been called the atherosclerotic aneurysm. Although these aneurysms show gross and microscopic evidence of atheromatous disease, the notion that atherosclerosis is the underlying cause of the arterial dilatation has become controversial. An alternative scenario is that as the vessel dilates, boundary layer separation occurs along the surface,[41] and hemodynamic forces stimulate subintimal proliferative changes resulting in plaque formation, as are known to occur in association with similar flow disturbances at curvatures and branch points. In support of this concept is evidence that atherosclerotic changes also occur in post-stenotic aneurysms.

The association with traditional atherosclerotic risk

factors[42] (i.e., smoking, hypertension, and hypercholesterolemia) is also subject to reinterpretation.[43] Elevated blood pressure may exert a direct dilating effect on a susceptible vessel independent of its effect on stimulating the myointimal proliferation that is a hallmark of atherosclerosis; smoking may play an independent role by inhibiting the activity of important antiproteolytic factors that protect the matrix (e.g., by methylating alpha$_1$-antitrypsin). Although elevated cholesterol levels appeared to be a risk factor in one large-scale study, approximately 60 per cent of the patients who had abdominal aortic aneurysms (AAAs) had serum cholesterol levels equal to or less than 240 mg/dl, and 40 per cent had levels equal to or less than 215 mg/dl.[42] The situation could be viewed in terms of overlapping Venn diagrams: smoking triggers atherosclerosis in some, promotes arterial dilatation in others, and stimulates both processes in those who have underlying genetic susceptibilities to both diseases. Accordingly, it is probably best at present to follow the recommendation of the SVS/ISCVS Subcommittee on Reporting Standards for Aneurysm Disease in referring to this group of aneurysms as nonspecific until the etiology is better understood.[1]

A phenomenon cited in support of the concept that aneurysms are simply the result of a lifetime of wear and tear is the steady increase in the incidence of the disease with aging. However, an autopsy study of 45,838 individuals found that in men the incidence peaks at age 80 and then declines.[44] This observation suggests that environmental factors may be important in the accumulated risk for AAA, but a point is reached at which the pool of genetically susceptible individuals has been exhausted. Women show a delay in the onset of the rising portion of the curve, and the rate is still on the rise at the end of the human life span. This observation may explain the rather dramatic male predominence of patients in the 6th and 7th decades of life, without implying, as some investigators once believed, that the genetic susceptibility factor is located on the X chromosome.[45]

Several investigators have concluded that there has been a true increase in the incidence of the disease over the last several decades. Melton and colleagues reported an increased incidence of approximately sevenfold in a well-studied Minnesota community.[46] This observation is interesting in light of the fact that there appears to be a general decrease in the incidence of atherosclerosis. The phenomenon cannot be explained on the basis of the fact that more and more people are living long enough to reach the age of risk because the increase in prevalence is age specific.[44, 47]

A final point on the general relationship of atherosclerosis to AAA is that aneurysms are like balloons, whereas atherosclerosis makes arteries hard and stiff. Martin was among the first to question whether dilating disease of the aorta was fundamentally different from stenosing disease.[48] Tilson and Stansel observed that in comparison with patients with atherosclerotic occlusive disease, the patients with aneurysms were older, represented a higher ratio of males:females, had less distal peripheral vascular disease, and had a superior long-term graft patency rate.[49] In addition, the generalized arteriomegaly of nonatherosclerotic segments,[45] the association with aneurysms of minimally atherosclerotic arteries (e.g., the popliteal), and the association with complex inguinal hernias and emphysema[50] all suggest that the disease involves unknown systemic or constitutional factors in addition to atherosclerotic stimuli.

Experimental Models

Models of aneurysmal disease may be divided into the following categories: spontaneous, pharmacologic, dietary, and surgical. *Spontaneous* aneurysms occur consistently in the blotchy mouse, which has a mutation on the X chromosome, and rarely in other species, such as horses (usually stallions) and turkeys. The blotchy mouse mutation interferes with copper metabolism, and copper is a cofactor for lysyl oxidase (the enzyme essential for cross-linking in collagen and elastin). Aneurysms of the mouse have been described in detail,[28, 29] but attempts to make correlations with the disease in humans have been disappointing. After Tilson presented preliminary data with the suggestion that copper deficiency might be important,[51] two studies reported that copper levels were normal,[52, 53] and one study reported that copper levels were elevated.[54]

Pharmacologic aneurysms may be induced by lathyrism or by steroid use. The most common lathyrogen in experimental use is beta-aminoproprionitrile, which has been studied extensively in turkeys.[55, 56] Corticosteroids have been used to induce aortic aneurysms or aortic ruptures in hamsters[57] and mice.[58]

Dietary models fall into two categories: copper deficiency and variations in cholesterol intake. The species that appears to be most susceptible to copper deficiency is the pig.[59] The induction of aneurysms by high-cholesterol feeding appears to occur only rarely, and it is not entirely clear whether this incidence is significantly greater than that due to chance alone. Strickland and Bond reported a single fusiform aortic aneurysm among 730 squirrel monkeys fed atherogenic diets,[60] and Zarins and coworkers reported five aneurysms among 443 animals.[61] DePalma and colleagues were the first to report aneurysms in association with experimental regression of atherosclerosis in dogs,[62] and more recently, Zarins and associates reported an increase of approximately twofold in the internal elastic lamella area (a 38 per cent increase in diameter) in the abdominal aorta of six monkeys receiving regression diets.[63] The diet used for induction of atherosclerosis contained 25 per cent peanut oil, which tends to induce an inflammatory variant of atherosclerosis. This factor may also be important in aneurysm pathogenesis (see the later section on the role of inflammation).

The *surgical* models are a mixed bag, including ex vivo variations, transplantation (immunologic), hemodynamic types, and direct injuries. Allografts of the aorta in inbred rats provide an interesting model for studying the relative importance of immunologic variables versus hemodynamic factors such as hypertension.[64] Post-stenotic dilatations are also being studied with renewed interest.[2] Perhaps the most interesting concepts at present are arising from studies of a new variation of arterial injury with direct infusion of pancreatic elastase into an isolated segment of the rat abdominal aorta.[65] Dobrin and colleagues had previously shown ex vivo that elastase-injured arteries tend to dilate, whereas collagenase-injured arteries tend to rupture.[66] Tilson and colleagues interpreted these data and concluded that the dilatation induced by elastase alone fails to reach aneurysmal proportions.[4] Only when collagenase was combined with elastase did aneurysmal dilatation occur, suggesting that collagen must also fail in order to produce an experimental aneurysm. Details of the in vivo model are being worked out in the authors' laboratory and by others. At present, the initial injury appears to trigger a cascade of events that activate a group of endogenous proteinases at the same time that inflammatory infiltration occurs. The aneurysm does not form immediately after elastase injury but only after biochemical interactions of significant complexity.[67, 68]

Role of Genetic Susceptibility

In 1977, Clifton reported on three brothers who had ruptured AAAs during the 7th decade of life.[69] Tilson and Seashore reported on 50 families in 1984 with two or more first-order relatives affected with AAAs.[70] Because about 25 per cent of the families had father-son patterns, the investigators concluded that if there was only one aneurysm gene, it would have to be autosomal. Interestingly, when this series was extended to 94 families, the male:female ratio of affected offspring of the 22 affected fathers was 62:2.[71]

Johansen and Koepsell also confirmed the familial incidence of AAA in their study of 250 patients and 250 atherosclerotic control subjects. They reported a sixfold increase in the risk : odds ratio for an AAA among first-degree relatives of probands (19 per cent) versus control patients.[72] Numerous other studies support the concept of an important genetic susceptibility factor.[73–78] Powell and Greenhalgh calculated the genetic component to be approximately 70 per cent in a multi-factorial model,[76] and subsequently Powell and coworkers suggested an association between AAA and polymorphisms of two genes on the long arm of chromosome 16.[79]

About 25 per cent of AAA patients will be aware of another first-order relative with the disease, and if the male siblings of a proband are screened with ultrasonography, approximately 20 to 30 per cent will have positive findings.[80–82] Because one must live a long time to pass through the age of risk, it has been speculated that the true lifetime incidence in a sibling surviving to old age might approach 50 per cent, which would be compatible with a single dominant gene. However, the most extensive genetic analysis reported to date, by Majumder and colleagues, proposes an autosomal recessive mode.[83]

Biochemistry of Aneurysmal Aorta

Structural Proteins

Sumner and colleagues reported decreases in the elastin and collagen contents of aneurysm walls in comparison with normal or atherosclerotic aortas in 1970.[84] The result with respect to elastin has been confirmed extensively,[85–88] but the collagen content appears to be more variable, with some groups reporting normal or elevated levels.[85, 86, 89] It is perhaps not surprising that this is the case, considering that the cells of connective tissue matrix have substantial potential for synthesis of new collagen after injury or destruction but the capacity for synthesis of new elastin is quite limited in adult life. The evidence has been summarized that collagen must fail in AAAs. However, smooth muscle cells have the capacity to regenerate collagen, although not necessarily with the substructural organization in relation to other matrix components that is necessary to maintain normal tensile strength.

Proteolytic Enzymes and Their Inhibitors

In separate studies in 1982, Busuttil and coworkers[90] and Cannon and Read[91] were the first to report increases in elastase activity in AAA disease. Cannon and Read attributed the increase to leukocyte elastase (a serine protease).[91] Studies by Dubick and colleagues also implicated a serine protease, showing a two- to threefold increase in elastolytic activity inhibited by phenylmethylsulfonylfluoride, which they attributed to pancreatic elastase.[92] Cohen and colleagues have also implicated a serine elastase, which they attribute to a smooth muscle cell elastase.[93] However, other studies, beginning with that of Brown and associates, have suggested that the elastase of interest is a "new," nonserine protease.[94] More recent work by Campa and associates also suggests that the principal elastase belongs to the metalloprotease rather than the serine protease family.[87] It does not cross-react immunologically with antibody to leukocyte elastase, and it is inhibited by ethylenediaminetetra-acetic acid (EDTA). Work from the authors' laboratory is consistent with this view. The principal elastase capable of degrading aortic elastin is inhibited by EDTA,[95] and it has an apparent molecular weight on substrate gel enzymography of approximately 80 kd.[96] Further studies have suggested that it is a member of the matrix metalloprotease family (MMP) that was originally described as a type IV collagenase and is now designated as MMP 9 in the nomenclature.[97, 98] Other investigators have shown that MMP 9 is a potent elastase.[99]

Interest in collagenolytic activity in AAA was initiated by Busuttil and associates in 1980.[100] Although Webster and coworkers confirmed that collagenolytic activity is present in AAAs,[101] other investigators have detected authentic mammalian collagenase (MMP 1) only in ruptured aneurysmal tissue.[102] This difficulty may relate to the binding of MMP 1 to its natural inhibitor, tissue inhibitor of metalloproteinases (TIMP), masking its detection. The authors have circumvented this problem by using Western blots, which separate MMP 1 from TIMP during the electrophoresis, and under these conditions, a protein is detected that is immunoreactive with antibody to MMP 1.[103]

The possibility of failure of antiproteolytic systems as a mechanism of disease in AAAs was suggested by Cannon and Read in 1982,[91] and Cohen and colleagues have suggested that there is an imbalance between serine elastase and alpha$_1$-antitrypsin levels.[104] Similarly, the authors' group suggested such an imbalance between the metalloprotease systems and TIMP, and there appears to be a relative deficiency in immunoreactive TIMP in AAA tissue.[105]

Histochemistry and Immunohistochemistry

Destruction of Matrix

Histologic studies confirm the extensive loss of elastin that has occurred in AAAs.[106] White and colleagues again confirmed the substantial loss of elastin, but they added the interesting finding that elastin depletion is essentially complete at the stage of relatively small aneurysms, implying that loss or reorganization of additional structural components is important as the AAA enlarges.[107] Because the mechanical strength of collagen is four orders of magnitude greater than that of elastin,[108] it is logical to infer that continuing destruction of collagen is significant. Synthesis of new but poorly organized collagen may account for the observation that collagen content is usually maintained.

Role of Inflammation

Beckman reviewed 156 specimens of AAA tissue and found that more than two thirds had a notable infiltration of chronic inflammatory cells in the adventitia.[109] Interestingly, this zone is the site of most of the structural collagen. It is well known clinically that aneurysms are most unusual after endarterectomy if the adventitia remains intact. The authors' group has confirmed a significant infiltration of the adventitia in AAAs with inflammatory cells,[110] and Koch and colleagues have taken initial steps to identify these cells immunohistochemically.[111] They reported significant numbers of macrophages and T-cells, and the authors' group has confirmed this finding by another technique based on fluorescence-activated cell sorting.[97] In addition, Brophy and associates demonstrated an increase in immunoglobulin by Western blot assay in the aneurysmal tissue.[110] These results suggest that the pathogenesis of AAA is a loop with several potential initiating events. If there is mutation in one of the structural components, allowing an inherently unstable matrix, the cleavage products (e.g., elastin degradation products)[112] are strongly chemotactic and may recruit an inflammatory reaction with a battery of proteolytic activities. Another entry point in theory would be deficiency of one of the antiproteolytic systems, which again would tip the balance toward destruction of the matrix. Finally, the initiating factor might be some process that promotes proteolytic activity directly. These three possibilities provide the basis for speculating about possible genetic predispositions.

Integration of These Concepts With Candidate Genes

The foregoing discussion leads to the consideration of several candidate genes that are presently under investigation. Tilson and Roberts suggested in 1988 that an abnormality in the primary structure of collagen might account for a subset of patients with AAA disease,[113] and in 1989, Powell and Greenhalgh identified a subset of patients with an apparently mild relative deficiency of type III collagen.[114] The first conclusive evidence of mutation in a gene for a structural protein in a family with AAA disease was presented by Kontusaari and coworkers.[20] There was a point mutation in the procollagen III gene, which resulted in the substitution of an arginine for the glycine at position 691. The presence of the small amino acid glycine at every third position in the helical portion of the fibrillar collagens is essential to permit normal coiling, so the substitution resulted in a collagen that was thermally unstable, with a lowered melting point. The family was not typical of most with clustering of AAAs because in two patients AAAs were detected at young ages. The family's disease also did not meet definitive criteria for assignment to a specific category of connective tissue disorders. Because mutations in type III collagen are associated with Ehlers-Danlos syndrome type IV (ED-IV), this family's disease may come in due course to be viewed as an ED-IV subtype, as was proposed earlier in this chapter. Another family has been found to have a mutation in the type III procollagen gene that causes a splicing error.[115]

On the theme of mutations that might stimulate aneurysm formation by promoting proteolysis, Powell and colleagues reported the association of AAA with an allele of the haptoglobin gene on chromosome 16, the product of which appears to promote elastolysis in vitro.[79] This illustrates the hypothesis that entry into the loop may occur at some site other than a structural abnormality of a matrix protein. The finding has not as yet been confirmed.[116]

A subset of patients (in the range of 10 per cent) may have a deficiency allele of alpha$_1$-antitrypsin, as reported by Cohen and colleagues,[117] illustrating the concept that the genetic predisposition is at the level of failure of protease inhibition. However, this finding also remains unconfirmed.[116] Along similar lines, Tilson and colleagues sequenced the *TIMP* gene in six patients. They found an identical point mutation at codon 101 in two patients, but the amino acid was conserved. At present, primary mutation in the *TIMP* gene does not appear to be the cause of its deficiency in AAA tissue, but further studies are required to rule out this gene conclusively.[118]

This brief discussion of candidate genes indicates the direction that research into the pathogenesis of AAA will probably take in the future.

Application of the Basic Science of AAA to Potential Pharmacologic Interventions for Prevention or Stabilization

The crescendo of interest in the basic biology of aneurysmal disease may have significant practical consequences in the near future. If a gene were discovered that accounted for a large subset of patients with AAAs, it could quickly become routine to screen for an etiologic mutation in the gene with a simple blood test. If patients were identified to be at risk, they could be advised to have periodic ultrasound examinations to detect potential problems before there was any risk of rupture. In addition, pharmacologic interventions may be developed to prevent the disease in those shown to be susceptible by the previously described approach or to stabilize the connective tissue matrix and prevent aneurysm enlargement in those with small AAAs.

One such potential intervention has already received some attention in experimental animals. Simpson and coworkers found that propranolol reduced the incidence of aortic aneurysms in the beta-aminoproprionitrile–induced turkey model, by some mechanism other than its hemodynamic effects on pulse and blood pressure.[55] Additional studies suggested that there was a direct stimulatory effect on the crosslinking of connective tissue components.[56] Similar findings have been confirmed in the aneurysm-prone blotchy mouse,[119, 120] and a small retrospective study in humans suggested that further study of this possibility should be considered.[121] The literature suggests that some beta-blocking agents may have direct connective tissue effects,[122] and in view of the fact that numerous drugs (e.g., phenytoin and tetracycline) have properties that affect the dynamics of matrix metabolism, there may be numerous candidates to be evaluated in the future for beneficial pharmacologic actions.[123, 124]

Inflammatory Aneurysms

The term *inflammatory aneurysm* was first used by Walker and colleagues to describe AAAs in 19 patients that showed excessive thickening of the walls and perianeurysmal adhesions to adjacent organs.[125] Numerous reports thereafter suggested that these aneurysms represented a variant of nonspecific aneurysms with distinct clinical, operative, and pathologic features.[126, 127] Most commonly involving the abdominal aorta, inflammatory aneurysms account for 5 per cent of AAAs. Clinically, most of these aneurysms are associated with symptoms of back pain and weight loss along with an elevation in the erythrocyte sedimentation rate. At laparotomy, the aneurysms are encased in a dense, shiny fibrotic reaction with frequent involvement of the duodenum, ureters, and inferior vena cava. Pathologic analysis of the wall demonstrates marked thickening of the media and adventitia. Varying degrees of infiltration into these two layers with lymphocytes, plasma cells, and mononuclear cells, along with endarteritis of the vasa vasorum, are usually present.

The etiology of this variant of nonspecific aneurysms is unknown. Advocates of the theory that separate etiologic factors are responsible for inflammatory aneurysm development have offered trauma, chronic leakage of blood or urine, intramural hemorrhage, and primary autoimmune disorder as possible initiators. Other investigators believe that the characteristic inflammatory process represents an extension of the inflammation observed in the nonspecific aneurysms. In support of this latter theory is the regression of the fibrotic process in the retroperitoneum after graft placement. However, why these patients respond with greater intensity and extension of the inflammatory response remains enigmatic. There must be a biochemical basis for this heightened response. One possibility might be the liberation of an elastin-derived degradation product with unique chemotactic characteristics, and another might be the abundant production by the inflammatory cells present of a cytokine with intense angiogenic properties.

ANASTOMOTIC AND GRAFT ANEURYSMS

When grafts are inserted to replace or bypass occluded or aneurysmal segments of the arterial tree, aneurysms can form at the junction between the graft and the host artery, as well as in the body of the graft itself. The former, anastomotic aneurysms, are essentially false aneurysms containing no elements of the original arterial wall. They are, in essence, a connective tissue sac communicating with the defect between graft and host artery. The fibrous capsule surrounding the anastomosis lacks the inherent strength to withstand the mechanical stresses of systemic arterial flow. Anything that causes a separation between graft and host artery can produce an anastomotic aneurysm. The use of silk sutures; suture line infection; inadequate suture purchase; and abnormal shearing forces bearing on the suture line because of joint flexion, compliance mismatch between prosthesis and artery, and turbulence due to junctional flow disturbances have all been implicated.

Aneurysms have developed in the body of almost every arterial substitute used to date.[128] Aneurysmal development was one of the main reasons for abandoning arterial homografts. Subsequently, heterografts, or more specifically, ficin-digested, formaldehyde-treated bovine carotid arteries, also showed a propensity for aneurysm formation.[129] The similarly modified human umbilical vein graft had to be reinforced with a circumferential Dacron mesh to prevent aneurysmal development. Despite this, up to 65 per cent aneurysmal degeneration is being reported in umbilical vein grafts patent for 5 years,[130] and histologic examination suggests that the collagen cross-linking process used is inadequate to prevent tissue digestion to a degree that can be compensated for even by an improved Dacron mesh. Arterial autografts do not become aneurysmal, but vein autografts placed in the systemic arterial tree do. Thin-walled deep veins are not used for arterial substitutes because almost all develop aneurysmal dilatation. The saphenous vein, because it must withstand gravitational pressures, is thicker walled and after implantation becomes even thicker by increased connective tissue deposition. Nevertheless, when used in extremity arterial reconstruction, it has a reported incidence of aneurysmal development of 4 per cent.[131] In addition, when this graft is placed in the aortorenal position, where the flows and pressures are generally higher, the rate of aneurysmal development is even higher. This complication has been partly attributed, although without proof, to forceful dilatation of the vein graft during its removal and preparation for implantation. This is no longer common practice, but no reports as yet have reflected any decrease in the development of these aneurysms.

Prosthetic grafts have been made of a number of materials, including Vinyon, nylon, Orlon, Teflon, Dacron, and polytetrafluoroethylene. The first three were quickly abandoned because of frequent complications, not the least of which was loss of tensile strength and aneurysm formation.[33] Teflon maintains its tensile strength best after implantation but lost its popularity as a "fabric" graft because of its lack of seating in the tissues. The overwhelming preference today in prosthetic grafts is Dacron or polytetrafluoroethylene. Knitted Dacron is more compliant than woven Dacron and may be less likely to contribute to anastomotic aneurysm formation. In addition, the knitted fabric has larger interstices through which capillary ingrowth can reach, nourish, and secure the neointima. In an effort to improve this ingrowth, knitted grafts were made progressively more porous until reports began to appear of diffuse dilatation or fragmentation and aneurysm formation.[132] Adoption of a velour construction and a tighter-warp knit may have solved this problem, for it has not been reported to date with any frequency with third-generation prostheses. Even the relatively solid expanded grafts, as originally constructed, were reported to have a significant incidence of aneurysm formation.[133] This has since been combatted either by adding an outer helical wrap or by increasing the thickness of the graft wall.

References

1. Johnston KW, Rutherford RB, Tilson MD, et al: Suggested standards for reporting on arterial aneurysms. J Vasc Surg 12:444, 1991.
2. Zarins CK, Runyon-Hass A, Zatina MA, et al: Increased collagenase activity in early aneurysmal dilation. J Vasc Surg 3:238, 1986.
3. Wolinsky H, Glagov S: A lamellar unit of aortic medial structure and function in mammals. Circ Res 20:99, 1967.
4. Tilson MD, Elefteriades J, Brophy CM: Tensile strength and collagen in abdominal aortic aneurysm disease. *In* Greenhalgh RM, Mannick JA, Powell JT (eds): The Cause and Management of Aneurysms. London, WB Saunders, 1990, pp 97–104.
5. Pyeritz RE: Marfan syndrome. N Engl J Med 323:987, 1990.
6. Kainulainen K, Pulkkinen L, Savolainen A, et al: Location on chromosome 15 of the gene defect causing Marfan syndrome. N Engl J Med 323:935, 1990.
7. McKusick VA: Mendelian Inheritance in Man. 5th ed. Baltimore, Johns Hopkins University Press, 1978.
8. Sakai LY, Keene DR, Engvall E: Fibrillin, a new 350-kD glycoprotein component of extracellular microfibrils. J Cell Biol 103:2499, 1986.
9. Hollister DW, Godfrey M, Sakai LY, Pyeritz RE: Immunohistologic abnormalities of the microfibrillar-fiber system in the Marfan syndrome. N Engl J Med 323:152, 1990.
10. Lee B, Godfrey M, Vitale E, et al: Linkage of Marfan syndrome and a phenotypically related disorder to two different fibrillin genes. Nature 352:330, 1991.
11. Dietz HC, Cutting GR, Pyeritz RE, et al: Marfan syndrome caused by a recurrent de novo missense mutation in the fibrillin gene. Nature 352:337, 1991.
12. vanMeekeren JA: De dilatabilitate extraordinaria cutis. As quoted by Sheiner NM, Miller N, Lachance C: Arterial complications of Ehlers-Danlos syndrome. J Cardiovasc Surg 26:291, 1985.
13. Barabas AP: Ehlers-Danlos syndrome. *In* Greenhalgh RM, Mannick JA, Powell JT (eds): The Cause and Management of Aneurysms. London, WB Saunders, 1990, pp 57–67.
14. Weber FP: The Ehlers-Danlos syndrome. Br J Dermatol 48:609, 1936.
15. Barabas AP: Heterogeneity of the Ehlers-Danlos syndrome. Br Med J 2:612, 1967.
16. Wesley JR, Mahour GH, Wooley MM: Multiple surgical problems in two patients with Ehlers-Danlos syndrome. Surgery 86:319, 1980.
17. Pope FM, Martin GR, McKusick VA: Patients with type IV EDS lack type III collagen. Proc Natl Acad Sci USA 72:1314, 1975.
18. Pope FM, Nicholls AC, Jones PM, et al: EDS IV (acrogeria): New autosomal dominant and recessive types. J R Soc Med 73:180, 1980.
19. Pope FM, Child AH, Nicholls AC, et al: Type III collagen deficiency with normal phenotype. J R Soc Med 76:518, 1983.
20. Kontusaari S, Tromp G, Kuivaniemi H, et al: A mutation in the gene for type III procollagen (COL3A1) in a family with aortic aneurysms. J Clin Invest 86:1465, 1990.
21. Tilson MD: Commentary on "Multiple aneurysms in a young man," by A Nemes and C Dzsinich. Postgrad Vasc Surg 2:14, 1991.
22. O'Hara PJ, Ratcliff NB, Grove RA, et al: Medial agenesis associated with multiple extracranial, peripheral and visceral arterial aneurysms. J Vasc Surg 2:298, 1985.
23. Hagood CA, Garvin DD, Lachina FM, et al: Abdominal aortic aneurysm and renal hamartoma in an infant with tuberous sclerosis. Surgery 79:713, 1976.
24. Allen DB, Hendricks SA, Levy JM: Aortic dilation in Turner syndrome. J Pediatr 109:302, 1986.
25. Lin AE, Lippe BM, Geffner ME, et al. Aortic dilation, dissection, and rupture in patients with Turner syndrome. J Pediatr 109:820, 1986.
26. Danks DM, Campbell PE, Walker-Smith G, et al: Menkes' kinky-hair syndrome. Lancet 1:1100, 1972.
27. Hunt DM: Primary defect in copper transport underlies mottled mutants in the mouse. Nature 249:852, 1974.
28. Andrews EJ, White WJ, Bullock LP: Spontaneous aortic aneurysms in blotchy mice. Am J Pathol 78:199, 1975.
29. Brophy CM, Tilson JE, Braverman IM, Tilson MD: Age of onset, pattern of distribution and histology of aneurysm development in a genetically predisposed mouse model. J Vasc Surg 8:45, 1988.
30. Roach MR: Hemodynamic factors in arterial stenosis and poststenotic dilation. *In* Stehbens WE (ed): Hemodynamics and the Blood Vessel Wall. Springfield, IL, Charles C Thomas, 1979.
31. Takayasu M: Patient who has peculiar changes in retinal central vessels. Acta Soc Ophthalmol Jpn 12:554, 1908.
32. Takagi A, Kajiura N, Tada Y, Ueno A: Surgical treatment of nonspecific inflammatory arterial aneurysms. J Cardiovasc Surg 27:117, 1986.
33. Klinkhoff AV, Reid GD, Moscovich M: Aortic regurgitation in giant cell arteritis. Arthritis Rheum 28:582, 1985.
34. Jorizzo J: Behçet's disease. Arch Dermatol 122:556, 1986.
35. Fukushige J, Bill MR, McNamara DG: Spectrum of cardiovascular lesions in mucocutaneous lymph node syndrome: Analysis of eight cases. Am J Cardiol 45:98, 1980.
36. Brown SL, Busuttil RW, Baker JD, et al: Bacteriologic and surgical determinants of survival in patients with mycotic aneurysms. J Vasc Surg 1:541, 1984.
37. Ernst CB, Campbell C, Daugherty ME, et al: Incidence and significance of intra-operative bacterial cultures during abdominal aortic aneurysmectomy. Ann Surg 185:626, 1977.
38. Barrett JM, Van Hooyclonk JE, Boehm FH: Pregnancy related rupture of arterial aneurysms. Obstet Gynecol Surg 37:557, 1982.
39. Williams GM, Gott VL, Brawley RK, et al: Aortic disease associated with pregnancy. J Vasc Surg 8:470, 1988.
40. Manalo-Estrella P, Barker AE: Histopathologic findings in human aortic media associated with pregnancy. Arch Pathol 83:336, 1967.
41. Scherer PW: Flow in an axisymmetrical glass model aneurysm. J Biomech 6:695, 1973.
42. Reed D, Reed C, Stemmermann G, Haysashi T: Are aortic aneurysms caused by atherosclerosis? Circulation 85:205, 1992.
43. Tilson MD: Aortic aneurysms and atherosclerosis [Editorial]. Circulation 85:378, 1992.
44. Bengtsson H, Bergqvist D, Sternby NH: Increasing prevalence of abdominal aortic aneurysms: A necropsy study. Eur J Surg 158:19, 1992.
45. Tilson MD, Dang C: Generalized arteriomegaly—A possible predisposition to formation of abdominal aortic aneurysms. Arch Surg 116:1030, 1981.
46. Melton L, Bickerstaff L, Hollier L, et al: Changing incidence of abdominal aortic aneurysms: A population based study. Am J Epidemiol 120:379, 1984.
47. Fowkes FGR, MacIntyre CCA, Ruckley CV: Increasing incidence of aortic aneurysms in England and Wales. Br Med J 298:33, 1989.
48. Martin P: On abdominal aortic aneurysms. J Cardiovasc Surg 19:597, 1978.
49. Tilson MD, Stansel HC: Differences in results for aneurysms vs. occlusive disease after bifurcation grafts: Results of 100 elective grafts. Arch Surg 115:1173, 1980.
50. Cannon DJ, Casteel L, Reed RC: Abdominal aortic aneurysms, Leriche's syndrome, inguinal herniation, and smoking. Arch Surg 119:387, 1984.
51. Tilson MD: Decreased hepatic copper levels—A possible chemical marker for the pathogenesis of aortic aneurysms in man. Arch Surg 117:1212, 1982.
52. Senapati A, Carsson L, Fletcher C, et al: Is tissue copper deficiency associated with abdominal aortic aneurysms? Br J Surg 72:352, 1985.
53. Dubick MA, Hunter GC, Casey SM, Keen CL: Aortic ascorbic acid, trace elements, and superoxide dismutase activity in human aneurysmal and occlusive disease. Proc Soc Exp Biol Med 184:138, 1987.
54. Alston J, Fody E, Couch L, et al: A prospective study of hepatic and skin copper levels in patients with abdominal aortic aneurysms. Surg Forum 24:466, 1983.
55. Simpson CF, Kling JM, Palemer RF: The use of propranolol for the protection of turkeys from the development of beta-aminoproprionitrile induced aortic rupture. Angiology 19:414, 1968.
56. Boucek RJ, Gunia-Smith Z, Noble NL, Simpson CF: Modulation by propranolol of the lysyl cross-links in aortic elastin and collagen of the aneurysm-prone turkey. Biochem Pharmacol 32:275, 1983.
57. Steffee CH, Snell KC: Dissecting aortic aneurysms in hamsters treated with cortisone acetate. Proc Soc Exp Biol Med 90:712, 1955.
58. Reilly JM, Brophy CM, Tilson MD: Hydrocortisone rapidly induces

aortic rupture in a genetically susceptible mouse. Arch Surg 125:707, 1990.
59. Coulson WF, Carnes WH: Cardiovascular studies on copper-deficient swine. Am J Pathol 43:945, 1963.
60. Strickland HL, Bond MG: Aneurysms in a large colony of squirrel monkeys (Samimi sciureus). Lab Anim Sci 33:589, 1983.
61. Zarins CK, Glagov S, Vesselinovitch D, Wissler RW: Aneurysm formation in experimental atherosclerosis: Relations to plaque evolution. J Vasc Surg 12:246, 1990.
62. DePalma R, Koletsky S, Bullon E, et al: Failure of regression of atherosclerosis in dogs with moderate cholesterolemia. Atherosclerosis 27:297, 1977.
63. Zarins CK, Xu C, Glagov S: Aneurysmal enlargement of the aorta during regression of experimental atherosclerosis. J Vasc Surg 15:90, 1992.
64. Schmitz-Rixen T, Colnin RB, Megerman J, et al: Immunosuppressive treatment of aortic allografts. J Vasc Surg 7:82, 1988.
65. Anidjar S, Salzmann JL, Gentric D, et al: Elastase induced experimental aneurysms in rats. Circulation 82:973, 1990.
66. Dobrin P, Baker W, Gley W: Elastolytic and collagenolytic studies of arteries. Arch Surg 119:405, 1984.
67. Anidjar S, Dobrin PB, Chejfec G: Progressive enlargement of experimental aortic aneurysms is associated with infiltration of inflammatory cells. J Cardiovasc Surg 32(Suppl):39, 1991.
68. Nackman GB, Halpern V, Gandhi R, et al: Induction of endogenous proteinases and alterations of extracellular matrix in a rat model of aortic aneurysm formation. Surg Forum 43:348, 1992.
69. Clifton M: Familial abdominal aortic aneurysms. Br J Surg 64:765, 1977.
70. Tilson MD, Seashore MR: Fifty families with abdominal aortic aneurysms in two or more first-order relatives. Am J Surg 147:551, 1984.
71. Tilson MD, Seashore MR: Ninety-four families with clustering of abdominal aortic aneurysms (AAA). Circulation 70 (Pt II): II-141, 1984.
72. Johansen K, Koepsell T: Familial tendency for abdominal aortic aneurysms. JAMA 256:1934, 1986.
73. Tilson MD, Seashore MR: Human genetics of the abdominal aortic aneurysm. Surg Gynecol Obstet 119:792, 1984.
74. Norrgard O, Rais O, Angquist KA: Familial occurrence of abdominal aortic aneurysms. Surgery 95:650, 1984.
75. Cole CW, Barber GG, Bouchard AG, et al: Abdominal aortic aneurysm: Consequences of a positive family history. Can J Surg 32:117, 1988.
76. Powell JT, Greenhalgh RM: Multifactorial inheritance of abdominal aortic aneurysm. Eur J Vasc Surg 1:29, 1987.
77. Darling RC III, Brewster DC, Darling RC, et al: Are familial abdominal aortic aneurysms different? J Vasc Surg 10:39, 1989.
78. Collin J, Walton J: Is abdominal aortic aneurysm a familial disease? Br Med J 299:493, 1989.
79. Powell JT, Bashir A, Dawson S, et al: Genetic variation on chromosome 16 is associated with abdominal aortic aneurysm. Clin Sci 78:13, 1990.
80. Collin J, Walton J, Araujo L, Lindsell D: Oxford screening programme for abdominal aortic aneurysm in men aged 65–74 years. Lancet 1:613, 1988.
81. Bengtsson H, Norrgard O, Angquist KA, et al: Ultrasonographic screening of the abdominal aorta among siblings of patients with abdominal aortic aneurysms. Br J Surg 76:589, 1989.
82. Webster MW, Ferrell RE, St. Jean PL, et al: Ultrasound screening of first-degree relatives of patients with an abdominal aortic aneurysm. J Vasc Surg 13:9, 1991.
83. Majumder PP, St. Jean PL, Ferrell RE, et al: On the inheritance of abdominal aortic aneurysm. Am J Hum Genet 48:164, 1991.
84. Sumner DS, Hokanson DE, Strandness DE: Stress-strain characteristics and collagen-elastin content of abdominal aortic aneurysms. Surg Gynecol Obstet 130:459, 1970.
85. Rizzo RJ, McCarthy WJ, Dixit SN, et al: Collagen types and matrix protein content in human abdominal aortic aneurysms. J Vasc Surg 10:365, 1989.
86. Hunter GC, Dubick MA, Keen CL, Eskelson CD: Effects of hypertension on aortic antioxidant status in human abdominal aneurysmal and occlusive disease. Proc Soc Exp Biol Med 196:273, 1991.
87. Campa JS, Greenhalgh RM, Powell JT: Elastin degradation in abdominal aortic aneurysms. Atherosclerosis 65:13, 1987.
88. Gandhi R, Keller S, Cantor J, et al: Analysis of elastin crosslinks in the insoluble matrix of aneurysmal abdominal aorta. FASEB J 6:A1914, 1992.
89. Menashi S, Campa JS, Greenhalgh RM, et al: Collagen in abdominal aortic aneurysm: Typing, content, and degradation. J Vasc Surg 6:578, 1987.
90. Busuttil RW, Rinderbriecht H, Flesher A, Carmack C: Elastase activity: The role of elastase in aortic aneurysm formation. J Surg Res 32:214, 1982.
91. Cannon DJ, Read RC: Blood elastolytic activity in patients with aortic aneurysm. Ann Thorac Surg 34:10, 1982.
92. Dubick MA, Hunter GC, Perez-Lizano E, et al: Assessment of the role of pancreatic proteases in human abdominal aortic aneurysms and occlusive disease. Clin Chem Acta 177:1, 1988.
93. Cohen JR, Mandell C, Wise L: Characterization of human aortic elastase found in patients with abdominal aortic aneurysms. Surg Gynecol Obstet 165:301, 1987.
94. Brown S, Backstrom B, Busuttil FW: A new serum proteolytic enzyme in aneurysm pathogenesis. J Vasc Surg 2:393, 1982.
95. Reilly JM, Brophy CM, Tilson MD: Preliminary characterization of an elastase from aneurysmal aorta. Surg Forum 40:283, 1989.
96. Brophy CM, Sumpio B, Reilly JM, Tilson MD: Electrophoretic characterization of protease expression in aneurysmal aorta: Report of a unique 80kDa elastolytic activity. Surg Res Commun 10:315, 1991.
97. Newman KM, Malon AM, Shin R, et al: Matrix metalloproteinases in abdominal aortic aneurysm disease. FASEB J 6:A1914, 1992.
98. Herron GS, Unemori E, Wong M, et al: Connective tissue proteinases and inhibitors in abdominal aortic aneurysms. Arterioscler Thromb 11:1667, 1991.
99. Senior RM, Griffin GL, Fliszar CJ, et al: Human 92- and 72-kilodalton type IV collagenases are elastases. J Biol Chem 266:7870, 1991.
100. Busuttil RW, Abou-Zamzam AM, Machleder HI: Collagenase activity of the human aorta: A comparison of patients with and without abdominal aortic aneurysms. Arch Surg 115:1373, 1980.
101. Webster MW, McAuley CE, Steed DL, et al: Collagen stability and collagenolytic activity in the normal and aneurysmal human abdominal aorta. Am J Surg 161:635, 1991.
102. Menashi S, Campa J, Greenhalgh R, et al: Collagen in abdominal aortic aneurysm: Typing, content, and degradation. J Vasc Surg 6:578, 1987.
103. Irizarry E, Newman K, Gandhi R, et al: Demonstration of interstitial collagenase in abdominal aortic aneurysms. J Surg Res 54:571, 1993.
104. Cohen JR, Mandell C, Margolis I, et al: Altered aortic protease and antiprotease activity in patients with ruptured aortic aneurysms. Surg Gynecol Obstet 164:355, 1987.
105. Brophy CM, Sumpio B, Reilly JM, Tilson MD: Decreased tissue inhibitor of metalloproteinases (TIMP) in abdominal aortic aneurysm tissue: A preliminary report. J Surg Res 50:653, 1991.
106. Tilson MD: Histochemistry of aortic elastin in patients with nonspecific aortic aneurysmal disease. Arch Surg 123:503, 1988.
107. White JV, Haas K, Phillips S, Comerota AJ: Adventitial elastolysis is a primary event in aneurysm formation. J Vasc Surg 17:371, 1993.
108. Dobrin PB: Mechanical properties of arteries. Physiol Rev 58:397, 1978.
109. Beckman EN: Plasma cell infiltrates in abdominal aortic aneurysm. Am J Clin Pathol 85:21, 1986.
110. Brophy CM, Reilly JM, Smith GJW, Tilson MD: The role of inflammation in nonspecific abdominal aortic aneurysm disease. Ann Vasc Surg 5:229, 1991.
111. Koch AE, Haines GK, Rizzo RJ, et al: Human abdominal aortic aneurysms: Immunophenotypic analysis suggesting an immune-mediated response. Am J Pathol 137:1199, 1990.
112. Senior RM, Griffin GL, Mecham RP: Chemotactic activity of elastin derived peptides. J Clin Invest 66:859, 1980.
113. Tilson MD, Roberts MP: Molecular diversity in the abdominal aortic aneurysm phenotype. Arch Surg 123:1202, 1988.
114. Powell J, Greenhalgh RM: Cellular, enzymatic, and genetic factors in the pathogenesis of abdominal aortic aneurysms. J Vasc Surg 9:297, 1989.
115. Kontusaari S, Tromp G, Kuivaniemi H, et al: Inheritance of an RNA splicing mutation (G+1 IVS200) in the type III procollagen gene (COL3AI) in a family having aortic aneurysms and easy bruisability: Phenotypic overlap between familial arterial aneurysms and Ehlers-Danlos syndrome type IV. Am J Hum Genet 47:112, 1990.

116. St. Jean PL, Ferrel RE, Majumder PP, et al: Abdominal aortic aneurysm (AAA): Association with alpha$_1$-antitrypsin, haptoglobin, and type III collagen. J Cardiovasc Surg (Torino) 32(Suppl):38, 1991.
117. Cohen JR, Sarfati I, Ratner L, Tilson MD: Alpha-1 antitrypsin phenotypes in patients with abdominal aortic aneurysms. J Surg Res 49:319, 1990.
118. Tilson MD, Brophy CM, Reilly JM, et al: Unpublished observations.
119. Brophy CM, Tilson JE, Tilson MD: Propranolol delays the formation of aortic aneurysms in the male blotchy mouse. J Surg Res 44:687, 1988.
120. Brophy CM, Tilson JE, Tilson MD: Propranolol stimulates the cross-linking of matrix components in the skin from the aneurysm-prone blotchy mouse. J Surg Res 46:330, 1989.
121. Leach SD, Toole AL, Stern H, et al: Effect of beta-adrenergic blockade on the growth rate of abdominal aortic aneurysms. Arch Surg 123:606, 1988.
122. Harty RF: Sclerosing peritonitis and propranolol. Arch Intern Med 138:1424, 1978.
123. Tilson MD: Propranolol versus placebo for small abdominal aortic aneurysms. J Vasc Surg 5:872, 1992.
124. Reilly JM, Tilson MD: The effects of pharmacologic agents on aortic aneurysm disease. *In* Veith FJ (ed): Current Critical Problems in Vascular Surgery. Quality Medical Publishing, 1990, pp 222–226.
125. Walker DI, Bloor K, Williams G, Gillie I: Inflammatory aneurysms of the abdominal aorta. Br J Surg 83:425, 1978.
126. Goldstone J, Malone JM, Moore WS: Inflammatory aneurysms of the abdominal aorta. Surgery 83:425, 1978.
127. Rose AG, Dent DM: Inflammatory variant of abdominal atherosclerotic aneurysm. Arch Pathol Lab Med 105:409, 1981.
128. Edwards WS: Arterial grafts: Past, present and future. Arch Surg 113:1225, 1978.
129. Dale WA, Lewis MR: Further experiences with bovine arterial grafts. Surgery 80:711, 1976.
130. Karkow WS, Cranley JJ, Cranley RD, et al: Extended study of aneurysm formation in umbilical vein grafts. J Vasc Surg 4:486, 1986.
131. Szilagyi EE, Elliot JP, Hageman JH, et al: Biologic fate of autogenous vein implants as arterial substitutes. Ann Surg 178:232, 1973.
132. Ottinger LW, Darling RC, Wirthlin LS, et al: Failure of ultra-lightweight knitted Dacron grafts in arterial reconstruction. Arch Surg 111:146, 1976.
133. Campbell CD, Brooks DH, Webster MW, et al: Aneurysm formation in expanded polytetrafluoroethylene prostheses. Surgery 74:491, 1976.

14

Arterial Fibrodysplasia

James C. Stanley, M.D., and Thomas W. Wakefield, M.D.

• • •

Arterial fibrodysplasia encompasses a heterogeneous group of nonatherosclerotic, noninflammatory vascular occlusive and aneurysmal diseases. Principal forms of arterial fibrodysplasic stenoses include intimal fibroplasia, medial hyperplasia, medial fibroplasia, and perimedial dysplasia.[101] The first two entities represent distinctly different pathologic processes, whereas the latter two appear to represent a continuum of disease. Compounding this classification are hypoplastic dysplastic vessels occurring as true developmental lesions. Various combinations of dysplastic lesions exist, as do other, less easily categorized vessel wall derangements. It is important to distinguish primary arterial disease from secondary fibrodysplasia occurring in vessels harboring other disease entities.

Dysplastic disease is known to affect the renal arteries; the extracranial and intracranial cerebral arteries; the axillary, subclavian, and brachial arteries; the celiac, superior mesenteric, and inferior mesenteric arteries and a number of their branches; the iliac, femoral, popliteal, tibial, and peroneal arteries; and the aorta. Venous involvement has been rare, having been reported in the superficial veins of the lower extremity as well as in the renal vein.[22, 39, 80] Complications of the dysplastic process, namely macroaneursym development, dissections, and the formation of arteriovenous fistulae, should be differentiated from the primary fibrodysplastic lesion. Arterial dysplasia represents a systemic arteriopathy in certain instances, although discussions on this subject usually focus on the specific vessels involved.[52, 53]

RENAL ARTERY FIBRODYSPLASIA

The precise incidence of renal artery dysplastic disease in the general population is unknown, but it is less than 0.5 per cent. The frequency among black hypertensive patients appears to be even lower. Renal artery dysplasia, first described in 1938,[45] is second only to atherosclerosis as the most common cause of surgically correctable hypertension. The entire spectrum of dysplastic stenoses affects the renal artery.[95, 96] The specific types of renal artery fibrodysplasia warrant separate consideration.

Intimal fibroplasia of the renal artery affects male and female patients with equal frequency. This lesion accounts for approximately 5 per cent of all dysplastic renal artery stenoses and is observed in infants, adolescents, and young adults more often than in the elderly. Primary intimal fibroplasia most often affects the main renal artery, usually occurring as a smooth focal stenosis (Fig. 14–1*A*). Segmental vessel involvement is a more uncommon manifestation of intimal disease that usually presents as a web-like lesion (Fig. 14–1*B*).

Irregularly arranged subendothelial mesenchymal cells within a loose matrix of fibrous connective tissue projecting into the vessel lumen characterize primary intimal fibroplasia (Fig. 14–2). The internal elastic lamina, although occasionally disrupted, is always indentifiable. Primary intimal proliferation is usually circumferential. The cause of primary intimal fibroplasia is unknown. In some cases, it appears to represent persistent neonatal arterial musculoelastic cushions, similar to the intimal cushions occurring at cerebral artery bifurcations in adults.[114] Lipid-containing foam cells and inflammatory cells are not part of this disease. Medial and adventitial tissues are usually normal in these dysplastic vessels.

Secondary intimal fibroplasia is often difficult to differentiate from primary intimal disease. Certain secondary lesions occur with developmental ostial lesions or advanced medial dysplasia, perhaps resulting from altered flow through these stenoses (Fig. 14–3). Blunt vascular trauma or intraluminal insults following thrombosis may contribute to other secondary lesions, with medial and adventitial structures in such cases appearing relatively uninvolved (Fig. 14–4). Long, tubular stenoses may be evidence of secondary disease occurring as a consequence of recanalization of a previously thrombosed artery (Fig. 14–5). In this regard, certain cases of intimal fibroplasia have been suggested to represent a resolved arteritis, such as might occur with rubella.[104] An infectious-immunologic etiology has been supported in certain cases by evidence of immunoglobulin deposition within intimal tissues of the stenotic vessels.[15]

Progression of intimal fibroplasia once a hemodynamically important arterial stenosis develops appears a likely consequence of abnormal surface blood flow, even if the initiating etiologic factors have resolved. The specific cellular messengers responsible for this tissue proliferation have not been identified. Intimal lesions appear to progress at a much slower rate than do medial fibroplastic stenoses.[63]

Medial hyperplasia without associated fibrosis is an unusual cause of renal artery stenosis. In fact, the existence of this particular dysplastic disease is subject to debate. In certain instances, oblique sections of the arterial wall or specimens near bifurcations may misleadingly portray an increase in medial thickness. Similarly, unusually large amounts of smooth muscle separated by recognizable excesses of ground substance represent medial fibrodysplasia,[9] not medial hyperplasia. Medial hyperplasia of the renal artery has been most often described in women during their 4th and 5th decades of life. If indeed this type of lesion actually exists, it will certainly account for less than 1 per

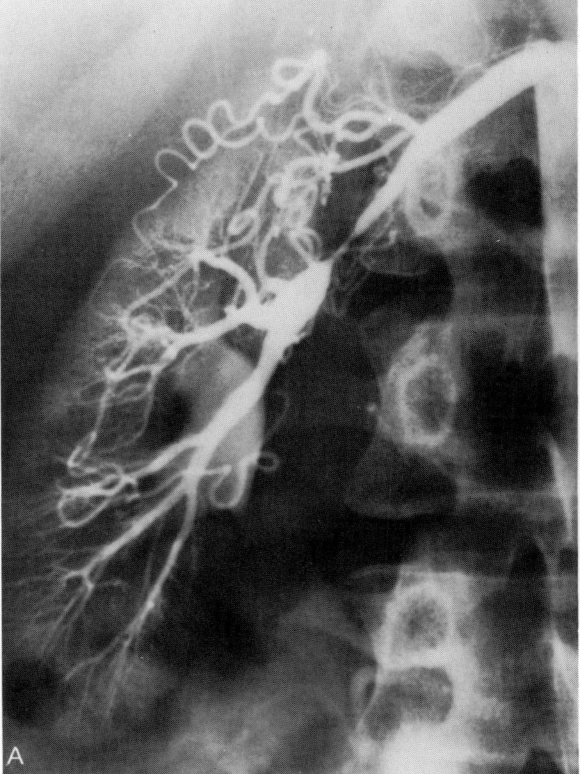

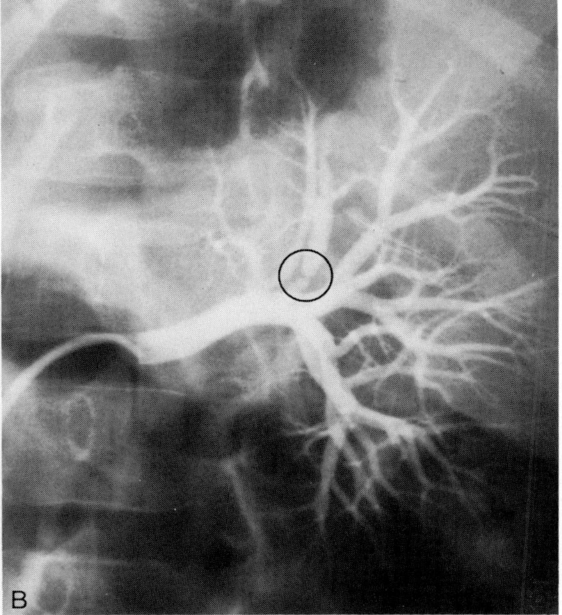

FIGURE 14–1. Primary intimal fibroplasia. *A*, Focal stenosis of the mid-portion of the main renal artery in a young adult. *B*, Intraparenchymal web-like stenosis of a segmental artery in a child. (*A*, From Stanley JC, Fry WJ: Renovascular hypertension secondary to arterial fibrodysplasia in adults: Criteria for operation and results of surgical therapy. Arch Surg 110:922–928, 1975. Copyright 1975, American Medical Association. *B*, From Stanley JC, Fry WJ: Pediatric renal artery occlusive disease and renovascular hypertension. Etiology, diagnosis and operative treatment. Arch Surg 116:669–676, 1981. Copyright 1981, American Medical Association.)

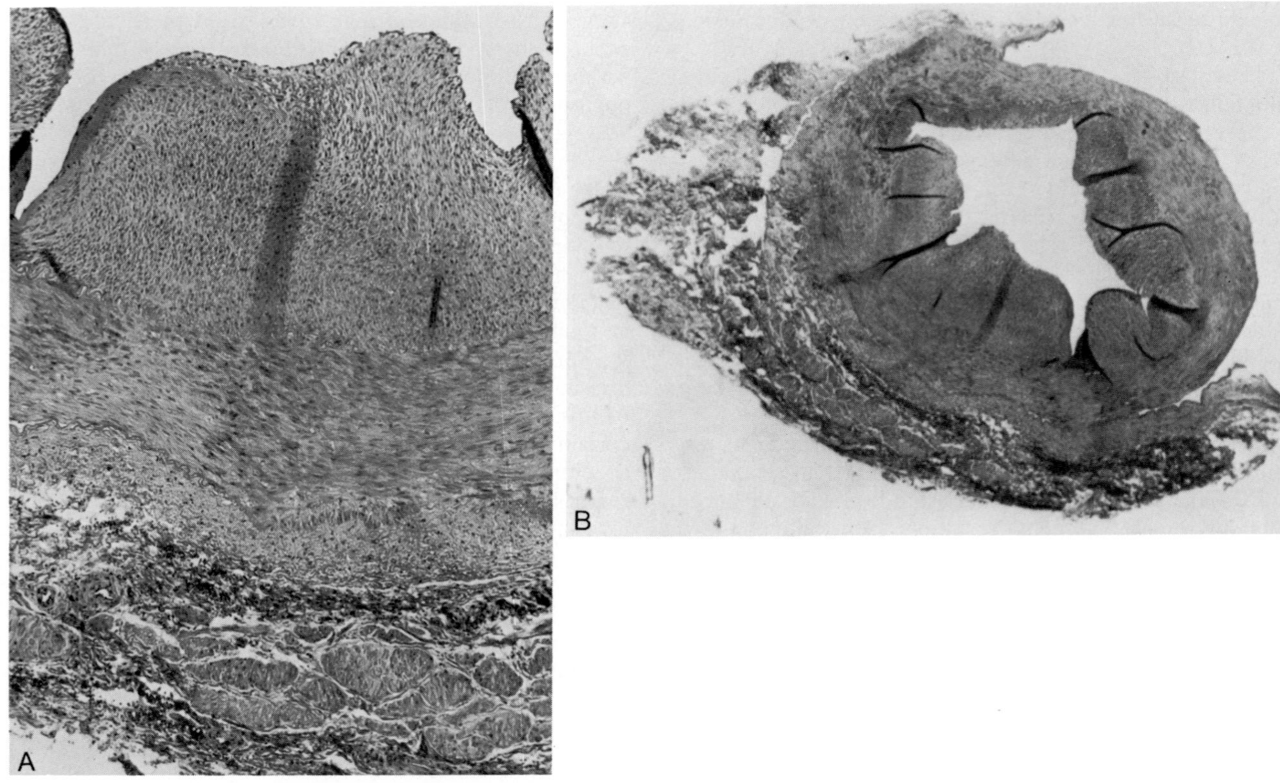

FIGURE 14–2. Primary intimal fibroplasia. *A*, Subendothelial mesenchymal cells within a loose fibrous connective tissue matrix are noted above an intact internal elastic lamina, a normal media, and normal adventitial tissues. (×100.) *B*, Luminal encroachments by this primary form of intimal fibroplasia are usually circumferential. (×35.) (*A* and *B*, H&E.) (*A*, From Stanley JC: Morphologic, histopathologic and clinical characteristics of renovascular fibrodysplasia and arteriosclerosis. *In* Bergan JJ, Yao JST [eds]: Surgery of the Aorta and Its Body Branches. New York, Grune & Stratton, 1979, pp 355–376. *B*, From Stanley JC: Pathologic basis of macrovascular renal artery disease. *In* Stanley JC, Ernst CB, Fry WJ [eds]: Renovascular Hypertension. Philadelphia, WB Saunders, 1984, pp 46–74.)

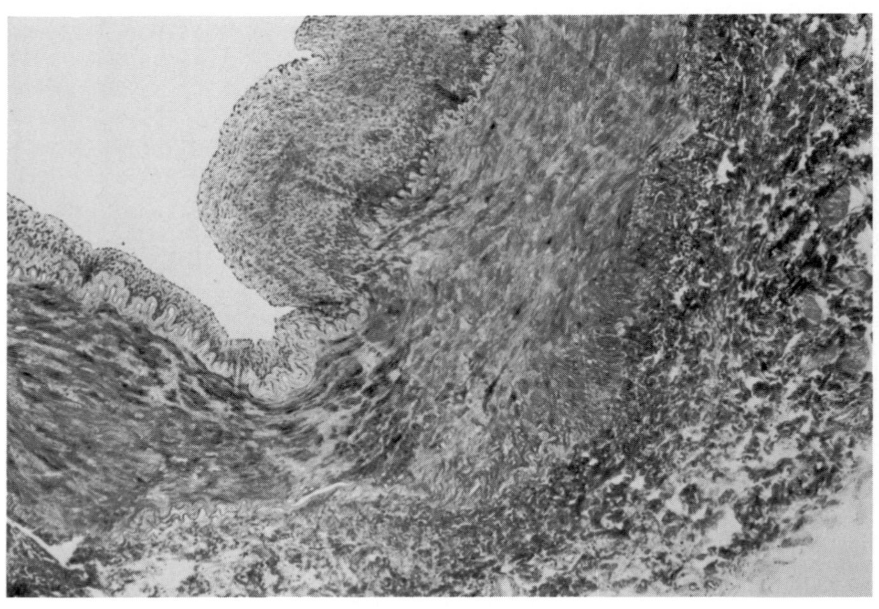

FIGURE 14–3. Secondary intimal fibroplasia. Cellular subendothelial tissue in an artery exhibiting advanced medial fibroplasia. (Masson, ×80.) (From Stanley JC: Pathologic basis of macrovascular renal artery disease. *In* Stanley JC, Ernst CB, Fry WJ [eds]: Renovascular Hypertension. Philadelphia, WB Saunders, 1984, pp 46–74.)

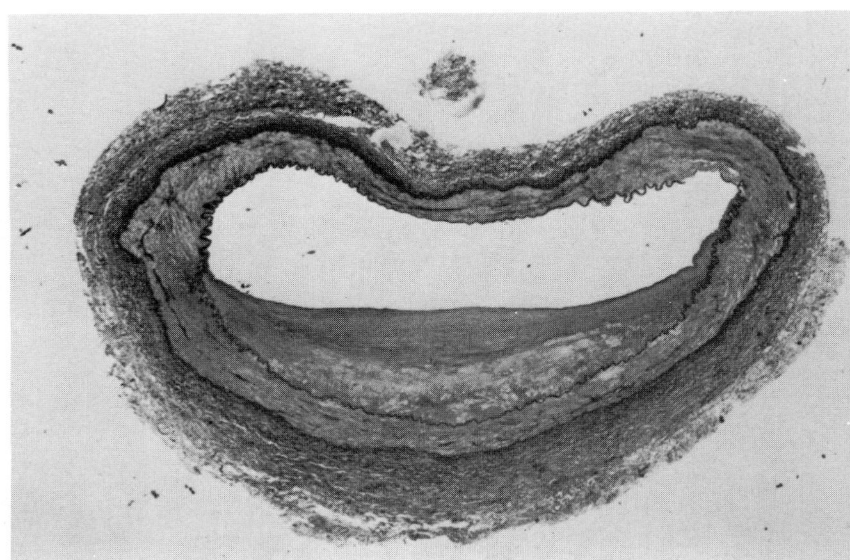

FIGURE 14–4. Secondary intimal fibrodysplasia. Marked intimal thickening in an otherwise relatively normal vessel, consistant with the organization of prior intraluminal thrombus. (Movat, ×40.)

cent of dysplastic renovascular lesions. Focal stenoses caused by medial hyperplasia usually involve the mid-portion of the renal artery, not its branchings or segmental vessels (Fig. 14–6). Increases in smooth muscle cell numbers with minimal disorganization and the absence of ground substance excesses characterize medial hyperplasia (Fig. 14–7). Intimal and adventitial structures are usually normal, although in severe stenoses subendothelial fibroplasia may occur as a secondary event. Medial hyperplasia of the renal artery has not been associated with any clearly recognized cause. Contributing to the controversy surrounding this lesion is the fact that a non-neoplastic increase in smooth muscle elsewhere within the vascular system is unusual.

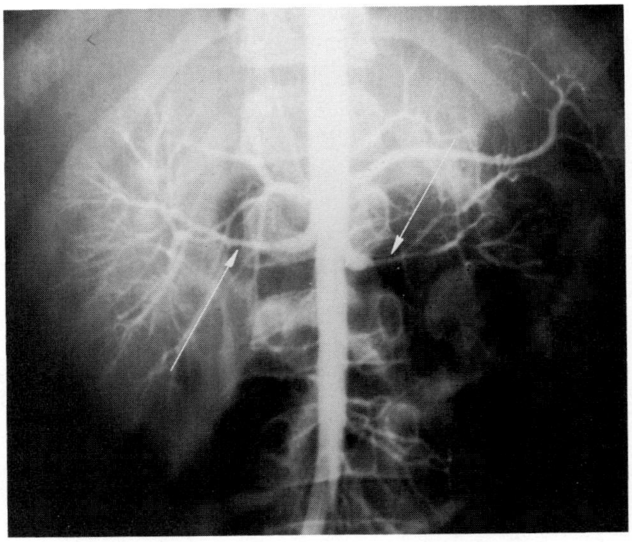

FIGURE 14–5. Secondary intimal fibroplasia. Long tubular stenoses (*arrows*) in the main distal renal arteries of an infant. (From Whitehouse WM Jr, Cho KJ, Coran AS, Stanley JC: Pediatric arterial disease. *In* Neiman HL, Yao JST [eds]: Angiography of Vascular Disease, pp 289–306. Churchill Livingstone, New York, 1985.)

Medial fibrodysplasia accounts for nearly 85 per cent of dysplastic renovascular disease. More than 90 per cent of patients with medial fibrodysplasia are female. This subgroup of disease is exceedingly uncommon among the black population. The disease is diagnosed most often during the 4th decade of life. Although medial fibrodysplasia is considered to be a systemic arteriopathy, clinically overt arterial involvement is usually limited to the renal, extracranial internal carotid, and external iliac vessels.

The morphologic appearance of renal artery medial fibrodysplasia ranges from a solitary focal stenosis to its more common presentation as a series of stenoses with intervening aneurysmal outpouchings (Fig. 14–8). The latter, which causes a string-of-beads appearance, has not been observed in female patients prior to menarche, with the exception of a single case report.[73] The thin-walled mural

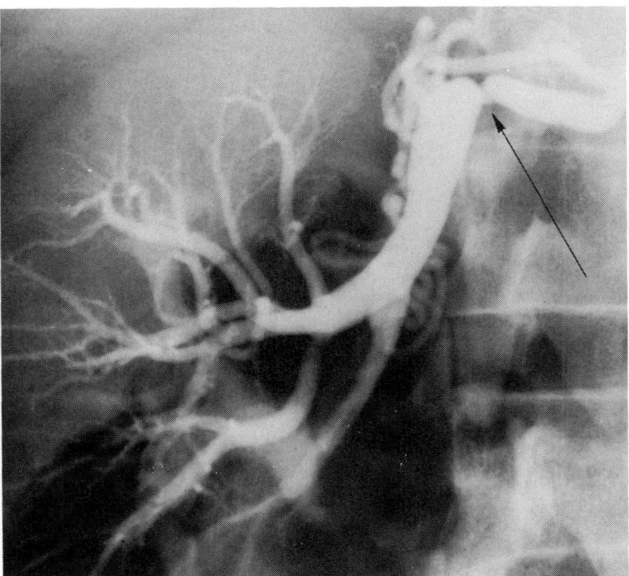

FIGURE 14–6. Medial hyperplasia. Focal stenosis (*arrow*) affecting the mid-portion of the main renal artery.

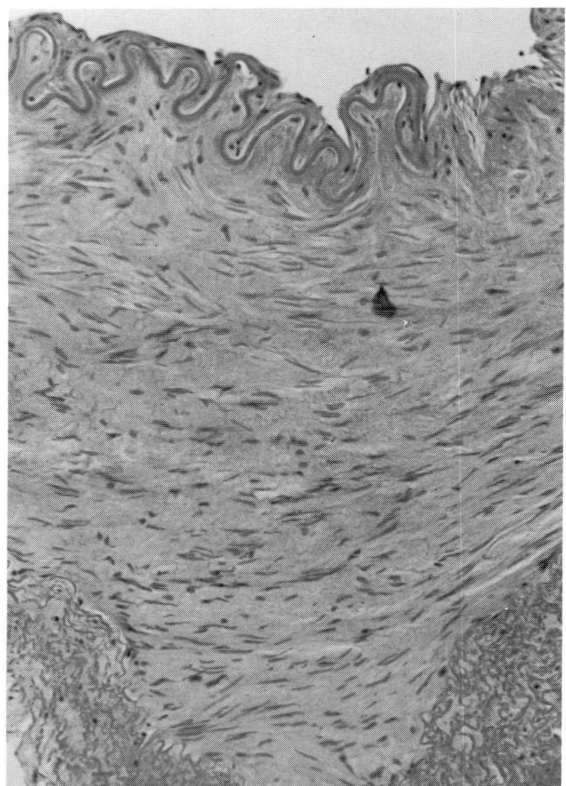

FIGURE 14–7. Medial hyperplasia. Unusual dysplastic lesion with excessive medial smooth muscle in an otherwise normal vessel. (H&E, ×120.) (From Stanley JC: Morphologic, histopathologic and clinical characteristics of renovascular fibrodysplasia and arteriosclerosis. *In* Bergan JJ, Yao JST [eds]: Surgery of the Aorta and Its Body Branches. New York, Grune & Stratton, 1979, pp 355–376.)

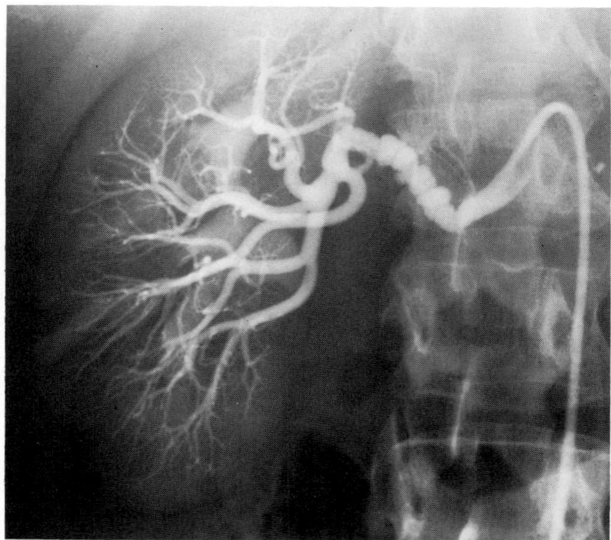

FIGURE 14–8. Medial fibrodysplasia. Serial stenoses alternating with mural aneurysms, producing a string-of-beads appearance in the mid-portion and distal main renal artery. (From Stanley JC, Graham LM: Renovascular hypertension. *In* Miller DC, Roon AJ [eds]: Diagnosis and Management of Peripheral Vascular Disease. Menlo Park, CA, Addison-Wesley, 1981, pp 231–235.)

aneurysms are usually evident grossly, as are distinct webs projecting internally (Fig. 14–9). Medial fibrodysplasia most commonly affects the distal main renal artery, with extensions into first-order segmental branches occurring in approximately 25 per cent of cases.

Progression of renal artery medial fibrodysplasia is less common than that associated with perimedial dysplasia.[26] Progression appears to occur in 12 to 66 per cent of patients with main renal artery lesions.[26, 63, 89, 98] Progression is generally thought to be more likely to affect premenopausal women, but some authors have noted no differences related to age.[87] Among a group of 71 potential kidney donors with angiographic evidence of renal artery fibrodysplasia, hypertension developed in 26 per cent over an average follow-up of 7½ years.[10] Hypertension developed in only 6 per cent of an age- and sex-matched group of control patients. Blood pressure increases in these instances were considered to be a reflection of progressive renal artery

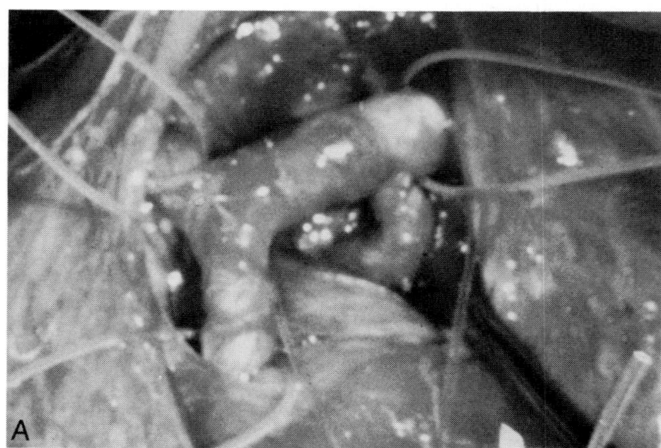

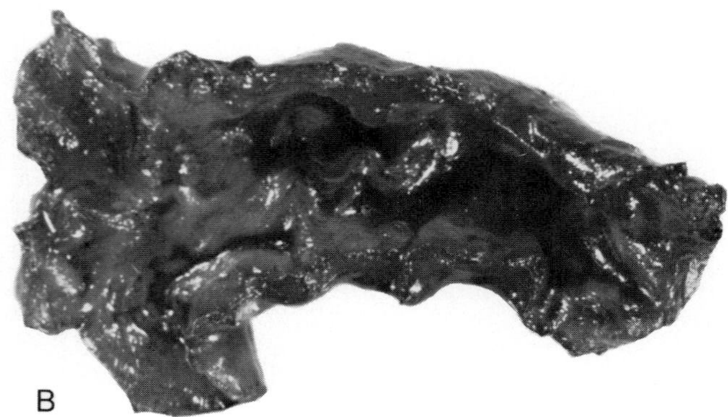

FIGURE 14–9. Medial fibrodysplasia. *A*, Gross appearance of a mural aneurysm characteristic of this type of renal artery dysplasia. *B*, Internal appearance of webs projecting into the lumen of an excised main renal artery specimen. (*A* and *B*, From Stanley JC: Pathologica basis of macrovascular renal artery disease. *In* Stanley JC, Ernst CB, Fry WJ [eds]: Renovascular Hypertension. Philadelphia, WB Saunders, 1984, pp 46–74.)

disease. Acute changes in fibrodysplastic renal vessels are relatively uncommon, although in one series 18 per cent had progressed to complete occlusion.[18] Regression of renal artery dysplastic stenoses has been reported,[69] although the validity of such an event has been challenged.[61]

Two histologic forms of renal artery medial fibrodysplasia are well recognized (Fig. 14–10). The first is evident by disease limited to the outer media (peripheral form). The second exhibits disease throughout the entire media (diffuse form). The latter is noted twice as often as the former. Gradations between these extremes have been observed in the same vessel, supporting the tenet that they represent the same disease process. The peripheral form of medial fibrodysplasia is usually encountered in younger patients. It is quite possible that with the passage of time, more advanced disease evolves to affect the entire media. Consistent with this hypothesis are observed changes in the arteriographic appearance of these lesions, with multiple severe stenoses in series and true macroaneurysms developing in many patients who initially had a solitary lesion or a few stenoses of minimal severity.

Peripheral medial fibrodysplasia is characterized by compact fibrous connective tissue replacing smooth muscle in the outer media. Less obvious findings are moderate accumulations of collagen and ground substances separating disorganized smooth muscle within the inner media. Intimal tissues and the internal elastic lamina are rarely affected in these peripheral lesions. Although continuity of the external elastic lamina is frequently lost, the adventitia is usually normal. Certain peripheral forms of medial fibrodysplasia were previously thought to represent perimedial or subadventitial disease.[30, 59, 60]

Diffuse medial fibrodysplasia is characterized by more severe disorganization and disruption of normal smooth muscle architecture. Occasionally, the diffuse form of dysplasia results in an amorphous-appearing media (Fig. 14–11). In other vessels, excessive medial accumulations of fibrous tissue alternate with areas of marked medial thinning (Fig. 14–12). In some instances, the media is nearly absent, and these regions account for the vessel's mural aneurysmal dilatations. Internal elastic lamina fragmentation and subendothelial fibrosis may also be evident. These latter two changes are considered secondary events in instances of more advanced medial fibrodysplasia. Adventitial tissues are relatively uninvolved in medial fibrodysplasia.

Extensive fragmentation and distortion of the internal elastic lamina occur in some renal arteries (Fig. 14–13). Deeper dissections may extend into middle and outer medial structures as limited dissections (Fig. 14–14*A*), or they

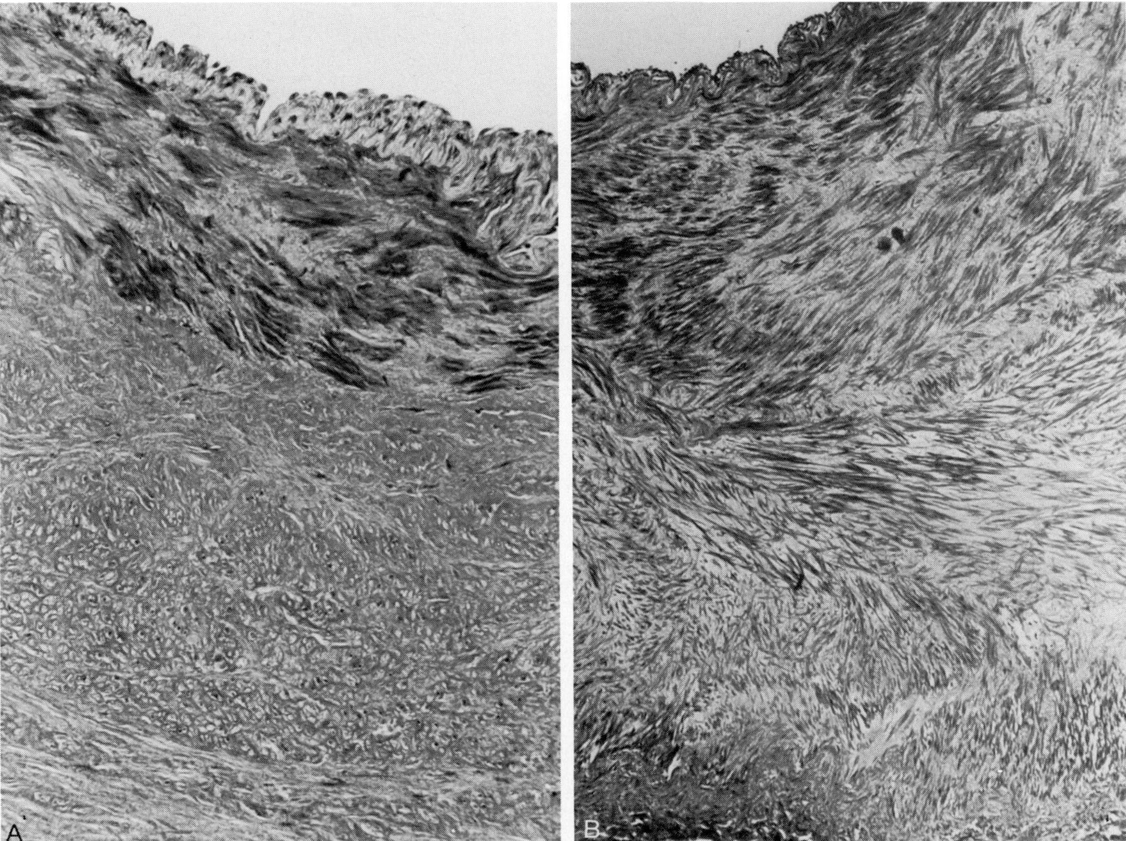

FIGURE 14–10. *A*, Peripheral form of medial fibrodysplasia. Dense fibrous connective tissue in the outer media, with disordered inner medial smooth muscle and normal intimal tissues. *B*, Diffuse form of medial fibrodysplasia. Total replacement of the media by disorganized cellular tissue (myofibroblasts) surrounded by fibrous connective tissue. (Masson, ×120.) (*A* and *B*, From Stanley JC: Morphologic, histopathologic and clinical characteristics of renovascular fibrodysplasia and arteriosclerosis. *In* Bergan JJ, Yao JST [eds]: Surgery of the Aorta and Its Body Branches. New York, Grune & Stratton, 1979, pp 355–376.)

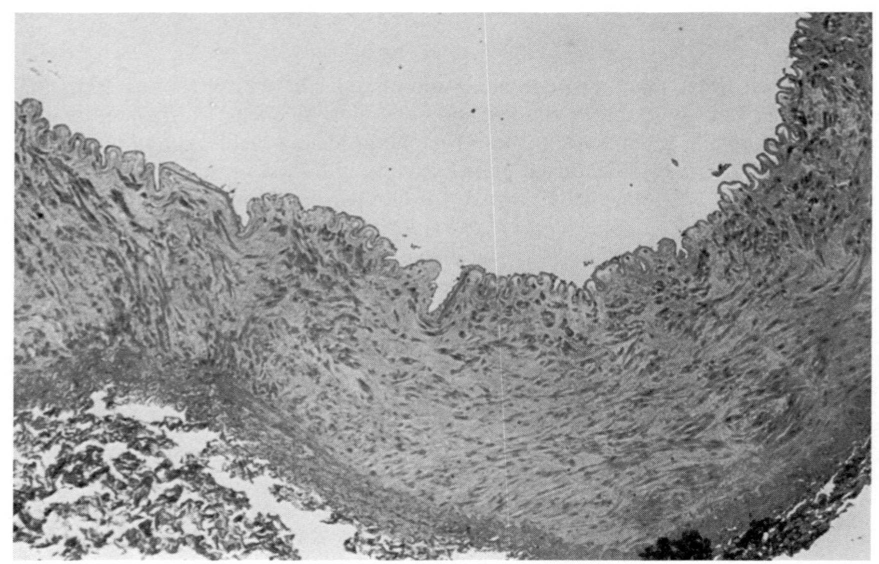

FIGURE 14–11. Diffuse form of medial fibrodysplasia. Amorphous appearance of excessive ground substances and fibrous connective tissue throughout the media. (Masson, ×80, longitudinal section.) (From Stanley JC: Pathologic basis of macrovascular renal artery disease. *In* Stanley JC, Ernst CB, Fry WJ [eds]: Renovascular Hypertension. Philadelphia, WB Saunders, 1984, pp 46–74.)

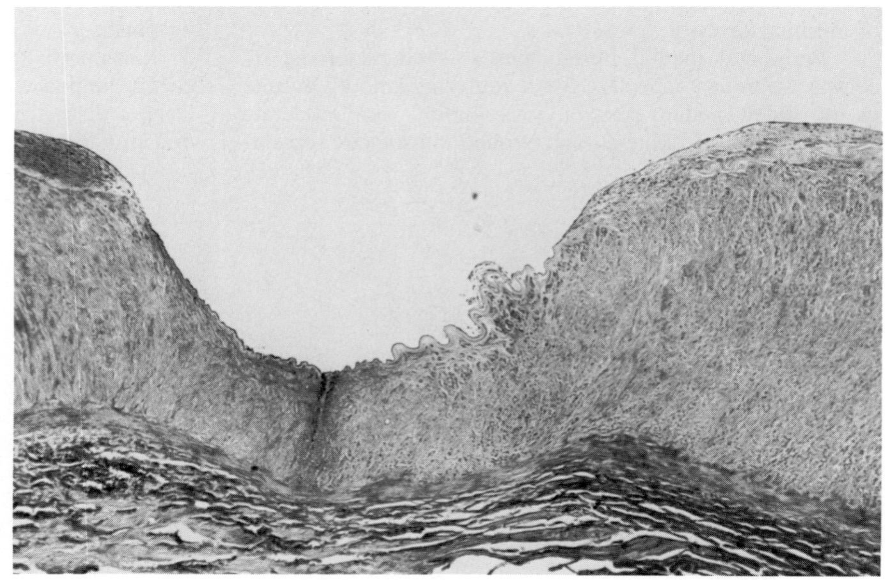

FIGURE 14–12. Diffuse form of medial fibrodysplasia. Regions of excessive fibroproliferation with intervening area of medial thinning. (Masson, ×60, longitudinal section.) (From Stanley JC: Morphologic, histopathologic and clinical characteristics of renovascular fibrodysplasia and arteriosclerosis. *In* Bergan JJ, Yao JST [eds]: Surgery of the Aorta and Its Body Branches. New York, Grune & Stratton, 1979, pp 355–376.)

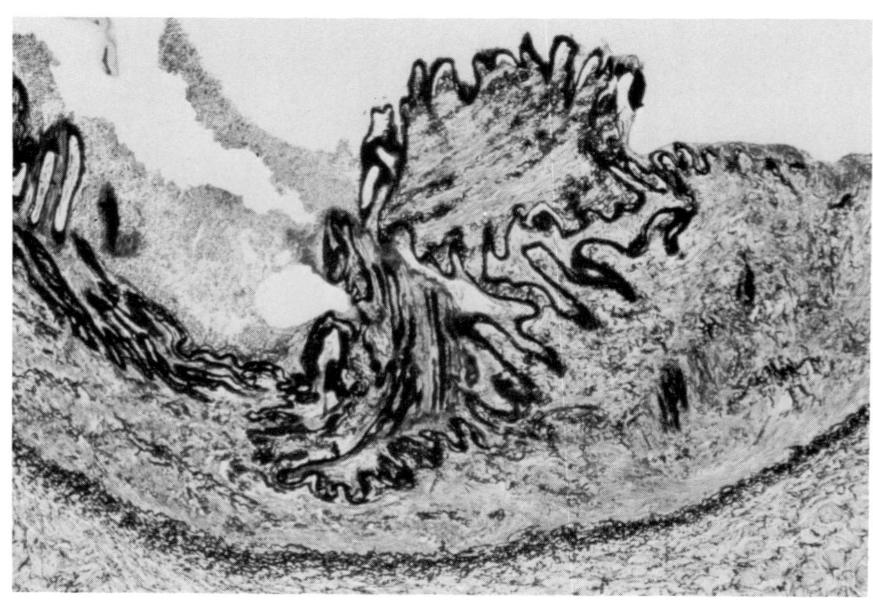

FIGURE 14–13. Medial fibrodysplasia. Extensive fragmentation and distortion of the internal elastic lamina with dissection. (Movat, ×160.)

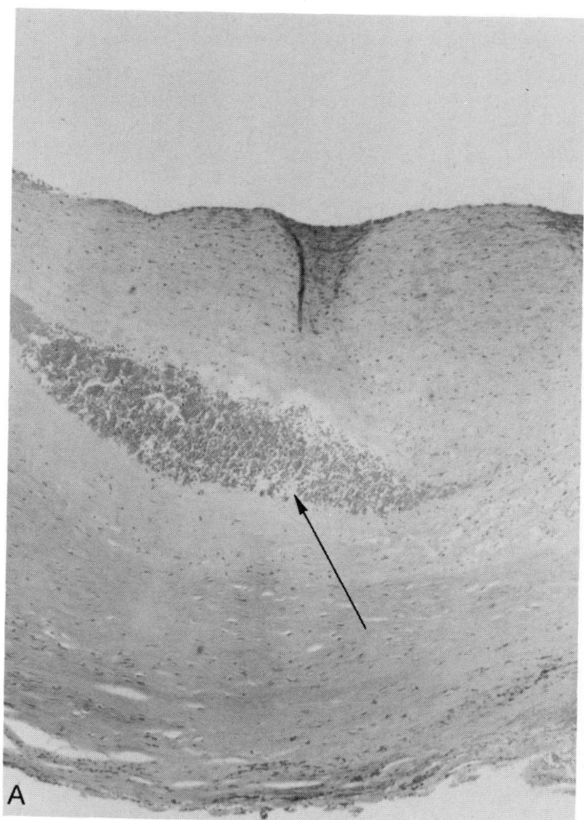

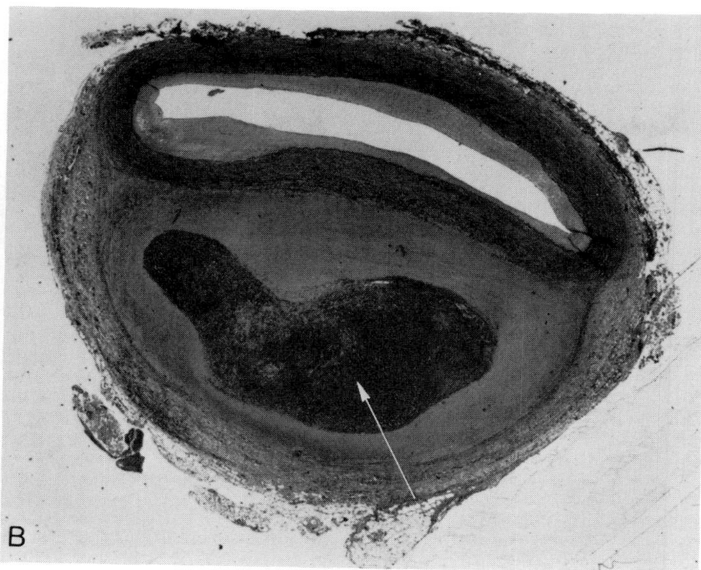

FIGURE 14–14. Dissections complicating medial fibrodysplasia. *A*, Intramedial dissection with limited hemorrhage (*arrow*). (×120.) *B*, Deep medial dissection with large intramural hematoma (*arrow*) compressing the vessel lumen. (×60.) (*A* and *B*, H&E.) (*A* and *B*, From Stanley JC: Pathologic basis of macrovascular renal artery disease. *In* Stanley JC, Ernst CB, Fry WJ [eds]: Renovascular Hypertension. Philadelphia, WB Saunders, 1984, pp 46–74.)

may progress as large intramural hematomas that compress the vessel lumen (Fig. 14–14*B*).[29] Loss of vessel integrity at bifurcations, with fragmentation of elastic tissue, is thought to lead to the development of renal artery macroaneurysms (Fig. 14–15).[103]

Perimedial dysplasia is the dominant abnormality affecting approximately 10 per cent of dysplastic renal arteries. It may coexist with medial fibrodysplasia. Most patients exhibiting perimedial dysplasia have been female, usually in their 4th or 5th decade of life. These lesions present as either focal stenoses or multiple constrictions involving the mid-portion of the main renal artery without mural aneurysms (Fig. 14–16*A*). Excessive elastic tissue at the junction of the media and the adventitia is the distinguishing feature of perimedial dysplasia (Fig. 14–16*B*). Minimal increases in medial ground substance surrounding intact smooth muscle cells, with little alteration of intimal tissues, characterize inner portions of the vessel wall in many of these dysplastic lesions whose dominant feature is the homogeneous collar of elastic tissue adjacent to the outer media (Fig. 14–17).

Certain ultrastructural features are common to medial fibrodysplasia and perimedial dysplasia.[94] Both exhibit accumulations of ground substance and fibrous elements. Perimedial dysplasia is differentiated by collections of amorphous material and elastic tissue at the adventitial-medial border. Most importantly, both manifest a spectrum of change within the cellular composition of the media, ranging from near-normal smooth muscle to myofibro-

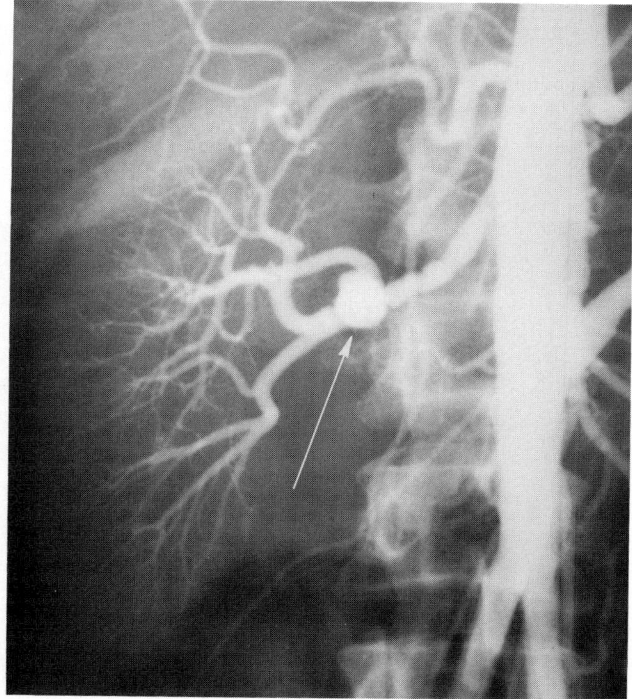

FIGURE 14–15. Macroaneurysms and medial fibrodysplasia. Large macroaneurysm (*arrow*) at a bifurcation of the renal artery. (From Ernst CB, Stanley JC, Fry WJ: Multiple primary and segmental renal artery revascularization utilizing autogenous saphenous vein. Surg Gynecol Obstet 137:1023, 1973.)

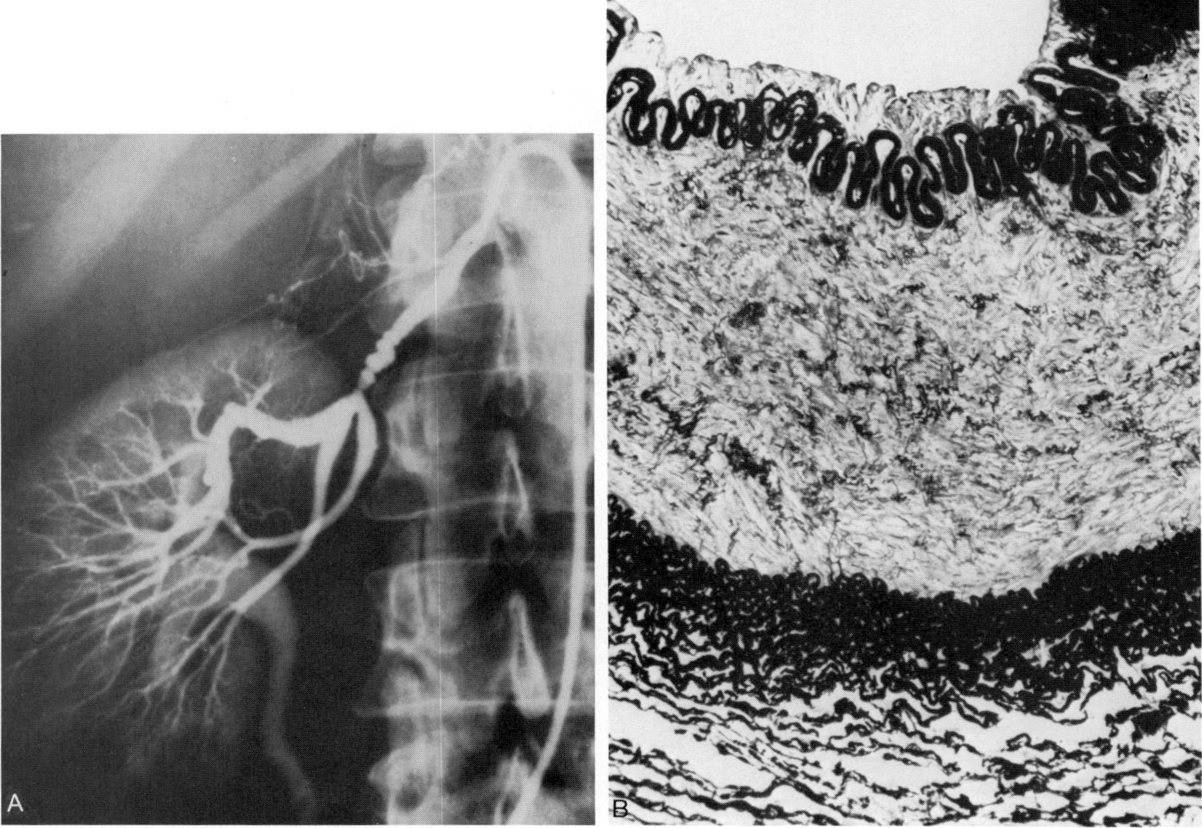

FIGURE 14–16. Perimedial dysplasia. *A*, Multiple stenoses without mural aneurysms in the mid-portion of the renal artery are characteristic of these lesions. *B*, These stenoses are due to excessive accumulations of elastic tissue at the medial-adventitial junction. (Verhoeff, ×120.) (*A* and *B*, From Stanley JC: Morphologic, histopathologic and clinical characteristics of renovascular fibrodysplasia and arteriosclerosis. *In* Bergan JJ, Yao JST [eds]: Surgery of the Aorta and Its Body Branches. New York, Grune & Stratton, 1979, pp 355–376.)

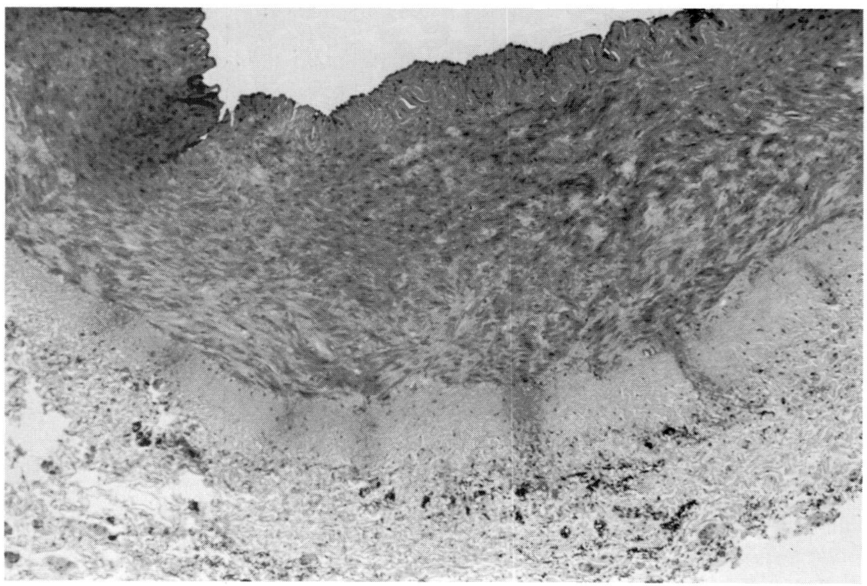

FIGURE 14–17. Perimedial dysplasia. Homogeneous collar of elastic tissue adjacent to the outer media is the dominant feature of this lesion. (H&E, ×80.) (From Stanley JC: Pathologic basis of macrovascular renal artery disease. *In* Stanley JC, Ernst CB, Fry WJ [eds]: Renovascular Hypertension. Philadelphia, WB Saunders, 1984, pp 46–74.)

blasts. Fibroblasts are not a usual component of the media and are infrequently observed in these diseased tissues. Similarly, macrophages and leukocytes, suggesting an inflammatory process, are not a relevant component of either medial fibroplasia or perimedial dysplasia. Normal smooth muscle cells are characterized by close apposition of cytoplasmic processes; a deeply indented and convoluted ovoid nucleus surrounded by a modest number of cellular organelles; orderly arranged thick and thin myofilaments parallel to the longitudinal cell axis, with electron-dense bodies at their attachment to the plasma lamina; basal laminations; and scattered micropinocytotic vesicles.

The earliest alterations in the smooth muscle ultrastructure of dysplastic vessels are focal myofilament reductions, as well as perinuclear sublemmal and cytoplasmic vacuolations (Fig. 14–18). In areas of advanced dysplasia, certain smooth muscle cells exhibit extreme deterioration, whereas others become fibroblast-like in appearance. The former are invariably isolated from surrounding cells by excessive amounts of ground substance (Fig. 14–19*A*). In these tissues, long, slender cytoplasmic processes reflect decreased cell volumes. Cell membranes are often indistinct, and the nucleus is usually pyknotic, containing dense chromatin material. Confluences of micropinocytotic vesicles are common, and subcellular organelles are sparse. Myofilaments appear dense and homogeneous in these cells. Modification of medial smooth muscle cells to fibroblast-type cells represents a continuum within dysplastic tissues. Alterations in nuclear contour; loss of myofilaments; and increases in free ribosomes, rough endoplasmic reticulum Golgi's complexes, and mitochondria seemingly parallel altered function from one of contractility to one of secretion.

Myofibroblasts are the end-product of smooth muscle transformation. Typical of these cells is a convoluted nucleus with numerous indentations and evaginations (Fig.

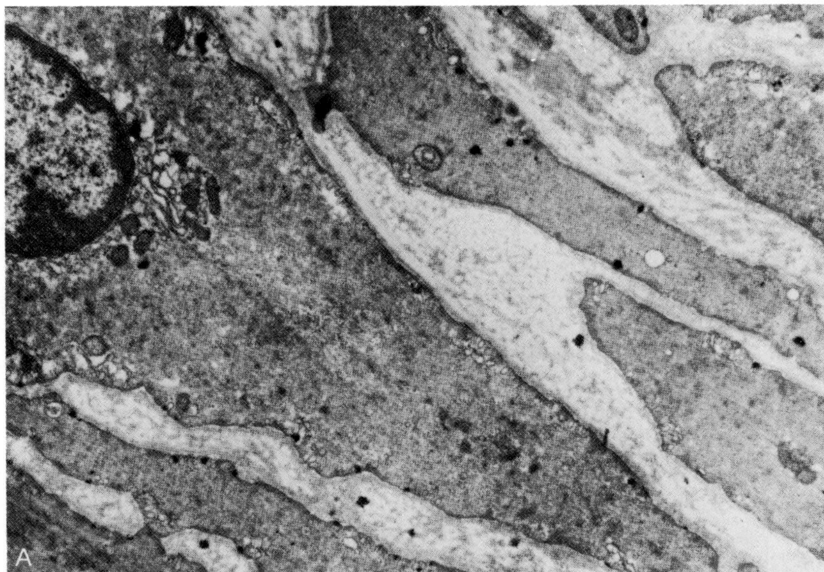

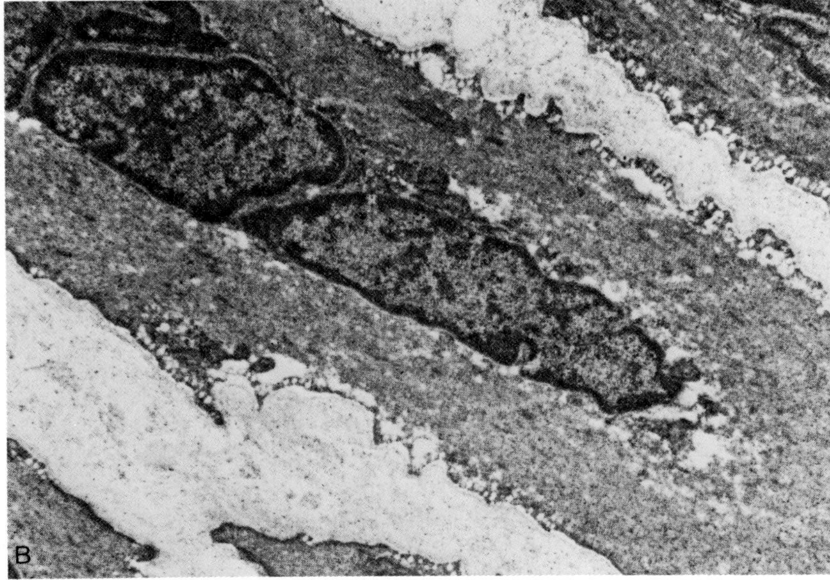

FIGURE 14–18. Smooth muscle cell. *A*, In a region of minimal fibrodysplasia, a relatively normal ultrastructure is seen, except for the focal reduction in myofilaments and the appearance of perinuclear, sublemmal, and cytoplasmic vacuoles. (×18,000.) *B*, In a region of moderate fibrodysplasia, more extensive perinuclear and peripheral vacuolation is evident. Loss of organelles and basement membrane and indistinct myofilaments characterize this type of cell. (×12,000.) (*A* and *B*, Transmission electron microscope [TEM].) (*A* and *B*, From Stanley JC: Pathologic basis of macrovascular renal artery disease. *In* Stanley JC, Ernst CB, Fry WJ [eds]: Renovascular Hypertension. Philadelphia, WB Saunders, 1984, pp 46–74.)

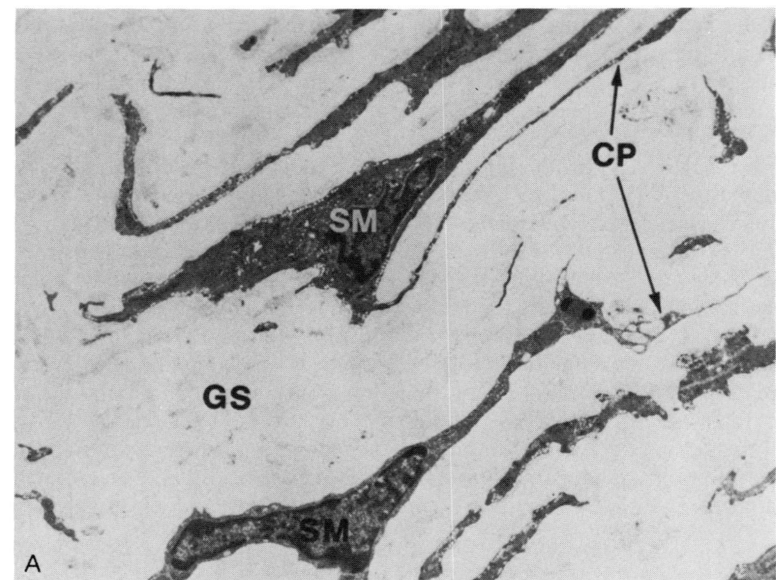

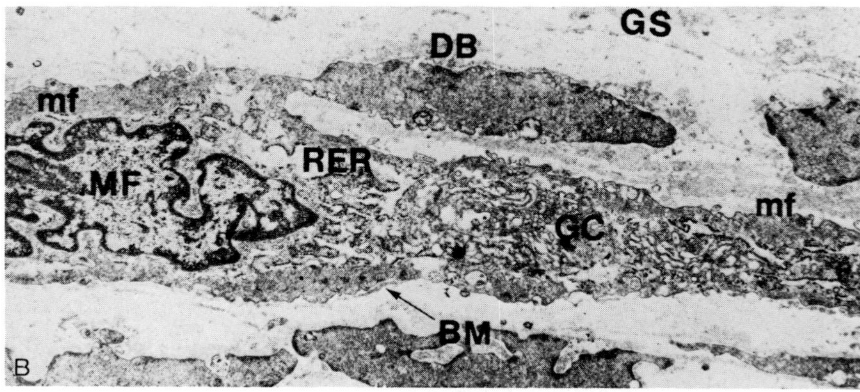

FIGURE 14–19. *A*, Smooth muscle cell. in an area of advanced fibrodysplasia. Isolation of slender cytoplasmic processes by excesses in ground substances, and pyknotic nuclei were typical of these markedly abnormal cells. (×6000.) *B*, Myofibroblast associated with medial fibroplasia. The convoluted nucleus is typical of smooth muscle, but increased numbers of centrally located organelles reflect the change in function from one of contractility to secretion. (×8000.) (*A* and *B*, TEM.) SM, smooth muscle; GS, ground substance; CP, cytoplasmic processes; mf, myofilament; DB, dense body; RER, rough endoplasmic reticulum; MF, myofibroblast; GC, Golgi complex; BM, basement membrane; (*A* and *B*, From Sottiurai VS, Fry WJ, Stanley JC: Ultrastructure of medial smooth muscle and myofibroblasts in human arterial dysplasia. Arch Surg 113:1280–1288, 1978. Copyright 1978, American Medical Association.)

14–19*B*). Major juxtanuclear increases in subcellular organelles and the presence of peripherally located cytoplasmic filaments are characteristic of myofibroblasts. Myofilaments are scant and poorly defined. Active exopinocytotic deposition of proteinaceous matter may be evident in some cells (Fig. 14–20).

Vasa vasorum within the media of diseased arteries are usually widely separated from adjacent cellular tissue by fibrous material and homogeneous mucoid substances. The type of surrounding connective tissue appears to be related to the category of arterial dysplasia. Vasa vasorum within medial fibrodysplasia are predominantly surrounded by collagen fibrous bundles, whereas those in perimedial dysplasia are usually surrounded by amorphous mucoid substances consistent with elastic tissue.

The *pathogenesis of medial fibrodysplasia and perimedial dysplasia* has been the subject of much speculation.[43, 101] Hormonal effects on smooth muscle, mechanical stresses on vessel walls, and the peculiar distribution of vasa vasorum in arteries exhibiting these lesions are all considered to be contributing factors. The exact relation of these factors to each other, or their association with other unrecognized pathogenic mechanisms, remains unknown. Because of the familial nature of this disease, a genetic-related autosomal dominant etiology with incomplete penetrance has been suggested. However, confirmatory arteriographic or histologic evidence to establish such a contention firmly has not been presented.[25, 56, 68, 82, 85] In fact, the absence of a female predilection in the data generated by those supporting a genetic etiology lessens the validity of their proposal.

Hormonal influences seem likely in view of arterial dysplasia's unusual female predilection. More than 95 per cent of patients exhibiting medial and perimedial disease are women. Pregnancy, although known to cause rather profound vascular wall changes, including alterations in medial structures, especially elastic tissue, is not an obvious etiologic factor in arterial fibrodysplasia. The reproductive histories of patients in a large series of patients with this arteriography did *not* reveal gravity or parity rates different from those in the general population.[101] Antiovulants are also known to have a significant effect on the arterial wall. However, the use of such drugs by less than half the female patients in the Michigan series does not support any obvious cause-and-effect association of progestins with arterial dysplasia.[101] A similar lack of association with oral contraceptive use was reported in a case-control study.[85] Certain smooth muscle cells and fibroblasts exposed to estrogens demonstrate increased synthesis of proteinaceous substances, including collagen.[81] It is speculated that physiologic preconditioning of vascular smooth muscle cells to

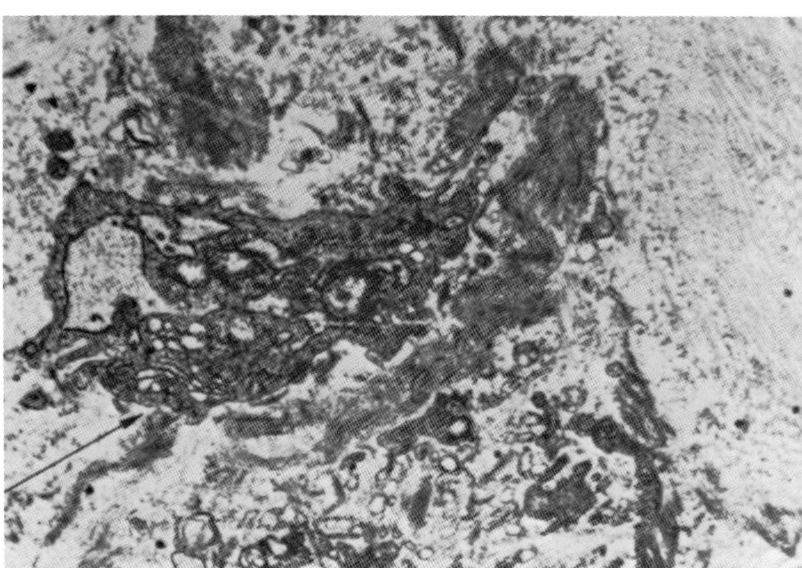

FIGURE 14–20. Myofibroblast in a region of extensive fibroplasia, exhibiting exopinocytotic secretion of proteinaceous matter (*arrow*). (TEM, ×25,000.) (From Stanley JC: Pathologic basis of macrovascular renal artery disease. *In* Stanley JC, Ernst CB, Fry WJ [eds]: Renovascular Hypertension. Philadelphia, WB Saunders, 1984, pp 46–74.)

a secretory state by normal circulating estrogens may account for the more frequent occurrence of medial dysplastic disease in females.

Unusual physical stresses due to ptosis of the kidneys may be associated with fibrodysplastic changes in the renal arteries (Fig. 14–21). Comparable stretch or traction forces are less likely to occur in similar-sized vessels unaffected by this disease. Ptotic kidneys are known to be common among patients with renal artery dysplastic lesions.[11, 42] In some cases, positional changes causing greater ptosis have been correlated with increases in blood pressure.[107] The fact that the right kidney is usually more ptotic than the left may account for the greater severity of right-sided disease in the majority of adults with bilateral medial fibroplasia. In addition, in the case of unilateral lesions, 80 per cent involve the right renal arteries. Cyclic stretching of smooth muscle cells in tissue culture causes an unusually large synthesis of collagen and certain acid mucopolysaccharides.[48] Although the existence of similar mechanisms in vivo is speculative, the predilection for dysplastic disease to occur most often in vessels subjected to peculiar mechanical forces may reflect an important pathogenic phenomenon. It is cautionary to note that in one recent case-control study, renal mobility was not greater in patients with renovascular fibrodysplasia.[85]

A final etiologic factor may be related to mural ischemia in dysplastic arteries. Vasa vasorum of muscular arteries usually originate from branchings of parent vessels.[4, 44] The renal, extracranial internal carotid, and external iliac arteries are the three vessels most likely to develop medial fibrodysplasia. The latter two arteries, in particular, have relatively few branches compared with similar-sized vessels. Compromise of vasa vasorum in these vessels, in which a sparsity of these nutrient channels may already exist, may lead to significant mural ischemia. Vasospasm may occur in these cases and further exacerbate vessel wall ischemia.[21, 74] The concept that insufficient vessel wall nourishment causes dysplastic changes is supported by the common involvement of the outermost part of the media in peripheral medial fibroplasia. It is precisely in this region that ischemia from inadequate vasa vasorum blood flow would be predictably greatest. Fibrodysplasia limited to the inner part of the media has never been reported. Vasa vasorum in these vessels have exhibited both dilatation[31] and isolation from adjacent medial smooth muscle cells.[55] Experimental occlusion of the vasa vasorum produces a dysplastic lesion in animals similar to that seen in humans, which supports the tenet that mural ischemia is a factor in the evolution of arterial dysplasia.[93]

Tissue hypoxia per se may be the inciting event in stimulating fibroplasia, but altered tissue pH, accumulation of metabolites, and other factors may be just as important.

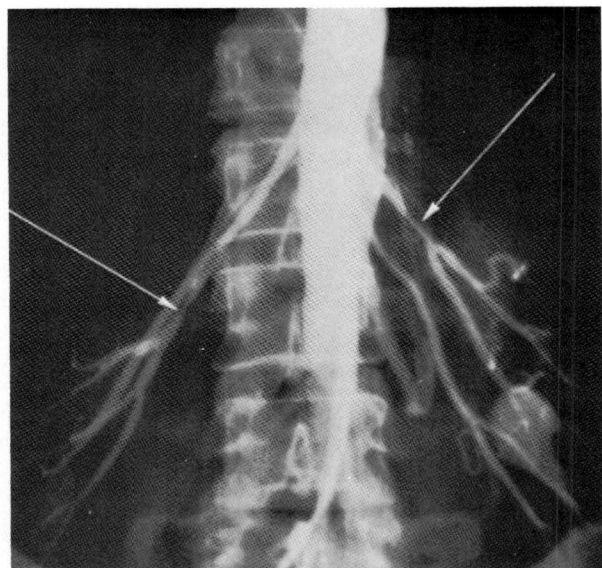

FIGURE 14–21. Medial fibrodysplasia manifest as irregular narrowings to ptotic kidneys (*arrows*) affecting the mid-portion of the main renal arteries, which appear stretched during upright aortography.

Cigarette smoking has been implicated as an important etiologic factor in this disease, although the mechanisms of this have not been defined.[85] Smooth muscle cells are central to the dysplastic process. Medial smooth muscle cells are considered by some investigators to represent multifunctional mesenchymal cells. The duration and exact degree of ischemia necessary to stimulate myofibroblasts are unknown. Myofibroblasts have been observed to develop in other tissues after very brief hypoxic events.[54] No evidence exists that myofibroblasts evolve from dormant mesenchymal cells, although this could be a remote possibility. Some investigators believe that myofibroblasts represent contractile fibroblasts rather than modified smooth muscle cells.[24] However, fibroblasts are not a normal part of artery media.

Developmental Renal Artery Stenoses

Developmental renal artery stenoses are a unique form of renal artery dysplasia. There is no apparent gender predilection for this entity, and its exact frequency is unknown. In a report on pediatric renovascular hypertension, nearly 40 per cent of children were considered to have developmental renal artery lesions.[99] Among adults with intimal fibroplastic renal artery disease, approximately 20 per cent have stenoses that appear to represent growth or developmental defects. Similarly, certain adults with isolated renal arteriosclerosis may have had preexisting developmentally narrowed vessels. Thus, developmental renal artery occlusive disease appears to be an uncommon but not rare entity in the general hypertensive population. Conversely, nearly 80 per cent of patients with abdominal aortic developmental lesions have coexisting renal artery stenoses and renovascular hypertension.[27] Developmental stenoses of the renal arteries are usually hypoplastic in character. As such, they have an external appearance of an hourglass constriction. Most developmental lesions occur at the origin of the vessel (Fig. 14–22).

The histologic character of the majority of these lesions, especially when they are recognized in pediatric patients, usually reveals abnormalities in more than one of the three layers of the vessel.[13, 99, 102] Sparse medial tissue and intimal fibroplasia are the most common histologic characteristics of these stenoses (Fig. 14–23*A*). Fragmentation and duplication of the internal elastic lamina is a frequent finding, and excesses in adventitial elastic tissue may be present (Fig. 14–23*B*). Similarly, irregular deficiencies in medial tissue may be observed in these diminutive vessels (Fig. 14–23*C*). In some cases, especially those associated with neurofibromatosis, abnormal proliferative changes within the media are apparent.[28, 65, 88] Occasionally, rather amorphous post-stenotic aneurysms affect the main renal artery in patients exhibiting central aortic coarctations and renal artery occlusive disease.

Developmental renal artery narrowings appear to be related to certain in utero events. Under normal circumstances, the paired dorsal aortas fuse and usually all but one of their lateral branches regress, leaving a solitary renal artery during the same period of embryonic development. Events that alter transition of mesenchyme to medial smooth muscle tissue at this time, or its later condensation and growth, may cause aortic or renovascular anomalies.

Several theories exist with regard to the cause of these lesions. One proposes that the constrictive lesions follow lack of, or unequal fusion of, the two dorsal aortas,[58] with subsequent obliteration of one of these channels and constriction of the associated renal artery. The basis for such an event is unknown. It may follow an acquired insult in utero or during early life that arrests the growth of an otherwise-normal aorta. In some instances, this insult may be viral. The fact that certain viruses, including the rubella virus, are cytocidal as well as inhibitory to cell replication supports this theory.[77] Examples of aortic hypoplasia and renal artery stenosis associated with gestational rubella have been observed.[91] In such instances, inhibition of smooth muscle cell mitoses may preclude normal aortic growth and produce renal artery ostial stenoses.

Renal arteries originate within mesenchymal tissue about the two dorsal aortas. They are initially represented by a caudally located group of vessels to the mesonephros that are replaced during fetal growth with a more cephalic group of vessels to the metanephros. A solitary artery to the primitive kidney usually evolves from each of these lateral vessel groups. Development of a single dominant vessel apparently occurs because of its obligate hemodynamic advantage over adjacent channels. Flow changes due to an evolving aortic coarctation in the region in which single renal arteries might normally arise may give coexisting polar channels hemodynamic advantages that cause their persistence. In support of such a hypothesis of renal artery occlusive disease in this subgroup of patients is the fact that central abdominal aortic coarctation and hypoplasia are frequently associated with multiple stenotic renal arteries.[27, 102]

CAROTID AND VERTEBRAL ARTERY FIBRODYSPLASIA

Arterial fibrodysplasia of the extracranial and intracranial cerebral vasculature is a clinical entity of potential importance, although controversy exists beyond the simple assertion that certain lesions cause cerebral ischemic symptoms. The precise incidence of this disease is poorly defined, although lesions of the extracranial internal carotid artery (ECICA) were noted in 0.42 per cent of 3600 patients undergoing cerebral arteriographic examinations at the authors' institution.[100] Many of these examinations were for suspected cerebrovascular disease, and thus the true frequency of ECICA fibrodysplasia in the general population would be expected to be lower. Vertebral artery disease is even less common, having been noted in approximately 20 per cent of patients manifesting ECICA fibrodysplasia.[92, 100]

Various pathologic processes have been categorized as ECICA fibrodysplasia.[70] This fact makes interpretation of the existing literature difficult. The two major subgroups of cerebrovascular lesions include intimal fibroplasia and medial fibrodysplasia. The former is often associated with elongation, kinking, and coiling of the carotid artery and appears for the most part to be a secondary rather than a primary dysplastic process. This seems particularly to be

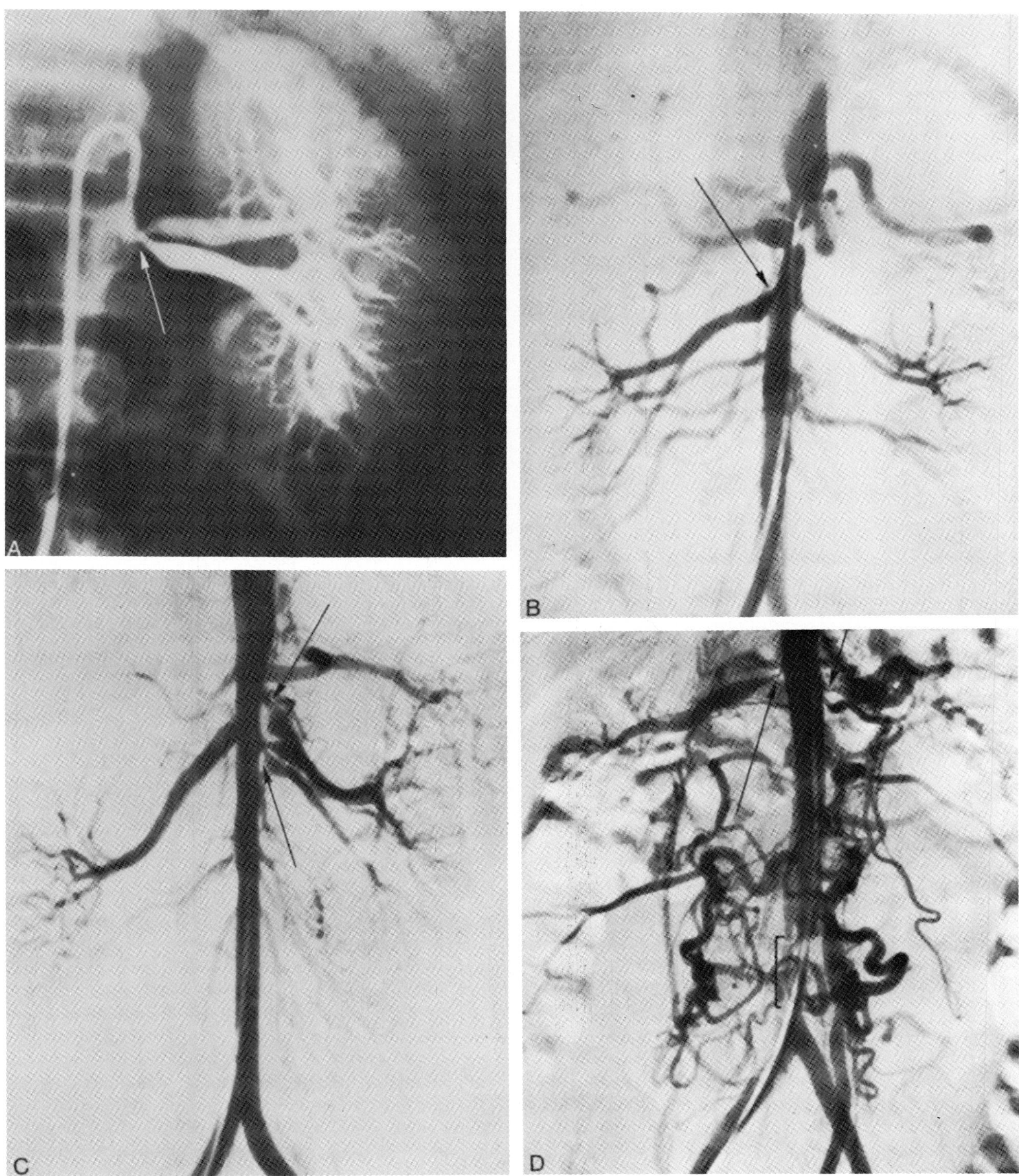

FIGURE 14–22. Developmental renal artery stenoses. *A*, Proximal stenosis (*arrow*) in a patient with neurofibromatosis. *B*, Proximal stenosis (*arrow*) in a patient with multiple renal arteries and mid-abdominal coarctation. *C*, Multi-vessel stenoses (*arrows*) in a patient with aortic hypoplasia. *D*, Bilateral proximal stenoses (*arrows*) in a patient with focal infrarenal aortic coarctation (*bracket*). (*A*, From Stanley JC, Fry WJ: Pediatric renal artery occlusive disease and renovascular hypertension. Etiology, diagnosis and operative treatment. Arch Surg 116:669–676, 1984. Copyright 1984, American Medical Association. *B* and *C*, From Graham LM, Zelenock GB, Erlandson EE, et al: Abdominal aortic coarctation and segmental hypoplasia. Surgery 86:519, 1979.)

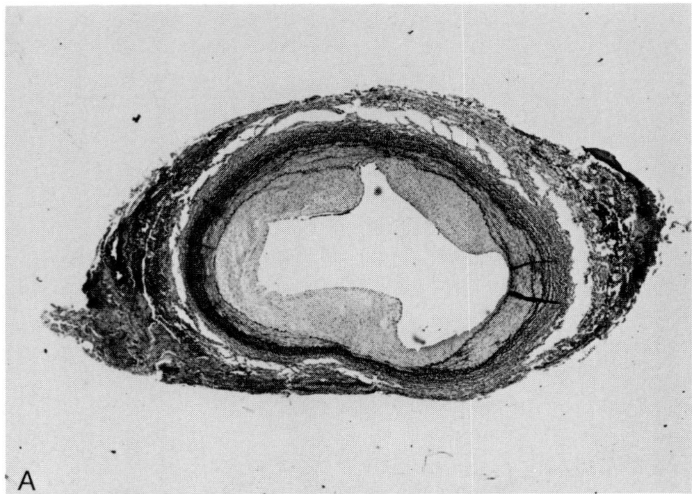

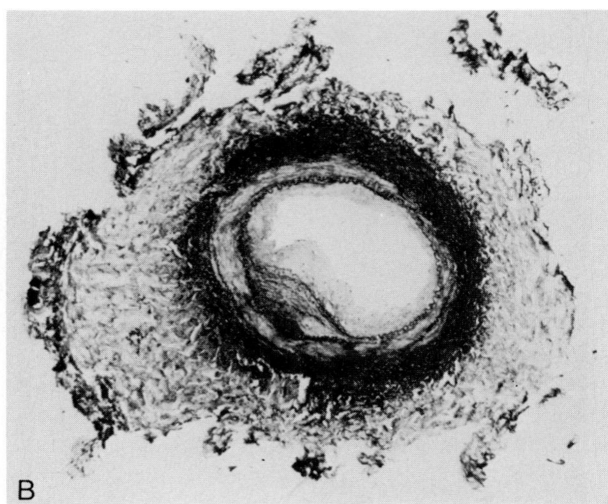

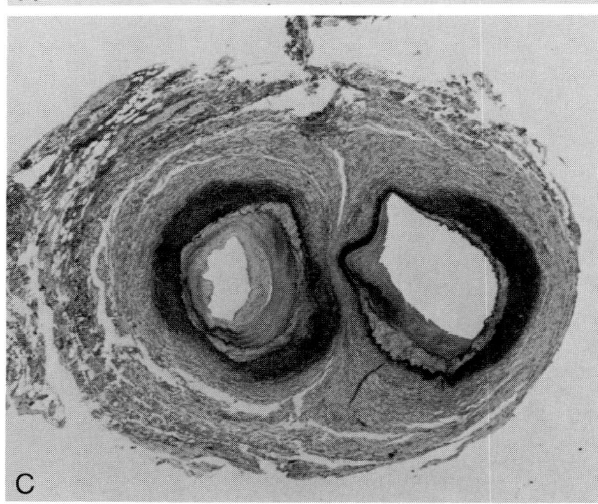

FIGURE 14–23. Hypoplastic developmental renal artery stenoses. *A*, Secondary intimal fibroplasia, fragmentation of the internal elastic lamina, and diminutions in medial tissue are typical features of this stenotic lesion. The greatest luminal dimension is 2 mm. (×80.) *B*, Marked fragmentation and duplication of the internal elastic lamina and attenuation of medial tissues characterize this vessel. Intimal fibroplasia encroaches on the vessel lumen, which is less than 1 mm in diameter. Adventitial elastic tissues appear excessive. (×100.) *C*, Diminutive paired renal arteries at their aortic origin exhibiting deficient media. (×100.) (*A–C*, Movat.) (*A* and *B*, From Stanley JC, Graham LM, Whitehouse WM Jr, et al: Developmental occlusive disease of the abdominal aorta, splanchnic and renal arteries. Am J Surg 142:190, 1981.)

FIGURE 14–24. Medial fibrodysplasia of the extracranial internal carotid artery adjacent to the second and third cervical vertebrae, with characteristic serial stenoses alternating with mural aneurysms. (From Stanley JC, Fry WJ, Seeger JF, et al: Extracranial internal carotid and vertebral artery fibrodysplasia. Arch Surg 109:215–222, 1974. Copyright 1974, American Medical Association.)

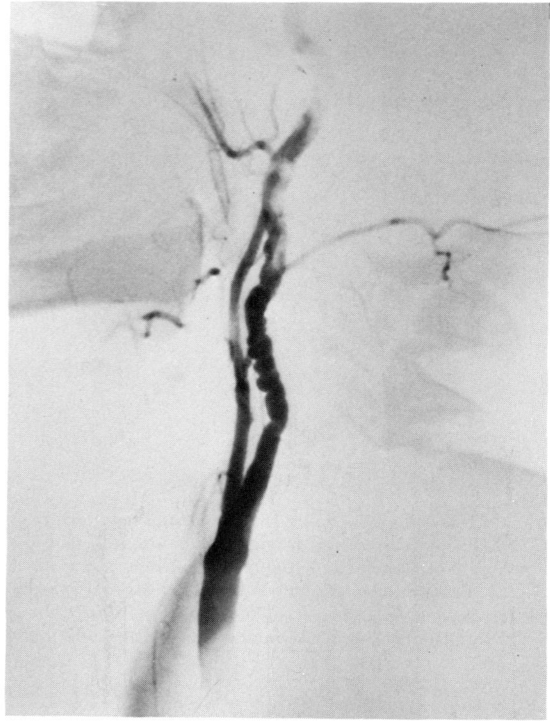

true of intracranial intimal fibroplasia.[34] Occasional atypical lesions appear as isolated webs of the ECICA.[113] Medial fibrodysplasia of the ECICA was first documented arteriographically and histologically more than 3 decades ago.[8, 72] These lesions invariably occur in female patients; mean patient age at the time of recognition is approximately 55 years.[7, 92, 100] Classic lesions of this type in childhood have been rare,[51] and when present, they are often noted to affect intracranial vessels.[46, 90] If previous definitions of medial fibrodysplasia are rigidly applied, this particular subgroup has rarely been described in men.[1] Similarly, these lesions, like those of the renal artery, have been infrequently recognized among black patients.[49, 66]

Medial fibrodysplasia of the ECICA typically involves a 2- to 6-cm segment of the mid–carotid artery adjacent to the second and third cervical vertebrae (Fig. 14–24). The serial stenoses are often evident on examination of the external surface of the artery (Fig. 14–25). Bilateral disease has been reported to occur in 35 to 85 per cent of patients with these lesions, with an average incidence of approximately 65 per cent.[7, 9, 92, 100, 105] Involvement of the ECICA at its origin with the classic form of this dysplastic lesion has not been described. Carotid arteries affected by medial fibrodysplasia are often elongated, and kinking occurs in approximately 5 per cent of cases (Fig. 14–26). Typical medial fibrodysplastic lesions of the anterior intracranial arteries are quite uncommon.[23, 46, 79] Similar lesions of the external carotid artery or its branches have been reported, but they are exceedingly rare.[33]

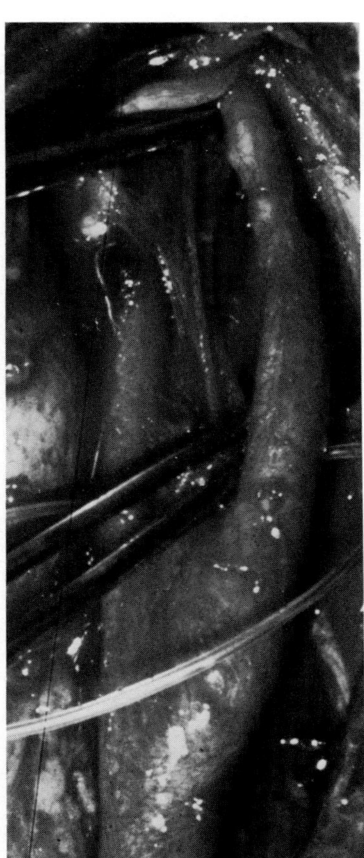

FIGURE 14–25. Medial fibrodysplasia of the extracranial internal carotid artery. Operative exposure of the artery reveals an external beaded appearance due to serial narrowings.

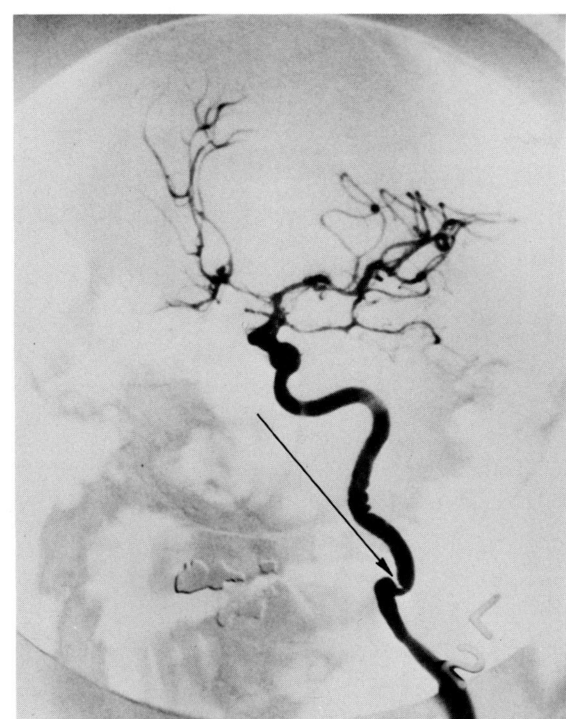

FIGURE 14–26. Medial fibrodysplasia of the extracranial internal carotid artery with angulation (*arrow*) affecting a tortuous elongated segment. (From Stanley JC, Fry WJ, Seeger JF, et al: Extracranial internal carotid and vertebral artery fibrodysplasia. Arch Surg 109:215–222, 1974. Copyright 1974, American Medical Association.)

Vertebral artery disease in the form of either multiple stenoses (Fig. 14–27) or nonocclusive mural aneurysms (Fig. 14–28) has often been overlooked. These lesions develop in the lower vertebral artery at the level of the fifth cervical vertebra, or higher, at the level of the second cervical vertebra. They exhibit marked irregularities and are often accompanied by eccentric mural aneurysms, but they do not manifest the typical string-of-beads appearance noted in other muscular vessels affected with medial fibrodysplasia. Dysplastic lesions of the basilar artery are an uncommon form of intracranial medial fibrodysplasia.[86]

Noncerebrovascular medial fibrodysplasia occurs in many patients with ECICA lesions. Renal artery involvement affects as many as 25 per cent of these individuals.[17, 100] The frequency of simultaneous ECICA and renal artery dysplasia may be even higher, and it has been reported to be 50 per cent in patients who underwent arteriographic assessments of both vessels.[19] Similar lesions have also been observed in the external iliac and superior mesenteric arteries.[17]

Coexistent intracranial aneurysms have been documented in 12 to 25 per cent of patients with ECICA medial fibrodysplasia.[9, 23, 66, 100, 112] Although intracranial arteries are occasionally the site of dysplastic disease, aneurysms do not necessarily develop in the involved vessel.[41] Instead, they may appear to evolve as a generalized dysplastic arte-

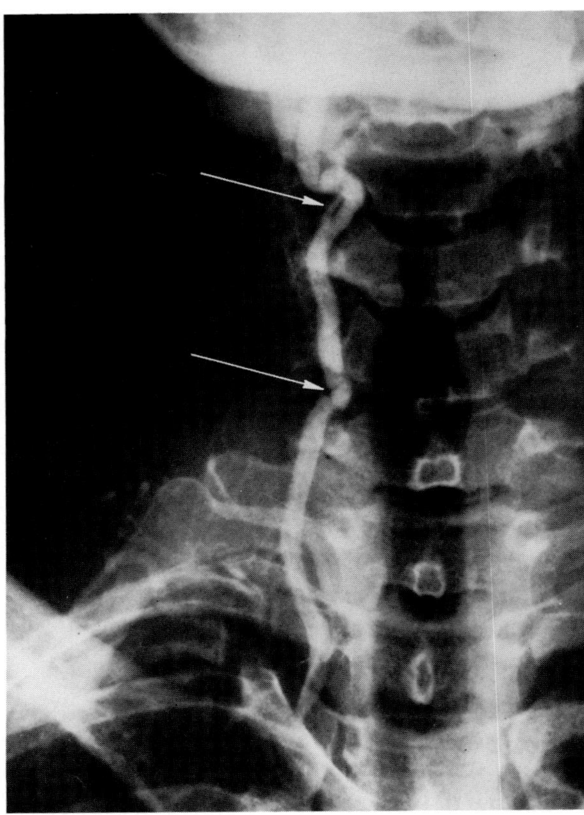

FIGURE 14–27. Medial fibrodysplasia of the vertebral artery with irregular stenoses (*arrows*).

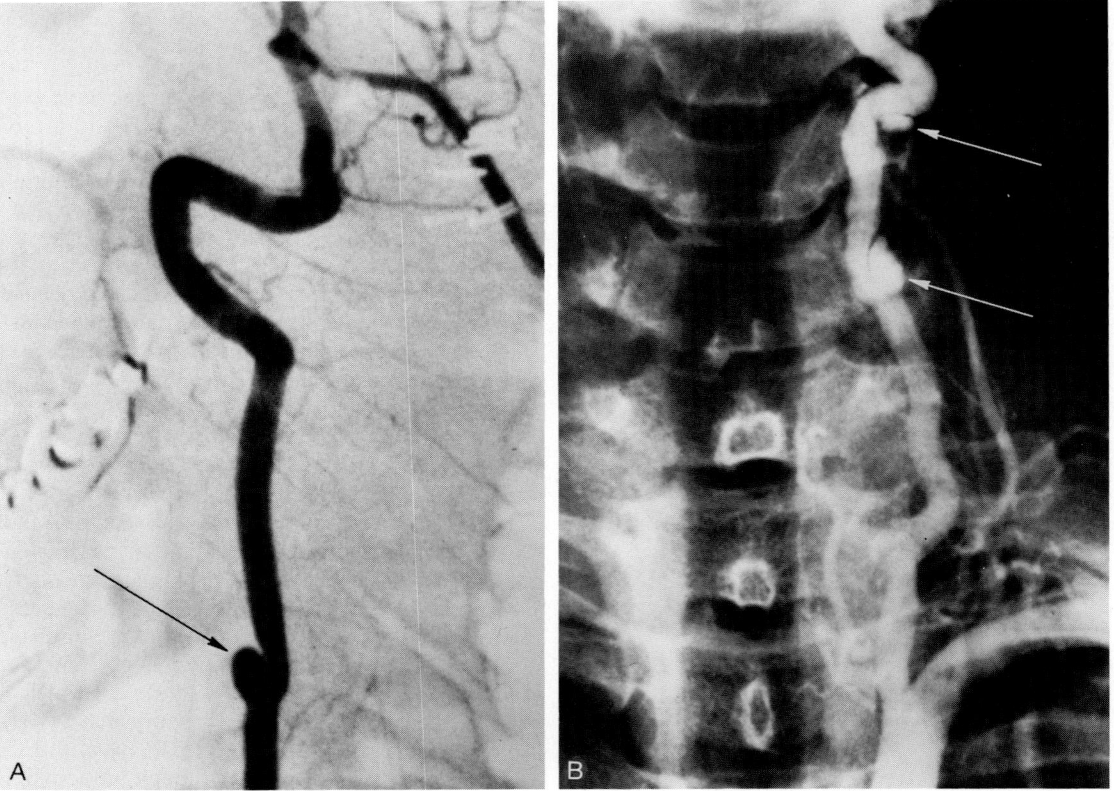

FIGURE 14–28. Medial fibrodysplasia of the vertebral artery. *A*, Isolated saccular intramural aneurysm (*arrow*). *B*, Multiple lesions (*arrows*) suggesting dissection and aneurysm formation. (*A* and *B*, From Stanley JC, Fry WJ, Seeger JF, et al: Extracranial internal carotid and vertebral artery fibrodysplasia. Arch Surg 109:215–222, 1974. Copyright 1974, American Medical Association.)

riopathy manifest by weakening in arterial branches, which increases the likelihood of berry aneurysm formation.[57, 71, 96, 103] A propensity of these aneurysms to occur on the same side as the ECICA disease has been reported.[67] The distribution of aneurysms in patients with medial fibrodysplasia is the same as that in patients not affected with dysplastic ECICA.[100] Hypertension may contribute to the evolution of these aneurysms but has not been identified as a dominant factor in their pathogenesis.

Complications occurring with medial fibrodysplasia of the ECICA appear to be related to encroachment on the lumen that causes flow reductions, occasional collection of thrombi[49, 76] within the cul-de-sacs, and potential distal embolization, as well as dissections and rupture with arteriovenous fistula formation.[6, 78] The precise incidence of these complications has not been determined, but they appear to occur in fewer than 10 per cent of cases. Frequently, the dissections obliterate clear evidence of the underlying fibrodysplastic process, and many individuals experiencing this complication are thought to have suffered only from spontaneous dissections.[2] Progression of ECICA medial fibrodysplasia may approach 30 per cent, but the exact rate has yet to be defined.[84, 92, 100, 104, 115] Complications occurring with medial fibrodysplasia of the vertebral arteries are rare and are usually related to thromboembolism or dissections.[75, 110]

The pathogenesis of ECICA medial fibrodysplasia is poorly understood, but it appears to be similar to that occurring in the renal vessels. The role of mural ischemia may be greater because very few muscular branches have origins from the extracranial portion of the internal carotid artery, thus reducing the number of intrinsic vasa vasorum in this vessel. Certainly, unusual traction or stretch stresses that occur with hyperextension rotation of the neck appear to be another dominant factor in the development of these lesions. Trauma has been cited as an etiologic factor in instances of vertebral artery fibrodysplasia.[37] In fact, unrecognized adventitial bleeding due to vertebral artery injury during birth may be important in the later development of these dysplastic lesions.[116]

ILIAC, FEMORAL, POPLITEAL, AND TIBIAL ARTERY FIBRODYSPLASIA

The third vessel most commonly affected with medial fibrodysplasia is the external iliac artery.[111] Serial stenoses with intervening mural aneurysms typically affect the proximal third of this vessel (see Fig. 14–28). These lesions are similar to those of the renal and ECICA vessels and may in fact occur in patients with these other lesions.[17, 108, 111] Fibroproliferative processes primarily involve the medial tissue adjacent to areas of relative thinning (Fig. 14–29). Occasional fibrodysplastic lesions of the iliac vessels appear as solitary dilatations. Complications of external iliac artery fibrodysplasia usually reflect encroachment on the lumen, with restriction of blood flow or the development of microthrombi that embolize peripherally.[64] Acute dissection may occur with these lesions, but it is rare.[5] Most individuals with medial fibrodysplasia of the iliac vessels have been female patients in their 5th or 6th decade of life (i.e., approximately 10 years older than those presenting with similar renovascular disease).[35, 36] This same lesion has been observed in an adolescent black male patient, albeit in association with a peculiar shortening of the affected lower extremity.[55]

Although exceedingly rare, similar lesions reflecting the systemic nature of medial fibroplasia have been reported to affect the femoral, popliteal, and tibial vessels of the lower extremity.[39, 109] In some instances, these extremity

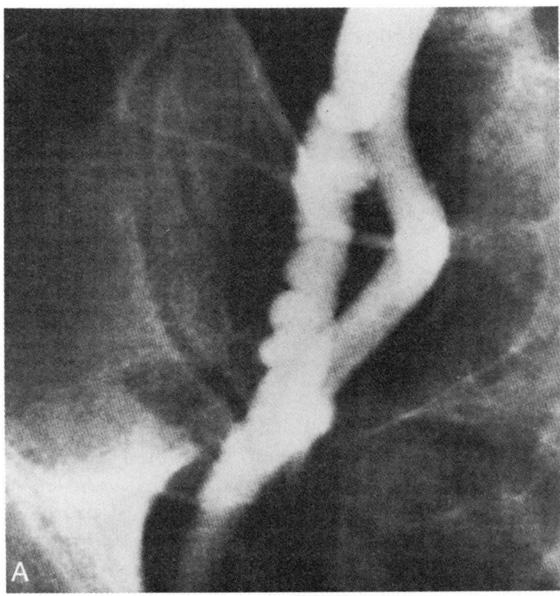

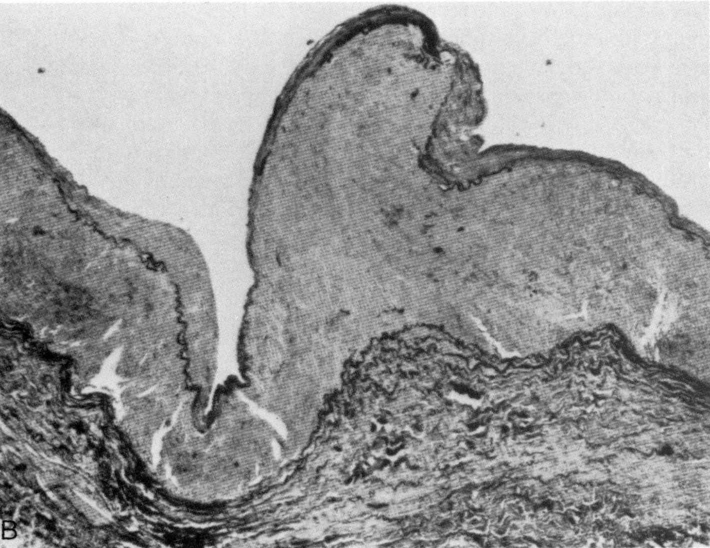

FIGURE 14–29. Medial fibrodysplasia of the external iliac artery. *A*, Multiple stenoses with intervening mural dilatations. *B*, Irregular proliferative changes within the media and minimal intimal fibroplasia. (Elastic van Gieson, ×20, longitudinal section.) (*A* and *B*, From Walter JF, Stanley JC, Mehigan JT, et al: External iliac artery fibrodysplasia. Am J Roentgenol 131:125, 1978.)

lesions have thrombosed,[109] and other have been reported to be associated with aneurysmal changes.[32, 106] The etiology of dysplastic lesions of the iliac or femoral arteries may be related more to the paucity of vasa vasorum than to any physical stretch or traction stresses. Indeed, the latter would be unlikely to affect any of these lower extremity muscular vessels. The incidence of external iliac artery fibrodysplasia is unknown, but this condition has been reported to occur in 1 to 6 per cent of patients with renal artery arterial fibrodysplasia.

Intimal fibroplasia of the external iliac artery as well as that of the femoral, popliteal, and tibial vessels is usually considered to be a secondary pathologic phenomenon rather than a primary etiologic process. Although most instances of intimal disease affecting these vessels may be the consequence of prior trauma, the result of thromboembolism with recannulation of intraluminal clot, or the sequela of a prior arteritis, certain cases appear to represent primary intimal fibroplasia.[20]

SUBCLAVIAN, AXILLARY, AND BRACHIAL ARTERY FIBRODYSPLASIA

The most common dysplastic lesion affecting upper extremity vessels appears to be intimal fibroplasia, which is usually manifest by smooth focal or long tubular stenoses. There is a slight predominance of women among patients with these dysplastic lesions. Speculation exists as to the etiology, although the most likely underlying cause is related to an arteritis, frequently affecting all mural elements. The difficulties in differentiating some of these lesions from resolved Takayasu's arteritis are considerable. Indeed, only in the presence of obvious aortic arch, brachiocephalic, or more distal abdominal aortic disease consistent with an inflammatory arteritis can the existence of this secondary form of transmural disease be easily considered. Other intimal fibroplastic lesions affecting the subclavian axillary vessels may be a consequence of injury, such as that associated with repetitive subclavian trauma at the thoracic outlet from costoclavicular entrapment, or may result from abnormal flow associated with anatomic bands causing vascular narrowing in the same region. Axillary artery involvement may also be the consequence of blunt trauma, with manifestations occurring many years after the actual vascular injury. Dysplastic disease compatible with medial fibroplasia, with characteristic dilatations and constrictions or histologic confirmation of this form of dysplasia, has been reported.[16, 39] However, information regarding this particular lesion affecting these upper extremity vessels is so rare as to be considered anecdotal.

SPLANCHNIC ARTERY FIBRODYSPLASIA

Intimal fibroplasia may affect the origins of the three principle splanchnic vessels: the celiac, superior mesenteric, and inferior mesenteric arteries. The basis for these lesions is unknown, but this fibrodysplasia may reflect a secondary phenomenon occurring in developmentally narrowed vessels. Ostial fibrodysplastic lesions are quite common in patients with intestinal angina and often exhibit associated atherosclerotic changes.[38] Intimal fibroplasia tends to occur more often in women than in men, with nearly equal involvement of the celiac and superior mesenteric arteries. The hepatic as well as the splenic and iliac vessels have all demonstrated fibrodysplastic tubular stenoses, which may represent the outcome of prior arteritis or resolved thrombosis. Occasional patients demonstrate more distal disease in the celiac or superior mesenteric circulatory beds. A dilatated appearance of the celiac artery just beyond an eccentric stenosis due to median ligament compression of this vessel is relatively common. Although earlier reports attributed this particular lesion to medial fibrodysplasia, it may simply represent chronic fibrosis of the "trapped" proximal vessel with post-stenotic dilatation.

Characteristic medial fibrodysplasia is rare within the splanchnic circulation, although histologic evidence of it has been reported.[62] When present, this form of splanchnic vascular disease is often associated with similar renal or carotid lesions.[62, 83] Histologic evidence of medial dysplasia is also common among patients developing splenic artery aneurysms.[97] In fact, the development of these aneurysms may be a reflection of compromised vascular integrity due to the disruptive dysplastic process. Similar aneurysms have been noted in other splanchnic vessels, including the superior mesenteric artery.[12] The proximal superior mesenteric artery may exhibit medial fibrodysplastic occlusive disease a few centimeters beyond its origin as it exists beneath the pancreas over the top of the duodenum. The basis for these latter lesions has not been established, although unusual stretch forces at the root of the mesentery may contribute to dysplastic changes.

Intestinal branch narrowings that have been considered dysplastic in character usually represent intimal lesions resulting from a prior inflammatory processes, be it part of the spectrum of an earlier arteritis or an adjacent inflammatory process such as pancreatitis. The occurrence of splanchnic artery fibrodysplasia is so uncommon as to prevent any firm conclusions about its natural history.

OTHER VASCULAR INVOLVEMENT WITH ARTERIAL FIBRODYSPLASIA

Most other vessels affected with dysplastic disease exhibit instances of intimal fibroplasia. Exceptions do exist: medial fibrodysplasia has been clearly documented to have affected coronary arteries, exhibiting dissections as well as thromboses.[3, 50] Other dysplastic lesions have been noted among patients ranging from neonates to the elderly, in large arteries the size of the aorta to very small vessels such as the coronary sinus node artery.[14, 33, 40] Certain of the aortic lesions may represent developmental webs or consequences of a prior intraluminal thrombotic event. Many of the latter do not appear arteriographically to be very distinct from focal arteriosclerosis.[47] It is unlikely that the changes in these vessels represent a systemic arteritis in its active stage, although they may represent an end-stage of an earlier arteritis. Again, experience with these rare forms of arterial dysplasia is so meager as to preclude rendering of any firm conclusions about their etiology or clinical relevance.

References

1. Abdul-Rahman AM, Salih A, Brun A, et al: Fibromuscular dysplasia of the cervico-cephalic arteries. Surg Neurol 9:216, 1978.
2. Andersen CA, Collins GJ Jr, Rich NM, McDonald PT: Bilateral internal carotid arterial occlusions associated with fibromuscular dysplasia. Vasc Surg 13:349, 1979.
3. Arey JB, Segal R: Fibromuscular dysplasia of intramyocardial coronary arteries. Pediatr Pathol 7:97, 1987.
4. Bader H: The anatomy and physiology of the vascular wall. *In* Hamilton WF (ed): Handbook of Physiology. Washington, DC, American Physiological Society, 1963, vol. 2, pp 865–889.
5. Burri B, Fontolliet C, Ruegsegger C-H, Mosimann R: External iliac artery dissection due to fibromuscular dysplasia. Vasa 12:76, 1983.
6. Canova A, Esposito S, Patricolo A, et al: Spontaneous obliteration of a carotid-cavernous fistula associated with fibromuscular dysplasia of the internal carotid artery. J Neurosurg Sci 31:37, 1987.
7. Collins GJ Jr, Rich NM, Clagett GP, et al: Fibromuscular dysplasia of the internal carotid arteries. Clinical experience and follow-up. Ann Surg 194:89, 1981.
8. Connett M, Lansche JM: Fibromuscular hyperplasia of the internal carotid artery—Report of a case. Ann Surg 162:59, 1965.
9. Corrin LS, Sandok BA, Houser OW: Cerebral ischemic events in patients with carotid artery fibromuscular dysplasia. Arch Neurol 38:616, 1981.
10. Cragg AH, Smith TP, Thompson BH, et al: Incidental fibromuscular dysplasia in potential renal donors: Long-term clinical follow-up. Radiology 172:145, 1989.
11. de Deeuw D, Donker AJM, Burema J, et al: Nephroptosis and hypertension. Lancet 1:213, 1977.
12. den Butter G, Bockel JH, Aarts JCNM: Arterial fibrodysplasia: Rapid progression complicated by rupture of a visceral aneurysm into the gastrointestinal tract. J Vasc Surg 7:449, 1988.
13. Devaney K, Kapur SP, Patterson K, Chandra RS: Pediatric renal artery dysplasia. A morphologic study. Pediatr Pathol 11:609, 1991.
14. Dominguez FE, Tate LG, Robinson MJ: Familial fibromuscular dysplasia presenting as sudden death. Am J Cardiovasc Pathol 2:269, 1988.
15. Dornfeld L, Kaufman JJ: Immunologic considerations in renovascular hypertension. Urol Clin North Am 2:285, 1975.
16. Drury JK, Pollock JG: Subclavian arteriopathy in the young patient. Br J Surg 68:617, 1981.
17. Effeney DJ, Ehrenfeld WK, Stoney RJ, Wylie EJ: Why operate on carotid fibromuscular dysplasia? Arch Surg 115:1261, 1980.
18. Ekelund L, Gerlock J, Molin J, Smith C: Roentgenologic appearance of fibromuscular dysplasia. Acta Radiol [Diagn] 19:433, 1978.
19. Ehrenfeld WK, Wylie EJ: Fibromuscular dysplasia of the internal carotid artery. Arch Surg 109:676, 1974.
20. Esfahani F, Rooholamini SA, Azadeh B, Daneshbod K: Arterial fibrodysplasia: A regional cause of peripheral occlusive vascular disease. Angiology 40:108, 1989.
21. Fievez ML: Fibromuscular dysplasia of arteries: A spastic phenomenon? Med Hypotheses 13:341, 1984.
22. Finley JL, Dabbs DJ: Renal vascular smooth muscle proliferation in neurofibromatosis. Hum Pathol 19:107, 1988.
23. Frens DB, Petajan JH, Anderson R, Deblanc HJ Jr: Fibromuscular dysplasia of the posterior cerebral artery: Report of a case and review of the literature. Stroke 5:161, 1974.
24. Gabbiani G, Majno G, Ryan GB: The fibroblast as a contractile cell. The myo-fibroblast. *In* Kulonen E, Pikkarainen J (eds): Biology of Fibroblast. New York, Academic Press, 1973, pp 139–154.
25. Gladstien K, Rushton AR, Kidd KK: Penetrance estimates and recurrence risks for fibromuscular dysplasia. Clin Genet 17:115, 1980.
26. Goncharenko V, Gerlock AJ, Shaff MI, Hollifield SW: Progression of renal artery fibromuscular dysplasia in 42 patients as seen on angiography. Radiology 139:45, 1981.
27. Graham LM, Zelenock GB, Erlandson EE, et al: Abdominal aortic coarctation and segmental hypoplasia. Surgery 86:519, 1979.
28. Halperin M, Currarino G: Vascular lesions causing hypertension in neurofibromatosis. N Engl J Med 273:248, 1965.
29. Harrison EG Jr, Hunt JC, Bernatz PE: Morphology of fibromuscular dysplasia of the renal artery in renovascular hypertension. Am J Med 43:97, 1967.
30. Harrison EG, McCormack LJ: Pathologic classification of renal artery disease in renovascular hypertension. Mayo Clin Proc 46:161, 1971.
31. Hata J-I, Hosoda Y: Perimedial fibroplasia of the renal artery. A light and electron microscopy study. Arch Pathol Lab Med 103:220, 1979.
32. Herpels V, Van de Voorde W, Wilms G, et al: Recurrent aneurysms of the upper arteries of the lower limb: An atypical manifestation of fibromuscular dysplasia—A case report. Angiology 38:411, 1987.
33. Hill LD, Antonius JI: Arterial dysplasia. Arch Surg 90:585, 1965.
34. Hirsch CS, Roessmann U: Arterial dysplasia with ruptured basilar artery aneurysm: Report of a case. Hum Pathol 6:749, 1975.
35. Horne TW: Fibromuscular hyperplasia of the iliac arteries. Aust NZ J Surg 45:415, 1975.
36. Houston C, Rosenthal D, Lamis PA, Stanton PE Jr: Fibromuscular dysplasia of the external iliac arteries: Surgical treatment by graduated internal dilatation technique. Surgery 85:713, 1979.
37. Hugenholtz H, Pokrupa R, Montpetit VJA, et al: Spontaneous dissecting aneurysm of the extracranial vertebral artery. Neurosurgery 10:96, 1982.
38. Insall RL, Chamberlain J, Loose HWC: Fibromuscular dysplasia of visceral arteries. Eur J Vasc Surg 6:668, 1992.
39. Iwai T, Konno S, Hiejima K, et al: Fibromuscular dysplasia in the extremities. J Cardiovasc Surg 26:296, 1985.
40. James TN: Morphologic characteristics and functional significance of focal fibromuscular dysplasia of small coronary arteries. Am J Cardiol 65:12G, 1990.
41. Kalyanaraman UP, Elwood PW: Fibromuscular dysplasia of intracranial arteries causing multiple intracranial aneurysms. Hum Pathol 11:481, 1980.
42. Kaufman JJ, Maxwell MH: Upright aortography in the study of nephroptosis, stenotic lesions of the renal artery, and hypertension. Surgery 53:736, 1963.
43. Kelly TF Jr, Morris GC: Arterial fibromuscular dysplasia. Observations on pathogenesis and surgical management. Am J Surg 143:232, 1982.
44. Lang J: Mikroskopische Anatomie der Arterien. Angiologica 2:225, 1965.
45. Leadbetter WF, Burkland CE: Hypertension in unilateral renal disease. J Urol 39:611, 1938.
46. Lemahieu SF, Marchau MMB: Intracranial fibromuscular dysplasia and stroke in children. Neuroradiology 18:99, 1979.
47. Letsch R, Kantartzis M, Sommer Th, Garcia M: Arterial fibromuscular dysplasia. Report of a case with involvement of the aorta and review of the literature. Thorac Cardiovasc Surg 28:206, 1980.
48. Leung DYM, Glagov S, Matthews MB: Cyclic stretching stimulates synthesis of matrix components by arterial smooth muscle cells in vitro. Science 191:475, 1976.
49. Levien LJ, Fritz VU, Lurie D, et al: Fibromuscular dysplasia of the extracranial carotid arteries. S Afr Med J 65:261, 1984.
50. Lie JT, Berg KK: Isolated fibromuscular dysplasia of the coronary arteries with spontaneous dissection and myocardial infarction. Hum Pathol 18:654, 1987.
51. Llorens-Terol J, Sole-Llelnas J, Tura A: Stroke due to fibromuscular hyperplasia of the internal carotid artery. Acta Paediatr Scand 72:299, 1983.
52. Luscher TF, Keller HM, Imhof HG, et al: Fibromuscular hyperplasia: Extension of the disease and therapeutic outcome. Results of the University Hospital Zurich cooperative study on fibromuscular hyperplasia. Nephron 44:109, 1986.
53. Luscher TF, Lie JT, Stanson AW, et al: Arterial fibromuscular dysplasia. Mayo Clin Proc 62:931, 1987.
54. Madden JW, Carlson EC, Hines J: Presence of modified fibroblasts in ischemic contracture of the intrinsic musculature of the hand. Surg Gynecol Obstet 140:509, 1975.
55. Madiba TE, Robbs JV: Fibromuscular dysplasia of the external iliac artery in association with congential short leg and mesodermal malformation. A case report. S Afr J Surg 27:139, 1989.
56. Major P, Genest J, Cariter P, Kuchel O: Heredity fibromuscular dysplasia with renovascular hypertension. Ann Intern Med 86:583, 1977.

57. Masuzawa T, Nakahara N, Kobayashi S: Intracranial multiple berry aneurysms associated with fibromuscular dysplasia and mixed connective tissue disease. Neurol Med Chir (Tokyo) 27:42, 1987.
58. Maycock Wd'A: Congenital stenosis of the abdominal aorta. Am Heart J 13:633, 1937.
59. McCormack LJ, Noto TJ Jr, Meaney TF, et al: Subadventitial fibroplasia of the renal artery: A disease of young women. Am Heart J 73:602, 1967.
60. McCormack LJ, Poutasse EF, Meaney TF, et al: A pathologic arteriographic correlation of renal arterial disease. Am Heart J 73:602, 1967.
61. McGrath TW: Fibromuscular dysplasia vs catheter-induced renal artery spasm [Letter]. Am J Roentgenol 148:651, 1987.
62. Meacham PW, Brantley B: Familial fibromuscular dysplasia of the mesenteric arteries. South Med J 80:1311, 1987.
63. Meaney TF, Dustan HF, McCormack LJ: Natural history of renal arterial disease. Radiology 91:881, 1968.
64. Mehigan JT, Stoney RJ: Arterial microemboli and fibromuscular dysplasia of the external iliac arteries. Surgery 81:484, 1977.
65. Mena E, Bookstein JJ, Holt JF, Fry WJ: Neurofibromatosis and renovascular hypertension in children. Am J Roentgenol 118:39, 1973.
66. Mettinger KL: Fibromuscular dysplasia and the brain. II. Current concept of the disease. Stroke 13:53, 1982.
67. Mettinger KL, Ericson K: Fibromuscular dysplasia and the brain. Observations on angiographic, clinical and genetic characteristics. Stroke 13:46, 1982.
68. Morimoto S, Kuroda M, Uchida K, et al: Occurrence of renovascular hypertension in two sisters. Nephron 17:314, 1976.
69. Nemcek AA, Holmburg CE: Reversible renal fibromuscular dysplasia. Am J Roentgenol 147:737, 1986.
70. Osborn AG, Anderson RE: Angiographic spectrum of cervical and intracranial fibromuscular dysplasia. Stroke 8:617, 1977.
71. Ouchi Y, Tagawa H, Yamakado M, et al: Clinical significance of cerebral aneurysm in renovascular hypertension due to fibromuscular dysplasia: Two cases in siblings. Angiology 40:581, 1989.
72. Palubinskas AJ, Ripley HR: Fibromuscular hyperplasia in extra-renal arteries. Radiology 82:451, 1964.
73. Park SH, Chi JG, Choi Y: Primary intimal fibroplasia with multiple aneurysms of renal artery in childhood. Child Nephrol Urol 10:51, 1990.
74. Paulson GW: Fibromuscular dysplasia, antiovulent drugs, and ergot preparations. Stroke 9:172, 1978.
75. Perez-Higueras A, Alvarez-Ruiz F, Martinez-Bermejo A, et al: Cerebrellar infarction from fibromuscular dysplasia and dissecting aneurysm of the vertebral artery. Stroke 19:521, 1988.
76. Perry MO: Fibromuscular dysplasia of the carotid artery. Surg Gynecol Obstet 134:57, 1972.
77. Plotkin SA, Boue A, Boue JG: The in vitro growth of rubella virus in human embryo cells. Am J Epidemiol 81:71, 1965.
78. Ramana Reddy SV, Karnes WE, Earnest F IV, Sundt TM Jr: Spontaneous extracranial vertebral arteriovenous fistula with fibromuscular dysplasia. J Neurosurg 54:399, 1981.
79. Rinaldi I, Harris WO Jr, Kopp JE, Legier J: Intracranial fibromuscular dysplasia: Report of two cases, one with autopsy verification. Stroke 7:511, 1976.
80. Rosenberger A, Adler O, Lichtig H: Angiographic appearance of the renal vein in a case of fibromuscular dysplasia of the artery. Radiology 118:579, 1976.
81. Ross R, Klebanoff SJ: Fine structural changes in uterine smooth muscle and fibroblasts in response to estrogen. J Cell Biol 32:155, 1967.
82. Rushton AR: The genetics of fibromuscular dysplasia. Arch Intern Med 140:233, 1980.
83. Salmon PJM, Allan JS: An unusual case of fibromuscular dysplasia. J Cardiovasc Surg 29:756, 1988.
84. Sandok BA: Fibromuscular dysplasia of the internal carotid artery. Neurol Clin 1:17, 1983.
85. Sang CN, Whelton PK, Hamper UM, et al: Etiologic factors in renovascular fibromuscular dysplasia. Hypertension 14:472, 1989.
86. Saygi S, Bolay H, Tekkok IH, et al: Fibromuscular dysplasia of the basilar artery: A case with brain stem stroke. Angiology 41:658, 1990.
87. Schreiber MJ, Pohl MA, Novick AC: The natural history of atherosclerotic and fibrous renal artery disease. Urol Clin North Am 11:383, 1984.
88. Schurch W, Messerli FH, Genest J, et al: Arterial hypertension and neurofibromatosis: Renal artery stenosis and coarctation of abdominal aorta. Can Med Assoc J 113:878, 1975.
89. Sheps SG, Kincaid OW, Hunt JC: Serial renal function and angiographic observations in idiopathic fibrous and fibromuscular stenoses of the renal arteries. Am J Cardiol 30:55, 1972.
90. Shields WD, Ziter FA, Osborn AG, Allen J: Fibromuscular dysplasia as a cause of stroke in infancy and childhood. Pediatrics 59:899, 1977.
91. Siassi B, Glyman G, Emmanouilides GC: Hypoplasia of the abdominal aorta associated with the rubella syndrome. Am J Dis Child 120:476, 1970.
92. So EL, Toole JF, Dalal P, Moody DM: Cephalic fibromuscular dysplasia in 32 patients. Clinical findings and radiologic features. Arch Neurol 38:619, 1981.
93. Sottiurai VS, Fry WJ, Stanley JC: Ultrastructural characteristics of experimental arterial medial fibrodysplasia induced by vasa vasorum occlusion. J Surg Res 24:169, 1978.
94. Sottiurai VS, Fry WJ, Stanley JC: Ultrastructure of medial smooth muscle and myofibroblasts in human arterial dysplasia. Arch Surg 113:1280, 1978.
95. Stanley JC: Morphologic, histopathologic and clinical characteristics of renovasuclar fibrodysplasia and arteriosclerosis. *In* Bergan JJ, Yao JST (eds): Surgery of the Aorta and Its Body Branches. New York, Grune & Stratton, 1979, pp 355–376.
96. Stanley JC: Pathologic basis of macrovascular renal artery disease. *In* Stanley JC, Ernst CB, Fry WJ (eds): Renovascular Hypertension. Philadelphia, WB Saunders, 1984, pp 46–74.
97. Stanley JC, Fry WJ: Pathogenesis and clinical significance of splenic artery aneurysms. Surgery 76:898, 1974.
98. Stanley JC, Fry WJ: Renovascular hypertension secondary to arterial fibrodysplasia in adults: Criteria for operation and results of surgical therapy. Arch Surg 110:922, 1975.
99. Stanley JC, Fry WJ: Pediatric renal artery occlusive disease and renovascular hypertension. Etiology, diagnosis and operative treatment. Arch Surg 116:669, 1981.
100. Stanley JC, Fry WJ, Seeger JF, et al: Extracranial internal carotid and vertebral artery fibrodysplasia. Arch Surg 109:215, 1974.
101. Stanley JC, Gewertz BC, Bove EL, et al: Arterial fibrodysplasia. Histopathologic character and current etiologic concepts. Arch Surg 110:561, 1975.
102. Stanley JC, Graham LM, Whitehouse WM Jr, et al: Developmental occlusive disease of the abdominal aorta, splanchnic and renal arteries. Am J Surg 142:190, 1981.
103. Stanley JC, Rhodes EL, Gewertz BL, et al: Renal artery aneurysms: Significance of macroaneurysms exclusive of dissections and fibrodysplastic mural dilatations. Arch Surg 110:1327, 1975.
104. Stewart DR, Price RA, Nebesar R, Schuster SR: Progressing peripheral fibromuscular hyperplasia in an infant. A possible manifestation of the rubella syndrome. Surgery 73:374, 1973.
105. Stewart MT, Moritz MW, Smith RB III, et al: The natural history of carotid fibromuscular dysplasia. J Vasc Surg 3:305, 1986.
106. Stinnett DM, Graham JM, Edwards WD: Fibromuscular dysplasia and thrombosed aneurysm of the popliteal artery in a child. J Vasc Surg 5:769, 1987.
107. Tsukamoto Y, Komuro Y, Akutsu F, et al: Orthostatic hypertension due to coexistence of renal fibromuscular dysplasia and nephroptosis. Jpn Circ J 52:1408, 1988.
108. Twigg HL, Palmisano PJ: Fibromuscular hyperplasia of the iliac artery. A case report. Am J Roentgenol 95:418, 1965.
109. van den Dungen JJAM, Boontje AH, Oosterhuis JW: Femoropopliteal arterial fibrodysplasia. Br J Surg 77:396, 1990.
110. Vles JSH, Hendriks JJE, Lodder J, Janevski B: Multiple vertebrobasilar infarctions from fibromuscular dysplasia–related dissecting aneurysm of the vertebral artery in a child. Neuropediatrics 21:104, 1990.
111. Walter JF, Stanley JC, Mehigan JJ, et al: Iliac artery fibrodysplasia. Am J Roentgenol 131:125, 1978.
112. Wesen CA, Elliott BM: Fibromuscular dysplasia of the carotid arteries. Am J Surg 151:448, 1986.
113. Wirth FP, Miller WA, Russell AP: Atypical fibromuscular hyperplasia. Report of two cases. J Neurosurg 54:685, 1981.

114. Wright I: Age changes in the peripheral arteries in man. Cardiovasc Anat Pathol 11:157, 1964.
115. Yamamoto I, Kageyama N, Usui K, Yoshida J: Fibromuscular dysplasia of the internal carotid artery. Unusual arteriographic changes with progression of clinical symptoms. Acta Neurochir (Wien) 50:293, 1979.
116. Yates PO: Birth trauma to the vertebral arteries. Arch Dis Child 109:215, 1974.

15

Pathologic Intimal Hyperplasia as a Response to Vascular Injury and Reconstruction

Alexander W. Clowes, M.D.

• • •

In the last 40 years, reconstruction has become the rule rather than the exception for the treatment of occlusive disease of major arteries. Techniques previously limited to the aorta and large branch vessels have been improved and extended to small vessels of the brain, heart, viscera, and extremities. Currently, these reconstructions cannot be expected to last indefinitely because they frequently develop stenosis and, ultimately, spontaneous thrombosis. Exactly why arterial reconstructions fail is not known, although one possibility is that narrowing of the lumen of a graft or endarterectomized artery is in essence a form of recurrent or continuing atherosclerosis superimposed on normal wound healing.[1, 2] We do know from studies of wound healing in animals and humans that luminal narrowing is due largely to smooth muscle proliferation and connective tissue deposition in the intima.

This chapter first defines a number of clinical conditions in which smooth muscle proliferation and intimal thickening play a significant part in the failure of vascular reconstructions. The mechanisms controlling smooth muscle growth are then considered in more detail. Finally, the operative and nonoperative approaches available for prevention and treatment of intimal thickening and luminal narrowing are evaluated.

EXAMPLES OF PATHOLOGIC INTIMAL HYPERPLASIA

A number of surgical procedures are in themselves disruptive of the normal vascular architecture. Simply passing an inflated *balloon embolectomy* catheter along a vessel denudes the surface of its endothelium, stretches the wall, and destroys some of the smooth muscle cells (SMC) in the media.[3, 4] In animal models of this procedure (described in more detail later), platelets accumulate in a thin layer on the denuded surface; they in turn are displaced by regenerating endothelium and proliferating intimal SMC. Ultimately, the intima thickens as a consequence of the accumulation of SMC and extracellular matrix. In small vessels in humans, this embolectomy catheter–induced intimal thickening can cause diffuse narrowing of the lumen;[5] in larger vessels, this process seems not to be of clinical importance.

Percutaneous transluminal angioplasty is used to dilate stenotic segments of atherosclerotic arteries and in so doing produces a rent in the plaque; the remaining media stretches but is not disrupted and maintains the structural integrity of the conduit.[6, 7] Thrombus forms in the disrupted portion of the plaque and over a period of weeks is remodeled into a fibrous lesion. As might be expected, this procedure yields the best results when the stenoses are discrete and are located in large vessels with high blood flow.[8–10] Although significant restenosis is only a modest problem in large vessels (e.g., iliac arteries), it is an important cause of ischemia and reduction in blood flow in small vessels such as the coronary and femoropopliteal arteries. Approximately 30 per cent of dilated coronary arteries develop marked restenosis by 6 months.[11, 12] This figure is derived from studies of patients who complain of new or recurrent symptoms and have ischemic changes on the electrocardiogram during treadmill testing performed prior to coronary angiography. Hence, the actual incidence of restenosis is likely to be even greater than 30 per cent. The lesions causing restenosis are largely fibrous and contain mostly SMC. In superficial arteries, restenosis is often adjacent to but not at the site of the dilation.[13, 14]

Endarterectomy is an equally traumatic form of vascular reconstruction and is also associated with the development of a hyperplastic intimal lesion that in some instances is sufficient to narrow the reconstructed lumen and reduce blood flow. The development of recurrent stenosis has been described in some detail in patients undergoing carotid endarterectomy.[15–20] Although the incidence of symptomatic recurrent stenosis appears to be low (about 1 per cent), the actual incidence of 50 per cent stenosis or more, as documented by duplex scanning or angiography, is between 10 and 20 per cent. These lesions have at least two kinds of morphology (Fig. 15–1); if examined within the first 2 years after surgery, they are smooth, white, firm, and fibrous and contain mostly SMC and extracellular matrix. Later, the lesions often have a friable and rubbery layer of thrombus at the luminal surface, with some underlying regions showing accumulations of lipid, calcium, and hemorrhage as well as foci of smooth muscle.

These results suggest that repair in severely traumatized vessels is effected by proliferation of SMC, derived perhaps from remnants of media or adjacent undamaged vessel. The new intimal lesion is further enlarged by synthesis and deposition of extracellular matrix by smooth muscle, including elastin, collagen, and proteoglycans. To what extent endothelium reestablishes a luminal surface is not known. Some of the details of this healing process have been defined in animal models and are reviewed later in this chapter.

All the examples of intimal hyperplasia complicating the restorative and reconstructive procedures described previously appear to be associated with extensive endothelial denudation and destruction of at least a part of the artery wall. In healing *vascular grafts*, the relationship between injury and intimal hyperplasia is not so obvious. It is certain that vigorous distention of a vein graft already in spasm or passage of a valvulotome can damage the endothelium and the graft wall, but because these defects are relatively small, endothelium should regenerate within a few days.[21–23] Nevertheless, such grafts may develop intimal thickening over a period of months. Significant stenosis in peripheral reconstructions develops in approximately 10 per cent of vein grafts and is usually apparent within 6 to 24 months.[24, 25] These lesions can be diffuse or limited and have been associated with scarring at the sites of vein valves or trauma. They have also been described in the less traumatized in situ vein grafts.[26] The lesions in these grafts are fibrous and smooth and resemble morphologically the early lesions of carotid restenosis.

At later times, some vein grafts develop frank atherosclerosis. These lesions are particularly prevalent in coronary artery bypass grafts (Fig. 15–2).[27, 28] A study of patients over a 10-year period following surgery at the Montreal Heart Institute demonstrated by serial angiography that 50 per cent of the grafts eventually developed thrombosis, and half of the remaining grafts had the angiographic appearance of advanced atherosclerosis.[29] There was a significant correlation between plasma low-density lipoprotein (LDL) apoprotein B levels, and graft atherosclerosis.[30] Why these grafts steadily deteriorate over time is not known. It is possible that the scarring process associated with the adaptation of vein grafts to the arterial circulation makes the grafts more susceptible to exogenous atherogenic stimuli. This hypothesis is supported by the observation that

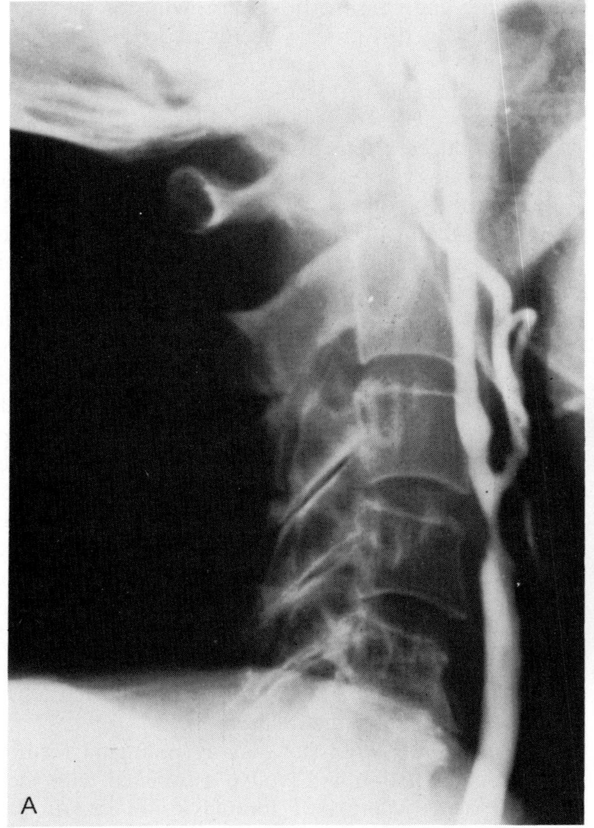

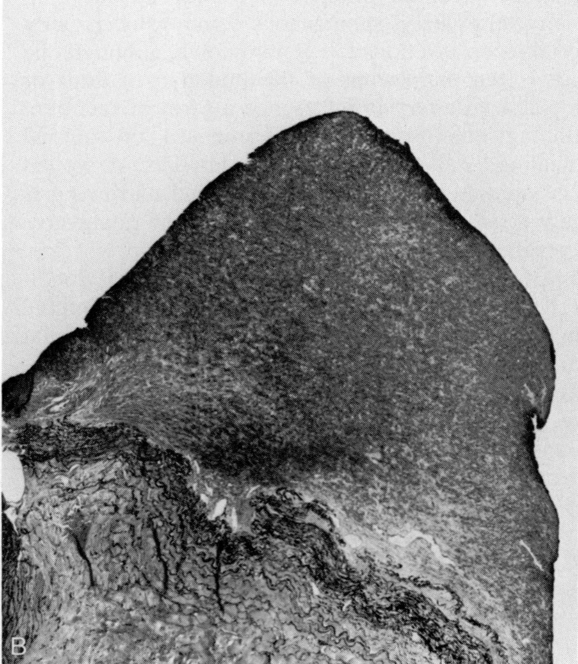

FIGURE 15–1. *A*, Arteriogram showing stenosis in the common carotid artery 6 months after endarterectomy. *B*, Histologic cross section of a recurrent carotid stenosis demonstrating massive accumulation of connective tissue. (*A*, Courtesy of R. Eugene Zierler, M.D. *B*, Courtesy of David Gordon, M.D.)

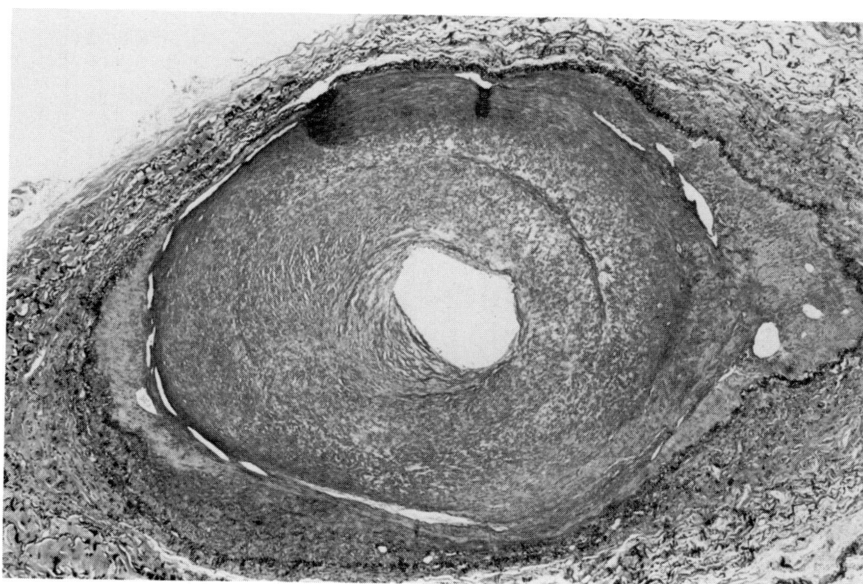

FIGURE 15–2. Histologic cross section demonstrating massive arteriosclerotic plaque in a saphenous vein coronary artery bypass graft. The patient had had bypass grafting 6 years earlier. (×45.) (Courtesy of David Gordon, M.D.)

coronary grafts made of internal mammary arteries, which do not need to adapt to the arterial circulation, also do not develop atherosclerotic plaques and do not exhibit the same high failure rates as vein grafts.[29]

In synthetic grafts, significant intimal thickening develops at the anastomoses or, just beyond, in the distal vessels (Fig. 15–3).[31–34] These lesions are similar to those found early on in vein grafts and usually appear within the first 2 years after surgery. In humans, coverage of the inner surface of synthetic grafts by endothelium and subendothelial connective tissue is limited to the first few centimeters at either end.[35, 36] It appears, then, that the adjacent artery serves as the only source of covering cells and that those cells have only a limited capacity to migrate along the graft. In contrast, lesions in vein grafts appear to be the result of proliferation of cells already residing in the graft.

We do not know to what extent injury plays a role in the healing of vascular grafts and the development of ex-

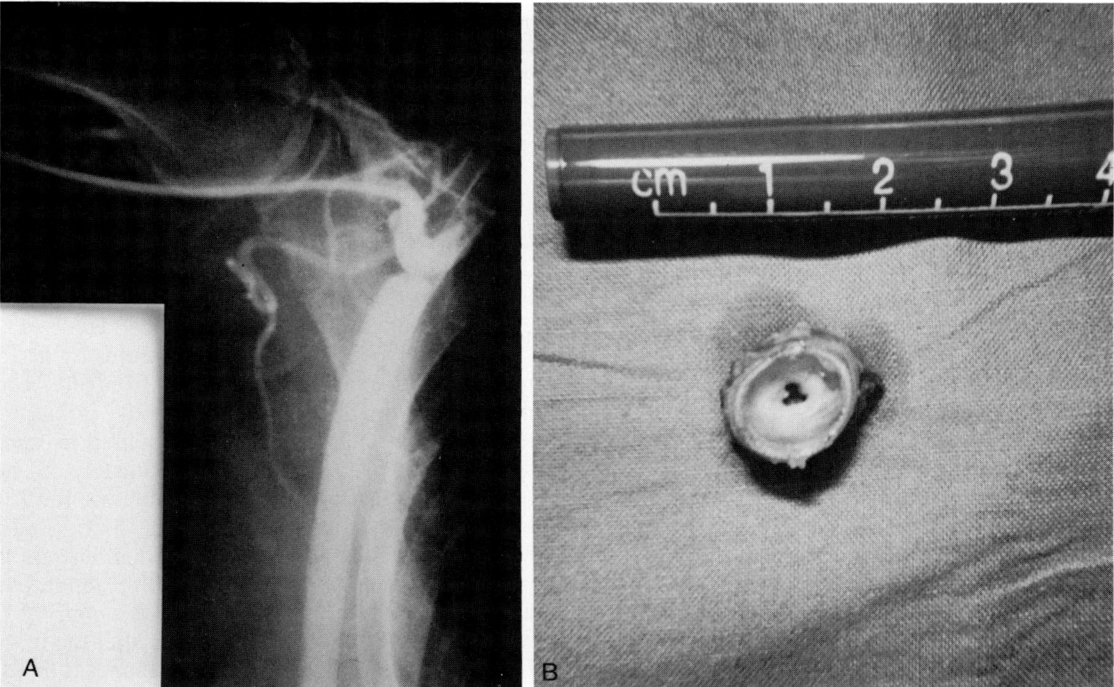

FIGURE 15–3. An elderly woman had a symptomatic decrease in right ankle blood pressure 2 years after right axillofemoral bypass with a Dacron graft. *A*, Right transaxillary arteriogram shows a buckle in the axillary artery and a thin, diaphragm-like stenosis at the anastomosis. The stenotic portion of the graft was resected. *B*, End-on view shows a pinhole opening. The lesion was composed of smooth muscle cells covered by endothelium. (*A* and *B*, From Clowes AW: Current theories of arterial graft failure. Vasc Diagn Ther 3:41, 1982.)

cessive intimal hyperplasia. In part, this is true because it is extremely difficult to document in humans the extent of endothelial denudation or wall disruption and the sequence of reparative events. In addition, we know now from animal studies that there may be a wide range of injurious insults; some cause disruption of the vascular architecture and others cause subtle loss of endothelium, which is repaired before denudation becomes apparent.

EXPERIMENTAL STUDIES ON INTIMAL HYPERPLASIA

Large undiseased arteries are made of layers of SMC alternating with layers of elastin and collagen in the media and are covered on the luminal surface by a continuous monolayer of endothelium. In adult animals, endothelium and SMC are in a state of quiescence, and turnover of these cells is barely detectable (in rat, approximately 0.06 per cent per day).[3] Once the surface has been denuded of endothelium, a stereotyped sequence of events ensues and leads to intimal thickening (Fig. 15–4). The denuded regions are immediately covered by a carpet of platelets. The platelets are then displaced over a period of days by an advancing front of regenerating endothelium. At the same time, SMC in the media begin to proliferate. They then migrate into the intima and continue to proliferate as well as to synthesize and secrete large amounts of extracellular matrix.

Even as the endothelial cells are being stripped away, platelets begin to adhere to the exposed subendothelium and to spread. The adherence and spreading are mediated by glycoproteins present in the platelet membranes and by exogenous substrate molecules such as von Willebrand's factor, fibrin, collagen, and thrombospondin.[37] It is surprising that the accumulation of platelets on the denuded surface of normal artery is a limited process, and if inhibited for a period of 8 hours by the infusion of prostacyclin (PGI_2) it does not occur at all.[38, 39] The reason for this change is not known; it might be related to some form of chemical adaptation that renders the denuded wall nonthrombogenic. Synthetic arterial surfaces lacking an endothelial covering do not exhibit this property and remain thrombogenic for years.[40]

As part of the process of adhesion, platelets release their granules. These granules contain not only vasoactive and thrombotic factors (serotonin, adenosine diphosphate [ADP], fibrinogen, von Willebrand's factor) but also growth factors (platelet-derived growth factor, transforming growth factor–beta, epidermal growth factor);[41] in theory, these growth factors may be the mitogenic stimulus for the initiation of smooth muscle growth because they are potent activators of SMC growth in vitro.

Endothelial cells regenerate from untraumatized sources adjacent to the damaged vessel and advance as a broad-growing edge.[42, 43] In damaged thoracic aorta, endothelial cells derived from intercostal vessel artery orifices migrate not only longitudinally but also transversely around the perimeter of the aorta. Migration begins within hours of injury, and proliferation begins by 24 hours. In most circumstances, the process goes to completion. However, if

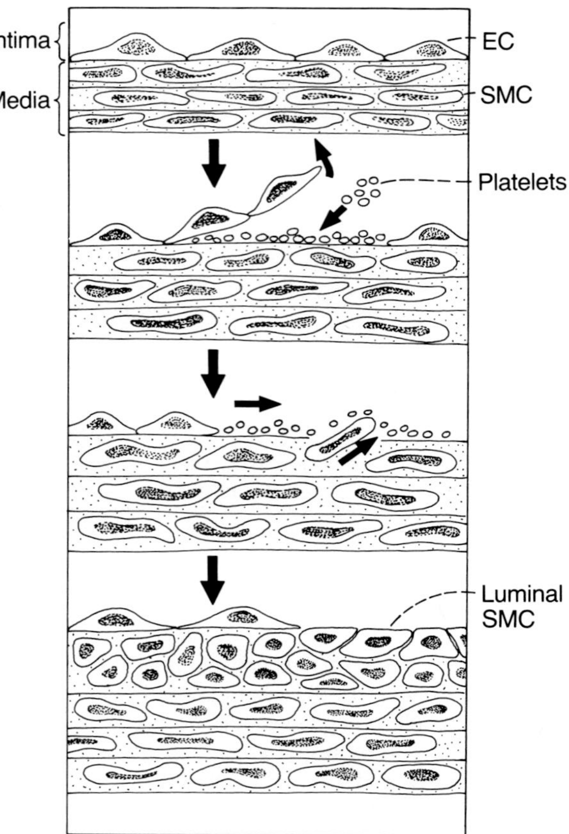

FIGURE 15–4. Schematic representation of arterial reaction to injury. A normal elastic artery is shown in cross section with endothelium (EC) on the luminal surface and smooth muscle cells (SMC) in the media *(top panel)*. When the endothelial layer is disrupted, platelets accumulate in the denuded region *(second panel)*. The surface layer is regenerated by an advancing endothelial front even as smooth muscle cells begin to proliferate in the media and migrate into the intima *(third panel)*. Smooth muscle cells continue to proliferate to form an intimal thickening. They also form a luminal surface (luminal SMC) where endothelium is absent *(bottom panel)*.

the distance between sources of endothelium is large, the denuded region may never become covered with endothelium.[44] The reason for the limited ability of endothelium to cover a denuded surface has yet to be identified.

SMC respond to the injury stimulus by first proliferating in the media, then migrating from the media to the intima, and finally proliferating in the intima to form an intimal thickening. In the balloon-injured rat carotid, SMC synthesize DNA (S-phase) approximately 27 hours after injury.[45] They then continue to proliferate for 7 to 14 days before stopping spontaneously (Fig. 15–5). Studies analyzing the early prereplicative events demonstrate that a limited cohort of cells enter the growth fraction (between 20 and 40 per cent) and do so shortly after injury.[46] The apparent growth fraction does not change after the first few days. Once committed to proliferation, it appears that these cells undergo three to four rounds of division and then stop dividing despite the absence of an overlying endothelium. In injured rat carotid, the central portion of the artery remains without endothelium for more than 12 months. In

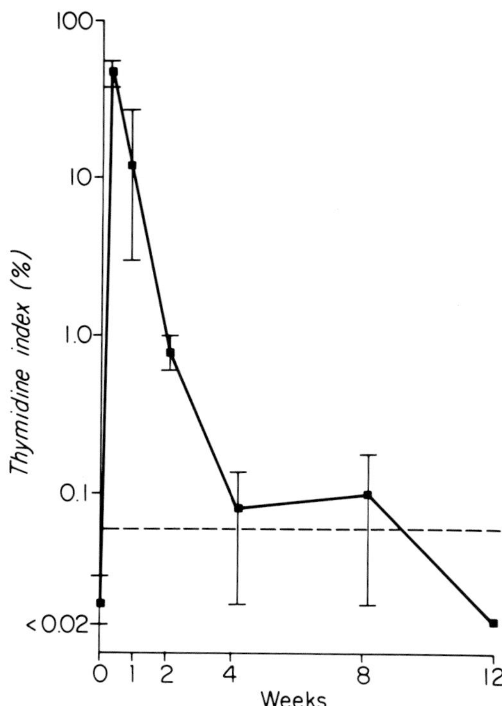

FIGURE 15–5. Schematic representation of the pattern of smooth muscle cell proliferation (thymidine index) as a function of time after injury. These cells start in the resting state, with a labeling index of approximately 0.06 per cent per day *(dashed line)*. After injury, the fraction of proliferating cells increases to 20–50 per cent per day and then returns to background levels by 4 weeks.

this region, SMC form a surface that is relatively nonthrombogenic but, unlike endothelium, is incapable of forming a layer of limited permeability to large molecules. SMC located at the luminal surface of chronically denuded regions continue to proliferate at levels (about 10- to 100-fold) above background even as late as 1 year after injury.[44] This proliferation of surface SMC appears to be matched by cell death because there is no net accumulation of smooth muscle within the wall after 2 weeks.

In the injured rat carotid, although the SMC content of the wall does not change after 12 weeks, the amount of intimal thickening nevertheless doubles between 2 and 12 weeks (Fig. 15–6).[4] The increase in intimal volume can be accounted for entirely by an increase in extracellular matrix, including elastin, collagen, and proteoglycan. In some circumstances, massive lipid accumulation is observed, particularly underneath the regenerated endothelium.[47]

Considered altogether, these observations support the concept that the process of injury-induced intimal thickening involves early thrombosis on the denuded wall followed by SMC proliferation and finally deposition of matrix by SMC. Hence, smooth muscle proliferation plays a central role in the development of the intimal lesion. Endothelium, in this model of intimal thickening, appears to modulate smooth muscle proliferation, accumulation of lipid, and to some extent vasomotor activity in the artery.[48] The "reaction-to-injury" hypothesis as originally stated suggested that the initial injury and the final intimal thickening might be linked by the early thrombotic events and the release of

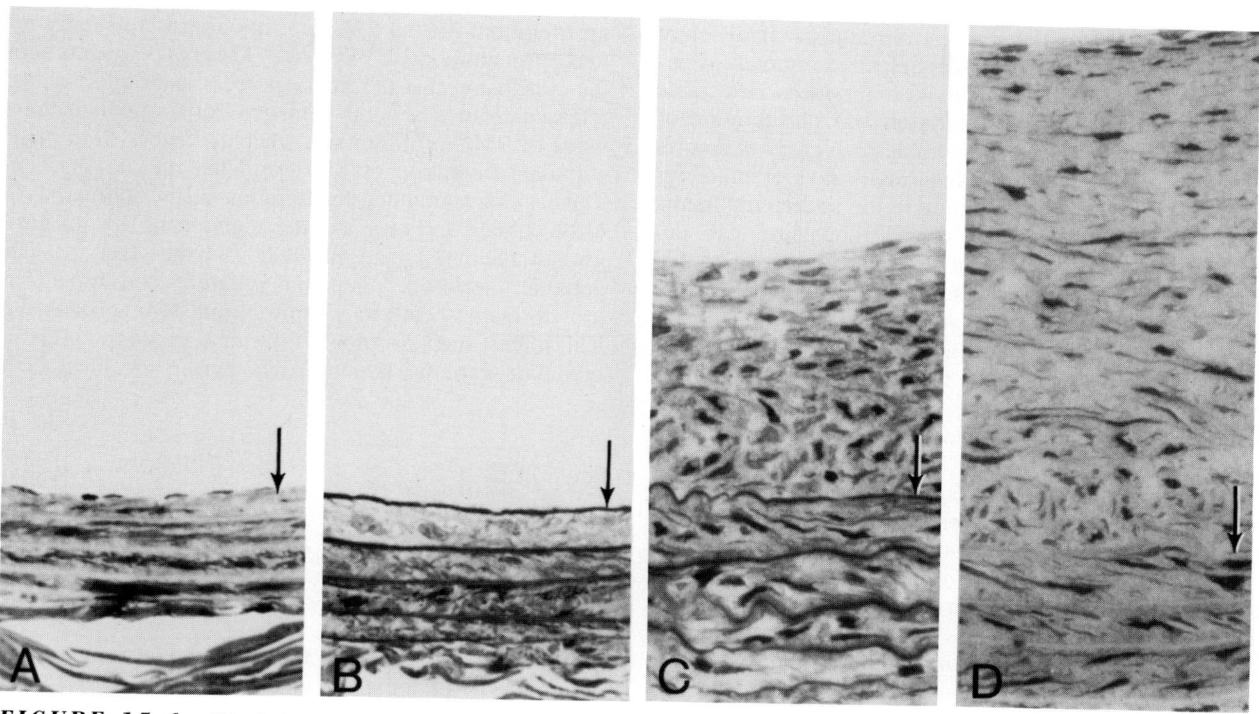

FIGURE 15–6. Histologic cross sections of rat carotid artery before injury *(A)*, immediately after endothelial denudation with a balloon catheter *(B)*, 2 weeks after injury *(C)*, and 12 weeks after injury *(D)*. Note the marked intimal thickening at 2 and 12 weeks. *Arrows* indicate the internal elastic lamina. The lumen is at the top. *(A–D*, From Clowes AW, Reidy MA, Clowes MM: Kinetics of cellular proliferation after arterial injury. I. Smooth muscle growth in the absence of endothelium. Lab Invest 49:327, © by U.S. and Canadian Academy of Pathology, Inc, 1983.)

smooth muscle growth factors from adherent platelets into the damaged artery.[48] This reaction-to-injury hypothesis was supported by early studies of arterial injury in animals. Injured aortas from rabbits rendered thrombocytopenic by administration of antiplatelet antibody appeared to develop smaller intimal thickenings.[49, 50] The effect of thrombocytopenia on intimal thickening has been confirmed in studies using the ballooned rat carotid model of arterial injury. However, the effect was shown to be due to inhibition of SMC migration. The magnitude of the first wave of SMC proliferation was the same in control and thrombocytopenic animals.[51] These somewhat unexpected results provide support for the conclusion that factors from thrombus are chemoattractants for SMC and fibroblasts. These factors are now being defined. One of the factors released from platelets, platelet-derived growth factor (PDGF), stimulates SMC migration from the media when infused in pharmacologic doses.[52] Injection of an antibody to PDGF blocks intimal thickening but not SMC proliferation.[53] Thus, it appears that platelets and PDGF from platelets (or possibly vascular wall cells) regulate SMC movement and thereby intimal thickening in damaged arteries. However, studies using pharmacologic inhibitors of platelet aggregation have not provided convincing support for the role of platelets in the intimal thickening process except in circumstances associated with massive accumulation of thrombus.[39, 54–59] An explanation for these negative results is that most antithrombotic drugs do not block platelet adhesion.

The thrombocytopenia experiments raise several disturbing questions. If platelet factors affect only SMC migration, what regulates SMC proliferation in injured arteries and vascular grafts? Furthermore, what is the importance, if any, of vessel and cellular injury in this process? Answers to these questions are emerging from studies of different animal models of vascular repair. Selective removal of endothelium with a fine filament loop produces detectable gaps, which are healed by migration and proliferation of adjacent endothelial cells. Nevertheless, even in examples of this kind of injury, which requires 7 days or more for full repair, little SMC proliferation in the underlying media is evident,[42] although some intimal thickening can develop.[60] Infusion of endotoxin also produces endothelial injury, but a form of injury that can be repaired by local migration and proliferation at sufficient speed to allow repair before dead and dying endothelial cells actually are liberated from the surface. In this latter circumstance, no gaps are apparent, and therefore no platelet accumulation is observed on the affected arteries. Also, no SMC proliferation is observed.

Several models have become available in which SMC proliferate in the absence of endothelial denudation. It is apparent that they will do so in response to hypertension, in the presence of a remote indwelling arterial catheter producing thrombosis, and over healing vascular grafts.[61–63] In all these examples, there has been no evidence of actual denudation, although the endothelial cells exhibit increased thymidine labeling. There has also been a rough correlation between medial smooth muscle and overlying endothelial proliferation. In each case, SMC proliferate *only* where endothelium is present. In the grafts, the endothelium is unlike regenerated endothelium in injured artery and continues to proliferate even though no gaps are apparent in the monolayer; this observation has suggested the possibility that the endothelium is subjected to a chronic but nondenuding form of injury.

In summary, these experiments support the hypothesis that SMC are able to proliferate whether or not endothelial cells are present. Furthermore, there may be a correlation between the extent of injury and the magnitude of the proliferative responses.[64] Medial damage and SMC proliferation are greater in balloon-injured than in filament loop–injured rat carotid arteries even though the endothelium is stripped completely in the two situations. Denudation alone is not sufficient to drive SMC proliferation, and therefore the effects of balloon catheter injury other than denudation, such as injury to the underlying media and distention of the vessel, must be important. In models of chronic endothelial proliferation without denudation, the factors responsible for stimulating SMC growth must come from the vascular wall cells themselves because platelets do not adhere to the endothelial lining.

We therefore arrive at the conclusion that something more than factors from platelets is required for smooth muscle growth. As suggested earlier, the vascular wall cells themselves or possibly small resident populations of macrophages appear to be the logical sources (Fig. 15–7). At present, we know that endothelial cells, SMC, and macrophages in culture can synthesize and secrete several defined growth factors, one of which resembles PDGF.[65–70]

Another such factor is basic fibroblast growth factor (bFGF). Basic fibroblast growth factor is stored in endothelial and smooth muscle cells, is released in response to injury, and is stored in the matrix.[71] It is a potent mitogen for endothelium and SMC. When administered to rats in pharmacologic amounts, it stimulates SMC and endothelial proliferation; medial SMC proliferation is markedly inhibited by an antibody to bFGF.[72–74] These experiments support the conclusion that the injury process itself and the factors released from dead and damaged cells stimulate the first wave of SMC proliferation, whereas factors from platelets stimulate migration of SMC into the intima (Fig. 15–8). The factors regulating proliferation in the intima have yet to be defined and may include angiotensin II,[75] insulin-like growth factor–I,[76] and PDGF.[77, 78] Other factors such as gamma interferon,[79] heparan sulfate,[80] and transforming growth factor–beta[81] may limit intimal SMC growth. Physical forces such as blood flow and blood pressure may modulate vascular structure by altering the local cellular

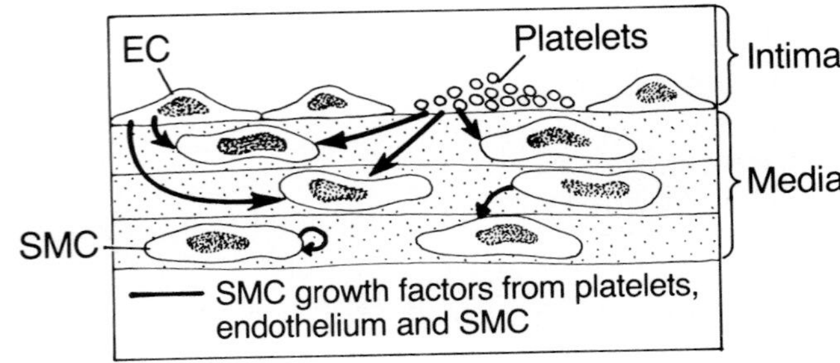

FIGURE 15–7. Diagrammatic representation of injured artery suggests that a variety of cell types, including platelets, endothelial cells (EC), and smooth muscle cells (SMC), might secrete growth factors for smooth muscle cells. Macrophages (not shown) also synthesize and secrete smooth muscle mitogens.

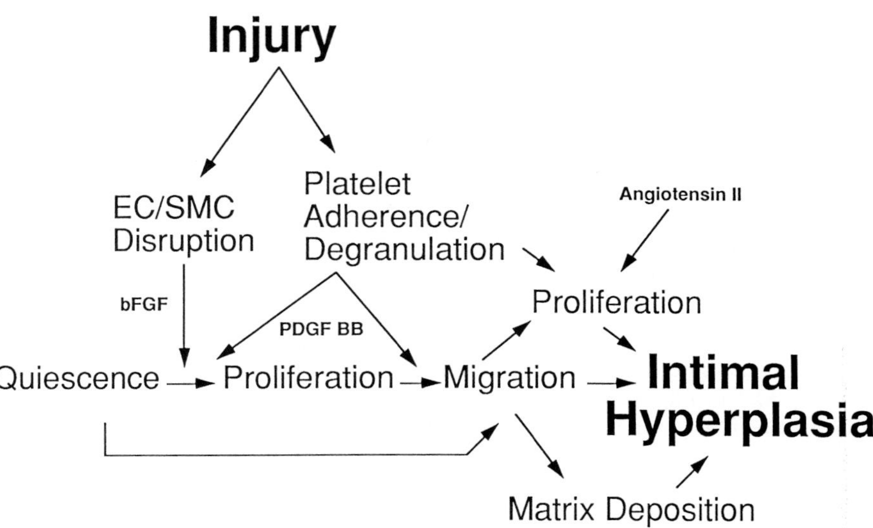

FIGURE 15–8. Illustration of how injury to the artery might cause endothelial cell (EC) and smooth muscle cell (SMC) disruption and release of intracellular mitogens such as basic fibroblast growth factor (bFGF). Fibroblast growth factor then stimulates medial smooth muscle proliferation. Factors from platelets, such as the BB isoform of platelet-derived growth factor (PDGF-BB), regulate movement of the smooth muscle cells from the media to the intima. Angiotensin II also affects the intimal thickening process. (From Clowes AW, Reidy MA: Prevention of stenosis after vascular reconstruction: Pharmacologic control of intimal hyperplasia—A review. J Vasc Surg 13:885, 1991.)

expression of one or more of these biochemical factors.[82, 83] In summary, we are forced to conclude that repair in even the simplest model of vascular injury is an exceedingly complex process; nevertheless, studies in such simple systems should continue to provide valuable insights for understanding vascular growth and development[84] as well as for designing pharmacologic strategies to control intimal thickening after arterial reconstruction.

CONTROL OF ABNORMAL INTIMAL THICKENING

The formation of a thickened intima is part of the normal reparative response of an artery and graft to injury. As noted earlier, under some circumstances, the amount of intima becomes excessive and produces marked luminal narrowing. This occurs in coronary arteries subjected to balloon angioplasty (30 per cent in 6 months),[11, 12] vein grafts used for peripheral arterial bypass (10 per cent in 6 to 24 months),[25] and coronary bypass grafts (52 to 75 per cent in 10 years)[29, 30] and is an important cause of low flow and eventual thrombosis. In large measure, the therapy for prevention or correction of excessive intimal thickening has taken one of two approaches: (1) antiplatelet (mainly aspirin and dipyridamole) and anticoagulant (warfarin [Coumadin]) drugs have been given based on the assumption that the accumulation of platelets and clotting factors plays a role in early and late thrombosis and might play a role in the development of intimal thickening;[56, 59] and (2) further surgical reconstruction has been undertaken based on the assumption that renewed or continued intimal thickening is unlikely.

Aspirin and dipyridamole have been effective in reducing coronary bypass graft failure by approximately 10 per cent in several clinical series.[56] It is important to note that these drugs are effective only if given at or within a short time after the surgery; if they are delayed more than 2 days, they are of no benefit when the grafts are evaluated by angiography later. This observation suggests that these drugs are preventing either acute graft occlusion or the early accumulation of thrombus that might later be remodeled into a fibrous lesion. Similar studies in patients receiving peripheral bypass grafts have been negative or have shown a weak effect.[56, 59] Studies in animals of the effects of antithrombotic drugs on intimal thickening in injured arteries and in vascular grafts have been both positive and negative.[54–58, 85] In view of what we know now about smooth muscle proliferation and intimal thickening, it seems logical that aspirin would only affect wound healing events associated with platelet aggregation and accumulation of large thrombi.

Further vascular reconstruction has remained the principal form of therapy for salvage of failing grafts and other vascular reconstructions. Several groups have demonstrated that assiduous follow-up of patients undergoing vein bypass reconstruction of femoropopliteal disease will allow discovery of stenoses due to intimal hyperplasia before these lesions actually cause graft thrombosis.[25, 26] If these lesions are reconstructed before they cause thrombosis, the long-term outcome is extremely good. On the other hand, if the grafts go on to thrombosis and the stenotic lesions are identified by arteriography only after the grafts have been subjected to thrombectomy, the reconstructions generally fail. These results tend to support the conclusion that the stenotic process, at least in peripheral bypass grafts, is limited and if corrected, does not recur; this conclusion fits very well with observations in animal models indicating that arterial intimal thickening in response to injury is a self-limited process. The difference in humans relates to the presence of significant atherogenic risk factors, which have a marked impact on the atherosclerotic process in proximal and distal vessels as well as in the grafts. The clinical experience with recurrent carotid stenoses is similar to the experience with peripheral bypass grafts; these arteries, when treated with vein patch grafts, remain patent. Stenotic lesions at anastomoses between synthetic grafts and arteries have proved to be more difficult to reconstruct because they tend to recur. No satisfactory approach has been developed to deal with this problem. In summary, it appears that frequent follow-up assessment of surgical reconstructions followed by appropriate further reconstruction provides optimal treatment for intimal hyperplastic lesions causing luminal stenosis of vascular reconstructions. Antithrombotic therapy seems to reduce the rate of occlusion in coronary bypass grafts and in certain massively thrombotic states such as angioplasty. The use of these drugs in preventing carotid restenosis and peripheral graft occlusion is not certain.

Several interesting and new forms of therapy are on the horizon. As has been obvious throughout this chapter, endothelium plays a pivotal and complicated role in the function of the normal artery and the artery undergoing repair. Regenerating endothelium over injured artery suppresses SMC proliferation and inhibits platelet accumulation on the artery wall.[86] Because of these observations, a number of investigators have been interested in the behavior of grafts deliberately seeded with endothelium.[87] These grafts, at least in animal models, tend to resist thrombosis and to develop lesser amounts of intimal thickening. Endothelial seeding also appears to improve graft patency in humans, although the studies are still quite preliminary.[88] We have pursued an alternative approach to solving the problem of endothelialization of synthetic grafts. By changing the porosity of polytetrafluoroethylene (PTFE) grafts (from 30 μm to 60 μm internodal distance) we have been able to produce spontaneous rapid endothelialization in animal experiments. This endothelial layer develops from multiple transmural capillaries arising from the granulation tissue surrounding the graft.[89] It is unfortunate that when placed in humans as femoropopliteal bypasses, the 60-μm PTFE grafts do not appear to develop an endothelial lining, although occasional intramural capillaries are seen.[36] Adjuvant pharmacology will be necessary to stimulate capillary ingrowth and endothelial coverage. Some form of endothelial chemoattractant (e.g., bFGF) might be inserted into the interstices of the graft. This approach to enhancing spontaneous endothelialization is being pursued actively in a number of laboratories.

Another alternative is to employ specific inhibitors of SMC proliferation, since, as we have seen, proliferation of SMC and subsequent deposition by SMC of extracellular matrix is central to the development of intimal hyperplasia. A number of drugs have been tried in animal models of arterial injury and in patients undergoing transluminal angioplasty of the coronary arteries. Although many drugs are inhibitory in the animal models, none have proved to be successful in preventing coronary restenosis in humans.[90]

The most completely characterized inhibitor of SMC growth is heparin (Fig. 15–9).[91–99] Heparin appears to inhibit SMC migration and proliferation both in vivo and in vitro, and its inhibitory capacity depends on a characteristic polysaccharide sequence with a high degree of sulfation. Of particular note, heparin inhibits SMC but not large-vessel endothelial proliferation. On the other hand, capillary endothelial cell proliferation and migration appear to be stimulated. The precise structure of heparin required for optimal activity has not yet been determined, although a pentasaccharide sequence with a unique 3–0 sulfate appears to be significantly more potent than other small fragments. Heparin appears to block SMC proliferation in the late G_1 stage (prereplicative state). Although the mechanism by which heparin inhibits SMC growth has not been defined, it is apparent from both cell culture and in vivo studies that the effect of heparin on proliferation and migration is specific for SMC and for heparin-like molecules; related glycosaminoglycans, such as chondroitin sulfate, do not affect cell growth. It has now become possible commercially to develop small fragments of heparin lacking anticoagulant activity. In vivo, a brief treatment with heparin of animals subjected to carotid injury produces inhibition of SMC proliferation and a decrease in the growth fraction.[94] If heparin treatment is stopped after 3 days, SMC proliferation does not resume normal levels. These observations support the concept that acute injury produces a single stimulatory event. If cells are not permitted to respond to the injury stimulus early, they do not do so later despite the fact that the arterial wall remains denuded of endothelium. Given that heparin treatment, at least for discrete injury situations,

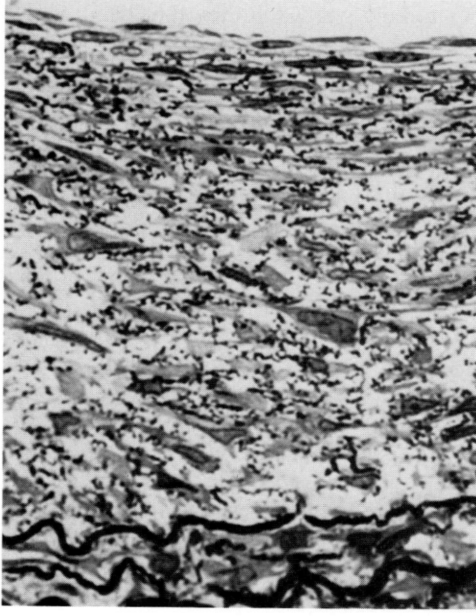

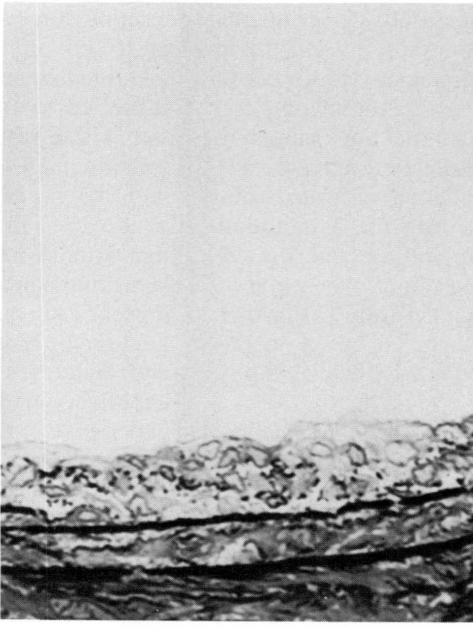

FIGURE 15–9. Histologic cross sections of injured carotid artery from control *(left)* and heparin-treated *(right)* animals. Note the marked reduction in intimal thickening in response to heparin. (From Clowes AW, Clowes MM: Kinetics of cellular proliferation after arterial injury. II. Inhibition of smooth muscle growth by heparin. Lab Invest 52:611, © by U.S. and Canadian Academy of Pathology, Inc, 1985.)

might be needed only for several days and the availability of nonanticoagulant fractions, it would seem reasonable to consider using a heparin-like drug for the treatment of injury-related intimal hyperplasia.

As the importance of other various cellular and molecular events is defined, new pharmacologic strategies for the control of intimal hyperplasia should emerge.[100] For example, inhibitors of bFGF and PDGF might be expected to suppress SMC proliferation and migration. These drugs might be given systemically, or they might be delivered directly into the arterial wall.[101] A new and potentially powerful approach to controlling SMC function is to introduce genetic material coding for specific SMC inhibitors directly into the vascular cells so that the gene product is released and acts locally.[102, 103] In principle, this approach should work because locally synthesized and released proteins such as gamma interferon inhibit SMC growth.[79, 104] Such gene therapy strategies for controlling intimal hyperplasia and restenosis are being actively developed.[105]

CONCLUSION

SMC proliferation and the formation of a thickened intima is part of normal wound healing in injured artery and vascular grafts. At times, this process becomes excessive and leads to luminal stenosis and eventual failure of vascular reconstructions. The growth factors and inhibitors that regulate the balance between normal healing and pathologic stenosis are now being defined. Nevertheless, the treatment of vascular stenosis due to intimal hyperplasia remains largely surgical. A detailed understanding of the biology of SMC growth and intimal hyperplasia should eventually lead to new forms of preventive adjuvant therapy.

References

1. Ross R, Glomset JA: The pathogenesis of atherosclerosis. N Engl J Med 295:369, 1976.
2. Clowes AW, Gown AM, Hanson SR, Reidy MA: Mechanisms of arterial graft failure. I. Role of cellular proliferation in early healing of PTFE prostheses. Am J Pathol 118:43, 1985.
3. Clowes AW, Reidy MA, Clowes MM: Kinetics of cellular proliferation after arterial injury. I. Smooth muscle growth in the absence of endothelium. Lab Invest 49:327, 1983.
4. Clowes AW, Reidy MA, Clowes MM: Mechanisms of stenosis after arterial injury. Lab Invest 49:208, 1983.
5. Chidi CC, DePalma RG: Atherogenic potential of the embolectomy catheter. Surgery 83:549, 1978.
6. Steele PM, Chesebro JH, Stanson AW, et al: Balloon angioplasty. Natural history of the pathophysiological response to injury in a pig model. Circ Res 57:105, 1985.
7. Zarins CK, Lu CT, Gewertz BL, et al: Arterial disruption and remodeling following balloon dilatation. Surgery 92:1086, 1982.
8. Gallino A, Mahler F, Probst P, Nachbur B: Percutaneous transluminal angioplasty of the arteries of the lower limbs: A 5-year follow-up. Circulation 70:619, 1984.
9. Lally ME, Johnston KW, Andrews D: Percutaneous transluminal dilatation of peripheral arteries: An analysis of factors predicting early success. J Vasc Surg 1:704, 1984.
10. Tegtmeyer CJ, Hartwell GD, Selby JB, et al: Results and complications of angioplasty in aortoiliac disease. Circulation Suppl 83, p I-53, 1991.
11. Holmes DR, Vlietstra RE, Smith HC, et al: Restenosis after percutaneous transluminal coronary angioplasty (PCTA): A report from the PTCA Registry of the National Heart, Lung, and Blood Institute. Am J Cardiol 53:77C, 1984.
12. Fanelli C, Aronoff R: Restenosis following coronary angioplasty. Am Heart J 119:357, 1990.
13. Kumpe DA, Jones DN: Percutaneous transluminal angioplasty—radiological viewpoint. Vasc Diag Ther 3:19, 1982.
14. Spence K, Freiman DB, Gatenby R: Long-term results of transluminal angioplasty of the iliac and femoral arteries. Arch Surg 116:1377, 1981.
15. Callow AD: Recurrent stenosis after carotid endarterectomy. Arch Surg 117:1082, 1982.
16. Clagett GP, Robinowitz M, Youkey JR, et al: Morphogenesis and clinicopathologic characteristics of recurrent carotid disease. J Vasc Surg 3:10, 1986.
17. Nicholls SC, Phillips DJ, Bergelin RO, et al: Carotid endarterectomy. Relationship of outcome to early restenosis. J Vasc Surg 2:375, 1985.
18. Stoney RJ, String ST: Recurrent carotid stenosis. Surgery 80:705, 1976.
19. Thomas M, Otis SM, Rush M, et al: Recurrent carotid artery stenosis following endarterectomy. Ann Surg 200:74, 1984.
20. Zierler RE, Bandyk DF, Thiele BL, Strandness DE Jr: Carotid artery stenosis following endarterectomy. Arch Surg 117:1408, 1982.
21. Cambria RP, Megerman J, Abbott WM: Endothelial preservation in reversed and in situ autogenous vein grafts. Ann Surg 202:50, 1985.
22. Fuchs JC, Mitchener JS 3d, Hagen PO: Postoperative changes in autologous vein grafts. Ann Surg 188:1, 1978.
23. LoGerfo FW, Quist WC, Cantelmo NL, Haudenschild CC: Integrity of vein grafts as a function of initial intimal and medial preservation. Circulation 68:II, 1983.
24. Szilagyi DE, Elliott JP, Hageman JH, et al: Biologic fate of autogenous vein implants as arterial substitutes. Ann Surg 178:232, 1973.
25. Whittemore AD, Clowes AW, Couch NP, Mannick JA: Secondary femoropopliteal reconstruction. Ann Surg 193:35, 1981.
26. Bandyk DF, Kaebnick HW, Stewart GW, Towne JB: Durability of the in situ saphenous vein arterial bypass: A comparison of primary and secondary patency. J Vasc Surg 5:256, 1987.
27. DePalma RG: Atherosclerosis in vascular grafts. Atherosclerosis Rev 6:146, 1979.
28. Spray TL, Roberts WC: Changes in saphenous veins used as aortocoronary bypass grafts. Am Heart J 94:500, 1977.
29. Grondin CM, Campeau L, Lesperance J, et al: Comparison of late changes in internal mammary artery and saphenous vein grafts in two consecutive series of patients 10 years after operation. Circulation 70:I, 1984.
30. Campeau L, Enjalbert M, Lesperance J, Bourassa MG: The relation of risk factors to the development of atherosclerosis in saphenous-vein bypass grafts and the progression of disease in the native circulation. N Engl J Med 311:1329, 1984.
31. Echave V, Koornick AR, Haimov M, Jacobson JH: Intimal hyperplasia as a complication of the use of the polytetrafluoroethylene graft for femoral-popliteal bypass. Surgery 86:791, 1979.
32. LoGerfo FW, Quist WC, Nowak MD, et al: Downstream anastomotic hyperplasia: A mechanism of failure in Dacron arterial grafts. Ann Surg 197:479, 1983.
33. Selman SH, Rhodes RS, Anderson JM, et al: Atheromatous changes in expanded polytetrafluoroethylene grafts. Surgery 87:630, 1980.
34. Szilagyi DE, Smith RF, Elliott JP, Allen HM: Long-term behavior of a Dacron arterial substitute: Clinical, roentgenologic and histologic correlations. Ann Surg 162:453, 1965.
35. Berger K, Sauvage LR, Rao AM, Wood SJ: Healing of arterial prostheses in man: Its incompleteness. Ann Surg 175:118, 1972.
36. Clowes AW, Kohler T: Graft endothelialization: The role of angiogenic mechanisms. J Vasc Surg 13:734, 1991.
37. George JN, Nurden AT, Phillips DR: Molecular defects in interactions of platelets with the vessel wall. N Engl J Med 311:1084, 1984.
38. Groves HM, Kinlough-Rathbone RL, Richardson M, et al: Platelet interaction with damaged rabbit aorta. Lab Invest 40:194, 1979.
39. Groves HM, Kinlough-Rathbone RL, Mustard JF: Development of nonthrombogenicity of injured rabbit aortas despite inhibition of platelet adherence. Arteriosclerosis 6:189, 1986.
40. Stratton JR, Thiele BL, Ritchie JL: Platelet deposition on Dacron aortic bifurcation grafts in man: Quantitation with indium-111 platelet imaging. Circulation 66:1287, 1982.
41. Bowen-Pope DF, Ross R, Seifert RA: Locally acting growth factors

for vascular smooth muscle cells: Endogenous synthesis and release from platelets. Circulation 72:735, 1985.
42. Reidy MA: A reassessment of endothelial injury and arterial lesion formation. Lab Invest 53:513, 1985.
43. Schwartz SM, Haudenschild CC, Eddy EM: Endothelial regeneration. I. Quantitative analysis of initial stages of endothelial regeneration in rat aortic intima. Lab Invest 38:568, 1978.
44. Clowes AW, Clowes MM, Reidy MA: Kinetics of cellular proliferation after arterial injury. III. Endothelial and smooth muscle growth in chronically denuded vessels. Lab Invest 54:295, 1986.
45. Majesky MW, Schwartz SM, Clowes MM, Clowes AW: Heparin regulates smooth muscle S phase entry in the injured rat carotid artery. Circ Res 61:296, 1987.
46. Clowes AW, Schwartz SM: Significance of quiescent smooth muscle migration in the injured rat carotid artery. Circ Res 56:139, 1985.
47. Falcone DJ, Hajjar DP, Minick CR: Lipoprotein and albumin accumulation in reendothelialized and deendothelialized aorta. Am J Pathol 114:112, 1984.
48. Ross R: Pathogenesis of atherosclerosis—an update. N Engl J Med 314:488, 1986.
49. Friedman RJ, Stemerman MB, Wenz B, et al: The effect of thrombocytopenia on experimental atherosclerotic lesion formation in rabbits. Smooth muscle cell proliferation and re-endothelialization. J Clin Invest 60:1191, 1977.
50. Moore S, Friedman RJ, Singal DP, et al: Inhibition of injury-induced thromboathero-sclerotic lesions by antiplatelet serum in rabbits. Thromb Haemost 35:70, 1976.
51. Fingerle J, Johnson R, Clowes AW, et al: Role of platelets in smooth muscle cell proliferation and migration after vascular injury in rat carotid artery. Proc Natl Acad Sci USA 86:8412, 1989.
52. Jawien A, Bowen-Pope DF, Lindner V, et al: Platelet-derived growth factor promotes smooth muscle migration and intimal thickening in a rat model of balloon angioplasty. J Clin Invest 89:507, 1992.
53. Ferns GAA, Raines EW, Sprugel KH, et al: Inhibition of neointimal smooth muscle accumulation after angioplasty by an antibody to PDGF. Science 253:1129, 1991.
54. Bomberger RA, DePalma RG, Ambrose TA, Manalo P: Aspirin and dipyridamole inhibit endothelial healing. Arch Surg 117:1459, 1982.
55. Clowes AW, Karnovsky MJ: Failure of certain antiplatelet drugs to affect myointimal thickening following arterial injury. Lab Invest 36:452, 1977.
56. Clowes AW: The role of aspirin in enhancing arterial graft patency. J Vasc Surg 3:381, 1986.
57. Faxon DP, Sanborn TA, Haudenschild CC, Ryan TJ: Effect of antiplatelet therapy on restenosis after experimental angioplasty. Am J Cardiol 53:72C, 1984.
58. Radic ZS, O'Mallery MK, Mikat EM, et al: The role of aspirin and dipyridamole on vascular DNA synthesis and intimal hyperplasia following deendothelialization. J Surg Res 41:84, 1986.
59. Clagett GP, Genton E, Salzman EW: Antithrombotic therapy in peripheral vascular disease. Chest 95:128S, 1989.
60. Fingerle J, Au YPT, Clowes AW, Reidy MA: Intimal lesion formation in rat carotid arteries after endothelial denudation in absence of medial injury. Arteriosclerosis 10:1082, 1990.
61. Owens GK, Reidy MA: Hyperplastic growth response of vascular smooth muscle cells following induction of acute hypertension in rats by aortic coarctation. Circ Res 57:695, 1985.
62. Reidy MA, Chao SS, Kirkman TR, Clowes AW: Endothelial regeneration. VI. Chronic nondenuding injury in baboon vascular grafts. Am J Pathol 123:432, 1986.
63. Reidy MA: In vivo proliferation of vascular smooth muscle cells in vessels with intact endothelial cover (Abstract). Fed Proc 45:683, 1986.
64. Clowes AW, Clowes MM, Fingerle J, Reidy MA: Regulation of smooth muscle cell growth in injured artery. J Cardiovasc Pharmacol 14 (Suppl 6):S12, 1989.
65. DiCorleto PE, Bowen-Pope DF: Cultured endothelial cells produce a platelet-derived growth factor-like protein. Proc Natl Acad Sci USA 80:1919, 1983.
66. Gajdusek C, DiCorleto P, Ross R, Schwartz SM: An endothelial cell-derived growth factor. J Cell Biol 85:467, 1980.
67. Nilsson J, Sjolund M, Palmberg L, et al: Arterial smooth muscle cells in primary culture produce a platelet-derived growth factor-like protein. Proc Natl Acad Sci USA 82:4418, 1985.
68. Seifert RA, Schwartz SM, Bowen-Pope DF: Developmentally regulated production of platelet-derived growth factor-like molecules. Nature 311:669, 1984.
69. Shimokado K, Raines EW, Madtes DK, et al: A significant part of macrophage-derived growth factor consists of at least two forms of PDGF. Cell 43:277, 1985.
70. Walker LN, Bowen-Pope DF, Reidy MA: Production of platelet-derived growth factor-like molecules by cultured arterial smooth muscle cells accompanies proliferation after arterial injury. Proc Natl Acad Sci USA 83:7311, 1986.
71. D'Amore PA: Modes of FGF release in vivo and in vitro. Cancer Metastasis Rev 9:227, 1990.
72. Lindner V, Majack RA, Reidy MA: Basic fibroblast growth factor stimulates endothelial regrowth and proliferation in denuded arteries. J Clin Invest 85:2004, 1990.
73. Lindner V, Lappi DA, Baird A, et al: Role of basic fibroblast growth factor in vascular lesion formation. Circ Res 68:106, 1991.
74. Lindner V, Reidy MA: Proliferation of smooth muscle cells after vascular injury is inhibited by an antibody against basic fibroblast growth factor. Proc Natl Acad Sci USA 88:3739, 1991.
75. Daemen MJAP, Lombardi DM, Bosman FT, Schwartz SM: Angiotensin II induces smooth muscle cell proliferation in the normal and injured rat arterial wall. Circ Res 68:450, 1991.
76. Bornfeldt KE, Arnqvist HJ, Capron L: In vivo proliferation of rat vascular smooth muscle in relation to diabetes mellitus insulin-like growth factor I and insulin. Diabetologia 35:104, 1992.
77. Majesky MW, Reidy MA, Bowen-Pope DF, et al: PDGF ligand and receptor gene expression during repair of arterial injury. J Cell Biol 111:2149, 1990.
78. Golden MA, Au YPT, Kirkman TR, et al: Platelet-derived growth factor activity and mRNA expression in healing vascular grafts in baboons. Association in vivo of platelet-derived growth factor mRNA and protein with cellular proliferation. J Clin Invest 87:406, 1991.
79. Hansson GK, Jonasson L, Holm J, et al: Gamma interferon regulates vascular smooth muscle proliferation and Ia espression in vitro and in vivo. Circ Res 63:712, 1988.
80. Castellot JJ, Jr, Addonizio ML, Rosenberg R, Karnovsky MJ: Cultured endothelial cells produce a heparin-like inhibitor of smooth muscle cell growth. J Cell Biol 90:372, 1981.
81. Majesky MW, Lindner V, Twardzik DR, et al: Production of transforming growth factor β_1 during repair of arterial injury. J Clin Invest 88:904, 1991.
82. Kraiss LW, Kirkman TR, Kohler TR, et al: Shear stress regulates smooth muscle proliferation and neointimal thickening in porous polytetrafluoroethylene grafts. Arteriosclerosis Thromb 11:1844, 1991.
83. Kohler TR, Kirkman TR, Kraiss LW, et al: Increased blood flow inhibits neointimal hyperplasia in endothelialized vascular grafts. Circ Res 69:1557, 1991.
84. Schwartz SM, Heimark RL, Majesky MW: Developmental mechanisms underlying pathology of arteries. Physiol Rev 70:1177, 1990.
85. Lovaas ME, Gloviczki P, Hollier LH, Kaye MP: Quantitative effects of antiplatelet therapy on healing of the endarterectomized canine aorta. Am J Surg 146:164, 1983.
86. Bush HL, Jr, Jakubowski JA, Sentissi JM, et al: Neointimal hyperplasia occurring after carotid endarterectomy in a canine model: Effect of endothelial cell seeding vs perioperative aspirin. J Vasc Surg 5:118, 1987.
87. Graham LM, Vinter DW, Ford JW, et al: Endothelial cell seeding of prosthetic vascular grafts. Early experimental studies with cultured autologous canine endothelium. Arch Surg 115:929, 1980.
88. Magometschnigg H, Kadletz M, Vodrazka M, et al: Prospective clinical study with in vitro endothelial cell lining of expanded polytetrafluoroethylene grafts in crural repeat reconstruction. J Vasc Surg 15:527, 1992.
89. Clowes AW, Kirkman TR, Reidy MA: Mechanisms of arterial graft healing. Rapid transmural capillary ingrowth provides a source of intimal endothelium and smooth muscle in porous PTFE prostheses. Am J Pathol 123:220, 1986.
90. Popma JJ, Califf RM, Topol EJ: Clinical trials of restenosis after coronary angioplasty. Circulation 84:1426, 1991.
91. Benitz WE, Lessler DS, Coulson JD, Bernfield M: Heparin inhibits proliferation of fetal vascular smooth muscle cells in the absence of platelet-derived growth factor. J Cell Physiol 127:1, 1986.
92. Castellot JJ, Jr, Choay J, Lormeau JC, et al: Structural determinants

of the capacity of heparin to inhibit the proliferation of vascular smooth muscle cells. II. Evidence for a pentasaccharide sequence that contains a 3–0 sulfate group. J Cell Biol 102:1979, 1986.
93. Castellot JJ, Jr, Cochran DL, Karnovsky MJ: Effect of heparin on vascular smooth muscle cells. I. Cell metabolism. J Cell Physiol 124:21, 1985.
94. Clowes AW, Clowes MM: Kinetics of cellular proliferation after arterial injury. IV. Heparin inhibits rat smooth muscle mitogenesis and migration. Circ Res 58:839, 1986.
95. Clowes AW, Clowes MM: Kinetics of cellular proliferation after arterial injury. II. Inhibition of smooth muscle growth by heparin. Lab Invest 52:611, 1985.
96. Clowes AW, Karnovsky MJ: Suppression by heparin of smooth muscle cell proliferation in injured arteries. Nature 265:625, 1977.
97. Hoover RL, Rosenberg R, Haering W, Karnovsky MJ: Inhibition of rat arterial smooth muscle cell proliferation by heparin. II. In vitro studies. Circ Res 47:578, 1980.
98. Majack RA, Clowes AW: Regulation of vascular smooth muscle cell migration by heparin-like glycosaminoglycans. J Cell Physiol 118:253, 1984.
99. Reilly CF, Fritze LMS, Rosenberg RD: Heparin inhibition of smooth muscle cell proliferation: A cellular site of action. J Cell Physiol 129:11, 1986.
100. Clowes AW, Reidy MA: Prevention of stenosis after vascular reconstruction: Pharmacologic control of intimal hyperplasia—A review. J Vasc Surg 13:885, 1991.
101. Nabel EG, Plautz G, Nabel GJ: Site specific gene expression in vivo by direct gene transfer into the arterial wall. Science 249:1285, 1990.
102. Wilson JM, Birinyi LK, Salomon RN, et al: Implantation of vascular grafts lined with genetically modified endothelial cells. Science 244:1344, 1989.
103. Nabel EG, Plautz G, Boyce FM, et al: Recombinant gene expression in vivo within endothelial cells of the arterial wall. Science 244:1342, 1989.
104. Lynch CM, Clowes MM, Osborne WRA, et al: Long-term expression of human adenosine deaminase in vascular smooth muscle cells of rats: A model for gene therapy. Proc Natl Acad Sci USA 89:1138, 1992.
105. Wu GY, Wu CH: Delivery systems for gene therapy. Biotherapy 3:87, 1991.

16

Uncommon Arteriopathies

John W. Joyce, M.D.

• • •

The approach to major arterial and venous disease states is an ingrained logic of the trained vascular specialist, based on understanding the etiology and usual behavior of these well-defined entities, and the constant refinement of their literature. In contrast to these repetitive experiences are the infrequently encountered problems that occur at random, perhaps only once or twice in a career, and that may require a literature search or tertiary consultation. Fortunately, such challenges often announce themselves by departing from the expected in tempo, location, age, setting, or particular clinical or laboratory features. Thus, one is best prepared for the uncommon by a sound knowledge of common problems and their variations.

Until recently, knowledge of fibromuscular dysplasia, popliteal and thoracic entrapments, femoral and popliteal cystic disease, thromboangiitis obliterans, nonspecific aortoarteritis (Takayasu's syndrome), and atherothrombotic microemboli was scattered throughout the medical literature. All are now well delineated and are discussed elsewhere in this text. Three additional diverse disease groups with vascular manifestations are presented in this chapter; the vasculitides, heritable disorders, and a selection of uncommon acquired lesions. Congenital and acquired clotting disorders warrant a separate chapter.

VASCULITIS

The term *arteritis* generically includes any arterial inflammatory response that radiation or direct, embolic, or contiguous infection may induce. In common usage, however, arteritis is usually applied to a diverse group of diseases of unknown or immunologic origin. Indeed, the term *vasculitis* is preferable because veins as well as arteries are involved in given entities.

The vasculitides can be classified by vessel size, microscopic features of tissue reaction (i.e., necrotizing, granulomatous, giant cell, infectious, radiation), or clinical features. Table 16–1 lists the vasculitides as defined clinical entities. It should be noted that the manifestations of periarteritis and the various hypersensitivity syndromes may overlap.

Acute or chronic inflammatory changes of small, medium, and large arteries or veins are the hallmarks of vasculitis. Most of the entities (those without asterisks in Table 16–1) involve small vessels. They present as characteristic, often multiple organ system dysfunctions, accompanied by systemic signs of fever, malaise, and weight loss. Associated rheumatologic and cutaneous lesions are common. Immune mechanisms are implicated in almost all entities.

Table 16–1. Clinical Classification of the Vasculitides

Periarteritis nodosa*	Giant cell arteritis
Hypersensitivity angiitis	Temporal*
Scleroderma*	Nonspecific aortoarteritis*
Systemic lupus erythematosus*	Miscellaneous
Serum sickness	Relapsing polychondritis*
Henoch-Schönlein purpura	Behçet's disease*
Essential mixed cryoglobulinemia	Mucocutaneous lymph node syndrome (Kawasaki's syndrome)*
Malignancy	Erythema nodosum
Churg-Strauss syndrome	Hypocomplementemic vasculitis
Wegener's granulomatosis	Rheumatoid syndromes*
Lymphomatoid granulomatosis	
Thromboangiitis obliterans*	

**Denotes entities that involve larger blood vessels.*

Known triggers of the reactions include drugs such as hydralazine, sulfonamides, procainamide, and amphetamines as well as infections (gonococcis, streptococcis, hepatitis B), inflammation (ulcerative colitis, biliary cirrhosis, serum sickness), and neoplasia (lymphoma, myeloma, cancer, chronic leukemia). In most instances, however, an inciting factor is not identified. Most are treated by steroids and cytotoxic or immunosuppressive agents, and the role of surgery is limited to biopsy and removal of necrotic tissue. Several excellent reviews consolidate the scattered literature on these diverse microcirculatory diseases, known immunologic observations, and their therapy.[1–6]

Major occlusive and aneurysmal disease of the aorta and its branches and of limb and neck arteries, as well as significant venous problems, all in the usual domain of the vascular surgeon, are hallmarks of several of the syndromes (marked by asterisks in Table 16–1). Thromboangiitis obliterans is discussed in Chapter 11, nonspecific aortoarteritis in Chapter 12, and scleroderma in Chapter 68. The remaining entities are presented in this chapter.

Giant Cell Arteritis

Some writers consider the term *giant cell arteritis* synonymous with temporal arteritis, but the author shares with others[1] a more generic usage that includes both temporal arteritis and nonspecific aortoarteritis (Takayasu's disease). The histology of each is identical in the acute phase, and both have as major manifestations the insidious development of occlusive disease of limb, carotid, visceral, and renal arteries, and inflammation, aneurysm, or dissection of the thoracic and abdominal aortas. They also share angiographic, laboratory, and systemic features. However, Takayasu's disease occurs predominantly in females under 50 years of age, whereas temporal arteritis is rare under 50 years of age, and the female distribution is less.

Arterial lesions occur in all patients with Takayasu's arteritis; aortic involvement is almost universal, and branch vessel stenosis is universal, predominantly near their aortic takeoff. In contrast, occlusive extracranial arterial lesions occur in about 9 per cent of temporal arteritis patients; these are usually more peripheral, and the aorta is involved only occasionally. Of importance, steroids suppress systemic symptoms and can reverse or arrest arterial lesions in the acute phase of both diseases.[7–10] However, the aneurysmal and stenotic lesions of Takayasu's arteritis frequently require operative management, whereas surgery is indicated only occasionally in temporal arteritis.

Temporal Arteritis

The name *temporal arteritis* does not fully describe the disease as it is now understood, yet other names such as cranial, granulomatous, Horton's, or systemic giant cell arteritis also lack specificity or overlap with other conditions. The original term is preferred by the author because of its historical origin[11] and common use.

A careful population-based study defined the average annual incidence of temporal arteritis as 17.4 cases per 100,000 persons over 50 years of age.[12] This incidence increases with age: 1.4 times the average for ages 50 to 59, 10.7 times for ages 60 to 69, 29.6 times for ages 70 to 79, and 28.9 times for those over 80. Females predominate by ratios of 2 : 1 to 4 : 1.

Arterial Lesions

Arterial lesions of the limbs in temporal arteritis are clinically quite characteristic. An insidious, bilaterally symmetric stenosis or occlusion occurs at a steady pace over only 1 to 3 months, producing limb claudication and absent distal pulses. Tissue necrosis is rare and usually reflects trauma superimposed on advanced occlusive disease in the author's experience. Raynaud's phenomenon is noted on occasion. When treated during the acute phase with adequate steroids, the lesions clear or improve significantly. The most common site of arterial involvement is the subclavian-axillary-brachial system. Indeed, it is axiomatic that patients in this age group (over 50 years) who develop bilateral arm claudication over a few weeks have temporal arteritis (Fig. 16–1). The second most common pattern is bilateral involvement of the profunda and superficial femoral arteries, with similar clinical behavior (Fig. 16–2). Presentation with symptoms in both upper and lower extremities in stages or of the legs alone also occurs. On occasion,

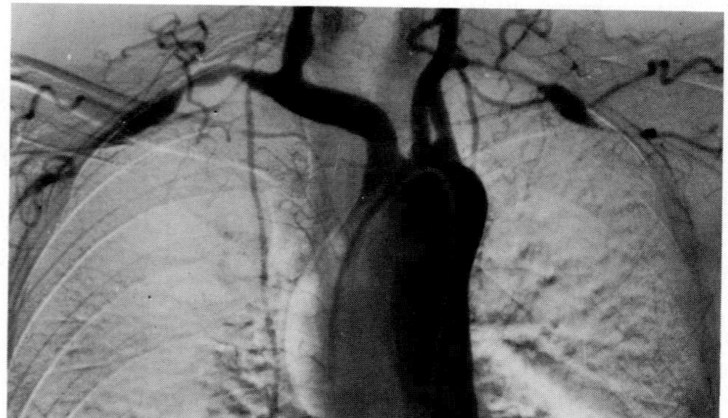

FIGURE 16–1. Focal tapered stenosis and post-stenotic dilatation in the axillary-subclavian system. This 67-year-old woman experienced 2 weeks of disabling occipital and neck pain; arm claudication was noted 15 weeks later. The erythrocyte sedimentation rate was 101 mm/hr. Blood pressure and pulses returned during the 10th week of steroid therapy.

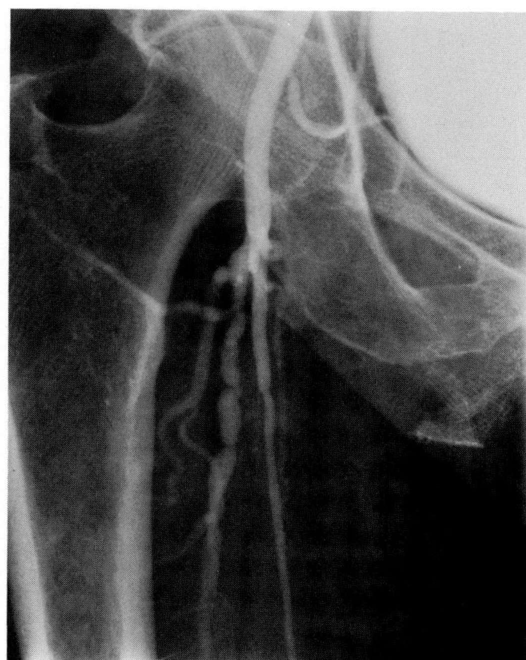

FIGURE 16–2. Arteritis of the right superficial and profunda femoral arteries. A similar lesion was seen on the left and in both subclavian arteries. This 65-year-old woman developed bilateral calf claudication following 2 months of malaise and arthralgias, and she subsequently developed bilateral arm claudication. Temporal artery biopsy results were positive. Steroid therapy restored pulses and full function in three limbs and improved the left leg.

additional focal lesions occur at the elbow and knee and in the arteries of the forearm and calf.[7, 12–14]

Rare sites of involvement include the celiac, superior mesenteric, iliac, renal, and coronary arteries. Myocardial infarction and death have been documented.[15] The common and internal carotid arteries, the latter chiefly in its petrous and cavernous portions, have shown modest, patchy lesions.[16] Extensive involvement of the vertebral artery to a point just above its dural entry can cause posterior circulation stroke from secondary thrombosis. A 12 per cent incidence of transient ischemic attack or stroke was noted in 166 cases of biopsy-proven temporal arteritis, 4 per cent involving events in the vertebrobasilar system and 8 per cent occurring in the carotid distribution.[17] Angiographic evidence of arteritis in the proximal portions of the anterior, middle, and posterior cerebral arteries has been documented.[18] Aneurysm of the ascending aorta, often with dissection and occasionally with aortic valve incompetence, and aneurysms of the proximal descending infrarenal abdominal aorta occur occasionally.[7, 15]

Angiographic Findings

Angiography demonstrates typical findings. Affected areas show multiple stenotic areas, almost always bilateral in paired arteries, often with post-stenotic dilatation (see Fig. 16–1). Stenotic segments may be short or long and tapering (Fig. 16–3). Occlusions occur at the end of a tapered area. The chronic nature of the occlusive process usually allows the development of generous collaterals, particularly in the upper extermity (Fig. 16–4). These same angiographic features are found in distal limb vessels involved with Takayasu's arteritis; the diagnosis is clarified by the difference in patient age and the associated proximal arterial and aortic lesions common to Takayasu's arteritis. Ergotism may also cause similar focal or long, tapered lesions. Proper inquiry about use of the drug and the absence of laboratory and clinical findings typical of arteritis establish the diagnosis.[19]

Clinical Picture

A typical case begins with a ''flu-like'' illness characterized by malaise, fever of 100 to 101°F, weight loss, scalp tenderness or headache, and myalgias, chiefly of the shoulder and hip girdles. After a period of 1 to 3 weeks, some of these symptoms may become quiescent or intensify. Tender, red, and elevated temporal or occipital arteries or disappearance of their pulse occurs in 45 to 60 per cent of patients. The girdle stiffness and pain may intensify (polymyalgia rheumatica) and dominate the symptoms. Jaw claudication develops in about two thirds of patients. Frank synovial reaction of wrist and knee joints occurs in a few. Major eye complications occur at about 3 months but may occur in a time span ranging from 3 days to 6 months after onset. These symptoms are predominantly unilateral or bilateral, partial or total blindness, amaurosis fugax, and on occasion, extraocular muscle dysfunction of sudden onset. These complications are explained by arteritis of the ophthalmic or posterior ciliary vessels and, to a lesser degree, by occlusion of the central retinal artery or vein.[16, 20] Large artery involvement, as delineated, occurs in about 9 per cent of patients at a median time of 8 months from onset (range, 0 to 84 months).[7] The untreated disease is self-limited to a course of 1 to 3 years and has a mortality of under 10 per cent,[21] with death caused by aortic dissection, aneurysm rupture, myocardial or cerebral infarction.[7, 15, 21] However, death and the significant morbidity of

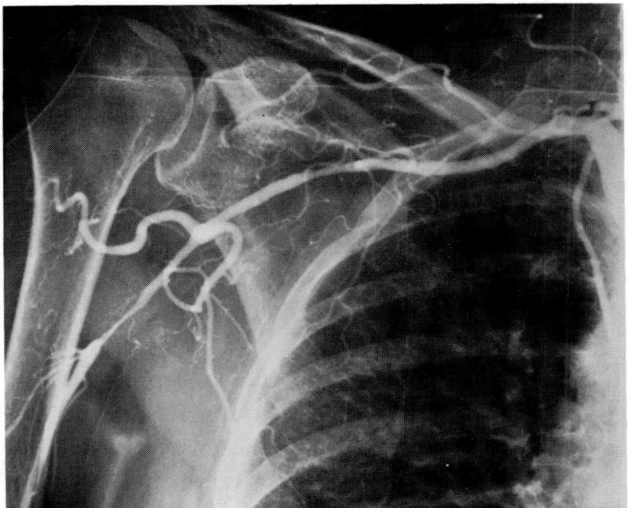

FIGURE 16–3. Multiple tapering stenosis and post-stenotic dilatation in the right brachial and axillary arteries. There is a similar distribution of lesions on the left. The temporal artery biopsy results were positive.

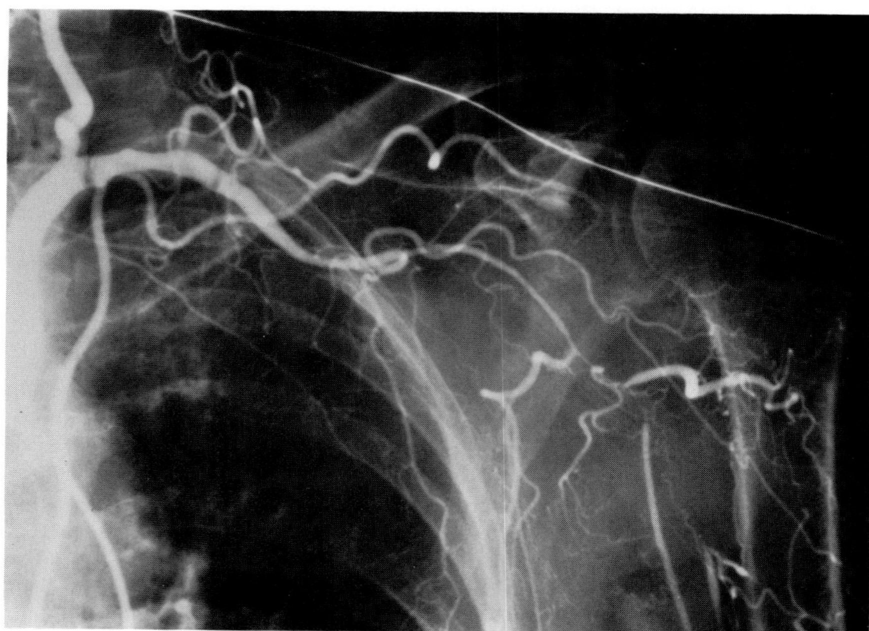

FIGURE 16–4. Long, tapering stenosis with terminal occlusion and well-developed collaterals. The right arm was also diseased but was not occluded. Pressure and pulses were normal on the right and improved on the left after steroid therapy.

the ocular and arterial complications can be prevented by adequate steroid therapy.[7, 20, 22]

Patients with such a typical course and an abnormal temporal artery are readily diagnosed. The usual tempo of the disease should allow early diagnosis and therapy, preventing the later ocular and vascular complications. However, the disease may be a diagnostic challenge. In rare instances the disease tempo is accelerated; blindness has been seen within 3 days,[17] and fatal aortic dissection has been noted within 2 weeks of onset.[7] Because the symptoms mimic other common illnesses and are scattered over several weeks time, correct correlation by patient or physician may not be made. Many older patients will not recall all events unless they and family members are carefully interrogated. Most noteworthy is the fact that any single feature of the syndrome may be so dominant that the presentation suggests obscure fever, occult malignancy, lymphoma, or various rheumatic diseases. Fevers of 103 to 104°F, shaking chills, drenching sweats, rapid loss of 20 to 30 pounds, and depression can contribute to the diagnostic problem.

Laboratory Findings

Elevation of the erythrocyte sedimentation rate (ESR) in the range of 40 to 140 mm/hr is characteristic of active temporal arteritis. A normal ESR rarely occurs, but one must be careful to exclude instances in which the ESR has been suppressed by anti-inflammatory agents given for the musculoskeletal or systemic symptoms.[23] Most patients have a mild normocytic anemia of about 11 gm/100 ml, though the levels may reach 7 to 9 gm/100 ml in some patients, and both mild hypochromic anemia and intravascular coagulopathy can occur. The leukocyte count and differential are normal in most patients, but in about a quarter of cases, leukocytosis of 10,000 to 19,000 is seen.[24] Mild thrombocytosis is not uncommon. Additional mild and nonspecific findings that clear promptly with treatment may include increase of alpha^2-globulin, transaminase elevation to one to two times normal, prothrombin time elevation of 1.2 to 1.5 times control, and elevation of alkaline phosphatase values to twice normal.[25]

Polymyalgia Rheumatica

Polymyalgia rheumatica is defined as a significant, often crippling pain and stiffness without local tenderness, involving the muscles of the neck, shoulder, and hip girdles in varying combinations. It has been present at least 1 month in patients over 50 years of age, is accompanied by a high ESR, and responds dramatically to steroids. Its incidence is almost four times that of temporal arteritis,[12, 26] yet it is a component of more than half of temporal arteritis cases.[5, 10] Although arteritis is not part of polymyalgia by definition, it is present silently in 5 to 40 per cent of such patients when routine biopsy of the temporal arteries is performed.[14, 27] The presence of arteritis is a critical question because high-dose steroids are essential to prevent ocular and arterial complications, whereas steroid complications can be minimal with the low-dose schedules that suffice to control uncomplicated polymyalgia.[26, 27] Of note, polymyalgia rheumatica on occasion may also be the prodrome of rheumatoid arthritis, periarteritis nodosa, systemic lupus erythematosus, occult infection, malignancy, and infectious endocarditis.[28]

Biopsy

The author advises biopsy in all cases of polymyalgia rheumatica in view of the preceding observations and because a palpably abnormal artery is found in only 45 to 60 per cent of biopsy-proven cases of temporal arteritis.[14, 29] Biopsy is also recommended when typically inflamed arteries are noted, to preclude the all too frequent late challenge of the initial diagnosis when steroid withdrawal causes confusing symptoms. Biopsy is performed with the patient under local anesthesia, and a 2- to 3-cm segment is adequate when the vessel is visibly diseased. As discussed, blind, diagnostic biopsy is often called for, and a generous 4- to 7-cm segment is advised. Also, multiple sections are examined because the pathology is often quite focal, with multiple, long skip areas. When such a biopsy specimen is negative, a similar contralateral biopsy is helpful in 10 to 15 per cent of cases. Following these guidelines, temporal artery biopsy was 94 per cent predictive of the need for high-dose steroids in a carefully followed population.[29]

Therapy

A major achievement of steroid therapy is the rapid suppression of symptoms and the prevention of blindness. Once adequate steroids have been given, no further blindness is seen.[20–22] Because the time between onset of arteritis and visual loss may be as little as 3 days, and the interval between involvement of a second eye after damage to the first may be 1 to 7 days, the author considers temporal arteritis a medical emergency.[20] Once the diagnosis is suspected, blood samples are taken and steroids begun immediately. Biopsy is accomplished on subsequent days, and steroids are tapered if the biopsy is negative. It is noteworthy that the incidence of blindness of 40 to 50 per cent given in early reports has dropped to a range of 10 to 20 per cent, attributable to early diagnosis and effective therapy.[13, 20, 29]

In the author's protocol, 60 mg of prednisone in divided, twice daily doses is given for a week and is then reduced to 45 mg/day in divided doses for an additional month. Systemic symptoms are suppressed in 24 to 72 hours, and the ESR normalizes in 1 to 2 weeks. When pulse deficits are present, improvement in Doppler systolic pressures begins after 4 to 6 weeks. The dosage is subsequently reduced by 5-mg increments/day at 2- to 3-week intervals, and when a level of 15 mg/day is reached, further reductions of 1 mg/day are made at similar intervals. The clinical status and ESR are monitored at each dose change. Ten to 15 per cent of patients require therapy into a second or even a third year. All patients eventually are taken off steroids. Recrudescence of disease is treated by doubling the dosage for 3 to 4 weeks and assessing suppression by means of the ESR and the presence of symptoms. A no-added-salt diet is advised, and acid suppression is given when there is a past history of peptic disease or if dyspepsia develops during treatment. The anticipated steroid side effects are explained. A prospective, randomized trial of alternate-day steroid therapy showed reduction of steroid side effects but incomplete disease suppression. Daily dosage is advised.[13]

The need for surgery occurs occasionally. Indications include significant aortic valve incompetence, aneurysmal disease, aortic dissection, and those rare cases in which claudication remains limiting after adequate steroid therapy has been given.[30, 31] We have seen bypass grafts become occluded in two patients when placed during the active phase of arteritis.[32]

Periarteritis Nodosa

Periarteritis nodosa may be seen from childhood on but is most common in the 4th through 6th decades of life. Males predominate by a ratio of 2 : 1. Lesions are characteristically focal, with skip zones, and affect small and medium arteries of almost all organs. The sequence of damage is acute inflammation, necrosis, secondary thrombosis, and late fibrosis. About 20 per cent of patients develop small aneurysms of visceral, renal, and, rarely, distal limb vessels. Lesions in different stages of evolution in a given organ or artery are typical, in contrast to the uniform age of lesions seen in hypersensitivity angiitis.[1, 2, 6]

Presentation is usually an insidious progression of multiple accumulating manifestations, but on occasion it is fulminant with death occurring in days or weeks. Systemic symptoms of fever, malaise, and weight loss are common. Many combinations of organ involvement occur, and the more common include mononeuritis multiplex (60 to 70 per cent), renal disease (microhematuria, glomerulitis in 50 to 60 per cent), gastrointestinal problems (50 per cent), arthralgias (50 per cent), and hypertension (40 per cent). Less common manifestations include severe myalgia, stroke, rash, skin infarctions, and orchitis. Pulmonary infiltrates and nodules, hemoptysis, and pleurisy occur, but the incidence is modest when those cases better classified as Churg-Strauss granulomatosis are excluded. Pericarditis, myocarditis, and inflammation of the coronary arteries are often noted at autopsy but are usually clinically silent. Elevation of the sedimentation rate, mild anemia, and moderate leukocytosis are usual.[1–2, 33–35]

Raynaud's phenomenon occurs in a few patients. Digital arteritis that may progress to infarction, livedo vasculitis of the legs that often ulcerates, and arteriolar ulcerations occur in less than 5 per cent; steroids often suppress these lesions.[33, 34] The major surgical challenge in periarteritis nodosa is the gastrointestinal and renal circulations, where lesions of the secondary and tertiary branches of the visceral, renal, and hepatic arteries either cause occlusion or become aneurysmal.[34, 36–38] Occluded vessels result in cholecystitis, appendicitis, or most commonly, gut perforation, gastrointestinal hemorrhage, or ischemic obstruction. Technical problems with gut viability in this multi-focal disease often dictate second-look surgery.[36, 39] Aneurysmal lesions often rupture, causing intrahepatic, perinephric, and intraperitoneal hemorrhage of significant magnitude. It is to be noted that these aneurysms often regress with vigorous steroid and cyclophosphamide therapy, and they should be so treated when asymptomatic.[37, 40]

Steroid therapy has increased the 5-year survival from less than 15 per cent of untreated patients to over 50 per cent of those treated.[1, 2, 34, 37] Cyclophosphamide is a valuable adjunct in acute, severe cases.[31] Vasculitis of the kidneys and gastrointestinal tract is the prime cause of mortality in the acute phase, and cardiovascular and cerebral events in long-standing cases, often from severe hypertension.[34]

Systemic Lupus Erythematosus

Systemic lupus erythematosus (SLE) is best considered an autoimmune disease that deposits damaging biologic substances via the microcirculation to specific tissues. Antibodies to DNA and other cellular components have been clearly identified.[1, 2] The resulting disease occurs chiefly in women in the 2nd through 4th decades of life. Multi-system manifestations such as arthritis, nephritis, pericarditis, pleuritis, cerebritis, lymphadenopathy, and hepatosplenomegaly occur in varying combinations. A characteristic facial rash occurs in 20 per cent. The sedimentation rate is significantly elevated, and leukopenia is common. The tempo may be smoldering, intermittent, or fulminant. A small subset of patients have additional findings suggesting periarteritis, scleroderma, or dermatomyositis, the so-called overlap syndromes. Antimalarial, nonsteroidal anti-inflammatory drugs, steroids, and both azothioprine and cyclophosphamide supplements can be effective in suppressing the disease, depending on its intensity.[1, 37]

Arteritis of small- and medium-sized vessels is an additional component of the basic mechanism in a significant number of patients. Major sites of vasculitis include the skin (livedo, nodules, infarcts); intestinal tract (ischemic perforation and hemorrhage of gut, pancreas, gallbladder, and appendix); and renal, pulmonary, and coronary circulations.

Although arteritis is not seen in larger vessels, the vascular surgeon may be the first to encounter certain cases. A circulating anticoagulant, or inhibitor, occurs in 5 to 10 per cent of cases, causing thrombosis of major arteries and veins, often as an early or even presenting event of SLE. Major thrombosis of the inferior vena cava and renal, retinal, and leg and arm veins, pulmonary embolism, and arterial thrombosis of the aortoiliac, femoral, axillary, carotid, cerebral, coronary, and retinal systems occur.[43–46] In a study of 205 patients with the lupus anticoagulant, 26 per cent experienced about equal numbers of arterial or venous thrombosis. The diathesis can be controlled by heparin and warfarin. The response of the circulating anticoagulant to steroids is unpredictable and slow: Anticoagulation is continued until the anticoagulant is suppressed.[46] Vascular surgery can be performed when indicated, under anticoagulant protection. Of note, hemorrhage is not a feature of the circulating anticoagulant. Further, this inhibitor is not specific to SLE nor diagnostic of it and can be seen primarily or in association with Behçet's disease, periarteritis, and other vasculitides.[43, 46]

Behçet's Disease

Recurrent aphthous ulcers of the mouth and genitalia, uveitis and recurrent hypopyon, and a variety of skin lesions including erythema nodosum, pustules, acne, and hypersensitivity to needle puncture are the major manifestations of this unusual disease. Additional lesions include nonerosive synovitis, recurrent meningoencephalitis, inflammatory bowel disease, and major arterial and venous problems. At least four schemes of criteria exist, each calling for various combinations of major or minor criteria to establish the diagnosis. And, except for aphthous lesions and ocular disease, there is disagreement about what constitutes major criteria. The disease is seen worldwide but occurs more commonly in Asian and Mediterranean countries. Blindness occurs in up to 25 per cent of patients with ocular involvement.[47, 48] The pathology is that of a vasculitis of both large and small arteries and veins. Immune complexes have been found in vessel walls. Cyclosporine, azathioprine, and chlorambucil have reduced the frequency of ocular attacks, and chlorambucil has shown benefit in treatment of meningoencephalitis. But these, and no other agents, including steroids, indomethacin, and colchicine, have been predictable in suppressing the disease completely.[49–51]

Major arterial and venous lesions occur in 6 to 25 per cent of cases and are the leading cause of death. Almost any superficial or deep vein can become thrombosed, including those of the legs, arms, and brain stem, and the axillosubclavian, hepatic, and portal veins, but most frequently the superior and inferior vena cava are affected, alone or together. Anticoagulation is effective in preventing further events, in the author's limited experience, but the duration of treatment is indeterminate and is guided by the quiescence of other manifestations of the disease.[52, 56]

Both focal arterial thrombosis and aneurysm formation can occur and may coexist in a given patient. Almost all named arteries have been involved in either process. The aneurysms are usually sacular and are often multiple.[47–48, 52–53, 56] Pulmonary arteries are often aneurysmal and can cause fatal hemoptysis with rupture.[54–55]

Tissue analysis has uniformly reported intimal hyperplasia, fragmentation of the internal elastic membrane, adventitial plasmacytosis, and infiltrates of the vasa vasorum. The lesions are random and focal. Bypass grafts or interposition grafts have been successful when they are sutured into healthy tissue. Anastomotic aneurysms and thromboses are not infrequent, however. Further, false aneurysm formation at sites of catheterization and needle puncture is a hazard.[51–53, 57–58] It has not been shown whether the medical agents listed suppress the vascular manifestations of Behçet's disease.

Kawasaki's Disease (Mucocutaneous Lymph Node Syndrome)

This unique syndrome of unknown origin affects chiefly infants in the 1st year of life, small children, and rarely, a few beyond 9 years of age. More than 63,000 patients had been diagnosed in Japan by 1984, after the first description by Kawasaki appeared in 1967.[59–60] Significant endemic groups have been studied in other parts of Asia, Europe, and North America. The illness begins with a week or more of high spiking fever, followed by conjunctivitis, truncal erythema, cricopharyngeal edema, cervical adenopathy, and erythema of the soles and palms. In the second phase, arthralgias, dry and cracking lips, and desquamation of involved skin occur. Laboratory findings are not specific and include mild anemia, neutrophilia, high ESR, and often marked thrombocytosis. Aseptic meningitis, hepatitis, pleurisy, and diarrhea may occur.[59]

The disease is self-limited, but about 0.5 per cent of patients die in the acute phase of an intense vasculitis, which has a distribution in the small and medium-sized arteries and veins indistinguishable from that of periarteritis nodosa.[61] However, the most common lethal lesions are multiple coronary artery aneurysms that become thrombosed or rupture. The incidence of coronary aneurysm formation is about 15 per cent;[62] it occurs usually in the 1st month but sometimes 6 to 48 months later. Echocardiography in the 1st month is highly sensitive in recognizing aneurysm formation.[63] No specific treatment has been identified. Aspirin suppresses systemic symptoms but has not been proved to reduce the vasculitis, and steroids may be life-saving for patients with myocarditis and shock but have failed to reduce the incidence of coronary artery stenosis and aneurysm.[64] However, studies have documented that high-dose gamma globulin given intravenously in the acute phase has had a significant impact on the occurrence of coronary disease.[66–67] Coronary artery angiography and surgery are fully incorporated into management.[61, 65] Spontaneous regression of aneurysms as well as late coronary occlusion occurs.[68]

Aneurysms of the abdominal aorta and brachial, axillary, iliac, renal, hepatic, and mesenteric arteries have been observed as occasional late sequelae, and when symptomatic or expanding, they can be successfully operated on using standard techniques of end-to-end anastomosis or saphenous interposition grafting.[65, 69–70] Just what the late incidence of arterial aneurysms will be, or whether acute-phase gamma globulin will minimize this risk, is still unknown.

Rheumatoid Disease With Vasculitis

A noninflammatory endarteritis may occur in patients with rheumatoid arthritis and may cause Raynaud's phenomenon, periungual infarcts, digital pad ulcers, or gangrene. In addition, an active vasculitis indistinguishable from periarteritis nodosa may be seen with rheumatoid arthritis, causing extensive digital gangrene, arteriolar ulcers of the legs, and mesenteric ischemic or bowel infarction. The syndrome occurs late in the course of rheumatoid arthritis, when patients have advanced joint changes, cutaneous nodules, positive antinuclear antibody test results, and high rheumatoid titers.[71–72] High-dose steroids often help such patients, unless mononeuritis is present.[73] Cyclophosphamide can be a valuable adjunct to steroids.[74] Gastrointestinal vascular catastrophies and renal disease are the usual terminal events.[73]

A small percentage of patients with rheumatoid arthritis, ankylosing spondylitis, Reiter's syndrome, juvenile rheumatoid arthritis, and the arthritis of inflammatory bowel disease may develop a proximal aortitis causing aneurysm of the ascending aorta or aortic valve incompetence. This is a late event in these diseases. Aneurysm of the descending and thoracoabdominal aorta has also been noted. The lesions can be surgically approached.[75–79] The role of adjunctive steroids is not clear.

Relapsing Polychondritis

Relapsing polychondritis, a rare disease, is easily diagnosed from a cluster of readily apparent defects. But all too often associated vascular problems that are a major source of mortality are overlooked, and an opportunity for corrective surgery is lost.[80–81]

Presentation is characterized by several major findings, all of which are at or exceed the 50th percentile in major reviews: auricular chondritis, nasal chondritis, respiratory tract chondritis, seronegative polyarthritis, ocular inflammation (episcleritis, conjunctivitis, uveitis), and audiovestibular damage. Malaise and fever are common, and the ESR is markedly elevated in most patients. Age of onset ranges from 13 to 84 years with a median of 51 years, and the sex ratio is about equal.[82]

Aneurysms of the ascending, descending, thoracoabdominal, or infrarenal aorta occur in about 10 per cent of cases. Aortic valve incompetence or dissection are frequent with ascending aortic aneurysms. All of the listed lesions have been successfully operated on, once identified.[80, 81] It can be asked whether regular screening of aortic lesions is justified. Tissue changes in the aorta include an increased level of collagen in the media, lymphocytic reaction of the adventitia, a decrease in mucopolysaccharide content, and inflammatory cells around the vasa vasorum.[80–82]

Further, other forms of vasculitis overlap with relapsing polychondritis in 20 to 30 per cent of cases. These include periarteritis, SLE, discoid lupus, Behçet's disease, and Reiter's syndrome; several of these are responsive to medical therapy.[82, 83]

Michet reports 5- and 10-year survival probabilities from the time of diagnosis as 74 per cent and 55 per cent, respectively. Of 41 deaths in 112 patients followed, 7 resulted from vasculitis and 5 resulted from cardiovascular pathology.[82] Steroids, aspirin, dapsone, and other agents suppress many manifestations of relapsing polychondritis, but it is not clear from the small populations described whether any agent prevents aortic damage.

CONGENITAL DISEASES WITH ARTERIAL INVOLVEMENT

These diverse disorders, each with multi-faceted presentations, are fortunately rare. However, dramatic and often devastating cardiovascular complications of spontaneous rupture, dissection, and aneurysm formation in the aorta and its major branches, and occlusive disease of the distal arteries are major components of these disorders. These vascular events occur in a young population, in the 2nd through 5th decades, but the age spectrum ranges from childhood through the 70s, depending on the intensity of expressivity of a specific deficit in a given patient.

Several of the diseases discussed are not only congenital but also hereditary. These include Marfan's syndrome, Ehlers-Danlos syndrome, pseudoxanthoma elasticum, homocystinurea, neurofibromatosis, and tuberous sclerosis. The genetic behavior of these diseases is well understood and detailed. Specific knowledge of their cellular and molecular deficits continues to emerge.[84–88]

Other well-defined arterial lesions that are congenital but not hereditary include cystic disease of the popliteal and femoral arteries (Chapter 60); popliteal artery entrapment syndromes (Chapter 61); thoracic outlet arterial compression, most often caused by congenital osseous and sometimes ligamentous abnormalities (Chapter 70); aortic coarctation; and persistent sciatic artery.

Marfan's Syndrome

Marfan's syndrome is characterized by an autosomal dominant defect in the cross-linking of collagen, caused by mutations of type I procollagen or its processing enzymes.[86–88] About 15 per cent of cases are de novo mutants. Defects in elastin have also been described, and studies have identified a mutation of the fibrillin gene on chromosone 15 as the cause of the syndrome.[89] At autopsy, tissue changes are confined to the ascending aorta, which is thickened but weakened, and show irregular muscle bundle patterns, increased collagen, decreased elastin, and sometimes vacuoles in the media.[84]

The diagnosis is clinical and is based on combinations of musculoskeletal, ocular, and hereditary features, all exceeding the 80th percentile in incidence, and the cardiovascular findings that occur in 95 per cent of patients.[84–91] Musculoskeletal abnormalities are multiple, but the most important involve limb length and proportions. Most but not all patients are tall, and critical measurements show that the arm span exceeds height and that upper segment length (pubes to crown) is 0.86 or less than lower segment length. The distal limbs are more affected, resulting in arachnodactyly. Body habitus changes of lesser specificity but considerable frequency include kyphoscoliosis, pectus carinatum and excavatum, genu recurvatum, pes planus, and hypermobile joints; recurrent patellar and hip dislocations; hernias, reduced body fat; and muscular hypotonia. At least 80 per cent of patients have ectopic lenses, sometimes requiring slit-lamp examination to identify; redundant or broken suspensory ligaments are the cause. Significant myopia is common, and spontaneous retinal detachment occurs in some.[84–91]

Mitral valve prolapse, ascending aortic aneurysm and dissection, and aortic valve incompetence are major cardiovascular manifestations. Mitral valve prolapse occurs in over 90 per cent of cases; it may be diagnosed only by echocardiography but is rarely florid enough to cause congestive heart failure and warrant repair. Aneurysms of the ascending aorta occur in at least 80 per cent of patients. The syndrome causes aortic valve incompetence in many, leading to congestive heart failure, and on occasion produces angina pectoris. Dissection in these aneurysms is the major cause of death in patients with Marfan's syndrome. Sometimes aneurysm formation is confined to the sinuses of Valsalva, where rupture and cardiac or pulmonary fistulae can follow. There have been a few documented cases of abdominal aortic aneurysm, both with and without involvement of the ascending aorta. Bacterial endocarditis may occur on the damaged valves. The average life expectancy of the patient with Marfan's syndrome is the mid-40s, and these cardiovascular dysfunctions cause most deaths. Fatalities have been recorded in the first 2 years of life, and a few patients survive past age 70 years.[84–91]

Initial diagnosis and management of the acute or chronic complications of aortic dissections and perhaps prophylaxis of Marfan's syndrome can involve the cardiovascular surgeon. Dissection is typically a major event with severe chest or abdominal pain, sometimes with shock, aortic branch vessel deficits, and findings of altered mediastinal or tracheal anatomy on chest x-ray. Branch vessel involvement may consist merely of reduced or absent pulses, but in a third of cases it is manifest by significant target organ dysfunction such as stroke, visceral or limb ischemia, accelerated hypertension, and occasionally myocardial ischemia.

However, dissection of the aorta may occur without recent diagnostic pain, or the sequence of events can be obscured by a cerebral deficit. Under these circumstances, dissection may first be diagnosed at the time of angiography or even surgery for ischemia of the brain, limbs, viscera, or kidney. At this juncture, the cardiovascular surgeon must determine whether a local repair is essential and can be effective and then direct medical or surgical efforts toward the primary tear to enhance survival.

In dissection of the ascending aorta, a common event in Marfan's patients, resection and graft of the primary site usually restore flow to the occluded limb vessels, and the need for direct revascularization or aortic fenestration is rare.[92–93] Focal stroke does not contraindicate life-protecting primary repair of the ascending aorta.[93–94] Visceral and partial renal ischemia may also improve when repair is prompt. Although rare in Marfan's syndrome patients, dissection of the descending aorta is problematic. In many hands, medical therapy has equaled or bettered the survival of primary surgical repairs.[94] However, residual limb and partial visceral or renal ischemia may require urgent fenestration or a bypass procedure. Salvage of a limb is reasonable, but mortality from visceral and renal ischemia is very high with this combined approach. For these reasons and to eliminate the basic danger of aortic rupture, primary descending aortic repair is preferred by other physicians.[92–93] In patients with chronic dissection, significant aortoiliac and descending aortic aneurysms and renovascular lesions warrant repair. Renovascular lesions may respond to revascularization or reimplantation, but nephrectomy may be required.[94–95]

In patients with Marfan's syndrome, there is evidence that beta-blockers started before aortic incompetence develops can retard the incompetence and aneurysm growth,[96] and that the incidence of fatal dissection is reduced by elective replacement of the aortic valve and ascending aorta when the transverse diameter exceeds 6 cm.[97]

Ehlers-Danlos Syndrome

The clinical features of Ehlers-Danlos syndrome (ED) as commonly described include joint laxity with a potential for recurrent effusions and dislocation; hyperextensible skin; and fragility of the skin that allows wide splitting or gross ecchymosis, producing "cigarette paper" scars after minor trauma. Fragility of the ocular globe, kyphoscoliosis, a tendency toward spontaneous rupture or large diverticuli of the gut, and, finally, catasrophic arterial complications in about 4 per cent of patients are additional uncommon components.[84–85, 98–99]

Accumulating observations, however, have defined eight and probably ten clinical types of ED, each with one or more features predominating.[88] Further, current knowledge of the genetics and biochemistry of collagen formation has delineated at least nine faults in gene formation or in the multiple enzymatic sequences that convert procollagen to collagen. These specific molecular defects now explain a few, but not all, of the variants of ED. Continued use of the clinical classification of ED, types I to X, remains appropriate until definitive biochemical data allow a complete etiologic nosology. ED is an autosomal dominant disorder, and an X-linked variant has been identified.[85–86]

Type I ED has varying combinations of the classic

skin and joint findings, a modest incidence of mitral valve prolapse, and occasional dilatation of the sinuses of Valsalva. The same lesions are randomly reported in all other types; the actual incidence awaits prospective, noninvasive screening of these small groups of patients over a prolonged period of time. Of note, an instance of aortic rupture has occurred in type VI ED, the ocular-scoliotic variant.[85]

Major arterial defects are the dominant findings in type IV ED, representing about 4 per cent of all ED patients.[99] At least three molecular defects in the formation of collagen III have been defined, but there have still not been clearly correlated with specific arterial syndromes.[88] In type IV of the syndrome, joint hypermobility may be absent or mild and may be confined to the fingers when present. Skin hyperelasticity is also minimal or absent, although translucent, thin truncal skin and premature aging of the facial and hand skin are typical when this sign is present. Easy, extensive bruisability from minor trauma is common, and type IV ED is often called the arterial-ecchymotic type.[84–85, 99]

Spontaneous arterial rupture, multiple aneurysms, and dissection of the aorta and arteriovenous fistulae result from a diffuse thinning of the media with reduced elastin and fragmented internal elastic membranes (Fig. 16–5).[85] An excellent report of five families and a careful literature review have summarized the vascular findings. Spontaneous hemorrhage occurred 38 times in the 36 patients analyzed, chiefly in the aorta and visceral, carotid, and calf arteries, but also in the iliac, femoral, and subclavian-axillary arteries, and occasionally in the coronary arteries. Twenty-nine aneurysms (including aortic dissection) were found in 15 patients at all the listed sites except the femoropopiteal segment; visceral, carotid, and aortic lesions were most frequent. Eight instances of arteriovenous fistulae, 5 at the carotid-cavernous site, were noted.[98]

These 36 patients underwent 29 vascular operations: ligation of 15 bleeding vessels, 5 aneurysms, and 4 carotid-cavernous fistulae, 1 thrombectomy, and 4 bypass procedures, only 1 of which was successful.[98] Other successful aortic grafts have been reported.[100–101] There were 7 surgical deaths, and 21 deaths were attributed to hemorrhage. Arteriography, performed in 12 patients, was complicated by significant hematoma 5 times, 1 femoral artery occlusion, and 2 deaths from bleeding.[98] Thus, the intrinsic arterial fragility of type IV ED frustrates both diagnostic and surgical efforts.[98]

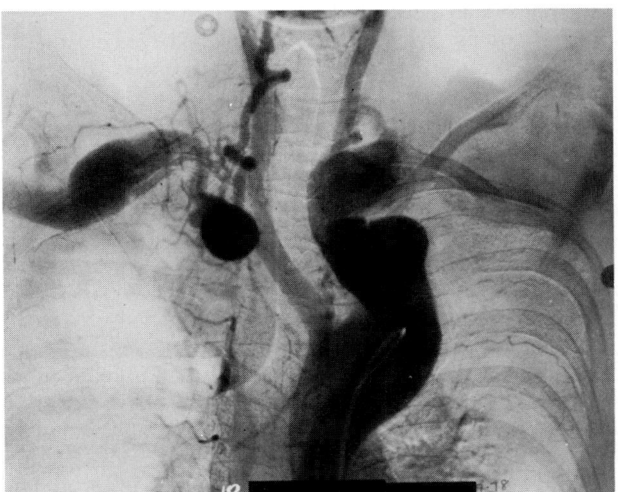

FIGURE 16–5. Bizarre, extensive ectasia and aneurysmal changes of the subclavian arteries. The patient was a 36-year-old woman with the long limbs, kyphoscoliosis, hyperelastic skin, and extensible joints typical of Ehlers-Danlos syndrome. There was lesser degree of ectasia and aneurysm formation of the ascending and thoracoabdominal aorta and the iliac and superior mesenteric arteries. Sudden death from dissection of the ascending aorta occurred 1 year later.

Ligation is the procedure of choice, when feasible, and reconstruction can be offered when essential only with due cautions to the patient; reinforcement of sutures and ligation sites is essential.[102] The use of intravenous digital subtraction angiography, computed tomography, and magnetic resonance imaging is preferred to direct, cautious angiography when possible. Specific therapy of the enzmatic defects is not to be expected. Genetic counseling and regular follow-up are of paramount importance for those affected.

Pseudoxanthoma Elasticum

Pseudoxanthoma elasticum (PXE) is the least common of these disorders, and the need for vascular surgery is rare. It is an autosomal recessive disorder, differing from ED in that the primary defect is in elastin rather than in collagen. The constellation of signs includes cutaneous, ocular, and cardiovascular manifestations and a significant incidence of upper intestinal and uterine hemorrhage. Diagnosis is made in patients in the 4th through 6th decades of life usually, but the disease can be apparent before age 10.[84, 103–105] Although the disorder predominates in females in most reports, this may reflect a concern with cosmetic signs because it prevails in males when no skin lesion is present.[103]

Ninety per cent or more of patients have the characteristic skin lesion or angioid retinal streaks, and all have one of the cardinal findings. Elevated plaques similar to xanthomas develop in the folds of the neck and axillae and to the lesser extent in those of the groin, cubital, popliteal, submammary, and umbilical areas. Reticulations and lax, redundant folds develop in time (Fig. 16–6). Biopsy findings are specific and demonstrate varying degrees of fragmentation and clumping of elastin.[84, 103–105] Angioid streaks are dark brown or red channels, usually wider than retinal vessels, that surround and radiate from the optic disc. They represent fractures in Bruch's membrane and may proceed to focal hemorrhages with late chorioretinal scarring and varying degrees of central blindness, usually bilateral. (Note: Angioid streaks also occur with Paget's disease of bone, sickle cell anemia, and hyperphosphatemia.) Upper intestinal hemorrhage occurs in up to one third of patients and is associated with marked thinning of vessels in the gastric mucosa and submucosa, and 7 of 11 women in another PXE population experienced significant uterine bleeding, leading to hysterectomy in 6.[105]

Cardiovascular problems of PXE include occlusive peripheral arterial disease, coronary occlusive disease, atrial subendocardiofibrosis, and renovascular hypertension.[103–105] Fifteen per cent to as much as 50 per cent of patients experience angina, and a few infarcts are seen in patients at an average age of 38 years and occasionally in the teens. Diffuse coronary calcification and triple vessel disease are common, and surgery has been successfully accomplished.

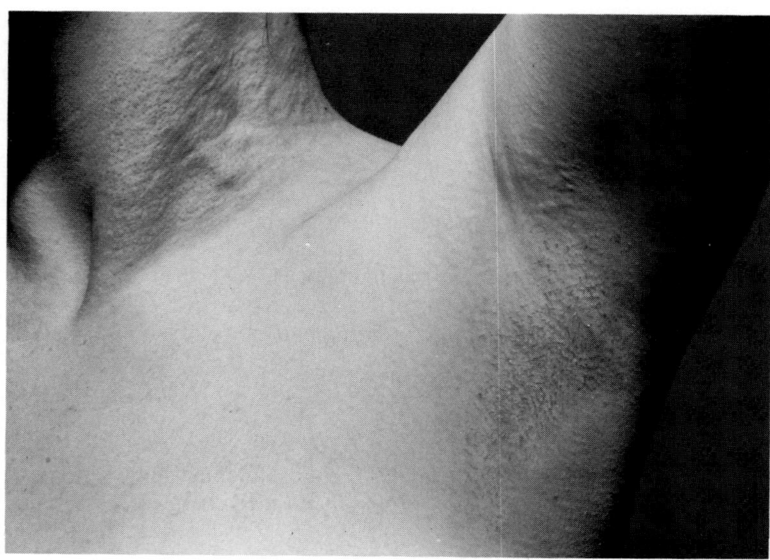

FIGURE 16–6. Soft, chamois-colored papules with the linear and reticular pattern typical of pseudoxanthoma elasticum seen in the neck and axillary folds of a 30-year-old woman. Similar lesions were seen across the popliteal spaces and in the groin folds. Angioid streaks in the retina were noted. The left radial and right posterior tibial pulses were not palpable. No arterial symptoms were noted. Angiography was not performed.

The renal lesion is noted in intrarenal arteries, and most attribute stroke in patients with PXE to long-standing hypertension.[105]

Reduced or absent limb pulses and premature arterial calcification have been noted in PXE for almost a century and have an incidence of 15 to 50 per cent, depending perhaps on attention to vascular assessment. The distal third of the radial and ulnar vessels is the most common site with preservation of the interosseous artery. Less common locations include the tibioperoneal, celiac, popliteal, and superficial femoral arteries. Contemporary studies utilizing noninvasive testing with exercise would be useful to define more fully the extent of peripheral arterial involvement.* Leg claudication is common, but ischemia of the hand or foot is rare. Of note, the aorta and its primary branches are spared.[103–106]

Standard techniques of reconstructive surgery can be successfully employed when indicated for rest pain, ischemic ulceration, or advanced claudication.[107] Patients presenting with modest claudication warrant regular follow-up to detect the coronary artery disease that develops with significant frequency.

Homocystinurea

Homocystinurea is a autosomal recessive error of methionine metabolism caused by a deficiency of cystathionine synthetase, homocysteine methyltransferase, or other enzymes, which allows homocystine to accumulate in body tissues and fluids. Patients early in life have a high degree of ocular defects (ectopic lens, acute glaucoma, retinal detachment, and cataract), mental retardation of varying degrees in up to 40 per cent of patients, and skeletal defects similar to those seen in Marfan's syndrome. In addition, accelerated fibrous arteriosclerosis causing arterial occlusive disease in the first 3 decades of life occurs, complicated by a propensity for acute thrombotic events in the arterial and venous systems. These are almost equally divided among acute venous thrombosis, peripheral occlusions, myocardial infarction, and stroke, and there is a significant incidence of premature death due to pulmonary embolism, myocardial infarction, and stroke.[108–112] Of importance, the defect can be corrected by administering cofactors such as pyridoxine, folate, and cobalamin in up to one half of this population, retarding subsequent progression of disease.[112, 114]

Increased levels of plasma homocysteine have been noted in patients with premature occlusive disease of the heart, brain, and peripheral systems, particularly after methionine loading. Ongoing studies suggest that plasma homocystine levels may be an independent risk factor for vascular disease. At present, testing has not consistently demonstrated a clear separation of the obligate heterozygote homocystinuric from a control population. Research remains active to ascertain whether homocystine is indeed a separate risk factor or a byproduct of the atherosclerotic process.[112–114]

Neurofibromatosis

Neurofibromatosis I is an autosomal dominant defect linked to chromosome 17 expressed in a broad mosaic of clinical patterns involving the skin and eye almost universally, the brain and spinal cord in up to half of the patients, and with occasional but distinctive involvement of the long bones by dysplasia and of major arteries by stenotic lesions and sometimes aneurysm formation. Cutaneous lesions may be subtle or extensive and include café-au-lait spots (six or more), neurofibromas, hypo- or hyperpigmentation, and freckling in the axillary or groin region. Small hamartomas are detected by magnetic resonance imaging of the brain in almost 50 per cent of patients, and cerebral neurofibromas,

---

**Editor's note:* This traditionally accepted distribution of lesions in PXE is, to a degree, based on angiographic follow-up of symptoms and pulse deficits. Routine screening of a large cohort of PXE patients by noninvasive methods (segmental limb pressures and plethysmography) indicates that partially occlusive and lower extremity lesions, especially of the femoropopliteal segment, are more common than has been realized and may even be more common than the more obvious, totally occlusive lesions of the distal upper extremity arteries (unpublished data).

optic gliomas, and both paraspinal and intradural neurofibromas and astrocytomas occur in 2 to 14 per cent of patients.[115]

The incidence of vascular involvement is unknown, but an evolving appreciation of arterial lesions is manifest by increasing case reports. The most frequently documented lesion is tubular coarctation of the pararenal aorta and proximal stenosis of the renal arteries, usually in combination but occasionally independent. Patients present in their 2nd or 3rd decades of life with significant hypertension and sometimes claudication. Aneurysm of the renal artery and its branches may occur. When available, tissue may show only intimal proliferation, but more commonly neurogenic cells are found in the media and adventia. Standard bypass procedures are effective.[116] Stenotic and aneurysmal lesions of the internal carotid and stenosis of the anterior and middle cerebral, superior mesenteric, and celiac arteries have also been reported.[117]

Tuberous Sclerosis

Tuberous sclerosis is an autosomal dominant defect characterized by multiple small angiofibromas involving almost any organ but chiefly the brain, face, and kidneys. It presents in the 1st decade of life with facial lesions, varying degrees of mental retardation, or seizures. Death can result from extensive replacement of the renal parenchyma and renal failure, malignant brain tumor, or rhabdomyoma of the heart with conduction disturbances, or from pneumonia and sepsis following status epilepticus.[118]

Aneurysm formation is a rare manifestation of the disease, which occurs from infancy through age 10. Less than a dozen such aneurysms have been reported, most in the infrarenal abdominal aorta. Prosthetic graft replacement has been successful and durable.[119–120] An axillary artery aneurysm has been associated with the disease,[121] and at the author's institution, a solitary ruptured thoracic aneurysm occurred in a series of more than 350 patients.[118] An abdominal aneurysm has been successfully repaired (Fig. 16–7).

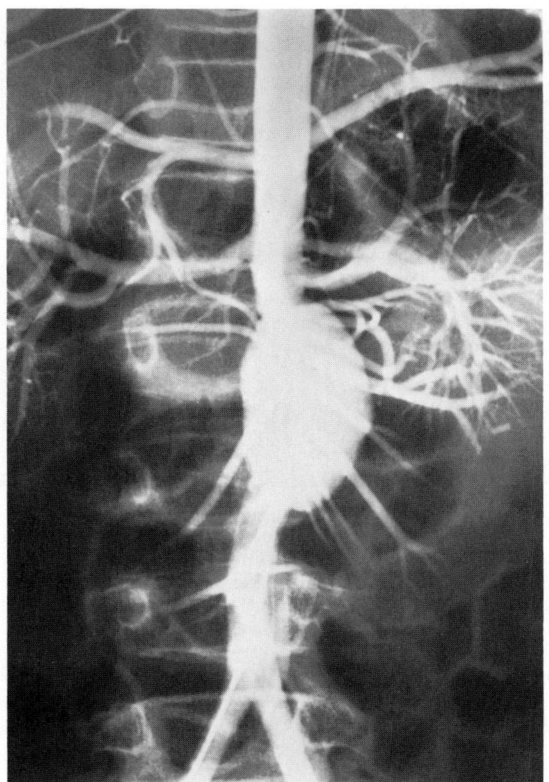

FIGURE 16–7. A 3-cm abdominal aortic aneurysm in a 9-year-old girl with tuberous sclerosis. The aneurysm was discovered during ultrasound imaging for assessment of a ventriculoperitoneal shunt placed because of recurrent astrocytoma. The aorta distal to the lesion measures 0.9 cm. The aneurysm was treated by conventional tube graft repair.

Most aneurysms of childhood are secondary to infection following umbilical artery catheterization.[119] Kawasaki's disease and nonspecific aortoarteritis are other causes of childhood aneurysms. Aneurysms caused by heritable connective tissue disorders and neurofibromatosis express themselves during the 2nd decade of life and often later.

Coarctation of the Abdominal Aorta

Abdominal aortic coarctation or hypoplasia is a nonhereditary lesion that is seen randomly and makes up only 0.5 to 2 per cent of all coarctations. The stenosis may be quite focal or may involve the entire intra-abdominal aorta. Most lesions occur above or at the level of the renal arteries. The proximal renal arteries are involved in about 80 per cent of cases, and the celiac and superior mesenteric arteries are affected on occasion (Fig. 16–8). Lesions are commonly detected in the 2nd or 3rd decade of life because of hypertension or claudication.[122–124] Hypertension is caused by activation of the renin-angiotension system.[123–124] Physical examination may show hypertension, an abdominal bruit, reduced or delayed femoral pulses, and sometimes palpable collateral arteries on the abdominal wall. Like patients with classic thoracic aortic coarctation, these patients are subject to cerebral vascular accidents, coronary disease, and congestive heart failure in their 3rd and 4th decades if control of hypertension is not timely.[123]

Repair follows established surgical principles. Depending on the extent of the lesion, hypertension can be treated by aortorenal bypass, splenorenal or hepatorenal shunts, reimplantation of the kidney, or nephrectomy, with or without aortic replacement as required by hypertension or claudication. The durability of autogenous vein or hypogastric artery grafts makes them preferable to prosthetic bypass to the renal arteries in these youthful patients. Staging of renal and aortic procedures is sometimes a prudent choice.[124]

Abdominal coarctation (the ''midaortic syndrome'') may also be associated with neurofibromatosis, radiation therapy (Fig. 16–9), focal atherosclerosis of the thoracic or abdominal aorta (all discussed in this chapter), and nonspecific aortoarteritis (see Chapter 12).

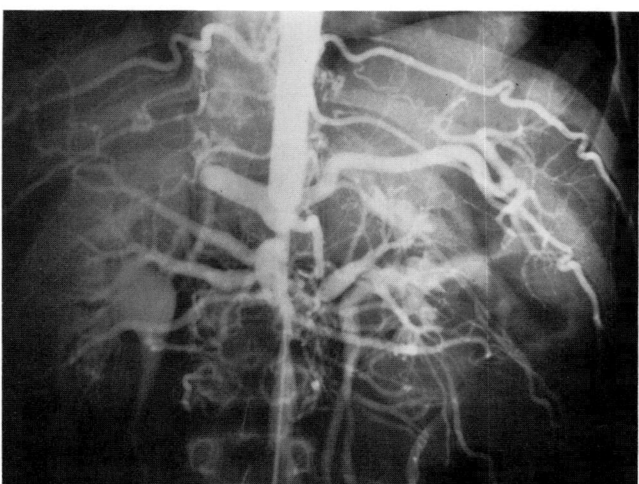

FIGURE 16–8. Multiple congenital stenoses of the abdominal aorta, the celiac and superior mesenteric arteries, two right renal arteries, and one left renal artery. When seen at age 11, this boy had reduced and delayed femoral and distal pulses bilaterally, claudication, and accelerated hypertension with serial values of 160–170/115–120 mmHg. Aortoaortic, renal, hepatic, and superior mesenteric Dacron bypass grafting were performed. The patient was normotensive and well at age 26, and all grafts were patent. Note the enlarged intercostal arteries that contributed to palpable collateral arteries for the legs.

Persistent Sciatic Artery

Persistence of the sciatic artery (axial artery) is rare, with less than a hundred reported cases and a prevalence of 0.25 per 1000 patients studied by angiography.[125] Knowledge of the lesion is important because it provides both a diagnostic and a therapeutic challenge. During early embryonic development, the femoral plexus is supplied both ventrally by the internal iliac (later to evolve into the femoropopliteal system) and dorsally by the axial artery, which later normally regresses to become the gluteal (sciatic) artery. In the complete form of this syndrome, the large embryonic sciatic vessel communicates directly with the popliteal artery, with or without an intact femoropopliteal vessel. In its incomplete form, the anomalous artery may terminate anywhere in the pelvis or thigh. Pillet and colleagues have provided a useful classification of the various variations.[126] An apparent paradox is created when the femoral pulse is absent, yet distal pulses are full, supplied by the persistent sciatic artery, entering the leg deeply through the sciatic notch; this is known as *Cowie's sign.*[127–128]

The syndrome is usually diagnosed at 50 years of age but may be noted throughout life. Sex distribution is almost equal, and the lesions are bilateral in a third of cases. More than a third of these lesions are noted incidental to angiographic or necropsy studies. Aneurysm formation, chiefly in the pelvic portion of the artery, accounts for most clinical signs. Manifestations include a pulsatile buttock mass, distal embolization, rupture, and compression of the sciatic nerve.[128] On occasion, aneurysm formation of an incomplete sciatic artery in the thigh may mimic a soft tissue tumor.[129]

Surgery is indicated for rupture and symptomatic aneurysms and those with ischemic complications. Both ligation and embolization are effective.[128, 130] Angiography of both legs is essential for diagnosis and surgical planning; bypass procedures must be added when the femoropopliteal system is not intact.

UNCOMMON ACQUIRED ARTERIOPATHIES

The generic categories of trauma, drugs, and occupational hazards are essential components of diagnostic logic, and their impact on the arterial system is detailed in Chapters 45 through 48 and 73. The microcirculation is subject to an additional diverse group of mechanisms that includes atheroembolism and environmental, hematologic, and immune processes, as delineated in Chapters 44 and 68. Four other uncommon problems warrant discussion.

Tumor

Only a few hundred primary vascular tumors have been recognized. Most are leiomyosarcomas and leiomyomas of the venous system, and only 20 per cent, numbering a few dozen cases, involve the arteries.[131–135] These are almost exclusively various sarcomas, including fibrosarcoma, myxosarcoma, fibroxanthoma, spindle and giant cell sarcoma, and leiomyosarcoma. Isolated instances of benign myxoma and fibromyxoma have been reported.[136] The sarcomas are located most commonly in the pulmonary arteries or any portion of the aorta, and occasionally in the femoral, popliteal, splenic, mesenteric, internal mammary, and other arteries.[133, 135] Local spread is usual, and metastases are common, chiefly to the skin, pleura, bones, lungs, adrenals, kidneys, liver, and spleen. Males are affected pre-

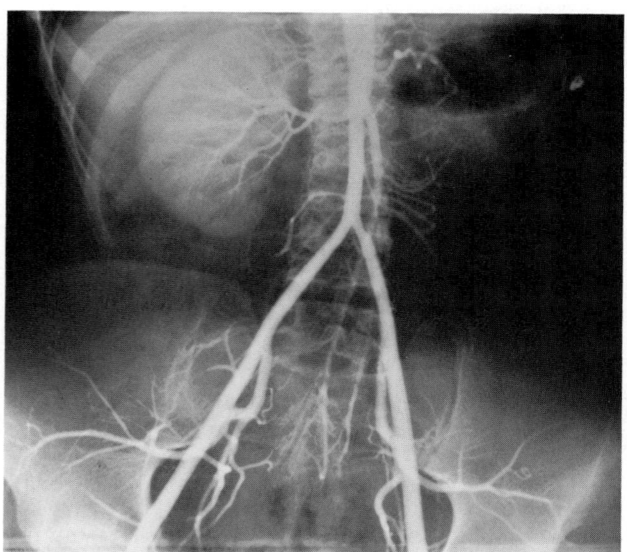

FIGURE 16–9. Hypoplastic abdominal aorta, solitary right renal artery, and splenic artery in a 24-year-old man given radiation therapy for left renal neuroblastoma at 6 months of age. The atrophic left kidney was removed and the patient's hypertension decreased at age 11. When seen at age 24, the patient described bilateral buttock, thigh, and calf claudication since age 6, and he had never run. He declined surgery and was normotensive and well at age 37 with antihypertensive drug therapy.

dominantly[133–135] in all except malignant fibrous histiocytoma,[132] and the diagnosis is usually made between the ages of 40 through 80 years.

Tumors may be intraluminal, intimal, or adventitial. Clinical presentation may be a mass found incidental to imaging or examination, claudication, acute ischemia from local thrombosis, distal embolization of tumor or thrombus, or a false aneurysm. Significant renovascular hypertension from aortic coarctation or renal artery involvement is not uncommon.[135]

Survival in all forms of sarcoma is usually measured in months, and recurrence is common after resection. Arterial repair is feasible for palliation. Aggressive adjunctive chemotherapy, currently evolving, offers hope of increased survival in selected cases.[132] The importance of careful histologic examination of resected material or emboli for identification of both primary tumors and those embolizing from other sources is self-evident.

Radiation

Massive radiation therapy from any source occasionally can cause early or late arterial lesions of clinical significance. These occur predominantly when the dosage has exceeded 5000 rads.[137–139] Radiation-induced arterial injury can be expressed many ways—acute thrombosis or arterial rupture in the early months of radiation arteritis, and later arterial fibrosis and stenosis, or accelerated local atherosclerosis 3 to 10 years following treatment.[137–138, 140–142]

Almost any artery can sustain damage. Presenting symptoms may include exsanguinating hemorrhage, acute carotid or peripheral arterial occlusion, claudication, transient ischemic attacks, stroke, and hypertension (see Fig. 16–9).[137, 139, 143]

Standard techniques of carotid endarterectomy and bypass as well as replacement or bypass of other arteries can be safely accomplished with some increased technical challenge from inflamed or fibrosed tissues.[139, 143] Of importance is a significant 25 per cent incidence of late graft infection in the area of prior radiation, which was recently reported. Successful reoperation was accomplished. This report recommended avoiding the radiated area, using autologous grafts when feasible, and performing regular surveillance of procedures performed in zones of radiation.[139]

Focal Calcific Aortic Obstruction

This unique localized manifestation of atherosclerosis causes significant obstruction of the abdominal or thoracic aorta and presents as advanced coarctation.[144–147] It is estimated to account for less than 1 per cent of operable aortic disease.[145] The lesion is only a few centimeters in length and consists of a heavily calcified thrombus that reduces the aortic lumen and produces a pressure gradient. The lesion is usually associated with other manifestations of atherosclerosis. Patients are more commonly female, almost always heavy smokers, and present from age 30 through 60 years. Both thoracic and abdominal calcific obstructive disease is easily overlooked when angiographic or ultrasound examination is used to assess more obvious pathology and is not extended to include these lesions.[146]

The abdominal form, often called ''coral reef'' atherosclerosis, predominates and is located in the celiac aorta, rarely in the infrarenal aorta. Renal and visceral artery stenosis may coexist, but the hemodynamics of the calcific lesion cause hypertension in almost all patients and claudication in most. Fatal acute thrombotic occlusion has been reported, but distal embolization is rare.[145] Thromboendarterectomy and occasionally bypass procedures eliminated the pressure gradient in 18 reported cases.[146]

Less than 10 cases of the thoracic form have been reported. The lesion is just distal to the left subclavian artery, and dense speckled calcification of the aortic knob is seen on chest roentgenograms or other images. Transesophageal echocardiography allows indirect measurement of the pressure gradient. These patients all present with severe hypertension and often with recurrent congestive heart failure or coronary events. Surgical resection and prosthetic replacement is the most common procedure and has been used in six reported cases with favorable results.[146] Severe calcification of the aortic arch and left subclavian artery may preclude this procedure, and successful bypass grafting was recently utilized at our institution.

Iliac Syndrome of Cyclists

An arterial lesion peculiar to competitive cyclists has been described and carefully analyzed.[148–149] A review of 23 cases is uniform in reporting clinical, angiographic, surgical, and pathology observations, defining a new entity. The cyclists had accumulated 50,000 to 150,000 km of high-level training and competition over several years, and symptoms began between the ages of 20 and 42. All complained of claudication, 21 characterizing it as buttock and thigh pain followed by numbness of the entire limb, and 2 as only heaviness and numbness. Symptoms occurred only under maximal stress such as ''hill climbing'' or sprinting, and quick relief was obtained as the pace was reduced. All but 1 of the patients were men, and only 1 patient had bilateral symptoms. Pulse and ankle systolic pressures were normal at rest but dropped when symptoms were reproduced by strenuous ergometric cycling. A lower quadrant bruit was noted at rest in 8 patients but only with the thigh flexed. Thus both history and examination are compatible with a subcritical stenosis that becomes hemodynamically significant only with maximal stress.[149]

Arteriography demonstrated modest narrowing of the midportion of the external iliac artery over 5 to 6 cm, with some lengthening and tortuosity when the thigh was flexed. At surgery, direct and angioscopic examination showed intimal hyperplasia confirmed by microscopy that was eccentrically located at the greatest curves produced in the artery by the cycling position. The stenoses were in the 40 to 60 per cent range. The authors explained the unilateral involvement by the observation that most cyclists have a dominant leg, confirmed by diameter measurements in some of the patients. All underwent segmental resection to shorten the artery, endarterectomy, and ligation of a prominent psoas arterial branch (felt to enhance iliac artery lengthening) when present. All patients returned to cycling.[149]

A solitary case in the author's experience (Fig. 16–10)

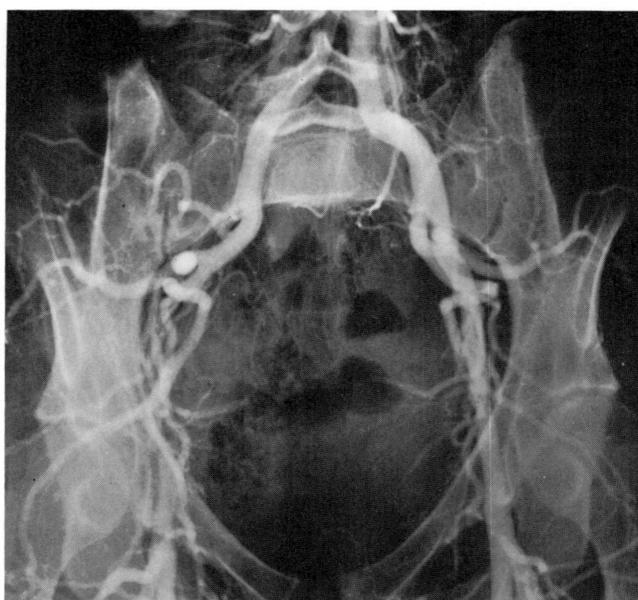

FIGURE 16–10. Complete occlusion of the right external iliac artery and remarkable collateral development in a 30-year-old woman. The patient, who was a high-level competitive cyclist for many years, experienced thigh and calf claudication during heavy workloads for 4 years and could identify an acute reduction in exercise capacity 6 months before diagnosis. Ten minutes on the treadmill at 4 mph and with a 15 per cent grade was required to duplicate her symptoms: ankle brachial indices were 0.71 at rest and 0.31 immediately after exercise. She was asymptomatic following bypass repair. Note, however, the early stenosis of the left external iliac artery, which became symptomatic at higher workloads after repair of the right.

differs in that complete thrombotic occlusion was superimposed on the basic lesion, and a contralateral lesion has become symptomatic since the initial repair.

References

1. Fauci AS, Haynes BF, Katz P: The spectrum of vasculitis: Clinical, pathologic, immunologic, and therapeutic considerations. Ann Intern Med 89:660, 1978.
2. Sheps SG, McDuffie FC: Vasculitis. *In* Juergens JL, Spittel JA, Fairbairn JF (eds): Peripheral Vascular Disease. Philadelphia, WB Saunders, 1980, p 493.
3. Hunder GG, Lie JT: The vasculitides. *In* Spittell JA Jr (ed): Clinical Vascular Disease. Philadelphia, FA Davis, 1983, p 261.
4. Paulus H, Kono D: Upper extremity manifestations of systemic vascular disorders. *In* Machleder HA (ed): Vascular Disorders of the Upper Extremity. Mount Kisco, NY, Future, 1989, p 305.
5. Churg A, Churg J: Systemic Vasculitides. New York, Igaku-Shoin, 1991.
6. Calabrese LH, Clough JD: Systemic vasculitis. *In* Young JR, Graor RA, Olin JW, et al (eds): Peripheral Vascular Disease. St. Louis, Mosby-Year Book, 1991, p 339.
7. Klein RG, Hunder GG, Stanson AW, Sheps SG: Large artery involvement in giant cell (temporal) arteritis. Ann Intern Med 83:806, 1975.
8. Fraga A, Mintz G, Valle L, Flores-Izquierdo G: Takayasu's arteritis: Frequency of systemic manifestations (study of 22 patients) and favorable response to maintenance steroid therapy with adrenocorticosteroids (12 patients). Arthritis Rheum 15(6):617, 1972.
9. Hall S, Barr W, Lie JT, et al: Takayasu's arteritis: A study of 32 North American patients. Medicine 64:89, 1985.
10. Shelhamer JH, Volkman DJ, Parrillo JE, et al: Takayasu's arteritis and its therapy. Ann Intern Med 103:121, 1985.
11. Horton BT, Magath TB, Brown GE: An undescribed form of arteritis of the temporal vessels. Proc Staff Meet Mayo Clin 7:700, 1932.
12. Huston KA, Hunder GG, Lie JT, et al: Temporal arteritis: A 25-year epidemiologic, clinical and pathologic study. Ann Intern Med 88:162, 1978.
13. Hunder GG, Sheps SG, Allen GL, Joyce JW: Daily and alternate-day corticosteroid regimens in treatment of giant cell arteritis: Comparison in a prospective study. Ann Intern Med 82:613, 1975.
14. Fauchald P, Rygvold O, Sytese B: Temporal arteritis and polymyalgia rheumatica: Clinical and biopsy findings. Ann Intern Med 77:845, 1972.
15. Save-Soderbergh J, Malmvall BE, Andersson R, et al: Giant cell arteritis as a cause of death: Report of nine cases. JAMA 255:493, 1986.
16. Wilkinson IMS, Russell RWR: Arteritis of the head and neck in giant cell arteritis: A pathologic study to show the pattern of arterial involvement. Arch Neurol 27:378, 1972.
17. Caselli RJ, Hunder GG, Whisnant JP: Neurologic disease in biopsy-proven giant cell (temporal) arteritis. Neurology 38:352, 1988.
18. Enzmann D, Scott WR: Intracranial involvement of giant-cell arteritis. Neurology 27:794, 1977.
19. Stanson AW, Klein RG, Hunder CG: Extracranial angiographic findings in giant cell (temporal) arteritis. Am J Roentgenol 127:957, 1976.
20. Hollenhorst RW, Brown JE, Wagener HP, et al: Neurologic aspects of temporal arteritis. Neurology 10:490, 1967.
21. Anderson T: Arteritis temporalis (Horton). A symptom of generalized vascular disease. Acta Med Scand 128:153, 1947.
22. Birkhead NC, Wagener HP, Shick RM: Treatment of temporal arteritis with adrenal corticosteroids: Results of fifty-five cases in which lesion was proved at biopsy. JAMA 163:821, 1957.
23. Wong RL, Korn JH: Temporal arteritis without an elevated erythrocyte sedimentation rate. Case report and review of the literature. Am J Med 80:959, 1986.
24. Whitaker JJ, Hagedorn AB, Pease GL: Anemia in temporal arteritis. Postgrad Med 40:35, 1966.
25. Dickson ER, Maldonado JE, Sheps SG, et al: Systemic giant cell arteritis with polymyalgia rheumatica: Reversible abnormalities of liver function. JAMA 224:1496, 1973.
26. Chuang TY, Hunder GG, Ilstrup DM, et al: Polymyalgia rheumatica: A 10-year epidemiologic and clinical study. Ann Intern Med 97:672, 1982.
27. Hunder GG, Allen GL: The relationship between polymyalgia rheumatica and temporal arteritis. Geriatrics 28:134, 1973.
28. Hunder GG, Disney TF, Ward LE: Polymyalgia rheumatica. Mayo Clin Proc 44:849, 1969.
29. Hall S, Lie JT, Kurland LT, et al: The therapeutic impact of temporal artery biopsy. Lancet 2:1217, 1983.
30. Austen WG, Blennerhassett JB: Giant cell aortitis causing an aneurysm of the ascending aorta and aortic regurgitation. N Engl J Med 272:80, 1965.
31. Halpin DP, Moran KT, Jewell ER: Arm ischemia secondary to giant cell arteritis. Ann Vasc Surg 2:381, 1988.
32. Joyce JW, Hollier LH: The giant cell arteritis: Temporal and Takayasu's arteritis. *In* Bergan JJ, Yao JST (eds): Evaluation and Treatment of Upper and Lower Extremity Circulatory Disorders. New York, Grune & Stratton, 1984, p 465.
33. Frohnert PP, Sheps SG: Long-term follow-up study of periarteritis nodosa. Am J Med 43:8, 1967.
34. Cohen RD, Conn DL, Ilstrup DM: Clinical features, prognosis, and response to treatment in polyarteritis. Mayo Clin Proc 55:146, 1980.
35. Rose GE, Spencer H: Polyarteritis nodosa. Q J Med 26:43, 1957.
36. McCauley RL, Johnston MR, Fauci AS: Surgical aspects of systemic necrotizing vasculitis. Surg 97:104, 1985.
37. Fauci AS, Katz P, Haynes BF, et al: Cyclophosphamide therapy of severe systemic necrotizing vasculitis. N Engl J Med 301:235, 1979.
38. Wold LE, Baggenstoss AH: Gastrointestinal lesions of periarteritis nodosa. Mayo Clin Proc 24:28, 1949.
39. Selke FW, Williams GB, Donovan DL, et al: Management of intraabdominal aneurysms associated with periarteritis nodosa. J Vasc Surg 4:294, 1986.
40. Mogle P, Hallerin Y, Kobrin K, et al: Rapid regression of aneurysms in polyarteritis nodosa. Br J Radiol 55:536, 1982.
41. Decker JL, Steinberg AD, Reinersten JL: Systemic lupus erythematosus: Evolving concepts. Ann Intern Med 91:587, 1979.

42. Donadio JV Jr, Holley KE, Ferguson RH, et al: Treatment of diffuse proliferative lupus nephritis with prednisone and combined prednisone and cyclophosphamide. N Engl J Med 299:1151, 1978.
43. Boey ML, Colaco CB, Gharavi AE, et al: Thrombosis in systemic lupus erythematosus: Striking association with the presence of circulating lupus anticoagulant. Br Med J 287:1021, 1983.
44. Gluek HI, Kent KS, Weiss MA, et al: Thrombosis in systemic lupus erythematosus: Relation to the presence of circulating anticoagulants. Arch Intern Med 145:1389, 1985.
45. Bowie EJW, Thompson JH, Cascuzzi PA, et al: Thrombosis in SLE despite circulating anticoagulants. J Lab Clin Med 62:416, 1963.
46. Gastineau DA, Kazmier FJ, Nichols WL, et al: Lupus anticoagulant: An analysis of the clinical and laboratory features of 219 cases. Am J Hem 19:265, 1985.
47. Shimizu T, Ehrlich GE, Inaba G, et al: Behçet disease (Behçet syndrome). Semin Arthritis Rheum 8:223, 1979.
48. O'Duffy JD: Vasculitis in Behçet's disease. Rheum Dis Clin North Am 16:423, 1990.
49. O'Duffy JE, Robertson DM, Goldstein NP: Chlorambucil in the treatment of uveitis and meningoencephalitis of Behçet's disease. Am J Med 76:75, 1984.
50. Masuda K, Nakajima A, Urayama A, et al: Double-masked trial of cyclosporin versus colchicine and long-term open study of cyclosporin in Behçet's disease. Lancet 1:1096, 1989.
51. Yazici H, Pazarli H, Barnes CG, et al: A controlled trial of azathioprine in Behçet's syndrome. N Engl J Med 322:281, 1990.
52. Plotkin GR: Cardiac, vascular, renal and pulomonary features. *In* Plotkin GR, Calabro JJ, O'Duffy JD (eds): Behçet's Disease: A Contemporary Synopsis. Mt. Kisco, NY, Futura, 1988, p 203.
53. Du LTH, Bletry O, Wechsler B, et al: Arterial manifestations in Behçet's disease: Fifteen cases in a series of 250 patients. *In* O'Duffy JD, Kokmen Emre (eds): Behçet's Disease: Basic and Clinical Aspects. New York, Decker, 1991, p 145.
54. Durieux P, Bletry O, Huchon G, et al: Multiple pulmonary artery aneurysms in Behçet's disease and Hughes-Stovin syndrome. Am J Med 71:736, 1981.
55. Grenier P, Bletry O, Cornud F, et al: Pulmonary involvement in Behçet disease. Am J Radiol 137:565, 1981.
56. Enoch BA, Castillo-Olivares JD, Khoo TCL, et al: Major vessel complications in Behçet's syndrome. Postgrad Med J 44:453, 1968.
57. Little AG, Zarins CG: Abdominal aortic aneurysm and Behçet's disease. Surgery 91:359, 1982.
58. Shefir A, Stewart P, Mendes DM: The repetitive vascular catastrophes of Behçet's disease: A case report with review of the literature. Ann Vasc Surg 6:85, 1992.
59. Yanagawa H, Kawasaki T, Shigematsu I: Nationwide survey on Kawasaki disease in Japan. Pediatrics 80:58, 1987.
60. Kawasaki T: Mucocutaneous lymph node syndrome: Clinical observation of 50 cases. Jpn J Allergy 16:178, 1967.
61. Nakamura Y, Yanagawa H, Kawasaki T: Mortality among children with Kawasaki disease in Japan. N Engl J Med 326:1246, 1992.
62. Kato H, Ichinose E, Yoshioka F, et al: Fate of coronary aneurysms in Kawasaki disease: Serial coronary angiography and long-term follow-up study. Am J Cardiol 49:1758, 1982.
63. Capannari TE, Daniels SR, Meyer RA, et al: Sensitivity, specificity and predictive value of two-dimensional echocardiography in detecting coronary artery aneurysms in patients with Kawasaki disease. J Am Coll Cardiol 7:355, 1986.
64. Bierman FZ, Gersony WM: Kawasaki disease: Clinical perspective. J Pediatr 111:789, 1987.
65. Sethi S, Ott DA, Nihill M: Surgical management of the cardiovascular complications of Kawasaki's disease. Texas Heart Inst J 10:343, 1983.
66. Newburger JW, Takahashi M, Burns JC, et al: The treatment of Kawasaki syndrome with intravenous gamma globulin. N Engl J Med 315:341, 1986.
67. Neuberger JW, Takahashi M, Beiser AS, et al: A single intravenous infusion of gamma globulin as compared with four infusions in the treatment of acute Kawasaki syndrome. N Engl J Med 324:1633, 1991.
68. Takahashi M, Mason W, Lewis AB: Regression of coronary aneurysms in patients with Kawasaki syndrome. Circulation 75:387, 1987.
69. Fukushige J, Nhill MR, McNamara DG: Spectrum of cardiovascular lesions in mucocutaneous lymph node syndrome: Analysis of eight cases. Am J Cardiol 45:98, 1980.
70. Caputo AE, Roberts WN, Yee YS, et al: Hepatic artery aneurysm in corticosteroid-treated, adult Kawasaki's disease. Ann Vasc Surg 5:533, 1991.
71. Rao SL, Misra RC, Chugh SK: Digital arteriopathy in rheumatoid arthritis. J Chron Dis 29:205, 1976.
72. Scott DGI, Bacon PA, Tribe CR: Systemic rheumatoid vasculitis: A clinical and laboratory study of 50 cases. Medicine 60:288, 1981.
73. Ferguson RH, Slocumb CH: Peripheral neuropathy in rheumatoid arthritis. Bull Rheum Dis 11:251, 1961.
74. Abel T, Andrews BS, Cunningham PH, et al: Rheumatoid vasculitis: Effect of cyclophosphamide on the clinical course and levels of circulating immune complexes. Ann Intern Med 93:407, 1980.
75. Gruickshank B: Pathology of ankylosing spondylitis. Bull Rheum Dis 10:211, 1960.
76. Ansell BM, Bywaters EGL, Doniach I: The aortic lesions of ankylosing spondylitis. Br Heart J 20:507, 1958.
77. Paulus HE, Pearson CM, Pitts W Jr: Aortic insufficiency in five patients with Reiter's syndrome. A detailed clinical and pathologic study. Am J Med 53:464, 1972.
78. Kean WF, Anastassiades TP, Ford PM: Aortic incompetence in HLA B27-positive juvenile arthritis. Ann Rheum Dis 39:294, 1980.
79. Duvernoy WFC, Schatz IJ: Rheumatoid spondylitis associated with aneurysmal dilation of the entire thoracic aorta. Henry Ford Hosp Med Bull 14:309, 1966.
80. Cipriano PR, Alonso DR, Baltaxe HA, et al: Multiple aortic aneurysms in relapsing polychondritis. Am J Cardiol 37:1097, 1976.
81. Esdaile J, Hawkins D, Gold P, et al: Vascular involvement in relapsing polychondritis. CMA Journal 116:1019, 1977.
82. Michet CJ, McKenna CH, Luthra HS, et al: Relapsing polychondritis: Survival and predictive roles of early disease manifestations. Ann Intern Med 104:74, 1986.
83. Hughes RAC, Berry CL, Seifert M, et al: Relapsing polychondritis: Three cases with a clinico-pathological study and literature review. Q J Med 41:363, 1972.
84. McKusick VA (ed): Heritable Disorders of Connective Tissue. 4th ed. St. Louis, CV Mosby, 1972.
85. Steinberg AG, Bearn AG, Motulsky AGH, et al (eds): Progress in Medical Genetics, New Series, vol. 5, Genetics of Cardiovascular Disease. Philadelphia, WB Saunders, 1983.
86. Prockop DJ, Kivirikk KI: Heritable disease of collagen. N Engl J Med 311:376, 1984.
87. McKusick VA: Mendelian Inheritance in Man. 6th ed. Baltimore, John Hopkins University Press, 1982.
88. Peyritz R: Ehlers-Danlos syndromes. *In* Steinberg AG, Bearn AG, Mofulsky AG, et al (eds): Progress in Medical Genetics, New Series, vol. 5, Genetics of Cardiovascular Disease. Philadelphia, WB Saunders, 1983.
89. Sarfarazi M, Tsipouras P, Del Mastro R, et al: A linkage map of 10 loci flanking the Marfan syndrome locus on 15q: Result of an international consortium study. Med Genet 29:75, 1992.
90. Abraham PA, Pereida AJ, Carnes WH, et al: Marfan syndrome: Demonstration of abnormal elastin in aorta. J Clin Invest 70:1245, 1982.
91. Peyritz RE, McKosick VA: The Marfan syndrome: Diagnosis and management. N Engl J Med 300:772, 1979.
92. DeBakey ME, McCollum CH, Crawford ES, et al: Dissecting aneurysms of the aorta. *In* Bergen J, Yao J (eds): Aneurysms: Diagnosis and treatment. New York, Grune and Stratton, 1982, pp 97–103.
93. Miller DC: Surgical management of aortic dissection: Medications, preoperative management, and long-term results. *In* Doroghazi RM, Slater EE (eds): Aortic Dissection. New York, McGraw-Hill, 1983, pp 197–243.
94. Cambria RP, Brewster DC, Gertler J, et al: Vascular complications associated with spontaneous aortic dissection. J Vasc Surg 7:199, 1988.
95. Adib K, Belzer FO: Renal autotransplantation in dissecting aortic aneurysm with renal artery involvement. Surgery 84:686, 1978.
96. Peyritz RE: Propranolol retards aortic root dilation in the Marfan syndrome [Abstract]. Circulation Suppl 3, p 111, 1983.
97. Gott VL, Pyeritz RE, Cameron DE, et al: Composite graft repair of Marfan aneurysm of the ascending aorta: Results in 100 patients. Ann Thorac Surg 52:38, 1991.

98. Cikrit DF, Miles JH, Silver D: Spontaneous arterial perforation: The Ehlers-Danlos spector. J Vasc Surg 5:248, 1987.
99. Beighton P: Lethal complications of the Ehlers-Danlos syndrome. Br Med J 3:656, 1968.
100. Luscher TF, Essandon LK, Lie JT, et al: Renovascular hypertension: A rare cardiovascular complication of the Ehlers-Danlos syndrome. Mayo Clin Proc 62:223, 1987.
101. Sherry C, Agomuoh OS, Goldin MD: Review of Ehlers-Danlos syndrome: Successful repair of rupture and dissection of abdominal aorta. J Cardiovasc Surg 29:530, 1988.
102. Bellenot F, Boisgard S, Kantelip B, et al: Type IV Ehlers-Danlos syndrome with isolated arterial involvement. Ann Vasc Surg 4:15, 1990.
103. Connor PJ Jr, Juergens JL, Perry HO, et al: Pseudoxanthoma elasticum and angioid streaks: A review of 106 cases. Am J Med 30:537, 1961.
104. Altman LK, Fialkow PJ, Parker F, et al: Pseudoxanthoma elasticum: An underdiagnosed genetically heterogeneous disorder with protean manifestations. Arch Intern Med 134:1048, 1974.
105. Mendelsohn G, Buckley BH, Hutchins GM: Cardiovascular manifestations of pseudoxanthoma elasticum. Arch Pathol Lab Med 102:298, 1978.
106. Carlborg V, Ejrup B, Gronglad E, et al: Vascular studies in pseudoxanthoma elasticum and angioid streaks. Acta Med Scand 350 (Suppl 166):3, 1959.
107. Carter DJ, Vince FP, Woodword DAK: Arterial surgery in pseudoexanthoma elasticum. Postgrad Med J 52:291, 1976.
108. Carson NAJ, Cusworth DC, Dent CE, et al: Homocystinurea: A new inborn error of metabolism associated with mental deficiency. Arch Dis Child 38:425, 1963.
109. Gibson JB, Carson NAJ, Neil DW: Pathologic findings in homocystinuria. J Clin Pathol 17:427, 1964.
110. Harker LA, Slichter SJ, Scott CR, et al: Homocystinemia: Vascular injury and arterial thrombosis. N Engl J Med 291:537, 1974.
111. Muss SH, Skouby F, Levy HL. The natural history of homocystinurea due to cystathionine beta synthetase deficiency. Am J Hum Genet 37:1, 1985.
112. Boers GHL, Smals AGH, Trijbels FJM: Heterozygote for homocystinuria in premature peripheral and cerebral arterial disease. N Engl J Med 313:709, 1985.
113. Clarke R, Daly L, Robinson K, et al: Hyperhomocystinemia: An independent risk factor for vascular disease. N Engl J Med 324:1149, 1991.
114. Harris EJ Jr, Taylor LM Jr, Malinow MR, et al: The association between elevated plasma homocysteine and symptomatic peripheral arterial disease. Surg Forum XL: 307, 1989.
115. Mulvihill JJ, Parry DM, Sherman JL, et al: Neurofibromatosis I (Recklinghausen disease) and neurofibromatosis II (bilateral ascoustic neurofibromatosis): An update. Ann Intern Med 113:39, 1990.
116. Halpern M, Currarino G: Vascular lesions causing hypertension in neurofibromatosis. N Engl J Med 273:248, 1965.
117. Riccardi VM: Neurofibromatosis: Phenotype, Natural History, and Pathogenesis. Baltimore, John Hopkins University Press, 1992, p 124.
118. Shepherd CW, Gomez MR, Lie JT, et al: Causes of death in patients with tuberous sclerosis. Mayo Clin Proc 66:792, 1991.
119. Roques X, Choussat A, Bourdeaud'hui A, et al: Aneurysms of the abdominal aorta in the neonate and infant. Ann Vasc Surg 3:335, 1989.
120. Van Reedt-Dortland RW, Bax NM, Huber J: Aortic aneurysm in a 5-year-old boy with tuberous sclerosis. J Pediatr Surg 26:1420, 1991.
121. Libby PA, Maitem AN, Strauss EB: Axillary artery aneurysm in a patient with tuberous sclerosis. Pediatr Radiol 20:94, 1989.
122. DeBakey MF, Garrett E, Howell JF, et al: Coarctation of the abdominal aorta with renal arterial stenosis: Surgical considerations. Ann Surg 165:830, 1967.
123. Onat T, Zeren E: Coarctation of the abdominal aorta: Review of 91 cases. Cardiology 54:140, 1969.
124. Hallett JW, Brewster DC, Darling RC, et al: Coarctation of the abdominal aorta: Current options in surgical management. Ann Surg 191:430, 1980.
125. Greebe J: Congenital anomalies of the iliofemoral artery. J Cardiovasc Surg 18:317, 1977.
126. Pillet J, Cronier P, Mercier PH, et al: The ischiopopliteal trunk. A report of two cases. Anat Clin 3:329, 1982.
127. Cowie TN, McKeller NJ, McLean, et al: Unilateral congenital absence of the external iliac and femoral arteries. Br J Radiol 33:520, 1960.
128. Noblet D, Gasmi T, Mikati A, et al: Persistent sciatic artery: Case report, anatomy and review of the literature. Ann Vasc Surg 2:390, 1988.
129. Simon MA, Scully RE, Springfield DS, et al: Case record of the Massachusetts General Hospital, Case 32, 1992. N Engl J Med 327:412, 1992.
130. Becquemin JP, Gaston A, Caubret P, et al: Aneurysm of persistent sciatic artery. Report of a case treated by endovascular occlusion and femoropopliteal bypass. Surgery 98:605, 1985.
131. Kevorkian Y, Cento DP: Leiomyosarcoma of large arteries and veins. Surgery 73:390, 1972.
132. Busby JR, Ochsner JL, Emory WB, et al: Malignant fibrous histiocytoma arising from descending thoracic aorta. Ann Vasc Surg 4:185, 1990.
133. Becquemin JP, Lebbe C, Saada F, et al: Sarcoma of the aorta. Report of a case and review of the literature. Ann Vasc Surg 2:225, 1988.
134. Briggs PJ, Poolry J, Malcolm AJ, et al: Popliteal artery leiomyosarcoma: A case report and review of the literature. Ann Vasc Surg 4:365, 1990.
135. Josen AS, Khine M: Primary malignant tumor of the aorta. J Vasc Surg 9:493, 1989.
136. Kattus AA, Longmire WP, Cannon JA, et al: Primary intraluminal tumor of the aorta producing malignant hypertension. N Engl J Med 262:694, 1960.
137. Marcial-Rojas RA, Castro JR: Irradiation injury to elastic arteries in the course of treatment for neoplastic disease. Ann Otol 71:945, 1962.
138. Poon TP, Kanshepolsky J, Tchertkoff V: Rupture of the aorta due to radiation injury. JAMA 205:875, 1968.
139. Phillips G, Peer RM, Upson JF, et al: Complications of bypass operations for radiation-induced arterial disease [Abstract]. J Vasc Surg 16:305, 1992.
140. Butler M, Lane R, Webster J: Irradiation injury to large arteries. Br J Surg 67:341, 1980.
141. Conomy J, Kellermeyer R: Delayed cerebrovascular consequences of therapeutic radiation. Cancer 36:1702, 1975.
142. Silverberg G, Britt R, Goffinet D: Radiation-induced carotid artery disease. Cancer 41:130, 1978.
143. Francfort JW, Gallager JF, Penmann E, et al: Surgery for radiation-induced symptomatic carotid atherosclerosis. Ann Vasc Surg 3:16, 1989.
144. Axilrod HD: Obstruction of the aortic isthmus by a calcified thrombus. Arch Pathol 41:63, 1946.
145. Qvarfordt PG, Reilly LM, Sedwitz MM, et al: "Coral reef" atherosclerosis of the supra-renal aorta: A unique clinical entity. J Vasc Surg 1:903, 1989.
146. Peillon C, Morlet C, Laissy JP, et al: Endoaortic calcific proliferation of the upper abdominal aorta. Ann Vasc Surg 3:181, 1989.
147. Coffin O, Maiza D, Alsweis S: Calcified obstructive disease of the aortic isthmus. Ann Vasc Surg 4:147, 1990.
148. Mosimann R, Walder J, VanMelle G: Stenotic intimal thickening of the external iliac artery: Illness of the competition cyclist. Vasc Surg 19:258, 1985.
149. Rousselet MC, Saint-Andre JP, L'Hoste P, et al: Stenotic intimal thickening of the external iliac artery in competition cyclists. Hum Pathol 21:524, 1990.

SECTION IV

Fundamental Therapeutic and Technical Considerations

Edited by Robert B. Rutherford, M.D.

17

Antithrombotic Therapy

Paul W. Humphrey, M.D., and Donald Silver, M.D.

• • •

The vascular surgeon, perhaps more than any other physician, must be intimately familiar with the principles of hemostasis and with ways to alter the hemostatic process to benefit the patient. The vascular surgeon should be able to reduce a patient's rate of coagulation, render a patient totally incoagulable, and when needed, enhance the patient's coagulation process. This chapter reviews the process of hemostasis and describes how the hemostatic process can be altered with antithrombotic therapy to reduce a patient's potential for arterial or venous thromboembolism. Although the fibrinolytic mechanism is closely related to the coagulation mechanism physiologically and therapeutically, fibrinolysis and thrombolytic therapy are discussed in Chapter 19.

HEMOSTASIS

Primary Hemostasis

Primary hemostasis consists of vasoconstriction and the formation of a platelet plug after vessel injury. The interactions of humoral, neurogenic, and myogenic responses lead to vascular smooth muscle cell (SMC) contraction in arteries and arterioles.[1] Once platelets adhere to the injured vessel they release adenosine diphosphate (ADP), serotonin, and thromboxane A_2, further stimulating SMC contraction. Local production of thrombin also contributes to SMC constriction. Vasoconstriction is additionally potentiated by the loss of endothelium, which produces vasodilatating mediators such as prostacyclin (PGI_2) and endothelium-derived relaxing factor (EDRF).[2]

Endothelium

The endothelium plays a critical role in the procoagulant and anticoagulant properties of blood.[3] Endothelial cells synthesize PGI_2, which, in addition to being a vasodilator, is an inhibitor of platelet aggregation. PGI_2 inhibits platelet activation by stimulating adenylate cyclase to increase cyclic adenosine monophosphate (cAMP) within the platelet. PGI_2 is synthesized by endothelial cells when they are stimulated by thrombin, ADP, adenosine triphosphate (ATP), histamine, and kallikrein.[4, 5] EDRF, released from the endothelial cells after stimulation by vasoactive peptides, adenine nucleotides, and acetylcholine, also inhibits platelet aggregation.[6]

The liver and the endothelium synthesize antithrombin III (AT III), the major naturally occurring anticoagulant. Endothelial cells also produce heparan sulfate, a cofactor of AT III.[7] Heparan sulfate significantly accelerates AT III inactivation of thrombin.

The endothelial cell synthesizes and expresses thrombomodulin, an endothelial cell membrane receptor for thrombin. Protein C activation is greatly accelerated when thrombin binds to thrombomodulin. Activated protein C inhibits activated factors V and VIII and enhances fibrinolytic activity. Protein S, a cofactor for protein C, is synthesized by the liver and endothelial cells. Protein S potentiates (up to 25-fold) protein C's inactivation of factor Va.[8]

The endothelial cell synthesizes the serine proteases urokinase and tissue plasminogen activator (tPA). Urokinase and tPA convert plasminogen to plasmin, the active fibrinolytic enzyme. Endothelial cells also synthesize a plasminogen activator inhibitor (PAI-1), which inactivates circulating tPA.[9]

Factor V, synthesized by the endothelial cell as well as by the liver, promotes the formation of the prothrombinase complex that leads to the production of thrombin. Endothelial cells are the primary producers of von Willebrand's factor (VIII : vWF), which is released into the circulation and the subendothelial matrix. Von Willebrand's factor is necessary for platelet binding to subendothelial collagen matrix.

Interleukin 1, endotoxin, and thrombin stimulate the expression of thromboplastin, a tissue factor, on the surface of the endothelial cells.[10] Thromboplastin promotes the activation of factor VII, which contributes to the activation of factor IX, which leads to thrombin formation via the intrinsic pathway. The endothelial cells also produce factor V, which promotes the binding of activated factor X to the endothelial cell with the formation of the prothrombinase complex.

Coagulation

The coagulation cascade consists of a series of reactions in which serine proteases are activated in sequence, the last step resulting in the conversion of fibrinogen to insoluble fibrin (Fig. 17–1).[11, 12] Factor Xa, the active form of factor X, is produced by the action of either the intrinsic pathway, which involves the sequential activation of factors XII, XI, and IX and their interaction with factor VIIIa, or the extrinsic pathway, which involves the activation of factor VII and a lipoprotein tissue factor (not usually present in blood and hence ''extrinsic''). Thrombin is produced from prothrombin by the action of factor Xa, with platelet and endothelial phospholipids providing a surface on which the clotting factor Va and calcium are concentrated. Thrombin cleaves two pairs of peptides (fibrinopeptides A and B) from fibrinogen. The resulting soluble fibrin monomer spontaneously polymerizes and forms a gel. The gel is cross-linked and stabilized by the action of factor XIIIa, which has also been activated by thrombin. The classic division between the extrinsic and the intrinsic pathways is not as sharp as once thought. Several zymogens from either pathway have been found to activate or inhibit aspects of the other.

Activation and Inhibition of Coagulation

Factor XII may be activated in vitro by kaolin, glass, proteolytic enzymes (such as plasmin, kallikrein, and trypsin), endotoxin, low pH, low temperature, and a variety of organic solvents. Factor XIIa initiates the coagulation cascade and contributes to the conversion of prekallikrein to kallikrein. Kallikrein cleaves high-molecular-weight kininogen (HMWK) to form bradykinin and activated HMWK. This latter substance accelerates the activation of both factors XII and XI.

Natural inhibitors of coagulation include alpha$_1$-antitrypsin, alpha$_2$-macroglobulin, AT III, and proteins C and S. The most important is AT III (heparin cofactor), a 65,000-dalton protein present in normal plasma at a concentration of about 300 μg/ml. AT III slowly binds and inactivates thrombin; however, this reaction is dramatically accelerated when heparin is present. Heparin induces a conformational change in the AT III molecule, which then reacts stoichiometrically with thrombin.[13] AT III also binds factors IXa, Xa, XIa, and XIIa. Antithrombin III has a major effect in inhibiting coagulation by inhibiting factor Xa (e.g., inhibition of 32 units of factor Xa prevents the potential activation of 1600 units of thrombin, a finding that led to trials of low-dosage heparin prophylaxis.[14]).

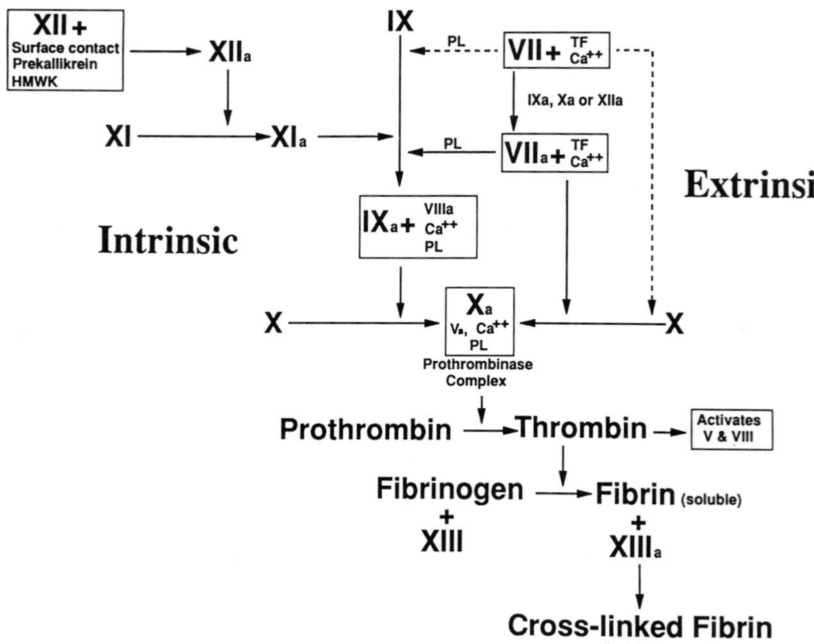

FIGURE 17–1. The two pathways of coagulation operate in conjunction to achieve hemostasis. The intrinsic pathway is initiated by surface contact, whereas the extrinsic pathway is initiated by the release of tissue factor (TF). Phospholipid (PL) is found on activated platelets and endothelial membranes. HMWK, high-molecular-weight kininogen. (From Humphrey PW, Hoch JR, Silver D: Hemostasis and thrombosis. *In* Moore WS [ed]: Vascular Surgery: A Comprehensive Review. 4th ed. Philadelphia, WB Saunders, 1993.)

Antithrombin III deficiency occurs as an inherited autosomal disorder. Afflicted individuals exhibit recurrent thrombotic episodes in early adult life. Widespread venous thrombosis is characteristic; thrombosis of the abdominal aorta has been observed.[15, 16] Heparin therapy is ineffective unless AT III is adequately restored by transfusions of fresh frozen plasma, cryoprecipitate, or AT III concentrate. AT III levels of 75 to 120 per cent are necessary for prophylactic and therapeutic heparin anticoagulation. Normal plasma contains one unit of AT III/ml, and the intravenous administration of 0.7 U/kg increases the level of AT III by 1 per cent. The dose of AT III concentrate is calculated by subtracting the patient's AT III level from the desired (100 to 120 per cent) level, multiplying this by the patient's weight in kilograms, and dividing the result by 1.4. Plasma AT III levels should be assayed at 12-hour intervals to ensure that the level remains at least 80 per cent.[17] AT III replacement should continue until the clinical condition being treated has resolved or oral anticoagulation has been achieved. Long-term administration of warfarin is recommended for AT III–deficient patients who have had thrombotic events. Antithrombin III deficiency is the best-defined congenital "hypercoagulable" disorder.

The thrombomodulin–protein C–protein S system has an important role in the regulation of hemostasis in vivo.[18] *Protein C* is a vitamin K–dependent proenzyme that is activated by thrombin to form a serine protease that inactivates factors Va and VIIIa and blocks platelet receptors for factor Xa. Thrombomodulin, a cofactor on the endothelial surface, enhances the activation of protein C by thrombin up to 20,000-fold. *Protein S*, a plasma cofactor for the protein C–mediated inactivation of factor Va, has no direct effect on coagulation but forms a complex with activated protein C to enhance the rate of inactivation of factor Va.[18]

Patients with hereditary deficiencies of either protein C or protein S may have recurrent venous, or, less frequently, arterial thromboembolism. Myocardial infarction, especially, has been noted in these patients. *Protein S deficiency* may be the most common congenital hypercoagulable syndrome. Acquired deficiencies of protein C or protein S, or both, can occur in patients with disseminated intravascular coagulation or severe hepatic dysfunction and in those taking vitamin K–inhibiting anticoagulants such as warfarin.

Platelets

Platelets are produced in the bone marrow by megakaryocytes. These anuclear discoid cells have a volume of 7 to 10 cubic microns and an average circulating life span of 8 to 12 days. The normal platelet count varies from 200,000 to 400,000 platelets/ml. When platelets are activated (Fig. 17–2), they become spherical, develop pseudopodia, secrete the contents of storage granules, and adhere to each other.

The platelet surface membrane is composed of a bilayer of phospholipids, glycoproteins, and proteins. There are platelet surface receptors for thrombin, serotonin, ADP, collagen, epinephrine, fibronectin, vasopressin, thromboxane A_2, platelet-activating factor, heparin, and the coagulation proteins V, VIII, and Xa.

The platelet cytoplasm contains several types of storage granules: (1) alpha granules, which contain factor V and VIII : vWF, fibronectin, HMWK, platelet-derived growth factor, beta-thromboglobulin, PAI-1, and platelet factor 4; (2) dense granules, which contain ADP, serotonin, and calcium; and (3) lysosomes, which contain proteases, acid hydrolases, and glycosidases.

Von Willebrand's factor is necessary for the binding of platelets to the areas of disrupted intima. *Glycoprotein Ib* is the primary platelet receptor for this factor. Exposed collagen fibrils are among the initial stimuli for platelet adherence. ADP, thrombin, collagen, and epinephrine inter-

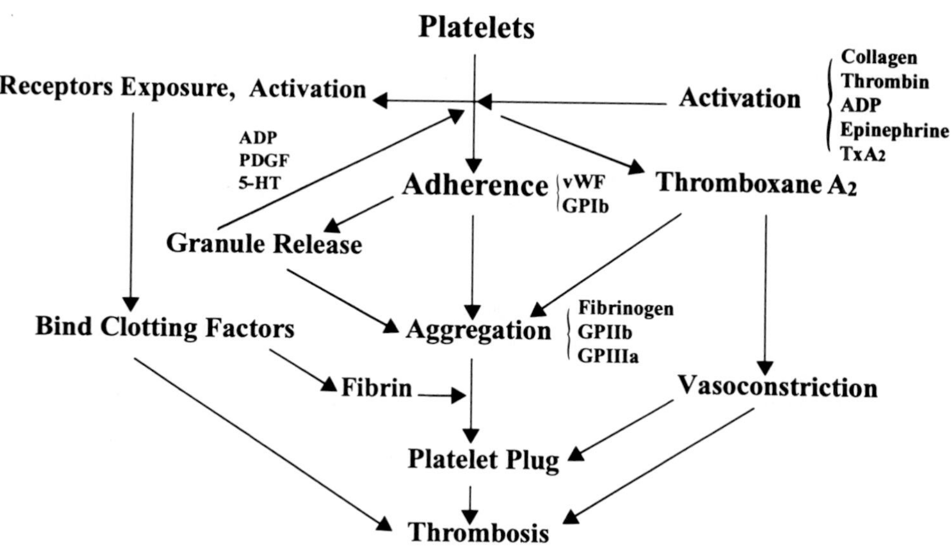

FIGURE 17–2. Mechanism of platelet activation. ADP, adenosine diphosphate; PDGF, platelet-derived growth factor; 5-HT, serotonin; GP, glycoprotein; TxA_2, thromboxane A_2.

act with specific platelet receptors, resulting in granule content release and stimulating platelet aggregation. ADP released from the dense granules initiates platelet-platelet interaction, which leads to a loose aggregation. Activation of membrane phospholipase results in arachidonic acid release, which stimulates additional platelet aggregation. Platelet cyclooxygenase converts arachidonic acid to the prostaglandin endoperoxides, PGG_2 and PGH_2. Thromboxane A_2 is generated by thromboxane synthetase's action on PGG_2. Thromboxane A_2, PGG_2, and PGH_2 stimulate additional platelet aggregation.[19]

Platelet activation exposes platelet surface fibrinogen receptors, which are instrumental in creating bridges between adjacent platelets. The binding sites consist of glycoproteins IIb and IIIa on the platelet surface. Binding sites for factor Va are also exposed with platelet activation. Factor Xa complexes with factor Va to form the *prothrombinase complex*, which leads to the final pathway of coagulation.

RISK FACTORS FOR THROMBOSIS

Recognition of risk factors remains the most practical method for identifying patients at risk for thrombosis. Patients with acquired risk factors for thrombosis have endothelial injury, stasis, hypercoagulability, or a combination of these factors. Acquired risk factors and their mechanisms of inducing thrombosis are listed in Table 17–1.

Tests have been developed to help detect patients with active thrombosis. These tests demonstrate thrombosis by measurement of fibrinopeptide A, prothrombin fragments 1 and 2, thrombin–antithrombin III complexes, D-dimers, or fibrin monomers, or a combination of these; all are increased during active thrombosis.[20] Platelet activation can be recognized by measurement of circulating platelet products (e.g., beta-thromboglobulin, platelet factor 4, and thromboxane B_2), by demonstration of shortened platelet survival, and by in vitro aggregation studies. Increases of platelet activation have been demonstrated in myocardial infarction,[21] unstable angina pectoris,[22] effort-induced angina,[23] transient cerebral ischemic attacks,[24] and recurrent venous thrombosis.[25]

Some patients are at risk for thrombosis because of congenital hypercoagulable states (Table 17–2). Many of these conditions can be detected with appropriate testing.[26] One should test for deficiencies of anticoagulation activities and deficiencies of fibrinolytic activities. When evaluating a patient for a congenital hypercoagulability we usually test for AT III, protein C (antigen and function), protein S (free and total), anticardiolipin antibody and lupus anticoagulant, and plasminogen and plasminogen activator inhibitors in addition to the prothrombin time (PT), activated partial thromboplastin time (aPTT), bleeding time, and platelet count.

Table 17–1. Acquired Risk Factors

Risk Factor	Mechanism
Soft tissue trauma, thermal injury, operative dissection, stroke	Tissue thromboplastin release
Sepsis	Platelet aggregation, activation of coagulation system
Malignancy	Tumor tissue thromboplastin release, increased coagulation factors, decreased AT III levels
Pregnancy/estrogen use	Increased coagulation factors, low AT III levels, decreased plasminogen activation
Intravascular hemolysis	Activation of intrinsic coagulation pathway by increased phospholipids
Lupus anticoagulant	Antiphospholipid antibodies
Hyperlipidemia, myeloproliferative diseases, diabetes mellitus, hemolytic uremic syndrome, thrombotic thrombocytopenic syndrome, heparin-induced thrombocytopenia	Platelet aggregation

Table 17–2. Congenital Hypercoagulable States

Antithrombin III deficiency
Protein C deficiency
Protein S deficiency
Plasminogen and plasminogen activator deficiencies
Increased plasminogen activator inhibitors
Fibrinogen abnormalities
Homocystinuria
Heparin cofactor II deficiency

PHARMACOLOGY

Heparin

Heparin is an effective agent for the prevention and management of thromboembolic disorders. Unfractionated heparin is a negatively charged, helical sulfated polysaccharide with a molecular weight that ranges between 4000 and 40,000 daltons. Commercial heparin is obtained from pork or beef lung or intestine. The greater part of pharmaceutical heparin is devoid of anticoagulant activity; only about 30 per cent of a heparin preparation is able to bind to antithrombin III.[27]

Heparin is administered either subcutaneously or intravenously. Intramuscular injection has an unacceptably high rate of hematoma formation. Slow absorption from subcutaneous sites may prolong the ''heparin effect'' to 8 to 12 hours.[28] Lower blood levels have been observed after subcutaneous administration of the heparin calcium salt compared with the sodium salt.[27] Heparin is bound by the plasma proteins and has a circulating half-life of approximately 90 minutes. Heparin clearance occurs primarily through the reticuloendothelial system. Secondary renal clearance occurs when the reticuloendothelial system becomes saturated with heparin. Heparin has no anticoagulant activity; its anticoagulant effect depends on the presence of adequate amounts of functionally active AT III. Heparin binds to AT III in a 1 : 1 ratio and induces a conformational change in the AT III that makes its active centers more available for binding to thrombin and the other serine proteases. The heparin–AT III complex irreversibly inhibits the active serine proteases IIa, IXa, Xa, XIa, and XIIa. After the serine proteases are bound to the heparin–AT III complex, heparin dissociates and is available to bind to other AT III binding sites.

Low-molecular-weight heparins (LMWH) are 4000 to 8000 molecular weight derivatives of unfractionated heparin. LMWHs have a renal clearance. They have smaller saccharide units (less than 18 to 20 saccharides), resulting in an inability to bind AT III and thrombin simultaneously. However, the smaller saccharide units of LMWHs are able to interact with AT III and factor Xa.[29] The antithrombotic effect of LMWHs is due to their inhibition of factor Xa. Because the LMWHs cannot bind to AT III and thrombin, they have decreased anticoagulant activity.

Large amounts of heparin are required to interfere with the coagulation process in patients with extensive thrombosis. Ineffective responses to heparin therapy may also occur in patients with congenital or acquired deficiencies of AT III. AT III levels are decreased in patients with intravascular coagulation or hepatic insufficiency and during heparin therapy. Patients who are deficient in AT III require fresh frozen plasma, cryoprecipitate, or AT III concentrates to raise their AT III level to at least 80 per cent of normal if they are to be anticoagulated with heparin. Platelet factor 4, released during platelet activation, may interfere with the binding of heparin to AT III.[30]

Administration. Intravenous heparin is administered either by continuous infusion or, less preferably, by intermittent injection. Prospective trials have indicated that there are fewer hemorrhagic complications when heparin is given by continuous infusion and that smaller doses are required for "adequate" anticoagulation.[31–33] When heparin is administered by continuous infusion, a loading dose of 100 to 200 U/kg is given to initiate therapy; this is usually followed by an infusion of approximately 1000 U/hr. The rate of infusion is adjusted to maintain the monitoring test value within a prescribed range. If the aPTT is used as the monitor, the recommended range for patients with active thrombosis is 1.5 to 1.8 times the control value. Spontaneous bleeding rarely occurs if the aPTT remains less than twice the control value.

When subcutaneous heparin is given prophylactically to surgical patients to prevent venous thromboembolism, it is injected in doses of 5000 units every 8 to 12 hours, starting 2 hours preoperatively. Therapeutic subcutaneous heparin usually requires 10,000 to 20,000 units every 8 to 12 hours; the dose is adjusted so that the aPTT will be 1.5 to 1.8 times the control value 30 minutes before the next dose. When heparin is given subcutaneously, concentrated solutions should be used to limit the administered volume. The injections are given carefully with a short needle in the subcutaneous tissue of the anterior abdominal wall or the anterior thigh.

Other tests available to regulate heparin therapy include the whole blood clotting time (two to three times control value), whole blood activated recalcification time (two to three times control value), and calcium thrombin time (two to six times control value). The therapeutic range of heparin as assayed by protamine titration or anti-Xa assay is 0.5 to 1.5 U/ml (0.5 U/ml usually provides adequate anticoagulation).

Before heparin therapy or heparin prophylaxis is commenced, a simple assessment of hemostasis should be performed (PT, PTT, platelet count) because hemorrhagic complications are common when preexisting coagulation defects are present.

Prophylaxis. The inhibition of factor Xa by antithrombin III and heparin prevents the potential generation of a considerably larger amount of thrombin. Thus, small doses of heparin should have a major antithrombotic effect. Sharnoff and DeBlasio first suggested that prophylactic small doses of heparin could reduce the incidence of fatal pulmonary embolism.[34] A large number of controlled studies have subsequently confirmed the efficacy of this method but have also shown the limitations of low-dose (5000 units subcutaneously every 8 to 12 hours) heparin prophylaxis. These studies have been summarized by Salzman and Davies.[35] Small subcutaneous doses of heparin reduced the incidence of venous thrombosis as detected by labeled fibrinogen in general surgical patients. In aggregate, the incidence of venous thrombosis was reduced from around 27 per cent (1173 of 4373 patients) to about 6 per cent (168 of 2570 patients; range, 0.8 to 13.5 per cent). Laboratory monitoring (apart from initial screening for bleeding disorders) does not appear to be required. The incidence of bleeding complications is low: 0.2 per cent of those given low-dose heparin died of bleeding, the same rate as in the control group.[36]

The effect of low-dose heparin on the incidence of pulmonary embolism has been more difficult to study because of the lack of standardized criteria for diagnosis. Kakkar and associates studied 4121 general surgical patients over 40 years of age who were randomized to receive either 5000 units of heparin or a placebo subcutaneously every 8 hours, starting 2 hours preoperatively and continuing for 7 days. There were 80 postoperative deaths in the heparin-treated group, of which 2 were attributed to pulmonary embolism; 16 of the 100 deaths in the control group were attributed to pulmonary embolism.[36] The study has been criticized because of a lower autopsy rate in the heparin-treated group (66 per cent as opposed to 72 per cent in the control group) and because of lax criteria for determining whether an embolus was the cause of death. Despite these criticisms, the results support the use of heparin in venous thromboembolism prophylaxis.

Low-dose heparin has been disappointing in patients undergoing hip surgery or open prostatectomy; however, heparin given in a dose that is titrated to a therapeutically prolonged PTT, rather than arbitrarily fixed, has been effective in these patients.[37, 38] Although there are reports of its use in neurosurgical patients, heparin has not gained wide acceptance because of the potential for disastrous bleeding complications in these patients.

LMWH has been advocated for the prophylaxis of venous thrombosis. LMWH was compared with unfractionated heparin (UH) by Kakkar and Murray in a controlled trial of patients undergoing abdominal surgery.[39] Patients received either 1850 units of LMWH daily or 5000 units of

UH twice daily. The LMWH group had a 2.5 per cent incidence of venous thrombosis, whereas the patients in the UH group had a 7.5 per cent incidence. The two groups did not differ in the number of bleeding episodes or wound hematomas. The incidence of bleeding complications has been reported to be higher as well as lower with LMWH compared with UH.[40, 41]

Heparin is routinely used in vascular surgery to prevent clotting in vessels and grafts during and after "clamping." Usually 5000 to 7000 units of heparin are administered intravenously prior to the application of the vascular clamps. Porous vascular grafts are "preclotted" prior to heparin administration. Many vascular surgeons are now using grafts that are impregnated with albumin or collagen to reduce the graft "leakage." One thousand to 2000 units of *additional* heparin are given each hour that the vascular clamps are in place. Heparin reversal is rarely necessary when adequate mechanical hemostasis has been achieved. Patients who have grafts that are at risk for early thrombosis (e.g., below-knee prosthetic grafts) are maintained on heparin intravenously (aPTT 1.5 to 1.7 times control value) until warfarin anticoagulation is satisfactory. In the postoperative period, for prophylaxis of deep venous thrombosis, our vascular patients who are immobile are maintained on 5000 units of subcutaneous heparin given every 8 hours until they are ambulatory.

Prior to the insertion of arterial and venous cannulas for cardiopulmonary bypass, patients receive 300 units heparin/kg. Additional heparin is administered periodically to maintain an activated coagulation time (ACT) of at least 400 seconds. The effect of heparin is often reversed at the end of cardiopulmonary bypass. The cardiopulmonary bypass pump return lines should be removed before the protamine is administered. The adequacy of heparin reversal is determined by the ACT, thrombin time, aPTT, or protamine titration test. Protamine sulfate administered intravenously in a dose of 1.0 mg/100 U heparin immediately reverses the anticoagulant effect of heparin. One third to one half of the calculated protamine dose should be infused slowly to avoid the risks of hypotension, bradycardia, and vasodilatation.[42] Protamine binds to heparin and interferes with its reaction with AT III. When large doses of heparin are given, as during cardiopulmonary bypass, "heparin rebound" may occur because of the dissociation of the heparin-protamine complex or because of further release of heparin from the microcirculation or extravascular sources. Additional protamine sulfate may be required in these instances. Excessive protamine administration may cause an anticoagulant effect because of the interaction of protamine with platelets and serum proteins.

Complications. Hemorrhagic complications have been observed in 10 to 20 per cent of patients who had normal hemostasis prior to receiving heparin and in up to 50 per cent of patients with thrombocytopenia or uremia.[43] Patients with active bleeding, intracranial hemorrhage, a recent neurologic procedure, or malignant hypertension may develop major bleeding complications during heparin therapy. Patients who have had recent operative procedures or a stroke are also at risk for bleeding if they receive heparin. Therapeutic doses of heparin in other patients are not likely to be associated with bleeding unless there is an underlying bleeding tendency. Bleeding complications can be reduced by closely monitoring the aPTT. The aPTT should be kept in the range of 1.5 to 1.7 times control. Concomitant administration of aspirin or other antiplatelet function–inhibiting drugs increases the risk of hemorrhage.

Approximately 4 to 5 per cent of patients receiving heparin develop heparin-associated antiplatelet antibodies. These antibodies lead to thrombocytopenia and thrombohemorrhagic complications. The heparin-induced thrombocytopenia syndrome (HIT) occurs after 4 to 15 days of therapy in those exposed to heparin for the first time. The development of HIT is independent of the type, dose, or route of administration of heparin. HIT may occur on the first day of reexposure to heparin; therefore, daily platelet counts should be obtained in all patients receiving heparin. HIT should be considered when a patient receiving any form of heparin has a falling platelet count or a platelet count of less than 100,000/ml, increasing resistance to anticoagulation with heparin, or new or progressive thrombohemorrhagic complications. HIT has been associated with a 23 per cent mortality and a 61 per cent morbidity.[44] Mortality and morbidity can be reduced to 12 per cent and 22.5 per cent, respectively, if the diagnosis is promptly established and heparin administration is stopped.[45] When the diagnosis is suspected, *all* heparin sources, including heparin-coated catheters, should be discontinued and platelet function inhibited. We administer aspirin 325 mg by mouth or 600 mg per rectum as soon as the diagnosis is suspected and then daily. The diagnosis is confirmed by an increasing platelet count following cessation of heparin, cessation of the thrombohemorrhagic complications, and positive platelet aggregometry or ^{14}C-serotonin release studies. Patients with heparin-associated antiplatelet antibodies should not receive heparin; alternate forms of anticoagulation (warfarin or dextran) are administered if needed. The antibodies may be present for a few weeks or, in our experience, up to 12 years. All patients with a history of HIT must test negative for the antibodies before receiving additional heparin.

Sensitivity reactions occur in 2 to 5 per cent of patients receiving heparin. Bronchiole constriction, urticaria, lacrimation, and rarely, anaphylaxis may occur. Alopecia and osteoporosis occur in fewer than 1 per cent of patients receiving long-term (more than 6 months) heparin. Hair growth resumes with the cessation of heparin therapy.

Warfarin

Oral anticoagulants interfere with the utilization of vitamin K by the liver during the synthesis of factors II, VII, IX, and X. Vitamin K is a cofactor in the reaction that converts glutamyl residues of clotting factor precursors to the carboxyglutamyl residues required for the binding of calcium. When oral anticoagulants are given, antigenically similar clotting factors are produced that are inactive because of their abnormal calcium binding characteristics. The rate at which anticoagulation occurs depends on the circulating half-lives of the factors. Although factor VII has a half-life of 6 hours, prothrombin has a half-life of 3 days. Anticoagulation is thus not complete for several days, although the PT may be in the therapeutic range within 36 hours because of a reduced level of factor VII. For this reason, therapy with heparin is advised for the first 2 to 4 days of anticoagulation with warfarin. An additional reason for a few days of heparin when initiating warfarin therapy is that warfarin suppresses the vitamin K–dependent protein C level (4- to 6-hour half-life), resulting in a transient procoagulant state and thus supporting the need for heparin anticoagulation during the first 2 to 4 days of anticoagulation with warfarin.

Administration. Warfarin is readily absorbed from the intestine, peak plasma concentrations being reached in 2 to 12 hours. Ninety-seven per cent of warfarin is bound to albumin and has a circulating half-life of 36 to 40 hours. The unbound fraction is responsible for the anticoagulant effect. Warfarin therapy is usually initiated with a daily dose of 7.5 to 10 mg. A reduced dose is given to the elderly, to patients with hepatic insufficiency, and to those receiving parenteral nutrition or broad-spectrum antibiotics. The maintenance dose of warfarin is determined by the PT, which should be maintained in the range of 1.4 to 1.7 times control. Hemorrhagic complications are infrequent when PT is maintained at this level. The PT should be monitored frequently until it stabilizes and then can be monitored infrequently (e.g., every 4 to 8 weeks). It is a misconception that patients receiving warfarin should not receive aspirin. Aspirin provides additional protection to the patient through its platelet inhibiting-function; the regulation of PT is not affected by daily doses of aspirin.

Prophylaxis. Warfarin anticoagulation during and after surgery is effective in preventing venous thrombosis and fatal pulmonary embolism. Sevitt and Gallagher's study of 300 patients with hip fractures demonstrated a reduction in the incidence of clinically diagnosed venous thrombosis from 29 per cent in control patients to 3 per cent in patients who received prophylactic warfarin anticoagulation.[46] At autopsy, the incidence of thrombosis was 83 per cent in the control group and 14 per cent in the group receiving anticoagulants. Pulmonary embolism was thought to be the cause of death in 10 per cent of the control patients but in none of those receiving anticoagulant therapy.[46] Several other studies have confirmed these findings. In the aggregate, warfarin reduces the rate of venographically detected thrombosis from 47.3 to 23.4 per cent and decreases the frequency of fatal pulmonary embolism from a range of about 2 to 10 per cent to approximately 0.4 per cent in patients undergoing hip surgery.

Long-term postoperative warfarin therapy may enhance infrapopliteal polytetrafluoroethylene (PTFE) graft patency. Flinn and colleagues[47] reviewed a series of patients who had femorotibial or femoropopliteal bypass with PTFE grafts while receiving perioperative heparin and postoperative warfarin anticoagulation. They noted a significant improvement in graft patency rates in the infrapopliteal position (37 per cent of patients had patent grafts after 4 years) compared with historical controls (who had a 12 per cent 4-year graft patency rate).[48] The PTs were maintained at twice the control values.

Complications. Bleeding occurs in 4 to 22 per cent of patients receiving warfarin. Fatal hemorrhage has been reported in 1.8 per cent of patients with arterial disease who received warfarin.[49] In the studies in which warfarin was used as the sole prophylactic agent during hip replacement, there was a 0.3 per cent incidence of fatal bleeding. The incidence of bleeding is less if the warfarin dosage is adjusted to cause less elevation of the PT (to 1.3 to 1.5 times control value).[50] Warfarin anticoagulation can be reversed and bleeding controlled with intramuscular or intravenous vitamin K in approximately 24 hours. If rapid reversal is needed, fresh frozen plasma should be given.

Less common complications of warfarin therapy include urticaria, dermatitis, alopecia, fever, nausea, diarrhea, abdominal cramping, and hypersensitivity reactions. Dermal gangrene of the breast, thigh, or buttocks is a rare complication. The dermal venous thrombosis and dermal gangrene have been related to the hypercoagulable state, which can occur with warfarin-induced decreases of protein C. It is not known why this event is limited to the skin.[18] Heparin should be administered for the first 2 to 4 days of warfarin therapy to avoid this complication.

Responsiveness to warfarin may be altered by drugs (Table 17–3) or by circumstances that (1) interfere with its absorption (e.g., cholestyramine); (2) displace it from albumin (e.g., aspirin, indomethacin, sulfinpyrazone, phenylbutazone, chloral hydrate, clofibrate, sulfonamides, and anabolic steroids); (3) reduce its metabolism in the liver, thus increasing its effect (e.g., chloramphenicol and tricyclic antidepressants); (4) enhance its metabolism, thus decreasing its effect (e.g., alcohol, glutethimide, and barbiturates); (5) and/or alter vitamin K absorption or availability (e.g., obstructive jaundice, diarrhea, parenteral nutrition, cholestyramine, neomycin, laxatives, or broad-spectrum antibiotics).

Warfarin should not be given during pregnancy, especially in the first trimester, because of its teratogenic effects. The risk of hemorrhagic birth injuries precludes its use near term. If antithrombotic therapy is required during pregnancy, heparin should be considered.

DEXTRAN

Dextran is a polysaccharide that was developed as a plasma volume expander in the early 1940s. Its antithrom-

Table 17–3. Drug Interactions With Oral Anticoagulants

Potentiate	Antagonize
Allopurinol	Antihistamines
Aminoglycosides	Carbamazepine
Anabolic steroids	Cholestyramine
Chloramphenicol	Glutethimide
Chlofibrate	Griseofulvin
Chlorpromazine	Haloperidol
Cimetidine	Oral contraceptives
Cotrimoxazole	Phenobarbital
Dipyridamole	Phenytoin
Disulfiram	Spironolactone
Metronidazole	Vitamin K
Oral hypoglycemic drugs	
Phenylbutazone	
Quinidine	
Salicylate	
Tricyclic antidepressants	

From Humphrey PW, Hoch JR, Silver D: Hemostasis and thrombosis. In *Moore WS (ed): Vascular Surgery: A Comprehensive Review. 4th ed. Philadelphia, WB Saunders, 1993.*

botic properties were noted in the 1960s and led to its use in the management of thromboembolic disorders in the 1970s. Two preparations are available for clinical use in the United States: dextran 70 (average molecular weight 70,000 daltons with 90 per cent in the range of 20,000 to 115,000 daltons) and dextran 40 (average molecular weight 40,000 daltons with 90 per cent in the range of 10,000 to 80,000 daltons). The two preparations seem to have equivalent antithrombotic effects.

Dextran decreases platelet aggregation and adhesiveness and causes prolongation of the bleeding time. Formation of a dextran complex with von Willebrand's factor has been demonstrated and may contribute to the decreased platelet function. The antithrombotic effect of dextran is enhanced by its interference with fibrin polymerization.

Administration. The dosage of dextran for antithrombosis is 500 ml given immediately preoperatively or intraoperatively followed by 500 to 1000 ml given daily during the postoperative period.

Prophylaxis. Dextran has been used to prevent venous and arterial thromboses. Pooled results of several randomized clinical trials using dextran as a prophylactic agent have demonstrated reductions in deep venous thromboses (15.6 per cent with dextran versus 24.2 per cent in controls) and pulmonary emboli (1.2 per cent with dextran versus 2.8 per cent in controls).[51] Dextran has provided effective venous thrombosis prophylaxis in patients undergoing hip surgery (resulting in a rate of approximately 6.5 per cent deep venous thrombosis).[52–55]

In an international multi-center prospective study of general surgical, gynecologic, urologic, and orthopedic patients undergoing elective operations lasting at least 30 minutes, prophylaxis with dextran 70 (given as three 500-ml doses, the first dose given during surgery) was compared with low-dose subcutaneous heparin (5000 units given every 8 hours, starting 2 hours before surgery and continuing for 6 days or until full mobility). There was no difference in the incidence of fatal pulmonary embolism in the two groups.[56] An equal number of bleeding complications occurred with both regimens, and serious allergic reactions occurred in 1.1 per cent of patients receiving dextran.

Complications. The most common complications of dextran infusions are hemorrhage and volume overload. These are reduced by limiting the volume of dextran infused to less than 10 per cent of the patient's blood volume daily. Other less common complications include allergic reactions (around 1 per cent of patients) and, rarely, anaphylactoid-type reactions (less than 0.1 per cent of patients). The preinfusion of short-chain dextrans (MW 3000 to 6000) to patients known to be sensitive to dextran prevents or diminishes allergic or anaphylactic reactions. Major complications such as volume overload and hemorrhage are more frequent with dextran 70 than with dextran 40.[57]

Ancrod

Ancrod, an amino acid compound with a molecular weight of 37,000, is derived from the venom of the Malayan pit viper *(Agkistrodon rhodostoma)*. The circulating half-life of ancrod ranges from 3 to 5 hours. Ancrod is excreted unchanged in the urine. Ancrod cleaves the A-fibrinopeptides (A, AY, and AP) from circulating fibrinogen. The resultant fibrin does not undergo cross-linking and therefore is more susceptible to fibrinolytic activity and to phagocytosis by the reticuloendothelial system than is normal fibrin. In addition to interfering with coagulation, the lowered fibrinogen concentration reduces the blood's viscosity and improves rheology. Platelets and the other coagulation proteins are unaffected by ancrod.

Ancrod is administered by the subcutaneous or intravenous route. The level of hypofibrinogenemia is more readily controlled by the intravenous route. It has been demonstrated that plasma fibrinogen concentrations of 0.2 to 0.6 gm/L are adequate for hemostasis but effectively prevent spontaneous thrombosis. Anticoagulation can be achieved by the infusion of 70 to 100 units (1 to 2 U/kg) over 12 to 36 hours; this usually results in a decline of fibrinogen to the level of 0.4 to 0.6 gm/L. Surgery can be safely performed with fibrinogen concentrations in this range. Serum fibrinogen levels should be measured every 12 hours for the initial 48 hours and then daily; the infusion rate is adjusted to maintain the fibrinogen level in the desired range. Resistance to ancrod may occur after 4 to 6 weeks of therapy because of the occurrence of serum proteinase inhibitors that bind and inactivate it.[58]

Ancrod is well suited for use in patients with heparin-induced thrombocytopenia who continue to require anticoagulation. Ancrod has been effectively used in patients with antithrombin III deficiency who are resistant to the effects of heparin and require anticoagulation.[59] Ancrod has been used successfully to manage patients with stroke, deep venous thrombosis, pulmonary embolism, and central retinal thrombosis. It has also been used as an anticoagulant in patients requiring hemodialysis, cardiopulmonary bypass, and peripheral vascular surgery.

The complications associated with ancrod use are fever, minor allergic reactions, and hemorrhage. If uncontrollable hemorrhage occurs, the administration of cryoprecipitate effectively reverses ancrod's effects. Surgical procedures can be performed while the patient is on ancrod with minimal risk of significant hemorrhage.

PLATELET FUNCTION INHIBITION

Many drugs alter platelet activity. Several have been evaluated in clinical trials as antithrombotic agents. Aspirin, dipyridamole, and ticlopidine have been investigated most extensively.

Aspirin

Aspirin irreversibly acetylates the cyclooxygenase of platelets, which interferes with the conversion of arachidonic acid to the prostaglandin endoperoxides, thus inhibiting platelet synthesis of thromboxane A_2. Because platelets are anucleate and cannot synthesize new enzymes, their functional inhibition is permanent. A single dose of aspirin results in defective platelet function that can be detected for several days.[60] The altered cyclooxygenase also reduces the production of prostacyclin in the endothelium. However, new cyclooxygenase is readily synthesized by the nucleated endothelial cells; hence, prostacyclin production by endothelial cells is restored to normal within a few hours. The net result of the administration of modest doses of aspirin (e.g., 600 mg or less once or twice a day) is an inhibition of thromboxane A_2 synthesis. It has been suggested that larger doses of aspirin might tilt the balance in favor of thrombosis by blocking endothelial prostacyclin production. However, no proof of a thrombotic effect of aspirin has been documented in humans.

Administration. We prescribe enteric-coated aspirin, 325 mg daily, usually with a meal, for platelet function inhibition. A few of our patients have received 80 mg of aspirin twice daily for platelet function inhibition.

Prophylaxis. Aspirin is ineffective in the management of ongoing thrombosis. Aspirin is helpful in maintaining vascular graft patency and in reducing the incidence of transient ischemic attacks (TIAs), stroke, myocardial infarction, and death.

Significant improvement in the early patency of both saphenous and PTFE grafts has been demonstrated in two randomized clinical trials when patients were given preoperative aspirin and dipyridamole.[61, 62] No proven difference in femoropopliteal bypass patency was found when aspirin and dipyridamole were begun 24 hours postoperatively.[63] We prescribe aspirin (325 mg daily) in the preoperative period for a femorodistal bypass and continue it indefinitely.

Improved graft patency has also been reported in patients receiving aspirin after coronary artery bypass. One clinical trial reported graft thrombosis in 10 per cent of patients submitting to coronary artery bypass who received a placebo, whereas graft thrombosis occurred in only 3 per cent of patients receiving aspirin and dipyridamole at the time of bypass.[64] Follow-up at 1 year revealed a 25 per cent occlusion rate in the placebo group and an 11 per cent occlusion rate in the treated group. Aspirin alone has proved to be as effective as a combination of aspirin and dipyridamole in patients undergoing coronary artery bypass.[65]

A significant reduction in the incidence of TIAs, stroke, and death in men taking aspirin was demonstrated by the Canadian Cooperative Study Group.[66] Several other clinical trials of aspirin alone or aspirin in combination with dipyridamole have shown reductions in the incidences of stroke and death.[67–69] A reduced incidence of fatal myocardial infarctions has also been demonstrated in studies in which patients received either aspirin alone or aspirin in combination with dipyridamole. The effective doses of aspirin for reducing graft thrombosis, TIAs, stroke, myocardial infarction, and progression of atherosclerotic occlusive disease have ranged from 80 mg once daily to 625 mg twice daily.[62, 69–72]

Complications. Contraindications to the use of platelet function–inhibiting agents include a bleeding tendency, peptic ulceration, and sensitivity to the agent. Care should be exercised when these agents are combined with warfarin or heparin because this combination results in an increased tendency toward bleeding. Chronic aspirin administration may be associated with elevation of blood urea and uric acid concentrations, but gout rarely occurs.

Dipyridamole

Dipyridamole suppresses platelet aggregation by inhibiting platelet phosphodiesterase, which causes an increase in intracellular cAMP. Elevated cAMP results in a decrease in cytoplasmic calcium with platelet aggregation inhibition. Other actions of dipyridamole may include inhibition of the synthesis of thromboxane A_2 and potentiation of the inhibition of platelet function by adenosine. The hypothesis that dipyridamole is synergistic with aspirin in its antithrombotic effect has not been proved by clinical trials.

Administration. Dipyridamole, 25 to 50 mg, is usually given by mouth three to four times daily.

Prophylaxis. Dipyridamole's effectiveness as a prophylactic vascular or cardiovascular agent alone or in combination with aspirin has yet to be proved.

Complications. Headache is the most common complication of dipyridamole administration, occurring in approximately 10 per cent of patients. Other complications include diarrhea, flushing, and rash.

Ticlopidine

Ticlopidine irreversibly alters the platelet membrane, inhibiting platelet aggregation induced by collagen, platelet-activating factor, adrenaline, and ADP.[73] It is administered orally in a dose of 125 mg twice a day. Ticlopidine reduces the event rate per year for stroke, myocardial infarction, or vascular death, considered together, by 23 per cent in patients who have had a previous stroke.[74] A clinical trial of ticlopidine in patients with intermittent claudication demonstrated only a 10 per cent improvement in distances walked compared with a placebo.[75] Complications of ticlopidine, which include neutropenia, pancytopenia, and agranulocytosis, have been described in 2 per cent of patients.[74] These complications usually resolve when the medication is stopped.

PHYSICAL MEASURES FOR THROMBOEMBOLISM PROPHYLAXIS

Physical measures for the prevention of thromboembolism are an attractive alternative to drug prophylaxis. They are noninvasive and are without major side effects or risks for bleeding. Early and aggressive mobilization provides a modest reduction, as determined by labeled fibrinogen studies, in the incidence of thrombosis in the elderly. Elastic stockings and venous pneumatic compression with inflatable leggings have successfully reduced the incidence of venous thrombosis.[76] A review of four randomized clinical trials evaluating the effectiveness of elastic stockings revealed a 9.3 per cent incidence of deep venous thrombosis in patients wearing stockings and a 24.5 per cent incidence in controls.[50]

The rate of postoperative venous thrombosis in surgical patients using pneumatic compression is about 8 per cent (25 of 270 patients), a rate comparable to that achieved with low-dose heparin.[35] Venous pneumatic compression has also been effective in preventing venous thrombosis in neurosurgical patients and patients undergoing open prostatectomy.[37, 76] In patients undergoing hip operations who have had previous thromboembolic events, pneumatic compression ''stockings'' have been shown to be as effective as warfarin if the preoperative venogram is normal.[77] The rate of clinically diagnosed pulmonary embolism in surgical patients using pneumatic compression was 0.9 per cent in one clinical trial.[35] A combination of low-dose heparin and pneumatic compression stockings may be more effective than either used alone for preventing venous thrombosis.[78]

The regimen of venous thrombosis prophylaxis should give the patient the most satisfactory protection with the least number of side effects. Young patients less than 40 years of age with no risk factors who undergo general surgery usually do not require specific measures. Low-dose subcutaneous heparin or pneumatic compression stockings are effective prophylactic measures in general surgical patients.[77] Pneumatic compression stockings are effective in neurosurgical and open prostatectomy patients in whom heparin is contraindicated or ineffective. Warfarin or dextran may be used in patients who are at a high risk for the occurrence of a thrombotic event. Patients in this category include those with prior thromboembolism, malignant disease, or hip fractures.

Thromboembolism is a serious problem in patients with major trauma. A reasonable approach to treatment of these patients includes pneumatic compression stockings or dextran, or both, in the immediate postinjury period. When the hazard of hemorrhage has abated, low-dose heparin may be prescribed in addition to pneumatic compression stockings if the risk of thromboembolism remains significant. If the trauma patient has bilateral lower extremity fractures prohibiting the use of pneumatic stockings and a contraindication to the use of low-dose heparin, duplex scanner surveillance (every 2 to 3 days) of the deep venous systems of the lower extremities is indicated. If deep venous thrombosis occurs under these circumstances and anticoagulation is prohibited, the insertion of a vena caval filter should be considered.

MAJOR ARTERIAL EMBOLISM

The management and prognosis of peripheral arterial embolism depends on the vessels that are occluded and the source of the emboli. The goals of management are to restore the circulation to normal and to prevent recurrences.

Heparin is administered promptly to patients with acute arterial thromboembolism to prevent thrombus propagation and to maintain the patency of collateral vessels. The patient is usually given a 5000 to 10,000 unit bolus of intravenous heparin while diagnostic or therapeutic measures are in process. If the patient has an embolectomy, additional intravenous heparin is usually given. In the postoperative period heparin is infused at a rate that will maintain the aPTT at 1.5 to 1.7 times control value. The heparin infusion should be continued for 3 to 4 days in the postoperative period while endothelial healing occurs. Postoperative bleeding complications are minimal if the aPTT is not allowed to exceed twice the control value. If warfarin therapy is indicated, it should be started in the immediate postoperative period to allow for a 3- to 4-day overlap with the heparin therapy.

Three retrospective studies compared reembolism and mortality rates in patients receiving and not receiving anticoagulation. The rate of reembolization was reduced by approximately 30 per cent, and this was associated with a lower overall mortality in those receiving anticoagulants.[79–81]

Anticoagulation with warfarin appears to reduce the incidence of recurrent cerebral emboli in patients with mitral valve stenosis.[82] Myocardial mural thromboses are common sources of peripheral emboli, and patients with these thromboses are usually anticoagulated first with heparin and then with warfarin. The threat of embolization from a mural thrombus associated with a myocardial infarct decreases with time, and it has been suggested that anticoagulants can be discontinued after 1 year in this circumstance.[83] Peripheral embolization related to ulcerated aortic plaques with thrombus is treated by endarterectomy or replacement of the involved segment of aorta. The role of thrombolytic therapy in acute thromboembolic occlusions of the extremities is discussed in Chapter 43.

CEREBROVASCULAR DISEASE

Antithrombotic therapy has been evaluated in the management of completed stroke, stroke-in-evolution, and TIAs. Anticoagulation is of no benefit in patients with a completed stroke. The value of anticoagulation in nonhemorrhagic evolving strokes is not clear. Anticoagulation does not reduce the number of deaths, but it may be of benefit in reducing the size of the infarction. Studies have suggested that anticoagulants reduce the frequency of TIAs, but this suggestion remains controversial.[82, 84] Anticoagulation may be useful in patients who have cerebral emboli from a cardiac source because of the approximately 15 per cent chance of repeat embolism within 2 weeks of the ischemic event.[82] Anticoagulant therapy may reduce the risk of early (within 2 weeks) recurrent cerebral embolism by two thirds.[85]

Attention has focused on the use of platelet function inhibition in the management of TIAs. Fields and coworkers reported a randomized double-blind trial of aspirin for the treatment of TIAs. Although there was no significant difference in the rates of death or cerebral or retinal infarction, there was a significant difference in favor of aspirin when death, cerebral infarction, and the occurrence of TIAs were considered together as an end-point.[86] The Canadian

Cooperative Study Group studied the effects of placebo versus aspirin alone or in combination with sulfinpyrazone in 585 patients who had TIAs. They found a striking reduction (48 per cent) in the ensuing risk of stroke or death in men treated with aspirin. No benefit was seen with aspirin in women or with sulfinpyrazone in either sex.[66] These studies and others have clearly established that aspirin therapy results in a 20 to 30 per cent reduction in the incidence of stroke among men with TIAs and minor strokes.[87, 88] The accepted dose of aspirin varies from 325 to 1300 mg/day. The authors currently use 325 mg daily. A British study showed that 325 mg/day compared with 1300 mg/day offered equal protection with few side effects from the occurrence of a stroke after a TIA.[88]

The recent North American Symptomatic Carotid Endarterectomy Trial (NASCET) study firmly documented the beneficial effect of carotid endarterectomy compared with medical (antiplatelet) therapy in symptomatic patients with high-grade (70 to 99 per cent) carotid stenosis. Patients who had carotid endarterectomies had significant reductions in the occurrence of minor, major, and fatal ipsilateral strokes. The cumulative risk of any ipsilateral strokes at 2 years was 26 per cent for the medically treated group and 9 per cent for the surgically treated group, a 17 per cent risk reduction. There was a 10.6 per cent reduction in the occurrence of major or fatal ipsilateral strokes with surgical therapy compared with medical therapy.[89]

THERAPEUTIC ANTITHROMBOSIS

Deep Venous Thrombosis

The therapeutic options available for the treatment of venous thrombosis include anticoagulation, fibrinolytic therapy, and surgery (venous filters/venous interruption or thrombectomy). Only anticoagulation therapy is discussed.

The management of an asymptomatic calf vein thrombosis is controversial. Surveillance alone, either by impedance plethysmography or, more recently, by duplex scanning,[90] has been advocated when a thrombus is confined to the calf because only 20 per cent of untreated calf thrombi propagate proximally to a point at which they pose the threat of a major pulmonary embolism.[26] However, one study has documented a 10 per cent incidence of pulmonary emboli originating from the deep calf veins.[91] A controlled prospective study of patients on a medical service also documented a 29 per cent recurrence of deep calf venous thrombosis within 90 days after a 5-day course of heparin, an 18 per cent rate of proximal extension of the calf thrombi, and a 3.6 per cent incidence of pulmonary emboli. In comparison, patients who received anticoagulant therapy for 3 months had none of these complications.[92] We recommend a minimum of 3 months of anticoagulation (initial intravenous heparin therapy followed by warfarin or subcutaneous heparin) for patients with deep calf vein thrombosis unless anticoagulation is contraindicated. When anticoagulant therapy is contraindicated, close surveillance with duplex scanning is recommended to identify patients with proximal extension of the thrombotic process. These patients may require a vena caval filter.

For deep venous thrombus, especially for thrombus extending above the calf, a bolus of heparin (200 to 300 U/kg body weight) is given, followed by a continuous infusion of heparin (approximately 1000 U/hr). The infusion is adjusted to maintain the aPTT at 1.5 to 1.7 times the control value. The continuous intravenous infusion method, compared with intermittent intravenous infusion or the subcutaneous administration of heparin, has a smaller incidence of hemorrhagic complication, is easier to monitor, requires less heparin, and provides a ''stable level'' of incoagulability. A study comparing subcutaneous LMWH to continuous intravenous heparin in the treatment of deep venous thrombosis reported that LMWH was as effective and safe as the continuous infusion of heparin. Six of 213 patients (2.8 per cent) who received LMWH and 15 of 219 patients (6.9 per cent) who received continuous intravenous heparin had new episodes of venous thromboembolism. Initial therapy resulted in major bleeding in 1 (0.5 per cent) patient receiving LMWH and in 11 (5.0 per cent) patients receiving continuous heparin.[93]

We recommend 5 to 7 days of intravenous heparin therapy for deep venous thrombosis. The heparin is continued longer if the symptoms do not resolve in this time period. Warfarin therapy is begun after 1 to 3 days of heparin therapy. The heparin is discontinued when the PT is approximately 1.5 times the control value. The optimal duration of oral anticoagulation therapy is not known. However, the recurrence rate of thrombosis is higher in patients who are anticoagulated for less than 3 months. We recommend at least 3 to 6 months of anticoagulant therapy. Recurrent thromboembolism occurs in 2 to 3 per cent of patients who are ''adequately'' treated with anticoagulants and is more common in patients with proximal thrombi than in those with thrombi confined to the calf.[49, 94]

Heparin is the drug of choice for the treatment of deep venous thrombosis during pregnancy because heparin does not cross the placenta. After 7 to 10 days of intravenous heparin therapy, the pregnant patient is managed with 10,000 to 15,000 units of subcutaneous heparin per day, given in divided doses, for continued inhibition of the coagulation mechanism. The heparin is usually stopped prior to delivery. Anticoagulation with heparin or warfarin is continued postdelivery.

Placement of an inferior vena caval filter is indicated in patients with deep venous thrombosis if anticoagulation is not possible because of active bleeding, intracranial hemorrhage, a recent neurosurgical procedure, or malignant hypertension or if extension of thrombosis occurs despite ''adequate'' anticoagulation (see Chapter 135).

Pulmonary Embolism

Anticoagulation, unless contraindicated (active bleeding), is the standard method of management for both major and minor emboli. Support for this practice was initiated by a randomized controlled trial undertaken by Barritt and Jordan.[95] After diagnosis of pulmonary embolism by clinical signs, electrocardiogram, and chest x-ray, patients were randomized to receive heparin in addition to an oral anticoagulant, or no treatment. Of the first 19 control patients, 5 died from recurrent embolism and 5 others had nonfatal recurrences. Among the first 16 patients receiving anticoagulants, there was 1 death from pneumonia and a bleeding duodenal ulcer. Among an additional 38 patients studied, all of whom received anticoagulation, 1 developed a nonfatal recurrent embolism. Despite its shortcomings, this trial emphasized the value of anticoagulation in the management of uncomplicated pulmonary embolism.

In patients with suspected pulmonary embolism, heparin is given promptly before the diagnosis is confirmed by arteriogram or ventilation-perfusion scanning. Once the diagnosis is established, anticoagulation is provided in a fashion similar to that employed for managing deep venous thrombosis. We continue warfarin or self-administered subcutaneous heparin anticoagulation for 3 to 6 months in patients who have had a pulmonary embolism. If a patient has recurrent pulmonary embolism after discontinuation of anticoagulant therapy, a longer period (12 months) of warfarin anticoagulation is recommended.

Vena caval filter placement is considered for patients who have recurrent pulmonary emboli despite adequate oral anticoagulation or if anticoagulation is contraindicated.

References

1. Vanhoutte PM: Platelets, endothelium, and vasospasm [Abstract]. Thromb Hemost 58:252, 1987.
2. Chesterman CN: Vascular endothelium, haemostasis, and thrombosis. Blood Rev 2:88, 1988.
3. Engleberg H: Endothelium in health and disease. Semin Thromb Hemost 14:1, 1988.
4. Pearson JD, Carlton JS, Hutchings A: Prostacyclin release stimulated by thrombin or bradykinin in porcine endothelial cells cultured from aorta and umbilical vein. Thromb Res 29:115, 1983.
5. Levin RI, Weksler BB, Marcus AJ, et al: Prostacyclin production by endothelial cells. *In* Jaffe EA (ed): Biology of Endothelial Cells. Boston, Martinus Nijhoff, 1984, pp 228–247.
6. Moncada S, Palma RMJ, Higgs EA: Prostacyclin and endothelium-derived relaxing factor: Biological interactions and significance. *In* Verstraete M, Vermylon J, Lijnen HR, Armout J (eds): Thrombosis and Hemostasis. Leuven, ISTH Leuven University Press, 1985, p597.
7. Bounassissi V: Sulfated mucopolysaccharide synthesis and secretion in endothelial cell cultures. Exp Cell Res 76:363, 1973.
8. Suzuki K, Nishioka J, Matsuda M, et al: Protein S is essential for the activated protein C-catalyzed inactivation of platelet-associated factor Va. J Biochem 96:455, 1984.
9. Kun-yu Wu K, Fasier-Scott K, Hatzakis H: Endothelial cell function in hemostasis and thrombosis. Adv Exp Med Biol 242:127, 1987.
10. Prydz H, Petterson KS: Synthesis of thromboplastin (tissue factor) by endothelial cells. Haemostasis 18:215, 1988.
11. Davie EW, Ratnoff OD: Waterfall sequence for intrinsic blood clotting. Science 145:1310, 1964.
12. McFarlane RG: An enzyme cascade in the blood clotting mechanism and its function as a biochemical amplifier. Nature 202:498, 1964.
13. Rosenberg RD: Actions and interactions of antithrombin and heparin. N Engl J Med 292:146, 1975.
14. Wessler S: Prevention of venous thromboembolism by low-dose heparin. Mod Concepts Cardiovasc Dis 45:105, 1976.
15. Egeberg O: Inherited antithrombin deficiency causing thrombophilia. Throm Diathes Haemorrh 13:516, 1965.
16. Shapiro ME, Rodvien R, Bauer KA, et al: Acute aortic thrombosis in antithrombin III deficiency. JAMA 245:1759, 1981.
17. Schwartz RS, Bauer KA, Rosenberg RD, et al: Clinical experience with antithrombin III concentrate in treatment of congenital and acquired deficiency of antithrombin. Am J Med 87 (Suppl 3B):53, 1989.
18. Crouse LH, Comp PC: The regulation of hemostasis: The protein C system. N Engl J Med 314:1298, 1986.
19. Silver MJ, Smith JB, Ingerman CM, et al: Arachidonic acid-induced human platelet aggregation and prostaglandin formation. Prostaglandins 4:863, 1973.
20. Estivals M, Pelzer H, Sie P, et al: Prothrombin fragment 1 + 2, thrombin-antithrombin III complexes and D-dimers in acute deep vein thrombosis: Effects of heparin treatment. Br J Haematol 78:421, 1991.
21. Guyton J, Willerson JT: Peripheral venous platelet aggregates in patients with unstable angina pectoris and acute myocardial infarction. Angiology 28:695, 1977.
22. Sobel M, Salzman EW, Davies GC, et al: Circulating platelet products in unstable angina pectoris. Circulation 63:300, 1981.
23. Green LH, Seroppian E, Handin RI: Platelet activation during exercise-induced myocardial ischemia. N Engl J Med 302:193, 1980.
24. Steele P, Carroll J, Overfield D, et al: Effect of sulfinpyrazone on platelet survival times in patients with transient cerebral ischemic attacks. Stroke 8:396, 1977.
25. Steele P, Ellis J, Genton E: Effects of platelet suppressant, anticoagulant and fibrinolytic therapy in patients with recurrent venous thrombosis. Am J Med 64:441, 1978.
26. Clayton JK, Anderson JA, McNicol GP: Preoperative prediction of postoperative deep vein thrombosis. Br Med J 2:910, 1976.
27. Coon W: Some recent developments in the pharmacology of heparin. J Clin Pharmacol 19:337, 1979.
28. Bentley PG, Kakkar V, Scully M, et al: An objective study of alternative methods of heparin administration. Thromb Res 18:177, 1980.
29. Lane DA, Denton J, Flynn AM, et al: Anticoagulant activities of heparin oligosaccharides and their neutralization by platelet factor 4. Biochem J 218:725, 1984.
30. Handin RI, Cohen HJ: Purification and binding properties of human platelet factor four. J Biol Chem 251:4273, 1976.
31. Glazier RL, Crowell EB: Randomized prospective trial of continuous versus intermittent heparin therapy. JAMA 236:1365, 1976.
32. Hull RD, Raskob GE, Hirsh J, et al: Continuous intravenous heparin compared with intermittent subcutaneous heparin in the initial treatment of proximal-vein thrombosis. N Engl J Med 315:1109, 1986.
33. Salzman EW, Deykin D, Shapiro R, et al: Management of heparin therapy: Controlled prospective trial. N Engl J Med 292:1042, 1975.
34. Sharnoff J, DeBlasio G: Prevention of fatal postoperative thromboembolism by heparin prophylaxis. Lancet 2:1006, 1970.
35. Salzman EW, Davies GC: Prophylaxis of venous thromboembolism: Analysis of cost effectiveness. Ann Surg 191:207, 1980.
36. International Multicentre Trial: Prevention of fatal postoperative pulmonary embolism by low doses of heparin. Lancet 1:45, 1975.
37. Coe N, Collins RE, Klein L, et al: Prevention of deep vein thrombosis in urological patients: A controlled randomized trial of low dose heparin and external pneumatic compression boots. Surgery 83:230, 1978.
38. Harris WH, Salzman E, Athanasoulis C, et al: Comparison of warfarin, low-molecular-weight dextran, aspirin, and subcutaneous heparin in prevention of venous thromboembolism following total hip replacement. J Bone Joint Surg (Am) 56:1552, 1974.
39. Kakkar VV, Murray WJG: Efficacy and safety of low-molecular weight heparin (CY216) in preventing postoperative venous thromboembolism: A co-operative study. Br J Surg 72:786, 1985.
40. Berqvist D, Burmark US, Frisell J, et al: Low molecular weight heparin once daily compared with conventional low dose heparin twice daily. Br J Surg 73:204, 1986.
41. Hirsch J: Rational for development of low molecular weight heparins and their clinical potential in the prevention of postoperative venous thrombosis. Am J Surg 161:512, 1991.
42. Hoch JR, Silver D: Complications and failures of anticoagulant therapy. *In* Bernhard VM, Towne JB, (eds): Complications in Vascular Surgery. St. Louis, Quality Medical Publishing, 1991, p 118.
43. Pitney WR, Pettit J, Armstrong L: Control of heparin therapy. Br Med J 4:139, 1970.
44. Silver D, Kapsch D, Tsoi E: Heparin induced thrombocytopenia, thrombosis, and hemorrhage. Ann Surg 198:301, 1983.
45. Lassiter J, Cikrit D, Silver D: The heparin-induced thrombocytopenia syndrome: An update. Surgery 102:763, 1987.
46. Sevitt S, Gallagher N: Prevention of venous thrombosis and pulmonary embolism in injured patients. Lancet 2:981, 1959.
47. Flinn WR, Rohrer MJ, Yao JST, et al: Improved long-term patency of infragenicular polytetrafluoroethylene grafts. J Vasc Surg 7:685, 1988.
48. Veith FJ, Gupta SK, Ascer E, et al: Six-year prospective multicenter randomized comparison of autologous saphenous vein and expanded polytetrafluoroethylene grafts in infrainguinal arterial reconstruction. J Vasc Surg 3:104, 1986.
49. Gallus AS, Hirsh J: Treatment of venous thromboembolic disease. Semin Thromb Hemost 2:291, 1976.

50. Hull R, Hirsh J, Jay R, et al: Different intensities of oral anticoagulant therapy in the treatment of proximal vein thrombosis. N Engl J Med 307:1676, 1982.
51. Clagett GP, Reisch JS: Prevention of venous thromboembolism in general surgical patients. Ann Surg 208:227, 1988.
52. Fearnley GR, Charkrabarti R, Hocking ED: Fibrinolytic effects of diguanides plus ethylestrenol in occlusive vascular disease. Lancet 2:1008, 1967.
53. Harris WH, Salzman EW, Athanasoulis C, et al: Aspirin prophylaxis of venous thromboembolism after total hip replacement. N Engl J Med 297:1246, 1977.
54. Berqvist D: Prevention of postoperative thromboembolism in Sweden. The development of practice during five years. Thromb Haemost 53:239, 1985.
55. Ljungstrom K-G: Prophylaxis of postoperative thromboembolism with dextran 70: Improvements of efficacy and safety. Acta Chir Scand 149 (Suppl 514):1, 1983.
56. Gruber UF, Saldeen T, Brokop T, et al: Incidences of fatal postoperative pulmonary embolism after prophylaxis with dextran 70 and low dose heparin. An international multicenter study. Br Med J 1:69, 1980.
57. Ring J, Messmer K: Incidence and severity of anaphylactoid reactions to colloid volume substitutes. Lancet 1:466, 1977.
58. Pitney WR, Bray C, Holt P, et al: Acquired resistance to ancrod. Lancet 1:79, 1969.
59. Cole CW, Bormanis J: Ancrod: A practical alternative to heparin. J Vasc Surg 8:59, 1988.
60. O'Brien JR: Effects of salicylates on human platelets. Lancet 1:779, 1968.
61. Goldman M, Hall C, Dykes J, et al: Does 111-indium platelet deposition predict patency in prosthetic arterial grafts? Br J Surg 70:635, 1983.
62. Green RM, Roedersheimer R, DeWeese JA: Effects of aspirin and dipyridamole on expanded PTFE graft patency. Surgery 92:1016, 1982.
63. Kohler TR, Kaufman JL, Kacoyanis G, et al: Effect of aspirin and dipyridamole on the patency of lower extremity bypass grafts. Surgery 96:462, 1984.
64. Chesebro JH, Fuster V, Elvback LR, et al: Effect of dipyridamole and aspirin on late vein-graft patency after coronary bypass operation. N Engl J Med 310:209, 1984.
65. Lorenz RL, Weber M, Lotzur J, et al: Improved aortocoronary bypass patency by low-dose aspirin (100 mg daily). Lancet 1:1261, 1984.
66. Canadian Cooperative Study Group: A randomized trial of aspirin and sulfinpyrazone in threatened stroke. N Engl J Med 299:53, 1978.
67. Turpie AGG: Antiplatelet therapy. Clin Hematol 10:497, 1981.
68. Bousser MG, Eschwege E, Haguenau M, et al: "AICLA" controlled trial of aspirin and dipyridamole in the secondary prevention of athero-thrombotic cerebral ischemia. Stroke 14:5, 1983.
69. Ramirez-Lassipas M: Platelet inhibitors for TIAs: A review of prospective drug trial results. Postgrad Med 75:52, 1984.
70. Harlan JM, Harker LA: Hemostasis, thrombosis, and thromboembolic disorders: The role of arachidonic acid metabolites in platelet-vessel wall interactions. Med Clin North Am 65:855, 1981.
71. Mustard JF, Kinlough-Rathbone RL, Packham MA: Aspirin in the treatment of cardiovascular disease: A review. Am J Med 74:43, 1983.
72. Lewis HD Jr, Davis JW, Archibald DG, et al: Protective effects of aspirin against acute myocardial infarction and death in men with unstable angina. N Engl J Med 309:396, 1983.
73. Brune JJ: The mechanism of action of ticlopidine. Thromb Res Suppl 4, p 59, 1983.
74. Gent M, Blakely JA, Easton JD, et al: The Canadian American Ticlopidine Study (CATS) in thromboembolic stroke. Lancet 1:1215, 1989.
75. Arcan JC, Blanchard J, Boissel JP, et al: Multicenter double blind study of ticlopidine in the treatment of intermittent claudication and the prevention of its complications. Angiology 39:802, 1988.
76. Skillman J, Collins RE, Coe N, et al: Prevention of deep vein thrombosis in neurosurgical patients: A controlled randomized trial of external pneumatic compression boots. Surgery 83:354, 1978.
77. Harris WH, Raines JK, Athanasoulis C, et al: External pneumatic compression versus warfarin in reducing thrombosis in high risk hip patients. *In* Madden J, Hume M (eds): Venous Thromboembolism: Prevention and Treatment. New York, Appleton-Century-Crofts, 1976, pp 51–60.
78. Torngren S: Optimal regimen of low dose heparin prophylaxis in gastrointestinal surgery. Acta Chir Scand 145:87, 1979.
79. Eriksson I, Holmberg JT: Analysis of factors affecting limb salvage and mortality after embolectomy. Acta Chir Scand 143:237, 1977.
80. Green RM, DeWeese J, Rob C: Arterial embolectomy before and after the Fogarty catheter. Surgery 77:24, 1975.
81. Holm J, Schersten T: Anticoagulant treatment during and after embolectomy. Acta Chir Scand 138:683, 1972.
82. Genton E, Barnett H, Fields WS, et al: Cerebral ischemia: The role of thrombosis and antithrombotic therapy. Stroke 8:150, 1977.
83. Carter AB: Prognosis of cerebral embolism. Lancet 2:514, 1965.
84. Millikan CH, McDowell FH: Treatment of transient ischemic attacks. Stroke 9:299, 1978.
85. Cerebral Embolism Task Force: Cardiogenic brain embolism. Arch Neurol 43:71, 1986.
86. Fields WS, Lemak NA, Frankowski RF, et al: Controlled trial of aspirin in cerebral ischemia. Stroke 8:301, 1977.
87. Riekkinen RJ, Lowenthal A, Googers FA: Main results of the European stroke prevention study. Neurology 37 (Suppl 1):103, 1987.
88. Grotta JC: Current medical and surgical therapy for cerebrovascular disease. N Engl J Med 317:1505, 1987.
89. North American Symptomatic Carotid Endarterectomy Trial Collaborators: Beneficial effect of carotid endarterectomy in symptomatic patients with high-grade stenosis. N Engl J Med 325:445, 1991.
90. Mattos MA, Gregg LL, Darr WL, et al: Color-flow duplex scanning for the surveillance and diagnosis of acute deep venous thrombosis. J Vasc Surg 15:366, 1992.
91. Kakkar VV, Howe CT, Nicolaides AN, et al: Deep vein thrombosis of the legs: Is there a high risk group? Am J Surg 120:527, 1970.
92. Lagerstedt CI, Olsson C-G, Faghr BQ, et al: Need for long term anticoagulant treatment in symptomatic calf-vein thrombosis. Lancet 2:515, 1985.
93. Hull RD, Raskob GE, Pineo GF, et al: Subcutaneous low-molecular weight heparin compared with continuous intravenous heparin in the treatment of proximal-vein thrombosis. N Engl J Med 326:975, 1992.
94. Hull R, Delmore T, Gento E, et al: Warfarin sodium versus low-dose heparin in the long term treatment of venous thrombosis. N Engl J Med 301:855, 1979.
95. Barritt DW, Jordan SC: Anticoagulant drugs in the treatment of pulmonary embolism. Lancet 1:1209, 1960.

18

Circulation-Enhancing Drugs

Young Wook Kim, M.D., Lloyd M. Taylor, Jr., M.D., and John M. Porter, M.D.

The practice of modern vascular surgery requires familiarity with an increasing number of drugs that have therapeutic actions specifically relevant to vascular disease. These agents may be broadly divided into two groups: the antithrombotic drugs, including anticoagulants, thrombolytic agents, and antiplatelet drugs, and a second group comprising drugs whose purpose is to improve circulation in ischemic areas. The antithrombotic drugs are discussed in Chapters 17 and 19.

As the indications for and expectations of reconstructive peripheral arterial surgery have become more realistically defined, clinicians have shown an increasing interest in pharmacologic treatment of occlusive vascular disease. Multiple new agents with widely differing mechanisms of action that appear to exert their beneficial effect by improving microcirculatory flow have become available in recent years. In this chapter we present our assessment of the role of the hemorrheologic agents pentoxifylline and dextran and of the metabolism-enhancing drugs naftidrofuryl and carnitine in the treatment of vascular disorders. We then describe the pharmacologic treatment of lower extremity ischemia including both intermittent claudication and impending tissue loss. The use of vasodilators in the treatment of both obstructive arterial disease and vasospastic disorders including Raynaud's syndrome, ergotism, and nonocclusive mesenteric ischemia is also described.

HEMORRHEOLOGIC DRUGS

Hemorrheology is the term applied to the study of the flow characteristics of blood. In large vessels the rheologic factor most important in determining blood flow is viscosity, as described in the Poiseuille equation (Fig. 18–1). Important factors influencing blood viscosity include plasma fibrinogen level and hematocrit. The number of platelets and leukocytes present in the blood is so small compared with the number of erythrocytes that viscosity is affected only when these cellular elements are present in extreme excess, as may occur in certain myeloproliferative disorders such as leukemia or thrombocytosis. Circulating platelets exist both singly and in aggregates of varying number. The same is true of leukocytes, although to a lesser degree. Because of their size, the presence of these aggregates can influence blood viscosity.

In the microcirculation, other rheologic factors in addition to viscosity may exert considerable influence on blood flow. One such factor is the ability of cellular elements, particularly erythrocytes and leukocytes, to undergo spherical deformation as they pass through the capillary network. The importance of this is obvious, because normal erythrocytes with a diameter of 8 to 9 microns must routinely undergo remarkable deformation to pass through capillaries that average 4 to 5 microns in diameter. Even greater degrees of deformation are necessary for the larger leukocytes to pass through capillaries. A second factor influencing microvascular flow is the degree of adhesiveness of platelets and leukocytes. This adhesion property is profoundly influenced by platelet and leukocyte activation instituted by coagulation factors or inflammatory mediators, or both. Activated platelets and platelet aggregates as well as activated leukocytes are capable of completely occluding capillaries and may have a profound negative influence on microcirculatory flow.

In 1976, several investigators independently reported that erythrocytes from patients with peripheral vascular disease were more rigid or less deformable than normal.[35, 71] These observations were based on studies of whole blood filterability as measured by the timed volume flow of blood under constant pressure through microporous material. Subsequent studies by other investigators using washed red blood cells failed to confirm impaired deformability of erythrocytes from patients with peripheral arterial disease.[53] It is now widely believed that the impairment in whole blood filterability observed in patients with severe peripheral vascular disease actually results from changes in the absolute number or aggregation of platelets and leukocytes or from changes in their adhesiveness.

In addition to impaired blood filterability, a number of observations confirming altered hemorrheologic factors in patients with peripheral arterial disease have been described, including elevated blood viscosity, increased platelet activation, elevated leukocyte count, and increased fibrinogen levels.[19, 30, 35, 38, 48, 53, 71] In recent years the role of leukocytes in the regulation of microcirculatory flow has

$$P_1 - P_2 = Q\frac{8L\eta}{\pi r^4}$$

FIGURE 18–1. Poiseuille's equation describing the factors influencing fluid flow in cylindrical tubes. (P1–P2, pressure gradient along the tube; Q, volume flow; L, length of the tube; η, viscosity of the fluid; r, radius of the tube.)

been widely recognized. An example is seen in studies demonstrating complete cessation of nailbed capillary flow caused by leukocyte capillary plugging in patients with septic shock.[95] A clear relationship has been demonstrated between absent reflow following prolonged ischemia and the presence of irreversible leukocyte capillary plugs.[37] Altered leukocyte rheology has been observed in patients with claudication.[57] Thus, considerable evidence indicates the presence of significant alterations in blood rheology in claudicants with all the observed changes in the direction of increased blood viscosity and decreased microcirculatory flow.

The consistent finding of an abnormal hemorrheologic state in patients with significant peripheral arterial occlusive disorders has led to intense interest in the development of pharmacologic agents intended to return the disordered microcirculation toward normal. Two drugs currently available have primarily hemorrheologic modes of action—pentoxifylline and dextran. There is evidence that some drugs classified currently as vasodilators, antiplatelet agents, and so on, may also have important hemorrheologic properties.

Pentoxifylline

Pentoxifylline is a theobromine derivative (see formula in Fig. 18–2) discovered in Germany in the 1930s. It was originally investigated as a potential vasodilator, but the drug does not produce systemic vasodilatation in humans, at least as indicated by its lack of effects on heart rate, blood pressure, and measured vascular resistance.[7] Hess and associates first showed in 1973 that pentoxifylline reduced whole blood viscosity,[50] and this observation has been confirmed in a number of studies since then.[4, 34, 80, 93] Pentoxifylline was also shown to improve the reduced whole blood filterability found in claudicants. As noted previously, this improvement was initially attributed to improved red blood cell deformability. Subsequently, pentoxifylline was shown to decrease plasma fibrinogen and platelet aggregation significantly, actions that decrease blood viscosity.[62, 71] Pentoxifylline does not improve the filterability of washed red blood cells as opposed to whole blood, but it does improve the rheologic characteristics of white blood cells.[57, 78] This action probably underlies the observed improvement with pentoxifylline of the filterability of whole blood taken from claudicants.

In normal subjects, pentoxifylline has been shown to increase both plethysmographically measured limb blood flow and xenon-133–determined capillary blood flow.[3, 5, 70, 75] Using direct micropipette techniques, Ehrly demonstrated improved calf muscle Po_2 in claudicants following pentoxifylline treatment.[33] Unfortunately, to date this important observation has not been confirmed by others.

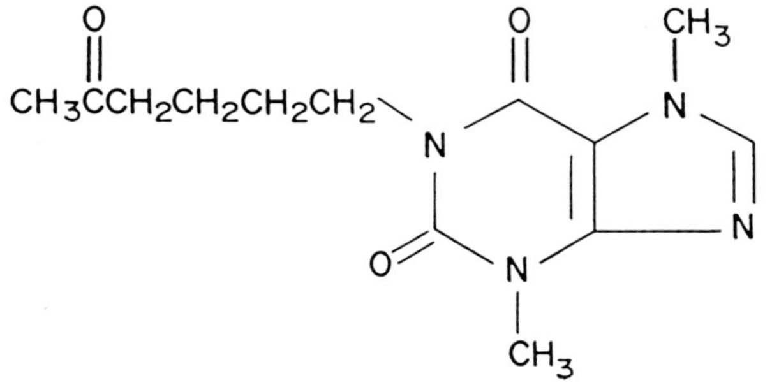

Use of the drug was based on the results of multiple blinded controlled trials conducted in Europe and the United States. The results of 11 controlled double-blind trials conducted in Europe are summarized in Table 18–1. These studies differed in pentoxifylline dosage, in the therapeutic end-points evaluated, in the duration of treatment, and in the nature of the control treatment. Despite these important differences, all these studies demonstrated significant patient benefit from treatment with pentoxifylline compared with controls.[3, 4, 12, 15, 29, 40, 54, 73, 79, 86, 91, 94] A large double-blind controlled trial of pentoxifylline treatment for claudication was conducted in the United States at multiple participating centers using treadmill walking as the therapeutic end-point.[68] This study demonstrated that pentoxifylline was significantly more effective than placebo in increasing walking distance as assessed by the initial appearance of pain and the absolute walking distance achieved. The benefit of the drug averaged only a 45 per cent improvement compared with a 23 per cent improvement with placebo. The side effects of pentoxifylline include gastrointestinal symptoms (nausea, vomiting, and bloating) and dizziness and require discontinuance of the drug in 3 to 5 per cent of patients.

CH3CCH2CH2CH2CH2 (=O) — N; O; CH3; N; N; N; O; N; CH3

FIGURE 18–2. Pentoxifylline.

Dextran

Dextrans are long-chain carbohydrates of varying molecular weight, the basic subunit of which is glucose. Two dextran preparations are available for clinical use: dextran 40 and dextran 70. The numbers refer to the mean molecular weight in thousands of the polymers. These products are commercially available as 6 per cent dextran 70 or 10 per cent dextran 40 in 5 per cent glucose or in normal saline solution. Dextrans are used clinically for three effects including plasma expansion, an antithrombotic effect, and microcirculatory flow improvement. The plasma expander effects of dextrans appear no different from those of any fluid containing macromolecules. The antithrombotic and microcirculatory enhancement properties of dextrans include coating of red blood cells, increasing the normal endothelial and blood cell electronegative membrane potential, and decreasing blood viscosity. In trauma victims, dextrans have been shown to lessen the abnormal decrease in plasma fibrinolytic activity that follows injury.[17] Dextran 70 has a half-life of 24 hours as opposed to 6 hours for dextran 40. The antithrombotic activity of the two preparations is similar. Because it is supplied as a 10 per cent solution, dextran 40 has a higher osmotic pressure and is more effective as a plasma expander. To date, the most frequent clinical use of dextrans has been in the prevention of venous thrombosis.

A small but definite benefit from the use of dextran in conjunction with arterial surgery has been repeatedly demonstrated. Experimentally, dextran improves the patency of small-caliber arterial grafts,[61] an observation supported by the clinical reports of Thomas and Silva[90] and of Bergentz

Table 18–1. European Studies on Efficacy of Pentoxifylline in Intermittent Claudication

Duration of Treatment (wk)	Dose of Pentoxifylline (mg)	No. of Patients/Clinical Observations	Reference
8	600	13 Pentoxifylline = 100% improved 13 Placebo = 8% improved	15
4	600	27 Pentoxifylline = 83% improved Treadmill walking + 126% 28 Placebo = 60% improved Treadmill walking + 38%	71
8	600	27 Pentoxifylline Walking + 208% 9 Placebo Walking + 52%	12
4–6	800	25 Pentoxifylline = 84% improved Walking + 120% 25 Placebo = 17% improved Walking + 20%	79
6–8	1200	20 Pentoxifylline Walking + 39% 29 Placebo Walking + 16%	54
4	1200	20 Pentoxifylline = 71% improved Walking + 45% 20 Placebo = 24% improved Walking + 28%	93
24	1200	8 Pentoxifylline = walking initial + 12% Walking absolute + 10% 8 Placebo = walking initial + 28% Walking absolute + 11%	73
8	1200	12 Pentoxifylline Walking + 38% 12 Placebo Walking + 3%	29
12	800	18 Pentoxifylline Walking + 46% 18 Placebo Walking + 4%	86
8	1200	18 Pentoxifylline = 83% improved Walking + 80% 18 Adenosine = 50% improved Walking + 6%	40
8	800–1200	25 Pentoxifylline = 73% improved Treadmill walking + 47% 24 Nylidrin = 46% improved Treadmill walking + 5%	3

From Taylor LM Jr, Porter JM: Drug treatment of claudication: Vasodilators, hemorrheologic agents, and antiserotonin drugs. J Vasc Surg 3:374, 1986.
+ indicates increase.

and colleagues.[10] In a randomized trial, Rutherford and colleagues demonstrated significantly improved patency of disadvantaged distal lower extremity bypass grafts when accompanied by perioperative dextran treatment.[76] Most of the patency advantage was lost after only a few months of follow-up, however, suggesting that the antithrombotic properties of dextran delay but do not ultimately prevent graft thrombosis.[77] Despite the modest underlying database, many clinicians use dextran in an attempt to improve the patency of arterial reconstructions. Dextrans can be given only by the intravenous route. As a general guideline, no more than 20 ml/kg body weight is given each 24 hours, and the drug is continued for no more than 72 hours.[25] Contraindications to the use of dextran include hypersensitivity, congestive heart failure, impaired renal function, and coagulopathy or active bleeding. Anaphylaxis can occur, usually at the beginning of the infusion, and may be prevented or diminished by preinfusion of short-chain dextrans (MW 3000 to 6000) in patients with a history of sensitivity. Abnormal bleeding from dextran can occur with excessive dosage or with concomitant anticoagulant or antiplatelet medications. Renal failure occurs rarely and is probably caused by osmotic damage to the tubular cells. Dextrans may interfere with blood typing and cross-matching.[74] Blood for this purpose should be obtained prior to administration of dextran.

METABOLISM-ENHANCING AGENTS

An alternative approach to improving the performance of ischemic muscles has nothing to do with increasing blood flow but rather with attempts to enhance ischemic muscle metabolism pharmacologically. Two drugs of current interest, carnitine and naftidrofuryl, appear to operate through such mechanisms. At present neither of these agents is approved for use by the United States Food and Drug Administration (FDA).

Carnitine

Carnitine is a naturally occurring substance that appears to be free of toxic effects at all doses.[6] The normal biochemical actions of carnitine are to facilitate the entry of pyruvate into the citric acid cycle and the transport of fatty acids. The net effect is one of increasing adenosine triphosphate (ATP) that would otherwise have been lost as lactate. Therefore, the available oxygen provides more energy in the presence of carnitine.[43] In theory, this results in greater work capacity by ischemic muscles.

Recent studies have indicated that ischemic muscle displays a relative carnitine deficiency and becomes especially inefficient during anaerobic metabolism. Brevetti and colleagues[14] gave carnitine to claudicants in a double-blind randomized trial and evaluated treadmill walking and popliteal vein lactate levels as well as muscle biopsy carnitine levels. They noted a significant increase in treadmill walking in patients treated with carnitine compared to those treated with placebo. Popliteal venous lactate was decreased and muscle biopsy carnitine was increased in patients receiving the drug compared to those receiving placebo. The results of this study have created considerable interest in the role of this nontoxic agent in the treatment of claudication.

At present, carnitine is not approved by the FDA for the treatment of claudication. Because it is a natural substance, carnitine can be sold and is available (although at considerable expense) in health food stores and similar outlets. A multicenter United States trial of carnitine is nearly complete, and a follow-up trial of *n*-propionylcarnitine, an analogue, is planned for the near future.

Naftidrofuryl

Naftidrofuryl (Praxilene) is an unusual drug available in Europe but not in the United States. The drug appears to stimulate the entry of carbohydrate and fat into the tricarboxylic acid cycle. This results in a net increase in ATP production and a decrease in lactate accumulation in areas of relative ischemia. Naftidrofuryl has been evaluated for the treatment of claudication, with most studies showing mixed results.[21, 95] It has also been evaluated for the treatment of ischemic rest pain. The results of this trial did not clearly establish a benefit of drug treatment.[46] In addition to its role in the treatment of ischemia, naftidrofuryl is currently being evaluated for a possible effect in reversing the protein wasting and negative nitrogen balance that may follow both trauma and major surgery.[16] Naftidrofuryl is widely prescribed in Europe, and United States physicians may encounter its use in their patients who have traveled abroad.

PHARMACOLOGIC TREATMENT OF CHRONIC LOWER EXTREMITY ISCHEMIA

Intermittent Claudication

The introduction of pentoxifylline as the first pharmacologic agent proved effective in the treatment of intermittent claudication marks the beginning of a new era in the treatment of lower extremity arterial insufficiency. This new era has been characterized both by a recognition that pharmacologic therapy of claudication is possible and may be beneficial and by better understanding of the natural history of claudication and the nature of the scientific evidence necessary to prove the efficacy of treatment. Currently, pentoxifylline is widely prescribed, and some data are becoming available about the effectiveness of this treatment. Many other agents have been and are being evaluated as possibly beneficial in the treatment of claudication.

Consistently, randomized trials have demonstrated that the benefit associated with pentoxifylline therapy is modest at best. In the United States randomized trial, the average differences in improvement in the distance achieved before the initial occurrence of claudication (45 per cent for the drug vs 23 per cent for placebo [Fig. 18–3]) and the absolute distance achieved with claudication (32 per cent for the drug vs 20 per cent for placebo [Fig. 18–4]) were statistically significant but small.[68] It is problematic whether such differences are clinically significant. Obviously, if a patient wishes to walk 150 meters to the mailbox, for example, and currently is stopped by claudication occurring at 100 meters, an increase in walking distance to 125 meters is of no value to the patient, although it is perhaps statistically significant. This issue of the difference between efficacy and clinical effectiveness has been partially addressed by several studies.

In an unblinded, nonrandomized trial, Green and McNamara[45] prescribed pentoxifylline for 130 consecutive patients with claudication and defined successful treatment as complete cessation of the symptoms of claudication. This result occurred in 23 patients (17 per cent), whereas no improvement was noted in 88 patients (67 per cent), the remainder having intermediate results or suffering side effects that required cessation of the drug (5 per cent of patients). There were no features, such as severity of initial symptoms or location of arterial lesions, for example, in this study that allowed prediction of which patients would or would not have a beneficial result.

AbuRahma and coworkers[2] evaluated 93 patients with all degrees of severity of arterial disease who were treated with pentoxifylline therapy for 8 weeks. They found no benefit in patients with severe disease (rest pain, ischemic ulcer, and so on) and no benefit in patients with mild claudication (able to walk more than 300 meters), but benefit did occur in patients with severe claudication (able to walk more than 50 meters but less than 300 meters).

A recent multicenter double-blind trial that included 150 patients with claudication from Scandinavia[55] confirmed the presence of a significant improvement in walking

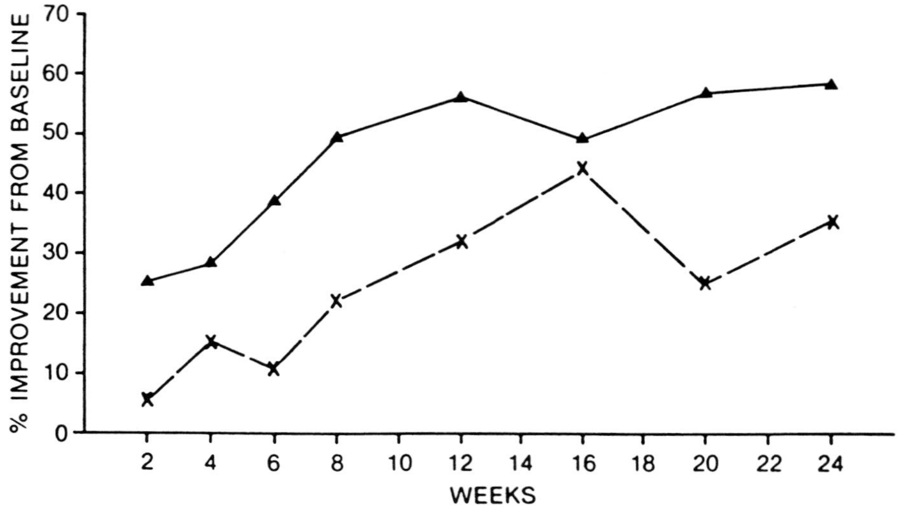

FIGURE 18–3. Initial claudication distance in placebo- and pentoxifylline-treated groups.

distance in patients treated with pentoxifylline. These authors noted that significant improvement was more likely in patients who had been symptomatic for more than 1 year and had an ankle-brachial pressure index of less than 0.80, whereas improvement was unlikely in patients with recent symptom onset and relatively mild ischemia.

It is important to remember that the modest benefits of pentoxifylline in regard to claudication cited earlier were derived from many patients in large multicenter trials. A careful review of the distribution of benefits within the treatment group reveals, unsurprisingly, that a moderate number of patients received considerable benefit, but about half received no benefit at all. Overall, 54 per cent of the treated patients achieved greater than or equal to a 50 per cent improvement in the claudication distance, a degree of improvement experienced by only 20 per cent of the placebo group. Thus, although the observation that pentoxifylline results in only a modest improvement of the entire claudication cohort is quite accurate, the drug greatly improves 30 to 35 per cent of claudicating patients. We do not recommend pentoxifylline for claudication without a preliminary trial of exercise and smoking cessation. In patients for whom pentoxifylline is elected, the drug should be continued for 6 to 8 weeks because this much time is required for maximal benefit. Interestingly, the United States drug company that markets pentoxifylline recognizes the uncertainty of the response pattern and offers a full purchase price refund to nonresponders.

Limb-Threatening Ischemia

Ischemic rest pain, ischemic ulcers, and gangrene are the end-stage manifestations of progressive lower extremity arterial occlusive disease. It has traditionally been assumed that the occurrence of these symptoms heralds an inevitable progression to limb loss if effective treatment is not instituted. Although surgical treatment is nearly always possible, most patients with limb-threatening ischemia are elderly and have multiple coexisting medical conditions that increase the risk and the practical and logistical difficulties accompanying surgery. The attractiveness of an effective drug therapy in this situation is obvious.

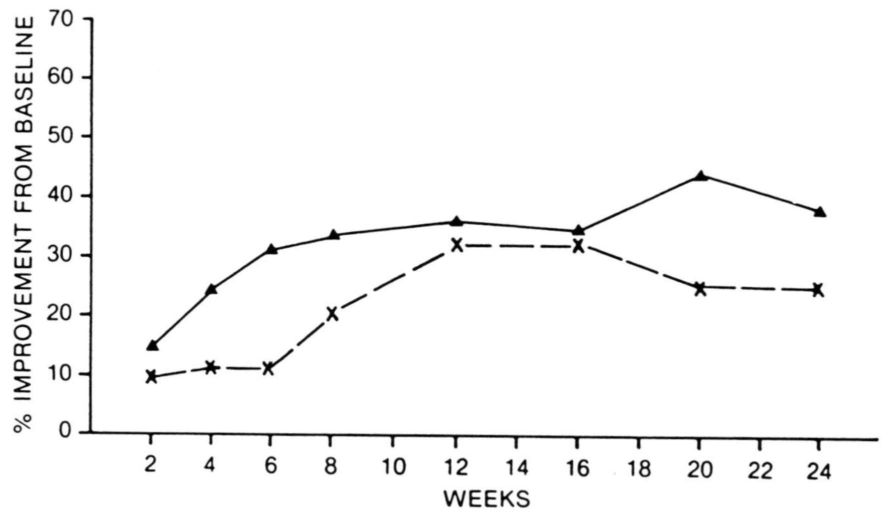

FIGURE 18–4. Absolute claudication distance in placebo- and pentoxifylline-treated groups.

Many drugs have been evaluated for the treatment of limb-threatening ischemia, most studies focusing on the treatment of ischemic ulceration. A partial list of such studies is given in Table 18–2. In these studies, all of which date from the 1980s, the drugs evaluated were all prostaglandins. To date, two observations have emerged from the collected studies. The first is that no drug has been shown to be clearly effective in the treatment of limb-threatening ischemia. In the few studies purporting to show benefit, the significant differences usually occurred in the areas of analgesic use or patients' perception of pain during the medication infusion rather than in durable healing of ischemic ulcers or avoidance of amputation. The second and perhaps more important observation is that a significant rate of spontaneous improvement in the symptoms of ischemic ulceration and ischemic rest pain is clearly shown in the placebo group in the drug studies and averages 25 to 40 per cent. Most studies used long hospitalization, bed rest, and assiduous wound care equally in both test and placebo groups. The observation that this treatment alone results in significant improvement in many patients with ischemic ulcers was brought to attention by Rivers and coworkers.[72] An obvious conclusion from these studies of limb-threatening ischemia is an emphasis on the critical requirement that any report claiming benefit for any treatment of limb-threatening ischemia include an appropriate randomized, placebo-treated control group. Studies that evaluate only the proposed treatment are obviously fatally flawed because they are based on the obviously false assumption that amputation is inevitable unless it is prevented by effective treatment.

VASODILATORS

For more than a century since Poiseuille first described the relationship between flow and the fourth power of the conduit radius, physicians have searched for effective vasodilating agents in the hope of improving blood flow to ischemic areas. Vasodilators currently in clinical use are listed in Table 18–3 and include adrenergic agents, direct-acting agents, calcium channel blockers, angiotensin-converting enzyme inhibitors, and prostaglandins. By far the most frequent clinical use of vasodilators has been in the treatment of hypertension and heart failure. In patients with peripheral vascular disease, vasodilators have been used for the treatment of obstructive arterial disease and vasospastic disorders. These indications for drug use are considered separately.

Obstructive Arterial Disease

In the past, clinicians observing the typically blanched feet of claudicants erroneously assumed that abnormal vasospasm was present in the ischemic areas. This assumption led to extensive use of vasodilators in attempts to treat lower extremity ischemia resulting from arterial obstruction. It is now well known that the pallor of the distal ischemic extremity results from redistribution, to the proximal muscle mass, of the limited blood flow entering the ischemic limb. Although anecdotal clinical benefit from the use of vasodilators in ischemia caused by fixed arterial obstructions has been described repeatedly, no control trial has ever shown consistent benefit.[22, 24, 48] The assumption that vasoconstriction exists in ischemic areas has been conclusively shown to be false.[24] Indeed, the products of ischemic anaerobic metabolism are potent vasodilators, and vessels in ischemic areas of limbs with proximal obstructive arterial disease are probably nearly maximally vasodilated, at least within the physiologic range. Treatment of such limbs with vasodilators may actually decrease blood flow in ischemic areas owing to a steal phenomenon resulting from dilatation of the normal vessels in nonischemic areas.[23] No vasodilator has ever been shown to increase blood flow in exercising muscle, a critical requirement for pharmacologic treatment of claudication.

Table 18–2. Controlled Studies of Prostaglandin Therapy of Limb-Threatening Ischemia

Reference	Number	Parameters	Drug	Result	Significance
65	30	Ischemic ulcer	PGI_2	Reduced size	$p < .02$
		Rest pain		No difference	n.s.
64	29	Ischemic ulcer	PGI_2	No difference	n.s.
		Rest pain		No difference	n.s.
36	24	Ischemic ulcer	PGE_1	No difference	n.s.
		Rest pain		No difference	n.s.
81	120	Ischemic ulcer	PGE_1	No difference	n.s.
		Rest pain		No difference	n.s.
88	30	Ischemic ulcer	PGE_1	No difference	n.s.
		Rest pain		No difference	n.s.
		Amputation		No difference	n.s.
8	28	Rest pain	PGI_2	Early benefit	n.s.
		Med cons		Sign improv	$p < .05$
		Ankle pressure		No difference	n.s.
27	26	Ischemic ulcer	PGI_2	No difference	n.s.
		Rest pain		No difference	n.s.
92	70	Ischemic ulcer	PGE_1	Reduced size	$p < .05$
		Rest pain		No difference	n.s.
		Med cons		Sign improv	$p < .005$
66	103	Ischemic ulcer	Iloprost	No difference	n.s.

Abbreviations: n.s., Not significant; med cons, consumption of analgesic medications; sign improv, significant improvement; PGI_2, prostacyclin; PGE_1, epoprostenol.

Table 18–3. Vasodilators in Clinical Use

Category	Drug	Indicated Uses
Alpha-adrenergic antagonists		
	Methyldopate	Hypertension
	Doxazosin	Hypertension
	Terazosin	Hypertension
	Prazosin	Hypertension
	Labetalol	Hypertension
	Guanfacine	Hypertension
	Phenoxybenzamine	Pheochromocytoma
Direct-acting agents		
	Hydralazine	Hypertension
	Minoxidil	Hypertension
	Papaverine	Cerebral ischemia, myocardial ischemia, peripheral ischemia
	Diazoxide	Hypertension
	Tolazoline	Pulmonary hypertension of the newborn
ACE inhibitors		
	Fosinopril	Hypertension
	Lisinopril	Hypertension
	Enalaprilat	Hypertension
	Captopril	Hypertension, heart failure
	Benazepril	Hypertension
	Enalapril	Hypertension, heart failure
Nitrates		
	Nitroprusside	Hypertension
	Erythrityl tetranitrate	Angina
	Nitroglycerin	Angina
	Isosorbide dinitrate	Angina
	Pentaerythritol tetranitrate	Angina
Calcium channel blockers		
	Ramipril	Hypertension
	Verapamil	Hypertension, angina, arrhythmias
	Nicardipine	Angina, hypertension
	Diltiazem	Angina
	Isradipine	Hypertension
	Nifedipine	Angina
	Nimodipine	Cerebral vasospasm
	Felodipine	Hypertension
	Bepridil	Angina
Ganglionic blockers		
	Trimethaphan	Hypertension, pulmonary edema caused by pulmonary hypertension
	Mecamylamine	Hypertension
	Guanethidine	Hypertension

Despite these considerations and despite the accumulation of a large number of controlled studies demonstrating no benefit from vasodilator treatment of arterial obstructive disease, considerable interest remains in the use of newer vasodilators for the treatment of ischemia. The agent currently undergoing evaluation is iloprost, a synthetic analogue of the prostaglandin prostacyclin, a potent vasodilator that also has strong platelet antiaggregant qualities. Iloprost can be administered intravenously or orally, a significant advantage in the treatment of chronic ischemia. A few studies have shown that treatment with iloprost in patients with severe lower extremity ischemia produces pain relief significantly more frequently than does placebo, although no advantage in prevention of the need for amputation or in healing of ischemic ulcers has been demonstrated.[8, 26, 65] The effectiveness of iloprost in achieving significant pain relief and healing of ischemic ulcers has also been demonstrated in patients with Buerger's disease compared with randomly chosen aspirin-treated controls.[41]

Most clinicians agree that at present there is little proven role for vasodilator treatment of obstructive arterial disorders. New agents are constantly being evaluated, and the principles of design of such studies, including objective quantification of the severity of ischemia and blind treatment using a carefully randomized control group, are well established. In the absence of such a study design, the extensively documented high rate of spontaneous improvement in patients with severe limb ischemia makes objective assessment of positive results impossible.

Specific Vasospastic Disorders

Emerging evidence suggests that abnormal vasospasm plays a role in many clinical disease states, only a few of which are well characterized. The most frequent and best characterized of these is Raynaud's syndrome. A much less frequent but clinically important vasospastic disorder is nonocclusive mesenteric ischemia, seen primarily as a complication of conditions accompanied by decreased cardiac output. Cerebral arterial spasm following subarachnoid hemorrhage and head trauma as well as coronary vasospasm are important clinical entities that are not further considered here because they are not primarily treated by vascular surgeons. Ergot intoxication results in symptomatic vasospasm that is easily mistaken for fixed arterial obstructive disease.

Raynaud's Syndrome

The underlying pathophysiology of Raynaud's syndrome remains unknown. At least two mechanisms are clearly operative, and patients can be conveniently grouped into two categories based on the underlying pathophysiology. In one category, Raynaud's symptoms result from a normal vasospastic response to cold in the digital arteries with reduced pressure caused by fixed obstructive disease (''obstructive Raynaud's syndrome''). Studies from our laboratory have shown an increased number of alpha-adrenoreceptors in the other category, that of patients with spastic Raynaud's syndrome,[32] perhaps providing an explanation for the ''local vascular fault'' originally proposed by Sir Thomas Lewis (1881–1945).

Most patients with Raynaud's syndrome require no therapy beyond simple cold avoidance and abstinence from tobacco. In our practice, only about 10 per cent of patients require pharmacologic therapy, and in the majority of these, the need for treatment is intermittent and confined to the colder months of the year. Predictably, patients with obstructive Raynaud's syndrome respond less favorably to drug therapy than do patients with spastic Raynaud's syndrome.

Initial therapy consists of nifedipine 10 mg/day, with a gradual increase in dosage up to 30 mg/day until improvement is noted. A sustained-release form of the medication is available, making once-daily dosage practical. The effectiveness of nifedipine therapy has been documented in controlled trials.[42, 84] If this single agent is ineffective, the addition of diltiazem 30 mg twice a day has been beneficial in some patients as assessed by a decrease in the temperature required to induce digital artery closure as well as the patient's subjective assessment of a reduction in the frequency and severity of vasospastic attacks. This regimen is based on the observation that diltiazem potentiates the binding of nifedipine to the calcium channel drug receptor.[85] Additional drug therapy for patients showing no improvement with calcium channel blockers includes prazosin and/or guanethidine.[69]

Patients with severe finger ischemia including ischemic finger ulcers and finger gangrene invariably have obstructive Raynaud's syndrome with minimal if any ischemia related to abnormal vasospasm.[59] Some of these patients can be successfully treated by performing arterial bypass to small vessels distal to the wrist,[28] a procedure previously performed infrequently. In the remaining patients, we have noted in the past anecdotal improvement in symptoms, particularly pain, following treatment with intravenous reserpine administered using the Bier block technique.[87] Reserpine is no longer available for injection, and our current regimen for the treatment of severe finger ischemia includes combined therapy with pentoxifylline and nifedipine. Again, we have noted anecdotal improvement. Many other agents have been evaluated for the treatment of severe Raynaud's syndrome, particularly prostaglandins. None has been proved effective in properly conducted controlled randomized trials.[9, 20, 31, 56, 60, 67]

Nonocclusive Mesenteric Ischemia

This important clinical syndrome appears to be caused by sustained severe mesenteric arterial spasm producing a marked reduction in intestinal blood flow. The syndrome typically occurs in two situations: The first is during administration of drugs known to produce splanchnic vasospasm, and the second is associated with a severe illness that produces a relative shock state with decreased cardiac output and reflex splanchnic vasoconstriction. Often the two settings coincide, as in patients receiving digitalis for the treatment of congestive heart failure or patients receiving vasopressors for the treatment of septic shock. Nonocclusive mesenteric ischemia caused by drugs has been reported after the ingestion of cocaine and following the use of ergot derivatives.[44, 63] Although drug-induced mesenteric ischemia may occur in otherwise normal patients, most cases of nonocclusive mesenteric ischemia occur in patients who are already severely ill from other causes, usually cardiac disease.

Treatment of nonocclusive mesenteric ischemia involves three components: First, correction of the underlying pathologic state responsible for the vasoconstriction; second, specific pharmacologic measures to reverse splanchnic vasoconstriction; and third, resection of necrotic bowel.

The use of specific drug therapy to relieve mesenteric vasospasm has been investigated by many authors. Various measures reported to improve mesenteric blood flow in this situation include systemic administration of the vasodilators phenoxybenzamine, isoproterenol, and tolazoline; use of epidural anesthetic block; and use of splanchnic anesthetic block.[1, 47, 52, 97] The direct injection of tolazoline through an angiographically placed catheter in the superior mesenteric artery was first reported by Bounos[13] in 1967. Ten years later Boley and associates described the treatment of 15 patients with nonocclusive mesenteric ischemia by continuous infusion of papaverine through a superior mesenteric artery catheter. In contrast to their previous experience, 9 of the 15 patients survived.[11] The dose of papaverine ranged from 30 to 60 mg/hr, and the infusions were continued for as long as 5 days.

At present, we favor the approach to nonocclusive mesenteric ischemia described in Chapter 96, the principal features of which are stabilization and improvement in cardiac function in an intensive care setting. The optimal role, if any, of vasodilator treatment is unknown. Interestingly, the incidence of this syndrome appears to be considerably decreased in recent years, perhaps reflecting the increasing use of hemodynamic monitoring to guide treatment of cardiac dysfunction and the use of vasodilator therapy to improve critically impaired cardiac output in contrast to the frequent use of pressors, which characterized such efforts in the past.

Ergotism

Ergot-induced vasospastic symptoms have been observed since antiquity in persons eating grain contaminated by the fungus *Claviceps purpurea*. The acrocyanosis, pain in the extremities, and gangrene that resulted was named St. Anthony's fire. Such outbreaks are currently rare. Most clinical episodes of ergotism result from ingestion of medications containing ergot derivatives prescribed for treatment of migraine or postpartum bleeding. The manifestations of ergot intoxication range from asymptomatic absence of pulses to severe ischemia of peripheral,[96] mesenteric,[51] renal,[39] and cerebral beds,[82] including the occurrence of extensive gangrene and limb loss.

Pharmacologic treatment of ergotism using many agents has been reported, including papaverine, tolazoline, ethyl alcohol, amyl nitrate, scopolamine, theophylline, ergoloid mesylates, phentolamine, sodium nicotinate, procaine, lidocaine, and various forms of epidural, spinal, and sympathetic anesthetic blocks.[58] However, all of these observations have been anecdotal, and the frequently repeated observation that simple cessation of ergot use results in rapid symptomatic improvement in most patients casts doubt on the validity of these therapeutic observations.[49]

In contrast to the questionable therapeutic benefit ascribed to the agents listed earlier, evidence has accumulated confirming a clear benefit in most patients with ergot-induced vasospasm treated with intravenous nitrates, either sodium nitroprusside or nitroglycerin. Successful therapy has been objectively demonstrated by angiography and vascular laboratory improvement.[18, 83, 89, 96] Most authors have emphasized the importance of simultaneous administration of heparin or dextran anticoagulation in conjunction with intravenous nitrate therapy.

References

1. Aakhus T, Brabrand G: Angiography in acute superior mesenteric arterial insufficiency. Acta Radiol Diagn 6:1, 1967.
2. AbuRahma AF, et al: Effects and limitations of pentoxifylline therapy in various stages of peripheral vascular disease of the lower extremities. Am J Surg 160:266, 1990.
3. Accetto B: Beneficial hemorrheologic therapy of chronic peripheral arterial disorders with pentoxifylline; Results of a double-blind study versus vasodilator-nylidrin. Am Heart J 113:864, 1982.
4. Angelkort B, Doppelfield E: Treatment of chronic arterial occlusive disease. Clinical study with a new galenic preparation of pentoxifylline. Trental 400. Pharmatherapeutica 3(Suppl I):18, 1983.
5. Angelkort B, Manion H, Bouteng K: Influence of pentoxifylline on erythrocyte deformability in peripheral occlusive arterial disease. Curr Med Res Opin 6:255, 1979.
6. Bahl JJ, Bresler RD: The pharmacology of carnitine. Ann Rev Pharmacol Toxicol 27:257, 1987.
7. Baumann JC: Erweiterte Moglichkeiten zur Konserviten. Behandlung arterieller. Durchblütungstor ungen. Therapiewoche 27:188, 1977.
8. Belch JJP, McKay A, McArdle B, et al. Epoprostenol (prostacyclin) and severe arterial disease: A double-blind trial. Lancet 1:315, 1983.
9. Belch JJP, Drury JK, Capell H, et al: Intermittent epoprostenol (prostacyclin) infusion in patients with Raynaud's syndrome: A double-blind controlled trial. Lancet 1:313, 1983.
10. Bergentz SE, Eiken O, Gelin LE: Rheomacrodex in vascular surgery. J Cardiovasc Surg 4:388, 1963.
11. Boley SJ, Sprayragan S, Siegelman SS, et al: Initial results from an aggressive roentgenological and surgical approach to acute mesenteric ischemia. Surgery 82:848, 1977.
12. Bollinger A, Frel C: Double-blind study of pentoxifylline against placebo in patients with intermittent claudication. Pharmatherapeutica 1:557, 1977.
13. Bounos G: Role of the intestinal contents in the pathophysiology of acute intestinal ischemia. Am J Surg 114:368, 1967.
14. Brevetti G, Chiariello M, Ferulano G, et al: Increases in walking distance in patients with peripheral vascular disease treated with L-carnitine: A double-blind, cross-over study. Circulation 77:767, 1988.
15. Buckert B, Hawart D: Trials of 3,7-dimethyl-1-(5′-oxohexyl)-xanthine (BL 191) in double-blind tests. Farmaco (Prat) 31:264, 1976.
16. Burns JG, Galloway DJ, Ledingham IM: Effect of naftidrofuryl on the metabolic response of surgery. Br Med J 283:7, 1981.
17. Cariin G, Modig J, Saldeen T: Effect of infusion of dextran 70 on fibrinolysis inhibition activity in human serum. Acta Clin Scand 145:129, 1979.
18. Carliner NH, Denune DP, Finsch CS Jr, et al: Sodium nitroprusside treatment of ergotamine-induced peripheral ischemia. JAMA 227:308, 1974.
19. Chesebro JH, Fuster V, Frye RL: Smoking, family history and shortened platelet survival in coronary disease patients age 50 and under. Circulation 58 (Suppl II):221, 1978.
20. Clifford P, Martin M, Sheddon E, et al: Treatment of vasospastic disease with prostaglandin El. Br Med J 281:1031, 1980.
21. Clyne CAC, Gallard RB, Fox MJ, et al: A controlled trial of naftidrofuryl in the treatment of intermittent claudication. Br J Surg 67:347, 1980.
22. Coffman JD, Mannick JA: Failure of vasodilator drugs in arteriosclerosis obliterans. Ann Intern Med 76:35, 1972.
23. Coffman JD: Pathophysiology of intermittent claudication. *In* Spittell JA, Jr (ed): Pharmacologic Approach to Treatment of Limb Ischemia. Philadelphia, American College of Clinical Pharmacology, 1983, pp 43–52.
24. Coffman JD: Vasodilator drugs in peripheral vascular disease. N Engl J Med 300:713, 1979.
25. Collins GJ, Bergentz SV: Dextrans. *In* Collins G (ed): Vascular Occlusive Disorders: Medical and Surgical Management. Mt. Kisco, NY, Futura Publ Co, 1981, pp 393–420.
26. Consensus Document. Chronic critical leg ischemia. Eur J Vasc Surg 6(Suppl A):S1, 1992.
27. Cronenwett JL, Zelenock GB, Whitehouse WM Jr, et al: Prostacyclin treatment of ischemic ulcers and rest pain in unreconstructable peripheral arterial occlusive disease. Surgery 100:369, 1986.
28. Dalman RL, Nehler MR, Harris EJ Jr, et al: Upper extremity bypass distal to the wrist. J Vasc Surg 16:633, 1992.
29. DiPerri T, Guerrini M: Placebo-controlled double-blind study with pentoxifylline of walking performance in patients with intermittent claudication. Angiology 34:40, 1983.
30. Dormandy JA, Hoare E, Colley J: Clinical hemodynamic and biochemical findings in 126 patients with intermittent claudication. Br Med J 4:576, 1973.
31. Dowd PM, Martin MPR, Cooke BD, et al: Treatment of Raynaud's phenomenon by intravenous infusion of prostacyclin (PGI_2). Br J Dermatol 106:81, 1982
32. Edwards JM, Phinney ES, Taylor LM Jr, et al: Alpha-$_2$ adrenoreceptor differences in obstructive and spastic Raynaud's syndrome. J Vasc Surg 5:38, 1987.
33. Ehrly AM: Effects of orally administered pentoxifylline on muscular oxygen pressure in patients with intermittent claudication. IRCS Med Sci 10:41, 1982.
34. Ehrly AM: Improvement of the flow properties of blood. A new therapeutic approach in occlusive arterial disease. Angiology 27:188, 1976.
35. Ehrly AM, Kohler HJ: Altered deformability of erythrocytes from patients with chronic occlusive arterial disease. Vasa 5:319, 1976.
36. Eklund AE, Eriksson G, Olsson AG: A controlled study showing significant short term effect of prostaglandin E1 in healing of ischaemic ulcers of the lower limb in man. Prostaglandins Leukot Med 8:265, 1982.
37. Engler RL, Dahlgren MD, Peterson MA, et al: Role of leukocytes in the response to acute myocardial ischemia and reflow in dogs. Am J Physiol 251:H93, 1986.
38. Ernst E, Hammerschmidt DE, Bagge U, et al: Leukocytes and the risk of ischemic disease. JAMA 257:2318, 1987.
39. Fedotin MS, Hartman C: Ergotamine poisoning producing renal arterial spasm. N Engl J Med 283:518, 1970.
40. Feine-Haake G: Assessment of therapeutic efficiency of Trental 400; double-blind trial in geriatric patients with vascular disorders. Pharmatherapeutica 30 (Suppl I):46, 1983.
41. Fiessinger JN, Schafer M, and the TAO Study Group: Trial of iloprost versus aspirin treatment for critical limb ischemia of thromboangiitis obliterans. Lancet 335:555, 1990.

42. Gjorup T, Kelback M, Hartling OJ, et al: Controlled double-blind trial of the clinical effect of nifedipine in the treatment of idiopathic Raynaud's phenomenon. Am Heart J 111:742, 1986.
43. Goa KL, Brogden RN: L-Carnitine: A preliminary review of its pharmacokinetics, and its therapeutic use in ischemic heart disease and primary and secondary carnitine deficiencies in relationship to its role in fatty acid metabolism. Drugs 34:1, 1987.
44. Green FC, Ariyan S, Stansel HC, Jr: Mesenteric and peripheral vascular ischemia secondary to ergotism. Surgery 81:176, 1977.
45. Green RM, McNamara JM: The effect of pentoxifylline on patients with intermittent claudication. J Vasc Surg 7:356, 1988.
46. Greenhalgh RM: Naftidrofuryl for ischemic rest pain: A controlled trial. Br J Surg 68:265, 1981.
47. Habboushe F, Wallace HW, Nusbaum M, et al: Non-occlusive mesenteric vascular insufficiency. Ann Surg 180:819, 1974.
48. Hansteen V, Lorensten E: Vasodilator drugs in the treatment of peripheral arterial insufficiency. Acta Med Scand 556 (Suppl 554):9, 1974.
49. Henry LG, Blackwood JS, Conley JE, et al: Ergotism. Arch Surg 110:929, 1975.
50. Hess HV, Franke I, Jauch M: Medikamentose Verbesserung der Flieseigenschaften des Blutes. Ein wirksames Prinzip zur Behandlung von arteriellen durchbluntungss Torungen. Fortschr Med 91:743, 1973.
51. Holmes G. Martin E, Tuba S: Mesenteric vascular occlusion in pregnancy: Suspected ergot poisoning. Med J Aust 2:1009, 1969.
52. Jackson BB, Lykins R: Serial epidural analgesia in mesenteric arterial failure. Arch Surg 90:177, 1965.
53. Johnson G, Jr, Keagy BA, Rodd DW, et al: Viscous factors in peripheral tissue perfusion. J Vasc Surg 2:530, 1985.
54. Kellner H: Treatment of chronic arterial circulatory disorders. Double-blind trial with Trental 400. Münch Med Wochenschr 118:1399, 1976.
55. Lindgarde F, Jelnes R, Bjorkman H, et al. Conservative drug treatment in patients with moderately severe chronic occlusive peripheral arterial disease. Circulation 80:1549, 1989.
56. Martin M, Dowd P, Ring E, et al: Prostaglandin El infusions for vascular insufficiency in progressive systemic sclerosis. Ann Rheum Dis 40:350, 1981.
57. Matrai A, Ernst E: Pentoxifylline improves white cell rheology in claudicants. Clin Hemorrheol 5:483, 1986.
58. Merhoff GC, Porter JM: Ergot intoxication. Ann Surg 180:773, 1974.
59. Mills JR, Friedman EI, Taylor LM, Jr, Porter JM: Upper extremity ischemia caused by small artery disease. Ann Surg 206:521, 1987.
60. Mohrland JS, Porter JM, Kahaleh MB, et al: A multiclinic, placebo-controlled, double-blind study of prostaglandin El in Raynaud's syndrome. Ann Rheum Dis 44:754, 1985.
61. Moncrief JA, Darin JC, Canizaro PC, et al: Use of dextran to prevent arterial and venous thrombosis. Ann Surg 158:553, 1963.
62. Muller R: Hemorrheology and peripheral vascular disease. A new therapeutic approach. J Med 12:209, 1981.
63. Nalbandran H, Sheth N, Dietrich R, et al: Intestinal ischemia caused by cocaine ingestion. Report of two cases. Surgery 397:374, 1985.
64. Negus D, Irving JD, Friedgood A: Intra-arterial prostacyclin compared to praxilene in the management of severe lower limb ischemia: A double-blind trial. J Cardiovasc Surg 28:196, 1987.
65. Nizandowski R, Krolikowski W, Beilatowicz J, Szczeklik A: Prostacyclin for ischemic ulcers in peripheral arterial disease: A random-assignment, placebo-controlled study. Thromb Res 37:21, 1985.
66. Norgren L, Alwmark A, Angqvist KA, et al: A stable prostacyclin analog (iloprost) in the treatment of ischaemic ulcers of the lower limb: A Scandinavian–Polish placebo-controlled, randomized multicenter study. Eur J Vasc Surg 4:463, 1990.
67. Pardy B, Hoare M, Eastcott H, et al: Prostaglandin El in severe Raynaud's phenomenon. Surgery 92:953, 1982.
68. Porter JM, Cutler BS, Lee BY, et al: Pentoxifylline efficacy in the treatment of intermittent claudication: Multicenter controlled double-blind trial objective assessment of chronic occlusive arterial disease patients. Am Heart J 104:66, 1982.
69. Porter JM, Rivers SP, Anderson CJ, et al: Evaluation and management of patients with Raynaud's syndrome. Am J Surg 142:183, 1981.
70. Pupita F, Rotatori P, Frausini G: Farmacologia clinica della sostanze vasoattive: Studi sulla pentoxifyllina. Ric Clin Lab II (Suppl I):293, 1981.
71. Reid JL, Dormandy JA, Barnes AJ, et al: Impaired red cell deformity in peripheral vascular disease. Lancet 1:666, 1976.
72. Rivers SP, Veith FJ, Ascer E, Gupta SK. Successful conservative therapy of severe limb-threatening ischemia: The value of nonsympathectomy. Surgery 99:759, 1986.
73. Rockaerts F, Deleers L: Trental 400 in the treatment of intermittent claudication. Angiology 35:396, 1984.
74. Rothermel JE, Wessinger JB, Stichfield FE: Dextran 40 and thromboembolism in total hip replacement surgery. Arch Surg 106:135, 1973.
75. Rudofsky G, Brock FE, Ulrich M, et al: Behandlung von Patienten mit arteriellar Verschulsskrankkheit (Stadium II) mit Pentoxifyllin. Hamodynamische und erogmetrische Befund. Med Klin 74:1093, 1979.
76. Rutherford RB, Jones DN, Bergentz SE, et al: The efficacy of dextran 40 in preventing early postoperative thrombosis following difficult lower extremity bypass. J Vasc Surg 1:765, 1984.
77. Rutherford RB, Jones DN, Bergentz SE, et al. Factors affecting the patency of infrainguinal bypass. J Vasc Surg 8:236, 1988.
78. Schumalzer EA, Chien S: Filterability of subpopulations of leukocytes: Effects of pentoxifylline. Blood 64:542, 1984.
79. Schubotz R: Double-blind trial of pentoxifylline in diabetes with peripheral vascular disorders. Pharmatherapeutica 1:172, 1976.
80. Schubotz R, Muhlfellner O: The effect of pentoxifylline on erythrocyte deformity in peripheral occlusive arterial disease. Curr Med Res Opin 6:255, 1979.
81. Schuler JJ, Flanigan DP, Holcroft JW, et al: Efficacy of prostaglandin El in the treatment of lower extremity ischemic ulcers secondary to peripheral vascular occlusive disease: Results of a prospective randomized double-blind, multi-center clinical trial. J Vasc Surg 1:160, 1984.
82. Senter HJ, Lieberman AN, Pinto R: Cerebral manifestations of ergotism. Stroke 7:88, 1976.
83. Skowronski GA, Tronson MD, Parkin WG: Successful treatment of ergotamine poisoning with sodium nitroprusside. Med J Aust 2:8, 1979.
84. Smith CD, McKendry RJ: Controlled trial of nifedipine in the treatment of Raynaud's phenomenon. Lancet 2:1299, 1982.
85. Snyder SH, Reynolds IJ: Calcium-antagonist drugs: Receptor interactions that clarify therapeutic effects. N Engl J Med 313:995, 1985.
86. Strano A, Davi G, Avellone G, et al: Double-blind, crossover study of the clinical efficacy and the hemorrheologic effects of pentoxifylline in patients with occlusive arterial disease of the lower limbs. Angiology 35:459, 1984.
87. Taylor LM Jr, Rivers SP, Keller FS, et al: Treatment of finger ischemia with Bier block reserpine. Surg Gynecol Obstet 154:39, 1982.
88. Telles GS, Campbell WB, Wood RFM, et al: Prostaglandin El in severe lower limb ischemia: A double-blind controlled trial. Br J Surg 71:506, 1984.
89. Tfelt-Hansen P, Ostergaard JR, Gothgen I, et al: Nitroglycerin for ergotism. Experimental studies in vitro and in migraine patients and treatment of an overt case. Eur J Clin Pharmacol 22:105, 1982.
90. Thomas JM, Silva J: Dextran 40 in the treatment of peripheral vascular diseases. Arch Surg 106:138, 1973.
91. Tonak J, Knechtk H, Groitl H: Treatment of circulatory disturbances with pentoxifylline. Double-blind trial with Trental. Pharmatherapeutica 46 (Suppl I):126, 1983.
92. Trubestein G, von Bary S, Breddin K, et al: Intravenous prostaglandin El versus pentoxifylline therapy in chronic arterial occlusive disease—a controlled randomized multicenter study. Vasa 28:44, 1989.
93. Volker D: Behandlung von Arteriopathien mit Trental 400: Ergebnisse einer doppelblid Studie. Med Welt 29:1244, 1978.
94. Volker D: Treatment of arteriopathies with Trental 400. Pharmatherapeutica 3 (Suppl I):154, 1976.
95. Waters KJ, Craxford AD, Chamberlain J: The effect of naftidrofuryl (Praxilene) on intermittent claudication. Br J Surg 67:349, 1980.
96. Wells KE, Steed DL, Zajko AB, et al: Recognition and treatment of arterial insufficiency from Cafergot. J Vasc Surg 4:8, 1986.
97. Williams LF, Anastasia LF, Hasiotis CA, et al: Experimental non-occlusive mesenteric ischemia: Therapeutic observations. Am J Surg 115:82, 1968.
98. Xiu, R-J: Studies on microcirculation in Institute of Basic Medical Sciences. Chinese Academy of Medical Sciences. Microvasc Res 2:371, 1980.

19

Principles of Thrombolytic Therapy

William J. Quiñones-Baldrich, M.D.

The most common indication for intervention in the practice of vascular surgery is occlusion of an arterial or venous segment by a thrombus or clot. Vascular techniques have evolved to the point at which most arterial occlusions and some venous thromboses can be successfully managed. Since the early 1980s, however, pharmacologic dissolution of these occlusive thrombi has become a clinical reality and is used successfully with increasing frequency. An understanding of the fibrinolytic system and how plasminogen activation affects both physiologic and pathologic thrombi is important for the appropriate use of thrombolytic therapy.

In both arterial and venous thrombosis the body's own system fails to maintain fluidity of the blood in the affected vessel. The imbalance resulting in thrombosis may be the result of vessel injury or other intrinsic vessel wall lesion, a low flow state, hypercoagulability of blood, or more frequently, a combination of these. Disordered progressive coagulation of blood in vivo is prevented during normal conditions by an intricate system of checks and balances that primarily involves the coagulation and fibrinolytic systems. To maintain homeostasis, abnormal depositions of fibrin (the end-product of the coagulation cascade) is rapidly followed by local stimulation of the fibrinolytic system. Nevertheless, the latter is easily overwhelmed in pathologic states, resulting in clinical thrombosis.

With the development of drugs capable of stimulating the fibrinolytic system, together with a better understanding of the components and interactions leading to fibrinolysis, it is now possible to treat pathologic intravascular thrombi with the goal of complete dissolution. The drugs available, although lacking precise control, have proved to be valuable and represent a significant advance when one is treating patients with difficult thrombotic problems. It is likely that newer, more specific fibrinolytic agents, combined with advanced drug delivery systems, will improve still further the outcome of appropriately selected patients.

This chapter focuses on the fibrinolytic system and available lytic agents. Current experimental and clinical experience with the use of fibrinolytic therapy for peripheral arterial and venous disease is discussed, keeping in mind that fibrinolytic therapy is still evolving. This chapter should provide the clinician with not only an understanding of the fibrinolytic system and the currently available fibrinolytic agents but also guidelines for patient selection.

THE FIBRINOLYTIC SYSTEM

Substantial progress has occurred since the early 1980s that has expanded our understanding of the intricate feedback control and activity mechanisms of the fibrinolytic system leading to safer and more effective use of fibrinolytic drugs. Although the fibrinolytic system is used to resolve pathologic thrombi, its vital physiologic role involves maintenance of blood fluidity. In 1958, Astrup proposed the concept of dynamic equilibrium for the coagulation and fibrinolytic systems.[9] In this delicate balance, fibrinolysis breaks down fibrin, which is continuously being deposited throughout the cardiovascular system as the result of limited activation of the coagulation system. This baseline fibrinolytic activity is under both local and systemic control mechanisms involving circulating inhibitors, cell-bound receptors, and other components of both the coagulation and the fibrinolytic systems. Under physiologic conditions, the process allows local, but not systemic, fibrinolysis. The coagulation and fibrinolytic systems interact through feedback mechanisms that are not fully understood. Nevertheless, some important feedback mechanisms have been elucidated, most of which may have clinical implications.

The key enzyme in the fibrinolytic system and the final common pathway is plasminogen (Fig. 19–1). This is a glycoprotein produced in the liver that consists of a heavy amino-terminal region made up of five homologous but distinct triple-disulfide bonded domains (kringles) joined to a lighter catalytic C-terminal domain. Activation of plasminogen occurs by the cleavage of an arginine-valine bond, which leads to changes in conformation, leading to an increased affinity for both substrate (fibrin) and activator.

Four forms of human plasminogen have been identified that depend on variation in the *N*-terminus and the degree of glycosylation. The two main forms in plasma are collectively known as glu-plasminogen, whereas the other two forms, found mostly absorbed or bound to fibrin, are collectively known as lys-plasminogen. Lys-plasminogen is formed rapidly from glu-plasminogen by the catalytic action of plasmin.[20] Treatment of either glu- or lys-plasminogen with various proteases results in lower-molecular-weight forms of human plasminogen. These have been observed in vivo in septic patients.[63]

The heavy chain of plasminogen (nonenzymatic portion) is composed of an activation peptide and five homologous domains known as *kringles.*[94] These kringles have a high degree of sequence homology with each other and with domains found in prothrombin, tissue plasminogen activator, urinary plasminogen activator, and factor XII. A repeating unit in apolipoprotein A has significant homology to kringle 4 of plasminogen. This may help to explain why patients with abnormalities of apolipoprotein A may exhibit

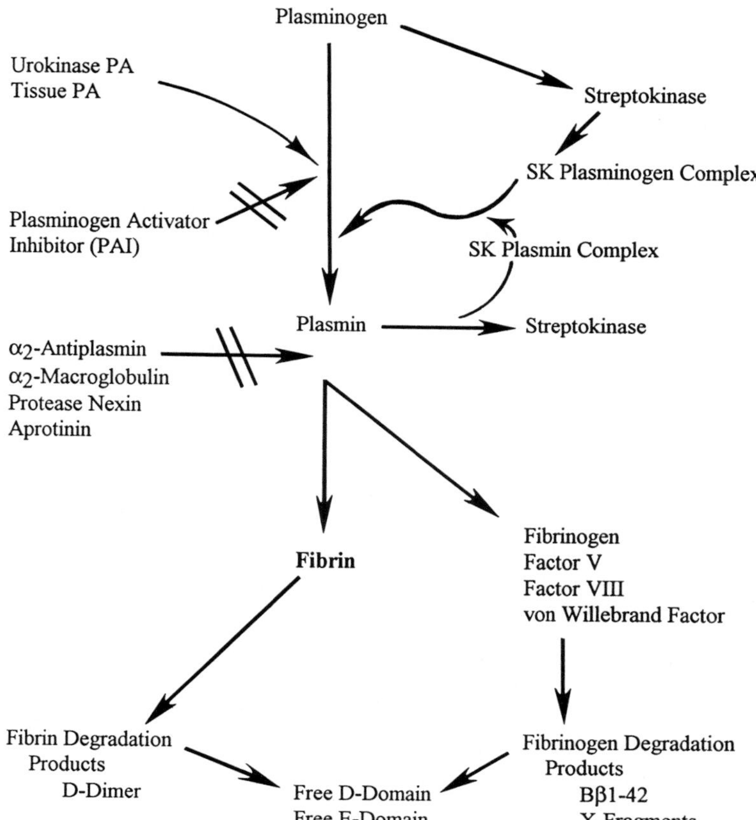

FIGURE 19–1. Simplified scheme of the fibrinolytic system. PA, plasminogen activator; SK, streptokinase.

a hypercoagulable condition. Kringles are responsible for the binding of plasminogen or plasmin to fibrin, alpha$_2$-antiplasmin, and other important macromolecules necessary for the process of fibrinolysis.[116, 148] In addition, the kringles of plasminogen have been implicated in mediating neutrophil adherence to endothelial cells.[70]

Plasminogen in its glu form usually exists in a closed structure. This conformation becomes open on the binding of lysine or lysine analogues. This conformational change produces a glu-plasminogen with properties similar to those of lys-plasminogen and, in many instances, is referred to as the *pseudo-lys form*. The main difference is that lys-plasminogen continues to have lysine binding sites that have a stable open conformation.[143] The open conformation of plasminogen renders the molecule much more readily cleaved, forming the active enzyme plasmin. The open conformation also binds more readily to the fibrin surface. The major binding of plasminogen to fibrin occurs through a strong lysine binding site in the first kringle.[135, 136] Lysine analogues, such as tranexamic acid or epsilon-aminocaproic acid, promote the open conformation of glu-plasminogen, thus potentially increasing fibrinolysis. However, they also prevent the binding of the open conformation of plasminogen to fibrin and therefore exert an antifibrinolytic effect.[123]

The primary substrates of plasmin are fibrinogen and fibrin. Circulating fibrinogen is composed of two identical subunits, each composed of three protein chains known as A alpha, B beta, and gamma chains.[28] The two subunits of fibrinogen are joined to form the E-domain of the molecule. Two arms extending from this E-domain form the D-domains of the molecule. D-domains have binding sites for plasminogen and plasmin. Fibrinogen in the circulation is complexed to various degrees with plasminogen through these binding sites. Small peptides also extend from the E-domain, forming part of the A alpha, B beta, and gamma chains. The peptides from the A alpha and B beta chains are known as *fibrinopeptides A* and *B* and are cleaved from the molecule by thrombin during conversion of fibrinogen to fibrin. Once these fibrinopeptides have been removed by thrombin, a fibrin monomer is formed. These monomers remain soluble until polymers are formed from the interaction between the E-domain of one monomer and the D-domains of two other monomers. These fibrin polymers have little strength or stability until factor XIII, activated by thrombin, cross-links adjacent fibrin monomers through adjacent D-domains. Plasminogen originally bound to fibrinogen becomes incorporated in the thrombus as this conversion occurs.

Plasmin cleaves both fibrin and fibrinogen between the D- and the E-domains. The result of this degradation is free D- and E-domains. Free D- and E-domains in plasma can be the result of degradation of both fibrinogen and fibrin monomers. The presence of D-dimers, however, implies degradation of cross-linked fibrin. D-dimers can be assayed, documenting fibrinolysis as opposed to fibrinogenolosis.[107] In contrast, attacks of plasmin on fibrinogen can produce end-terminal peptide-B beta 1–42, which is a measure of plasmin action on fibrinogen.[102]

An understanding of the action of plasmin on fibrinogen may help to clarify the clinical responses noted during fibrinolytic therapy. As cleavage of fibrinogen proceeds, residual polypeptides, collectively known as X-fragments, are formed. These fragments are not distinguishable by standard laboratory assays for fibrinogen. Loss of sites responsible for cross-linking leads to formation of fibrin that is relatively weak. These X-fragments may be incorporated into both newly forming and existing thrombi, causing them to be more fragile and sensitive to the action of plasmin. Large amounts of these X-fragments can be produced during thrombolytic therapy. The newly formed fibrin, which contains these fragments, is more sensitive to the action of plasmin. This may help to explain why a decrease in bleeding complications has not been seen with fibrin-specific agents such as tissue plasminogen activator. Recent clinical evidence suggests that bolus therapy, as opposed to continuous intravenous infusion, of tissue plasminogen activator may be associated with a decrease in bleeding tendencies. Incorporation of these X-fragments during therapy into newly formed fibrin may represent a lesser risk because of the lower plasma levels of the activator seen during intermittent bolus therapy[2] compared with the constant high levels seen during continuous intravenous infusion.

Fibrinogen is somewhat protected from the actions of plasmin in circulation by powerful and fast-acting plasmin inhibitors. These inhibitors neutralize free plasmin but are not as effective on fibrin-bound plasmin. During thrombolytic therapy, however, circulating plasmin levels exceed the capacity of plasmin inhibitors, and therefore fibrinogenolysis occurs.

Plasmin attacks other proteins in the plasma and extracellular spaces. The list of substrates for plasmin continues to increase and includes coagulation factors such as factors V and VIII and von Willebrand's factor. In addition, plasmin may reduce the effect of thrombin intermediates, further interfering with the coagulation cascade.[52]

Plasmin can also lead to the release of kinin from high-molecular-weight kininogen. It can activate prekallikrein, both directly and indirectly,[17] and this may also induce further kinin formation. Plasmin attacks the protein components of the basement membrane and also activates other proteases within the extracellular matrix. Therefore, it may affect fibronectin, collagen, and laminin. Many of these secondary effects of plasmin are not fully understood, and their clinical implications are unknown. Understanding the control mechanisms of this protease involves a familiarity with its activators and inhibitors.

Activators of Plasminogen

Two main types of plasminogen activator have been identified in humans. The first one was isolated from human urine by MacFarlane and Pilling in 1946.[74] It was named urokinase, or urinary plasminogen activator (u-PA). It is a serine protease with a limited substrate specificity. It consists of a serine protease region B chain and a short A chain. The protease portion, known as single-chain urokinase-type plasminogen activator (scu-PA), is responsible for the activation of plasminogen to plasmin. This portion of the activator has homology to domains on tissue plasminogen activator and other proteins involved in coagulation. It does not, however, contain lysine-binding sites and thus has no fibrin-binding properties.[69] High-affinity receptors for u-PA that recognize the molecule have been demonstrated in several cell types,[10, 12, 91] and its focal concentration on cell surfaces might be a mechanism by which cells invade the intracellular matrix and play a role in both normal and pathologic states. Both urokinase plasminogen activator (urokinase) and pro–urokinase plasminogen activator (pro-urokinase) are available commercially (see later).

Plasminogen is rapidly activated by urokinase plasminogen activator through cleavage of the susceptible site of plasminogen when it is in the open conformation (lys-plasminogen), but it is much less efficient with the closed form of plasminogen (glu-plasminogen).[119] Physiologic concentrations of chloride ions stabilize the closed conformation of glu-plasminogen and therefore may inhibit activation.[131] Pro-urokinase is activated by plasminogen to form a two-chain activator. Questions remain about the intrinsic activity of pro-urokinase before its conversion to the two-chain form. The low intrinsic activity of pro-urokinase may be sufficient to act as a primer for the fibrinolytic system, particularly by activation of fibrin-bound plasminogen. Although without intrinsic fibrin-binding ability, pro-urokinase may be converted to the two-chain form by fibrin-bound plasmin. Because this activation most likely occurs on the surface of the clot, the apparent fibrin specificity of pro-urokinase may be explained. In addition, pro-urokinase appears to have enhanced activity in the presence of lys-plasminogen, mostly found bound to thrombus.

A second plasminogen activator distinct from u-PA was discovered in melanoma cells in 1980 and was found to be the product of vascular endothelial cells.[66] Tissue-type plasminogen activator (t-PA) has been cloned and found to have a similar structure to u-PA.[37] It is secreted as a single-chain protein with activity equal to the two-chain t-PA formed by the action of its own substrate, plasmin. In circulation, t-PA is found mostly in the single-chain form.[124]

t-PA seems to bind to the clot surface in the presence of fibrin, enhancing the affinity of t-PA for plasminogen by 1000-fold.[54] This affinity is significantly affected by removal of the second kringle from the plasminogen molecule, suggesting a role for this kringle.[56]

t-PA binds to other surfaces in addition to fibrin. Extracellular matrix components such as collagen and gelatin can activate t-PA in the absence of fibrin.[114] t-PA is also bound and activated on the surface of platelets, which may help target the action of t-PA, leading to cleavage of glycoprotein-Ib (GPIb) and loss of platelet binding. This antiplatelet effect has been observed with t-PA administration. Others have suggested that platelet aggregation is inhibited by affecting GPIIb/IIIa receptors. In contrast, increased platelet aggregability has been observed early in therapy, followed by reduced aggregation later in therapy.[106]

Partly digested fragments (X-fragments) and clots incorporating these fragments bind more aggressively with t-PA than do fresh undigested clots.[53] This may be the result of conformational changes that optimize the presentation of the stimulator region of fibrin.

Inhibitors of Fibrinolysis

Inhibitors of fibrinolysis are composed of two main groups: proteins that exhibit antiactivator activity and those that exhibit antiplasmin activity. Both play a significant role in controlling otherwise disordered lytic activity. Whereas plasminogen activator inhibitor occurs both in plasma and at the cellular level, antiplasmins occur mostly in circulating plasma.

Plasminogen activator inhibitor (PAI-1) controls the physiologic activity of both u-PA and t-PA. PAI-1 is synthesized in the liver and vascular endothelial cells and is normally present in trace amounts in plasma. Plasma insulin appears to be the major physiologic regulator of PAI-1 activity in plasma.[4, 134] Plasma insulin levels correlate with PAI activity and body mass index. In addition, experimental studies suggest that release of platelet-derived growth factors may attenuate fibrinolysis in vivo by augmenting endothelial cell syntheses and release of PAI-1 locally in the vicinity of thrombi and by increasing the hepatic secretion of PAI-1 into the circulation.[38, 39, 73] In plasma, PAI-1 circulates in a stable complex with a binding protein, recently identified as vitronectin. Platelet activation may falsely elevate PAI-1 antigen levels because of release of inactive PAI from platelets.[31, 113, 133]

Diurnal fluctuations of both t-PA and PAI-1 have been described. t-PA activity is lowest in the early morning and highest in the afternoon. Plasma PAI activity peaks in the early morning and passes through a trough in the afternoon. Overall, there is decreased fibrinolytic activity in the morning.[5, 6, 19, 46] Differences in patterns have also been seen between men and women, suggesting a hormonal influence.[132] PAI activity may also vary with diet.[90] Caffeine-containing beverages may enhance fibrinolytic activity. On the other hand, smoking induces an acute increase in t-PA. This increase in t-PA induced by smoking may deplete normal stores, paradoxically decreasing fibrinolytic activity. Increased levels of PAI-1 are frequently combined with a decreased capacity to release t-PA, are probably related to depleted stores,[50] and can be demonstrated in up to 40 per cent of patients with deep vein thrombosis.[48, 59, 89, 149] Increased plasma PAI activity may also be part of an acute phase reaction seen in postoperative patients, which in part may explain their propensity to develop deep vein thrombosis. Impaired fibrinolytic function caused by elevated plasma PAI activity is the most commonly observed disturbance of the hemostatic system in patients with thrombotic disease, both venous and arterial.[146]

The other group of important inhibitors of the fibrinolytic system is plasmin inhibitors. Plasmin inhibitors include alpha$_2$-antiplasmin, alpha$_2$-macroglobulin, protease nexin, and aprotinin. These proteins inhibit plasmin once it is formed.

Alpha$_2$-antiplasmin is a protease inhibitor single-chain glycoprotein and is a member of the serpin family. It is the main physiologic inhibitor of plasmin. Inhibition of plasmin by alpha$_2$-antiplasmin is a two-step process. The first step is reversible and is followed by formation of a covalent complex involving the active sites of plasmin. The half-life of alpha$_2$-antiplasmin and plasmin complex is approximately 12 hours.[23] Abnormal concentrations of alpha$_2$-antiplasmin have been documented in some clinical disorders[24, 76] and have been found useful in the evaluation of patients with disseminated intravascular coagulation.[120]

Alpha$_2$-macroglobulin is a nonspecific inhibitor of endoproteases. It forms a covalent complex with plasmin at various ratios.[25] The most important mechanism of alpha$_2$-macroglobulin inhibition is a molecular trap process. Cell surface receptors for clearance of the complex have been demonstrated in fibroblasts.[86, 141]

Protease nexin is also a member of the serpin family and is secreted by anchored human fibroblasts. Protease nexin has been categorized according to its affinity for heparin. High-affinity protease nexin is the major form found in human fibroblasts.[109] It is a broad-spectrum inhibitor of trypsin-like serine proteases, which include trypsin, thrombin, urokinase, plasmin, and one-chain and two-chain t-PA. Once the proteases are bound to protease nexin, degradation occurs through internalization via nexin receptors on the cell surface.[72]

Aprotinin is a serine protease inhibitor obtained from bovine organs. It is also known as basic pancreatic trypsin inhibitor and is a potent inhibitor of trypsin, plasma kallikrein, urinary kallikrein, and plasmin. Aprotinin is thought to play an important physiologic role in the maintenance of hemostasis.[35] It does not appear to be a major inhibitor of plasmin. However, clinical grade material is now commercially available under the name of Trasylol (Miles, Inc., West Haven, CT). This compound has been shown to reduce postoperative bleeding after major surgery.[105] In animal models it has been shown to serve as an antidote for bleeding induced by administration of recombinant t-PA.[21] It acts as an inhibitor of plasmin, not an activator, so it is postulated that it would work with other plasminogen activators.

Other inhibitors of fibrinolysis exert their antifibrinolytic effect by blocking the binding of plasmin to fibrin. These antifibrinolytic agents are lysine analogues and are commercially available as epsilon-aminocaproic acid and tranexamic acid. As mentioned earlier, conformational changes are produced by these agents on plasmin, inducing an increased affinity for fibrin. Sufficient amounts of the antifibrinolytic agent, however, block the lysine binding sites, thus exerting their antifibrinolytic effect.

Other Biologic Roles

Biologic functions other than those involving coagulation have now been firmly established for several components of the fibrinolytic system. These components are thought to be actively involved in biologic functions at the cellular level, such as embryogenesis, neuronal growth, ovulation, muscle regeneration, wound healing, angiogenesis, and tumor growth and invasion. Expression of certain components of the system has been observed in cells in culture and in tissues.

In certain malignancies, expression of u-PA has been correlated with an unfavorable clinical prognosis. Tumor cell invasion as well as migration may be specifically linked to the expression of u-PA, t-PA, and their inhibitors in endothelial cells and smooth muscle cells. This observation may be relevant, not only in thrombosis and atherogenesis but also specifically during reparative processes following vascular injury.[64] Expression of these components is modulated by transcriptional regulation of cytokines, interferon, tumor necrosis factor, and hormones (e.g., corticosteroid and gonadotropins).[41, 67, 92, 115, 140] Growth factors, including those found in fibroblasts, platelets, and endothelial cells, may also control the expression of certain components of the fibrinolytic system at the cellular level.

Cell movement through the extracellular membrane is a pivotal step in many physiologic and pathophysiologic processes. Focal proteolysis of the extracellular components may be accomplished in part by metalloproteinases that are activated primarily by plasmin.[26, 108, 122] Thus, generation of u-PA or t-PA is an important step in cell migration. Although both t-PA and u-PA are plasminogen activators, their cellular function may be different owing to their respective inhibition by PAI. u-PA, for example, is secreted in a single-chain form, which is resistant to inhibition by PAI. u-PA has been found to be a growth stimulant for epidermal tumor cell lines and is mitogenic for malignant renal cells.[61] Its mitogenic potential may have implications in the proliferation of endothelial and smooth muscle cells during both repair of vascular injury and atherogenesis. Receptors for u-PA may allow this protein to be localized on the cell surface in high concentrations at focal points where activation of plasminogen takes place during cell migration. PAI is present on cell surfaces and is uniformly distributed in the cell substratum.[68, 98] This differential distribution may allow focal points of proteolysis on the cell surface with inhibition in the cell substratum, providing a foothold for the migrating cell.

It is evident that the fibrinolytic system has now been identified as playing an increasingly pivotal role in both physiologic and diseased states. With the development of specific inhibitor, it may well be possible to utilize some of these mechanisms to favor resolution of pathologic processes. These appear to encompass a large variety of pathologic states, well beyond those limited to thromboembolic disorders.

It is now recognized that certain specific thromboembolic disorders are due to impaired fibrinolysis. Congenital disturbances of the fibrinolytic system associated with deep vein thrombosis and pulmonary embolism have been described. These are generally caused by plasminogen deficiencies including both dysplasminogenemias and hypoplasminogenemias.[146] The genetic defect responsible for these variants seems to be more common in Japan but is virtually absent among white Americans.[7] In addition, approximately 15 per cent of patients with dysfibrinogenemias appear to have an increased risk of thrombosis. This may also involve impaired fibrinolytic function. The abnormal fibrin formed may not stimulate t-PA–mediated plasminogen activator or, alternatively, it may not be readily digested by the plasmin form.

Lipoprotein-a is a low-density lipoprotein (LDL)–like protein with a unique glycoprotein called apolipoprotein-a. There is a striking homology between apolipoprotein-a and one of the kringles of the plasminogen molecule.[79] It has been postulated that lipoprotein-a might mediate a prothrombotic function by interfering with the physiologic functions of plasminogen. It competitively inhibits the binding of plasminogen to fibrinogen or fibrin[51, 71] and to plasminogen receptors on endothelial cells.[43, 49, 83] Elevated levels of apolipoprotein-a have been associated with thrombotic disorders.

A relationship between PAI and thrombotic disorders has also been suggested. Experimentally, release of platelet-associated growth factors may decrease fibrinolysis in vivo by increasing endothelial cell syntheses and release of PAI and increasing hepatic secretion of PAI into the circulation.

Impaired fibrinolytic function is the most common biochemical or hemostatic disturbance seen in patients with idiopathic deep vein thrombosis. It has been shown that 30 to 40 per cent of patients with idiopathic deep vein thrombosis have impaired fibrinolytic function.[146] This impairment seems to be related to increased plasma levels of PAI combined with a decreased capacity to release t-PA. It has been postulated that continuous release of t-PA, perhaps induced by increased PAI activity, may lead to depleted endothelial stores of t-PA, thus hampering fibrinolytic response.[50]

Well-established risk factors for coronary heart disease (e.g., cigarette smoking, diabetes, obesity, age, hypertension, and hyperlipoproteinemia) are associated with decreased fibrinolytic activity.[147] There is also a negative association between the intake of vegetables, fruits, and root vegetables and plasma PAI activity.[90] There is a strong relationship between serum triglycerides and PAI levels in plasma.[50, 58, 82] This raises the possibility that hypertriglyceridemia may lead to a predisposition to thrombosis through an increase in PAI concentration.

PAI activity is increased in plasma in the postoperative period. This appears to be part of an acute phase reaction and may be secondary to platelet release of PAI.[42]

Syndrome X, a cluster of hypertriglyceridemia, hypertension, central obesity, and insulin resistance with hyperinsulinemia, has gained interest because of its potential association with impaired fibrinolytic function. PAI activity is increased in plasma, probably as a result of the hyperinsulinemic state.[146] This suggests that insulin may be an added risk factor for coronary heart disease, exerting its effects through modification of other risk factors including triglyceride-rich lipoproteins and plasma PAI activity.

FIBRINOLYTIC AGENTS

Drugs used to activate the fibrinolytic system pharmacologically may be divided into direct and indirect activators. Indirect activators achieve increased fibrinolytic activity in vivo without acting directly in vitro on plasminogen. These indirect activators include a long list of drugs whose mechanism of action is variable and has not been elucidated. Chronic enhancement of fibrinolytic activity is attractive, although of unproven clinical value. Most indirect fibrinolytic drugs lose their effectiveness with time, as is the case with nicotinic acid and adrenalin. Both of these cause an abrupt but transient increase in activity by release of endothelial t-PA. Antidiuretic hormone is capable of stimulating the fibrinolytic system at the expense of severe cardiovascular side effects. A more prolonged response may be obtained with desamino-D-arginine vasopressin (DDAVP), although this response seems clinically insignificant compared with the procoagulant effects of this agent. Steroids and diguanides (phenformin) have been the most promising of these compounds. Stanozol, an anabolic steroid, is capable of producing sustained stimulation of the fibrinolytic system for periods of over 5 years with daily administration.[144]

Evidence of the clinical usefulness of indirect fibrinolytic agents is mostly anecdotal. The long-term benefits of an enhanced fibrinolytic system remain to be established. Increased fibrinolytic activity may occur in patients whose baseline activity is depressed. In other instances, no clinical benefit is observed despite a sustained drug effect. Importantly, fibrinolytic capacity may be decreased by chronic stimulation, thus rendering the system incapable of responding adequately to a thrombotic stimulus.[148] Further investigation is necessary before the value of chronic manipulation of the fibrinolytic system is established.

Direct fibrinolytic agents are capable of converting plasminogen to plasmin, thus exerting their lytic activity through the final common pathway of the fibrinolytic system. They do not have fibrinolytic activity themselves and require plasminogen to exert their lytic action. These direct fibrinolytic activators, of which streptokinase and urokinase are prime examples, achieve their lytic effect to a great extent by overwhelming the circulating plasmin inhibitors and generating an abundance of plasmin (exogenous fibrinolysis).

It is well known that thrombus contains plasminogen within its substance. Activation of thrombus-bound plasminogen to plasmin results in local fibrinolysis, and importantly, this process is partially protected from circulating inhibitors (endogenous fibrinolysis). Thrombolysis without systemic lytic activity can thus be achieved. Current investigations are concentrating on producing agents with a high affinity for thrombus-bound plasminogen with little activation of the circulating proenzyme. t-PA obtained from melanoma cell lines and, more recently, through use of recombinant DNA technology has undergone initial clinical and experimental trials with encouraging results.[45, 78, 126] Systemic fibrinolysis still occurs with these agents but to a lesser extent than with streptokinase and urokinase.

Streptokinase

Streptokinase is a *nonenzymatic* protein produced by Lancefield's group C strains of beta-hemolytic streptococci. The fibrinolytic activity of a filtrate of beta-hemolytic streptococci was discovered in 1933 by Tillett and Garner.[125] It initially combines with plasminogen on an equimolar basis (1 : 1 stoichiometric ratio) to form the activator complex. This streptokinase-plasminogen complex then activates the fibrinolytic mechanism by converting uncomplexed plasminogen to plasmin. As the process evolves, the streptokinase-plasminogen complex is gradually converted to the streptokinase-plasmin form, which can also activate and convert plasminogen. Because this conversion takes place slowly, initial activity is due to the streptokinase-plasminogen complex, whereas later activity is due to the streptokinase-plasmin form. With streptokinase, the supply of fibrin-bound plasminogen may be exhausted by combining it with streptokinase to form the activator complex. As a result, insufficient plasminogen may remain to be activated. Thus, there is a decrease in thrombolytic effect with concentrations of streptokinase above 2500 to 5000 U/ml.[85] The kinetics of these reactions have been studied mostly in vitro. A more complicated series of reactions occurs in vivo following an infusion of streptokinase. Initially, the drug is neutralized by circulating antistreptococcal antibodies. Any remaining drug combines with circulating plasminogen forming the activator complex, which converts plasminogen to plasmin. Plasmin combines with excess free streptokinase, is neutralized by circulating antiplasmin, or binds to preformed fibrin. The latter effect produces the desired thrombolytic action. The two half-lives that are detected at 16 and 83 minutes underscore the complexity of these reactions and have a significant impact on the concentration and activity of the drug.

Streptokinase is a foreign protein and therefore is antigenic. Human plasma usually contains antibodies directed against streptokinase that have developed as a result of prior infections with beta-hemolytic streptococci. When streptokinase is infused, an antigen-antibody complex is formed, thus rendering it biochemically inert. Therefore, sufficient amounts of streptokinase must be infused to neutralize the antibodies before fibrinolytic activation is obtained.[57] Minor (and occasionally major) allergic reactions to streptokinase are not uncommon and have been reported at a frequency range of 1.7 to 18 per cent.[110] Serum sickness, with leukocytoclastic vasculitis, is another potential rare complication and is attributed to a delayed hypersensitivity reaction to the foreign protein streptokinase.[130]

Urokinase

Urokinase is a direct activator that is capable of initiating fibrinolysis without forming an activator complex. It is a trypsin-like serine protease isolated from human urine or cultured from human embryonic kidney cells. It was isolated from human urine by MacFarlane and Pilling in 1946.[74] In 1967, it was successfully isolated from tissue cultures of human embryonic kidney cells.[14] Urokinase is nonantigenic, and its pyrogenicity is low. Urokinase requires an initial high loading dose, and like streptokinase, it possesses little specific affinity for fibrin[78] and therefore does not discriminate between circulating plasminogen and fibrin-bound plasminogen.

Urokinase cleaves plasminogen (its only known protein substrate) by first-order reaction kinetics to plasmin. It is relatively pH and temperature stable. No neutralizing antibodies are present, and its direct mechanism of action allows for a better dose response relationship compared with streptokinase. Urokinase does not contain lysine-binding sites, which explains its lack of affinity for fibrin.[69] Receptors for urokinase have been demonstrated in several cell types, as mentioned earlier, and these are postulated as a mechanism for cellular movement in the extracellular matrix.

Activation of plasminogen by urokinase occurs through proteolysis of its substrate. On intravenous administration, it is rapidly removed from the circulation via hepatic clearance. The half-life of urokinase in humans has been estimated to be about 14 minutes. Urokinase also reacts with other proteins, including fibrinogen. The lys-form of plasminogen is much more readily cleaved by urokinase, and this activation may be enhanced by the presence of fibrin.[145]

Laboratory findings in patients treated with urokinase have shown a lesser fibrinogenolytic response compared with streptokinase.[81] Endogenous lytic activity is thus proposed, although results in clinical practice have paralleled those of streptokinase. A decreased incidence of bleeding complications has been suggested by several investigators and may be explained by reduced plasminemia.[13, 121, 138]

Tissue Plasminogen Activator

t-PA, a serine protease present in most body tissues,[3, 8] can cause in vivo activation of the fibrinolytic system. It is similar in nature to plasminogen activator produced by human vascular endothelial cells.[1, 16] t-PA is a poor enzyme in the absence of fibrin, but the presence of fibrin strikingly enhances the activation rate of plasminogen. The high affinity of t-PA for plasminogen in the presence of fibrin allows efficient activation on the fibrin clot without significant conversion by t-PA of plasminogen in circulating plasma.[100, 101] Under normal physiologic conditions, fibrin-bound t-PA activates the conversion of fibrin-bound plasminogen to plasmin. The plasmin thus formed on the fibrin surface rapidly induces thrombolysis. t-PA circulating in the blood has a low affinity for circulating plasminogen; therefore, plasmin is not formed in the circulation. Circulating alpha$_2$-antiplasmin is not consumed, fibrinogen is not degraded, and a systemic lytic state is avoided.

Although t-PA was identified in the 1940s, its isolation and purification proceeded slowly until the 1980s, when it became possible to extract it from uterine tissue. Subsequently, the Bowes melanoma cell line was found to secrete a plasminogen activator similar to human uterine t-PA.[22] Through the use of recombinant DNA technology, the human t-PA gene has been cloned. The recombinant human tissue–type plasminogen activator (rt-PA) appears to be biologically identical to plasminogen activator derived from the melanoma cell line.

t-PA is a direct plasminogen activator. Commercially available rt-PA is a combination of two types of t-PA. A single-chain form is cleaved by plasminogen to yield two-chain t-PA. Both the one- and two-chain forms of t-PA are comparable in activity, the one-chain activator being quickly converted to the two-chain type as lysis proceeds. The half-life of t-PA has been estimated at between 4 and 7 minutes in vivo.[111]

Because it is a fibrin-selective agent, most of the thrombolytic effect of t-PA is secondary to fibrin-bound plasminogen converted to plasmin. Recently, however, the importance of a fresh supply of plasminogen to maintain the fibrin-bound plasminogen pool has been emphasized. Experimental studies have suggested that clot lysis induced by activation of plasminogen is dependent on clot-associated plasminogen, which in turn depends on the concentration of plasminogen in plasma. Depletion of both contributes to a lower frequency and rapidity of recanalization, which is more noticeable with nonfribin-selective agents compared with fibrin-selective agents, probably as the result of depletion of plasminogen induced by nonselective agents.[128]

Systemic bleeding complications in clinical trials of rt-PA have been similar to those seen with other lytic agents, despite a milder hemostatic defect demonstrated by laboratory evaluation.[126] Questions regarding dosage and method of administration still exist, with bolus infusion of rt-PA suggested as a method of decreasing bleeding complications.

rt-PA may also bind and be activated on platelet surfaces. Owing to binding to platelet receptors, platelets may direct the action of rt-PA on their surfaces, leading to rapid cleavage of GPIb and loss of platelet binding to von Willebrand's factor. This may explain why concentrations of t-PA achieved early in therapy may inhibit platelet aggregation.

Results of the limited experience available with the use of rt-PA in patients with peripheral vascular occlusions have suggested the occurrence of fewer systemic complications with increased effectiveness of therapy and decreased infusion times. Several controlled randomized trials of t-PA compared with other fibrinolytic agents in the acute phase of myocardial infarction have suggested a slight but important increase in intracranial bleeding. The incidence appears to be increased in patients who have been on oral anticoagulants prior to therapy, patients weighing less than 70 kg, and patients older than 65 years of age.[27]

Acylated Streptokinase Plasminogen Complex

Attempts to produce fibrin-specific agents have led to derivatives of streptokinase that not only change its biologic activity but also the duration of such activity. p-Anisoylated human plasminogen streptokinase activator complex (APSAC) is the most studied and the most frequently used derivative of streptokinase. It is an acylated complex of streptokinase with human lys-plasminogen. Acylation of the catalytic site of the plasminogen molecule delays the formation of the active fibrinolytic enzyme plasmin but leaves the lysine-binding sites necessary to bind the complex to fibrin. In addition, acylation prevents activation of circulating plasminogen by streptokinase, delaying such activation for the interval necessary for the complex to bind to fibrin. Deacylation of the molecule then leads to activation of the streptokinase moiety, a large percentage of the drug being bound to fibrin at the time of deacylation. Any deacylation occurring in the circulation is rapidly deactivated by antiplasmins.[84]

The potency of APSAC has been found to be 10 times that of streptokinase in vivo. This increased activity is dependent on both fibrin binding and the deacylation process. The half-life of APSAC has been estimated to be around 105 minutes. This prolonged half-life is desirable in patients with acute myocardial infarction and, combined with its increased fibrin selectivity, is a welcomed improvement over the parent drug, streptokinase. It shares, however, the same side effects characteristic of streptokinase because antistreptococcal antibodies have a significant inhibitory effect on APSAC. Antibodies form in patients treated with APSAC, and therefore retreatment with either the parent drug (streptokinase) or APSAC should not be done within 6 months.

The prolonged half-life of APSAC may be a disadvantage in patients needing regional infusion. In patients with peripheral vascular disease, the possibility of having to proceed with surgical intervention shortly after failed fibrinolytic therapy is an important consideration in the selection of the appropriate lytic agent. Thus, shorter-acting drugs may be preferable in the treatment of arterial thrombosis.

Plasmin B-Chain Streptokinase Complex

By utilizing the smallest derivative of plasmin that retains enzymatic activity (plasmin B-chain), another derivative of streptokinase has been produced known as plasmin B-chain streptokinase complex. The half-life of this preparation is estimated at 4.5 hours, which is prolonged compared with that of streptokinase. Its efficiency in lysing fibrin is four times that of streptokinase, its activity falling somewhere between that of streptokinase and that of urokinase.[117] This complex may have certain advantages over streptokinase because of its prolonged half-life and its increased affinity for fibrin-bound plasminogen. Its advantages over other currently available lytic agents, such as u-PA or t-PA, must await clinical trials.

Pro-Urokinase

Different molecular weight forms of urokinase with variable activity are recognized. A single-chain form of urokinase of about 55,000 daltons was isolated by Husain and colleagues in 1979.[55] It has superior fibrin specificity and lytic activity compared with urokinase.

Pro-urokinase is highly effective in the conversion of lys-plasminogen to plasmin. It has little or no activity in the conversion of glu-plasminogen to plasmin. High concentrations of lys-plasminogen are present in thrombus, which gives pro-urokinase fibrin-specific properties. Plasminogen that has been absorbed in thrombus changes its configuration to a pseudo–lys-form that is also attacked by pro-urokinase, converting it to lys-plasmin. Circulating pro-urokinase is stable in plasma because of its resistance to plasma inhibitors and ionized calcium.[93]

Pro-urokinase has a prolonged half-life that, in some instances, has been estimated to be several days.[47] Such a prolonged half-life may have disadvantages in clinical situations in which patients may require surgery shortly after failed lytic therapy.

Immunofibrinolysis

In an attempt to develop fibrin-specific agents, monoclonal antifibrin antibodies have been bonded to urokinase or streptokinase, rendering these agents fibrin selective. A marked increase in in vitro fibrinolysis has been demonstrated compared with unmodified drug. These monoclonal antibodies do not appear to cross-react with fibrinogen, which may explain the enhanced activity.[15] Repeat therapy, however, would require different monoclonal antibodies to avoid adverse immunologic reactions. The clinical applicability of these agents remains to be determined.

FIBRINOLYTIC THERAPY

Generally, two clinical approaches are used in modern practice for the administration of lytic agents. Systemic lytic therapy involves intravenous administration of the drug, the goal being establishment of a systemic lytic state capable of dissolving fibrin wherever deposited. This method of administration is currently limited to patients with acute venous thromboembolism. Regional administration of thrombolytic agents seems to enhance their effectiveness and decreases systemic complications. This is accomplished by catheter-directed administration into the thrombotic material. Regional fibrinolytic therapy is the preferred method of managing arterial thromboses, some venous thrombotic disorders (e.g., axillosubclavian vein thrombosis), and selected patients with iliofemoral venous thrombosis.

The principles of systemic and regional fibrinolytic therapy are discussed separately. It must be kept in mind that complications and side effects may be similar, regardless of the method of administration, because of the systemic effects that may be seen, even with regional administration.

The discussion is limited to general principles of both systemic and regional fibrinolytic therapy. The reader is referred to specific chapters covering the various clinical entities for which fibrinolytic therapy may be recommended.

Thrombolytic Therapy

Guidelines

This section discusses the use of thrombolytic agents for the treatment of venous and peripheral arterial occlusions. Treatment of acute coronary thrombosis is specifically omitted.

Two delivery methods of thrombolytic agents are currently used. Systemic therapy is achieved by infusing large doses of the thrombolytic agent intravenously with the goal of establishing a systemic lytic state. Although peripheral arterial occlusions have been treated with systemic therapy, results have been disappointing owing to a significant incidence of bleeding complications. Currently, systemic therapy is reserved for venous thromboembolic states. Local intravascular infusion of the lytic agent avoids some of the systemic complications and is largely used for peripheral arterial and graft occlusions. Occasionally, localized venous disorders, such as axillary vein thrombosis, may be treated by local intravenous instillation of the lytic agent. Collateral pathways rapidly develop following venous thrombosis, making local infusion less advantageous and systemic therapy remains the delivery method of choice for the treatment of infrainguinal venous thrombosis and pulmonary embolism.

Patient selection is important in obtaining good results with either systemic or local fibrinolytic therapy. The various sections that follow offer guidelines for selecting patients for lytic therapy, administering and monitoring therapy, and dealing with complications, as well as some perspective on the expected outcome. Most of the available clinical experience has been with streptokinase and urokinase, and therefore the discussion emphasizes these two agents. The early experience with t-PA is also presented, emphasizing its differences with streptokinase and urokinase.

Systemic Therapy

Patient Selection

The goal of systemic thrombolytic therapy is to establish a systemic lytic state characterized by a prolongation of the thrombin time (twice normal) and the presence of detectable fibrin degradation products. During a systemic lytic state, fibrin is degraded wherever it has been deposited throughout the body. Hemostatic plugs are as vulnerable to lysis as the clot and thrombus for which therapy has been initiated. Selection of patients for systemic lytic therapy is based on the documented presence of an accepted indication and the absence of absolute contraindications (Table 19–1).

Careful evaluation for the presence of contraindications to systemic lytic therapy is of paramount importance in avoiding serious bleeding complications. Contraindications to systemic thrombolytic therapy[88] are listed in Table 19–1. Absolute contraindications are active internal bleeding and recent (within 2 months) cerebrovascular accident or other intracranial pathology. Relative major contraindications include left heart thrombus, recent (less than 10 days) major surgery, trauma, obstetric delivery, organ biopsy or puncture of a noncompressible vessel, recent gastrointestinal bleed, and severe uncontrolled hypertension. In these circumstances, patients are at a significant risk of peripheral embolization or bleeding and thus the indication for thrombolytic therapy must be carefully weighed against the hazards of bleeding. The use of systemic thrombolytic therapy under these circumstances should essentially be reserved for life-threatening pulmonary emboli.

Table 19–1. Contraindications for Systemic Lytic Therapy

Absolute
Active internal bleeding
Recent (<2 mo) cerebrovascular accident
Intracranial pathology
Relative: Major
Recent (<10 days) major surgery, obstetric delivery or organ biopsy
Left heart thrombus
Active peptic ulcer or gastrointestinal pathology
Recent major trauma
Uncontrolled hypertension
Relative: Minor
Minor surgery or trauma
Recent cardiopulmonary resuscitation
Atrial fibrillation with mitral valve disease
Bacterial endocarditis
Hemostatic defects: e.g., renal or liver disease
Diabetic hemorrhagic retinopathy
Pregnancy
Contraindications for Streptokinase
Known allergy
Recent streptococcal infection
Previous therapy within 6 mo

Data from NIH Consensus Development Conference: Thrombolytic therapy in treatment. Ann Intern Med 93:141, 1980.

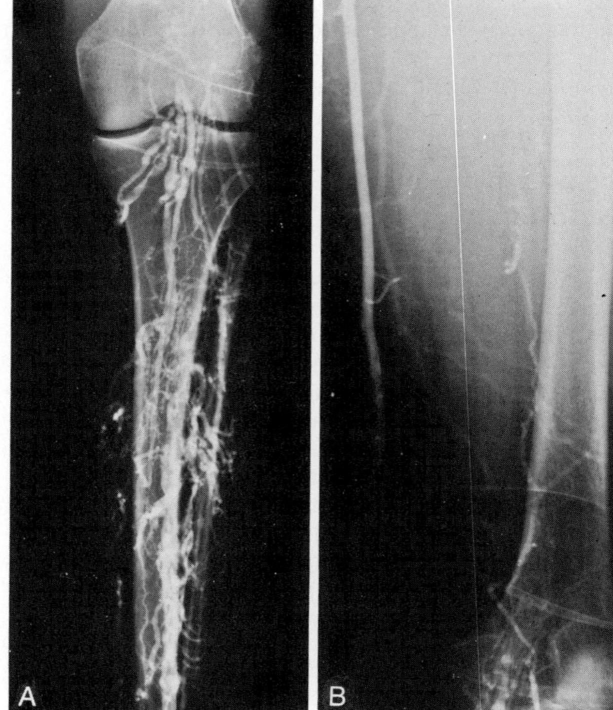

FIGURE 19–2. A 57-year-old woman with phlegmasia cerulea of the left lower extremity. Venogram after streptokinase therapy. *A*, Incomplete clearance of calf thrombi. *B*, Persistent occlusion of the deep femoral system. The superficial system is patent. This was sufficient to achieve limb salvage (see text).

Relative minor contraindications carry a higher risk of complications, but the benefits of therapy may still outweigh the hazards. Peripheral embolization from a central source is a potential hazard of systemic lytic therapy. Therefore, valvular heart disease or atrial fibrillation without demonstrable left heart thrombus on echocardiography and a previous history of emboli represents a minor contraindication to systemic lytic therapy. Severe liver disease will delay metabolism of the drug and, in addition, may compound a preexisting coagulopathy. This makes the response to thrombolytic drug infusion less predictable. During pregnancy, a systemic lytic state may precipitate abruptio placentae or may lead to hypofibrinogenemia in the fetus with an increased risk of bleeding. Antistreptococcal antibodies can neutralize streptokinase, blocking the formation of the activator complex. For these reasons, streptokinase is specifically contraindicated in patients with recent streptococcal infection, previous streptokinase therapy within 6 months, known allergy to streptokinase, or high titers of antistreptococcal antibodies. In these situations, urokinase is the agent of choice.

Systemic administration of thrombolytic agents in current clinical practice is usually limited to the management of deep vein thrombosis (Fig. 19–2) or pulmonary embolism. The reader is referred to the sections in this book that deal specifically with these entities. Doses of the three agents more commonly used for this purpose are shown in Table 19–2.

Systemic administration of fibrinolytic drugs creates a

Table 19–2. Systemic Administration of Common Thrombolytic Agents

Drug	Dose	
	Systemic	*Regional*
Streptokinase	250,000 U IV/30 min 100,000 U IV/hr	5000–10,000 U/hr
Urokinase	2000 U/lb/10 min 2000 U/lb/hr	1000–4000 U/min
Tissue-type plasminogen activator	40–50 mg IV/2 hr	0.05–0.1 mg/kg/hr

significant hemostatic defect. Thus, patients should be monitored appropriately, and invasive procedures should be avoided. Intramuscular injections are contraindicated. Fibrinogen levels are usually monitored not only to document the presence of a systemic lytic state but also to alert the clinician of levels that may predispose the patient to significant bleeding. Although fibrinogen levels do not correlate precisely with the risk of bleeding, bleeding more frequently occurs when fibrinogen levels fall below 100 mg/dl.

In view of the significant contraindications to lytic therapy frequently encountered in patients presenting with deep vein thrombosis or pulmonary embolism, the impact of lytic therapy in the management of these patients is limited. Documentation of the diagnosis is essential before thrombolytic therapy is initiated for either deep vein thrombosis or pulmonary embolism. Noninvasive studies during therapy are useful. The duration of therapy is best guided by the clinical response, and noninvasive studies with repeat invasive angiographic studies are best reserved to evaluate the final outcome. As a rule, if no improvement is seen within 24 hours, it may be best to either discontinue therapy or use an alternative agent.

Method

The goal of intravenous administration of thrombolytic agents is to establish a lytic state. This is evidenced by prolongation of the thrombin time or partial thromboplastin time (PTT) and by the presence of fibrin degradation products. Once the diagnosis is objectively established and the patient is thought to be a suitable candidate for lytic therapy, informed consent should be obtained. Pretreatment fibrinogen level, thrombin time, prothrombin time (PT), PTT, hematocrit, and platelet count should be obtained. If heparin is being administered, it is discontinued.

The thrombolytic agent is then given intravenously with a loading dose (urokinase 2000 U/lb given over 10 minutes, or streptokinase 250,000 units given over 30 minutes) aimed at establishing a lytic state rapidly. These doses have been estimated to establish such a state in approximately 95 per cent of patients. The lytic state is then maintained by a continuous infusion of the agent (urokinase 2000 U/lb/hr, or streptokinase 100,000 U/hr). When streptokinase is chosen, we prefer to administer 100 mg of hydrocortisone prior to initiation of therapy to prevent or decrease some of the allergic reactions that may occur.

Invasive procedures, intramuscular injections, and cutdowns should be avoided. When arterial blood gases are needed, they should be obtained from the wrist, followed by at least a 20-minute compression of the artery. Puncture of noncompressible arteries is contraindicated.

Three to 4 hours after starting the infusion, thrombin time (or PTT if thrombin time is not available), fibrinogen level, and fibrin degradation products are obtained. These will document the presence of a systemic lytic state. A drop in fibrinogen level is to be expected and, in the absence of bleeding complications, is accepted. However, the hematocrit should be followed every 6 hours. If a lytic state is not seen after the initial 4 hours, another bolus dose is given and the hourly dose increased. Alternatively, if streptokinase has been used, a change to urokinase may be advisable.

Following completion of therapy, anticoagulants should be started 2 to 3 hours after discontinuation of the lytic agent. No heparin loading dose is necessary and should be avoided. Warfarin therapy should follow in a conventional manner.

Complications of Systemic Lytic Therapy

Clearly, bleeding is the most feared and frequent complication of systemic thrombolytic therapy. The incidence of major bleeding (requiring discontinuation of therapy or blood transfusions) has been estimated at between 7 and 45 per cent.[30, 87] The number and type of invasive procedures and the duration of therapy appear to influence significantly the incidence of bleeding complications. Superficial bleeding at invaded sites is easily controlled with pressure. Avoidance of unnecessary procedures with preservation of an intact vascular system is the best preventive measure. Internal bleeding, evidenced by an unexplained drop in hematocrit, is usually localized in the gastrointestinal tract. This may be the result of poor patient selection or unknown risk factors. Intracranial bleeding is the most serious hemorrhagic complication. As a rule, any change in the neurologic status of a patient receiving fibrinolytic therapy should be considered an intracranial bleed until proved otherwise. The infusion should be discontinued immediately and appropriate diagnostic and therapeutic measures instituted. Reversal of the lytic state by rapid administration of fresh frozen plasma or cryoprecipitate is advisable. Administration of epsilon-aminocaproic acid (plasmin inhibitor) is *not* recommended and carries a significant risk of aggravating the process for which lytic therapy was instituted. Increasing the dose of streptokinase to decrease its proteolytic effect is theoretically correct but has been abandoned as a clinical option.

Superficial bleeding, which can be controlled by local measures, can be tolerated in the final stages of therapy. If it occurs at the beginning of therapy, or if bleeding is significant enough to require transfusion, the drug should be discontinued and the systemic lytic state reversed.

Bleeding can occur during the lag period between the termination of lytic therapy and the administration of anticoagulant.[30, 34] Thus, it is advisable to delay heparin administration until the thrombin time or the PTT is less than twice normal, and heparin should be initiated without a loading dose. It is unclear why bleeding could occur with urokinase. With streptokinase, however, as plasma levels of the drug decrease, more plasminogen is available for activation of the already formed streptokinase-plasminogen complex.

Intermittent administration of the lytic agent, allowing for plasminogen repletion, has been advocated by some investigators but is cumbersome and has shown no improvement of the results of continuous administration.

Generally, laboratory parameters correlate poorly with the risk of bleeding. However, extremely low fibrinogen levels (less than 20 per cent of baseline) in the presence of an otherwise minor bleeding complication increase the chance of significant bleeding enough to require cessation of therapy. An alternative, in these instances, is to discontinue the drug, correct the coagulopathy, and restart the infusion several hours later.

Pulmonary embolism can occur during treatment for deep vein thrombosis. However, the evidence suggests that it is no more frequent than with conventional heparin therapy. In the absence of bleeding complications, continuation of therapy appears advisable. However, if recurrent emboli are observed, discontinuation of the fibrinolytic agent, heparin administration, and insertion of a caval filter may be life-saving.

Serious allergic reactions are extremely rare with streptokinase and are not a problem with urokinase. However, febrile allergic reactions can occur in up to 30 per cent of patients receiving streptokinase and have been increasingly recognized in patients receiving urokinase. These allergic reactions are well tolerated and generally are of no clinical consequence, but if a serious allergic reaction is evident, immediate discontinuation of the drug is mandatory. Pretreatment of patients with antihistamines, steroids, or meperidine usually avoids allergic and pyretic side effects.

Regional Thrombolytic Therapy

Systemic fibrinolytic therapy has been utilized for the treatment of thrombotic and embolic disease of the systemic arteries. It has been shown to be effective in acute arterial thrombosis that has been present for less than 10 days.[110] The results of intravenous infusion of thrombolytic agents in patients with chronic arterial thrombotic occlusions have not been encouraging.[97, 142] Martin, using a titrated loading dose of streptokinase and a 72-hour infusion of 100,000 U/hr, reported successful treatment in only 8.9 per cent of patients with chronic femoral occlusions, 19.5 per cent of those with chronic iliac occlusions, and 24.4 per cent of those with chronic aortic occlusions.[77] Enthusiasm for this approach was further dampened by the high incidence of hemorrhagic complications.

In an attempt to circumvent the hemorrhagic problems, Dotter and coworkers[29] proposed the administration of low-dose thrombolytic therapy through an angiographically placed catheter. The purpose of this technique was to increase the rate of fibrinolysis and decrease the systemic effect and its associated complications. Katzen and Von Breda[60] and others have evaluated and recommended this low-dose regimen.

In the standard technique a 5-Fr angiographic catheter is advanced so that its tip is near or just within the thrombus. Streptokinase, usually in a dose of 5000 to 8000 U/hr, or urokinase in a dose of 1000 to 4000 U/min, is then infused. Patients are restudied at varying intervals of 6 to 12 hours. Treatment times vary from 1 to 48 hours, with exceptional patients requiring longer infusion times. The concomitant use of heparin is controversial but is often used to avoid pericatheter thrombosis (Fig. 19–3).

The results of several series are summarized in Table 19–3. Despite localized infusion, systemic fibrinolysis occurs within 12 to 24 hours with degradation of fibrinogen, plasminogen, factor V, and factor VIII. Major or minor complications have occurred in 15 to 30 per cent of patients in most series.[85] If the catheter does not properly penetrate the thrombus, lysis is slowed and inefficient because the lytic agent is "washed out" through collaterals, the fibrinolytic effect being the result of the systemic lytic state.

McNamara and Fischer[80] reported complete clot lysis in 75 per cent of patients using a high-dose intra-arterial urokinase regimen. The method described involves making a passageway through the clot with a guidewire or catheter and then instilling urokinase at 4000 U/min for 2 hours. If patency is restored, the catheter is withdrawn proximal to the remaining clot, and the urokinase is infused at 1000 to 2000 U/min until complete lysis is accomplished. Using this technique, the mean infusion time was 18 hours, and the incidence of bleeding complications was low despite the use of heparin to prevent pericatheter thrombosis. The higher cost of urokinase relative to streptokinase can be justified on the basis of the shorter infusion time and fewer bleeding complications.

In general, with both the low-dose regimen and the high-dose urokinase regimen, the likelihood of serious bleeding increases if fibrinogen is decreased to less than 100 mg/dl.[80, 129] When heparin is used with low-dose streptokinase, the PTT should be limited to two times normal.[11, 85] With the shorter duration, high-dose urokinase technique, a PTT of three to five times normal was found to prevent new thrombus formation effectively without increased risk of bleeding. Most applications of regional fibrinolytic therapy have been in the management of extremity arterial disease.[62]

Table 19–3. Results of Thrombolytic Therapy

Reference	Total No. Infusions	Complete Lysis (%)	Duration Infusion (hr)	Major Bleeding (%)
Low-Dose Streptokinase				
Dotter[29]	17	35	71	24
Katzen[60]	12	92	7	17
Totty[129]	19	38	44	19
Becker[11]	57	47	*	12
Mori[85]	50	44	38	8
High-Dose Urokinase				
McNamara[80]	93	83	18	4

**Duration of infusion not reported.*

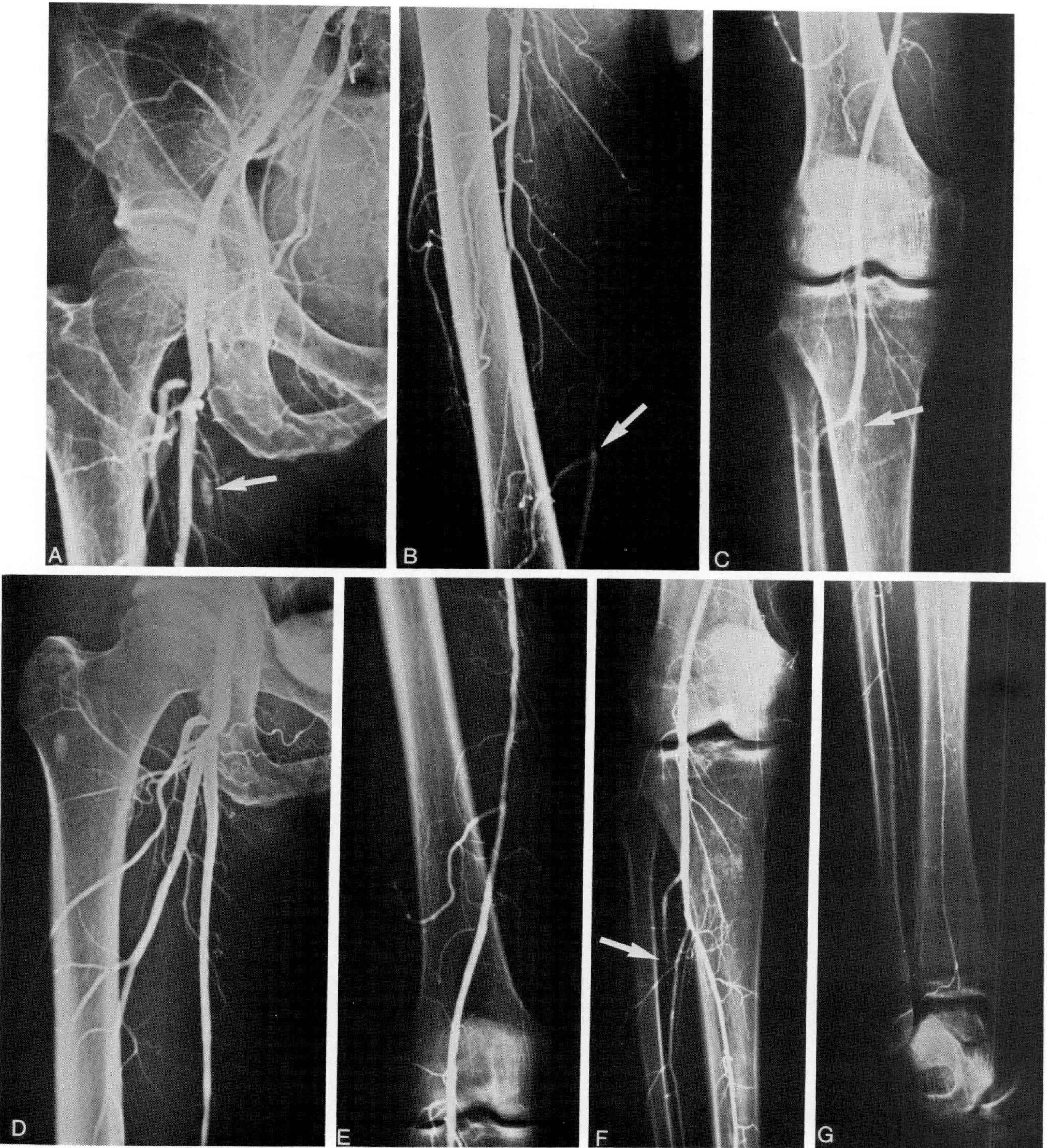

FIGURE 19–3. This 54-year-old man was admitted to the hospital with rest pain and ischemic changes in his right foot and a history suggestive of embolic episodes. An aortogram showed moderate atherosclerotic changes. Runoff study shows the following: *A*, Occlusion of the right superficial femoral artery (SFA) at its origin with delayed filling of a short interrupted segment of the right SFA proximally (*arrow*). *B*, The right SFA reconstitutes at the adductor hiatus (*arrow*). *C*, There is abrupt occlusion of the tibioperoneal trunk proximally, suggesting embolic occlusion (*arrow*). The anterior tibial artery terminated abruptly in the mid-calf. A catheter was advanced to the level of the thrombus, and low-dose intra-arterial streptokinase infusion was started. After 24 hours of therapy, the right SFA and tibioperoneal trunk were patent; however, there was evidence of extensive thrombus sheathing in the infusion catheter proximally. Despite the presence of fever, the streptokinase infusion was increased to systemic doses for 16 additional hours, at which time the patient developed major bleeding from the catheter entry site, with a drop in hematocrit necessitating transfusion and cessation of lytic therapy. An arteriogram was performed at cessation of thrombolytic therapy. Recanalization of the right SFA (*D*) and patency of the popliteal artery (*E*). *F*, The tibioperoneal trunk is patent. The anterior tibial artery remained occluded proximally (*arrow*). *G*, In the calf, the posterior tibial and peroneal arteries are patent to the ankle. A short, interrupted segment of the anterior tibial artery is seen in the mid-calf. One week later he underwent an aortoiliac bypass to remove the site of embolism and subsequently did well.

Acute thrombosis occurring immediately following percutaneous transluminal angioplasty usually is a result of fresh thrombi. These thrombi respond well to thrombolytic therapy, and the success rate for treatment is high in this situation.[75, 129, 137]

Local low-dose streptokinase or urokinase fibrinolytic therapy has also been used successfully in the treatment of occluded grafts (Fig. 19–4).[11] The catheter tip should be inserted into the clot or as close to it as possible. With the catheter in such a position, there are no collaterals to bypass the occlusion, so all of the fibrinolytic agent is directed into the thrombus. Becker and coworkers[11] reported complete lysis in 71 per cent of grafts, Van Breda and associates[139] in 60 per cent, and Gardiner and colleagues in 59 per cent.[40] Perler and associates[95] obtained successful lyses in only 3 of 10 (33 per cent) patients. Concomitant heparin was used sporadically in Perler and associates' series. In the series reported by McNamara and Fischer,[80] one third of the

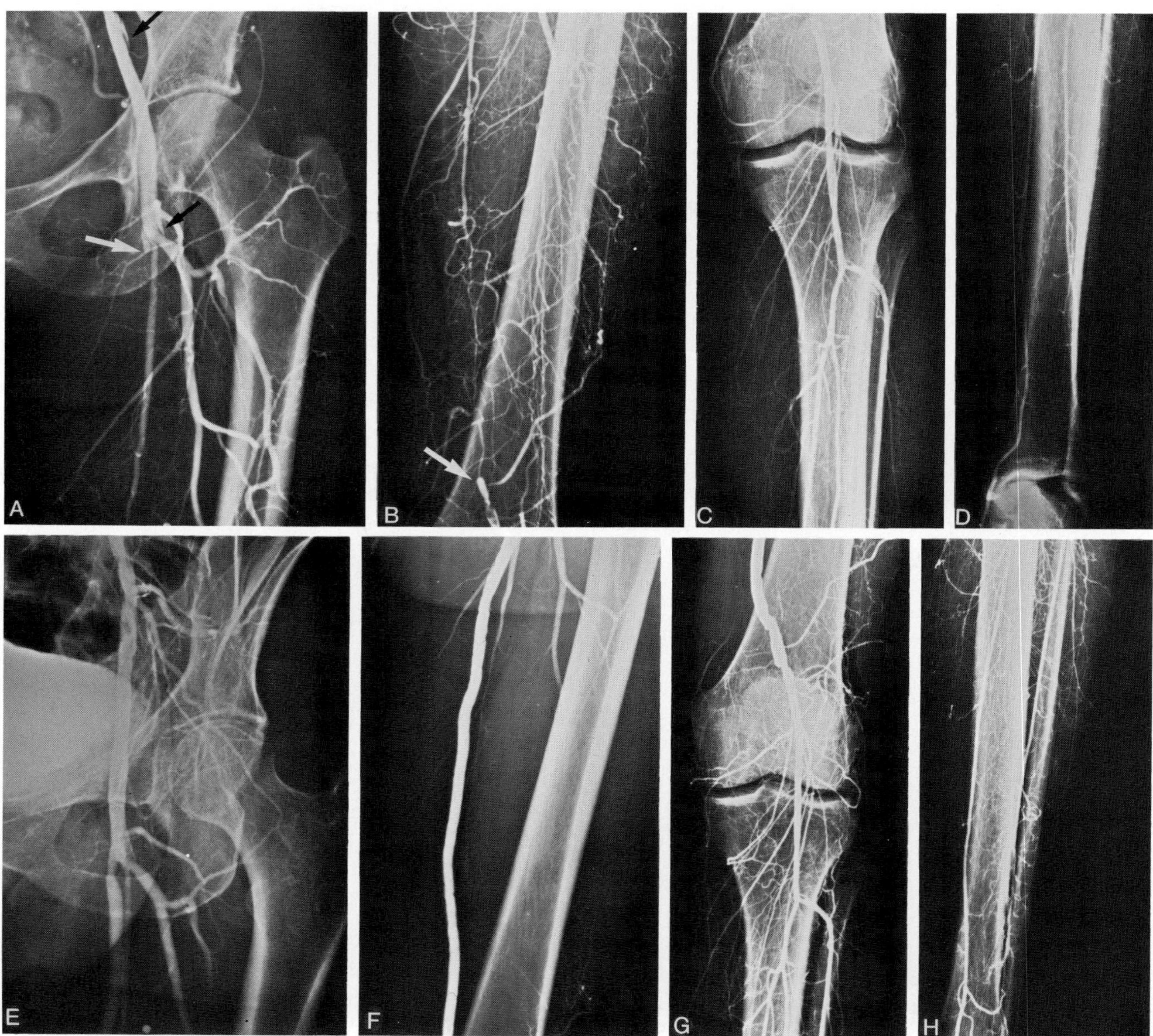

FIGURE 19–4. This 56-year-old woman had recently undergone thrombectomy of her femoropopliteal bypass graft and returned with recurrent ischemic symptoms in the left lower extremity. An arteriogram showed *A*, complete occlusion of the graft at its proximal anastomosis (*white arrow*). Also noted is an incidental post-thrombectomy dissection of the left common femoral artery (*black arrows*). *B*, The left superficial femoral artery is occluded in the mid-thigh. Multiple collaterals reconstitute the proximal popliteal artery, which contains a thrombus (*arrow*). *C*, The distal popliteal artery is patent as is the anterior tibial artery and the tibioperoneal trunk. A small thrombus is seen in the tibioperoneal trunk. *D*, Three-vessel runoff is present in the lower leg. The catheter was advanced to the level of the graft and urokinase infusion was instituted at 4000 U/min for several hours followed by 1000 U/min with concomitant low-dose heparin. Total infusion time was 19 hours. The postinfusion arteriogram shows that the graft is patent proximally (*E*). Residual postoperative narrowing is seen at the proximal anastomosis. *F*, The graft is widely patent in the thigh. *G*, The distal graft anastomosis is recanalized, and the previously seen thrombus in the popliteal artery is lysed. *H*, Three-vessel runoff to the ankle is present. No hemorrhagic complications occurred, and the patient did well.

thrombotic occlusions treated were graft thrombi. Given the excellent results of early surgical thrombectomy of prosthetic grafts, the role of lytic agents in the treatment of acute graft occlusions remains in doubt, particularly with the risk of bleeding if the bypass procedure was recent (i.e., 10 to 14 days).

Fibrinolytic agents may dissolve fibrin in the interstices of knitted Dacron or, less commonly, polytetrafluoroethylene grafts.[99, 104, 139] This can lead to perigraft extravasation, which does not usually cause significant symptoms[99] but may result in marked bleeding.[139]

Acute and subacute hand ischemia resulting from thromboembolic events has also been treated successfully with low-dose intra-arterial regional streptokinase therapy. Good results were reported in 9 of 10 patients in one series.[127] Becker and coworkers[11] reported successful thrombolysis in 71 per cent of patients with renal dialysis shunts but in none of five patients with fistulae. The better results with shunts were attributed to the lack of collateral pathways through which fibrinolytic therapy is washed away.

Occlusions of the celiac, superior mesenteric, and renal arteries have also been successfully treated with intra-arterial fibrinolytic therapy.[36, 96, 150] The technique has not gained widespread use because the poor tolerance of these organs to ischemia imposes time limitations, and changes in their circulatory status cannot be easily monitored. When fibrinolytic therapy is used, frequent angiographic surveillance of clot dissolution is required because clinical parameters alone are unreliable in detecting worsening visceral ischemia.

The fear of embolization and hemorrhagic infarction has limited the use of fibrinolytics in cerebrovascular occlusive disease. In a study in which six dogs were given intracarotid urokinase after varying times of embolic occlusion of the carotid artery, hemorrhagic infarction resulted in all of the animals. This occurred even when fibrinolytic therapy was given within 15 minutes of occlusion.[32] Zeumer and colleagues[151] reported rapid recanalization of the carotid artery in a clinical series in which a balloon occlusion catheter was placed in the carotid artery and urokinase was administered at 50,000 U/hr. Use of fibrinolytic therapy in occlusion of the cerebral arteries remains highly controversial.

Because a systemic lytic state may occur with prolonged regional intravascular fibrinolytic therapy, patient selection is guided by criteria similar to those used for systemic therapy. Absolute contraindications include active internal bleeding, recent surgery or trauma to the area to be perfused, recent cerebrovascular accident, or documented left heart thrombus. Relative contraindications include recent surgery, gastrointestinal bleeding or trauma, severe hypertension, mitral valve disease, endocarditis, hemostatic defects, or pregnancy.[129] Patients who have had recent vascular surgery can be treated in the postoperative setting;[18] however, because of perigraft extravasation, Dacron graft occlusions should not be treated in the early postoperative period (less than 4 to 6 weeks).[118, 139]

In addition, and of particular importance, thrombolysis should not be attempted in any patient whose ischemia has been of sufficient severity or duration to cause severe motor or sensory impairment or in patients whose ischemia cannot be tolerated for the anticipated duration of the infusion. Serious sequelae and high mortality, similar to those associated with operative revascularization of a limb with advanced ischemia, can also occur with fibrinolytic therapy.[80, 85]

It was initially thought that thrombotic occlusions more than 1 to 2 weeks old were unlikely to respond to fibrinolytic therapy. However, it has been shown that intrathrombotic injections of streptokinase or urokinase can effect complete fibrinolysis in occlusions up to several years old. Lammer and coworkers[65] reported success in 75 per cent of 47 patients with chronic occlusions. The fact remains that earlier thrombi are more sensitive to lysis, as evidenced by the experience with postangioplasty thrombosis.

There is no consensus regarding laboratory monitoring during local fibrinolytic therapy. The therapeutic effect of local fibrinolytic therapy is most accurately determined by serial angiography.[62] Hemorrhagic complications occur primarily at sites of vascular cannulation as a result of lysis of hemostatic thrombi but cannot be correlated or predicted from specific laboratory values. Bleeding complications are usually associated with increasing duration of therapy rather than with the dose of the agent. Baseline studies to identify existing hemostatic defects should be performed. These include hemoglobin, hematocrit, platelet count, PTT, PT, bleeding time, serum fibrinogen level, and fibrin degradation products. During therapy, in order of decreasing value, the fibrinogen level, thrombin time, fibrinogen degradation products, and PTT may be monitored at intervals. If heparin is used, the thrombin time is inaccurate, and the PTT may be used to determine heparin dose.[62] Although hematologic monitoring cannot regularly predict the safety or efficacy of thrombolytic infusion, a low fibrinogen level (i.e., less than 100 mg/dl) correlates sufficiently well with the occurrence of bleeding complications that it should not be ignored, even if there is no evidence of active bleeding.

Local thrombolytic therapy with streptokinase or urokinase has several major drawbacks. It does not always result in complete lysis. There is no predictor of successful infusion, and it is not possible to predict how long an infusion may be necessary to restore patency. Ease of passage of the guidewire through the occlusion remains the best predictor of potential success.

The approach chosen for access to the arterial system needs to maximize access to the occluding segment and minimize morbidity. Arterial punctures distal to the presumed occlusion should be avoided. Sites where bleeding may cause serious morbidity, such as axillary or translumbar approaches, should also be avoided. Contralateral puncture with the catheter passed around the aortic bifurcation is preferred and is associated with a lower risk of complications compared with antegrade ipsilateral puncture. Occlusions distal to the mid-superficial femoral artery may be approached with an antegrade ipsilateral puncture. Infusions into the upper extremity or aortic branches are best carried out through a transfemoral approach. End-hole catheters are usually used for infusion with the tip embedded in the thrombus. Multiple-hole catheters are preferred for longer occlusions.

The dosage chosen will depend largely on the length and volume of the thrombus and the location and clinical importance of the vascular territory. Small volume, short thrombi in important territories (e.g., renal) are best treated with high-dose infusions aimed at rapid resolution. Creation of a channel into the thrombus with the angiographic guidewire is of prognostic significance and is technically necessary. Failure to pass the guidewire through the occlusion implies either plaque or a well-organized thrombus, which may be resistant to fibrinolysis. On the other hand, easy passage of the guidewire through the occlusion not only establishes a channel in which the fibrinolytic agent will have the opportunity to concentrate but also implies a soft lysable thrombus. Lacing the thrombus with 50,000 units of urokinase so that the agent is distributed within the thrombus itself and then retrieving the catheter for infusion is frequently practiced and seems effective. Switching to a low-dose regimen is appropriate when prolonged infusions seem necessary; however, angiography is repeated within 12 to 16 hours to document progress. Bleeding complications appear to correlate most closely with duration of therapy rather than with the total dosage of the agent. Thus, high-dose short-term infusions are better tolerated than long-term low-dose infusions.

Administration of heparin during regional thrombolytic therapy remains controversial. Patients with profound ischemia who are found to have very low flow in the extremity and those in whom pericatheter thrombus formation is significant (e.g., when 3 to 4 cm of the catheter extends into a vessel with low or no flow) will benefit from heparin administration. Heparin may have an enhancing effect in increasing thrombolysis and minimizing the adverse consequences of a potential episode of distal clot migration or embolization. Heparin therapy, however, may increase the incidence and severity of pericatheter bleeding during lytic therapy and may increase the risk of distant bleeding. When administered, it is usually best to use it as a continuous infusion to maintain a prolonged PTT of 1.5 to 2.0 times the control value. A bolus infusion prior to initiation of continuous therapy is used in the presence of acute severe ischemia or when low-flow states are identified. In a coaxial system, a lower dose of heparin may be administered through the larger sheath, usually 500 U/hr. It is important that the PTT not exceed 60 seconds at the time of catheter and sheath removal. Heparin may then be restarted without a bolus. The procedure is technically demanding and requires substantial labor and resource commitment.[137]

The relatively new fibrin-specific thrombolytic agent rt-PA has been approved by the Food and Drug Administration for clinical trials. Risius and coworkers[103] have reported the use of this agent in 25 patients with thrombosed peripheral arteries or bypass grafts. The mean age of the occlusions ranged from 1 hour to 21 days (mean, 6.5 days). Thrombolysis occurred in 23 of 25 patients (92 per cent). The failures occurred in two patients with thrombosed femoropopliteal grafts in whom the grafts could not be catheterized. Time to lysis ranged from 1 to 6.5 hours (average, 3.6 hours), with the total dose ranging from 4.5 to 58 mg. Thrombus age had no effect on the infusion time or on the total dose infused. Six patients (24 per cent) experienced profound decreases in plasma fibrinogen levels, and absolute values were less than 100 mg/dl. Complications occurred in three patients (12 per cent). Decreases in plasma fibrinogen, plasminogen, and alpha$_2$-antiplasmin indicative of a systemic lytic state occurred with longer infusion times, suggesting that the fibrin specificity of rt-PA is relative. Nonetheless, with the total doses and infusion durations employed, rt-PA exerted a lesser systemic lytic effect than did streptokinase or urokinase. It appears that rt-PA is a potent and potentially highly effective thrombolytic agent, but additional clinical studies are necessary to determine the ultimate role of rt-PA and other new fibrinolytic agents.

Regardless of the type of agent used, fibrinolytic therapy should not be considered as curative. Although lysis alone can be quite successful in initially restoring patency to a vessel or graft, more often lysis allows delineation of an underlying arterial stenosis or graft abnormality that then must be treated by operation or angioplasty to maintain patency.[118, 129] Long-term patency of native arteries managed in this manner is reasonably good, as is patency of proximal grafts, but late patency in infrainguinal bypasses is disappointing (i.e., less than 20 per cent [see Chapter 35]).

The intraoperative use of thrombolytic agents is now supported by both experimental and clinical experience. The reader is referred to specific sections in this book that discuss this potentially valuable method of administration.

Complications of Regional Lytic Therapy

Complications of local thrombolytic therapy include hemorrhage, distal embolization, pericatheter thrombosis, graft extravasation, fever, and allergic reactions. In addition, all complications discussed earlier under Systemic Therapy may be seen when prolonged regional infusions are necessary.

Distal embolization of clot fragments may cause temporary worsening of symptoms in the treated region. The emboli often disappear with continued fibrinolytic therapy; however, occasionally embolectomy may be required.[80] Pericatheter thrombosis is common and may be avoided by the use of heparin, either systemically or through coaxial systems.[11, 33]

Fever is common with streptokinase and may occur in up to 30 per cent of patients. Severe allergic reactions with improved purification, however, are rare. Retreatment with streptokinase within 6 months should be avoided.

As with any form of lytic therapy, bleeding is the most feared and frequent complication of regional fibrinolytic therapy. The risk of major bleeding (requiring cessation of therapy or blood transfusions) ranges from 5 to 15 per cent, even when appropriate precautions are observed.[44, 80] Bleeding is usually related to systemic effects of the drug, and management has been discussed earlier under Complications of Systemic Lytic Therapy.

The most recent experience seems to indicate that the risk of bleeding correlates more with the duration of therapy than with the actual dose of the agent used. It is preferable to use higher-dose protocols, especially in circumstances in which a shortened duration of infusion may be anticipated. Although specific coagulation parameters do not correlate with the risk of bleeding, the presence of a systemic lytic state decidedly increases this risk. The presence of such systemic effects may help determine the most appropriate course of action in the presence of a minor bleeding complication. A systemic lytic state is heralded by a 50 per cent drop in fibrinogen from baseline or a prolongation of the thrombin time to two times normal, or both. If significant progress is being made in the presence of systemic effects, continuation of therapy is warranted. If, on the other hand, no significant improvement is noted within the last interval of observation, reassessment should be based on weighing the risks and benefits of the alternative.

Treatment of hemorrhagic complications depends on the severity of the process and progress made during lytic therapy. Oozing around the catheter entry site without hematoma formation during the late stages of the infusion may be locally controlled, keeping the patient under observation. A similar situation in the early stages of the infusion, when more than 12 to 24 hours of therapy are anticipated, should lead to discontinuation of the drug. Development of a significant hematoma or bleeding at a remote site requires cessation of therapy. Replacement of fibrinogen with components (e.g., cryoprecipitate or fresh frozen plasma) usually suffices because the half-lives of urokinase, streptokinase, and t-PA are relatively short.

Pseudoaneurysm formation is rare but may occur secondary to bleeding from an arterial puncture site. Current methods of management of pseudoaneurysm are applicable.

Intracranial bleeding is perhaps the most feared complication of any form of lytic therapy. This has been discussed under Systemic Therapy, but any change in the neurologic status of a patient during thrombolytic therapy should be viewed as a complication of treatment and the agent discontinued.

Fatal pulmonary emboli have been reported during intra-arterial fibrinolytic therapy.[112] A potential mechanism for this complication implies decreased venous circulation in the ischemic extremity with formation of clot, partial lysis, and eventual embolization. Treatment options include cessation of lytic therapy with heparinization, or maintaining or increasing the dose of the plasminogen activator. If the latter course is chosen, leaving the intra-arterial catheter in place may decrease the risk of bleeding though the puncture site.

Conversion of an ischemic myocardial infarction into a hemorrhagic infarct has been reported as a complication of lytic therapy. No relationship between the lytic agent and the few reported cases can be made. Nevertheless, deterioration of cardiac function in the presence of an acute myocardial infarction during thrombolytic therapy should lead the clinician to consider this possibility. Therapy may need to be discontinued until the etiology of the cardiac decompensation has been determined.

SUMMARY

A knowledge and understanding of the fibrinolytic system is likely to improve the clinical results obtained with thrombolytic drugs. It is evident that this powerful system, which ensures the fluidity of blood under physiologic conditions, may be utilized as part of the therapy in thromboembolic disorders and perhaps even in other pathologic states controlling cell migration and proliferation.

References

1. Aastad B: Purification and characterization of human vascular plasminogen activator. Biochim Biophys Acta 621:241, 1980.
2. Agnelli G, Parise P: Bolus thrombolysis in venous thromboembolism. Chest 101(4):172S, 1992.
3. Albrechtson OK: The fibrinolytic activity of human tissue. Br J Haematol 3:284, 1957.
4. Alessi MC, Juhan-Vague I, Kooistra T, et al: Insulin stimulates the synthesis of plasminogen activator inhibitor 1 by hepatocellular cell line Hep G2. Thromb Haemost 60:491, 1988.
5. Andreotti F, Davies GJ, Hackett DR, et al: Major circadian fluctuations in fibrinolytic factors and possible relevance to time of onset of myocardial infarction, sudden cardiac death and stroke. Am J Cardiol 62:635, 1988.
6. Angleton P, Chandler WL, Schmer G: Diurnal variation of tissue-type plasminogen activator and its rapid inhibition. Circulation 79:101, 1989.
7. Aoki N, Takeno K, Sakata Y: Differences of frequency distributions of plasminogen phenotypes between Japanese and American populations: New methods for the detection of plasminogen variants. Biochem Genet 22:871, 1984.
8. Astrup T: Stage A. Isolation of a soluble fibrinolytic activator from animal tissue. Nature 170:929, 1952.
9. Astrup T: The haemostatic balance. Thromb Diath Haemost 2:347, 1958.
10. Barnathan ES, Kuo A, Rosenfeld L, et al: Interaction of single-chain urokinase-type plasminogen activator with human endothelial cells. J Biol Chem 265:2865, 1990.
11. Becker GJ, Rabe FE, Richmond BD, et al: Low-dose fibrinolytic therapy. Radiology 148:663, 1983.
12. Behrendt N, Ronne E, Plough M, et al: The human receptor for urokinase plasminogen activator. NH_2-terminal amino acid sequence and glycosylation variants. J Biol Chem 265:6453, 1990.
13. Belkin M, Belkin B, Bucknam CA, et al: Intraarterial fibrinolytic therapy: Efficacy of streptokinase versus urokinase. Arch Surg 121:769, 1986.
14. Bernik MB, Kwaan HC: Origin of fibrinolytic activity in cultures of the human kidney. J Lab Clin Med 70:650, 1967.
15. Bode C, Matsueda G, Haber E: Targeted thrombolysis with a fibrin-specific antibody urokinase conjugate. Circulation 72:111, 1985.
16. Booyse FM, Scheinbuks JR, Radek J, et al: Immunological identification and comparison of plasminogen activator forms in cultured normal human endothelial cells and smooth muscle cells. Thromb Res 24:495, 1981.
17. Burrowes CE: Activation of human prekallikrein by plasmin. Fed Proc 30:451, 1971.
18. Chaise L, Comerota AJ, Soulen RC, et al: Selective intraarterial streptokinase in the immediate postoperative period. JAMA 247:2397, 1982.
19. Chandler WL, Trimble SL, Loo S-C, Mornin D: Effect of PAI-1 levels on the molar concentrations of active tissue plasminogen activator (t-PA) and t-PA/PAI-1 complex in plasma. Blood 76:930, 1990.
20. Claeys H, Molla A, Verstraete M: Conversion of NH_2-terminal glutamic acid to NH_2-terminal lysine human plasminogen by plasmin. Thromb Res 3:515, 1973.
21. Clozel JP, Banken L, Roux S: Aprotinin: An antidote for recombinant tissue-type plasminogen activator (rt-PA) active in vivo. J Am Coll Cardiol 16:507, 1990.
22. Collen D: Human tissue type plasminogen activator: From the laboratory to the bedside [editorial]. Circulation 72:18, 1985.
23. Collen D, Wiman B: Turnover of antiplasmin, the fast-acting plasmin inhibitor of plasma. Blood 53:313, 1979.
24. Cucuianu M, Crisnic I, Knauer O, et al: Severe bleeding in heterozygous α_2 plasmin inhibitor deficiency. Rev Roum Biochim 26:273, 1989.
25. Cummings H, Castellino F: Interaction of human plasmin with human α_2-macroglobulin. Biochemistry 23:105, 1984.
26. Dairbairn S, Gilbert R, Ojakian G, et al: The extracellular matrix of normal chick embryo fibroblasts. Its effect on transformed chick fibroblasts and its proteolytic degradation by the transformation. J Cell Biol 101:1790, 1985.
27. De Jaegere PP, Arnold AA, Balk AH, Simoons ML: Intracranial

hemorrhage in association with thrombolytic therapy: Incidence and clinical predictive factors. J Am Coll Cardiol 19:289, 1992.
28. Doolittle RF: Fibrinogen and fibrin. Ann Rev Biochem 53:195, 1984.
29. Dotter CT, Rosch J, Seaman AJ: Selective clot lysis with low-dose streptokinase. Radiology 11:31, 1974.
30. Elliot MS, Immelman EJ, Jeffery P, et al: A comparative randomized trial of heparin vs. streptokinase in the treatment of acute proximal venous thrombosis. An interim report of a prospective trial. Br J Surg 66:838, 1979.
31. Erickson LA, Hekman CM, Loskutoff DJ: The primary plasminogen-activator inhibitors in endothelial cells, platelets, serum and plasma are immunologically related. Proc Natl Acad Sci USA 82:8710, 1985.
32. Eskridge JM, Becker GJ, Rabe FE, et al: Carotid occlusion in a canine model. Semin Intervent Radiol 2:405, 1985.
33. Eskridge JM, Becker GJ, Rabe FE, et al: Catheter related thrombosis and fibrinolytic therapy. Radiology 149:429, 1983.
34. Feissinger JN, Vayssiairat M, Juillet Y, et al: Local urokinase in arterial thromboembolism. Angiology 31:715, 1980.
35. Fioretti E, Angeletti M, Citro G, et al: Kunitz-type inhibitors in human serum. Identification and characterization. J Biol Chem 262:3586, 1987.
36. Flickinger EG, Jonnsrude IS, Osburn HL, et al: Local streptokinase infusion for superior mesenteric artery thromboembolism. AJR 140:771, 1983.
37. Friezner Degen SJ, Rajput B, Reich E: The human tissue plasminogen activator gene. J Biol Chem 261:6972–6985, 1986.
38. Fujii S, Lucore CL, Hopkins WE, et al: Potential attenuation of fibrinolysis by growth factors released from platelets and their pharmacologic implications. Am J Cardiol 63:1505, 1989.
39. Fujii S, Sobel BE: Induction of plasminogen activator inhibitor by products released from platelets. Circulation 82:1485, 1990.
40. Gardiner GA, Koltun W, Kandarpa K, et al: Thrombolysis of occluded femoropopliteal grafts. AJR 147:621, 1986.
41. Gelehrter TD, Sznycer-Laszuk R, Zeheb R, et al: Dexamethasone inhibition of tissue-type plasminogen activator (t-PA) activity; paradoxical induction of both t-PA antigen and plasminogen activator inhibitor. Mol Endocrinol 1:97, 1987.
42. Gomez MJ, Carroll RC, Hansard MR, et al: Regulation of fibrinolysis in aortic surgery. J Vasc Surg 8:348, 1988.
43. Gonzales-Gronow M, Edelberg JM, Pizzo SV: Further characterization of the cellular plasminogen binding site: Evidence that plasminogen 2 and lipoprotein(a) compete for the same site. Biochemistry 28:2374, 1989.
44. Graor RA, Risius B, Denny KM, et al: Local thrombolysis in the treatment of thrombosed arteries, bypassed grafts, and arteriovenous fistulas. J Vasc Surg 2:406, 1985.
45. Graor RA, Risius B, Young JR, et al: Peripheral artery and bypass graft thrombolysis with recombinant human tissue type plasminogen activator. J Vasc Surg 3:115, 1986.
46. Grimaudo V, Hauert J, Bachmann F, et al: Diurnal variation of the fibrinolytic system. Thromb Haemost 59:495, 1988.
47. Gurewich V, Pannell R, Louie S, et al: Effective and fibrin specific clot lysis by a zymogen precursor form of urokinase (pro-urokinase): A study in vitro and two animal species. J Clin Invest 73:1731, 1984.
48. Häggroth L, Mattson C, Felding P, et al: Plasminogen activator inhibitors in plasma and platelets from patients with recurrent venous thrombosis and pregnant women. Thromb Res 42:585, 1986.
49. Hajjar KA, Gavish D, Breslow JL, et al: Lipoprotein(a) modulation of endothelial cell surface fibrinolysis and its potential role in atherosclerosis. Nature 339:303, 1989.
50. Hamsten A, Wiman B, de Faire U, Blömback M: Increased plasma levels of a rapid inhibitor of tissue plasminogen activator in young survivors of myocardial infarction. N Engl J Med 313:1557, 1985.
51. Harpel PC, Gordon BR, Parker TS: Plasmin catalyzes binding of lipoprotein(a) to immobilized fibrinogen and fibrin. Proc Natl Acad Sci USA 86:3847, 1989.
52. Henkin J, Marcotte P, Yang H: The plasminogen-plasmin system. Prog Cardiovasc Dis 34(2):135, 1991.
53. Higgins D, Vehar G: Interaction of one-chain tissue plasminogen activator with intact and plasmin-degraded fibrin. Biochemistry 26:7786, 1987.
54. Hoylaerts M, Rijken DC, Lijnen HR, et al: Kinetics of the activation of plasminogen by human tissue plasminogen activator. J Biol Chem 257:2912, 1982.
55. Husain SS, Gurewich V, Lipinski B: Purification and partial characterization of a single chain, high molecular weight form of urokinase from human urine. Arch Biochem Biophys 220:31, 1983.
56. Ichinose A, Takio K, Fujikawa K: Localization of the binding site of tissue-type plasminogen activator in fibrin. J Clin Invest 78:163, 1986.
57. Johnson AJ, McCarty WR: The lysis of artificially induced intravascular clots in man by infusions of streptokinase. J Clin Invest 38:1624, 1959.
58. Juhan-Vague I, Vague PH, Alessi MC, et al: Relationships between plasma insulin, triglyceride, body mass index, and plasminogen activator inhibitor 1. Diabetes Metab 13:331, 1987.
59. Juhan-Vague I, Valadier J, Alessi M-C, et al: Deficient t-PA release and elevated PA inhibitor levels in patients with spontaneous deep venous thrombosis. Thromb Haemost 57:67, 1987.
60. Katzen BT, Van Breda A: Low-dose streptokinase in treatment of arterial occlusions. AJR 136:1171, 1981.
61. Kirchheimer JC, Wojta J, Christ G, et al: Proliferation of a human epidermal tumor cell line stimulated by urokinase. FASEB J 1:125, 1987.
62. Klatte EC, Becker GJ, Holden RE, et al: Fibrinolytic therapy. Radiology 159:619, 1986.
63. Kordich L, Porterie V, Lago O, et al: Mini-plasminogen–like molecule in septic patients. Thromb Res 47:553, 1987.
64. Kwaan HC: The biologic role of components of the plasminogen-plasmin system. Prog Cardiovasc Dis 34(5):309, 1992.
65. Lammer J, Pilger E, Justich E, et al: Fibrinolysis in chronic arteriosclerotic occlusions: Intrathrombotic injection of streptokinase. Radiology 157:45, 1985.
66. Levin EG: Latent tissue plasminogen activator produced by human endothelial cells in culture: Evidence for an enzyme-inhibitor complex. Proc Natl Acad Sci USA 80:6804, 1983.
67. Levin EG, Loskutoff DJ: Regulation of plasminogen activator production by cultured endothelial cells. Ann NY Acad Sci 401:184, 1982.
68. Levin EG, Santell L: Association of a plasminogen activator inhibitor (PAI-1) with the growth substratum and membrane of human endothelial cells. J Cell Biol 105:2543, 1987.
69. Lijnen HR, Zamarron C, Blaber M, et al: Activation of plasminogen by pro-urokinase. I. Mechanism. J Biol Chem 261:1253, 1986.
70. Lo SK, Ryan TJ, Gilboa N, et al: Role of catalytic and lysine-binding sites in plasmin-induced neutrophil adherence to endothelium. J Clin Invest 84:793, 1989.
71. Loscalzo J, Weinfeld M, Fless GM, et al: Lipoprotein (a), fibrin binding and plasminogen activation. Arteriosclerosis 10:240, 1990.
72. Low DA, Baker JB, Koonce WC: Released protease-nexin regulates cellular binding, internalization, and degradation of serine proteases. Proc Natl Acad Sci USA 78:2340, 1981.
73. Lucore CL, Fujii S, Wun T-C, et al: Regulation of the expression of type 1 plasminogen activator inhibitor in Hep G2 cells by epidermal growth factor. J Biol Chem 263:15845, 1988.
74. MacFarlane RG, Pilling J: Observations on fibrinolytic plasminogen, plasmin and antiplasmin content of human blood. Lancet 2:562, 1946.
75. Marder VJ, Soulen RL, Atichartakarn V, et al: Quantitative venographic assessment of deep vein thrombosis in the evaluation of streptokinase and heparin therapy. J Lab Clin Med 89:1018, 1977.
76. Marongiu F, Conti M, Mameli G, et al: Is the imbalance between thrombin and plasmin activity in diabetes related to the behavior of antiplasmin activity? Thromb Res 58:91, 1990.
77. Martin M: Thrombolytic therapy in arterial thromboembolism. Prog Cardiovasc Dis 21:351, 1979.
78. Matsuo O, Rijken DC, Cullen D: Thrombolysis by human tissue plasminogen activator and urokinase in rabbits with experimental pulmonary embolus. Nature 291:590, 1981.
79. McLean JW, Tomlinson JE, Kuang W-J, et al: cDNA sequence of human apolipoprotein (a) is homologous to plasminogen. Nature 300:132, 1987.
80. McNamara TO, Fischer JR: Thrombolysis of peripheral arterial and graft occlusions: Improved results using high dose urokinase. AJR 144:769, 1985.
81. McNicol GP, Gale SB, Douglas AS: In vitro and in vivo studies of a preparation of urokinase. Br Med J 1:909, 1963.

82. Mehta J, Mehta P, Lawson D, et al: Plasma tissue plasminogen activator inhibitor levels in coronary artery disease: Correlation with age and serum triglyceride concentrations. J Am Coll Cardiol 9:263, 1987.
83. Miles LA, Fless GM, Levin EG, et al: A potential basis for the thrombotic risks associated with lipoprotein(a). Nature 339:301, 1989.
84. Monk JP, Heel RC: Anisoylated plasminogen streptokinase activator complex (APSAC): A review of its mechanism of action, clinical pharmacology, and therapeutic use in acute myocardial infarction. Drugs 34:25, 1987.
85. Mori KW, Bookstein JJ, Heeney DJ, et al: Selective streptokinase infusion: Clinical and laboratory correlates. Radiology 148:677, 1983.
86. Mosher DF, Vaheri A: Binding and degradation of α_2-macroglobulin by cultured fibroblasts. Biochim Biophys Acta 627:113, 1980.
87. National Heart and Lung Institute Cooperative Study Group: Urokinase pulmonary embolism trial: Phase I results. JAMA 214(12): 2163, 1970.
88. NIH Consensus Development Conference: Thrombolytic therapy in treatment. Ann Intern Med 93:141, 1980.
89. Nilsson IM, Ljungner H, Tengborn L: Two different mechanisms in patients with venous thrombosis and defective fibrinolysis: Low concentrations of plasminogen activator or increased concentration of plasminogen activator inhibitor. Br Med J 290:1453, 1985.
90. Nilsson TK, Sundell B, Hellsten G, et al: Reduced plasminogen activator inhibitor activity in high consumers of fruits, vegetables and root vegetables. J Intern Med 227:267, 1990.
91. Nykjaer A, Petersen CM, Christensen EI, et al: Urokinase receptors in human monocytes. Biochim Biophys Acta 1052:399, 1990.
92. Ohlsson M, Peng XR, Liu YX, et al: Hormone regulation of tissue-type plasminogen activator gene expression and plasminogen activator-mediated proteolysis. Semin Thromb Hemost 17:286, 1991.
93. Pannell R, Gurewich V: Pro-urokinase: A study of its stability in plasma and of a mechanism for its selective fibrinolytic effect. Blood 67:1215, 1986.
94. Patthy L, Trexler M, Vali Z, et al: Kringles: Modules specialized for protein binding. Homology of the gelatin-binding region of fibronectin with the kringle structures of proteins. FEBS Lett 171:131, 1984.
95. Perler BA, White RI, Ernst CG, et al: Low-dose thrombolytic therapy for infrainguinal graft occlusions: An idea whose time has passed? J Vasc Surg 2:799, 1986.
96. Pillari G, Doscher W, Fierstein J, et al: Low-dose streptokinase in the treatment of celiac and superior mesenteric artery occlusion. Arch Surg 118:1340, 1983.
97. Poliwoda H, Alexander K, Buhl V, et al: Treatment of chronic arterial occlusions with streptokinase. N Engl J Med 280:689, 1969.
98. Pollanen J, Saksela O, Salonen EM, et al: Distinct localizations of urokinase-type plasminogen activator and its type 1 inhibitor under cultured human fibroblasts and sarcoma cells. J Cell Biol 104:1085, 1987.
99. Rabe FE, Becker GJ, Richmond BD, et al: Contrast extravasation through Dacron grafts: A sequela of low-dose streptokinase therapy. AJR 138:917, 1982.
100. Rijken DC, Collen D: Purification and characterization of the plasminogen activator secreted by human melanoma cells in culture. J Biol Chem 256:7035, 1981.
101. Rijken DC, Hoylaerts M, Collen D: Fibrinolytic properties of one-chain and two-chain human extrinsic (tissue type) plasminogen activator. J Biol Chem 257:2920, 1982.
102. Ring M, Butman S, Bruck D, et al: Fibrin metabolism in patients with acute myocardial infarction during and after treatment with tissue-type plasminogen activator. Thromb Haemost 60:428, 1988.
103. Risius B, Graor RA, Geisinger MA, et al: Recombinant human tissue–type plasminogen activator for thrombolysis in peripheral arteries and bypass grafts. Radiology 60:183, 1986.
104. Rosner NH, Dous PE: Contrast extravasation through Dacron grafts: A sequela of low-dose streptokinase therapy. AJR 148:668, 1984.
105. Royston D: Review paper: The serine antiprotease aprotinin (Trasylol™): A novel approach to reducing postoperative bleeding. Blood Coagul Fibrin 1:55, 1990.
106. Rudd MA, George D, Amarante P, et al: Temporal effects of thrombolytic agents in platelet function in vivo and their modulation by prostaglandins. Circ Res 67:1175, 1990.
107. Rylatt DB, Blake LE, Cottis DA, et al: An immunoassay for human D-dimer using monoclonal antibodies. Thromb Res 31:767, 1983.
108. Salo T, Liotta LA, Keski-Oja J, et al: Secretion of basement membrane collagens degrading enzyme and plasminogen activator by transformed cells—Role in metastasis. Int J Cancer 30:669, 1982.
109. Scott RW, Bergman BL, Bajpai A, et al: Protease nexin: Properties and a modified purification procedure. J Biol Chem 260:7029, 1985.
110. Sharma GV, Cella G, Parisi AF, et al: Thrombolytic therapy. N Engl J Med 306:1268, 1982.
111. Sherry S: Tissue plasminogen activator (t-PA): Will it fulfill its promise? N Engl J Med 313:1014, 1985.
112. Sicard GA, Schier JJ, Totty WG, et al: Thrombolytic therapy for acute arterial occlusion. J Vasc Surg 2:65, 1985.
113. Sprengers ED, Akkerman JWN, Jansen BG: Blood platelet plasminogen activator inhibitor: Two different pools of endothelial cell type plasminogen activator inhibitor in human blood. Thromb Haemost 55:325, 1986.
114. Stack S, Gonzalez-Gronow M, Pizzo S: Regulation of plasminogen activation by components of the extracellular matrix. Biochemistry 29:4966, 1990.
115. Strickland S, Beers WH: Studies on the role of plasminogen activator in ovulation. J Biol Chem 18:5694, 1976.
116. Sugiyama N, Iwamoto M, Abiko A: Effects of kringles derived from human plasminogen on fibrinolysis in vitro. Thromb Res 47:459, 1987.
117. Summaria L: The plasmin b-chain streptokinase complex. *In* Comerota AJ (ed): Thrombolytic Therapy. Orlando, FL, Grune & Stratton, 1988.
118. Sussman B, Dardik H, Ibrahim IM, et al: Improved patient selection for enzymatic lysis of peripheral arterial and graft occlusions. Am J Surg 148:244, 1984.
119. Takada A, Sugawara Y, Takada Y: Enhancement of the activation of glu-plasminogen by urokinase in the simultaneous presence of tranexamic acid or fibrin. Haemostasis 1:26, 1989.
120. Takahashi H, Hanano M, Takizawa S, et al: Plasmin-α_2-plasmin inhibitor complex in plasma of patients with disseminated intravascular coagulation. Am J Haematol 28:162, 1988.
121. Tennant SN, Dixon J, Venable TC, et al: Intracoronary thrombolysis in patients with acute myocardial infarction: Comparison of the efficacy of urokinase versus streptokinase. Circulation 69:756, 1984.
122. Testa JE, Quigley JP: The role of urokinase-type plasminogen activator in aggressive tumor cell behavior. Cancer Metastasis Rev 9:355, 1990.
123. Thorsen S: Differences in the binding to fibrin of native plasminogen and plasminogen modified by protolytic degradation influence of ω-aminocarboxylic acids. Biochim Biophys Acta 393:55, 1975.
124. Thorsen S, Philips M, Selmer J, et al: Kinetics of inhibition of tissue-type and urokinase-type plasminogen activator by plasminogen-activator inhibitor type 1 and type 2. Eur J Biochem 175:33, 1988.
125. Tillett WS, Garner RL: The fibrinolytic activity of hemolytic streptococci. J Exp Med 58:485, 1933.
126. TIMI Study Group: Thrombolysis in myocardial infarction (TIMI) trial. Phase I findings. N Engl J Med 312:932, 1985.
127. Tisnado J, Cho S, Beachley MC, et al: Low-dose fibrinolytic therapy in hand ischemia. Semin Intervent Radiol 2:367, 1985.
128. Torr SR, Nachowiak DA, Fujii S, Sobel BE: "Plasminogen steal" and clot lysis. J Am Coll Cardiol 19(5):1085, 1992.
129. Totty WG, Gilula LA, McClennan BL, et al: Low-dose intravascular fibrinolytic therapy. Radiology 143:59, 1982.
130. Totty WG, Romano T, Benian GM, et al: Serum sickness following streptokinase therapy. AJR 138:143, 1982.
131. Urano T, Chibber B, Castellino F: The reciprocal effects of ϵ-aminohexanoic acid and chloride ion on the activation of human [Glu^1] plasminogen by human urokinase. Proc Natl Acad Sci USA 84:4031, 1987.
132. Urano T, Sumiyoshi K, Nakamura M, et al: Fluctuation of tPA and PAI-1 antigen levels in plasma: Difference in their fluctuation patterns between male and female. J Thromb Res 60:55, 1990.
133. Urden G, Chmielewska J, Carlsson T, et al: Immunological relationship between plasminogen activator inhibitors from different sources. Thromb Haemost 57:29, 1987.
134. Vague P, Juhan-Vague I, Alessi MC, et al: Metformin decreases the high plasminogen activator inhibition capacity, plasma insulin and triglyceride levels in non-diabetic obese subjects. Thromb Haemost 57:326, 1987.

135. Vali Z, Patthy L: Locations of the intermediate and high-affinity ω-aminocarboxylic acid-binding sites in human plasminogen. J Biol Chem 257:2104, 1982.
136. Vali Z, Patthy L: The fibrin-binding site of human plasminogen. Arginines 32 and 34 are essential for fibrin affinity of the kringle 1 domain. J Biol Chem 259:13690, 1984.
137. Van Breda A, Katzen BT: Thrombolytic therapy of peripheral vascular disease. Semin Intervent Radiol 2:354, 1985.
138. Van Breda A, Katzen BT, Deutsch AS: Urokinase versus streptokinase in local thrombolysis. Radiology 165:109, 1987.
139. Van Breda A, Robison JC, Feldman L, et al: Local thrombolysis in the treatment of arterial graft occlusions. J Vasc Surg 1:103, 1984.
140. Van Hinsberg VWM, van den Berg EA, Fiers W, et al: Tumor necrosis factor induces the production of urokinase-type plasminogen activator by human endothelial cells. Blood 75:1991, 1990.
141. Van Leuven F, Cassiman JJ, Van Den Berghe H: Demonstration of an α_2-macroglobulin receptor in human fibroblasts, absent in tumor-derived cell lines. J Biol Chem 254:5155, 1970.
142. Verstraete M, Vermylen J, Donati MB: The effect of streptokinase infusion on chronic arterial occlusion and stenoses. Ann Intern Med 74:377, 1971.
143. Violand BN, Sodetz JM, Castellino FJ: The effect of ϵ-amino caproic acid on the gross conformation of plasminogen and plasmin. Arch Biochem Biophys 170:300, 1975.
144. Walker ID, Davidson JF: Long-term fibrinolytic enhancement with anabolic steroid therapy: A five-year study. *In* Davidson JF, Rowan RM, Samama MM, Desnoyers PC (eds): Progress in Chemical Fibrinolysis and Thrombolysis. New York, Raven Press, 1978, vol. 3, pp 491–500.
145. Watahiki Y, Takeda Y, Takeda A: Kinetic analyses of the activation of glu-plasminogen by urokinase in the presence of fibrin, fibrinogen or its degradation products. Thromb Res 46:9, 1987.
146. Wiman B, Hamsten A: Impaired fibrinolysis and risk of thromboembolism. Prog Cardiovasc Dis 34(3):179, 1991.
147. Wiman B, Hamsten A: The fibrinolytic enzyme system and its role in the etiology of thromboembolic disease. Semin Thromb Haemost 16:207, 1990.
148. Wiman B, Lijnen HR, Collen D: On the specific interaction between the lysine-binding sites in plasminogen and complementary sites in α_2-antiplasmin and in fibrinogen. J Biochim Biophys Acta 579:142, 1979.
149. Wiman B, Ljungberg B, Chmielewska J, et al: The role of the fibrinolytic system in deep vein thrombosis. J Lab Clin Med 105:267, 1985.
150. Zajko AB, McLean GK, Grossman RA, et al: Percutaneous transluminal angioplasty and fibrinolytic therapy for renal allograft arterial stenoses and thrombosis. Transplantation 33:447, 1982.
151. Zeumer H, Hundgren R, Ferbert A, et al: Local intra-arterial fibrinolytic therapy in inaccessible internal carotid occlusion. Neuroradiology 26:315, 1984.

20

Percutaneous Transluminal Angioplasty and Other Endovascular Technologies

David A. Kumpe, M.D., and Gary J. Becker, M.D.

Percutaneous Transluminal Angioplasty

David A. Kumpe, M.D.

• • •

HISTORICAL BACKGROUND

In a landmark publication in 1964, Dotter and Judkins reported a new therapeutic approach to superficial femoral artery occlusion in which an angiographic technique rather than surgery was used.[1] Their treatment, which they called percutaneous transluminal angioplasty, achieved marked clinical improvement in 6 of 11 ischemic extremities and averted amputation in four. Their work was greeted with considerable skepticism, owing in part to preconceived notions that it could not possibly work and to the inability of others to duplicate their results.

Over the next decade, few angioplasties were performed in the United States except by Dotter. In Europe, however, a number of investigators, including van Andel, Zeitler, and Porstmann and Wierny, developed and refined the procedure and accumulated substantial experience demonstrating its effectiveness and the durability of its results.[2–4] In 1968, Staple proposed using a single tapered catheter instead of the coaxial Dotter system.[5] This was subsequently modified by van Andel and is commonly called the van Andel catheter. Dotter tried to use Fogarty's balloon catheters to dilate iliac lesions, but their soft latex balloons exerted relatively weak lateral force, were too easily deformed by many lesions, and had no maximum diameter.[6] The first effective balloon dilating catheter was developed by Porstmann, who enclosed a latex balloon inside a stiff Teflon catheter with longitudinal slits at the balloon site.[7]

This "corset catheter" allowed lesions to be dilated to larger diameters than the catheter shaft, but it was quite stiff and thrombogenic.

The modern era of percutaneous arterial dilation began in 1974 with the development by Grüntzig and Hopff of a nonelastomeric, double-lumen balloon catheter of polyvinyl chloride that would expand to a predetermined maximum diameter and no further.[8] The catheter could be introduced into an artery by using routine Seldinger technique and was considerably more flexible and less thrombogenic than the corset catheter. The balloon could be manufactured in different lengths and with maximum expanded diameters. It quickly became apparent that such balloon catheters could be placed in virtually any major artery or vein, where balloon expansion then produced only radial pressures on the lesion with none of the axial force exerted on the vessel wall by the Dotter and van Andel catheters. Grüntzig's balloon catheters became widely available commercially in 1978. Figure 20–1 shows examples of early dilatation catheter designs.

Coronary artery dilatation was first performed in September 1977 by Grüntzig using a coaxial catheter system that he developed, with an outer guiding catheter being used to direct a smaller balloon catheter to the dilatation site.

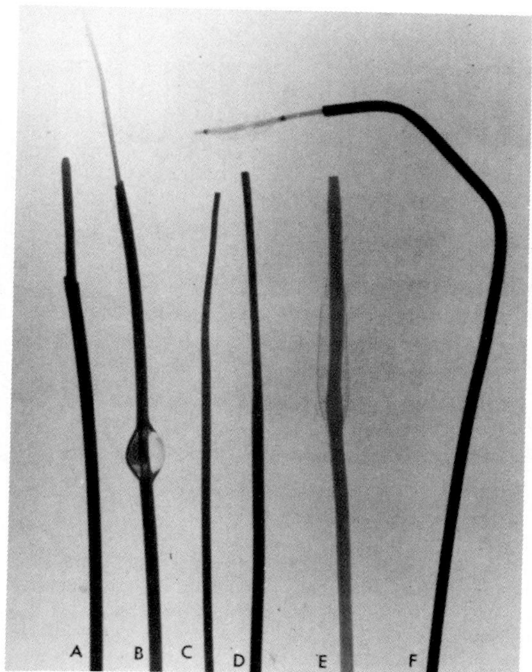

FIGURE 20–1. Early dilatation catheter designs include the Dotter coaxial (*A*) and the Staple-van Andel catheters (*C* and *D*). The Porstmann "caged balloon" (*B*) was an early latex balloon catheter. The Grüntzig catheter (*E*), used in most peripheral dilatations, was developed in 1974. The Grüntzig coaxial balloon catheter (*F*), introduced in 1977, has an outer guiding and an inner balloon dilatation catheter and is used in coronary and some renal artery dilatations. (From Sos TA, Pickering TG, Saddekni S, et al: The current role of renal angioplasty in the treatment of renovascular hypertension. Urol Clin North Am 11:503, 1984.)

CURRENT EQUIPMENT

Previously, most standard balloon catheters for peripheral (noncoronary) angioplasty had a 7 Fr catheter shaft, although they have now been replaced with similar catheters having a 5 Fr shaft. Most balloon catheter shafts for balloon diameters ranging from 4 to 8 mm are now 5 Fr. Percutaneous transluminal coronary angioplasty (PTCA) catheters and small vessel peripheral balloon catheters for tibial arteries and for renal branch stenoses are now available with shafts of 3 Fr and smaller.[9] Standard balloon lengths employed in peripheral percutaneous transluminal angioplasty (PTA) vary from 2 to 10 cm, and maximum balloon diameters range from 4 to 30 mm. Although the first commercially available balloons were made from polyvinyl chloride, this material has now essentially been abandoned in favor of polyethylene because the latter's lower compliance prevents overexpansion beyond the maximum intended diameter before the balloon ruptures. More recently, balloons made from reinforced polyurethane, strengthened polyvinyl chloride, nylon, polyamide, and new composites have become available. All allow higher dilating pressures.

Coaxial outer guiding catheters and inner balloon catheter systems are used almost exclusively in coronary angioplasty but are occasionally helpful in renal and tibial angioplasty as well. Modified coronary angioplasty balloon catheters, designed for use without an outer guiding catheter, have become available for angioplasty of tibial arteries and branch stenoses in renal arteries. These catheters have shafts with diameters of 3 to 4.2 Fr and have maximum balloon diameters of 2 to 6 mm.

MECHANISM OF BALLOON ANGIOPLASTY

In their original report of percutaneous transluminal angioplasty, Dotter and Judkins also put forth a brief description of the proposed mechanism.[1] It was their belief that the atherosclerotic plaque underwent compression and elongation during serial coaxial (bougie) dilatation—a kind of "cold flow" as might occur with a putty-like substance—that resulted in the increased luminal diameter they had observed. With some minor variations, the same mechanism was held to be operative in balloon angioplasty until 1980, when Castañeda-Zúñiga and colleagues set forth the currently accepted model of balloon angioplasty.[10] These authors have summarized their human cadaver and animal research.[11–14] Their work has subsequently been supported by others, and pathologic correlation has been obtained in both humans and animals.[15–22]

Castañeda-Zúñiga and coworkers contended that atherosclerotic plaque is essentially incompressible and does not undergo remodeling during transluminal angioplasty. Instead, the radial forces exerted by the expanding balloon lead to a cracking and partial shearing of the rigid plaque from the elastic media of the arterial wall (Fig. 20–2), accounting for the subintimal tracking of contrast material often seen on angiograms immediately following dilatation.

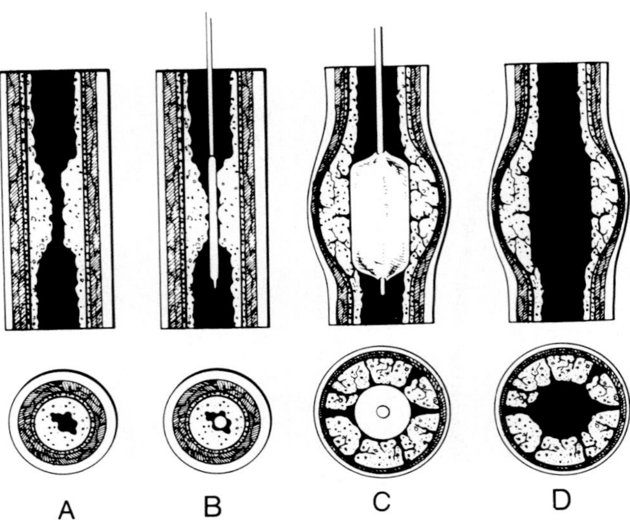

FIGURE 20–2. Proposed mechanism of angioplasty. Expansion of the balloon splits the atherosclerotic plaque and stretches the media and adventitia, partially shearing the plaque from its attachment to the media. The plaque is essentially incompressible. It does not embolize because it remains attached to the media. (From Castañeda-Zúñiga WR, Formanek A, Tradavarthy M, et al: The mechanism of balloon angioplasty. Radiology 135:565, 1980.)

Because this separation of plaque and media is only partial, clinically significant embolization of the plaque is rare, occurring in less than 1 per cent of patients during balloon angioplasty. With further dilatation, the media is irreversibly stretched, as evidenced histologically by the "corkscrew" appearance of the smooth muscle nuclei in specimens obtained following balloon angioplasty.[10] When the media has been freed from the restraints of the rigid atherosclerotic plaque, it can then adapt to local circulatory needs, possibly accounting for the further dilatation ("remodeling") that has been observed on repeat arteriography following some angioplasties (Fig. 20–3).[10, 23] A similar phenomenon has also been observed after surgical removal of atherosclerotic intima by endarterectomy.

Balloon dilatation of an artery was termed a "controlled injury" by Grüntzig. Histologic studies after dilatation and during healing have shown the following sequence of events in each layer of the anterial wall:

1. *Intima.* Immediately following dilatation, the endothelial layer of the intima is completely abraded, exposing an underlying, fractured, and partially destroyed internal elastic lamina. Within 30 minutes, platelets begin to deposit on the denuded intima. By 1 week, a neointima can be identified with endothelial cells appearing on the luminal surface. Reendothelialization is complete by 1 to 2 months, with a mature endothelium apparent at 2 months. However, reconstruction of the disrupted internal elastic lamina does not occur.

2. *Media.* The media of the vessel wall is made of elastin, collagen, and muscle fibers. During dilatation, the media is overstretched, causing widespread destruction as well as loss of elastic properties of the various components of this layer. The muscle fibers of the media are especially affected because the myocytes are extensively damaged. Stretching and fragmentation of the elastic fibers also occur. By 3 days, debris from dead and damaged myocytes is removed, leaving empty spaces and edematous ground substance in the media. At the end of the first week, rebuilding of the media is under way with invasion by myofibroblasts, which play an important part in any wound healing in the body. New myocytes form, and collagen proliferation occurs and continues for 3 to 6 months. The fibers of the media, particularly the muscle fibers, remain permanently overstretched, an essential part of the mechanism of angioplasty.[10] If the artery is overdilated further, the media is ruptured as well as the intima, leaving only the adventitia to contain the blood. In this circumstance, the media is repaired by scar formation.[10]

3. *Adventitia.* The adventitia of medium-sized arteries consists of fibroblasts, strands of elastin, and bundles of collagen. The adventitial layer remains intact after dilatation, although presumably it is stretched, the predominant changes occurring in the intima and media rather than in the adventitia. If the artery is overdilated sufficiently, the adventitia ruptures, with extravasation of blood and formation of a false aneurysm. Fortunately, rupture of an artery during dilatation is very rare.

The changes just described in the three layers of the arterial wall have been accepted as the major events that occur during balloon dilatation and subsequent healing. However, evidence also exists that plaque remodeling by elongation (particularly "soft" plaque) may contribute slightly to the final result in the dilatation of some lesions.[24] Kinney and colleagues showed that extrusion of fluid from the plaque accounted for 6 to 12 per cent of the overall lumen increase, compaction of the plaque for 1 to 1.5 per cent of the increase, and plaque and arterial wall disruption for 87 to 93 per cent of the luminal increase.[25]

Fibromuscular Dysplasia. Dilatation is also effective in fibromuscular dysplasia.[23] During PTA there is delamination of the endothelium, stretching of the wall with dehiscence of the fibrous bands and collagenous tissues, and stretching or disruption of the muscle. Healing occurs by fibrosis of the media and by neointima formation.[89]

MECHANISM OF POSTANGIOPLASTY RESTENOSIS

Clinical failures or recurrence of symptoms and signs late after balloon angioplasty (weeks to 1 year) may be due to either (1) restenosis or occlusion at the original PTA site, or (2) progression of disease proximal or distal to the original treatment site. A discussion of progressive atherosclerosis remote from the treatment site is beyond the scope of this chapter. The following discussion is limited to restenosis at the site of previous balloon PTA.

Intimal Hyperplasia

Restenosis due to intimal hyperplasia is considered by some to be the Achilles' heel of PTA. Liu and colleagues summarized much of the important research in this area in

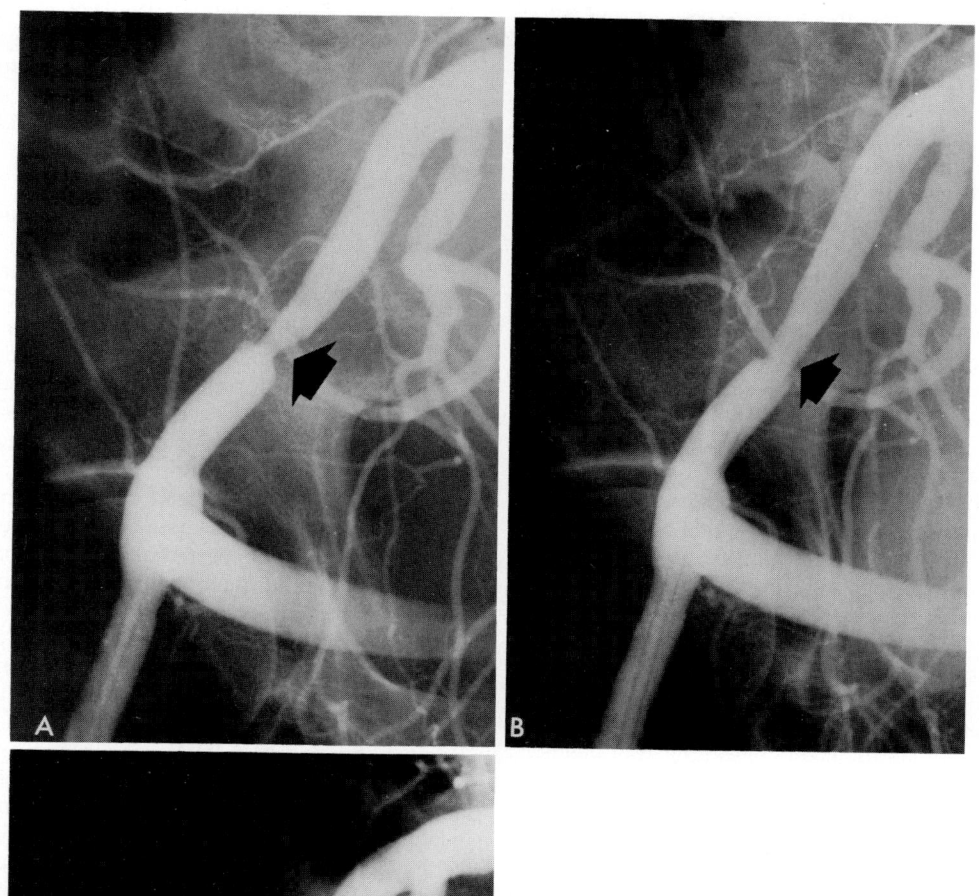

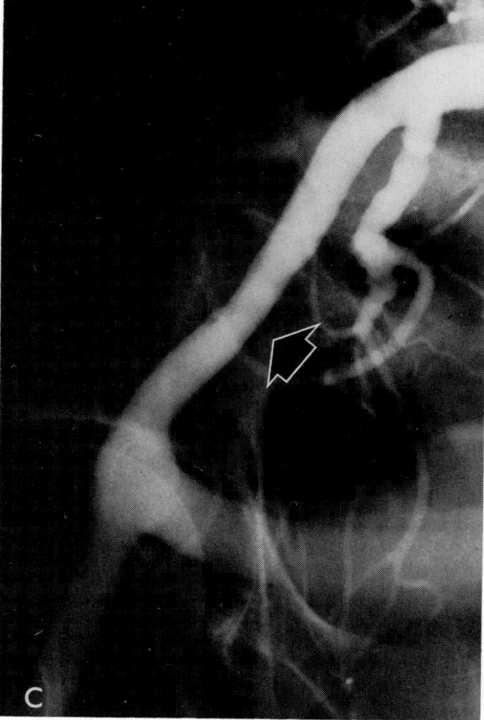

FIGURE 20–3. *A*, External iliac stenosis proximal to a femorofemoral graft in a 66-year-old man. *B*, Immediately after percutaneous transluminal angioplasty (PTA) there was only a modest increase in diameter at the stenosis site, although hemodynamics in both legs became normal. *C*, Three years later, the dilatation site is wider and smoother. This "remodeling" phenomenon is thought to be due to further stretching of the media and adventitia in response to local hemodynamic requirements after these layers have been freed from being bound to the underlying atherosclerotic plaque by the expanded balloon (see Fig. 20–1). (From Kumpe DA, Jones DN: Percutaneous transluminal angioplasty—Radiological viewpoint. Appl Radiol 11:29, 1982.)

their excellent review article.[26] Much of our present knowledge about intimal hyperplasia derives from necropsy studies of human coronary arteries, angiographic studies, studies of atherosclerotic vessels in animals, and studies of normal vessels in animals following injury. In clinical PTA, intimal hyperplasia is nearly impossible to predict, nearly impossible to prevent, and difficult to treat. It detracts significantly from the economic advantage of PTA compared with surgical bypass grafting and has become the focus of intense investigation worldwide.

Platelet-derived growth factor (PDGF) is thought to play a pivotal role in the development of intimal hyperplasia. Ferns and coworkers[27] recently reported that a polyclonal antibody to PDGF inhibited formation of intimal hyperplasia in carotid arteries of athymic nude rats; intimal hyperplasia is otherwise induced in this model by de-endothelialization of the arterial wall by a balloon catheter.

The most widely held theory of the etiology of intimal hyperplasia (fibrous cellular intimal proliferation) involves the response of damaged vessel endothelium and media. Platelet deposition on damaged endothelial cells and exposed media produces release of thromboxane A_2, further platelet deposition, and subsequent release of PDGF. However, it appears that the platelet granule contents that are subsequently found in the subjacent vessel wall[28] are derived almost exclusively from the adhering layer of platelets that are deposited initially on the area of injury, and not from the platelets that subsequently aggregate on this initial layer of platelets.[29–31] The adhering platelet layer therefore seems to be much more important in the pathogenesis of intimal hyperplasia than the layers of aggregating platelets, and thus a shadow of doubt is cast upon studies examining the association between indium-platelet scintigraphic results on the one hand and the likelihood or severity of restenosis on the other. A scintigraphic study specific for activated platelets seems to have great potential value. Recently, an agent for this purpose has been proposed and tested.[32]

As important as adhering platelets may be in the early pathogenesis of intimal hyperplasia, they are not a necessary condition for its development. Following arterial injury, intimal hyperplasia occurs even in the presence of extreme thrombocytopenia.[33]

Vessel endothelium also releases various growth factors such as endothelial and fibroblast growth factors, which lead to migration, proliferation, and alteration of vessel wall smooth muscle cells, so that they reproduce as fibrous cellular intimal proliferation.[26, 34–39] Johnson and associates showed that intimal hyperplasia occurs in lesions of restenosis but not in primary stenoses. They evaluated atherectomy specimens from 218 peripheral arteries in 100 patients.[40–41] One hundred and seventy were lesions treated by primary atherectomy, and 48 were restenosis lesions that occurred following previous balloon angioplasty (n = 15), atherectomy (n = 29), or combined angioplasty and atherectomy (n = 4). The histologic categorization of the lesions fell into two groups: atherosclerotic plaque plus thrombus, and intimal hyperplasia. Among the stenoses treated with primary atherectomy, all specimens consisted of atherosclerotic plaque, fibrous thickening, or thrombus. None had intimal proliferation. On the other hand, tissue from the excised restenosis lesions consisted of atherosclerotic plaque plus thrombus with no intimal hyperplasia in 25 per cent, and of intimal hyperplasia in 75 per cent. The atherosclerotic plaque in these lesions was not histologically different from de novo atherosclerotic plaque. The excised intimal hyperplasia specimens post angioplasty and post atherectomy were identical. Waller[42] and other investigators[43–44] also had previously found that myointimal hyperplasia identical to that associated with postcarotid-endarterectomy restenosis[45] occurs following PTA, but the percentages were not known.

Other Mechanisms of Restenosis

At least one mechanism other than intimal hyperplasia—elastic recoil—also causes restenosis. Waller and colleagues, in a study of 20 necropsy patients who had undergone coronary balloon angioplasty more than 30 days prior to death, made a histologic study of all dilated sites and reported both apparent mechanisms of restenosis.[38] Histologic findings of a response to PTA, including intimal fibrous proliferation, occurred in 60 per cent of patients, whereas chronic elastic recoil without intimal fibrous proliferation was found in 40 per cent of patients. The 40 per cent of lesions with chronic elastic recoil showed the presence of plaque, but there was absolutely no evidence that a PTA had previously occurred (i.e., there was no intimal hyperplasia, no previous plaque fracture, and no evidence of new immature plaque formation).[37–39] The lack of immature plaque formation in both these and the other 60 per cent of lesions with intimal hyperplasia provides evidence against theories that PTA can accelerate atherosclerosis. Moreover, the lack of evidence of a prior PTA in the 40 per cent group suggests that (1) mechanisms other than plaque fracture may be important in a high percentage of technically successful PTAs, and (2) elastic recoil, recovery of myocyte function, and perhaps other processes yet to be delineated are important in a high percentage of cases of restenosis detected clinically and angiographically. The finding that not all restenosis is due to intimal hyperplasia suggests that stents, thermal molding of the vessel wall, and other efforts to optimize lumen geometry may offer a promise of both improved technical success and longer term patency. These newer therapeutic modalities are discussed in a later section in this chapter.

Morphologic, Hemodynamic, and Clinical Factors Associated With Restenosis

A wealth of information gained from angiographic studies of the coronary circulation has provided valuable insights and theories about the importance of lumen geometry, hemodynamics, and restenosis. Restenosis following coronary angioplasty occurs with increased frequency in arteries with relatively low flow[46–47] or with 35 per cent or more stenosis remaining after angioplasty, at PTA sites with a residual gradient of 15 mmHg (systolic) or greater, in vessels with marked tortuosity, and in still other specific morphologic circumstances, such as extensive disease and eccentric lesions.[26] Investigators have also postulated that there is a relationship between shear stress and restenosis. Shear stress is greatest when flow velocity is high. Fluctuation in shear stress is great in post-stenotic areas with turbulent flow or reversal of flow (areas of flow separation), such as the area beyond a residual stenosis following PTA. The theory is that when lumen geometry and flow are optimal, shear stress is high and fluctuation in shear stress is low. In such circumstances there is little or no restenosis; when lumen geometry and/or flow are suboptimal, shear stress is low and fluctuation in shear stress is great. Under these circumstances, there is a high likelihood of restenosis.[48] In any case, the concept lends credence to the strategy of optimizing both lumen geometry and the hemodynamic result of PTA.

In addition to these factors, there are certain clinical risk factors that are known to predispose the patient to a higher likelihood of restenosis following (coronary) angioplasty. These include the following: diabetes mellitus (particularly if the current PTA is being done for treatment of restenosis), continued cigarette smoking, absence of a previous myocardial infarction (MI), and unstable angina.[35] A high total cholesterol : high-density lipoprotein (HDL)-cholesterol ratio has been reported to be an important predictor of restenosis,[49] but some investigators have disagreed.[50–51]

Differences in the mechanism of restenosis between coronary arteries and the larger peripheral arteries, if any, have not yet been defined.

Strategies for Prevention of Restenosis

Mechanical (technical) approaches have involved the removal or remolding of the stenotic plaque with laser heat-probe thermal angioplasty,[52] thermal balloon angioplasty with a heated balloon (simple thermal balloon angioplasty [TBA][53]; radiofrequency balloon angioplasty [RFBA][54–56]; and laser balloon angioplasty [LBA][57–58]), atherectomy, and stents. The thermal approaches have thus far failed to show any reduction in the incidence of restenosis. Atherectomy cuts deep enough to include the media (presumably associated with more smooth muscle cell injury) are associated with a greater frequency of restenosis.[40] Atherectomy and stents have some utility, as discussed below, but in specific situations rather than as general replacements for PTA.

Pharmacologic maneuvers attempted thus far have been numerous but likewise have failed to reduce the incidence of restenosis. Aspirin and other platelet inhibitors have been used nearly universally following angioplasty to decrease platelet deposition at the dilatation site in the hope of decreasing intimal proliferation and the chance of restenosis. However, antiplatelet drugs have their greatest impact in preventing the accretion of new platelet layers (platelet aggregation) after platelet adhesion to the exposed connective tissue has already occurred. As detailed above, growth factors from these additional platelet layers seem to have little if any effect on smooth muscle cells in the media. A meta-analysis of several studies employing aspirin following coronary angioplasty has failed to reveal a significant reduction in restenosis.[59] Growth factors from the adherent platelet layer probably enter the vessel wall extremely rapidly after PTA.

Other pharmacologic substances that have been and are being investigated include (1) hirudin, a leech enzyme that has antithrombin effects and, unlike heparin, is capable of abolishing the growth of an acute thrombus;[60] (2) PPACK (D-phenylalanyl-prolyl-arginine chloromethyl ketone), a synthetic hirudin-like compound;[60] (3) ciprostene, a synthetic prostacyclin analogue (prostacyclin[60] [PGI_2] is a naturally occurring prostaglandin produced by endothelial cells that is known to be a potent vasodilator, potent inhibitor of platelet aggregation, and potent disaggregator of platelet clumps); (4) calcium channel antagonists, which have antiproliferative effects on smooth muscle cells but have been clinically ineffective in preventing restenosis;[61–62] (5) low-molecular-weight heparin compounds, which have antiproliferative properties but few or no anticoagulant properties are beginning to prove efficacious in reducing restenosis in animal studies[63] and are under study in clinical trials; (6) colchicine, which causes metaphase arrest in mitosis, has proved capable of inhibiting DNA synthesis in vascular smooth muscle cells and of reducing restenosis in laboratory studies;[64–65] however, it has so far failed to reduce restenosis in clinical trials;[64–67] (7) antineoplastic drugs, which in low doses in animal studies of arterial injury have proved effective in decreasing the early smooth muscle cell proliferative response;[68] whether the results will have longer term benefit or eventual clinical application is not known; (8) corticosteroids, which in animal studies have been shown to inhibit smooth muscle cell proliferation, growth, chemotaxis, and possibly even PDGF production;[69–71] (9) combinations of corticosteroids and heparin, which in vitro have antiproliferative effects on smooth muscle cells that are additive;[72] however, thus far clinical trials have not shown a significant reduction in restenosis.[73]

Other potential pharmacologic agents include antagonists to platelet membrane glycoprotein IIb/IIIa receptor complex that could effectively prevent platelet adhesion to exposed collagen[74]; angiopeptin, a somatostatin analogue that inhibits smooth muscle cell hyperplasia in response-to-injury animal models[75]; and cilazapril, an angiotensin-converting enzyme inhibitor that also inhibits smooth muscle cell hyperplasia in animals.[76] Interest in fish oils was prompted by their antiaggregatory effects on platelets, antimitogenic qualities, and lipid effects. However, clinical trials (five studies in all) have failed to demonstrate a clear reduction in restenosis.[59] One final pharmacologic strategy is that of giving cholesterol-lowering agents to reduce total cholesterol and the total cholesterol : HDL cholesterol ratio. The angiographic results of the two best studies are at odds with one another. One claims a marked reduction in restenosis following cholesterol control on a regimen of diet and cholesterol-lowering agents following coronary angioplasty,[77] and the other shows no advantage at all.[78]

Combined technical and pharmacologic approaches are not in common use and have not been tried in any large-scale trial but have been explored in limited feasibility studies. An interventional device is used to deliver drugs or bioengineered growth factor inhibitors to the vessel wall. Examples of such devices include local infusion angioplasty balloon catheters that achieve pressures adequate for PTA, yet have microholes in the balloon surface for drug delivery,[79–81] and bioresorbable stents,[82] in which the drug is incorporated for timed release.

Molecular biologic manipulations are the newest and perhaps most exciting potential avenue of attack on intimal hyperplasia. The idea is to identify and isolate genes that are important in intimal hyperplasia (those that lead to smooth muscle cell proliferation and migration, those that lead to elaboration of matrix, and so on) and then either block them or inhibit their effects. Such blocking strategies likely involve direct transfer of oligonucleotides and/or protein products directly to the vessel wall. One such strategy, known as ''antisense,'' involves transferring to vascular smooth muscle cells an oligodeoxyribonucleotide (single-stranded DNA fragment) that is complementary to an mRNA known to be important in proliferation, migration, and matrix synthesis. In this form of therapy, the effect of the mRNA (growth factor production or other effect) is blocked (usually partially).

Nabel and colleagues have shown that direct gene transfer to the vessel wall is feasible.[83] In their early experiments, the *Escherichia coli* gene that encodes for the synthesis of beta-galactosidase was successfully transferred to the iliac arteries of swine by perfusion of the experimental iliac segments (in vivo), using a double-balloon catheter. The perfusion fluid carried the genes in the replication-defective retrovirus directly into the intima, media, and adventitia of the vessel wall. Weeks to months after perfusion, the gene was proved by means of a histochemical staining assay to be present and functioning in the vessel wall. Subsequently, the investigators also transferred the gene to porcine iliac arteries in vivo using liposomal transfection (no viruses). Another group of investigators transferred the gene that encodes for firefly luciferase to canine coronary and carotid arteries.[84] Using an assay for luminescence, they proved that the gene was present and expressing (producing luciferase) in the vessel wall. The implications are obvious. Transfer of desirable genes, mRNA, or peptides to vessel walls in humans is really possible. Delivery of such genes or products to the target site at the time of PTA is the next step in intravascular therapy. In vitro and animal studies continue.[85–87] As Nabel and colleagues point out, the implications for the future of gene therapy are even farther reaching and include the possibilities of preventing atherosclerosis and treating nonatherosclerotic conditions. For instance, isolation of the gene encoding for clotting factor VIII would render a cure for hemophilia possible using similar transfer methods. More than 20 investigational protocols utilizing gene transfer for various conditions are now under way.

Finally, in an editorial review, Schwartz and colleagues have proposed a different mechanism to explain the development of intimal hyperplasia. They posit that almost all therapies aimed at preventing clinical restenosis have failed because the fundamental processes involved have not been recognized.[88] Based upon extensive clinical observations, all of the available histopathologic studies, and the results of response-to-injury experiments in a porcine model of intimal hyperplasia, they proposed an alternative theory that includes three stages: In stage I, thrombus occurs at the injury site. In stage II, the thrombus is covered by endothelium. A mononuclear leukocytic infiltrate then begins to develop on the luminal side of the vessel. Monocytes migrate into the subendothelial space, secrete fibrinolytic substances that begin to cause resorption of thrombus, and secrete additional substances that are responsible for more cellular recruitment. Finally, in the proliferative stage (stage III), a cap of actin-positive cells accumulates on the luminal surface. The cap thickens as additional cells are recruited and additional matrix is deposited. The remainder of the thrombus is resorbed. The cells do *not* arise from the vascular media. In their theory, ''intimal hyperplasia'' grows toward the site of injury (i.e., outward from the luminal surface). The authors assigned major importance to thrombus, which is viewed as providing the matrix for smooth muscle cell proliferation. This new theory will probably explain some but not all of the features of and phenomena associated with postangioplasty restenosis in humans.

TECHNIQUE OF ANGIOPLASTY

The technique of percutaneous transluminal angioplasty has been described in detail and is now familiar to most physicians treating vascular disease. It should be performed in a well-equipped angiographic suite that has facilities for monitoring intra-arterial pressures. Additional physiologic monitoring should include electrocardiography and pulse oximetry. The angiography suite should be equipped with a defibrillator and other resuscitative equipment and medications. It should be staffed by individuals who are experienced or knowledgeable in resuscitation. A wide variety of diagnostic catheters with different shapes and shaft thicknesses (profiles) as well as guidewires, balloon catheters, vascular stents, and infusion catheters for fibrinolysis should all be available to deal with the problems that will be encountered during the performance of an angioplasty.

For iliac lesions, a straight angiographic catheter or a catheter with a hockey-stick tip configuration is inserted via an ipsilateral or contralateral puncture. For femoropopliteal lesions, ipsilateral antegrade (''downhill'') insertion of the catheter is preferable. An axillary approach for renal, abdominal aortic, iliac, and even femoropopliteal lesions can be used if the patient's anatomy or habitus dictates, though extreme care should be used in following the patient afterward to avoid brachial plexus palsy from an axillary hematoma, and this condition must be surgically corrected immediately by axillary decompression if it does develop (see Chapter 7).

After the tip of the catheter has been positioned near the stenosis or occlusion, an appropriate guidewire is passed across the lesion. In patients with complete occlusions or eccentric stenoses in tortuous arteries, this maneuver requires considerable angiographic skill and judgment. Digital fluoroscopy with roadmapping and a variety of steerable wires coated with hydrophilic polymers are recent developments that are of great value in crossing a complex lesion. Once the guidewire tip has crossed the lesion, the catheter is advanced over the wire so that the collapsed balloon straddles the lesion. The balloon is expanded with a mixture of equal amounts of saline and contrast agent for

60 seconds at an appropriate pressure. This pressure, in the range of 4 to 17 atmospheres, is judged by observing balloon deformation and can be measured by an external manometer attached to the catheter hub. For renal artery and supra-aortic lesions, shorter expansion times are sometimes used. Intra-arterial pressures are measured across the lesion before and after dilatation. Arteriography is performed following dilatation to document the final result and to reveal local thrombus formation or distal emboli. Clot formation and distal embolization are rare. If either occurs it can usually be treated successfully with transcatheter infusion of a fibrinolytic agent.[90–91] (See later section, Complications of Angioplasty and Their Management.)

If possible, balloon length should correspond to the length of the lesion so that only one balloon expansion is necessary, although lesions longer than the balloon can be treated by multiple stepwise balloon expansions. Catheters with long balloons (8 to 10 cm in length) are now available for treating longer lesions with a single balloon expansion. For stenoses in the abdominal aorta, two or three balloons positioned at the same level may still occasionally be necessary, although the larger angioplasty balloons (up to 30 mm in diameter) can usually be employed.[92–93]

Maximal balloon diameter can be equal to but should not exceed the angiographic luminal diameter adjacent to the lesion, as measured on an angiographic film. This measurement has an intrinsic 20 to 30 per cent magnification factor; therefore, balloon diameter as determined by measurement from the film will slightly exceed the actual arterial luminal diameter. With current digital subtraction angiographic techniques, the exact arterial luminal diameter may be available if a reference object of known size (e.g., the angiographic catheter) is included in the field of view. This exact diameter, lacking intrinsic magnification, is smaller than the apparent luminal diameter as measured on an angiographic film, and a balloon diameter about 20 per cent larger can be chosen for concentric lesions. Eccentric stenoses should be dilated with balloons smaller than the measurement of the adjacent arterial luminal diameter because only a portion of the arterial wall is available to be stretched by the expanding balloon. Many investigators, including the authors,[94] believe that one should not dilate adjacent uninvolved segments of artery beyond the atheroma because the splitting of the intima spreading into this region may lead to recurrent stenosis away from the site of the original lesion.

The configuration of the proximal end of the occlusion is also important. If the proximal collateral vessel arises at a relatively acute angle, giving a "pocket" configuration at the proximal end of the occlusion, the appropriate pathway for initial passage of the guidewire into the occlusion is entered relatively easily (Fig. 20–4). If, on the other hand, the collateral vessel at the proximal end of the occlusion arises in a nearly straight line with the axis of the parent artery, the guidewire tends to pass into the collateral vessel rather than into the proximal end of the occlusion. Creation of a passageway through the occlusion is still possible but is much more difficult. In crossing occlusions, care must be taken not to disturb the collaterals at the proximal and distal ends of the occlusion. Preservation of these collaterals ensures that no extension of the occlusion will occur even if there is a technical failure of recanalization.

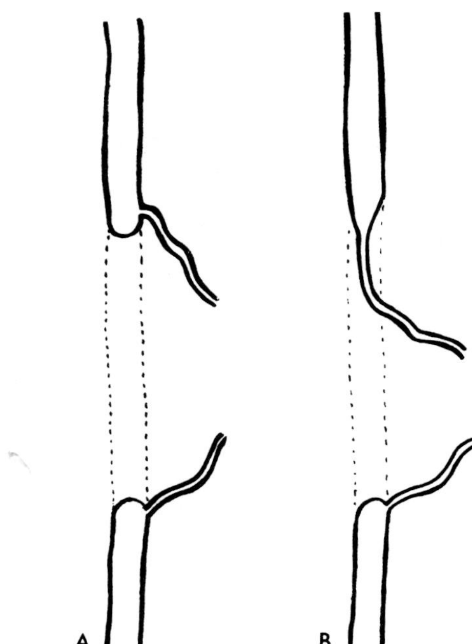

FIGURE 20–4. *A*, "Pocket" configuration at the proximal pole of an arterial occlusion is due to the acute angle of takeoff of the collateral artery. Such configurations are amenable to PTA because the pathway for passage of the guidewire through the obstructed lumen is obvious. *B*, Unfavorable configuration of the proximal collateral vessel arises in the same axis as the main arterial lumen. The guidewire passes easily into the collateral. It is more difficult to pass the wire through the obstructed lumen.

It is often difficult to judge the age of an occluding thrombus angiographically. Accordingly, in the last several years the author's technique has been modified with occlusions. If the occlusion is "hard"—difficult to pass a guidewire through—it is treated with angioplasty primarily. If, on the other hand, the guidewire passes through the occlusion with little or no resistance, suggesting that the occluding thrombus is acute or subacute, the patient is treated with intra-arterial transcatheter urokinase to lyse the clot before dilating the underlying stenosis.

FOLLOW-UP EVALUATIONS

Clinically, the highest frequency of recurrent stenosis or new stenosis in the treated segment occurs during the "healing phase" in the first 12 months following angioplasty. Therefore, any angioplasty patient, but particularly one who has a graft distal to the dilated segment, should be followed closely by noninvasive vascular laboratory surveillance at least every 3 months during the first year after dilatation and every 6 months thereafter. A deterioration of the ankle-brachial index of more than 0.15 is an indication for repeat arteriography. When this protocol is followed, recurrent stenoses are detected relatively early and can be easily treated by repeat dilatations. Another cause of recurrent symptoms and deterioration in the results of noninvasive studies is progression of atheromatosis, particularly if it is distal to the site of the original PTA.

COMPLICATIONS OF ANGIOPLASTY AND THEIR MANAGEMENT

The complication rate for angioplasty is significantly higher than that for diagnostic arteriography, but most angioplasty complications are of minor consequence, do not require surgical intervention, and can be minimized by experience and judgment. Total complications usually range from 4 to 22 per cent, and the complication rate will, of course, vary with who determines what constitutes a complication.[95] Complications of angioplasty requiring surgery rarely exceed 5 per cent. The incidence of complications appears to be higher in patients in whom angioplasty is unsuccessful[96] and in cases in which the angiographer is inexperienced.[97] In our own initial series, as many complications occurred in the first 15 procedures as in the subsequent 95 dilatations. Zeitler and coworkers[98] showed a progressive decline in the complication rate over three time periods, from 14 to 4 per cent; for complications requiring surgical intervention, the rate decreased from 2.3 to 0.45 per cent.

Mortality

Deaths following percutaneous transluminal angioplasty are extremely rare, with most series having mortalities of less than 0.5 per cent.[99] Mortalities occur almost universally in patients with severe widespread atheromatosis who are not surgical candidates because of poor outflow and complicating medical conditions such as myocardial infarction or ventricular arrhythmias.

Puncture Site Complications

The majority of complications at the catheter introduction site are due to hematomas, but large hematomas requiring transfusion or surgical evacuation are rare, occurring in 2 to 8 per cent of cases.[99] Other significant puncture site complications requiring surgery occur in less than 1 per cent of cases and include false aneurysms, thromboses, and arteriovenous fistulae.

Dilatation Site Complications

The most common serious complication at the dilatation site is acute occlusion, which occurs in 1 to 7 per cent of cases.[99] Occlusion is usually attributed to thrombosis but may also be due to raising of intimal flaps or to local spasm. Development of an acute occlusion seems to be unrelated to the severity or location of the lesion. The use of heparin during the dilatation of large arteries with rapid flow may not be necessary, but systemic anticoagulation during angioplasty is important with smaller arteries and in low-flow situations.[100] Vasodilators (nifedipine 10 mg orally or sublingually and nitroglycerin 100 to 600 μg intra-arterially) may help to avoid acute occlusions and are employed especially during tibial artery PTA. When acute thrombosis occurs during angioplasty, it can usually be treated by means of an intra-arterial fibrinolytic infusion given through the catheter followed by repeat dilatation, or by percutaneous aspiration of the embolus through a catheter,[101–103] or by percutaneous Fogarty embolectomy[104–106] rather than by surgery.

Subintimal dissection and/or perforation at the lesion site with a guidewire or catheter occurs in 1 to 5 per cent of cases and is one principal cause of technical failure to perform angioplasty. In most instances, the event is of no clinical consequence if care is taken to recognize the dissection early, before the severity of stenosis or occlusion is made worse. One can repeat the PTA at a later time (one to several weeks). Guidewire dissection is often an avoidable complication that is related to operator inexperience.[99]

More recently, roadmapping and steerable guidewires have rendered this type of dissection during PTA even less consequential. Often the procedure can be completed despite subintimal passage of the guidewire. For flow-limiting dissections that occur during PTA (usually as a consequence of dilatation rather than of subintimal passage of the guidewire), directional atherectomy and stents have proved to be valuable adjuncts. These will be discussed in more detail below.

Complications of balloon inflation include arterial dissection and rupture. Nonobstructive intimal flaps occur commonly after PTA and are a result of the previously described mechanism of PTA, in which there is tearing and partial detachment of the atherosclerotic intima from the media. Acute subtotal and total occlusions after angioplasty may be due to a partially or completely obstructing intimal flap. Dissections do not automatically lead to technical failure. High-grade partially obstructing flaps that compromise flow can be managed by redilatation as soon as they are recognized, in the hope of compressing the offending flap against the vessel wall. The hemodynamic effect of such flaps sometimes resolves spontaneously within several hours to a day. Another maneuver is to remove the persistent flap by performing directional atherectomy (Fig. 20–5).[107–108] In iliac segments, placement of one or multiple stents into the dissected segment now appears to be the treatment of choice (Fig. 20–6).[109–111] Stent insertion for postangioplasty flow-limiting dissections of the femoropopliteal segment will reestablish flow but has a less favorable long-term patency rate because of a high incidence of intimal hyperplasia at the stented site.[112–117] Surgery is performed only if the patient is acutely worse after the above maneuvers fail.

Arterial rupture during balloon dilatation is quite rare when appropriately sized balloons are used, but it may be a greater danger among patients receiving corticosteroids on a chronic basis for an underlying illness.[118]

Other Complications

Distal embolization of clinical significance is quite rare, occurring in less than 1 per cent of cases. Some investigators have reported that distal embolization is more common in patients being treated for long chronic iliac occlusions.[119] More recent experience, however, suggests that

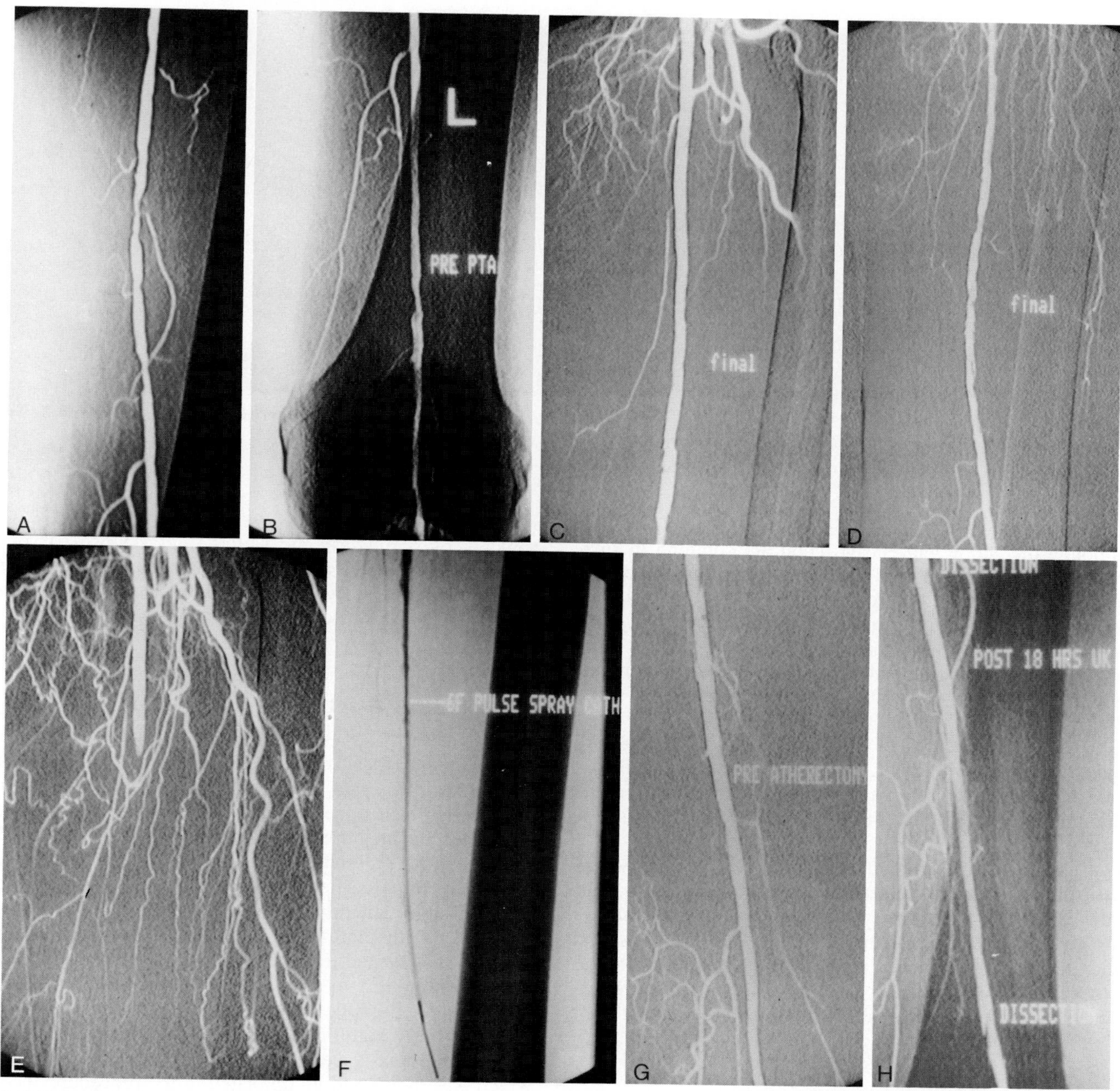

FIGURE 20–5. Use of atherectomy to remove PTA-related intimal flap. *A* and *B*, Pretreatment selective superficial femoral artery (SFA) angiogram in a woman with severe claudication shows stenoses in the SFA and popliteal artery. *C* and *D*, Angiogram following PTA. *E*, Angiogram 24 hours after the patient's leg and foot turned cold, her pulses disappeared, and her pulse volume recordings were shown to be flat. The SFA is thrombosed. *F*, Thrombolytic therapy is initiated. *G* and *H*, Following thrombolysis, dissections in the SFA and popliteal artery are revealed.

Illustration continued on following page

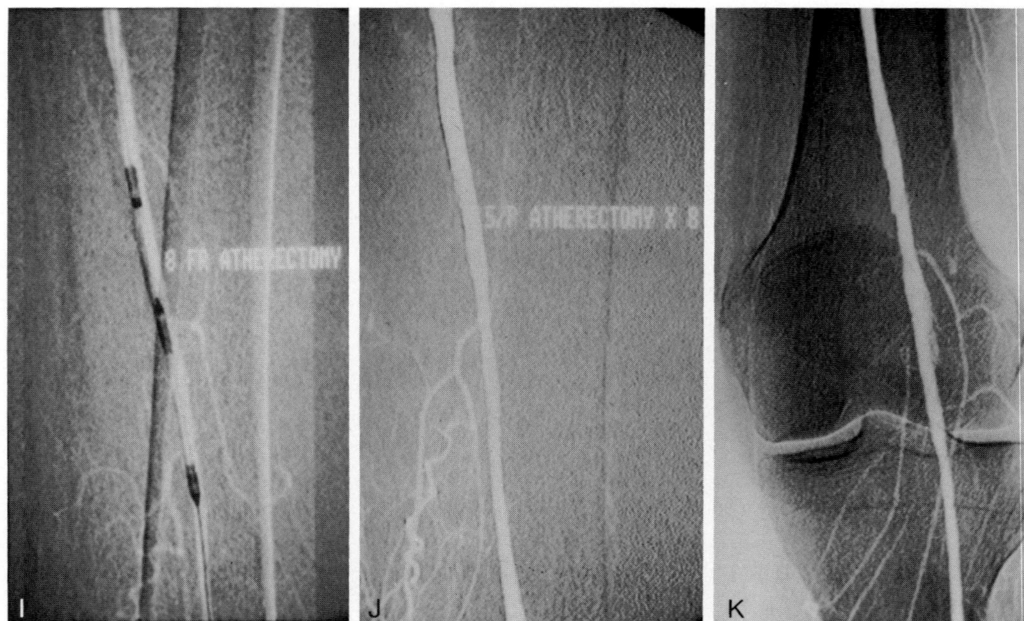

FIGURE 20–5 Continued *I*, An 8 F, atherectomy catheter is used to retrieve the atherosclerotic material causing the flap. *J* and *K*, The SFA and popliteal artery are patent again after atherectomy.

although dissection and elastic recoil are common in such cases, embolization is unusual. Such long chronic occlusions can be treated percutaneously either by primary stenting[112, 120–123] or by fibrinolysis followed by PTA, with or without a stent. It is not established which is the most appropriate percutaneous therapy and whether a percutaneous approach for long chronic iliac occlusions is a satisfactory alternative to standard surgical procedures.

Microembolization of no clinical significance occurs more frequently in femoropopliteal dilatations; such microemboli were seen in 8 per cent of our first 50 femoropopliteal dilatations, though none had any clinical manifestation.

The incidence of contrast-induced renal failure varies depending on patient selection, criteria for diagnosis, and how carefully it is sought. It occurs more frequently following renal angioplasty, usually in 3 to 6 per cent of cases,[124] and does not represent a problem in angioplasty in the extremities, provided that the usual preangiographic precautions are observed, particularly adequate hydration.

OTHER APPLICATIONS OF TRANSLUMINAL ANGIOPLASTY

The role of angioplasty in lower extremity ischemia as well as renal artery stenosis is discussed elsewhere in this text. However, application of percutaneous angioplasty to other arteries is also increasing, including treatment of stenotic lesions of the abdominal aorta, the mesenteric and celiac arteries, and the brachiocephalic arteries. In addition, balloon angioplasty has been employed in treating venous and arterial stenoses associated with dialysis shunts, narrowings of portal-systemic shunts, and stenoses of both synthetic and venous arterial bypass grafts and their anastomoses. The efficacy of angioplasty in coronary artery stenoses is not discussed in this chapter.

Abdominal Aorta

Although focal stenosis of the infrarenal abdominal aorta is relatively rare, five different reports of dilatation of such lesions have appeared in the literature in which angioplasty results in more than 10 patients (range, 12 to 32 patients) were presented.[125–129] Of a total of 96 patients in these five reports, technical and clinical success was achieved in all patients. Follow-up ranged from a mean of 16 to 38 months with a range of 7 to 70 months. Primary patency rates ranged from 100 per cent with a mean follow-up of 16 months[128] to a cumulative patency of 70 per cent at 5 years.[125] Complications were few. Among the 96 patients the only significant complication was one death in the postangioplasty period due to a myocardial infarction, which was thought to be unrelated to the procedure. There is a single report of delayed aortic rupture occurring some 8 hours after successful balloon dilatation of a stenosis of the distal abdominal aorta, which was then successfully repaired by venous patch graft.[130] The authors believe that balloon angioplasty is the treatment of choice for discrete, concentric stenoses of the abdominal aorta that are not heavily calcified. Eccentric or heavily calcified focal stenoses and more diffuse stenoses of the abdominal aorta are still best managed surgically, although intravascular stenting has emerged as a treatment alternative for distal aortic and bifurcation disease in selected patients.

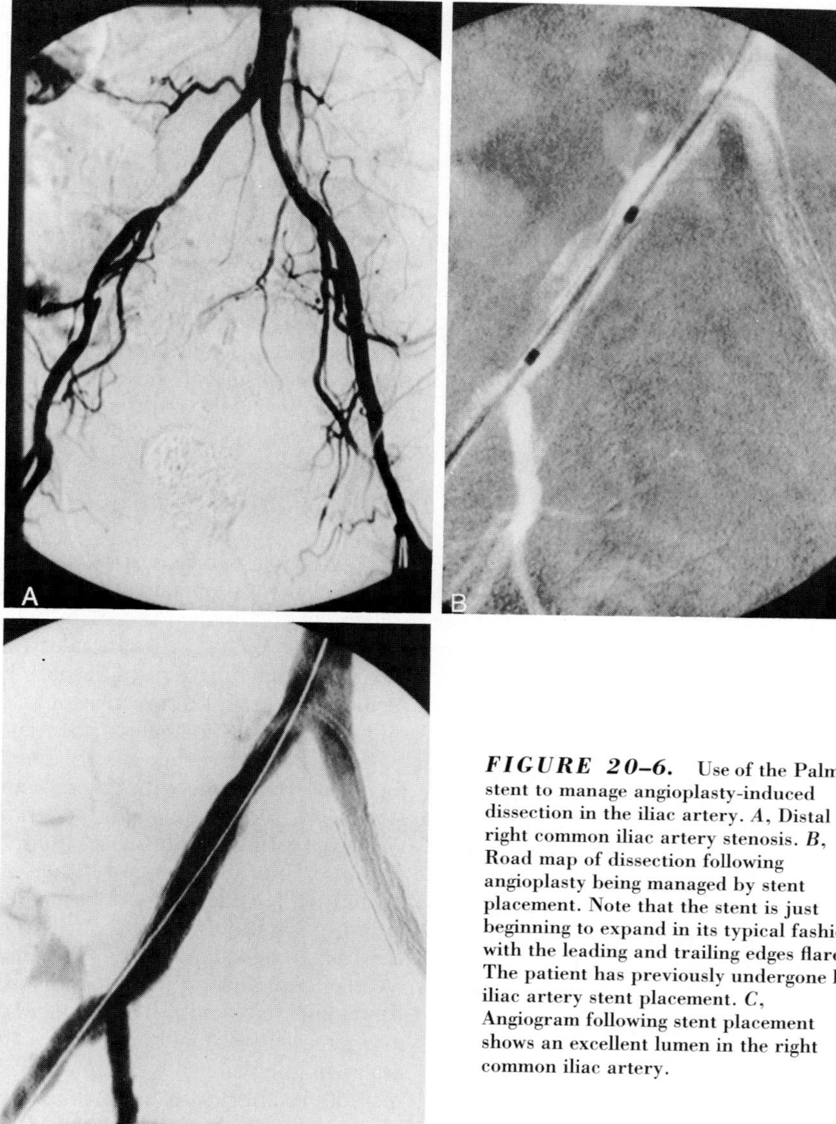

FIGURE 20–6. Use of the Palmaz stent to manage angioplasty-induced dissection in the iliac artery. *A*, Distal right common iliac artery stenosis. *B*, Road map of dissection following angioplasty being managed by stent placement. Note that the stent is just beginning to expand in its typical fashion, with the leading and trailing edges flared. The patient has previously undergone left iliac artery stent placement. *C*, Angiogram following stent placement shows an excellent lumen in the right common iliac artery.

Brachiocephalic Arteries

Subclavian Artery

The widest experience with dilatation of the brachiocephalic arteries has accrued in patients who have proximal subclavian stenoses with either subclavian steal syndrome or arm claudication.[131–155] The initial success rates are reported to be 88 to 100 per cent, with the majority of patients experiencing no recurrence of symptoms during follow-up periods ranging from 4 months to 5 years. In one nonrandomized, retrospective comparison of the follow-up of subclavian PTA versus carotid-subclavian surgical reconstruction, the patency of the surgical reconstruction was found to be superior.[156] Complications have been few, ranging from 0 to 8.6 per cent. There were three neurologic complications and one death among 402 patients with 423 dilated subclavian and innominate arteries summarized by Becker and associates.[157] Two strokes in the carotid artery distribution occurred on the *contralateral* side, one an extension of a contralateral stroke and the second occurring during a follow-up arch aortogram. Significantly, there are *no* reported cases of embolism in the vertebral artery distribution on the side dilated. The lack of vertebral artery emboli is explained at least in part by observations by two groups of investigators using Doppler ultrasound that retrograde flow in the vertebral artery in a patient with subclavian steal syndrome does not instantaneously revert to normal antegrade flow after dilatation but does so gradually over a period of 20 seconds to 20 minutes (and occasionally longer).[149, 151] The continued retrograde flow in the vertebral artery after subclavian PTA protects the vertebral circulation from emboli. The intrinsically low incidence of embolism during balloon angioplasty is, no doubt, also a factor.

Vertebral Artery

Patients who are candidates for surgical treatment of vertebral and innominate artery lesions have undergone successful dilatation without experiencing significant cerebral embolism.[134–138, 140–142, 148, 151, 153–155, 158–161] Included in these reports are at least 66 patients undergoing attempted PTA for ostial stenosis of the vertebral artery in the presence of vertebrobasilar insufficiency.[157] The initial technical success rate was high (greater than 95 per cent). For example, in Courtheoux' series,[158] 24 of 26 attempted PTAs in 24 patients were technically successful (92 per cent), with resolution of the symptoms in 21 patients (88 per cent); one patient experienced temporary blindness, and one had vertebral artery occlusion after PTA with resolution of the symptoms of vertebrobasilar insufficiency. Overall, for the reported experience, data on complications and follow-up are insufficient to determine the proper role of vertebral artery angioplasty in the treatment of symptoms of vertebrobasilar insufficiency.

Carotid Artery

Because of the fear of stroke, balloon angioplasty of atherosclerotic stenoses at the carotid bifurcation has been applied very cautiously. Nonetheless, enough experience has accumulated to suggest that carotid PTA is safe and needs further investigation.[137, 140, 144, 153, 155, 159, 162–169] For example, Kachel and associates[137] reported the performance of PTA in 112 stenotic or occluded supra-aortic arteries in 105 patients, including 35 stenoses of the internal carotid and two stenoses of common carotid arteries. One hundred and four patients were symptomatic. All patients were symptom-free after angioplasty. There were four minor complications (two hematomas, one transient ischemic attack, and one small thrombus of the internal carotid artery detected by indium-111 platelet scintigraphy and treated with thromboendarterectomy before the appearance of any neurologic symptoms). In a follow-up period ranging from 3 to 109 months (average, 58 months) there were two patients with restenosis after 44 subclavian angioplasties. These authors also summarized the results of PTA of the supra-aortic arteries in more than 700 patients in personal and published studies and suggested that the complication rate for angioplasty of the supra-aortic arteries is unlikely to be higher than that of operative treatment.

Venous and Synthetic Grafts for Arterial Bypass

Balloon angioplasty has been successfully applied to late stenoses associated with surgical bypass grafts, either venous or synthetic. Stenoses associated with synthetic grafts occur predominantly at the graft to native artery anastomosis and can occur as a result of scarring, intimal hyperplasia, or progression of atherosclerotic disease in the vessel at the anastomosis.[170–171] The stenoses usually occur at the distal anastomosis. Surgical repair of these lesions can be difficult owing to scarring, and balloon angioplasty offers an alternative method of treatment; however, balloon angioplasty of graft lesions may produce inferior results to dilatation of atherosclerotic occlusive lesions.

Stenosis of arterial bypass grafts that have been constructed from in situ or reversed saphenous veins may be caused by intimal thickening, fibrosis of a valve, fibrosis due to surgical trauma, a suture stenosis, or an atherosclerotic-like lesion within the vein graft.[172] The mechanism of angioplasty in these venous graft lesions is probably an overstretching of the wall of the vein graft[172] rather than the cracking and partial dehiscence that occurs in dilatation of atherosclerotic lesions. Because of this, recurrent stenosis is more common in balloon dilatation of graft (synthetic and vein) narrowings compared with arterial atherosclerotic stenoses, and repeat dilatations are often necessary.

Mesenteric Arteries

Although numbers are small and follow-up is short, there are reports of patients with symptomatic mesenteric ischemia being treated successfully by percutaneous angioplasty.[173–184] Balloon dilatation of the superior mesenteric artery is theoretically risky because bowel infarction could result from arterial thrombosis at or embolization from the dilatation site. Nonetheless, the reported experience suggests that the procedure is safe. The largest reported series included 10 patients with chronic mesenteric ischemia and stenosis of the celiac and/or superior mesenteric artery.[185] PTA was technically unsuccessful in two patients. In eight patients, 17 of 19 arteries (90 per cent) were successfully dilated with relief of symptoms lasting from 6 to 24 months. Symptoms recurred in five patients but were successfully relieved in three by redilatation. Three patients were asymptomatic 7 to 9 months after PTA, one of them following redilatation. The only complication was an asymptomatic intimal dissection of the superior mesenteric artery in one patient. A complete occlusion of the superior mesenteric artery was recanalized by percutaneous angioplasty.[178] In the series of Rapp and colleagues,[186] thromboendarterectomy and bypass grafting yielded a very high clinical success rate. However, as in other series reporting the results of surgery for abdominal angina, coronary comorbidity proved to be the most important cause of perioperative and late mortality. Because coronary comorbidity is prevalent in patients with abdominal angina, PTA should be considered an acceptable treatment alternative in select cases.

Narrowing caused by compression of the celiac axis by the crus of the diaphragm seems to be less likely to respond to angioplasty than an atherosclerotic lesion of the same vessel. Although the treatment of choice of chronic intestinal ischemia continues to be surgical reconstruction, balloon angioplasty should be considered in the poor-risk patient who has a proximal mesenteric artery stenosis that is favorable for dilatation.

Dialysis Fistulae and Shunts

Although the traditional method of surgical revision of a failing or thrombosed hemodialysis access site is reasonably effective in prolonging the life of the access site, the problems of loss of usable vein by the revision, the need for interim placement of a subclavian catheter until the revision is healed, the recognition that repeated surgical revisions will be necessary to maintain patency in most patients, and the expense of surgical revision has led to the exploration of alternative means of maintaining vascular access. Percutaneous balloon angioplasty of arterial anastomotic and venous outflow stenoses can be performed in 20 to 30 minutes on an outpatient basis after dialysis, using the indwelling dialysis needles. Schwab and colleagues used prophylactic angioplasty to correct stenotic lesions in patients who had rising venous pressures indicating that their polytetrafluoroethylene (PTFE) access grafts were failing.[187] The incidence of fistula thrombosis/patient-year decreased threefold compared with that in patients from the same institution before these measures were instituted. Replacement of fistulae decreased 3.5-fold during the same period. Patients with elevated venous pressures who underwent elective fistulography and outpatient percutaneous angioplasty of the venous stenoses had the same rate of fistula thrombosis as patients who had normal venous pressures (0.13 thromboses/patient-year and 0.15 thromboses/patient-year, respectively), whereas patients with elevated pressures who had no treatment had an incidence of 1.4 thromboses/patient-year—a 10-fold difference ($p < .001$).

Three different groups of investigators compared the results of surgical revision with angioplasty and drew different conclusions. In a series of patients who had failing or failed hemodialysis access sites, both PTFE and autogenous arteriovenous fistulae (AVF), Dapunt and coworkers[188] performed a retrospective analysis of the cumulative patencies of those sites treated with angioplasty compared with those treated with surgical revision. For angioplasty and surgical revision, respectively, the cumulative patency rates were 94.5 and 78.1 per cent after 1 week, 72.3 and 64.1 per cent at 1 month, 41.2 and 28.9 per cent at 5 months, and 31.3 and 19.3 per cent at 1 year ($p < .001$). The differences were due mainly to the early reocclusions that occurred after operation. The authors concluded that transluminal angioplasty achieved at least as good results as surgical revision. Cada and coworkers[189] performed 47 angioplasties in 40 patients with a variety of failing fistula sites, principally native AVF, and reported a 91.5 per cent initial success rate and a mean patency after angioplasty of 10.5 months. In comparison, patients treated with surgical revision had a slightly shorter functional patency (9.93 months) and a higher need for repeat surgical intervention (56 per cent of patients) after surgical revision than after angioplasty. The percentage of fistulae with long-term functional patency after angioplasty was almost twice that following surgical revision. They also favored balloon angioplasty as the method of choice for correcting failing fistulae. In contrast, Brooks and colleagues, in a prospective study on PTFE and bovine graft stenoses treated with inpatient angioplasty or surgical revision, found significantly longer patencies with surgical revision.[190]

Failing Brescia-Cimino fistulae have been treated with transluminal angioplasty to correct stenoses and occlusions. Balloon dilatation of poorly functioning fistulae appears to be beneficial when the malfunctioning fistula is mature and when poorly functioning AVF (with primary flow rates of less than 150 ml/min) are excluded. Success in the hands of Gmelin and associates,[191] defined as patency of the shunt for at least 1 month, was achieved in 70 per cent of cases overall and was higher with stenoses (89 per cent) than with occlusions (46 per cent). Although follow-up patency rates among the two groups were similar, they also favored the stenosis group. Patency rates at 6 months, 1 year, and 2 years were 93 per cent, 91 per cent, and 57 per cent for stenoses, and 80 per cent, 50 per cent, and 14 per cent for occlusions. Among patients whose initial treatment was successful, 52 per cent required only one angioplasty, whereas 48 per cent required two to five repeat dilatations during follow-up. Surgical repair of equivalent lesions is difficult at best.

There is a low incidence of complications of angioplasty for treatment of arterial and venous stenoses associated with AVF and PTFE grafts. In almost all series the reported complication rate is less than 8 per cent and is usually 0 to 2 per cent.[189, 191–196]

Angioplasty can be repeated many times in patients with venous and arterial stenoses. Because such stenoses have a high likelihood of recurrence with either surgical revision or balloon dilatation, the authors and others[187–189, 195] have concluded that outpatient angioplasty is the preferred treatment to preserve the failing dialysis access.

References

1. Dotter CT, Judkins MP: Transluminal treatment of arteriosclerotic obstruction. Description of a new technique and a preliminary report of its application. Circulation 30:654, 1964.
2. Porstmann W, Wierny L: Intravasale Rekanalisation inoperabler arterieller Obliterationen. Zentralbl Chir 92:1586, 1967.
3. van Andel CJ: Percutaneous Transluminal Angioplasty: The Dotter Procedure. Amsterdam, Excerpta Medica, 1976.
4. Zeitler E: Die percutane Rekanalisation arterieller Obliterationen mit Katheter nach Dotter (Dotter-Technik). Dtsch Med Wochenschr 97:1392, 1972.
5. Staple TW: Modified catheter for percutaneous transluminal treatment of arteriosclerotic obstruction. Radiology 91:1041, 1968.
6. Dotter CT: Transluminal angioplasty: A long view. Radiology 135:561, 1980.
7. Porstmann W: Ein neuer Korsett-Ballonkatheter zur transluminalen Rekanalisation nach Dotter unter besondere Berücksichtigung von Obliterationen an den Beckenarterien. Radiol Diagn (Berl) 14:239, 1973.
8. Grüntzig A, Hopff H: Perkutane Rekanalisation chronischer arterieller Verschlusse mit einem neuen Dilatations-Katheter. Dtsch Med Wochenschr 99:2502, 1974.
9. Abele J: Balloon catheter technology. *In* Castañeda-Zúñiga WR, Tadavarthy SM (eds): Interventional Radiology. 2nd ed. Baltimore, Williams & Wilkins, 1992, vol. 1, pp 345–350.
10. Castañeda-Zúñiga WR, Formanek A, Tradavarthy M, et al: The mechanism of balloon angioplasty. Radiology 135:565, 1980.
11. Zollikofer C, Cragg A, Hunter D, et al: Mechanism of transluminal angioplasty. *In* Castañeda-Zúñiga WR, Tadavarthy SM (eds): Interventional Radiology. 2nd ed. Baltimore, Williams & Wilkins, 1992, vol. 1, pp 249–297.
12. Castañeda-Zúñiga WR, Formanek A, Tradavarthy M, et al: The mechanism of balloon angioplasty. Radiology 135:565, 1980.
13. Laerum F, Vlodaver Z, Castañeda-Zúñiga WR, et al: The mechanism of angioplasty: Dilatation of iliac cadaver arteries with intravascular pressure control. ROFO 136:573, 1982.
14. Zollikofer CL, Chain J, Salomonowitz E, et al: Percutaneous transluminal angioplasty of the aorta. Radiology 151:355, 1984.
15. Faxon DP, Sanborn TA, Haudenschild CC, Ryan TJ: Effect of antiplatelet therapy on restenosis after experimental angioplasty. Am J Cardiol 53:72C, 1984.
16. Faxon DP, Sanborn TA, Weber JV, et al: Restenosis following trans-

luminal angioplasty in experimental atherosclerosis. Arteriosclerosis 4:189, 1984.
17. Sanborn TA, Faxon DP, Haudenschild C, et al: The mechanism of intraluminal angioplasty: Evidence for formation of aneurysms in experimental atherosclerosis. Circulation 68:1136, 1983.
18. Faxon DP, Weber VJ, Haudenschild C, et al: Acute effects of transluminal angioplasty in three experimental models of atherosclerosis. Arteriosclerosis 2:125, 1982.
19. Block PC, Myler RK, Stertzer S, Fallon JT: Morphology after transluminal angioplasty in human beings. N Engl J Med 305:382, 1981.
20. Hoffman MA, Fallon JT, Greenfield AJ, et al: Arterial pathology after percutaneous transluminal angioplasty. AJR 137:147, 1981.
21. Clouse ME, Tomashefski JF Jr, Reinhold RE, et al: Mechanical effect of balloon angioplasty: Case report with histology. AJR 137:869, 1981.
22. Saffitz JE, Totty WG, McClennan BL, et al: Percutaneous transluminal angioplasty: Radiological-pathological correlation. Radiology 141:651, 1981.
23. Castañeda-Zúñiga WR: Transluminal Angioplasty. New York, Thieme-Stratton, 1983.
24. Wolf GL, LeVeen RF, Ring, EJ: Potential mechanisms of angioplasty. Cardiovasc Intervent Radiol 7:11, 1984.
25. Kinney TB, Chin AK, Rurik GW, et al: Transluminal angioplasty: A mechanical-pathological correlation with its physical mechanisms. Radiology 153:85, 1984.
26. Liu MW, Roubin GS, King SB: Restenosis after coronary angioplasty. Potential biologic determinants and role of intima hyperplasia. Point of view. Circulation 79:1374, 1989.
27. Ferns GA, Raines EW, Sprugel KH, et al. Inhibition of neointimal smooth muscle accumulation after angioplasty by an antibody to PDGF. Science 253(5024):1129, 1991.
28. Goldberg ID, Stemerman MB: Vascular permeation of platelet factor 4 after endothelial injury. Science 209:611, 1980.
29. Serruys PW, Luijten HE, Beutt KJ, et al: Incidence of restenosis after successful coronary angioplasty: A time-related phenomenon. A quantitative angiographic follow-up study in 342 patients at 1, 2, 3, and 4 months. Circulation 77:361, 1988.
30. Baumgartner HR, Muggli R: Adhesion and aggregation: Morphological demonstration and quantitation in vivo and in vitro. *In* Gordon JL (ed): Platelets in Biology and Pathology. Amsterdam, Elsevier, 1976, pp 23–60.
31. Ross R, Raines EW, Bowen-Pope DF: The biology of platelet-derived growth factor. Cell 46:155, 1986.
32. Rivera FJ, Miller DD, Garcia OJ, et al: Noninvasive detection of platelet activation at human postangioplasty sites with S-12 monoclonal antibody imaging [Abstract]. J Vasc Interv Radiol 2:31, 1991.
33. Guyton JR, Karnovsky MJ: Smooth muscle cell proliferation in the occluded rat carotid artery: Lack of requirement for luminal platelets. Am J Pathol 94(3):585, 1979.
34. Myler RM, Shaw RE, Stertzler SH, et al: Recurrence after coronary angioplasty. Cathet Cardiovasc Diagn 13:77, 1987.
35. Califf AR, Ohman EM, Frid DJ, et al: Restenosis: The clinical issues. *In* Topol EJ (ed): Textbook of Interventional Cardiology. Philadelphia, WB Saunders, 1990, pp 363–394.
36. Blackshear JL, O'Callaghan WG, Califf RM: Medical approaches to prevention of restenosis after coronary angioplasty. J Am Coll Cardiol 9:834, 1987.
37. Waller BF, Orr CM, Pinkerton CA, et al: Morphologic observations late after coronary balloon angioplasty. Mechanisms of acute injury and relationship to restenosis. Radiology 174:961, 1991.
38. Waller BF, Pinkerton CA, Orr CM, et al: Restenosis 1 to 24 months after clinically successful coronary balloon angioplasty: A necropsy study of 20 patients. J Am Coll Cardiol 17:58B, 1991.
39. Waller BF, Orr CM, Pinkerton CA, et al: Balloon angioplasty restenosis: Intimal proliferation and chronic elastic recoil. *In* Castañeda-Zúñiga WR, Tadavarthy SM (eds): Interventional Radiology. 2nd ed. Baltimore, Williams & Wilkins, 1992, vol. 1, pp 451–460.
40. Johnson DE, Hinohara T, Selmon MR, et al: Primary peripheral arterial stenosis and restenosis excised by transluminal atherectomy: A histopathologic study. J Am Coll Cardiol 15:419, 1990.
41. Johnson DE: Directional peripheral atherectomy: Histologic aspects of a new interventional technique. J Vasc Interv Radiol 1:29, 1990.
42. Waller BF, McManus BM, Garfinkel HJ, et al: Status of the major epicardial coronary arteries 80 to 150 days after percutaneous transluminal coronary angioplasty: Analysis of 3 necropsy patients. Am J Cardiol 51:81, 1983.
43. Essed CE, Van Den Brand M, Becker AE: Transluminar coronary angioplasty and early restenosis: Fibrocellular occlusion after wall laceration. Br Heart J 49:393, 1983.
44. Giraldo A, Esposo OM, Meis JM: Intimal hyperplasia as cause of restenosis after percutaneous transluminal coronary angioplasty. Arch Pathol Lab Med 109:173, 1985.
45. Stoney RJ, String ST: Recurrent carotid stenosis. Surgery 80:705, 1976.
46. Faulkner SL, Fisher RD, Conkle DM, et al: Effect of blood flow rate on subendothelial proliferation in venous autografts used as arterial substitutes. Circulation 51 & 52 (Suppl. I):I-163, 1975.
47. Zarins CK, Bomberger RA, Glagov S: Local effects of stenoses: Increased flow velocity inhibits atherogenesis. Circulation 64(Suppl. II):II-221, 1981.
48. Ku DN, Giddens DP, Zarins CK, Glagov S: Pulsatile flow and atherosclerosis in human carotid bifurcation: Positive correlation between plaque location and low and oscillating shear stress. Arteriosclerosis 5:292, 1985.
49. Bergelson BA, Jacobs AK, Small DM: Lipoproteins predict restenosis after PTCA [Abstract]. Circulation 80 (Suppl. II):II-65, 1989.
50. Austin GE, Hollman J, Lynn MJ, Meier B: Serum lipoprotein levels fail to predict postangioplasty recurrent coronary artery stenosis. Cleve Clin J Med 56:509, 1989.
51. Hearn JA, Donohue BC, King SB, et al: Does serum LP(a) predict restenosis after PTCA? [Abstract]. J Am Coll Cardiol 15 (Suppl. A): 205A, 1990.
52. Sanborn T, Cumberland D, Greenfield A, et al: Percutaneous laser thermal angioplasty: Initial results and 1-year follow-up in 129 femoropopliteal lesions. Radiology 168:121, 1988.
53. Gleason T, Cragg AH, Smith TP, et al. Thermal balloon angioplasty in a canine model: Preliminary results. J Vasc Interv Radiol 1:121, 1990.
54. Becker GJ, Lee BI, Waller BF, et al: Radiofrequency balloon angioplasty: Rationale and proof of principle. Invest Radiol 23:810, 1988.
55. Becker GJ, Lee BI, Waller BF, et al: Potential of radiofrequency balloon angioplasty: Weld strengths, dose response relationships, and correlative histology. Radiology 174:1003, 1990.
56. Lee BI, Becker GJ, Waller BJ, et al: Thermal compression and molding of atherosclerotic vascular tissue with use of radiofrequency energy: Implications for radiofrequency balloon angioplasty. J Am Coll Cardiol 13:1167, 1989.
57. Spears JR, Reyes VP, James LM, Sinofsky EL: Laser balloon angioplasty: Initial clinical experience. Circulation 78 (Suppl. II):II-296, 1988.
58. Ferguson JJ, Dear WE, Leatherman LL, et al: A multi-center trial of laser balloon angioplasty for abrupt closure following PTCA [Abstract]. J Am Coll Cardiol 15 (Suppl. A):25A, 1990.
59. Ohman EM, Califf RM, Lee KL, et al: Restenosis after angioplasty: Overview of clinical trials using aspirin and omega-3 fatty acids [Abstract]. J Am Coll Cardiol 15 (Suppl A):88A, 1990.
60. Badimon L, Badimon J, Lassila R, et al: Thrombin inhibition by hirudin decreases platelet thrombus growth on areas of severe vessel wall injury [Abstract]. J Am Coll Cardiol 13:145A, 1989.
61. Knudtson ML, Flintoft VA, Roth DL, et al: Effect of short-term prostacyclin administration on restenosis after percutaneous transluminal coronary angioplasty. J Am Coll Cardiol 15:691, 1990.
62. Whitworth HB, Roubin GS, Hollman J, et al: Effect of nifedipine on recurrent stenosis after percutaneous transluminal coronary angioplasty. J Am Coll Cardiol 8:1271, 1986.
63. Currier JW, Pow TK, Haudenschild CC, et al: Low molecular weight heparin (Enoxaparin) reduces restenosis after iliac angioplasty in the hypercholesterolemic rabbit. J Am Coll Cardiol 17:118B, 1991.
64. Currier JW, Pow TK, Minihan AC, et al: Colchicine inhibits restenosis after iliac angioplasty in the atherosclerotic rabbit [Abstract]. Circulation 80 (Suppl. II):II-66, 1989.
65. March K, Mohanraj S, Ho P, et al: Biodegradable microspheres containing a colchicine analog inhibit DNA synthesis in vascular smooth muscle cells. Circulation 86(4):I-381, 1992.
66. Muller DWM, Ellis SG, Topol EJ: Colchicine and antineoplastic therapy for the prevention of restenosis after percutaneous coronary interventions. J Am Coll Cardiol 17:126B, 1991.
67. O'Keefe JH, McCallister BD, Bateman TM, et al: Colchicine for the prevention of restenosis after coronary angioplasty [Abstract]. J Am Coll Cardiol 17:181A, 1991.
68. Barath P, Arakawa K, Cao J, et al: Low dose of antitumor agents

prevents smooth muscle cell proliferation after endothelial injury [Abstract]. J Am Coll Cardiol 13:252A, 1989.
69. Berk BC, Vallega G, Griendling KK, et al: Effect of glucocorticoids on Na/H exchange and growth in clutured vascular smooth muscle cells. J Cell Physiol 137:391, 1988.
70. Berk BC, Raines EW: Vascular smooth muscle growth inhibition by hydrocortisone is associated with decreased PDGF. A chain expression [Abstract]. FASEB J 3:A611, 1989.
71. Longnecker JP, Kilty LA, Johnston LK: Glucocorticoid influence on the growth of vascular wall cells in culture. J Cell Physiol 113:197, 1982.
72. Gordon JB, Berk BC, Bettmann MA, et al: Vascular smooth muscle cell proliferation following balloon injury is synergistically inhibited by low molecular weight heparin and hydrocortisone [Abstract]. Circulation 76 (Suppl. IV):IV-213, 1987.
73. Pepine CJ, Hirshfeld JW, Macdonald RG, et al: A controlled trial of corticosteroids to prevent restenosis after coronary angioplasty [Abstract]. Circulation 81:1753, 1990.
74. Ellis SG, Bates ER, Schaible T, et al: Prospects for the use of antagonists to the platelet glycoprotein IIB/IIIa receptor to prevent postangioplasty restenosis and thrombosis. J Am Coll Cardiol 17:89B, 1991.
75. Lundergan CF, Foegh ML, Ramwell PW: Peptide inhibition of myointimal proliferation by angiopeptin, a somatostatin analogue. J Am Coll Cardiol 17:132B, 1991.
76. Powell JS, Muller RK, Baumgartner HR: Suppression of the vascular response to injury: The role of angiotensin-converting enzyme inhibitors. J Am Coll Cardiol 17:137B, 1991.
77. Sahni R, Maniet AR, Moci G, Banka VS: Prevention of restenosis by lovastatin [Abstract]. Circulation 80 (Suppl. II):II-65, 1989.
78. Hollman J, Konrad K, Raymond R, et al: Lipid lowering for the prevention of recurrent stenosis following coronary angioplasty [Abstract]. Circulation 80 (Suppl. II):II-65, 1989.
79. Hong MK, Farb A, Unger EF, et al: A new PTCA balloon catheter with intramural channels for local delivery of drugs at low pressure. Circulation 86(4):I-380, 1992.
80. Lambert CR, Leone J, Rowland S: The microporous balloon: A minimal-trauma local drug delivery catheter. Circulation 86(4):I-381, 1992.
81. Wolinsky H, Lin C-S: Use of the perforated balloon catheter to infuse marker substances into diseased coronary artery walls after experimental postmortem angioplasty. J Am Coll Cardiol 17:174B, 1991.
82. Slepian MJ, Schindler A: Polymeric endoluminal paving/sealing: A biodegradable alternative to intracoronary stenting. Circulation 78 (Suppl. II):II-409, 1988.
83. Nabel EG, Plautz G, Nabel GJ: Gene transfer into vascular cells. J Am Coll Cardiol 17:189B, 1991.
84. Lim CS, Chapman GD, Gammon RS, et al: Direct in vivo gene transfer into the coronary and peripheral vasculatures of the intact dog. Circulation 83:2007, 1991.
85. Pickering JG, Jekanowski J, Weir L: Demonstration that gene transfer may be successfully accomplished in human vascular smooth muscle cells obtained from atherosclerotic lesions by directional atherectomy. Circulation 86(4):I-798, 1992.
86. Takeshita S, Leclerc G, Gal D, Weir L: In vivo arterial gene transfer: Effect of angioplasty on transfection efficiency in atherosclerotic arteries. Circulation 86(4):I-799, 1992.
87. Hutchinson HG, Shi Y, Sigman S, et al: Inhibition of human vascular smooth muscle cell proliferation using c-myc antisense oligonucleotides. Circulation 86(4):I-226, 1992.
88. Schwartz RS, Holmes DR, Topol EJ: The restenosis paradigm revisited: An alternative proposal for cellular mechanisms. J Am Coll Cardiol 20:1284, 1992.
89. Castañeda-Zúñiga WR: Transluminal angioplasty. Semin Intervent Radiol I(4), 1984.
90. van Breda A, Katzen BT, Picus D, et al: Intraarterial urokinase infusion for treatment of acute and chronic arterial occlusions. Seventy-second Annual Meeting, Radiological Society of North America. Chicago, December 1, 1986.
91. Horvath L: Percutaneous transluminal angioplasty: Importance of anticoagulant and fibrinolytic drugs. AJR 135:951, 1980.
92. Velasquez G, Castañeda-Zúñiga W, Formanek A, et al: Non-surgical aortoplasty in Leriche syndrome. Radiology 134:359, 1980.
93. Kumpe DA: Percutaneous dilatation of an abdominal aortic stenosis. Three-balloon-catheter technique. Radiology 141:536, 1985.
94. Kumpe DA, Jones DN: Percutaneous transluminal angioplasty—Radiological viewpoint. Appl Radiol 11:29, 1982.
95. Mahler F, Triller J, Weidmann P, et al: Complications in percutaneous dilatation of renal arteries. Nephron 44(Suppl 1):60, 1986.
96. Glover JL, Bendick PJ, Dilley RS, et al: Efficacy of balloon catheter dilatation for lower extremity atherosclerosis. Surgery 91:560, 1982.
97. Health and Public Policy Committee, American College of Physicians: Percutaneous transluminal angioplasty. Ann Intern Med 99:864, 1983.
98. Zeitler E, Richter EI, Roth FJ, et al: Results of percutaneous transluminal angioplasty. Radiology 146:57, 1983.
99. Gardiner GA, Meyerowitz MF, Stokes KR, et al: Complications of transluminal angioplasty. Radiology 159:201, 1986.
100. Horvath L: Percutaneous transluminal angioplasty: Importance of anticoagulant and fibrinolytic drugs. AJR 135:951, 1980.
101. Starck E, McDermott JC: Advantages of percutaneous aspiration thromboembolectomy. *In* Zeitler E, Seyferth W (eds): Pros and Cons in PTA and Auxiliary Methods. Berlin, Springer-Verlag, 1989, pp 241–247.
102. Starck EE, McDermott JC, Crummy AB: Percutaneous aspiration thromboembolectomy. Radiology 156:61, 1985.
103. Starck E, Wagner H: Percutaneous aspiration thromboembolectomy. *In* Wilfrido R, Castañeda-Zúñiga M, Tadavarthy S (eds): Interventional Radiology. 2nd ed. Baltimore, Williams & Wilkins, 1992, vol. 1, pp 652–659.
104. Schwarten DE, Tadavarthy SM, Castañeda-Zúñiga WR: Aortic, iliac, and peripheral arterial angioplasty. *In* Castañeda-Zúñiga WR, Tadavarthy SM (eds): Interventional Radiology. 2nd ed. Baltimore, Williams & Wilkins, 1992, vol. 1, pp 378–422.
105. Hayden W: Presented at a round table discussion on distal percutaneous transluminal angioplasty. American Heart Association Annual Meeting, Washington, DC, November 1984.
106. Train JS, Dan SJ, Mitty HA, et al: Occlusion during iliac angioplasty: A salvageable complication. Radiology 168:131, 1988.
107. Maynar M, Reyes R, Pulido-Duque JM, et al: Directional atherectomy with the Simpson atherocath. *In* Castañeda-Zúñiga WR, Tadavarthy SM (eds): Interventional Radiology. 2nd ed. Baltimore, Williams & Wilkins, 1992, vol. 1, pp 527–543.
108. Saddenkni S, Sniderman KW, Hilton S, Sos TA: Percutaneous transluminal angioplasty of nonatherosclerotic lesions. AJR 135:975, 1980.
109. Bonn J, Gardiner B, Shapiro M, et al: Palmaz vascular stent: Initial clinical experience. Radiology 174:741, 1990.
110. Becker G, Palmaz J, Rees C, et al: Palmaz balloon expandable intraluminal stents in the management of angioplasty-induced dissections in human iliac arteries. Radiology 176:31, 1990.
111. Castañeda-Zúñiga WR, Tadavarthy SM: Part 2. Palmaz balloon expandable stent. *In* Castañeda-Zúñiga WR, Tadavarthy SM (eds): Interventional Radiology. 2nd ed. Baltimore, Williams & Wilkins, 1992, vol. 1, pp 556–563.
112. Günther R, Vorwerk D, Bohndorf K, et al: Iliac and femoral artery stenoses and occlusion: Treatment with intravascular stents. Radiology 172:725, 1989.
113. Liermann D, Strecker E, Peters J: The Strecker stent: Indications and results in iliac and femoropopliteal arteries. Cardiovasc Intervent Radiol 15:298, 1992.
114. Sapoval M, Long A, Raynaud A, et al: Femoropopliteal stent placement: Long-term results. Radiology 184:833, 1992.
115. Zollikofer C, Antonucci F, Pfyffer M, et al: Arterial stent placement with use of the Wallstent: Midterm results of clinical experience. Radiology 179:449, 1991.
116. Rousseau H, Raillat C, Joffre F, et al: Treatment of femoro-popliteal stenoses by means of self expandable endoprostheses: Midterm results. Radiology 172:961, 1989.
117. Joffre F, Rousseau H, Chemali R: Part 3. Self-expandable intravascular stent: Long-term results in the iliac and superficial femoral arteries. *In* Castañeda-Zúñiga WR, Tadavarthy SM (eds): Interventional Radiology. 2nd ed. Baltimore, Williams & Wilkins, 1992, vol. 1, pp 563–569.
118. Lois JF, Takiff H, Schechter MS, et al: Vessel rupture by balloon catheters complicating chronic steroid therapy. AJR 144:1073, 1985.
119. Ring EJ, Freiman DB, McLean GK, et al: Percutaneous recanalization of common iliac artery occlusions: An unacceptable complication rate? AJR 139:587, 1982.
120. Palmaz JC: Part 1. Intravascular stents: Experimental observations and anatomopathologic correlates. *In* Castañeda-Zúñiga W, Tadavar-

thy SM (eds): Interventional Radiology. 2nd ed. Baltimore, Williams & Wilkins, 1992, vol. 1, pp 553–556.

121. Vorwerk D, Günther R: Stent placement in iliac arterial lesions: Three years of clinical experience with the Wallstent. Cardiovasc Intervent Radiol 15:285, 1992.
122. Raillat C, Rousseau H, Joffre F, et al: Treatment of iliac artery stenoses with the Wallstent prosthesis. AJR 154:613, 1990.
123. Rees CR, Palmaz JC, Garcia O, et al: Angioplasty and stenting of completely occluded iliac arteries. Radiology 172:953, 1989.
124. Tegtmeyer CJ, Kellum CD, Ayers C: Percutaneous transluminal angioplasty of the renal artery. Radiology 153:77, 1984.
125. Odurny A, Colapinto RF, Sniderman KW, Johnston KW: Percutaneous transluminal angioplasty of abdominal aortic stenoses. Cardiovasc Intervent Radiol 12(1):1, 1989.
126. Yakes WF, Kumpe DA, Brown SB, et al: Percutaneous transluminal aortic angioplasty: Techniques and results. Radiology 172:965, 1989.
127. Belli AM, Hemingway AP, Cumberland DC, Welsh CL: Percutaneous transluminal angioplasty of the distal abdominal aorta. Eur J Vasc Surg 3(5):449, 1989.
128. Charlebois N, Saint GG, Hudon G: Percutaneous transluminal angioplasty of the lower abdominal aorta. AJR 146(2):369, 1986.
129. Gross-Fengels W, Steinbrich W, Pichlmaier H, Erasmi H: Die perkutane transluminale Angioplastie (PTA) der infrarenalen Aorta abdominalis. [Percutaneous transluminal angioplasty of the infrarenal abdominal aorta]. Radiologe 30(5):235, 1990.
130. Berger T, Sorensen R, Konrad J: Aortic rupture: A complication of transluminal angioplasty. AJR 146:373, 1986.
131. Bachman DM, Kim RM: Transluminal dilatation for subclavian steal syndrome. AJR 135:995, 1980.
132. Damuth HJ, Diamond AB, Rappoport AS, Renner JW: Angioplasty of subclavian artery stenosis proximal to the vertebral origin. Am J Neuroradiol 4(6):1239, 1983.
133. Motarjeme A, Keifer JW, Zuska AJ, Nabawi P: Percutaneous transluminal angioplasty for treatment for subclavian steal. Radiology 155:611, 1985.
134. Vitek JJ, Keller FS, Duvall ER, et al: Brachiocephalic artery dilation by percutaneous transluminal angioplasty. Radiology 158:779, 1986.
135. Burke DR, Gordon RL, Mishkin JD, et al: Percutaneous transluminal angioplasty of subclavian arteries. Radiology 164:699, 1987.
136. Insall RL, Lambert D, Chamberlain J, et al: Percutaneous transluminal angioplasty of the innominate, subclavian, and axillary arteries. Eur J Vasc Surg 4(6):591, 1990.
137. Kachel R, Basche S, Heerklotz I, et al: Percutaneous transluminal angioplasty (PTA) of supra-aortic arteries, especially the internal carotid artery. Neuroradiology 33(3):191, 1991.
138. Tesdal IK, Jaschke W, Haueisen H, et al: Percutaneous transluminal angioplasty (PTA) of the arteries of the arm in brachial and cerebral ischemia. ROFO 155(4):363, 1991.
139. Andresen JH, Henneberg EW: Percutaneous transluminal angioplasty of the brachiocephalic arteries. Ugeskr Laeger 151(23):1468, 1989.
140. Kachel R, Endert G, Basche S, et al: Percutaneous transluminal angioplasty (dilatation) of carotid, vertebral, and innominate artery stenoses. Cardiovasc Intervent Radiol 10(3):142, 1987.
141. Erbstein RA, Wholey MH, Smoot S: Subclavian artery steal syndrome: Treatment by percutaneous transluminal angioplasty. AJR 151:291, 1988.
142. Theron J: Angioplasty of supra-aortic arteries. Semin Intervent Radiol 4:331, 1987.
143. Theron J, Melancon D, Ethier R: ''Pre'' subclavian steal syndromes and their treatment by angioplasty: Hemodynamic classification of subclavian artery stenoses. Neuroradiology 27:265, 1985.
144. Hodgins GW, Dutton JW: Subclavian and carotid angioplasties for Takayasu's arteritis. J Can Assoc Radiol 33(3):205, 1982.
145. Galichia JP, Bajaj AK, Vine DL, Roberts RW: Subclavian artery stenosis treated by transluminal angioplasty: Six cases. Cardiovasc Intervent Radiol 6:78, 1983.
146. Kobinia GS, Bergmann H Jr: Angioplasty in stenosis of the innominate artery. Cardiovasc Intervent Radiol 6:82, 1983.
147. Gordon RL, Haskell L, Hirsch M, et al: Transluminal dilatation of the subclavian artery. Cardiolovasc Intervent Radiol 8:14, 1985.
148. Wilms G, Baret A, Dewaele D, et al: Percutaneous transluminal angioplasty of the subclavian artery: Early and late results. Cardiovasc Intervent Radiol 10:123, 1987.
149. Ringelstein EB, Zeumer H: Delayed reversal of vertebral artery blood flow following percutaneous transluminal angioplasty for subclavian steal syndrome. Neuroradiology 26:189, 1984.
150. Moore TS, Russell WF, Parent AD, et al: Percutaneous transluminal angioplasty in subclavian steal syndrome: Recurrent stenosis and retreatment in two patients. Neurosurgery 11:512, 1982.
151. Tournade A, Zenglein JP, Braun JP, et al: Percutaneous transluminal angioplasty of the vertebral and subclavian arteries: An angiographic-velocimetry comparison. J Neuroradiol 13:95, 1986.
152. Kodera K: Percutaneous transluminal angioplasty for subclavian steal syndrome. Nippon Acta Radiol 47:1, 1987.
153. Pavone P, Castrucci M, Cavallaro A, Rossi P: PTA of subclavian artery: Comparative study with surgical procedures [Abstract]. Cardiovascular and Interventional Radiology Society of Europe, Porto Cervo, Sardinia, Italy, May 27, 1987, pp 85–86.
154. Mathias K: Catheter treatment of cerebrovascular disease [Abstract]. Cardiovascular and Interventional Radiology Society of Europe, Porto Cervo, Sardinia, Italy, May 27, 1987, pp 84–85.
155. Motarjeme A: Percutaneous transluminal angioplasty of the brachiocephalic vessels: An update report [Abstract]. Cardiovascular and Interventional Radiology Society of Europe, Porto Cervo, Sardinia, Italy, May 27, 1987, p 83.
156. Farina C, Mingoli A, Schultz RD, et al: Percutaneous transluminal angioplasty versus surgery for subclavian artery occlusive disease. Am J Surg 158(6):511, 1989.
157. Becker GJ, Katzen BT, Dake MD: Noncoronary angioplasty: State of the art. Radiology 170:921, 1989.
158. Courtheoux P, Tournade A, Theron J, et al: Transcutaneous angioplasty of ventebral artery atheromatous ostial stricture. Neuroradiology 27:259, 1985.
159. Theron J, Raymond J, Casasco A, Courtheoux F: Percutaneous angioplasty of atherosclerotic and postsurgical stenosis of carotid arteries. Am J Neuroradiol 8(3):495, 1987.
160. Vitek JJ, Raymon BC, Oh SJ: Innominate artery angioplasty. Am J Neuroradiol 5:113, 1984.
161. Motarjeme A: Percutaneous transluminal angioplasty of the vertebral artery. *In* Castañeda-Zúñiga W (ed): Transluminal Angioplasty. New York, Thieme-Stratton, 1983.
162. Tsai FY, Matovich V, Hieshima G, et al: Percutaneous transluminal angioplasty of the carotid artery. Am J Neuroradiol 7:349, 1986.
163. Courtheoux P, Tournade A, Theron J, et al: Percutaneous endoluminal angioplasty of post endarterectomy carotid stenoses. Neuroradiology 29:186, 1987.
164. Tievsky AL, Dury EM, Mardiat JG: Transluminal angioplasty in post surgical stenosis of the extracranial carotid artery. Am J Neuroradiol 4:800, 1983.
165. Smith DC, Smith LL, Hasso AN: Fibromuscular dysplasia of the internal carotid artery treated by operative transluminal balloon angioplasty. Radiology 155:645, 1985.
166. Hasso AN, Bird CR, Zinke DE, Thompson JR: Fibromuscular dysplasia of the internal carotid artery: Percutaneous transluminal angioplasty. Am J Neuroradiol 2:175, 1981.
167. Bockenhemer SAM, Mathias K: Percutaneous transluminal angioplasty in arteriosclerotic internal carotid artery stenosis. Am J Neuroradiol 4:791, 1983.
168. Wiggli U, Gratzl O: Transluminal angioplasty of stenotic carotid arteries: Case reports and protocol. Am J Neuroradiol 4(3):793, 1983.
169. Kerber CW, Cromwell LD, Loehden OL: Catheter dilatation of proximal carotid stenosis during distal bifurcation endarterectomy. Am J Neuroradiol 1:348, 1980.
170. Alpert JR, Ring EJ, Berkowitz HD, et al: Treatment of vein graft stenosis by balloon catheter dilatation. JAMA 242:2769, 1979.
171. Mitchell SE, Kadir S, Kaufman SL, et al: Percutaneous transluminal angioplasty of aortic graft stenosis. Radiology 149:439, 1983.
172. Roth FJ, Cappius G, Krings W: Seldom indications for angioplasty. Inter Angio 4:101, 1985.
173. Roth FJ, Cappius G, Krings W: Seldom indications for angioplasty. Inter Angio 4:101, 1985.
174. Uflacker R, Goldany MA, Constant S: Resolution of mesenteric angina with percutaneous transluminal angioplasty of a superior mesenteric artery stenosis using a balloon catheter. Gastrointest Radiol 5:367, 1980.
175. Furrer J, Gruntzig A, Kugelmeier J, et al: Treatment of abdominal angina with percutaneous dilatation of an arteria mesenterica superior stenosis. Cardiovasc Intervent Radiol 5:367, 1980.

176. Golden DA, Ring EJ, McLean GK, et al: Percutaneous transluminal angioplasty in the treatment of abdominal angina. AJR 139:247, 1982.
177. Freitag G, Freitag J: Percutaneous transluminal angioplasty in abdominal angina—stenosis of the celiac-mesenteric trunk. Vasa 17(1):47, 1988.
178. Warnock NG, Gaines PA, Beard JD, Cumberland DC: Treatment of intestinal angina by percutaneous transluminal angioplasty of a superior mesenteric artery occlusion. Clin Radiol 45(1):18, 1992.
179. Mee C: Intestinal angina: Percutaneous transluminal angioplasty of the celiac and superior mesenteric arteries. Radiology 167(1):59, 1988.
180. Fuochi C, Moser E, Dalla PF, Picetti C: Treatment of chronic mesenteric ischaemia by percutaneous transluminal angioplasty. Radiogr Today 55(620):19, 1989.
181. Picetti C, Fuochi C, Moser E, Dalla PF: Percutaneous angioplasty of the superior mesenteric artery in the treatment of abdominal angina. Radiol Med (Torino) 80(6):926, 1990.
182. Freitag G, Freitag J: Abdominal angina: Percutaneous transluminal angioplasty of the superior mesenteric artery. Vasa 19(3):260, 1990.
183. Fuochi C, Moser E, Dalla PF, Picetti C: Percutaneous angioplasty of the superior mesenteric artery in the treatment of abdominal angina. Radiol Med (Torino) 80(6):926, 1990.
184. Picetti C, Fuochi C, Moser E, Dalla PF: Abdominal angina: Percutaneous transluminal angioplasty of the superior mesenteric artery. Vasa 19(3):260, 1990.
185. Odurny A, Sniderman KW, Colapinto RF: Intestinal angina: Percutaneous transluminal angioplasty of the celiac and superior mesenteric arteries. Radiology 167(1):59, 1988.
186. Rapp JG, Reilly LM, Qvarfordt PG, et al: Durability of endarterectomy and antegrade grafts in the treatment of chronic visceral ischemia. J Vasc Surg 3:799, 1986.
187. Schwab SJ, Raymond JR, Saeed M, et al: Prevention of hemodialysis fistula thrombosis. Early detection of venous stenosis. Kidney Int 36:707, 1989.
188. Dapunt O, Feurstein M, Rendl K, Prenner K: Transluminal angioplasty versus conventional operation in the treatment of haemodialysus fistula stenosis: Results from a 5-year study. Br J Surg 74:1004, 1987.
189. Cada E, Karnel F, Mayer G, et al: Percutaneous transluminal angioplasty of failing arteriovenous dialysis fistulae. Nephrol Dial Transpl 4:57, 1989.
190. Brooks JL, Sigley RD, May KJ, Mack RM: Transluminal angioplasty versus surgical repair for stenosis of hemodialysis grafts. Am J Surg 153:530, 1987.
191. Gmelin E, Winterhoff R, Rinast E: Insufficient hemodialysis access fistulas: Late results of treatment with percutaneous balloon angioplasty. Radiology 171:657, 1989.
192. Glanz S, Gordon DH, Butt KMH, et al: The role of percutaneous angioplasty in the management of chronic hemodialysis fistulas. Ann Surg 206(6):777, 1987.
193. Hunter DW, Castañeda-Zúñiga WR, Coleman CC, et al: Failing arteriovenous dialysis fistulas: Evaluation and treatment. Radiology 152:631, 1984.
194. Smith TP, Cragg AH, Castañeda F, Hunter DW: Thrombosed polytetrafluoroethylene hemodialysis fistulas: Salvage with combined thrombectomy and angioplasty. Radiology 171:507, 1989.
195. Saeed M, Newman GE, McCann RL, et al: Stenoses in dialysis fistulas: Treatment with percutaneous angioplasty. Radiology 164:693, 1987.
196. Rodriguez-Perez JC, Maynar M, Rams A, et al: Percutaneous transluminal angioplasty as best treatment in stenosis of vascular access for hemodialysis. Nephron 51:192, 1989.

Limitations of Peripheral Angioplasty and the Role of New Devices

Gary J. Becker, M.D.

• • •

The limitations of modern PTA include (1) unsuitability of some lesions for percutaneous therapy, (2) acute failures, and (3) late failures due to restenosis and progressive disease. Some of the problems are unique to specific vascular distributions; others are common to all. Guidelines for the appropriate application of PTA in specific clinical and morphologic circumstances have been developed.[1] Even as the guidelines are being gradually accepted, modern transluminal devices developed to deal with the limitations of PTA are being increasingly applied. The most important of these devices are atherectomy catheters and stents. Therefore, most of this discussion concerns these two categories of devices.

THE ROLE OF ATHERECTOMY

General Principles

Atherectomy is a procedure in which a specially designed catheter (most often motor-driven) is used to remove atherosclerotic plaque material from the path of blood flow inside the vessel lumen. In theory, removal of plaque results in debulking that should prevent recurrent symptoms or significantly delay the onset of clinically apparent restenosis.

The term atherectomy has actually been applied rather generically to a wide variety of procedures, each of which falls into one of two categories: atherectomy or atheroablation. McLean has termed these two categories of procedure extirpative atherectomy and ablative atherectomy, respectively.[2] In both, the plaque is removed from the path of bloodflow. However, in the former it is removed from the body; in the latter technique it is pulverized or microfragmented and allowed to embolize distally, where in theory the particles are disposed of by the reticuloendothelial system.

Specific Atherectomy Devices

Simpson Directional Atherectomy Catheter

The Simpson device was the first major atherectomy catheter to be used clinically in the peripheral vascula-

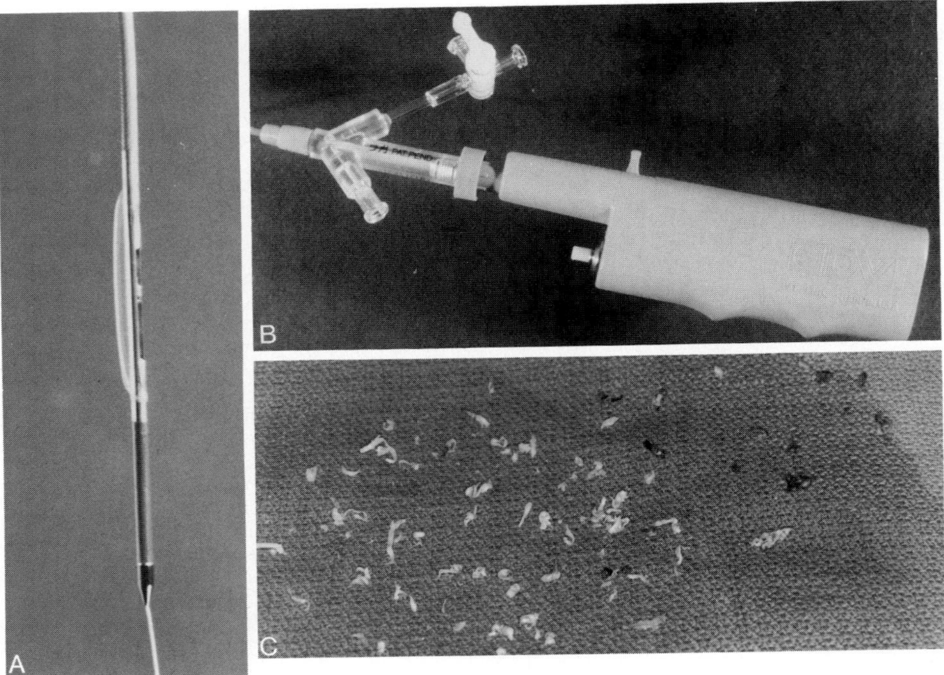

FIGURE 20–7. Simpson atherectomy catheter. *A*, Catheter with positioning balloon in profile opposite the cutting window. Note extended housing and leading guidewire. *B*, Motor drive unit. *C*, Atherectomy specimens obtained with use of the Simpson device.

ture.[3–5] The device (Fig. 20–7) consists of a rotating cutter blade driven by a cutter torque cable that is connected to the motor drive. At the working end of the catheter there is a cutting window that opens toward the atheroma that is to be cut. Opposite the cutting window is a low-pressure positioning balloon that is eccentrically placed and is not intended to dilate but rather to force the cutting window against the plaque. In operation, the operator advances the cutter from the trailing edge to the leading edge of the cutting window by pushing a lever on the motor-drive unit. The plaque is literally shaved into a collecting chamber beyond the cutting window. Currently, the Atherocath (fixed-wire device) and the Atherotrac (over-the-wire device) have an extended housing for the collection of larger quantities of atheromatous material. This enables the operator to rotate the catheter sequentially to obtain more material before removing the catheter from the sheath each time. The catheters are available in sizes from 6 to 11 Fr and can treat arteries ranging from 3.5 to 9.7 mm in diameter.

Transluminal Endarterectomy Catheter (TEC)

This is an over-the-wire device that, like the directional atherectomy catheter, removes plaque from the arterial wall (Fig. 20–8). The shape of the cutting window is conical. Housed inside the cutting window are two triangular blades that rotate at 700 rpm. Vacuum bottles apply suction by way of a hollow drive shaft attached to the drive unit, so that all material cut by the triangular blades is aspirated into the bottles. The TEC device, as it is known, was first introduced in 1989.[4–5] Although it is available in sizes ranging from 5 to 11 Fr, it is not expandable and cannot be positioned eccentrically against one wall because it lacks a positioning balloon. Therefore, the actual lumen size that can be achieved is only the same diameter as that of the cutting head and thus the size of the lumen of the insertion sheath. For example, the 9 Fr system can produce a maximum lumen diameter of 3 mm. Consequently, adjunctive balloon angioplasty must be used most of the time.

Pullback Atherectomy Catheter (PAC)

This is an investigational over-the-wire device (Fig. 20–9) that removes atheroma by cutting in a retrograde fashion.[6] The cutter, a circular blade that rotates with use of a motor drive, is exposed when it is advanced to reveal the cutting window after the catheter has been positioned at the target location. Although it does not have a positioning balloon or an expandable tip, it is capable of producing a lumen significantly larger than the catheter shaft. The

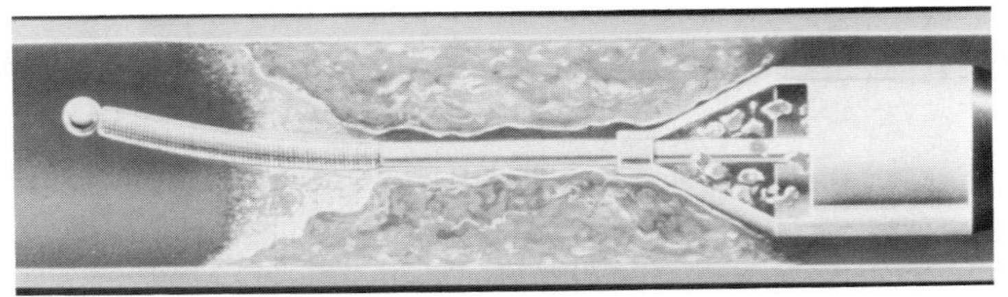

FIGURE 20–8. Transluminal endarterectomy catheter.

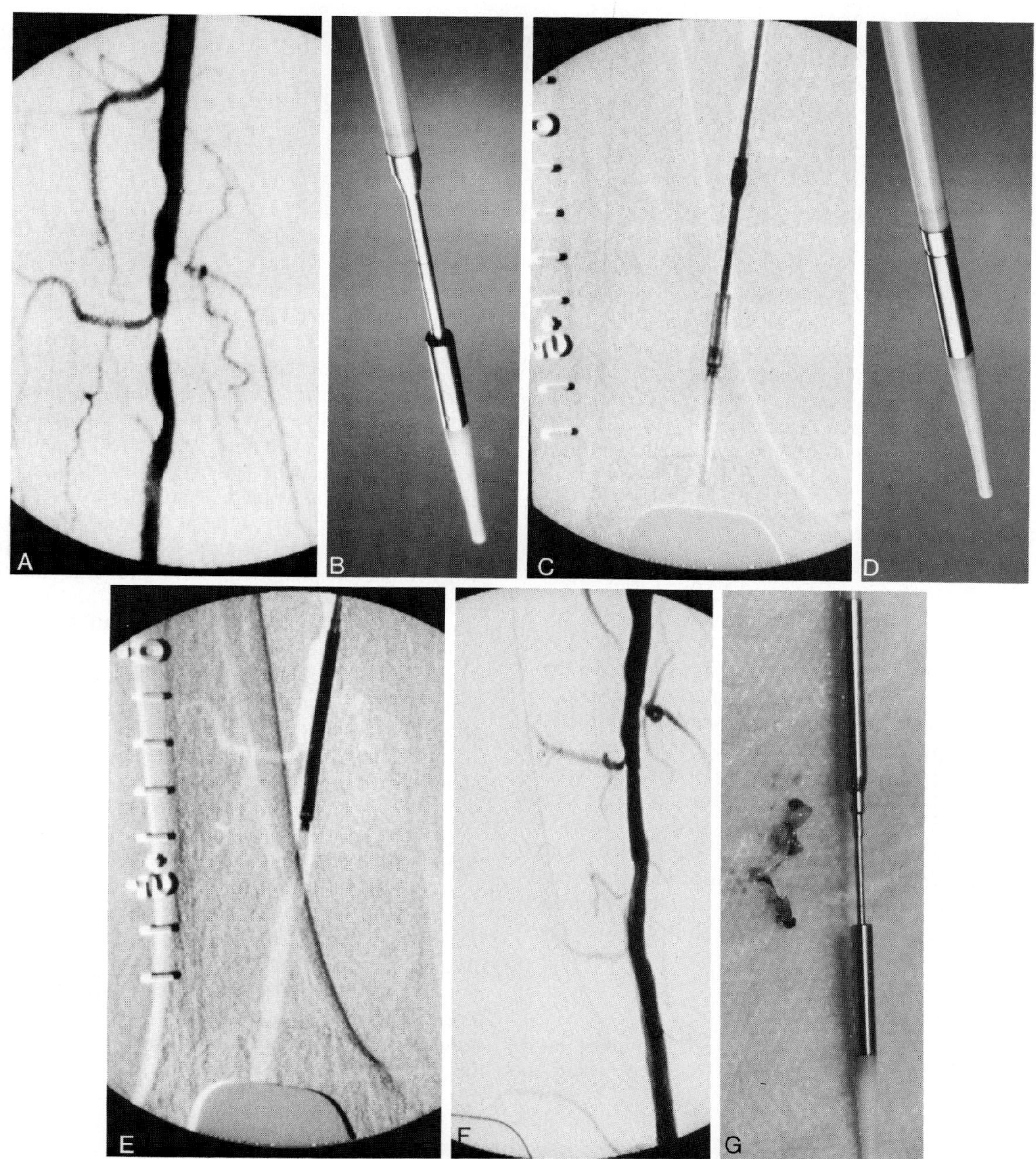

FIGURE 20–9. Pullback atherectomy catheter (PAC). *A*, SFA stenosis. *B*, PAC with cutter open. *C*, PAC with cutter open in the SFA lesion. *D*, PAC with cutter closed. *E*, PAC with cutter closed in SFA lesion. *F*, SFA angiogram immediately after pullback atherectomy. *G*, Specimen of atheroma removed by PAC.

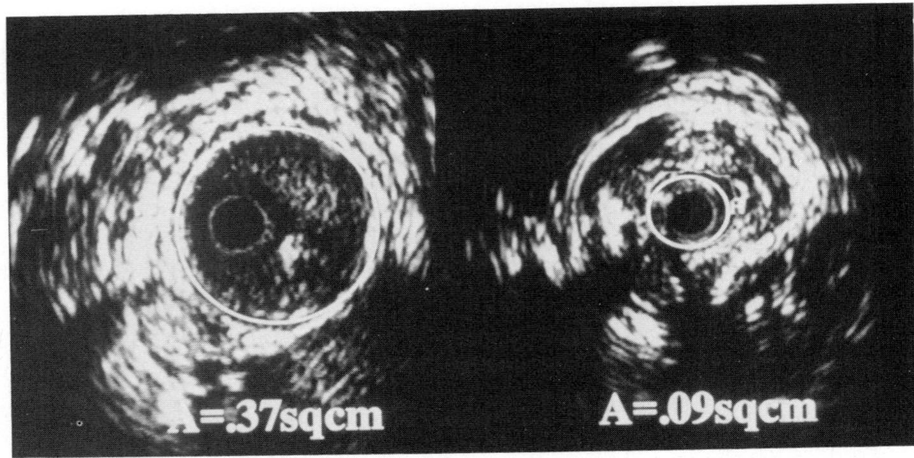

FIGURE 20–10. Intravascular sonogram obtained without cuff application (*left*) and with a suprasystolic cuff in place (*right*). Note that vessel yields unevenly to external pressure because of mineralized atheroma.

method of atherectomy involves placing a cuff on the limb segment and inflating it to suprasystolic pressures. This technique forces atheroma into the cutting window. Intravascular ultrasound (IVUS) studies during cuff inflation prove that this does in fact occur; however, atheromatous vessels are often compressed eccentrically (Fig. 20–10). Both 8 Fr and 9 Fr PACs are being evaluated in clinical trials.

Auth Device: Rotablator

This is an extremely high speed (up to 190,000 rpm) rotating, over-the-wire atheroablation device whose working end consists of a football-shaped burr, in which fine diamond chips are embedded (Fig. 20–11). Rotation of the diamond-studded burr produces an abrasive effect. In theory, plaque, which is unyielding, is ablated by the device, whereas softer, nonatherosclerotic tissue is unaffected. Embolization of plaque material does occur, as expected. Most of the particles are in the 5- to 10-μ size range, though some reach 15 to 20 μ.[7] Burr diameters range from 1.25 to 4.5 mm. Obviously, the larger sizes can only be used with a surgical approach. Because the device is not expandable, percutaneous use must often be complemented with balloon angioplasty. Destruction of red blood cells due to the action of the rotating burr can result in hemoglobinuria.[8]

Kensey Catheter (Trac-Wright)

This was the first atheroablation device to come into clinical use.[9] A high-pressure water jet is used to rotate a smooth, elliptical cam at variable speeds up to approximately 100,000 rpm (Fig. 20–12). The fluid vortex created by this high-speed rotation draws the plaque fragments or particles back into the rotating cam. Theoretically, this recirculation pulverizes plaque into tiny fragments that are harmlessly embolized downstream, where they will be ultimately engulfed by the body's reticuloendothelial cells. Also, the smooth cam was originally thought to be self-centering and most applicable to "impassable" occlusions, to which it was proposed that it could be applied without a significant risk of perforation. Now there is experimental evidence that the plaque fragments are larger than originally anticipated (most greater than 7 μ),[10] and there is documented clinical evidence of a substantial perforation rate when the device is applied to complete occlusions.[11–15] As with most of the other atherectomy devices, the Trac-Wright is not expandable. It is available in 5, 8, and 10 Fr sizes. The largest device achieves a maximum diameter of 3.3 mm. Therefore, adjunctive balloon angioplasty is frequently necessary.

Applications of Atherectomy

In order to understand the current role of atherectomy in the management of occlusive disease in any vascular distribution, one must first understand the results and limitations of angioplasty in the same distribution and the appropriate utilization of angioplasty. Indeed, PTA is the gold standard for evaluating new transluminal treatment modalities.

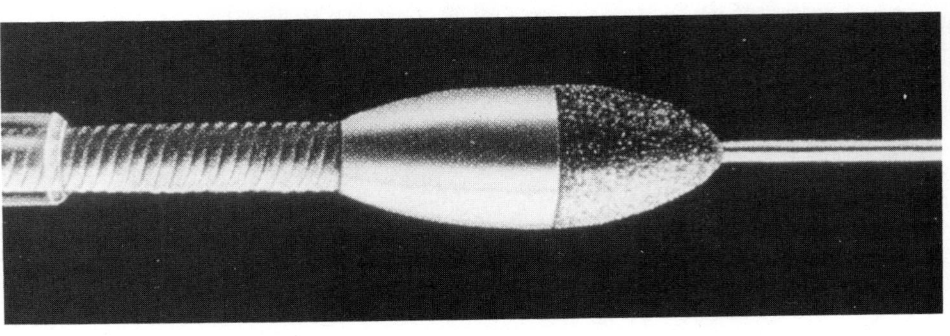

FIGURE 20–11. Close-up of the diamond-studded burr of the Rotoblator.

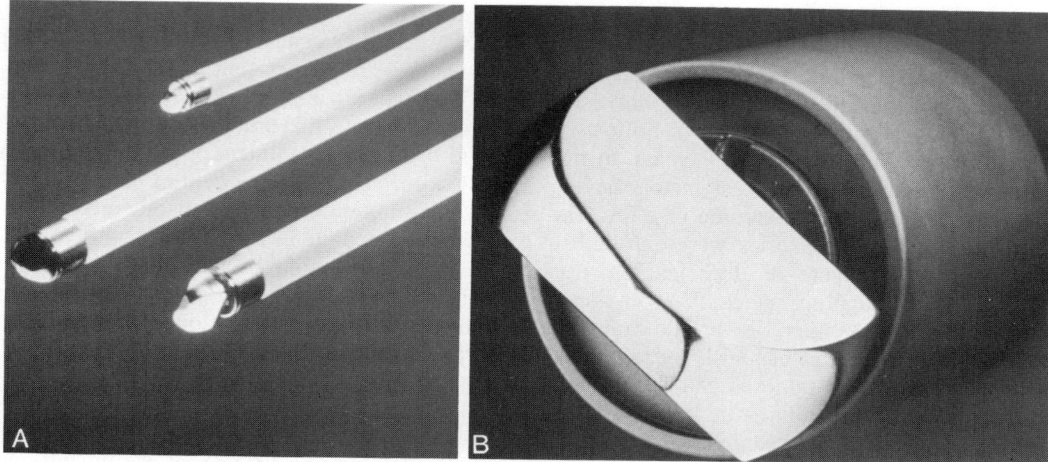

FIGURE 20–12. Kensey (Trac-Wright) catheter. *A*, Several catheters with rotating cams. *B*, Close-up of rotating cam at the end of one catheter.

As stated above, the best resource available to date that details the appropriateness of PTA for each clinical and morphologic setting in most major circulations is the Guidelines for Percutaneous Transluminal Angioplasty, formulated by the Standards of Practice Committee of the Society of Cardiovascular and Interventional Radiology.[1] In creating this document, the committee utilized the available literature and the consensus of experts to categorize lesions according to the applicability of PTA.

Category 1. Balloon angioplasty is the procedure of choice, and treatment by PTA results in a high rate of technical success and complete obliteration of pressure gradients with complete relief of symptoms generally expected.

Category 2. Generally well suited for PTA; complete relief or improvement can be expected. This category includes patients whose PTA is to be followed by bypass to treat multi-level disease.

Category 3. Amenable to PTA, but in general because of location, disease extent, or severity, surgery offers a better chance of technical success and lasting patency.

Category 4. Surgical options are superior to PTA. PTA plays a minor role in selected cases.

In general, PTA is more successful when lesions are (1) short instead of long, (2) single instead of multiple, (3) concentric instead of markedly eccentric, (4) nonostial, and (5) stenoses rather than occlusions (given equal lesion length).

Importantly, it is understood that these guidelines will require updating. As technology advances and our scientific database increases, changes in recommendations are likely to evolve. Also, the committee realized that no two health care facilities are completely alike. In some hospitals, the operating skills of the surgeons may provide the most experience with a disease process, and the operating suites may offer the most advanced technology and the safest procedural environment. In such cases, no matter what the suitability of a lesion for PTA, surgery may be the safest approach. Conversely, even a category 3 lesion should be approached by the skilled and knowledgeable interventionalist if in his or her hospital, the angiography suite and his or her level of experience offer the patient the best and safest alternative.

Femoropopliteal Disease

In femoropopliteal disease in particular, *category 1* lesions are single stenoses up to 3 cm in length not at the origin of the superficial femoral artery (SFA) or the distal popliteal artery; *category 2* lesions are (1) single stenoses (3 to 10 cm long) not involving the distal popliteal, (2) heavily calcified stenoses up to 3 cm in length, (3) multiple lesions each less than 3 cm (stenoses or occlusions), (4) single or multiple lesions in the absence of continuous tibial runoff to improve inflow for distal surgical bypass; *category 3* lesions are (1) single (3 to 10 cm long) lesions involving the distal popliteal, (2) multiple (each 3 to 5 cm) and with or without heavy calcification, or (3) single stenoses or occlusions more than 10 cm long; and *category 4* lesions are complete common femoral artery (CFA) or SFA occlusions or complete popliteal or proximal trifurcation occlusions.

Three very important studies of femoropopliteal PTA have appeared in the literature since the late 1980s. The first was a report by Morgenstern and colleagues from Columbia Presbyterian in New York that documents a 95 per cent success rate in crossing femoropopliteal occlusions 1 to 4 cm in length and an 86 per cent success rate in crossing occlusions 5 to 10 cm long using modern imaging methods and catheters together with a variety of steerable and special-function guidewires.[16] Overall, technical success with balloon PTA for these occlusions was achieved in 64 of 70 patients (91 per cent). These figures update the authors' experience to a total of 160 femoropopliteal recanalizations. Importantly, this 91 per cent initial success rate, which was achieved with standard guidewires and catheters, represents an expected frequency of success in clinical practice today. Considering the costs involved in utilizing any of the new recanalization devices, Morgenstern and colleagues have made it clear that substantial advantages in safety, technical success, or long-term benefit will be required to justify the increased expenditures of the new devices.

In the second important study, Capek and associates reported the long-term results of 217 PTA procedures in the superficial femoral and popliteal arteries over an 8-year period.[17] Patients were followed with serial noninvasive studies and, in 71 cases, with angiography. Follow-up ranged from 2 to 11 years, with a mean of 7 years. In this study, life table analysis was used to assess factors having a potential impact on the long-term outcome of PTA. The greatest number of patients in this series were enrolled in 1979 and 1980 before the advent of digital subtraction angiography (DSA), roadmapping, steerable soft-tipped guidewires, calcium channel blockers, low-profile catheters, and several other important advances. Still, the technical success rate was 93 per cent for stenoses and 82 per cent for occlusions. Excluding initial failures in 10 per cent of patients, the patencies at 1, 3, and 5 years were 81, 61, and 58 per cent, respectively. Inclusion of the initial failures according to the new standards (i.e., accounting for all patients subjected to this form of therapy) results in overall patencies at 1, 3, and 5 years of 73, 55, and 52 per cent, respectively. Complications occurred in 10 per cent of cases, but one quarter of these were technical "complications" that were without clinical consequences. Clinical factors that were found to influence long-term patency negatively included diabetes mellitus (p = .04), diffuse atherosclerotic cardiovascular disease (p = .05), and threatened limb loss at the time of initial presentation for treatment (p = .01). Morphologic factors found to influence long-term outcome negatively included long lesion length (overall, p = .004; for lesions of 0 to 2 cm vs. those greater than 2 cm, p = .001; for those 0 to 2 cm vs. greater than 10 cm, p = .007; for those 2 to 5 cm vs. greater than 10 cm, p = .015); moderate eccentricity (p = .04); and residual stenosis on post-PTA angiogram (p = .02).

The third important study was Johnston's reanalysis of data from the femoropopliteal angioplasty subgroup in the Toronto series.[18] The author analyzed data from 254 femoropopliteal PTAs that were performed for chronic ischemia of all levels of severity. Cumulative clinical success was measured by standard objective criteria, and the Kaplan-Meier method was used to recalculate the data. Cox multiple regression analysis was used to determine variables predictive of late results. For stenoses with good runoff, the 5-year cumulative clinical success rate was 53 per cent; with poor runoff it was 31 per cent. For occlusions, the cumulative clinical success rate was 36 per cent at 5 years for patients with good runoff and 16 per cent for those with poor runoff. Occlusion may have been a confounding variable in this study, just as it was in the study of Capek and associates. In other words, in the Capek study, patients with femoropopliteal occlusion who underwent successful recanalization and PTA were just as likely to have lasting patency as those who began with stenoses. The differences in cumulative clinical success rate were almost all due to the differences in technical success from the very beginning. The data in Johnston's reanalysis suggest a similar phenomenon. In the overall study group, cumulative clinical success ± standard error (SE) was 88.8 ± 2.0 per cent at 1 month, 62.5 ± 3.2 per cent at 1 year, 52.6 ± 3.5 per cent at 2 years, 50.7 ± 3.5 per cent at 3 years, 44.1 ± 4.0 per cent at 4 years, and 38.1 ± 4.4 at 5 years. When only initially successful cases were included, the cumulative clinical success rates were 70.4 ± 3.3 per cent at 1 year, 59.4 ± 3.7 per cent at 2 years, 57.1 ± 3.8 per cent at 3 years, 49.7 ± 4.3 per cent at 4 years, 42.9 ± 4.9 per cent at 5 years, and 40.2 ± 5.3 per cent at 6 years. It seems from these data that initial success portends a high likelihood of long-term clinical benefit. Importantly, initial success occurred in 88.8 per cent of cases in the study.

The *potential* benefits of atherectomy over PTA that have been sought in the femoropopliteal segment include (1) improved technical success of recanalization in cases of occlusion, (2) a smoother post-treatment lumen that may minimize platelet aggregation and, ultimately, intimal hyperplasia and restenosis, (3) minimal injury to the media so that the stimulus for restenosis is minimized or removed, and (4) effective debulking, which should set back the starting point of luminal narrowing due to intimal hyperplasia, thereby delaying the onset of clinically apparent restenosis.

Concerning devices intended to enhance the success of recanalization, we must include laser heat probes, sapphire tip Nd:YAG lasers, and the Kensey (Trac-Wright) catheter. The over-the-wire atherectomy devices do not enhance recanalization, since the guidewire must be passed across the occlusion before the device can be used. Lasers have been uniformly disappointing in that they have failed to demonstrate superiority over conventional recanalization techniques.[19–23] Clinical studies of the Kensey catheter have also been disappointing in this regard.[11–15]

Regarding the smoothness of the post-treatment lumen, there has been no evidence to date that a smooth appearance on angiography or angioscopy confers any long-term advantage such as improved patency. The Kensey (Trac-Wright) catheter even fails in this regard, since reports of procedure-related dissection have been quite frequent,[11–15] ranging from 9 to 24 per cent. The Simpson directional atherectomy catheter and the Auth Rotablator typically do leave a smooth angiographic appearance, the latter even more than the former. However, long-term benefits have not yet been realized. Long-term results are discussed below.

Completeness of debulking with atherectomy is difficult to measure. Angiographic appearances notoriously underestimate the completeness of an atherectomy. IVUS has been somewhat helpful in this regard (Fig. 20–13). Still, there has been no carefully performed, prospective, lesion-by-lesion study of long-term atherectomy results as a function of the completeness of atherectomy.

Long-term results of atherectomy have not proved superior to those achieved with angioplasty alone. For directional atherectomy, 2-year patency rates of 37 to 86 per cent have been reported,[11–15, 24–28] and adjunctive PTA has been used in several of the studies. For TEC atherectomy, virtually no long-term results are available, and, as expected, in all of the reported series, balloon PTA has been a required adjunct.[4–5, 29]

For the Auth Rotablator, patencies at 6 months range from 37 to 90 per cent, and long-term follow-up is not available.[8, 30–32] Hemoglobinuria has occurred in one third to two thirds of cases in some series,[30–32] and total complications range from 0 to 46 per cent.

Considering the added costs of atherectomy compared to those of balloon PTA, the larger sheath required, the

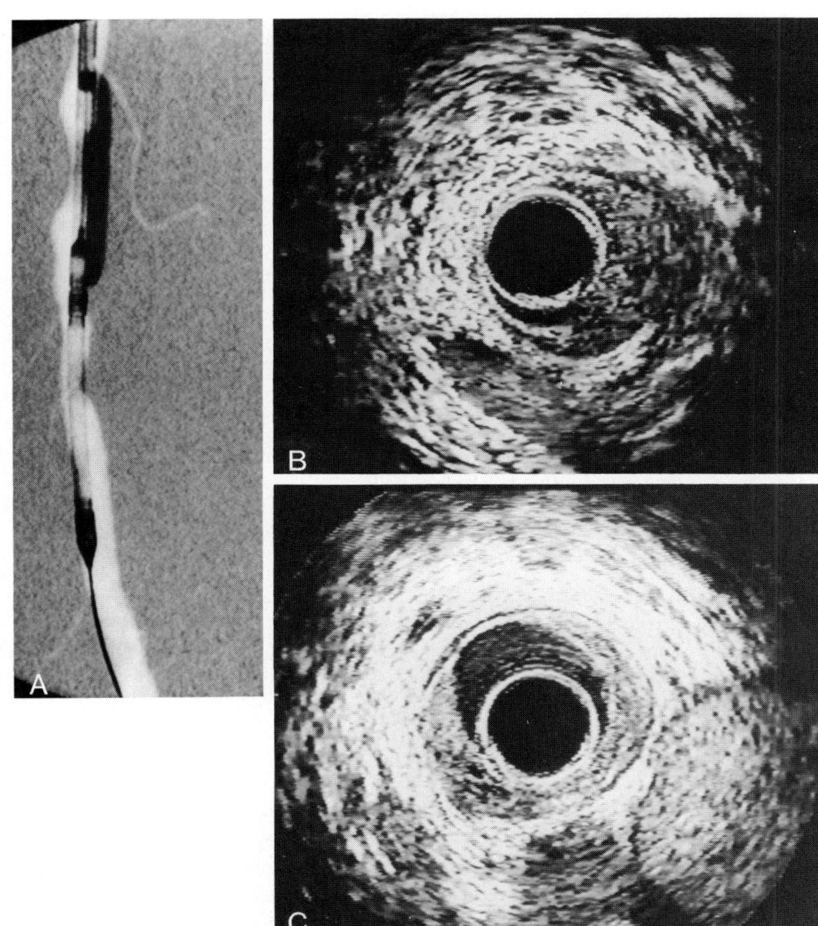

FIGURE 20–13. Intravascular ultrasound (IVUS). *A*, Road map of an SFA stenosis being treated with Simpson atherectomy. *B*, Immediately prior to atherectomy, IVUS reveals that probe (*dark area, center*) nearly obstructs the lumen (*dark crescent beneath probe*) because of large eccentric atheroma (*gray, homogeneous, moon-shaped material to the right of the probe in this illustration*). *C*, Lumen is larger following atherectomy. Although the completion angiogram (not shown) in this case indicated less than 20 per cent residual stenosis (single diameter), considerable atheroma still remains. Orientation of atheroma on the image changes if the catheter is rotated by the operator.

relatively high frequency of complications compared to those reported for PTA, and the lack of demonstrable long-term benefit, atherectomy in the femoropopliteal segment should be reserved for cases in which PTA has failed and those for which PTA is associated with results inferior to those of atherectomy. These include cases of eccentric plaque, flow-limiting angioplasty-induced dissections that have failed to respond to prolonged balloon inflation, and the presence of intimal hyperplasia at graft anastomoses.

Aortoiliac Disease

Although directional atherectomy has been employed in iliac atherosclerosis, the size of the device and sheath required to treat human iliac arteries and the aorta is prohibitive. Therefore, atherectomy in iliac arteries has been almost completely abandoned. Most iliac interventions involve balloon angioplasty with or without stent placement. As will be discussed below, the availability of balloon expandable stents for iliac arteries has had a major impact on the interventionalist's ability to correct suboptimal angioplasty results.

Stenoses in Dialysis Access Fistulae

One area in which directional atherectomy may prove useful is in the management of the stenotic dialysis access fistula, including those that have failed to respond to balloon angioplasty and those including lesions in the subclavian and brachiocephalic veins.[30–34] Twenty-six of 28 lesions in the series of Gray and colleagues[33] were found to consist of intimal hyperplasia.

THE ROLE OF INTRAVASCULAR STENTS

General Principles

Amazingly, the potential benefits of intravascular stenting were first described by Dotter and Judkins in their original article on angioplasty in 1964.[35] In 1969, Dotter reported his laboratory experience with a spring-coil prosthesis in canine popliteal arteries.[36] In the United States, no further interest was demonstrated until 1983.[37–38] Since that time, many stents have been designed and evaluated in laboratory and clinical studies. Table 20–1 lists the characteristics of an ideal intravascular stent. No stent is ideal. Rather, each has its own strengths and weaknesses. Each stent may be categorized as balloon-expandable or self-expanding. Here we take a closer look at the characteristics of the most important stents.

Table 20–1. Ideal Characteristics of a Metallic Stent

The ideal stent should:
Be deployed with familiar percutaneous transluminal angioplasty
Be delivered on a very low profile catheter
Have a very high expansion ratio
Be available in a range of lengths and diameters
Be highly radiopaque
Permit consistently precise delivery to the target site
Be retrievable in the event of errant placement
Have high hoop strength to resist recoil
Not permanently deform in response to two-point compression
Be flexible for use in tortuous vessels
Not embolize or migrate
Be thromboresistant
Be incorporated into the vessel wall with thin neointima and a functional endothelial coat on luminal surface
Be isocompliant with adjacent vessel segments
Be biologically inert or prevent restenosis
Provide long-term patency
Maintain structural integrity after hundreds of millions of cardiocirculatory cycles
Permit noninvasive imaging follow-up, including magnetic resonance imaging
Be inexpensive

Balloon-Expandable Stents

Palmaz Balloon-Expandable Intraluminal Stent

The Palmaz balloon-expandable intraluminal stent (BEIS) (Johnson & Johnson Interventional Systems, Warren, NJ) (Fig. 20–14) is the only stent thus far approved for peripheral arterial use in the United States.[39] It has been approved by the United States Food and Drug Administration for deployment in iliac angioplasty cases with suboptimal results. It provides endovascular support by balloon-mediated expansion, which results in a plastic deformation of the metallic endoprosthesis beyond its elastic limit. Each stent is a single tube of 316L stainless steel with etched rectangular slots oriented in the long axis of the stent and arranged in staggered rows around the entire circumference of the tube. For delivery, the stent-balloon assembly is introduced to the target site over a guidewire and within a protective outer sheath. When the target site is reached, the sheath is withdrawn, and the stent is deployed by balloon inflation. The balloon is then deflated, the catheter is rotated to be certain that the balloon is free from the stent, and the catheter is removed. In the deployed condition, the openings in the stent appear as diamond-shaped rather than rectangular. The major positive attributes of the Palmaz BEIS are its hoop strength and its high expansion ratio. It is intermediate in radiopacity and lacks longitudinal flexibility (although additional, more flexible permutations of this design with connecting segments are under study), and therefore it cannot readily be inserted from the contralateral groin over the aortic bifurcation. It is also susceptible to permanent deformation by two-point compression. Various sizes of this stent are being tested in different applications. Renal stents and coronary stents have undergone clinical testing in the United States.

Strecker Stent

The Strecker stent (Medi-Tech, Watertown, MA) is a highly radiopaque, balloon-expandable tantalum stent (Fig. 20–15).[40] It is a cylindrical, interwoven-wire mesh stent with a wire diameter that may be varied to change such properties as hoop strength but with an impact on profile. The method of deployment is slightly different from that of the Palmaz BEIS. In the unexpanded state, the stent is secured on the balloon surface by leading and trailing edge retainer sleeves made of silicone. As the balloon is inflated at the target site, the stent expands and shortens slightly as it is freed from the retainer sleeves. The major strengths of this stent are its high radiopacity and its intermediate flexibility. It has a lower hoop strength than the Palmaz BEIS. Clinical trials of this device in peripheral arterial applications are underway in the United States.

Cordis Stent

Cordis Corporation (Miami, FL) has developed a flexible, balloon-expandable, tantalum zigzag stent that is

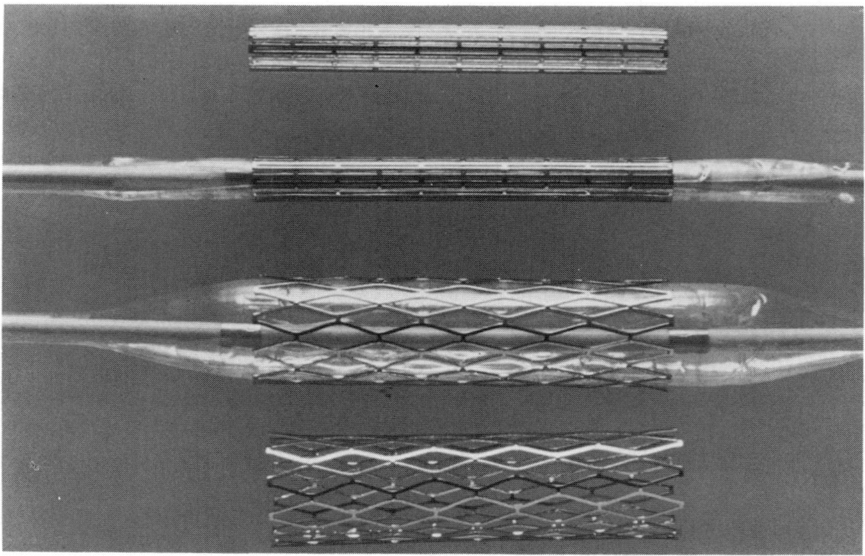

FIGURE 20–14. Palmaz balloon expandable intraluminal stent.

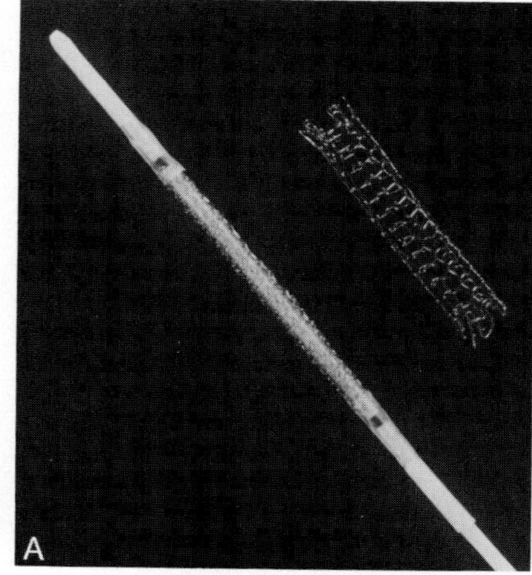

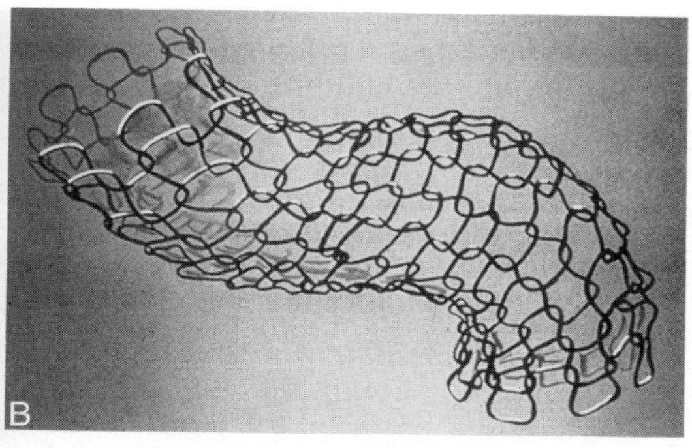

FIGURE 20–15. Strecker balloon expandable stent. *A*, Mounted on balloon (*left*) and after deployment (*right*). *B*, Flexibility of the device allows it to conform to curved vessels.

wrapped on the balloon surface in a helical coil.[41] Originally designed as a coronary stent, it is currently undergoing modifications for peripheral vascular and other applications. The stent already has very high radiopacity and excellent flexibility. The new modifications are aimed at increasing hoop strength. This stent has not yet been used in clinical trials anywhere in the world.

Wiktor and Fontaine-Dake Stents

Other investigational balloon-expandable stents with characteristics similar to the Cordis stent are the Wiktor stent (Medtronics Corp., Minneapolis, MN) and the Fontaine-Dake stent (Cook, Inc., Bloomington, IN). They also have single tantalum wire zigzag designs.

Gianturco-Roubin Bookbinder Stent

One final balloon-expandable stent is the Gianturco-Roubin or ''bookbinder'' stent, so named because it resembles the binding of a spiral notebook (Fig. 20–16).[42] It is a flexible, stainless steel, small vessel stent (Cook, Inc., Bloomington, IN) made of surgical suture wire (0.0006 inch or 0.15 mm in diameter). The wire is wrapped cylindrically with the bends adopting alternating U and inverted U configurations every 360 degrees. The major strengths of this stent are its simplicity and its flexibility. It is minimally radiopaque. Of all the stents mentioned thus far, this one has the least potential for peripheral vascular applications because of its low expansion ratio. Because of the low ratio, stenting an iliac or femoral artery would require a large-bore catheter and therefore a prohibitively large arterial sheath. Therefore, although it may ultimately find applications in the tibial arteries, its principal intended use is in the coronary circulation.

Self-Expanding Stents

Each self-expanding stent works by one of the following mechanisms: (1) a spring action triggered by unloading the device from a constraining delivery catheter, or (2) thermal memory alloys that cause the stent to assume the proper configuration when warmed to body temperature.

Nitinol Spring Coil Stents

Thermal memory stents are composed of nitinol, a nickel-titanium alloy with a thermally triggered shape memory.[43] Because of this property they may be loaded into or onto a catheter in a relatively elongated state for delivery, yet they regain their useful configuration, such as a spring coil, upon deployment at body temperature. The two interchangeable shapes correspond to two distinct crystalline structures possessed by the alloy at different temperatures. The actual thermal trigger point for shape change can be controlled metallurgically by varying the proportions of nickel and titanium and by varying the annealing temperature. Although these stents have been used extensively in Russia, they are just beginning clinical trials in the United States.

Schneider Wallstent

The most widely used self-expanding stent, the Schneider WallStent (Schneider Stent Division, Pfizer, Minneapolis, MN), is a stainless-steel spring-loaded stent that has undergone clinical trials in the iliac and superficial femoral arteries in the United States (Fig. 20–17) but has not yet received market approval from the U.S. Food and

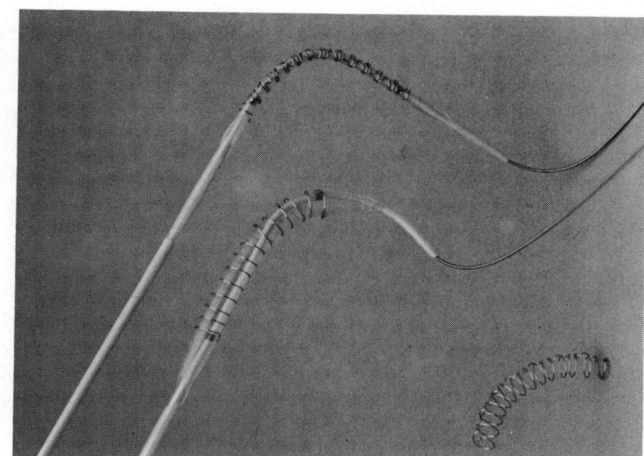

FIGURE 20–16. Gianturco-Roubin balloon expandable stent.

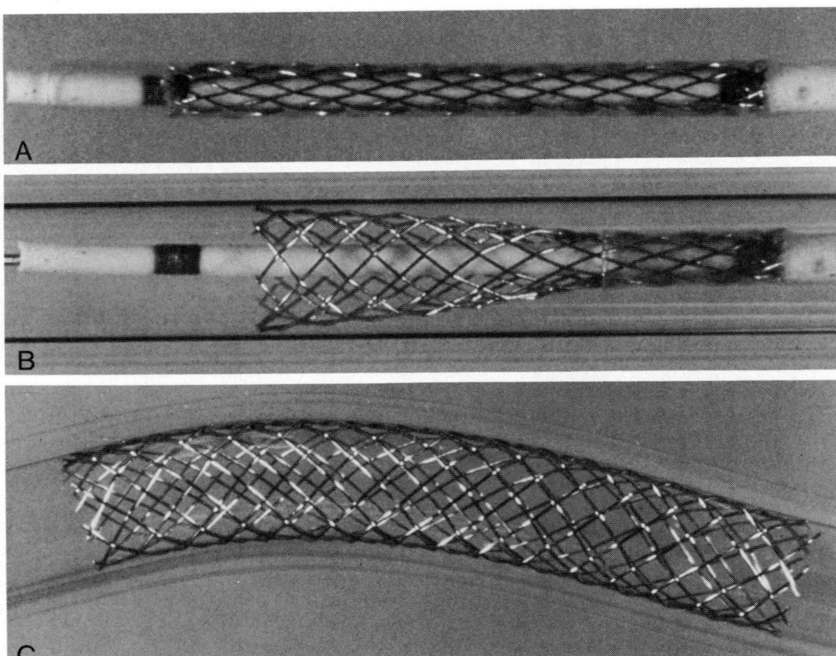

FIGURE 20–17. Schneider WallStent. *A*, Before deployment. *B*, During deployment as membrane is retracted. *C*, Following deployment.

Drug Administration.[44] These stents have been manufactured in a range of sizes from 2.5 mm (expanded diameter) to 35 mm. Each stent comprises 16 to 20 spring-steel filaments (surgical grade stainless steel alloy) woven into a tubular, flexible, self-expanding braid configuration. Hoop strength varies with the number and gauge of the wires. Filaments of the smallest stents are 0.075 to 0.100 mm in diameter; those of the larger stents are 0.12 to 0.17 mm in diameter. At the crossing points, the filaments are free to pivot. This allows for excellent longitudinal flexibility, the most outstanding characteristic of this stent. The smaller stents for coronary applications are delivered on 5 Fr catheters over 0.014-inch guidewires. The larger stents for peripheral applications are delivered on 7 Fr catheters over 0.035-inch guidewires. In the original design, the stent was mounted on the delivery catheter in such a way that it was stretched to a very low profile under a constraining rolling membrane. To deploy the stent, it is first positioned within the target site. A separate port that connects to the rolling membrane is injected with a 30 per cent weight per volume mixture of contrast material under 3 atmospheres of pressure. As the catheter is pulled back steadily against a stable pushing rod, the rolling membrane is retracted, and the stent is deployed by self-expansion. In an updated design (known as Unistep), there is no rolling membrane to be pressurized in the deployment process. Instead, the outer constraining catheter is simply withdrawn to expose the stent. This latter design has not yet been used for vascular applications in the United States. The WallStent has a high hoop strength (though not as high as that of a Palmaz BEIS), excellent flexibility, and marginal radiopacity. Also, because it shortens substantially as it is deployed, it is often difficult to position the ends of the stent precisely. As an aside, the WallStent is the most frequently used device for transjugular intrahepatic portosystemic shunt (TIPS) procedures.[45]

Gianturco Z Stent

Another type of self-expanding stainless-steel stent is the Gianturco zig-zag (Z stent) (Cook, Inc, Bloomington, IN).[46] In this design, a wire is bent into a zigzag pattern, and its ends are connected to form a cylinder (Fig. 20–18). The stent is compressed radially and loaded into a non-tapered delivery catheter. At the target site, the outer catheter is withdrawn against an inner pusher catheter without altering the position of the pusher or the stent. This deploys the stent in its unconstrained configuration. In an experi-

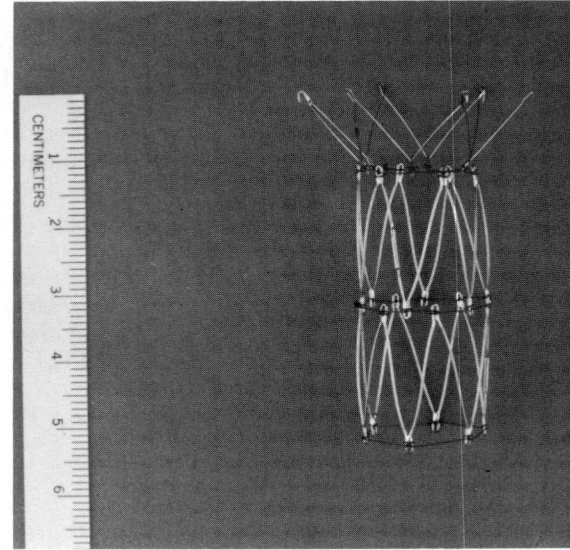

FIGURE 20–18. Gianturco-Rosch Z-stent with skirts and anchor hooks. This device is suitable for use in superior vena caval stenoses.

mental study of Z-stent properties, Fallone and colleagues used a "tire-wrap" device and a simple spring gauge to describe a coefficient of stiffness for each Z stent.[47] The value of the coefficient is independent of the original fully expanded radius, linearly dependent on the caliber of the stent wire, and inversely related to stent length. Small radial displacements are linearly related to the force required to compress the stent, and the coefficient of stiffness is the proportionality constant. Vascular applications of this device have been limited primarily to the treatment of vena cava syndromes. Various modifications[48] of the original design have been made, including multi-segmented stents, stents with skirts to prevent embolization and migration, and barbs for anchoring. Monofilament lines made of nylon suture (Ethicon, Inc., Somerville, NJ) may be placed through "eyes" at each of the bends to prevent overexpansion of the stent and overdistention of the stented vessel.

Noncoronary Vascular Applications of Stents

Atherosclerotic Aortoiliac Disease

The procedure of choice for diffuse atherosclerotic occlusive disease of the infrarenal abdominal aorta and iliac arteries is aortobifemoral bypass grafting. It is the most durable procedure, and in properly selected elective cases it has a very low morbidity and mortality.

PTA has been applied to more focal disease of the infrarenal abdominal aorta, common iliac arteries, and external iliac arteries for the past 14 years. Most of the collective experience has derived from aortoiliac and iliac artery PTA.

The previously published Guidelines for Percutaneous Transluminal Angioplasty[1] have categorized iliac lesions as follows:

Category 1. Noncalcified, concentric stenoses less than 3 cm in length.

Category 2. Stenoses 3 to 5 cm in length or calcified or eccentric stenoses less than 3 cm in length.

Category 3. Stenoses 5 to 10 cm in length or chronic occlusions less than 5 cm in length after thrombolytic therapy.

Category 4. a. Stenoses more than 10 cm in length.
b. Chronic occlusions more than 5 cm in length after thrombolytic therapy.
c. Extensive aortoiliac disease.
d. Iliac stenoses in a patient with an abdominal aortic aneurysm or other lesion requiring aortic or iliac surgery.

The technical and initial clinical success in all series exceeds 90 per cent, and for focal iliac stenosis it approaches 100 per cent. Reported long-term patencies have ranged from 50 per cent to almost 100 per cent. Only a few studies have carefully documented clinical results over a long period of follow-up using standard life table methods. Most of the authors have been guilty of frontloading, as described by Rutherford. A recent report by Tegtmeyer and colleagues of 340 aortoiliac lesions treated in 200 patients utilized standard life table methods.[49] The mean follow-up was approximately 29 months, and cumulative patency at 7.5 years was found to be 85 per cent of patients when only initially successful procedures were included and 79 per cent of patients overall (SE = 3 per cent). Complications occurred in 10.5 per cent of patients. In a reanalysis of 667 balloon angioplasties of the iliac arteries from the University of Toronto series, Johnston examined variables associated with success or failure by Kaplan-Meier, Cox regression, and logistic regression analysis.[50] Cumulative clinical success was measured rather than cumulative patency by angiography. Among 82 iliac occlusions, there were 15 technical failures and 1 complication. In initially successful cases, the cumulative clinical success rate ± SE was 91.0 ± 3.5 per cent at 1 month and 58.8 ± 7.1 per cent at 3 years. In 580 iliac stenoses, there were only eight technical failures. In 313 common iliac PTAs, the cumulative clinical success rate was 97.1 ± 0.9 per cent at 1 month, 81.1 ± 2.3 per cent at 1 year, 70.6 ± 2.9 per cent at 2 years, 67.8 ± 3.0 per cent at 3 years, 64.9 ± 3.3 per cent at 4 years, 60.2 ± 4.0 per cent at 5 years, and 52.0 ± 5.7 per cent at 6 years. In 209 external iliac PTAs, the predicted 3-year cumulative clinical success rate was 57 per cent for men and 34 per cent for women. In 58 PTAs of common and external iliac arteries combined, the predicted 3-year cumulative clinical success rate was 73 per cent for patients with good runoff and 30 per cent for those with poor runoff. Adverse events included death in 0.3 per cent of patients, complications requiring surgery in 1.0 per cent, and delayed hospital discharge in 2.6 per cent.

It is imperative to recognize here that the definition of an acceptable immediate result in aortoiliac PTA is changing now that intraluminal stenting has become part of the percutaneous armamentarium. Stents improve the immediate hemodynamic results of iliac PTA, effectively manage elastic recoil and flow-limiting dissections resulting from PTA, allow more effective treatment of complete iliac artery occlusions, and probably have substantially higher long-term patencies than those with PTA alone.

In regard to the hemodynamic superiority of stenting compared with PTA alone, in a limited study by Bonn and colleagues at Thomas Jefferson University in Philadelphia, patients undergoing PTA followed by immediate intraluminal stenting with the Palmaz BEIS were studied as follows.[51] The translesional pressure gradient was found to average 52 mmHg (peak systolic) and 66 mmHg after vasodilation and prior to PTA. Following PTA, the gradients were found to have decreased to a mean of 11 mmHg (personal communication). Following intraluminal stenting, the gradients were found to have decreased to a mean of 2 mmHg. These differences in pressure gradient have been consistent across several studies done since that time. In a large prospective randomized clinical trial comparing iliac PTA to primary iliac stenting with the Palmaz BEIS, Richter found that the mean gradient across the treatment site in the PTA group was 6 mmHg (peak systolic), whereas in the stent group it was 1 mmHg.[52]

Stents are superior to PTA in the treatment of PTA-induced iliac artery dissection.[53] In a previous series, the author reported that the frequency of flow-limiting PTA-related dissection in the iliac arteries was probably not less than 4.8 per cent, and possibly significantly higher. It was noted that extensively calcified iliac artery lesions seemed prone to PTA-induced dissection but that these lesions were readily managed by intraluminal stent placement. Long-term patency was documented in that series. Since that report, intraluminal stenting has become the standard treatment for PTA-induced, flow-limiting iliac artery dissection (Fig. 20–19).

Stents also improve significantly the percutaneous treatment of complete occlusions of the iliac arteries. Prior to 1988, the sum of the available literature (what limited amount there was) was overwhelmingly negative on the use of PTA for iliac artery occlusions. Then Rees and colleagues reported the use of recanalization techniques and PTA followed by intraluminal stenting as an improved way to manage iliac artery occlusions percutaneously.[54] In that series, 12 patients with complete iliac occlusion underwent percutaneous treatment. Five of those were judged to have chronic iliac occlusion. More recently, Palmaz and colleagues reported the long-term follow-up results on 587

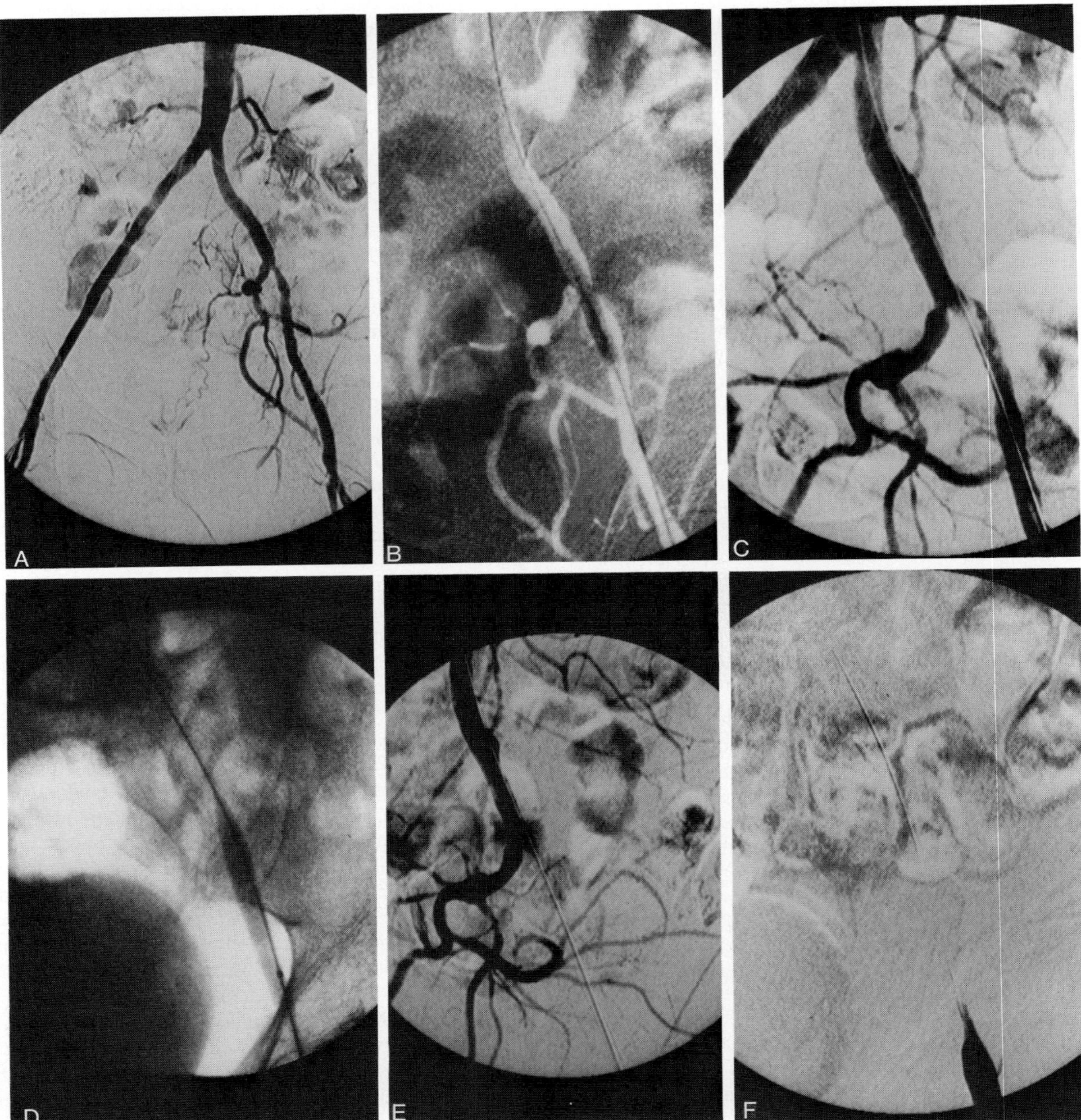

FIGURE 20–19. Use of the WallStent to manage a PTA-induced dissection that occurred in the external iliac artery following angioplasty from a contralateral approach. *A*, Left external iliac artery stenosis. *B*, Balloon angioplasty. *C*, Focal dissection shown in proximal external iliac artery on angiogram immediately following PTA. *D*, Prolonged balloon inflation done in an attempt to "tack down" the dissection. *E*, After prolonged inflation failed to open the dissected segment, a repeat angiogram disclosed complete occlusion of the external iliac artery. *F*, With wire still across the lesion, catheter was advanced to end of dissection, where injection through a Y-adaptor revealed a widely patent common femoral artery.

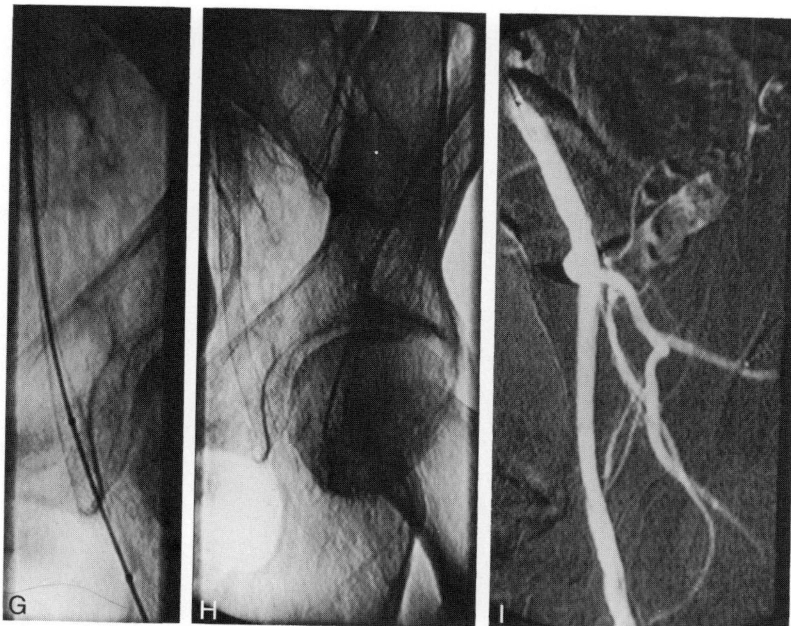

FIGURE 20–19 *Continued* *G* and *H*, Deployment of WallStents. *I*, Arteriogram immediately after stent deployment shows a widely patent external iliac artery.

stent procedures in 486 patients.[55] In that series, the ongoing clinical success rate was 87.8 per cent at 40 months in the group originally treated for iliac occlusion and only 66.6 per cent for those with iliac stenosis. Long and colleagues reported long-term follow-up in 49 consecutive patients treated with iliac artery stents.[56] Twenty-eight per cent of 53 lesions in that series were iliac occlusions. Both Strecker stents and WallStents were included in the series. Primary patencies were 85.3 per cent at 12 months and 80.9 per cent at 18 months. Secondary patencies were 96.1 per cent at 12 and 18 months. Vorwerk and Günther reported a 3-year experience with the use of WallStents for iliac artery disease.[57] Eighty-five of their initial 147 patients presented with iliac artery occlusions, and 62 had stenoses. Failure to recanalize occurred in 22 per cent of occlusions; therefore, only 63 patients underwent stenting for iliac artery occlusion. Complications occurred in 4 per cent of the entire group, but all of the complications occurred in patients with iliac artery occlusion rather than stenosis. Importantly, three of the complications were embolic (one ipsilateral and two contralateral). Only two complications required surgical or percutaneous intervention. Cumulative patency at 2 years in this series was 89.4 per cent. In the author's experience at the Miami Vascular Institute, using angiography, intraluminal pressure measurements, and intravascular ultrasound, at least two major reasons why PTA alone often fails in cases of iliac occlusion have been identified: dissection with residual gradient and marked elastic recoil with residual gradient (Fig. 20–20). Each of these limitations is readily overcome with use of stents.

Does PTA plus stenting provide a more durable result than PTA alone? The answer is a resounding ''probably.'' In a prospective randomized trial of iliac artery stenting versus PTA conducted by Richter in Heidelberg, patients matched for risk factors and disease severity have been enrolled in the trial for treatment. In the most recent analysis of the data, 92 patients had been enrolled in the stent group and 93 in the PTA group.[52] Long-term patency has been documented by angiography in some but by clinical and noninvasive hemodynamic follow-up criteria in all except for a small number of patients lost to follow-up. According to life table analysis, cumulative patencies at 3 years of follow-up were 68 per cent for PTA and 96 per cent for stenting. In a review by Palmaz and colleagues of 587 procedures in 486 patients, ongoing clinical success was defined as the retention of at least one stage improvement in the ischemic ranking system.[55] Using this definition, ongoing clinical success was present in 99.2 per cent immediately post treatment, 90.9 per cent at 1 year, 84.1 per cent at 2 years, and 68.6 per cent at 43 months. Angiographic follow-up was not available in the majority of cases, but in those in whom studies were obtained there was an angiographic patency rate of 91.9 per cent. The mean loss of lumen diameter was 15 per cent, including the few who had developed total occlusions. The Wilcoxon test revealed significantly better long-term clinical success in nondiabetics than in diabetics ($p < .00001$), and in patients with good runoff versus those with poor runoff ($p = .0013$).

Long-term follow-up for stents not available in the United States for intra-arterial use (i.e., all stents other than the Palmaz BEIS) is more scant. Liermann and colleagues have reported their experience with placement of more than 100 Strecker stents in the iliac and femoral arteries.[58] Follow-up, which ranged from 8 to 48 months with a mean of 20 months, included noninvasive testing and intravenous DSA. Thirty iliac stenoses and 22 iliac occlusions were included in the report, and at a mean follow-up of 20 months only 1 vessel had developed a restenosis. The long-term follow-up after treatment of iliac stenoses and occlusions with the WallStent, as reported by Vorwerk and Günther, is indicated earlier.

The preceding discussion demonstrates how profoundly stents have influenced modern aortoiliac PTA by providing a means of opposing elastic recoil, treating PTA-related dissections, managing total iliac artery occlusions,

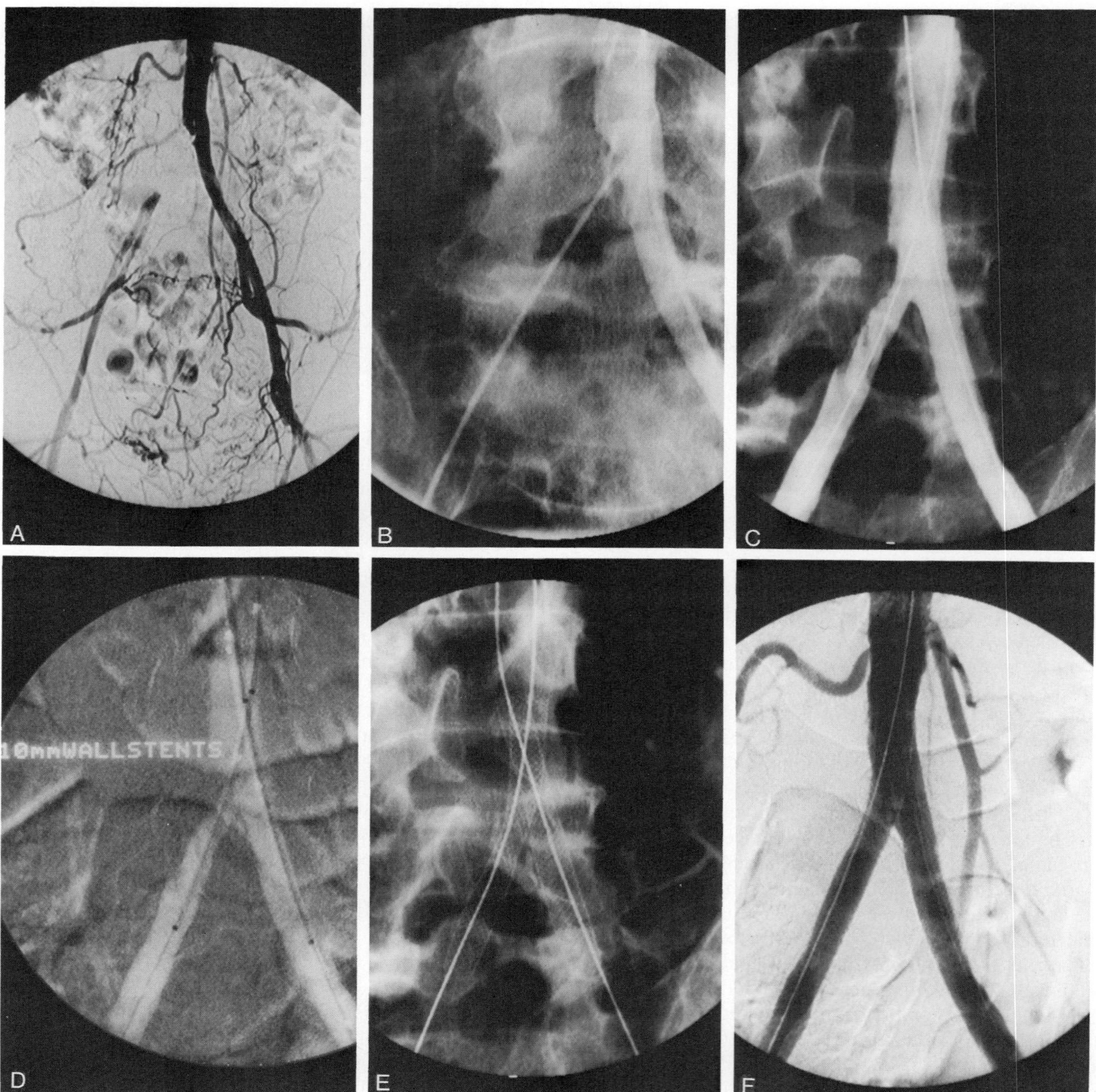

FIGURE 20–20. Use of stents in chronic iliac artery occlusion. *A*, Occlusion of the right common iliac artery in a patient with chronic claudication. *B*, Wire across occlusion. *C*, Angiogram immediately following balloon angioplasty shows evidence of recoil (compare sizes of right and left common iliac arteries) and PTA-induced dissection (*spiral linear lucencies in right common iliac artery*). *D*, Road map during placement of bilateral WallStents. *E*, WallStents after deployment. *F*, Aortoiliac arteriogram immediately following stent placement.

and possibly improving the long-term clinical patency rate. In addition to these benefits, stents have also provided a way to deal with category 3 and category 4 aortoiliac bifurcation disease in selected patients (Fig. 20–21).[59] For an area of vascular practice as seemingly established as aortoiliac surgery and iliac angioplasty for occlusive disease, developments are still occurring rapidly. A more complete understanding of the various roles of stents in this area awaits further investigation and longer term follow-up.

Atherosclerotic Femoropopliteal Disease

The guidelines for femoropopliteal angioplasty have been outlined earlier. The most troublesome lesions for percutaneous intervention include eccentric stenoses, long-segment occlusions, long-segment stenoses, obstructing intimal flaps after PTA, and stenoses due to intimal hyperplasia at graft anastomoses. Not surprisingly, stents have been applied to all of these problems. In general, the immediate and early results have been spectacular, but intimal hyperplasia has resulted in a very high frequency of restenosis.

Most of the experience has been accumulated with the WallStent and Strecker stent. The Palmaz BEIS has been used for these indications in Europe but is just now beginning clinical trials in the United States. Examples of use of the WallStent in a superficial femoral artery occlusion resistant to PTA and another for treatment of an occlusive post-PTA intimal flap are shown in Figures 20–22 and 20–23, respectively.

Preliminary studies using a variety of stents show less than promising results due to intimal hyperplasia and occlusion. In a study of 22 femoropopliteal lesions in 21 patients, Sapoval and associates used the WallStent and found a primary patency of 49 per cent at 1 year.[60] In a study of 26 patients, Do-dai-Do and colleagues reported a secondary patency rate of 69 per cent at 1 year using the same device.[61] Zollikofer and co-workers used WallStents in 15 patients who showed an inadequate response to recanalization and angioplasty for femoropopliteal occlusion.[62] At a mean follow-up of 20 months in 11 patients available for follow-up, only 6 arteries were patent. Using the Strecker stent, Liermann and colleagues found a patency rate of 70.8 per cent at a mean follow-up of 19 months.[58] Thus far, anticoagulant regimens have failed to improve the long-term results.

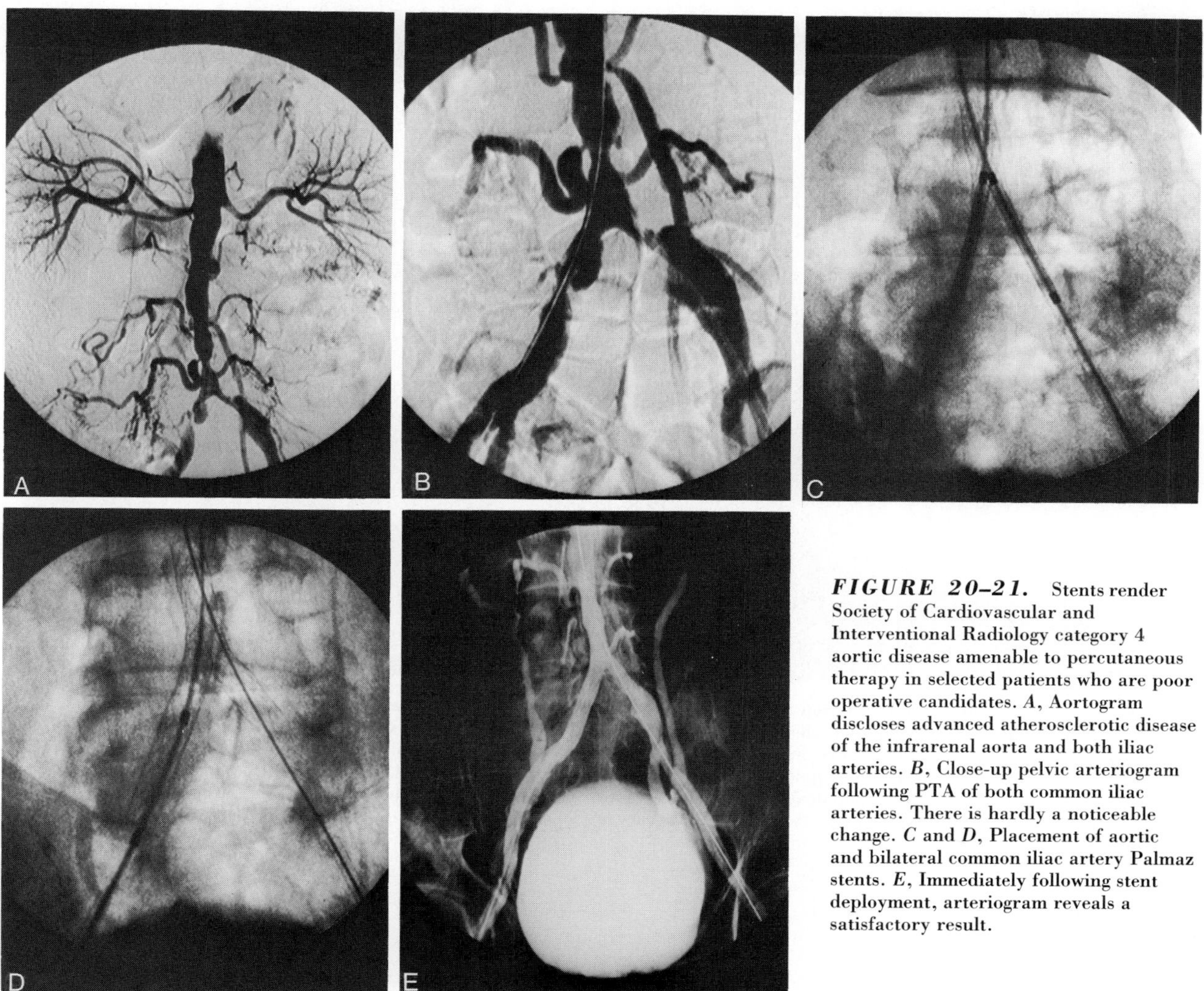

FIGURE 20–21. Stents render Society of Cardiovascular and Interventional Radiology category 4 aortic disease amenable to percutaneous therapy in selected patients who are poor operative candidates. *A*, Aortogram discloses advanced atherosclerotic disease of the infrarenal aorta and both iliac arteries. *B*, Close-up pelvic arteriogram following PTA of both common iliac arteries. There is hardly a noticeable change. *C* and *D*, Placement of aortic and bilateral common iliac artery Palmaz stents. *E*, Immediately following stent deployment, arteriogram reveals a satisfactory result.

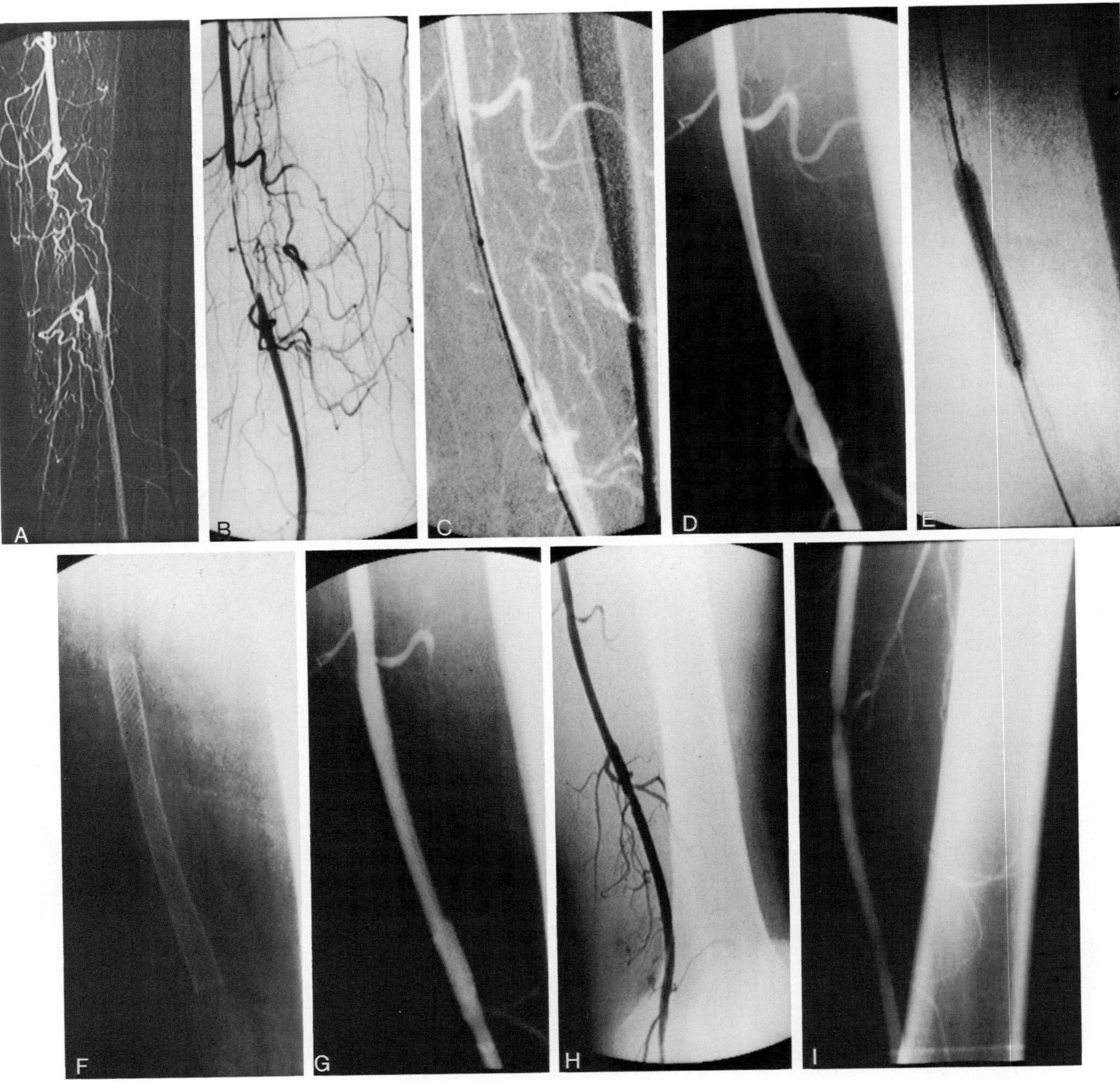

FIGURE 20–22. Stent for SFA occlusion that is refractory to PTA alone. *A*, Selective angiogram showing SFA occlusion and reconstitution by collaterals. *B*, Arteriogram following recanalization and PTA shows effect of marked elastic recoil in this very firm occlusion of the SFA. *C*, Road map during WallStent deployment. *D*, Angiogram immediately following deployment shows persistent effect of elastic recoil. *E*, Balloon expansion inside WallStent. *F*, Final appearance of WallStent. *G* and *H*, Selective SFA angiogram immediately following PTA inside of stent shows a widely patent lumen and a popliteal artery stenosis distally. *I*, Angiogram at 6 months shows a thin neointima (*thin radiolucent line*) within stent and outside contrast column. Most important, there is a stenosis (most likely due to intimal hyperplasia) immediately above the stented segment.

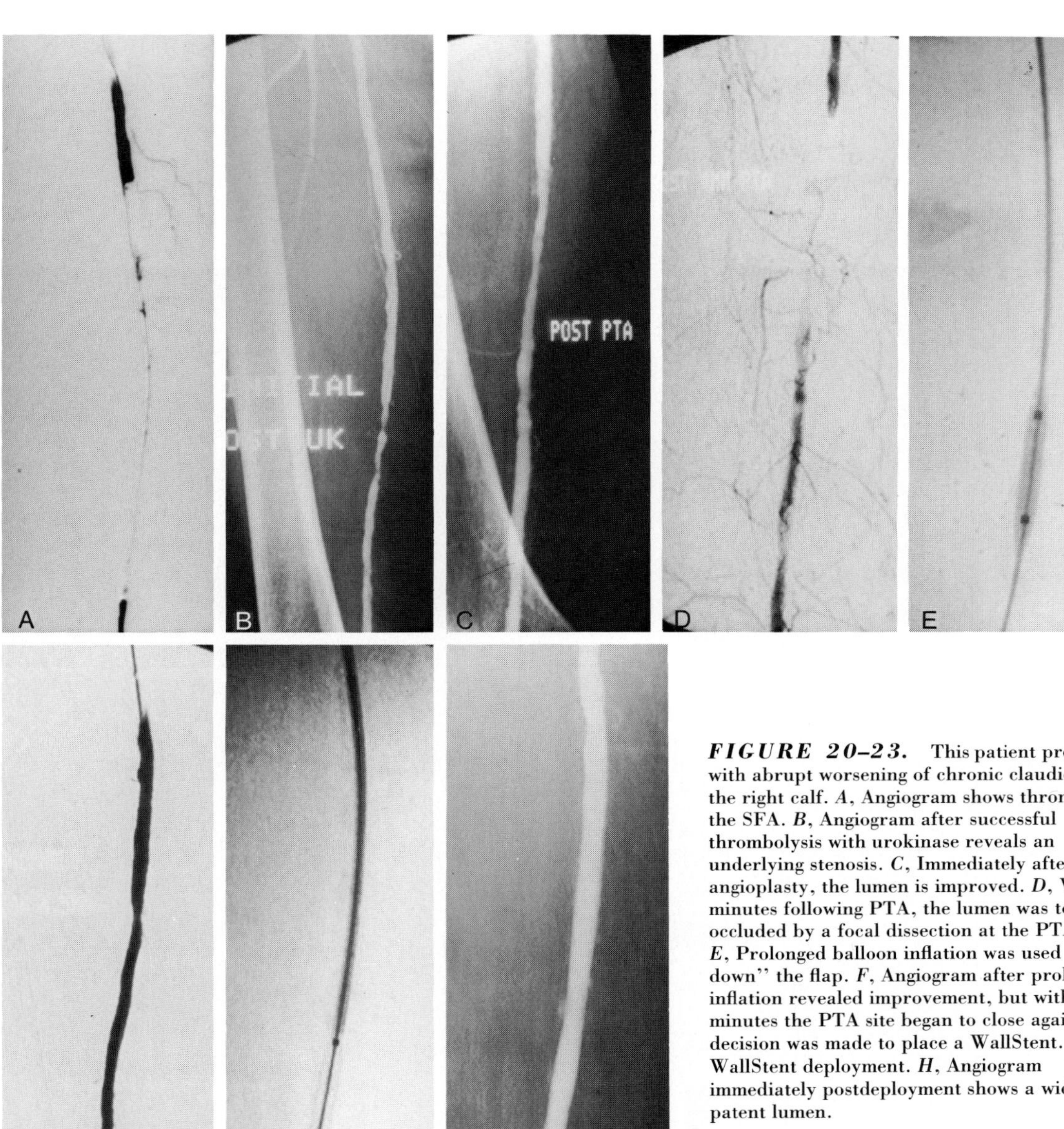

FIGURE 20–23. This patient presented with abrupt worsening of chronic claudication in the right calf. *A*, Angiogram shows thrombosis of the SFA. *B*, Angiogram after successful thrombolysis with urokinase reveals an underlying stenosis. *C*, Immediately after angioplasty, the lumen is improved. *D*, Within 5 minutes following PTA, the lumen was totally occluded by a focal dissection at the PTA site. *E*, Prolonged balloon inflation was used to "tack down" the flap. *F*, Angiogram after prolonged inflation revealed improvement, but within minutes the PTA site began to close again. A decision was made to place a WallStent. *G*, WallStent deployment. *H*, Angiogram immediately postdeployment shows a widely patent lumen.

Renal Artery Disease

Percutaneous transluminal renal angioplasty (PTRA) is covered in Chapter 107. PTRA is the treatment of choice for fibromuscular dysplasia and nonostial atherosclerotic renal artery stenoses. Recurrent stenoses are about twice as frequent in the atherosclerotic group (one third of patients) as in the fibromuscular group. The situation is not as favorable for ostial renal artery lesions (true aortic renal artery ostial plaque), in which acceptable immediate anatomic results of PTRA are achieved in less than half the cases and in which lasting benefit for control of hypertension occurs in 0 to 24 per cent.[63] In general, surgical bypass grafting is the procedure of choice in such patients. In addition, PTA-induced dissection can be a problem in the renal arteries, as it is in the coronaries and the iliacs.

Two of the most significant problems associated with the management of renal artery stenosis and renovascular hypertension are post-PTRA restenosis and aortic renal ostial atheromatous stenoses, which are associated with elastic recoil and are generally refractory to PTRA. Stent trials have been undertaken to attempt to address these problems, utilizing the Palmaz BEIS,[64] the WallStent,[65] and the Strecker stent.[66] Stents have shown benefit in patients who had poor results from conventional PTRA for ostial atheroma (Fig. 20–24). However, restenosis after stenting has occurred in more than 43 per cent with the Palmaz stent. The reported experience with the Strecker and WallStents is too small at this writing to assess the frequency of restenosis with these devices. In addition, a specific renal artery WallStent is now in development.

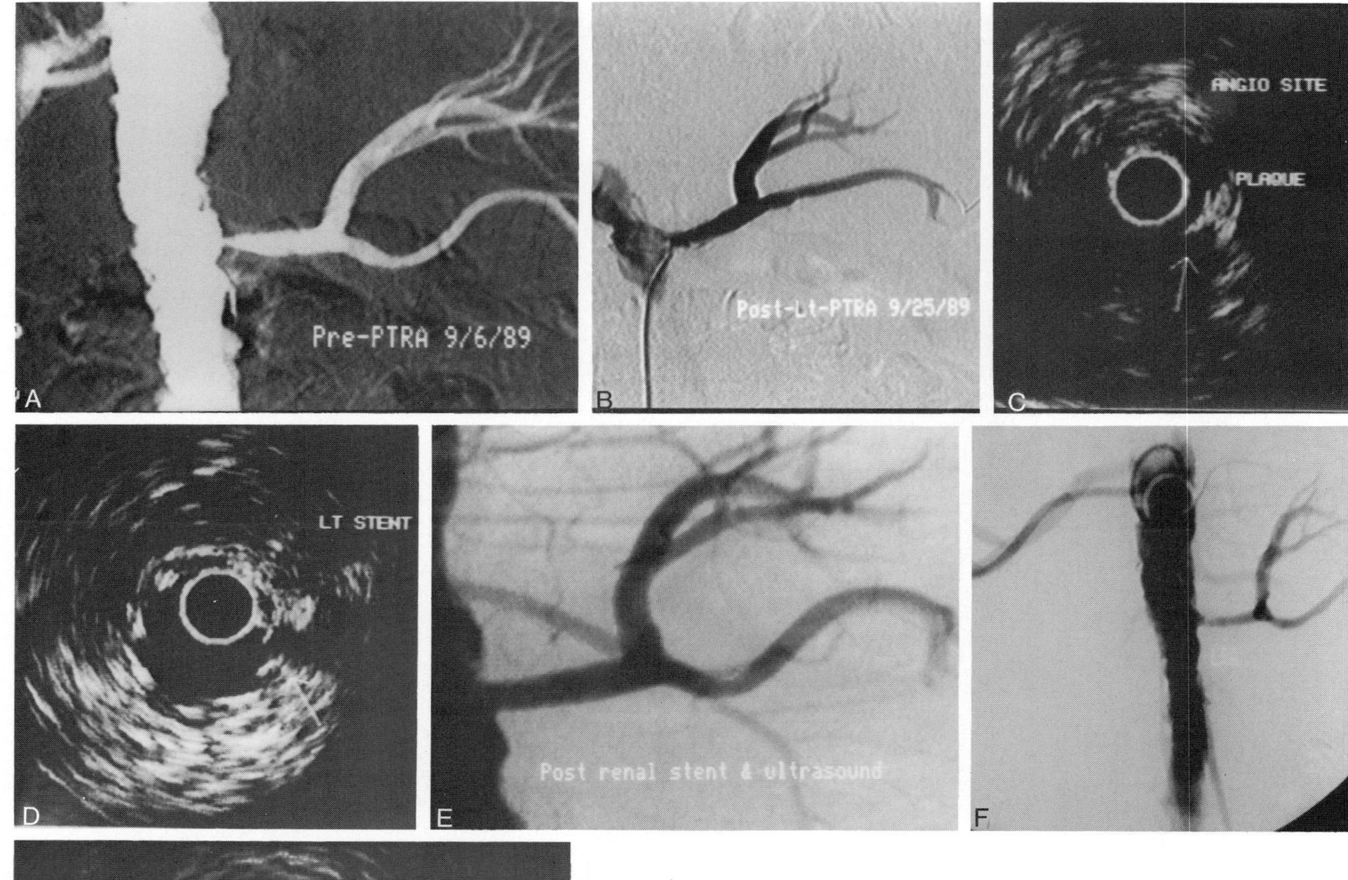

FIGURE 20–24. Use of a Palmaz stent for ostial renal artery stenosis in a patient with hypertension. *A*, Aortogram reveals extensive atheroma with an ostial left renal artery stenosis. *B*, Angiogram immediately following PTA shows improvement. *C*, IVUS at the left renal ostium shows extensive plaque surrounding the probe. *D*, IVUS after stent deployment shows much improvement in the lumen. Also seen are the brightly echogenic stent struts. *E*, Aortogram immediately following stent procedure shows marked improvement. *F*, Patient experienced blood pressure improvement, which was stable at the time of this 18-month follow-up arteriogram. *G*, IVUS at time of 18-month arteriogram shows homogeneous echoes of the thin neointima (*outside the probe*).

Two exciting areas of stent application that have been recently added to our experience include the management of post-PTRA dissection (Fig. 20–25) and acute renal artery closure due to spontaneous dissection of the aorta (Fig. 20–26). The Palmaz stent has proved extremely effective in both of these situations in limited case experience.

Clearly, experience with renal artery stents is still preliminary. Stents should be reserved for clinical studies and for situations in which conventional options are precluded by other factors. In all cases, stents should be deployed only in a proximal position that will avoid limiting the patient's surgical options in the event of a failure.

Malignant Superior Vena Cava Syndromes

A variety of additional applications of stents have extended the bounds of percutaneous therapy. These include stenting of stenoses in dialysis access fistulae,[67] stenting of the central veins in dialysis fistula patients, stenting of the superior and inferior vena cavae in patients with benign conditions, and finally, stenting for malignant vena cava syndromes. Only the last situation is described here.

Benign and malignant venous stenoses occur in both the superior vena cava (SVC) and the inferior vena cava (IVC). The SVC is involved much more commonly and therefore will comprise most of this discussion. The IVC will be mentioned briefly later. SVC obstruction produces superior vena cava syndrome. This consists of (1) facial and upper extremity swelling, edema, and cyanosis, (2) the appearance of superficial thoracic venous collaterals on physical examination, (3) neck swelling, (4) headache, and (5) conjunctival injection. Sometimes the above symptoms are accompanied by orthopnea and a feeling of impending doom. Patients with the most severe symptoms are generally miserable and frightened.

Iatrogenic SVC syndrome is most prominent among the offending etiologies. Of true de novo cases of SVC syndrome, 80 per cent are malignant in origin and 20 per cent are benign. Benign SVC syndrome, which is not the major topic considered here, may be due to histoplasmosis or other fungal disorder, radiation therapy, idiopathic fi-

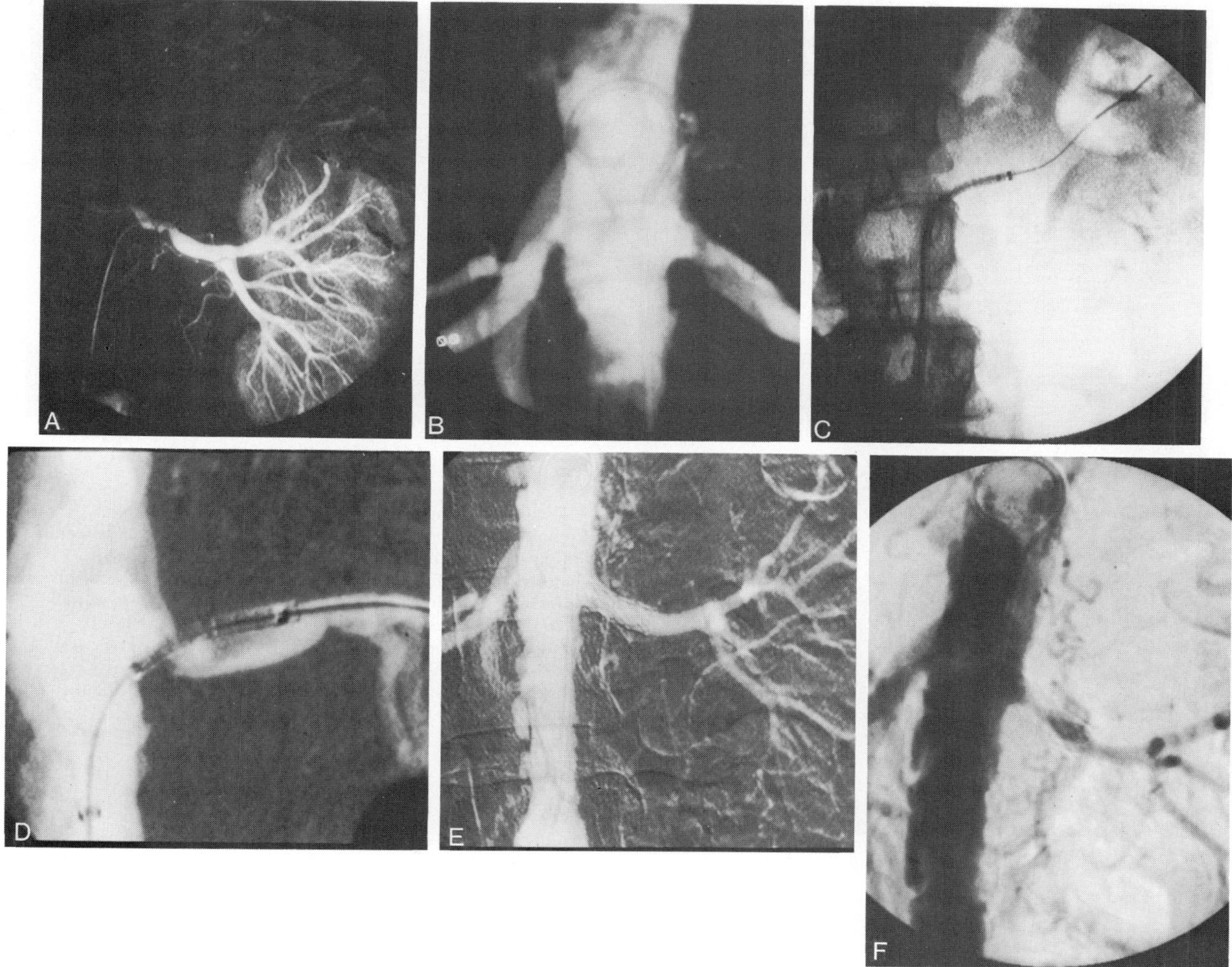

FIGURE 20–25. Use of the Palmaz stent for renal angioplasty–related dissection. *A*, Left renal artery stenosis. *B*, Left renal artery dissection following PTA. *C*, Guiding catheter across dissected segment contains balloon-mounted stent. *D*, Close-up of aortic injection at time of stent positioning for deployment. *E*, After deployment the aortogram shows a widely patent left renal artery lumen. *F*, At 6 months, restenosis (most likely due to intimal hyperplasia) has caused recurrent hypertension and this angiographic picture.

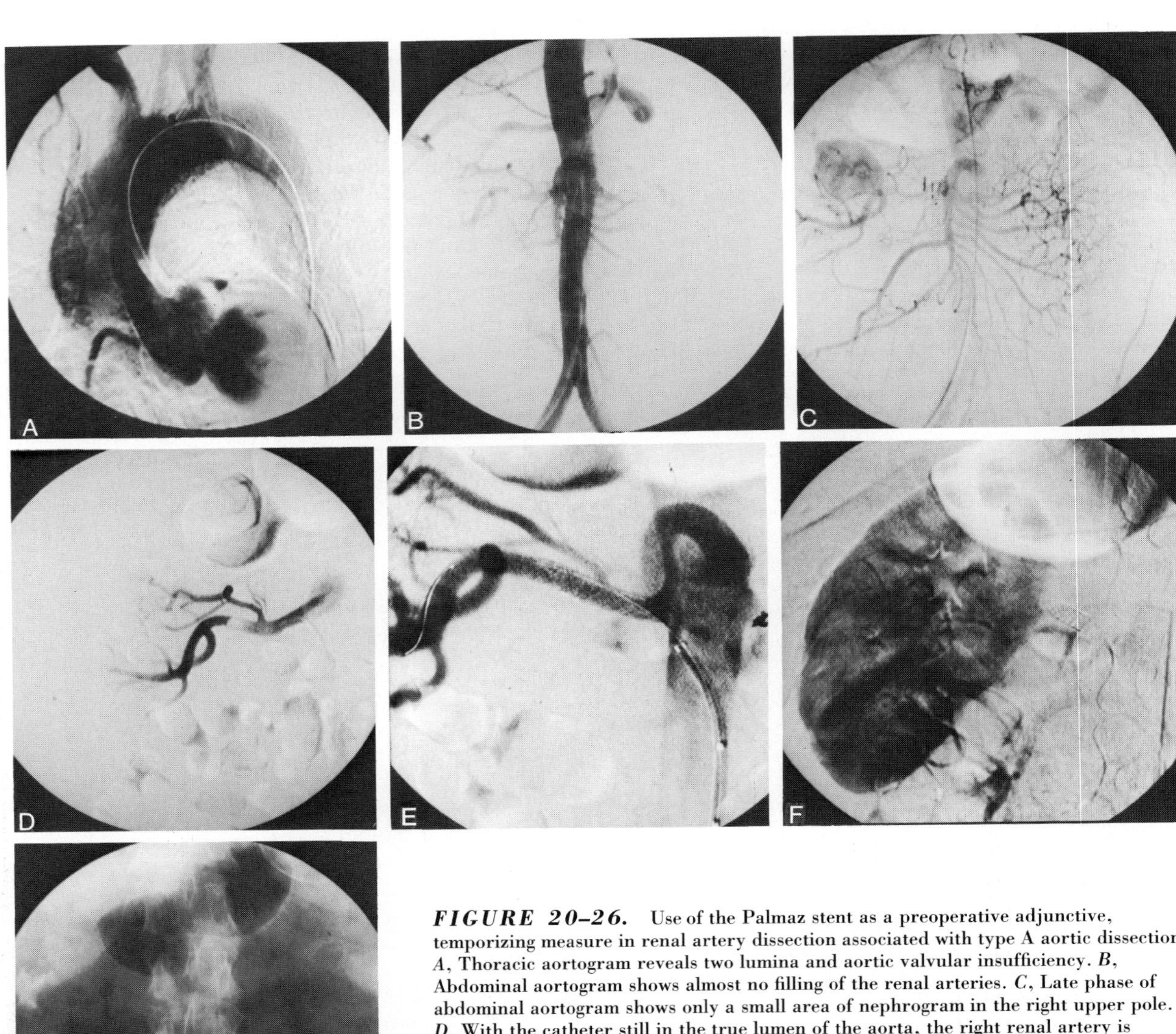

FIGURE 20–26. Use of the Palmaz stent as a preoperative adjunctive, temporizing measure in renal artery dissection associated with type A aortic dissection. *A*, Thoracic aortogram reveals two lumina and aortic valvular insufficiency. *B*, Abdominal aortogram shows almost no filling of the renal arteries. *C*, Late phase of abdominal aortogram shows only a small area of nephrogram in the right upper pole. *D*, With the catheter still in the true lumen of the aorta, the right renal artery is selected. *E*, After placement of two Palmaz stents, flow in the right renal artery is normal. *F*, Normal nephrogram following selective injection into the right renal artery. *G*, Calyceal filling confirms that the right kidney is now functioning as the patient is taken to the operating room for repair of aortic dissection.

brosing mediastinitis, Behçet's syndrome, or extrinsic compression by neighboring structures. In the past, ascending aortic aneurysm due to luetic aortitis was the most common cause of benign SVC syndrome in the United States.

Malignant SVC syndrome is most often due to bronchogenic carcinoma. It may also be due to lymphoma, metastatic disease, or, rarely, to direct extension of neoplasm from the right atrium into the SVC or from the pericardium to the SVC (e.g., angiosarcoma). In the past, radiation and chemotherapy for the underlying malignant obstruction have been the mainstays of treatment for malignant SVC syndrome. However, several limitations of these approaches must be mentioned. First, not all tumors are radiosensitive. Next, chemotherapy may be successful in some cases, but even those require a finite response time. Neither of these approaches is particularly well suited to patients who have the most severe symptoms of SVC syndrome. The final problem, which is the one that originally gave interventional radiologists a role in the management of these patients, is that even in patients who respond to chemotherapy or radiation, there are maximum dosage limits.

Angioplasty was used initially in patients who had already reached or exceeded their dose limits of radiation or chemotherapy. Unfortunately, despite sometimes dramatic initial responses, patients typically presented with recurrence of the syndrome within 2 to 3 weeks. This is not surprising, since elastic recoil of the tumor mass should be expected. Vessels narrowed by neoplasm are not amenable to the same pathophysiologic responses to angioplasty as those narrowed by atherosclerotic plaque.

Surgical bypass of the obstructed SVC has merit in many cases of benign disease. However, malignancy and postirradiation fibrosis with SVC obstruction are often associated with increased surgical risk and diminishing benefits. A few innovative surgical methods have been reported in the past 10 years, but as a rule, all surgical approaches to malignant SVC syndrome have too high a risk : benefit ratio.

Expandable metallic stents came into use because of the limitations of surgical, radiotherapeutic, and combined treatments of malignant (and benign) SVC syndrome. At first, they were employed only in situations in which radiation and chemotherapy doses had been maximized and angioplasty had failed. Now they are increasingly being employed as a first-line approach to SVC syndrome. Virtually all of the suitable metallic stent types have been employed. Some of the results of the Gianturco-Rösch expandable Z stents, Palmaz balloon-expandable intraluminal stents, and the WallStent endoprostheses are presented later.

Of 22 patients treated with Z stents for SVC syndrome by Rösch and colleagues, 20 had malignant obstruction.[68] All had advanced SVC syndrome and had received maximum radiation. Because of complete obstruction with thrombosis, urokinase (UK) thrombolysis was used adjunctively to establish a channel in five of the patients. The same authors have also reported use of adjunctive urokinase in a total of 13 patients with SVC syndrome.[69] Heparin anticoagulation was followed by long-term anticoagulation with warfarin in each case. Stent deployment was followed by balloon expansion as a rule. Patients experienced chest pain during balloon expansion. There was one case of intraprocedural thrombosis that resolved with urokinase. All patients experienced relief of their SVC syndrome, with most of the severe symptoms resolving within 24 hours, and truncal and upper extremity edema resolving by 2 to 3 days. Follow-up radiographs at 2 months showed continued expansion of the stents to near maximum diameters. Seventeen patients died 1 to 11 months after stent placement (median, 5.2 months). Only one had recurrence of the SVC syndrome, and he had stopped taking warfarin. After thrombolysis, intravascular biopsy of remaining masses showed ingrowth of malignant tumor. At the time of the report, the remaining patients were alive without recurrent symptoms.

Of 25 patients treated with Z stents for SVC syndrome and other central venous obstructions by Irving and colleagues, 17 SVC syndromes were due to malignancy (lung carcinoma, 15; malignant thymoma, 1; lymphoma, 1) that was recurrent after maximum radiation or chemotherapy.[70] Stent sizes ranged from 15 to 35 mm in diameter. Thirteen patients died from 10 days to 3 months after treatment without recurrence of SVC syndrome. Another 3 patients experienced relief of symptoms and were still alive 7 to 25 months after treatment at the time of the report. One patient died 3 days after treatment.

In 18 patients treated by Zollikofer and colleagues with WallStents for a variety of venous stenoses, five stenoses were due to malignancy.[67] Two were obstructions of the SVC. Stents from 10 to 14 mm in diameter were used. One additional patient had a malignant obstruction of the IVC (25 mm diameter stents were used). The iliac veins and upper extremity veins were involved in the remainder. Three died 6 weeks to 9 months after treatment without recurrent symptoms. The patient with malignant IVC obstruction was still asymptomatic, but the one with upper extremity venous obstruction due to metastatic disease had recurrent stenosis at the time of this report.

Elson and colleagues reported on the use of Palmaz BEIS in the management of seven patients who had vena caval and central venous obstructions, all of which failed to respond satisfactorily to balloon PTA.[71] Six obstructions (SVC, 5; IVC, 1) were due to malignancy, although in two patients the occlusion occurred remotely in time after irradiation, and recurrence of tumor could not be established at the time of presentation. Adjunctive UK thrombolysis was necessary in five of the patients. All patients experienced relief of symptoms. The patient with IVC obstruction underwent placement of several stents at the bifurcation in a Y configuration. The left iliac portion thrombosed owing to two-point compression between the common iliac artery and the spine. The occlusion caused only minimal symptom persistence in the left lower extremity.

Dake and colleagues reported the use of metallic stents in the management of 98 patients with venous occlusive disease.[72] Although 25 of these were malignant SVC obstructions, thus far details in regard to the subgroup are lacking. For instance, the data have not been separated for outcome according to underlying disease (benign vs. malignant), nor have they been analyzed according to which type of stent was placed. These investigators also used an oral anticoagulant regimen. Similarly, Vereycken and colleagues reported on 35 patients who underwent stent placement for malignant obstruction of the SVC (n = 20) and

IVC (n = 15).[73] Eighteen patients experienced complete relief of symptoms, but one of these developed a late recurrence. Seventeen experienced improvement. Complications occurred in 23 per cent. The specific stents used in this study were not mentioned. Figure 20–27 depicts a case in which metallic stents were used to manage a malignant obstruction of the SVC.

Two final comments must be made in regard to the use of stents in patients with malignant superior vena cava syndrome. First, of all the patients the author has treated in his career, no other group is as grateful as those with successfully stented malignant SVC obstructions. The nearly immediate and complete relief of symptoms that derives from successful stenting is dramatic. Second, in the vast majority of cases, the patency that derives from successful stenting lasts for the remainder of the patient's lifetime. Therefore, the goal of palliation is achieved.

Malignant obstruction of the IVC,[73] although much less commonly encountered than SVC obstruction, can also be managed by stenting, as shown in Figure 20–28.

LASERS

Lasers came and went between the last edition of this textbook and the current one. The initial hope was that lasers would improve the recanalization success of occlusions not satisfactorily treated with current endovascular techniques and would lead to better long-term patency of a successfully recanalized artery. The ability to apply an enormous amount of energy to a precise spot within a vessel should eventually prove useful. Unfortunately, none of the laser devices utilized so far have offered any advantage over the results of balloon PTA using current technologies (steerable guidewires, lytic therapy, DSA, roadmapping, low-profile balloon catheters) to justify their great

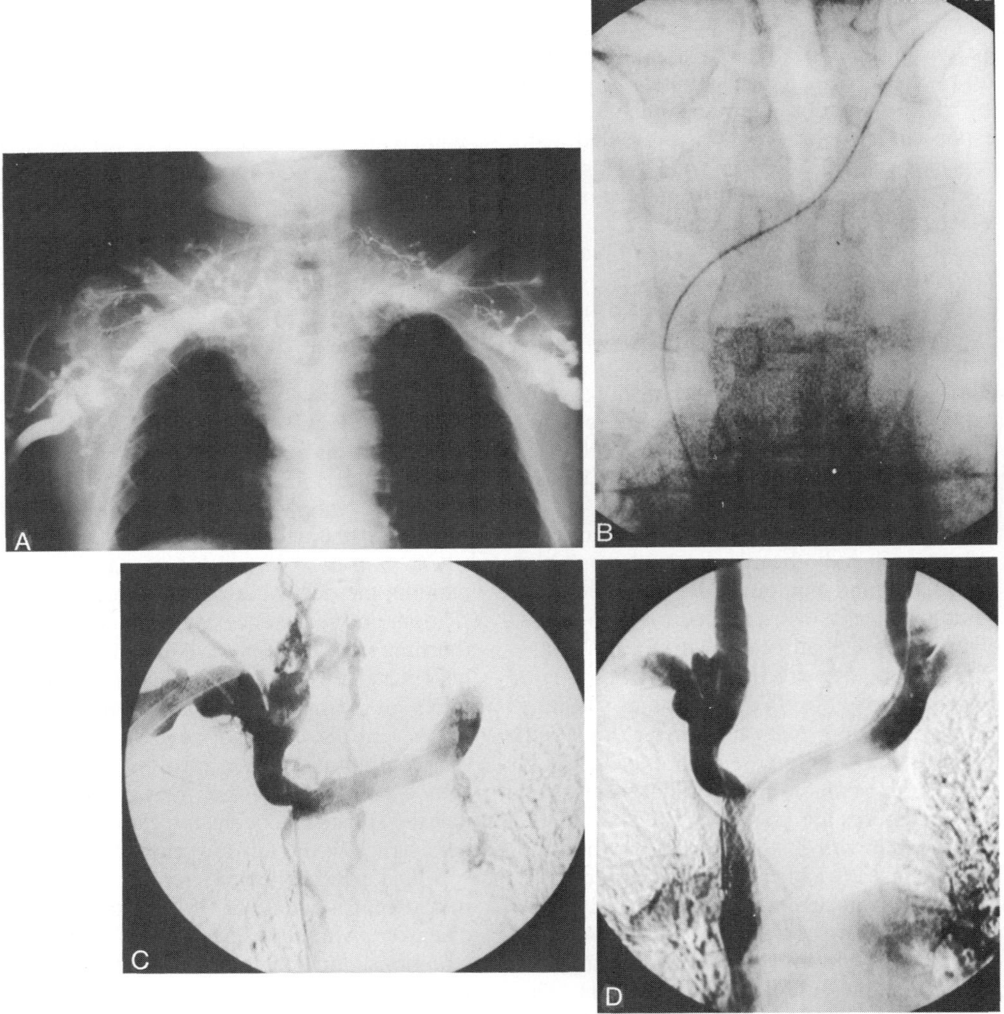

FIGURE 20–27. Stents for malignant superior vena cava obstruction. This patient had marked facial swelling, cyanosis, orthopnea, and superficial venous collaterals. *A*, Superior venacavogram (bilateral upper extremity injections) shows extensive occlusion involving not only the superior vena cava but also both brachiocephalic veins. *B*, Two multi-sidehole infusion devices are placed for simultaneous urokinase thrombolysis of both brachiocephalic veins and the superior vena cava. *C*, Venogram after thrombolysis (following day) shows widely patent brachiocephalic veins and severely stenotic superior vena cava (due to malignant obstruction). *D*, Injection following stent placement shows that superior vena cava patency has been restored.

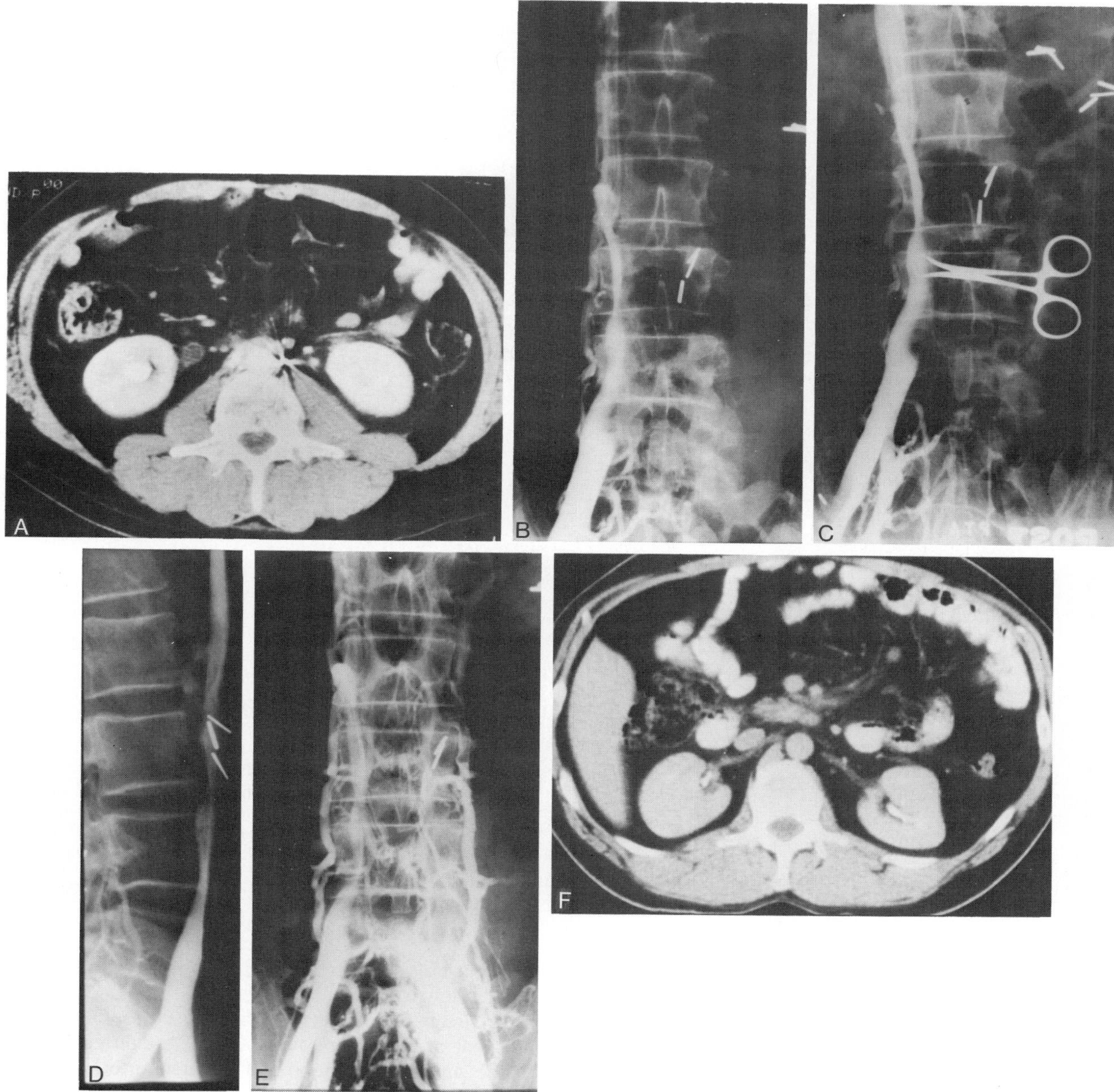

FIGURE 20–28. Use of the Palmaz stent in an inferior vena cava obstruction. This 44-year-old man had a history of Hodgkin's lymphoma and abdominopelvic irradiation. He presented with scrotal and penile swelling, lower extremity edema, and pain. *A*, Computed tomography (CT) shows a very small mantle of tissue around the aorta and an almost imperceptible inferior vena cava. *B*, Inferior venacavogram shows severely narrowed lumen. *C* and *D*, After angioplasty the lumen is minimally improved. There was no clinical improvement. *E*, Bilateral femoral venous injections on the day of stent placement show extensive ascending lumbar and epidural venous collaterals. *F*, CT strongly suggests that the inferior vena cava above the level of the renal veins is normal and that the only segment warranting treatment is infrarenal.

Illustration continued on following page

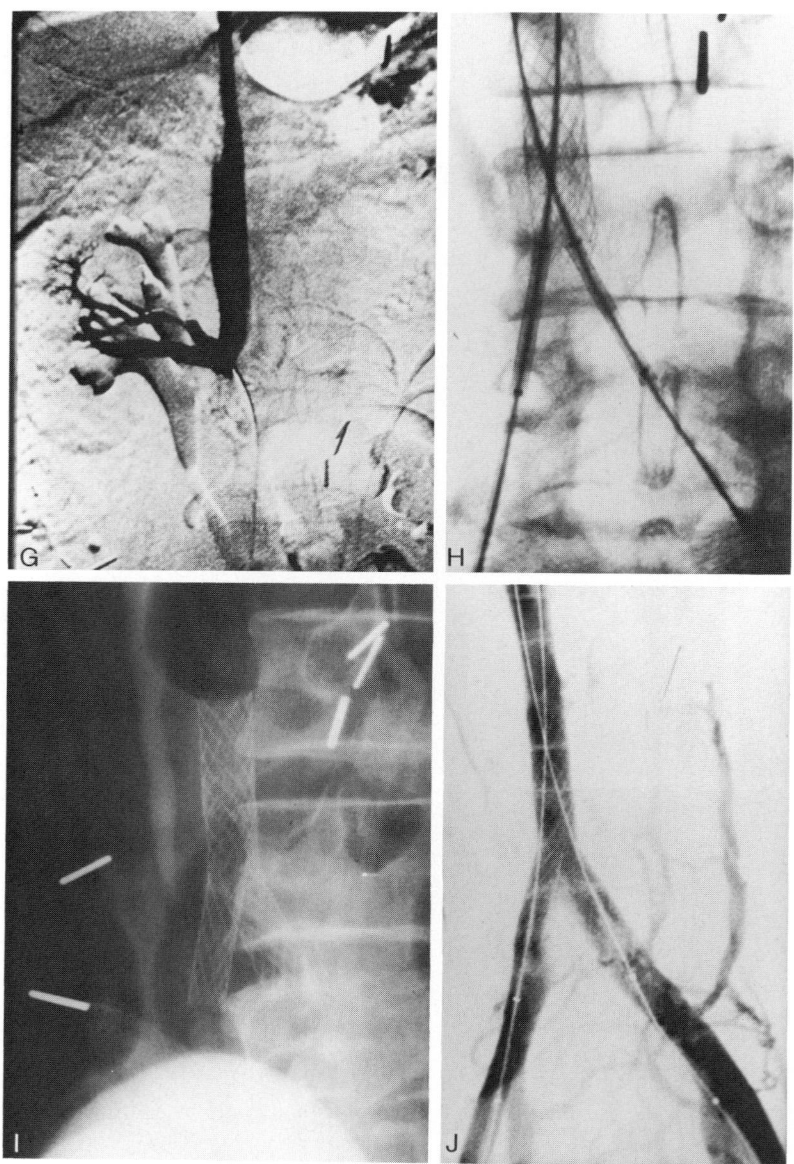

FIGURE 20–28 Continued *G*, Selective right renal vein injection shows patency of renal vein and suprarenal inferior vena cava. *H* and *I*, Stent deployment in distal inferior vena cava and both common iliac veins. *J*, Inferior venacavogram following stent deployment.

expense. It will not be surprising if further development of new laser technologies does eventually lead to a clinically useful device. At the present writing, however, the currently available laser systems are uniformly disappointing and have no place in the endovascular management of peripheral arterial occlusions. They have therefore not been considered in this chapter.

SUMMARY

PTA is an established, safe, and effective method of revascularization that is useful in a variety of clinical conditions. The safety and efficacy of PTA have been improved through advances in imaging, catheter and guidewire technology, and pharmacologic adjuncts. Conventional guidewire and catheter methods have resulted in technical success rates of recanalization that are equal to or greater than those of sophisticated recanalization devices and have a much lower cost.

Directional atherectomy has proved useful in the management of eccentric lesions and PTA-induced dissections of the superficial femoral and popliteal arteries as well as in the management of femoropopliteal graft anastomoses narrowed by intimal hyperplasia. The role of directional atherectomy and other atherectomy devices in primary atherosclerotic lesions below the inguinal ligament is still uncertain.

Initial technical, hemodynamic, and clinical successes in iliac angioplasty have been improved by the addition of stents for the management of elastic recoil, refractory eccentric lesions, and PTA-induced dissections. Stents have also enhanced the interventionalist's ability to treat chronic iliac artery occlusions and some category 3 and category 4 aortoiliac bifurcation lesions percutaneously. Stents have improved the immediate results of renal angioplasty, particularly in patients with ostial lesions, and of superficial femoral artery angioplasty, particularly when occlusions or PTA-related dissections are involved. On the other hand, long-term patency rates following stenting in the renal and superficial femoral arteries thus far do not appear to be improved over those of angioplasty alone.

Stents have proved to be an important adjunct in the management of malignant superior vena cava syndrome, particularly in patients whose dosage limits for chemotherapy and irradiation have been reached. Stents provide a much more durable effect than PTA under these circumstances and therefore almost always succeed in achieving lifelong palliation.

Intimal hyperplasia, the process responsible for the majority of restenosis at prior PTA sites, remains the target of investigative efforts. Technical strategies have failed to prevent intimal hyperplasia. Almost all drug regimens attempted have failed, but some have still been inadequately tested. Drugs that interfere with platelet adhesion or thrombus propagation at the angioplasty site may represent an important new class of agents for the prevention of intimal hyperplasia. Local delivery of drugs or oligonucleotides with the potential to inhibit smooth muscle cell growth or migration or to inhibit the elaboration of matrix by smooth muscle cells is a focus of current investigation. Local infusion balloons and biodegradable or bioresorbable stents are among the delivery systems being developed.

All of the newer alternatives in the endovascular management of arterial occlusions are more costly than balloon angioplasty. The cost effectiveness of the application of these devices has not been rigorously evaluated. Increasing cost controls in the future will clearly play a major role in determining which technologies ultimately reach clinical application in the management of the patient who has symptomatic peripheral vascular disease.

References

1. Standards of Practice Committee of the Society of Cardiovascular and Interventional Radiology: Guidelines for percutaneous transluminal angioplasty, formulated by the Standards of Practice Committee of the Society of Cardiovascular and Interventional Radiology. J Vasc Interv Radiol 1:5, 1990.
2. McLean GK: Percutaneous peripheral atherectomy. J Vasc Interv Radiol (In press).
3. Simpson JB, Zimmerman JJ, Selmon RM, et al: Transluminal atherectomy: Initial clinical results in 27 patients. Circulation 74 (Suppl. II):II-203, 1986.
4. Wholey MH, Jarmolowski CR: New reperfusion devices: The Kensey catheter, the atherolytic reperfusion wire device, and the transluminal extraction catheter. Radiology 172:947, 1989.
5. Wholey MH, Jarmolowski CR, Fein D, et al: Multicenter trial with the transluminal endarterectomy catheter in 200 patients with peripheral vascular occlusive disease. Radiology 173(P):267, 1989.
6. Fischell TA, Fischell RE, White RI, et al: In-vivo results using a new pullback atherectomy catheter (PAC). Cathet Cardiovasc Diagn 21(4):287, 1990.
7. Ahn SS, Auth D, Marcus DR, et al: Removal of focal atheromatous lesions by angioscopically guided high-speed rotary atherectomy. J Vasc Surg 7(2):292, 1988.
8. Ahn SS: The rotablator—High-speed rotary atherectomy: Indications, technique, results and complications. *In* Moore WS, Ahn SS (eds): Endovascular Surgery. Philadelphia, WB Saunders, 1989, pp 327–335.
9. Kensey RR, Nash JE, Abrahams C, et al: Recanalization of obstructed arteries with a flexible rotating tip catheter. Radiology 165(2):387, 1987.
10. Coleman CC, Posalaky IP, Robinson JD, et al: Atheroablation with the Kensey catheter: A pathologic study. Radiology 170:391, 1989.
11. Snyder SO, Wheeler JR, Overlie PA, et al: Kensey catheter, a mechanical recanalization device: Use in 113 patients with 157 lesions in the peripheral circulation. Radiology 177:203, 1990.
12. Desbrosses D, Petit H, Torres E, et al: Percutaneous atherectomy with the Kensey catheter: Early and midterm results in femoropopliteal occlusions unsuitable for conventional angioplasty. Ann Vasc Surg 4(6):550, 1990.
13. Dyet JF: High speed rotational angioplasty in occluded peripheral arteries. J Interv Radiol 7:1, 1992.
14. Triller J, Do DD, Maddern G, et al: Femoropopliteal artery occlusion: clinical experience with the Kensey catheter. Radiology 182:257, 1992.
15. Cull DL, Feinberg RL, Wheeler JR, et al: Experience with laser-assisted balloon angioplasty and a rotary angioplasty instrument: Lessons learned. J Vasc Surg 14(3):332, 1991.
16. Morgenstern BR, Getrajdman GI, Laffey KJ, et al: Total occlusions of the femoropopliteal artery: High technical success rate of conventional balloon angioplasty. Radiology 172:937, 1989.
17. Capek P, McLean GK, Berowitz HD: Femoropopliteal angioplasty: Factors influencing long-term success. Circulation 83 (Suppl. I):I-70, 1991.
18. Johnston KW: Femoral and popliteal arteries: Reanalysis of results of balloon angioplasty. Radiology 183:767, 1992.
19. Lammer J, Pilger E, Karnel F, et al: Laser angioplasty: Results of a prospective multicenter study at 3-year follow-up. Radiology 178:335, 1991.
20. Spies JB, LeQuire MH, Brantley SD, et al: Comparison of balloon angioplasty and laser thermal angioplasty in the treatment of femoropopliteal atherosclerotic disease: Initial results of a prospective randomized trial. Work in progress. J Vasc Interv Radiol 1:39, 1990.
21. Nordstrom LA, Castañeda-Zúñiga WR, Von Seggern KB: Peripheral arterial obstructions: Analysis of patency 1 year after laser-assisted transluminal angioplasty. Radiology 181:515, 1991.
22. Belli A-M, Cumberland DC, Procter AE, Welsh C: Follow-up of conventional angioplasty versus laser thermal angioplasty for total femoropopliteal artery occlusions: Results of a randomized trial. J Vasc Interv Radiol 2:485, 1991.
23. Odink HF, de Valois HC, Eikelboom BC: Femoropopliteal arterial occlusions: Laser-assisted versus conventional percutaneous transluminal angioplasty. Radiology 181:61, 1991.
24. Dorros G, Lyer S, Lewin R, et al: Angiographic follow-up and clinical outcome of 126 patients after percutaneous directional atherectomy (Simpson AtheroCath) for occlusive peripheral vascular disease. Cathet Cardiovasc Diagn 22:79, 1991.
25. Graor RA, Whitlow P: Directional atherectomy for peripheral vascular disease: Two year patency and factors influencing patency. J Am Coll Cardiol 17(2):106A, 1991.
26. Katzen BT, Becker GJ, Benenati JF, et al: Long-term follow-up of directional atherectomy in the femoral and popliteal arteries. J Vasc Interv Radiol 3:38, 1992.
27. Kim D, Gianturco LE, Porter DH, et al: Peripheral directional atherectomy: 4-year experience. Radiology 183:773, 1992.
28. VonPolnitz A, Nerlich A, Berger H, et al: Percutaneous peripheral atherectomy: Angiographic and clinical follow-up of 60 patients. J Am Coll Cardiol 15(3):682, 1990.
29. Jarmolowski CR, Wholey MH, Lim CL: Efficacy of transluminal endarterectomy catheter atherectomy in peripheral vascular disease. J Vasc Interv Radiol 3:39, 1992.
30. Dorros G, Lyer S, Zaitoun R: Acute angiographic and clinical outcome of high speed percutaneous rotational atherectomy (Rotablator). Cathet Cardiovasc Diagn 22:157, 1991.
31. Ginsburg R, Jenkins N, Wright A, et al: Transluminal rotational atherectomy: Clinical experience in 20 patients. Circulation 78 (Suppl. II):II-4, 1988.
32. Zacca NM, Raizner AE, Noon JP: Treatment of symptomatic peripheral atherosclerotic disease with a rotational atherectomy device. Am J Cardiol 63:77, 1989.
33. Gray JR, Dolmatch BL, Buick MK: Directional atherectomy treatment for hemodialysis access: Early results. J Vasc Interv Radiol 3:497, 1992.
34. Zemel G, Katzen BT, Dake MD, et al: Directional atherectomy in the treatment of stenotic dialysis access fistulas. J Vasc Interv Radiol 1:35, 1990.

35. Dotter CT, Judkins MP: Transluminal treatment of arteriosclerotic obstructions: Description of a new technique and a preliminary report of its application. Circulation 30:654, 1964.
36. Dotter CT: Transluminally-placed coilspring endarterial tube grafts: Long-term patency in canine popliteal artery. Invest Radiol 4:327, 1969.
37. Dotter CT, Bluschmann RW, McKinney MK, Rosch J: Transluminally expandable nitinol coil stent grafting: Preliminary report. Radiology 147:259, 1983.
38. Cragg A, Lund G, Rysavy J, et al: Nonsurgical placement of arterial endoprosthesis: A new technique using nitinol wire. Radiology 147:261, 1983.
39. Palmaz JC, Richter GM, Noeldge G, et al: Intraluminal stents in atherosclerotic iliac artery stenosis: Preliminary report of a multicenter study. Radiology 168:727, 1988.
40. Strecker EP: Flexible, balloon expandable percutaneously insertable vascular prosthesis: Experimental and clinical results. Radiology 169:388, 1988.
41. Muhlstein JB, Quigley PJ, Mikat EM, et al: Percutaneous removal of endovascular stents: Initial experimental results. Circulation 80 (Suppl. II):II-259, 1989.
42. Duprat G Jr, Wright KC, Charnsangavej C, et al: Flexible balloon-expanded stent for small vessels. Radiology 162:276, 1987.
43. Rabkin JE, Matevosov AL, Gothman LN: Roentgenovascular surgery. *In* Moscow, Medicine, 1987, pp 176–198.
44. Rousseau H, Puel J, Joffre F, et al: Self-expanding endovascular prosthesis: An experimental study. Radiology 164:709, 1987.
45. Ring EJ, Lake JR, Roberts JP, et al: Percutaneous intrahepatic portosystemic shunts to control variceal bleeding prior to liver transplantation. Ann Intern Med 166:304, 1992.
46. Charnsangavej C, Carrasco CH, Wallace S, et al: Stenosis of the vena cava: Preliminary assessment of treatment with expandable metallic stents. Radiology 161:295, 1986.
47. Fallone BG, Wallace S, Gianturco C: Elastic characteristics of the self-expanding metallic stents. Invest Radiol 23:370, 1988.
48. Uchida BP, Putman JS, Rosch J: Modifications of Gianturco expandable wire stents. Am J Roentgenol 150:1185, 1988.
49. Tegtmeyer CJ, Harwell GD, Selby JB, et al: Results and complications of angioplasty in aortoiliac disease. Circulation 83 (Suppl. I):I-53, 1991.
50. Johnston KW: Iliac arteries: Reanalysis of results of balloon angioplasty. Radiology 186:207, 1993.
51. Bonn J, Gardiner B, Shapiro M, et al: Palmaz vascular stent: Initial clinical experience. Radiology 174:741, 1990.
52. Richter GM, Roeren TK, Noeldge G, et al: Balloon-expandable stent placement versus PTA in iliac artery stenoses and occlusions: Long-term results of a randomized trial. J Vasc Interv Radiol 3(1):9, 1992.
53. Becker GJ, Palmaz JC, Rees CR, et al: Angioplasty-induced dissections in human iliac arteries: Management with Palmaz balloon-expandable intraluminal stents. Radiology 176:31, 1990.
54. Rees CR, Palmaz JC, Garcia O, et al: Angioplasty and stenting of completely occluded iliac arteries. Radiology 172:953, 1989.
55. Palmaz J, Laborde J, Rivera F, et al: Stenting of the iliac arteries with the Palmaz stent: Experience from a multicenter trial. Cardiovasc Intervent Radiol 15:291, 1992.
56. Long AL, Page PE, Raynaud AC, et al: Percutaneous iliac artery stent: Angiographic long-term follow-up. Radiology 180:771, 1991.
57. Vorwerk D, Günther R: Stent placement in iliac arterial lesions: Three years of clinical experience with the Wallstent. Cardiovasc Intervent Radiol 15:285, 1992.
58. Liermann D, Strecker E, Peters J: The Strecker stent: Indications and results in iliac and femoropopliteal arteries. Cardiovasc Intervent Radiol 15:298, 1992.
59. Palmaz JC, Encarnacion C, Garcia OJ, et al: Aortic bifurcation stenosis: Treatment with intravascular stents. J Vasc Interv Radiol 2:319, 1991.
60. Sapoval M, Long A, Raynaud A, et al: Femoropopliteal stent placement: Long-term results. Radiology 184:833, 1992.
61. Do DD, Triller J, Walpoth BH, et al: A comparison study of self-expandable stents vs balloon angioplasty alone in femoropopliteal artery occlusions. Cardiovasc Intervent Radiol 15:306, 1992.
62. Zollikofer C, Antonucci F, Pfyffer M, et al: Arterial stent placement with use of the Wallstent: Midterm results of clinical experience. Radiology 179:449, 1991.
63. Martin LG, Price RB, Casarella WJ, et al: Percutaneous angioplasty in clinical management of renovascular hypertension: Initial and longl-term results. Radiology 155:629, 1985.
64. Rees CR, Palmaz JC, Becker GJ, et al: Palmaz stent in atherosclerotic stenoses involving the ostia of the renal arteries: Preliminary report of a multicenter study. Radiology 181:507, 1991.
65. Joffre F, Rousseau H, Bernadet P, et al: Midterm results of renal artery stenting. Cardiovasc Intervent Radiology 15:313, 1992.
66. Strecker E-P, Liermann D, Wolf HRD, et al: Part 4. Strecker intravascular flexible tantalum stent. *In* Castañeda-Zúñiga WR, Tadavarthy SM (eds): Interventional Radiology. 2nd ed. Baltimore, Williams & Wilkins, 1992, vol. 1, pp 570–575.
67. Zollikofer CL, Antonucci F, Stuckmann G, et al: Use of the WallStent in the venous system including hemodialysis-related stenoses. Cardiovasc Intervent Radiol 15:334, 1992.
68. Rösch J, Uchida BT, Hall LD, et al: Gianturco-Rösch expandable Z stents in the treatment of superior vena cava syndrome. Cardiovasc Intervent Radiol 15:319, 1992.
69. Lakin PC, Petersen BD, Barton RE, et al: Combined local urokinase thrombolysis with expandable Z-stents in the treatment of major venous obstruction [Abstract]. J Vasc Interv Radiol 4(1):42, 1993.
70. Irving JD, Dondelinger RF, Reidy JF, et al: Gianturco self-expanding stents: Clinical experience in the vena cava and large veins. Cardiovasc Intervent Radiol 15:328, 1992.
71. Elson JD, Becker GJ, Wholey MH, Ehrman KO: Vena caval and central venous stenoses: Management with Palmaz balloon-expandable intraluminal stents. J Vasc Interv Radiol 2:215, 1991.
72. Dake MD, Semba CP, Enstrom RJ, et al: Percutaneous treatment of venous occlusive disease with stents [Abstract]. J Vasc Interv Radiol 4(1):42, 1993.
73. Vereycken HA, Oudkerk M Sr, de Wit R, Stoter G: Results of stent placement in the superior and inferior vena cava in cases of malignant obstruction [Abstract]. J Vasc Interv Radiol 4(1):43, 1993.

21

Fundamental Techniques in Vascular Surgery

Basic Vascular Surgical Techniques

Robert B. Rutherford, M.D.

• • •

To avoid unnecessary repetition elsewhere in this book, this chapter reviews some of the basic technical principles on which vascular surgery is based: e.g., the dissection, exposure, and control of vessels; intraoperative hemostasis and anticoagulation; vascular incisions and closures; basic anastomotic techniques; and specialized technical considerations, such as microsurgical techniques, thromboembolectomy, and endarterectomy.

HISTORICAL BACKGROUND

The first recorded vascular reconstruction was reported by Lambert in 1762. He described Hallowell's closure in 1759 of a small opening in a brachial artery, performed with a pin around which a thread was twisted. This was a historic step because prior to that time restoration of flow had always been sacrificed for the sake of hemostasis, and ligation was essentially the only vascular procedure practiced. Unfortunately, Asman's subsequent failures to achieve patency following vascular repair by similar techniques in experimental animals discouraged the surgeons of the day, and for almost a century it was believed that suture material entering the lumen of a vessel would invariably produce an obliterating thrombosis.

By 1882, Schede had accomplished the first successful lateral vein repair. The first direct vascular anastomosis probably was Nicolai Eck's lateral anastomosis in 1877 between the inferior vena cava and the portal vein in dogs. The opposing surfaces of the two vessels were sutured together by two rows of interrupted sutures. A suture at one corner was left untied temporarily to allow a special instrument to be inserted to slit open each vessel in order to allow cross-flow through the anastomosis. Although this was technically a lateral, or side-to-side, anastomosis, it was converted into an end-to-side portacaval shunt by subsequently ligating the hepatic limb of the portal vein. It is interesting to reflect on Eck's enduring fame as a result of this experiment, considering that he had only one survivor and produced no other significant contributions to surgery.

In 1899, Kummell performed the first end-to-end anastomosis of an artery in a human, if one discounts Murphy's invagination anastomosis 2 years earlier. As a background to these and other sporadic clinical successes, the decades surrounding the turn of this century witnessed numerous experimental studies evaluating almost every conceivable suture technique. Absorbable versus nonabsorbable suture and continuous versus interrupted, simple versus mattress, and everting versus edge-to-edge approximation techniques all were tried. These endeavors culminated in the classic studies of Carrel and Guthrie, which established the principles and techniques of the modern vascular anastomosis.[2, 5] These investigators also were the first to achieve significant experimental success with fresh and preserved homografts and heterografts for vascular replacement and bypass.[3]

In 1906, Goyanes used a segment of popliteal vein to bridge a defect caused by the excision of an aneurysm of the accompanying artery. The next year, Lexer used the saphenous vein for arterial reconstruction following excision of an axillary artery aneurysm. Although the stage appeared to be set by the aforementioned experimental studies and by continuing, though sporadic, clinical successes such as these, widespread clinical application of these principles and techniques did not occur for almost 40 years. The reasons for this delay are not entirely clear, but the development of better diagnostic techniques, especially angiography and cardiac catheterization, the evolution of vascular prostheses and homograft storage methods, and the development of techniques that allowed thoracotomy to be performed at reasonable risk, plus the availability of heparin and type-specific, cross-matched blood were probably all important in the final launching of the "golden era of cardiovascular surgery," which began after World War II.

Prior to the technical explosion that followed in the 1950s, arterial ligation for vascular trauma, arteriovenous fistulae, or aneurysm; simple vascular repair with or without local thrombectomy for acute occlusion; sympathectomy for chronic ischemia; and a variety of amputations were the mainstays of surgery for peripheral vascular disease. The implantation, first of arterial homografts, then of a succession of plastic prostheses culminating in the porous, knitted Dacron graft of today; the emerging preference for fresh venous and arterial autografts for smaller arterial replacement; and finally the additional availability of the human umbilical vein allograft and the expanded polytetrafluoroethylene graft have now provided the vascular surgeon with an adequate array of arterial substitutes for most situations. Unfortunately, the concomitant development and refinement of vascular suture materials, atraumatic vascular clamps, and other mechanical devices such as vena cava filters and embolectomy catheters have received almost better coverage in manufacturers' brochures than in the formal surgical literature.

The development of microsurgical technique began in 1960 when Jacobson and Suarez used the operating microscope to suture blood vessels 1.4 mm in diameter, achieving consistent patency in the animal.[6] Buncke and Schultz continued Jacobson's work and developed a metalized microneedle on a 12-μ suture. They were able to anastomose blood vessels 1 mm in diameter and successfully replanted a rabbit's ear.[1] The clinical application of these techniques soon followed with the first digital replantation by Komatsu and Tamai in 1965.[7] The elective use of microvascular surgery began with the transfer of a groin flap to the lower extremity in 1972 by Daniel and Taylor.[4] Since that time, a large variety of composite tissue transfers have been performed using microsurgical techniques. With current technology, it is possible to achieve consistent patency of vessels as small as 0.35 mm using 11–0 nylon sutures on 50-μ needles.

INSTRUMENTS AND SUTURE MATERIAL

The instruments required for simple vascular procedures, in addition to the standard instruments used in any operative dissection, essentially include only vascular forceps, a fine-pointed diamond-jawed needle holder, a right-angled clamp, vascular scissors, and an assortment of atraumatic vascular clamps. Vascular forceps usually have fine teeth or serrations that interdigitate, allowing them to grip the vessel wall without crushing, as exemplified by the DeBakey or Swan-Brown forceps shown in Figure 21–1. Similar requirements pertain to vascular clamps, and although there are many different designs available, most achieve their nonslipping, noncrushing, occlusive grip by means of several longitudinal rows of serrations or teeth on the inside of the jaw or clamp, which are offset so that they interdigitate as shown in Figure 21–2. An assortment of such vascular clamps, of different sizes and shapes, is necessary to accommodate differences in degree of exposure, depth of wound, size of vessel, and angle of application (i.e., transverse, oblique, or tangential) (Fig. 21–3).

In addition to these vascular clamps, which have handles that allow them to be held and with which vessel position can be manipulated, there are smaller vascular clamps without handles, the jaws of which are held in the occlusive position by a spring. These so-called bulldog clamps, or large neurosurgical ''aneurysm'' clips, are useful when working on smaller vessels or in controlling branches or tributaries, particularly when the exposure is limited (Fig. 21–4). Moistened umbilical tapes, Silastic loops, or thin rubber catheters are used to encircle vessels and their major tributaries during dissection and manipulation. A heavy silk suture, doubly looped around a small branch or tributary, can, by the weight of a hemostat clamped to its end, control intraoperative bleeding from these branches without crowding the operative field with additional vascular clamps. During maneuvers to dissect, free, and encircle vessels, a right-angled clamp with fine (but not too pointed) tips is invaluable. Small Metzenbaum scissors or (on smaller, more delicate vessels) plastic scissors are particularly suitable for dissection on or around the vessels because they do not have sharp-pointed tips and are less likely to injure the vessel inadvertently. On the other hand, curved, straight, or angled Pott scissors are preferable for incising or excising the vessel wall itself because they do have delicately pointed tips. An assortment of balloon and irrigating catheters is useful for many purposes in addition to that of removing intravascular thrombus (see later discussion).

To some extent, the selection of vascular suture material, like that of vascular instruments, is an individual mat-

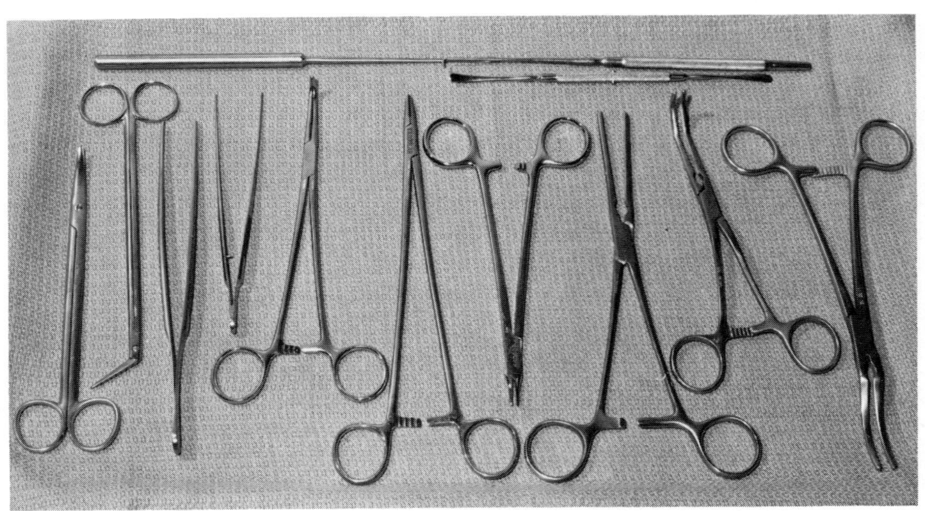

FIGURE 21–1. Some basic vascular instruments, including, from left to right: Metzenbaum and angled Pott scissors; DeBakey and Swan-Brown forceps; a right-angle clamp; long and short vascular needle holders; straight, Satinsky, and spoon-shaped vascular clamps; and at top, a blunted nerve hook and a Penfield and a Freer dissector for endarterectomy.

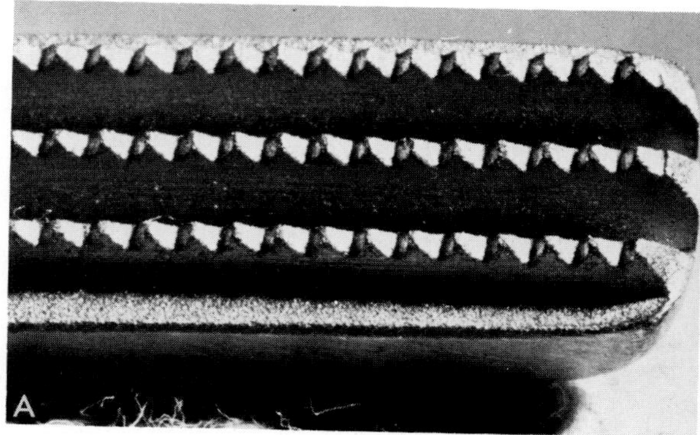

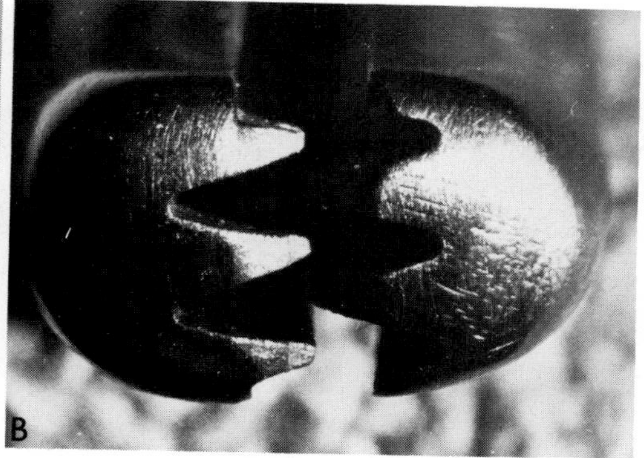

FIGURE 21–2. Magnified views show the multiple "teeth" of a typical vascular clamp. *A*, Side view of one jaw. *B*, End-on view of the jaws interdigitating.

ter, and every surgeon has favorites. The caliber of the suture used should be as fine as possible, short of risking suture line disruption (and anastomotic aneurysm formation), to minimize hemorrhage through suture holes and the amount of suture material in contact with the vessel lumen. As a frame of reference, a range from 2–0 to 7–0 is used in most clinical practice as the surgeon progresses from the aorta centrally to the radial or crural arteries peripherally. For most peripheral anastomoses, 5–0 or 6–0 sutures usually are preferred. All vascular sutures should be swaged onto fine one-half or three-eighths circle, round needles with tapered or slightly beveled tips. Flattening of the body of such a fine needle parallel with the radius of its curve and placing a tapered cutting edge on the side of its tip facilitate penetration through hard arteriosclerotic plaques and avoid bending the body of the needle during the anastomosis. Braided silk, lubricated with sterile mineral oil or bone wax, handles well and is satisfactory for autogenous tissues, especially venous anastomoses, but Teflon-coated Dacron and monofilament polypropylene usually are preferred for arterial work because of their greater strength and durability and their reduced tissue reactivity. Absorbable monofilament suture with a long half-life (e.g., polydiaxanone suture) is now being used instead of interrupted sutures in pediatric vascular surgery to allow anastomotic growth. It is common practice to use doubled swaged-on vascular suture (i.e., with a needle on each end) to allow more flexibility and speed in performing vascular anastomoses.

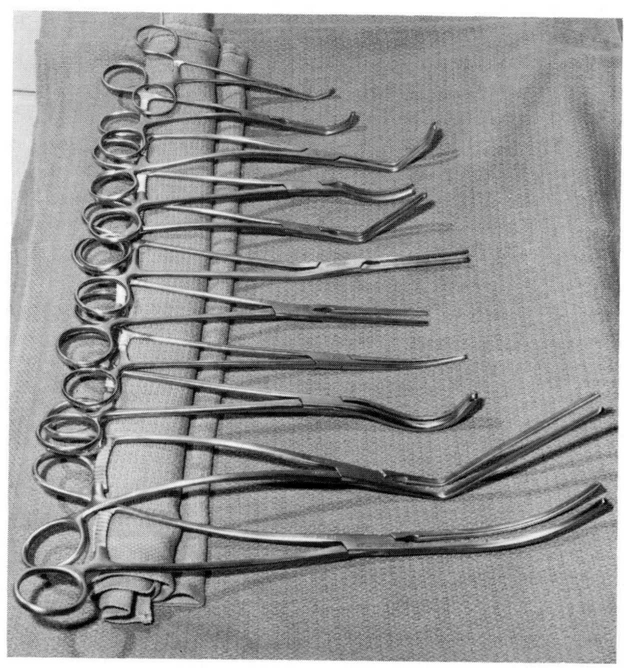

FIGURE 21–3. An assortment of vascular clamps demonstrating variety of shape and size.

VASCULAR EXPOSURE AND CONTROL

Vascular exposure and control usually are the first order of business during any vascular operation. They are completed before systemic anticoagulation is instituted, to facilitate the dissection and minimize blood loss. A clear knowledge of the anatomic relationships among the involved vessels, their major collaterals or tributaries, and the surrounding structures is essential, since the procedure often is performed for occlusive disease and the luxury of dissecting toward a palpable pulse is not afforded the surgeon. However, in such a situation, it may be possible to detect the location of a firmly thrombosed or hardened arteriosclerotic artery by rolling it with the fingertip from side to side in the underlying tissues. A patent though pulseless artery can be located using a sterile Doppler probe. This device may be particularly helpful when dissecting through scarred or inflamed tissues.

Major vessels usually are enclosed in an identifiable fascial envelope or sheath, incision of which normally is the final step in obtaining exposure because the characteristic pattern of the vasa vasorum will immediately identify an exposed artery, and the bluish-white color and the almost ballotable sensation (imparted by the rapid refilling following the quick application and release of pressure) usually makes the accompanying vein easy to recognize. Smaller, more peripheral vessels, such as may be encountered at the wrist or ankle, may go into spasm during the dissection. This, or the lack of arterial pulsations below an obstructive

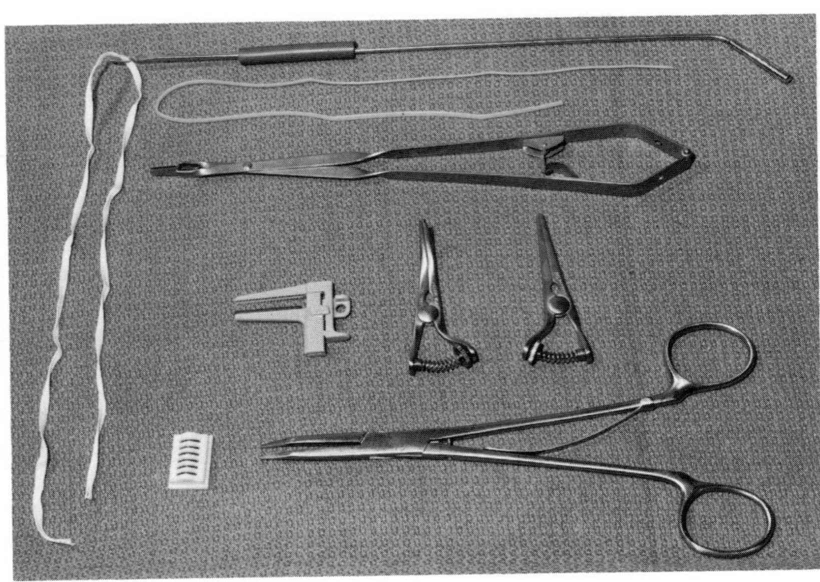

FIGURE 21–4. **A variety of instruments used to control or occlude smaller arterial branches. Included, from the top down, are: a modified Rummel tourniquet using umbilical tape; a Silastic rubber "loop"; a Heifitz aneurysm clip with applicator; a Fogarty and two DeBakey bulldog clamps; and metal "ligaclips" with applicator.**

lesion, may make difficult the distinction between an adjacent artery and vein. Observing the direction of blood flow following temporary occlusion or comparing the color of microaspirates of blood taken with a tuberculin syringe and 25-gauge needle can be helpful maneuvers in these situations.

In the presence of arterial or venous occlusive disease, there may be considerable inflammatory reaction and connective tissue surrounding the vessels. In this situation, the standard advice to dissect off the looser outer adventitial layers and stay "close" to the artery is particularly worthwhile. Arteries are usually approached from the direction of their closest proximity to the skin, and because they rarely give off major branches in that direction, the nearest, or uppermost, surface of the artery normally is devoid of branches, or "free." Once in the correct plane inside the loose outer investiture of the artery and after its upper surface has been exposed fully, the surgeon should dissect a convenient segment of the artery free circumferentially in this same plane by gently spreading the tissues with a right-angle clamp and taking care not to puncture the accompanying vein, which may be closely adherent to the opposite surface, especially near bifurcations. Next, an umbilical tape or Silastic loop is passed around the artery, and its loose ends are clamped with a hemostat. Traction on this, and on each additional encircling tape, progressively draws the arterial structures up out of their bed, allowing restricting points of fixation and major branches to be identified, thus making the dissection progressively easier. One should proceed in this manner until an adequate length of arterial segment and all its major branches are completely free and encircled with tapes. Small branches may represent potentially significant future collaterals; therefore, rather than divide them, they should be controlled temporarily with a double loop of heavy braided silk or a small cerebral aneurysm clip. In obtaining control of the vessels, even in elective procedures, it is best first to dissect out the major inflow and then the main outflow vessels before proceeding with lesser collaterals. Depending on the operative procedure planned, exposure and control of one or more such arterial segments may be necessary, and if a bypass graft between such segments is to be constructed, the intervening "tunnel" or passage for the graft should be prepared before heparin is given.

HEMOSTASIS AND ANTICOAGULATION

The processes of hemostasis and anticoagulation lie at the very foundation of vascular surgery. Only the simplest, most abbreviated vascular surgical procedures can be undertaken without the need to interrupt the flow of blood temporarily. In doing so, one must avoid the two opposing complications of vascular surgery: exsanguinating hemorrhage and intravascular thrombosis.

Hemostasis. Hemostasis, produced spontaneously by spasm and platelet thrombi in smaller vessels and by clamping and ligature in larger vessels, is an integral part of almost every surgical dissection. However, whenever the operation involves the direct transgression of major blood vessels, as is characteristic of vascular surgery, blood flow will need to be either temporarily or permanently interrupted. The former requires the application of atraumatic vascular clamps or double-looped Silastic tapes after exposure and control of the vessels have been achieved, as illustrated in Figure 21–5. A valuable alternative during bypass to small calcified distal arteries, to avoid crushing or otherwise traumatizing them, is the application of a sterile pneumatic tourniquet during the distal anastomosis.

Anticoagulation. With ligation or division of major vessels, it is not ordinarily necessary to take any measures to prevent thrombus formation in the interrupted vessel. Thrombus formation usually occurs eventually within the blind end of the vessel and propagates back as far as the "take-off" of the last major collateral. However, in most vascular procedures the vessels are not simply divided but are explored, replaced, or bypassed; also, to ensure restora-

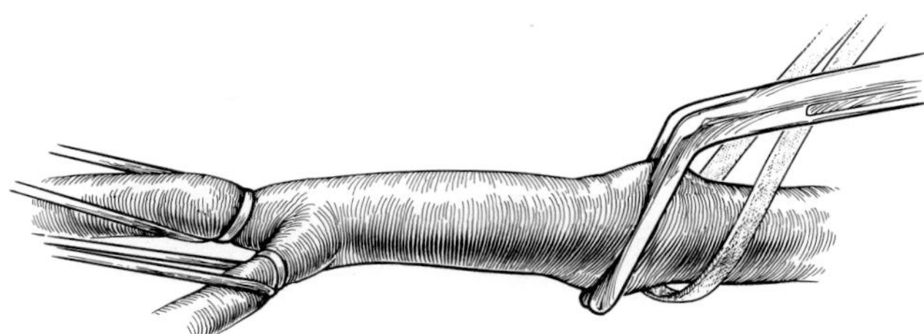

FIGURE 21–5. Two methods for obtaining temporary vascular control. A standard vascular clamp occludes the proximal inflow vessel, while less traumatic Silastic loops are adequate for the smaller distal branches. (From Rutherford RB: Basic vascular techniques. *In* Atlas of Vascular Surgery: Basic Techniques and Exposures. Philadelphia, WB Saunders, 1993, p 16.)

tion of flow *after* an arteriotomy or venotomy has been closed or an anastomosis has been performed, one must either prevent intravascular thrombus formation while flow is interrupted or remove the accumulated thrombus immediately prior to completion of the final suture line. If a vessel, such as the external jugular vein of the dog, is occluded temporarily between two adjacent vascular clamps or nooses, the blood trapped in the intervening segment ordinarily will not clot. However, if, in addition, this same vessel is simply opened and closed with fine silk sutures, thrombosis commonly will occur. Understandably, such segmental vascular thrombosis is even more likely to occur in diseased vessels during the more extensive manipulations required in vascular surgery.

If the procedure is relatively simple, accumulated thrombus may be extracted with forceps or balloon catheters just before placement of the final sutures, and flow thus restored before further clotting occurs. Although still used as an expedient in selected circumstances, this practice carries a small but definite risk of failure that has been made unnecessary by the introduction of heparin anticoagulation. This is used in all but the simplest vascular procedures, the only major exception being thoracoabdominal aneurysm repair in which, because of large anastomoses, high flows, and the risk of creating a bleeding diathesis, timely flushing and irrigation are preferred to heparinization.

Although spontaneous clotting may be retarded by aspirin, dextran, dipyridamole, and other drugs that reduce platelet aggregation, and by coumarin drugs that reduce the circulating levels of clotting factors II, VII, IX, and X, none of these drugs can be relied on to prevent intravascular thrombosis during the performance of a major vascular procedure. On the other hand, in sufficient dosage, heparin will render blood uncoagulable at normal temperatures and pH. The action of heparin is complex, affecting platelet adhesiveness, the endothelial cells' negative charge (or zeta potential), and the early phases of clotting by inhibiting the activation of factors IX and X. However, its major action is believed to result from its union with a cofactor in the blood to form an antithrombin that inhibits the conversion of fibrinogen to fibrin. Given intravenously, it has an effective action for 3 to 4 hours, or even longer with higher or repeated dosage. A satisfactory level of anticoagulation may be achieved within 5 minutes after the intravenous injection of 100 units (approximately 1.0 mg) per kg body weight of aqueous sodium heparin. For continued, sustained anticoagulation, as required during longer vascular procedures, one third to one half of this dose may be repeated at hourly intervals. During procedures in which the blood will be exposed to large surface areas of foreign material, as during cardiopulmonary bypass, larger heparin doses (up to 300 units/kg) usually are advisable. Using larger doses also significantly lengthens the half-life of heparin. Rendering the blood completely incoagulable is not without its disadvantages. Wound surfaces that would remain naturally hemostatic may bleed profusely, and spontaneous bleeding may occur elsewhere in the body, but fortunately these complications are extremely rare during most vascular operations. Although the greatest risk of segmental thrombosis during a vascular procedure lies in the static circulation distal to the point of occlusion, regional heparinization cannot be achieved practically. Therefore, after dissection and exposure of the vessel has been carried out, including "tunneling," and after a porous knitted Dacron graft (if it is to be used) has been preclotted, the appropriate systemic dosage of heparin (usually 100 units/kg) is injected intravenously by the anesthesiologist at the direction of the surgeon. The time is noted so that half of this dose can be repeated at 1 to 1½ hours in longer procedures. Whenever large tissue surfaces have been exposed during the course of the dissection or whenever there is extensive oozing of blood from the tissues or prosthesis following completion of the anastomosis, the heparin effect may be reversed prior to wound closure by using an equivalent dose of protamine sulfate, e.g., milligram for milligram, allowing for the temporal decay of heparin that was given earlier. It is important to remember that protamine may cause hypotension if it is injected too rapidly and that it may produce the opposite of the intended effect, namely hypocoagulability, if it is administered in a dose in excess of that needed to counteract the heparin. For this reason, the anesthesiologist usually is asked to give half of the calculated dose over the first 5 minutes, and then an additional 5 mg every few minutes until the surgeon notes a decrease in oozing or the appearance of clots in the operative field. In most vascular procedures, however, protamine need not be given; instead, the effects of administered heparin are simply allowed to wear off.

VASCULAR INCISIONS AND CLOSURES

Entering a vessel through a simple lateral incision ranks only slightly above vessel ligature in degree of complexity. This maneuver is used clinically to introduce catheters or cardiac bypass cannulas and to remove thrombi, emboli, or atheromatous deposits. Only two aspects deserve special consideration here: the direction of the incision and the manner of closure. Closure of either longitudinal or transverse incisions usually produces some reduction in the cross-sectional area of the vessel. At normal systemic pressures, a reduction of almost 50 per cent in diameter is required to produce a significant hemodynamic effect or gradient in most peripheral arteries. However, there may be some turbulence with lesser degrees of stenosis, particularly in low-flow, high-resistance situations. Furthermore, there is a tendency toward hypercoagulability in the immediate postoperative period, and these factors, combined with the

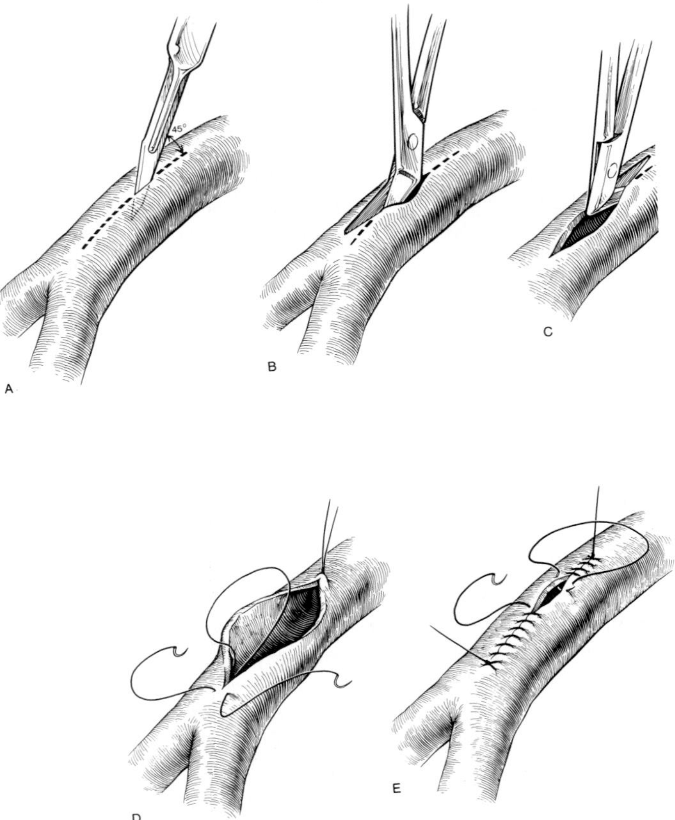

FIGURE 21–6. Longitudinal arteriotomy is begun with a sharp scalpel blade and completed with Pott scissors. Closure is done with continuous suture, run from each end toward the middle. (From Rutherford RB: Basic vascular techniques. *In* Atlas of Vascular Surgery: Basic Techniques and Exposures. Philadelphia, WB Saunders, 1993, p 31.)

break in intimal continuity and the presence of foreign (suture) material at the site of closure, may lead to thrombosis. For these reasons, care must be taken to minimize this narrowing.

Longitudinal incisions offer good exposure and can be extended readily (Fig. 21–6). They have the additional advantage of being convertible into an end-to-side anastomosis. However, closure of a longitudinal incision in *smaller* (i.e., less than 4 mm) vessels is likely to narrow the lumen over a greater distance and therefore is more likely to produce significant stenosis and turbulence and lead to thrombosis than is a transverse incision. For this reason, a trans-

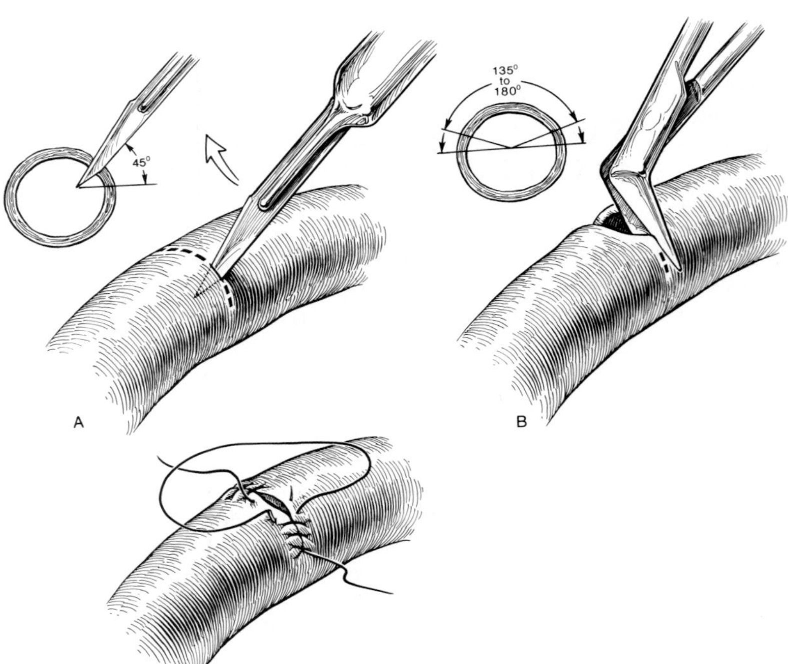

FIGURE 21–7. Transverse arteriotomy is performed first with a scalpel blade followed by enlargement to 135 to 180 degrees of the circumference using Pott scissors. Continuous closure, from both ends toward the middle, is most commonly employed. (From Rutherford RB: Basic vascular techniques. *In* Atlas of Vascular Surgery: Basic Techniques and Exposures. Philadelphia, WB Saunders, 1993, p 30.)

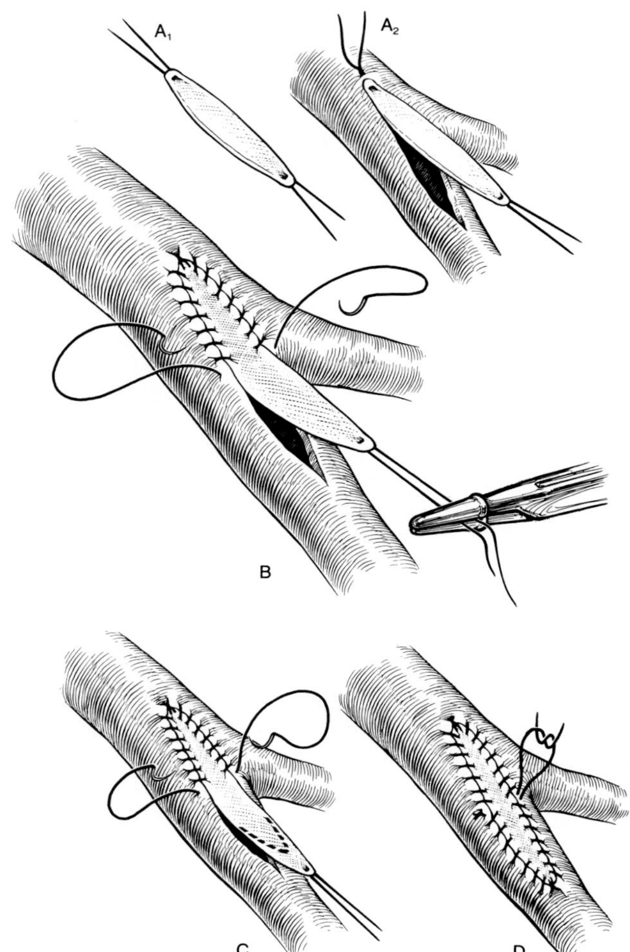

FIGURE 21–8. Patch angioplasty. A thin elliptical patch is fashioned, and mattress sutures are placed in both tips. One is carried into the corner of the arteriotomy and is tied to begin closure, aided by traction on the other suture. The closure is continued from each end, along the sides of the arteriotomy, toward the middle, where the sutures are tied to each other. Before beginning the second corner, the tip may need to be trimmed for better fit. (From Rutherford RB: Basic vascular techniques. *In* Atlas of Vascular Surgery: Basic Techniques and Exposures. Philadelphia, WB Saunders, 1993, p 33.)

verse arteriotomy or venotomy usually is preferable in smaller vessels (Fig. 21–7). When a longitudinal incision is necessary, narrowing of its closure may be obviated by the insertion of an elliptical patch graft of vein or Dacron into the arteriotomy (Fig. 21–8).

Placement of Vascular Sutures

Regardless of the manner in which the vascular suture is placed, two rules always should be observed: (1) excess adventitial tissue should be excised from the outer surface of the vessel so that it will not be dragged into the anastomosis and promote suture line thrombus formation; and (2) the suture should pass through all layers, particular care being taken always to include the intima. Interrupted sutures are still popular in very small anastomoses. A simple over-and-over suture usually is chosen for most arterial closures or anastomoses, with ''bites'' taken 1 mm apart and 1 mm from the edges, unless the vessels are large, thick-walled, or diseased. Eversion of the edges in order to produce a smooth, sutureless internal surface by the placement of continuous or interrupted horizontal mattress sutures has lost much of its original popularity, mainly because the theoretical advantages have not been manifested in major arterial reconstructions and because it tends to produce a greater narrowing at the closure or anastomosis. Even with the simpler, over-and-over continuous suture, some degree of eversion usually can be achieved in most anastomoses by starting each ''corner'' with a horizontal mattress suture (Kunlin's technique) and by gently holding out the edges of the vessel or graft with forceps as they are being sutured together. Whenever possible, the direction of penetration of vessels should be from the inside out, with care being taken to include the intima. This is particularly important in suturing arteriosclerotic arteries, in which penetration in the reverse direction may push a hard plaque inward rather than penetrating it, creating an intimal flap that may be dissected further by arterial flow and leading to occlusion. The vascular suture must be pulled taut continuously to avoid suture line bleeding at slack points. In this regard, it should be pointed out that most vascular suture line bleeding will stop with finger tamponade, a little patience, and occasionally the help of a fine, superficially placed suture that draws more adventitia over the leak. If deeper sutures are required, flow should be interrupted again while they are placed; otherwise, new suture holes will be created that may bleed more vigorously than the old. Care must be taken as one nears the corner, or end, of an anastomosis to ensure that the opposite side of the vessel or graft is not being caught by the suture. Inserting a fine nerve hook with blunted point through the opening in the anastomosis as each stitch is placed is a useful precaution against this error. Another safeguard is the practice of always beginning at and sewing away from the corners and toward the ''middle'' of each suture line, using two separate sutures that are tied together there.

Methods of Vascular Interruption

The permanent interruption of flow through a major vessel may be accomplished in several ways, as illustrated in Figure 21–9. Smaller arteries or veins may be divided between two hemostats before ligature and release of the clamps or, preferably, if there is adequate exposure, doubly ligated before division. In the latter approach, a curved or right-angle clamp usually is passed under the vessel after it has been dissected free, and a ligature, held taut by a clamp at its distal end, is ''fed'' into the grasp of the right-angle clamp and pulled around the vessel as the latter is withdrawn. This maneuver is repeated, the two ligatures then are tied, and the vessel between them is divided.

Because of the potential danger that pulsations, thrusting against the blind end of an artery that has been simply ligated and divided, eventually may force the ligatures off, it usually is advisable to ligate larger arteries doubly on *both* sides of the point of division, with the central one of each of these pairs of ligatures being a ''transfixion,'' or

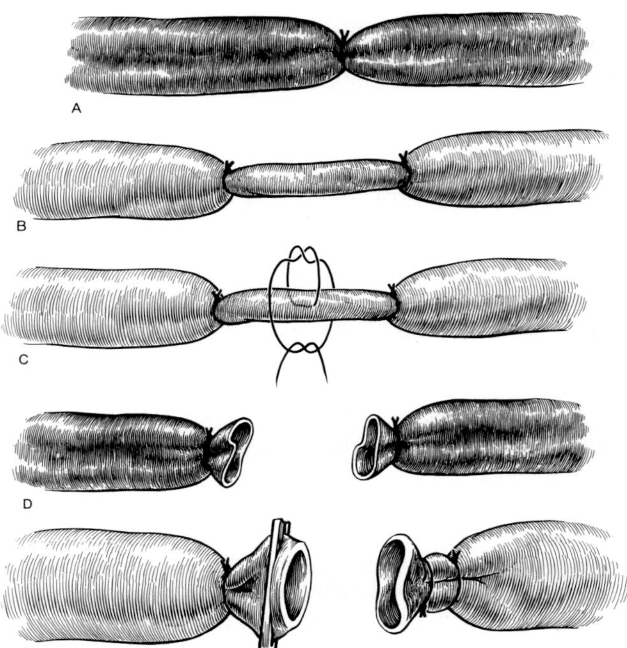

FIGURE 21–9. Vascular interruption techniques for small arteries and veins. *A*, Single ligation. *B*, Double ligation in continuity. *C*, Double ligation with intervening transfixion suture. *D*, Double ligation and division. *E*, Reinforcing ligatured ends with a transfixion suture or metal clip. (From Rutherford RB: Basic vascular techniques. *In* Atlas of Vascular Surgery: Basic Techniques and Exposures. Philadelphia, WB Saunders, 1993, p 26.)

''suture ligature,'' that is placed through the lumen of the vessel and tied on either side of it. Another alternative, which usually is reserved for the largest of vessels, is division between vascular clamps, followed by a formal closure of the cut ends by continuous vascular suture. If, on the other hand, interruption of flow is all that is desired and division of the vessel is not required, ligation-in-continuity is an acceptable alternative to the maneuvers just mentioned; furthermore, if the vessel in question is short and difficult to control with vascular clamps, this may be not only the most expedient but also the safest approach. The recommended technique for ligation-in-continuity is to place two heavy ligature circumferences around the vessel, thereby interrupting flow, and then to place a transfixion suture between them to destroy intimal continuity and promote an organized thrombotic occlusion of that segment. This precaution is designed to prevent later recanalization, the major objection to simple ligation-in-continuity. The clinical situation that best illustrates the application of the foregoing principles is that used in correcting a patent ductus arteriosus. Indeed, the early history of cardiovascular surgery was enriched and enlivened by studies and debates centering on the most appropriate technical approach for closing this congenital anomaly.

VASCULAR ANASTOMOSES

End-to-End Anastomosis

The end-to-end anastomosis is usually begun with two corner sutures placed 180 degrees apart. Although these may be placed as simple sutures, a horizontal mattress suture results in slight eversion of the suture line and facilitates intima-to-intima approximation. If double-ended vascular sutures are used, these corner sutures are tied, both ends being left of equal length. One needle from each corner is then used to ''run'' the suture line in a simple over-and-over fashion to the middle of each side of the anastomosis. There the ends of the two sutures are tied together, completing the anterior half of the anastomosis. The vessel ends are then rotated 180 degrees by moving the vascular clamps, thus exposing the previous ''posterior'' half of the anastomosis. The suture line is then continued in an identical fashion to complete the anastomosis (Fig. 21–10). If the vessel ends are not sufficiently mobile for this technique, one may perform the ''posterior'' half of the suture line transluminally, or place the corner sutures directly anteriorly and posteriorly, instead of laterally, and sew from the posterior midline around each side to the anterior midline. With this approach, only minimal rotation of the vascular clamps will be necessary to make the suture line readily visible.

If the vessels to be joined are relatively small (e.g., 2 to 5 mm in diameter), the anastomosis may be enlarged by beveling the ends 45 degrees in opposite directions; or, if the vessel is thin-walled and flexible, the opposing ends may be slit longitudinally for a length approximating the vessel's diameter but 180 degrees out of phase from each other and rounding off the corners (Fig. 21–11). These flanged or beveled anastomoses are designed to avoid the

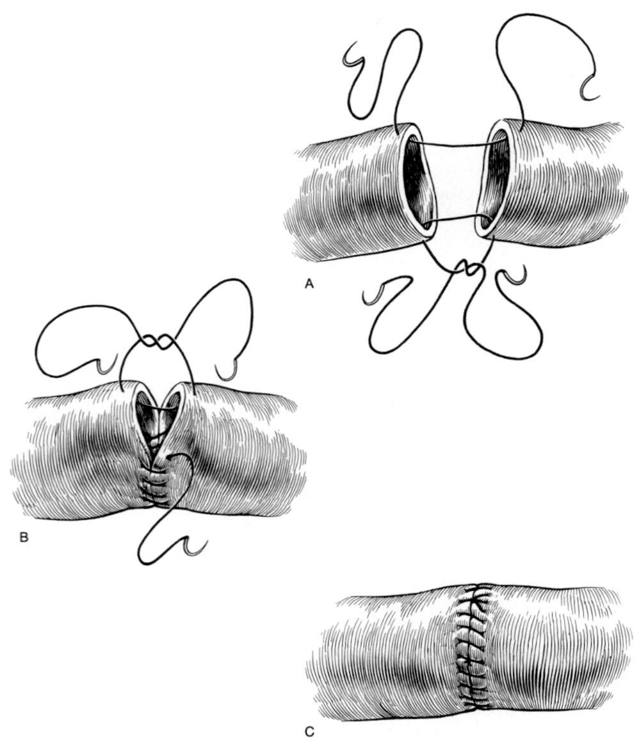

FIGURE 21–10. A simple perpendicular end-to-end anastomosis begun with two sutures 180 degrees apart and run continuously toward each other. (From Rutherford RB: Basic vascular techniques. *In* Atlas of Vascular Surgery: Basic Techniques and Exposures. Philadelphia, WB Saunders, 1993, p 35.)

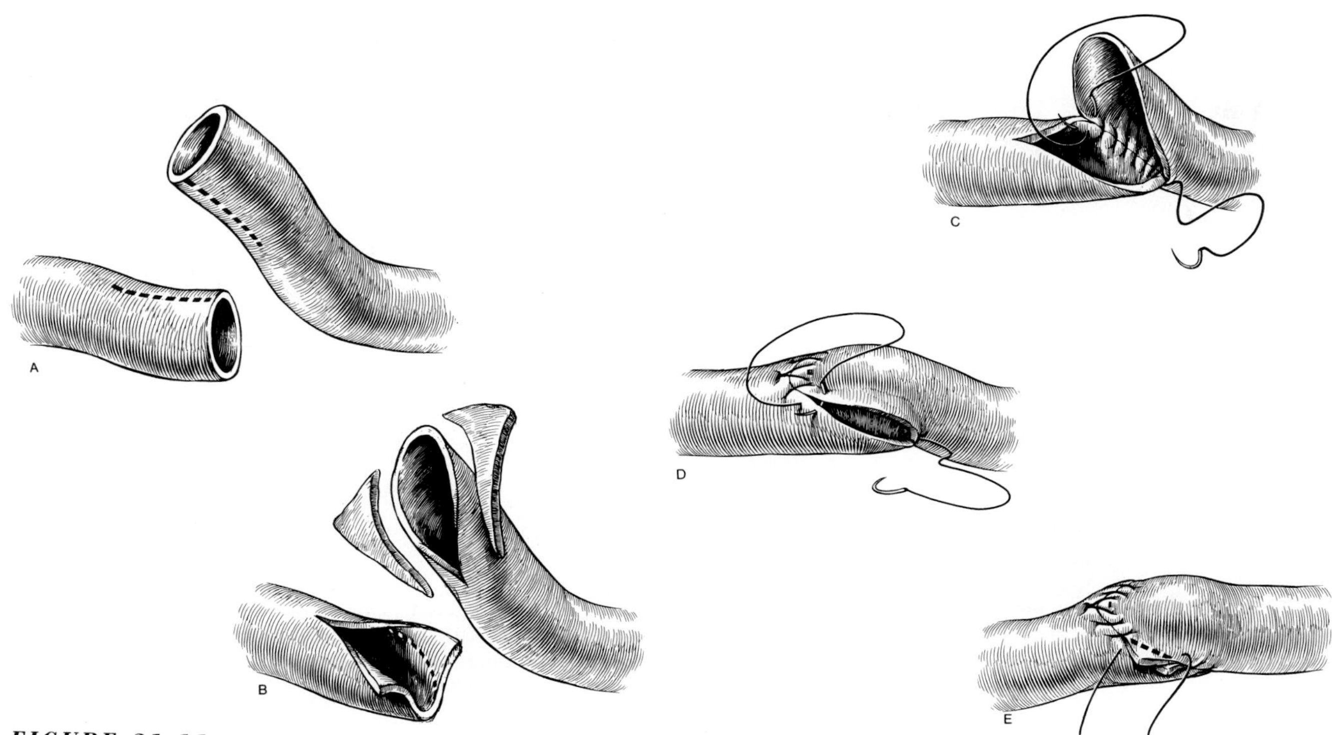

FIGURE 21–11. Technique of oblique end-to-end anastomosis. *A*, The two ends are slit 180 degrees apart. *B*, The resultant corners and adjacent lateral edges are trimmed conservatively. *C*, Anastomosis is begun in one corner (head-to-toe) and *(D)* run to and around the opposite end and back toward the starting point. *E*, The other suture is run up to meet it in the middle, trimming any remaining "angles" to avoid "dog ears." (From Rutherford RB: Basic vascular techniques. *In* Atlas of Vascular Surgery: Basic Techniques and Exposures. Philadelphia, WB Saunders, 1993, pp 40–41.)

circumferential, constricting effect that may be produced by a simple perpendicular end-to-end anastomosis in smaller vessels.

In addition, because a continuous suture, when used for end-to-end anastomosis, may result in "purse stringing" or circumferential narrowing of the anastomosis, interrupted sutures may be preferred for end-to-end anastomosis of smaller vessels. If smooth, monofilament vascular sutures with doubled swaged-on needles are used, the sutures can be placed and left untied prior to completion of the anastomosis. Then the vascular clamps can be slowly released, allowing the lumen to expand and the suture to slide slightly to accommodate this expansion (Fig. 21–12). The sutures are then tied while the clamps are briefly reapplied. These techniques apply as well to the direct interposition of a segment of vein or prosthetic graft as they do to a direct end-to-end anastomosis.

End-to-Side Anastomosis

The end-to-side anastomosis has wide clinical use in placing arterial bypass grafts. The side of the "recipient" vessel may be prepared by elliptical excision or simple longitudinal incision, and the end of the donor vessel usually is beveled to produce an acute angle of entry and to minimize turbulence. Although the optimal angle of entry for an end-to-side anastomosis depends on the velocity of flow across it, it should be 30 to 45 degrees or less for arterial anastomosis. This will result in a functional approximation and minimal turbulence. As illustrated in Figure 21–13, the end of the donor vessel (vein or prosthetic graft) is fashioned (cut, beveled, or trimmed) to fit into the lateral opening in the recipient artery or vein, whose length is at least twice the diameter of the donor vessel. The "heel" of the anastomosis is started first, using a running suture carried part way along each side. Then the "toe" of the anastomosis is started, using continuous sutures brought along each side to meet the other sutures in the middle on both sides. This heel-first, toe-last technique is the safest end-to-side technique. It ensures good hemostasis at the most inaccessible aspect (the heel), allows accurate suture placement at the most critical point to avoid narrowing (the toe), allows adjustments to be made in the fit of the anastomosis by trimming the graft tip or lengthening the arteriotomy (see Fig. 21–14), and allows the final sutures to be placed quickly and accurately along the sides. Although it must be modified, depending on the nature of the host and donor vessels, it is equally applicable to the anastomosis of prosthesis to artery, vein to artery, vein to vein, and artery to artery. It is one of the most commonly used techniques in reconstructive vascular surgery.

Side-to-Side Anastomosis

Although the side-to-side anastomosis is not commonly used in clinical vascular surgery, the best known

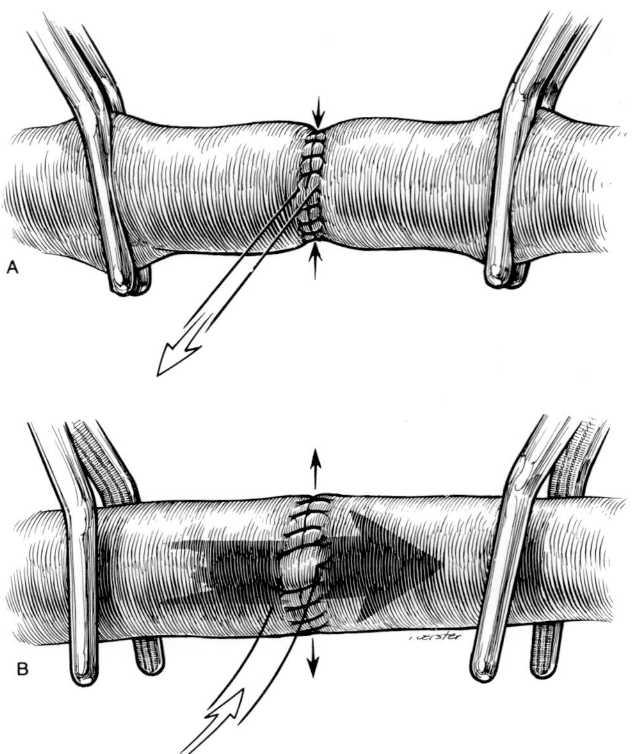

FIGURE 21–12. Pulling up and tying a continuous suture in a perpendicular end-to-end anastomosis may cause an anastomotic stricture *(top)*. Briefly releasing the clamps before tying allows the monofilament suture to slide and the anastomosis to expand to a fuller diameter *(bottom)*. (From Rutherford RB: Basic vascular techniques. *In* Atlas of Vascular Surgery: Basic Techniques and Exposures. Philadelphia, WB Saunders, 1993, p 36.)

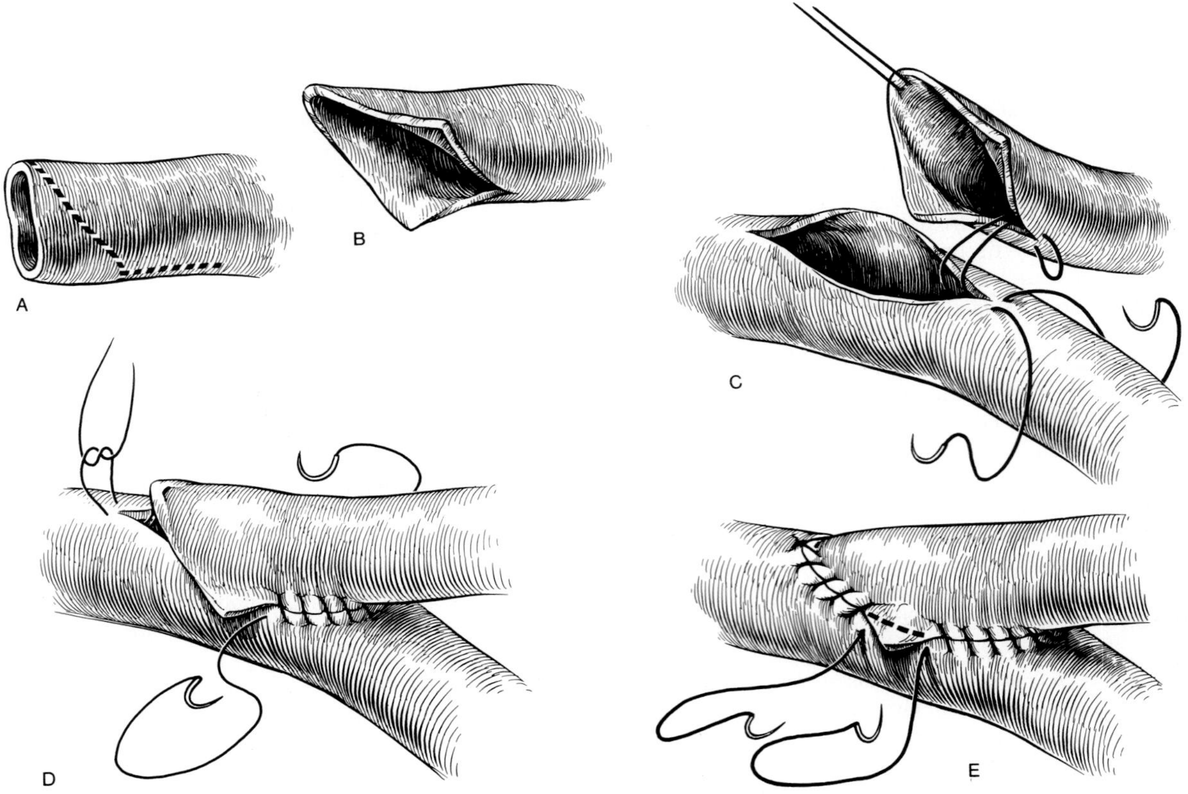

FIGURE 21–13. Typical end-to-side, prosthesis-to-recipient artery anastomosis. *A* and *B*, Trimming the graft. *C*, Starting the "heel" of the anastomosis with a mattress suture. *D*, With the heel completed, the "toe" is begun with another horizontal mattress suture. *E*, Excess edges require trimming before completion. (From Rutherford RB: Basic vascular techniques. *In* Atlas of Vascular Surgery: Basic Techniques and Exposures. Philadelphia, WB Saunders, 1993, pp 50–51.)

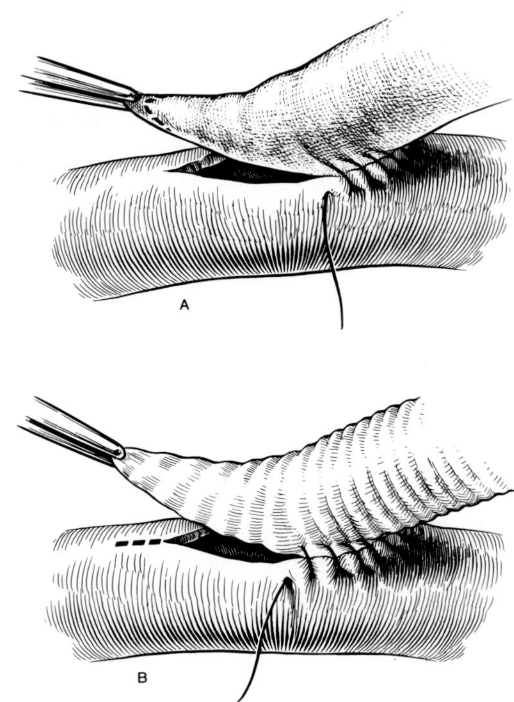

FIGURE 21–14. **The advantages of the heel-first, toe-last sequence is illustrated. It allows a final length adjustment by either trimming the tip (toe) *(A)* or extending the arteriotomy *(B)*. (From Rutherford RB: Basic vascular techniques. *In* Atlas of Vascular Surgery: Basic Techniques and Exposures. Philadelphia, WB Saunders, 1993, p 53.)**

examples of this technique probably are the side-to-side portacaval shunt, the Potts and Waterston aortopulmonary anastomosis, and arteriovenous fistulae. For this anastomosis, a curved, spoon-shaped, or angled Satinsky's vascular clamp may be placed laterally on adjacent segments of the two vessels to be anastomosed, and then, after matching longitudinal incisions are made in (or equal ellipses removed from) each segment, the adjacent openings can be sutured together with continuous suture, the posterior line being performed intraluminally.

There are many varieties of each of these basic techniques. Knowledge of these and a knowledge of vascular exposures are the two major foundations of operative technique in vascular surgery. For further details, the reader is referred to the companion Atlas.[8]

References

1. Buncke HJ, Schultz WP: Total ear reimplantation in the rabbit utilizing microminiature vascular anastomoses. Br J Plast Surg 10:15, 1966.
2. Carrel A: The surgery of blood vessels. Johns Hopkins Med J 18:18, 1907.
3. Carrel A: Heterotransplantation of blood vessels preserved in cold storage. J Exp Med 9:226, 1907.
4. Daniel RK, Taylor GI: Distant transfer of an island flap by microvascular anastomoses. Plast Reconstr Surg 52:111, 1973.
5. Guthrie CG: Heterotransplantation of blood vessels. Am J Physiol 19:482, 1907.
6. Jacobson JH, Suarez EL: Microsurgery in the anastomosis of small blood vessels. Surg Forum 11:243, 1968.
7. Komatsu S, Tamai S: Successful replantation of a completely cut off thumb: Case report. Plast Reconstr Surg 42:374, 1968.
8. Rutherford RB: An Atlas of Vascular Surgery: Basic Techniques and Exposures. Philadelphia, WB Saunders, 1993.

Microvascular Surgery

Lawrence L. Ketch, M.D., F.A.C.S., F.A.A.P.

• • •

Microsurgery is the technique of performing routine surgical procedures on otherwise inoperably small structures by the aid of a surgical microscope. Chapters in earlier editions have emphasized extracranial and intracranial bypass and reimplantation of severed distal parts, but this chapter focuses on the role of the free flap transfer in limb salvage. Microvascular free tissue transfer is the technique of transplanting healthy, well-vascularized, undamaged tissue (flap) with its dominant vascular pedicle from one anatomic region to another using the surgical microscope to reconnect precisely the small blood vessels (usually less than 2 mm in diameter) that provide circulation to this tissue. This chapter emphasizes the unique aspects of this application of microvascular surgery and is intended to acquaint the vascular surgeon with its potential applications in achieving limb salvage in the complex situation.

TRAINING IN MICROVASCULAR SURGERY

A formal period of animal laboratory instruction is needed with graduation to clinical cases under the watchful eye of an experienced operator. Attained skills must be maintained constantly, if not by clinical performance then by continuing laboratory practice. Free tissue transfer must be performed by a *team* well versed in technical aspects of the surgery. Surgical assistants must be almost as well trained and as technically competent as the primary surgeon.

INSTRUMENTATION

Surgical instruments differ from those used in peripheral vascular surgery in both design and size (Fig. 21–15). The delicate instruments are controlled primarily with the thumb and index finger and are an extension of these two digits. Hemostasis in a microsurgical field is achieved with wet field bipolar coagulation to prevent damage caused by current extension along blood vessels in the path of the grounding pad. Microvascular clamps, unlike standard peripheral vascular instruments, have a predetermined closing pressure that is applied over a broad flat surface. These clamps are often attached to a sliding rail that will allow the ends of the microvessels to be drawn into accurate alignment, avoiding tension at the suture line until the anastomosis has been completed. Suture material consists of monofilament nylon ranging in size from 9–0 for larger vessels to 11–0 for very small anastomoses. Effective needle sizes range from 139 to 50 μ in diameter. Very sophisticated microscopes are available with continuous zoom magnification from 6 to 40 power, foot control in multiple axes, remote control, and capable of photography and video camera documentation.

TECHNIQUE

For a complete description of technique the reader is referred to an excellent laboratory manual by Ackland.[1] The essential highlights are briefly discussed here.

Patient positioning is paramount because accessability to the operative field and the comfort of the surgeon are critically important to success. The elbows and forearms must be well supported to allow fine manipulations with optimal steadiness. The microscope must be in good working order and should be adjusted to provide optimal vision. The surgeon and the assistant must be very familiar with the mechanical operation of the instrument. Strict attention must be paid to both the anesthetic control of the patient and the temperature of the operating room environment to minimize vasospasm, a major difficulty when dealing with vessels of such small size. Preparation of the recipient zone requires removal of necrotic and contaminated tissue. In certain circumstances this is better accomplished in a separate preceding procedure. Hemostasis is critical because the smallest amount of ooze may obscure minute structures in the surgical field. Dissection of vessels prior to microsurgical anastomosis should be performed under loupe magnification. The recipient site should be selected in a zone where there is a flexible, normal vessel wall outside of the area of injury. When damaged vessels must be resected back to normal vital tissue or when the vascular pedicle of the transfer is not long enough to reach the donor vessel easily, interposition vein grafts may be necessary. These vessels should be harvested under loupe magnification with all side branches carefully ligated or coagulated at a distance removed from the main vessel. No synthetic bypass grafts are used. The techniques of end-to-end (Fig. 21–16) and end-to-side (Fig. 21–17) anastomosis have changed little from the time of Alexis Carrel and are essentially the same as those used in macrovascular technique. However, the application of these principles is far more demanding, and attention to detail must be much more precise to produce an

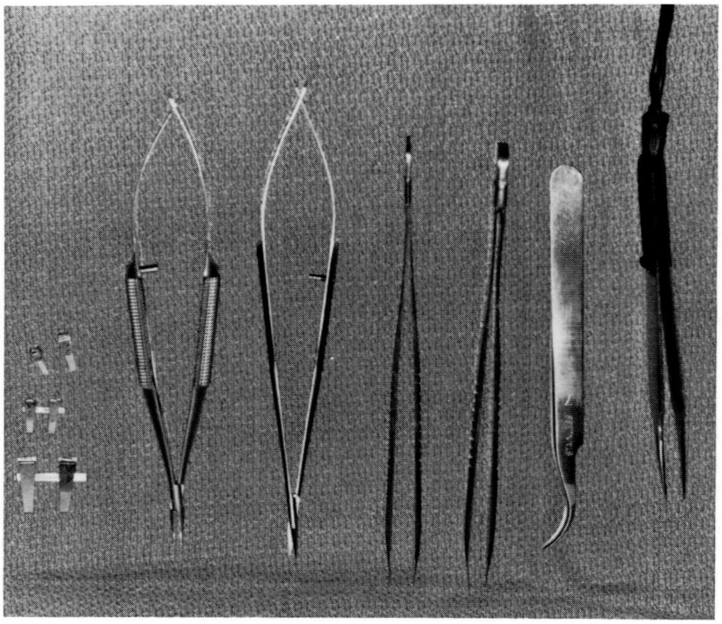

FIGURE 21–15. Basic microsurgical instruments. *Left to right*, Double and single clamp approximators, Barraquer needle holder, straight microscissors, straight and curved jeweler's forceps, bipolar coagulating forceps.

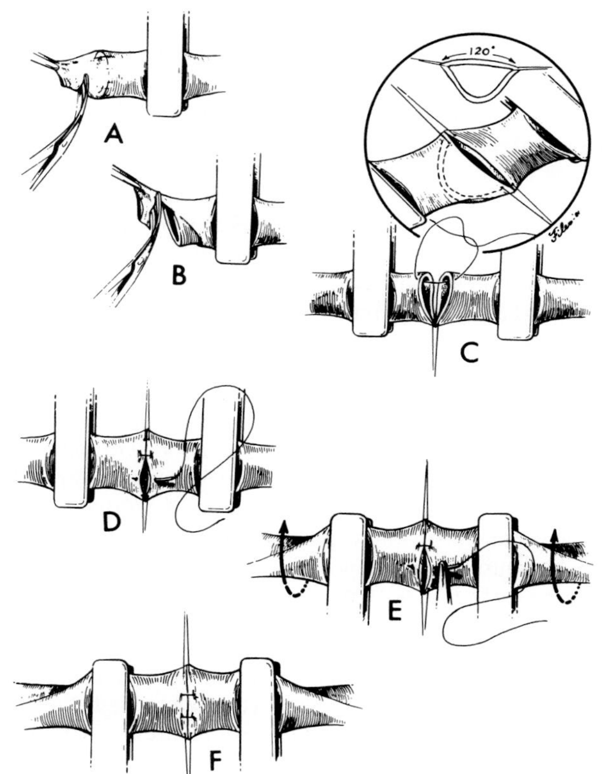

FIGURE 21-16. The end-to-end anastomosis. *A* and *B*, Trimming the adventitia from the vessel end. *C*, Guide sutures placed 120 degrees apart. *D*, Completion of the front wall. *E*, Clamp turned 180 degrees for completion of back wall. *F*, Back wall completed.

acceptable success rate. Like macrovascular reconstruction, the most significant factor required for consistent patency of the anastomosis is impeccable surgical technique. Owing to the size and delicacy of the vessels, however, the margin for error is considerably less. Although the risk of arterial thrombosis may be reduced with use of vasodilatating and antiplatelet agents, little effect on venous patency has been achieved with these agents. Unlike the situation in macrovascular surgery, heparin has limited usefulness and in fact can add the risk of bleeding at sites of extensive dissection in flap donor areas and can cause obstruction of the microanastomoses by even small hemorrhages at the transfer site. No prospective, randomized, double-blind studies have shown any benefit in postoperative anticoagulation by any pharmacologic agent; however, aspirin is routinely administered pre- and postoperatively. Postoperative low-molecular-weight dextran is favored by some surgeons. Anastomotic failure may result not only from poor technique but also from poor preoperative planning, flawed intraoperative judgment, and failure to control the postoperative environment appropriately.

MICROVASCULAR FREE TISSUE TRANSFER FOR PERIPHERAL VASCULAR DISEASE

In 1973 the advent of microvascular free tissue transfer created a major impact on lower extremity reconstruction,[2] particularly in trauma cases involving the distal third of the leg and foot. It was inevitable that these initial applications would evolve to use in chronic infection.[3] Until recently, traditional thought has excluded extension of this technology to limb salvage in patients with diabetes or severe ischemic conditions with inadequate arterial inflow. The convergence of macrovascular and microvascular reconstructive techniques for limb salvage was signaled by the report of Allen and colleagues in 1981 on their use of free tissue transfer to salvage severely traumatized limbs by providing reconstruction of bony and soft tissue defects following traditional arterial reconstruction.[4] Previously, many such injuries resulted in amputation because of the inability to produce a closed wound in the face of compound soft tissue loss. This initial series of patients underwent revascularization after severe trifurcation injuries with reverse saphenous vein grafts and subsequent coverage of their complex distal wounds, which could not be managed by conventional techniques, by free flap transfer. This procedure preserved the extremities neurologically intact that otherwise would have progressed ultimately to amputation without provision of locally well-vascularized tissue. Obviously, a denervated extremity or multiple life-threatening injuries may preclude use of such a simultaneous combined approach.

In 1985 this concept was extended with reports of enhanced limb salvage in patients with chronic ulceration by means of combined arterial reconstruction and subsequent free tissue transfer. Employment of this technique in limbs threatened by severe atherosclerotic occlusive disease

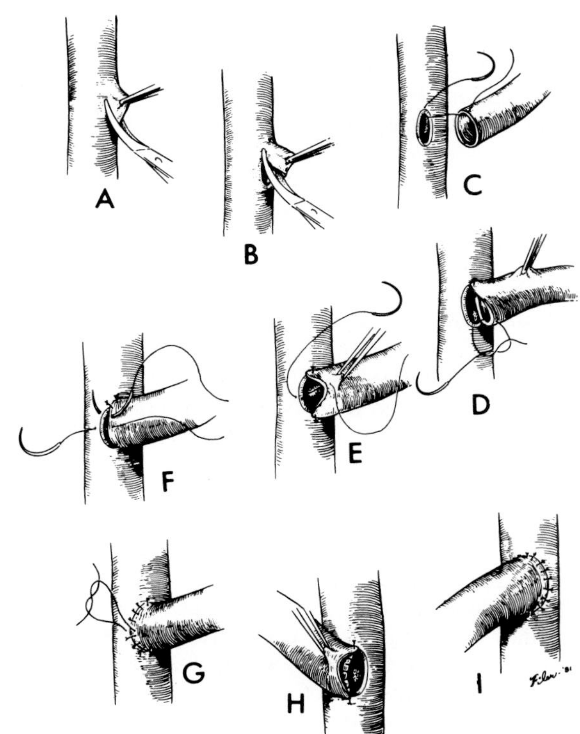

FIGURE 21-17. End-to-side anastomosis. *A* and *B*, Arteriotomy performed. *C* and *D*, Corner sutures placed. *E–G*, Left side wall sutured. *H*, Inspection of left side wall. *I*, Right side wall completed.

produced salvage of the extremity and healing of ischemic lesions rather than amputation. Briggs and associates, employing distal revascularization followed by free tissue transfer for the coverage of ulcerative or necrotic lower extremity defects, produced healed wounds and successful ambulation in three of four diabetic patients.[5] Conventional therapy, consisting of skin grafts or local pedicle flaps, may be contraindicated in this situation owing to lack of adequate recipient vessels, local factors including neuropathy, or systemic disease such as diabetes, as well as exposed tendon or bone with or without infection. Despite aggressive distal revascularization by inframalleolar bypass, 20 to 40 per cent of patients ultimately come to amputation because advanced ischemic or infected ulcerations fail to heal.[6–8] It is now possible to heal many of these lesions, return the patient to ambulation, and forestall amputation.

Diabetes. The myth of small vessel occlusive disease and an abnormal reactivity and resistance in diabetic vessels persists despite evidence to the contrary. It has been shown that diabetes does not intrinsically affect the microcirculation, and there has been no confirmation of a reported increased incidence of intimal hyperplasia in the disease. There are functional permeability abnormalities of the vessel wall that may contribute to tissue breakdown and ulceration, but it is likely that these microvascular abnormalities (i.e., basement membrane thickening) are minor compared to the role played by concomitant neuropathy.[9–13]

In 1987, this knowledge led Colen to the application of microsurgical free tissue transfers to salvage feet with nonhealing neurotrophic ulcers, some of which were associated with osteomyelitis.[14] Many such patients underwent prior distal revascularization, and all but 1 of 10 extremities were salvaged. Application of this technique is invaluable in patients who have undergone or are at risk for contralateral amputation. Extensive tissue loss secondary to gangrene in diabetic patients traditionally has precluded salvage by conventional techniques despite the ability to bypass infrapopliteal occlusive disease. Many such patients progress to amputation despite arterial reconstruction because they have large heel or ankle ulcers with exposed and infected tendon or bone.

Peripheral Arterial Occlusive Disease. The combination of arterial bypass with microvascular free tissue transfer or the use of free tissue transfer alone when arterial inflow is adequate can reliably result in ischemic limb salvage. The pathophysiologic basis for such efforts has recently been explained by the introduction of the concept of the "nutrient flap."[15] Postoperative arteriograms of patients with severely atherosclerotic lower limbs who have undergone free tissue transfer demonstrate the local proliferation and progressive development of new capillary networks (beds). It is notable here that no attempt was made at distal revascularization prior to the use of free flap transfers. Such treatment is effective not only in the absence of patent leg arteries or in the presence of a single patent artery but also in the absence of a patent plantar arch.

Owing to the small number of cases reported, the indications for and success rate of this approach have not been adequately defined. The hypothesis of enhanced neovascularization promoted by a perfusion gradient between the flap and the wound margin has been accepted. Extending this concept, Shestak and colleagues have reported successful limb salvage, in patients deemed incapable of reconstruction by distal bypass, by means of "indirect" revascularization of ischemic ulcers using a proximal vein graft as a conduit for the tissue transfer. Not only are the wounds healed, but the patients report resolution of rest pain and claudication as well.[16, 17] This is not a new concept. However, the phenomenon of neovascularization of the extremity has now been confirmed by postoperative arteriography. It has been assumed but has not been proved that failure of such attempts should not result in a higher level of amputation than that which would have been performed primarily. Experience with several patients in this series suggests that perhaps a free flap alone can serve as the sole outflow source for a bypass graft in patients with otherwise unacceptable "runoff." A rabbit model has been devised to investigate this concept in the laboratory.[18] Subsequently, it has been shown by microsphere injection that the flap does increase muscle perfusion in the ischemic limb (comparing those treated with a flap versus sham controls) and that permanent, hemodynamically significant connections do develop between a well-perfused muscle flap and an ischemic hind limb. This augmentation of perfusion has been quantified.[19] Clinical observations suggest that the high blood flow of such a flap induces neorevascularization, but eventually flow equilibrates with the circulation of the surrounding tissue. Similar principles are applicable to "stump salvage" following major amputation in severely ischemic limbs.[20, 21]

In the early 1990s, microsurgical femoral–epiploic artery anastomotic techniques were used to place free omental grafts in severely ischemic lower limbs.[22] Despite low late patency rates, relief of claudication and rest pain and healing of ulcers were reported, again presumably due to neovascularization. This approach may be even more advantageous if anastomoses can be performed at multiple levels between omental branches and focal areas of ischemia. However, at present, this should be viewed as an experimental salvage procedure.

PREOPERATIVE ASSESSMENT

From the preceding discussion, it should be apparent that severe atherosclerosis and diabetes per se are not contraindications, nor do they preclude microsurgical reconstruction. Poor inflow through an atherosclerotic artery is a potentially limiting factor, not the vessel wall disease itself. Thorough preoperative assessment and careful patient selection are extremely important. The obvious major criterion for success in microvascular transfer is the presence of an acceptable recipient vessel.* Preoperative arteriography is essential as is hemodynamic assessment by noninvasive testing. The ankle-brachial index (ABI) is useful as an initial screening criterion. Extremities with ABIs of 0.5 or less should undergo preliminary proximal revascularization to

*There is a conflict of terminology between specialties with regard to this definition. Vascular surgeons prefer to classify the recipient vessel as the donor vessel (source of inflow) because it *receives* the flap but donates the blood supply.

improve inflow. Those with indices of more than 0.7 may undergo isolated flap transposition providing that the Doppler waveform in the recipient artery is of good quality (biphasic or triphasic) and is suitable for anastomosis. Obviously, noncompressibility of diseased arteries, seen typically in diabetics, may render these measurements inaccurate. Duplex scanning with Doppler waveform analysis will allow qualitative assessment of flow and the localization of focal obstructive plaques as well as identification of nonsclerotic segments suitable for anastomosis.[23] Neuropathy should be assessed because its presence negates the construction of a sensate flap. It is obvious also that the general status of all patients in regard to the operative risk of reconstruction versus amputation must be critically assessed.

The need for adequate hydration to achieve optimal systemic hemodynamics, antibiotics based upon bacterial cultures and sensitivities, and thorough surgical débridement of all devitalized tissue prior to bypass is well established. If a vein graft is required, preoperative duplex mapping may be helpful in identification of the vessel at the time of surgery. Lengthening of the overall operative time as a consequence of superimposing the microsurgical procedure should not be a consideration. It has been shown that increased duration of operation does not increase risk in patients of any age.[24]

SURGICAL TECHNIQUE

A team approach is used in which flap design and elevation are performed at the same time as the "recipient" site is prepared. A distal bypass may be indicated in patients who do not have conventional indications for arterial reconstruction to provide a conduit for free flap anastomosis. The choice between simultaneous versus staged reconstruction is controversial, and the decision must be made on an individual basis by each surgical team themselves. Those who advocate a two-stage procedure cite the advantages of better bacterial control of the wound and the security of documented patency of the distal arterial reconstruction prior to risking expenditure of a flap donor site. The recipient artery and vein should be exposed and dissected free for at least 5 to 6 cm. Anastomosis should be completed under 15- to 20-power magnification with interrupted 9–0 or 10–0 nylon suture. Its location may be at a native artery, distal to a reversed or in situ saphenous vein bypass graft, or distal to the autogenous vein graft itself if no native artery is available.[5, 14, 17] Vein grafts up to 40 cm in length have been successfully used in free flap transfers, and their length does not appear to correlate with patency.[25] The steal phenomenon has not been documented in free flap transfers because average flow rates of 2 to 10 ml/min are determined by the resistance of the vascular bed of the flap and are inconsequential relative to the potential recipient vessel inflow.[5]

Choice of flap is dictated by the size, depth, and location of the wound and the pedicle length required. Because of the rarity of atherosclerotic disease in the upper extremities, donor sites ordinarily should be chosen from regions above the waist. A meticulous anastomosis must be performed, to a nonsclerotic segment if possible. The arterial anastomosis should be performed end-to-side, whereas venous anastomoses are usually done end-to-end to a *deep* venous recipient. With the use of in situ saphenous vein grafts, intraoperative arteriography must be performed to ensure patency and to locate and interrupt perforators that would otherwise develop into significant postoperative arteriovenous fistulae. If distal pedal bypass is necessary, it should be performed using the operative microscope and standard microsurgical technique.[26, 27] After microvascular bypass has been performed, direct arterial anastomosis to the graft is preferable unless the revascularization level is too far proximal.[28]

POSTOPERATIVE CARE

Epidural blocks relieve pain and enhance circulation by mitigating vasospasm. The extremity should be elevated to minimize swelling, and the patient should be kept at bed rest for 10 days to 2 weeks. High-molecular-weight dextran (500 ml/day) is often used for 3 days, and 325 mg aspirin is administered by mouth daily for 2 weeks to enhance anastomotic patency, although the scientific basis of these interventions has never been proved. The flaps are serially monitored for color, temperature, capillary refill, flap artery Doppler signals, and laser Doppler flow assessment. Serial surveillance with flow velocity determinations by means of duplex scanning should be carried out at 3-month intervals for 1 year and at 6-month intervals thereafter. Any deterioration in flow velocity warrants repeat angiography. Judicious reoperation contributes to improved tissue preservation with higher secondary patency rates and long-term limb salvage.

SUMMARY

Microsurgery has become an important adjunct to limb salvage in patients with either trauma or atherosclerosis and should be considered the procedure of choice in many cases in which amputation would otherwise be required. Patients with ischemic limbs often present with complex wound problems, including exposed or infected tendon and bone, that are insoluble with conventional techniques using skin grafts or local flaps. Microvascular free tissue transfer has proved to be an important alternative to amputation in such difficult circumstances. Obviously, this approach should not be considered in patients with insensate limbs or multiple life-threatening injuries. However, advanced age and multisystem disease may be only relative contraindications, and concomitant diabetes per se is *not* a contraindication. These techniques require a team approach. Transferred viable free flaps appear to provide additional vascularity to the surrounding tissue, aiding in wound healing, combating chronic infection, and relieving rest pain. Free flap transfer can be successfully combined with autogenous or in situ saphenous vein bypass procedures and may be indicated alone when adequate circulation exists or a single leg artery is patent but primary or secondary pedal arcades are occluded.

Experience with more patients with more long-term patency data is needed to assess these techniques and their indications completely, but morbidity and mortality rates appear to be equal to those achieved with amputation or bypass alone. Bypass grafts should be patent for at least 1 year to be cost effective.

There is no evidence that failure of such reconstructions causes a higher level of amputation than would otherwise result. Patient selection is of utmost importance, but in experienced hands success rates can be expected to exceed 80 per cent. Close collaboration between plastic and vascular surgeons is essential to undertake these complex extremity salvage procedures.

References

1. Acland RD: Microsurgery Practice Manual. Louisville, Louisville School of Medicine, Department of Surgery, 1977.
2. Daniel RK, Taylor GI: Distant transfer of an island flap by microvascular anastamosis. Plast Reconstr Surg 52:111, 1973.
3. May JW Jr, Gallico GG III, Lukash FN: Microvascular transfer of free tissue for closure of bone wounds of the distal lower extremity. N Engl J Med 306:253, 1982.
4. Allen TR, Franklin JD, Withers EH, Davis LJ: Extremity salvage utilizing microvascular free tissue transfer. Surgery 90:1047, 1981.
5. Briggs SE, Banis JC Jr, Kaebnick H, et al: Distal revascularization and microvascular free tissue transfer: An alternative to amputation in ischemic lesions of the lower extremity. J Vasc Surg 2:806, 1985.
6. Stoney RJ: Ultimate salvage for the patient with limb threatening ischemia. Realistic goals and surgical considerations. Am J Surg 136:228, 1978.
7. Yeager RA, Hobson RW, Jamil Z, et al: Differential patency and limb salvage for polytetrafluoroethylene and autogenous saphenous vein in severe lower extremity ischemia. Surgery 91:99, 1982.
8. Bergan JJ, Veith FJ, Bernhard VM, et al: Randomization of autogenous vein and polytetrafluoroethylene grafts in femoral-distal reconstruction. Surgery 92:921, 1982.
9. Goldberg S, Alex M, Joshi RA, Blumenthal HT: Nonatheromatous peripheral vascular disease of the lower extremity in diabetes mellitus. Diabetes 8:261, 1959.
10. LoGerfo FW, Coffman JD: Vascular and microvascular disease of the foot in diabetes. N Engl J Med 311(25):1615, 1984.
11. Strandness DE, Priest RE, Gibbons GE: Combined clinical and pathologic study of diabetic and nondiabetic peripheral arterial disease. Diabetes 13:366, 1964.
12. Conrad MC: Large and small artery occlusion in diabetics and nondiabetics with severe vascular disease. Circulation 36:83, 1967.
13. Barner HB, Kaiser GC, William VL: Blood flow in the diabetic leg. Circulation 43:391, 1971.
14. Colen LB: Limb salvage in the patient with severe peripheral vascular disease: The role of microsurgical free-tissue transfer. Plast Reconstr Surg 79(3):389, 1986.
15. Mimoun M, Hilligot P, Baux S: The nutrient flap: A new concept of the role of the flap and application to the salvage of arteriosclerotic lower limbs. Plast Reconstr Surg 84(3): 458, 1989.
16. Shestak KC, Fitz DG, Newton ED, et al: Expanding the horizons in treatment of severe peripheral vascular disease using microsurgical techniques. Plast Reconstr Surg 85(3): 411, 1990.
17. Shestak KC, Hendricks DL, Webster MW: Indirect revascularization of the lower extremity by means of microvascular free-muscle flap—A preliminary report. J Vasc Surg 12:581, 1990.
18. Pevec WC, Hendricks D, Rosenthal MS, et al: Revascularization of an ischemic limb by use of a muscle pedicle flap: A rabbit model. J Vasc Surg 13:385, 1991.
19. Lai CS, Lin SD, Chou CK, et al: Limb salvage of infected diabetic foot ulcers with microsurgical free-muscle transfer. Ann Plast Surg 26(3):212, 1991.
20. Shenag SM, Krouskop T, Stal S, et al: Salvage of amputation stumps by secondary reconstruction utilizing microsurgical free tissue transfer. Plast Reconstr Surg 79:861, 1987.
21. Gallico GG III, Ehrlichman RJ, Jupiter J, et al: Free flaps to preserve below-knee amputation stumps: Long-term evaluation. Plast Reconstr Surg 79:871, 1979.
22. Herrera HR, Geary J, Whitehead P, et al: Revascularization of the lower extremity with omentum. Clin Plast Surg 18(3):491, 1991.
23. Colen L, Musson A: Preoperative assessment of the peripheral vascular disease patient for free tissue transfers. Plast Reconstr Surg 82(6):112, 1988.
24. Goldman L, Caldera DL, Southwick FS, et al: Cardiac risk factors and complications in non-cardiac surgery. Medicine 57:357, 1978.
25. Shaw WW: Microvascular free flaps. The first decade. Clin Plast Surg 10:3, 1983.
26. Gloviczki P, Morris SM, Bopwer TC, et al: Microvascular pedal bypass for salvage of the severely ischemic limb. Mayo Clinic Proc 66:243, 1991.
27. Klamer TW, Lambert GE Jr, Richardson JD, et al: Utility of inframalleolar arterial bypass grafting. J Vasc Surg 11:164, 1990.
28. Chowdary RP, Celani VJ, Goodreau JJ, et al: Free-tissue transfers for limb salvage utilizing in situ saphenous vein bypass conduit as the inflow. Plast Reconstr Surg 87(3): 529, 1991.

Fogarty Catheter Thrombectomy

Thomas J. Fogarty, M.D.

• • •

Catheter thrombectomy is a simple and effective method for the treatment of acute arterial occlusion.[2] Its correct usage restores arterial circulation with minimal arterial trauma, in normal as well as atherosclerotic vessels. The embolectomy balloon is designed to deform in response to arterial narrowing when it is withdrawn from a diseased vessel (Fig. 21–18). This decreases the possibility of arterial damage during thrombectomy.

GENERAL CATHETER USE

Specific points that apply to the use of the embolectomy catheter include the following: first, a sufficient length of the artery must be exposed to allow control both proximal and distal to the catheter introduction site. For aortic embolectomy, bilateral groin incisions are made, and vessel loops are placed around the exposed common, superficial, and deep femoral arteries. For femoropopliteal embolectomy, control of the common femoral artery is gained prior to embolectomy catheter cannulation. A transverse arteriotomy is made to avoid stricture formation upon arterial closure. In some situations a longitudinal or tangential incision may be needed owing to the pattern of atherosclerotic disease.

Second, the balloon catheter is prepared for use. The embolectomy catheter is inflated with saline and checked

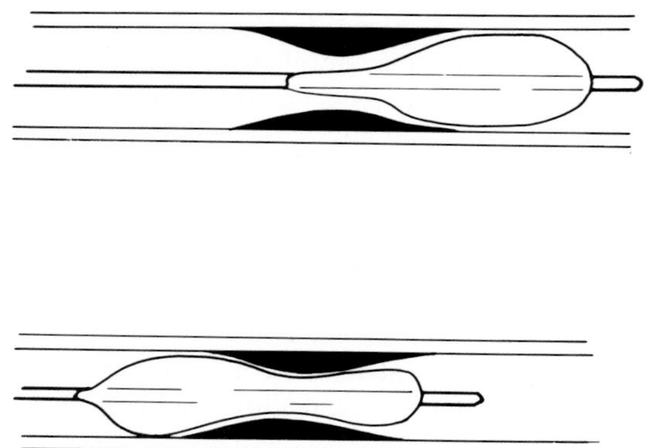

FIGURE 21–18. The compliance of the embolectomy balloon.

for concentricity and leaks. Concentricity of the balloon about the catheter body is important. An eccentric balloon tends to displace the catheter tip and body toward one side of the arterial wall, thereby increasing catheter drag and friction.[1] Sequential inflation and deflation of the balloon are then performed until the balloon is pliable and easily inflated. This increases balloon control during the embolectomy procedure. Smaller bore syringes are used for balloon inflation: 3-cc syringes for the larger balloons and 1-cc syringes for the smaller 2 Fr embolectomy catheters. When one is using the 2 Fr embolectomy balloon, the 1-cc syringe should be dipped in saline prior to catheter attachment. Wetting the syringe tip in this fashion ensures that an airtight seal is achieved between the syringe and the catheter. Air is used to inflate the 1 Fr embolectomy catheter. The inflation lumen of the catheter is too tiny to permit quick adjustments in balloon size if saline inflation is performed. If the 2 Fr embolectomy catheter is applied in situations in which even tiny amounts of air from a ruptured balloon may pose problems, as in the cerebral vasculature, carbon dioxide is used for inflation.

A third point regarding embolectomy catheter use is the importance of distal cannulation. The only guarantee of distal patency is direct catheter passage into the distal vasculature. Distal thrombus may be discontinuous with proximal thrombus. Removal of only the proximal thrombus may generate vigorous blood backflow, giving false assurance of distal patency. Failure to continue embolectomy catheter passage will result in retained thrombus, which will propagate proximally to cause reocclusion.

Fourth, although the pliable embolectomy catheter is designed to facilitate passage, cannulation of specific vessels may be difficult at times. In the lower extremity, the most common site of difficulty is the popliteal artery. Varying the angle of knee flexion usually allows the catheter to pass. If this does not work, partial inflation and deflation of the balloon may recenter the catheter within the lumen and permit catheter advancement. The embolectomy catheter tip may be preformed with a bend, and the catheter body rotated at the point of difficult passage. Persistent inability to pass the catheter indicates atherosclerotic obstruction of the vessel. Evaluation of this area using intraoperative arteriography or angioscopy is preferable to continued vigorous attempts at catheter passage. The latter may lead to regrettable vascular damage and complications.[3]

Last, catheter retrieval must be performed in a gentle manner. If a large amount of pull force is required to remove the catheter, it indicates that the balloon has been overinflated. On the other hand, when withdrawing the balloon embolectomy catheter from a vessel with an increasing taper, addition of saline may be required for the balloon to maintain arterial wall contact. Balloon overinflation causes an inordinate amount of shear force to be exerted on the arterial endothelium. Endothelial injury and plaque dislodgment may occur. Experimentally, shear force values of 30 gm and less resulted in the absence of electron microscopic evidence of endothelial damage in canine carotid arteries.[15] In general, clot extraction[3] should be performed with the least possible amount of shear force.

EMBOLECTOMY IN SPECIFIC VESSELS

Aortic Embolectomy. Removal of emboli and thrombi from the aorta is performed via an arteriotomy in the common femoral artery, just proximal to the bifurcation of the deep femoral artery. Bilateral proximal and distal exploration with the balloon catheter is necessary in aortic thromboembolism to rule out embolization that may have occurred to either side (Fig. 21–19). Distal exploration is conducted first, with passage of the entire length of a 2 or 3 Fr embolectomy catheter. Following distal embolectomy, a heparin solution is infused into the femoral system, and the common femoral artery is clamped. Embolectomy of the aorta and the ipsilateral iliac artery is performed, followed by closure of the arteriotomy. The contralateral distal system is explored as before, followed by contralateral proximal exploration.

Femoropopliteal Embolectomy. A groin incision is made, and the common, superficial, and deep femoral arte-

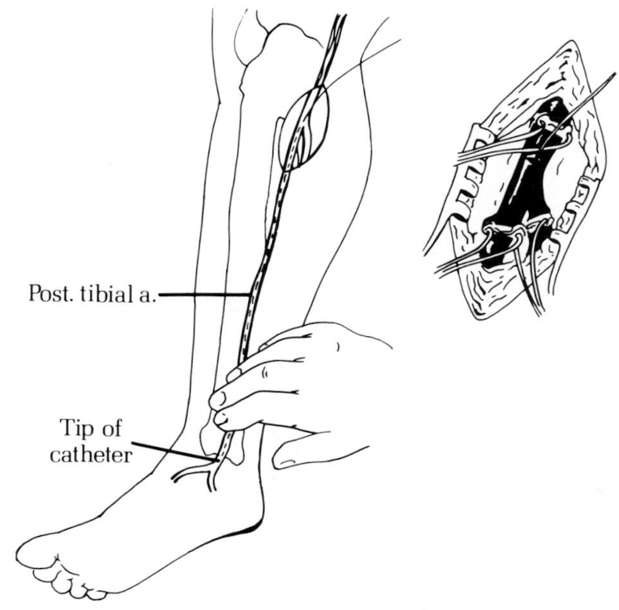

FIGURE 21–19. Embolectomy of the tibial vessels.

ries are isolated. Control of these arteries is established with vessel loops. Both the superficial and the deep femoral systems are explored. Cannulation of the deep system is limited to 25 cm owing to the rapid tapering of this vessel. Catheters of 2 or 3 Fr are simultaneously passed into the distal lower extremity. The first catheter usually passes into the peroneal or posterior tibial artery. Introduction of additional embolectomy catheters allows cannulation of the remaining crural arteries.

The retrieved thrombus should be carefully examined. A sharp cutoff indicates incomplete removal, and catheter passage must be repeated. If no additional clot can be retrieved on a second passage, angioscopy is helpful in delineating the pathology. Residual thrombus on the arteriogram is an indication for a second incision at the knee to expose the distal popliteal artery. The anterior and posterior tibial arteries are isolated and looped with Silastic tapes. An arteriotomy is made in the distal popliteal artery, and 2 or 3 Fr catheters are passed into the anterior and posterior tibial arteries (Fig. 21–20). In previously undiseased vessels, the 2 Fr catheters should pass beyond the ankle joint. If this is impossible, even upon varying the plantar flexion at the foot, and the arteriogram shows evidence of obstruction, direct exposure of the anterior and posterior tibial arteries at the ankle is indicated. Manipulation of the isolated anterior and posterior tibial arteries through the incision may allow catheter passage. If necessary, an arteriotomy just large enough to admit a 2 Fr catheter is made. Following clot removal, heparin flush solution is used to irrigate the distal arterial system.

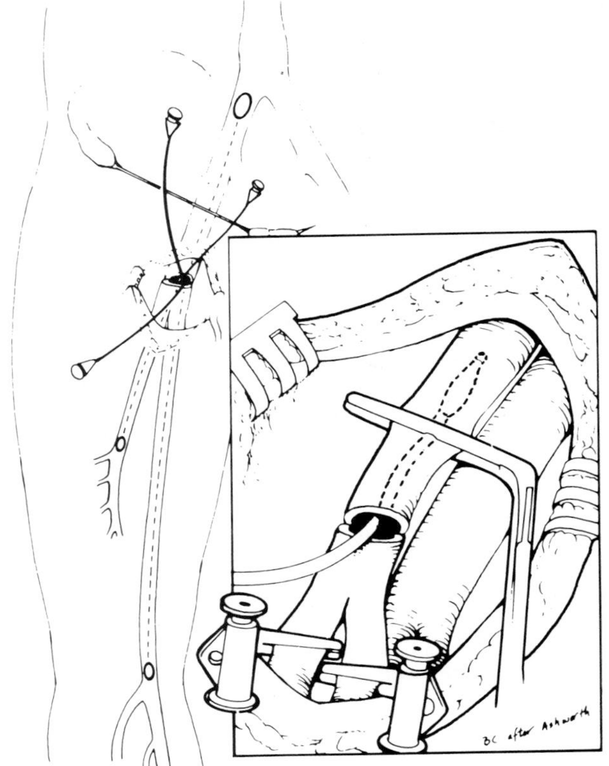

FIGURE 21–20. Cannulation of both proximal and distal vessels in aortoiliac embolectomy.

Venous Thrombectomy. Ineffective clot removal and serious complications may result from the use of arterial catheters in the venous system. Tip pliability and body flexibility of venous and arterial catheters differ, although the basic concepts of their use are similar. The soft, pliable tip of the venous catheter bends upon itself when the valve leaflet is encountered, acting as a J-guidewire to facilitate passage across the valve. Other techniques may aid venous thrombectomy catheter passage. Forceful distal calf or thigh compression may open the valve leaflets, allowing catheter advancement. Partial inflation of the balloon above the valve may distend the vein and allow the tip of the catheter to penetrate the open leaflets.[4]

Venous thrombosis is often associated with arterial occlusion in cases of advanced ischemia. A lower extremity that presents in rigor following acute arterial occlusion should be examined for concomitant venous thrombosis following arterial embolectomy. The venous outflow system of the involved extremity is clamped. The extremity is tightly wrapped with an elastic bandage, and repeated extension and dorsiflexion of the foot are performed to increase the resting venous pressure. Upon clamp removal, the venous clot is expelled from the vein. If additional venous thrombectomy is needed, a 6 Fr venous catheter is introduced. In advanced ischemia, phlebotomy of an additional 300 to 500 ml of venous effluent should be performed to avoid metabolic complications. This effluent is passed through a cell saver to reduce the need for transfusion.

In the patient who requires venous thrombectomy for iliofemoral venous occlusion, the following sequence is observed: first, preoperative descending venography is performed to determine the proximal extent of the clot. An 8/22 Fr venous catheter is introduced via the right cephalic vein at the shoulder, passed proximal to the clot, and inflated to occlude the vena cava. An 8/10 Fr venous catheter is passed into the vena cava from the involved side, inflated, and withdrawn. Deflation is necessary as the catheter enters the iliac vein. Valves located above the inguinal ligament offer resistance to the extraction of thrombi. Effective clot removal can be accomplished by alternate inflation and deflation of the balloon at valve locations.

Graft Thrombectomy. Additional catheters have been developed to address the problem of removing the adherent thrombus that is frequently encountered in artificial conduits for both bypass and angioaccess. These two new devices, one called an adherent clot catheter and the other a graft thrombectomy catheter (Baxter V. Mueller, Niles, IL) are described in more detail in a subsequent chapter (see Chapter 43). The catheters are designed to remove the adherent material that is left behind after use of the conventional balloon embolectomy catheter.

The technique for use of both of these catheters is similar to that of the standard balloon embolectomy catheter. The catheter is passed in the low profile configuration until the retrieval end of the catheter is positioned within the region of the adherent material. To effect removal, the pitch of the spiral retrieval element is adjusted via a control knob on the handle of the catheter. This maneuver engages the adherent material within the retrieval element, and the

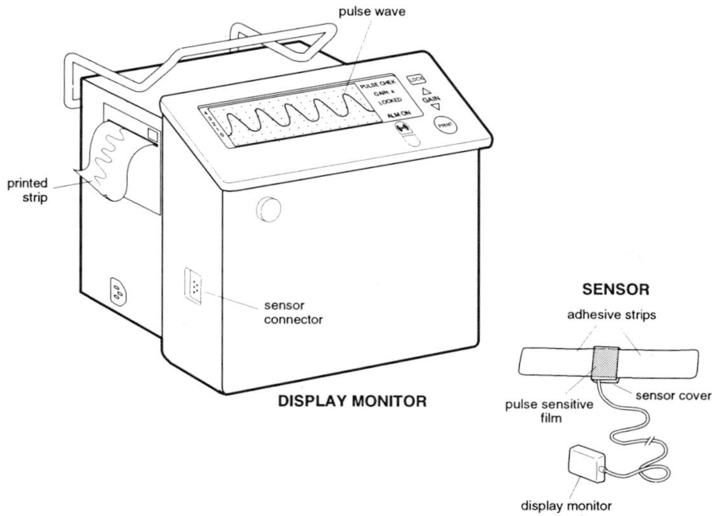

FIGURE 21–21. Pulse amplitude monitor system: portable display monitor and piezoelectric sensor.

catheter is withdrawn through the arteriotomy or graftotomy.

Another new instrument that is useful during the thrombectomy of aortoiliac and femoral bypass grafts is a pulse amplitude monitor. It consists of a portable display monitor and a piezoelectric sensor (Fig. 21–21). The sensor, which is applied intraoperatively over the dorsalis pedis, quantitatively monitors the amplitude of the mechanical oscillations of the pulsing distal artery before, during, and after the thrombectomy procedure. The amplitude of the waveform displayed in real-time on the monitor is an indicator of perfusion. This monitoring system serves as an expedient alternative to arteriography in the operating room and, when left in place postoperatively, permits continuous monitoring of the status of the reperfused extremity during recovery.

OTHER USES FOR BALLOON CATHETERS

Temporary Vessel Occlusion. The balloon embolectomy catheter may be used during reconstructive procedures to occlude flow in vessels with marked atherosclerotic narrowing. Mechanical clamps have a tendency to fracture calcified plaque and cause dissection. The pliable embolectomy balloon is advantageous in this situation. McCaughan and Young reported on an extensive clinical experience, supplying histologic and physiologic data that supported the advantages of intraluminal occlusion with balloon catheters during arterial reconstruction.[6]

Balloon catheter tamponade is used in several situations. The most common of these involves emergent aortic occlusion to control hemorrhage due to a ruptured abdominal aortic aneurysm.[5, 8] An 8/22 Fr balloon catheter is introduced via a cutdown in the left brachial artery, near the antecubital fossa. The catheter is threaded 35 cm and inflated with 6 to 10 ml of 60 per cent angiographic contrast material. The partially inflated balloon catheter is advanced a total distance of 60 cm, guided by the flow in the descending aorta. At this point, the balloon is inflated to a volume of 43 ml and is then withdrawn until the aorta is occluded at the neck of the aneurysm. Total or partial occlusion can be ascertained by palpation of the femoral pulses. Fluoroscopy, although not necessary, is recommended for this procedure.

Temporary balloon vessel occlusion may be applied in other circumstances. For example, balloon tamponade for repair of damage to the heart chambers and aorta often obviates cardiopulmonary bypass. The take-down of the Potts anastomosis in preparation for total surgical correction of tetralogy of Fallot can be simplified by introducing the balloon catheter through the anastomosis from the pulmonary artery side, thus eliminating the need for profound hypothermia, periods of low perfusion, and the danger of air embolization. Merkel described an intraluminal technique for arterial occlusion during renal transplantation.[7] In cases of high abdominal aortic aneurysm in which the surgical neck extends to the renal arteries, temporary retrograde balloon occlusion using 8/22 Fr catheters above the renal arteries affords safe limited dissection control during the completion of proximal anastomoses. Some very high carotid endarterectomies may require balloon tamponade for safe visualization of end-points. A 3 Fr arterial catheter filled with saline closely approximates the vessel diameter and gives excellent safe occlusion.

Permanent Vessel Occlusion. In the patient receiving long-term dialysis, a previously created internal arteriovenous fistula can be obliterated simply by percutaneous balloon occlusion. It is important that the puncture site be downstream from the site of balloon occlusion so that hemorrhage at the puncture site may be avoided. Thrombosis of the fistula occurs within 24 hours. The catheter is removed after documentation of permanent thrombotic occlusion. Permanent occlusion of carotid–cavernous sinus fistulae with a balloon catheter has been described by Prolo and Hanbery.[9]

Calibration. The Fogarty balloon catheter may be used to derive valuable information about vessel size and about the degree and location of lesions in the vascular system. If significant stenoses are present, air or fluid must be withdrawn from the balloon for easy catheter removal, thus establishing a relative lumen diameter.

When a more accurate measurement of lumen diameter is desired, the catheter is inflated with fluid until the balloon just contacts the vessel wall. The volume of fluid used for injection is noted, and the balloon catheter is deflated and removed. Reinflation of the balloon with the same volume of fluid, followed by measurement of the balloon diameter with a ruler or a circular template, yields the calibrated lumen diameter.

The distance of a stenosis from an arteriotomy site may also be determined. A balloon catheter is inserted into the arteriotomy, partially inflated with saline, and advanced until it meets the leading edge of the stenosis. The distance is noted using length markers on the catheter body. Measurements of stenosis location and vessel diameter are particularly useful for determining correct angioplasty balloon sizes for intraoperative balloon dilatation procedures.

References

1. Dobrin PB, Jorgensen RA: Balloon embolectomy catheters in small arteries. III. Surgical significance of eccentric balloons. Surgery 93:402, 1983.
2. Fogarty TJ, Cranley JJ, Krause RJ, et al: A method of extraction of arterial emboli and thrombi. Surg Gynecol Obstet 116:241, 1963.
3. Foster JH, Carter JW, Edwards WH, et al: Arterial injuries secondary to the use of the Fogarty catheter. Ann Surg 171:971, 1970.
4. Haimov M, Jacobson JH: Auxiliary applications of the Fogarty catheter. Surg Gynecol Obstet 133:666, 1971.
5. Hyde GL, Sullivan DM: Fogarty catheter tamponade of ruptured abdominal aortic aneurysms. Surg Gynecol Obstet 154:197, 1982.
6. McCaughan JJ Jr, Young JM: Intra-arterial occlusion in vascular surgery. Ann Surg 171:695, 1970.
7. Merkel FK: An intraluminal technique for arterial occlusion during renal transplantation. Arch Surg 110:348, 1975.
8. Ng AC, Ochsner EC: Use of Fogarty catheter tamponade for ruptured abdominal aortic aneurysms. Am J Roentgenol 128:31, 1977.
9. Prolo DJ, Hanbery JW: Intraluminal occlusion of a carotid–cavernous sinus fistula with a balloon catheter. J Neurosurg 35:237, 1971.

Endarterectomy

Ronald J. Stoney, M.D., and Robert W. Thompson, M.D.

• • •

The possibility of directly removing occlusive arterial lesions that impair blood flow became a clinical reality 45 years ago, when Dos Santos of Lisbon successfully restored patency to the superficial femoral artery of a man with a threatened limb.[15] He named this operation "arterial disobstruction," or "disobliteration," and attributed its feasibility to the use of the new anticoagulant drug heparin. Bazy and Reboul[2] later described this procedure as endarterectomy, and Leriche[31] chose the more comprehensive term thromboendarterectomy to indicate removal of obstructing thrombus as well as the diseased arterial intima. There is no truly precise term to describe this technique completely because, when properly performed, the inner media is also removed, but the terms endarterectomy and thromboendarterectomy, used interchangeably, are used most commonly.

Three years after Dos Santos' operation, Wylie of San Francisco performed the first thromboendarterectomy in the United States in an epic attempt to relieve aortoiliac obstruction.[46] Shortly thereafter, Wylie reported a large experience with this technique at the University of California Medical Center in San Francisco (UCSF).[44] Since the 1950s, at UCSF, continuing use of endarterectomy as one of the preferred therapeutic options for patients with occlusive vascular disease has resulted in a significant experience with this operation in every extracranial arterial site where such lesions occur.

The critical feature that makes endarterectomy feasible is the pathologic localization of atherosclerotic plaque to the intima and subjacent media of the diseased artery. The outer media and adventitia are spared by atherosclerosis; therefore, a cleavage plane can be readily developed between the diseased and nondiseased zones of the arterial wall. Such a cleavage plane is marked by poor adherence between the two zones, and it is macroscopically continuous throughout the length of the lesion. With localized regions of atherosclerotic stenosis, the tapering distal termination of the lesion or "end-point" coincides with a gradual lessening of medial involvement. This allows removal of obvious disease smoothly or with only a minimal residual ledge of thickened intima that is adherent to the underlying media. When such an intimal ledge is present, it can be transected on a bevel to minimize the risk of an obstructing flap becoming elevated after restoration of flow. If the distal end-point is not adherent to the underlying media or adventitia, it can be secured with fine "tacking" sutures tied externally. Nearly all anatomic patterns of occlusive atherosclerosis are suitable for endarterectomy, whether the disease is localized, diffuse, calcific, or otherwise degenerative.

The immediate success of endarterectomy is also dependent on the characteristics of arteries that allow them to resist dilation and eventual disruption following restoration of pulsatile flow at systemic blood pressures. It has always been of great interest that the residual outer media and adventitia left after endarterectomy have sufficient tensile strength to support the vessel wall; this is true even in the aorta, where the medial myoelastic lamellae are thought to be so important to vascular integrity. This feature of arteries is destroyed if any degree of dilating or aneurysmal degeneration is present. Interestingly, current information suggests that aneurysmal degeneration involves an activation of degradative protease activities throughout the arterial wall, perhaps most importantly in the adventitia, and that this process may be biochemically distinct from the atherosclerotic changes evident in occlusive disease patterns (see Chapter 13). Endarterectomy of such an artery, even if initially successful, will predictably lead to aneurysmal dilation of the endarterectomized segment over time. For this reason, the presence of aneurysmal disease is the only contraindication to endarterectomy for the management of occlusive arterial disease.

PATTERNS OF ATHEROSCLEROSIS

There are three distinct patterns of occlusive atherosclerosis, which can be characterized according to (1) site in the arterial tree, (2) relation to sites of arterial fixation, and (3) proximity to sites of turbulence. Each pattern is associated with particular arterial lesions amenable to endarterectomy.

Sites Within the Arterial Tree

Lesions in the ten major aortic branches are predictably located near the origin of the vessel from the aorta, are short in length, and terminate with a smooth transition to a nearly normal lumen within the arterial branch. Only rarely is the aortic ostia of an involved aortic branch spared, with the obstructing lesion originating within the proximal artery and extending distally for a variable length.

These features of aortic branch atherosclerosis make transaortic endarterectomy an important technique for improving perfusion in all vascular beds supplied by these branches, with the exception of the three branches of the transverse aortic arch. A proximal aortic cross-clamp cannot be applied in these locations. Therefore, transvessel retrograde endarterectomy is necessary, but the proximal occluding clamp must include the orifice of the branch (e.g., the innominate artery). The five major abdominal aortic branches (three viscerals, two renals) are ideally suited for transaortic endarterectomy. Disease affecting the two terminal aortic branches, the iliac arteries, consistently extends to the iliac bifurcation or further. Therefore, in addition to the transaortic approach, transiliac endarterectomy is needed to facilitate safe and complete removal of these lengthy lesions.

Sites of Arterial Fixation

The superficial femoral artery traverses the adductor canal in the lower third of the thigh. At this site it is confined by the adductor magnus muscle and is locally fixed by the adductor tendon at the hiatus through which it passes as it enters the popliteal space. This normal anatomic configuration favors the development of atherosclerotic disease at this particular site in the femoropopliteal arterial segment. Osseous or myofascial anomalies may also cause fixation of arteries in other locations, particularly near active joints. The subclavian artery near the thoracic outlet and the popliteal artery adjacent to the knee are typical examples. A cervical rib or gastrocnemius muscle entrapment produces arterial compression and eventually injury. Repeated arterial injury of the subclavian artery produces poststenotic aneurysm or focal atherosclerotic intimal ulceration. These can produce upper extremity micro- or macroembolization. The focal occlusive and ulcerated lesions of the subclavian arterial tree are quite amenable to thromboendarterectomy through the affected artery. However, when either subclavian or popliteal aneurysms are present, they are preferably replaced with a graft.

Sites of Turbulence

Turbulent blood flow may enhance the deposition of intimal atheromatous lesions. The carotid bifurcation may be the most common example, although the bifurcations of the common femoral and popliteal arteries are also important in relation to lower extremity ischemia. The carotid bifurcation is the undisputed site for preferential use of endarterectomy in vascular surgery as it is practiced currently, and in many surgeons' practices, it is the *only* place where this technique is employed!

TECHNIQUE

When analyzed closely, atheromatous lesions comprise a heterogeneous spectrum of disease. Most vascular surgeons are familiar with the lesion in the carotid bifurcation and perhaps portions of lesions removed to facilitate the implantation of grafts in other sites in the arterial tree. The pathologist dutifully reports the segment of atherosclerotic plaque and describes the microscopic features in relatively bland terms. However, to the surgeon who regularly uses the technique of endarterectomy it becomes obvious that different lesions require different endarterectomy techniques. The variation in the composition of these lesions is in part the result of metabolism of the arterial wall and the response to injury and repair, and certainly the result of systemic and local factors currently unknown. Activity within an atherosclerotic plaque, such as hemorrhage, alters the composition of the lesion and its intimal surface. Finally, the location, distribution, luminal size, and contour of the atheroma vary significantly and affect not only the conduct of the endarterectomy but also the short- and long-term results.

Five specific techniques of endarterectomy are available to the surgeon, depending on the type, extent, and location of the lesion to be removed and on his or her experience.

Open Endarterectomy

This is the most commonly employed technique, originally advocated by Bazy and Reboul[2] and performed through a longitudinal arteriotomy. It exposes the extent of the lesion to be removed and allows direct separation of the disease from the subjacent arterial wall. An elevator or clamp is the instrument usually selected to separate the atheroma from the arterial wall. The most common example is carotid bifurcation endarterectomy (Fig. 21–22).

Semi-Closed Endarterectomy

This technique was originally performed by Dos Santos[16] and requires either transverse or longitudinal arteriotomies placed at the proximal and distal extent of the lesion within the artery. A distal end-point is established, and retrograde separation of the atheromatous plaque or core from the uninvolved artery proceeds in a proximal direction through the unopened vessel (Fig. 21–23). One or more intervening arteriotomies may be used to disobliterate long arterial segments. This procedure is continued to the proximal arteriotomy, where the lesion is detached and then removed; a hand-held loop stripper[4] or gas- or electric-powered strippers that oscillate[32] are available and may be used to traverse long distances between arteriotomies. These devices maintain the separation plane between the atheroma and the residual arterial wall. This technique is commonly used in the iliac or superficial femoral artery. It avoids the use of a long segmental patch, which would generally be required if the endarterectomy were performed in an open manner through a longitudinal arteriotomy.

Extraction Endarterectomy

The technique of extraction endarterectomy requires either retrograde or antegrade removal of an atheroma through a single arteriotomy, either transverse or longitudinal, in the involved vessel. It is performed using straight or slightly curved long-jawed clamps or an elevator. If the

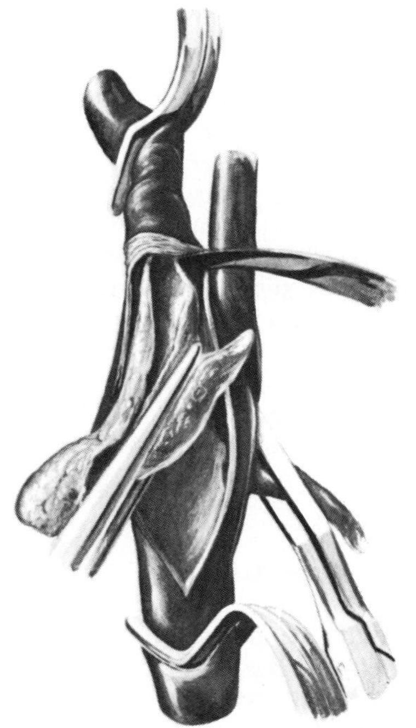

FIGURE 21–22. Eversion endarterectomy of distal internal carotid lesion beyond end of the arteriotomy.

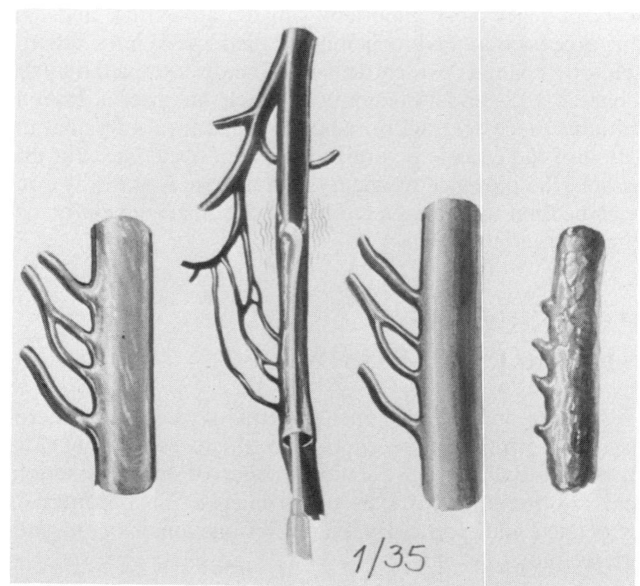

FIGURE 21–23. Semi-closed endarterectomy. Retrograde separation of plaque with loop stripper yields atheromatous core with branch artery orifices.

endarterectomy is performed retrograde, the proximal end-point is separated by clamping the artery, which fractures or crushes the plaque. This technique is used in performing common femoral and distal external iliac endarterectomy. If the endarterectomy is performed in an antegrade direction, the distal end-point is identified by external palpation of the artery. The atheromatous termination is gently controlled and removed by grasping it in the jaws of the clamp—in effect, operating *beyond* the surgeon's direct vision. This technique may be particularly useful in endarterectomies of lesions of hypogastric or profunda femoris origin (Fig. 21–24).

When performing transaortic endarterectomy (open) that involves the removal of lesions from the orifices of major arterial branches (renal or visceral), the portion of the endarterectomy conducted in the branch artery uses the extraction principle. The dissection plane is carried from the aorta into the branch circumferentially and extended beyond the orifice. Within 1.5 to 3 cm the thickened intima returns to a normal thin layer and separates cleanly. The well-mobilized branch is prolapsed toward the aorta, and simultaneous traction on the specimen permits visualization of the end-point. Special angled extraction clamps (Figs. 21–25 and 21–26) facilitate the endarterectomy and removal of the occlusive lesion in the proximal aortic branch (Figs. 21–27 and 21–28).

Eversion Endarterectomy

This technique, originally described by Harrison and associates,[23] requires distal transection of the artery beyond the site of disease and eversion or turning back of the residual proximal arterial wall upon itself as traction is applied to the atheromatous core. The core of disease can be transected at its origin after the eversion is complete and

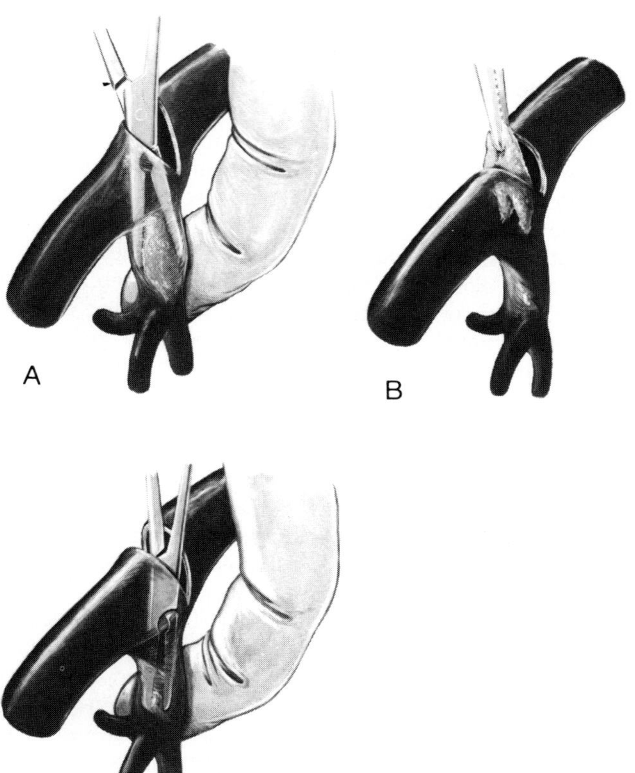

FIGURE 21–24. Hypogastric endarterectomy. *A*, Development of intimal core with hemostat. *B*, Extraction of specimen (incomplete). *C*, Removal of residual fragments.

the atheroma removed. The arterial wall is then drawn back distally into a normal position, restoring the now patent artery to its normal location where it can be reanastomosed to the distal arterial segment. This technique can also be used to disobliterate totally occluded excised arterial segments, which can then be employed in remote sites as arterial autografts. A common example is the use of the internal or external iliac arteries or the occluded superficial femoral artery.

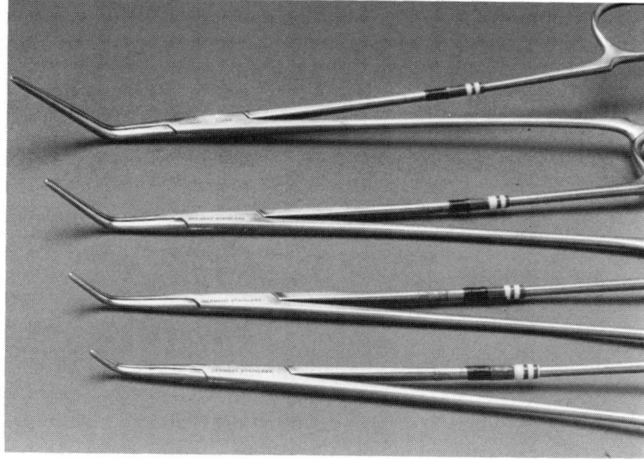

FIGURE 21–25. Special angled extraction clamps facilitate extraction endarterectomy.

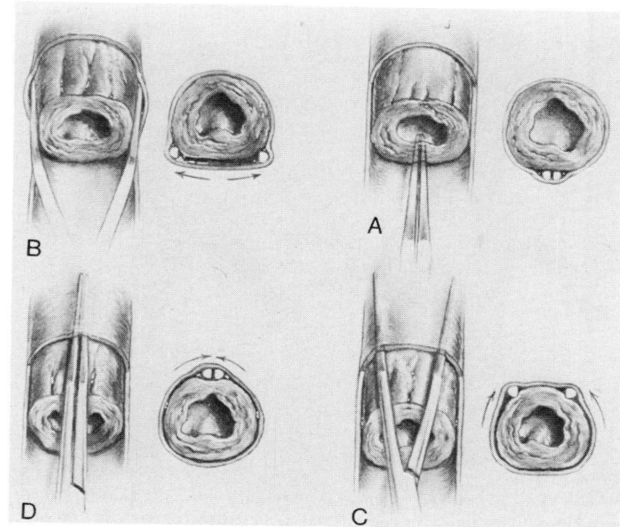

FIGURE 21–26. Use of angled extraction clamp to separate atheromatous core from arterial wall during extraction endarterectomy.

Selective Endarterectomy

This technique is a modification of the semi-closed endarterectomy and is used to remove discontinuous atheromatous lesions in one arterial segment. It is performed in a retrograde manner through a distal arteriotomy. It requires precise sizing of the arterial loop stripper to the artery to be treated. The operator is guided during careful retrograde advancement of this instrument by the *feel* of resistance as the loop engages, separates, and then disengages the discontinuous lesion in the artery. This type of endarterectomy is used often in the external iliac artery.

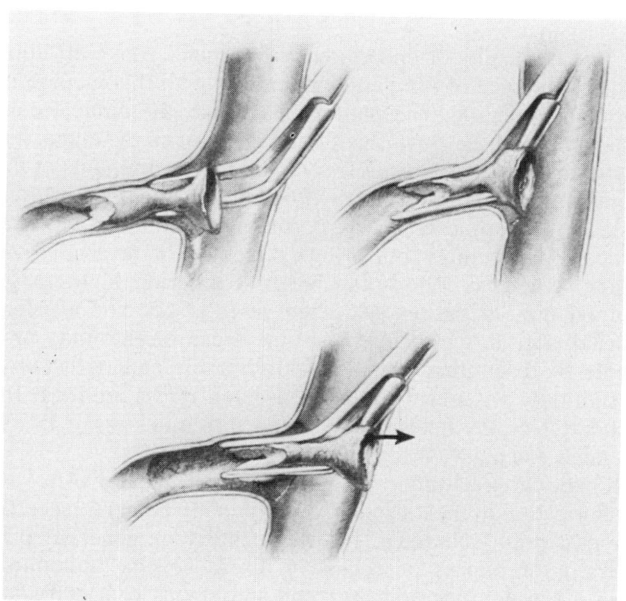

FIGURE 21–27. Angled extraction clamps allow endarterectomy of branch vessels to a disease-free end-point.

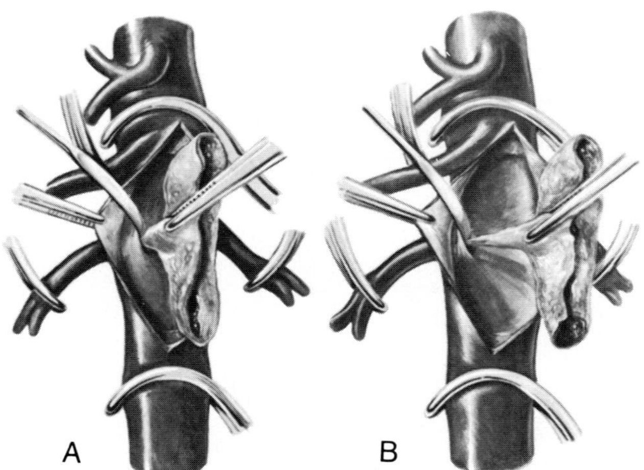

FIGURE 21–28. Removal of renal lesions. *A*, Dissection in endarterectomy plane in right renal artery after aortic portion has been completed. *B*, End-point of renal endarterectomy.

Selective endarterectomy can be performed within the diseased arterial segment itself (e.g., superficial femoral artery), through the parent artery (e.g., the aortorenal region), or both (e.g., the carotid or common femoral bifurcation). In endarterectomy performed from the parent artery the disease in the parent artery should always be separated before the endarterectomy plane is extended into the diseased branch (e.g., transaortic renal thromboendarterectomy) (Fig. 21–28). In cases of disease contained in both the parent artery and its bifurcation branches, it is usually preferable to separate the disease first from the parent (proximal artery) and next from the less critical bifurcation branch, completing the endarterectomy finally in the critical bifurcation branch. An example is carotid bifurcation endarterectomy.

RESULTS

The results of endarterectomy depend above all upon the experience of the vascular surgeon with this method of revascularization. The pattern of disease, the clinical consequences of the flow-obstructing lesion, and the characteristics of the atheroma are less important determinants of the outcome. Localized lesions with short terminations or transitions to normal or nearly normal distal arteries are ideal for endarterectomy. As in every method of revascularization, a normal inflow capable of delivering high-energy blood flow to the reconstructed vascular bed and a patent distal arterial tree that perfuses the organ or extremity provide the best characteristics for a durable endarterectomy. High-flow vascular beds (i.e., visceral, renal) are ideal for endarterectomy because their high flow rates result in extended patency.[39, 42, 45]

Endarterectomy, once the preferred method of revascularization in most centers, has gradually been replaced by bypass graft techniques. Prosthetic grafts are generally preferred for bypass of occlusive disease of the abdominal aorta and the iliac branches, and autologous vein grafts are favored for the distal arteries supplying the lower extremities. Aortofemoral and femoropopliteal bypass procedures replaced endarterectomy for revascularization in the early 1960s, and by the mid-1970s femorotibial bypass was developed to revascularize ischemic limbs with distal tibial disease.

There are several reasons for the abandonment of lengthy endarterectomy procedures: to minimize the dissection, to shorten the procedure, and to use the available reliable prosthetic material. The original technique of long endarterectomy was less than ideal. Crude devices were designed to disobliterate diseased vessels, but no standardized technique or training was available to young vascular surgeons trying to acquire the skill to perform such procedures. Only reports by Inahara[26] in Oregon and Imparato and colleagues[25] in New York emphasized the excellent results that endarterectomy could achieve when precisely performed in the superficial femoral and popliteal arterial segments. However, early and late patency rates of femoropopliteal endarterectomies performed by others were found to be inferior to comparable bypass grafts, and the bypass graft became firmly established as the preferred method for revascularization in these arterial beds.

Although prosthetic textile grafts have performed admirably in proximal sites, namely the aorta and its terminal branches, the results with prosthetics remain inferior to those achieved with autogenous saphenous vein grafts in the lower extremity itself. Because the greater saphenous vein is suitable in only about 80 per cent of patients, other autogenous revascularization techniques must frequently be sought. The use of autologous cephalic or lesser saphenous veins (see Chapter 28) is one alternative, and another is superficial femoropopliteal endarterectomy performed by open or semi-closed techniques (see Chapter 56).

It is therefore appropriate to consider new technologic contributions that may overcome those factors reported to cause poor results. Extensive circumferential mobilization of long segments of the arterial tree has been considered mandatory to facilitate semi-closed endarterectomy when disobliterating these long occlusions. Circumferential fibrosis can develop throughout the length of the endarterectomized segment, causing narrowing and eventual occlusion, and this has contributed to the low late patency rate of endarterectomy. Because endarterectomy is a controlled arterial injury that ideally heals by intimal regrowth, it requires an optimal environment for this healing to occur. Extensive mobilization of the entire length of the artery to be treated may in fact devascularize the artery, stimulating postoperative periarterial fibrosis, impaired metabolism of the arterial wall, and therefore compromised arterial healing.

To eliminate these possible local problems arising from previous endarterectomy techniques, we have begun to evaluate new instruments and exposures that minimize trauma during semi-closed endarterectomy of long arterial segments. The air-driven oscillating loop device developed by Lerwick and Amsco-Hall has certain attractive features.[32] However, it is unwieldy and awkward because of its weight, inflexibility, and immobility. Its air hose tethers the instruments and makes its use somewhat restrictive. The authors have designed and developed an electric loop endarterectomy stripper that is light and flexible and adapts to various anatomic sites in the arterial tree. This device is battery-powered and can be sterilized.

Studies are now underway to assess the immediate and long-term patency rates of these technological modifications for superficial femoral-popliteal semi-closed endarterectomy. Minimal dissection and the reduced intimal trauma using the power-driven loop to create the endarterectomy cleavage plane are obvious immediate benefits of this method compared with older techniques using the hand-held or even the oscillating Lerwick loop instruments. The early results are encouraging, and the regulation of arterial healing and the myointimal response to injury may support increasing future use of this potentially valuable technique.

As noted above, the healing of arteries subjected to endarterectomy involves a number of favorable and unfavorable cellular responses. In the past, the late development of neointimal hyperplasia was responsible for the occlusive failure of many long-segment endarterectomy techniques. Research into the cellular and molecular biology of arterial healing may now make it feasible to consider novel pharmacologic adjuncts to the performance of endarterectomy to modulate these events. For example, investigation using a well-established animal model of intimal injury has allowed Clowes and associates to categorize arterial healing into three phases of myointimal cell response: cellular *migration* into the neointimal layer, myointimal cell *proliferation*, and deposition of *extracellular matrix*[9] (also see Chapter 15). The precise factors regulating each of these phases are now becoming more clear, and this may allow the use of pharmacologic adjuncts such as heparin,[10] angiotensin-converting enzyme (ACE) inhibitors,[11] and growth factor antagonists[17, 33] to improve the results of endarterectomy. Limited clinical trials are now underway to evaluate the potential of heparin-like agents to limit myointimal cell migration and proliferation, ACE inhibitors to modulate myointimal cell proliferation, and other agents to limit the deposition of matrix materials. It may also be possible, owing to the exciting developments in gene transfer technology currently underway, to use these methods to manipulate the healing response of the arterial wall following endarterectomy. With the availability of these new adjunctive therapies, it would not be surprising to see endarterectomy become the preferred technique of arterial reconstruction for occlusive disease during the next decade.

A technically perfect endarterectomy depends on a number of factors now available to the vascular surgeon. Improved illumination of the field using fiberoptic headlights will aid in detection and elimination of technical defects that could adversely affect the healing of the endarterectomy site. The use of angioscopy may further aid in inspecting segments of the disobliterated artery at sites remote from the arteriotomies and therefore may improve the precision with which a smooth endarterectomy plane is achieved throughout the entire length of the vessel. Finally, we have now accumulated considerable experience with intraoperative duplex scanning with spectral analysis to confirm the adequacy of endarterectomy in various locations and are quite pleased with its accuracy in intraoperative assessment of the repair compared with operative arteriography.

The benefits of endarterectomy for the vascular surgeon who has mastered the technique and has the knowledge and skill to utilize it appropriately in the practice of vascular surgery are immeasurable. It documents the individual's understanding of atherosclerotic occlusive disease and its potential for management. This knowledge extends the vascular surgeon's ability to improve perfusion for any patient even under conditions in which the alternative, the bypass graft procedure, is either contraindicated or impossible.

Dos Santos knew the problems he faced in the battle to manage occlusive arterial disease successfully with this technique when he wrote, "At the beginning failure was usual, success occasional."[15] The proper use of endarterectomy, after more than 40 years, is still not without controversy. However, as technical refinements, improved instrumentation, training programs offering technical opportunities in endarterectomy, and pharmacologic regulation of arterial injury and healing are perfected, it is the authors' opinion that endarterectomy will assume an increasingly important role for the vascular surgeon.

References

1. Acland RD: Microsurgery Practice Manual. Louisville, Louisville School of Medicine, Department of Surgery, 1977.
2. Bazy L, Reboul H: Technique de l'endarterectomie desobliterate. J Int Chir 65:196, 1950.
3. Buncke HJ, Schultz WP: Total ear reimplantation in the rabbit utilizing microminiature vascular anastomoses. Br J Plast Surg 10:15, 1966.
4. Cannon JA, Barker WF: Successful management of obstructive femoral atherosclerosis by endarterectomy. Surgery 38:48, 1955.
5. Carrel A: The surgery of blood vessels. Johns Hopkins Med J 18:18, 1970.
6. Carrel A: Heterotransplantation of blood vessels preserved in cold storage. J Exp Med 9:226, 1907.
7. Carrel A: Results of the transplantation of blood vessels, organs, and limbs. JAMA 51:1662, 1968.
8. Chang WH, Petry J: Platelets, prostaglandins, and patency in microvascular surgery. J Microsurg 2:27, 1980.
9. Clowes AW, Reidy MA: Prevention of stenosis after vascular reconstruction: Pharmacologic control of intimal hyperplasia—A review. J Vasc Surg; 13:885, 1991.
10. Clowes AW, Clowes MM: Kinetics of cellular proliferation after arterial injury. IV. Heparin inhibits rat smooth muscle mitogenesis and migration. Circ Res 58:839, 1986.
11. Clowes AW, Clowes MM, Vergel SC, et al: Heparin and cilazapril together inhibit injury-induced intimal hyperplasia. Hypertension 18(Suppl):II 65, 1991.
12. Daniel RK, Taylor GI: Distant transfer of an island flap by microvascular anastomoses. Plast Reconstr Surg 52:111, 1973.
13. Daniel RK, Terzis JK (eds): Reconstructive Microsurgery. Boston, Little, Brown, 1977.
14. Dobrin PB, Jorgensen RA: Balloon embolectomy catheters in small arteries. III. Surgical significance of eccentric balloons. Surgery 93:402, 1983.
15. Dos Santos JC: Sur la desobstuction des thrombus arterielles anciennes. Mem Acad Chir 73:409, 1947.
16. Dos Santos JC: Late results of reconstructive arterial surgery (restoration, disobliteration, replacement with the establishment of some operative principles). J Cardiovasc Surg 5:445, 1964.
17. Ferns GAA, Raines EW, Sprugel KH, et al: Inhibition of neointimal smooth muscle accumulation after angioplasty by an antibody to PDGF. Science 253:1129, 1991.
18. Fogarty TJ, Cranley JJ, Krause RJ, et al: A method of extraction of arterial emboli and thrombi. Surg Gynecol Obstet 116:241, 1963.
19. Foster JH, Carter JW, Edwards WH, et al: Arterial injuries secondary to the use of the Fogarty catheter. Ann Surg 171:971, 1970.
20. Godina M: Preferential use of end to side arterial anastomoses in free flap transfers. Plast Reconstr Surg 64:673, 1970.
21. Guthrie CG: Heterotransplantation of blood vessels. Am J Physiol 19:482, 1907.

22. Haimov M, Jacobson JH: Auxiliary applications of the Fogarty catheter. Surg Gynecol Obstet 133:666, 1971.
23. Harrison JH, Jordan WD, Perez AR: Eversion thromboendarterectomy. Surgery 61:26, 1967.
24. Hyde GL, Sullivan DM: Fogarty catheter tamponade of ruptured abdominal aortic aneurysms. Surg Gynecol Obstet 154:197, 1982.
25. Imparato AM, et al: Comparison of three techniques for femoropopliteal arterial reconstruction. Ann Surg 117:375, 1973.
26. Inahara T: Eversion endarterectomy for aorto-ilio-femoral occlusive disease. Am J Surg 138:196, 1979.
27. Jacobson JH, Suarez EL: Microsurgery in the anastomosis of small blood vessels. Surg Forum 11:243, 1968.
28. Jorgensen RA, Dobrin PB: Balloon embolectomy catheters in small arteries. IV. Correlation of shear forces with histologic injury. Surgery 93:798, 1983.
29. Ketchum LD, Wennen WW, Masters FW, et al: Experimental use of pluronic F68 in microvascular surgery. Plast Reconst Surg 53:288, 1974.
30. Komatsu S, Tamai S: Successful replantation of a completely cut off thumb: Case report. Plast Reconstr Surg 42:374, 1968.
31. Leriche R, Kunlin J: Essais de désobstruction des enteres thromboses suivant la technique de Jean Cid Dos Santos. Lyon Chir 42:475, 1947.
32. Lerwick ER: Oscillating loop endarterectomy for peripheral vascular reconstruction. Surgery 97:574, 1985.
33. Lindner V, Reidy MA: Proliferation of smooth muscle cells after vascular injury is inhibited by an antibody against basic fibroblast growth factor. Proc Nat Acad Sci USA 88:3739, 1991.
34. McCaughan JJ Jr, Young JM: Intra-arterial occlusion in vascular surgery. Ann Surg 171:695, 1970.
35. Merkel FK: An intraluminal technique for arterial occlusion during renal transplantation. Arch Surg 110:348, 1975.
36. Nam DA, Roberts T, Ackland R: An experimental study of end to end anastomoses. Surg Gynecol Obstet 147:339, 1978.
37. Ng AC, Ochsner EC: Use of Fogarty catheter tamponade for ruptured abdominal aortic aneurysms. Am J Roentgenol 128:31, 1977.
38. Prolo DJ, Hanbery JW: Intraluminal occlusion of a carotid-cavernous sinus fistula with a balloon catheter. J Neurosurg 35:237, 1971.
39. Rapp JH, Reilly LM, Quarfordt PG, et al: Durability of endarterectomy and antegrade grafts in the treatment of chronic visceral ischemia. J Vasc Surg 3:799, 1986.
40. Schumacker HB Jr, Muhm HY: Arterial suture techniques, past, present and future. Surgery 66:419, 1969.
41. Starzl TE, Groth CG, Brettschneider L: An everting technique for intraluminal vascular suturing. Surg Gynecol Obstet 127:125, 1968.
42. Stoney RJ, Ehrenfeld WK, Wylie EJ: Revascularization method in chronic visceral ischemia. Ann Surg 186:468, 1977.
43. Swartz WM, Brink RR, Buncke HJ: Prevention of thrombosis in arterial and venous microanastomoses using topical agents. Plast Reconstr Surg 58:478, 1976.
44. Wylie EJ: Thromboendarterectomy for arteriosclerotic thrombosis of major arteries. Surgery 23:275, 1952.
45. Wylie EJ: Endarterectomy and autogenous arterial grafts in the surgical treatment of stenosing lesions of the renal artery. Urol Clin North Am 2:351, 1975.
46. Wylie EJ, Kerr E, Davis O: Experimental and clinical experiences with the use of fascia lata applied as a graft about major arteries after thromboendarterectomy and aneurysmorrhaphy. Surg Gynecol Obstet 93:257, 1951.

22

Preoperative Cardiac Evaluation of Patients for Vascular Surgery

Denis D. Bensard, M.D., and William C. Krupski, M.D.

• • •

There is a great deal to be said for the conservative management of arteriosclerosis and being content to allow patients to grow old gracefully.

A. M. Boyd[7]

Atherosclerosis is a systemic disease affecting one in four adults in Western cultures. The annual mortality of cardiovascular disease in the United States exceeds 1 million, more than all other diseases combined.[49] Although a patient may present with a ''peripheral vascular disorder,'' in reality the patient suffers from a systemic illness that will ultimately determine both the early and the late outcome. As a result, the cornerstone of clinical vascular surgery is the evaluation of risk-benefit in patients being considered for operative intervention.

The specific indications for various operative procedures are discussed elsewhere. The purpose of this chapter is to review the current approach to preoperative evaluation of the vascular surgery patient with respect to coexisting health disorders. The degree of cardiac, pulmonary, and renal comorbidity detected by careful preoperative screening must be weighed carefully against the natural history of the underlying vascular disorder, so that the benefits of intervention exceed the risk of surgery. Although decisions must be individualized, estimates of patient longevity, operative risk, improvement in quality of life, and durability of the planned arterial reconstruction direct the decision to operate or not to operate on a given patient.

BACKGROUND

Adverse late outcomes after vascular surgery illustrate the systemic nature of atherosclerotic vascular disease. For example, the risk of amputation due to vascular insufficiency is significantly less than the risk of death during the same time interval.[38] Principal causes of late death in patients undergoing vascular reconstruction are coronary artery disease (40 to 60 per cent), malignancy (7 to 23 per cent), and cerebrovascular disease (2 to 15 per cent).[2] Thus, the systemic complications of atherosclerosis constitute the leading causes of death in patients with peripheral vascular disease.

This concept was recognized more than three decades ago by Boyd, who emphasized the ominous implications of peripheral vascular disease.[7] In a natural history study of patients suffering from intermittent claudication he reported that 39 per cent suffered a nonfatal myocardial infarction or stroke within 10 years of the onset of extremity symptoms; remarkably, only 22 per cent of patients remained alive 15 years after the onset of symptoms.[7] Similarly, Kallero found that patients 55 to 69 years of age with abnormal segmental limb pressure measurements had a twofold increased risk of death and a 14-fold increased risk of myocardial infarction at 10 years.[43] In a series of 871 patients requiring vascular reconstruction, Hertzer demonstrated that cumulative cardiac mortality (30 per cent) at 10 years was markedly increased in patients with suspected but uncorrected coronary artery disease (CAD) compared with patients without evidence of synchronous CAD or those who had undergone myocardial revascularization.[38] Based on these observations, one can anticipate that half of those patients with severe CAD at the time of diagnosis of peripheral vascular disease will sustain a fatal cardiac complication within the ensuing 5 years (Fig. 22–1).

Because the prevalence of cardiovascular disease increases with age and the average age of the population in the United States is increasing, it is projected that nearly 9 million people over the age of 65 will develop symptomatic atherosclerosis by the year 2010. Confounding these projections is the recognition that "silent" or asymptomatic myocardial ischemia, which is prognostically similar to clinically manifest CAD, is frequently underappreciated. In a recent review, Cohn concluded that (1) 2.5 to 10 per cent of middle-aged men who have never had signs or symptoms of CAD, (2) 18 per cent of asymptomatic patients after myocardial infarction, and (3) 40 per cent of patients with angina demonstrate episodic silent ischemia as documented by ambulatory electrocardiographic (ECG) monitoring (Holter) or exercise electrocardiography.[12] As a result, current statistics underestimate the true incidence of CAD in the general population. In 1988 more than 25 million patients required noncardiac surgery, 7 to 8 million of whom were considered at risk for cardiac morbidity or mortality by standard criteria; it is likely that a substantially higher number of patients were at increased risk.[49]

In patients with peripheral vascular disease the incidence of severe CAD (30 per cent, documented angiographically) is independent of the extent of peripheral arterial

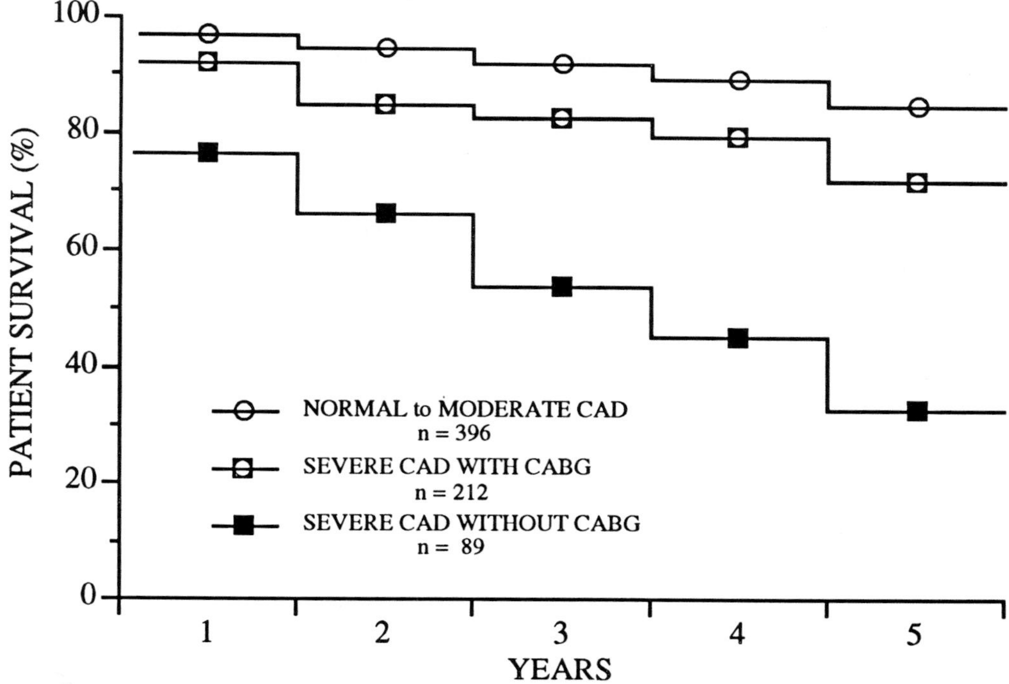

FIGURE 22–1. Cumulative 5-year survival of patients following elective vascular reconstruction stratified according to angiographic severity of coronary artery disease. CABG, coronary bypass prior to elective vascular reconstruction. (Adapted from Hertzer NR: The natural history of peripheral vascular disease: implications for its management. Circulation 83 [Suppl I]:I–12, 1991. Reproduced with permission. Copyright 1991 American Heart Association.)

occlusive disease.[40] The accuracy of clinical detection of CAD is often handicapped by the limitations in activity imposed by peripheral vascular disease.[37] Furthermore, the Cleveland Clinic series demonstrates that in patients scheduled for elective vascular procedures normal coronary arteriograms were found in only 4 per cent of patients with and 14 per cent of patients without clinically suspected CAD. Coronary artery bypass grafting (CABG) was performed in 70 of 250 patients (28 per cent) with infrarenal abdominal aortic aneurysms (AAA), 63 of 295 (21 per cent) of those with cerebrovascular disease, and 70 of 381 (18 per cent) of those with lower extremity vascular insufficiency prior to the planned vascular reconstruction.[40] Of these 216 patients with surgically correctable CAD who subsequently underwent coronary artery bypass, 72 per cent were alive 5 years postoperatively. In contrast, only 15 of 35 patients (43 per cent) who were considered candidates but never received CABG and 12 of 54 (22 per cent) with severe, uncorrectable CAD remained alive at 5 years (Fig. 22–1).[38] Regardless of the merits of vascular reconstruction, these studies emphasize the striking prevalence of concurrent coronary artery disease in patients with peripheral vascular disease and confirm that CAD is a major determinant of long-term survival following vascular reconstruction.

Predictably, associated cardiovascular disease similarly affects the early morbidity and mortality of vascular reconstructions. Perioperative cardiac morbidity, defined as the occurrence of myocardial infarction, unstable angina, congestive heart failure, serious dysrhythmia, or cardiac death during the intraoperative or in-hospital postoperative period, is the leading cause of death following anesthesia and surgery.[49] Cardiac morbidity is often heralded by the onset of myocardial ischemia. Yet perioperative myocardial ischemia is typically silent, occurs with unexpected frequency, and is often suggested only by persistent tachycardia, making detection difficult.[51–53] Patients are vulnerable throughout the perioperative period, and, because accurate detection is difficult, the reported rates of adverse cardiac outcomes vary markedly.

Comparison of cardiac morbidity between different studies is often misleading because the frequency of occurrence of cardiac complications depends on the vigor with which the diagnosis is pursued. Retrospective reviews generally report perioperative myocardial infarction rates of about 3 per cent, whereas more intensive prospective surveillance leads to detection rates of 10 to 15 per cent.[77] Unless cardiac enzymes and ECGs are routinely obtained, postoperative myocardial infarction is substantially underestimated.[11] Moreover, in a series of patients with known CAD undergoing vascular surgery, 63 per cent were found to have clinically silent postoperative myocardial ischemia by ambulatory ECG monitoring, and more than half of these patients subsequently experienced a clinically significant adverse outcome (myocardial infarction, congestive heart failure, or unstable angina).[59]

The Coronary Artery Surgery Study (CASS) provided additional useful information about the risk of noncardiac surgery in patients with defined coronary disease. The risk of postoperative cardiac death in the general population is 0.5 per cent, but this increases nearly fivefold (to 2.4 per cent) in patients with CAD.[27] Foster and colleagues reported an 8.7 per cent incidence of postoperative chest pain in patients with CAD undergoing noncardiac surgery, nearly double that of patients without CAD or with previous CABG.[27] Given the silent nature of most postoperative ischemia, this small percentage of patients with postoperative chest pain probably underestimates the true incidence and represents only a fraction of clinical events. Certainly the observation that 50 to 90 per cent of postoperative ischemic events detected by ambulatory ECG (Holter) monitoring are silent supports this contention.[51, 55, 59, 60] The incidence of myocardial infarction (MI) after noncardiac surgery ranges from 0 to 0.7 per cent, but the incidence increases substantially to 2 to 6.4 per cent in patients undergoing elective vascular reconstruction, and nearly half of these are fatal.[77]

Although reinfarction rates vary from 5 to 8 per cent in patients with a history of prior MI, these rates increase to 15 per cent in patients undergoing vascular surgery and to 37 per cent in patients who have had a recent MI.[49] However, current studies suggest that implementation of risk stratification, aggressive intraoperative monitoring, and extended stay in the intensive care unit (ICU) can substantially reduce reinfarction rates in patients with a previous history of MI who are undergoing vascular reconstruction.[3, 65]

In summary, postoperative cardiac morbidity is the primary cause of death following anesthesia and surgery. Approximately 50,000 patients per year sustain a perioperative MI, and 20,000 of these are fatal.[49] The cardiac risk associated with noncardiac surgery is due primarily to clinically silent or apparently stable CAD that is unmasked by the stress of surgery. To be sure, all patients undergoing vascular reconstruction require careful preoperative evaluation with attention paid to all organ systems, but cardiac morbidity is the overwhelming determinant of both early and late outcome. The risk of neurologic events associated with noncardiac vascular surgery is surprisingly low (0.4 to 0.9 per cent),[36, 39] and, although preexisting pulmonary or renal disease may contribute to postoperative morbidity, these conditions, like carotid disease, are rarely the primary cause of postoperative death.[9, 35, 66] A thoughtful approach must consider the type of surgery, the likelihood of an adverse event, the relative usefulness of confirmatory tests, and the therapeutic options for patients at risk.

RISK ASSESSMENT

The likelihood that cardiac morbidity will occur during noncardiac surgery can be predicted partly on the basis of simple clinical information.[19] Identification of a subset of patients at high cardiac risk can be used to recommend prophylactic CABG or percutaneous transluminal coronary angioplasty. In addition, risk stratification allows selection of alternative methods of patient management (e.g., percutaneous endovascular procedures, (extra-anatomic bypass, or a combination of lower risk modalities) instead of conventional revascularization. On occasion, surgery should be avoided altogether in patients with less than compelling indications.

Taylor and colleagues described their results after the implementation of a conservative preoperative screening program in 513 patients referred for vascular surgery (aortic, 105; carotid, 87; infrainguinal, 207; extra-anatomic, 51; other, 84).[70] All patients underwent basic cardiac evaluation including history, physical examination, and resting ECG. In patients with severe symptomatic CAD (5.8 per cent), defined as unstable angina, uncontrolled arrhythmia, congestive heart failure (CHF), or MI within the preceding 6 months), further evaluation was performed using one or more of the following: cardiology consultation, dipyridamole thallium scanning, multi-gated cardiac blood pool scanning, cardiac echocardiography, or coronary arteriography. The method of risk stratification of these authors was based on clinical criteria and resulted in a postoperative MI rate of only 4.2 per cent and a death rate of 2.2 per cent (0.8 per cent cardiac deaths). However, enthusiasm for such an approach should be tempered by the fact that one fourth of the patients in the study had undergone previous myocardial revascularization, the postoperative period was limited to 72 hours, and no long-term follow-up of patients was provided. The latter criticisms are relevant considering the observations that up to 50 per cent of ischemic events occur after the third postoperative day.[53] Furthermore, in patients who develop postoperative myocardial ischemia the risk of an acute MI in the subsequent 2 years is increased twofold, and in those who develop unstable angina the risk of a cardiac complication is increased 20-fold during the following 2-year interval.[50]

An equally effective approach to preoperative risk assessment has been outlined by Bunt.[8] Six hundred and thirty consecutive patients scheduled for elective vascular surgery were entered into a prospective protocol for preoperative risk assessment. All patients underwent a detailed history and physical examination, radionuclide cardioangiography, and resting electrocardiogram. If no abnormalities were detected on the initial examination, elective surgery followed (32 per cent); however, if abnormalities were detected in one component of the initial examination (68 per cent), dipyridamole thallium scans (DTS) were performed. Patients with normal DTS (no perfusion defect, 93 per cent) proceeded to surgery, whereas those with fixed or reversible perfusion defects (7 per cent) underwent coronary angiography. This detailed cardiac risk protocol resulted in a perioperative MI rate of 0.7 per cent, ranging from 0 per cent in patients undergoing aortic or carotid surgery to 1.6 per cent in patients undergoing infrainguinal revascularization. The algorithm described by Bunt resulted in nearly a fourfold reduction in perioperative MI relative to the more conservative approach described by Taylor and colleagues.[70] Nevertheless, the studies of Bunt and Taylor and colleagues illustrate that an organized and thoughtful approach to preoperative screening of vascular surgery patients can succeed in achieving meaningful cardiac risk reduction.

RISK FACTORS

Age, previous MI, angina, CHF, diabetes mellitus, and peripheral vascular disease have been implicated as important risk factors for postoperative cardiac morbidity.[40] In the last two decades numerous studies have attempted to identify which clinical risk factors are most predictive of perioperative cardiac risk.[49] Few, however, have had more influence on this topic than the seminal work of Goldman and associates.[34] They were among the first investigators to demonstrate that estimates of perioperative cardiac risk could be derived from information available in a careful history and physical examination. Of the clinical variables examined, (1) recent MI and (2) CHF were the strongest predictors of adverse cardiac outcome; additional factors identified included (in order of decreasing importance): (3) abnormal rhythm; (4) more than five premature ventricular contractions per minute; (5) intra-abdominal, intrathoracic, or aortic surgery; (6) age greater than 70 years; (7) significant aortic valvular stenosis; (8) emergency operation; and (9) poor general medical condition. Although no current consensus exists on the best cardiac risk indicators, the following discussion will review several that are consistently proposed as important.

Previous Myocardial Infarction. In 1964, Topkins and Artusio reported the first comprehensive, large-scale study relating previous MI to the cardiac risk of subsequent noncardiac surgery.[71] They found that the incidence of postoperative MI in patients without previous MI was 0.66 per cent compared with 6.5 per cent in patients with documented prior MI. The mortality of postoperative MI in patients without previous MI was 26.5 per cent but increased to a staggering 72 per cent in patients who had had an antecedent MI! Reinfarction occurred in 54.5 per cent of patients when a previous MI had occurred within 6 months of surgery compared to 4.5 per cent in patients who suffered an MI more than 6 months earlier. Thus, both the history of a prior MI and its temporal relationship to the planned operative procedure determine susceptibility to postoperative adverse cardiac events. These trends are corroborated in a contemporary series that reports reinfarction rates of 36 per cent at 3 months or less, 26 per cent at 3 to 6 months, and 5 per cent at more than 6 months.[65] Overall, following vascular surgery postoperative reinfarction rates average 2 to 6.4 per cent, and more than half of these patients die as a consequence.[77]

Congestive Heart Failure. In 1988, 2.3 million Americans developed CHF. The incidence of CHF doubles in each decade of life after age 45 years, and less than half of these patients remain alive 5 years after the time of diagnosis.[49] Nonsurgical patients who retain normal left ventricular (LV) function after MI have a 7 per cent 1-year mortality; in contrast, 1-year mortality increases to 44 per cent in those whose ejection fraction deteriorates to less than 30 per cent or who cannot complete an exercise test after MI.[22] Similar data have led some to suggest that it is the degree of myocardial dysfunction, not the time from infarction or the extent of CAD, that determines perioperative mortality.[20, 67] Furthermore, in most cardiac risk indexes, CHF is among the most heavily weighted predictors.[34, 76] Yet, CHF is a constellation of clinical symptoms rather than a specific disease. There is controversy over which marker of heart failure is most predictive of cardiac prognosis. Pathologic heart sounds (S_3, S_4 gallop), jugular venous distention,[33, 76] alveolar pulmonary edema,[27] dyspnea on exertion, LV wall motion abnormalities, and LV ejection fraction of less than 50 per cent[47, 62] have been proposed as predictors of adverse outcome. Arguably, the most objective finding is quantification of LV dysfunction by measurement of ejection fraction. In patients undergoing either aortic surgery[61] or lower extremity revascularization,[62] Pasternack and colleagues demonstrated that the degree of LV dysfunction as measured by radionuclide angiography correlated with the risk of perioperative MI. In these studies 80 per cent of patients undergoing aortic surgery and 70 per cent of patients undergoing infrainguinal operations sustained an adverse perioperative cardiac event when the ejection fraction was found to be less than 30 per cent.[61, 62] Although these findings have been challenged by some,[28, 56] Bunt has demonstrated that the detection of CHF by physical examination and the quantification of LV function by ejection fraction helps to stratify the perioperative cardiac risk and further directs the decision to proceed directly to surgery or to obtain additional tests.[8]

Myocardial Ischemia. By analyzing the pooled data of angiographically confirmed CAD and autopsies, Diamond and Forrester estimated that 90 per cent of males over 40 years of age and 90 per cent of females over 60 years of age with angina have significant CAD.[19] Surprisingly, he suggested that up to 20 per cent of similarly aged *asymptomatic* patients have significant CAD. Goldman and associates' studies determined that angina was conspicuously absent as a significant predictor of perioperative cardiac morbidity either by univariate or multivariate analysis.[33, 34] These results should not be viewed as contradictory if we consider that most perioperative ischemia is clinically silent.[51, 53] Whereas the existence of occlusive CAD places the patient at increased risk from ischemia, the presence of angina per se confers no additional risk.

Cardiac Rhythm Disturbance. Cardiac arrhythmias are not uncommon, and in the patient without significant heart disease they are normally benign. However, if significant CAD is present or LV function is compromised, the development of rhythm disturbances can be lethal.[4] Rhythm disturbances that arise in patients with acute MI or concurrent hypokalemia and ischemia are frequent causes of sudden death.[57, 68] Although few studies have adequately addressed the importance of postoperative arrhythmias, the available data do suggest that frequent premature ventricular contractions or rhythms other than normal sinus rhythm on preoperative ECG are independent predictors of outcome in patients undergoing noncardiac surgery.[27, 33, 34]

Diabetes Mellitus. An unquestionable association exists between diabetes and the development of atherosclerosis.[44] Patients with diabetes appear to be particularly susceptible to CAD, MI, and premature death compared to nondiabetics.[44, 74] Although controversial, recent studies suggest that diabetics are at increased cardiac risk following noncardiac surgery.[27, 37] Indeed in our experience, diabetics requiring infrainguinal operations have a markedly increased risk of developing myocardial ischemia that is consistent with a more advanced stage of systemic atherosclerosis.[45]

Operative Procedure. The anatomic location of the planned vascular operation has little bearing on postoperative cardiac morbidity. The reported incidence of MI following vascular surgery is fairly consistent regardless of the type of procedure performed, ranging from 2 to 6 per cent. For example, in patients undergoing infrainguinal reconstruction we observed that the number of postoperative cardiac events (cardiac death, MI, unstable angina, CHF, ventricular tachycardia) was similar to that seen in patients undergoing major abdominal procedures (Fig. 22–2).[45] Further, 57 per cent of patients undergoing infrainguinal operations had documented ischemia on ambulatory ECG monitoring compared to 31 per cent of patients undergoing aortic reconstruction ($p = .005$). Interestingly, the ischemia was clinically silent in nearly all (98 per cent) patients, consistent with previous reports suggesting that most postoperative ischemia is asymptomatic.[51, 53]

RISK STRATIFICATION

Risk stratification has three purposes: (1) to identify patients for whom the cardiac risks outweigh the potential benefits of therapy, (2) to identify patients with clinical problems that might be corrected before surgery, (3) to identify those who are most likely to benefit from risk-reducing interventions. In addition to clinical risk indexes, methods of risk stratification include exercise stress testing, cardiac nuclear imaging (DTS, gated blood pool scans), ambulatory ECG (Holter) monitoring, and coronary angiography. These tests attempt to quantify risk in patients who are in danger of perioperative coronary events.

RISK INDEXES

The history alone will detect CAD with a sensitivity and specificity ranging from 80 to 90 per cent. Physical examination may reveal signs of CHF, cardiac dysrhythmia, or valvular heart disease; it also helps to clarify the patient's general medical status. The physical examination together with a careful history form the basis of all clinical risk indexes. In fact, features elicited by the history and physical examination alone account for 35 of 53 points in the Goldman cardiac risk index (GCRI), with the remaining points derived from simple laboratory tests and an electrocardiogram (Fig. 22–3).[34] As noted previously, Goldman and associates were among the first to attempt to quantify the relative risks of cardiac morbidity and mortality in patients undergoing noncardiac surgical procedures by clinical markers.[34] Multivariate analysis of 39 clinical variables in 1001 surgical patients identified nine features that were predictive of perioperative cardiac morbidity. Points were assigned to each variable to reflect its statistical weight in the analysis, and the GCRI thus was formulated.[34] Subsequently, the GCRI was validated in several studies.[11, 17, 69, 79] For example, Shah and coworkers, using stepwise logistic regression, retrospectively analyzed 24 preoperative variables in 688 patients undergoing noncardiac operations who either had cardiac disease (which they defined as previous MI, unstable or stable angina, previous CABG, CHF, valvular heart disease, or ECG abnormality) or were older than 70 years of age.[69] They identified eight variables predictive of perioperative cardiac morbidity (age more than 70 years, emergency operation, chronic stable angina, previous MI,

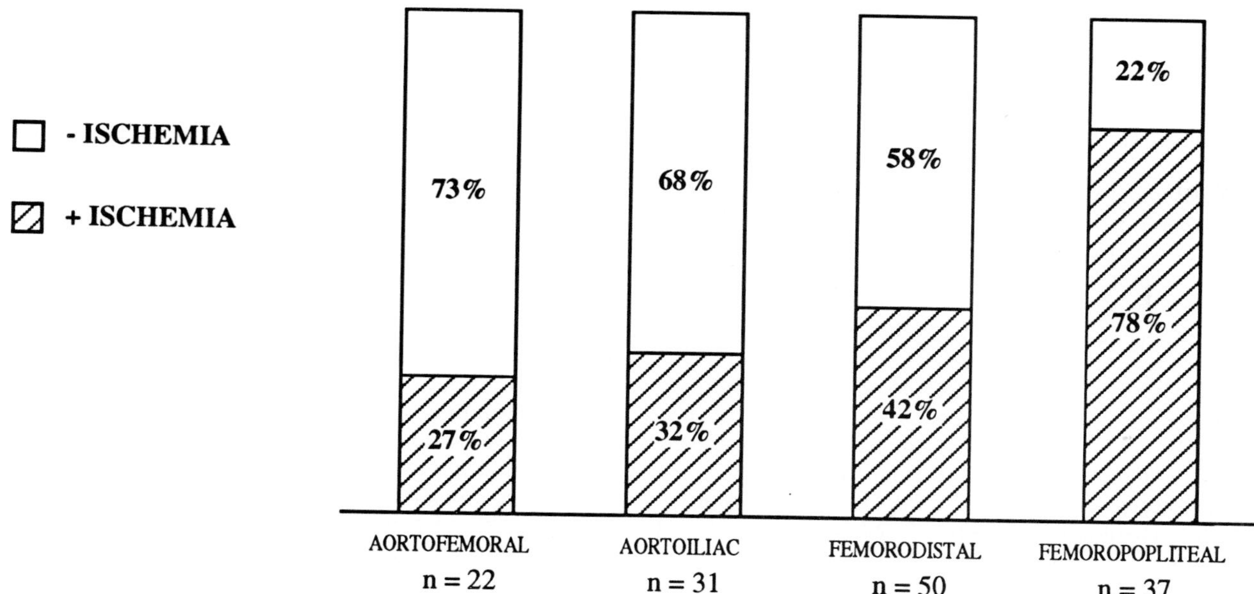

FIGURE 22–2. Incidence of postoperative myocardial ischemia documented by continuous ambulatory electrocardiography in patients undergoing aortic or infrainguinal vascular reconstruction. (Adapted from Krupski WC, Layug EL, Reilly LM, et al: Comparison of cardiac morbidity between aortic and infrainguinal operations. Study of Perioperative Ischemia [SPI] Research Group. J Vasc Surg 15:354, 1992.)

	GOLDMAN CRI	DETSKY CRI	EAGLE CRITERIA
RISK FACTOR	*WEIGHTED RISK FACTOR SCORE*		
AGE >70	5	5	1
MI			1
< 6 months	10	10	
> 6 months		5	
ANGINA			
Class III		10	1
Class IV		20	
Unstable		10	
DIABETES			1
OPERATION			
Emergency	4	10	
Aortic, Abdominal, Thoracic	3		
CHF	11		1
≤ 1 week		10	
> 1 week		5	
ELECTROCARDIOGRAM			
Rhythm other than sinus	7	5	
> 5 PVC / min	7	5	
POOR MEDICAL STATUS	3	5	
CARDIAC RISK	*SUMMED RISK FACTOR SCORES*		
LOW	0-12	0-15	0
INTERMEDIATE	13-25	16-30	1-2
HIGH	> 25	> 30	≥ 3

FIGURE 22–3. Comparison of clinical cardiac risk indexes (CRI) commonly employed in the preoperative risk assessment of patients scheduled for noncardiac surgery. (Adapted from Detsky AS, Abrams HB, Forbath N, et al: Cardiac assessment for patients undergoing noncardiac surgery: A multifactorial clinical risk index. Arch Intern Med 146:2131–2134, Copyright 1986, American Medical Association; Eagle KA, Strauss HW, Boucher CA: Dipyridamole-thallium scanning in patients undergoing vascular surgery. Optimizing preoperative evaluation of cardiac risk. JAMA 257:2185–2189, Copyright 1987, American Medical Association; and Goldman L, Caldera DL, Nessbaum SR, et al: Multifactorial index of cardiac risk in noncardiac surgical procedures. Reprinted with permission from *The New England Journal of Medicine* 297:845, 1977.)

ECG signs of ischemia, type of surgical procedure, hypokalemia). Of these eight variables, only two (chronic stable angina and ECG signs of ischemia) do not have a counterpart on the GCRI.

Unfortunately, uniform agreement on the utility of a predictive preoperative risk index has yet to be reached, particularly when applied to vascular surgery patients. In a study by Lette and colleagues, 125 consecutive patients undergoing vascular reconstruction were evaluated with cardiac risk indexes and DTS.[48] All clinical scoring systems studied (Dripps ASA,[21] CRI,[34] Detsky cardiac risk index,[18] Eagle criteria,[25] Yeager criteria,[78] Cooperman probability[13]) failed to predict adverse perioperative outcome (cardiac death or postoperative MI). Wong and Detsky reexamined Lette and colleagues' conclusions using Bayesian logic (see paper for discussion) and reached different conclusions.[76] Their analysis suggests that a higher GCRI score (class 3) was accurate in predicting increased perioperative cardiac risk, but all clinical indexes appear to lack sufficient sensitivity to identify very low risk subsets of patients. Thus, their analysis suggests that clinical risk indexes appear to be useful in predicting perioperative cardiac complications that are of intermediate or high risk.

Despite the lack of a consensus, these studies support the application of risk indexes, like the GCRI, to stratify patients according to estimated perioperative cardiac morbidity. As a result, patients who may potentially benefit from further preoperative evaluation, changes in the planned operative procedure, or modification of the planned perioperative management can be identified. Although a universally accepted risk index has not been developed, the evolution of prognostic indexes demonstrates that useful information can be obtained by a thorough history and physical examination.

DIAGNOSTIC TESTING PREDICTORS

Rational recommendations for additional preoperative tests for patients with suspected CAD must be based on several assumptions: (1) perioperative cardiac complications occur sufficiently frequently to justify commitment of significant resources in an attempt to lower their incidence; (2) the proposed tests accurately identify patients at risk; (3) effective treatment exists to lower the risk of complications significantly in the selected patients.[70] Historical predictors and clinical risk indexes are relatively insensitive in patients with vascular disease whose exercise tolerance is limited either by intermittent claudication or previous amputation. The impairment in ambulation imposed by occlusive vascular disease may mask symptoms of exertional angina or CHF, resulting in risk scores that do not accurately reflect the degree of risk of CAD present. Lette and colleagues' finding that vascular surgery patients classified as Goldman or Detsky class 1 (i.e., lowest risk) have a 10.4 per cent incidence of perioperative cardiac morbidity underscores these limitations.[48]

As a result, more recent attention has focused on the development of adjunctive preoperative cardiac testing that may enhance the sensitivity and specificity of preoperative risk assessment (Fig. 22–4). Clearly, surgical patients who have either symptomatic ischemic heart disease or global LV dysfunction are at greatest risk for perioperative com-

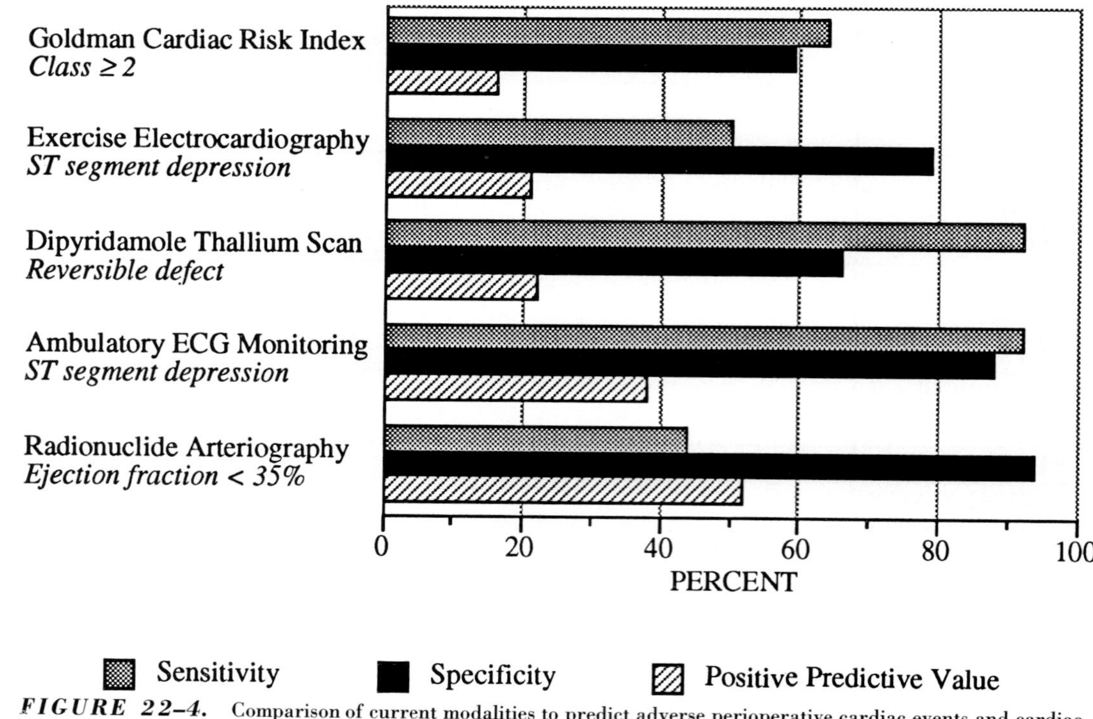

FIGURE 22–4. Comparison of current modalities to predict adverse perioperative cardiac events and cardiac death in patients undergoing vascular reconstruction. (Adapted from Yeager RA: Basic data related to cardiac testing and cardiac risk associated with vascular surgery. Ann Vasc Surg 4[2]:193–197, 1990. Reprinted by permission of Blackwell Scientific Publications, Inc.; and Raby KE, Goldman L, Creager MA, et al: Predictive value of preoperative electrocardiographic monitoring. Reprinted with permission from *The New England Journal of Medicine* 322:931, 1990.)

plications and are usually easily identified.[8, 34, 49, 76] Conversely, a significant number of patients appear to be at significant risk due to occult cardiac disease unmasked only by the stress of surgery.[40] The proliferation of adjunctive tests to help quantify cardiac risk has further complicated the evaluation of these intermediate-risk patients. Information from a test alters the estimate of an individual patient's risk for developing a cardiac complication. Patients who have a positive test result are expected to have a higher than average chance of having a cardiac complication, whereas those with a negative test result are expected to have a lower than average risk.[76] However, the procedures are expensive, of uncertain utility, and sometimes risky, either as a direct result of the procedure or because of how the information is subsequently used.[42] In reviewing their own data, Eagle and associates suggested that an adverse cardiac event rate of 10 to 15 per cent may be expected in vascular surgery patients who are determined to be at intermediate or high risk following clinical assessment,[23–25] whereas less than 5 per cent of vascular patients in the low-risk category may experience an adverse cardiac event. These figures represent the pretest probability of an adverse cardiac event. Additional testing should be performed only if the post-test probability is increased significantly compared to the pretest probability.[76] In patients already deemed to be at low or high risk, additional tests (and subsequent clinical management) are unlikely to change these pretest probabilities substantially enough to justify their use (when post-test probability is equal to or less than pretest probability). Conversely, in patients considered to be at intermediate risk, adjunctive tests may provide sufficient information to alter their clinical management enough to justify screening (post-test probability greater than pretest probability).

The most commonly employed screening tests include ECG, exercise ECG, ambulatory ECG (Holter) monitoring, DTS, and coronary angiography. However, it must be emphasized that a consensus regarding the best test or approach to be used for preoperative risk assessment of vascular surgery patients has not been reached. Furthermore, studies of adjunctive tests must be reviewed with caution and analyzed with respect to the following critical limitations: (1) only selected patients had the recommended diagnostic procedure; (2) the *degree* of ischemia could not be quantified by the diagnostic study; (3) patients were excluded for poorly defined reasons; (4) patients enrolled in the study had undergone prior myocardial revascularization; (5) studies were not blinded and therefore physicians could employ therapeutic interventions that altered outcome; (6) data were retrospectively analyzed; (7) interpretation of the diagnostic test was arbitrary; and (8) length of the postoperative period (typically less than or equal to 72 hours) precluded identification of adverse cardiac events occurring later in the postoperative course.

Resting Electrocardiogram

Data on the predictive value of preoperative resting ECG are conflicting. Considering the prevalence of CAD in vascular surgery patients specifically, it is hard to justify *not* obtaining a baseline ECG.[72] Electrocardiographic abnormalities are common. Numerous studies have documented that an abnormal preoperative ECG is a statistically significant predictor of adverse cardiac outcome.[10, 72, 73] An abnormal resting ECG has been associated with up to a threefold increase in perioperative cardiac complications. Hertzer and associates found that 44 per cent of patients with a clinical history of cardiac disease and an abnormal ECG (evidence of previous MI; ST-T segment changes) had *severe* CAD by angiography (more than 70 per cent stenosis of one or more coronary arteries) compared with only 22 per cent of those with normal ECGs.[40] In a study of 12,654 patients undergoing major noncardiac surgery, 214 patients with ECG patterns suggestive of previous MI, LV hypertrophy or strain, or myocardial ischemia were studied prospectively.[73] Von Knorring found that of these 214 patients with abnormal preoperative ECGs, 17.7 per cent sustained a postoperative MI with a cardiac mortality of 32 per cent. Type of surgery, anesthetic techniques or duration, and patient factors such as history of chest pain, diabetes, age, or sex were not predictive.

Although an abnormal ECG suggests underlying CAD, a normal resting ECG may be misleading. Twenty-five to 50 per cent of previous MIs are missed on ECG because they are misread or lack the pathognomonic findings of old MI. Using findings from routine coronary arteriograms, Hertzer and colleagues reported that 37 per cent of vascular patients with *normal* resting ECGs had significant stenosis (more than 70 per cent) of one or more coronary arteries.[40] Similarly, Benchimol and associates found angiographic evidence of significant three-vessel coronary artery disease in 15 per cent of patients with completely normal ECGs.[1] These studies illustrate that an abnormal ECG may denote the presence of significant underlying CAD, but a normal ECG should not reassure the physician that significant CAD is absent. Thus, resting ECG cannot be used as the sole diagnostic test to estimate perioperative cardiac risk.

Special Cardiac Screening Tests

A decision to obtain additional tests should be made only after the operative indications, the patient's general health status, and the cardiac risk profile have been considered. Several investigators have suggested that special preoperative testing should be employed for stratifying cardiac risk only in patients considered to be at intermediate or high clinical risk.[6, 24, 63] In their studies of patients undergoing noncardiac surgical procedures, only 4 per cent of patients clinically identified as low risk suffered nonfatal cardiac events. In contrast, 9 to 21 per cent of patients identified as intermediate or high clinical risk suffered adverse perioperative cardiac events. Patients with previous MI, angina pectoris, or CHF warrant periodic testing on their own merits regardless of the requirement for noncardiac surgery. In the absence of these criteria, subsets of patients or operative procedures in which the perioperative cardiac event rate exceeds 10 per cent benefit from additional screening tests. Numerous studies illustrate that patients with high scores on clinical cardiac risk indexes (GCRI greater than 12 or Detsky index greater than 15) or more than three of the five Eagle criteria (age over 70 years, diabetes mellitus, angina, Q waves on ECG, or ventricular arrhythmias) are at the greatest risk for MI or cardiac death following vascular surgery.[17, 18, 24, 25, 34, 63] Patients identified clinically to be at low cardiac risk and not limited by their peripheral vascular disease or general medical condition are unlikely to benefit from further testing. It is doubtful whether additional tests in this subset of patients would provide additional information sufficient to alter management. Alternatively, patients considered to be at high risk by clinical criteria are unlikely to benefit from further risk stratification because the clinical evidence of increased perioperative cardiac morbidity is overwhelming.[76] Most such patients require intervention for their heart disease in preparation for an elective peripheral vascular procedure. Therefore, the remaining discussion will focus on methods of further stratifying patients categorized as *intermediate* risk by clinical scoring.

Stress Electrocardiography

The enhanced respiratory, metabolic, and cardiovascular work required in the postoperative period increases myocardial stress. In patients with the physical capacity to exercise, ECG stress testing is an inexpensive, noninvasive, and suitable method of predicting postoperative cardiac morbidity. Inability to exercise at low cardiac workloads or the presence of ST-segment abnormalities on ECG during exercise correlates with an increased risk of adverse postoperative cardiac outcomes. Gerson and coworkers found that an inability to exercise was 80 per cent sensitive and 53 per cent specific for postoperative cardiac morbidity.[32] Exercise-induced ST-segment changes clearly predict cardiac risk; Cutler and colleagues reported the occurrence of perioperative MI in 37 per cent of vascular patients with positive results on stress ECGs compared to an incidence of 1.5 per cent in those with normal studies.[16]

Stress ECG is the most popular study method of unmasking myocardial ischemia, but it has less applicability in vascular surgery patients. Patients with vascular disease are often older and deconditioned and are therefore unable to exercise adequately. Submaximal effort leads to an increased frequency of false-negative results.[24] Gage and associates found that patients screened by exercise treadmill testing prior to noncardiac surgery were often unable to complete the examination owing to dyspnea or claudication (24 per cent), and the results were often unreliable owing to the increased false-positive (40 per cent) and false-negative (15 per cent) rates.[29] Analysis of the CASS registry revealed that of 2045 patients with a history of angina pectoris, 65 per cent of men and 33 per cent of women with angiographically documented significant CAD had *normal* exercise treadmill tests (ETT).[75] Subset analysis of men and women matched for age, presence (31 per cent), and extent of CAD demonstrated that the false-positive (44 per cent vs. 51 per cent) and false-negative (12 per cent vs. 14 per cent) rates were the same regardless of sex. Thus, the electrocardiographic response to exercise when used as an objective finding to confirm or exclude CAD will be affected by the prevalence of the disease in the population studied, and in a population in whom the prevalence of CAD is high, a positive ETT only slightly increases the likelihood of CAD, whereas a negative stress test correlates poorly with the absence of CAD.[75] Therefore, ECG stress tests have limited application in elderly patients with diffuse atherosclerosis, in those whose claudication or medical condition precludes maximum exercise, and in those who are strongly suspected to have CAD on the basis of the cardiac history or baseline ECG.

Ambulatory Electrocardiographic (Holter) Monitoring

Holter monitoring is commonly used to evaluate cardiac dysrhythmia. During the 1980s it was employed in preoperative risk analysis of patients undergoing noncardiac surgical procedures.[5, 30, 51, 53, 55, 60, 64] Approximately 18 to 40 per cent of surgical patients with or at risk for CAD demonstrate frequent ischemic episodes during the 48-hour interval preceding surgery. Most (more than 75 per cent) ischemic episodes are clinically silent.[45] In a prospective study Raby and colleagues found that preoperative ischemia as diagnosed by ambulatory ECG was the most significant predictor of postoperative cardiac events by multivariate analysis.[63] Ischemia on Holter monitoring remained an independent predictor of adverse cardiac events even after all other preoperative risk factors were controlled. Less than 1 per cent of patients without detectable ischemia suffered perioperative cardiac morbidity.[63]

Similarly, Pasternack and associates reported that silent ischemia detected by Holter monitoring occurred in over 60 per cent of patients undergoing vascular surgical procedures.[60] Patients who sustained postoperative MI had a prolonged duration of perioperative ischemic time, an increased number of perioperative ischemic episodes, and an increased duration of perioperative ischemic time (per cent of total monitoring time). Only preoperative silent MI and angina at rest proved to be predictive of perioperative MI. No patient experienced perioperative cardiac morbidity in the absence of preoperative evidence on Holter monitoring of ischemia.

In studies of patients undergoing noncardiac surgery Mangano and colleagues found that 28 per cent of patients had documented preoperative ischemia on Holter monitoring, and the incidence of ischemia nearly doubled in the postoperative period.[51, 53] Most (94 per cent) ischemic episodes were silent and peaked in severity on the third postoperative day. Ischemia occurred throughout the postoperative week-long monitored period (7 days), further emphasizing the underestimated incidence of perioperative cardiac morbidity. All adverse cardiac outcomes (unstable angina, MI, cardiac death) were heralded by postoperative ischemia detected on Holter monitoring, but due to the blinded design of the study, no interventions were performed on the basis of these findings.[51, 53]

The advantages of ambulatory ECG monitoring over other noninvasive methods to determine cardiac risk, such as DTS, include its wider availability and lower cost. Its disadvantages include the fact that 10 per cent or more of patients have underlying ECG abnormalities that limit or preclude the interpretation of ST-segment depression, and ECG patterns such as LV hypertrophy may lead to false-positive evidence of ST-segment depression that is not due to CAD.[24]

Stress Thallium Imaging (Dipyridamole Thallium Scintigraphy)

Stress thallium imaging, performed under conditions of near-maximal coronary blood flow (exercise or injection of dipyridamole [Persantine]), is more sensitive than resting imaging and can detect heterogeneous perfusion due to stenoses as small as 50 per cent.[25] Boucher and coworkers first reported DTS as an accurate, safe, and noninvasive alternative to exercise stress testing for patients in whom claudication precluded exercise.[6]

Thallium-201 is taken up by myocardial cells in proportion to blood flow. Intravenous dipyridamole dilates coronary vessels, thus increasing blood flow to parts of the myocardium supplied by nonstenotic vessels. Dipyridamole acts by inhibiting myocardial cellular reuptake and endothelial transport of endogenously produced adenosine, a potent coronary vasodilator. As adenosine accumulates in the interstitium, coronary vasodilation ensues. Administration of dipyridamole, through its adenosine effect, results in an increase in coronary flow by two- to threefold.[26, 54] However, myocardium supplied by stenotic vessels has poor uptake on early scintigraphic scans, resulting in relative absence of thallium uptake in that portion of the heart. In effect, intravenous dipyridamole produces a *steal* phenomenon because nonstenotic arteries enjoy enhanced flow, whereas stenotic arteries cannot vasodilate. Later, this defect resolves if viable myocardium is present, suggesting the presence of an area of myocardium that is potentially at risk during periods of increased stress; late uptake of thallium-201 in areas of myocardium that are initially underperfused is termed redistribution. In contrast, a persistent defect on thallium scan suggests an area of prior myocardial infarction and therefore, myocardium that is already irreversibly injured (myocardial scarring).[26]

Several studies have suggested that normal findings on DTS in a patient scheduled for vascular surgery indicate low risk for cardiac complications.[6, 14, 15, 24–26, 46] The prognostic implications of a scan that detects either a fixed or reversible defect is less certain. When DTS is used as a guide to selection of patients for preoperative diagnostic angiography, it may be possible to identify subsets of patients at risk for ischemic complications of noncardiac vascular operations.[31] Lette and colleagues studied 125 consecutive patients with DTS prior to elective vascular surgery and found that no clinical risk index (GCRI, Dripps-ASA, Detsky cardiac risk index, Eagle criteria, Yeager criteria, Cooperman probability) accurately predicted adverse perioperative outcomes, whereas 21 per cent of patients with reversible defects suffered a postoperative cardiac event.[48] If the defects were further quantified by the severity and extent of reversibility of defects (i.e., myocardium at risk), 85 per cent of patients with a substantial amount of myocardium at risk by DTS suffered cardiac death or MI. The failure of clinical indexes to be predictive in part reflects the study design (retrospective) and study end-points (cardiac death, MI). Furthermore, the low specificity of DTS when interpreted only as positive (reversible defect) or negative (''normal'' or fixed defect) illustrates the low yield if it is applied to all patients referred for vascular surgery. Such a conclusion is supported by our findings in a prospective study of 60 patients undergoing elective vascular surgery.[52] Dipyridamole thallium scanning was performed preoperatively in all patients, and treating physicians were blinded to the results. No association could be found between redistribution defects and adverse cardiac outcomes, risk of adverse outcome with redistribution defect, or risk of perioperative ischemia (Holter monitoring, ETT) with redistribution defect. These results lead us to conclude that routine use of DTS for preoperative screening is unwarranted.

The selective use of preoperative DTS in vascular surgery patients has been investigated by Eagle and colleagues.[24, 25] In the initial study, five clinical markers (age over 70 years, Q waves, diabetes mellitus, angina, and arrhythmias requiring treatment) identified in a retrospective analysis of 61 patients scheduled for vascular surgery predicted perioperative cardiac morbidity (see Fig. 22–3).[25] These clinical variables were then applied prospectively to 50 consecutive patients undergoing vascular surgery. Only 3 per cent of those who had no clinical indicators sustained an adverse postoperative cardiac event. In this low-risk group 52 DTS were performed; nine revealed reversible defects, and only one patient had an adverse ischemic event (angina). In contrast, 29 per cent of patients with one or more clinical markers suffered an adverse cardiac event, and a reversible defect was present in 33 of 59 (56 per cent) patients. In a subsequent study, Eagle and colleagues corroborated their initial findings and were able to identify further an intermediate-risk group in whom DTS was most useful.[24] Again, in the low-risk group (no clinical markers) a 3 per cent postoperative cardiac event rate was noted. Patients considered to be at intermediate risk (one to two clinical predictors) and high risk (three or more clinical predictors) had cardiac event rates of 33 per cent and 50 per cent, respectively. Performance of DTS in the intermediate-risk group demonstrated that in patients with normal thallium scans the cardiac event rate (3.2 per cent) approximated that of the low-risk group, whereas 30 per cent of those with thallium redistribution suffered postoperative cardiac morbidity. Therefore, DTS appears to add little to the preoperative evaluation of the low- and high-risk groups because accurate cardiac risk assessment is possible by clinical criteria alone. The identification of an intermediate-risk group by clinical criteria allows selective application of DTS and permits additional stratification—that is, the absence of thallium redistribution suggests a 3 per cent probability of an adverse cardiac event, whereas the presence of thallium redistribution increases the probability of an adverse cardiac event to 30 per cent. The findings of Eagle and colleagues support our contention that routine preoperative DTS is not justified. Dipyridamale thallium scanning appears to be most useful in patients deemed to be at intermediate risk by clinical analysis, who may benefit from coronary revascularization prior to elective vascular surgery.[76]

Coronary Angiography

Angiographic confirmation of significant left main or multi-vessel CAD correlates with both early and late survival, as established in CASS.[58] Similar findings have been reported in patients undergoing vascular surgery.[27] The largest experience with preoperative coronary angiography in vascular patients has been accumulated at the Cleveland Clinic.[38, 40, 41] Hertzer and associates found that significant three-vessel CAD was present in 57 per cent of patients with clinical evidence of CAD.[40] Moreover, 31 per cent of those in whom severe CAD was unsuspected had significant CAD. Yet, the presence of significant coronary stenosis does not necessarily imply that MI is unavoidable or that invasive intervention is necessary, particularly if the involved artery supplies an area of myocardial scar or is compensated by intracoronary collaterals. Notably, in the study of Hertzer and associates some degree of LV impairment existed in more than one fourth of the study group, including nearly half of those patients in whom CAD was clinically suspected. The data of Hertzer and associates support the identification and treatment of significant CAD prior to vascular reconstruction by reducing postoperative MI and prolonging life.[38]

Accordingly, some centers recommend routine preoperative coronary angiography, followed, when indicated, by CABG or angioplasty before peripheral vascular surgery is done. However, such an approach is not without inherent risk. For example, in the study by Hertzer and associates the operative mortality of CABG before elective vascular surgery exceeded 5 per cent.[40] Thus, the benefit of risk reduction by prophylactic coronary revascularization is realized only by those who survive bypass surgery *and* subsequent vascular reconstruction. Cutler and Leppo further illustrate this point: One hundred and sixteen patients scheduled for aortic surgery underwent DTS; based on the results, 6 per cent of patients were referred for CABG. No operative deaths occurred in the patients undergoing aortic surgery without CABG, but two deaths resulting from the screening and treatment of CAD led to an overall mortality of 1.7 per cent.[14] These results remind us that to make risk reduction meaningful the planned procedure must be associated with a relatively high risk, or the cure may become worse than the disease. Clearly, routine application of preoperative cardiac catheterization and prophylactic bypass is unrealistic owing to the excessive cost and the risks of the procedure. However, the optimal approach to the assessment and treatment of patients with severe CAD and peripheral vascular disease sufficient to warrant multiple surgical procedures is unresolved.

SUMMARY

The patient with vascular disease has a systemic disease—*atherosclerosis.* Unequivocally, the greatest perioperative risk to such a patient is intimately related to the extent of involvement of other organ systems, in particular the degree of underlying cardiac disease, which may or may

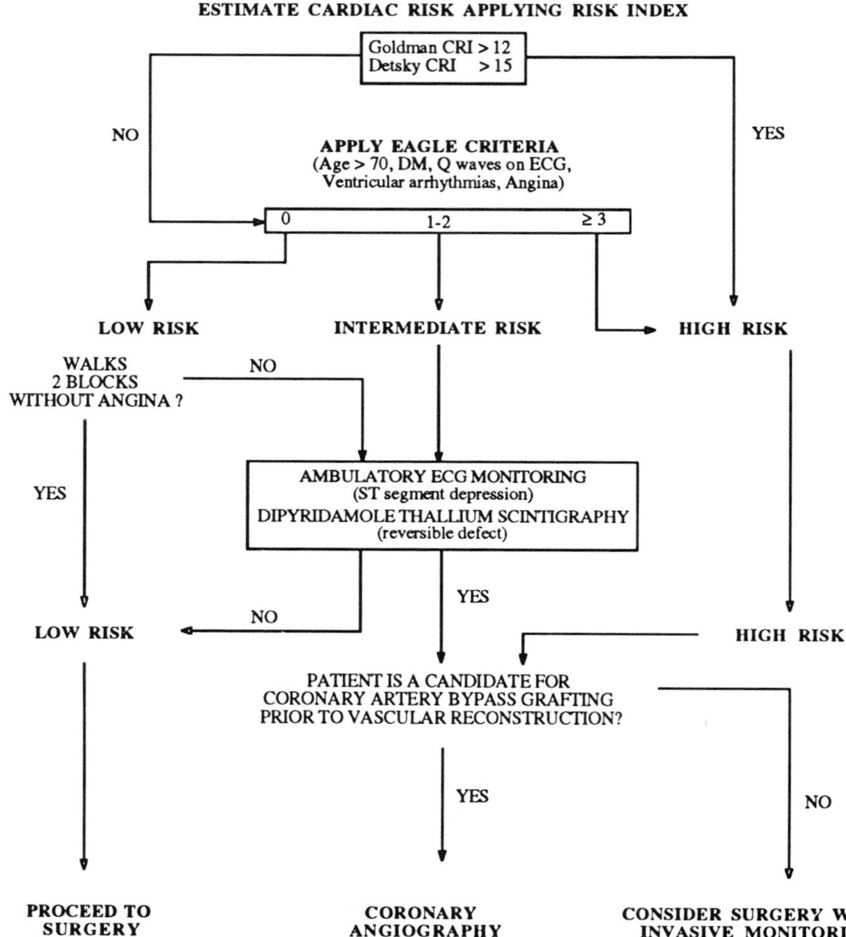

FIGURE 22–5. Proposed algorithm for the evaluation of preoperative cardiac risk in patients scheduled for elective vascular reconstruction. (Adapted with permission, from Wong T, Detsky AS: Preoperative cardiac risk assessment for patients having peripheral vascular surgery. Ann Intern Med. 1992; 116:743.)

not be obvious. Although the optimal strategy of identifying this risk remains controversial, a careful preoperative evaluation is necessary to assist in a rational selection of therapy.

The preceding studies suggest that improved results following vascular reconstruction may be achieved through careful preoperative evaluation, risk assessment, and risk reduction. A modification of the algorithm proposed by Wong and Detsky[76] illustrates and incorporates many of the principles of preoperative evaluation that have emerged from studies conducted during the last two decades (Fig. 22–5).

Risk assessment begins by the use of a clinical scoring system. An estimate of perioperative risk (low, intermediate, or high) is assigned. Although estimates of low risk do not preclude the presence of perioperative complications, further testing adds little additional information to the estimates obtained by the clinical scoring system. Conversely, patients with high cardiac risk scores are clearly at increased risk of experiencing postoperative complications, but further investigations are needed only if knowledge of the functional severity or degree of myocardial ischemia will alter subsequent management. In these patients, ambulatory ECG, DTS, or coronary arteriography may be useful if the vascular surgery can be delayed until myocardial revascularization is completed. Otherwise, the additional information provided is unlikely to alter the perioperative management. Patients identified as intermediate risk by clinical scoring benefit most from additional tests. Although a consensus has not yet been reached, DTS has emerged as the most popular noninvasive test for evaluating the intermediate-risk patient. Alternatively, we as well as others have demonstrated that ambulatory ECG monitoring is an equally effective noninvasive method of determining cardiac risk. Coronary artery bypass surgery should be recommended only on the basis of the patient's cardiac symptoms and anatomy, not necessarily on its potential for reducing perioperative risk or the complications associated with the proposed vascular procedure.

Many therapeutic options exist for both intermediate-risk and high-risk patients, including proceeding with surgery, instituting aggressive perioperative monitoring and anti-ischemic therapy, performing coronary arteriography and myocardial revascularization before the elective operation, selecting a lower risk surgical procedure, or canceling the planned procedure. Recent advances in surgical and anesthetic techniques as well as intraoperative and postoperative monitoring have resulted in lower morbidity and mortality in elective noncardiac procedures, but none can substitute for sound surgical judgment.

References

1. Benchimol A, Harris CL, Desser KB, et al: Resting electrocardiogram in major coronary artery disease. JAMA 224:1489, 1973.
2. Bergan JJ, Wilson SE, Wolf G, et al: Unexpected, late cardiovascular effects of surgery for peripheral artery disease. Arch Surg 127:1119, 1992.
3. Berlauk JF, Abrams JH, Gilmour IJ, et al: Preoperative optimization of cardiovascular hemodynamics improves outcome in peripheral vascular surgery. A prospective, randomized clinical trial. Ann Surg 214:289, 1991.
4. Bigger JTJ, Fleiss JL, Kleiger R, et al: The relationship among ventricular arrhythmias, left ventricular dysfunction, and mortality in the 2 years after myocardial infarction. Circulation 69:250, 1984.
5. Boucher CA, Brewster DC, Darling RC, et al: Correlation between preoperative ischemia and major cardiac events after peripheral vascular surgery. N Engl J Med 321:1296, 1989.
6. Boucher CA, Brewster DC, Darling RC, et al: Determination of cardiac risk by dipyridamole-thallium imaging before peripheral vascular surgery. N Engl J Med 312:389, 1985.
7. Boyd AM: The natural course of arteriosclerosis of the lower extremities. Angiology 11:10, 1960.
8. Bunt TJ: The role of a defined protocol for cardiac risk assessment in decreasing perioperative myocardial infarction in vascular surgery. J Vasc Surg 15:626, 1992.
9. Bush HL: Renal failure following abdominal aortic reconstruction. Surgery 93:107, 1983.
10. Carliner NH, Fisher ML, Plotnick GD, et al: Routine pre-operative exercise testing in patients undergoing major non-cardiac surgery. Am J Cardiol 56:51, 1985.
11. Charlson ME, MacKenzie CR, Ales K, et al: Surveillance for postoperative myocardial infarction after noncardiac operations. Surg Gynecol Obstet 167:407, 1988.
12. Cohn PF: Silent myocardial ischemia. Ann Intern Med 109:312, 1988.
13. Cooperman M, Pflug B, Martin EW, et al: Cardiovascular risk factors in patients with peripheral vascular disease. Surgery 84:505, 1978.
14. Cutler BS, Leppo JA: Dipyridamole thallium 201 scintigraphy to detect coronary artery disease before abdominal aortic surgery. J Vasc Surg 5:91, 1987.
15. Cutler BS, Hendel RC, Leppo JA: Dipyridamole-thallium scintigraphy predicts perioperative and long-term survival after major vascular surgery. J Vasc Surg 15:972, 1992.
16. Cutler BS, Wheeler HB, Paraskos JA, et al: Applicability and interpretation of electrocardiographic stress testing in patients with peripheral vascular disease. Am J Surg 141:501, 1981.
17. Detsky AS, Abrams HB, Forbath N, et al: Cardiac assessment for patients undergoing noncardiac surgery: A multifactorial clinical risk index. Arch Intern Med 146:2131, 1986.
18. Detsky AS, Abrams HB, McLaughlin JR, et al: Predicting cardiac complications in patients undergoing non-cardiac surgery. J Gen Intern Med 1:211, 1986.
19. Diamond GA, Forrester JS: Analysis of probability as an aid in the clinical diagnosis of coronary artery disease. N Engl J Med 300:1350, 1979.
20. Dirksen A, Kjoller E: Cardiac predictors of death after non-cardiac surgery evaluated by intention to treat. Br Med J 297:1011, 1988.
21. Dripps RD, Lamont A, Eckenhoff JE: The role of anaesthesia in surgical mortality. JAMA 178:261, 1961.
22. Dwyer EMJ, Greenberg HM, Steinberg G: Clinical characteristics and natural history of survivors of pulmonary congestion during acute myocardial infarction. The Multicenter Postinfarction Research Group. Am J Cardiol 63:1423, 1989.
23. Eagle KA, Boucher CA: Cardiac risk of noncardiac surgery. N Engl J Med 321:1330, 1989.
24. Eagle KA, Coley CM, Newell JB, et al: Combining clinical and thallium data optimizes preoperative assessment of cardiac risk before major vascular surgery. Ann Intern Med 110:859, 1989.
25. Eagle KA, Singer DE, Brewster DC, et al: Dipyridamole-thallium scanning in patients undergoing vascular surgery. Optimizing preoperative evaluation of cardiac risk. JAMA 257:2185, 1987.
26. Eagle KA, Strauss HW, Boucher CA: Dipyridamole myocardial perfusion imaging for coronary heart disease. Am J Cardiac Imaging 2:292, 1988.
27. Foster ED, Davis KB, Carpenter JA, et al: Risk of noncardiac operation in patients with defined coronary disease: The coronary artery surgery study (CASS) registry experience. Ann Thorac Surg 41:42, 1986.
28. Franco CD, Goldsmith J, Veith FJ, et al: Resting gated pool ejection fraction: A poor predictor of perioperative myocardial infarction in patients undergoing vascular surgery for infrainguinal bypass grafting. J Vasc Surg 10:656, 1989.
29. Gage AA, Bhayana JN, Balu V, et al: Assessment of cardiac risk in surgical patients. Arch Surg 112:1488, 1977.
30. Gardine RL, McBride K, Greenberg H, et al: The value of cardiac monitoring during peripheral arterial stress testing in the surgical management of peripheral vascular disease. J Cardiovasc Surg (Torino) 26:258, 1985.

31. Gersh BJ, Rihal CS, Rooke TW, et al: Evaluation and management of patients with both peripheral vascular and coronary artery disease. J Am Coll Cardiol 18:203, 1991.
32. Gerson MC, Hurst JM, Hertzberg VS, et al: Cardiac prognosis in noncardiac geriatric surgery. Ann Intern Med 103:832, 1985.
33. Goldman L: Cardiac risks and complications of noncardiac surgery. Ann Intern Med 98:504, 1983.
34. Goldman L, Caldera DL, Nessbaum SR, et al: Multifactorial index of cardiac risk in noncardiac surgical procedures. N Engl J Med 297:845, 1977.
35. Halperin BD, Feeley TW: The effect of anesthesia and surgery on renal function. Int Anesthesiol Clin 22:157, 1984.
36. Harris EJ, Moneta GL, Yeager RA, et al: Neurologic deficits following noncarotid vascular surgery. Am J Surg 163:537, 1992.
37. Hertzer NR: Myocardial ischemia. Surgery 83:97, 1983.
38. Hertzer NR: The natural history of peripheral vascular disease: Implications for its management. Circulation 83 (Suppl I): I-12, 1991.
39. Hertzer NR, Beven EG, Young JR, et al: Incidental asymptomatic carotid bruits in patients scheduled for peripheral vascular reconstruction: Results of cerebral and coronary angiography. Surgery 96:535, 1984.
40. Hertzer NR, Beven EG, Young JR, et al: Coronary artery disease in peripheral vascular patients: A classification of 1000 coronary angiograms and results of surgical management. Ann Surg 199:223, 1984.
41. Hertzer NR, Young JR, Beven EG, et al: Late results of coronary bypass in patients with infrarenal aortic aneurysms. Ann Surg 205:360, 1986.
42. Isner JM, Rosenfield K: Reducing the cardiac risk associated with vascular surgical procedures: Balloons as prophylactics. Mayo Clin Proc 67:95, 1992.
43. Kallero KS: Mortality and morbidity in patients with intermittent claudication as defined by venous occlusion plethysmography: A ten-year follow-up study. J Chronic Dis 34:455, 1981.
44. Kannel WB, McGee DL: Diabetes and cardiovascular risk factors: The Framingham study. Circulation 59:8, 1979.
45. Krupski WC, Layug EL, Reilly LM, et al: Comparison of cardiac morbidity between aortic and infrainguinal operations. Study of Perioperative Ischemia (SPI) Research Group. J Vasc Surg 15:354, 1992.
46. Lane SE, Lewis SM, Pippin JJ, et al: Predictive value of quantitative dipyridamole-thallium scintigraphy in assessing cardiovascular risk after vascular surgery in diabetes mellitus. Am J Cardiol 64:1275, 1989.
47. Lazor L, Russell JC, DaSilva J, et al: Use of the multiple uptake gated acquisition scan for the preoperative assessment of cardiac risk. Surg Gynecol Obstet 167:234, 1987.
48. Lette J, Waters D, Lassonde J, et al: Multivariate clinical models and quantitative dipyridamole-thallium imaging to predict cardiac morbidity and death after vascular reconstruction. J Vasc Surg 14:160, 1991.
49. Mangano DT: Perioperative cardiac morbidity. Anesthesiology 72:153, 1990.
50. Mangano DT, Browner WS, Hollenberg M, et al: Long-term cardiac prognosis following noncardiac surgery. JAMA 268:233, 1992.
51. Mangano DT, Hollenberg M, Fegert G, et al: Perioperative myocardial ischemia in patients undergoing noncardiac surgery. I. Incidence and severity during the 4 day perioperative period. The Study of Perioperative Ischemia (SPI) Research Group. J Am Coll Cardiol 17:843, 1991.
52. Mangano DT, London MJ, Tubau JF, et al: Dipyridamole thallium-201 scintigraphy as a preoperative screening test: A reexamination of its predictive potential. Circulation 84:493, 1991.
53. Mangano DT, Wong MG, London MJ, et al: Perioperative myocardial ischemia in patients undergoing noncardiac surgery. II. Incidence and severity during the 1st week after surgery. J Am Coll Cardiol 17:851, 1991.
54. Mays AE, Cobb FR: Relationship between regional myocardial blood flow and thallium 201 redistribution in the presence of coronary artery stenosis and dipyridamole-induced vasodilation. J Clin Invest 73:1359, 1984.
55. McCann RL, Clements FM: Silent myocardial ischemia in patients undergoing peripheral vascular surgery: Incidence and association with perioperative cardiac morbidity and mortality. J Vasc Surg 9:583, 1989.
56. McEnroe CS, O'Donnell TFJ, Yeager A, et al: Comparison of ejection fraction and Goldman risk factor analysis to dipyridamole-thallium 201 studies in the evaluation of cardiac morbidity after aortic aneurysm surgery. J Vasc Surg 11:497, 1990.
57. McGovern B: Hypokalemia and cardiac arrhythmias. Anesthesiology 63:127, 1985.
58. Myers WO, Gersh BJ, Fisher LD, et al: Medical versus early surgical therapy in patients with triple vessel disease and mild angina pectoris: A CASS registry study of survival. Ann Thorac Surg 44:471, 1987.
59. Ouyang P, Gerstenblith G, Furman WR, et al: Frequency and significance of early postoperative silent myocardial ischemia in patients having peripheral vascular surgery. Am J Cardiol 64:1113, 1989.
60. Pasternack PF, Grossi EA, Baumann FG, et al: The value of silent myocardial ischemia monitoring in the prediction of perioperative myocardial infarction in patients undergoing peripheral vascular surgery. J Vasc Surg 10:617, 1989.
61. Pasternack PF, Imparato AM, Bear G, et al: The value of radionuclide angiography as a predictor of perioperative myocardial infarction in patients undergoing abdominal aortic aneurysm resection. J Vasc Surg 1:320, 1984.
62. Pasternack PF, Imparato AM, Riles TS, et al: The value of radionuclide angiogram in the prediction of perioperative myocardial infarction in patients undergoing lower extremity revascularization procedures. Circulation 72 (Suppl II): II-13, 1985.
63. Raby KE, Goldman L, Creager MA, et al: Correlation between preoperative ischemia and major cardiac events after peripheral vascular surgery. N Engl J Med 321:1296, 1989.
64. Raby KE, Goldman L, Creager MA, et al: Predictive value of preoperative electrocardiographic monitoring. N Engl J Med 322:931, 1990.
65. Rao TL, Jacobs KH, El-Etr AA: Reinfarction following anesthesia in patients with myocardial infarction. Anesthesiology 59:499, 1983.
66. Sachs RN, Tellier P, Larmignat P, et al: Risk factors of postoperative pulmonary complications after vascular surgery. Surgery 105:360, 1989.
67. Sanz G, Castaner A, Betriu A: Determinants of prognosis in survivors of myocardial infarction. N Engl J Med 306:1065, 1982.
68. Schultz RAJ, Strauss HW, Pitt B: Sudden death in the year following myocardial infarction: Relation to ventricular premature contractions in the late hospital phase and left ventricular ejection fraction. Am J Med 62:192, 1976.
69. Shah KB, Kleinman BS, Rao TL, et al: Angina and other risk factors in patients with cardiac diseases undergoing noncardiac operations. Anesth Analg 70:240, 1990.
70. Taylor LJ, Yeager RA, Moneta GL, et al: The incidence of perioperative myocardial infarction in general vascular surgery. J Vasc Surg 15:52, 1992.
71. Topkins MJ, Artusio JF: Myocardial infarction and surgery: A five-year study. Anesth Analg 43:716, 1964.
72. Velanovich V: The value of routine preoperative laboratory testing in predicting postoperative complications: A multivariate analysis. Surgery 109:236, 1991.
73. von Knorring J: Postoperative myocardial infarction: A prospective study in a risk group of surgical patients. Surgery 90:55, 1981.
74. Waller BF, Palumbo PJ, Lie JT, et al: Status of the coronary arteries at necropsy in diabetes mellitus with onset after age 30 years: Analysis of 229 diabetic patients with and without clinical evidence of coronary heart disease and comparison to 183 control subjects. Am J Med 69:498, 1980.
75. Weiner DA, Ryan TJ, McCabe CH, et al: Correlations among history of angina, ST-segment response and prevalence of coronary artery disease in the coronary artery surgery study (CASS). N Engl J Med 301:230, 1979.
76. Wong T, Detsky AS: Preoperative cardiac risk assessment for patients having peripheral vascular surgery. Ann Intern Med 116:743, 1992.
77. Yeager RA: Basic data related to cardiac testing and cardiac risk associated with vascular surgery. Ann Vasc Surg 4:193, 1990.
78. Yeager RA, Weigel RM, Murphy ES, et al: Application of clinically valid cardiac risk factors to aortic aneurysm surgery. Arch Surg 121:278, 1986.
79. Zeldin RA: Assessing cardiac risk in patients who undergo noncardiac surgical procedures. Can J Surg 27:402, 1984.

23

Blood Replacement and Autotransfusion in Major Vascular Surgery

Roy L. Tawes, Jr., M.D.

• • •

The 1980s have witnessed a progressive growth in cardiovascular procedures, transplantation, trauma, and other major operations that have burdened the nation's blood supply. Over 12 million units of blood are transfused annually in the United States, of which two thirds are used for surgery. During this period there has been serious concern about the safety of the blood supply with a subsequent dramatic change in attitude toward homologous blood transfusions (HBT). The advent of transfusion-related human immunodeficiency virus (HIV) and acquired immunodeficiency syndrome (AIDS) in the early 1980s, as well as the even greater risk of hepatitis transmission, provided the impetus for a conservative attitude toward HBT and the search for alternatives. Otherwise, it is doubtful whether blood banks could have met the increasing demands for blood transfusions.

Several trends have emerged consequently. Component therapy, the transfusion of packs of red blood cells, platelets, and fresh frozen plasma (FFP) separately as indicated, has essentially replaced the previously whole blood transfusion. Stricter indications for transfusion and the realization that patients will tolerate lower hemoglobin Hgb levels than previously thought necessary for oxygen transport have decreased the demand for banked blood.

New technology led the shift from homologous to autologous blood transfusions (ABT) with the development of rapid, safe autotransfusion (AT) machines that salvage blood usually lost or shed at operation and process it for reinfusion. In major vascular surgery AT is becoming the standard of care. Other technologic advances provide autologous platelet-rich plasma (PRP) using a technique of perioperative plasmapheresis for vascular operations associated with large anticipated blood losses. Also, advanced infusion systems are now available for rapid normothermic, large-volume replacement, making thoracoabdominal aortic procedures and other major vascular operations safer as well as conserving the supply of blood by avoiding the coagulopathies often associated with these major procedures.

Other trends in blood banking and transfusion therapy involve biogenetic engineering. The development of recombinant erythropoietin (EPO) decreases the need for later transfusion. New research directed toward producing genetically engineered Hgb and the continued effort to develop artificial blood are making progress. Other relatively recent approaches to conserving blood through improved hemostasis have been directed toward decreasing blood loss in cardiovascular surgery through the use of blood products and medications. For example, aprotinin (popular in Europe), desmopressin, fibrin glue, and single-donor platelets (apheresis) should all contribute to progress in this field, since better hemostasis will result in fewer transfusions.

Finally the recent focus on medicolegal and economic aspects as well as risk benefit analyses have contributed to changing attitudes toward transfusion therapy. The following sections address these subjects.

HISTORICAL OVERVIEW

Historical perspective gives us a better understanding of our major advances. Modern blood typing and blood banks to facilitate transfusion did not become available until 1936. Therefore, early transfusion efforts were essentially rudimentary AT techniques. The development of these techniques and the chronology of the stages of AT were covered by Maddox in the previous edition's chapter on blood replacement in major vascular surgery.[1] That literature review is summarized, augmented, and updated here. The early history of blood transfusion is characterized by innovative but largely unsuccessful attempts to salvage blood for reinfusion, followed by novel attempts to collect and reinfuse it. Heterologous transfusion was attempted in the 17th century by surgeons Tower, Denis, and Purmann.[2–3] Blundell later reported the first homologous transfusion in 1818 in London and also attempted AT in women with postpartum hemorrhage.[4] The first American credited with AT was Brainard in 1860, who salvaged blood lost during an amputation for reinfusion.[5] Highmore emphasized the merits of AT in 1864 and urged its acceptance.[6] Subsequent cases were reported, but AT remained rare during the 19th century.[7] At this stage, transfusion was more experimental than therapeutic.

The early 20th century produced more advocates of using the patient's own blood in surgery. Blood banking and blood typing still had not been developed, so surgeons were confronted with the need for a suitable means of blood replacement. The patient's own blood seemed to be the only reasonable source. Thies is credited with coining the word autotransfusion in 1914 after reporting successful treatment of a woman with an ectopic pregnancy.[8] During World War I Elmendorf attempted AT using blood from a patient's hemothorax for reinfusion.[9] Despite the strong support for AT offered by famous contemporary surgeons (Halsted, Cushing, and Davis), only 272 cases had been reported in the American literature by 1936.[10]

Landsteiner's major contribution to blood transfusion in the early 1900s was the first description of A, B, and O blood types.[11] He emphasized the importance of blood typing prior to transfusion. The fourth blood type, AB, was reported in 1902 by DeCastello and Sturli.[12] Investigations by Hektoen,[13] Ottenberg and Kaliski,[14] and their colleagues led to the development of cross-matching of donors and the detection of blood incompatibility. Landsteiner subsequently developed the standard international nomenclature for blood typing, cold agglutinins, Rh factors, and M and N factors,[15, 16] but there was almost a 40-year lag before this knowledge was translated into practical modern-day blood banking.

This development of practical and safe blood typing techniques made large-scale homologous transfusion and blood banking feasible by 1936. By 1940, with cross-typing available, whole blood transfusions became the state of the art in civilian practice and in World War II, the Korean War, and during the early development of heart surgery in the 1940s and 1950s. In 1953 Gibbon developed the first cardiopulmonary bypass machine,[17] and open heart surgery escalated the use of HBT to new levels. Meanwhile, AT techniques fell into relative disuse until the late 1960s, when surgeons during the Vietnam conflict experienced acute blood shortages. Attention then focused again on AT techniques and further fostered the development of ABT. The first generation of ABT methods was innovative but unsophisticated. Under combat conditions blood was salvaged by every method imaginable, filtered through gauze, and then reinfused by every conceivable route: subcutaneous, intramuscular, intravenous, even per rectum.[18]

In 1966, Dyer introduced significant refinements. They designed collection techniques using a special suction tip with plastic tubing and a collection chamber connected to a wall vacuum suction.[19] Two years later Dyer collaborated with Klebanoff and colleagues to develop the basic concept for the first effective AT machine used in wartime conditions.[20, 21] Klebanoff borrowed cardiac surgery technology, replacing the vacuum suction with a roller pump to reduce hemolysis and replacing the collecting chamber with a cardiotomy reservoir. Bentley Laboratories (Santa Ana, CA) further developed these design concepts into the Bentley ATS-100 device (Fig. 23–1), which was used extensively from 1968 to the mid-1970s.

The early AT machines were large, cumbersome, and plagued with many of the same problems that affected the early cardiopulmonary bypass machines, particularly air embolism and hemolysis. Additionally, coagulopathies resulted from reinfusing blood that was high in fibrin degradation products (FDP), complement, and activated clotting factors. The concept of washing the red blood cells (RBC) and more sophisticated filtration techniques evolved in the early 1970s, but the technology did not become refined until the mid seventies. During this period, third-generation collection-reinfusion systems became universal, and some are still in use today.

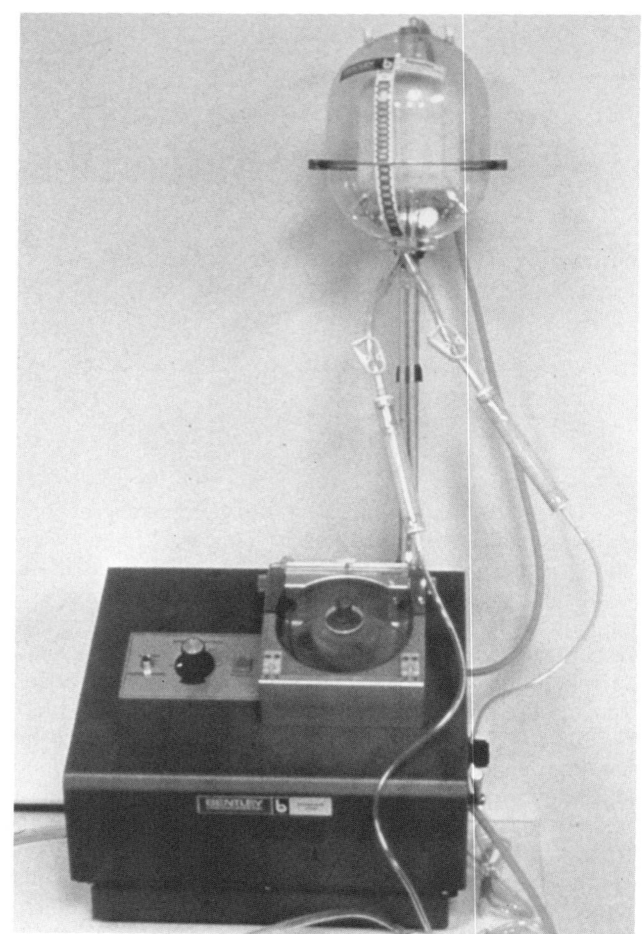

FIGURE 23–1. Bentley ATS-100 autotransfusor.

The third-generation AT devices collected shed blood in sterile plastic disposable containers. The Sorenson device (Sorenson Research Co., Salt Lake City, UT) has been used extensively in postoperative salvage of blood from mediastinal and chest tubes. Similar commercially available AT devices are the Socotrans, Autovac, and Pleura-Vac devices. However, the trend now is away from reinfusing unwashed blood because newer, fourth-generation AT technology is available.

Technologic advances by Haemonetics Corporation (Braintree, MA) in 1974 introduced AT machines that salvaged blood from the operative field, filtered it in a collection reservoir containing anticoagulant, and then washed the RBCs free by differential centrifugation, processing them for rapid, safe reinfusion. The Haemonetics Cell Saver became synonymous with the term autotransfusion (AT).

The 1980s witnessed a major shift from predominantly HBT to alternatives that included ABT because of concern about the safety of the blood supply. The main impetus was the discovery of HIV (AIDS) transmission in 1982. By the mid-1980's, about 2 per cent of AIDS cases resulted from transmission through HBT. This caused widespread public reaction bordering on hysteria. HIV antibody screening tests became available by late 1984 but were not completely accurate or effective. During the late 1980s laws were passed in many states requiring "informed consent" for blood transfusions. The Gann law in California was the first of these and served as a model for others.

By the late 1980s technology had advanced to the point where autologous platelets and plasma could be processed during surgery using the technique of perioperative plasmapheresis. The Haemonetics Corporation developed the Plasma Saver, which was approved by the United States Food and Drug Administration (FDA) in 1988 for clinical use. Not only had complete autologous perioperative transfusion become feasible, but because freshly processed PRP had hemostatic value, it often decreased the need for blood bank transfusion.[22]

A final advance in transfusion therapy in the late 1980s was the development of a system capable of *rapid* infusion of large volumes of blood, colloid, and crystalloids at *normothermia.* This technology helps to avoid shock, coagulopathy, and acidosis during vascular surgery involving large-volume losses. These newer devices further retard the depletion of blood bank supplies. Two currently available machines for this process are the Rapid Infusion System (RIS, made by Haemonetics), and Level-I Technologies (Marshfield, MA). The evolution of AT devices is depicted in Figure 23–2.

Summarizing the history of blood transfusion, the highlights are the development of blood typing in 1936, the development of practical AT machines by the 1960s, and a series of technologic advances during the 1970s and 1980s. However, it was the contamination of the blood supply in the early 1980s by HIV that led to a serious reappraisal of our blood supply and forever changed our attitude toward homologous transfusion therapy.

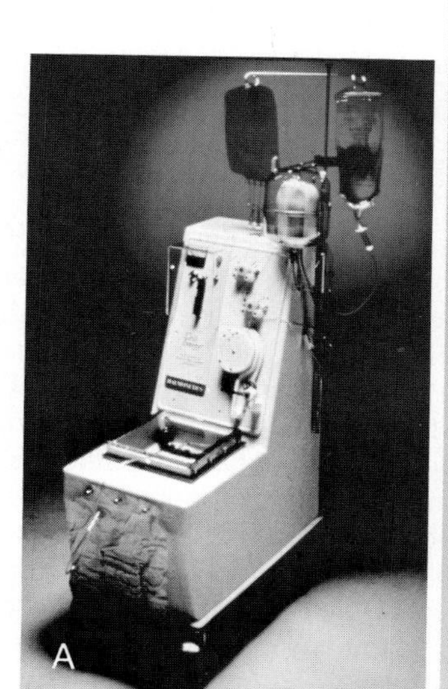

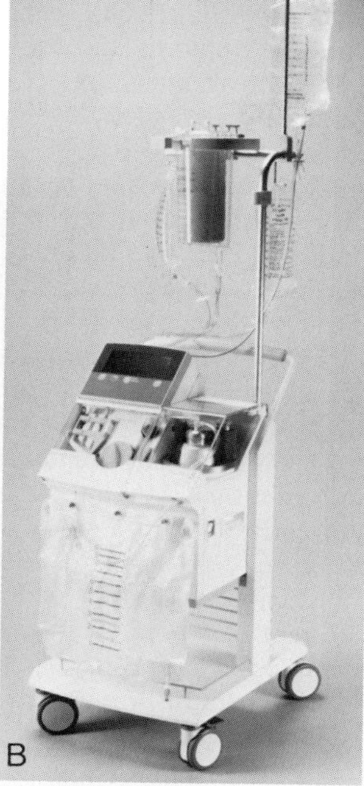

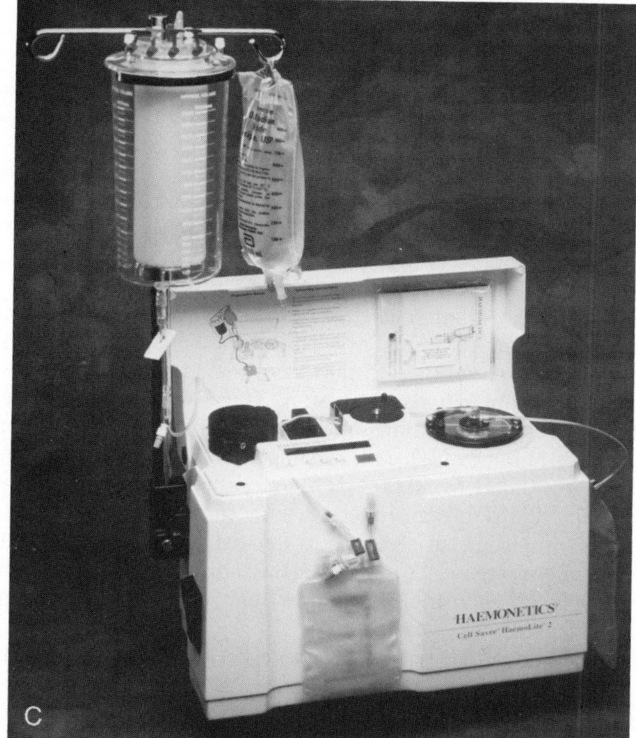

FIGURE 23–2. Evolution of autotransfusion devices. *A*, Cell Saver 1. *B*, Cell Saver 5. *C*, HaemoLite 2.

RISKS OF HOMOLOGOUS BLOOD TRANSFUSION

Human error infrequently results in transfusion mismatches, which are fatal in a small number of cases owing to acute hemolysis.[23] The risk of delayed hemolysis from an immune response related to sensitization by a prior transfusion or pregnancy is about 1 in 6000, resulting in death in approximately 1 in 100,000.[24, 25] However, the great majority of transfusion reactions are not fatal and are manifest by fever or urticaria in response to leukocyte antigens or plasma proteins.[26] Anaphylactic shock is the most severe transfusion reaction but fortunately is rare. It occurs when patients who are IgA-deficient receive blood transfusions in which IgA is present.[27] Other unusual complications associated with HBT include graft-versus-host disease in immunosuppressed patients and septic shock due to bacterial contamination. In addition, recent literature has indicated an association of HBT with earlier than expected cancer recurrence and an increase in septic complications.[23, 28–30]

At present, the major concern in transfusion therapy is still the risk of transmissible diseases. During the late 1970s the increased prevalence, morbidity, and mortality associated with transmission of hepatitis through transfusions should have initiated a greater effort among surgeons and blood banks toward blood conservation and the use of alternatives to HBT. Transfusion-related hepatitis was described in 1943 by Beeson.[31] Subsequent screening of asymptomatic carriers for hepatitis B (HBsAg) excluded some prospective donors, but failed to eliminate post-transfusion hepatitis or even significantly reduce its incidence[23] because the majority of cases were non-A, non-B (NANB) hepatitis. Even with the HBsAg screening the incidence of hepatitis is 3 to 12 per cent in the U.S. population receiving transfusion,[32, 33] with about 1 per cent of these patients showing clinical symptoms and the others abnormal liver function tests. But as many as 50 per cent of this asymptomatic subgroup may later develop chronic active hepatitis and cirrhosis.[34] Between 1988 and 1990 hepatitis C (HCV) antibody screening tests became available.[35, 36] Most patients with transfusion-related non-A, non-B hepatitis have antibodies to HCV, so this may lead to more effective screening that could decrease the risk of hepatitis to 1 per cent or less.[37]

Other viruses transmitted by HBT are the Epstein-Barr virus, associated with a chronic fatigue syndrome, and cytomegalovirus (CMV), which causes a range of clinical presentations from mononucleosis to hepatitis, pneumonia, and enteritis. CMV infection was reported in 1966 by Kreel and colleagues in a study of patients with "postperfusion syndrome" following cardiopulmonary bypass and multiple transfusions.[38] CMV is endemic in healthy donors, 40 to 90 per cent of whom are seropositive. The risk to the patient receiving a seropositive transfusion is 3 to 12 per cent for development of primary infection, which is usually mild or asymptomatic.[23] However, immunosuppressed patients, such as transplant recipients receiving immunosuppressive therapy, are likely to develop serious manifestations. Therefore, CMV-negative blood is advisable when possible, particularly for these patients.

Currently, the major public concern about HBT is the risk of AIDS. Although *antibody* screening tests for HIV have decreased the risk of disease transmission with transfusion, they are not entirely reliable because the unpredictable "window period" for seroconversion ranges from months to as much as 10 years.[39] Furthermore, current tests that screen for HIV *antigens* lack the sensitivity to detect seronegative infected donors.[40] As of June 1992, 6014 patients in the United States had developed transfusion-related AIDS, and approximately two thirds of these had died. It is estimated that another 15,000 have become HIV seropositive following blood transfusion. The Centers for Disease Control and Prevention reports the risk to be about 1 in 153,000,[41] but in high-risk urban centers it may be as much as 1 in 40,000 to 50,000. It is important to note that this risk increases proportionately with multiple transfusions. For example, in an area where the risk is 1 in 150,000, if the patient receives 3 units of HBT (components included), the risk of HIV transmission is then approximately 1 in 50,000.

For completeness, it should be noted that malaria, syphilis, and HTLV virus have also been reported as complications of HBT. At present, these diseases pose no major threat to the U.S. blood supply.

ALTERNATIVES TO HOMOLOGOUS BLOOD TRANSFUSIONS

Strict Criteria for Transfusion

The simplest method of decreasing the risk of transmission of diseases by transfusion is to decrease the need for transfusion. This may be accomplished by limiting the indications for transfusion, promoting better intraoperative hemostasis, and judiciously selecting alternatives to transfusion.

It is common practice to initiate transfusion if the hemoglobin falls below 10 gm or the hematocrit falls below 30 per cent. These levels are arbitrary. It has been shown by rheologic studies that patients do quite well with hematocrits as low as 20 to 24 per cent. Perfusion and oxygenation of tissue is adequate and well tolerated at these levels. Additional experiences with Jehovah's Witnesses and renal failure patients who are severely anemic have reinforced this impression.[23] Therefore, the decision to begin transfusion should be based on clinical assessment of oxygen delivery to the tissues (e.g., tachycardia, decreased blood pressure, decreased Po_2, and decreased cardiac output).[23] No study has conclusively shown that moderate anemia increases wound infection or impairs recuperation. A list of the current indications for appropriate blood usage followed in the author's hospital is presented in Table 23–1.

The other alternatives to HBT are listed in Table 23–2. In addition to stricter transfusion indications, a number of other options are available. Acute isovolemic hemodilution is widely practiced and is discussed below. Perhaps the best resource is the patient's own blood.[42] ABT is possible

Table 23–1. Blood Use Review

Appropriate transfusion of homologous and autologous whole blood or packed RBCs
- For homologous transfusions
  - a. Hemoglobin <9 gm
  - b. Mean corpuscular volume (MCV) >75 and <115 gm
- For autologous transfusions
  - a. Hemoglobin <10 gm
  - b. MCV >75 and <115 gm
  - Excludes:
    - a. Patients with congestive heart failure
    - b. Patients with myocardial ischemia, angina, or past myocardial infarction
    - c. Patients with cerebrovascular accident or cerebrovascular insufficiency
    - d. Patients with chronic obstructive pulmonary disease
    - e. Patients with acute blood loss of >600 ml (homologous) or >450 ml (autologous)

Appropriate transfusion of platelet concentrate
- Platelet count <75,000/mm^3 and bleeding present
  - or
- Platelet count <20,000/mm^3 and no bleeding present

Appropriate transfusion of fresh frozen plasma
- Prothrombin time >18 sec
  - or
- Partial thromboplastin time >45 sec
  - or
- More than 1 unit given

Appropriate transfusion of cryoprecipitates
- Patients requiring heat-labile coagulation factors (II, XIII, VII) in addition to treatment of disseminated intravascular coagulation and von Willebrand's disease

Appropriate transfusion of leukocyte-poor packed cells
- Patients who have undergone more than two documented febrile transfusion reactions or other leukocyte-related reactions
- Excludes:
  - a. Patients with chronic anemia.
  - b. Patients requiring multiple transfusions.
  - c. Patients undergoing chemotherapy.

Table 23–2. Alternatives to Homologous Blood Transfusion

Strict criteria for transfusion
Acute isovolemic hemodilution
Preoperative autologous donation
Intra-operative autotransfusion
Postoperative autotransfusion
Promotion of hemostasis
Blood substitutes

by ensuring preoperative donation and by using intraoperative and postoperative salvage. Another categorical approach is through promoting hemostasis. This can be accomplished by using autologous platelet-rich plasma (PRP) and fibrin glue or administering medications such as aprotinin and desmopressin. Rapid infusion systems that ensure normothermic, high-volume replacement greatly aid hemostasis.[43] Blood substitutes are a final consideration.[44] Each of these options is now discussed.

ISOVOLEMIC HEMODILUTION

Up to 20 per cent of the patient's blood volume can be safely removed after the induction of anesthesia and replaced with crystalloid or saline (2 ml saline/1 ml blood). This blood is anticoagulated with citrate-phosphate-dextrose (CPD) and given back at the end of the operation. The advantage of this method is that the blood loss during surgery has a much lower hematocrit and is more easily replaced.[45–47] The patient's cardiac output and ventricular function can be safely monitored using a Swan-Ganz catheter and transesophageal echocardiography, respectively.

AUTOLOGOUS BLOOD TRANSFUSION

Preoperative Donation

Patients scheduled to undergo major procedures are requested to donate 1 to 3 units of blood 1 to 3 weeks before the operation. Preoperative hematocrit values of 33 per cent are acceptable and well tolerated. Routinely, patients are given supplemental iron therapy.[42, 48–50] This is an excellent but underutilized option to HBT. A multi-center study by Toy and associates reported only a 5 per cent compliance rate among eligible patients in 18 predeposit programs.[51] The safety of this method has been tested in high-risk patients,[52] children,[53] and third-trimester pregnant women.[54–55] Its efficacy in avoiding HBT by preoperative autologous donation is well documented.[56–58] Goodnough and colleagues reported increasing preoperative collection of autologous blood in conjunction with recombinant erythropoietin therapy with no apparent side effects.[57] This is becoming a popular practice in Japan.[59]

Designated donors are another appealing approach taken by patients concerned about the risk of HBT. Cordell and coworkers reported no statistical difference between designated donors and volunteer homologous donors with regard to seropositivity for syphilis, hepatitis, or HIV.[60] They concluded that designated donor blood was as safe, but no safer, than homologous blood based on 12,000 studied patients. In fact, the risk of graft-versus-host disease may increase with transfusion of blood from first-degree relatives, somewhat decreasing the attraction of this approach.

Autotransfusion

The advantages of ABT are listed in Table 23–3. Aside from logistic considerations, autologous salvaged RBCs are physiologically and biochemically superior or equal to homologous RBCs. First, the logistic considerations noted in Table 23–3 are persuasive. Blood retrieved at operation by AT techniques is not only a ready source of RBCs but may also be rapidly reinfused after processing. This is life saving in emergency cases such as a ruptured aortic aneurysm. In terms of conservation, it does not deplete blood bank supplies. Recycling is simple and straightforward and obviates problems with blood typing and cross-matching (rare blood types or antibody problems), autoimmunization, and transfusion reactions. A major advantage is the absence of risk of transfusion-related diseases such as AIDS and hepatitis. Finally, it is acceptable by most religious groups including Jehovah's Witnesses.[1, 42] Second, the biochemical, physiologic, and morphologic characteristics of salvaged autologous RBCs make them superior or equal to homologous RBCs.

Red Cell Survival. RBC survival has been measured by various investigators.[61, 64] Ansel and colleagues found no significant difference in the survival of RBCs salvaged by AT methods compared to predonated autologous RBCs using double-isotope studies.[63] Thorley and associates, using dual-isotope techniques, demonstrated no significant loss in RBC survival with salvaged red blood cells compared to the patient's own cells.[64]

Morphologic Changes. Paravicini and colleagues used scanning electron microscopy to show little or no morphologic changes between RBCs processed by a Cell-Saver and nonprocessed cells.[65] Cell detritus was eliminated by microfiltration. These investigators concluded that survival and morphologic alteration of RBCs by the intraoperative AT system of washing and separating the cells appeared to be superior to transfusion of homologous blood.

Physiology of Washed RBC by Intraoperative Autotransfusion. Orr and Blenko demonstrated that washing of

Table 23–3. Advantages of Autotransfused Blood

Ready and rapid availability
No incompatibility
No autoimmunization
No risk of disease transmission
Conserves blood bank supply
Answers religious objections
Net blood loss reduced
Blood quality superior

shed blood in the autotransfusor removed virtually all contaminants, including activated clotting factors, cell debris, and free Hgb.[66] Washed cells had a better than average 2,3-diphosphoglycerate (DPG) and osmotic fragility index. The AT technique did not significantly compromise effectiveness compared with existing procedures in this study, and it decreased the use of homologous blood by 25 per cent. Other studies at the Mayo Clinic[67] and at Duke University[68] have reported reduced use of homologous transfusions by 40 to 75 per cent after the implementation of effective AT techniques. This has also been our experience.[63] McShane and associates evaluated the quality of blood prepared with an RBC processing device and reported normal 2,3-DPG levels and physiologic pH and potassium concentrations.[70] Aaron and coworkers[71] and Schaff and colleagues[72] independently compared serum electrolytes and arterial blood gases in AT blood with those in homologous blood and found them to be within normal limits in ex vivo autotransfused blood.[73]

Disadvantages, Potential Problems, and Relative Contraindications. Table 23–4 enumerates the potential negative aspects of AT techniques. It should be noted that many of these problems can be avoided by proper management of the AT equipment, whereas in other instances a relative contraindication exists, or the risk of potential complication is so high, that the use of AT can be justified only in life-threatening circumstances.

Hemolysis can result from improper suction tips, reaction to the tubing and plastic surfaces, or too high a rate of centrifugation or roller-pump action. Suction greater than 30 psi will cause excessive turbulence leading to RBC damage. Plasma-free hemoglobin counts are high (more than 1000 mg/100 ml) in *unwashed* blood retrieved by all AT systems.[71–75] But after *washing*, free hemoglobin levels of less than 100 mg/100 ml) have been reported by Orr,[76] which are comparable to those present in banked blood[74] and are not harmful with reinfusion into the patient.[77]

Air embolism plagued the early AT machines, much like the early cardiopulmonary bypass machines, but newer devices are equipped with air traps and warning devices that automatically combat this potential problem.

Coagulopathy may occur in conjunction with AT. The cause is complex and may be related to several factors: shock, multiple transfusions, hypothermia, cardiopulmonary bypass, and inadequate heparin neutralization. The AT technique itself may be implicated. Because clotting factors and platelets are removed by the Cell-Saver technique, a dilutional coagulopathy may result. Also, poor management of cell washing, lack of proper filtration, and reinfusion of "residual heparin" may all play a role.[78] The activated clotting time (ACT) should be closely monitored in the patient[79] and a protocol implemented for homologous or autologous platelet and plasma replacement.[78]

Table 23–4. Negative Aspects of Autotransfusion

Hemolysis
Air embolism
Coagulopathy
Protein loss
Sepsis, contamination
Cancer dissemination
Sickle cell disease

Protein loss is a normal and unavoidable problem because the cell washing technique salvages the RBCs and discards the plasma proteins.

Sepsis and contamination of AT blood is an obvious contraindication for reinfusion into a patient receiving a prosthetic graft.[80] Successful reinfusion of contaminated blood has been reported in desperate, life-saving *trauma* cases.[81–83]

Cancer dissemination is rarely a concern during vascular surgery using an AT system but should be recognized as a contraindication if encountered.[84–85]

Sickle cell disease is a relative contraindication unless a preoperative exchange transfusion has been performed.[86, 87]

Obviously, the advantages of AT far outweigh the disadvantages, and this method can be enthusiastically advocated as the vascular surgeon's best resource.[42, 69]

Indications

The intraoperative AT technique is generally indicated in all patients undergoing major cardiovascular procedures with anticipated blood losses of more than 2 units. The technique is used in conjunction with preoperative donation of autologous blood and postoperative salvage.[42] With the newer impervious prosthetic grafts blood conservation is becoming more efficient.[88] AT may be used during and after cardiopulmonary bypass and during elective and emergency operations for occlusive and aneurysmal disease—thoracic, thoracoabdominal, and abdominal. It is especially useful in "re-do" procedures, major vascular trauma, and operations for portal hypertension. Because of the potential threat of transmissible diseases with HBT, the AT is becoming standard operating procedure.

Technique. The author has had extensive experience with the Cell-Saver and other devices since 1978.[69] The current technique he uses differs somewhat from the standard commercial protocol. The two essential components of RBC salvage are *cell separation and hemofiltration.* The author advocates *ultrafiltration* with a 25-μ screen in the collection (cardiotomy) reservoir and a 40-μ *microfilter* in the reinfusion line to the patient. This method, in conjunction with cell separation accomplished by a differential centrifugation washing technique, produces optimal results.[78] Otherwise, the author's AT technique is standard.[89]

Blood is salvaged from the operative field through a special heparinized tube with a large-bore suction tip (see Fig. 23–3 on Color Plate I) into a collection (cardiotomy) reservoir. As emphasized, the author uses a 25-μ COBE filter to achieve ultrafiltration of microaggregates rather than the large screen (120 to 150 μ) filter provided by several AT companies. The suction line is anticoagulated with heparin (10,000 units), and the reservoir with an additional 20,000 units. After collection of 500 to 1000 ml of blood from the operative field, the salvaged blood is then processed in a Latham-design centrifuge bowl. The RBCs are then washed and separated by differential centrifugation in normal saline (9 per cent sodium chloride). The wash cycle must follow the standard protocol to be maximally effective. The author routinely uses 3 to 6 volume washing

(1 to 2 liters of physiologic saline) in his cell separation technique. Operations for ruptured abdominal aortic aneurysms and other emergency procedures for trauma may require more extensive washing, particularly if ultrafiltration is not employed in the collection reservoir. Washing removes any particulate matter or soluble procoagulants not filtered by the 25-μ screen in the reservoir, such as circulating fibrin, debris from the operative field, plasma, platelets, white blood cell (WBC) clumps and other microaggregates, procoagulants, and activated clotting factors. These are collected in the waste bag and discarded. Most heparin is washed out, but some residual heparin persists.[78] The ACT is closely monitored to ensure adequate anticoagulation and reversal.

Depending on the urgency of the case and the speed of processing, 1 unit of washed packed RBCs with a hematocrit of 40 to 60 per cent can be obtained in a 3- to 7-minute wash cycle. One unit consists of 225 to 250 ml of packed RBCs. An in-line 40-μ filter with a blood warmer is used for reinfusion of the blood to the patient. Near the completion of the procedure, the operative field is irrigated with saline and checked for hemostasis. At this point, the author switches to wall suction. The AT is not used at this stage of the operation, especially if local hemostatic agents (e.g., thrombin-soaked Gelfoam) have been used.

The Cell-Saver may be operated in the auto or manual mode. A dedicated technician, registered nurse, or person who is thoroughly familiar with the AT technique is recommended as an operator. In emergency cases, blood may be collected in the reservoir containing anticoagulant and processed later, if indicated, avoiding "standby" technician costs.

Postoperative Salvage

Postoperative blood loss from chest or mediastinal tubes may be retrieved by the Sorenson system and reinfused.[42] However, the author now advocates washing the shed blood with a Haemolite, a small, portable AT device, prior to reinfusion. The reasons for this approach will be discussed later in the section on unresolved issues and controversies.

PROMOTION OF HEMOSTASIS

Autologous platelet-rich plasma (PRP) may be obtained perioperatively by means of plasmapheresis.[22] In 1988 the FDA approved the Plasma-Saver, a second-generation, rapid plasmapheresis device that may be used in the operating room as well as the blood bank, obviating the need for homologous components. Figures 23–4 and 23–5 (see Color Plate I) demonstrate the technique of perioperative plasmapheresis. The chief advantage of the Plasma-Saver is that it can rapidly collect and process donor blood in half the time needed by the older machines, making it practical for surgery. In about the time it takes to dissect, anticoagulate, and cross-clamp the aorta for bypass (approximately 30 minutes), 600 to 1000 ml of PRP can be collected (see Fig. 23–4 on Color Plate I). This amount is approximately equivalent to 2 units of fresh frozen plasma and 6 packs of platelets. The packed RBCs resulting from the differential centrifugation technique are returned to the patient after each 10- to 15-minute cycle of PRP collection (see Fig. 23–5 on Color Plate I).

The amount of PRP collected depends on the patient's weight, body build, hematocrit, and cardiovascular compliance. Collection of up to 20 per cent of total blood volume (600 to 1000 ml) usually causes no untoward effects. Collection set-up usually takes about 5 minutes. Experienced technicians, registered nurses, and anesthesiologists have a short learning curve because of the simplicity of the equipment.

Cycling continues with the draw-return steps until the programming collection weight is met. Processing takes approximately 10 to 15 minutes for every 250 ml of PRP collected. During the processing, RBC loss is minimal. After each cycle the RBCs are reinfused into the patient. Additional technical safeguards include a donor pressure sensor in the machine to avoid build-up of pressure; this sensor automatically stops the pump until the pressure situation is corrected. Four air detectors are incorporated. The PRP can be stored at room temperature until it is transfused, usually after protamine reversal of the anticoagulant effect of heparin. It is recommended that the collected product be placed on a rocker until infusion and that pH be held constant. It should be wrapped in a blanket to maintain a temperature of 36 to 37°C.[89] The anticoagulant used in the system is citrate but hypocalcemic responses to the PRP product infusion have been rare thus far. In the event of a hypocalcemic reaction, slowing down the transfusion rate or administering calcium will quickly alleviate the problem. The amount of citrate in PRP product is less than that found in equivalent homologous products from the blood bank.

It is important to note that in patients with cardiac or vascular problems, the PRP is not returned to the patient until reversal of the heparin action with protamine. In the author's patients, ACT is monitored with a Hemochron device[79] during the procedure to ensure both adequate anticoagulation and reversal. The author advises using ACD rather than heparin in the Plasma-Saver as the anticoagulant because heparin may activate platelets and could potentially cause a hypercoagulable state.[89, 90]

Current technology has reached the point where complete autotransfusion of major blood components (RBCs and PRP) is a reality with proper planning and experience. In addition, perioperative plasmapheresis has been shown in early studies to restore hemostasis significantly by the infusion of fresh autologous PRP, increasing the patient's platelet count and clotting proteins. This reduces blood loss and consequently the requirement for transfusion of homologous blood components. This observation has been documented in other studies worldwide.[91–95]

Local measures to promote hemostasis include the use of new impervious grafts that do not require preclotting and feature decreased needle hole bleeding.[88] Particularly effective in vascular trauma patients is the use of hemostatic agents such as Avetine (Alcon-Biochem-Medchem), thrombin-soaked Gelfoam (Upjohn), and Surgical (Johnson & Johnson) as adjuvants to hemostasis. Nothing replaces a well-placed suture, however. A separate suction system (not the AT system) should be used when these hemostatic agents are on the operative field to avoid triggering clotting in the system.

Fibrin glue may be the perfect hemostatic agent for operative use because it has no tissue toxicity, seals in minutes, reabsorbs, and promotes local tissue growth and repair.[96–101] Since Matras and colleagues[102] first successfully used fibrin glue in surgery in 1972, this sealant has been used extensively in Europe for various indications.[96] Use in the United States has been limited, however, because of lack of commercially prepared materials,[100] lack of a concentrated source of fibrinogen, and, in the last decade, concern about hepatitis transmission in pooled *homologous* plasma and cryoprecipitate-based methods.[103]

The cryoprecipitate mechanism of fibrin glue involves application of thawed cryoprecipitate to the bleeding surface followed by application of topical thrombin[104–107] plus ionized calcium chloride.[108] Current research in the United States is directed towards autologous or single-donor cryoprecipitate as the source of fibrinogen.[96, 100, 104–109] An autologous source eliminates the threat of viral transmission. Modification of the European methods by centrifugation yields increased concentrations of fibrinogen,[100, 109, 110] as does repeat freeze-thaw recycling with centrifugation.[111] INSTACOOL (Sacramento, CA) has recently developed a heat transfer technology that allows rapid freezing and thawing of cryoprecipitate, achieving an average of 5000 ml/dl of fibrinogen concentrate with 6- to 8-hour-old plasmapheresis plasma within 3 hours. It is anticipated that even higher yields are possible using perioperative plasmapheresis in conjunction with freeze-thaw recycling technology.[112] The chief advantage of this technology is that it is autologous.

Numerous positive reports have indicated that fibrin glue has wide clinical applications in cardiothoracic and vascular surgery.[96, 113–119] With newer technology fibrin glue may achieve wider applicability and acceptance in the United States.

Medications to promote hemostasis and conserve blood loss have received attention in the past few years. Aprotinin, a promising polypeptide serine proteinase inhibitor derived from bovine lung, is widely used in cardiovascular surgery in Europe and Japan. Its mechanism of reducing blood loss is unclear but is suspected to be suppression of the fibrinolytic system, probably by blocking the conversion of plasminogen to plasmin. In recently reported series,[120–123] operative blood loss was reduced by approximately 50 per cent. Anecdotal cases of hypercoagulopathy have led to using aprotinin in conjunction with heparin. Also, because of potential sensitivity problems, the major indication for its use has been in revision cardiac surgery, although Thompson has reported a controlled series of aneurysm resections in which blood loss was significantly reduced.[124] Aprotinin is currently not approved by the FDA in the United States.

Desmopressin (DDAVP) is a synthetic vasopressin analogue that is believed to exert its hemostatic effect by releasing endogenous von Willebrand's factor[125, 126] and increasing platelet aggregation.[127, 128] Salzman and colleagues[129] and Czer and associates[130] reported substantial reduction of blood loss and transfusion requirements in cardiac procedures when DDAVP was used. However, this observation was not substantiated in later studies by Hackmann and colleagues,[131] Hedderich and colleagues,[132] Rocha and colleagues,[133] and Seear and colleagues.[134] Desmopressin has been shown to produce beneficial effects in congenital and acquired hemostatic disorders such as von Willebrand's disease,[135] hemophilia,[135–137] and uremia.[138] Also, DDAVP is effective in the treatment of intrinsic qualitative defects in platelets as well as in those induced by aspirin.[139]

Contribution of AT Technology to Hemostasis. One of the most important considerations in promoting hemostasis is the need to avoid hypothermia, shock, and acidosis and the resultant coagulopathy which necessitates multiple transfusions and blood component therapy (fresh frozen plasma and platelet). When these complications are present, despite adequate volume replacement and massive transfusions, significant bleeding and clotting difficulties persist and result in a high mortality.[78, 140] The underlying pathophysiology is complex and multi-faceted and involves an intricate interplay of tissue hypoperfusion and hypothermia.[141–155] Ideally, these factors may be prevented and must be corrected. Several technologic developments in the past 5 years in AT systems have contributed to progress in this direction. Haemonetics Corporation has developed the Rapid Infusion System (RIS), and Level 1 Technologies has developed a high-efficiency blood warmer. The RIS provides rapid normothermic volume replacement of up to 1500 ml of fluid *per minute*. Clinically, this capability has offered a number of advantages and been led to a decrease in morbidity but has not yet demonstrated a significant reduction in mortality in severely injured patients.[156] In liver transplantations and major vascular surgery, however, there has been a significant reduction in both mortality and morbidity with the use of the RIS.[157]

Applications. The major applications for the RIS are in liver transplantation patients and in those with trauma, burns, and high blood loss situations such as abdominal aortic aneurysms, dissecting thoracoabdominal aortic aneurysms, major orthopedic surgeries, vena cava tumors, and liver resections. The RIS may be used in conjunction with the Cell-Saver and the Plasma-Saver. The technology has been described earlier[43] and is depicted in Figure 23–6.

ARTIFICIAL BLOOD

Artifical blood is the final alternative to HBT considered here. Winslow has nicely summarized its current status in recent review.[44] RBC substitutes must be sterile, free of endotoxin, nontoxic, stable, biologically efficacious and must have optimal colloid osmotic pressure, low viscosity, and minimal immunogenicity. RBC substitutes must have the capability for large-scale commercial production with minimal lot-to-lot variation and must have close to 100 per cent purity. Another important consideration involves the indications for use and the contrast between the requirements for acute and chronic blood loss. In this respect, the two major considerations are colloid osmotic pressure and duration of plasma retention. For acute resuscitation the ideal characteristics are high colloid osmotic pressure but short plasma retention time because blood is soon available for transfusion.[44] For the treatment of chronic refractory anemia the requirements are the reverse. The minimal safe oxygen-carrying capacity is probably 8 gm/dl.[158] Essential

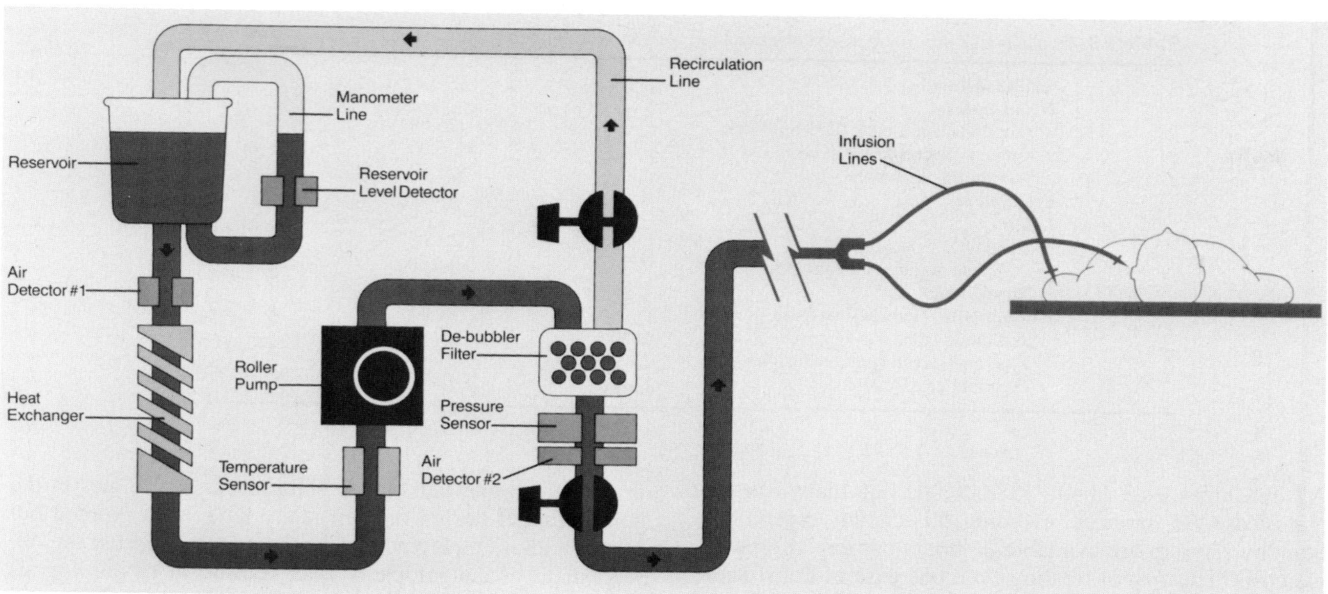

FIGURE 23–6. Rapid infusion system (RIS).

criteria for a red cell substitute are a capability to bind oxygen cooperatively (P_{50} of about 28 mmHg +/−), exhibit a Bohr effect, and transport carbon dioxide.[159]

Perfluorocarbons (PFC) are similar to Teflon, inert, and insoluble in water. The oxygen content of PFC has a linear dependence on Po_2, requiring a very high oxygen tension to transport physiologic amounts of oxygen. This factor, plus a propensity by the reticuloendothelial system to trap PFC, has limited the development of clinically useful PFC blood substitutes.[44] As early as 1966 it was shown that laboratory mice could survive total immersion in PFC solutions.[160] Some investigators have developed water-soluble emulsions that can be mixed with blood,[161] and others have replaced the total blood volume of rats with PFC solutions; with long-term survival in an atmosphere of 90 to 100 per cent oxygen.[162] Newer emulsions, like PerfluoroOctal Bromide (PFOB), have been developed to provide higher concentrations of dissolved oxygen. One new product, Fluosol-DA, a 20 per cent emulsion, has been approved for use during coronary angioplasty to increase myocardial oxygen perfusion with a low-viscosity PFC.[163]

Hemoglobin is an obvious choice for a red cell substitute because of its capacity to carry oxygen and its oncotic property. According to Winslow,[44] the many attempts to harness its potential during the last 70 years have failed because of three major problems. First, the kidney rapidly clears Hgb in dilute solution. Second, dilute Hgb has such an affinity for oxygen that little bound oxygen is released in the tissue capillary beds. Third, even small amounts of cell membrane contaminants can be toxic.

Moss and colleagues reported on DLP-polyhemoglobin, the first modified Hgb to be used in human trials, in 1989.[164] Encapsulated Hgb has been used successfully in exchange transfusions in experiments in animals.[165] Progress in the development of artificial Hgb for humans has been slow because of reticuloendothelial and macrophage reactions, difficulties with sterility, and endotoxin contamination.[44] It is difficult to create a product with 100 per cent purity.

The latest research thrust has been directed toward recombinant Hgb technology. Somatogen Corporation (Boulder, CO) is in the process of developing such a product (rHb 1), which is designed to replace blood lost in surgery. Genetic engineering techniques potentially offer a safe and effective alternative to HBT with no risk of disease transmission and universal compatibility (no blood typing and cross-matching required). Its other advantage over modified Hgb is fewer toxic reactions. Somatogen plans large-scale production of rHb 1 using conventional bacterial expression techniques similar to those used with recombinant human insulin. The ultimate test will be the quality of purification attained. Even a minute fraction of impurity may cause adverse reactions. Realistically, this research product is at least 2 to 3 years from clinical application.

MISCELLANEOUS CONSIDERATIONS AND CONTROVERSIES

The balance between risk and benefit will determine the final choice of options for blood transfusion. Other considerations include cost-effectiveness (in an economy with less room for expanding the health care budget), medicolegal and religious implications, and the ultimate choice between washed and unwashed blood cells for transfusion. Finally, there is the unsettled controversy about the existence of a "salvaged blood syndrome."[166–168] The following sections address these issues.

Cost-Effectiveness. The current costs involved in intraoperative use of AT versus HBT in our medical center are compared in Table 23–5. The AT technique becomes cost-effective at and beyond 2 units of blood transfused.

Table 23–5. Cost Comparison of Autotransfusion Versus Homologous Transfusion

Autotransfusion	
Disposables	
Autotransfusion pack (225 ml bowl)	$100–125.00
Filtered cardiotomy reservoirs	$115.00
Suction line assembly	$23.50
Equipment	$38,000.00
Labor	
Standby	$125.00
Complete autotransfusion	$240.00
After 4 hours	$35.00 per hour
Homologous Transfusion (cost per unit)	
Red blood cells	$110.00
Type and screen (pretransfusion)	$70.00
Type and cross-match	$108.00

AT machines cost about $38,000.00, but many surgical units lease AT services, avoiding this capital expenditure. Standby services are available 24 hours per day at reasonable costs. The cost of treating even one case of transfusion-related AIDS or hepatitis justifies these modest expenses. Many patients now request autotransfusion. It is rapidly becoming a standard of care in certain settings, carrying with it medicolegal implications.

Medicolegal Implications. Many states have passed "informed consent" laws regarding blood transfusion. California's Gann law led the way in the late 1980s. An example of such a consent form is shown in Figure 23–7. A copy is required in each surgical patient's chart. Furthermore, blood banks are now being sued for inadequate screening of contaminated blood in the early and mid-1980s. Screening tests were under development then and even now may miss some instances of potential contamination because of the "window period" in seroconversion. Transfusion is no longer considered a routine procedure in surgery, even though the United States' blood supply is relatively safe, especially when compared to that of Africa.

Washed Versus Unwashed Blood. There is an emerging trend toward washing *all* salvaged blood before reinfusion, with some good reason.[169] Although AT devices that collect unwashed (shed) blood are fast, easy to use, and inexpensive, the end-product contains activated complement[170] and activated clotting factors as well as fibrin degradation products (FDP), which cannot be removed by a microaggregate filter. Only washing the shed blood will remove the FDPs.[171] The question arises, Why have there not been more cases of disseminated intravascular coagulopathy (DIC) after reinfusion of unwashed blood? The answer appears to be dose-related.[172] In this regard, most patients can tolerate up to 2 units of unwashed blood. Some authors have advocated washing *all* blood products prior to reinfusion.[173] This may be the next step in transfusion therapy to avoid coagulopathy.

The "Salvaged Blood Syndrome." Some surgeons perceive AT as exacerbating, aggravating, or causing a coagulopathy. Anecdotal cases of this are not infrequent. Bull and colleagues coined the term salvaged blood syndrome and attributed this effect to retained platelet-leukocyte deposits in the centrifuge bowl that produce a variety of procoagulant and leukotactic substances.[166–168] Flaws in the animal model design of their study have been pointed out by the author.[174] Nevertheless, others have reported the development of coagulopathy after reinfusion of autologous scavenged RBCs.[175] Although various bleeding and clotting disorders of some extent occur in patients undergoing cardiovascular operations, in the author's experience coagulopathy occurs infrequently. Duvall reviewed the author's cardiovascular experience as well as that of the orthopedic, gynecologic, and general surgery-trauma services from 1978 to 1992.[176] In more than 32,000 autotransfusions only 16 documented cases of DIC were found, most in the early years of the Cell-Saver experience. Complex factors played a role in all of these cases: shock, hypothermia, multiple transfusions, cardiopulmonary bypass, or a combination of these. If not properly managed, AT techniques may be implicated in the development of coagulopathy secondary to the *dilutional effect* of removing platelets and clotting factors during the RBC washing. Failure to perform ultrafiltration or wash out all particulate and soluble procoagulants are a further consideration. Inadvertent reinfusion of "residual heparin" with washed RBCs and failure to monitor the patient's ACT as recommended previously may also contribute to a bleeding and clotting diathesis.[78] When platelets and white blood cells are damaged they tend to clump, averaging about 45 μ in size. This is why the author advocates ultrafiltration in the collection reservoir of incoming blood from the operative field with a 25-μ filter screen and use of a 40-μ filter in the outgoing line carrying RBCs salvaged for reinfusion. The benefits of fine-screen filtration were demonstrated in the early 1970s by DeBakey, Reul, and others.[177–178] Renewed interest in ultrafiltration has been reported by Boldt and colleagues.[179] Ultrafiltration plus liberal heparinization plus washing of the RBCs account for the low incidence of coagulopathy encountered in the author's experience. Pulmonary insufficiency adult respiratory distress syndrome caused by reinfusion of microaggregates (platelets and white blood cell clumps, cellular debris, aspirated foreign bodies, hemolyzed cell membranes) can be prevented in most cases.[177] Therefore, fine-screen ultrafiltration is recommended in conjunction with proper cell washing techniques to achieve optimal results.

Autologous Blood—Always Give It Back? Most patients consider only the risks of viral transmission with

TRANSFUSION INFORMATION FORM

(Paul Gann Blood Safety Act, Health & Safety Code #1645)

Patient Name: ____________________________________

I have provided the patient with information concerning the advantages, disadvantages, risks and benefits of autologous blood and of directed and non-directed homologous blood from volunteers. I have also allowed adequate time prior to surgery for the patient to pre-donate his/her own blood for transfusion purposes.

__ The patient has waived allowing adequate time for pre-donation.

I have not provided the patient with the above information for the following reason:

__ 1. There is a life-threatening emergency as follows: ______________

____

__ 2. There are medical contraindications as follows: ______________

____

__ 3. There is a minimal possibility that a blood transfusion may be necessary for this procedure.

Date:________________ Physician's Signature: ________________

FIGURE 23–7. Transfusion information sheet, in compliance with Paul Gann Blood Safety Act.

blood transfusion, which are zero if they receive their own blood. But clerical errors do occur, as does bacterial contamination. The patient may have had an occult infection at the time of donation and during storage bacterial growth and endotoxin production occur. Fatal cases of *Yersinia enterocolitica* infection secondary to septic shock have been reported in patients who received their own predonated blood transfusion.[180] Other hazards exist. Acute intravascular hemolysis has been reported following infusion of inadequately deglycerolized, previously frozen RBCs.[181] AuBuchon has reported that only 50 to 70 per cent of autologous units are reinfused.[182] Although the criteria for transfusion of autologous blood, are not as strict as those for HBT, blood transfusions should *not* be administered without good indication and not just because the patient requests his or her own blood.

Summary

The threat of transfusion-related HIV in the past decade led to a dramatic transformation of transfusion therapy and a search for alternatives to homologous blood transfusions. Technologic advances have resulted that offer practical and safe alternatives and have led to the development of efficient AT devices for salvage of operative blood loss. The patient's own blood is his or her best and safest resource.

References

1. Mattox KL: Blood Replacement in Major Vascular Surgery. *In* Rutherford RB (ed): Vascular Surgery. Philadelphia, WB Saunders, 1984, pp 430–439.
2. Hoff HE, Guillemin R: The first experiments on autotransfusion in France. J Hist Med 18:103, 1963.
3. Hutchin P: History of blood transfusion with a tercentennial look. Surgery 64:685, 1968.
4. Blundell J: Experiments on the transfusion of blood. Med Chir Trans 9:56, 1818.
5. Brainerd D: Cited in Intraoperative autotransfusion. Contemp Surg 3:30, 1973.
6. Highmore W: Overlooked source of blood supply for transfusion in postpartum haemorrhage. Lancet 1:89, 1874.
7. Duncan J: On reinfusion of blood in primary and other amputations. Br Med J 1:192, 1886.
8. Thies HJ: Zur Behandlung der Extrauteringraviditat. Zentralbl Gynaekol 38:1191, 1914.
9. Elmendorf F: Veber Wiederinfusion nach Punktion eines frishen Haemathorax. Münch Med Wochenschr 64:36, 1917.
10. Watson CM, Watson JR: Autotransfusion: Review of American literature with report of two additional cases. Am J Surg 33:232, 1936.
11. Landsteiner K: Zur Kenntniss der Antifermentativen, Lytischen und Agglutinierenden Wirkungen des Blutserums und der Lymphe. Zentralbl Bakt 27:357, 1900.
12. Decastello A, Sturli A: Ueber die Isoagglutinine im Serum gesunder und kranker Menschen. Münch Med Wochenschr 49:1090, 1902.
13. Hektoen L: Iso-agglutination of human corpuscles. JAMA 48:1739, 1907.
14. Ottenberg R, Kaliski DJ: Accidents in transfusion, their prevention by preliminary blood examination. JAMA 61:2138, 1913.
15. Landsteiner K, Wiener AS: An agglutinable factor in human blood recognized by immune sera for Rhesus blood. Proc Soc Exp Biol Med 43:223, 1940.
16. Levine P, Katzin EM: Iso-immunization in pregnancy and the varieties of isoagglutinins observed. Proc Soc Exp Biol Med 45:343, 1940.
17. Gibbon JH: Application of a mechanical heart-lung apparatus to cardiac surgery. Minn Med 37:171, 1954.
18. Glover JL: Panel on present use of blood and blood products. J Trauma 21:1005, 1981.
19. Dyer RH: Intraoperative autotransfusion: A preliminary report and new method. Am J Surg 112:874, 1966.
20. Klebanoff G, Watkins D: A disposable autotransfusion unit. Am J Surg 116:345, 1968.
21. Klebanoff G, Phillips J, Evans W: Use of a disposable autotransfusion unit under varying conditions of contamination. Am J Surg 120:351, 1970.
22. Tawes RL, Sydorak GR, DuVall TB: The plasma collection system: A new concept in autotransfusion. Ann Vasc Surg 3:304, 1989.
23. Kang S: Complications of blood transfusion in surgery. Curr Surg p 48, 1992.
24. Sazama K: Reports of 355 transfusion-associated deaths: 1976–1985. Transfusion 30:583, 1990.
25. National Institutes of Health Consensus Conference: Perioperative red blood cell transfusion. JAMA 260:2700, 1988.
26. Churchill WH: Transfusion reactions. *In* Churchill WH, Kurtz SR (eds): Transfusion Medicine. Boston, Blackwell Scientific Publications, 1988, pp 91–106.
27. Koistinen J: Selective IgA deficiency in blood donors. Vox Sang 29:192, 1975.
28. Anderson KC, Weinstein HJ: Transfusion-associated graft-versus-host disease. N Engl J Med 373:315, 1990.
29. Brunson ME, Alexander JW: Mechanisms of transfusion-induced immunosuppression. Transfusion 30:651, 1990.
30. Tartter PL: Blood transfusion and infectious complications following colorectal cancer surgery. Br J Surg 75:789, 1988.
31. Beeson PB: Jaundice occurring one to four months after transfusion of blood or plasma: Report of seven cases. JAMA 121:1332, 1943.
32. Bove JR: Transfusion-associated hepatitis and AIDS: What is the risk? N Engl J Med 317:242, 1987.
33. Goodnough LT, Shuck JM: Risks, options and informed consent for blood transfusion in elective surgery. Am J Surg 159:603, 1990.
34. Alter MJ, Sampliner RE: Hepatitis C: and miles to go before we sleep. N Engl J Med 321:1538, 1989.
35. Choo QL, Kuo G, Weiner AJ, et al: Isolation of a cDNA clone derived from non-A, non-B viral hepatitis genome. Science 244:359, 1989.
36. Kuo G, Choo QL, Alter HJ, et al: An assay for circulating antibodies to a major etiologic virus of human non-A, non-B hepatitis. Science 244:362, 1989.
37. Alter HJ, Purcell RH, Shih JW, et al: Detection of antibody to hepatitis C virus in prospectively followed recipients with acute and chronic non-A, non-B hepatitis. N Engl J Med 321:1494, 1989.
38. Kreel I, Zaroff LI, Canter JW, et al: A syndrome following total body perfusion. Surg Gynecol Obstet 111:317, 1960.
39. Ranki AM, Valle SL, Krohn M, et al: Long latency precedes overt seroconversion in sexually transmitted human immunodeficiency virus infection. Lancet 2:589, 1987.
40. Alter HJ, Epstein JS, Swenson SG, et al: Prevalence of human immunodeficiency virus type 1 p24 antigen in U.S. blood donors—an assessment of the efficacy of testing in donor screening. N Engl J Med 323:1312, 1990.
41. Cumming PD, Wallace EL, Schoor JB, et al: Exposure of patients to human immunodeficiency virus through the transfusion of blood components that test antibody-negative. N Engl J Med 321:941, 1989.
42. Tawes RL, Scribner RG, DuVall TB, et al: The cell-saver and autotransfusion: An under-utilized resource in vascular surgery. Am J Surg 152:105, 1986.
43. Tawes RL, Duvall TB: The Rapid Infusion System. *In* Braverman M, Tawes RL (eds): Surgical Technology International. London, Century Press, 1991, pp 112–113.
44. Winslow RM: Blood substitutes. *In* Braverman M, Tawes RL (eds): Surgical Technology International. London, Century Press, 1991, pp 97–101.
45. DePalma L, Luban NL: Autologous blood transfusion in pediatrics. Pediatrics 85:125, 1990.
46. The use of autologous blood: The National Blood Resource Education Program Expert Panel. JAMA 263:414, 1990.
47. Dietrich W, Barankay A, Dilthey G, et al: Reduction of blood utili-

zation during myocardial revascularization. J Thorac Cardiovasc Surg 97:213, 1989.
48. Simon TL, Smith KJ: The issues in autologous transfusion. Hum Pathol 20:3, 1989.
49. Axelrod FB, Pepkowitz SH, Goldfinger D: Establishment of a schedule of optimal preoperative collection of autologous blood. Transfusion 29:677, 1989.
50. Pittman RD, Inahara T: Eliminating homologous blood transfusions during abdominal aortic aneurysm repair. Am J Surg 159:522, 1990.
51. Toy PTCY, Strauss RG, Stehling LC, et al: Predeposited autologous blood for elective surgery: A national multicenter study. N Engl J Med 316:517, 1987.
52. Mann M, Sacks HJ, Goldfinger D: Safety of autologous blood donation prior to elective surgery for a variety of potentially "high-risk" patients. Transfusion 23:229, 1983.
53. Silvergleid AJ: Safety and effectiveness of predeposit autologous transfusions in preteen and adolescent children. JAMA 257:3403, 1987.
54. McVay PA, Hoag RW, Hoag MS, et al: Safety and use of autologous blood donation during the third trimester of pregnancy. Am J Obstet Gynecol 160:1479, 1989.
55. Kruskall MS: Controversies in transfusion medicine: The safety and utility of autologous donations by pregnant patients: pro. Transfusion 30:168, 1990.
56. Owings DV, Kruskall MS, Thurer RL, et al: Autologous blood donations prior to elective cardiac surgery: Safety and effect on subsequent blood use. JAMA 262:1963, 1989.
57. Goodnough LT, Rudnick S, Price TH, et al: Increased preoperative collection of autologous blood with recombinant human erythropoietin therapy. N Engl J Med 321:1163, 1989.
58. Graf H, Watzinger U, Ludvik B, et al: Recombinant human erythropoietin as adjuvant treatment for autologous blood donation. Br Med J 300:1627, 1990.
59. Yuasa S: Department of Transfusion Medicine, Juntendo University School of Medicine, Tokyo, personal communication.
60. Cordell RR, Yalon VA, Cigahn-Haskell C, et al: Experience with 11,916 designated donors. Transfusion 26:484, 1986.
61. Bennett SH, Geelhoed GW, Gralnick HR, et al: Effects of autotransfusion on blood elements. Am J Surg 125:257, 1972.
62. Symbal PN: Autotransfusion from hemothorax: Experimental and clinical studies. J Trauma 12:689, 1972.
63. Ansel J, Parrila N, King M, et al: Survival of autotransfused red blood cells recovered from the surgical field during cardiovascular operations. J Thorac Cardiovasc Surg 85:387, 1982.
64. Thorley PJ, Shaw A, Kent P, et al: Dual tracer technique to measure salvaged red cell survival following autotransfusion in aortic surgery. Nucl Med Commun 11:369, 1990.
65. Paravicini D, Wasylewski AH, Rassap J, et al: Red blood cell survival in morphology during and after intraoperative transfusion. Acta Ananesthesiol Belg 35:43, 1984.
66. Orr MD, Blenko J: Autotransfusion of concentrated, selected washed red cells from the surgical field: A biochemical and physiological comparison with homologous cell transfusion. Proceedings of the Blood Conservation Institute, 1978.
67. McCarthy PM, Popovsky MA, Schaff HV, et al: Effect of blood conservation efforts in cardiac operations at the Mayo Clinic. Mayo Clin Proc 63:225, 1988.
68. Tyson GS, Sladen RN, Spainhour V, et al: Blood conservation in cardiac surgery: Preliminary results with an institutional commitment. Ann Surg 209:736, 1989.
69. Tawes RL, Sydorak GR, DuVall TB, et al: Autotransfusion: An overview of a ten-year experience with the cell-saver. *In* Matsumoto A, DeBakey ME, Kondo J (eds): Advances in Cardiovascular Surgery. New York, Elsevier Science Publishers, 1991, pp 383–384.
70. McShane AJ, Power C, Jackson JF, et al: Autotransfusion: Quality of blood prepared with a red cell processing device. Br J Anaesthesiol 59:1035, 1987.
71. Aaron RK, Beazlery RM, Riggle GC: Hematologic integrity after intraoperative allotransfusion. Arch Surg 108:831, 1974.
72. Schaff HV, Hauer JM, Beall WR, et al: Autotransfusion of shed mediastinal blood after cardiac surgery: A prospective study. J Thorac Cardiovasc Surg 75:632, 1978.
73. Mattox KL: Blood replacement in major vascular surgery. *In* Rutherford RB (ed): Vascular Surgery. Philadelphia, WB Saunders, 1984, p 308.
74. Noon GNP, Solis RT, Natelson EA: A simple method of intraoperative autotransfusion. Surg Gynecol Obstet 143:65, 1976.
75. McKenzie FN, Heimbecker RO, Wall W, et al: Intraoperative autotransfusion in elective and emergency vascular surgery. Surgery 83:470, 1978.
76. Orr M: Autotransfusion: The use of washed red cells as an adjunct to component therapy. Surgery 84:728, 1978.
77. Greenberg AG, Hayashi R, Siefert I, et al: Intravascular persistence and oxygen delivery of pyridoxalated, stroma-free hemoglobin during gradations of hypotension. Surgery 86:13, 1979.
78. Tawes RL, Sydorak GR, DuVall TB, et al: Avoiding coagulopathy in vascular surgery. Am J Surg 160:212, 1990.
79. Mattox KL, Guinn GA, Rubio PA, et al: Use of activated coagulation time in the intraoperative heparin reversal for cardiopulmonary surgery. Ann Thorac Surg 19:634, 1975.
80. Schweiger IM, Gallagher CJ, Finlayson DC, et al: Incidence of Cell-Saver contamination during cardiopulmonary bypass. Ann Thorac Surg 48:51, 1989.
81. Glover JL, Braodia TA: Intraoperative autotransfusion. World J Surg 11:60, 1987.
82. Rumisek JD, Waeddle RL: Autotransfusion in penetrating abdominal trauma. *In* Hauer JM, Thurer RL, Dawson RB (eds): Autotransfusion. New York, Elsevier/North-Holland, 1981, pp 105–113.
83. Timberlake GA, McSwain NE Jr: Autotransfusion of blood contaminated by enteric contents: A potentially life-saving measure in the massively hemorrhaging trauma patient? J Trauma 28:855, 1988.
84. Dale RF, Kipling RM, Smith MF, et al: Separation of malignant cells during autotransfusion. Br J Surg 75:581, 1988.
85. Klimber I, Sirois R, Wajsman Z, et al: Intraoperative autotransfusion in urologic oncology. Arch Surg 121:1326, 1986.
86. Brajtbord D, Paulsen AW, Ramsay MA: Potential problems with autotransfusion during hepatic transplantation. Transplant Proc 21:2347, 1989.
87. Cook A, Hanowell LH: Intraoperative autotransfusion for a patient with homozygous sickle cell disease. Anesthesiology 73:177, 1990.
88. Kempczinski RF: Prosthetic vascular grafts: The state of the art in the 90's. *In* Braverman MH, Tawes RL (eds): Surgery Technology International. London, Century Press, 1991, pp 144–445.
89. Tawes RL, DuVall TB: Autotransfusion: Cell-Saver and Plasma-Saver. *In* Braverman MH, Tawes RL (eds): Surgery Technology International. London, Century Press, 1991, pp 110–111.
90. Vertrees RA, Delrossi AJ, Cernaianu AC, et al: The contribution of anticoagulants to platelet dysfunction with extracorporeal circulation. J Thorac Cardiovasc Surg 72:735, 1976.
91. Giordano GF, Rivers SL, Chung GKT, et al: Autologous platelet-rich plasma in cardiac surgery: Effect on intraoperative and postoperative transfusion requirements. Ann Thorac Surg 46:416, 1988.
92. Giordano GF, Giordano GF, Rivers SL, et al: Determinants of homologous blood usage utilizing autologous platelet-rich plasma in cardiac operations. Ann Thorac Surg 47:897, 1989.
93. Jones JW, McCoy TA, Rawitscher RA, et al: Effect of intraoperative plasmapheresis on blood loss and homologous transfusion in cardiac surgery. J Cardiovasc Surg (Torino) (in press).
94. Halden MD, Hultman J: Effect of autotransfused platelet-rich plasma on blood clot formation assessed by thromboelastrography. Thorac Anaesthesiol Univ Hospital S–751, Uppsala, Sweden.
95. Boldt J, vonBorman B, Kling D, et al: Preoperative plasmapheresis in patients undergoing cardiac surgery procedures. Anesthesia 72:282, 1990.
96. Gibble JW, Ness PM: Fibrin glue: The perfect operative sealant? Transfusion 30:741, 1990.
97. Ellis DAF, Pelausa EO: Fibrin glue in facial plastic and reconstructive surgery. J Otolaryngology 17:74, 1988.
98. Matras H: Fibrin seal: The state of the art. J Oral Maxillofac Surg 43:605, 1985.
99. Kram HB, Nathan RC, Mackabee JR, et al: Clinical use of nonautologous fibrin glue. Am Surg 54:570, 1988.
100. Dresdale A, Rose EA, Jeevanandam V, et al: Preparation of fibrin glue from single-donor fresh-frozen plasma. Surgery 97:750, 1985.
101. Weisman RA, Torsiglieri AJ, Schreiber AD, et al: Biochemical characterization of autologous fibrinogen adhesive. Laryngoscope 97:1186, 1987.
102. Matras H, Dinges HP, Lassmann H, et al: [Suture-free interfascicular nerve transplantation in animal experiments]. Wien Med Wochenschr 122:517, 1972.

103. Bove JR: Fibrinogen—is the benefit worth the risk? Transfusion 19:129, 1978.
104. Moront MG, Katz NM, O'Connell J, et al: The use of topical fibrin glue at cannulation sites in neonates. Surg Gynecol Obstet 166:358, 1988.
105. Kennedy JG, Saunders RL: Use of cryoprecipitate coagulum to control tumor-bed bleeding. Case report. Neurosurg 60:1099, 1984.
106. Lupinetti FM, Stoney WS, Alford WC, et al: Cryoprecipitate-topical thrombin glue. Initial experience in patients undergoing cardiac operations. J Thorac Cardiovasc Surg 90:502, 1985.
107. Rousou JA, Engelman RM, Breyer RH: Fibrin glue: An effective hemostatic agent for nonsuturable intraoperative bleeding. Ann Thorac Surg 38:409, 1984.
108. Spotnitz WD, Mintz PD, Avery N, et al: Fibrin glue from stored human plasma. An inexpensive and efficient method for local blood bank preparation. Am Surg 53:460, 1987.
109. Dresdale A, Bowman FO, Malm JR, et al: Hemostatic effectiveness of fibrin glue derived from single-donor fresh frozen plasma. Ann Thorac Surg 40:385, 1985.
110. Moretz WH Jr, Shea JJ Jr, Emmett JR, et al: A simple autologous fibrinogen glue for otologic surgery. Otolaryngol Head Neck Surg 95:122, 1986.
111. Wan HL, Huang ST, Floyd DM, et al: Is the amount of fibrinogen in cryoprecipitate adequate for fibrin glue? Introducing an improved recycled cryoprecipitate method [Abstract]. Transfusion Suppl 29, p 41S, 1989.
112. Oz MC, Jeevanandam V, Smith CR, et al: Autologous fibrin glue from intraoperatively collected platelet-rich plasma. Ann Thorac Surg 53:530, 1992.
113. Wolner E: Fibrin gluing in cardiovascular surgery. Thorac Cardiovasc Surg 30:236, 1982.
114. Siedentop KH, Harris DM, Sanchez B: Autologous fibrin tissue adhesive. Laryngoscope 95:1074, 1985.
115. Silberstein LE, Williams LJ, Hughlet MA, et al: An autologous fibrinogen-based adhesive for use in otologic surgery. Transfusion 28:319, 1988.
116. Gundry SR, Behrendt DM: A quantitative and qualitative comparison of fibrin glue, albumin and blood as agents to pretreat porous vascular grafts. J Surg Res 43:75, 1987.
117. Borst HG, Haverich A, Walterbusch G, et al: Fibrin adhesive: An important hemostatic adjunct in cardiovascular operations. J Thorac Cardiovasc Surg 84:548, 1982.
118. Kram HB, Shoemaker WC, Hino ST, et al: Tracheal repair with fibrin glue. J Thorac Cardiovasc Surg 90:771, 1985.
119. Jessen C, Sharma P: Use of fibrin glue in thoracic surgery. Ann Thorac Surg 39:521, 1985.
120. Korfer R, Minami K, Arusoglu L, et al: Reduction of postoperative blood loss in patients with "re-do" heart transplantation by application of high dose aprotinin. Proceedings of IX Congress of ME DeBakey International Surgery Society, Frankfurt, Germany, June 1992, p 20.
121. Riess H, Neuhaus P: Effects of aprotinin on hemostasis in liver transplantation. Proceedings of IX Congress of ME DeBakey International Surgery Society, Frankfurt, Germany, June 1992, p 37.
122. Ueyama K, Kawasuji M, Sakakibara N, et al: Clinical study about effect of aprotinin on reduction of blood loss during the extracorporeal circulation. Proceedings of IX Congress of ME DeBakey International Surgery Society, Frankfurt, Germany, June 1992, p 43.
123. Vigelius U, Rauch R, Neuhof, et al: Blood saving with aprotinin in open heart surgery. Proceedings of IX Congress of ME DeBakey International Surgery Society, Frankfurt, Germany, June 1992, p 44.
124. Thompson J: Decreased blood loss in aortic aneurysmectomy with aprotinin. Proceedings of IX Congress of ME DeBakey International Surgery Society, Frankfurt, Germany, June 1992.
125. Mannucci PM, Pareti FI, Holmbert L, et al: Studies on the prolonged bleeding time in von Willebrand's disease. J Lab Clin Med 88:662, 1976.
126. De la Fuente B, Kasper CK, Rickles FR, et al: Response of patients with mild and moderate hemophilia A and von Willebrand's disease to treatment with desmopressin. Ann Intern Med 103:6, 1985.
127. Holmberg L, Nilsson IM, Borge L, et al: Platelet aggregation induced by 1-desamino-8-D-arginine vasopressin (DDAVP) in Type IIB von Willebrand's disease. N Engl J Med 309:816, 1982.
128. Manucci PM, Remuzzi G, Pusineri F, et al: Deamino-8-D-arginine vasopressin shortens the bleeding time in uremia. N Engl J Med 308:8, 1983.
129. Salzman EW, Weinstein MJ, Weintraub RM, et al: Treatment with desmopressin acetate to reduce blood loss after cardiac surgery. A double-blind randomized trial. N Engl J Med 314:1402, 1986.
130. Czer LS, Bateman TM, Gray RJ, et al: Treatment of severe platelet dysfunction and hemorrhage after cardiopulmonary bypass: Reduction in blood product usage with desmopressin. J Am Coll Cardiol 9:1139, 1987.
131. Hackmann T, Gascoyne RD, Naiman SC, et al: A trial of desmopressin to reduce blood loss in uncomplicated cardiac surgery. N Engl J Med 321:1437, 1989.
132. Hedderich GS, Petsikas DJ, Cooper BA, et al: Desmopressin acetate in uncomplicated coronary artery bypass surgery: A prospective randomized clinical trial. Can J Surg 33:3336, 1990.
133. Rocha E, Llorens R, Paramo JA, et al: Does desmopressin acetate reduce blood loss after surgery in patients on cardiopulmonary bypass? Circulation 77:1319, 1988.
134. Seear MD, Wadsworth LD, Rogers PC, et al: The effect of desmopressin acetate (DDAVP) on postoperative blood loss after cardiac operations in children. J Thorac Cardiovasc Surg 98:217, 1989.
135. Lupinetti FM, Stoney WS, Alford WC Jr, et al: Cryoprecipitate-topical thrombin glue. Initial experience in patients undergoing cardiac operations. J Thorac Cardiovasc Surg 90:502, 1985.
136. Manucci PM, Ruggeri ZM, Pareti FI, et al: 1-deamino-8-D-arginine vasopressin: A new pharmacological approach to the management of haemophilia and von Willebrand's disease. Lancet 12:869, 1977.
137. Warrier AI, Lusher JM: DDAVP: A useful alternative to blood components in moderate hemophilia A and von Willebrand disease. J Pediatr 102:228, 1983.
138. Manucci PM, Remuzzi G, Pusiner F, et al: DDAVP vasopressin shortens the bleeding time in uremia. N Engl J Med 308:8, 1983.
139. Kobrinsky NL, Israels ED, Gerrard JM, et al: Shortening of bleeding time by 1-deamino-8-D-arginine vasopressin in various bleeding disorders. Lancet 1:1145, 1984.
140. Ferrara A, MacArthur JD, Wright HK, et al: Hypothermia and acidosis worsens coagulopathy in patient requiring massive transfusion. Am J Surg 160:515, 1990.
141. Rutledge R, Sheldon GF, Collins MI: Massive transfusion. Crit Care Clin 2:791, 1986.
142. Collins JAA: Recent developments in the area of massive transfusion. World J Surg 11:75, 1987.
143. Martin DJ, Lucas CE, Ledgerwood AM, et al: Fresh frozen plasma supplement to massive red blood cell transfusion. Ann Surg 202:505, 1985.
144. Harrigan C, Lucas CE, Ledgerwood AM, et al: Serial changes in primary hemostasis after massive transfusion. Surgery 98:836, 1985.
145. Reed RI, Ciaverella D, Heimbach DM, et al: Prophylactic platelet administration during massive transfusion. Ann Surg 203:40, 1986.
146. Counts RB, Haisch C, Simon TI, et al: Hemostasis in massively transfused trauma patients. Ann Surg 190:91, 1979.
147. Phillips TF, Soulier G, Wilson RF: Outcome of massive transfusions exceeding two blood volumes in trauma and emergency surgery. J Trauma 27:903, 1987.
148. Valeri CR, Feingold H, Cassidy G, et al: Hypothermia-induced reversible platelet dysfunction. Ann Surg 205:175, 1987.
149. Flanchbaum I, Trooskin S, Pedersen H: Evaluation of blood-warming devices with the apparent thermal clearance. Ann Emerg Med 18:355, 1989.
150. Boyan CP: Cold or warmed blood for massive transfusions. Ann Surg 190:282, 1964.
151. Luna GK, Maier RV, Pavlin EG, et al: Incidence and effect of hypothermia in seriously injured patients. J Trauma 27:1014, 1987.
152. Jurkovich GJ, Greiser WB, Luterman A, et al: Hypothermia in trauma victims: An ominous predictor of survival. J Trauma 27:1019, 1987.
153. Sori AJ, El-Assuooty A, Rush BF, et al: The effect of temperature on survival in haemorrhagic shock. Am Surg 53:706, 1987.
154. Fried SF, Satiani CT, Zeeb P: Normothermic rapid volume replacement for hypovolemic shock: An in vivo and in vitro study utilising a new technique. J Trauma 26:183, 1986.
155. Satiani B, Fried SJ, Zeeb P, et al: Normothermic rapid volume replacement in traumatic hypovolemia. Arch Surg 122:1044, 1987.
156. Dunham MC, Belzberg H, Lyles R, et al: The rapid infusion system: A superior method for the resuscitation of hypovolemic trauma patients. Maryland Institute Emergency Medicine, 1990.
157. Winter P, Kang YG: Hepatic Transplantation. New York, Praeger, 1986.

158. National Institutes of Health Consensus Conference: Perioperative red cell transfusion JAMA 260:2700, 1988.
159. Winslow RM, Monge CC: Hypoxia, Polycythemia and Chronic Mountain Sickness. Baltimore, Johns Hopkins University Press, 1987.
160. Clark LC, Golan F: Survival of mammals breathing organic liquids equilibrated with oxygen at atmospheric pressure. Science 152:1755, 1966.
161. Sloviter HA, Kamimoto T: Erythrocyte substitutes for perfusion of brain. Nature 216:458, 1967.
162. Geyer RP, Momoe RG, Taylor K: Survival of rats having red cells totally replaced with emulsified fluorocarbon. Fed Proc 27:386, 1968.
163. Rossen JD, Snyder SR, Kerber RE, et al: Coronary perfusion with a modified haemoglobin prevents myocardial dysfunction during coronary occlusion [Abstract]. Midwest AFCR Cardiovasc 4:837, 1987.
164. Moss GS, Gould SA, Rosen AL, et al: Results of the first clinical trial with a polymerised haemoglobin solution. Biomater Artif Cells Artif Organs 17:633, 1989.
165. Hess JR, Fadare SO, Tolentino LSL, et al: The intravascular persistence of cross-linked human haemoglobin. *In* Brewer G (ed): The Red Cell: Seventh Ann Arbor Conference. New York, Alan R. Liss, 1989, pp 351–360.
166. Bull MH, Bull BS, Var Arsdell GS, et al: Clinical implications of procoagulant and leukoattractant formation during intraoperative blood salvage. Arch Surg 123:1073, 1988.
167. Bull BS, Bull MH: Enhancing the safety of intraoperative blood salvage. J Trauma 28:320, 1988.
168. Bull BS, Bull MH: The salvaged blood syndrome: A sequel to mechanochemical activation of platelets and leukocytes? Blood Cells 16(5):223, 1990.
169. McCarthy JC, Turner RH, Renten JJ, et al: The effect of cell washing on the quality of shed blood in major reconstructive surgery [Abstract]. Presented at Orthopaedic Research Society, Washington DC, February 17–20, 1992.
170. Blaylock R: Autotransfusion and orthopedic surgery: An overview and research study. Electromedics Blood Conversation Update 4(2):6, 1990.
171. Bhavnanii JM: A haematological evaluation of the Solcotrans intraoperative blood salvage system. Excerpt from American Society of Hematology Meeting, Boston 1990.
172. Abbott W, Maloney RD, Valeri CR: Symposium: Intraoperative autotransfusion. Contemp Surg 28, 1986.
173. Sieunarine K, Brown MMD, Brennan D, et al: The quality of blood used for transfusion. J Cardiovasc Surg 33:98, 1992.
174. Tawes RL: In discussion of Bull MH, Bull BS, Van Arsdell GS, et al: Clinical implications of procoagulant and leukoattractant formation during intraoperative blood salvage. Arch Surg 123:1077, 1988.
175. Murray DJ, Gress K, Weinstein SL: Coagulopathy after reinfusion of autologous scavenged red blood cells. Anesth Analg 75:125, 1992.
176. Duvall TB: Unpublished data, personal communication.
177. Reul GJ, Greenberg SD, Lefrak EA, et al: Prevention of posttraumatic pulmonary insufficiency with fine screen filtration of blood. Arch Surg 105:386, 1973.
178. Reul GJ, Solis RT, Greenberg SD, et al: Experience with autotransfusion in the surgical management of trauma. Surgery 76:546, 1974.
179. Boldt J, Kling D, Von Bormann B, et al: Blood conservation in cardiac operations. Cell separation versus hemofiltration. J Thorac Cardiovasc Surg 97:832, 1989.
180. Tipple MA, Bland LA, Murphy JJ, et al: Sepsis associated with transfusion of red cells contaminated with *Yersinia enterocolitica*. Transfusion 30:207, 1990.
181. Cregan P, Donegan E, Gotelli G: Hemolytic transfusion reaction following transfusion of frozen and washed autologous red cells. Transfusion 31:172, 1991.
182. AuBuchon JP: Autologous transfusion and directed donations: Current controversies and future directions. Transfusion Med Rev 3:290, 1989.

24

Intraoperative Assessment of Technical Adequacy

Jack L. Cronenwett, M.D., and Daniel B. Walsh, M.D.

• • •

Technical perfection is a requirement of any arterial reconstruction if complications are to be avoided. Although other factors, such as hypercoagulability or inadequate outflow are also important, correctable technical defects cause 15 to 25 per cent of early graft failures.[1, 2] It follows that improved results of arterial surgery require not only precise techniques but also accurate intraoperative assessment of technical adequacy. A variety of modalities are now available for this assessment, which has revealed defects requiring operative correction in 5 to 48 per cent of arterial reconstructions.[3, 4] The choice of these modalities and their application to specific arterial procedures is the subject of this chapter.

TECHNIQUES OF ASSESSMENT

Physical Examination

The most basic methods of assessing technical adequacy are inspection and pulse palpation. The former includes not only examination of a bypass graft itself for kinks, twists, or stenoses but also inspection of a distal extremity for return of color and capillary refill following revascularization. This is facilitated by including the entire extremity in the operative field or by covering the foot with a sterile, clear plastic bag to allow easy visualization. Pulse palpation is the most traditional physiologic method of evaluation of arterial function, but, like inspection, it can be quite subjective. This technique can erroneously indicate poor flow if calcification is present in the distal arteries that reduces transmural pulse palpation. Furthermore, proximal extremity reconstructions do not always result in palpable distal pulses despite their adequacy. More importantly, false-negative results can occur when a graft has a strong pulse, yet no blood flow exits owing to a severe outflow restriction. Because of their low sensitivity for detecting technical defects, pulse palpation and inspection can be used reliably only in conjunction with other, more precise methods.

Blood Flow Measurement

The development of electromagnetic flowmeters stimulated vascular surgeons to measure graft flow directly at the completion of an arterial bypass in an attempt to identify defects. Although this technique provides a numerical, physiologic assessment, it is difficult to interpret because graft flow is influenced not only by potential graft problems but also by variations in inflow and outflow that may result during general or regional anesthesia. Furthermore, small graft defects that are not hemodynamically significant cannot be detected but may cause postoperative thrombosis. Although the finding of very low or absent blood flow reliably identifies a problem, such a finding is rare. Since flow measurement does not localize a potential graft defect without an accompanying anatomic study, it has largely been supplanted by newer assessment modalities. Studies using an ultrasound flowmeter have confirmed the inability of graft flow alone to predict outcome.[5] When combined with pressure measurements and resistance calculations made during pharmacologic hyperemia, this technique becomes more accurate, but it has been used infrequently.

Arteriography

Since its introduction, intraoperative arteriography has been the gold standard for evaluating anatomically the technical adequacy of arterial procedures. It is uniquely capable of assessing the anatomy of outflow arteries, which is important in patients in whom preoperative studies have been inadequate. Although this is an invasive procedure associated with potential complications due to the arterial puncture (intimal injury, dissection), injection (air embolism), radiographic contrast (renal failure, anaphylaxis), or radiation exposure, the actual observed complication rate has been negligible in large series.[3,6,7] The technique varies according to individual application, but involves the insertion of an 18- to 20-gauge plastic angiocatheter into the artery or graft to allow the subsequent injection of 10 to 30 ml of a radiographic contrast agent. Temporary occlusion of the arterial inflow in high-flow settings maximizes the concentration of the contrast agent without the need for an excessively rapid injection. A portable x-ray generator can be used, but in application in the extremity, the use of a permanent overhead generator at a greater height above the operating table allows the entire leg to be filmed in a single exposure using one long cassette (Fig. 24–1).

Arteriography does have several inherent weaknesses. In lower extremity bypass grafts the proximal anastomosis is frequently not evaluated with this technique. Air bubbles or overlying structures may lead to false-positive interpretations. A potential source of false-negative studies is the use of a single plane to analyze a multidimensional artery, which can underestimate stenoses or miss small defects such as intimal flaps or platelet aggregates.[9] To avoid this problem, intraoperative digital subtraction arteriography (DSA) used with a portable C-arm imaging device can more easily obtain views from different angles.[8] Such technology is more expensive but is often available in modern operating rooms because it is used during other procedures as well. This technique also allows the use of smaller amounts of contrast agent and real-time video replay after the injection, which sometimes highlights flow defects better than cut-film arteriograms. It is more applicable to a localized area, such as that associated with carotid endarterectomy, than to an entire extremity. However, an entire leg can be filmed using repeated injections of small amounts of contrast to obtain sequential images.

Doppler Ultrasound

The advent of Doppler ultrasound techniques led to the use of these noninvasive modalities for intraoperative

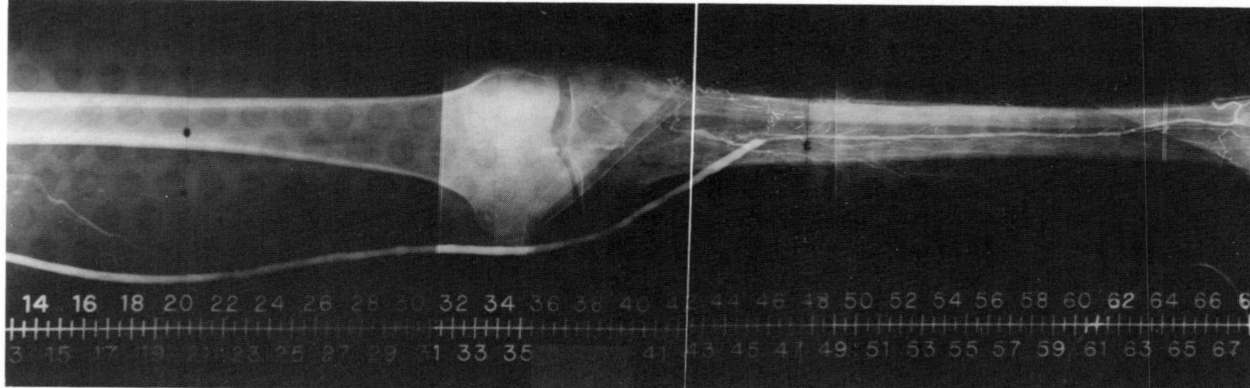

FIGURE 24–1. Normal intraoperative completion arteriogram of a femoral-peroneal in situ saphenous vein graft. A ceiling-mounted x-ray generator allows visualization of nearly the entire leg with a single exposure. A radiopaque ruler facilitates the localization of any graft defects.

assessment of arterial reconstructions. The simplest and least expensive such device is a continuous-wave (CW) Doppler with an 8- to 10-mHz pencil probe. A major advantage of these probes is that they are easily sterilized by gas and thus are readily available for intraoperative use. Furthermore, their small size allows insonation of arteries in areas that are less accessible to larger probes. Using saline as an acoustic coupling, the probe is successively passed along the graft or endarterectomy site, where a localized increase in the audible sound frequency or a turbulent sound indicates a potential defect. Similarly, patent residual vein branches after an in situ saphenous vein graft (ISSVG) can be identified by the presence of a locally increased frequency, diastolic flow, and flow outside the graft boundary. Successively compressing the graft from the proximal to the distal end while listening for residual proximal flow with the Doppler can also localize these arteriovenous fistulas. Unfortunately, use of the audible CW Doppler is quite subjective and operator dependent and requires considerable experience to be used accurately. Although its sensitivity is relatively high, potential false-positive studies make it more useful as a screening method to guide the selective use of a more precise technique. If no flow is detected owing to a major defect or thrombosis, CW Doppler information alone is sufficient to warrant reexploration. This occurs infrequently, however, and sufficient anatomic information is usually not provided to recommend reexploration without a more definitive determination of the severity of the underlying defect.

To increase the objectivity of the CW Doppler, it is possible to use a fast-Fourier transform spectral analysis computer to quantitate changes in frequency or velocity. A further potential refinement is the use of a high-frequency (20 mHz) pulsed Doppler device contained in a small needle probe that allows easy access to all operative sites.[9] Considerable experience with a pulsed-Doppler probe is required to achieve accurate results, however, and the technique fails to provide anatomic images that are reassuring to most surgeons considering arterial reexploration.

B-Mode Ultrasound

To obtain anatomic imaging noninvasively, B-mode ultrasound has been used intraoperatively. Initial experimental studies established the ability of B-mode ultrasound to detect small arteriographic defects and suggested its superiority compared with arteriography.[10] With arterial defects created in dogs, arteriography and B-mode ultrasound were both nearly 100 per cent specific in excluding arterial defects. However, ultrasound had a significantly greater sensitivity in detecting defects (92 per cent overall) compared with a sensitivity of 70 per cent for serial byplane arteriography and only 50 per cent for portable arteriography. These techniques had comparable accuracy in detecting stenoses. Since it does not evaluate blood flow, B-mode ultrasound cannot differentiate fresh thrombus from flowing blood, which has the same echogenicity. In comparison with Doppler pencil probes, B-mode ultrasound probes are larger and cannot be sterilized. Thus, their use is somewhat more cumbersome. They must be used with a sterile covering containing a gel to maintain an appropriate acoustic interface, and more operator experience is required to obtain optimal images. In clinical situations, the greatest problem with this technique is the difficulty of determining the significance of the many small defects that are identified but may not require repair.

Duplex Ultrasound

To add flow-measuring capability to B-mode ultrasound, duplex scanning may also be used intraoperatively (Fig. 24–2). Like B-mode ultrasound, these probes are larger, cannot be sterilized, and require considerable operator skill, not only to obtain an accurate image but also to position the Doppler probe appropriately within the arterial lumen. In this regard, duplex color flow technology provides continuous Doppler signals along the artery at multiple points and is easier to use intraoperatively, albeit more expensive.[11] It is still sometimes difficult to manipulate these larger probe heads into small operative fields to obtain very proximal or distal images. Examination of the outflow arteries is less precise than with arteriography but can be done transcutaneously. Duplex scanning appears to be better than arteriography for identifying defects in a proximal leg anastomosis because the arteriogram is often poorly exposed in this region owing to inadequate penetration or is obtained through a more distally placed catheter, which prevents imaging the proximal anastomosis.[12] Furthermore, duplex scanning can identify low graft velocities that are undetectable by arteriography. Importantly, duplex scanning is unable to assess polytetrafluoroethylene (PTFE) grafts immediately after placement because they contain air that prevents ultrasound penetration.

Angioscopy

Intraoperative angioscopy has become an attractive technique for evaluating bypass grafts and arterial procedures since the introduction of small flexible catheters with high-resolution optical systems. Angioscopy requires irrigation with saline accompanied by inflow and sometimes outflow occlusion to provide a visually clear image. The use of a specifically designed infusion pump with high and low flow rates has greatly facilitated this visualization.[4] Experience is required to manipulate properly the angioscope within a bypass graft to obtain complete visualization. It has been most widely used to inspect ISSVG, to ensure complete valve lysis, and to exclude unligated venous branches (Fig. 24–3). We employ a 1.4-mm diameter angioscope in such grafts, introducing the angioscope through a sheath placed through the most proximal branch of the saphenous vein, which is left unligated for this purpose. Saline irrigation is administered through the sheath. Prior to angioscopy it is useful to identify and ligate as many venous side branches as possible to optimize distal irrigation and visualization. Angioscopy can be used in other sites if blood flow can be temporarily excluded, which sometimes requires the use of balloon occlusion catheters if proximal control is not surgically accessible.

Because angioscopy is an invasive intraluminal procedure it has several possible complications including endo-

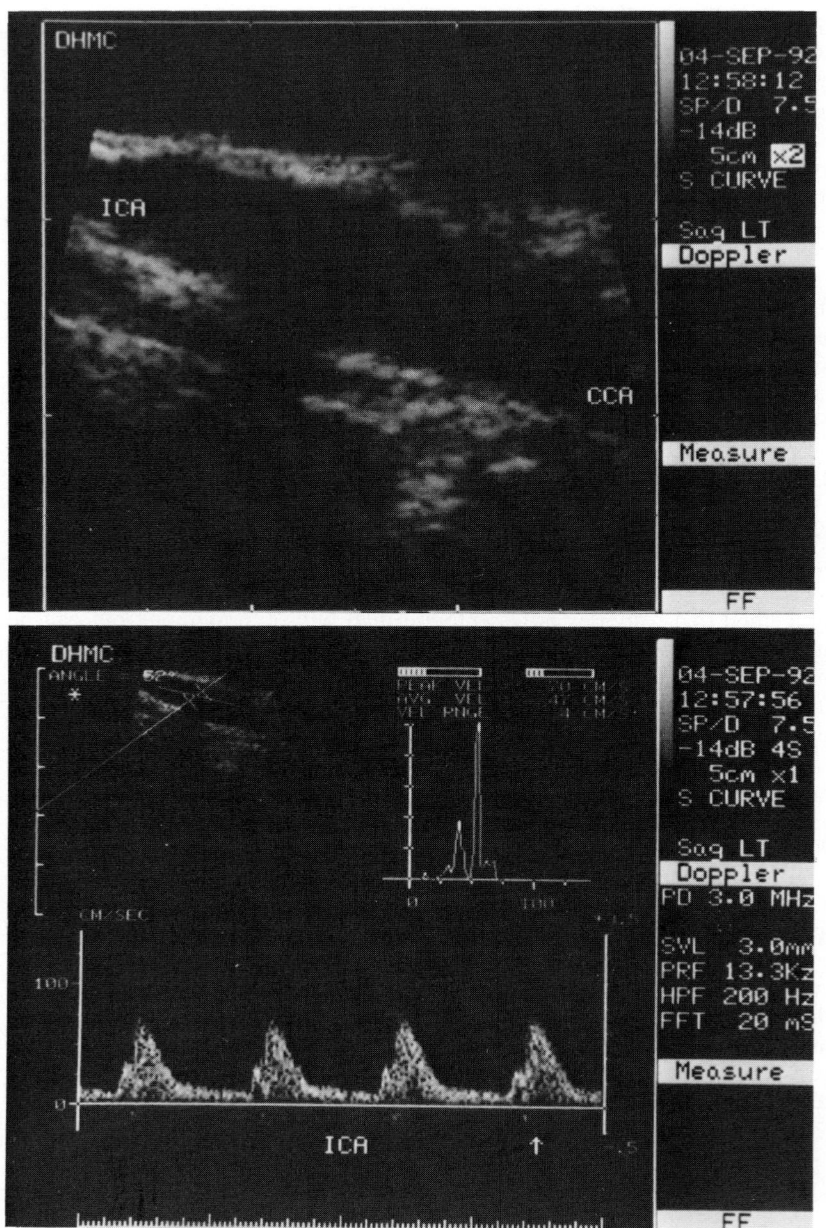

FIGURE 24–2. Normal intraoperative duplex ultrasound scan at the completion of a carotid endarterectomy. *Upper panel* demonstrates the B-mode image of the endarterectomy site. If present, intimal flaps may be seen moving during real-time scanning. *Lower panel* shows pulsed Doppler spectral analysis from the distal endarterectomy, revealing a normal low-velocity waveform without spectral broadening.

thelial injury leading to late hyperplasia, creation of intimal flaps, and fluid overload due to excess irrigation. Experimental studies have documented that mild intimal injury does occur but only after multiple, repeated passages of larger diameter angioscopes.[13] In canine veins, mild endothelial injury after simulated angioscopic trauma heals after 1 month, when normal prostacyclin synthesis is then restored.[14] The long-term effects of this mild trauma are not firmly established, but there do not appear to be late detrimental consequences of clinical angioscopy using few passes of small-diameter (~1.4 mm) angioscopes in human vein grafts. Several studies have shown that the irrigation solution can be limited to 500 ml in most patients, an amount that has not caused complications, especially when planned as part of the overall fluid administration.[4, 15]

Intravascular Ultrasound

The newest potential modality for intraoperative evaluation of arterial procedures is intravascular ultrasound. These devices are based on a flexible, catheter-based system and generate two-dimensional cross-sectional images by circumferential rotation of a miniaturized (10 to 30 mHz) ultrasound crystal at the catheter tip. In experimental studies, this technique has proved to be quite accurate for measuring lumen diameter and for identifying stenoses caused by atherosclerosis or anastomotic hyperplasia.[16] As expected, this ultrasound technique is insensitive for detecting thrombus owing to the equivalent echogenicity of flowing blood. Both intravascular ultrasound and angioscopy were found to be 100 per cent accurate in detecting 2-mm intimal

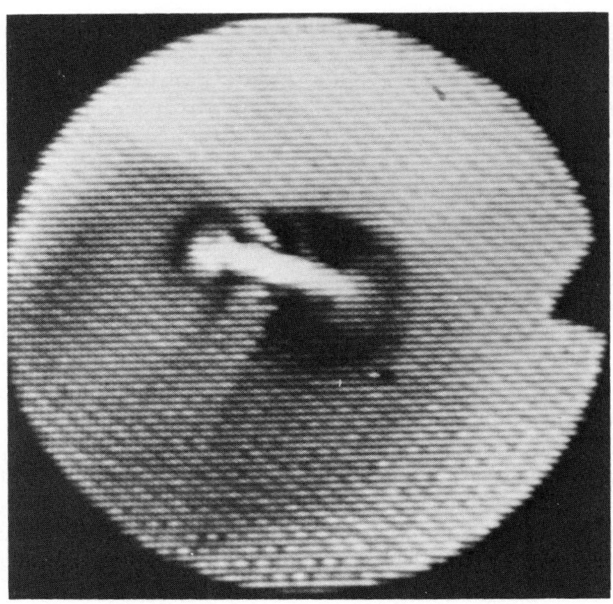

FIGURE 24–3. Angioscopic visualization of a residual valve cusp after completion of an in situ vein graft bypass. Not only can the angioscope identify the valve cusp but also allows direct observation of the subsequent valve lysis as shown here, where a retrograde valvulotome engages the retained cusp.

flaps in canine femoral arteries, compared with only 60 per cent accuracy for single-plane arteriography.[17] Clinical studies of this device are required to establish its efficacy and potential role in comparison with other intraoperative modalities.

Indirect Methods

In addition to the direct methods described above for evaluating arterial reconstructions intraoperatively, it is also possible to evaluate adequate blood flow restoration, especially in the extremities. This is most easily accomplished intraoperatively by using a CW Doppler probe placed over a distal artery, listening for an audible augmentation in waveform after release of a temporary graft occlusion. A more quantitative assessment can be obtained by measuring the distal extremity pressure (e.g., the ankle-brachial index) using a sterile blood pressure cuff intraoperatively. In patients with more proximal reconstruction with residual abnormalities in the outflow arteries, the ankle pressure may not be maximal intraoperatively and may gradually increase postoperatively. Thus, this intraoperative pressure measurement does not have an absolute criterion but must be selectively interpreted based on the preoperative arteriographic anatomy of each patient. Other similar modalities including pulse volume recording, strain-gauge plethysmography, photoplethysmography, or even transcutaneous oxygen tension can be used intraoperatively to evaluate restoration of distal flow, looking for a significant change in magnitude with and without graft occlusion.

Although not a direct method of assessing operative technique, *outflow resistance* has been measured intraoperatively to predict subsequent graft failure in the extremities. This technique calculates outflow resistance based on the pressure measured while injecting saline into the distal end of a bypass graft at a known rate. Ascer and colleagues found that grafts with an outflow resistance of more than 1.2 resistance units (mmHg pressure ÷ ml/min flow) all experienced failure within 30 days.[18] Other groups, however, have not confirmed this observation and have reported long-term patency in grafts with high outflow resistance, especially vein grafts.[19] Like other indirect methods, this technique does not provide anatomic information sufficient to isolate the cause of high outflow resistance and thus requires a subsequent anatomic study of the graft and outflow to identify a potentially correctable problem. In most cases, high outflow resistance is due to severe distal disease and can usually not be improved. In a few cases, this technique may lead to the identification of a distal anastomotic stenosis or the need for extension of a proximal graft to a more distal site for improved outflow.

CLINICAL APPLICATIONS

Cerebrovascular Reconstructions

The efficacy of cerebrovascular surgery for preventing stroke is predicated upon a low operative complication rate. The technical requirements of these procedures, including the most frequently performed procedure, carotid endarterectomy, are demanding. The need for improved technical performance is best assessed by the operative complication rate, which for carotid endarterectomy is indexed by the rate of postoperative stroke, residual stenosis, and late stenosis or stroke. Given that most reports describe postoperative stroke rates of less than 5 per cent, one would expect the detection rate for intraoperative technical defects during carotid endarterectomy to be similarly low. Surprisingly, this has not been the case using both arteriography and ultrasonography. In a collected review of more than 2000 endarterectomies evaluated intraoperatively, an average of 12 per cent were found to have residual defects, with a range of 5 to 43 per cent.[20] Although most defects are found in the external carotid artery (due to the "blind" nature of this portion of the endarterectomy), defects were found in the common and internal carotid artery in 6.5 per cent of these collected cases, usually at the distal end of the endarterectomy. In a similar review of 1500 carotid endarterectomies, the average frequency of residual defects found by postoperative arteriography or noninvasive testing was 5.7 per cent, with the lowest incidence reported in series employing some type of intraoperative evaluation.[20] Since the early and late stroke rate in these patients was considerably less than the rate of technical defects detected, it is clear that not all residual carotid defects will cause symptoms. Nonetheless, it is axiomatic that technical defects should be eliminated if possible, which has led most surgeons to use some form of intraoperative assessment after carotid, vertebral, or subclavian reconstructions. Although there is usually some hesitation to reexplore a completed carotid endarterectomy because of a *possible* technical defect, there is widespread agreement that this step does not increase morbidity.[21, 22] Reluctance to reexplore an artery is more easily overcome if the surgeon has confidence in the method of assessing technical adequacy.

Use of intraoperative *arteriography* has led to carotid reexploration in 2.4 to 26 per cent of reported series.[6] After introducing routine intraoperative carotid arteriography, Courbier and colleagues found a reduction in the rate of stroke from 8.2 to 2 per cent compared with historical controls not undergoing arteriography.[6] Using this approach, these authors found that 5 per cent of patients with carotid endarterectomy required reexploration to correct a significant technical defect. They further noted that intraoperative arteriograms helped to refine their techniques of endarterectomy, progressively reducing the incidence of defects detected. A unique advantage of carotid arteriography compared with other assessment techniques is the capability of obtaining intracranial images if needed to exclude distal problems such as residual thrombus after a carotid occlusion. Using DSA techniques in 50 consecutive patients, Bredenberg and associates found that 12 per cent of their patients with carotid endarterectomy required reexploration to correct defects in the internal carotid artery (end-point stenosis or nonocclusive platelet thrombi).[8] Although the use of DSA may enhance carotid imaging intraoperatively, it has not been objectively compared with conventional arteriography in a prospective study.

CW Doppler ultrasound alone has been used to assess carotid endarterectomy and in experienced hands it appears to be quite sensitive. Seifert and Blackshear detected 4.3 per cent residual defects in 229 carotid endarterectomies by CW Doppler inspection, of which 70 per cent were confirmed by reexploration or arteriography.[23] No false-negative studies were reported. Barnes and coworkers reported the detection of internal carotid artery stenoses in 8 per cent of 125 endarterectomies, although only 30 per cent of these were found to require exploration as judged by subsequent arteriography, since 70 per cent were related only to spasm at the distal clamp site.[20] Thus, CW Doppler appears to be sensitive but not specific enough to justify reexploration without a confirmatory additional study.

Using *pulsed-Doppler spectral analysis*, Bandyk and associates found that 20 (8 per cent) of 250 patients undergoing carotid endarterectomy had severe flow defects using the criterion of a focal velocity increase of more than 150 cm/sec with uniform spectral broadening.[24] Of these, half had a confirmatory arteriogram and were reexplored for end-point stenosis, intimal flaps, or platelet aggregates. The other 10 patients had less than 30 per cent stenosis as shown on intraoperative arteriography and were not reexplored. Two of these latter patients developed postoperative neurologic deficits and were found to have thrombosis due to platelet aggregates. An additional three patients who were not reexplored developed a residual carotid stenosis of more than 50 per cent within 3 months following surgery. This suggested that pulsed-Doppler spectral analysis detected some important residual lesions (especially platelet aggregates) that were missed by arteriography. The authors noted that 10 per cent of their arteriograms were of inadequate quality and concluded that pulsed-Doppler ultrasound was more accurate in their hands.

Flanigan and colleagues used *B-mode ultrasound* to evaluate 155 carotid endarterectomies and found that 19 per cent had a common or internal carotid artery defect, of which most (73 per cent) were intimal flaps, with stenosis being next most frequent.[21] In only 7 per cent of these cases was a decision made to reexplore the endarterectomy, using the criterion of a stenosis of 30 per cent diameter reduction or more or an intimal flap at least 3 mm long. Although this study emphasized the sensitivity of B-mode ultrasound for identifying arterial defects after carotid endarterectomy, it detected a large number of apparently insignificant defects. The same authors addressed these in a subsequent study, which demonstrated that such "lesser" defects did not result in either early or late stroke or residual stenosis after late follow-up using duplex ultrasound.[25] They concluded that "minor" defects (see under "B-Mode Ultrasound") detected by B-mode ultrasound after carotid endarterectomy are benign and do not need reexploration. In a direct comparison using both arteriography and B-mode ultrasound, Dilly and Bernstein found significant defects requiring reexploration in 8.3 per cent of 158 patients undergoing carotid endarterectomy.[22] They noted that both techniques had a false-negative rate of 5 to 8 per cent and that combining the techniques improved accuracy. These authors concluded that the use of intraoperative assessment helped to improve their technique of endarterectomy but that no assessment technique is likely to be perfect.

Using gray-scale *duplex ultrasound* intraoperatively, Schwartz and associates found arterial defects requiring reexploration in 11 per cent of 76 patients undergoing carotid endarterectomy.[26] The authors used Doppler velocity criteria to differentiate significant from trivial intimal flaps that were observed with B-mode imaging, and concluded that this technique represents a major advantage over B-mode ultrasound alone. In their experience using duplex ultrasound to evaluate 131 carotid endarterectomies, Reilly and coworkers found that 11 per cent of arteries required reexploration to correct technical defects, of which 5 per cent involved the external carotid, 5 per cent the internal carotid, and 1 per cent the common carotid.[27] They found it difficult to obtain adequate images in 14 per cent of the arterial segments but noted a positive correlation between the size of the unrepaired intraoperative defects and the severity of later restenosis. These authors agree that minor anatomic defects visualized with B-mode ultrasound but not accompanied by Doppler flow alterations are benign and should not be repaired.

Limited experience using intraoperative *angioscopy* following carotid endarterectomy has been reported.[28] Insufficient patients have been evaluated to reach conclusions, but some defects have been clearly visualized. Unfortunately, this technique has the potential complications of an invasive procedure, and, like B-mode ultrasound, it may provide an anatomic image of small intimal defects without a physiologic demonstration of their significance.

When used routinely, these various methods of intraoperative evaluation of carotid endarterectomy have led to reexploration rates of 4 to 10 per cent in medical centers of excellence and have improved the technical results in most series. The need for intraoperative assessment of technical adequacy clearly depends on each surgeon's complication rate. Given the frequency of this procedure and its high visibility, most surgeons would benefit from one of these techniques. Our practice is to use a CW Doppler probe routinely following carotid endarterectomy and then to employ either duplex ultrasound or intraoperative arteriography if any focally increased frequency is detected along the endarterectomy site. We apply the same technique in vertebral and subclavian reconstructions.

Extremity Revascularization

Although intraoperative assessment techniques can be applied equally well after arterial endarterectomy, thrombectomy, embolectomy, or intraoperative balloon angioplasty, most experience has been acquired with lower extremity bypass grafts. Despite improved overall results, the early failure rate in contemporary series of infrainguinal vein grafts varies from 5 to 10 per cent, often due to correctable graft or anastomotic defects.[1] Since it is difficult to salvage failed extremity vein grafts, efforts to prevent these defects are certainly justified.[2]

Early studies using completion *arteriography* found that the introduction of this technique reduced the early thrombosis rate from 18 to 0 per cent due to its ability to defects in 27 per cent of patients undergoing extremity endarterectomies.[29] Using intraoperative arteriography in more than 1800 arterial reconstructions, Corbier and investigators detected significant technical problems in 4.6 per cent.[3] Similarly, Liebman and colleagues found that intraoperative arteriography identified defects in 5.2 per cent of 250 lower extremity bypass grafts and had a false-positive rate of less than 0.1 per cent.[7] These early reports demonstrate the impact of intraoperative arteriography on the development of better techniques for vascular surgery as well as the evaluation of individual procedures.

To evaluate *pulsed-Doppler spectral analysis*, Schmitt and coworkers assessed 83 lower extremity ISSVG intraoperatively.[30] By measuring the peak systolic velocity (PSV) in the smallest diameter of the distal vein, they found that 93 per cent of patients had a PSV of greater than 40 cm/sec, and there were no postoperative failures in this group. In the 7 per cent of grafts with slower velocities, however, two-thirds failed early or required intraoperative correction of a defect identified with a confirmatory arteriogram. They found this low velocity to be quite specific for a graft luminal defect, a sclerosed vein segment, or a large vein diameter (greater than 5 mm). In previous reports these authors also found that a focal increase in Doppler velocity indicated a potential graft or endarterectomy stenosis.[9] They recorded a 40 per cent incidence of false-positive detection of small, insignificant defects, however, and thus recommend this method as a companion for intraoperative arteriography.

Sigel and associates used real time *B-mode ultrasound* imaging during 165 vascular reconstructions and compared their results with those achieved with intraoperative arteriography.[31] Defects were detected by ultrasound in 29 per cent of the cases, but only 8 per cent were judged significant enough to warrant reexploration. In a subset of patients who underwent simultaneous intraoperative arteriography, the authors determined that the accuracy of ultrasound and arteriography was 96 per cent and 85 per cent, respectively. They concluded that the sensitivity of ultrasound in detecting potential defects is high but that many insignificant abnormalities are also detected that do not require repair. They substantiated this conclusion by noting the lack of subsequent graft failure in patients with small defects that were not corrected. However, B-mode ultrasound still resulted in unnecessary reexplorations in 14 per cent of patients due to false-positive studies. This illustrates the major difficulty with this technique—namely, the selection of defects that are significant enough to warrant reexploration, since many small abnormalities are identified.

In an attempt to define the hemodynamic severity of defects detected by B-mode ultrasound, Cull and colleagues studied 56 lower extremity bypass grafts using *duplex scanning* intraoperatively.[12] They considered a lesion hemodynamically significant if the PSV increased focally by more than 50 per cent or was lower than 45 cm/sec at any point along the graft, excluding increases in PSV immediately beyond the distal anastomosis, where a significant diameter reduction occurs. Duplex scanning identified technical defects in 39 per cent of these grafts, of which half were judged clinically to warrant reexploration. Four of these defects were missed by completion arteriography, and one defect identified by arteriography was missed by duplex scanning. Interestingly, half of the grafts with uncorrected defects that were detected by duplex scanning became occluded within 1 month of surgery, suggesting that these duplex-identified defects were more significant than originally judged on clinical grounds. Unlike B-mode ultrasound used alone, duplex scanning was not overly sensitive because it resulted in only one false-positive study that led to unnecessary graft exploration. The authors concluded that both arteriography and duplex scanning had good sensitivity (88 per cent for both) for identifying graft defects but the combination of both modalities was even more accurate. Thus, they concluded that these techniques are complimentary. Despite the combination of both techniques, however, the authors reported a 9 per cent early graft failure rate, a rate similar to that reported by other authors who have not used duplex scanning to evaluate their grafts. Our own experience (described below) suggests that gray-scale duplex scanning is not sensitive for detecting residual valve cusps in ISSVG grafts. Color flow scanning may be more accurate in this regard and is certainly faster.[11] Further evaluation of these techniques is required before a definitive conclusion can be reached about their general utility.

Considerable experience in the use of *angioscopy* to evaluate lower extremity reconstructions has been reported. Graft defects that require surgical correction, including stenoses, webs and bands resulting from recannalization, intimal flaps, thrombus, anastomotic strictures, and kinks, have been identified in 10 to 20 per cent of these cases.[32–34] The largest experience with angioscopy has been obtained during evaluation of infrainguinal vein grafts, especially the detection of residual valve cusps or unligated vein branches of ISSVG.[4] The incidence of angioscopically detected defects has been significantly higher in these grafts, residual valve cusps being found in 19 to 47 per cent and unligated vein side branches in 37 to 75 per cent.[4, 15, 34] Arm vein grafts seem to be particularly prone to defects of recannalization (webs or bands), which were detected in 74 per cent of these grafts, perhaps due to the trauma of previous venipuncture.[35] Several reports have now compared angioscopy with arteriography in the same patients, and all agree that angioscopy is more sensitive in detecting small defects. Baxter and colleagues found that arteriography was 95 per cent as specific as angioscopy but only 67 per cent as sensitive.[32] They reported a 20 per cent false-positive rate of arteriography related to small filling defects that could not be substantiated, and a 7 per cent false-negative rate for detecting intimal flaps. Stonebridge and associates found that neither CW Doppler or arteriography could identify webs or bands in recannalized arm veins and that introduction of angioscopy reduced the early failure rate of these veins from 11 to 0 per cent.[35] In the largest reported experience with angioscopy used for vein graft inspection, Miller and coworkers found that nearly half of 259 angioscopies led to important surgical decisions.[4] They pointed out the utility of angioscopy for monitoring the correction of defects after they are detected intraoperatively. Furthermore, they noted that even after considerable experience with in situ techniques, 10 per cent of their recent ISSVG grafts had residual valve cusps, which presumably will increase the risk of graft failure. This conclusion has not been firmly established, however, since studies using angioscopy have detected far more defects than studies using arteriography without obvious changes in the rate of early graft failure. Thus, the remaining key question concerning small defects detected only by angioscopy is the extent to which they affect subsequent graft failure, which would determine the appropriate criteria for repairing them intraoperatively. Although the need for repair of all defects detected by angioscopy has not been firmly proved, it is clear that this is the most sensitive modality for detecting such defects.

In an attempt to resolve questions about determining the optimal method of intraoperative ISSVG graft evaluation, we performed a blinded prospective comparison of *arteriography*, *angioscopy*, and *duplex ultrasound* in 20 patients using prospectively defined criteria for defects detected by each modality.[15] Sensitivity in detecting residual unligated vein branches was highest for angioscopy (66 per cent) and arteriography (44 per cent), whereas gray-scale duplex scanning detected only 12 per cent of these vein branches. Angioscopy was significantly more sensitive (100 per cent) than either duplex scanning (11 per cent) or arteriography (22 per cent) in detecting residual valve leaflets. No anastomotic stenoses were confirmed in our study, although six were suggested, yielding a false-positive rate for erroneous detection of stenosis of 20 per cent for arteriography, 10 per cent for duplex ultrasound, and 0 per cent for angioscopy. The time required to complete these studies was 17 to 20 minutes and did not vary among the three modalities. No stenoses, occlusions, or arteriovenous fistulae have been detected in any of these grafts by postoperative duplex surveillance during a 10-month mean follow-up interval. In this study, arteriography or duplex ultrasound used alone would have missed more than 75 per cent of the actual residual valve cusps, which occurred in 30 per cent of these bypass grafts. Based on this experience, we now use angioscopy combined with CW Doppler ultrasound to evaluate our ISSVG.

In addition to bypass grafts or endarterectomy, intraoperative assessment can also yield important information after *arterial embolectomy or thrombectomy.* Although these procedures are often performed without intraoperative assessment of adequacy, we found that completion arteriography detected 87 per cent of complications occurring after balloon catheter usage compared with only 23 per cent of complications that were recognized without arteriography.[36] Since many of these complications led to the need for subsequent operation or even limb loss, some intraoperative technique is needed to identify distal pseudoaneurysms, arteriovenous fistulae, arterial disruption, intimal injury, or inadequate thrombus extraction. Several recent studies have reported the efficacy of intraoperative angioscopy to confirm the adequacy of graft arterial thromboembolectomy by direct inspection to identify residual thrombus. This inspection led to repeat thrombectomy or alterations in the surgical procedure in more than 80 per cent of these cases, and the authors believed that it contributed substantially to the success of the procedure.[37, 38] They also pointed out the usefulness of angioscopy in directing subsequent attempts at thrombus retrieval, including the ability to guide a balloon catheter selectively into tibial branches.

Abdominal Reconstruction

Due to the large size of *aortoiliac reconstructions*, small technical defects causing flow disturbances that affect graft patency are much less frequent than they are in carotid or extremity reconstructions. However, because iliac intimal flaps may occasionally cause immediate or delayed graft limb thrombosis, they require intraoperative assessment. When aortoiliac bypass or endarterectomy has been uneventful, we rely on the palpation of a normal distal iliac or femoral pulse, supplemented with CW Doppler insonation of the anastomoses or endarterectomy end-point, looking for a focal increase in frequency or marked turbulence. If a major defect is found, the site should be immediately explored. In less certain cases, we then employ intraoperative duplex ultrasound. We find that duplex scanning provides more accurate and precise information than arteriography in the abdomen, where the large volume of contrast needed requires a very rapid injection to obtain an adequate study, which is often further limited by the inadequate penetration afforded by portable x-ray generators. In practice, it is infrequent that anything more than pulse palpation plus CW Doppler examination is required in the aortoiliac system, a conclusion supported by the low incidence of postoperative stenoses or thromboses in this region.

For an *aortofemoral graft*, especially if it is extended onto the profunda femoris artery, a more precise determination of technical adequacy is required because the smaller diameter of the femoral arteries is more easily influenced by minor imperfections. Accordingly, we routinely employ CW Doppler in this area, supplementing it with intraoperative duplex ultrasound as required. Good quality intraoperative arteriography is also easier to obtain at this site by injecting the contrast agent into the aortofemoral graft limb using a temporary proximal graft occlusion to maximize contrast concentration in the femoral graft. We do not advocate this procedure routinely but believe that duplex ultrasound or arteriography should be used liberally if any question is raised about an anastomotic stricture by CW Doppler, especially at the profunda femoris anastomosis.

As in the femoral location, *renal and mesenteric* arterial reconstructions also require a careful intraoperative evaluation because small technical defects are more likely to lead to failure. The major difficulty associated with evaluation of these endarterectomies or reconstructions is the anatomic location of the arteries, which are often difficult to approach with anything but a small Doppler probe. We have had difficulty in obtaining optimal arteriograms of these arteries because the reconstruction usually requires examination of an aortic anastomosis, making it difficult to achieve sufficient contrast concentration and good x-ray penetration. Furthermore, intraoperative arteriography for the evaluation of renal artery reconstructions has a major potential disadvantage, in that the majority of these patients have some degree of renal insufficiency that may be exacerbated by concentrated radiographic contrast injection. Accordingly, we rely initially on CW Doppler inspection followed by frequent use of intraoperative duplex scanning.

To assess intraoperative *duplex ultrasound* after renal artery repair, Hansen and colleagues evaluated 57 renal artery reconstructions, including both bypass grafts and thromboendarterectomy.[39] They found defects on B-mode scanning in 23 per cent of these repairs, of which half (11 per cent) were confirmed as major defects by an increase in PSV of 200 cm/sec or greater. This change corresponded to a stenosis with an estimated 60 per cent or greater reduction in diameter. The defects consisted of vein graft anastomotic stenoses and flaps or residual disease in the endarterectomized segment. Postoperatively, duplex and arteriographic evaluation indicated that 98 per cent of their patients without major intraoperative duplex abnormalities had patent arteries that were free of critical stenoses, demonstrating the specificity of duplex assessment. Of the six renal arteries that were revised because of major defects detected on duplex scanning, four remained patent, one became stenotic, and one became occluded. The authors were confident that all the major defects that they explored based on intraoperative duplex evaluation were significant and would have led to the failure of the revascularization, suggesting a low false-positive rate. Renal artery procedures that have only minor B-mode ultrasound defects without Doppler spectral changes do not require revision based on this experience.

In a similar study using intraoperative duplex ultrasound after 83 renal and mesenteric reconstructions, Okuhn and coworkers found minor duplex defects in 31 per cent of their repairs and major defects that required reexploration in 5 per cent based on obviously abnormal Doppler signals.[40] They determined that intraoperative duplex ultrasound had a sensitivity of 85 per cent and a specificity of 75 per cent in the evaluation of these visceral artery repairs. These authors also found arteriography to be suboptimal in this location but reported excellent results using duplex ultrasound assessment.

SUMMARY

A variety of modalities are now available for accurate intraoperative assessment of technical adequacy after arterial reconstructions. Intraoperative arteriography is most widely used and remains an appropriate gold standard. However, angioscopy and Doppler or duplex ultrasound offer significant advantages in specialized cases. In practice, these techniques are complementary rather than competitive. Individual surgeons will choose different modalities for specific procedures depending on their own experience. It is clear, however, that some type of intraoperative assessment of technical adequacy is the current standard for arterial surgery and that it has led to gratifyingly good results.

References

1. Stept LL, Flinn WR, McCarthy WJ III, et al: Technical defects as a cause of early graft failure after femorodistal bypass. Arch Surg 122:599, 1987.
2. Walsh DB, Zwolak RM, McDaniel MD, et al: Intragraft drug infusion as an adjunct to balloon catheter thrombectomy for salvage of thrombosed infragenicular vein grafts: A preliminary report. J Vasc Surg 11:753, 1990.
3. Courbier R, Jausseran JM, Reggi M: Detecting complications of direct arterial surgery. The role of intraoperative arteriography. Arch Surg 112:1115, 1977.
4. Miller A, Stonebridge PA, Jepsen SJ, et al: Continued experience with intraoperative angioscopy for monitoring infrainguinal bypass grafting. Surgery 109:286, 1991.
5. Beard JD, Scott DJA, Skidmore R, et al: Operative assessment of femorodistal bypass grafts using a new Doppler flowmeter. Br J Surg 76:925, 1989.
6. Courbier R, Jausseran JM, Reggi M, et al: Routine intraoperative carotid angiography: Its impact on operative morbidity and carotid restenosis. J Vasc Surg 3:343, 1986.
7. Liebman PR, Menzoian JO, Mannick JA, et al: Intraoperative arteriography in femoropopliteal and femorotibial bypass grafts. Arch Surg 116:1019, 1981.
8. Bredenberg CE, Iannettoni M, Rosenbloom M, et al: Operative angiography by intraarterial digital subtraction angiography: A new technique for quality control of carotid endarterectomy. J Vasc Surg 9:530, 1989.
9. Bandyk DF, Zierler RE, Thiele BL: Detection of technical error during arterial surgery by pulsed Doppler spectral analysis. Arch Surg 119:421, 1984.
10. Coelho JCU, Sigel B, Flanigan DP, et al: An experimental evaluation of arteriography and imaging ultrasonography in detecting arterial defects at operation. J Surg Res 32:130, 1982.
11. Machi J, Sigel B, Roberts A, et al: Operative color Doppler imaging for vascular surgery. J Ultrasound Med 11:65, 1992.
12. Cull DL, Gregory RT, Wheeler JR, et al: Duplex scanning for the intraoperative assessment of infrainguinal arterial reconstruction: A useful tool? Ann Vasc Surg 6:20, 1992.
13. Lee G, Beerline D, Lee MH, et al: Hazards of angioscopic examination: Documentation of damage to the arterial intima. Am Heart J 116:1530, 1988.
14. Hashizume M, Yang Y, Galt S, et al: Intimal response of saphenous vein to intraluminal trauma by simulated angioscopic insertion. J Vasc Surg 5:862, 1987.
15. Gilbertson JJ, Walsh DB, Zwolak RM, et al: A blinded comparison of angiography, angioscopy, and duplex scanning in the intraoperative evaluation of in situ saphenous vein bypass grafts. J Vasc Surg 15:121, 1992.
16. Siegel RJ, Ariani M, Fishbein MC, et al: Histopathologic validation of angioscopy and intravascular ultrasound. Circulation 84:109, 1991.
17. Neville RF Jr, Yasuhara H, Watanabe BI, et al: Endovascular management of arterial intimal defects: An experimental comparison by arteriography, angioscopy, and intravascular ultrasonography. J Vasc Surg 13:496, 1991.
18. Ascer E, Veith FJ, Morin L, et al: Components of outflow resistance and their correlation with graft patency in lower extremity arterial reconstructions. J Vasc Surg 1:817, 1984.
19. Peterkin GA, LaMorte WW, Menzoian JO: Runoff resistance and early graft failure in infrainguinal bypass surgery. Arch Surg 123:1199, 1988.
20. Barnes RW, Nix ML, Nichols BT, et al: Recurrent versus residual carotid stenosis. Incidence detected by Doppler ultrasound. Ann Surg 203:652, 1986.
21. Flanigan DP, Douglas DJ, Machi J, et al: Intraoperative ultrasonic imaging of the carotid artery during carotid endarterectomy. Surgery 100:893, 1986.
22. Dilly RB, Bernstein EF: A comparison of B-mode real-time imaging

and arteriography in the intraoperative assessment of carotid endarterectomy. J Vasc Surg 4:457, 1986.
23. Seifert KB, Blackshear WM Jr: Continuous-wave Doppler in the intraoperative assessment of carotid endarterectomy. J Vasc Surg 2:817, 1985.
24. Bandyk DF, Kaebnick HW, Adams MB, et al: Turbulence occurring after carotid bifurcation endarterectomy: A harbinger of residual and recurrent carotid stenosis. J Vasc Surg 7:261, 1988.
25. Sawchuk AP, Flanigan DP, Machi J, et al: The fate of unrepaired minor technical defects by intraoperative ultrasonography during carotid endarterectomy. J Vasc Surg 9:671, 1989.
26. Schwartz RA, Peterson GJ, Noland KA, et al: Intraoperative duplex scanning after carotid artery reconstruction: A valuable tool. J Vasc Surg 7:620, 1988.
27. Reilly LM, Okuhn SP, Rapp JH, et al: Recurrent carotid stenosis: A consequence of local of systemic factors? The influence of unrepaired technical defects. J Vasc Surg 11:448, 1990.
28. Mehigan JT, Olcott C IV: Video angioscopy as an alternative to intraoperative arteriography. Am J Surg 152:139, 1986.
29. Renwick S, Royle JP, Martin P: Operative angiography after femoropopliteal arterial reconstruction—Its influence on early failure rate. Br J Surg 55:134, 1968.
30. Schmitt DD, Seabrook GR, Bandyk DF, et al: Early patency of *in situ* saphenous vein bypasses as determined by intraoperative velocity waveform analysis. Ann Vasc Surg 4:270, 1990.
31. Sigel B, Coelho JCU, Flanigan DP, et al: Detection of vascular defects during operation by imaging ultrasound. Ann Surg 196:473, 1982.
32. Baxter BT, Rizzo RJ, Flinn WR, et al: A comparative study of intraoperative angioscopy and completion arteriography following femorodistal bypass. Arch Surg 125:997, 1990.
33. White GH, White RA, Kopchok GE, et al: Intraoperative video angioscopy compared with arteriography during peripheral vascular operations. J Vasc Surg 6:488, 1987.
34. Grundfest WS, Litvack F, Glick D, et al: Intraoperative decisions based on angioscopy in peripheral vascular surgery. Circulation 78:I-13, 1988.
35. Stonebridge PA, Miller A, Tsoukas A, et al: Angioscopy of arm vein infrainguinal bypass grafts. Ann Vasc Surg 5:170, 1991.
36. Cronenwett JL, Walsh DB, Garrett HE: Tibial artery pseudoaneurysms: Delayed complication of balloon catheter embolectomy. J Vasc Surg 8:483, 1988.
37. Segalowitz J, Grundfest WS, Treiman RL, et al: Angioscopy for intraoperative management of thromboembolectomy. Arch Surg 125:1357, 1990.
38. White GH, White RA, Kopchok GE et al: Angioscopic thromboembolectomy: Preliminary observations with a recent technique. J Vasc Surg 7:318, 1988.
39. Hansen KJ, O'Neil EA, Reavis SW, et al: Intraoperative duplex sonography during renal artery reconstruction. J Vasc Surg 14:364, 1991.
40. Okuhn SP, Reilly LM, Bennett JB III, et al: Intraoperative assessment of renal and visceral artery reconstruction: The role of duplex scanning and spectral analysis. J Vasc Surg 5:137, 1987.

25

Evaluation of Results, Standard Reporting Practices, and the Computerized Vascular Registry

Darrell N. Jones, Ph.D., and Robert B. Rutherford, M.D.

• • •

The published literature should provide a yardstick against which individual surgical practices can be measured and a common forum for the comparison of different operative approaches. However, owing to a lack of accepted standards in reporting the results of vascular surgical procedures, one could question whether the yardstick is accurate and whether the forum, in fact, provides any commonality to diverse clinical experiences. This consideration begs the larger question of whether the published literature provides a true measure of the vascular surgical experience.

This chapter outlines the potential causes of variance and confusion in reports from the literature. A number of suggested reporting standards that could help to alleviate these problems are offered. Finally, computer-based vascular registries will be discussed on the premise that, once the manner in which we assess our results is standardized, such registries may provide a more accurate overall view of the practice of vascular surgery as well as a means of studying certain problems cooperatively and with significantly large numbers of cases, larger than would be possible in individual or group experiences.

EVALUATION OF RESULTS

When the results of different surgical procedures or different surgical practices are compared, there are a number of potential reasons for the observed differences in surgical outcome. Certainly the most obvious reason and the commonly offered conclusion is that the particular procedure, graft, or some other feature of the therapeutic approach being studied is intrinsically superior. However,

Table 25–1. Factors Affecting Observed Differences in the Results of Surgical Procedures

- Intrinsically superior approach
- Technical differences
  - Superior surgical skills or experience
  - Differing use of adjunctive and adjuvant therapies
- Statistical artifacts and abuses
  - Simple misuse/abuse of statistical testing
  - Artifacts of the life table
- Differences in patient populations
  - Duration of follow-up
  - Patient exclusions
  - Prevalence of disease
  - Associated risk factors
  - Patient selection/indications for surgery
- Differing criteria for success or failure
  - Technical/angiographic success
  - Hemodynamic success
  - Symptomatic/functional success
  - Primary/secondary patency

other factors may play a significant if not the major role in producing the reported differences. The essential problem lies in identifying these other factors and either avoiding them, when possible (as in a prospective trial), or uniformly reporting them to allow their potential influence to be gauged objectively.

Some of these factors have been identified by category and are listed in Table 25–1. They include (1) technical differences (superior surgical skill or experience, use of adjunctive procedures and adjuvant therapies); (2) statistical artifacts and abuses, particularly with respect to life table estimates; (3) differences in patient populations (differences in referral patterns leading to differences in prevalence of disease and associated risk factors, and differences in the indications for surgery producing differences in severity of disease and associated risk factors); and (4) differing criteria for success or failure (patency, symptomatic relief, hemodynamic improvement, extremity function, mortality, amputation rate, etc.). Each of these aspects is illustrated in the following discussion.

Technical Differences

Superior surgical skill or judgment by one group that produces better results than those reported by another group is very difficult to assess. Nevertheless, it is a factor that cannot be dismissed. For example, the controversy over the value of carotid endarterectomy is ultimately a risk:benefit analysis that primarily weighs the mortality and morbidity rates of the procedure against the protection offered against stroke, observed from a comparison of the operated and unoperated patients. However, these success rates vary from institution to institution (and from surgeon to surgeon) to such a degree that the surgical skill of particular surgeons or groups of surgeons must be conceded to be an important factor, one that significantly alters the risk: benefit analysis. Similarly, part of the controversy over the claimed superiority of in situ versus reversed vein graft for femorodistal bypass revolves around significant differences in surgical skill, not only between groups practicing either technique but also between the initial and ultimately acquired skills of the same group.[36, 13]

Factors that are more easily documented include the use of adjunctive procedures or therapeutic adjuvants that might influence outcome. Examples include the use of profundaplasty in association with aortobifemoral bypass performed in the presence of superficial femoral artery occlusion, the routine use of completion arteriography, dextran 40, and antiplatelet drugs, and frequent vascular laboratory surveillance after femorodistal bypass. Such variations may reflect technological advances more than philosophical differences in technique, making it important to consider the time span covered by each study. Exemplary of this are the contrasting results initially reported for extra-anatomic bypass (Table 25–2). Consider, for example, two articles published within 4 years of each other by Eugene and Ray and their respective colleagues.[9, 25] Although there are other reasons for the twofold differences in patency and mortality for both axillo-unifemoral and axillobifemoral bypass (discussed later), it is worth noting that the former series covers a period from 1960 to 1975, whereas the latter series reports on the results of operations performed between 1970 and 1979. Thus, there is only a 5-year overlap between the older 15-year and the more recent 9-year experience. Obviously, significant technical advances can emerge during such a time span; for example, in the former series, there was a demonstrated effect on patency of improving arterial prostheses and only 7 of the study's 92 extra-anatomic bypasses utilized the double velour knitted Dacron graft, which is currently in widespread use and which was exclusively used in the latter series. The same could be said for more recent reports. El Massry and colleagues[44] have reported later results from the same center as Ray and associates.[25] The prosthesis used has *not* significantly changed, although the results have continued to improve. On the other hand, Harris and colleagues[45] have reported very sig-

Table 25–2. Variation in Reported Results for Extra-anatomic Bypass

Procedure	Authors	Operative Mortality (per cent)	Five-year Patency (per cent)
Axillounifemoral	El-Massry et al	5	76*
	Ray et al	3	67
	Hepp et al	5	46
	Ascer et al	5	44*
	LoGerfo et al	8	37
	Chang	NR	33*
	Eugene et al	8	30*
	Rutherford et al	13	19*
Axillobifemoral	El-Massry et al	5	79*
	Ray et al	5	77
	Johnson et al	2	76
	Chang	NR	75*
	LoGerfo et al	8	74
	Hepp et al	5	73
	Rutherford et al	11	62*
	Ascer et al	5	50*
	Eugene et al	8	33*

NR = not reported.
** = Primary patency; all others are secondary patency or not defined.*

nificant improvements in their results with axillofemoral bypass grafting that they credit to the use of a ringed polytetrafluoroethylene (PTFE) prosthesis, and yet there are major differences in case selection, and presumably of technique and postoperative care as well, between their earlier and later experiences. The reported results with extra-anatomic bypass will be referred to again later to illustrate other reasons for reported differences in surgical procedures.

Statistical Artifacts and Abuses

It is likely that a substantial portion of the medical literature contains errors in the use of statistical methods. This portion has been estimated to range from 40 to 60 per cent, based on samples reviewed from American, British, and Canadian medical journals.[11] The more common abuses include multiple comparisons between population stratifications and the reliance on the *t*-test as a universal "test of significance." Although a critique of statistical techniques is beyond the scope of this discussion, the life table analysis or the Kaplan-Meier estimate of survival curves deserves examination. Life table analysis was originally proposed as a means of measuring survival of patients with cancer and the effect of therapeutic intervention on that survival.[42, 43] It has subsequently been adopted by vascular surgeons, among others, to measure other outcome criteria, especially patency. It may well have been an appropriate choice because survival in patients with systemic atherosclerosis is often reduced, and this method accommodates patient losses from death or disappearance from follow-up surveillance.

Because it is now common practice to use the life table method to assess patency, one might assume that two reports employing this method would be comparable. However, a known artifact of this method is the better projected patency rates when a series is "front loaded" with many recent cases. This results in a characteristic leveling off of the declining patency curve near the end, the final plateau representing a relatively small number of grafts remaining patent during the later time periods. Patency projections during the first 2 to 3 years of a bypass graft experience by the life table method are notoriously misleading. For example, Veith and colleagues[35] published a "14-month" comparison of PTFE and autologous saphenous vein (ASV) grafts in "high risk, limb salvage" cases. There were 45 cases of each type of reconstruction. Figure 25–1 shows projected 14-month patencies that are greater for PTFE than ASV though admittedly not statistically significant. The mean follow-up times were also admittedly different, as might have been suspected from the gradually declining curve for ASV and the flat line for PTFE. Furthermore, it was not stated in the text describing this "comparable series of patients" whether the grafts were performed over the same time span, what proportion were below the knee, whether runoff was comparable, or whether the reported patencies were aided by thrombectomy or revision. More will be said later of such considerations.

As DeWeese and Robb have pointed out, the life table method tends to overestimate the actual patency rate, i.e., that measured at the *end* of a given time period.[8] In an

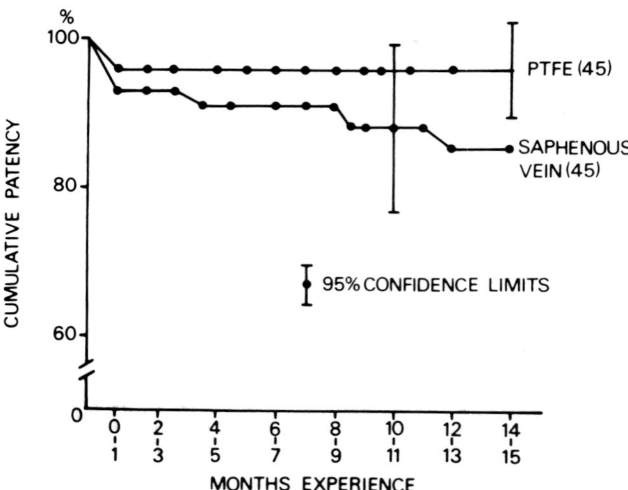

FIGURE 25–1. Life table comparison of projected 14-month patencies for polytetrafluoroethylene (PTFE) and saphenous vein grafts used in the femoropopliteal position. (From Veith FJ, Moss CM, Fell SC, et al: Surg Gynecol Obstet 147:749, 1978. By permission of Surgery Gynecology & Obstetrics.)

analysis of "autogenous venous grafts ten years later," they noted that 58 per cent of their femoropopliteal grafts were "patent at the time of death or last follow-up" (once the most common method of projecting patency). The cumulative patency of the same grafts using the life table method was 45 per cent at 10 years, but the *actual* patency of grafts in patients surviving 10 years or beyond graft occlusion was only 38 per cent.

Conversely, the effect of the declining population at risk over the duration of the study can result in secondary patency rates that are lower than the primary patency rates. This results from simply moving an early failure, which represents a small percentage of the initial population at risk, to a later failure, where it represents a larger percentage of the residual population at risk and thus has a larger effect on the cumulative patency rate. This artifact is a direct result of small populations, limited follow-up, and extrapolation of patency rates beyond what the data will support.

Finally, it is not unusual for comparisons to be made between series of cases with significantly different follow-up. For example, in the previously cited report by Ray and colleagues, 84 axillobifemoral grafts with a mean implant time of 30 months were compared with 105 aortobifemoral grafts with a mean implant time of 44 months.[25] Similarly, comparison was made between axillounifemoral and axillobifemoral grafts based on "mean implant times" of only 20.4 and 9.4 months, respectively, in a study that covered 9 years! The series with the much shorter mean implant times are thus "front loaded" compared with the longer series and have a more rapidly declining population at risk.

The preceding observations are not made to impugn the life table method nor deny the trends it is used to demonstrate but rather to point out how it may suggest differences that are more apparent than real and to emphasize that the technique provides an estimate, not an actual measure. For a more explicit critique of the method, the reader is referred to the classic article by Underwood and Charlesworth.[34]

Differences in Patient Populations

As noted previously, the declining numbers of patients at risk over the duration of a study can have detrimental effects on the accuracy of the patency estimates. In addition to the simple loss of numbers of patients, lack of diligent follow-up also biases the data. In some cases, one is more likely to receive bad news rather than good news, i.e., patients are more likely to come or be referred back when their graft fails than when they continue to be asymptomatic. Periodic surveillance of bypass grafts by noninvasive testing has been demonstrated to detect, and, by allowing timely intervention, prevent impending graft failure.[4] Thus, a reasonable degree of follow-up should be required of published reports, and a poorly followed large series, as indicated by those lost to follow-up in the life table, may not provide as valid an estimate as a well-followed small one.

Patients excluded from a report are often as important, if not more important, as those included in it. For example, it has been common practice for interventional radiologists to exclude from their projected success rates for transluminal angioplasty those patients on whom the procedure was attempted but not successfully completed. Although this technical failure rate is low with proximal dilations, it is much higher with dilations of smaller distal vessels (3 vs. 17.5 per cent, respectively, in the authors' experience).[30] Similarly, some vascular surgeons have eliminated from their patency projections those reconstructions that thrombosed during the immediate postoperative period if patency was not restored and have included as patent those clotted grafts that were successfully reopened. This may represent a significant proportion of cases; for example, the early postoperative thrombosis rate after ''difficult'' distal bypasses may exceed 20 per cent.[28] Also not included in the patency calculations of most bypass series are cases in which the procedure was abandoned because of technical difficulties. This may constitute a significant number of in situ or reverse vein bypasses to tibial or peroneal arteries, being as high as 14 per cent of cases in one early experience with the latter bypass.[26] In two reports concerning axillobifemoral bypasses from the same affiliated institutions and appearing within 4 months of each other,[18, 14] mortality rates of 8 per cent and less than 2 per cent were claimed. There were 10 fewer cases and 1 more year covered by the latter study. The apparent explanation for the fourfold difference in mortality reported from the same institutions is the elimination of ''emergency'' operations from consideration in the second report.

Patient mix is clearly one of the most important contributors to the wide variance in mortality and patency rates between reported series of arterial reconstruction. There may be differences in disease severity and risk factors affecting outcome that reflect intrinsic group differences in disease prevalence, severity, or relative distribution of occlusive lesions. On the other hand, such differences may reflect conscious philosophical differences in indications for operation. For example, patients operated on for the indication of claudication are, as a group, younger; have less coronary, carotid, and visceral artery atherosclerotic involvement; and less frequently have diabetes, multi-level disease, and poor ''runoff'' than patients operated on for ''limb salvage.'' This is apparent from Table 25–3, which compares two reports of 100 consecutive femoropopliteal vein bypasses each, performed for claudication and for limb salvage by vascular surgeons at the University of Pennsylvania.[20, 21] Even within the category of limb salvage, there are better results for those with ischemic rest pain than for those with nonhealing ulcers, and both, in turn, are better than results for those with digital gangrene. Furthermore, the amputation rates are progressively higher in each of these three categories if the bypass graft fails.[31]

Table 25–3. Comparison of 100 Consecutive Femoropopliteal Bypasses Performed for Claudication and for "Limb Salvage"

	Claudication (per cent)	Limb Salvage (per cent)
Risk factors		
Cardiac disease	36	56
Diabetes	22	44
Transient ischemic attack, stroke	5	10
Pulmonary disease	19	29
Outcome		
Operative mortality	0	3
Survival (5-year)	74	60
Limb loss	3	30
Patency (5-year)	69	46

Thus, the indications for surgery, represented in different proportions in different series, can, by associated differences in severity of disease and risk factors, significantly influence outcome. For example, in the San Francisco experience with extra-anatomic bypass reported by Eugene and coworkers and cited previously, only 12 per cent of patients were operated on for claudication.[9] In contrast, in the Seattle series reported by Ray and colleagues, almost two-thirds of patients were claudicators.[25] Similarly, in the San Francisco series, axillofemoral bypass graft was limited, for the most part, to extremely poor risk patients, whereas in the Boston series, axillobifemoral bypass was liberally applied because the authors ''seldom recommended conventional aortoiliac reconstruction in patients over the age of 65, regardless of risk.''[14] Thus, the higher mortality and lower patency rates reported by the San Francisco group are not surprising. However, an even greater contribution to these differences in patency rates was made by the criteria used in their estimation. (see later). Whenever there are major differences in the ratio between claudicators and limb salvage patients, one should also expect differences in survival and patency. In a comparison of recent and earlier experiences with axillofemoral bypass, in which improved results were attributed to changing to an externally supported prosthesis, the proportion of limb salvage cases also changed from 60 to 24 per cent![45]

Differing Criteria for Success or Failure

In some articles, the patency of an arterial bypass or reconstruction is considered to end with its occlusion. Other reports treat as patent any graft that is still open even if this has been achieved by thrombectomy, thrombolysis, transluminal angioplasty, local revision, extension, or a new inflow source. More recently, these differences have been designated primary patency and secondary patency, but only recently have the majority of reports made this distinction clear. For example, the "bottom line" 5-year patency rates quoted in the two contrasting reports on axillobifemoral bypass by Ray and Eugene and their colleagues were 77 per cent and 33 per cent, respectively, but the former is a secondary and the latter a primary patency rate.[25, 9] Johnson and associates, in comparing axillobifemoral with aortobifemoral bypass, noted essentially identical patency rates (76.4 per cent vs. 76.9 per cent),[14] but the former was achieved with a 43 per cent rate of thrombectomy or revision compared with 9 per cent for the latter. It is not possible to tell if any of the 20 successful thrombectomies in the 56 axillobifemoral grafts reported in the companion series by LoGerfo and associates were multiple procedures performed on the same graft, but if they were not (as implied by the term "successful"), the primary 5-year patency rate in this experience from Boston University–affiliated hospitals would not be 76 per cent but would be very close to the 33 per cent patency rate reported by Eugene and coworkers from the San Francisco Veterans Hospital.[9]

Why should we argue opposing points of view which maintain either that a thrombosed graft has clearly failed or that a graft whose patency has been maintained by thrombectomy, dilation, or revision is open and functioning? One reflects the unmodified natural history of the graft or procedure and the other the ultimate utility that can be achieved by the surgeon's close surveillance and persistent efforts. No surgeon likes to report a low patency rate, lest it be considered a personal reflection on his or her ability. Once it becomes more widely appreciated that primary patency mainly reflects the intrinsic merits of the procedure or graft and not the surgeon's skill, and that surgeons need to know about the risks of postoperative occlusion from early graft-surface thrombogenicity and the need to intervene for neointimal fibroplasia to prevent occlusion or to resect a graft aneurysm in a heterograft or homograft, and so forth (all of which are commonly excluded when estimating patency), vascular surgeons will accept the stricter definitions of primary patency and be content to let the secondary patency rate speak for their efforts. But clearly, *both rates should be reported*, as in more recent articles on extra-anatomic bypass by Ascer[1] and Rutherford[46] and their respective colleagues, in which the large differences between primary and secondary patency rates are readily apparent.

Finally, reports on arterial reconstructive surgery are often unclear about the manner in which patency was determined. The acceptance of the lack of return of limb-threatening ischemia, or clinic notes of "palpable pulses" or "patient not bothered by claudication" by a junior resident or other indirect evidence of graft patency are inappropriate. Scientific articles deserve more objective data, and acceptable criteria are recommended later in this discussion.

Some overall clinical measure of success is needed, commonly the combination of continued relief of symptoms or limb salvage. The former would apply to the claudicator, the latter to those with ischemic ulcers and digital gangrene, with both applying to those with ischemic rest pain. Flanigan and associates reported an 81 per cent 5-year "success" rate for femorofemoral bypass grafts, considering failure to be graft thrombosis, amputation, or failure to relieve symptoms.[10] This dual requirement of clinical improvement *and* patency is admirable, to be sure, but it brings out the need for objective patency criteria because both symptomatic relief and credit for avoidance of amputation may be quite subjective, and patency is not usually confirmed arteriographically or by some other direct imaging technique.

The noninvasive vascular laboratory offers objective means of monitoring graft function and supplying confirmatory evidence of both hemodynamic improvement and patency. Because a difference of 0.10 in the ankle-brachial index (ABI) is within the range of observer error, surgeons should demand at least this degree of improvement as evidence of continued graft patency. However, when an aortobifemoral bypass or iliac balloon angioplasty is performed for aortoiliac occlusive disease associated with a significant distal lesion (e.g., superficial femoral artery occlusion), the evaluation of "success" becomes more difficult (Table 25–4). One may have a significantly higher rate of patency, as reflected by persistent elevation of the thigh-brachial index (TBI), than of symptomatic relief, which correlates better with the ABI. Those who require both symptomatic relief and an elevation of the ABI as criteria for success following intervention for aortoiliac occlusive disease, rather than elevation of the TBI, may have contributed to the impression that percutaneous transluminal angioplasty (PTA) for iliac stenoses is not very effective or durable.[15] In contrast are reports in which technical failures are eliminated and an increased TBI is accepted as the ultimate criterion of continued success regardless of the ABI and the patient's symptoms. Using data from a personal experience with PTA, the authors found that, depending on the criteria chosen, the projected 3-year success rate for iliac dilations varied between 52 and 86 per cent, and similarly, with distal dilations, a rate of success as high as 63 per cent or as low as 27 per cent could be claimed.[30]

In fairness, the same can be said for reported experiences with surgical attacks on aortoiliac disease, namely that the patency rates do not reflect the degree of hemodynamic improvement or symptomatic relief attained. In a review of 265 aortobifemoral graft limbs in which the initial patency rate was 97.7 per cent and the late patency rate 88 per cent, the authors found that in spite of excellent patency, 7.3 per cent of grafts failed to have improved inflow (TBI increase less than 0.10) because the iliac dis-

Table 25–4. Comparison of "Success" Rate of Iliac Dilations as Judged by Different Criteria (per cent)

Criterion	All Cases (n = 66)	Initial Successes Only
Thigh-brachial index increased >0.10	84	89
As above, but sustained	74	79
Ankle-brachial index increased >0.10	64	68
As above, but sustained	54	58
As above, plus symptomatic improvement	52	54

ease on the better side was not very significant in the first place (preoperative TBI greater than 0.95), and 9.4 per cent failed to improve the ABI because of the severity of distal occlusive disease.[29]

In the past, carotid reconstructions have been judged almost exclusively on the basis of continued symptomatic relief; thus, silent restenosis has not until recently been reported. The vascular laboratory and, particularly, the use of duplex scanning have changed surgeons' perspective of progression of disease and restenosis of carotid endarterectomies.[39, 22]

It should be clear from the preceding discussion that although the reader may wish to carry away a simple "bottom line" result, such as a mortality and a patency rate, there are a number of other different but valid measures of success or failure, all adding to the overall perspective. These include primary and secondary patency; technical failure and hemodynamic failure; postoperative mortality and late survival rates; permanent procedure-related morbidity; and some overall gauge of clinical outcome, i.e., symptomatic relief or "limb salvage."

RECOMMENDED STANDARD REPORTING PRACTICES

Because of the problems outlined previously, the Society for Vascular Surgery (SVS) and the North American Chapter of the International Society for Cardiovascular Surgery (ISCVS) appointed an ad hoc committee on "reporting standards," currently chaired by the senior author. Subcommittees have been appointed to recommend reporting standards for lower extremity ischemia,[27] cerebrovascular disease,[2] venous disease,[24] aneurysms,[40] mesenteric and renovascular disease, and noninvasive testing.[41] The first of five subcommittees have reported recommendations that have been published. These reports have several suggestions in common. They define essential terms and make recommendations regarding clinical classification; criteria for improvement, deterioration, and failure; a grading system for risk factors; a categorization of operations; and the complications encountered with grades for severity and/or outcome. *Some* of the recommendations that are most pertinent to the problems discussed previously are summarized here.

Estimating Patency Rates

The life table (LT) method for survival (patency) estimation is the type of analysis recommended by the SVS/ISCVS ad hoc committee for estimating patency rates,[17] but the Kaplan-Meier method also deserves consideration. Both methods require clear criteria for withdrawal and failure. The point of "lost to follow-up" or "dead with patent revascularization" occurs at the last *objective* evaluation. The committee recommends that patients whose grafts have failed since their last evaluation be treated as having failure dates halfway between the two examination points. This latter criterion is consistent with LT methods, although it does not define the LT method.

The LT method has two characteristic features worth noting here. The first is that events on the survival curve, e.g., graft failures, are grouped into intervals. Survival rates are then calculated for each of these intervals and used to generate cumulative patencies that describe the survival curve. The second important feature is the assumption that any withdrawals during an interval occur at the midpoint of the interval. It is this assumption that leads to the characteristic correction to the calculated failure rate in a given interval:

$$R = \frac{F}{N - w/2}$$

where F is the number of failures, N is the number at risk at the beginning of the interval, and w is the number withdrawn during the interval. This reduces the number at risk by half of the withdrawals and is *equivalent* to increasing the interval failure rate by the number of expected failures in the withdrawal group (L):

$$R = \frac{F}{N} + \frac{R^* \, w/2}{N}$$

Somewhat hidden in the mathematics is the further consequence that the failure rate is assumed to be uniform over the interval. With this perspective, the use of the stair-step graphic presentation of the LT survival curve, as recommended by the SVS/ISCVS ad hoc committee, is inappropriate. The LT graph (but not the Kaplan-Meier graph) is better represented by straight line connections between the patency estimates located at the *end* of each interval. In this presentation the only intervals with level lines are those with no failures.

There has been mild controversy over the "classic" vs. the "traditional" approach in calculating the LT.[52] The classic method assigns the cumulative patency calculated in an interval to the subsequent interval. The traditional method assigns the cumulative patency to the same interval. This should not be an issue and results primarily from the confusion fostered by using the stair-step graphic presentation. The cumulative patency is the resulting conditional probability at the *end* of the interval based on the failure rate over the entire interval. In this regard the classic method[42, 43] is correct.

The Kaplan-Meier (KM) survival estimate, which is also called the product-limit method, is different from the LT estimate in that data are *not* grouped into intervals. Events on the survival curve occur only at individual failure points. One can conceptualize the KM method as an LT method with intervals containing a single observation and the intervals being very small. Consequently, no corrections are needed for the effect of withdrawals. In contrast to the LT method, graphic presentation of the KM survival curve *should* use the stair-step method because, between events on the KM curve, nothing is known or assumed about the failure rate.

The LT method is a technique that makes calculations easier for large amounts of data, and this may be the main justification for using it rather than the KM method. Indeed, the LT method is not valid for numbers of less than 30, whereas the KM method remains appropriate for any data size.[53] Either method is acceptable if used properly and documented.

Complete life table data should be submitted with each report, even though it may be the choice of the editor to print only the graph. Numbers for the patients at risk at the start of each interval (periodically for the KM) or the standard error for each estimate of patency must be displayed. When the standard error of the patency estimate exceeds 10 per cent, the curve should not be drawn or should be represented by a dotted line or some other means of indicating lack of reliability of the estimate. Comparisons of patency curves should be performed using the log-rank test of significance.[17]

Associated Risk Factors

Standardized grading codes for several factors that modify the outcome of procedures performed for arteriosclerotic occlusive disease have been developed and previously published.[27] These factors include diabetes; tobacco use; hypertension; hyperlipidemia; and cardiac, renal, and pulmonary status. In every case, although specific and detailed guidelines have been identified, the severity code can be reduced to four simple levels: 0 = absent, 1 = mild, 2 = moderate, and 3 = severe. Similar severity coding and risk factors have been developed for acute lower extremity deep vein thrombosis.[24] The detailed analysis of risk factors may not be appropriate for all or even most reports, but it is recommended for any report claiming that such factors do, or do not, affect outcome.

Reporting Deaths and Complications

Both early and late mortality rates following revascularization procedures should routinely be reported. The latter may be included as an additional column in the life table entitled "cumulative mortality." Late deaths should be categorized as due to the underlying disease (e.g., atherosclerosis), to delayed complications of surgical management, or to unrelated factors. In certain peripheral vascular procedures, it may be valuable to include "systemic/remote" and "local nonvascular" complications, as well as "local vascular" complications, categorizing them as to type and grading them as to severity and outcome.[27] These are discussed in more detail in Section VI, particularly Chapter 30. In addition, the senior author has published an article on the reporting of complications in vascular surgery that includes a grading of disability, a complications severity grading, and, to allow comparison between groups or others' experiences, a complications severity score.[47] The comparable reporting practice in cerebrovascular procedures involves reporting stroke-related and non-stroke-related deaths separately as well as separating neurologic morbidity due to stroke from that due to cranial nerve injury. For many clinical trials, a stroke severity scale is recommended.[2]

Lower Extremity Arterial Disease

Clinical Classification

The categories, or clinical classifications, recommended for stratifying limbs with *chronic* ischemia are outlined in Table 25–5. The asymptomatic category (grade 0/category 0) and a breakdown of claudicators (grade I) into three categories (1 to 3) according to duration of treadmill exercise *and* the degree of ankle pressure drop it produces are included to gauge degrees of improvement. These categories are primarily intended for clinical research; for most clinical practices, the classic grades I to III are adequate.

An ankle pressure of 40 mmHg or a toe pressure of 30 mmHg, as an objective criterion of diffuse pedal ischemia, is required to place the patient in category 4 (grade II)—ischemic rest pain. Because healing requires an additional inflammatory response, these levels are *increased* to 60 mmHg ankle pressure and 40 mmHg toe pressure in the presence of infection, nonhealing ulceration, loss of tissue, or gangrene (category 5, grade III). The term "foot salvage" applies only to cases fulfilling both the clinical and the noninvasive testing criteria for categories 4 and 5. Absence of rest pain and no amputation or at most a minor amputation qualify for the designation "limb/foot salvage." Neither a Symes amputation nor amputation at a below-knee rather than an (anticipated) above-knee level qualifies for inclusion. Cases of atheroembolism, or the

Table 25–5. Clinical Categories of Chronic Limb Ischemia

Grade	Category	Clinical Description	Objective Criteria
0	0	Asymptomatic: no hemodynamically significant occlusive disease	Normal treadmill/stress test
I	1	Mild claudication	Completes treadmill exercise,* AP after exercise >50 mmHg, but 25 mmHg less than BP
	2	Moderate claudication	Between categories 1 and 3
	3	Severe claudication	Cannot complete treadmill exercise, and AP after exercise <50 mmHg
II	4	Ischemic rest pain	Resting AP <40 mmHg, flat or barely pulsatile ankle or metatarsal PVR; TP <30 mmHg
III	5	Minor tissue loss: nonhealing ulcer, focal gangrene with diffuse pedal ischemia	Resting AP <60 mmHg, ankle or metatarsal PVR flat or barely pulsatile; TP <40 mmHg
	6	Major tissue loss: extending above TM level, functional foot no longer salvageable	Same as category 5

Key: *AP = ankle pressure; BP = brachial pressure; PVR = pulse volume recording; TP = toe pressure; TN = transmetatarsal.*
**Five minutes at 2 mph on a 12 per cent incline.*

''blue toe syndrome,'' should ordinarily be considered separately. They should *not* be included in the ''threatened'' or ''limb salvage'' categories without objective evidence of diffuse forefoot ischemia. Many of these issues have been dealt with recently in a consensus article on chronic critical ischemia.[48]

Outcome Criteria

The following criteria are recommended for gauging change in limb status:

+3 *Markedly improved*: asymptomatic with ABI increased to normal limits (> 0.95).
+2 *Moderately improved*: still symptomatic but at least single category* improvement; ABI increase greater than 0.10, but not normalized.
+1 *Minimally improved*: greater than 0.10 increase in ABI but either no categorical improvement or an upward categorical shift without an increase in ABI of greater than 0.10.
0 *No change*: no categorical shift and less than 0.10 change in ABI.
−1 *Mildly worse*: no categorical worsening but either ABI decreased more than 0.10 or a downward categorical shift with an ABI decrease of less than 0.10.
−2 *Moderately worse*: one category worse or *unexpected* minor amputation (skin intact, preoperatively).
−3 *Markedly worse*: more than one category worse or *unexpected* major amputation.

Criteria for Patency

Articles in scientific journals should not accept patency rates that are not based on objective findings; ''no evidence of occlusion'' cannot be equated with patency for reporting purposes, nor can ''palpable pulses'' recorded from a clinic visit, considering the inaccuracy of pulse palpation by *relatively* inexperienced health care professionals. A bypass graft or otherwise reconstructed arterial segment may be considered patent when any of the following criteria are met:

1. Demonstrably patent by conventional arteriography or other established imaging techniques (e.g., digital subtraction arteriography, duplex ultrasound, contrast-enhanced CT scan, magnetic resonance imaging, or radionuclide study).
2. Maintenance of the achieved improvement in the appropriate segmental pressure index, which, if not normalized, must be at least 0.10 above the preoperative index and no more than 0.10 less than the maximum postoperative index. (The former without the latter qualifies as deterioration rather than failure.)
3. Maintenance of a plethysmographic tracing distal to the reconstruction that is significantly greater in magnitude than the preoperative value, e.g., +5 mm or +50 per cent for PVR. This criterion is acceptable *only* when segmental limb pressures *cannot* be accurately measured, as in many diabetics.
4. The presence of a palpable pulse or the recording of a biphasic or triphasic Doppler waveform at two points directly over a superficially placed graft.
5. Direct observation of patency at operation or postmortem examination.

Manner of Reporting Patency Status. A graft is considered to have *primary patency* if it has had uninterrupted patency with either no procedures performed on it or a procedure (such as transluminal dilation or distal extension from the graft) to *deal with disease progression in the adjacent native vessel.* Dilations or minor revisions performed for anastomotic or graft stenoses, graft dilations, or other structural defects *before occlusion* do not constitute exceptions in defining primary patency because they are intended to prevent eventual graft failure. Because the outcome of such interventions to preserve patency of the ''failing'' graft is markedly different from the outcome of interventions used to restore patency to a thrombosed graft, an *assisted* primary patency rate may be quoted as long as the pure primary patency rate is also noted. If graft patency is restored *after occlusion* by thrombectomy or thrombolysis, or if problems with the graft itself or one of its anastomoses require transluminal angioplasty revision or reconstruction, it must then be listed under *secondary patency*. However, a ''redo'' operation, specifically one that does not preserve flow through most of the original graft and at least one of its anastomoses, does *not* contribute to secondary patency.

*Refers to categories in Table 25–5.

Cerebrovascular Disease

Clinical Classification

A scheme for clinical classification of cerebrovascular disease is presented in Table 25–6. This system is called CHAT, based on categories of *Clinical* status, *History*, the responsible *Arterial* lesion, and the pathologic status of the *Target* organ, i.e., the brain or eye.

The clinical portion of the system includes both current clinical status and past clinical status or history (C and H). The cutoff between current and past has been selected to be 1 year. The primary clinical categories are as follows: (0) asymptomatic; (1) brief stroke: full recovery in less than 24 hours (internationally more acceptable than transient ischemic attack [TIA]); (2) temporary stroke: full recovery in 24 hours to 1 month (often called resolving ischemic neurologic deficit [RIND]); and (3) permanent stroke: symptoms/signs lasting longer than 1 month. In addition to these primary clinical categories, the category of (4) nonspecific dysfunction allows identification of patients who do not fit into the precise classifications, a regrettable but necessary concession to the realities of clinical medicine. Finally, in the current clinical presentation, a category of (5) changing stroke (formerly stroke-in-evolution) is allowed for those patients in whom therapeutic intervention is applied before the outcome of their current episode is known. In each of the primary clinical classifications 1 to 3, an additional coding can be used to identify the vascular territory involved: carotid-ocular, carotid-hemispheric, ver-

Table 25–6. Clinical Classification Scheme for Cerebrovascular Disease (CHAT)

C: Current Clinical Presentation (< 1 yr)	H: Past History	A: Artery	T: Target Organ (Brain)
		Territory	
0. *Asymptomatic* 1. *Brief* (stroke (<24 hr) a. Carotid-ocular b. Carotid-cortical c. Vertebrobasilar d. Other focal e. Diffuse	0. *Asymptomatic* 1. *Brief* stroke (< 24 hr) a. Carotid-ocular b. Carotid-cortical c. Vertebrobasilar d. Other focal e. Diffuse	0. No lesion 1. Appropriate lesion for symptom 2. Lesion only in other vascular territory 3. Combination 1 + 2	0. No lesion 1. Appropriate lesion for symptom 2. Lesion only in other vascular territory 3. Combination 1 + 2
		Pathology	
2. *Temporary* stroke with full recovery (24 hr–1 month); a, b, c, d, e, same as # 1 3. *Permanent* stroke (> 1 month); a, b, c, d, e, same as # 1 4. *Nonspecific* dysfunction 5. *Changing* stroke a. Improving b. Stable or fluctuating c. Deteriorating	2. *Temporary* stroke with full recovery (24 hr–1 month); a, b, c, d, e, same as # 1 3. *Permanent* stroke (> 1 month); a, b, c, d, e, same as # 1 4. *Nonspecific* dysfunction	a. Arteriosclerotic plaque c. Cardiogenic (embolic) d. Dissection (spontaneous) e. Aneurysm f. Fibromuscular dysplasia r. Arteritis t. Trauma o. Other	h. Hemorrhage i. Infarct l. Lacuna m. Arteriovenous malformation n. Neoplasm o. Other

tebrobasilar, other focal, or diffuse. For the changing stroke category, additional coding identifies the nature of the stroke-in-evolution as improving, fluctuating, or deteriorating. After 1 month, a ‘‘changing stroke’’ with residual neurologic signs/symptoms must be reclassified as a ‘‘permanent stroke.’’

The artery and brain (target) involvement is coded simply by whether or not identifiable lesions are associated with the appropriate territory to match symptoms, i.e., 0 = no lesion, 1 = appropriate lesion, 2 = lesion in other vascular territory, and 3 = combination of 1 and 2. Subcoding allows identification of the pathology such as arteriosclerosis or fibromuscular dysplasia (etc.) for the artery and hemorrhage or infarct (etc.) for the brain (or eye) (see Table 25–6).

Diagnostic and Clinical Criteria

The severity of the residual neurologic deficit can be simply classified as either minor or major, depending on whether or not independence is maintained. For more detailed classification, the stroke severity scale in Table 25–7 is recommended. This is a graded scale of 1 to 11 depending on the impairment in any one or more of five domains, i.e., swallowing, self-care, ambulation, communication, and comprehension. This more detailed classification allows risk-benefit assessments of carotid endarterectomy and the outcome of intervention for stroke.

Contrast arteriography remains the gold standard for definition of the severity of arterial lesions. Classification of lesions is based primarily on the per cent diameter reduction *measured* from the view showing the greatest luminal reduction and using the normal outflow vessel as the comparison (e.g., the internal carotid artery beyond the upper extent of disease). The physiologic arguments for using cross-sectional area or residual lumen are valid, but those measures cannot be used as standards as long as current arteriographic methods are widely used. The suggested classification of lesions uses four divisions of stenosis ranges: 0 to 19 per cent = normal, 20 to 59 per cent = mild, 60 to 79 per cent = moderate, 80 to 99 per cent = severe, plus 100 per cent = occluded. A second aspect of categorization of lesions is the description of the surface irregularity and ulceration. Here, the recommendation is as follows: 0 = normal, smooth surface; 1 = small ulcer less than 2 mm deep by 5 mm long; 2 = moderate ulcer;

Table 25–7. Neurologic Event Severity Scale

Severity Grade	Impairment*	Neurologic Symptoms	Neurologic Signs
1	None	Present	Absent
2	None	Absent	Present
3	None	Present	Present
4	Minor, in one or more domains	Present	Present
5	Major, in only one domain	NA†	NA
6	Major, in any two domains	NA	NA
7	Major, in any three domains	NA	NA
8	Major, in any four domains	NA	NA
9	Major, in all five domains	NA	NA
10	Reduced level of consciousness	NA	NA
11	Death	NA	NA

From the EC/IC Bypass Study Group: The International Cooperative Study of Extracranial/Intracranial Arterial Anastomosis (EC/IC Bypass Study): Methodology and entry characteristics. By permission of the American Heart Association, Inc. Stroke 16:397–406, 1985.

**Impairment in the domains of swallowing, self-care, ambulation, speech, and comprehension. If independence is maintained despite the impairment, deficit is classified as minor; if independence is lost, it is classified as major.*

†Neurologic signs and symptoms are integrated into the higher grades of impairment.

3 = large ulcer more than 4 mm deep or 10 mm long; and 4 = complex ulceration.

Reporting Results

The results of therapeutic intervention for extracranial arteries are best measured by the occurrence (or absence) of stroke (including transient or temporary cerebrovascular symptoms) in the distribution of the artery operated upon and the recurrence (or relief) of preoperative symptoms. If the overall postoperative stroke rate were applied, estimates of benefit could be adversely affected by progression of disease in the contralateral, untreated carotid artery. However, when surgical intervention is intended to relieve hypoperfusion in the contralateral hemisphere, recurrence of those symptoms must also be considered a treatment failure. Carotid patency is not a valid criterion because almost all stenoses are patent preoperatively. Carotid restenosis (i.e., more than 50 per cent) is an appropriate yardstick, but if used, the relative incidence of symptomatic versus silent restenosis should be stated.

Further measures of postoperative status include grading the severity of strokes using the aforementioned stroke severity scale (see Table 25–7) and categorizing the timing of stroke into (1) intraoperative stroke; (2) perioperative stroke: worsening of neurologic status after the initial postoperative evaluation up to a period of 30 days; and (3) late postoperative stroke (after 30 days).

Venous Disease

Deep Venous Thrombosis

The recommended clinical classification of lower extremity venous thrombosis is made on the basis of location and extent of thrombus. Six segments are identified in the deep venous system affecting the lower extremities: tibial-soleal veins, popliteal vein, common and superficial femoral veins, profunda vein, iliac vein, and the vena cava. (The greater and lesser saphenous veins can also be classified when relevant to the case report.) Each segment is graded on a 4-point scale of 0 to 3: 0= patent, 1 = nonocclusive thrombus, 2 = subsegmental occlusive thrombus, and 3 = occlusive thrombus throughout the segmental length. Traditionally, this classification required detailed phlebography, but duplex ultrasound is now used with accuracies equal to or exceeding phlebography (particularly for nonocclusive thrombi).

Associated risk factors for deep venous thrombosis (DVT) are substantially different from those used for other vascular conditions and are listed in Table 25–8. Also included in the table is a severity scale for each risk factor. Overall, the maximum point total is 28, and it has been proposed that this total score can be used to stratify patients in comparative studies of prophylaxis or therapies.[24] Although this approach may be empirically useful, the extent to which these risks are in any sense additive is debatable, and the assignment of relative risk under this scoring system awaits further research. Nevertheless, the consistent identification and grading of individual risk factors allow assessment of population comparability and indeed generation of the data necessary for relative risk assessment.

Table 25–8. Associated Risk Factors for Deep Venous Thrombosis (DVT)

Risk Factor	Severity Scale	
Prior DVT	0–3	None/suspected/proved/multiple
Immobilization	0–3	None/1–3 days/>3 days/paraplegia
Anesthesia	0–3	Local/45 minutes general/>45 minutes general/> 3 hr
Age	0–2	<40 yr/40–70 yr/>70 yr
Malignancy	0–3	None/recurrence/extensive regional tumor/metastatic
Malignant tissue type	0–1	where 1 = adenocarcinoma
Cardiac disease	0–3	NY Heart Assn: class 1, class 2, class 3, class 4
Limb trauma	0–4	None/soft tissue injury/fracture of tibia and/or fibula/fracture of femur/fracture of hip or pelvis
Thrombotic tendency	0–3	None suspected/suspected, proved treated/proved untreated
Hormonal therapy	0–1	No/yes
Pregnancy	0–1	Absent/present
Obesity	0–1	Normal to + 175 per cent ideal body weight/>175 per cent ideal body weight

The results of therapy for treatment of DVT, e.g., thrombolytic therapy or thrombectomy, must specify both the patency and the valvular competence (using vascular laboratory venous refilling time [VRT] determinations—see later discussion), with the exception of the larger veins such as the vena cava, in which valvular competency is irrelevant. There is no benefit to reporting partial clot resolution.

Chronic Venous Insufficiency

The classification of chronic venous insufficiency (CVI) by clinical severity is outlined in Table 25–9. This system is reminiscent of the CHAT system proposed for cerebrovascular disease, with categories for *C*urrent clinical classification, prior clinical classification or *H*istory, *A*natomic location, and *E*tiology. Both current and prior clinical classifications use a 4-point severity scale: 0 = asymptomatic; 1 = mild ankle swelling or painful varicosities, usually limited to superficial veins; 2 = moderate CVI with hyperpigmentation in the gaiter area, moderate brawny edema, and subcutaneous fibrosis without ulceration; and 3 = severe CVI with chronic distal leg pain associated with ulcerated or pre-ulcerative skin changes. The anatomic area

Table 25–9. Overall Classification for Chronic Venous Insufficiency

	Clinical			
Class	*Current*	*Prior*	Anatomic Location	Etiology
0	Asymptomatic	Same	0 Unknown	0 Unknown
1	Mild	Same	1 Superficial veins	1 Congenital
2	Moderate	Same	2 Perforators	2 Post-thrombotic
3	Severe (ulceration)	Same	3 Deep calf	
			4 Deep thigh	
			5 Deep iliofemoral	
			6 Deep caval	
			7 Combination of 2–5 (any)	

Table 25–10. Clinical Outcome for Chronic Venous Insufficiency

The final clinical outcome should be classified as follows:

+3	Asymptomatic. Improved at least one clincial class. Improvement of VRT and AVP to normal or at least +5 seconds, and −10 torr, respectively.
+2	Moderate improvement. Continuing mild symptoms with same clinical and VL improvement as in +3.
+1	Mild improvement. Improvement in either clinical class or VL tests, but not both.
0	Unchanged clinically or by laboratory tests.
−1	Mild worsening. Worsening of either clinical outcome by one category or VL tests.
−2	Significant worsening. Both clinical and VL worsening.
−3	Marked worsening. Same as −2 accompanied by either new or worsening ankle ulceration.

Key: *VRT = venous refilling time; AVP = ambulatory venous pressure; VL = vascular laboratory.*

is coded as six isolated segments, and code 7 = combined segments. Etiology is coded simply as unknown, congenital, or post-thrombotic.

Functional documentation of CVI historically has used ambulatory venous pressures, which are still considered the gold standard by many. Normal ambulatory foot venous pressure is less than 50 per cent of standing pressure. The noninvasive correlate of these measures is obtained by photoplethysmographic (PPG) assessment of VRT, which is the time needed for return to baseline PPG levels following venous emptying by plantar flexion (this test is described in Chapter 133).[3] Normal VRT is greater than 20 seconds, mild CVI = 15 to 20 seconds, moderate CVI = 5 to 15 seconds, and severe CVI is less than 5 seconds. However, it should be remembered that in many patients a normal VRT is considerably longer (e.g., 25 to 40 seconds), and, if one leg is normal, its VRT can be used as that patient's normal value.

Reporting results of therapy and surgical intervention for relief of CVI must include functional assessment as well as symptomatic assessment. A scheme for gauging clinical outcome is listed in Table 25–10. A major shortcoming of reports on surgical interventions, particularly valvuloplasty and valve interposition, has been the lack of objective venous hemodynamic measurements (see Chapter 133).

Arterial Aneurysm

Classification

Arterial aneurysms are defined as focal arterial dilatations with a diameter at least 50 per cent greater than that of the proximal normal arterial segment. Aneurysms may be classified by several factors including site, etiology, morphology, and clinicopathology. Each of these classifiers may be more appropriate than others, depending on the circumstances. For example, etiology is particularly relevant to anastomotic aneurysms but is indeed unknown for arteriosclerotic aneurysms (see also Chapter 13).

Evaluation of Result

Patency is not the most valid measure of long-term success following prosthetic repair of major or central arterial aneurysms. Patient survival and freedom from significant complications are more important factors. The evaluation of complications was discussed previously for lower extremity arterial disease and cerebrovascular disease. However, recurrent aneurysm formation should also be included as a major index of long-term success.

It is hoped that adopting precise definitions of essential terms, developing objective criteria by which the various measures of success or failure can be judged, and establishing a standardized scheme by which severity of disease, degrees of improvement or deterioration, and risk factors that affect outcome can be graded will improve the quality of published reports of the results of vascular surgical procedures.

COMPUTER-BASED VASCULAR REGISTRY

The need for accurate and uniform reporting standards existed prior to the advent of computer database technologies, but the microcomputer provides both impetus and a medium for achieving that goal. The requirement by computer data management software for precise, codifiable clinical data should provide some additional impetus to establishing such standards. The availability of powerful but relatively inexpensive hardware and software means that this medium for information is now accessible to the smallest surgical practice.

The clinical databases or "vascular registries" of individuals and well-circumscribed group practices have, in fact, formed the basis of the vast majority of published reports in vascular surgery.[16] Several groups have advocated the establishment of regional or even national vascular registries.[23] The benefits of such a database could be significant in providing a true picture of vascular surgical practices, prevalence of disease, and prognosis under varying therapies and in the presence of concomitant risk factors. Such a registry could allow the study of relatively rare problems.

The use of databases for tracking patients and, in particular, in retrospective studies has the potential for misuse. The major concern is one of scientific method and the associated statistical caveat that such data are indeed retrospective and nonrandomized with respect to any prognostic factors that might be studied.[7] This potential problem is not unique to computer-based "registries"; it is an ongoing issue in clinical research and medicine that is due in large part to the fact that the practice of clinical medicine is not performed in a controlled experimental setting. Ethics and cost are major considerations in conducting prospective randomized trials. It is also true that the randomized controlled clinical trial does not guarantee unbiased data, nor can the experimental design balance more than a few important prognostic factors. Considering the cost and effort of the randomized clinical trial and the focus imposed by randomization, the use of (vascular) registries as a source for observational studies should be viewed as a major opportunity to improve the design and focus of the limited number of randomized trials that actually occur.

The utility of the vascular registry in an observational or retrospective study is dependent on the quality and uniformity of its data. In addition to the reduction of bias by use of randomization, the randomized controlled trial also benefits from a strict protocol that standardizes definitions and assessment criteria among participating investigators and over time. It is this standardization that allows rational use of stratification by prognostic factors in an attempt to balance the study groups of the experimental population. It is essential that the individual, regional, or national registry use standardized definitions and criteria.

Considerations in the Design of a Vascular Registry

Collection of data is not synonymous with information. Information may be better described as a process than as a commodity,[5] i.e., the end result of data processing. Philosophically, it can be argued that until data are utilized, information does not exist,[6] but it is certainly true that data that will not or cannot be utilized represent wasted time, effort, and money. Thus, effective retrieval and integration of data begin with an effective storage scheme.

Computer software for data management is usually known as a database management system (DBMS). These application software programs perform two separate tasks: data filing (the record-keeper) and data management (the information generator).

Primarily, there are two types of macrostructures used to store data: hierarchical and relational. With the panoply of DBMS software now available[32, 33] and the expanding emphasis on ease of use, the storage structure becomes increasingly unimportant to the end user. Nevertheless, most DBMS software for use with micro (personal) computers uses relational structures (if not flat-file) because they are more easily modified and more easily understood.[19, 37]

Relational databases are often explained using the analogy of office file cabinets in which the database is a drawer in the cabinet, a file is a folder in the drawer, a record is a page in the folder, a field is a concise item on the page, and a byte is one character of the item. Data relationships are established by this macrostructure and by so-called keys, or unique data items in each record. Relationships among records are best visualized if each file is considered to be a table with rows of records and columns of fields (Table 25–11). When a computer database is being planned, the data should be given a contextual structure that is compatible with this tabular representation.

Data storage is easy; data management is the difficult part, but the processes are not independent. It may seem obvious that data retrieval and integration are easier when the amount of data is small. On the other hand, these processes are meaningless without pertinent data. Which data should be stored is a difficult decision. An all too common approach is the storage of too much data in an attempt to ensure that all the necessary data will be available. The balance between too little and too much is more easily determined if the purpose of collecting the data has been identified.[38]

Data are also more easily accessed if the storage is logically encoded. Although the future holds the promise of

Table 25–11. Example of Relational Table Structures

File #1.

Social Security #	Name	Sex	Date of Birth
111–22–3333	Doe, Jane	F	03/01/39
123–45–6789	Doe, John	M	02/01/39
222–22–2222	Doe, Jack	M	01/01/39

Related Records

File #2.

Social Security #	Clinic Date	CHAT Score
111–22–3333	01/01/87	2b-1a-1a-li
111–22–3333	01/01/88	0-2b-0-0
222–22–2222	01/01/88	0-0-0-0

efficient text-based data storage, made possible by faster processors and cheap, vast amounts of storage area (memory), current techniques utilize data encoding for efficient storage and access. As an illustration of encoding, Table 25–12 shows a list of indications for surgery, a list of operative procedures, and a list of anatomic sites taken from the vascular surgical registry in use at the University of Colorado. A femoropopliteal bypass performed for rest pain is encoded by five discrete codes: 11 = rest pain, 16 = single bypass, L = left, 7 = primary/inflow site at common femoral, and 10 = outflow site at AK popliteal. Other vascular registries similarly use encoding schemes; this is true of the registry of the Cleveland Vascular Society,[23] Albany Medical College,[16] and Montefiore Medical Center.[12]

The most difficult aspect of a good vascular registry is data entry and maintenance of patient records. For example, when one is interested in follow-up on a 5-year perspective of carotid endarterectomy, the registry would not be very useful if 20 per cent of the cases were missing at random—or worse, at some specific biased time over the period of interest. A major cost of computers in general and databases in particular is the associated labor cost. In this instance, some knowledgeable individual must aid in coding and entering data, or the data will not only be incomplete but also unreliable. The vascular surgeon must participate in the design, creation, and maintenance of the vascular registry.

Multi-center studies are usually the result of either corporate-sponsored research in support of Food and Drug Administration (FDA) applications or government-sponsored research on very specific questions (e.g., current Veterans Administration cooperative studies) and occur relatively infrequently. Yet when multi-center reports appear in the literature, they are usually referenced as definitive studies. This perception of the larger importance of multi-center studies as compared with individual experiences is a direct result of the increased reliability of larger sample sizes incorporating different patient populations, different surgeons, and so forth, but also of standardizing clinical data such as clinical classifications, risk factors, and outcome. In effect, the multi-center trial as a well-designed, experimental clinical design benefits from standardized reporting practices. The vascular registry cannot replace the multi-center or randomized trial, but with the incorporation of standardized reporting practices it provides a means of studying certain problems cooperatively and with larger numbers than would be possible in individual or group

Table 25–12. Example of Codes for Describing Operative Procedure

Indication	Procedure	Anatomic Site
1: Aneurysm—no sx	1: Not applicable	1: Thoracic aorta
2: Aneurysm—ruptured/dissecting	2: Exploration	2: Suprarenal aorta
3: Aneurysm—thromboembolic	3: Ligation	3: Infrarenal aorta
4: Aneurysm—false	4: Excision	4: Common iliac
5: Aneurysm—infected	5: Repair	5: Internal iliac
6: Arteriovenous (AV) fistula—congenital	6: Vascular decompression	6: External iliac
7: AV fistula—acquired	7: Neurolysis	7: Common femoral
8: Hemangioma/congenital vascular malformation (CVM)	8: Fasciotomy	8: Superficial femoral
9: Acute ischemia—thromboembolic	9: Sympathectomy	9: Profunda femoral
10: Claudication	10: Thromboembolectomy	10: Popliteal above knee (AK)
11: Rest pain	11: Thrombolysis	11: Popliteal below knee (BK)
12: Nonhealing ulceration	12: Luminal dilatation	12: Per-tib trunk
13: Distal gangrene	13: Patch angioplasty	13: Posterior tibial
14: Blue digit/embolism	14: Endarterectomy	14: Anterior tibial
15: Occlusion—acute postoperative	15: Replacement graft	15: Peroneal
16: Occlusion/stenosis—late postoperative	16: Single bypass	16: Subclavian
17: Graft infection	17: Composite bypass	17: Innominate
18: Diabetic foot	18: Sequential bypass	18: Axillary
19: Asymptomatic cartoid disease	19: Operative a′gram (arteriogram)	19: Brachial
20: Transient ischemic attack (TIA)	20: Amputation	20: Ulnar
21: Resolve ischemic neuro deficit (RIND)	21: Wrap aneurysm	21: Radial
22: Amaurosis fugax	22: Temp AV fistula	22: Common carotid
23: Stroke	23: Angioaccess fistula	23: Internal carotid
24: Other cardiovascular (CV)—VBI/global sx	24: Angioaccess graft	24: External carotid
25: Trauma—blunt	25: Angioaccess catheter	25: Vertebral
26: Trauma—penetrating	26: Valvuloplasty	26: Superficial temporal
27: Trauma—iatrogenic	27: Venous system bypass	27: Renal
28: Thoracic outlet syndrome	28: Venous valve	28: Superior mesenteric artery (SMA)
29: Carpal tunnel syndrome	29: Peritoneal shunt	29: Inferior mesenteric artery (IMA)
30: Compartment syndrome	30: Clip/filter	30: Splenic
31: Popliteal entrapment/cyst	31: Other	31: Celiac
32: Dialysis access		32: Hepatic
33: Acute intestinal ischemia		33: Superior vena cava (SVC)
34: Chronic intestinal ischemia		34: Inferior vena cava (IVC)
35: Lymphatic disorder		35: Pulmonary artery
36: Portal hypertension		36: Greater saphenous
37: Renal hypertension		37: Lesser saphenous
38: Renal ischemia		38: Perforators
39: Pulmonary embolus		39: Cephalic
40: Varicose veins		40: Basilic
41: Venous insufficiency/obstruction		41: Portal
42: Acute venous obstruction		42: Azygous
43: Vasospastic/Raynaud's		43: Internal jugular
44: Causalgia/reflex sympathetic dystrophy (RSD)		44: External jugular
45: Complication of previous procedure		45: Thoracic duct
46: Other		46: Brachial plexus
		47: Median nerve
		48: Ulnar nerve
		49: First rib
		50: Other

experiences. The well-defined vascular registry, at the least, should provide the practitioner with a means of assessing his or her experience and realistically comparing that experience to similarly well-defined published studies.

References

1. Ascer E, Veith FJ, Gupta SK, et al: Comparison of axillounifemoral and axillobifemoral bypass operations. Surgery 97:169, 1985.
2. Baker JD, Rutherford RB, Bernstein EF, et al: Suggested standards for reports dealing with cerebrovascular disease. J Vasc Surg 8:721, 1988.
3. Barnes RW: Noninvasive techniques in chronic venous insufficiency. *In* Bernstein EF (ed): Noninvasive Diagnostic Techniques in Vascular Disease. 3rd ed. St. Louis, CV Mosby, 1985, p 839.
4. Berkowitz HD, Hobbs CL, Roberts B, et al: Value of routine vascular laboratory studies to identify vein graft stenosis. Surgery 90:971, 1981.
5. Blois MS: Information and Medicine. Berkeley and Los Angeles, University of California Press, 1980, pp 1–17.
6. Ibid, pp 22–24.
7. Dambrosia JM, Ellenberg JH: Statistical considerations for a medical data base. Biometrics 36:323, 1980.
8. DeWeese JA, Rob CG: Autogenous venous grafts five years later. Am Surg 174:346, 1971.
9. Eugene J, Goldstone J, Moore WS: Fifteen-year experience with subcutaneous bypass grafts for lower extremity ischemia. Ann Surg 186:177, 1976.
10. Flanigan DP, Pratt DG, Goodreau JJ, et al: Hemodynamic and angiographic guidelines in selection of patients for femoro-femoral bypass. Arch Surg 113:1257, 1978.
11. Glantz SA: Primer of Biostatistics. New York, McGraw-Hill, 1981, p 7.
12. Gupta SK, Veith FJ, White-Flores SA, et al: System for wide-spread

application of microcomputers to vascular surgery. J Vasc Surg 1:601, 1984.
13. Harris PL, Jones D, How T: A prospective randomized clinical trial to compare in situ and reversed vein grafts for femoro-popliteal bypass. Br J Surg 74:252, 1987.
14. Johnson WC, LoGerfo FW, Vollman RW: Is axillobilateral femoral graft an effective substitute for aortobilateral iliac femoral graft? Ann Surg 186:123, 1976.
15. Johnston KW, Colapinto RF, Baird RJ: Transluminal dilation. An alternative. Arch Surg 117:1604, 1982.
16. Karmody AM, Fitzgerald K, Branagh BS, et al: Development of a computerized registry for large-scale use. J Vasc Surg 1:594, 1984.
17. Lawless JF: Statistical Models and Methods for Lifetime Data. New York, John Wiley & Sons, 1982.
18. LoGerfo FW, Johnson WC, Corson JD, et al: A comparison of the late patency rates of axillobilateral femoral and axillounilateral femoral grafts. Surgery 81:33, 1977.
19. Martin J: Principles of Data-base Management. Englewood Cliffs, NJ, Prentice-Hall, 1976.
20. Naji A, Barker CF, Berkowitz HD, et al: Femoropopliteal vein grafts for claudication: Analysis of 100 consecutive cases. Ann Surg 188:79, 1978.
21. Naji A, Jennifer C, McCombs PR, et al: Results of 100 consecutive femoropopliteal vein grafts for limb salvage. Ann Surg 188:162, 1978.
22. Ouriel K, Green RM: Clinical and technical factors influencing recurrent carotid stenosis and occlusion after endarterectomy. J Vasc Surg 5:702, 1987.
23. Plecha FR, Avellone JC, Beven GC, et al: A computerized vascular registry. Experience of The Cleveland Vascular Society. Surgery 86:826, 1979.
24. Porter JM, Clagett GP, Cranley J, et al: Reporting standards in venous disease. J Vasc Surg 8(2):172, 1988.
25. Ray LI, O'Connor JB, Davis CC, et al: Axillofemoral bypass: A critical reappraisal of its role in the management of aortoiliac occlusive disease. Am J Surg 138:117, 1979.
26. Reichle FA, Tyson RR: Bypasses to tibial or popliteal arteries in severely ischemic lower extremities: Comparison of long-term results in 233 patients. Ann Surg 176:315, 1972.
27. Rutherford RB, Flanigan DP, Gupta SK, et al: Suggested standards for reports dealing with lower extremity ischemia. J Vasc Surg 4:80, 1986.
28. Rutherford RB, Jones DN, Bergentz SE, et al: The efficacy of dextran-40 in preventing early postoperative thrombosis following difficult lower extremity bypass. J Vasc Surg 1:765, 1984.
29. Rutherford RB, Jones DN, Martin MS, et al: Serial hemodynamic assessment of aortobifemoral bypass. J Vasc Surg 4:428, 1986.
30. Rutherford RB, Patt A, Kumpe DA: The current role of percutaneous transluminal angioplasty. *In* Greenhalgh KM, Jamieson CW, Nicolaides AN (eds): Vascular Surgery: Issues in Current Practice. London, Grune & Stratton, 1986, pp 229–244.
31. Sanders RJ: Personal communication.
32. Seymour J: Programmable databases. Byte 7(9):93, 1988.
33. Seymour J: Relational databases. Byte 7(8):153, 1988.
34. Underwood CG, Charlesworth D: Uses and abuses of life table analysis in vascular surgery. Br J Surg 71:495, 1984.
35. Veith FJ, Moss CM, Fell SC, et al: Comparison of expanded polytetrafluoroethylene and autologous saphenous vein grafts in high risk arterial reconstructions for limb salvage. Surg Gynecol Obstet 147:749, 1978.
36. Veith FJ, Gupta SK, Ascer E, et al: Six-year prospective multicenter randomized comparison of autologous saphenous vein and expanded polytetrafluoroethylene grafts in infrainguinal arterial reconstructions. J Vasc Surg 3:104, 1986.
37. Walters RF: Database Principles for Personal Computers. New York, Prentice-Hall Press, 1987.
38. Wasserman AI: Personal computers in the health care environment. *In* Lindberg DAB, Collen MF, Van Brunt EE (eds): Computer Applications in Medical Care. New York, Masson Publishing, 1982, pp 51–55.
39. Zeirler RE, Bandyk DF, Thiele BL, et al: Carotid artery stenosis following endarterectomy. Arch Surg 117:1408, 1982.
40. Johnston KW, Rutherford RB, Tilson MD, et al: Suggested standards for reporting on arterial aneurysms. J Vasc Surg 13:444, 1991.
41. Thiele BL, Jones AM, Hobson RW, et al: Standards in noninvasive cerebrovascular testing. J Vasc Surg 15:495, 1992.
42. Peto R, Pike MC, Armitage P, et al: Design and analysis of randomized trials requiring prolonged observations of each patient. I. Introduction and design. Br J Cancer 34:585, 1976.
43. Peto R, Pike MC, Armitage P, et al: Design and analysis of randomized trials requiring prolonged observations of each patient. II. Analysis and examples. Br J Cancer 35:1, 1977.
44. El-Massry S, Saad E, Sauvage LR, et al: Axillofemoral bypass using externally supported, knitted dacron grafts: A followup through twelve years. J Vasc Surg 17:107, 1993.
45. Harris EJ, Taylor LM, McConnel DB, et al: Clinical results of axillobifemoral bypass using externally supported polytetrafluoroethylene. J Vasc Surg 12:416, 1990.
46. Rutherford RB, Patt A, Pearce WH: Extra-anatomic bypass: A closer view. J Vasc Surg 5:437, 1987.
47. Rutherford RB: Suggested standards for reporting complications in vascular surgery. *In* Towne JB, Bernhard WM (eds): Complications in Vascular Surgery. 3rd ed. St. Louis, Quality Medical Publishing, 1991, pp 1–10.
48. Dormany J, et al: Second European consensus document on chronic critical leg ischaemia. Circulation 84(4 Suppl.): IV-1 1991.
49. Chang JB: Current state of extra-anantomic bypasses. Am J Surg 152:202, 1986.
50. Hepp W, de Jonge K, Pallua N: Late results following extra-anatomic bypass procedures for chronic aortoiliac occlusive disease. J Cardiovasc Surg 29:181, 1988.
51. Colton T: Statistics in Medicine. Boston, Little, Brown, 1974, pp 244–246.
52. Mehta S, Rutherford RB: Reply to letters to the editors. J Vasc Surg 5:501, 1987.
53. Lee ET: Statistical Methods for Survival Data Analysis. Belmont, CA, Wadsworth, 1980, pp 75–92.

Vascular Grafts

Edited by Richard F. Kempczinski, M.D.

26

Overview

Richard F. Kempczinski, M.D.

• • •

Although an arterial aneurysm was successfully treated by Matas in 1888 and a vascular anastomosis was performed by Murphy in 1897, the real birth of vascular surgery occurred more than 50 years later with the introduction of the first practical arterial prosthesis. In the intervening half century, a variety of potential vascular grafts had been tested and rejected.

During these early years of vascular prosthetic development, the characteristics of the *ideal graft* were defined.[30] It must be readily available in a variety of sizes and lengths and suitable for use throughout the body. It must be durable in long-term implantation in humans, nonreactive, and free of toxic or allergic side effects. Its handling characteristics must include elasticity, conformability, pliability, ease of suturing, and absence of fraying at cut ends or kinking at flexion points. Its luminal surface must be smooth, minimally traumatic to formed blood elements, resistant to infection, and nonthrombogenic. It must be available at a reasonable cost and be capable of being repeatedly sterilized without alteration.

Although no current prosthetic material satisfies all these requirements, a number of very satisfactory alternatives are available. This and the following eight chapters review the characteristics and biologic behavior of various arterial substitutes, the clinical considerations in their handling, and the complications encountered with their use.

HISTORICAL BACKGROUND

Table 26–1 briefly summarizes the history of materials that have been used as vascular grafts. Although Carrel initially demonstrated the suitability of homologous and heterologous artery and vein as arterial substitutes in dogs, and Goyanes confirmed that autologous vein transplants in man could serve as a suitable arterial replacement, most early graft development focused on the use of impervious nonbiologic tubes.[5, 14] Although these functioned adequately as short-term passive conduits, they were never incorporated by the host and ultimately were subject to suture line disruption, distal embolization, and thrombosis. In 1948, Gross returned to the arterial allograft and launched the modern era of vascular surgery.[16] With the introduction of Vinyon-N in 1952, the concept of a porous, fabric arterial prosthesis was born.[3] Three years later, the introduction of "crimping" brought added flexibility and elasticity to the fabric grafts and extended their use.[10] Over the years, stronger and more durable textiles such as Dacron have been developed, and numerous modifications of fabrication have been introduced, but the basic principle that so revolutionized vascular surgery has stood the test of time (see Chapter 29).[6]

In 1966, the bovine heterograft ushered in a new generation of vascular prostheses, i.e., the tanned collagen tube.[24] Although this particular graft has been abandoned because of its tendency to aneurysmal dilation and thrombosis, it was the prototype for the human umbilical cord vein allograft (HUCVAG). The HUCVAG is available in a variety of lengths, but its 5- to 8-mm diameters limit its application to the replacement of small to medium-sized vessels. Because all its living elements are killed during the fixation process, it gradually loses compliance as it is replaced by host collagen. The original HUCVAG was reinforced with a thin external Dacron mesh to prevent aneurysmal dilatation. However, virtually all such grafts have become dilated or developed frank aneurysm if they remained patent for more than 5 years.[17] The graft has recently been modified by increasing the strength of its surrounding Dacron mesh, but only long-term follow-up will determine whether this has corrected the problem (see Chapter 29).

Polytetrafluoroethylene (Teflon, PTFE) was first used as a vascular prosthesis in 1957.[9] It was found to be extremely durable and has been widely used as a woven arterial substitute. In the late 1960s, a process was developed for extruding PTFE (ePTFE) to create a nonfabric

Table 26–1. History of Vascular Grafts

1906 Carrel	Homologous and heterologous artery and vein transplant in dogs
1906 Goyanes	First autologous vein transplant in man
1915 Tuffier	Paraffin-lined silver tubes
1942 Blakemore	Vitallium tubes
1947 Hufuagel	Polished methyl methacrylate tubes
1948 Gross	Arterial allografts
1949 Donovan	Polyethylene tubes
1952 Voorhees	Vinyon-N, first fabric prosthesis
1955 Egdahl	Siliconized rubber
1955 Edwards and Tapp	Crimped nylon
1957 Edwards	Teflon
1960 DeBakey	Dacron
1966 Rosenberg	Bovine heterograft
1968 Sparks	Dacron-supported autogenous fibrous tubes
1972 Soyer	Polytetrafluoroethylene (PTFE)
1975 Dardik	Human umbilical cord vein (HUCVAG)

graft that enjoyed all the advantages of Teflon without several of its disadvantages. This prosthesis was first used clinically in 1972 and has subsequently been widely applied as a small and medium-sized vessel replacement (see Chapter 29).[31]

BIOLOGIC BEHAVIOR OF VASCULAR GRAFTS

Although most discussions of vascular grafts emphasize the physical characteristics of the prosthesis, numerous factors other than graft composition are equally important in determining its clinical success. Paramount among these is the realization that bypass grafts fail to halt progression of the underlying disease process, which ultimately appears responsible for most graft failure. In addition, patient selection and choice of operative procedures are tremendously important in determining long-term clinical success and may explain some of the variation in reported results.

Furthermore, since most grafts are initially tested in various experimental animal models, it must be appreciated that there are wide interspecies variations in the host response to an implanted vascular graft. In humans, spread of the endothelial pannus that originates at the anastomoses is very limited when compared with its extent in the pig, calf, or baboon. Furthermore, the ingrowth of fibroblasts through the wall of the prosthesis and the ability to "heal" the inner lining is rudimentary compared with that in various other species in which healing occurs very rapidly and may be complete in 4 to 8 weeks.[29] The behavior of prostheses in dogs most closely parallels that in humans, thus explaining the emergence of the dog as the favorite animal model for evaluation of vascular grafts. These differences must be remembered when reviewing reported results.

The fabric prosthetic grafts represented a radical departure from the rigid metal and plastic tubes that preceded them. Virtually all arterial prostheses develop a layer of fibrin of varying thickness on their luminal surfaces. In addition, endothelium grows across each anastomosis in an attempt to bridge the defect and cover the graft's luminal surface. In nonporous prostheses, this luminal fibrin cannot be organized by the ingrowth of connective tissue, and the spreading endothelial pannus does not become adherent, thus predisposing to distal embolization of fibrin fragments or intimal proliferation and graft occlusion. In contrast, the porous fabric prostheses develop a thin layer of luminal fibrin that is gradually replaced by mature collagen growing in from the outer surface of the prosthesis, resulting in a stable, relatively nonthrombogenic luminal surface. In many experimental animals, this layer is then rapidly covered by endothelium spreading from the anastomoses. The advantages of such "healing" of prosthetic grafts, in addition to those already described, include an increased resistance to late hematogenous infection and improved patency in low-flow situations (see Chapter 29).[21, 27]

Unfortunately, increasing the porosity of grafts to facilitate this healing was accompanied by an increased incidence of both early and late hemorrhage as well as increased fiber fragmentation and aneurysm formation.[4] Thus, it is necessary in the design of any prosthesis to strike a balance between a relatively low implantation porosity and a high biologic porosity to tissue ingrowth.

Some modifications of graft construction have improved graft healing by employing a loose, filamentous yarn in the entire graft or by adding a textured velour surface to standard Dacron grafts.[28] Such veloured, knitted Dacron prostheses develop a thinner fibrin lining and are more likely to undergo transmural healing, thus creating the most favorable situation for endothelialization of the luminal surface. Despite these modifications, complete endothelialization of long grafts is yet to be observed in the human subject.[2] Yet another technique used to combine low implant and high biologic porosity is the coating of a high-porosity knitted Dacron graft with bovine collagen. Such grafts require no "preclotting" with the patient's own blood at the time of implantation but still permit the ingrowth of tissue into and around the graft fibers as the coating is gradually replaced by autologous collagen.[11] In addition to facilitating graft placement and reducing perioperative blood loss, such grafts may provide a better substrate for ingrowth of host endothelium.

There are two major unresolved problems with the clinical use of prosthetic arterial grafts: (1) a persistently higher thrombosis rate compared with autologous grafts when they are used for small vessel replacement in a low-flow runoff bed, and (2) an increased risk of graft infection, especially when they are sutured to the common femoral artery.

One of the major differences between prosthetic vascular grafts and autologous grafts is the absence of a living endothelial layer on the luminal surface. Despite all previous efforts to modify the structure and composition of vascular prostheses to foster the ingrowth of an endothelial lining, no vascular prosthesis implanted in a human being has ever developed a documented, complete endothelial layer. Because endothelium poses unique thromboresistant properties and may also help to protect the underlying vascular wall from secondary infection, a large body of research has focused on techniques designed to foster the development of such a lining. The most promising of these involves the "seeding" of autologous endothelial cells into the graft prior to implantation.[15] Host endothelial cells are harvested from a small segment of vein and are either added to the blood used to "preclot" the graft prior to implantation or are used to coat grafts that would not otherwise require preclotting. Although such "seeded" endothelial cells have been shown to replicate and completely cover the flow surface of both fabric and ePTFE grafts in a number of different animal models, human endothelial cells are much more easily traumatized and may behave differently. Thus far, no "endothelium-seeded" vascular prosthesis has developed a confluent endothelial lining in man.

Other mechanical approaches being studied to render the flow surface of small-diameter vascular prostheses thromboresistant involve coating the luminal surface of such grafts with colloidal graphite.[7] Although this approach appears to increase the thromboresistance of various grafts in animal models, its clinical applicability remains to be proved. When such a colloidal graphite surface is rinsed with a cationic, surface-active agent, it is capable of bonding heparin, which may further increase its thromboresistance. This ability to bind heparin to its surface may be the most important anticoagulant property of a carbon-lined graft. At the moment, no carbon-coated graft is approved for clinical use.

Finally, because infection of a vascular prosthesis is such a disastrous and feared complication, a new procedure for the bonding of antibacterial agents directly to the graft has been developed.[22] In the past, attempts to coat grafts directly with antibiotics have failed because of the poor penetration of drugs into the graft material. However, the use of metals such as silver in the bonding process increases retention of the antibiotic on the graft fabric but allows its gradual release into the surrounding tissue. No antibiotic-coated vascular grafts have yet been approved for use in humans.

One additional characteristic of prosthetic grafts that may significantly influence their long-term function is *compliance*. Although many current prostheses have an initial compliance that is similar to that of the host artery, virtually all of them undergo fibrous ingrowth and become rigid. The exceptions to this generalization are the autograft artery and vein, which maintain essentially normal compliance even on long-term implantation. This decrease in compliance has been implicated in the loss of the graft's ability to "self-cleanse" its intimal surface and may be responsible for the progressive deposition of luminal fibrin that occurs in most grafts.[8] In addition, the disparity in compliance that develops between the implanted graft and the host artery creates stress at the anastomoses, which has been implicated in the formation of an anastomotic false aneurysm and the development of neointimal fibroplasia.[8, 13]

SELECTION AND HANDLING OF VASCULAR GRAFTS

No graft currently available is suitable for every clinical application, and grafts must be selected on an individual basis for each case. Table 26–2 lists the vascular grafts that are currently used clinically and indicates the preferred and alternate choices for various clinical applications. Autogenous artery is an almost ideal vascular replacement (see Chapter 27).[33] Few large arteries in the body are expendable, however, and thus its limited availability makes it suitable only for short segmental replacements of small and medium-sized arteries. Autogenous vein, on the other hand, specifically the greater saphenous vein, is usually available in longer segments. Although subject to some medial fibrous intimal proliferation and long-term degeneration, it has proved to be a durable and amazingly serviceable replacement, especially for extremity bypass grafting.[32] Unfortunately, in 20 to 30 per cent of patients, the reversed saphenous vein will be either unavailable, of inadequate caliber, or of poor quality, and alternate substitutes must be found.[19] The resurgence of interest in using the saphenous vein in situ for lower extremity bypass grafting has resulted in a much greater utilization (more than 90 per cent) of the vein and may also improve long-term patency (see Chapter 28).[20]

Table 26–2. Vascular Grafts in Use at Present and Their Clinical Application

	Type of Graft*							
	Biologic				*Prosthetic*			
	Autograft		Allograft	Heterograft	Fabric		Nontextile	
					Dacron		Teflon	
Clinical Application	Artery	Vein	HUCVAG	Bovine	Knitted	Woven	Woven	PTFE
Thoracic aorta or ruptured aneurysm						P	P	A
Infrarenal aorta					P	A	A	A
Aortovisceral	P	P			A			A
Femoropopliteal		P	A		A			A
Femorotibial		P	A					A
Axillofemoral					P			P
Femorofemoral					P			P
Extrathoracic bypass of arch vessel occlusion					P			P
Coronary artery		P						
Arteriovenous fistula			A	P	A			P
Carotid	P	P			A			A
Venous replacement		P			A			A

P = preferred; A = alternate; PTFE = polytetrafluoroethylene.

The bovine heterograft was initially used for a variety of clinical applications. Because of frequent late complications, however, its usefulness is presently limited to vascular access. The HUCVAG was reinforced with an external mesh of Dacron to prevent aneurysmal dilatation, and it functioned quite satisfactorily as a small and medium-sized vessel replacement. However, as long-term clinical experience with this graft has accumulated, it now appears that more than a third of such *patent* grafts have become significantly dilated or frankly aneurysmal, thus raising serious questions regarding their future clinical application (see Chapter 29).

Although PTFE has been most widely used in replacement of small to medium-sized extremity vessels, it is also available as a bifurcated prosthesis for aortic replacement that appears particularly suitable for the management of ruptured aneurysms. It has also become very popular for vascular access.

The choice of a graft is based not only on its physical characteristics but also on clinical considerations. The size of the vessel to be bypassed or replaced is obviously of importance. Since no autograft is large enough to replace the aorta or vena cava, prosthetic grafts are necessary, and because of their large caliber and high flow they have performed satisfactorily. Conversely, because of the frequent thrombosis of most prosthetic grafts in small-vessel replacement, autogenous tissue is generally preferable for such situations.

Placement of oversized grafts will result in an exuberant layer of luminal fibrin, impaired healing, and ultimately an increased frequency of graft thrombosis.[25] The aim of surgery should therefore be to choose a graft large enough to deliver the increased blood flows that will be required during reactive hyperemia but still small enough to maintain the velocity of blood flow at rest that will prevent the formation of excessive luminal fibrin. Sauvage has demonstrated that this "thrombotic threshold velocity" varies, depending on the graft material and the time after implantation.[27] No prosthetic flow surface yet developed can remain patent at the low flow rates possible with endothelium-lined autogenous grafts, thus explaining the rationale behind their use when outflow is limited.

The age of the patient must also be considered. Grafts used in children or young adults must be capable of growth. Under such circumstances, autogenous tissue should be used whenever possible, and interrupted sutures should be employed for at least a portion of the anastomosis.

In the presence of infection or heavy contamination, such as frequently occurs in arterial trauma, prosthetic grafts should be avoided because of the risk of infection. It may be necessary in such cases to harvest a viable artery from a remote, clean field, replace it with a prosthetic graft, and then use the autograft within the contaminated field to restore arterial continuity (see Chapters 27 and 29).

Expediency and reduced operating time occasionally may be considerations in the selection of graft materials. Elderly patients with limited life expectancy and with a serious medical condition may not tolerate prolonged operations. Under such circumstances, one might consider choosing a prosthetic graft to avoid the additional time required to harvest an autogenous saphenous vein.

Once the graft has been selected, the surgeon must create the most favorable environment for its incorporation. This includes the avoidance of perigraft hematoma, which would prevent fibrous ingrowth and coverage of the graft with viable tissue. The graft must not be placed in proximity to the serosal surface of the bowel, since this may result in vascular enteric fistula formation. In addition, the perioperative use of prophylactic antibiotics for 24 to 72 hours is generally advised to minimize the risk of graft infection.

Upon completion of the procedure, the operating surgeon should carefully record the precise type and lot number of the implanted graft. If complications later develop, this information will be vital in determining whether failure of the graft represented an isolated occurrence or was part of a widespread pattern, suggesting a flaw in graft design.

Since atherosclerosis is a progressive disease and since bypass grafting does not alter its course, the vascular surgeon must accept the responsibility for following patients indefinitely. One must be alert not only to the early detection of impending graft failure—and act promptly to prevent it—but also to the development of arterial occlusions in sites remote from the original surgery.

COMPLICATIONS

The history of vascular grafts is replete with examples of prostheses that initially functioned quite well only to develop late complications. Graft failure may not occur for several years after implantation, and all new grafts should be tested and proved durable for at least 5 years before widespread clinical acceptance.

Two basic categories of graft complications occur: *direct* complications involving failure of the graft itself; and *indirect* complications related to the graft but not impairing its function.

The most common direct graft complication is thrombosis. Although this is occasionally idiopathic and responds to simple thrombectomy, it is usually a consequence of disease progression and requires some form of remedial surgery. Most grafts have been shown to undergo some dilation in response to arterial pressure.[23] Occasionally, this reaches the proportions of a true aneurysm and may rarely result in graft disruption.[1] Autogenous vein undergoes gradual medial fibrosis as well as intimal proliferation in response to arterial pressure.[12] In addition, it may develop atherosclerosis, which can lead to graft stenosis and thrombosis.

Indirect complications may require additional surgery despite continued graft patency. Perhaps the most common of these is a false aneurysm at one or more suture lines (see Chapter 37). Graft infection is usually a disastrous complication and requires removal of the entire graft if suture lines are involved (see Chapter 36). Late infection in the midbody of a graft may occasionally respond to local therapy and permit salvage of the graft.[18] Distal emboli may result from either poor fixation of the luminal fibrin or aneurysmal dilatation of the graft. If the graft has not been adequately covered by viable tissue, it can erode into adjacent hollow viscera, such as the bowel or bladder, causing septicemia or bleeding (see Chapter 38).

CONCLUSIONS

Although a variety of suitable prosthetic grafts are available for nearly every clinical situation, clearly no ideal prosthesis has yet been developed. Large-diameter grafts with high flow have excellent patency rates but remain subject to infection. On the other hand, smaller diameter prostheses, as used in the lower extremity, continue to become thrombosed at unacceptable rates. In addition to the search for newer graft materials, current prosthetic research has centered on the creation of infection-resistant conduits by binding antibiotics to the graft itself and to rendering small grafts less thrombogenic by the addition of endothelial cells to the preclot used to prepare them for implantation.[15,22] Modification of the graft's luminal surface by pretreating it with various substances such as fibronectin and basement membrane gel is also being explored as another approach to facilitate endothelial cell coverage of these grafts. Such work offers hope that a prosthetic material will be found that is readily available in a variety of sizes, resistant to both infection and thrombosis, and suitable for replacement of large to small arteries throughout the body.

References

1. Berger K, Sauvage LR: Late fiber deterioration in Dacron arterial grafts. Ann Surg 193:477, 1981.
2. Berger K, Sauvage LR, Rao AM, et al: Healing of arterial prostheses in man: Its incompleteness. Ann Surg 175:118, 1972.
3. Blakemore AH, Voorhees AB Jr: Use of tubes constructed from vinyon "N" cloth in bridging arterial defects: Experimental and clinical. Ann Surg 140:324, 1954.
4. Blumenberg RM, Gelfand ML: Failure of knitted Dacron as an arterial prosthesis. Surgery 81:493, 1977.
5. Carrel A, Guthrie CG: Uniterminal and biterminal venous transplantations. Surg Gynecol Obstet 2:266, 1906.
6. DeBakey ME, Cooley DA, Crawford ES, et al: Clinical application of a new flexible knitted Dacron arterial substitute. Am Surg 24:862, 1958.
7. Debski R, Borovetz H, Haubold A, Hardesty R: Polytetrafluoroethylene grafts coated with ULTI carbon. Trans Am Soc Artif Intern Organs 28:456, 1982.
8. Edwards WS: Arterial grafts. Past, present, and future. Arch Surg 113:1225, 1978.
9. Edwards WS, Lyons C: Three years' experience with peripheral arterial grafts of crimped nylon and Teflon. Surg Gynecol Obstet 107:62, 1958.
10. Edwards WS, Tapp JS: Chemically treated nylon tubes as arterial grafts. Surgery 38:61, 1955.
11. Freischlag JA, Moore WS. Clinical experience with a collagen-impregnated knitted Dacron vascular graft. Ann Vasc Surg 4:449, 1990.
12. Fuchs JCA, Mitchener JS, Hagen P: Postoperative changes in autologous vein grafts. Ann Surg 188:1, 1978.
13. Gaylis H: Pathogenesis of anastomotic aneurysms. Surgery 90:509, 1981.
14. Goyanes DJ: Substitution plastica de las arterias por las venas, ó arterioplastia venosa, aplicada, como nuevo metodo, al tratamiento de los aneurismas. El Siglo Medico, Sept. 1, 1906, p 346; Sept. 8, 1906, p 561.
15. Graham LM, Burkel WE, Ford JW, et al: Immediate seeding of enzymatically derived endothelium in Dacron vascular grafts. Arch Surg 115:1289, 1980.
16. Gross RE, Hurwitt ES, Bill AH Jr, et al: Preliminary observations on the use of human arterial grafts in the treatment of certain cardiovascular defects. N Engl J Med 239:578, 1948.
17. Karkow WS, Cranley JJ, Cranley RD, et al: Extended study of aneurysm formation in umbilical vein grafts. J Vasc Surg 4:486, 1986.
18. Kwaan JHM, Connolly JE: Successful management of prosthetic graft infection with continuous povidone-iodine irrigation. Arch Surg 116:716, 1981.
19. Leather RP, Shah DM, Karmody AM: Infrapopliteal arterial bypass for limb salvage: Increased patency and utilization of the saphenous vein used "in situ." Surgery 90:1000, 1981.
20. Leather RP, Shah DM, Buchbinder D, et al: Further experience with the saphenous vein used in situ for arterial bypass. Am J Surg 142:506, 1981.
21. Malone JM, Moore WS, Campagna G, et al: Bacteremic infectability of vascular grafts: The influence of pseudointimal integrity and duration of graft function. Surgery 78:211, 1975.
22. Moore WS, Chvapil M, Seiffert G, et al: Development of an infection-resistant vascular prosthesis. Arch Surg 116:1403, 1981.
23. Nunn DB, Freeman MH, Hudgins PC: Postoperative alterations in size of Dacron aortic grafts. Ann Surg 189:741, 1979.
24. Rosenberg N, Gaughran ERL, Henderson J, et al: The use of segmental arterial implants prepared by enzymatic modification of heterologous blood vessels. Surg Forum 6:242, 1955.
25. Sanders RJ, Kempczinski RF, Hammond W, et al: The significance of graft diameter. Surgery 88:856, 1980.
26. Sauvage LR, Berger K, Beilin LB, et al: Presence of endothelium in an axillary femoral graft of knitted Dacron with an external velour surface. Ann Surg 182:749, 1975.
27. Sauvage LR, Berger K, Mansfield PB, et al: Future directions in the development of arterial prostheses for small and medium caliber arteries. Surg Clin North Am 54:213, 1974.
28. Sauvage LR, Berger K, Nakagawa Y, et al: An external velour surface for porous arterial prostheses. Surgery 70:940, 1971.
29. Sauvage LR, Berger K, Wood SJ, et al: Interspecies healing of porus arterial prostheses: Observations, 1960–1974. Arch Surg 109:698, 1974.
30. Scales JT: Tissue reactions to synthetic materials. Proc R Soc Med 46:647, 1953.
31. Soyer T, Lempinen M, Cooper P, et al: A new venous prosthesis. Surgery 72:864, 1972.
32. Szilagyi DE, Elliott JP, Hageman JH, et al: Biologic fate of autogenous vein implants as arterial substitutes: Clinical, angiographic and histopathologic observations in femoro-popliteal operations for atherosclerosis. Ann Surg 178:232, 1973.
33. Wylie EJ: Vascular replacement with arterial autografts. Surgery 57:14, 1965.

27

The Arterial Autograft

Ronald J. Stoney, M.D., and Daniel P. Connelly, M.D.

• • •

Arterial autografts for vascular replacement were introduced in 1964 at the University of California Medical Center in San Francisco.[1] The past 28 years have provided an opportunity to examine the usefulness and durability of this graft, which has been employed for a wide range of arterial problems.[2–5] The results of over 400 autograft reconstructions support the contention that it is the ideal arterial graft because it retains its viability, demonstrates proportional arterial growth when used in children, does not degenerate with time, heals in an infected field, and exhibits normal flexibility at points of joint motion.

Experimental results showing that an optimal compliance match at an arterial graft anastomosis leads to a reduction in graft thrombosis may help to explain the excellent patency seen with arterial autograft reconstruction.[6]

PROCUREMENT

Autografts can be procured from various donor sites in the arterial system (Fig. 27–1). Whenever possible, the autograft selected should closely approximate the size of the artery being replaced (Table 27–1). Often, the autograft can be obtained from a donor site within the same surgical field in which the arterial reconstruction is to be performed. The splenic artery should be avoided for use as an autograft in older patients because it is frequently kinked or coiled, making it unsuitable for transplantation (Fig. 27–2).

Reconstruction of the donor site when the common or external iliac artery segments are used may be performed satisfactorily with prosthetic grafts. Excised internal iliac arterial segments, frequently used as renal artery grafts, do not require replacement. Arterial autografts also may be constructed from an arterial segment previously occluded by atherosclerosis. The thrombosed superficial femoral artery has been the most commonly used donor vessel of this type (Fig. 27–3). Normal patency is restored by an eversion or semi-closed endarterectomy. Such a segment can be used as a conduit for revascularization after removal of an infected synthetic graft. The vessel is also suitable for use as a patch or bypass graft for distal reconstruction of the profunda femoris artery (Fig. 27–4).

Although most arterial autografts are used in the abdomen or groin, more remote arteries (e.g., carotid, popliteal) occasionally may require an autograft for repair. When arterial autografts are used in these positions, donor artery is seldom available within the same operative field. In these cases donor artery may be harvested from the iliac vessels using an oblique lower abdominal incision and a retroperitoneal approach. This incision is well tolerated by the patient and allows for harvest of 4 to 7 cm of internal iliac artery. Increased conduit length may be obtained by removing the common and external iliac arteries and reconstructing these vessels with synthetic material (see Table 27–1).

In patients with internal carotid artery occlusion and symptomatic ipsilateral external carotid artery disease, the

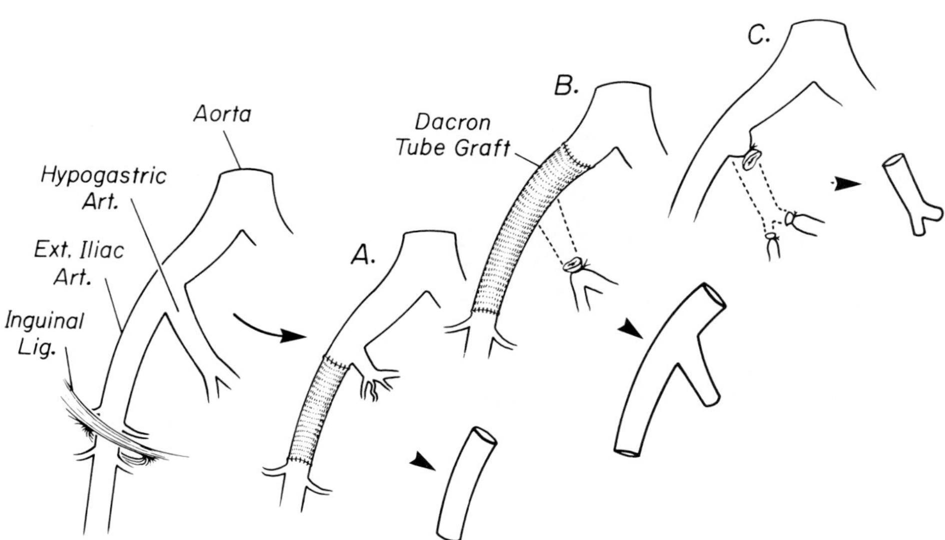

FIGURE 27–1. Procurement of iliac autografts. As depicted here, the iliac arteries are the best source of arterial autografts that can be obtained in grafts of various diameters and lengths, with or without distal branches.

Table 27–1. Arterial Autograft Sizes and Recipient Arterial Sites

Autograft	Size: Length (cm)	Size: Diameter (mm)	Recipient Site
Internal iliac	4–5	7–8	Renal Visceral
External iliac	7–10	6–8	Carotid Renal Common femoral Popliteal
Superficial femoral	10–20	5–6	Common femoral Profunda Cross-femoral subcutaneous bypass

occluded internal carotid artery may be utilized to facilitate external carotid endarterectomy. This can be accomplished by harvesting the internal carotid artery and using it as a patch angioplasty (see Fig. 27–4) or by leaving the internal carotid artery attached and rolling it over onto the external carotid artery as a patch (Fig. 27–5).[7]

PLACEMENT

End-to-end autograft anastomoses, using interrupted sutures, are recommended whenever circumferential arterial defects are repaired. Partial defects in the circumference of an artery are covered with an opened arterial autograft used as a patch or gusset, and the anastomosis is performed with a continuous suture (see Fig. 27–5). When coverage of the autograft is not possible because of infection or inadequate skin flaps, secondary wound healing will consistently occur, leading to granulation over the exposed functioning autograft. No thrombosis, impairment in autograft healing, or secondary hemorrhage has occurred under these circumstances of delayed wound healing.

INDICATIONS

Although an arterial autograft is the ideal arterial substitute, size and availability preclude its use in most circumstances requiring aortic replacement (i.e., abdominal aortic aneurysm or aortoiliac femoral occlusive disease). Nevertheless, autografts are used preferentially for certain primary vascular repairs as well as in secondary repairs to reconstruct defects in arterial continuity following the removal of an infected prosthesis.

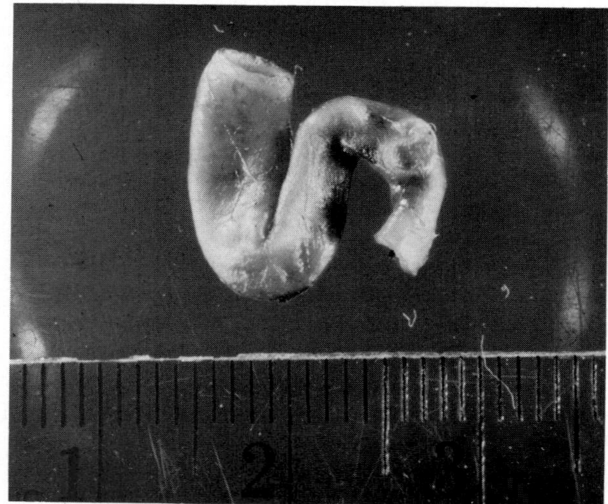

FIGURE 27–2. Photograph of a harvested splenic artery. The obvious tortuosity makes this an unacceptable vessel for use as an autograft.

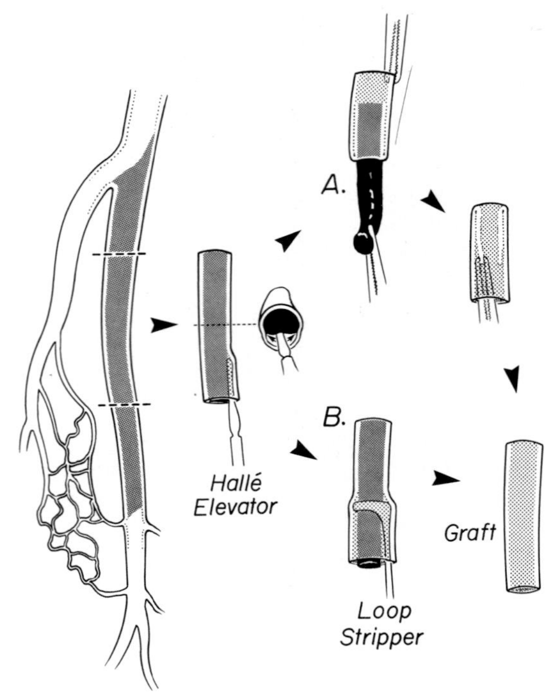

FIGURE 27–3. An occluded superficial femoral artery is an alternative source of arterial autograft, which can be prepared by either of the techniques depicted here. *A*, Eversion endarterectomy. *B*, Loop endarterectomy.

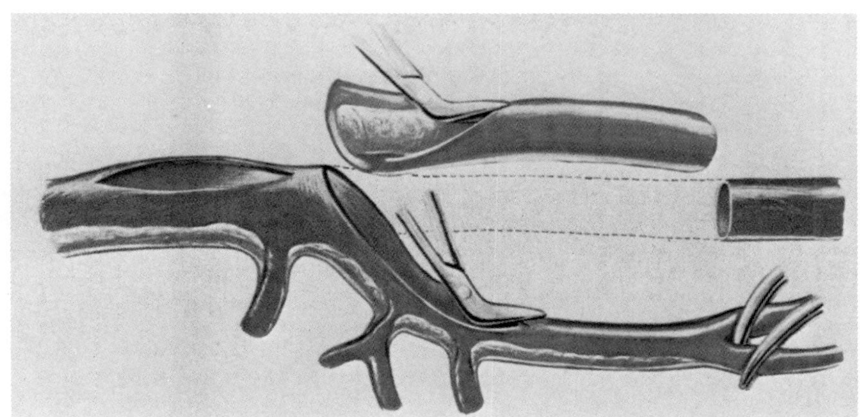

FIGURE 27–4. A chronically thrombosed superficial femoral artery has been removed and is being prepared for placement as a patch onto the profunda femoris artery. (From Wylie EJ, Stoney RJ, Ehrenfeld WK, et al: Manual of Vascular Surgery. New York, Springer-Verlag, 1986, vol. 2, p 15.)

PRIMARY ARTERIAL RECONSTRUCTIONS

Renal Artery Fibrous Dysplasia

Renal artery occlusive lesions involving portions of the main renal artery and its branches produce renovascular hypertension. The fibromuscular dysplastic lesions of the renal arteries are particularly amenable to arterial autograft reconstruction. The hypogastric artery is the same diameter as the renal artery, and its branches closely approximate those of the renal artery branches in size and configuration (Fig. 27–6). Durable results have been achieved in 135 patients who underwent 143 aortorenal arterial autograft reconstructions.[3, 8] Arteriographic follow-up over 20 years has revealed only one late graft occlusion, one anastomotic stenosis, and one aneurysmal dilatation (this aneurysm has remained arteriographically stable for more than 10 years). Hypertension was cured or improved in 96 per cent of the patients, supporting our view that this is the preferred graft for patients with nonatherosclerotic renal artery lesions of the primary, secondary, or tertiary branches causing renovascular hypertension.

Peripheral Aneurysms

Carotid, popliteal, and femoral artery aneurysms are ideal sites for arterial autografts: The lengths of the diseased

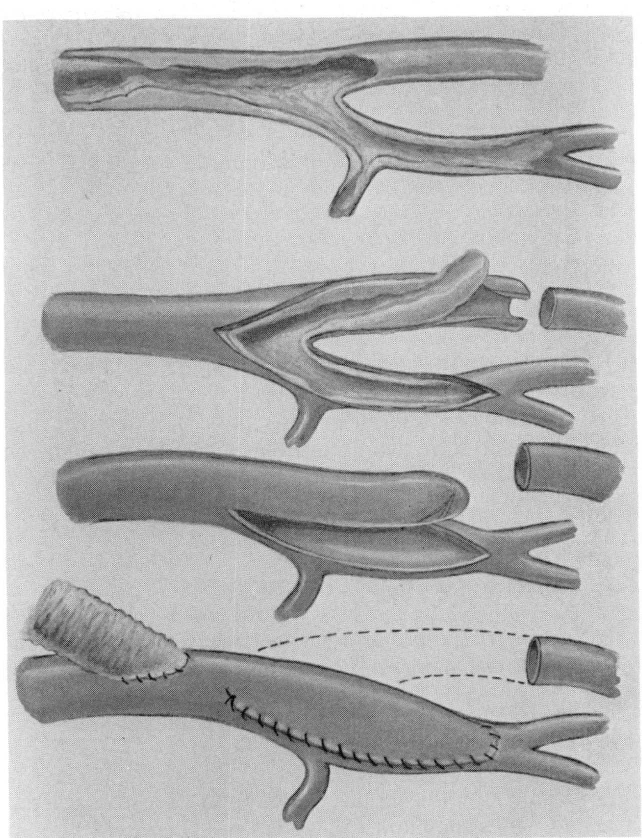

FIGURE 27–5. Profunda femoral endarterectomy utilizing the occluded superficial femoral artery as a transposed patch angioplasty. This allows autogenous hinge-flap closure. (From Stoney RJ, Effeney DJ: Wylie's Atlas of Vascular Surgery—Basic Considerations and Techniques. Philadelphia, JB Lippincott, 1992.)

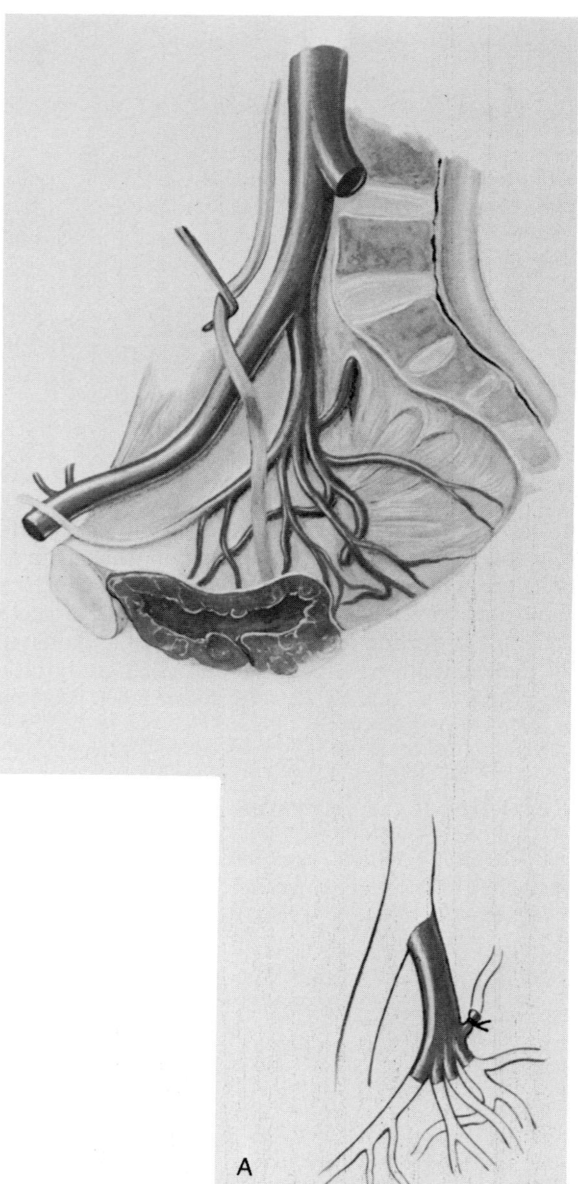

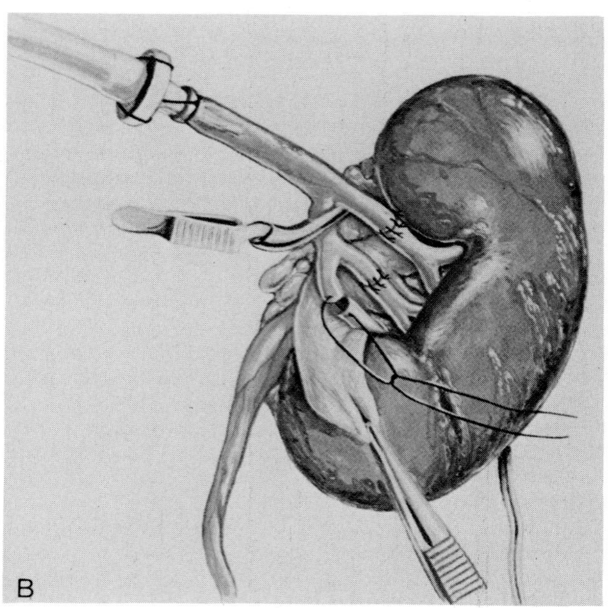

FIGURE 27–6. Illustration of a hypogastric artery demonstrating its terminal branches *(A)*, which make this vessel ideal for use when branched renal artery reconstruction is required *(B)*. (*A* and *B*, From Wylie EJ, Stoney RJ, Ehrenfeld WK, et al: Manual of Vascular Surgery. New York, Springer-Verlag, 1986, vol. 2, p 221.)

segments are short, and their normal diameter closely approximates that of the external iliac artery (Fig. 27–7). For common femoral artery aneurysms, the donor external iliac artery segment is frequently tortuous and can be mobilized and extended to the femoral bifurcation for repair of these aneurysms (Fig. 27–8).[9]

Renal and Visceral Aneurysms

The internal iliac artery is an ideal replacement for renal or visceral aneurysms requiring resection (Fig. 27–9).

Arterial Trauma

Prosthetic grafts should not be used to restore arterial continuity after trauma if the wound has been heavily contaminated and infection appears likely. In such circumstances, an autogenous graft of artery or vein may be harvested from a remote clean field and used as a satisfactory substitute. The resulting defect in donor arterial continuity is repaired with a suitable prosthetic conduit.

SECONDARY ARTERIAL RECONSTRUCTIONS

Infected Prostheses

When planning the removal of a patent infected prosthesis, another source of perfusion is usually necessary to supply the limbs. Although extra-anatomic bypass techniques that avoid the septic field are available, in the authors' experience, the infected graft-artery segment in the

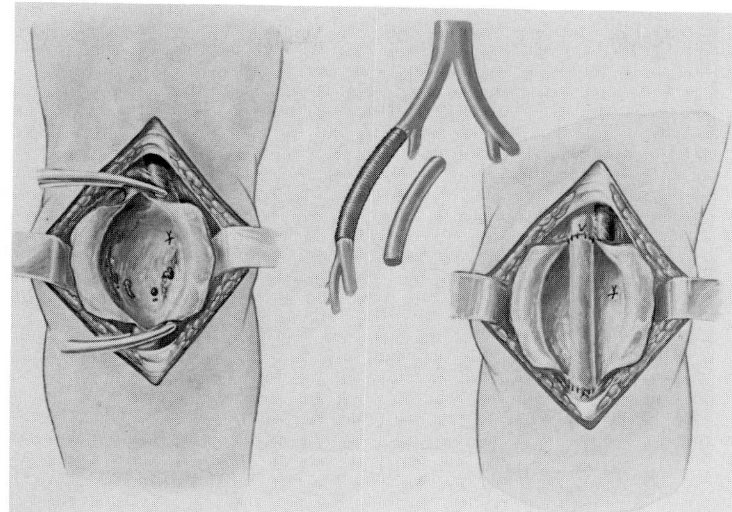

FIGURE 27–7. An exposed and opened popliteal artery aneurysm being replaced with an external iliac artery autograft. The harvest site is reconstructed with a prosthetic graft. (From Wylie EJ, Stoney RJ, Ehrenfeld WK, et al: Manual of Vascular Surgery. New York, Springer-Verlag, 1986, vol. 2, p 58.)

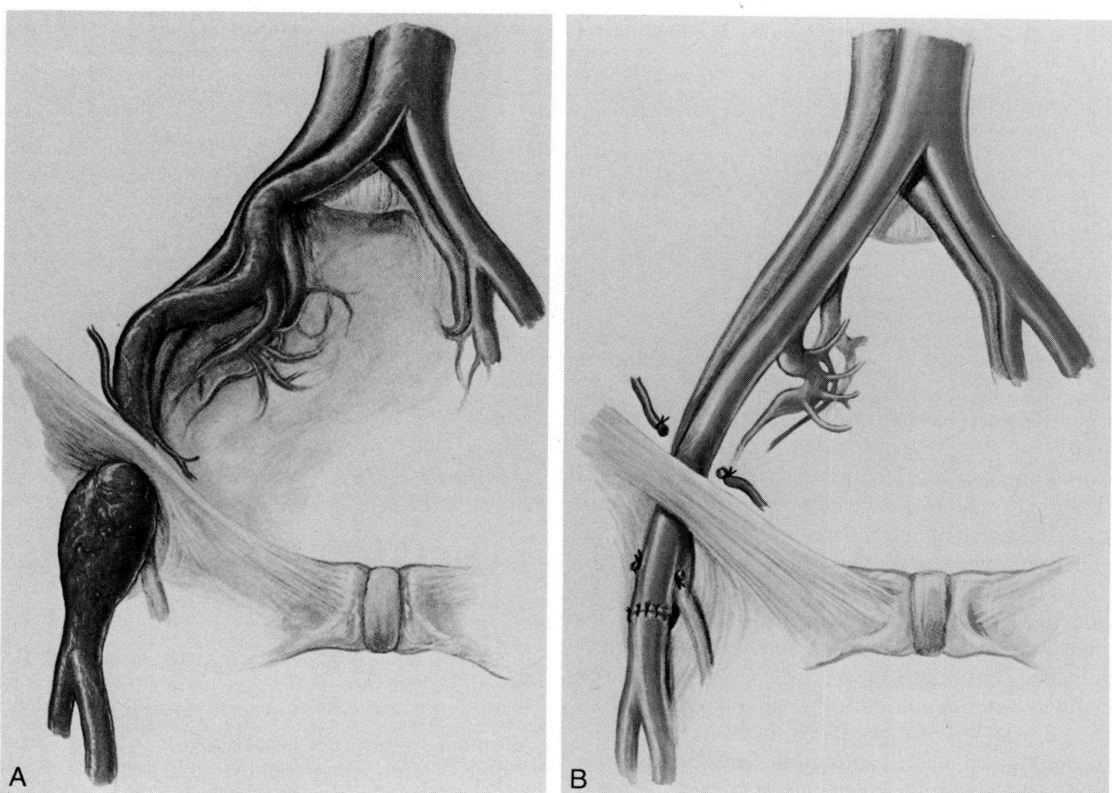

FIGURE 27–8. A femoral artery aneurysm before *(A)* and after *(B)* reconstruction with external iliac artery. (*A* and *B*, From Wylie EJ, Stoney RJ, Ehrenfeld WK, et al: Manual of Vascular Surgery. New York, Springer-Verlag, 1986, vol. 2, p 61.)

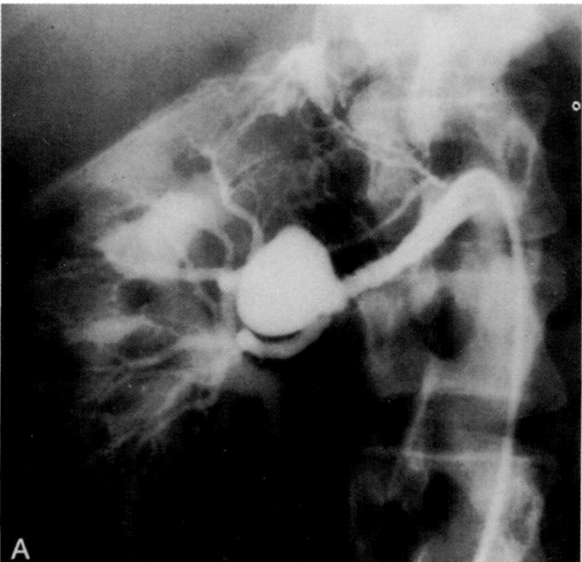

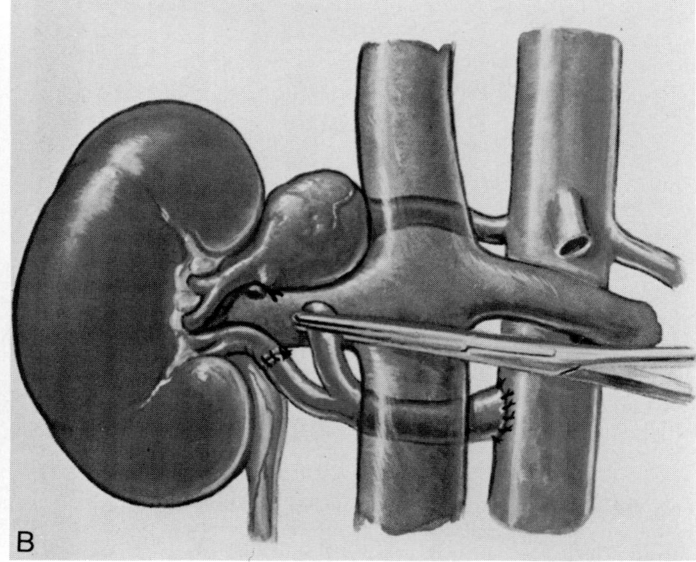

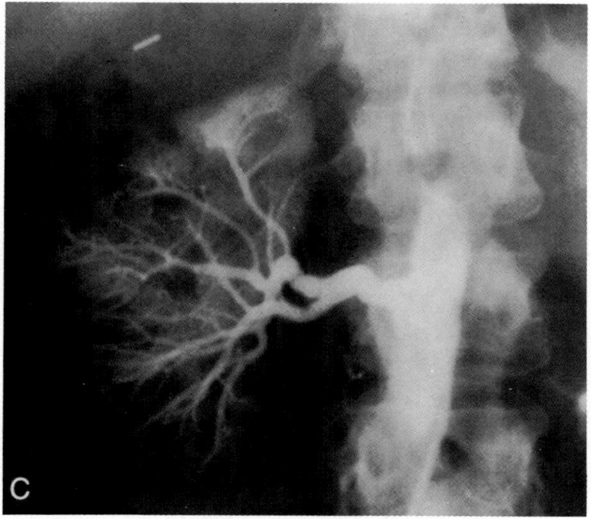

FIGURE 27–9. *A*, Arteriogram demonstrating a renal artery aneurysm at the bifurcation of the renal artery. *B*, In situ branched autograft repair. *C*, Postoperative arteriogram demonstrating a patent reconstruction. (*A–C*, From Wylie EJ, Stoney RJ, Ehrenfeld WK, et al: Manual of Vascular Surgery. New York, Springer-Verlag, 1986, vol. 2, p 61.)

groin can be reconstructed in situ using an autogenous cross-femoral graft. We prefer a conduit of arterial autograft obtained from either occluded superficial femoral artery or, if needed, the previously bypassed external iliac artery (Fig. 27–10). No subsequent infections of the cross-femoral autograft repair have appeared in patients in whom this technique has been used.[10]

Mycotic aneurysms or primarily infected arterial repairs in other sites (e.g., popliteal artery–carotid bifurcation) occur rarely, but when they do they can be excised and replaced with arterial autograft. Thus, when excision of any infected arterial segment produces distal ischemia and remote bypass is not feasible, autografts from the iliac arteries can be used and may be expected to heal without failure.

Anastomotic False Aneurysms

This complication of graft healing, often due to suture or arterial wall degeneration, usually appears at sites of active motion near a major joint. Autogenous artery segments can be useful as interposition grafts to repair the defect after excision of the aneurysms.[11]

LATE FAILURES OF ARTERIAL RECONSTRUCTION

Any late complication following an arterial reconstruction may threaten its function or contribute to its subsequent failure. Therefore, reoperative arterial repairs are indicated to manage late complications of arterial reconstruction. These complications include progression of the original disease, false aneurysm formation whether anastomotic or primary, altered healing of the arterial repair or prosthetic implant, and deterioration of the host artery or prosthesis.

The objective of a reoperative arterial repair is to reestablish or preserve arterial or prosthetic graft patency. Patch and conduit arterial autografts have proved suitable for accomplishing these objectives. Since many reoperative

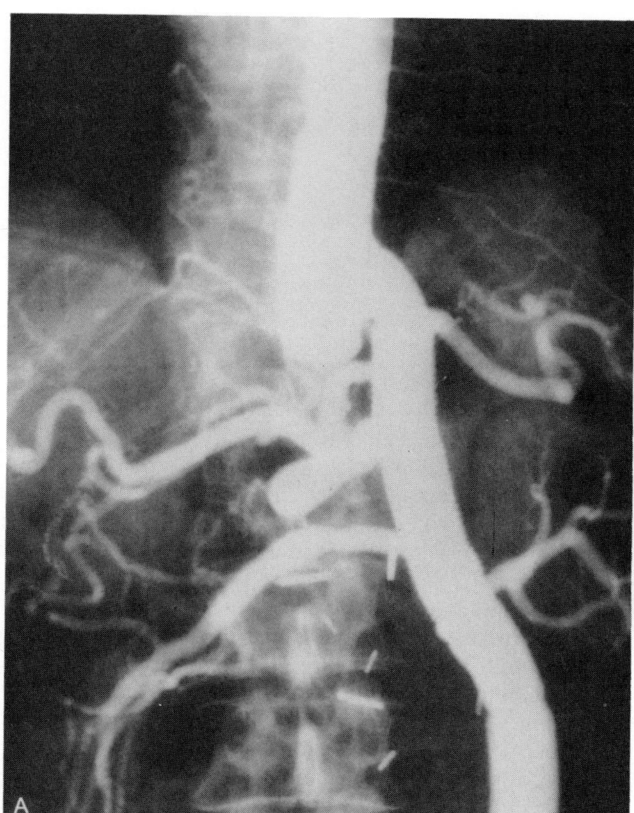

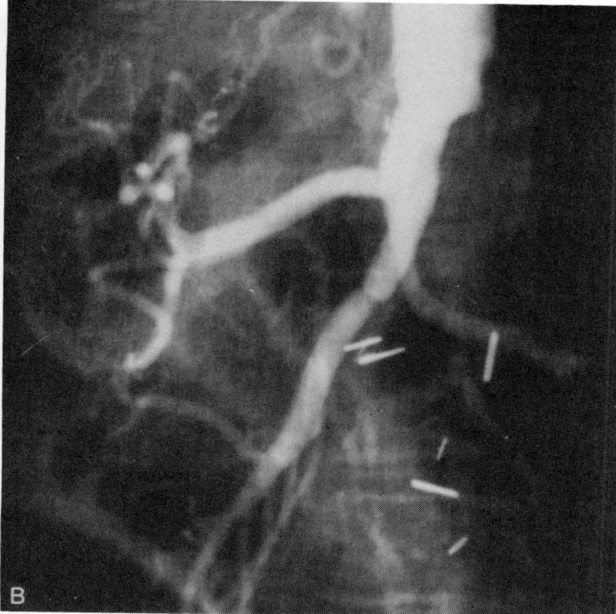

FIGURE 27–10. *A*, Radiograph of an infected aortobifemoral bypass graft originating from the thoracic aorta. Contaminated synthetic grafts to the visceral circulation originated from this prosthesis. *B*, Radiograph showing the completed reconstruction after graft excision. Harvested right common, internal, and external iliac arteries were utilized to reconstruct the visceral circulation. The proximal anastomosis originates from the stump of the aorta. The origin of the excised graft was repaired using a patch from the residual common iliac artery. (*A* and *B*, From Stoney RJ, Effeney DJ: Wylie's Atlas of Vascular Surgery—Complications Requiring Reoperation. Philadelphia, JB Lippincott, 1991.)

arterial repairs are required because of late failure of an original revascularization of the lower extremity, repair in the limb (usually the groin region) is common. Conduit or patch autografts are easily harvested from the chronically occluded superficial femoral artery within the same operative field (see Fig. 27–3). A suitable length of the artery can be reclaimed as illustrated to provide an autograft for a variety of revascularization requirements. Of more than 400 arterial autograft reconstructions performed at the University of California Medical Center in San Francisco over the past 28 years, nearly a quarter (98) were used in cases of late failure of a previous arterial repair.[12] Most of these were either combined with in situ thromboendarterectomy or used alone to repair defects in vascular continuity. Successful secondary repairs with durable results were achieved in nearly every patient.

Summary

The arterial autograft is an ideal arterial substitute, since it retains its function as an artery despite its transplantation to a new site. The suitability of the arterial autograft for certain primary aortic branch reconstructions, arterial repair in growing children, complex distal renal artery reconstructions, and complications of vascular reconstructions, including sepsis, makes it an essential part of the armamentarium of the complete vascular surgeon.

Acknowledgments: *This chapter was supported in part by the Pacific Vascular Research Foundation, San Francisco, California.*

References

1. Wylie EJ: Vascular replacement with arterial autografts. Surgery 57:14, 1965.
2. Stoney RJ, Wylie EJ: Arterial autografts. Surgery 67:18, 1970.
3. Lye CR, String ST, Wylie EJ, et al: Aortorenal arterial autografts. Arch Surg 110:1321, 1975.
4. Stoney RJ, DeLuccia N, Ehrenfeld WK, et al: Aortorenal arterial autografts. Arch Surg 116:1416, 1981.
5. Ehrenfeld WK, Stoney RJ, Wylie EJ: Autogenous arterial grafts. *In* Stanley JC, et al (eds): Biologic and Synthetic Vascular Prostheses. New York, Grune & Stratton, 1982.
6. Abbott WM, Megerman J, Hasson JE, et al: Effect of compliance mismatch on vascular graft patency. J Vasc Surg 5:376, 1987.
7. Kent CG, Salvatierra O, Reilly LM, et al: Evolving strategies for the repair of complex renovascular lesions. Ann Surg 206:272, 1987.
8. Inahara T: Aneurysms of the common femoral artery: reconstruction with the mobilized external iliac artery. Am J Surg 111:795, 1966.
9. Qvarfordt PG, Reilly LM, Ehrenfeld WK, et al: Surgical management of vascular graft infections—local treatment, graft excision, and methods of revascularization. *In* Bernhard VM, Towne JB (eds): Complications in Vascular Surgery. New York, Grune & Stratton, 1985, pp 499–511.
10. Stoney RJ, Albo RJ, Wylie EJ: False aneurysms occurring after arterial grafting operations. Am J Surg 110:157, 1965.
11. Qvarfort PG, Stoney RJ: Arterial Autografts. Acta Chir Scand 529(Suppl):37, 1985.
12. Wylie EJ, Stoney RJ, Ehrenfeld WK, et al: Manual of Vascular Surgery, vol. II. New York, Springer-Verlag, 1986.

28

The Autogenous Vein

Jonathan B. Towne, M.D.

• • •

For revascularization of the lower extremity, the autogenous vein is the conduit of choice for small-caliber arterial bypass. This superiority of autogenous conduits has been repeatedly documented in the vascular surgical literature.[1–4] Since the 1970s there has been a progressive improvement in the results of lower extremity bypass, which is attributed to better vein harvest techniques, improvements in operative technique, including the use of small-caliber sutures, and optical magnification. Intraoperative assessment of the vascular repair with angiography, duplex imaging, and Doppler flow studies has become routine, and patients are followed with postoperative surveillance protocols. As a result of these improvements, the type of conduit used now remains the primary determinant of long-term graft patency.

With the development of cellular biology research techniques, a new understanding about the function of the autogenous vein is evolving. Instead of serving as a passive conduit, the vein graft actively participates in keeping blood fluid as it passes over the endothelium. This chapter will review our current knowledge of the structure and function of the autogenous vein and the reasons for its high quality as a conduit for lower limb arterial reconstruction.

ANATOMY

The greater saphenous vein is the longest vein in the body; it begins at the medial aspect of the dorsum of the foot and terminates in the femoral vein just distal to the inguinal ligament. Classically, it ascends anterior to the medial malleolus along the medial side of the leg in relationship to the saphenous nerve.[5] It passes posterior to the medial condyle of the tibia and femur and usually traverses the medial thigh, gaining access to the common femoral vein at the fossa ovalis. There are significant variations in normal saphenous vein anatomy that are of interest to surgeons who use the vessel for arterial reconstruction.

In a classic study from Albany, Shah and his group evaluated the greater saphenous venous system in 385 legs of 331 patients.[6] Their findings comprise the most detailed account of the greater saphenous vein anatomy and its variations that is available in the literature. Only 38.2 per cent of their venograms demonstrated a conventional saphenous vein that had a continuous trunk arising anterior to the ankle and ending in the common femoral vein. The other 61.8 per cent of venograms demonstrated significant variations, which the authors studied by anatomic region. In the thigh, the vein presented as a single trunk in 65 per cent of patients. This was the classic medially located trunk in 60 per cent. However, in 5 per cent the trunk of the saphenous vein was located in a more lateral position. A complete double system was present in 11 per cent of patients, and an additional 15 per cent had portions of a double system. Less common variations occurred in 9 per cent. Usually the double trunks in the thigh rejoined and formed a single trunk within 10 cm of the knee joint. However, occasionally the junction occurred more proximally. In the leg, the saphenous vein had a single trunk in only 45 per cent of patients. The usual location of the saphenous vein was 1 to 2 cm posterior to the medial border of the tibia. The vein also occurred in a more posterior position, which Shah and colleagues defined as 4 to 6 cm posterior to the medial border of the tibia. In 46 per cent of patients a well-defined double trunk was present, of which the anterior branch was the most dominant. The bifurcation of the saphenous vein usually occurred within 5 cm of the knee joint but occasionally occurred at the midthigh level. Vieth and associates, in an earlier study using the preoperative saphenous venography in 100 extremities in 60 patients, noted an absence of the saphenous vein in 4 per cent.[7] The exact incidence of total absence of the saphenous vein is not known, but it is important to realize that this anomaly can occur, and the surgeon needs to be prepared to deal with such eventualities.

The valves in the saphenous vein are classically bicuspid valves and on occasion may have only one cusp. The valve cusps are oriented parallel to the surface of the skin. The physiologic basis for this was described by Edwards, who demonstrated that if the valves are parallel to the surface of the skin, they remain competent when external pressure is applied to the leg.[8] Shah and colleagues encountered an average of 6.3 valves in each saphenous vein bypass that they performed. There usually is a valve at the fossa ovalis and one 5 cm distally. The number of valves in the remainder of the vein is variable and ranges from as few as one and to as many as 13.

Knowledge of the vagaries of the saphenous system is particularly important for surgeons who plan to prepare the vein for in situ bypass using angioscopic guidance to avoid exposing the entire vein. When a segment of identified vein does not appear to be of adequate caliber for a bypass, it may often be found in parallel with a totally or partially double system. By utilizing the best quality segments of the saphenous system, an autogenous conduit can usually be constructed.

ALTERNATIVE SOURCES OF AUTOGENOUS VEIN

There are many reasons why the saphenous vein is not usable. Most commonly, it has been harvested previously for coronary artery bypass or peripheral vascular surgery. On occasion, it may be congenitally absent or may have suffered the ravages of superficial phlebitis. The incidence of patients without an intact usable saphenous vein was 22 per cent in the series of Taylor and coworkers.[2] However, by using alternative sources of autogenous vein, they were able to perform lower extremity revascularization with autogenous material in 94 per cent of their patients.

The most obvious alternative source for a missing or inadequate saphenous vein is the saphenous vein in the contralateral leg. However, some surgeons are reluctant to resort to the contralateral saphenous vein because such a use removes the potential to use that vein for bypass vascular surgery in that limb; they believe that for limb salvage each leg should contribute its own autogenous conduit. An alternative source of autogenous vein is the lesser saphenous vein, which originates posterior to the lateral malleolus as a continuation of the lateral marginal vein.[5] It ascends proximally along the lateral margin of the Achilles tendon, coursing medially to reach the middle of the popliteal fossa, where it perforates the fascia and joins the popliteal vein. The lesser saphenous vein is accompanied through much of its course by the sural nerve. There are multiple variations in the lesser saphenous vein. It may perforate the fascia in the middle portion of the calf and then proceed in the proximal third of the calf in the subfascial position. The lesser saphenous vein may also be unusable for bypass because of previous episodes of phlebitis. The patency, size, and course of the lesser saphenous can be determined by duplex scanning prior to harvesting of the vein. Initially, intraoperatively, the patient is placed prone on the operating table to allow both lesser saphenous veins to be removed simultaneously. The incisions are closed, and the patient is turned to the supine position, reprepared, and draped. Although this approach takes more time, it allows the precise and gentle vein dissection that is necessary to obtain the optimum conduit. If the lesser saphenous vein is patent in both lower extremities, these two segments can be spliced together to perform most distal tibial bypasses.

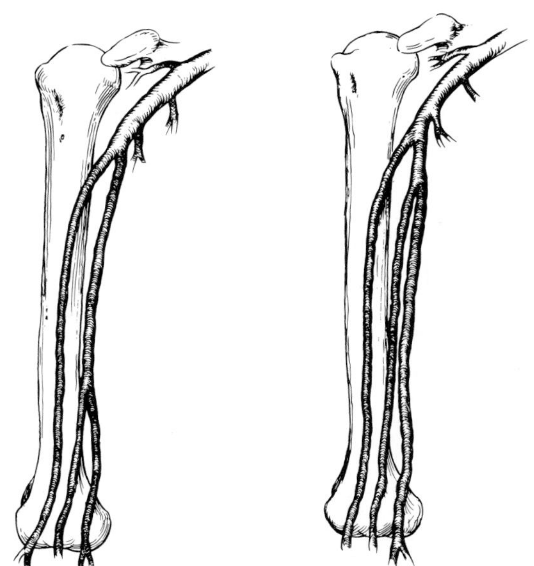

FIGURE 28–2. Variations in the confluence of the basilic and brachial veins. (From Andrus G, Harris RW: The place of arm veins in arterial revascularization. *In* Bergen J, Yao JST [eds]: Arterial Surgery: New Diagnostic and Operative Techniques. Orlando, FL, Grune & Stratton, 1988, p 526.)

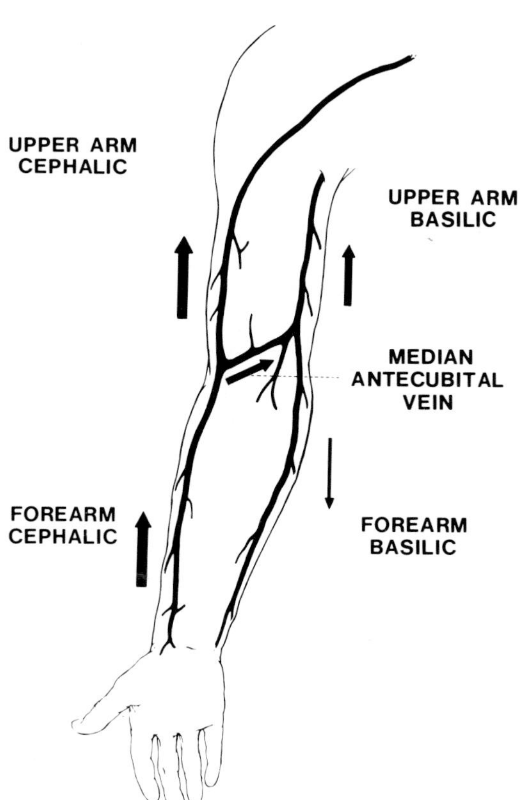

FIGURE 28–1. Order of preference of arm veins for alternative autogenous grafts: 1, cephalic (forearm and arm); 2, forearm cephalic–median antecubital–arm basilic; 3, basilic (forearm and arm); 4, composite (lower and upper extremity veins).

The cephalic vein also represents an alternative source of autogenous vein for use in vascular reconstructive surgery, and among some practitioners it is the favored alternative (Fig. 28–1).[9] The cephalic vein courses from the anatomic snuff box on the radial side of the wrist to the deltopectoral groove, where it joins the axillary vein. As with the saphenous vein in the leg, there are many anatomic variations in the arm veins (Figs. 28–2 and 28–3).[10] A dominant secondary branch may arise on the dorsum of the hand, joining the primary cephalic vein in the forearm. Double cephalic veins in the forearm may course in parallel and join together proximal to the antecubital fossa. Occasionally there may be an accessory cephalic vein that remains on the radial side of the cephalic vein and usually joins it at the elbow.

The basilic vein may also be used as an arterial conduit. It begins in the ulnar part of the dorsal venous network

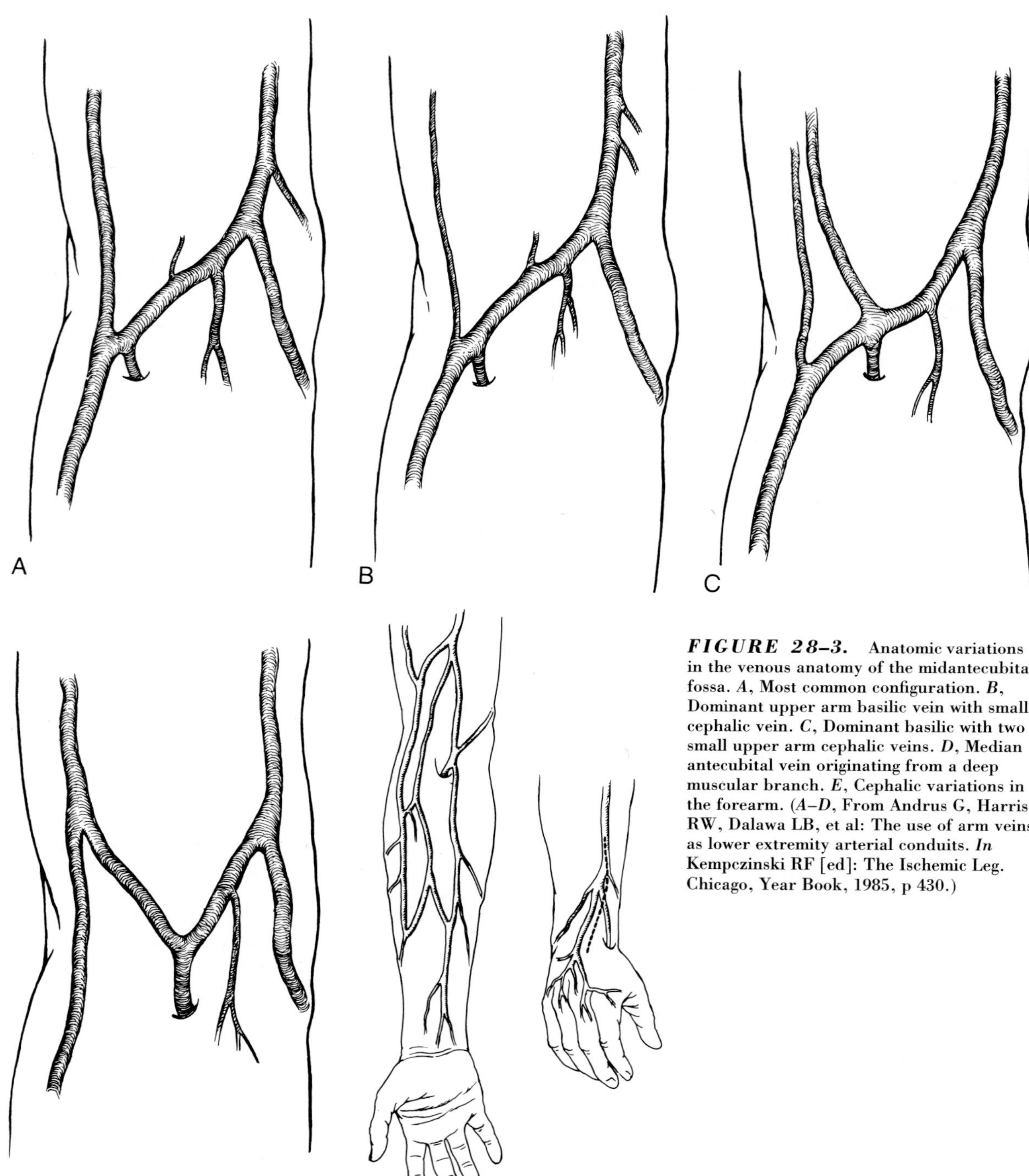

FIGURE 28–3. Anatomic variations in the venous anatomy of the midantecubital fossa. *A*, Most common configuration. *B*, Dominant upper arm basilic vein with small cephalic vein. *C*, Dominant basilic with two small upper arm cephalic veins. *D*, Median antecubital vein originating from a deep muscular branch. *E*, Cephalic variations in the forearm. (*A–D*, From Andrus G, Harris RW, Dalawa LB, et al: The use of arm veins as lower extremity arterial conduits. *In* Kempczinski RF [ed]: The Ischemic Leg. Chicago, Year Book, 1985, p 430.)

of the hand and runs proximally on the posterior surface of the ulnar side of the forearm, inclining toward the anterior surface distal to the elbow, where it is joined by the medial antecubital vein. Proximal to the elbow it ascends obliquely, crossing in the groove between the biceps and the pronator teres, and then crosses the brachial artery from which it is separated by the bicipital aponeurosis. It then runs proximally along the medial border of the biceps brachia, perforating the deep fascia distal to the middle of the arm. It ascends to the distal border of the teres major muscle, where it joins the brachial vein to form the axillary vein. There is great variation in the superficial veins of the forearm, and often a reciprocal relationship exists between the cephalic and basilic veins. One or the other may predominate with the other being absent. Because many patients with vascular occlusive disease have had multiple prior hospitalizations, the cephalic and basilic veins and their branches in the arm are often damaged because of previously placed intravenous lines and the need for many venipunctures for drawing blood.

Other potential sources of autogenous vein are the internal jugular vein, which can be used when a short segment of a large-caliber conduit is needed, as in injuries of the common femoral vein. The internal jugular vein is a better size match than the contralateral saphenous vein. It has been reported that the superficial femoral vein can be used as a conduit; however, this vein has never gained favor because of the difficulty of dissecting it and concerns about compromising the deep venous circulation of the leg.

MICROSCOPIC ANATOMY

The intima is a thin endothelial layer on the luminal surface of the vessel, lying on a fenestrated basement membrane.[11] In cross section, the intimal layer lies in folds along the inner surface of the vessel. Owing to poor cytoplasmic uptake of histologic stains, only the nuclei are seen distinctly. With en face sectioning, the orderly distribution of the nuclei in the endothelial cells can be appreciated. The smooth muscle cells are arranged in inner longitudinal and outer circumferential directions and are interlaced with collagen and elastic fibrils. Elastic fibrils appear to be oriented predominantly in the longitudinal direction.[11] The adventitia forms the outer layer of the vein wall and is frequently thicker than the media; it consists of a loose collagen network interspersed with vasa vasorum. Longitudinal or spirally arranged smooth muscle cells may appear in the portion of the adventitia adjacent to the media.[11]

PHYSIOLOGY

The autogenous vein serves as a superior conduit because it is a living structure that actively participates in keeping the flowing stream of blood liquid as it crosses its surface. A variety of molecules secreted by the vein wall have been identified. These include the glycosaminoglycans, which serve as cofactors for antithrombin III, and heparin cofactor II.[12] Thrombomodulin, protein C, and protein S are also secreted and together participate in inactivation of coagulant antihemophilic factor (factor VIII) and proaccelerin (factor V).[13] The endothelial cells also synthesize prostacyclin, a potent inhibitor of platelet aggregation and a stimulus for platelet disaggregation.[14, 15] More recently, Ratnoff and his group have demonstrated that endothelial cells secrete in addition a substance that inactivates Hageman factor, which prevents the first steps of the intrinsic pathway of thrombus formation.[12] Additional work has identified another potent, locally vasoactive substance known as endothelium-derived relaxing factor (EDRF).[16, 17] EDRF mediates vascular relaxation tonically in response to increased flow and to a variety of agonists (adenosine triphosphate, 5-hydroxytryptamine) that may be released by activated platelets. EDRF is also a potent inhibitor of platelet aggregation and adhesion. The chief function of EDRF is to restrict vasoconstriction and thrombus propagation at sites of vascular injury. Iba and associates have evaluated the ability of the vein endothelium to secrete tissue plasminogen activator, which triggers the fibrolytic cascade to maintain blood in a fluid state.[18]

TECHNIQUES OF VEIN HARVEST AND PREPARATION

There are three variables to be evaluated in the harvesting of autogenous veins: the pressure at which the vein is distended, the temperature at which the vein is stored, and the use of vasoactive agents to dilate the vein. A variety of reports have demonstrated the deleterious effect of high pressures in distending the saphenous vein prior to bypass. Kurusz and colleagues showed that the morphology of the endothelium of venous specimens was preserved when the distending pressure was limited to 200 mmHg.[19] In contrast, veins distended without pressure controls showed massive endothelial disruption. The control of pressure was a greater factor in endothelial preservation than the type of distending solution used (blood, saline, cardioplegic solution). Bonchek, in a similar study, demonstrated in a primate model that veins distended at high pressures (700 mmHg) showed severe damage to the endothelium and increased lipid uptake by the vein wall.[20] He stated that the upper limit of pressures used for vein distention and preparation should be in the 300- to 400-mmHg range. It is universally accepted that pressure needs to be carefully controlled in the distention of veins. Lawrie and associates also showed that pressurization of veins to 400 mmHg lessened EDRF relaxation compared with control veins.[16] This work basically provides functional evidence that substantiates the morphologic findings of previous investigators. Malone and his group detected changes in venous endothelial fibrolytic activity with increased pressures. As the pressure increased from control levels to 700 mmHg, fibrolytic activity progressively decreased, demonstrating the adverse effects of pressure on venous function.[21] Abbott and colleagues likewise demonstrated that hydrostatic dilatation is associated with a stiffening of the vein wall.[22]

The second factor affecting vein harvest is the use of papaverine to dilate veins either prior to or after vein harvest. LoGerfo and coworkers recommended percutaneous infiltration with papaverine along the course of the vein prior to making an incision to dissect the vein.[23] Endothelial morphology was best preserved when veins were treated with papaverine before they were excised and when a warm solution was used for the dilatation of the vein grafts. In addition to preservation of intimal morphology, dilatation of the veins with papaverine made them resistant to the adverse effects of pressure up to 500 mm of mercury. Similar findings were noted by Baumann and colleagues, who demonstrated that veins preserved with a combination of plasmalyte and papaverine showed the least degree of endothelial cell contraction, the best endothelial preservation, and no microaggregates of leukocytes on the surface.[24] They hypothesized that vigorous prolonged contracture of a vein leads to endothelial protrusion and sloughing. As the vein wall continues to contract beyond a certain critical limit, the total area of luminal surface upon which the endothelial lining rests becomes reduced to less than the total area of the endothelial cell layer. Because of their tight interendothelial junctions, the endothelial cells are unable to reorient themselves or slide over one another as do the smooth muscle cells in the media of the contracting wall, and they herniate into the lumen as they are disrupted from the vessel wall.

Sottiurai and his group studied the effects of high and low pressure vein distention and the effect of papaverine on a long-term canine jugular vein model.[25] They noted that mechanical distention of the vein to 150 mmHg or more induced endothelial damage, subendothelial leukocyte infiltration, and excessive intimal and medial fibroplasia. Papaverine protected the mural myoblast during mechanical distention, reduced medial fibroplasia, and enhanced intimal hyperplasia and elastic tissue formation in the media. Papaverine was useful in vein preparation because it protected the endothelium and smooth muscle cells and prevented leukocyte infiltration and medial fibrosis.

The temperature at which an excised vein should be stored is controversial. LoGerfo and coworkers suggested that optimum storage occurs at 4°C.[23] More recent studies in which the function of the vein graft was examined, either by the elaboration of molecules such as prostacyclin or by the graft's ability to dilate in response to a variety of agonists have suggested that cold storage is deleterious. Gundry and colleagues initially demonstrated that cold blood or saline immersion fully preserved the endothelium and that cold saline immersion produced medial edema.[26] Using prostacyclin as a metabolic marker of endothelial functional capacity, Bush and associates noted that normothermia (37°C) during vein graft storage was the optimal temperature for preserving prostacyclin production.[15] Hypothermic storage markedly impaired the subsequent capacity of the endothelium to produce prostacyclin. A progressive decrease in storage temperature resulted in a stepwise decrease in prostacyclin production following ex vivo storage. This work suggests that hypothermia induced direct and persistent metabolic injury in the endothelial cell. Lawrie and colleagues studied the effect of the storage solution on the activity of EDRF using an open ring preparation of fresh human saphenous veins.[16] They noted that veins stored at 2 to 4°C had severe depression of EDRF relaxation compared with those stored at 37°C. At this time the author recommends careful distention of the harvested veins with papaverine and storage at room temperature until the veins are inserted into the circulation.

OPERATIVE TECHNIQUES

It is essential in the harvesting of veins to use meticulous delicate techniques. Multiple incisions can be made in harvesting the saphenous vein if care is taken not to exert undue traction or pressure in moving the vein from beneath the skin bridges. When harvesting a lesser saphenous vein and arm veins, the author believes that a continuous incision makes the process easier. This is particularly true in dealing with arm veins because they are thin and easily injured. Prior to dissection, papaverine is injected along the course of the vein. Side branches are carefully mobilized and ligated so that the ligature does not impinge on the lumen of the vessel (Figs. 28–4 and 28–5). Previous mapping of the veins by duplex ultrasonography helps in placement of incisions. It is important to close vein harvest sites meticulously, avoiding suture techniques that create skin ischemia. Particularly in diabetic patients these wounds can become necrosed and slough, resulting in prolonged convalescence following the arterial bypass.

CONTROVERSIES IN AUTOGENOUS VEIN GRAFTING

There is probably no greater area of disagreement among vascular surgeons than that concerning the selection of techniques for lower extremity bypass. In patients who have intact saphenous veins there are three options: to perform a reverse vein graft, usually tunneled anatomically; to perform an in situ bypass; or to remove the vein, incise the valves, and place it in an antegrade fashion. The difficulty in resolving this issue lies in the fact that comparison of various series is difficult owing to several common variables: the smallest size of vein that is considered usable, the different proportions of limb salvage and claudication patients, and differences in operative technique. Excellent results have been reported with all techniques. Approximately 10 years ago, a variety of reports were published that indicated that the in situ technique was superior because it allowed better endothelial preservation. Buchbinder and colleagues published the results of canine carotid bypasses with jugular vein using both the in situ and the reverse technique.[27] They demonstrated that with the reverse technique there was extensive endothelial sloughing and denuding of the flow surface, whereas with the in situ technique a normal endothelium was retained. The biochemical basis of this was presented by Bush and coworkers who, also in a canine model, noted higher levels of prostacyclin from in situ grafts compared to veins that were reversed.[28] Cambria and associates compared in situ grafts with atraumatically dissected, nondistended reverse grafts and with grafts that were distended to a pressure of 500 mmHg. They noted that endothelial denudation was least, on average, in the in situ grafts, intermediate in the reverse grafts, and most severe in the reverse and distended grafts.[29] Perhaps of greater significance, there was no difference in endothelial fibrolytic activity between the in situ and the gently handled reverse grafts at 24 hours or 6 weeks after surgery. Batson and Sottiuri, also using a canine model, compared nonreversed, reversed, and in situ grafts and could distinguish no

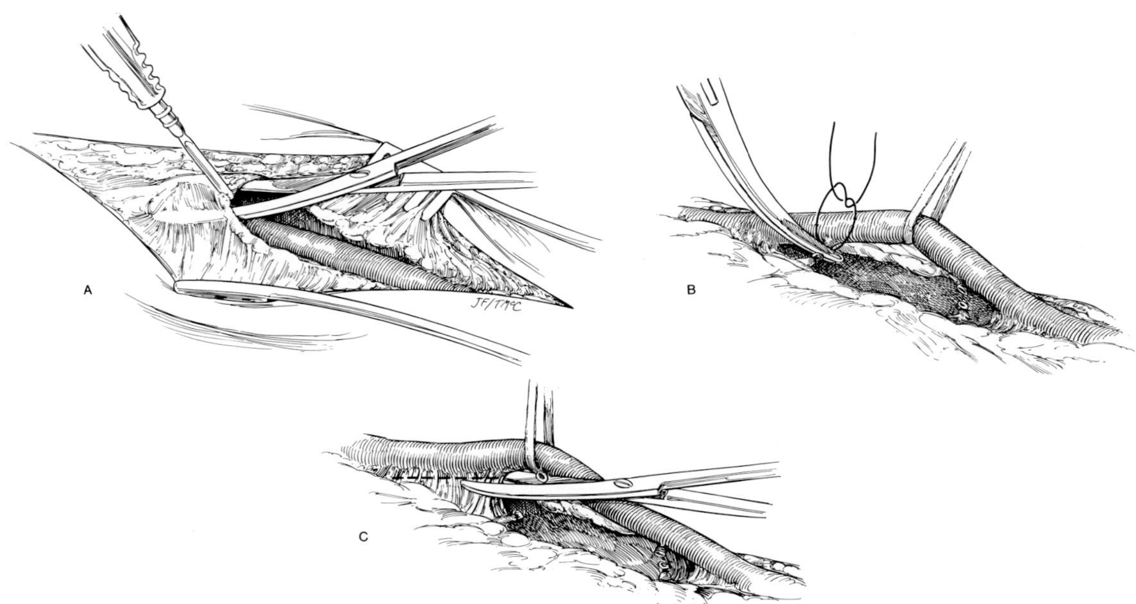

FIGURE 28–4. Vein harvest. *A*, the vein is exposed through the use of upward traction on the overlying tissues by spread scissor blades (or clamp) to protect the underlying vein from injury. *B*, Traction with a Silastic loop often reveals the location of tributaries, which are then ligated and divided with 1-mm ends. *C*, Trimming away tissue 2–3 mm from the vein allows small tributaries inadvertently cut to be later clamped and tied. (*A–C*, From Rutherford R: Atlas of Vascular Surgery. Philadelphia, WB Saunders, 1993, p 75.)

discernible morphologic differences in the translocated and in situ grafts.[30]

To date there has been no clinical study showing conclusively which bypass technique is better. Selection of one technique over another involves a series of trade-offs. With the in situ technique, there is a learning curve during which the unique techniques of the procedure must be mastered. The valves need to be incised, and patent side branches need to be ligated. There is an inherent incidence of reoperation because of residual competent valve cusps and missed arteriovenous fistulae. The advantages of the in situ technique are that the large end of the saphenous vein is anastomosed to the common femoral artery and the small end, which is a better size match, is anastomosed to the distal artery. With the in situ technique, the smaller veins have a potential use as bypass conduits. In the author's experience, conduits as small as 2 mm in diameter have been used in situ, and excellent long-term patency has been obtained. With the in situ technique, 2 mm is the lower limit of venous diameter that is usable for long bypasses owing to technical problems with valve ablation in the small veins. Precise data on vein diameter are currently absent from the literature originating from the major centers that champion the use of the reverse vein technique. Once this information is forthcoming, the disparity in results can be resolved. Whichever technique is used, the most important aspect is that the procedure be done well and the vein be of good quality.

Stratification of vein graft diameter has failed to produce statistically significant data for early and long-term

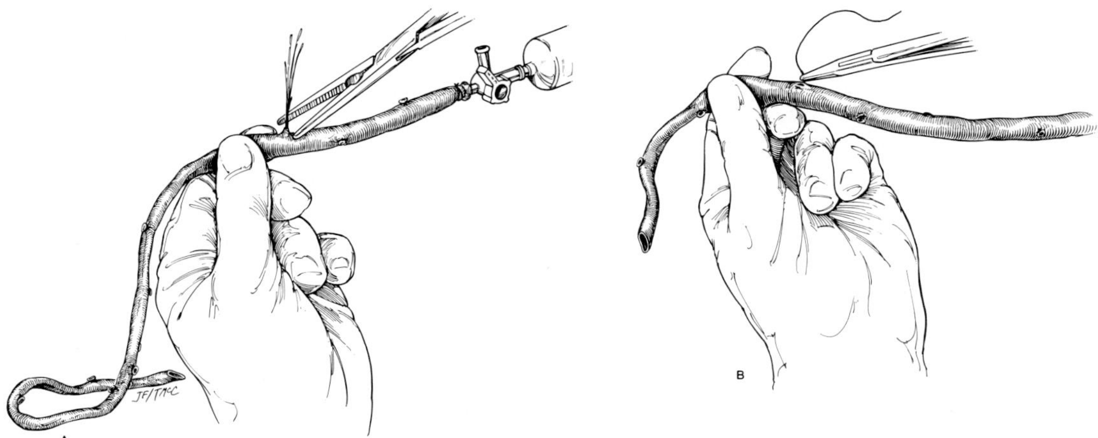

FIGURE 28–5. *A*, Gentle segmental dilatation of the vein may reveal leaks from small tributaries that were inadvertently cut. *B*, Avulsed tributaries must be repaired with fine sutures. (*A* and *B*, From Rutherford R: Atlas of Vascular Surgery. Philadelphia, WB Saunders, 1993, p 77.)

patency rates. The author noted that veins with a diameter of less than 3 mm had a 30-day patency (86 per cent), which was lower than that of veins 3 to 3.9 mm in diameter (97 per cent) or of those greater than 4 mm in diameter (98 per cent).[31] Sonnenfeld and Cronestrand, in a study of reversed veins used for femoral popliteal bypass, noted no difference in patency between veins less than 3 mm and those greater than 3 mm in diameter.[32] Because 82 per cent of their grafts were with the above-knee popliteal artery, and 70 per cent were in patients whose operative indication was claudication, it is hard to compare their results with the author's series. In a series in which all grafts were made to infrapopliteal arteries in limb salvage patients, Wengerter and colleagues noted decreased patency in reverse vein grafts of less than 3.5 mm in diameter.[33] It is the author's impression that the in situ technique allows the use of smaller diameter veins for distal bypass.

It is very difficult to evaluate the quality of the vein. Small diameter veins may be the result of previous phlebitic processes that have caused thickening of the valve wall, scarring of the vein endothelium, and loss of distensibility. These poor quality veins are not suitable for use as arterial conduits. Small veins that can be used for arterial bypasses must be thin walled and distensible. Some of the poor results reported by previous authors using small veins may have been due to the fact that the veins were of poor quality. When small veins are used for in situ bypass, meticulous surgical technique is required to prevent vein injury. Early in the author's experience the endothelium of small veins was lacerated during valve lysis because the small vein contracted around the valvotome. To prevent vein spasm in the small conduits, the author now infuses a solution of 500 ml of dextran, 60 mg of papaverine, and 500 international units of heparin into the distal vein to dilate it prior to inserting the valvotome. This technique prevents the smooth muscle of the vein from constricting around the valvotome.

Two-, three-, and four-year patency rates of small-diameter veins in the author's series were no different from the rates reported with larger diameter conduits, demonstrating the durability of small conduits.[31] Patients with small-diameter conduits may not have hemodynamically normal limbs. The function and flow characteristics of a graft can be quantitated by measuring graft flow velocity. For smaller-diameter grafts to carry the same volume of blood, the velocity of flow must be increased proportionately. In a previously reported study, the author noted that 23 per cent of bypasses had flow restrictive venous conduits.[34] These were characterized by small-diameter vein grafts, increased graft flow velocity, and smaller postoperative increases in ankle-brachial indices, which averaged 0.67 on the first postoperative day and increased to 0.89 at 1 week. Since these bypass grafts are utilized for patients who have limb-threatening ischemia, there is, nonetheless, sufficient blood flow to heal ulcers and prevent rest pain. The good quality small saphenous vein is a suitable conduit and should be considered for use in lower limb bypasses, particularly with the in situ technique.

The principal determinant of success with vein bypass surgery is the quality of the conduit. Portions of the vein may be absent because of previous coronary artery bypass or arterial bypass surgery, or the vein may have suffered previous phlebitic processes, rendering portions of the vein unusable. Regardless of which technique is used, modification of the conduit is necessary, ranging from localized repair of short stenotic segments to imposition of long segments in order to have sufficient graft to perform the autologous bypass. In addition, technical errors occurring during vein harvest or graft preparation by valve lysis can require vein modification. In a series of 361 consecutive bypasses, modifications were required in 23 per cent of the grafts.[35] Ten per cent of these were needed because of a sclerotic segment, a small-diameter vein, the presence of varicosities, or previous utilization. Modification in 13 per cent was necessitated by technical errors related to the in situ technique. These included vein injury, anastomotic stenosis, retained valves, and torsion of the graft. It is significant that this modification affected both the short- and long-term patency of the grafts, with 3-month patencies in the unmodified group being 20 per cent better. These data emphasize the need for meticulous dissection of the veins to avoid technical errors and illustrate the fact that, if multiple repairs of the vein are required, the results are still reasonable but not as good as if a virgin, continuous length of vein had been used.

LONG-TERM CHANGES IN VEIN GRAFTS

Because the vein is a biologic conduit, it has a dynamic life. Deterioration of the vein graft can occur throughout its life and is related to specific processes at various time intervals. Most changes that occur in a graft during the first 30 days are related to technical errors in the construction of the bypass, patient selection, or quality of the conduit (Fig. 28–6). Problems that occur in the interval between 30 days and 2 years are usually attributed to fibrointimal hyperplasia, which occurs at sites of anastomosis, areas of vein repair, and sites of valve incisions (Fig. 28–7). After 24 months, changes are primarily due to the progression of atherosclerosis. Excellent short- and long-term patency rates and limb salvage rates are now achievable. Technical success has outpaced physiologic and anatomic knowledge of the mature arterialized vein graft. Using color duplex ultrasonography, the author found that only 43 per cent of lower extremity bypass grafts, which had been patent for a median of 79 months, were normal and that nearly half of the normal grafts had needed either conduit revisions or correction of inflow or outflow disease progression to maintain patency. In addition, nearly one in five grafts harbored lesions that would pose a threat to continued long-term patency.

Atherosclerotic degeneration of saphenous vein grafts was first described in 1947, when a femoral interposition graft, which had been in place for 22 years, was removed and found to contain atheromatous plaques.[37] In 1973 Szilagyi and associates reported their experience with lower extremity saphenous vein grafts that had been followed by arteriography.[38] They described eight different morphologic findings in grafts of varying ages. Several of these were related to surgical technique, including suture stenosis caused by tying side branches too closely, long venous side

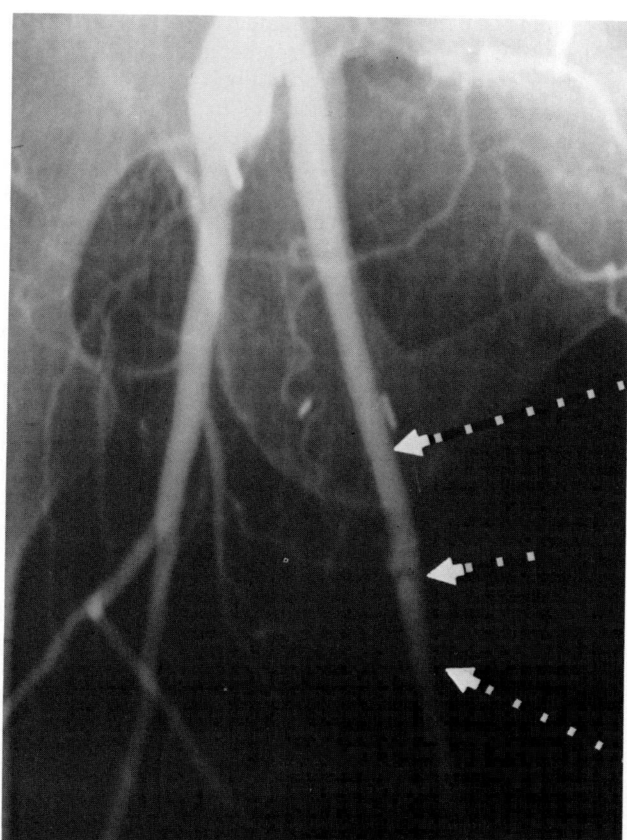

FIGURE 28–6. Retained valve *(arrows)* following in situ bypass.

branch stumps, and traumatic stenosis caused by clamps. They also described the changes that occur later, including intimal thickening, mild intimal hyperplasia at valve sites, arterial sclerotic irregularity, and aneurysmal dilatation. In the author's study, autogenous grafts were examined at least 4½ years after construction. The early postoperative changes noted by Szylagyi and associates were not detectable. However, the author's group did find three distinct atherosclerotic abnormalities: wall plaque, aneurysmal dilatation, and discrete stenosis. The most prevalent finding was wall plaque, which was present in all the abnormal grafts, although this was frequently overshadowed by more impressive stenosis or aneurysms. Typically, plaques were several centimeters long, multi-centric, ectogenic, and slightly raised from the normal wall. These are a mild form of atherosclerotic degeneration. In Szilagyi and associates' series, atherosclerotic changes developed in approximately 45 months. Atkinson and colleagues looked at coronary artery saphenous vein grafts at autopsy and found atherosclerotic changes in 21 per cent, which had been in place an average of 62.7 months.[39] However, when DeWeese and Rob followed long-term grafts using arteriography, they noted atherosclerotic changes in only 3 of 18 patients studied after 5 years, and two grafts did not develop changes until after 10 years.[40] The author's group used color duplex ultrasonography to interrogate the grafts and were able to visualize changes in the arterial wall, such as thickening and wall plaque, that are not necessarily seen on contrast arteriography, which only defines the column of flowing blood. Thus, this group found a high incidence of atherosclerotic changes, with evidence of it in over half the grafts at a median postoperative follow-up time of 74 months (see Figs. 28–8 and 28–9 on Color Plate II).

Aneurysmal degeneration in saphenous vein grafts is a more dramatic late development (Fig. 28–10). It is infrequent, only 29 cases having been described in the literature. The author's group found eight grafts harboring 16 segments with aneurysmal change. Five (63 per cent) of these grafts had occluded and undergone either thrombectomy or thrombolysis many months prior to diagnosis of the vein graft aneurysm. Three grafts with aneurysms had no history of occlusion, and two of these were reversed saphenous vein grafts. The author postulates that transmural ischemic injury occurs at the time of graft thrombosis or vein harvest. This alters the integrity of the vein graft wall, allowing subsequent aneurysmal formation. Vein graft aneurysms have been described as atherosclerotic in nature, but this may be a result of the ongoing reparative changes rather than the cause of the aneurysm.

The site of the autogenous graft has some effect on its tendency to develop aneurysmal degeneration. Stanley and coworkers, in studying aortorenal vein grafts, noted that one third exhibited uniform expansion with an 18 per cent mean increase in diameter. Eight of these grafts expanded

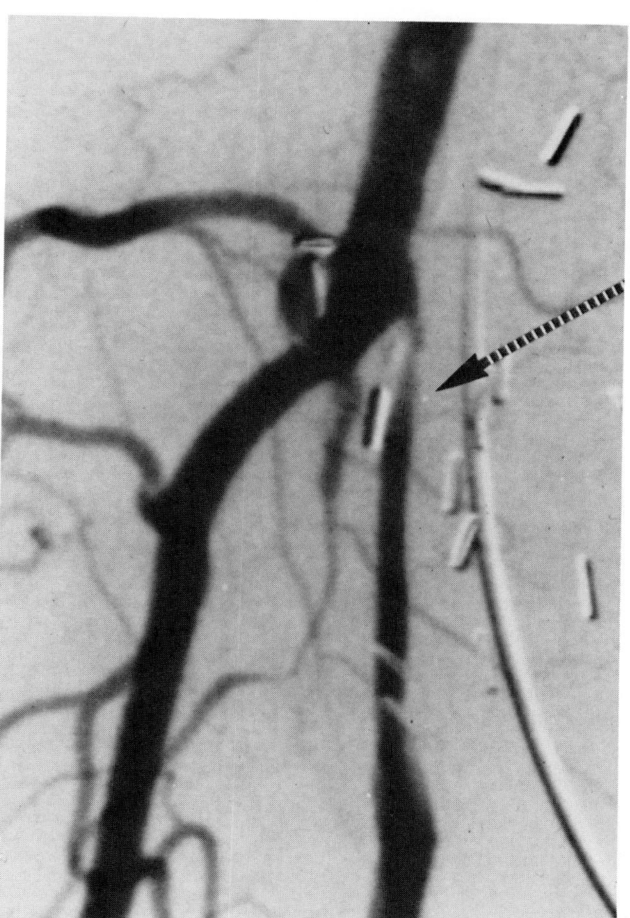

FIGURE 28–7. Postoperative stenosis *(arrow)* occurring in vein graft 8 months after operation.

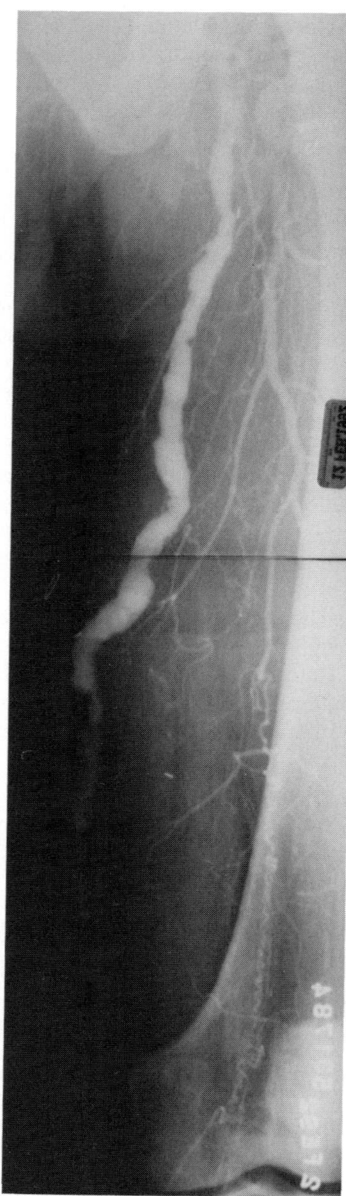

FIGURE 28–10. Arteriogram of aneurysmal vein graft. Stenotic areas and aneurysmal areas exist in same graft. (From Reifsnyder T, Towne JB, Seabrook GR, et al: Biology of long-term autogenous vein grafts. J Vasc Surg 17:207, 1993.)

25 to 47 per cent, and six grafts showed aneurysmal dilatation manifested by concentric dilatations that averaged 114 per cent and ranged from 62 to 150 per cent.

Vein grafts are prone to the development of atherosclerotic changes. Development of these lesions is accelerated because the graft develops changes in several years whereas decades are needed for the same result in native vessels. Changes in long-term vein grafts are usually combinations of fibrointimal hyperplasia and atherosclerosis (see Figs. 28–11 and 28–12 on Color Plate III). Atherosclerotic changes that threatened graft survival were noted in 11 extremities in the author's study. These lesions were always very discrete and short and were surrounded by a normal vein graft proximally and distally. Half of these stenoses were at the site of a previous defect, and the other half developed in the nondisturbed segments de novo. One of the author's patients had nine different procedures in an attempt to correct recurrent stenoses in the distal third of the femoral anterior tibial graft. Even when the stenosis plus 10 cm of normal graft on either side was replaced, a new stenosis occurred in the midportion of the replacement graft within a few months. Why stenosis developed in some grafts while others developed only wall plaque is unknown.

The relationship between risk factors and the development of vein graft atherosclerosis has been examined by Campeau and colleagues, who studied saphenous vein grafts in the coronary circulation and documented the development of new stenoses or changes in old stenoses over 10 years.[42] They found that patients who developed new or changing stenoses had significantly higher lipid levels. In their necropsy study Atkinson and colleagues found that atherosclerotic lesions in coronary saphenous vein grafts were related to hypercholesterolemia.[39] In this study there were no risk factors (hypertension, coronary artery disease, diabetes mellitus, smoking, treated hyperlipidemia) that significantly predicted the occurrence of graft lesions, but lipid levels were not prospectively evaluated. A prospective study correlating lipids and lower extremity graft morphology would help to elucidate further the natural history of autogenous bypasses. Vein grafts used for lower extremity bypass are ideally suited for this kind of study. Unlike grafts used in the coronary circulation, lower extremity bypasses can be sequentially studied noninvasively using the color duplex scanner without risk or discomfort to the patient.

Long-term graft morphology is affected by postoperative revisions. In the author's study, 38 (53 per cent) of the grafts underwent at least one revision either to repair the conduit or to protect inflow and outflow. Revised conduits contained 12 of the 15 graft-threatening lesions, whereas the grafts that had never been modified tended to be normal in appearance. During the early postoperative period revisions involved the conduit and were necessary to correct technical errors such as retained valves, arteriovenous fistulae, a twisted graft, or the use of an unsuitable vein segment. These revisions did not condemn the graft because 7 of 11 (64 per cent) were normal at the time of long-term follow-up. Between 1 and 24 months postoperatively, grafts were most commonly revised because of stenotic lesions at the anastomoses and valve sites that microscopically demonstrated fibrointimal hyperplasia. These revisions tended to portend future problems, and only 17 per cent of these conduits were normal on color duplex scanning at late follow-up. After 2 years the grafted extremities were more affected by the ongoing atherosclerotic process. Inflow and outflow disease progression necessitated two thirds of the late revisions. Thus, the cause of impending graft failure varies with the length of time the graft has been in place. More important, the ravages of atherosclerosis are incessant. The need for perpetual graft surveillance cannot be emphasized enough. Our surveillance protocol now consists of seeing patients with mature grafts twice yearly. The 6-month visit is brief, consisting of a physical examination, ankle-brachial index, and a single determination of graft flow velocity. Each year, in addition to the tests, we now scan the entire graft.

When a good vein conduit is used and no intraoperative problems are encountered, grafts do not develop intrinsic conduit lesions that threaten patency. Nonetheless, many of these grafts do develop atherosclerotic changes, as evidenced by the high incidence of wall plaque. In less than optimal circumstances, graft-threatening lesions in the conduit and in the inflow and outflow vessels develop continually. If identified and corrected in a timely manner, prolonged patency is obtained. The autogenous lower extremity bypass can be durable but requires diligent surveillance by the vascular surgeon.

References

1. Bergamini TM, Towne JB, Bandyk DF, et al: Experience with in situ saphenous vein bypasses during 1981–1989: Determinant factors of long-term patency. J Vasc Surg 13:137, 1991.
2. Taylor LM, Edwards JM, Porter JM: Present status of reversed vein bypass grafting: Five-year results of a modern series. J Vasc Surg 11:193, 1990.
3. Leather RP, Shah DM, Chang BB, Kaufman JL: Resurrection of the in situ saphenous vein bypass: 1000 cases later. Ann Surg 208:435, 1988.
4. Veith FJ, Gupta SK, Ascer E, et al: Six-year prospective multicenter randomized comparison of autologous saphenous vein and expanded PTFE grafts in infrainguinal arterial reconstructions. J Vasc Surg 3:104, 1986.
5. Goss CM (ed): Gray's Anatomy of the Human Body, 29th ed. Philadelphia, Lea & Febiger, 1975, pp 717–719.
6. Shah DM, Chang BB, Leopold PW, et al: The anatomy of the grater saphenous venous system. J Vasc Surg 3:273, 1986.
7. Veith FJ, Moss CM, Sprayregen S, Montefusco C: Preoperative saphenous venography in arterial reconstructive surgery of the lower extremity. Surgery 85:253, 1979.
8. Edwards EA: The orientation of venous valves in relation to body surfaces. Anat Rec 64:369, 1986.
9. Andrus G, Harris RW, Salles-Cunha SX, et al: Arm veins for arterial revascularization of the leg: Arteriographic and clinical observations. J Vasc Surg 4:416, 1986.
10. Goss CM (ed): Gray's Anatomy of the Human Body, 29th ed. Philadelphia, Lea & Febiger, 1975, pp 700–703.
11. Fuchs JCA, Mitchener JS III, Hagen P: Postoperative changes in autologous vein grafts. Ann Surg 188:1, 1978.
12. Ratnoff OD, Everson B, Embury P, et al: Inhibition of the activation of Hageman factor (factor XII) by human vascular endothelial cell culture suppurates. Proc Natl Acad Sci USA 88:10740, 1991.
13. Marlar RA: Protein C in thromboembolic disease. Semin Thromb Hemost 2:387, 1985.
14. Eldor A, Falcone DJ, Hajjar DP, et al: Recovery of prostacyclin production by de-endothelialized rabbit aorta. J Clin Invest 67:735, 1981.
15. Bush HL, McCabe ME, Nabseth DC: Functional injury of vein graft endothelium. Arch Surg 119:770, 1984.
16. Lawrie GM, Weilbacher DE, Henry PD: Endothelium-dependent relaxation in human saphenous vein grafts. J Thorac Cardiovasc Surg 100:612, 1990.
17. Angelini GD, Christie MI, Bryan AJ, Lewis MJ: Surgical preparation impairs release of endothelium-derived relaxing factor from human saphenous vein. Ann Thorac Surg 48:417, 1989.
18. Iba T, Shin T, Sonoda T, et al: Stimulation of endothelial secretion of tissue-type plasminogen activator by repetitive stretch. J Surg Invest 50:457, 1991.
19. Kurusz M, Christman EW, Derick JR, et al: Use of cold cardioplegic solution for vein graft distention and preservation: A light and scanning electron microscopic study. Ann Thorac Surg 32:68, 1981.
20. Bonchek LI: Prevention of endothelial damage during preparation of saphenous veins for bypass grafting. J Thorac Cardiovasc Surg 79:911, 1980.
21. Malone JM, Kischer CW, Moore WS: Changes in venous endothelial fibrinolytic activity and histology with in vitro venous distention and arterial implantation. Am J Surg 142:178, 1981.
22. Abbott WM, Wieland S, Austin WG: Structural changes during preparation of autogenous venous grafts. Surgery 76:1031, 1972.
23. LoGerfo FW, Quist WC, Crawshaw HM, Haudenschild C: An improved technique for preservation of endothelial morphology in vein grafts. Surgery 90:1015, 1981.
24. Bauman FG, Catinella FP, Cunningham JNJ, Spencer FC: Vein contraction and smooth muscle cell extensions as causes of endothelial damage during graft preparation. Ann Surg 194:199, 1981.
25. Sottiurai VS, Sue SL, Batson RC, et al: Effects of papaverine on smooth muscle cell morphology and vein graft preparation. J Vasc Surg 2:834, 1985.
26. Gundry SR, Jones M, Ishihara T: Optimal preparation techniques for human saphenous vein grafts. Surgery 88:785, 1980.
27. Buchbinder D, Singh JK, Karmody AM, et al: Comparison of patency rate and structural change of in situ and reversed vein arterial bypass. J Surg Res 30:213, 1981.
28. Bush HL, Jakubowski JA, Curl GR, et al: The natural history of endothelial structure and function in arterialized vein grafts. J Vasc Surg 3:204, 1986.
29. Cambria RP, Megerman J, Abbott WM: Endothelial preservation in reversed and in situ autogenous vein grafts. Ann Surg 202:50, 1985.
30. Batson RC, Sottiurai VS: Nonreversed and in situ vein grafts. Ann Surg 201:771, 1985.
31. Towne JB, Schmitt DD, Seabrook GR, Bandyk DF: The effect of vein diameter on patency of in situ grafts. J Cardiovasc Surg 32:192, 1991.
32. Sonnenfeld T, Cronestrand R: Factors determining outcome of reversed saphenous vein femoropopliteal bypass grafts. Br J Surg 67:642, 1980.
33. Wengerter KR, Veith FJ, Gupta SK, Ascer E: Influence of vein size (diameter) on intrapopliteal reversed vein graft patency. J Vasc Surg 11:525, 1990.
34. Bandyk DF, Kaebnick HW, Bergamini TM, et al: Hemodynamics of in situ saphenous vein arterial bypass. Arch Surg 123:477, 1988.
35. Bergamini TM, Towne JB, Bandyk DF, et al: Experience with in situ saphenous vein bypasses during 1981 to 1989: Determinant factors of long-term patency. J Vasc Surg 13:137, 1991.
36. Reifsnyder T, Towne JB, Seabrook GR, et al: Biologic characteristics of long-term autogenous vein grafts: A dynamic evolution. J Vasc Surg 17:207, 1993.
37. Batzner IC: Über die Chirurgie der arterien Verlotzungen und die Frage des Venentransplantats. Chirurg 17:345, 1947.
38. Szilagyi DE, Elliott JP, Hagerman JH, et al: Biologic fate of autogenous vein implants as arterial substitutes. Ann Surg 178:232, 1973.
39. Atkinson JB, Forman MB, Vaughn WK, et al: Morphologic changes in long-term saphenous vein bypass grafts. Chest 88:341, 1985.
40. DeWeese JA, Rob C: Autogenous venous grafts ten years later. Surgery 82:775, 1977.
41. Stanley JC, Ernst CB, Fry WJ: Fate of 100 aortorenal vein grafts: Characteristics of late graft expansion, aneurysmal dilatation, and stenosis. Surgery 74:931, 1973.
42. Campeau L, Enjulbert M, Lesperance J, et al: The relation of risk factors to the development of atherosclerosis in saphenous vein bypass grafts and the progression of disease in the native circulation. N Engl J Med 311:1329, 1984.

29

Prosthetic Grafts

David C. Brewster, M.D.

• • •

Although autogenous arterial or venous grafts currently represent the nearest approximation of the ideal blood vessel substitute and are acknowledged to provide the best current results of vascular reconstruction, it is evident that such autologous grafts may not always be expendable, are often difficult to procure, or may in fact be unavailable due to prior use or a diseased condition of their own. Similarly, autogenous tissue conduits may be inadequate in size or length for use in a particular anatomic position or clinical situation. Obvious examples of such circumstances are the unsuitability of saphenous vein grafts for large-vessel reconstruction for aortoiliac aneurysmal or occlusive disease, or the not uncommon difficulty of obtaining a vein graft of adequate length and caliber for long distal small-vessel bypass procedures.

For these reasons, the need for substitute vascular grafts has been an important and continuing concern in the field of vascular surgery. Indeed, development of a variety of prosthetic grafts has been a vital factor in the extraordinary advances and achievements in vascular reconstructive surgery made during the past four decades, along with other notable achievements such as the control of blood coagulation, the study of diseased vessels by angiography, and so on.[1,2]

Although currently available synthetic grafts are generally satisfactory for large-vessel reconstruction of the aortoiliac segment of the arterial tree, the limitations and less than optimal results of prosthetic grafts utilized for medium- and small-vessel (less than 6 mm) procedures below the inguinal ligament are well recognized and continue to represent a major challenge. Recurring problems related to prosthetic grafts, principally thrombosis, anastomotic problems such as anastomotic aneurysm and intimal hyperplasia, a tendency toward structural deterioration, healing abnormalities, and susceptibility to infection continue to occur and result in the need for reoperation.

Intensive laboratory and clinical research since the 1950s has led to a wealth of data on the basic biologic mechanisms of blood and tissue reactions to foreign materials in replacement grafts. Yet much remains unknown about such interactions and the consequences of these interactions within the graft itself and the vascular bed downstream. Although it is now appreciated that a successful vascular graft is far more than an inert conduit carrying blood from one area to another, there is continuing controversy about the importance and relevance of specific structural, mechanical, and electrochemical features of the graft and its flow surface that ultimately determine its long-term behavior and clinical effectiveness. A lack of consensus about the optimal design features of the ideal vessel substitute has led to a sometimes bewildering array of vascular grafts of different materials, as well as frequent modifications of grafts of even the same prosthetic material by means of alterations in the specific composition and production techniques utilized in their manufacture. Such alterations have been proposed in the hope of improving the performance and characteristics of the graft, usually in terms of patency, durability, healing and incorporation within host tissues, resistance to infection, reduced blood loss through the graft, and better handling qualities. Various claims about the benefits of one type of prosthetic graft over another have been made, though it is often difficult to discern science from salesmanship. Past clinical studies have often lacked adequate controls to allow accurate conclusions to be reached, leading to confusing, often conflicting results. Laboratory investigation is frequently hampered by species variability and recognized differences in the behavior of grafts between man and various laboratory animals.[3] Commercial pressures and interests often result in the clinical availability of new prostheses before adequate experience with its anticipated performance and behavior is available. Hence, it is often difficult for the practicing vascular surgeon who is not a chemical engineer, polymer chemist, or laboratory biologic scientist to evaluate the vast amount of data and claims and make informed choices regarding the proper use of prosthetic grafts.

In this chapter a broad classification of prosthetic grafts is outlined, together with a brief discussion of some design concepts and principles important to a basic understanding of vascular grafts. The specific features, physical properties, and the known biologic behavior of various blood vessel substitutes currently in common usage are examined, with emphasis on the particular advantages and potential limitations unique to each type of graft. The applicability and recommended use of specific prosthetic grafts for various clinical problems are summarized, and finally the potential direction of future development is examined.

CLASSIFICATION

A prosthesis is defined as an artificial device meant to replace a missing or malfunctioning body part. In the case of vascular prosthetic grafts, the intent is obviously to substitute the graft for a segment of the arterial tree whose

Table 29–1. Classification of Prosthetic Grafts

Synthetic	Biologic	Composite
Textile	Allografts	End-to-end straight grafts
Woven Dacron	Arterial homografts	Sequential grafts
Knitted Dacron	Venous allografts	
Velour	Umbilical vein	
Biologically coated	Xenografts	
Nontextile	Bovine carotid	
Teflon (ePTFE)	Canine carotid	
Polyurethane	Fibrocollagenous tubes	
Bioabsorbable	Autogenous	
	Heterogenous	

function is compromised by injury, occlusive disease, or aneurysmal degenerative changes. The prosthetic graft provides a substitute conduit for blood flow, allowing the diseased segment to be repaired, excised, or bypassed.

As shown in Table 29–1, prosthetic grafts may be classified according to their method of construction and basic component. The blood vessel substitute may be entirely manufactured or synthetic, or it may be derived from various naturally occurring tissues (biologic grafts). Almost all currently available synthetic grafts are constructed from polymers. In textile or fabric grafts, typically varieties of current Dacron prostheses, the basic polymer is first made into a yarn, which is then used to construct a graft by various methods of knitting or weaving. Nontextile grafts, for example, polytetrafluoroethylene (PTFE), and polyurethane, are manufactured by techniques of precipitation or extrusion of the polymer from solutions or sheets of the material. In contrast to synthetic grafts, biologic prosthetic grafts are composed of actual tissues, most often blood vessels (arteries and veins) themselves, taken from other humans (allografts or homografts) or other animal species (xenografts or heterografts). Although vascular grafts using artery or vein from the patient himself can certainly be considered biologic grafts, such autogenous (autologous) conduits have been previously discussed in prior chapters and are not pertinent to this section concerning prosthetic substitutes.

A third broad category of vascular grafts that are appropriate to a discussion of prosthetic grafts is composite grafts. Such grafts are constructed by combining segments of a prosthetic with autogenous material to form a substitute vessel conduit, occasionally a consideration when the available length of an autogenous tissue graft is inadequate for the required reconstruction.

GRAFT DESIGN CONCEPTS AND PRINCIPLES

There is general agreement on the desirable characteristics of a vessel substitute that will contribute to its function as an optimal vascular graft (Table 29–2). As initially enumerated by Scales in 1953,[4] a primary prerequisite is the need for a prosthesis to be *biocompatible* with the host into which it is implanted. Its material must be free of significant toxic, allergic, or carcinogenic side effects. Since all prosthetic grafts are foreign material to the body, some tissue reaction is to be expected and, in fact, is probably desirable in terms of generating a healing response leading to incorporation within host tissue. Yet this tissue reactivity and subsequent ''healing'' response must not be excessive or otherwise detrimental in terms of excessive thickness of perigraft fibrous tissue formation or the inner graft cellular or tissue lining. Similarly, overly reactive responses at graft-host vessel anastomoses are undesirable because they may progressively compromise graft flow and ultimately result in graft closure.

It is obvious that a graft should be *physically durable*, free from deleterious dimensional instability over time, which would result in significant dilatation, aneurysm formation, rupture, or excessive elongation that could promote tortuosity, kinking, and eventual thrombosis. The graft should be as *resistant to infection* as possible and be capable of being adequately *sterilized* without deterioration and *conveniently stored* in a sterilized condition for prolonged periods. A graft should be *readily available* in a variety of sizes and lengths as required by different clinical situations.

From a surgeon's perspective, a graft should be *easy to implant*. This characteristic is principally determined by various properties that, in aggregate, determine the so-called handling characteristics of the conduit. The graft should have adequate flexibility or pliability, that is, the ability to bend without significant kinking, a quality that is especially important in long grafts across joints or grafts that must follow curved or irregular pathways. In addition, the graft should be sufficiently conformable or able to coapt satisfactorily to diseased irregular vessel ends or arteriotomies at anastomotic sites. Similarly, the graft should have good suturability, that is, suture needles should be able to penetrate the graft without undue resistance, and the graft should retain sutures adequately without their pulling

Table 29–2. Characteristics of Ideal Prosthetic Graft

Biocompatible with host
Physically durable
Resistant to infection
Easy to sterilize and store
Available in variety of sizes
Easy to implant
Impervious to blood leakage
Nonthrombogenic
Compliant
Low cost : ease of manufacturing

through the wall and should not fray when cut to required lengths or shapes. Handling characteristics of a graft are closely related to and determined by the material used to construct the graft and, in the case of textile grafts, its porosity.

When implanted, a vascular graft clearly needs to be relatively *impervious to blood leakage* through the graft wall to prevent potentially life-threatening hemorrhage and limit perigraft hematoma formation, which may not only hinder the desired healing responses by the host but also foster possible graft infection. Imperviousness is closely related to graft porosity. All grafts may be thought of as a combination of a porous scaffold or framework and a material that closes the interstices of the framework if they are large enough to allow blood to escape. Macroporous interstices of autografts or biologic prostheses are closed by nature with a cellular parenchyma that is viable in autografts and preserved in a nonviable state by aldehyde processing or similar methodology in various biologic prosthetic grafts.[5] In microporous grafts, the interstices are so small owing to the manufacturing method or nature of the graft material that the cohesive forces of the blood (viscosity and surface tension) are stronger than intraluminal pressure, thereby preventing or limiting significant perigraft bleeding. Examples of such microporous grafts are those composed of extruded PTFE (ePTFE) or tightly woven Dacron, in which no preclotting is necessary. In contrast, macroporous synthetic grafts, typically knitted Dacron or more loosely woven Dacron, have porosities that require preclotting by the surgeon prior to implantation, with closure of graft interstices by a fibrin matrix deposited during the preclotting process.

Beginning with the early phases of development of textile synthetic grafts, *porosity* has long been considered an important characteristic of a successful vascular substitute. The concepts of porosity and ''healability'' of vascular grafts are closely intertwined. The cellular response by which the host attempts to incorporate (heal) a foreign body (the graft) has two components: pannus ingrowth of smooth muscle cells and endothelial cells from the ends of the artery itself, and vascularized fibrous tissue invading the wall of the prosthesis. Pannus ingrowth is closely limited to the area of anastomotic union, but fibrous encapsulation of the graft occurs along the entire outer surface of the conduit from perigraft areolar tissue. Awareness of the potential value of porous grafts followed observation of the high failure rate of impermeable synthetic conduits. It was hoped that porous grafts would allow autogenous tissue ingrowth through such pores that would initiate and provide adherence for a stable intimal lining. This hypothesis was strengthened experimentally by Edwards in 1957, who showed a higher rate of thrombosis in dogs with tightly woven Teflon grafts compared with knitted or more porous woven Teflon prostheses.[6] This correlated with clinical observations of higher failure rates of low-porosity, tightly woven aortic Teflon grafts owing to separation and dissection of their poorly adherent pseudointimal lining.[7, 8]

The concept that larger pore size correlated well with improved patency and long-term function was emphasized by Weslowski and colleagues.[9] Rapid and unencumbered ingrowth of areolar tissue from perigraft sources through the interstices of porous grafts during the process of incorporation and encapsulation of the graft by the host was thought to be a vital component in achieving a ''healed'' graft with an organized cellular, hypothrombogenic flow surface.[10, 11] The stability of such an inner lining was enhanced by nourishment of its cells not only by diffusion from luminal blood but also by its own vasa vasorum, and its attachment improved by actual connection to the invading fibrous tissue. The greater the porosity or the thinner the graft wall, the better such a process could be achieved, and the more favorable the handling characteristics of the graft. Extension of this ''gossamer'' concept led eventually to creation of a highly porous, very thin walled Dacron graft. Such ultralightweight grafts, however, proved to have other negative features such as structural deterioration, to be discussed subsequently.

Acceptable limits of porosity, of course, are dictated by increasing time requirements, the difficulty in adequately preclotting a high porosity graft, and the occasional but potentially disastrous loss of an initially adequate preclot with subsequent transgraft hemorrhage, perhaps related to a fibrinolytic reaction. Whereas woven Dacron grafts are easier to preclot and some require no effort in this regard, their handling characteristics are recognized to be less desirable, and their healing potential is thought to be reduced. Therefore, as with most prosthetic grafts, the mechanical properties of the end product often represent a compromise between engineering and design concepts and functional requirements. In the case of currently employed textile grafts, ease of preclotting is balanced against handling qualities and healing potential, with different varieties of textile grafts favoring one consideration over another by virtue of different components and fabrication techniques. This diversity, of course, provides the surgeon with various options of graft selection in different clinical circumstances.

Increasing laboratory and clinical experience with more recently developed grafts, however, has led to reexamination of the importance of graft porosity. With ePTFE grafts it has been shown that, in fact, smaller pore sizes correlate with better patency.[12, 13] Sustained patency and generally adequate healing of other varieties of grafts has therefore challenged the traditional idea that porosity of the graft is an indispensable quality for satisfactory function. Although mechanical porosity may be desirable for fabric grafts, this type of porosity is not necessary to the same extent for ePTFE grafts and unnecessary to any extent for autogenous tissue grafts or other forms of biologically derived grafts. Hence, obligatory porosity for all types of grafts does not seem to be an absolute graft design concept. The conclusion is inevitable that the degree of thrombogenicity of the inner graft surface is a more important functional determinant.[14]

The concept of *graft thrombogenicity* is obviously of pivotal importance in the design of a clinically useful and successful prosthetic graft, but it is incompletely understood and difficult to measure or quantify. The key to understanding graft thrombogenicity is appreciation of the extremely complex and dynamic biologic events occurring at the blood-graft interface. A requirement of a successful graft is that its inner flow surface not provoke a significant thrombotic reaction to blood flowing over it. Many characteristics of the material used to construct the prosthesis, including its chemical composition, electrical charge, surface texture, elasticity, and porosity, all effect a host of complex responses at the interfaces with blood, adjacent artery, and surrounding tissue.[15, 16] On exposure to blood flow following implantation, the luminal surface of a vascular prosthesis is immediately coated with a layer of serum proteins, principally fibrinogen. The characteristics of the particular graft surface, both chemical and physical, affect protein absorption. Differences in fibrinogen absorption have been shown to be related to characteristics of a graft surface; surfaces that are irregular and have many electrochemically active sites tend to absorb proteins more rapidly than do relatively smooth and inert surfaces.[16] Within minutes, platelets adhere to the flow surface, usually to a degree directly proportional to the concentration of adherent fibrinogen.[15] With platelet adhesion, contact ''activation'' rapidly occurs with release of various bioactive substances such as adenosine diphosphate and thromboxane A_2. These in turn cause aggregation and activation of other platelets, deposition of leukocytes, and activation of the intrinsic coagulation system with deposition of fibrin and red blood cells. If this process is controlled or limited, the graft surface will remain patent and will become lined with a relatively thin layer of proteinaceous material and compacted fibrin, traditionally referred to as neointima or pseudointima. If not, graft thrombosis will occur as the graft lumen is obliterated by continued deposition of cellular elements and fibrin.

If a graft flow surface has little platelet contact–activating capacity, it is said to be passive. If it has the additional ability, like that of endothelium-lined native vessels, to deactivate platelets, neutralize thrombin, and lyse fibrin, it is said to possess antithrombotic capacities.[5] The confluent, living, and functioning endothelial surface of a vascular autograft, when procured properly and atraumatically, has enormous advantages over the flow surface of any synthetic or biologic prosthesis because of its powerful antithrombotic capabilities. These antithrombotic characteristics of endothelial cells result from the generation of prostacyclin, plasminogen activators, antithrombin III, and other antithrombotic compounds. To emphasize comparison with any current prosthetic graft, it is useful to recall that the endothelial surface maintains the patency of human capillaries at a caliber of 4 μ, smaller than the caliber of red blood cells that must elongate to traverse them. In contrast to this is the fact that no truly satisfactory prosthetic graft below a caliber of 6000 μ (6 mm) currently exists.[5] Although the luminal surface of prosthetic grafts in various laboratory animal species does ultimately become covered with a confluent layer of viable endothelial cells, this process unfortunately has not been demonstrated to occur in the human with any available prosthetic graft.[17] In humans, endothelialization is seen only within 1 to 2 cm of the ends of the graft from transanastomotic pannus ingrowth or occasionally in focal patches within the body of a graft.[18] This observation of ''incomplete healing'' in humans, of course, has keyed interest in endothelial cell seeding of grafts, to be discussed in a later section.

The likelihood of thrombosis of a vascular graft is related not only to the inherent thrombogenicity of the material from which it is constructed but also to the velocity and nature of blood flow (e.g., turbulent versus laminar) over its surface. Differences in the propensity of thrombus formation also undoubtedly vary in individual patients, but our ability to determine high- and low-risk profiles preoperatively by some battery of tests is currently ill defined and quite limited.[19] Regardless of the thrombotic potential of the graft or patient, the faster blood flows through a graft, the less opportunity there is for thick fibrin deposition and platelet adherence and aggregation to occur on the flow surface. Sauvage and associates termed this the *thrombotic threshold velocity*.[20] The lower the thrombogenicity of a surface, the lower the flow a graft can tolerate. Undoubtedly, this is a crucial factor in the long-term superior patency of autogenous vein grafts for long lower extremity revascularization extending below the knee, where hemodynamic conditions are often unfavorable. At low flow rates, or as sheer stresses and exposure times increase, thrombotic consequences limit the applicability of many materials. The size of the conduit is a related factor because deposition of a relatively thick graft lining (Fig. 29–1) will logically have a greater adverse impact on a small-caliber substitute as opposed to a large-sized graft utilized for aortoiliac reconstruction. The interplay of thrombogenicity, graft size, and flow rates is dramatically illustrated by the marked difference in results with the same prosthetic material when utilized in different anatomic positions. For instance, Sauvage's group, using similar Dacron grafts, reported a 99 per cent patency at 5 years in the aortoiliac position, about 50 per cent at a similar period in the femoropopliteal position, and a patency rate of only 15 to 20 per cent in a location distal to the calf.[21] Long-term function of low-porosity, tightly woven, crimped Dacron prostheses is generally good in a position such as the thoracic aorta. In this high-flow location, the importance of transmural healing and thrombogenicity of the flow surface is minimal. Similarly, the relationship and importance of graft caliber and flow velocity are important in understanding the potential adverse effects of late graft dilation, or the generally inferior results with initial implantation of too large a prosthesis in comparison to native vessels.[22]

The mechanical properties of vascular grafts have also received considerable attention. Logically, it would seem to be appropriate to attempt to match the biophysical characteristics of the artery that the graft is meant to replace. Considerable controversy has developed around the issue of *compliance* and its importance. Compliance may be defined as the percentage of radial change per unit of pressure. It is a convenient index of vessel wall distensibility as a reflection of a pressure pulse.[23] The viscoelastic nature of

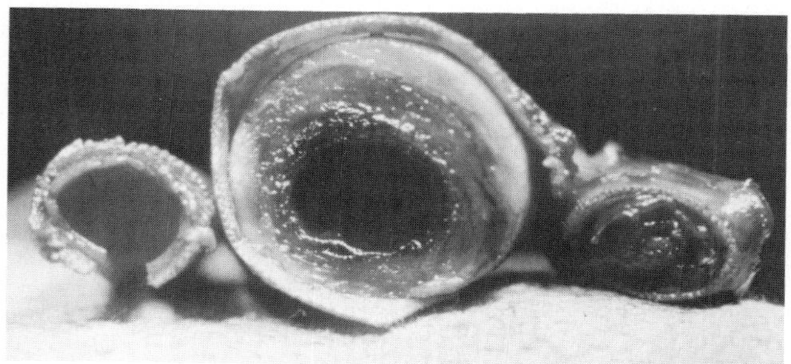

FIGURE 29–1. Deposition of chronic thick pseudointima in Dacron graft in response to reduced flow and small capacity of diseased outflow tract.

arteries is derived principally from their structural proteins collagen and elastin, with other components such as smooth muscle, endothelium, and ground substance contributing to a lesser extent. The disadvantage of noncompliant materials that lack such viscoelastic components is loss of elastic recoil that normally occurs during diastole and thereby provides energy to maintain prograde flow during the diastolic portion of the cardiac cycle. The consequence of a compliance mismatch at artery-graft interfaces is thought to be regional hemodynamic disturbances, which result in turbulent blood flow and shear forces that are imparted to adjacent flow surfaces. Such flow disruption has been implicated in the pathophysiology of perianastomotic intimal hyperplasia, anastomotic aneurysms, and acceleration of downstream atherosclerotic changes.[24–26] Obviously, these factors, and hence compliance, may therefore play a significant part in graft thrombosis and may explain, in part, the inferior performance of prosthetic grafts for medium- and small-vessel replacement.

All currently available prosthetic grafts are less compliant than host arteries, with arterial or venous autografts most nearly approaching normal values, modified biologically derived grafts such as human umbilical vein and Bovine heterografts in the intermediate range, and Dacron and ePTFE grafts relatively noncompliant. Abbott and coworkers have demonstrated a close relationship between compliance and patency of grafts, both in the laboratory and in the human.[23, 27, 28]

It is difficult to separate the biophysical effects of compliance from other factors relating to graft thrombogenicity, and experimental models are therefore sometimes imperfect. Certainly events occurring at the anastomotic interface are complex, and establishing a cause and effect relationship of a single variable such as compliance may not be possible. For instance, it is recognized that the pathogenesis of intimal hyperplasia is very complex indeed, with a host of biomechanical, hemodynamic, and biochemical mediators all contributing to the cellular proliferation characteristic of this lesion. In addition, one must also remember that diseased arteries are not necessarily compliant, and that although a graft may have desirable compliance upon implantation, the inevitable stiffening that occurs with the healing process likely alters its compliance. Nonetheless, it seems reasonable to conclude that attempting to approximate the compliance of native arteries is, in general, a valuable graft design concept.

A final mechanical factor that has been suggested as potentially important in graft design is that of *external support*. By the use of relatively stiff rings or coils placed around the outside of the graft, it is hoped to eliminate or minimize potential adverse events such as kinking or mechanical compression that might compromise graft flow and function. Such external supports may be constructed of the same material as the graft or from other biocompatible substances. Evidence of the potential benefit of this concept will be discussed subsequently.

TEXTILE SYNTHETIC GRAFTS

Development of prosthetic grafts was spawned in 1952 with the seminal observation by Voorhees and colleagues that a silk thread lying loose within the right ventricle of an experimental dog being used for investigation of homograft valve leaflets had become covered over its entire length with a smooth, glistening, endothelial-like coating, free of macroscopic thrombi, within a period of several months.[29] This observation led these investigators to reason that fine-mesh synthetic fabrics might therefore be used to bridge arterial defects, with fibrin plugs in the fabric interstices preventing initial hemorrhage, and the material ultimately becoming covered with a similar tissue coating. Tubes 1 to 6 cm in length, constructed from Vinyon-N cloth, were placed in the abdominal aorta of dogs. At sacrifice within several months, it was noted that the luminal surface of these grafts was indeed covered by a thin, shiny layer that on histologic examination was seen to be composed of collagen fibers and flattened fibroblasts, without significant foreign body reaction or giant cell formation. Fibroblasts growing into and through the interstices of the graft wall were evident. The architecture of the graft lining was strikingly similar to that of the normal aorta except for the absence of elastic and smooth muscle elements.[29] Within 2 years, in 1954, they reported implantation of such synthetic grafts in 18 patient to treat 17 abdominal aneurysms and one popliteal aneurysm, and the development of prosthetic grafts was launched.[30]

A wide variety of synthetic materials were investigated as possible fabric grafts, including Vinyon-N, nylon, Teflon, Ivalon, Orlon, and Dacron.[31–35] It became apparent that many of these basic materials lose significant tensile strength following implantation, whereas Dacron (polyethylene terephthate) and Teflon (polytetrafluoroethylene) remain essentially unchanged in tensile strength even after long periods after insertion.[36] Hence, these polymers became predominant in the further development of textile prostheses. Although Teflon is slightly less reactive than Dacron, this property may in fact be less desirable because it reduces tissue incorporation.[37] The important contributions of DeBakey and others eventually led to the emergence of Dacron as the standard material for virtually all textile synthetic grafts in current usage.[38] Teflon is no longer used as a fabric but rather in its nontextile extruded form, ePTFE.

Fabrication

Dacron yarn may be fashioned into a prosthetic graft by weaving, knitting, or braiding methods. The Dacron yarn is a multi-filament yarn that contains many small continuous filaments and is generally texturized with spiral and coil-spring shapes to impart greater elasticity and softness and better handling qualities than can be achieved by nontexturized or monofilament yarns.

In woven grafts, fabric threads are interlaced in a simple over-and-under pattern (Fig. 29–2), both in lengthwise (warp) and circumferential (weft) directions. Many variations are possible; for example, the weft yarn may go over two or three warp yarns and then under only one warp fiber before repeating the pattern. However, such variations in the weave pattern have not been shown to yield any significant advantages or differences compared with the existing simple structure.[39] Woven fabric grafts, in general, have

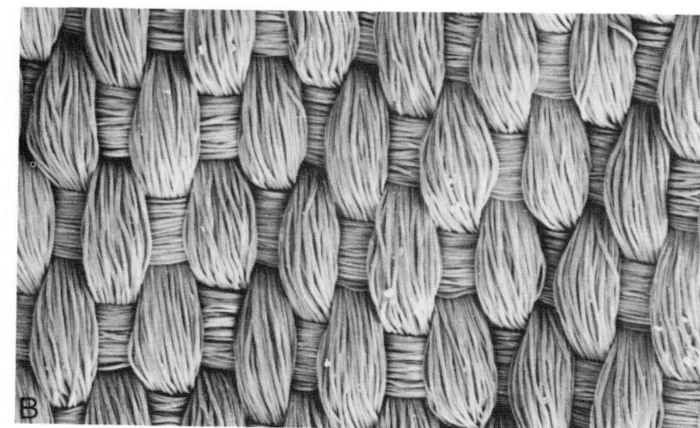

FIGURE 29–2. Woven Dacron graft. *A*, Schematic drawing of typical over-and-under interlacing weave pattern of woven vascular grafts. *B*, Scanning electron micrograph (SEM) ×50 of surface of woven Dacron graft.

little to no stretch in any direction. Since loosely woven cloth tends to fray when cut, and the yarn tends to slide and gather, woven grafts are generally tightly constructed because the permissible looseness of the weave is limited. Therefore, woven grafts are typically of low porosity, very strong, and relatively stiff. The advantages of such grafts are reduced bleeding through the smaller interstices and less likelihood of dilatation or structural deformation over time. These features are a trade-off for the disadvantages of less desirable handling features, reduced compliance, and a tendency to fray at cut edges. Because of their construction, it is often recommended that woven vascular grafts be cut with a cautery to prevent unraveling of the cut edge. Because of their reduced porosity, woven grafts have a potential for reduced tissue incorporation, transmural tissue ingrowth, and less cellular organization and secure attachment of the inner flow surface.

In a knit structure, the yarns may be oriented in either a predominantly longitudinal (warp knitting) or circumferential (weft knitting) direction. Warp-knitted grafts have more dimensional stability, and most current knit grafts are manufactured in this fashion. Knit fabrics are constructed by looping yarns around a needle to form a continuous interlocking chain of loops (Fig. 29–3). The spacing of the yarns, and therefore the pore dimensions, is related to the size of the needles used and the radius of the curvature taken by the yarn as it bends around the needles.[39] Thus knitted grafts have a greater range of possible porosities than woven grafts and possess, in general, a higher porosity than woven grafts. The ability of the loops to rotate with respect to one another also produces more stretch in all directions. These features create the recognized advantages and disadvantages of knitted Dacron grafts. Better theoretic healing characteristics owing to greater porosity, greater

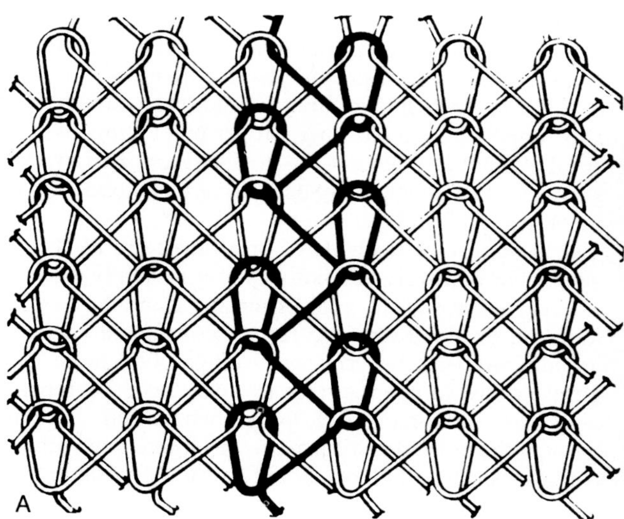

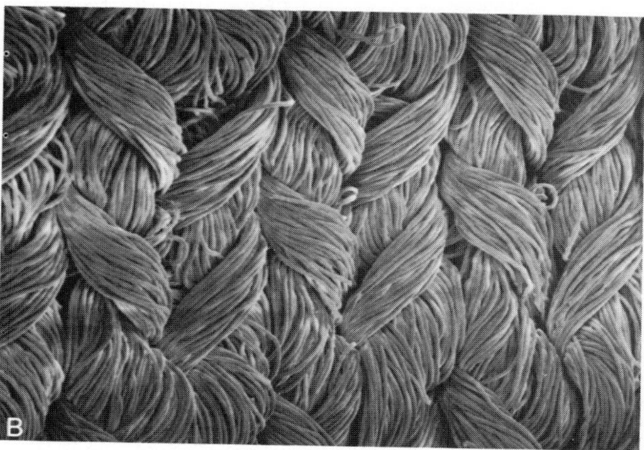

FIGURE 29–3. Knitted Dacron graft. *A*, Schematic drawing of yarn configuration for warp knitting with interlocking loops. *B*, Surface of graft knitted from texturized Dacron yarn. SEM, original magnification ×50.

mechanical compliance, and acknowledged superior handling features such as suturability, flexibility, conformability, and a lesser tendency to fray are balanced against the time requirement and potential difficulty of the need to preclot the graft to make it impervious to blood loss through the graft wall upon implantation. In addition, knitted grafts are less strong than woven textile grafts and hence subject to more frequent structural changes following implantation. Braided fabrics are no longer used because they require heavier yarn, fray easily, and are bulky and relatively nonporous.[40]

A frequently employed variation or modification of textile synthetic grafts is the addition of a velour finish to the inner, outer, or both graft surfaces. Velour fabrics are constructed with loops of yarn extending upward at right angles to the fabric's surface, giving it a plush, velvety texture (Fig. 29–4). As first described by Hall and colleagues,[41] and Lindenauer and coworkers,[42] and later emphasized by Sauvage and associates,[43] velour can be formed on a woven or knitted structure. The porosity and thickness of the pile surface can be varied with the choice of yarn, the number of loops, whether the loops are uncut or cut, and so on. It is also possible to fabricate a velour-like surface by vigorously brushing a standard knit or woven textile, resulting in broken or cut filaments on the surface rather than loops.[39]

Velour fabrication imparts improved elasticity and handling features to knitted or woven grafts, but its primary purpose is to provide a superior environment of lattices or a so-called trellis, to which fibrin may adhere and fibroblasts can attach to and "crawl on."[44] It is hoped that this process will facilitate initial preclotting and thereby enable more porous grafts to be used and will subsequently promote healing of the prosthesis by the host as well.[5] Grafts with external velour surfaces are thought to produce a graft that is better incorporated by adjacent host fibrous tissue and achieves better tissue ingrowth into the graft wall (Fig. 29–5). Internal velour surfaces are thought to yield better cellular organization and a firmer anchorage for the fibrinothrombus material that initially lines a synthetic graft. Neither internal, external, nor "double" velour grafts have been conclusively shown to result in differences in thrombogenicity or long-term performance, however, compared with standard Dacron grafts.[45] The uncertainty of the benefit of velour surfaces is illustrated by the fact that even advocates of external velour grafts such as Sauvage and associates feel that internal velour surfaces are undesirable owing to their tendency to promote formation of a thicker inner lining with its potentially increased thrombogenicity.[5, 44, 46]

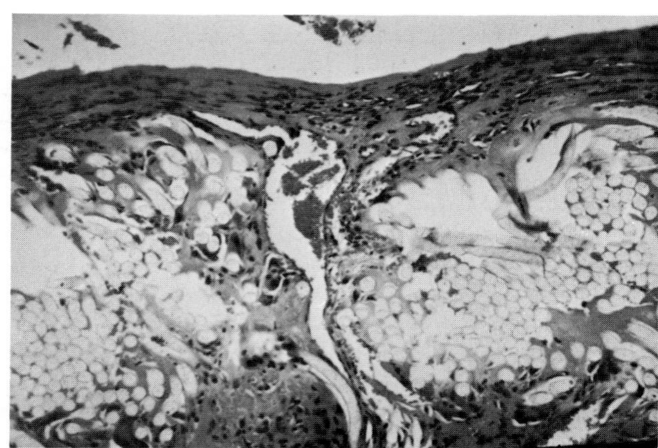

FIGURE 29–5. Light micrograph of velour Dacron prosthesis 13 months after implantation in a human. Tissue ingrowth through graft interstices is seen, with the luminal surface *(top)* covered by a relatively thin, well-organized layer of fibrin and collagen, synthesized by fibroblasts present within the tissue. Capillaries, such as the one in the center of this photomicrograph, are clearly evident and contribute to the organization and maintenance of the pseudointimal tissue. H&E, original magnification ×40.

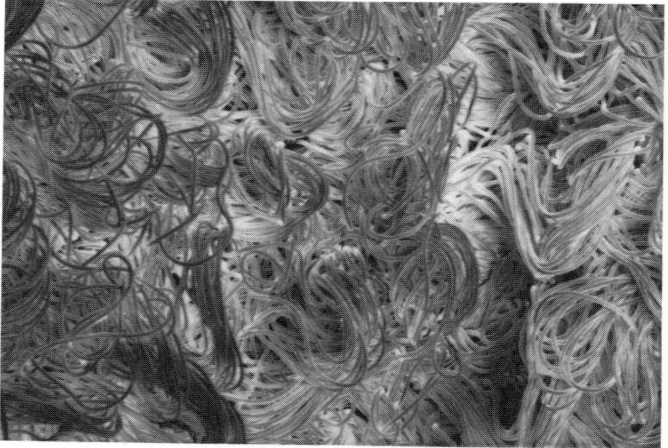

FIGURE 29–4. Outer surface of velour knitted Dacron graft. Note thick, rough, plush surface achieved by loops of yarn extending perpendicular to fabric's surface. SEM, original magnification ×50.

All standard or velour knitted Dacron grafts require preclotting prior to insertion to seal the interstices of the porous fabric and decrease implantation bleeding. Obviously, higher porosity grafts are more difficult to preclot, whereas many woven low-porosity grafts require little or no preclotting in normal circumstances. Although it has been suggested that, from a healing perspective, grafts with a porosity of 10,000 ml/cm^2/min would be ideal,[9, 37] this level of porosity is unrealistic because of the inordinate difficulties of achieving satisfactory preclotting of such a graft. Grafts with a porosity of approximately 4000 ml/cm^2/min can be used, but most knitted grafts commonly employed in clinical practice have porosities in the range of 1200 to 1900 ml/cm^2/min. In addition to rendering the graft impervious to bleeding, proper preclotting, as emphasized by Sauvage, renders the flow surface of a raw Dacron graft less thrombogenic by depositing a compacted hypothrombogenic fibrin layer.[5]

A variety of methods of preclotting are used by surgeons. For relatively low porosity grafts, simply wetting the external surface of the graft or placing it in a basin with 50 to 60 ml of blood obtained from a convenient vessel prior to administering heparin will suffice. For more porous grafts, many surgeons prefer to flush the graft repeatedly with the nonheparinized withdrawn blood, forcing it through the graft interstices until they tighten up with fibrin. Any excess clotted blood should be carefully suctioned out, but further flushing with saline will tend to negate the effects of preclotting and is not recommended. Preclotting with heparinized blood may well be difficult and tedious.

The addition of a small amount of thrombin to the withdrawn blood can help considerably. Yates, Sauvage, and colleagues have recommended a more complex three-stage process, emphasizing the need for a terminal flushing with heparinized blood to neutralize thrombin on the flow surface,[47] but evidence of the benefits of this technique is uncertain, and it is certainly more complex and time-consuming than the more widely applied preclotting methods.

Crimping of fabric grafts is done to impart flexibility, elasticity, and shape retention (kink resistence) with bending. Almost all current textile grafts employ this feature. It is recognized, however, that much of the initial elasticity is lost with the stretching that occurs during implantation as well as the inevitable stiffening that occurs with later tissue incorporation. Crimping has a number of potential disadvantages. It increases the thickness of the graft wall and reduces the effective internal diameter of the prosthesis. Furthermore, the unevenness of the inner graft surface interferes with smooth laminar flow and leads to increased fibrin deposition in convexities of the graft and a potential increase in surface thrombogenicity.[40] Although such considerations may not cause problems in large-caliber grafts, significant adverse consequences may result in small arterial replacements. This has prompted some investigators to abandon crimping and use noncrimped grafts for which external support is provided by means of rings or coils to avoid kinking with bending and foster dimensional stability.[48] Perhaps the smooth noncrimped surface of ePTFE grafts, supported or not, is advantageous in this respect as well.

There has been increasing interest in the use of biologically coated Dacron grafts. Porous textile grafts may be rendered impervious by coating or impregnating them during the process of manufacture with various absorbable biologic materials such as xenogenic bovine dermal collagen, allogeneic albumin, or gel. This process has the appealing feature of providing grafts with zero or low implantation porosity without the time needed for preclotting while retaining the subsequent potential healing advantages of relatively high porosity fabrics.[49] Although the process may stiffen the graft slightly, the favorable handling characteristics of the basic material, generally knitted Dacron, are largely retained and are superior to low-porosity woven grafts. The protein matrix is gradually resorbed within several months, allowing normal or even enhanced healing responses.[50–52] Some evidence suggests that early thrombogenicity of the graft surface may be lessened by such graft coatings.[49, 53–55] Although concern about possible immune reponses or allergic reactions to the coating substances exists, low antigenicity and no evidence of clinically adverse effects have been noted.[52, 56, 57] Although implantation of a Dacron aortic prosthesis has been found to activate the complement system significantly, collagen-impregnated grafts have not been found to provoke any greater complement activation than their nonsealed conventional Dacron counterparts.[58]

Albumin or fibrin glue may be applied by the surgeon in the operating room to render porous grafts impervious,[59, 60] but most interest currently centers on commercially produced collagen- or albumin-coated grafts with "off-the-shelf" availability. Early clinical experience with collagen-impregnated grafts (Hemashield-Meadox Medicals, Oakland, NJ) for thoracic and abdominal aortic reconstructions has been favorable, with no apparent graft-related problems reported.[61–63] Albumin-impregnated grafts (Bard Cardiovascular, Billerica, MA) have been temporarily removed from commercial availability in the United States to await further studies required by the United States Food and Drug Administration (FDA), but are in clinical use abroad. Initial experience in canine studies[51, 64–66] suggests similar benefits, and Brancherau and colleagues have reported good short-term clinical results with such albumin-impregnated grafts in 120 patients during the years 1987 to 1989.[67] Gelatin, or soluble collagen, has been similarly used as a sealant in Dacron grafts. Gelatin-impregnated grafts (Gelseal-Vascutek, Glasgow, Scotland; Uni-Graft DV-B, Braun, Melsungen, Germany) are currently available commercially in Europe, and reports of early laboratory and clinical experience with such prostheses are optimistic.[68–70]

The principal advantages of this design concept are expediency in terms of saving time by eliminating the need for preclotting and reducing the operative blood loss related to transgraft bleeding. Most clinical experience has been obtained in large vessel reconstructions; whether the possible laboratory evidence of lower flow surface thrombogenicity in the early postimplant period is in fact real or will translate into improved long-term patency in medium- or small-vessel reconstructions must await further experience and data. These grafts appear to be safe, although one must realize that resorption of the protein matrix will eventually unmask the underlying basic fabrication of the graft. If this is prone to dilatation or adverse performance in any other fashion, the initial implantation advantages of biologically coated grafts will obviously be dissipated. In addition, all such grafts are more expensive (approximately double the price) than standard textile grafts. In view of the current pressures for cost control and economic constraints in medicine, one wonders if the expediency of such grafts justifies their greater expense, especially in large-vessel reconstructions, where conventional textile synthetic grafts have provided generally satisfactory long-term results.

The most common inherent complication of fabric Dacron prostheses is the propensity for some varieties of such grafts to dilate in size over time. Dilatation may be diffuse and may involve the entire graft, or it may be confined to more limited portions of the graft, resulting in enlargement of the graft body, limb, or areas of focal aneurysmal change.[71–78] Generalized dilation is by far the most prevalent manifestation. Although the incidence of structural deterioration in Dacron grafts was formerly thought to be low (1 to 3 per cent), these data are undoubtedly inaccurate because much of the data predated the availability of comprehensive imaging of grafts during late follow-up, and often only symptomatic patients were studied.[79] Such changes have been observed in increasing numbers of more recent reports. Dilatation has been noted to occur immediately, with implantation and restoration of arterial pressure to the graft, and may possibly be progressive at later follow-up intervals. A variety of knitted Dacron grafts have been shown to measure 10 to 20 per cent more than the alleged manufacturers' box size at declamping in the operating room.[80, 81] Progressive dilatation may continue, although the rate of change decreases with the passage of time.[82, 83] Late studies by ultrasound or CT scan follow-up

1 to 20 years after implantation have shown mean increases of 23 to 94 per cent compared with initial implant size.[81, 84]

The likelihood of such altered dimensional stability has been closely related to the method of fabrication. Woven grafts with interlacing yarns have a high initial modulus and strength, and therefore exhibit little to no dilatation. Because of their looped structure, knitted fabrics have much less resistance to extension as their interlocking loops straighten in the line of highest stress. Weft-knitted grafts are less dimensionally stable than warp-knitted constructions.[84, 85] Very thin, highly porous, ultralightweight knitted grafts have been noted to manifest the greatest structural problems.[86]

In addition to simple structural slippage of the knit pattern, other factors have occasionally been implicated as causative.[79, 87] These include mechanical fatiguing or actual fracture of yarn fibers, damage to the material by the manufacturing process (heating, crimping, and so on), improper or excessively frequent sterilization procedures, or damage caused by traumatic handling, clamp applications to the graft, use of cutting-tipped needles, and so on. Although generally considered biologically stable, some evidence suggests that biodegradation of Dacron fibers may occur over time owing to the degradative effects of tissue fluids and enzymes.[82] Nunn and colleagues have noted an increased incidence of dilatation in hypertensive patients.[80]

Although a considerable number of previously reported instances involved varieties of grafts that are no longer manufactured, the potential dimensional instability of knitted Dacron grafts appears to be a consideration in even current generations of such prostheses.[81] The clinical impact of graft dilatation remains uncertain but is a concern. Modest dilatation does not necessarily imply graft failure, and no clear association between graft dilatation and graft complications has been directly established.[81] Nonetheless, structural defects have led on occasion to delayed bleeding through the graft or to actual rupture. More important, dilatation has been imputed as a major etiologic factor in the subsequent development of anastomotic aneurysms.[88, 89] Finally, deposition of mural thrombus and the lower velocity of flow through such dilated conduits may well contribute to an increased frequency of thrombosis. This suggests that it is advisable for the surgeon to select a slightly ''undersized'' graft if she or he elects to employ a knitted Dacron prosthesis. Because evidence suggests that dimensional alterations may be progressive and may lead to potentially serious late complications, lifetime patient follow-up with periodic CT scan evaluation of the entire graft appears advisable.[84]

NONTEXTILE SYNTHETIC GRAFTS

Expanded Teflon (ePTFE) Grafts

Despite generally satisfactory function of early synthetic grafts for aortoiliac reconstruction, the frequently disappointing long-term performance of Dacron grafts for more peripheral procedures involving smaller arteries, particularly those below the inguinal ligament, was a strong impetus for the development of other prosthetic materials and fabrication methods. Although textile Teflon grafts had been largely abandoned and replaced with Dacron as the material of choice for fabric prostheses, a method of extruding the Teflon polymer was discovered in 1969 by Robert W. Gore.[90] Used only for industrial purposes at first, in 1972 Soyer and colleagues described the use of ePTFE to replace the inferior vena cava in experimental animals.[91] Shortly thereafter, Matsumoto and coworkers reported good patency of such grafts as an arterial substitute in dogs.[92] Campbell and colleagues reported the first clinical use of ePTFE arterial grafts in 1976.[93]

The expanded polymer is manufactured by a heating and mechanical stretching process and extruded through a die, producing a porous material of a characteristic structure that has solid nodes interconnected by fine fibrils (Fig. 29–6). Fibril length can be varied and determines the pore size, which in standard ePTFE grafts currently available commercially measures 30 μ. The result is a unique nontextile material that can be fashioned into a tubular vascular graft. The material is chemically inert, highly electronegative, and hydrophobic. Initial observation of aneurysmal change in early grafts[94] led to addition of a thin outer reinforcing wrap of ePTFE material to provide circumferential strength in Gore-Tex grafts (W.L. Gore and Associates, Flagstaff, AZ), or a thicker wall and application of an external coil support in Impra ePTFE grafts (Impra, Inc., Tempe, AZ). Such modifications have eliminated the structural instability of current ePTFE prostheses.

Although ePFTE is considered a porous material, the behavior of ePTFE grafts in terms of implantation bleeding through the graft wall is considerably different from that of conventional porous textile prostheses. The node-fibril structure of ePTFE material occupies only about 15 to 20 per cent of the total volume of the expanded polymer. The void space is filled with air. Although the porosity (ratio of pores to material) of ePTFE is greater than that of textile Dacron grafts, the void spaces are smaller in comparison with the voids between the fiber bundles of fabric materials. The hydrophobicity of ePTFE material also limits bleeding. For these reasons, porosity is difficult to determine by methods such as the Weslowski water porosity test, which is used to characterize the porosity of textile grafts.[90] In

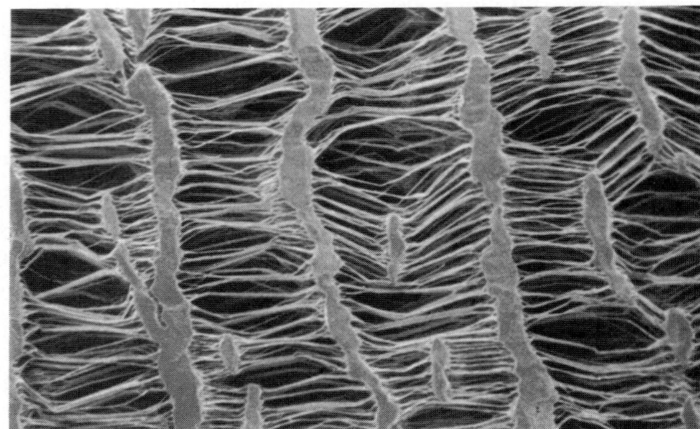

FIGURE 29–6. **Luminal surface of a Gore-Tex extruded polytetrafluoroethylene (ePTFE) graft, demonstrating the characteristic node-fibril microstructure. SEM, original magnification ×1000.**

essence, ePTFE grafts can be thought of as a microporous framework that requires no material to close its tiny interstices and can be used without preclotting.

Although the luminal surface of ePTFE grafts is negatively charged, immediately on exposure to blood events and interactions occur that are common to other synthetic polymers. Proteins adhere rapidly to the surface within 30 to 60 seconds, followed by platelet aggregation. If the process is limited and flow sufficient, the graft eventually becomes lined with a thin, relatively acellular protein film. Although the graft is incorporated by the surrounding tissues, little tissue grows into the PTFE wall even at 6 months in the dog.[5, 95] This is probably due to the microporous nature of the material and the external reinforcing wrap.[96] As a consequence, in ePTFE grafts any endothelialization is restricted to pannus ingrowth within 1 to 2 cm of each anastomosis. In the baboon model, Clowes and associates were able to demonstrate improved capillary ingrowth from surrounding granulation tissue and production of an endothelial lining in ePTFE grafts by making the grafts more porous.[97, 98] Such experimental, higher porosity ePTFE grafts (mean internodal distance, 60μ) lack an external wrap and are not available for clinical use, however. The relationship of pore size to graft performance remains uncertain. Early work on ePTFE grafts by Campbell and colleagues actually correlated increasing fibril length (pore size) with inferior patency in dogs, which was thought to be due to development of a thicker neointima.[12] Indeed, the general success of microporous ePTFE as an arterial substitute has seriously challenged the previously accepted Weslowski concept of higher porosity as a desirable if not indispensable quality for function of an arterial substitute.[14]

A variety of modified Gore-Tex ePTFE grafts have become available. In addition to the standard ePTFE prosthesis, grafts with a thinner wall construction (still retaining the outer wrap, however) have been constructed, resulting in easier handling characteristics, better conformability, and perhaps improved compliance. Recently, processing alterations have also produced a "stretch" ePTFE graft, which has some inherent elasticity absent from the original grafts. Longitudinal extensibility, the stretch feature of the graft, is achieved by a "microcrimping" of the fibrils of the tube (Fig. 29–7). Despite such microcrimping of the fibrils, the luminal surface remains smooth. No additional materials, such as elastimers, are used to produce the stretch characteristic. The actual internodal spacing, or fibril lengths, are similar in nonstretch and extended stretch ePTFE grafts. When the stretch graft is extended, with tensioning achieved either manually or by arterial pressure distention, the tented fibrils are extended to their full length. At that point, no further elongation is possible, and the microstructure of the stretch graft is identical to that of any Gore-Tex prosthesis. This has certainly provided a conduit with a softer, more conformable wall and excellent handling qualities, possibly less tendency to kink across joints, and less necessity for the surgeon to cut the graft to precise required lengths. The short time elapsed since introduction of such modified ePTFE grafts has not provided sufficient follow-up to ensure that such alterations in the basic material will not have an adverse impact in terms of structural deterioration and similar properties, but the evidence thus far accumulated is that resistance to radial dilatation and longitudinal elongation is identical to that of conventional Gore-Tex vascular grafts. However, there are also no data to suggest improved patency or any other outcome benefits other than improved handling features and ease of implantation.

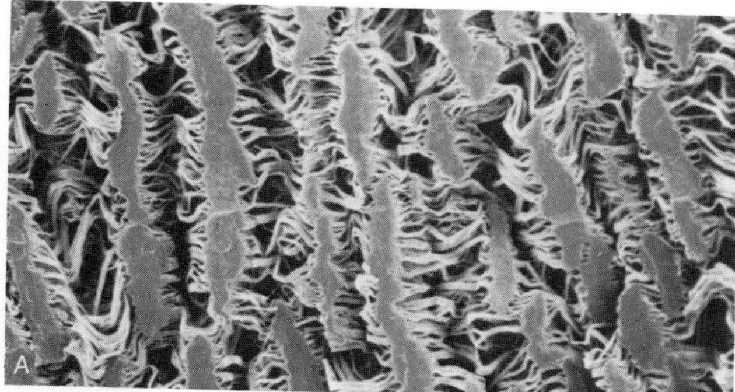

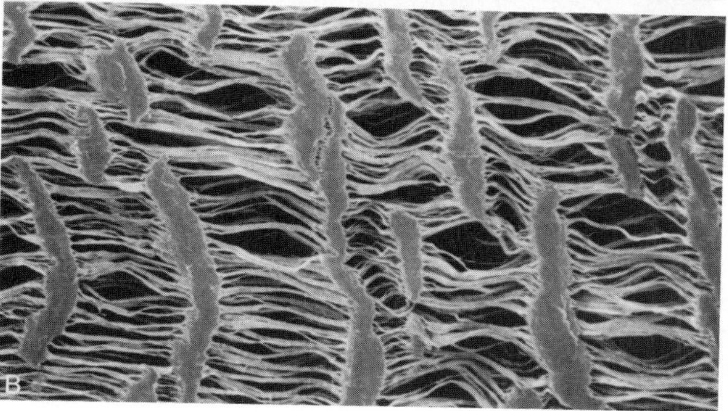

FIGURE 29–7. Scanning electron photomicrograph ×1000 of the luminal surface of Gore-Tex ePTFE stretch vascular graft. *A*, Relaxed microstructure demonstrating "micro-crimping" of internodal fibrils. *B*, Moderately tensioned graft, with longitudinal extensibility achieved by extending crimped or tented fibrils. Microstructure is now identical to that of conventional ePTFE graft (Fig. 29–6), with internodal spacing (fibril length) of approximately 25 μ.

Like several other prosthetic Dacron grafts, a variety of externally supported ePTFE grafts are currently available (Fig. 29–8). It is hoped that external support rings or coils will lessen possible mechanical compression, particularly in subcutaneously placed extra-anatomic grafts. Although conflicting results of prior studies of external graft compression have been previously reported,[99–101] the newer, much improved results (compared to historic controls) of externally supported Dacron and ePTFE grafts in the axillofemoral and femoropopliteal positions suggest that this may indeed be a valuable concept for these types of reconstructions.[102, 103] In addition, external support may help to reduce the possible kinking of ePTFE grafts across the knee joint, which has been suggested as a contributing factor in the less-than-optimal performance of below-knee ePTFE grafts.[48, 99, 104] Several reports[48, 105–107] have suggested that improved patency results when externally supported ePTFE grafts are used for femoropopliteal or tibial revascularization, although results of a randomized prospective study by Gupta and colleagues did not demonstrate any statistically significant benefit.[108]

In addition to external support, several other treatment adjuncts or technical modifications have been suggested to improve the late results of ePTFE grafts. Flinn and cowork-

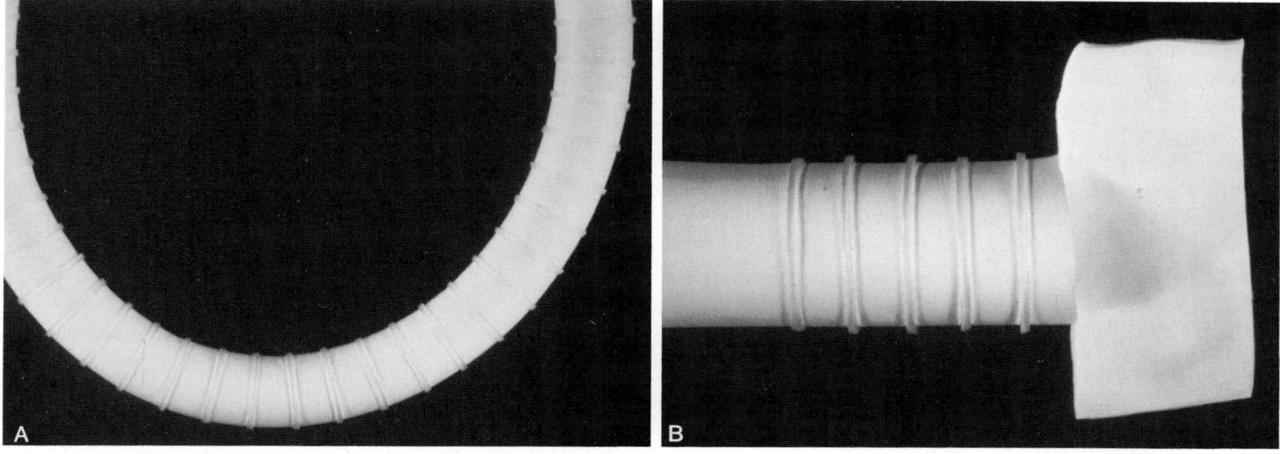

FIGURE 29–8. *A*, Example of externally supported ePTFE graft. *B*, Close-up view of detachable external rings; end of the prosthesis has been opened, demonstrating standard smooth inner graft surface. (*A* and *B*, Gore-Tex, WL Gore and Associates.)

ers reported improved late patency of infrageniculate ePTFE grafts when patients were maintained indefinitely on postoperative warfarin.[109] In addition, several reports have described significant improvements in patency when a vein cuff or patch is inserted at the distal anastomosis.[110–113] Although variations of the specific technique exist, the results of these studies suggest that this may be a useful technical adjunct during insertion of PTFE grafts, particularly grafts to small crural arteries. Laboratory evidence suggests that this technique may help to reduce the potential of compliance mismatch to stimulate neointimal hyperplasia, lessen mechanical distortions at the anastomosis, and actually result in improved hemodynamics and blood flow through anastomoses constructed in such a manner.[114–117]

Although the great majority of clinical experience with ePTFE has involved relatively small caliber tubular grafts for infrainguinal or extra-anatomic arterial reconstructions, within the 1980s a Gore-Tex ePTFE aortic bifurcation graft has become available. Recent technological changes in production have resulted in a stretch bifurcation prosthesis that has a thinner wall and some longitudinal extensibility, considerably reducing the stiffness of the graft that was previously noted by many surgeons. The current prosthesis is softer and more flexible and has improved handling characteristics and conformability. Although reported experience with the current version of the ePTFE aortic graft is scant, several reports of the clinical use of prior generations of such grafts have been favorable. Corson and colleagues have described its use in aortic aneurysm repair in 216 patients from 1980 to 1987.[118] Thirty-one per cent of grafts were carried to the femoral level. Although no significant difference in short-term patency or complication rates between ePTFE and a concurrent equal number of Dacron grafts was detected during a mean follow-up of 22 months, the authors stressed the lack of any graft dilatation or anastomotic false aneurysms and the advantages associated with the implantation imperviousness of the ePTFE grafts. In a somewhat later follow-up report extending the experience of this group, no graft limb thromboses or false aneurysms were noted with ePTFE grafts, and only one infection occurred.[119]

Cintora and colleagues compared ePTFE and Dacron grafts in a nonrandomized, nonprospective series of 312 patients undergoing aortofemoral bypass graft for aortoiliac occlusive disease.[120] They found no significant difference in patency (cumulative 4-year patency, Dacron 90 per cent vs. ePTFE 97 per cent) but noted that complications affected 13 per cent of the Dacron group and only 4 per cent of the ePTFE group. All 6 graft infections and all 7 double-limb thromboses occurred in Dacron grafts. Anastomotic aneurysms, amputations, and late graft revisions were more frequent with Dacron grafts. Forty-four per cent of patients with Dacron grafts required blood transfusion compared with 7 per cent of patients in the ePTFE group. Burke and associates[121] reviewed retrospectively Dacron and ePTFE aortic bifurcation grafts in 42 patients with a hypoplastic aorta (external diameter of infrarenal aorta, less than 14 mm). They found much improved patency with ePTFE grafts compared with a historical control group in which Dacron grafts of a similar size were employed, and concluded that ePTFE bifurcation grafts were preferred in patients with small aortic and iliac vessels. Other studies have reported favorable results with ePTFE aortic grafts as well.[122, 123] Hence, these reports seem to suggest an emerging role for ePTFE grafts for aortic reconstruction as well as for more standard applications. However, one recent prospective randomized study from Vienna reported no difference in patency between Dacron and ePTFE aortic grafts and a higher complication rate in the PTFE group, thus failing to confirm the alleged advantage of ePTFE grafts in terms of infection, frequency of anastomotic aneurysm, and so on.[124] Further experience must be accumulated.

There are several potential advantages of ePTFE grafts as a prosthetic vessel substitute. They do not require preclotting, do not leak, are resistant to dilatation in their current form, and are biocompatible. Most surgeons believe that they are easier to thrombectomize than vein grafts or Dacron conduits if graft thrombosis has occurred.[125] There is some clinical and laboratory evidence that ePTFE grafts are more resistant to infection,[126–130] perhaps due to their smoother surfaces, which have less chance of bacterial adherence.[131, 132] Several investigators have reported less platelet deposition, and hence potentially less thrombogenicity of the flow surface, compared with Dacron grafts.[133–136] Grafts of ePTFE have also been shown by Shepard and associates to cause substantially less complement activation than Dacron grafts following implantation, with less corresponding polymorphonuclear leukocyte infiltration and release of potent and potentially damaging inflammatory mediators.[137] Such mechanisms may better foster potential endothelial cell growth and contribute to a less thrombogenic flow surface, which is necessary for successful smaller vessel grafting. Healing at ePTFE-native vessel anastomoses has also been demonstrated to result in a stronger bond with greater anastomotic tensile strength than that achieved with Dacron grafts;[138] this has implications for a potentially lower rate of anastomotic aneurysm formation and may explain why the observed incidence of such pseudoaneurysms has been low with ePTFE grafts. Finally, ePTFE grafts are clearly easier to use than autogenous vein grafts. Reduced operating time, more limited incisions and dissection, and similar considerations may be a factor in some elderly high-risk patients.[139]

The principal disadvantage of ePTFE grafts is their less compliant nature compared with that of autogenous materials or even other prosthetic grafts, including Dacron. As emphasized by Abbott and others, such viscoelastic mechanical discrepancies between a prosthetic material and the native artery to which it is attached may foster development of energy and flow disturbances at the interface, potentially contributing to graft failure or anastomotic aneurysm formation.[23, 25, 27, 28, 140] Compliance mismatch may play an important role in the frequent development of perianastomotic healing abnormalities, neointimal hyperplasia, and acceleration of distal arteriosclerosis, which are so often causative factors in failure of ePTFE grafts.[26, 141–143] Although such processes are common modes of graft failure in general, ePTFE grafts appear to be particularly vulnerable, most likely due to their poor compliance (Fig. 29–9). Experimental studies have shown that anastomotic narrowing may occur with ePTFE grafts owing to surface thrombus formation or chronic endothelial injury.[144, 145] Antiplatelet agents have been demonstrated to reduce platelet adherence to ePTFE grafts and decrease intimal hyperplasia in experimental models, but the clinical utility of such pharmaceutical agents in enhancing the long-term function of ePTFE grafts has not been as promising.[146–148]

A propensity for troublesome bleeding through needle holes at sutured anastomoses of ePTFE grafts is also commonly recognized by many vascular surgeons. This may be obviated to a substantial degree by using fine-caliber suture material with small needles. Topical hemostatic agents such as oxidized cellulose, powdered collagen, or fibrin glue may also be applied after completion of anastomoses to hasten sealing of needle holes with fibrin and platelets.[149] Use of sutures made of ePTFE by W.L. Gore and Associates, which are especially designed for this problem and have a near one-to-one suture-to-needle diameter ratio, may also help to minimize such bleeding.[150] There are also anecdotal comments by some vascular surgeons that the recently introduced stretch ePTFE grafts may have less propensity to needle hole bleeding, perhaps due to the ability of this modified material to constrict around suture material to a greater degree than the standard nonextensible graft.

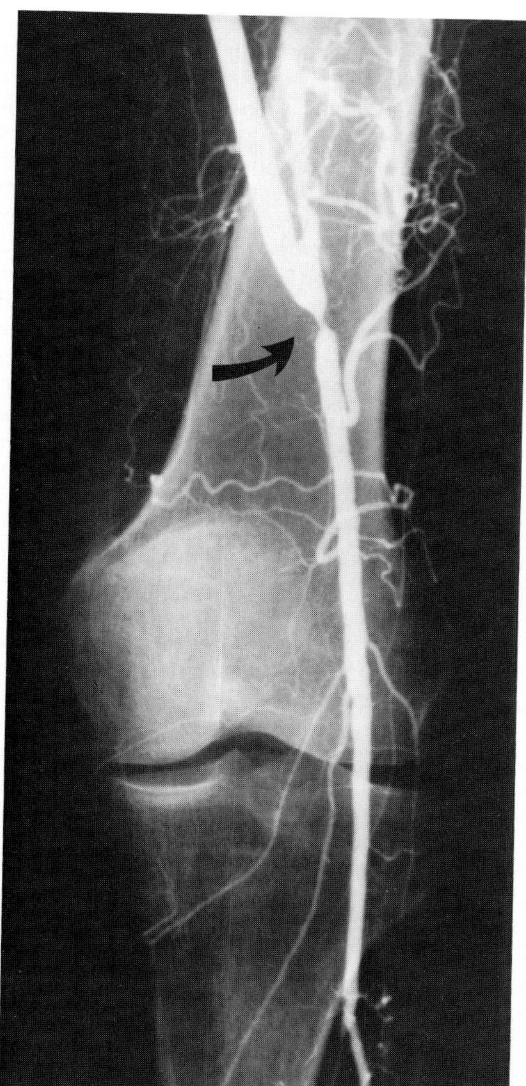

FIGURE 29–9. Neointimal hyperplasia *(arrow)*, just beyond distal anastomosis of above-knee ePTFE femoropopliteal bypass graft, threatens graft function and patency 9 months after implantation.

The greater cost of ePTFE grafts compared with vein grafts or standard Dacron synthetic grafts is also a relative disadvantage. However, the moderately increased expense of the prosthesis itself does not reflect the possible savings of expensive operating room time with the use of ePTFE grafts rather than vein grafts, or the potentially improved long-term patency compared with historical control series of standard Dacron conduits for lower limb revascularization if a vein graft is not possible.

BIOLOGIC PROSTHETIC GRAFTS

Arterial and Venous Allografts

Fresh or preserved arterial segments from human cadaver donors as arterial substitutes were initially used in the

1940s and early 1950s because of the lack of other suitable artificial conduits. Beginning with the first successful repair of a thoracic aortic coarctation by Gross and coworkers in 1948,[151] arterial allografts (homografts) enabled vascular surgeons to utilize developing surgical capabilities for large-vessel repair or replacement in cases not otherwise suitable for thromboendarterectomy. Indeed, the first aortic aneurysm repairs and aortoiliac grafts for occlusive disease were done with aortic homografts.[152, 153] Initially, aortic segments were harvested sterile and stored in cold tissue culture medium. Subsequent modifications included sterilization by irradiation, freeze-drying for preservation, storage in a vacuum or beta-propriolactone, and development of artery banks. Within a short time, however, follow-up indicated serious drawbacks in the use of arterial homografts in addition to their relatively short supply and the difficulties of procurement. Szilagyi, Meade, Deterling, and their colleagues, as well as others, all reported a high incidence of late occlusions, severe calcification, and particularly aneurysmal degenerative changes.[154–156] Much of the functional and structural deterioration was attributed to the nonviability of tissue imparted by preservation and also to immunologic responses to the antigenicity of the allograft tissue. At present, arterial allografts are not employed in clinical practice, although a recent report by Kieffer and associates of Paris suggests that in situ replacement of infected prosthetic aortic grafts with fresh cadaver aortic allografts provides the best outcome for this difficult problem.[157]

Recognition of the unfortunately rather common problem of the absence or inadequacy of the autogenous saphenous vein as a vascular graft for smaller vessel reconstruction led to interest in the use of venous allografts in the late 1960s and early 1970s.[158–160] Cadaver human saphenous veins functioned fairly well for up to 2 years, but late patency was relatively poor, and general interest in such prosthetic substitutes waned as other substitutes became available. Again, immunologic factors seemed to be important, and somewhat more favorable results were reported when ABO compatibility existed.[161] Interest in venous allografts has been revived somewhat in recent years with the development of techniques of cryopreservation with dimethylsulfoxide (DMSO) and liquid nitrogen, which promises to retain wall viability, decrease host immunologic responses, and increase long-term function of such allografts.[162–164] Clinical data and experience to date are very preliminary, however, and do not allow current evaluation of this modified allograft.

Human Umbilical Vein Allografts

Human umbilical cords average approximately 50 cm in length and normally contain one vein and two arteries in a mucopolysaccharide matrix called Wharton's jelly. The vessels are of uniform diameter, without branches or valves. The vein is larger and may be dilated up to 7 mm in diameter.[165]

Interest in umbilical cord veins as a potential arterial graft has been present for over 30 years. Initial efforts produced poor results, due largely to inadequate preservation, and such grafts were abandoned in the early 1960s.[166] Dardik and coworkers[1] renewed interest in the mid-1970s in umbilical veins showed similar rejection and degenerative phenomena in unmodified grafts placed in baboons.[167] Encouraged by methods of tanning and preservation then being applied to other vascular and cardiac valve heterografts, Dardik and coworkers then investigated the effects of both dialdehyde starch and glutaraldehyde tanning on umbilical cord vessels prior to implantation. Glutaraldehyde was determined to be superior as a tanning agent and resulted in an encouraging initial experience with such modified human umbilical vein (HUV) grafts.[168, 169]

Preparation of these conduits begins in the delivery room, where umbilical cords are cleaned and refrigerated. At the manufacturing plant, individual cords are further cleaned, and all cord tissue surrounding the vein is manually stripped. Cord veins are then placed on mandrils and tanned with a buffered 1 per cent glutaraldehyde solution. The tanning process establishes cross-links between the amino groups of the polypeptide chains of collagen, which are important for strength and preservation. Glutaraldehyde appears to produce better collagen cross-linking and a less antigenic biologic material compared with dialdehyde starch, which had been used for tanning bovine carotid artery heterografts.[165, 170, 171] The grafts next undergo multiple ethanol extractions to remove excess Wharton's jelly and soluble proteins from the structure. The conduit is covered by a polyester (Dacron) mesh to improve tensile strength because a high rate of degenerative changes and rupture was noted in baboon implants without the mesh.[167] The result is a musculocollagenous tube, relatively nonantigenic and lined by a somewhat thromboresistant basement membrane.[165] Subsequent manufacturing refinements have utilized computer-controlled mechanical lathes to produce HUV grafts with a somewhat thinner and more uniform wall thickness than the original version of the graft. In addition, a more tightly knitted Dacron mesh, stronger than that originally used, has been placed around the graft (Fig. 29–10).

The great majority of clinical experience with HUV grafts has been gained in lower extremity revascularization procedures when the autogenous saphenous vein is unavail-

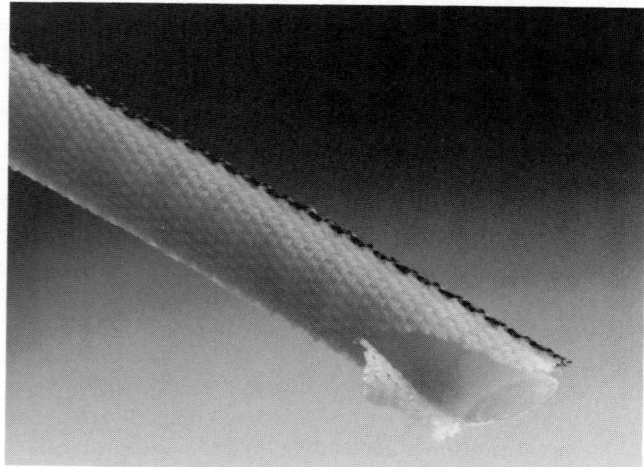

FIGURE 29–10. **Current version of modified human umbilical vein graft (Dardik Biograft Human Umbilical Vein, Bio-Vascular, Inc.), demonstrating a somewhat thinner, more uniform wall and a denser mesh covering with a guideline (partially removed at right end of graft).**

able or unsuitable for use, or in cases in which the surgeon wishes to perform a quicker and more expeditious operation than a vein bypass procedure. Although HUV grafts have been employed for axillofemoral and other extra-anatomic bypasses, aortorenal grafts, or grafts in other anatomic positions, they seem to have little advantage over other prosthetic grafts in these situations and have been seldom applied. The principal potential advantage of HUV grafts over other possible arterial substitutes for infrainguinal bypass is their possible better later patency rates, which are perhaps attributable to the physical and electrochemical features of their flow surface and their better implantation compliance.[23] Long-term experience has been carefully analyzed by Dardik and associates in over 900 cases, approximately half of which were grafts to the popliteal artery and half were to crural vessels. Approximately 60 per cent of grafts were performed for limb salvage indications. One-year patency rates for femoropopliteal, femorotibial, and femoroperoneal bypasses were 79 per cent, 58 per cent, and 58 per cent, respectively. Five-year patency rates for the same bypasses were 53 per cent, 26 per cent, and 28 per cent, respectively.[172] Other reports have noted similar, generally satisfactory patency results.[173–175]

Although some investigators[176, 177] have found that HUV grafts have equivalent patency rates for above-knee femoropopliteal bypass compared with saphenous vein grafts in this position, virtually all studies show a clear superiority of vein grafts at the below-knee level, and especially for bypass below the popliteal level. The important question is whether when a vein graft is not feasible, HUV grafts might be a better alternative than the more widely utilized ePTFE prosthetic grafts. Several prospective randomized studies have revealed statistically significant better patency rates of HUV grafts compared with ePTFE prostheses for above- or below-knee femoropopliteal bypasses.[178, 179] Other reports, however, show no significant difference between the two grafts, and this appears to be the current consensus among most vascular surgeons.[176, 177, 180, 181]

HUV grafts have some distinct disadvantages. They are more difficult to implant properly, and certain technical maneuvers must be observed.[182] They must be handled quite gently because intimal fracture or mural dissection can occur with rough handling or clamp application. Their relatively thick wall and sometimes uneven wall thickness as well as the surrounding mesh may present technical difficulties, particularly for anastomosis to small crural vessels. Tunneling of the graft may be difficult owing to friction of the outer mesh with adjacent tissues, leading to potential fracture of the graft wall or disruption of the factory suture line joining two HUV segments. Management of graft thrombosis is also considerably more difficult; redissection may be very challenging owing to inflammatory reactions secondary to the mesh and the somewhat fragile nature of the graft wall. Balloon catheters must be used with great care lest the graft lining be disrupted.

By far the principal liability of HUV grafts is their tendency toward biodegeneration (Fig. 29–11), a phenomenon that has plagued all biologic grafts to date. The incidence of structural deterioration appears to increase sharply after 5 years.[183] At 5 years, Dardik and associates reported a 36 per cent incidence of aneurysms and 21 per cent dilatation, and numerous other studies have also documented a 33 to 57 per cent incidence of frank aneurysmal change in grafts implanted longer than 3 years.[172, 184–189] Such changes may be readily detected by duplex imaging.[190] Such aneurysmal change or diffuse dilatation is likely to lead to thrombosis or potential rupture. Although segmental repair may be possible, this is often difficult, and suturing to the original biomaterial is sometimes hazardous. Our own experience supports Dardik and associates' contention that this is not as significant a problem as it might appear because the actual number of patients surviving with patent grafts 3 to 5 years after implantation is considerably reduced.[172, 185] It is not known whether the current generation of HUV grafts covered with a tighter mesh has a lower dilation potential. Nonetheless, real concern about such po-

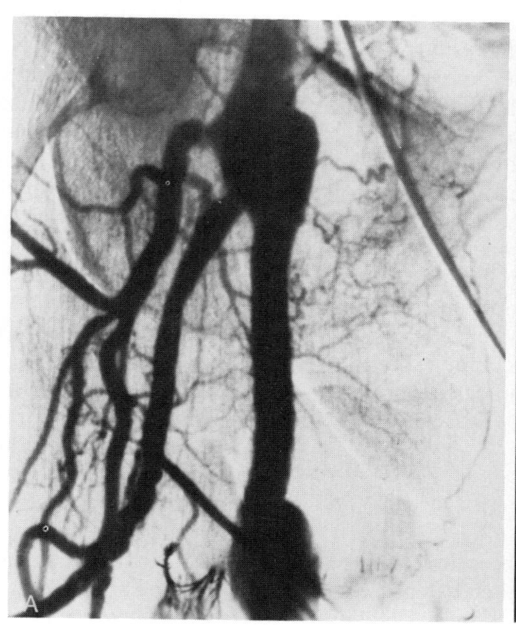

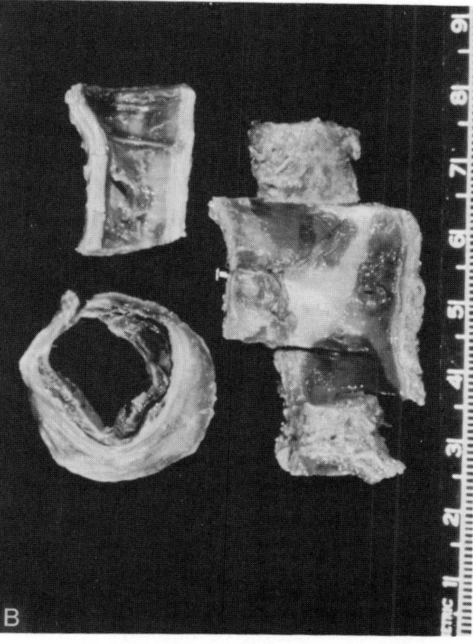

FIGURE 29–11. Example of degenerative aneurysmal changes in umbilical vein graft. *A*, Angiogram demonstrating graft aneurysms just distal to proximal anastomosis and in midgraft, 54 months after implantation. *B*, Photograph of gross appearance of sections of the graft shown in *A* following its surgical removal. Laminated thrombus is evident in the frankly aneurysmal portion, and wall irregularity, ulceration, and areas of intramural hemorrhage and lipid deposition are noted in adjacent ectatic or nondilated graft segments. (From Hasson JE, Newton WD, Waltman AC, et al: Mural degeneration in the glutaraldehyde-tanned umbilical vein graft: Incidence and implications. J Vasc Surg 4:243, 1986.)

tential biodegradation, the lack of any clearly established patency superiority of HUV grafts, plus the acknowledged technical difficulties and inconvenience of their implantation have sharply curtailed current usage of the Dardik-modified HUV graft in current practice.

Xenografts

Possible use of substitute grafts constructed from the vessels or tissues of other animal species was first investigated experimentally in the early 1950s during the initial era of prosthetic graft development. Untreated arterial heterografts demonstrated poor performance. Later in the decade, work began with the use of ficin, a protease derived from the fig tree, to remove smooth muscle, elastica, and other immunoreactive tissue enzymatically from the cow carotid artery, leaving a relatively nonantigenic collagen tube.[191] This tube then underwent dialdehyde starch tanning to cross-link its collagen and strengthen the conduit. The first implantation of such a graft in a human was done in 1962 in a femoropopliteal bypass. Fairly widespread utilization followed and led to accumulated experience that showed patency rates resembling those achieved with fabric prostheses, being only approximately 40 to 50 per cent for above-knee femoropopliteal grafts. Further, the grafts were noted to have a propensity for both aneurysm formation and infection.[192, 193] For these reasons, this type of graft is currently used only for possible angioaccess, where it has performed fairly well.[192, 194] Even for such purposes its use has been restricted owing to the growing popularity and success of ePTFE for arteriovenous fistula construction for patients undergoing hemodialysis.

Modifications of the bovine heterograft have been developed. Based on evidence of the superiority of glutaraldehyde as a tanning agent, an alternative bovine carotid heterograft treated in this fashion has been developed.[195] This negatively charged glutaraldehyde-tanned (NCGT) graft has shown promise in a series described by its developers, Sawyer and colleagues.[196] However, use of the NCGT (St. Jude Medical Biopolymeric, St. Paul, MN) graft by others has been very limited, and further study is required. Other tanning modifications of the bovine carotid artery and coverage with an external mesh, similar to that used for HUV grafts, have been used in the Solcograft. Again, clinical implantation experience is quite limited, but one series from Germany noted a significant incidence of loss of structural stability similar to that characteristic of other biologic prosthetics.[197] A final experimental variation of heterografts is the treatment of canine carotid arteries with detergents to extract their cellular components, leaving behind an acellular skeleton of collagen and elastin, including a basement membrane.[198] Although encouraging results have been noted in the labortory, no clinical experience with this type of graft is available.

Fibrocollagenous Tubes

A variant of biologic grafts that has been investigated in the laboratory and used in man to a limited extent is the concept of creating or actually ''growing'' an autologous or heterologous tissue tube for use as a vascular graft. Peirce, in 1953, first reported production and implantation of an aortic fibrocollagen tube.[199] He had observed that polyethylene implanted subcutaneously in dogs resulted in formation of a fibroserous membrane surrounding the material. He subsequently inserted polyethlene tubes in the canine rectus sheath; 5 weeks later, the tube and its surrounding fascia were removed en bloc and anastomosed into the dog aorta as a straight graft; the grafts remained patent for up to 30 months. A decade later, Eiken and Norden[200] described satisfactory results in dogs with connective tissue tubes as vascular grafts that were formed around subcutaneously implanted polyvinyl rods (mandrils). However, they noted a high incidence of aneurysm formation and rupture. Further work[201, 202] culminated in the clinical introduction of the Sparks mandril autogenous tissue tube graft and its use for femoropopliteal reconstruction.[203, 204] This device was formed over a silicone mandril covered by a two-layer knitted Dacron support mesh implanted into subcutaneous tissue adjacent to the site of usage. Five to 6 weeks later, when the mesh-supported fibrocollagen tube had matured, the mandril was removed, only the proximal and distal ends of the newly formed subcutaneous conduit mobilized, and the tube used as an in situ bypass conduit.

Initially favorable laboratory and early clinical results led to a commercially available mandril and some popularity of the method. Unfortunately, subsequent clinical results reported poor long-term function.[205, 206] Based on these studies, mandril-grown autogenous fibrocollagen grafts have been eliminated from clinical use. In 1981, however, such concepts led to laboratory investigation and limited clinical use of a mandril-grown, glutaraldehyde-tanned fibrocollageous ovine heterograft covered by a polyester mesh.[207] Silicone rubber rods with a single layer of loosely knitted polyester mesh were implanted subcutaneously in sheep. Twelve weeks later the fibrous capsule was excised and tanned in 2.5 per cent glutaraldehyde solution, and subsequently implanted in laboratory animals and in 28 patients (27 lower limb grafts, 1 aortocoronary graft). Satisfactory function in relatively brief follow-up periods (2 to 19 months) was reported. No further clinical experience has subsequently appeared in the literature.

Although not clinically employed at present, such grafts illustrate the continued interest in attempts to develop a biologic substitute as opposed to a synthetic vascular prosthesis, and in the application of several previously used design concepts to the creation of an improved vascular graft.

COMPOSITE GRAFTS

It is well established that 20 to 30 per cent of patients undergoing primary infrainguinal revascularization procedures do not have a suitable ipsilateral greater saphenous vein for the entire bypass.[208–210] In some of these patients, the saphenous vein has been used in prior cardiac or peripheral vascular procedures or has been previously stripped because of varicosities. In others, intrinsic vein abnormalities including small size, early multiple branching, areas of sclerosis, or varicosities, limit the length of usable vein.

The problem is of even greater magnitude in the 40 to 50 per cent or more of patients who require secondary revision procedures, in whom a suitable vein is not available.[211]

In such situations, the contralateral saphenous vein may be employed, but it often has the same problems of size, quality, and length that have afflicted the ipsilateral vein. In addition, clinically significant occlusive disease in the contralateral limb may be a cause of concern about taking the vein from this leg. The lesser saphenous vein or arm veins are valuable alternatives, but often such veins are too short for a long below-knee popliteal or tibial pulse.

The acknowledged inferior performance of prosthetic conduits for such long grafts is believed to reflect the consequences of the greater thrombogenicity of the prosthetic graft flow surface and the lower flow rates in grafts to those smaller vessels with frequently compromised runoff. In addition, the adverse effects of possible kinking of the stiffer prosthetic material as it crosses the knee joint, and the potentially greater impact of neointimal hyperplasia developing at the distal anastomosis of a prosthetic graft to a small distal vessel, may also pose important limits to sustained function of infrageniculate prosthetic bypasses.[24, 28, 99, 104, 141]

Composite grafts have been suggested to help overcome some of these problems. Such grafts are defined as vascular conduits made up of two or more distinct portions. Although some authors[212–214] have used the term autogenous composite graft to refer to a graft constructed by splicing together two or more segments of autogenous vein, composite grafts are commonly understood to refer to a combination of both prosthetic material and autogenous vein composing a vascular graft of adequate length. Typically, the proximal segment is a prosthetic material such as Dacron or ePTFE, whereas the distal segment of the graft utilizes an available portion of autologous vein (greater saphenous, lesser saphenous, arm vein). In direct composite grafts (Fig. 29–12*A*), the prosthetic and vein components are joined by some variety of end-to-end anastomosis. As originally suggested by Edwards and associates,[215] a "sequential graft" implies use of a single graft with several points of distal anastomoses to different runoff beds. A composite sequential graft (Fig. 29–12*B*) refers to a graft composed of a proximal prosthetic conduit inserted into an isolated segment of patent popliteal artery, above or below the knee, which possesses some runoff of its own via geniculate collateral branches. The distal portion of the graft is a vein graft, usually arising end-to-side from the distal portion of the proximal prosthetic graft, which continues distally to a patent tibial or peroneal vessel in the calf or, on occasion, in the ankle or foot. Such a configuration suggests that even if the distal vein segment should occlude, the proximal prosthetic bypass to the isolated popliteal segment might retain patency on its own. Through the addition of the second distal bypass segment it is hoped to increase flow through the prosthetic component, thereby improving its patency and augmenting the extent of overall revascularization of the extremity.[215–217]

The theoretic advantage of either form of composite graft is the use of the more flexible and kink-resistant vein segment to traverse the knee joint. Even if the length of available autogenous tissue is insufficient for this purpose, use of a distal vein segment may facilitate anastomosis to a small diseased distal vessel, potentially reducing the chance of later compromise due to perianastomotic intimal hyperplasia. This is similar to the rationale for the use of an interposition vein cuff with prosthetic grafts, which has been suggested by several authors to improve significantly the late patency of below-knee or tibial ePTFE grafts.[110–113] Potential disadvantages of composite grafts are the time and difficulty involved in obtaining a suitable vein segment from some other remote area as well as the need to perform a third anastomosis to join the prosthetic vein segments. This composite anastomosis may be difficult owing to a size discrepancy between the two graft segments, and difficulties with kinking, rotation, or excessive angulation may occur at this point. Obviously, compliance mismatch and turbulent flow may also occur at this junction, although the greater caliber of the two conduits at this point may lessen its potential impact compared with the smaller distal anastomosis. Finally, anastomotic aneurysms may develop over time at this location; we have seen several.

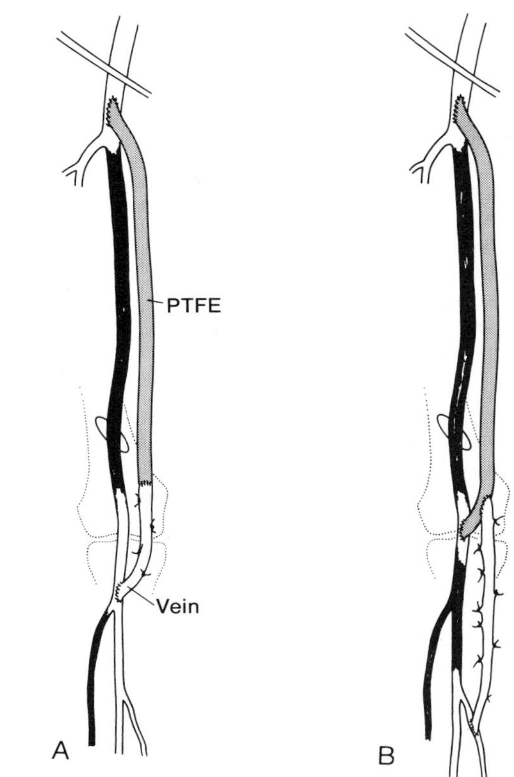

FIGURE 29–12. Types of composite grafts. *A*, Direct composite graft, with end-to-end anastomosis of graft components. *B*, Composite sequential bypass graft, with insertion of proximal prosthetic graft into isolated popliteal artery segment and continuation of distal vein segment to a tibial artery.

Conflicting results regarding the benefits of composite grafts have been reported, some investigators[218–221] finding no better patency rates than those achieved with standard all-prosthetic grafts, whereas other earlier reports[222, 223] have suggested improved late function. Our own results at the Massachusetts General Hospital have been described by LaSalle and colleagues.[224] There was no statistical difference in late patency between 39 composite grafts and 79 prosthetic grafts of various types to the below-knee popliteal artery. The length of vein relative to prosthesis did not appear to influence the late function of composite grafts. The results of both alternative grafts was markedly inferior to the results of vein grafts (73 per cent cumulative patency at 5 years). Because of the added difficulties of constructing such grafts and the lack of conclusive evidence of better performance compared with currently available prosthetic grafts, we found little support for the use of composite graft reconstructions. Femorotibial grafts were not included in this analysis, however.

In contrast, several other recent reports have indicated better outcome and continued enthusiasm for composite graft reconstructions.[225–231] In general, however, patency rates of such grafts have been only approximately 50 per cent at the 3-year interval, although advocates emphasize that such results are superior to the function of straight prosthetic grafts, most commonly ePTFE grafts, inserted in such below-knee popliteal or tibial positions, often with poor runoff. Most favorable are reports of composite sequential grafts. Flinn and colleagues obtained an 80 per cent cumulative patency rate at 2 years for 30 composite PTFE–vein femoropopliteal-tibial sequential grafts, which is indistinguishable from the rate for a group of 12 similar grafts done entirely with vein and much superior to the 47 per cent 2-year patency of sequential grafts done with PTFE grafts alone.[217] These investigators found that such grafts utilizing an otherwise inadequate segment of saphenous vein were a sound alternative revascularization procedure if the arteriographic configuration was suitable to sequential grafting. McCarthy and associates recently reported longer term follow-up data on such grafts at Northwestern University, noting generally acceptable results that are superior to results obtained with all-prosthetic tibial bypass grafts.[232] Similarly, Verta reported excellent long-term results of 54 composite sequential bypass grafts of PTFE and saphenous vein to the distal tibial or pedal vessels.[233] Patency rates by the life table method were 81.4 per cent at 2 years and 72.4 per cent at 4 years. Verta believed that the use of vein distally allowed the creation of anastomoses to delicate distal vessels with a graft material of more appropriate viscoelastic properties that is better able to tolerate low flow states (34.8 ml/min in his series). The major drawback to the technique noted in Verta's report was the additional time required (an average of 51 minutes) compared with that needed for direct femorotibial vein grafts. Again, a patent segment of popliteal artery is required for construction of a composite sequential graft.

Firm conclusions about the utility of composite grafts are difficult to arrive at based on available clinical data. Prior series are hard to compare owing to variability in factors such as severity of ischemia, primary versus redo operations, popliteal versus tibial anastomoses, and differences in techniques and actual materials used in fashioning the composite grafts. Overall, it seems fair to acknowledge the often unsatisfactory performance of prosthetic grafts in distal revascularizations, and therefore composite grafts remain a reasonable alternative. Although fairly equivalent results in the femoropopliteal position may not justify the additional time and difficulty of composite grafts compared with the use of straight prosthetic bypasses, real advantages may well exist for tibial bypass, especially if a composite sequential configuration is possible.

GRAFT SELECTION

In selecting a graft for a particular vascular reconstructive procedure, the surgeon considers the performance characteristics of various conduits in relation to the requirements imposed by the specific clinical problem. After weighing such variables, a rational choice of a graft appropriate for the circumstances unique to the individual patient can be made. It is obvious, however, that no single graft is always optimal for a certain operation, nor is there a consensus of opinion about the available options in many situations. Considerable controversy exists about certain aspects of graft selection, due in part to the substantial variation in reported long-term performance of grafts in the literature and in part to the personal preferences of individual surgeons.

From a surgeon's perspective, certain features are most important. These include patency, convenience, absence of complications, and cost. Desire for long-term patency is obvious. Although this in part reflects the thrombogenicity of a graft, sustained graft function is also heavily dependent upon its position as well as design. The term convenience refers to the presence of desirable handling qualities that facilitate graft implantation, ease of preclotting or lack of such a need entirely, and the ready availability of a graft in the needed size and configuration. The surgeon naturally wishes a graft to be free of subsequent complications, such as structural degeneration, infection, or healing abnormalities. Finally, if anticipated performance of a graft is thought to be relatively equivalent to another option in all these aspects, the less expensive alternative may be the most appropriate choice in this cost-conscious era.

Although uncertainty and controversy are acknowledged, the attributes or weaknesses of currently available blood vessel substitutes can be considered for general areas of application, and several preferred alternatives can be identified.

Aortic Reconstruction

Size and length requirements preclude the use of autogenous venous or arterial grafts, and aortic allografts are unsatisfactory given the existing methods of procurement and preservation as well as continued immunologic phenomena. Hence, a prosthetic graft is required. Fortunately, a variety of prostheses are available that function quite adequately in these large-diameter, high-flow positions, in which graft thrombogenicity is a consideration of much lower priority.

For procedures on the thoracic aorta or extensive thoracoabdominal aortic reconstructions, bleeding is often a prime consideration, particularly if the patient requires cardiopulmonary bypass, high-dose systemic heparinization, and so on. In these instances, tightly woven Dacron grafts of relatively low porosity are certainly an appropriate choice. Their long-term patency and dimensional stability

COLOR PLATES

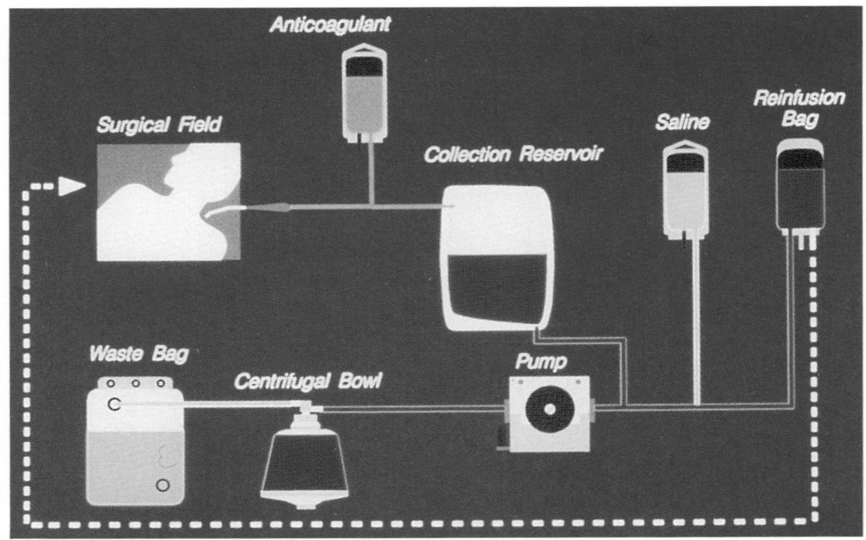

FIGURE 23–3. Cell Saver technique.

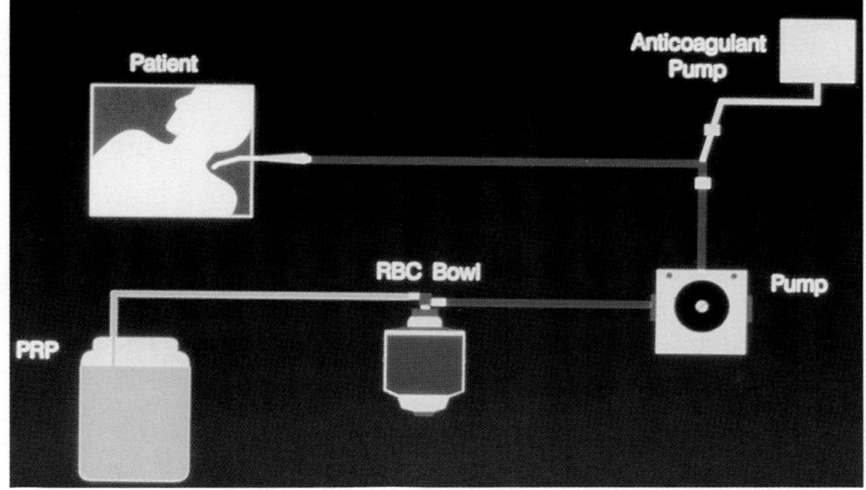

FIGURE 23–4. Plasma Saver technique (draw cycle). PRP, platelet-rich plasma; RBC, red blood cell.

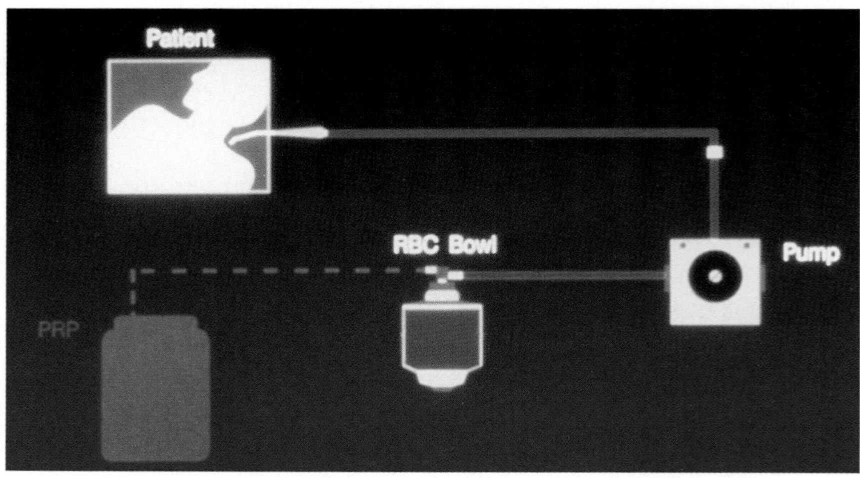

FIGURE 23–5. Plasma Saver technique (return cycle). PRP, platelet-rich plasma; RBC, red blood cell.

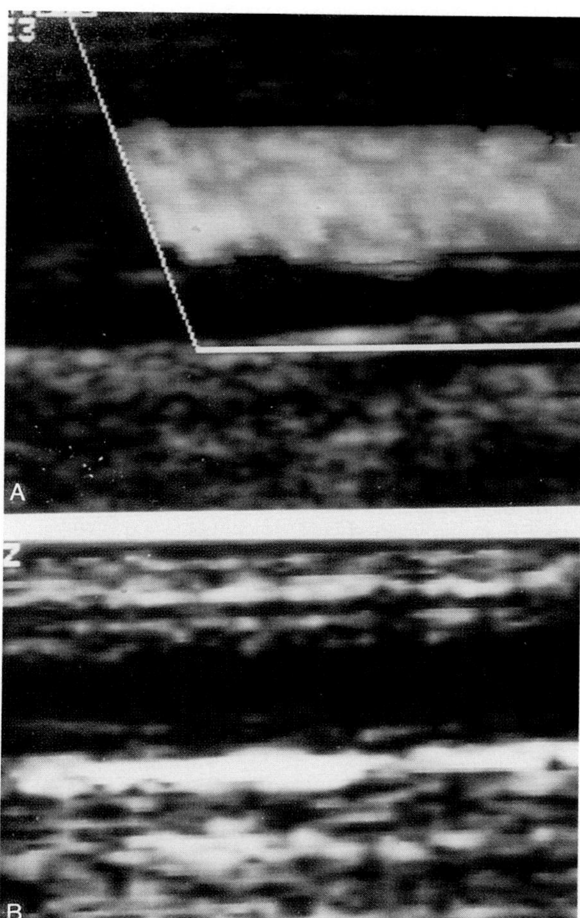

FIGURE 28–8. *A*, Color duplex scan of normal saphenous vein graft. There is uniform homogeneous color saturation of flow stream. *B*, Gray scale image of the same segment reveals smooth luminal surface. (*A* and *B*, From Reifsnyder T, Towne JB, Seabrook GR, et al: Biology of long-term autogenous vein grafts. J Vasc Surg 17:207, 1993.)

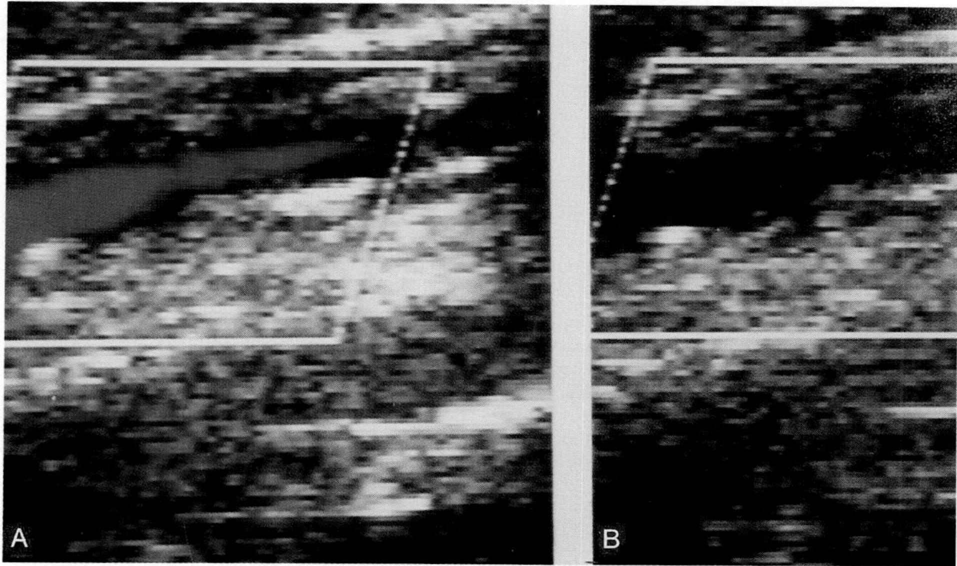

FIGURE 28–9. *A*, Color duplex scan of saphenous vein graft with atherosclerotic wall plaque. Color pattern displays uniform velocity, but irregular vessel wall surfaces are present. *B*, Gray scale image of same segment provides better definition of wall irregularity. (*A* and *B*, From Reifsynder T, Towne JB, Seabrook GR, et al: Biology of long-term autogenous vein grafts. J Vasc Surg 17:207, 1993.)

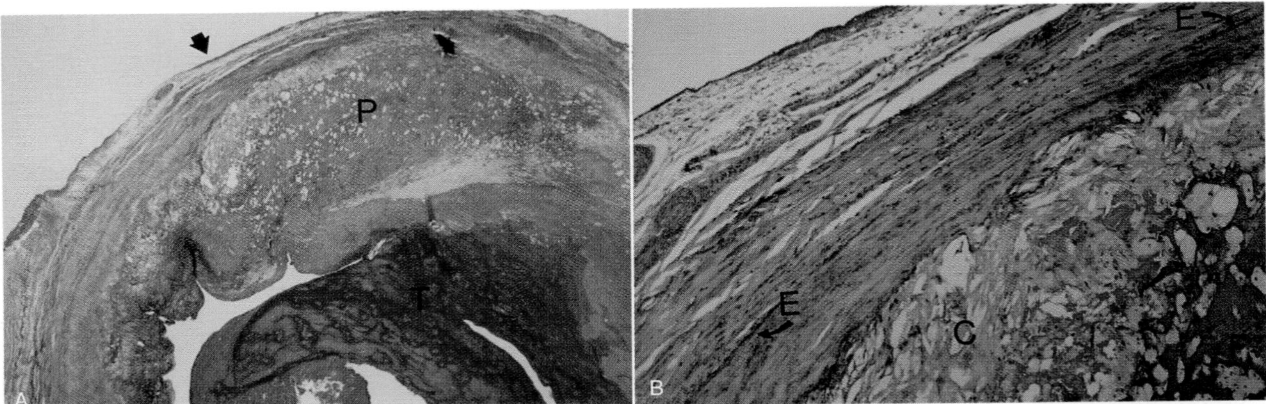

FIGURE 28–11. *A*, Photomicrograph of transverse section of aneurysmal saphenous vein graft. There is adherent intraluminal thrombus (T). Wall of graft is thinned *(arrow)* and covers a thick atherosclerotic plaque (P). Movat technique stains elastic fibers black, easily identifying remnants of internal elastic lamina. (Original magnification, ×20.) *B*, Photomicrograph (detail of *A*) of thin, aneurysmal vein graft wall show disrupted elastic lamina (E), cholesterol clefts (C), and multiple foam cells (F). (Original magnification, ×100.) (*A* and *B*, Movat pentachrome stain.) (*A* and *B*, From Reifsnyder T, Towne JB, Seabrook GR, et al: Biology of long-term autogenous vein grafts. J Vasc Surg 17:207, 1993.)

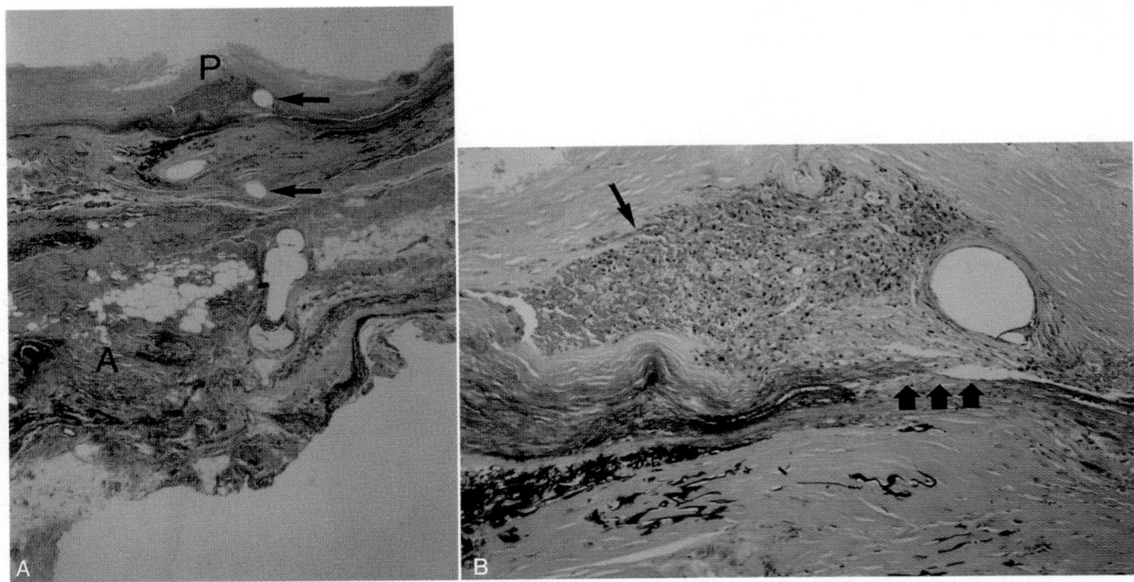

FIGURE 28–12. *A*, Photomicrograph of segment of saphenous vein graft where stenosis had occurred at site of previous modification. Suture sites are present *(arrows)*. Atherosclerotic plaque (P) and fibrotic adventitia (A) are revealed. (Original magnification, ×20.) *B*, Photomicrograph (detail of *A*) of vessel wall at site of stenosis demonstrates area devoid of smooth muscle cells and collagen proliferation typical of atherosclerosis. Small interplaque hemorrhage is filled with red cells and macrophages *(thin arrow)*. There is poor replacement of elastic tissue at site of previous surgical manipulation *(wide arrows)*. (Original magnification, ×100.) (*A* and *B*, Movat pentachrome stain.) (*A* and *B*, From Reifsnyder T, Towne JB, Seabrook GR, et al: Biology of long-term autogenous vein grafts. J Vasc Surg 17:207, 1993.)

have been highly satisfactory, overcoming their chief drawbacks of poor surgical handling characteristics, tendency to fray, and limited tissue ingrowth. These disadvantages become more important, however, in complex thoracoabdominal aortic reconstructions using the method of Crawford[234] as opposed to simple tube grafts for large vessel aneurysm repair. In the former instance, "buttons" must be cut in the graft and sutured from within the aneurysm around orifices of critical visceral or intercostal vessels. The stiffness and poor conformability of conventional low-porosity woven Dacron grafts may be a significant impediment in this regard. Therefore, use of higher porosity woven grafts, perhaps soaked in plasma and autoclaved just prior to implantation to augment their imperviousness, may be considered.[59, 60] Or, one of the several varieties of biologically coated knitted Dacron grafts may be advantageous. ePTFE tubular grafts have similar appeal and are currently available in sizes up to 24 mm in diameter. Similar considerations regarding imperviousness apply to patients with ruptured abdominal aortic aneurysms or those with a coagulation disorder of some sort.

For elective infrarenal aortoiliac replacement or bypass, Dacron prostheses have long been a conventional and successful choice and show excellent long-term results that are well documented.[21, 235–240] Many surgeons prefer knitted grafts owing to their advantages of better handling and healing characteristics. Such features are thought by many to be particularly important for aortofemoral grafts done for occlusive disease that must cross the inguinal ligament, often with anastomoses made to a diseased femoral artery or profunda femoris branch alone.[235] However, the long-term patency advantages of knitted versus woven grafts have not been conclusively established, and several currently manufactured, more porous woven Dacron grafts have acceptable handling qualities. The recently introduced biologically coated knitted Dacron grafts are quite appealing owing to the convenience of their low implant porosity, which precludes the need for preclotting, while they retain much of their flexibility, conformability, suturability, and so on.[49] Their greater cost, approximately double that of a conventional Dacron prosthesis, is a relative drawback, however, and further experience must be accumulated to ensure that the coating process does not prove detrimental in some fashion in later years. The recently introduced version of the ePTFE bifurcation graft has potential attributes that warrant serious consideration for its use. In addition to imperviousness, it has adequate handling features, and may be more resistant to infection or development of late anastomotic aneurysm formation.[118–123, 126–132, 138] In addition, it appears to have excellent structural stability in contrast to knitted Dacron grafts, which are increasingly recognized to be prone to dilatation. The increased cost of ePTFE bifurcation grafts is a relative disadvantage, as with coated grafts. The relatively poor compliance of ePTFE grafts is probably of lesser importance in terms of late patency rates in the larger caliber, higher flow aortoiliofemoral position. Indeed, the generally good patency of many varieties of available prosthetic grafts for aortic reconstruction makes it unlikely that this will be a primary discriminating feature of graft selection for such procedures; issues of convenience and diminished late complications will probably assume greater importance.

Infrainguinal Reconstruction

It is well established that for lower extremity bypass grafts autogenous saphenous vein is the preferred choice, particularly for grafts with very low points of distal anastomosis and very long grafts.[139, 173, 176, 208, 241–245] Two major areas of disagreement remain, however. First, some authorities propose that prosthetic grafts are, in fact, the graft of choice when bypass to the above-knee popliteal level is feasible. Second, if a below-knee bypass is required and no autogenous vein is available, controversy persists about the best choice between ePTFE, HUV, and Dacron grafts or whether prosthetic grafts are in fact superior to primary amputation.

Proponents of preferential use of prosthetic grafts for above-knee femoropopliteal reconstruction emphasize that numerous studies, including some well-controlled, randomized, and prospective series, have not detected statistically significant differences in patency or limb salvage rates between vein and prosthetic grafts in this position, particularly at shorter follow-up intervals and in patients undergoing operation for claudication.[139, 176, 177, 246–253] The advantages of initial use of prosthetic grafts are the shorter operative time and the need for less dissection and only two small incisions–factors that may be advantageous in the high-risk elderly patient population. The compromised long-term survival of many of these patients may also reduce the importance of truly long-term graft patency. It is reasoned that even if patency rates with prosthetic conduits are slightly lower, the saphenous vein will still be available for use in reoperation if this is required.[254] Graft failure is also anticipated in a significant number of patients who have primary vein grafts. It is well recognized that reoperations using autogenous vein result in much higher long-term patency rates than reoperations using prosthetic grafts.[211, 251, 255, 256] Hence, it is reasoned that the fairly similar primary patency rates of above-knee vein and prosthetic grafts plus the much superior results of reoperation if the vein is still available will ultimately lead to a better long-term outcome. Or, in other words, the management sequence of initial preferential use of a prosthetic graft for above-knee reconstruction followed by autogenous saphenous vein for patients who do ultimately require secondary repair is preferable.[257]

Michaels[258] has done an extensive literature review and constructed a mathematical model to test this hypothesis. He concluded that there was a clear overall advantage to using vein for the initial graft, whereas the alternative strategy of prosthetic graft first, vein later if necessary increases the number of additional operations and results in a lower 5-year patency rate when both first and second grafts are considered. Although this is an interesting work, it must be remembered that it is only a model and is limited, as he points out, by a lack of sufficient data from well-controlled trials. Other studies have shown that the argument sometimes advanced for saving the saphenous vein for possible future use in coronary revascularization is, in fact, rarely necessary.[251, 259] Furthermore, although use of prosthetic grafts is quicker, a corresponding reduction in mortality and morbidity has not been conclusively demonstrated by any study. If a greater number of second operations is indeed required with initial use of prosthetic grafts, the morbidity and possible associated complications such as graft infection, which are clearly greater with reoperations, must also be considered.[258] As is obvious, this remains a debated and controversial topic. My own personal belief is that initial use of prosthetic grafts is indeed an appropriate strategy in certain patients, particularly older patients undergoing operation for noncritical ischemia with fairly good runoff.

As previously noted, autogenous vein may not be available or may be inadequate for use in infrainguinal bypass in 10 to 40 per cent of patients, depending on the length of the graft and whether or not it is a primary or secondary operation. In these circumstances, controversy continues about the best substitute conduit. Dacron grafts were initially utilized for lower extremity grafts in the early era of arterial reconstructive surgery, but mediocre late results, with 5-year patency rates in the range of 50 to 60 per cent, were generally noted, and even more discouraging results were reported in grafts extending below the knee.[260–263] Such outcomes and the attractive features of ePTFE grafts, such as the absence of the need for preclotting and the promise of potential lower thrombogenicity, led to a rapid decline in the use of Dacron grafts for femoropopliteal reconstruction. Yet, as recently pointed out by Pevec and associates, no contemporary comparative study of these grafts has been done that really establishes the superiority of ePTFE.[264, 265] Kenney and coworkers reported a 78 per cent 4-year patency rate for externally supported, noncrimped Dacron grafts to the above-knee popliteal artery, which is certainly equivalent to the results of any series of ePTFE grafts.[48]

Nonetheless, ePTFE grafts have clearly emerged as the most widely utilized alternative to autogenous vein for lower extremity revascularization procedures. Despite reports of early good experiences,[221, 266–268] their long-term function in below-knee or, particularly, tibial bypasses has been far from ideal.[139, 269–271] With development of the modified HUV graft by Dardik and coworkers, debate began about the best alternative graft, and this remains an unsettled issue. Some studies have shown improved patency of HUV grafts compared to ePTFE bypasses.[173, 178, 179] Our own results in a series of 99 HUV grafts showed no significant differences between HUV and ePTFE grafts for above-knee anastomoses or good runoff situations, but there was an advantage in late cumulative patency rates for HUV used in below-knee grafts and poor runoff situations.[175]

Despite their possible advantages in long grafts or in situations of compromised outflow, the disadvantages of HUV grafts weigh heavily against their use. They are clearly more cumbersome to deal with from a technical standpoint, and most important, they are subject to a significant incidence of biodegradative changes as previously detailed. For these reasons, unless further modifications in graft production can be shown to reduce the frequency of loss of structural integrity, umbilical vein grafts will be infrequently employed by vascular surgeons. ePTFE conduits are currently the most acceptable alternative to the saphenous vein for lower extremity revascularization procedures. Although the long-term patency of ePTFE grafts to infrapopliteal vessels is rather poor, surprisingly good results can sometimes be achieved. Veith and colleagues[139] noted a limb salvage rate of 38 per cent at 4 years, similar to that of several other reports. Certainly if a patent tibial vessel exists and no autogenous material of any sort is available, bypass to a tibial or peroneal artery is justified in selected patients for attempted limb salvage as opposed to primary amputation.[139, 272] It is hoped that concepts such as vein cuff interposition or long-term maintenance of warfarin therapy may improve the long-term performance of such grafts. A realistic appraisal of available experience, however, reemphasizes that all efforts to utilize autogenous tissue for infrageniculate grafts should be made, serving as a continued stimulus to develop new and improved small calibre prosthetic grafts.

Extra-anatomic Grafts

Few comparative data exist on the use of Dacron or ePTFE grafts for the variety of remote subcutaneously implanted grafts collectively referred to as extra-anatomic reconstructions. HUV grafts have little to recommend them in this position. Currently, most vascular surgeons regard ePTFE grafts as the graft of choice for axillofemoral, femorofemoral, or axillo-axillary grafts. Although patency rates may not be demonstrably higher, the lack of implantation bleeding with ePTFE grafts may be particularly helpful in avoiding hematoma formation in the subcutaneous tunnels compared with knitted Dacron grafts, even when careful preclotting is done. In addition, the relative resistance of ePTFE to compression or kinking and ease of thrombectomy are valuable features.[103, 273–275] In these subcutaneous positions, the use of externally supported grafts seems logical, although it is of unproven benefit. Sauvage's group has also described good long-term patency of externally supported Dacron conduits for axillofemoral grafts.[48, 102] For carotid-subclavian grafts, some authors have documented higher long-term patency rates with ePTFE or Dacron grafts than with vein grafts.[276–278] The relatively small diameter of vein grafts and their potential for kinking and shortening secondary to neck flexion and mobility in contrast to the larger and more rigid prostheses may be factors.

Other Locations

Visceral or renal arterial reconstructions may be performed with prosthetic grafts with good results and are used in preference to vein grafts by many surgeons in these locations. Satisfactory patency is no doubt related to the fact that these are generally short grafts with high blood flow and are not subjected to mechanical stresses around body joints. An exception may be distal renal artery grafts in young patients with fibromuscular disease or visceral or renal procedures that involve bypass to diseased vessels with compromised distal arterial beds. Most previous experience has been gained with Dacron grafts. Preclotted knitted Dacron seems to be the preferred choice, although currently use of a coated Dacron graft represents an appealing possibility. Grafts of ePTFE have similar potential benefits and are an equally acceptable choice. However, extensive experience with ePTFE grafts for renal or mesenteric revascularization procedures has not been accumulated to date.[279]

Grafts of ePTFE may also be employed for large-caliber venous replacements in unusual circumstances, and their use has been described for replacement or bypass of the inferior or superior vena cava,[280–282] jugular,[283] and portal[284] veins, or for construction of portosystemic shunts for portal hypertension.[285] Stented grafts appear to be advisable for venous grafts.[286] The moderate success of large-caliber supported ePTFE venous grafts may attest to their reduced thrombogenicity and ability to remain patent in lower flow states. Very limited experience with venous reconstructions employing other prosthetic materials has been generally unsuccessful.

When a primary arteriovenous fistula for hemodialysis cannot be performed or has failed, ePTFE grafts have become the prosthetic vessel of choice for angioaccess in the opinion of most authorities, in contrast to bovine heterografts or other possible alternatives. Its resistance to infection, reasonable long-term patency, ease of revision, satisfactory tissue incorporation, and ability to withstand repeated puncture with less pseudoaneurysm formation have been documented.[287–289]

THE FUTURE

Considerable research is currently in progress in the development of improved vascular substitutes, particularly for small vessel replacement. Such efforts are directed at both the potential use of new biomaterials with better surface properties and compliance, and continued modification of substances already in use in an attempt to lower their flow-surface thrombogenicity.[290] Much current emphasis is appropriately focused on a better understanding of the biologic phenomena at the cellular level that occur at the blood-prostheses interface. It is hoped that better knowledge of the cellular, humoral, and enzymatic processes that control the interdependent interactions of platelets, endothelial cells, smooth muscle cells, and other blood and tissue components will allow favorable modification of the graft flow surface, better control of neointimal hyperplasia, and more specific and successful pharmacologic control of the clotting process. Ultimately, a true biologic era of grafts may result because efforts to develop a biologic graft using cell culture technology are already underway.[291]

Endothelial Cell Seeding

Appreciation of the integral role played by living endothelial cells, with their diverse and dynamic biochemical functions, in maintaining a thrombus-free flow surface in normal vessels or autogenous tissue vascular grafts has quite logically stimulated efforts to produce a similar antithrombogenic lining in prosthetic grafts (Fig. 29–13). It is now clearly established that endothelial regeneration in synthetic vascular grafts, as often demonstrated in various experimental animals, does not occur in the human except within several centimeters of each anastomosis of a graft. Hence, efforts have been directed toward ''seeding'' prosthetic grafts with mechanically or enzymatically derived autologous endothelial cells at the time of graft implantation in the expectation that subsequent attachment and proliferation of these cells will produce a confluent monolayer of living endothelial cells that will cover the entire graft flow surface and render it less prone to thrombosis (Fig. 29–14).

The concept of endothelial cell seeding was first introduced in 1970 by Mansfield,[292] who employed granulation tissue as a cell source to seed a mixture of endothelial cells, fibroblasts, and macrophages onto Dacron patches implanted into the hearts of dogs. At excision 3 weeks later, the patches seeded with autogenous cells exhibited a surface completely free of thrombus. Since this observation, a voluminous amount of laboratory work has attempted to develop techniques of lining prosthetic grafts with a functional endothelial cell layer, and progress has been made in methods of harvesting, culturing, and seeding techniques.[293]

In the pioneering work of Herring and colleagues,[294] reported in 1978, endothelial cells derived from mechanically scraping veins with steel wool pledgets were used to seed Dacron grafts in a canine model. The cells were mixed with blood to preclot the grafts, which were immediately implanted in a single-stage technique. When explanted, the seeded grafts showed greater thrombus-free surface over

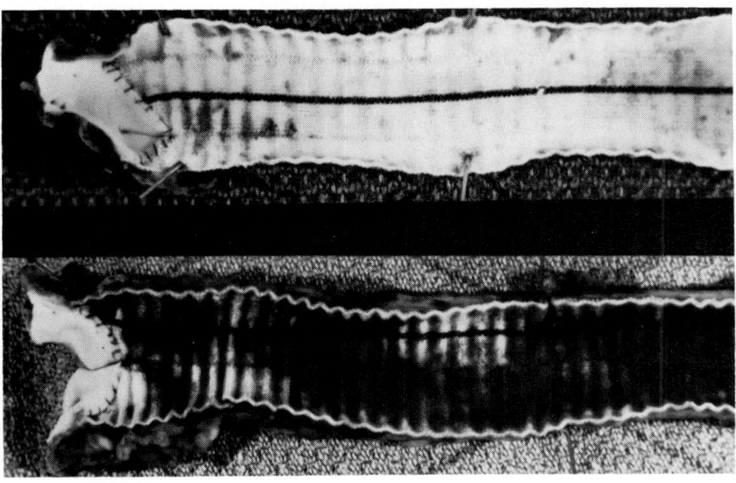

FIGURE 29–13. Endothelial cell–seeded *(upper)* and -unseeded *(lower)* Dacron prosthesis 4 weeks following canine thoracoabdominal implantation. Note thrombus-free surface of seeded graft compared with typical appearance of inner surface of the unseeded graft.

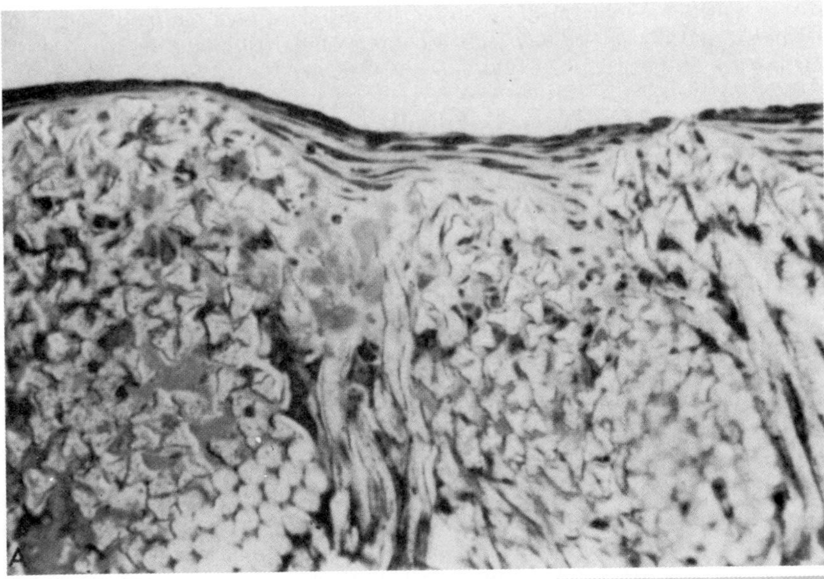

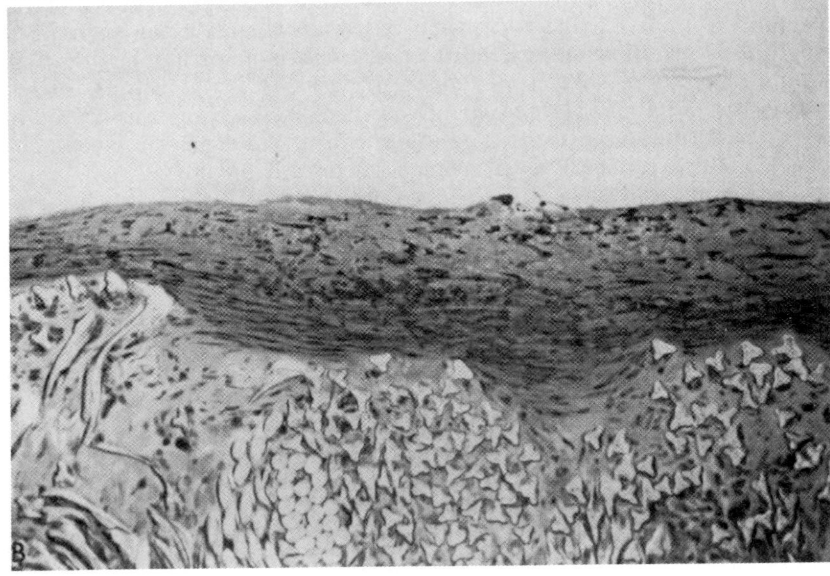

FIGURE 29–14. Photomicrographs of midportion of Dacron prosthesis 4 weeks after canine implantation. *A*, Endothelial cell–seeded graft. Note thin endothelium-lined flow surface (×64). *B*, Thick fibrin-lined surface in unseeded graft (×40, methylene blue-basic fuchsin stain).

time compared with unseeded controls and also demonstrated significantly thinner inner capsules. Subsequent work confirmed the endothelial nature of the graft lining and showed that seeded ePTFE grafts developed endothelial linings significantly sooner than similar Dacron grafts.[295] This fact suggests that less porous grafts may be better for seeding or that Dacron is a ''less hospitable'' material for the endothelial cell. Because mechanical débridement of cells is relatively cumbersome and inefficient and produces a mixture of smooth muscle as well as endothelial cells, Graham and colleagues developed methods of enzymatic derivation with collagenase.[296] These investigators noted more efficient harvesting using enzymes rather than mechanical scraping. They also cultured the cells before later adding them to blood used to preclot Dacron grafts. Good results in terms of the degree of endothelialization of both seeded Dacron and ePTFE grafts were noted.[297]

Subsequent work in laboratory animals has suggested that small-caliber endothelial cell–seeded grafts have better early patency, less platelet deposition, greater tolerance to low flow states, confirmed prostacyclin-generating capacity, and other functional attributes similar to those of the flow surfaces of native vessels.[298–304] Seeded grafts have also been demonstrated to have greater resistance to bacteremic infection due to decreased bacterial adherence to endothelialized graft surfaces as opposed to areas of accumulated surface thrombus.[305]

Although the potential benefits of endothelial cell seeding have been documented, more recent experimental work has focused on maximizing the number of cells harvested and improving their adherence to the graft surface. Large numbers of microvascular endothelial cells may be obtained from adipose tissue, but such endothelial cells may not be a pure enough population for successful growth.[306–309] Culture of enzymatically derived cells may provide a larger number of cells for high-density seeding at a later interval, but this process requires considerable time for their growth and increases the risk of bacterial contamination with subsequent inoculation into the host. Rosenman and associates have characterized the difficulties encountered with satisfactory adherence of seeded endothelial cells to graft surfaces of ePTFE conduits with exposure to blood flow.[310] They noted a 30 per cent detachment of cells within the first 30 minutes, which decreased to 2 per cent per hour over the next 24 hours. However, only about 5 per cent of harvested cells remained attached to the graft 72 hours after seeding. Seeger[311, 312] demonstrated that precoating ePTFE grafts with fibronectin significantly improved endothelial cell adherence, and Kempczinski's group confirmed a sixfold increase in cell retention in ePTFE grafts pretreated with fibronectin.[313]

Limited clinical experience with results of endothelial cell seeding in humans is available. In 1984, Herring and coworkers described seeding of Dacron femoropopliteal, axillofemoral, and femorofemoral grafts. No difference in patency was observed between seeded and nonseeded grafts, although early patency of seeded grafts was worse in patients who continued to smoke.[314] Herring and coworkers also reported the first documented evidence of endothelialization in a human with a seeded ePTFE graft.[315] Ortenwall and colleagues found significantly less platelet deposition in seeded limbs of Dacron aortic bifurcation grafts compared with unseeded opposite limbs, seeming to imply an antiplatelet effect.[316, 317] In a subsequent series of 23 lower extremity grafts, these investigators seeded half of each ePTFE implant with autogenous endothelial cells. Seeded segments accumulated significantly fewer platelets at 1 and 6 months after surgery compared with unseeded portions, suggesting a reduced surface thrombogenicity in the seeded areas.[318] Several small clinical series of seeded femoropopliteal grafts have shown short-term results appearing to favor seeded versus unseeded grafts, although they were not statistically significant.[319, 320] Another clinical trial failed to show any significant patency differences.[321]

It is clear that successful practical application in humans of the wealth of promising animal and laboratory results remains a presently unfulfilled prospect. The ability to harvest cells and seed the graft in the operating room requires simplified methods. The ability of seeded cells to adhere and grow on a particular graft surface and resist the sheer surface of flowing blood needs to be improved. It remains to be established conclusively that seeded cells will maintain their anticoagulant and other favorable biologic functions in ways that will translate into better late patency of small vessel grafts. This work remains an exciting and potentially valuable concept for prosthetic grafts, however, and the use of recombinant gene technology to allow genetic modification of the function of seeded endothelial cells is perhaps a revolutionary influence on the horizon.[322]

Biodegradable Prostheses

Recognition of the advantages of autogenous tissue vascular grafts and the potential adverse long-term mechanical and biochemical effects of blood and tissue interaction with prosthetic materials has continually spurred efforts to develop satisfactory biologically derived tissue conduits. A relatively recent example of this is the development of an absorbable prosthetic graft. In theory, subsequent tissue ingrowth and incorporation would eventually result in a conduit whose functional attributes were those of the regenerated host tissues themselves. The concept of using a totally biodegradable mesh prosthesis with acceptable implant porosity was initially investigated in several laboratories.[323, 324] Animal studies demonstrated the capabilities of many components of an animal artery to regenerate over a scaffold of material such as an absorbable woven polyglactin acid (Vicryl) prosthesis. Microscopic studies showed that the polyglactin prostheses had almost entirely disappeared after several months and were replaced by regenerating endothelialized vessels containing smooth muscle–like myofibroblasts and dense fibroplasia, without thrombosis or infection. A tendency toward dilation or frank aneurysm was noted, however. The clinical efficacy of bioresorbable vascular prostheses depends in part upon the development of adequate strength of the regenerated tissue prior to loss of strength of the absorbable prosthesis itself.[325] If this is a problem in potential human implantation, as appears likely, "compound" grafts might be constructed from yarns containing both bioresorbable and more permanent inert materials, or prostheses can be constructed of a mix of different biodegradable components that are resorbed at slower rates, thereby promoting early tissue ingrowth while the more slowly resorbed component remains as a mechanical strut. Laboratory work along these lines has been reported.[326–328] Although intriguing and potentially clinically useful, at present bioresorbable vascular prostheses remain an experimental example of a "bioprosthetic compound" vascular graft.

Impregnated Grafts

In addition to coating or impregnating grafts with albumin, collagen, or gelatin to reduce implantation porosity and bleeding, efforts have been directed toward incorporating substances within grafts or on their flow surfaces that might improve some aspect of their performance.

Although infection following implantation of vascular prostheses is relatively infrequent (2 to 6 per cent) in current practice, such problems continue to occur despite use of prophylactic systemic antibiotics or local irrigation with antibiotic solutions, and they remain a challenging complication. An appealing concept is a process that would render grafts more resistant to infection. Conventional antibiotic usage or soaking a prosthetic graft in an antibiotic solution immediately prior to implantation is relatively ineffective owing to the brief residence of the drug at the implantation site. In contrast, direct *incorporation of antibacterial agents* into the graft can theoretically prolong residence of drugs at the immediate graft site. In 1974, Clark and Margraff described experimental treatment of prosthetic grafts with a silver-allantoin-heparin complex that significantly resisted infection in dogs.[329] Further work on the bonding of antibiotics to Dacron and ePTFE grafts, employing carriers such as a benzalkonium-oxacillin complex, tridodecylmethylammonium chloride (TDMAC), and other compounds, has been reported with promising laboratory results.[330–335] Incorporation of silver along with the antibiotic appears to enhance antibacterial activity and prolong retention of the antibiotic in the graft, slowing the washout effect of blood flow and allowing a slower steady diffusion.[336] Moore and associates[337] have used collagen as the vehicle for bonding amikacin to knitted Dacron grafts. Such grafts were found to be much more resistant than controls implanted in the canine aorta to intravenously administered bacterial challenges. This line of work remains experimental, and further efforts need to be directed toward finding the best method of affixing antibiotics to grafts and improving their retention and release. Furthermore, translation of results of animal studies to humans may be difficult. Nonetheless, this developmental approach remains promising.

In related work, *heparin bonding* as a means of reducing the thrombogenicity of prosthetic materials and potentially improving their function as small-diameter vessel substitutes has been investigated. Gott and associates described the direct binding of heparin to prosthetic surfaces using benzalkonium chloride and graphite as absorbed anchoring molecules.[338] Refinement of this concept led to development of the Gott shunt for bypass of the thoracic aorta without systemic heparinization in repair of thoracic aneurysms. Esquival and associates[339] have described covalent bonding of heparin to ePTFE and polyurethane prostheses, noting a significant reduction of thrombogenicity in a sheep laboratory model. Bonding of antithrombotic pharmacologic agents other than heparin, such as urokinase, and affixation of endothelial cell mitogens such as growth factor in order to enhance potential endothelialization have also been studied, but such studies are in their early stages, and results are inconclusive thus far.[16, 52, 340]

Alternative Grafts

Building upon both theoretic concepts and prior laboratory and clinical experience with prosthetic grafts continues to lead to introduction of new graft materials and designs. Most have been investigated only in the laboratory and remain experimental; a few have had limited clinical application.

Alternative polymers for construction of small-caliber synthetic grafts have included various polyurethanes. Despite their promise of low thrombogenicity and relatively high implant compliance, the patency rates of such grafts have not been as good when tested in vivo.[341, 342] These and other polymers have also exhibited a disturbing tendency toward later degeneration and aneurysm formation.[343]

A unique replamineform graft has been described by White and colleagues.[344, 345] This conduit is formed using the sea urchin spine as a cast of uniform microporosity. The structure is impregnated with polyurethane and polymerized. Finally, the urchin bioskeleton is dissolved with 5 per cent hydrochloric acid, yielding a polyurethane tube with uniform pores measuring 15 to 20 μ. Any advantage of this uniform pore size and geometric arrangement over that of microporous ePTFE grafts remains to be established.

Attempts to modify interactions favorably at the blood-prosthesis interface on the graft flow surface have also been attempted. It has been shown that the normal intraluminal polarity of the normal blood vessel is negative. Because blood cells are also negatively charged, it is logical that a repulsive negative charge interface normally exists between the vessel wall and the blood components, resulting in decreased thrombogenicity.[342] Emphasis on such electrochemical forces to produce an "ion cloud" that will help make a graft surface "invisible" to blood has been promulgated by Sawyer and associates.[195, 196, 346] This effort resulted in the NCGT heterograft previously described, whose flow surface was modified by attachment of an organic diphatic acid to the amino acid side chain of the collagen helix to impart an increased negative charge. Coating grafts with carbon or bioelectric polyurethane to impart a negative intraluminal charge has also been utilized but with limited success.[347–349] Coating of grafts with carbon or other compounds may also alter other important physical characteristics of the basic prosthetic material, such as porosity, and needs further investigation.

Conclusion

Nearly five decades of clinical experience with arterial reconstruction have demonstrated the importance of prosthetic grafts in the treatment of patients with vascular disease. A variety of synthetic and biologically derived conduits have been developed, often by innovative vascular surgeons in response to a particular clinical need. When vessel reconstruction with autogenous tissue grafts is not feasible, a number of generally satisfactory alternative prosthetic grafts exist for each specific clinical requirement. Although no consensus on the optimal prosthetic choice for a particular procedure exists, the vascular surgeon can make a reasoned selection based on the particular advantages and disadvantages unique to each type of prosthesis. Considerations include the attributes of each material in a particular location, anatomic requirements, patient status, handling characteristics of the material, cost, and of course, individual preferences of each surgeon.

As some of the biologic mysteries of prosthesis-host interactions are unraveled, a better understanding of the events occurring at these interfaces will undoubtedly lead to new concepts and designs of prosthetic grafts. Whether the ultimate ideal prosthetic graft—that is, a vessel substitute with a live intima and a permanently stable and compliant wall that truly parallels the complex dynamic functions of an artery—will ever be developed is uncertain. In striving for this goal, it is important to emphasize Szilagyi's admonition that any clinical introduction of newly modified prostheses should be preceded by careful and extended laboratory studies and that commercial introduction should occur only after a period of controlled clinical use with careful and thorough analysis by critically minded and unbiased investigators.[1]

References

1. Szilagyi DE: Vascular substitutes, 1981: Achievements, disappointments, prospects. J Cardiovasc Surg 23:183, 1982.
2. Callow AD: Historical overview of experimental and clinical development of vascular grafts. *In* Stanley JC (ed): Biologic and Synthetic Vascular Prostheses. New York, Grune & Stratton, 1982, pp 11–26.
3. Sauvage LR, Berger KE, Wood SJ, et al: Interspecies healing of porous arterial prostheses. Arch Surg 109:698, 1974.
4. Scales JT: Tissue reactions to synthetic materials. Proc R Soc Med 46:647, 1953.

5. Sauvage LR: Biologic behavior of grafts in arterial system. *In* Haimovici H (ed): Vascular Surgery: Principles and Techniques, 3rd ed. Norwalk, CT, Appleton & Lange, 1989, pp 136–60.
6. Edwards WS: The effect of porosity in solid plastic grafts. Surg Forum 8:446, 1957.
7. Boyd DP, Midell AI: Woven Teflon aortic grafts: An unsatisfactory prosthesis. Vasc Surg 5:148, 1971.
8. Fry WJ, DeWeese MS, Kraft RO, et al: Importance of porosity in arterial prostheses. Arch Surg 88:836, 1964.
9. Weslowski SA, Fries CC, Karlson KE, et al: Porosity: Primary determinant of ultimate fate of synthetic vascular grafts. Surgery 50:91, 1961.
10. Weslowski SA: The healing of vascular prostheses. Surgery 57:319, 1965.
11. Mathisen SR, Wu H-D, Sauvage LR, et al: The influence of denier and porosity on performance of a warp-knit Dacron arterial prosthesis. Ann Surg 203:382, 1986.
12. Campbell CD, Goldfarb D, Roe A: A small arterial substitute: Expanded microporous PTFE: Patency vs. porosity. Ann Surg 182:38, 1975.
13. White RA: Evaluation of small diameter graft parameters using replamineform vascular prostheses. *In* Wright CB (ed): Vascular Grafting. Littleton, MA, John Wright PSG, 1983, pp 315–325.
14. Szilagyi DE: Arterial substitutes: Current problems and preferences. *In* Najarian JS, Delaney JP (eds): Advances in Vascular Surgery. Chicago, Year Book Medical, 1983, pp 81–90.
15. Greisler HP: Vascular graft healing—Interfacial phenomena. *In* Greisler HP: New Biologic and Synthetic Vascular Prostheses. Austin, TX, RG Landes, 1991, pp 1–19.
16. Esquivel CO, Blaisdell FW: Why small caliber vascular grafts fail: A review of clinical and experimental experience and the significance of the interaction of blood at the interface. J Surg Res 41:1, 1986.
17. Berger K, Sauvage LR, Rao AM, et al: Healing of arterial prostheses in man: Its incompleteness. Ann Surg 175:118, 1972.
18. Sauvage LR, Berger K, Beilin LB, et al: Presence of endothelium in an axillary femoral graft of knitted Dacron with an external velour surface. Ann Surg 186:749, 1975.
19. Kaplan S, Marcoe KF, Sauvage LR, et al: The effect of predetermined thrombotic potential of the recipient on small-caliber graft performance. J Vasc Surg 3:311, 1986.
20. Sauvage LR, Walker MW, Berger K, et al: Current arterial prostheses: Experimental evaluation by implantation in the carotid and circumflex coronary arteries of the dog. Arch Surg 114:687, 1979.
21. Sauvage LR, Smith JC, Davis CC: Dacron arterial grafts: Comparative structures and basis for successful use of current prostheses. *In* Kambic HE, Kantrowitz A, Sung P (eds): Vascular Graft Update: Safety and Performance. Philadelphia, American Society of Testing and Materials, 1986, pp 16–24.
22. Sanders RJ, Kempczinski RF, Hammond W, DiClementi D: The significance of graft diameter. Surgery 88:856, 1980.
23. Abbott WM, Cambria RP: Control of physical characteristics (elasticity and compliance) of vascular grafts. *In* Stanley JC (ed): Biologic and Synthetic Vascular Prostheses. New York, Grune & Stratton, 1982, pp 189–220.
24. Imparato AM, Bracco A, Kim GE, Zeff R: Intimal and neointimal fibrous proliferation causing failure of arterial reconstructions. Surgery 72:1007, 1972.
25. Gaylis H: Pathogenesis of anastomotic aneurysms. Surgery 90:509, 1981
26. O'Donnell TF, Mackey W, McCullough JL, et al: Correlation of operative findings with angiographic and noninvasive hemodynamic factors associated with failure of polytetrafluoroethylene grafts. J Vasc Surg 1:136, 1984.
27. Kidson IG, Abbott WM: Low compliance and arterial graft occlusion. Circulation 58(Suppl I):1, 1978.
28. Walden R, L'Italien G, Megerman J, et al: Matched elastic properties and successful arterial grafting. Arch Surg 115:1166, 1980.
29. Voorhees AB Jr, Jaretzke AL III, Blakemore AH: The use of tubes constructed from Vinyon-"N" cloth in bridging arterial defects. Ann Surg 135:332, 1952.
30. Blakemore AH, Voorhees AB Jr: The use of tubes constructed from Vinyon-N cloth in bridging arterial defects: Experimental and clinical. Ann Surg 140:324, 1954.
31. Edwards WS, Tapp JS: Chemically treated nylon tubes as arterial grafts. Surgery 38:61, 1955.
32. Edwards WS, Tapp JS: A flexible aortic bifurcation graft of chemically treated nylon. Surgery 41:723, 1957.
33. Edwards WS: Progress in synthetic graft development: An improved crimped graft of Teflon. Surgery 45:298, 1959.
34. Deterling RA, Bhonslay SB: An evaluation of synthetic materials and fabrics suitable for blood vessel replacement. Surgery 38:71, 1955.
35. Harrison JH: Synthetic materials as vascular prostheses: A comparative study in small vessels of nylon, Dacron, Orlon, Ivalon sponge and Teflon (I and II). Am J Surg 95:3, 1958.
36. Creech O Jr, Deterling RA Jr, Edwards WS, et al: Vascular prostheses: Report of Committee for Study of Vascular Prostheses for the Society of Vascular Surgery. Surgery 41:62, 1957.
37. Weslowski SA, Dennis C: Fundamentals of Vascular Grafting. New York, McGraw-Hill, 1963.
38. DeBakey ME, Jordan GL Jr, Abbott JP, et al: The fate of Dacron vascular grafts. Arch Surg 89:757, 1964.
39. Snyder RW, Botzko KM: Woven, knitted, and externally supported Dacron vascular prostheses. *In* Stanley JC (ed): Biologic and Synthetic Vascular Prostheses. New York, Grune & Stratton, 1982, pp 485–508.
40. Lindenauer SM: The fabric vascular prosthesis. *In* Rutherford RB (ed): Vascular Surgery, 3rd ed. Philadelphia, WB Saunders, 1989, pp 450–460.
41. Hall CW, Liotta D, Ghidoni JJ, et al: Velour fabrics applied to medicine. J Biomed Mater Res 1:179, 1967.
42. Lindenauer SM, Lavanway JM, Fry WJ: Development of a velour vascular prosthesis. Curr Top Surg Res 2:491, 1970.
43. Sauvage LR, Berger K, Wood SJ, et al: An external velour surface for porous arterial prostheses. Surgery 70:940, 1971.
44. Sauvage LR, Berger KE, Mansfield PB, et al: Future directions in the development of arterial prostheses for small and medium caliber arteries. Surg Clin North Am 54:213, 1974.
45. Goldman M, McCollum CN, Hawker RJ, et al: Dacron arterial grafts: The influence of porosity, velour, and maturity on thrombogenicity. Surgery 92:947, 1982.
46. Wu H-D, Zammit M, Sauvage LR, Steicher MD: The influence of inner wall filamentousness on the performance of small- and large-caliber arterial grafts. J Vasc Surg 2:255, 1985.
47. Yates SG, Barros D'Sa AAB, Berger K, et al: The preclotting of porous arterial prostheses. Ann Surg 188:611, 1978.
48. Kenney DA, Sauvage LR, Wood SJ, et al: Comparison of non-crimped, externally supported (EXS) and crimped, non-supported Dacron prostheses for axillo-femoral and above-knee femoropopliteal bypass. Surgery 92:931, 1982.
49. Quinones-Baldrich WJ, Moore WS, Ziomek S, Chvapil M: Development of a "leak-proof," knitted Dacron vascular prosthesis. J Vasc Surg 3:895, 1986.
50. Ruhland D, Wigger J, Botleher K, et al: Fate of collagen following implantation of Microvel Hemashield grafts in the dog. Angio Archiv 9:22, 1985.
51. McGee GS, Shuman TA, Atkinson JB, et al: Long-term assessment of a damp-stored, albumin-coated, knitted vascular graft. Ann Surg 55:174, 1989.
52. Greisler HP: Biohybrids—Biological coatings in synthetic grafts. *In* Greisler HP: New Biologic and Synthetic Vascular Prostheses. Austin, TX, RG Landes, 1991, pp 33–46.
53. Chang TMS: Platelet-surface interaction: Effect of albumin coating on heparin complexing on thrombogenic surfaces. Can J Phys Pharmacol 52:275, 1974.
54. Kottke-Marchant K, Anderson JM, Umemura Y, et al: Effect of albumin coating on the in vitro compatibility of Dacron arterial prostheses. Biomaterials 110:147, 1989.
55. Lyman DJ, Klein KG, Brosh JJ, et al: Platelet interaction with protein coated surfaces. Thromb Diath Hemor 42 (Suppl):109, 1970.
56. Canadian Multicenter Hemashield Study Group: Immunological response to collagen-impregnated vascular grafts: A randomized prospective study. J Vasc Surg 12:741, 1990.
57. Norgren L, Holtas S, Persson G, et al: Systemic response to collagen-impregnated versus non-treated Dacron velour grafts for aortic and aortofemoral reconstructions. Eur J Vasc Surg 4:379, 1990.
58. De Mol Van Otterloo JCA, Van Bockel JH, Ponfoort ED, et al: The effects of aortic reconstruction and collagen impregnation of Dacron prostheses on the complement system. J Vasc Surg 16:774, 1992.

59. Cooley DA, Romagnoli A, Milam JD, Bossart NI: A method of preparing woven Dacron aortic graft to prevent interstitial hemorrhage. Dis Bull Tex Heart Inst 8:48, 1981.
60. Rumisek JD, Wade CE, Brooks DE, et al: Heat-denatured albumin coated Dacron vascular grafts: Physical characteristics and in vivo performance. J Vasc Surg 4:136, 1986.
61. Stegmann TH, Haverich A, Borst HG: Clinical experience with a new collagen-coated Dacron double-velour prosthesis. Thorac Cardiovasc Surg 34:54, 1986.
62. Reigel MM, Hollier LH, Pairolero PC, Hallett JW Jr: Early experience with a new collagen-impregnated aortic graft. Am Surg 54:134, 1988.
63. Freischlag JA, Moore WS: Clinical experience with a collagen-impregnated knitted Dacron vascular graft. Ann Vasc Surg 4:449, 1990.
64. Guidoin R, Snyder R, Martin L, et al: Albumin coating of a knitted polyester arterial prosthesis: An alternative to preclotting. Ann Thorac Surg 37:457, 1984.
65. Guidoin R, Marois Y, Rao TJ, et al: An albumin-coated polyester arterial prosthesis made ready to anastomose: In vivo evaluation in dogs. Clin Mater 3:119, 1988.
66. Cziperle DJ, Joyce KA, Tattersall CW, et al: Albumin impregnated vascular grafts: Albumin resorption and tissue reactions. J Cardiovasc Surg 33:407, 1992.
67. Branchereau A, Rudondy P, Gournier J-P, Espinoza H: The albumin-coated knitted Dacron aortic prosthesis: A clinical study. Ann Vasc Surg 4:138, 1990.
68. Jonas RA, Ziemer G, Schoen FJ, et al: A new sealant for knitted Dacron prostheses: Minimally cross-linked gelatin. J Vasc Surg 7:414, 1988.
69. Sottiurai VS, Sue SL, Rau DJ, Tran AB: Comparative analysis of pseudointimal biogenesis in Gelseal coated Dacron knitted graft versus crimped and noncrimped graft. J Cardiovasc Surg 30:902, 1989.
70. Drury JK, Ashton TR, Cunningham JD, et al: Experimental and clinical experience with a gelatin impregnated Dacron prosthesis. Ann Vasc Surg 1:542, 1987.
71. Cooke PA, Nobis PA, Stoney RJ: Dacron aortic graft failure. Arch Surg 108:101, 1974.
72. Perry MO: Early failure of Dacron prosthetic grafts. J Cardiovasc Surg 16:318, 1975.
73. Haywood RH, Korompai FL: Degeneration of knitted Dacron grafts. Surgery 79:581, 1976.
74. Blumenberg RM, Gelfand ML: Failure of knitted Dacron as an arterial prosthesis. Surgery 81:493, 1977.
75. May J: Multiple aneurysms in Dacron velour graft. Arch Surg 113:320, 1978.
76. Watanabe T, Kusaka A, Kuma H, et al: Failure of Dacron arterial prostheses caused by structural defects. J Cardiovasc Surg 24:95, 1983.
77. Lundqvist B, Almgren B, Bowald S, et al: Deterioration and dilation of Dacron prosthetic grafts. Acta Chir Scand Suppl 29:81, 1985.
78. Sladen JG, Gerein AN, Miyagishima RT: Late rupture of prosthetic aortic grafts. Am J Surg 153:453, 1987.
79. Berger K, Sauvage LR: Late fiber deterioration in Dacron arterial grafts. Ann Surg 193:477, 1981.
80. Nunn DB, Freeman MH, Hudgins PC: Postoperative alterations in size of Dacron aortic grafts. Ann Surg 189:741, 1979.
81. Blumenberg RM, Gelfand ML, Barton EA, et al: Clinical significance of aortic graft dilation. J Vasc Surg 14:175, 1991.
82. King MW, Guidoin R, Blais P, et al: Degeneration of polyester arterial prostheses: A physical or chemical mechanism? *In* Fraker AC, Griffin CD (eds): Corrosion and Degradation of Implant Materials: Second Symposium, ASTM STP 859. Philadelphia, American Society for Testing and Materials, 1985, pp 295–307.
83. Pourdeyhimi B, Wagner D: On the correlation between the failure of vascular grafts and their structural and material properties: A critical analysis. J Biomed Mater Res 20:375, 1987.
84. Nunn DB, Carter MM, Donohue MT, et al: Postoperative dilation of knitted Dacron aortic bifurcation graft. J Vasc Surg 12:291, 1990.
85. Hunter GC, Bull DA: The healing characteristics, durability, and long-term complications of vascular prostheses. *In* Bernhard VM, Towne JB (eds): Complications in Vascular Surgery. St. Louis, Quality Medical Publishing, 1991, pp 65–86.
86. Ottinger LW, Darling RC, Wirthlin LS, Linton RR: Failure of ultralightweight knitted Dacron grafts in arterial reconstruction. Arch Surg 111:146, 1976.
87. Yashar JJ, Richmond MH, Dyckman J, et al: Failure of Dacron prostheses caused by structural defect. Surgery 84:659, 1978.
88. Kim GE, Imparato AM, Nathan I, et al: Dilatation of synthetic grafts and junctional aneurysms. Arch Surg 114:1296, 1979.
89. Claggett GP, Salander JM, Eddleman WL, et al: Dilation of knitted Dacron aortic prostheses and anastomotic false aneurysms: Etiologic considerations. Surgery 93:9, 1983.
90. Boyce B: Physical characteristics of expanded polytetrafluoroethylene grafts. *In* Stanley JC (ed): Biologic and Synthetic Vascular Prostheses. New York, Grune & Stratton, 1982, pp 553–561.
91. Soyer Y, Lempinen M, Cooper P, et al: A new venous prosthesis. Surgery 72:864, 1972.
92. Matusmoto H, Hasegawa T, Fuse K: A new vascular prosthesis for a small caliber artery. Surgery 74:518, 1973.
93. Campbell CD, Brooks DH, Webster MW, et al: The use of expanded microporous polytetrafluoroethylene for limb salvage: A preliminary report. Surgery 79:485, 1976.
94. Campbell DC, Brooks DH, Webster MW, et al: Aneurysm formation in expanded polytetrafluoroethylene prostheses. Surgery 79:491, 1976.
95. Mathisen SR, Wu HD, Sauvage LR, et al: An experimental study of eight current arterial prostheses. J Vasc Surg 4:33, 1986.
96. Kohler TR, Stratton JR, Kirkman TR, et al: Conventional versus high-porosity polytetrafluoroethylene grafts: Clinical evaluation. Surgery 112:901, 1992.
97. Clowes AW, Kirkman TR, Reidy MA: Mechanisms of arterial graft healing. Rapid transmural capillary ingrowth provides a source of intimal endothelium and smooth muscle in porous PTFE prostheses. Am J Pathol 123:220, 1986.
98. Zacharias RK, Kirkman TR, Clowes AW: Mechanisms of healing in synthetic grafts. J Vasc Surg 6:429, 1987.
99. Kempczinski RF: Physical characteristics of implanted polytetrafluoroethylene grafts: A preliminary report. Arch Surg 114:917, 1979.
100. Jarowenko MV, Buchbinder D, Shah DM: Effect of external pressure on axillo-femoral bypass grafts. Arch Surg 193:274, 1981.
101. Cavallaro A, Sciacca V, DiMarzo L, et al: The effect of body weight compression on axillo-femoral bypass patency. J Cardiovasc Surg 29:476, 1988.
102. Schultz GA, Sauvage LR, Mathisen SR, et al: A five- to seven-year experience with externally supported Dacron prostheses in axillofemoral and femoropopliteal bypass. Ann Vasc Surg 1:214, 1986.
103. Harris JE, Taylor LM, McConnell DB, et al: Clinical results of axillofemoral bypass using externally supported polytetrafluoroethylene. J Vasc Surg 12:416, 1990.
104. Burnham SJ, Flanigan DP, Goodreau JJ, et al: Ankle pressure changes in distal bypass grafts during knee flexion. Surgery 87:652, 1980.
105. Taylor RS, McFarland RJ, Cox MI: An investigation into the causes of failure of PTFE grafts. Eur J Vasc Surg 1:335, 1987.
106. Hurwitz RL, Johnson JM, Hufnagel CE: Femoropopliteal bypass using externally supported polytetrafluoroethylene grafts: Early results in a multi-institutional study. Am J Surg 150:574, 1985.
107. Dunn MM, Robinette DR, Peoples JB: Comparison between externally stented and unstented PTFE vascular grafts. Am Surg 54:324, 1988.
108. Gupta SK, Veith FJ, Kram HB, Wengerter KR: Prospective, randomized comparison of ringed and nonringed polytetrafluoroethylene femoropopliteal bypass grafts: A preliminary report. J Vasc Surg 13:162, 1991.
109. Flinn WR, Rohrer MJ, Yao JST, et al: Improved long-term patency of infragenicular polytetrafluoroethylene grafts. J Vasc Surg 7:685, 1988.
110. Miller JH, Foreman RK, Ferguson L, Faris I: Interposition vein cuff for anastomosis of prosthesis to small artery. Aust NZ J Surg 54:283, 1984.
111. Batson RC, Sottiurai VS, Craighead CC: Linton patch angioplasty: An adjunct to distal bypass with polytetrafluoroethylene grafts. Ann Surg 199:684, 1984.
112. Tyrrell MR, Wolfe JHN: New prosthetic venous collar anastomotic technique: Combining the best of other procedures. Br J Surg 78:1016, 1991.
113. Taylor RS, Loh A, McFarland RJ, et al: Improved technique for polytetrafluoroethylene bypass grafting: Long-term results using anastomotic vein patches. Br J Surg 79:348, 1992.
114. Beard JD, Benveniste GL, Miller JH, et al: Hemodynamics of the interposition vein cuff. Br J Surg 73:823, 1986.

115. Suggs WD, Henriques HF, DePalma RG: Vein cuff interposition prevents juxta-anastomotic neointimal hyperplasia. Ann Surg 207:717, 1988.
116. Tyrrell MR, Chester JF, Vipond MN, et al: Experimental evidence to support the use of interposition vein collars/patches in distal PTFE anastomoses. Eur J Vasc Surg 4:95, 1990.
117. Wolfe JHN, Tyrrell MR: Justifying arterial reconstruction to crural vessels—even with a prosthetic graft. Br J Surg 78:897, 1991.
118. Corson JD, Reinhardt R, von Grondell A, et al: Clinical and experimental evaluation of aortic polytetrafluoroethylene grafts for aneurysm replacement. Arch Surg 123:453, 1988.
119. Corson JD, Baraniewski HM, Shah DM, et al: Large diameter expanded polytetrafluoroethylene grafts for infrarenal aortic aneurysm surgery. J Cardiovasc Surg 31:702, 1990.
120. Cintora I, Pearce DE, Cannon JA: A clinical survey of aortobifemoral bypass using two inherently different graft types. Ann Surg 208:625, 1988.
121. Burke PM Jr, Herrmann JB, Cutler BS: Optimal grafting methods for the small abdominal aorta. J Cardiovasc Surg 28:420, 1987.
122. Avramov S, Petrovic P, Fabri M: Bifurcated grafts (Dacron vs PTFE) in aortoiliac reconstruction: Five years follow-up. J Cardiovasc Surg 28:33, 1987.
123. Lord RSA, Nash PA, Raj PT, et al: Prospective randomized trial of polytetrafluoroethylene and Dacron aortic prosthesis. I. Perioperative results. Ann Vasc Surg 3:248, 1988.
124. Polterauer P, Prager M, Holzenbein TH, et al: Dacron versus polytetrafluoroethylene for Y-aortic bifurcation grafts: A six-year prospective randomized trial. Surgery 111:626, 1992.
125. Veith FJ, Gupta S, Daly V: Management of early and late thrombosis of expanded polytetrafluoroethylene (PTFE) femoropopliteal bypass grafts: Favorable prognosis with appropriate reoperation. Surgery 87:581, 1980.
126. Bergamini TM, Bandyk DF, Govostis D, et al: Infection of vascular prostheses caused by bacterial biofilms. J Vasc Surg 7:21, 1988.
127. Bandyk DF, Bergamini TM, Kinney EV, et al: In situ replacement of vascular prostheses infected by bacterial biofilms. J Vasc Surg 13:575, 1991.
128. Shah PM, Ito K, Clauss RH, et al: Expanded microporous polytetrafluoroethylene (PTFE) grafts in contaminated wounds: Experimental and clinical study. J Truama 23:1030, 1983.
129. Stone KS, Walshaw R, Sugiyama GT, et al: Polytetrafluoroethylene versus autogenous vein grafts for vascular reconstruction in contaminated wounds. Am J Surg 147:692, 1984.
130. Feliciano DV, Mattox KL, Graham JM, Bitondo CG: Five-year experience with PTFE grafts in vascular wounds. J Trauma 25:71, 1985.
131. Schmitt DD, Bandyk DF, Pequet AJ, Towne JB: Bacterial adherence to vascular prostheses. J Vasc Surg 3:732, 1986.
132. Harris JM, Martin LF: An in vitro study of the properties influencing *Staphylococcus epidermidis* adhesion to prosthetic vascular graft materials. Ann Surg 207:612, 1987.
133. Hamlin GW, Rajah SM, Crow MJ, et al: Evaluation of the thrombogenic potential of three types of arterial grafts studied in an artificial circulation. Br J Surg 65:272, 1978.
134. Goldman M, Hall C, Dykes J, et al: Does 111-indium platelet deposition predict patency in prosthetic arterial grafts? Br J Surg 70:635, 1983.
135. Allen BT, Sicard GA, Welch MJ, et al: Platelet deposition in vascular grafts: The accuracy of in vivo quantification and the significance of in vivo platelet reactivity. Ann Surg 203:318, 1986.
136. Shoenfeld NA, Connolly R, Ramberg K, et al: The systemic activation of platelets by Dacron grafts. Surg Gynecol Obstet 166:454, 1988.
137. Shepard AD, Gelfand JA, Callow AD, O'Donnell TF Jr: Complement activation by synthetic vascular prostheses. J Vasc Surg 1:829, 1984.
138. Quiñones-Baldrich WJ, Ziomek S, Henderson T, Moore WS: Primary anastomotic bonding in polytetrafluoroethylene grafts? J Vasc Surg 5:311, 1987.
139. Veith FJ, Gupta SK, Ascer E, et al: Six-year prospective multicenter randomized comparison of autogenous saphenous vein and expanded polytetrafluoroethylene grafts in infrainguinal arterial reconstruction. J Vasc Surg 3:104, 1986.
140. Mehigan DG, Fitzpatrick B, Browne HI, Boucher-Hayes DJ: Is compliance mismatch the major cause of anastomotic arterial aneurysms? Analysis of 42 cases. J Cardiovasc Surg 26:147, 1985.
141. Echave V, Koornick AR, Haimov M, et al: Intimal hyperplasia as a complication of the use of the polytetrafluoroethylene graft for femoropopliteal bypass. Surgery 86:791, 1979.
142. Sottiurai VS, Yao JS, Flinn WR, et al: Intimal hyperplasia and neointima: An ultrastructural analysis of thrombosed grafts in humans. Surgery 93:809, 1983.
143. Sladen JG, Maxwell TM: Experience with 130 polytetrafluoroethylene grafts. Am J Surg 141:546, 1981.
144. Clowes AW, Gown AM, Hanson SR, Reidy MA: Mechanisms of arterial graft failure: 1. Role of cellular proliferation in early healing of PTFE prostheses. Am J Pathol 118:43, 1985.
145. Kuwano H, Hashizume M, Yang Y, et al: Patterns of pannus growth of the expanded polytetrafluoroethylene vascular graft with special attention to the intimal hyperplasia formation. Am Surg 52:663, 1986.
146. Oblath RW, Buckley FO, Green RM, et al: Prevention of platelet aggregation and adherence to prosthetic grafts by aspirin and dipyridamole. Surgery 84:37, 1978.
147. Hagen PO, Wang ZG, Mikat EM, Hackel DB: Antiplatelet therapy reduces aortic intimal hyperplasia distal to small diameter vascular prostheses (PTFE) in nonhuman primates. Ann Surg 195:328, 1982.
148. Green RM, Roedersheimer R, DeWeese JA: Effects of aspirin and dipyridamole on expanded polytetrafluoroethylene graft patency. Surgery 92:1016, 1982.
149. Barbalinardo RJ, Citrin P, Franco CD, et al: A comparison of isobutyl 2-cyanoacrylate glue, fibrin adhesive, and oxidized regenerated cellulose for control of needle hole bleeding from polytetrafluoroethylene vascular prostheses. J Vasc Surg 4:220, 1986.
150. Miller CM, Sangiolo P, Jacobson JH II: Reduced anastomotic bleeding using new sutures with a needle-suture diameter ratio of one. Surgery 101:156, 1987.
151. Gross RE, Hierwitt ES, Bill AH Jr, Pierce EC: Preliminary observations on the use of human arterial grafts in the treatment of certain cardiovascular defects. N Engl J Med 239:578, 1948.
152. Dubost C, Allerg M, Deconomos N: Resection of an aneurysm of the abdominal aorta—re-establishment of the continuity by a preserved human arterial graft, with results after five months. Arch Surg 64:405, 1952.
153. Oudot J, Beaconsfield P: Thrombosis of aortic bifurcation treated by resection and homograft replacement. Report of five cases. Arch Surg 66:365, 1953.
154. Szilagyi DE, McDonald RT, Smith RF, et al: Biologic fate of human arterial homografts. Arch Surg 75:506, 1957.
155. Deterling RA, Clauss RH: Long-term fate of aortic arterial homografts. J Cardiovasc Surg 11:35, 1970.
156. Meade JW, Linton RR, Darling RC, Menendez CV: Arterial homografts: A long-term clinical follow-up. Arch Surg 173:933, 1971.
157. Kieffer E, Bahnini A, Koshas F, et al: In situ allograft replacement of infected infrarenal aortic prosthetic grafts: Results in 43 patients. J Vasc Surg 17:349, 1993.
158. Ochsner JL, DeCamp PT, Leonard GL: Experience with fresh venous allografts as an arterial substitute. Ann Surg 173:933, 1971.
159. Tice DA, Zerbino V: Clinical experience with preserved human allografts for vascular reconstruction. Surgery 72:260, 1972.
160. Piccone VA, Sika J, Ahmed N, et al: Preserved saphenous vein allografts for vascular access. Surg Gynecol Obstet 147:385, 1978.
161. Ochsner JL, Lawson JD, Eskind SJ, et al: Homologous veins as an arterial substitute: Long-term results. J Vasc Surg 1:306, 1984.
162. Showalter D, Durham S, Sheppeck R, et al: Cryopreserved venous conduits in canine carotid arteries. Surgery 106:652, 1989.
163. Sellke FW, Meng RC, Rossi NP: Cryopreserved saphenous vein homografts for femoral-distal vascular reconstruction. J Cardiovasc Surg 30:836, 1989.
164. Brockbank KG, Donovan TJ, Ruby ST, et al: Functional analysis of cryopreserved veins. Preliminary report. J Vasc Surg 11:94, 1990.
165. Dardik H: Modified human umbilical vein allograft. *In* Rutherford RB (ed): Vascular Surgery, 3rd ed. Philadelphia, WB Saunders, 1989, pp 474–480.
166. Nabseth DC, Wilson JT, Tan B, et al: Fetal arterial heterografts. Arch Surg 81:929, 1960.
167. Dardik I, Dardik H: The fate of human umbilical cord vessels used as interposition arterial grafts in the baboon. Surg Gynecol Obstet 140:567, 1975.
168. Dardik H, Ibrahim IM, Dardik I: Successful arterial substitution with modified human umbilical vein. Ann Surg 183:252, 1976.
169. Dardik H, Ibrahim IM, Sprayregen S, et al: Clinical experience with

modified human umbilical cord vein for arterial bypass. Surgery 79:618, 1976.
170. Weinberg SL, Cipolletti GB, Turner RJ: Human umbilical vein grafts: Physical evaluation criteria. *In* Stanley JC (ed): Biologic and Synthetic Vascular Prostheses. New York, Grune & Stratton, 1982, 433–449.
171. Rosenberg N, Martinez A, Sawyer PN, et al: Tanned collagen arterial prosthesis of bovine carotid origin in man. Preliminary studies of enzyme-treated heterografts. Ann Surg 164:247, 1966.
172. Dardik H, Miller N, Dardik A, et al: A decade of experience with the glutaraldehyde-tanned human umbilical cord vein graft for revascularization of the lower limb. J Vasc Surg 7:336, 1988.
173. Cranley JJ, Hafner CD: Revascularization of the femoropopliteal arteries using saphenous vein, polytetrafluoroethylene, and umbilical vein grafts. Five- and six-year results. Arch Surg 117:1543, 1982.
174. Hirsch SA, Jarrett F: The use of stabilized human umbilical vein for femoropopliteal bypass: Experience with 133 operations with 5-year follow up. Ann Surg 200:147, 1984.
175. Robison JG, Brewster DC, Abbott WM, Darling RC: Femoropopliteal and tibioperoneal artery reconstruction using human umbilical vein. Arch Surg 118:1039, 1983.
176. Rutherford RB, Jones DN, Bergentz S-E, et al: Factors affecting the patency of infrainguinal bypass. J Vasc Surg 8:236, 1988.
177. Johnson WC, Lee KK, Bartle E, et al: Comparative evaluation of PTFE, HUV, and saphenous vein bypasses in femoropopliteal above-knee vascular reconstruction. Presented at International Society of Cardiovascular Surgery, 40th Annual Meeting, Chicago, June 9, 1992. J Vasc Surg (in press).
178. Eickhoff JH, Broome A, Ericsson BF, et al: Four years' results of a prospective randomized clinical trial comparing polytetrafluoroethylene and modified human umbilical vein for below-knee femoropopliteal bypass. J Vasc Surg 6:506, 1987.
179. Aalders GJ, van Vroonhoven TJMV: Polytetrafluoroethylene versus human umbilical vein in above-knee femoropopliteal bypass: Six-year results of a randomized clinical trial. J Vasc Surg 16:816, 1992.
180. Johnson WC, Squires JW: Axillo-femoral (PTFE) and infrainguinal revascularization (PTFE and umbilical vein). J Cardiovasc Surg 32:344, 1991.
181. McCollum C, Kenchington G, Alexander C, et al: PTFE or HUV for femoropopliteal bypass: A multi-centre trial. Eur J Vasc Surg 5:435, 1991.
182. Dardik H: Technical aspects of umbilical bypass to the tibial vessels. J Vasc Surg 1:916, 1984.
183. Dardik H, Ibrahim IM, Sussman B, et al: Biodegradation and aneurysm formation in umbilical vein grafts: Observation and a realistic strategy. Ann Surg 199:61, 1984.
184. Boontje AH: Aneurysm formation in human umbilical vein grafts used as arterial substitutes. J Vasc Surg 2:524, 1985.
185. Hasson JE, Newton WD, Waltman AC, et al: Mural degeneration in the glutaraldehyde-tanned umbilical vein graft: Incidence and implications. J Vasc Surg 4:243, 1986.
186. Cranley JJ, Karkow WS, Hafner CD, et al: Aneurysmal dilation in umbilical vein grafts. *In* Bergan JJ, Yao JST (eds): Reoperative Arterial Surgery. New York, Grune & Stratton, 1986, pp 343–358.
187. Karkow WS, Cranley JJ, Cranley RD, et al: Extended study of aneurysm formation in umbilical vein grafts. J Vasc Surg 4:486, 1986.
188. Guidoin R, Gagnon Y, Roy E-P, et al: Pathologic features of surgically excised human umbilical vein grafts. J Vasc Surg 3:146, 1986.
189. Julien S, Gill F, Guidoin R, et al: Biologic and structural evaluation of 80 surgically excised human umbilical vein grafts. Can J Surg 32:101, 1989.
190. Nevelsteen A, Smet G, Wilms G, et al: Intravenous digital subtraction angiography and duplex scanning in the detection of late human umbilical vein degeneration. Br J Surg 75:668, 1988.
191. Rosenberg N, Gaughram ERL, Henderson J, et al: The use of segmental implants prepared by enzymatic modification of heterologous blood vessls. Surg Forum 6:242, 1956.
192. Rosenberg N, Thompson JE, Keshishian JM, VanderWerf BA: The modified bovine arterial graft. Arch Surg 111:222, 1976.
193. Dale WA, Lewis MR: Further experiences with bovine arterial grafts. Surgery 80:711, 1976.
194. Brems J, Castaneda M, Garvin PJ: A five-year experience with the bovine heterograft for vascular access. Arch Surg 121:941, 1986.
195. Sawyer PN, O'Shaughnessy AM, Sophie Z: Patency of small-diameter negatively charged glutaraldehyde-tanned (St. Jude Medical Biopolymeric) grafts. *In* Sawyer PN (ed): Modern Vascular Grafts. New York, McGraw-Hill, 1987, pp 163–180.
196. Sawyer PN, Fitzgerald J, Kaplitt MJ, et al: Ten year experience with the negatively charged glutaraldehyde-tanned vascular graft in peripheral vascular surgery. Initial multicenter trial. Am J Surg 154:533, 1987.
197. Schroder A, Imig H, Peiper U, et al: Results of a bovine collagen vascular graft (Solcograft-P) in infra-inguinal positions. Eur J Vasc Surg 2:315, 1988.
198. Malone JM, Brendel K, Duhamel RC, et al: Detergent-extracted small-diameter vascular prostheses. J Vasc Surg 1:181, 1984.
199. Peirce EC: Autologous tissue tubes for aortic grafts in dogs. Surgery 33:648, 1953.
200. Eiken O, Norden G: Bridging small artery defects in the dog with in situ preformed autologous connective-tissue tubes. Acta Chir Scand 121:90, 1961.
201. Schilling JA, Schurley HM, Joel W, et al: Abdominal aortic grafts: Use of in vivo structured autologous and homologous fibrocollagenous tubes. Ann Surg 159:819, 1964.
202. Parsonnet V, Alpert J, Brief DK: Autogenous polypropylene-supported collagen tubes for long-term arterial replacement. Surgery 70:935, 1971.
203. Sparks CH: Autogenous grafts made to order. Ann Thorac Surg 8:104, 1969.
204. Sparks CH: Silicone mandril method for growing reinforced autogenous femoropopliteal artery grafts in situ. Ann Surg 177:293, 1973.
205. Hallin RW, Sweetman WR: The Spark's mandril graft. Am J Surg 132:221, 1976.
206. Parsonnet V, Tino AC, Brief DK, et al: The fibrocollagenous tube as a small arterial prosthesis. *In* Dardik H (ed): Graft Materials in Vascular Surgery. Miami, Symposia Specialists, 1978, pp 249–262.
207. Perloff LJ, Christie BA, Ketharanathan V, et al: A new replacement for small vessels. Surgery 89:31, 1981.
208. Brewster DC, LaSalle AJ, Robison JG, et al: Factors affecting patency of femoropopliteal bypass grafts. Surg Gynecol Obstet 157:437, 1983.
209. Dale WA: Alternatives for femoropopliteal reconstruction. *In* Dale WA (ed): Management of Vascular Surgical Problems. New York, McGraw-Hill, 1985, pp 166–189.
210. Veith FJ, Moss CM, Sprayregen S, Montefusco C: Preoperative saphenous venography in arterial reconstructive surgery of the lower extremity. Surgery 85:253, 1979.
211. Brewster DC, LaSalle AJ, Robison JG, et al: Femoropopliteal graft failures: Clinical consequences and success of secondary reconstructions. Arch Surg 118:1043, 1983.
212. Graham JW, Lusby RJ: Infrapopliteal bypass grafting: Use of upper limb vein alone and in autogenous composite grafts. Surgery 91:646, 1982.
213. Harris RW, Andros F, Salles-Cunha SX, et al: Totally autogenous venovenous composite bypass grafts. Arch Surg 121:1128, 1986.
214. Taylor LM Jr, Edwards JM, Brant B, et al: Autogenous reversed vein bypass for lower extremity ischemia in patients with absent or inadequate greater saphenous vein. Am J Surg 153:505, 1987.
215. Edwards WS, Gerety E, Larkin J, et al: Multiple sequential femoral tibial grafting for severe ischemia. Surgery 80:722, 1976.
216. Jarrett F, Berkoff HA, Crummy AB, Belzer FO: Femorotibial bypass grafts with sequential technique. Arch Surg 116:709, 1981.
217. Flinn WR, Ricco JB, Yao JST, et al: Composite sequential grafts in severe ischemia: A comparative study. J Vasc Surg 1:449, 1984.
218. Dale WA, Pridgen WR, Shoulders HH Jr: Failure of composite (Teflon and vein) grafting in small human arteries. Surgery 51:258, 1962.
219. Hobson RW II, O'Donnell JA, Jamil Z, Mehta K: Below-knee bypass for limb salvage: Comparison of autogenous saphenous vein, polytetrafluoroethylene, and composite Dacron-autogenous vein grafts. Arch Surg 115:833, 1980.
220. Baker WH, Hadcock MM, Littooy FN: Management of polytetrafluoroethylene graft occlusions. Arch Surg 115:508, 1980.
221. Burnham SJ, Flanigan DP, Goodreau JJ, et al: Nonvein bypass in below-knee reoperation for lower limb ischemia. Surgery 84:417, 1978.
222. Linton RR, Wirthlin LS: Femoropopliteal composite Dacron and autogenous vein bypass grafts: A preliminary report. Arch Surg 107:748, 1973.
223. Lord JW Jr, Sadranagani B, Bajwa G, Rossi G: New technique for

construction of composite Dacron vein grafts for femoro-distal popliteal bypass in the severely ischemic leg. Ann Surg 181:670, 1975.
224. LaSalle AJ, Brewster DC, Corson JD, Darling RC: Femoropopliteal composite bypass grafts: Current status. Surgery 92:36, 1982.
225. Snyder SO Jr, Gregory RT, Wheeler JR, Gayle RG: Composite grafts utilizing polytetrafluoroethylene-autogenous tissue for lower extremity arterial reconstructions. Surgery 90:881, 1981.
226. Gregory RT, Raithel D, Snyder SO Jr, et al: Composite grafts: An alternative to saphenous vein for lower extremity arterial reconstruction. J Cardiovasc Surg 24:53, 1983.
227. Wheeler JR, Gregory RT, Snyder SO Jr, Gayle RG: Gore-Tex autogenous vein composite grafts for tibial reconstruction. J Vasc Surg 1:914, 1984.
228. Rosenfeld JC, Savarese RP, Friedman P, DeLaurentis DA: Sequential femoropopliteal and femorotibial bypasses: A ten-year follow-up study. Arch Surg 116:1538, 1981.
229. Hall RG, Coupland GAE, Lane R, et al: Vein, Gore-Tex or a composite graft for femoropopliteal bypass. Surg Gynecol Obstet 161:308, 1985.
230. Lundqvist B, Bowald S, Eriksson I: Composite grafts for femoro-distal bypass surgery. Acta Chir Scand 529 (Suppl):69, 1985.
231. Scribner RG, Beare JP, Harris EJ, et al: Polytetrafluoroethylene vein composite grafts across the knee. Surg Gynecol Obstet 157:237, 1983.
232. McCarthy WJ, Pearce WH, Flinn WR, et al: Long-term evaluation of composite sequential bypass for limb-threatening ischemia. J Vasc Surg 15:761, 1992.
233. Verta MJ: Composite sequential bypasses to the ankle and beyond for limb salvage. J Vasc Surg 1:381, 1984.
234. Crawford ES: Thoraco-abdominal and abdominal aortic aneurysms involving renal, superior mesenteric, and celiac arteries. Ann Surg 179:763, 1974.
235. Brewster DC, Darling RC: Optimal methods of aortoiliac reconstruction. Surgery 84:739, 1978.
236. Brewster DC, Cooke JC: Longevity of aortofemoral bypass grafts. *In* Yao JST, Pearce WH (eds): Long-Term Results in Vascular Surgery. Norwalk, CT, Appleton & Lange, 1993, pp 149–161.
237. Crawford ES, Bomberger RA, Glaeser DH, et al: Aortoiliac occlusive disease: Factors influencing survival and function following reconstructive operation over a twenty-five year period. Surgery 90:1055, 1981.
238. Szilagyi DE, Elliott JP Jr, Smith RF, et al: A thirty-year survey of the reconstructive surgical treatment of aortoiliac occlusive disease. J Vasc Surg 3:421, 1986.
239. Crawford ES, Saleh SA, Babb JW, et al: Infrarenal abdominal aortic aneurysm: Factors influencing survival after operation performed over a 25-year period. Ann Surg 193:699, 1981.
240. Cronenwett JL: Factors influencing the long-term results of aortic aneurysm surgery. *In* Yao JST, Pearce WH (eds): Long-Term Results in Vascular Surgery. Norwalk, CT, Appleton & Lange, 1993, pp 171–179.
241. Tilanus HW, Obertop H, Urk HV: Saphenous vein or PTFE for femoropopliteal bypass. A prospective randomized trial. Ann Surg 202:780, 1985.
242. Veterans Administration Cooperative Study Group 141: Comparative evaluation of prosthetic, reversed, and in situ vein bypass grafts in distal popliteal and tibial-peroneal revascularization. Arch Surg 123:434, 1988.
243. Bennion RS, Williams RA, Stabile BE, et al: Patency of autogenous saphenous vein versus polytetrafluoroethylene grafts in femoropopliteal bypass for advanced ischemia of the extremity. Surg Gynecol Obstet 160:239, 1985.
244. Budd JS, Brennan J, Beard JD, et al: Infrainguinal bypass surgery: Factors determining late graft patency. Br J Surg 77:1382, 1990.
245. Weisel RD, Johnston KW, Baird RJ, et al: Comparison of conduits for leg revascularization. Surgery 89:8, 1981.
246. Bergan JJ, Veith FJ, Bernhard VM, et al: Randomization of autogenous vein and polytetrafluoroethylene grafts in femoro-distal reconstruction. Surgery 92:921, 1982.
247. Quiñones-Baldrich WJ, Martin-Paredero V, Baker JD, et al: Polytetrafluoroethylene grafts as first-choice arterial substitute in femoropopliteal revascularization. Arch Surg 119:1238, 1984.
248. Quiñones-Baldrich WJ, Busuttil RW, Baker JD, et al: Is the preferential use of polytetrafluoroethylene grafts for femoropopliteal bypass justified? J Vasc Surg 8:219, 1988.
249. O'Donnell TF, Farber SP, Richmond DM, et al: Above-knee polytetrafluoroethylene femoropopliteal bypass graft: Is it a reasonable alternative to the below-knee reversed autogenous vein graft? Surgery 94:26, 1983.
250. Rosen RC, Johnson WC, Bush HL, et al: Staged infrainguinal revascularization: Initial prosthetic above-knee bypass followed by a distal vein bypass for recurrent ischemia: A valid concept for extending limb salvage. Am J Surg 152:224, 1986.
251. Sterpetti AV, Schultz RD, Feldhaus RJ, Peetz DJ: Seven-year experience with polytetrafluoroethylene as above-knee femoropopliteal bypass graft. Is it worthwhile to preserve the autologous saphenous vein? J Vasc Surg 2:907, 1985.
252. Patterson RB, Fowl RJ, Kempczinski RF, et al: Preferential use of ePTFE for above-knee femoropopliteal bypass grafts. Ann Vasc Surg 4:338, 1990.
253. Prendiville EJ, Yeager A, O'Donnell TF, et al: Long-term results with above-knee popliteal expanded polytetrafluoroethylene graft. J Vasc Surg 11:517, 1990.
254. Budd JS, Langdon I, Brennan J, Bell PRF: Above-knee prosthetic grafts do not compromise the ipsilateral long saphenous vein. Br J Surg 78:1379, 1991.
255. Whittemore AD, Clowes AW, Couch NP, Mannick JA: Secondary femoropopliteal reconstruction. Ann Surg 193:35, 1982.
256. Edwards JM, Taylor LM, Porter JM: Treatment of failed lower extremity bypass grafts with new autogenous vein bypass grafting. J Vasc Surg 11:136, 1990.
257. Moore WS: The preferential use of PTFE for initial femoropopliteal bypass. *In* Veith FJ (ed): Current Critical Problems in Vascular Surgery, vol. 2. St. Louis, Quality Medical Publishing, 1990, pp 59–61.
258. Michaels JA: Choice of material for above-knee femoropopliteal bypass graft. Br J Surg 76:7, 1989.
259. Houser SL, Hashmi FH, Jaeger VJ, et al: Should the greater saphenous vein be preserved in patients requiring arterial outflow reconstruction in the lower extremity? Surgery 95:467, 1984.
260. Stephen M, Loewenthal J, Little JM, et al: Autogenous veins and velour Dacron in femoropopliteal arterial bypass. Surgery 81:314, 1977.
261. Christenson JT, Eklof B: Sparks mandril, velour Dacron and autogenous saphenous vein grafts in femoropopliteal bypass. Br J Surg 66:514, 1979.
262. Yashar JJ, Thompson R, Burnhard RJ, et al: Dacron vs vein for femoropopliteal arterial bypass. Arch Surg 116:1037, 1981.
263. Rosenthal D, Evans D, McKinsey J, et al: Prosthetic above-knee femoropopliteal bypass for intermittent claudication. J Cardiovasc Surg 31:462, 1990.
264. Pevec WC, Darling RC, L'Italien GJ, Abbott WM: Femoropopliteal reconstruction with knitted, non-velour Dacron versus expanded polytetrafluorethylene. J Vasc Surg 16:60, 1992.
265. Pevec WC, Abbott WM: Femoropopliteal Dacron graft: Five- to ten-year patency. *In* Yao JST, Pearce WH (eds): Long-Term Results in Vascular Surgery. Norwalk, CT, Appleton & Lange, 1993, pp 273–277.
266. Campbell CD, Brooks DH, Webster MW, et al: Expanded microporous polytetrafluoroethylene as a vascular substitute: A two-year follow-up. Surgery 85:177, 1979.
267. Veith FJ, Moss CM, Fell SC, et al: Comparison of expanded polytetrafluoroethylene and autologous saphenous vein grafts in high-risk arterial reconstructions for limb salvage. Surg Gynecol Obstet 147:749, 1978.
268. Haimov M, Giron F, Jacobson JH: The expanded polytetrafluoroethylene graft. Arch Surg 114:673, 1979.
269. Hallett JW, Brewster DC, Darling RC: The limitations of polytetrafluoroethylene in reconstruction of femoropopliteal and tibial arteries. Surg Gynecol Obstet 152:189, 1981.
270. Charlesworth PM, Brewster DC, Darling RC, et al: The fate of polytetrafluoroethylene grafts in lower limb bypass surgery: A six-year follow-up. Br J Surg 72:896, 1985.
271. Whittemore AD, Kent KC, Donaldson MC, et al: What is the proper role of polytetrafluoroethylene grafts in infrainguinal reconstruction? J Vasc Surg 10:299, 1989.
272. Davies MG, Feeley TM, O'Malley MK, et al: Infrainguinal polytetrafluoroethylene grafts: Saved limbs or wasted effort? A report on ten years' experience. Ann Vasc Surg 5:519, 1991.
273. Connolly JE, Kwan JHM, Brownell D, et al: Newer developments of extraanatomic bypass. Surg Gynecol Obstet 158:415, 1984.

274. Chang JB: Current status of extraanatomic bypasses. Am J Surg 152:202, 1986.
275. Garcia-Rinaldi R, Revuelta JM, Vaughan GD III, et al: The versatility of Gore-Tex grafts for extra-anatomic bypass. Vasc Surg 18:294, 1984.
276. Craido FJ: Extrathoracic management of aortic arch syndrome. Br J Surg 69 (Suppl):45, 1982.
277. Ziomek S, Quiñones-Baldrich WJ, Busuttil RW, et al: The superiority of synthetic arterial grafts over autogenous veins in carotid-subclavian bypass. J Vasc Surg 3:140, 1986.
278. Perler BA, Williams GM: Carotid-subclavian bypass—A decade of experience. J Vasc Surg 12:716, 1990.
279. Langneau P, Michel JB, Charrat JM: Use of polytetrafluoroethylene grafts for renal bypass. J Vasc Surg 5:738, 1987.
280. Dale WA, Harris J, Terry RB: Polytetrafluoroethylene reconstruction of the inferior vena cava. Surgery 95:625, 1984.
281. Chan EL, Bardin JA, Bernstein EF: Inferior vena cava bypass: Experimental evaluation of externally supported grafts and initial clinical application. J Vasc Surg 1:675, 1984.
282. Fujiwara Y, Cohn LH, Adams D, et al: Use of Gore-Tex grafts for replacement of the superior and inferior venae cavae. J Cardiovasc Surg 67:774, 1974.
283. Comerata AJ, Harwick RD, White JV: Jugular venous reconstruction: A technique to minimize morbidity of bilateral radical neck dissection. J Vasc Surg 3:322, 1986.
284. Norton L, Eiseman B: Replacement of portal vein during pancreatectomy for carcinoma. Surgery 77:280, 1975.
285. Sarfeh IJ, Rypins EB, Mason GR: A systematic appraisal of portacaval H-graft diameters. Clinical and hemodynamic perspectives. Ann Surg 204:356, 1986.
286. Robinson RJ, Peigh PS, Fiore AC, et al: Venous prostheses: Improved patency with external stents. J Surg Res 36:306, 1984.
287. Raju S: PTFE grafts for hemodialysis access. Techniques for insertion and management of complications. Ann Surg 206:666, 1987.
288. Palder SB, Kirkman RL, Whittemore AD, et al: Vascular access for hemodialysis. Patency rates and results of revision. Ann Surg 202:235, 1985.
289. Hurt AV, Batello-Cruz M, Skipper BJ, et al: Bovine carotid artery heterografts versus polytetrafluoroethylene grafts. A prospective randomized study. Am J Surg 146:844, 1983.
290. Taylor DEM: How may vascular grafts be modified to improve patency? *In* Greenhalgh RM, Jamieson W, Nicolaides AN (eds): Vascular Surgery: Issues in Current Practice. London, Grune & Stratton, 1986, pp 175–186.
291. Weinberg CB, Bell E: A blood vessel model constructed from collagen and cultured vascular cells. Science 231:397, 1986.
292. Mansfield PB: Tissue cultured endothelium for vascular prosthetic devices. Rev Surg 27:291, 1970.
293. Welch M, Durrans D, Car HMH, et al: Endothelial cell seeding: A review. Ann Vasc Surg 6:473, 1992.
294. Herring MB, Gardiner A, Glover JL: A single-staged technique for seeding vascular grafts with autogenous endothelium. Surgery 84:498, 1978.
295. Herring MB, Baughman S, Glover JL, et al: Endothelial seeding of Dacron and polytetrafluoroethylene grafts: The cellular events of healing. Surgery 96:745, 1984.
296. Graham LM, Vinter DW, Ford JW, et al: Endothelial cell seeding of prosthetic vascular grafts—early experimental studies with cultured autologous canine endothelium. Arch Surg 115:929, 1980.
297. Graham LM, Burkel WE, Ford JW, et al: Expanded polytetrafluoroethylene vascular prostheses seeded with enzymatically derived and cultured endothelial cells. Surgery 91:550, 1982.
298. Stanley JC, Burkel WE, Ford JW, et al: Enhanced patency of small-diameter externally supported Dacron iliofemoral grafts seeded with endothelial cells. Surgery 92:994, 1982.
299. Allen BT, Long JA, Welch MJ, et al: Influence of endothelial cell seeding on platelet deposition and patency in small-diameter Dacron arterial grafts. J Vasc Surg 1:224, 1984.
300. Clagett GP, Burkel WE, Sharefkin JB, et al: Platelet reactivity in vivo in dogs with arterial prostheses seeded with endothelial cells. Circulation 69:632, 1984.
301. Schmidt SP, Hunter TJ, Sharp WV, et al: Endothelial cell-seeded four millimeter Dacron vascular grafts: Effects of blood flow manipulation through the grafts. J Vasc Surg 1:434, 1984.
302. Sicard GA, Allen BT, Long JA, et al: Prostaglandin production and platelet reactivity of small diameter grafts. J Vasc Surg 1:774, 1984.
303. Shepard AD, Eldrup-Jorgensen J, Keough EM, et al: Endothelial cell seeding of small-caliber synthetic grafts in the baboon. Surgery 99:318, 1986.
304. Sharp WV, Schmidt SP, Donovan DL: Prostaglandin biochemistry of seeded endothelial cells on Dacron prostheses. J Vasc Surg 3:256, 1986.
305. Birinyi LK, Douville EC, Lewis SA, et al: Increased resistance to bacteremic graft infection after endothelial cell seeding. J Vasc Surg 5:193, 1987.
306. Jarrell BE, Williams SK, Stokes G, et al: Use of freshly isolated capillary endothelial cells for the immediate establishment of a monolayer on a vascular graft. Surgery 100:392, 1986.
307. Sterpetti AV, Hunter WJ, Schultz RD: Seeding with endothelial cells derived from the microvessels of the omentum and from the jugular vein: A comparative study. J Vasc Surg 7:677, 1988.
308. Rupnick MA, Hubbard FA, Pratt K, et al: Endothelialization of vascular prosthetic surfaces after seeding or sodding with human microvascular endothelial cells. J Vasc Surg 9:788, 1989.
309. Williams SK, Jarrell BE, Rose DG, et al: Human microvessel endothelial cell isolation and vascular graft sodding in the operating room. Ann Vasc Surg 3:146, 1989.
310. Rosenman JE, Kempczinski RF, Pearce WH, et al: Kinetics of endothelial cell seeding. J Vasc Surg 2:778, 1985.
311. Seeger JM: Improved endothelial cell seeding density after flow exposure in fibronectin-coated grafts. Surg Forum 36:450, 1985.
312. Seeger JM: Improved endothelial cell seeding efficiency with cultured cells and fibronectin coated grafts. J Surg Res 38:641, 1985.
313. Ramalanjaona G, Kempczinski RF, Rosenman JE, et al: The effect of fibronectin coating on endothelial cell kinetics in PTFE grafts. J Vasc Surg 3:264, 1986.
314. Herring MB, Gardner A, Glover JL: Seeding human arterial prostheses with mechanically derived endothelium: The detrimental effect of smoking. J Vasc Surg 2:279, 1984.
315. Herring MB, Baughman S, Glover JL: Endothelium develops on seeded arterial prosthesis. A brief clinical report. J Vasc Surg 2:727, 1985.
316. Ortenwall P, Wadenvik H, Kutti J, et al: Reduction in deposition of indium-111–labelled platelets after autologous endothelial cell seeding of Dacron aortic bifurcation grafts in humans: A preliminary report. J Vasc Surg 6:17, 1987.
317. Ortenwall P, Wadenvik H, Kutti J, et al: Endothelial cell seeding reduces thrombogenicity of Dacron grafts in humans. J Vasc Surg 11:403, 1990.
318. Ortenwall P, Wadenvik H, Risbert B: Reduced platelet deposition on seeded versus unseeded segments of expanded polytetrafluoroethylene grafts: Clinical observations after a 6 month follow-up. J Vasc Surg 10:374, 1989.
319. Herring MB, Compton RS, Legrand DR, et al: Endothelial seeding of polytetrafluoroethylene popliteal bypasses: A preliminary report. J Vasc Surg 6:114, 1987.
320. Zilla P, Fasol R, Deutsch M, et al: Endothelial cell seeding of polytetrafluoroethylene vascular grafts in humans: A preliminary report. J Vasc Surg 6:535, 1987.
321. Walker MG, Thompson GJL, Shaw JW: Endothelial cell seeded versus non-seeded ePTFE grafts in patients with severe peripheral vascular disease: Preliminary results. *In* Zilla P, Fasol R, Deutsch M (eds): Endothelialization of Vascular Grafts. Basel, S Karger, 1987, pp 245–248.
322. Callow AD: The vascular endothelial cell as a vehicle for gene therapy. J Vasc Surg 11:793, 1990.
323. Bowald S, Busch C, Eriksson I: Arterial regeneration following polyglactin 910 suture mesh grafting. Surgery 86:722, 1979.
324. Greisler HP: Arterial regeneration over absorbable prostheses. Arch Surg 177:1425, 1982.
325. Greisler HP: Bioresorbable vascular grafts. *In* Greisler HP: New Biologic and Synthetic Vascular Prostheses. Austin TX, RG Landes, 1991, pp 70–86.
326. Greisler HP, Endean ED, Klosak JJ, et al: Polyglactin 910/polydioxanone biocomponent totally resorbable vascular prostheses. J Vasc Surg 7:697, 1988.
327. Van der Lei B, Nieuwenhuis P, Molenaar I, Wildevuur Ch RR: Long-term biologic fate of neoarteries regenerated in microporous, compliant, biodegradable, small-caliber vascular grafts in rats. Surgery 101:459, 1987.
328. Galletti PM, Aebischer P, Sashen HF, et al: Experience with fully bioresorbable aortic grafts in the dog. Surgery 103:231, 1988.

329. Clark RE, Margraff HW: Antibacterial vascular grafts with improved thrombo resistance. Arch Surg 109:159, 1974.
330. Harvey RA, Alcid DV, Greco RS: Antibiotic bonding to polytetrafluoroethylene with tridodecylmethylammonium chloride. Surgery 92:504, 1982.
331. Greco RS, Harvey RA: The role of antibiotic bonding in the prevention of vascular prosthetic infection. Ann Surg 195:168, 1982.
332. Greco RS, Harvey RA, Smilow PC, et al: Prevention of vascular prosthetic infection by a benzalkonium-oxacillin–bonded polytetrafluoroethylene graft. Surg Gynecol Obstet 155:28, 1982.
333. White JV, Benvenisty A: Simple methods for direct antibiotic protection of synthetic vascular grafts. J Vasc Surg 1:372, 1984.
334. Webb LX, Myers RT, Cordell AR, et al: Inhibition of bacterial adhesion by antibacterial surface pretreatment of vascular prostheses. J Vasc Surg 4:16, 1986.
335. Shue WB, Worosilo SC, Donetz AP, et al: Prevention of vascular prosthetic infection with an antibiotic-bonded Dacron graft. J Vasc Surg 8:600, 1988.
336. Modak SM, Sampath L, Fox CL Jr, et al: A new method for the direct incorporation of antibiotic in prosthetic vascular grafts. Surg Gynecol Obstet 164:143, 1987.
337. Moore WS, Chvapil M, Sieffert G: Development of an infection resistant vascular prosthesis. Arch Surg 116:1403, 1981.
338. Gott VL, Whiffen JD, Dutton RC: Heparin bonding on colloidin graphite surfaces. Science 142:1927, 1963.
339. Esquivel CO, Bjorck C-G, Bergentz S-E, et al: Reduced thrombogenic characteristics of expanded polytetrafluoroethylene and polyurethane arterial grafts after heparin bonding. Surgery 95:102, 1984.
340. Greisler HP, Klosak JJ, Dennis JW, et al: Biomaterial pretreatment with ECGF to augment endothelial cell proliferation. J Vasc Surg 2:393, 1987.
341. Geeraert AJ, Callaghan JC: Experimental study of selected small calibre arterial grafts. J Cardiovasc Surg 18:155, 1977.
342. Cronenwett JL, Zelenock GB: Alternative small arterial grafts. *In* Stanley JC (ed): Biologic and Synthetic Vascular Prostheses. New York, Grune & Stratton, 1982, pp 595–620.
343. Yeager A, Callow AD: New graft materials and current approaches to an acceptable small-diameter vascular graft. Trans Am Soc Artif Organs 34:88, 1988.
344. White RA, White EW, Hanson EL, et al: Preliminary report: Evaluation of tissue ingrowth into experimental replamineform vascular prostheses. Surgery 79:229, 1976.
345. White RA, Klein SR, Shors EC: Preservation of compliance in a small diameter microporous, silicon rubber vascular prosthesis. J Cardiovasc Surg 28:485, 1987.
346. Sawyer PN, Sophie Z, O'Shaughnessy A: Vascular prostheses: Innovative properties. *In* Kambic HE, Kantrowitz A, Sung P (eds): Vascular Graft Update: Safety and Performance. ASTM Spec Tech Publ 898. Philadelphia, American Society of Testing and Materials, 1986, pp 290–305.
347. Haubold A: Carbon in prosthetics. Ann NY Acad Sci 283:383, 1977.
348. Sharp WV, Teague PC, Scott DL: Thromboresistance of pyrolytic carbon grafts. Trans Am Soc Artif Organs 24:223, 1978.
349. Scott SM, Gaddy LR, Parra S: Pyrolytic carbon-coated vascular prostheses. J Surg Res 29:395, 1980.

SECTION VI

Common Complications of Vascular Surgery: Prevention and Management

Edited by K. Wayne Johnston, M.D., F.R.C.S.(C.)

30

Overview

K. Wayne Johnston, M.D., F.R.C.S.(C.)

The complications associated with vascular surgery can be classified as (1) nonvascular systemic, (2) nonvascular local, (3) vascular local, and (4) remote ischemic vascular complications (see Tables 30–1 to 30–4). Their incidence and severity can be reduced by paying attention to preventive measures, early recognition, and specific treatment.

Meticulous attention to detail is the most important aspect of *prevention.* The initial step is the establishment of an accurate vascular diagnosis by appropriate clinical assessment, noninvasive studies, and angiography. Patient selection should be based on knowledge of the untreated natural history of the underlying disease process and the indications for and limitations of surgery. The preoperative work-up should include careful assessment of the severity and risks of coexisting medical problems, especially cerebrovascular, cardiac, respiratory, hepatic, renal, and hematologic diseases, and detailed preoperative preparation for surgery. The operation and operative approach, based on the indications for surgery and the patient's general status, should be considered carefully. The surgery should be conducted meticulously to avoid errors in technique; in particular, it is important to recognize that congenital anomalies may complicate dissection, diseased vessels can be damaged easily, equipment such as vascular clamps or Fogarty catheters must be used with care, and hemostasis should be complete. Intraoperative objective assessment may be necessary to confirm the success of the procedure. Specific measures to prevent vascular complications, including thrombosis and infection, and general complications such as atelectasis, myocardial infarction, and thromboembolism should be considered. When a complication arises, *early recognition* and *prompt treatment* offer the best opportunity for a good result.

The complications specific to the surgical management of lower extremity arterial disease are described in various chapters throughout the book. This section of the book includes chapters on the complications that warrant individual consideration either because they are inherent risks of any vascular surgery operation or because they are serious and warrant individual consideration.

The following paragraphs summarize the pathogenesis, diagnosis, and management of the complications included in this section of the book. They are intended to serve as both a synopsis and brief overview of the material covered.

CARDIAC COMPLICATIONS

(Chapter 31)

All patients with occlusive and aneurysmal arterial disease have some degree of coronary artery disease (CAD). The complications of CAD are the most common cause of early and late mortality. Preoperative screening by history and electrocardiography (ECG) is of practical value in assessing the operative risk of cardiac mortality, but objective screening tests are necessary to identify all patients with hemodynamically significant CAD who might benefit from coronary angiography and angioplasty or bypass grafting to reduce their risk of myocardial infarction and death. Of the available screening tests, including exercise electrocardiography, radionuclide ventriculography,

Table 30–1. Nonvascular Complications, Systemic

0. None
1. Cerebrovascular
2. Cardiac
    - 2.1 Myocardial infarction
        - 2.1.1 Enzyme changes only
        - 2.1.2 ST-T wave changes; positive CPK-MB
        - 2.1.3 Q waves or loss R waves
        - 2.1.4 Death
    - 2.2 Arrhythmia
        - 2.2.1 Atrial
        - 2.2.2 Ventricular
        - 2.2.3 Heart block
    - 2.3 Congestive heart failure
3. Pulmonary
4. Renal
    - 4.0 No change renal function
    - 4.1 Creatinine increase less than 2 times baseline
    - 4.2 Creatinine increase more than 2 times baseline
    - 4.3 Temporary dialysis
    - 4.4 Permanent dialysis
5. Gastrointestinal including hepatobiliary and pancreatic
6. Venous thromboembolism
    - 6.1 Deep vein thrombosis
        - 6.1.1 Suspected
        - 6.1.2. Proved
    - 6.2 Pulmonary embolism
        - 6.2.1 Suspected
        - 6.2.2 Proved
7. Coagulation complications
8. Drug/blood reaction
9. Other

Modified from Rutherford RB, Flanigan DP, Gupta SK, et al: Suggested standards for reports dealing with lower extremity ischemia. J Vasc Surg 4:80, 1986.

Table 30–2. Nonvascular Complications, Local

0. None
1. Fluid accumulation (early or persistent)
    - 1.1 Sterile
    - 1.2 Infected
2. Wound
    - 2.1 Infection (record specific organisms)
        - 2.1.1 Superficial
        - 2.2.2 Deep, not involving graft
        - 2.3.3 Deep, involving graft
    - 2.2 Separation
    - 2.3 Evisceration
    - 2.4 Hematoma
    - 2.5 Pain
3. Lymphatic disruption
    - Peripheral site
        - 3.1 Lymphocele
        - 3.2 Lymph fistula
    - Central site
        - 3.3 Chylothorax
        - 3.4 Chylous ascites
4. Vascular injury
    - 4.1 Artery
    - 4.2 Vein
5. Ureteric injury
6. Pleural, pneumothorax
7. Nerve injury
8. Sexual dysfunction
    - 8.1 Neurogenic
    - 8.2 Vasculogenic

Modified from Rutherford RB, Flanigan DP, Gupta SK, et al: Suggested standards for reports dealing with lower extremity ischemia. J Vasc Surg 4:80, 1986.

continuous ECG monitoring, and dipyridamole thallium scintigraphy, the last is the most widely used. Most studies have demonstrated that dipyridamole thallium scintigraphy is quite sensitive for predicting perioperative cardiac morbidity and mortality and late survival but has limited specificity.

Based on clinical and objective assessment, the patient's risk of surgery may be reduced by using maximum medical management, considering an alternative vascular surgical procedure, or considering coronary revascularization by angioplasty or bypass. Intraoperative management requires careful surgical technique to minimize blood loss and hemodynamic changes due to aortic clamping, invasive monitoring, and optimal choice of anesthetic technique.

RESPIRATORY COMPLICATIONS

(Chapter 32)

In the vascular surgery population of elderly patients who often require major surgery and may have underlying pulmonary disease, it is important to identify which patients are at risk by a careful history, physical examination, chest x-ray, and, when indicated, pulmonary function tests. In some cases, preoperative therapy with vigorous chest physiotherapy, cessation of smoking, bronchodilators, and antibiotics may be of benefit. If postoperative ventilation is necessary, standard cardiovascular monitoring provides appropriate surveillance of the multiple factors that influence ventilation and the balance between oxygen delivery and consumption.

Management of respiratory complications depends upon recognition of the specific cause. Nonpulmonary parenchymal causes include central nervous system depression, mechanical problems of ventilation, or upper airway obstruction. Parenchymal causes include atelectasis, pneumonia, pulmonary edema, adult respiratory distress syndrome, and pulmonary embolus. Pulmonary complications may prove to be rapidly fatal, but in most cases they are

Table 30–3. Vascular Complications, Local

0. None
1. Hemorrhage
    - 1.1 Intraoperative
    - 1.2 Postoperative, not requiring reoperation; record blood loss/time
    - 1.3 Postoperative, requiring reoperation
2. Infection graft (record specific organisms)
    - 2.1 Suspected
    - 2.2 Proved
3. Pseudoaneurysm
4. Graft
    - 4.1 Dilatation
    - 4.2 Degeneration/aneurysm
    - 4.3 Stenosis, intimal hyperplasia
    - 4.4 Stenosis, atherosclerosis
    - 4.5 Elongation/kinking
5. Thrombosis or unsatisfactory hemodynamic result
6. Fistulization
    - 6.1 Vein
    - 6.2 Bowel
    - 6.3 Biliary tract
    - 6.4 Ureter
7. Injury artery or vein

Modified from Rutherford RB, Flanigan DP, Gupta SK, et al: Suggested standards for reports dealing with lower extremity ischemia. J Vasc Surg 4:80, 1986.

Table 30–4. Ischemic Vascular Complications, Remote (i.e., Due to Effects of Ischemia, Thromboembolism, Steal, or Dissection on Limb or End Organ)

0. None
1. Limb ischemia (see ref. 1)
2. Bowel ischemia
3. Renal ischemia (see below)
4. Spinal cord and cauda equina ischemia
5. Cerebral ischemia (Use stroke severity scale)
   - 5.0 Asymptomatic
   - 5.1 Transient ischemic attack (<24 hours)
   - 5.2 Temporary stroke with full recovery (24 hours to 3 weeks)
   - 5.3 Permanent stroke, minor (>3 weeks)
   - 5.4 Permanent stroke, major (>3 weeks)
   - 5.5 Nonspecific dysfunction
6. Nerve ischemia and dysfunction
7. Muscle (compartment syndrome)
8. Other

Modified from Rutherford RB, Flanigan DP, Gupta SK, et al: Suggested standards for reports dealing with lower extremity ischemia. J Vasc Surg 4:80, 1986.

self-limited and, if properly recognized, respond to treatment.

RENAL COMPLICATIONS (Chapter 33)

Associated with angiography and arterial reconstructive surgery, renal dysfunction may range from minor abnormalities of function to anuric acute renal failure. Of the prerenal causes (hypovolemia, low cardiac output, septic shock, and renal artery occlusion) in the patient with diffuse atherosclerosis and impaired cardiac function, the distinction between hypovolemia and cardiogenic causes can be problematic even with the use of invasive hemodynamic monitoring. Postrenal causes (obstruction of ureter, bladder, or catheter) of oliguria are the easiest to correct when diagnosed correctly. Parenchymal causes of renal failure may be the result of ischemic injury or toxic injury by angiographic contrast agents, drugs, or myoglobin. Following aortic surgery, the incidence of renal impairment depends upon the patient's preoperative renal function, intraoperative technical management (juxtarenal cross-clamping, left renal vein ligation), and postoperative complications. Approaches to protect renal function include preoperative fluid hydration, limiting the period of warm renal ischemia, careful aortic clamping to prevent direct renal artery damage and atheromatous embolization, and maintenance of optimum blood volume and cardiac function. The consequences of renal ischemia may be minimized by mannitol or other diuretic administration, regional renal hypothermia, or other investigation methods.

PERIOPERATIVE HEMORRHAGE (Chapter 34)

Prevention of hemorrhage begins in the *preoperative* period. Prior to any vascular surgery, patients should be asked if they have a history of easy bruising, bleeding, or petechiae or a family history of a coagulopathy, and coagulation screening tests should be performed (bleeding time, prothrombin time, activated partial thromboplastin time). This chapter outlines the specific preoperative treatment of abnormalities detected by these tests, including coagulopathies related to vitamin K antagonist oral anticoagulants, thrombocytopenia and abnormal platelet function, azotemia, von Willebrand's disease, antiplatelet drugs, liver disease, heparin, inactivating inhibitors, and deficiencies of individual coagulation factors.

Intraoperative prevention is directed toward technical details, including the use of blended electrocautery dissection, minimal arterial dissection, avoidance of excessive heparin and reversal of its effect with protamine at the end of the procedure, selection of the appropriate graft, suture of the anastomosis with appropriate deep bites and tension, evaluation of the proximal anastomosis by declamping, and caution in applying clamps to the graft to minimize the chances of disrupting the fabric. If large amounts of blood must be transfused, 1 or 2 units of fresh frozen plasma should be administered for every 4 to 6 units of blood transfused, and all the platelets harvested from 6 units of fresh plasma should be administered after 6 to 8 units of blood have been given. When an autotransfusion device is used, platelets and plasma are removed in the washing process, and if large volumes of blood are reinfused, platelets and fresh frozen plasma should be administered to prevent a coagulopathy.

Intraoperative bleeding is usually controlled by local pressure, suture, or both, but in some cases topical hemostatic agents are required (gelatin sponge, oxidized cellulose, microfibrillar collagen, thrombin). Systemic consumptive coagulopathy (disseminated intravascular coagulation, DIC) can usually be prevented by administering fresh frozen plasma and platelets during a prolonged operation. DIC is associated with tissue hypoperfusion, shock, and multiple transfusions. The initial phase of hypercoagulation and thrombosis results in the production of intravascular microthrombi that trigger fibrinolysis. If the initial stimulus continues, the reserves of coagulation factors are consumed and hemostasis fails. During the initial phase, anticoagulation may be indicated; during the later phase, replacement therapy is necessary.

GRAFT THROMBOSIS (Chapter 35)

Early graft thrombosis is most often due to a technical error. Other contributing causes include thrombogenicity of the graft surface, low flow rate due to poor inflow, poor runoff, hypotension or venous obstruction, and, rarely, hypercoagulability (low antithrombin III, circulatory lupus anticoagulant, protein C or protein S levels, heparin-induced platelet aggregation, or hyperfibrinogenemia). Preventive measures include accurate operative technique; use of intraoperative angiography, Doppler sonography, duplex Doppler ultrasonography, or angioscopy to detect operative errors; hemodynamic monitoring to avoid hypotension; and, in high-risk cases, administration of dextran 40. Other antithrombotic drugs are rarely used; heparin is associated with a risk of postoperative hemorrhage, warfarin has a slow onset of action, and the efficacy of antiplatelet drugs has been disappointing. Prompt detection of graft occlusion requires careful perioperative monitoring by clinical and noninvasive Doppler methods. Treatment consists of reoperation with thrombectomy, intraoperative angiography, and correction of technical errors.

Late graft thrombosis is due to anastomotic neointimal hyperplasia, progression of atherosclerosis, changes in an in situ or reversed saphenous graft (e.g., intimal thickening, fibrous stenosis), and a prosthetic graft. Noninvasive surveillance may allow early detection and treatment before graft thrombosis occurs. Treatment depends on the severity of the ischemia. If the limb is viable but symptomatic, thrombolytic therapy may clear the vessel, and if no underlying lesion is demonstrated, long-term anticoagulant therapy is indicated. If arterial stenosis is present, management is achieved by operation or dilatation, depending on the site and nature of the lesions. If limb viability is threatened, thrombectomy, angiography, and repair of the underlying stenoses are indicated. Reoperation and revision or replacement of bypass grafts can significantly increase the long-term success rate.

Intraoperative embolization of thrombus or atheromatous debris can have serious ischemic sequelae. The following details are important in prevention: minimal manipulation of arteries during dissection, especially aneurysmal vessels, gentle application of clamps at sites with the least atherosclerosis, heparinization, judicious flushing, and unclamping in sequence so that flow is first directed into the least important vessel. Early diagnosis in the operating room by clinical and Doppler evaluation of the pedal circulation is important. Since emboli may lodge in distal or side branches, direct surgical removal or intra-arterial thrombolytic therapy is difficult but remains the most important method of treatment.

INFECTION IN PROSTHETIC VASCULAR GRAFTS (Chapter 36)

Early and late graft infection is a very serious complication of arterial reconstructive surgery because of the high rates of amputation and mortality. Microorganisms can infect the prosthesis through direct implantation at the time of surgery, through the wound if there is a complication of healing, or through hematogenous or lymphatic routes from remote sites of infection. The environment around and within the interstices of biomaterials is conducive to the formation of a bacterial biofilm, which tends to protect the bacteria from both host defenses and antibiotics. Although the inflammatory response stimulated by the bacteria may localize the infection, alternatively, the combined inflammatory response to the infection and biomaterial may result in spread along the graft, involvement of adjacent structures, or significant local tissue damage with possible arterial wall or anastomotic disruption and hemorrhage.

The pathologic consequences depend on the virulence of the organism, the host responses, and the site of graft infection. Early graft infections are relatively uncommon and are usually associated with virulent pathogens and serious complications (e.g., systemic sepsis, infected false aneurysm, enlargement and erosion into bowel, or external drainage). On the other hand, late-appearing graft infections are commonly the result of less virulent bacteria (e.g., *Staphylococcus epidermidis*), which may grow within a biofilm and may remain indolent.

Preventive measures include administration of prophylactic antibiotics, attention to meticulous sterile technique, careful multi-layer wound closure, early recognition and aggressive treatment of wound infection, education of the patient that late graft colonization is possible at the time of certain procedures (e.g., dental work, cystoscopy) and that prophylactic antibiotics are recommended.

The diagnosis is often difficult and may be delayed but can be made on the basis of the clinical presentation or routine laboratory studies; however, late graft infections may require investigations including ultrasound, computed tomography (CT), magnetic resonance imaging (MRI), contrast sinography, aspiration and culture, white blood cell scans, or angiography. Operative exploration may be necessary. Routine culture techniques may not recover organisms of low virulence; mechanical or ultrasonic disruption of the bacteria from the surface of the graft may be necessary.

Depending on the extent of involvement, the infected graft limb or the entire graft is removed, and the arteriotomy is closed with monofilament suture and an autogenous patch if it is necessary to maintain patency of the artery at the site of arteriotomy. The perigraft tissues and arterial wall should be débrided and the area drained. Extra-anatomic bypass grafts are usually necessary. Culture-specific antibiotics are indicated. In selected cases of infection with low-virulence organisms that are presumably confined to the ''slime'' layer around the prosthesis, local graft removal and in situ replacement can be considered.

ANASTOMOTIC ANEURYSMS (Chapter 37)

The risk of a false aneurysm can be minimized by using synthetic sutures, taking relatively large bites in the artery, preventing hematomas by paying careful attention to hemostasis and obliteration of dead space, avoiding excessive tension on the anastomosis, not performing an excessive endarterectomy, and administering prophylactic antibiotics to prevent graft infection. It may not be possible to protect these aneurysms against stress from joint movement or atherosclerotic degeneration of the wall.

The clinical presentation depends on the site (intra-abdominal versus extremity) and the presence of complications (expansion and pressure on surrounding nerves and veins, distal emboli from a mural thrombus, thrombosis of the aneurysm with concomitant occlusion of the native artery or bypass graft, or rupture into soft tissues or adjacent hollow viscera). Diagnosis is confirmed by a combination of ultrasound scan, CT scan, and angiography.

Although the natural history of an untreated anastomotic aneurysm has not been documented, it is generally agreed that most will continue to enlarge and therefore should be repaired surgically. Dissection of the aneurysm is avoided. Proximal and distal control are obtained; often it is safer to obtain distal control by using intraluminal balloon catheters. Although it may be possible to simply resuture the anastomosis, most often a short segment of the graft is removed, healthy arterial wall tissue identified, and a new segment of graft reanastomosed.

AORTOENTERIC FISTULA
(Chapter 38)

An aortoenteric fistula is one of the most serious complications that can follow aortic surgery. The fistula can occur between the bowel and the suture line, or the side of the body, or limb of the prosthetic graft (paraprosthetic). When the suture line is involved, recurrent significant bleeding episodes eventually result in massive hemorrhage, whereas a paraprosthetic fistula is usually associated with minor bleeding through the interstices of the graft or from the edge of the bowel, leading to anemia. In either case, there may be evidence of local or systemic infection.

If time permits, investigations include endoscopy to rule out other causes of gastrointestinal bleeding and occasionally to visualize the mucosal abnormality associated with the fistula; arteriography to demonstrate a false aneurysm and rarely the site of bleeding; and multiple cultures along the aortic graft at the time of angiography, CT scan, or gallium scan.

Prevention is directed toward elimination of the common etiologic factors: direct erosion (which is prevented by separation of the prosthesis and bowel by interposing an appropriate retroperitoneal tissue layer), false aneurysm, graft redundancy, and primary graft infection. Treatment includes high-dose broad-spectrum antibiotics; control of the aorta by cross-clamping, usually at the level of the diaphragm; removal of the aortic graft; suture of the aortic stump and coverage with omentum; closure of the defect in the bowel; and revascularization by extra-anatomic bypass if necessary.

ISCHEMIC NEUROPATHY (Chapter 39)

Ischemic neuropathy is the term used to describe any injury of peripheral nerve caused by reduction in blood supply and may follow acute or chronic ischemia. If acute ischemia is of short duration or is mild, function in peripheral nerve is impaired in a transient manner; however, with prolonged or severe ischemia, damage may be permanent. With chronic arterial insufficiency, nerves show a combination of segmental demyelination and axonal degeneration, and there may be evidence of remyelination and axonal regeneration.

With chronic ischemia, sensory symptoms (burning pain, hyperesthesia, hyperalgesia) are seen in a stocking distribution or involve patchy localized areas in the foot and must be distinguished from symptoms caused by persistent ischemia. Small muscles of the foot may be wasted and weak, and there may be slight ankle weakness and depression of the ankle reflex compared with the normal side. The diagnosis is confirmed by electromyography. Symptoms associated with chronic ischemia are often mild and improve after arterial reconstruction; however, the symptoms may be severe and persist even after adequate revascularization. In this situation, it is important to recognize that the patient's symptoms are neuropathic in origin and that further arterial reconstructive surgery will not be of benefit. The more severe cases require treatment with analgesics or amitriptyline.

Following correction of acute ischemia, the symptoms of ischemic neuropathy usually improve spontaneously. However, if flow is not reestablished within several hours, symptoms and signs of neurogenic dysfunction may persist when circulation is restored, and the deficit may be permanent.

Ischemia may cause neuropathy of individual nerves: peroneal, femoral, and lumbosacral plexus. It is important to distinguish lumbosacral plexus involvement from lesions of the lower spinal cord or cauda equina, which have a very poor prognosis for recovery.

LYMPHATIC COMPLICATIONS OF VASCULAR SURGERY (Chapter 40)

Several causes may contribute to the development of postbypass leg edema; however, the major factors are increased production of interstitial fluid associated with successful revascularization (increased lymphatic load) and lymphatic interruption or compression. In the femoral and popliteal incisions, lymphatic interruption can be minimized by limiting the extent of arterial dissection, using a femoral incision that is slightly lateral to the femoral pulse to allow medial retraction of the lymphatics, and opening the popliteal vascular sheath directly over the artery.

Lymphatic fistulae and lymphoceles can be prevented by the aforementioned methods and, in addition, by cauterizing and ligating any divided lymphatic tissue and carefully closing the incision in layers. A conservative approach is justified if the lymphatic drainage is of low volume and subsides quickly; otherwise, operative ligation of the divided lymphatics should be considered to shorten the hospital stay and reduce the possibility of a graft or wound infection. Small lymphoceles can be observed because they may be reabsorbed spontaneously; however, enlarging or symptomatic lymphoceles are considered indications for operation.

Special considerations are given to the management of thoracic duct lymph fistulae in the neck, retroperitoneal lymphoceles, chylous ascites, and chylothorax.

POSTOPERATIVE SEXUAL DYSFUNCTION FOLLOWING AORTOILIAC REVASCULARIZATION (Chapter 41)

Sexual dysfunction can result from any of the following major causes: impaired pelvic blood supply, sympathetic or parasympathetic nerve damage, psychogenic causes, drugs, and endocrine disorders. Following abdominal aortic surgery, erectile and ejaculatory dysfunction can result if the bypass reduces pelvic blood flow or the parasympathetic or sympathetic nerve plexuses are damaged in the para-aortic plexus, superior hypogastric plexus (inferior mesenteric artery region), or common iliac artery plexus. The incidence of sexual dysfunction can be reduced by planning the bypass to maintain or improve the pelvic blood flow and by avoiding damage to the autonomic nerve plexuses by using minimal aortic dissection, which is best achieved through a right lateral aortic approach just below the renal arteries.

URETERAL OBSTRUCTION

This section is included to cover the problem of ureteral obstruction that may be seen after abdominal aortic reconstructive surgery.

Etiology

Ureteral obstruction and hydronephrosis and consequent urinary sepsis and renal failure may follow an aortobifemoral bypass or abdominal aortic aneurysm surgery. Obstruction may be caused by direct operative trauma to the ureter, ischemic damage to the ureter, kinking of the ureter during tunneling by inadvertently grasping the periureteric tissue, or formation of a dense fibrotic reaction around the prosthesis that invades the muscular wall of the ureter. Although the ureter may be trapped by a graft placed anterior to it, this mechanism does not appear to be a major factor. Following early reports of patients with ureteral obstruction following aortic surgery, most vascular surgeons accepted the theory that direct compression of the ureter between the prosthetic graft and the iliac artery is the principal cause of late obstruction. However, recent reports by Sant and colleagues[2] and Kaufman and coworkers[3] have concluded that the ureter is most commonly bound down in localized fibrosis around the graft and that direct compression by an anteriorly placed graft is an important factor in only half the reported cases.

Clinical Pathology

The consequences of ureteral damage following aortic surgery consist of three clinical types. Early transient hydronephrosis occurs in 10 to 15 per cent of these cases owing to edema from the dissection and is of no clinical significance because it usually resolves.[4] Early persistent hydronephrosis is uncommon, occurring in approximately 1 to 2 per cent of aortic cases.[4] These patients require continued follow-up, but operation is necessary only for those who develop further complications. Ernst and colleagues[5] clarified the pathology associated with delayed-onset hydronephrosis, which occurred in 1.2 per cent of their series. In half the cases, delayed ureteral obstruction was due to a dense local fibrotic reaction, the etiology of which is unknown. To detect this complication, during late follow-up, patients should be studied by ultrasound, CT scan, or intravenous pyelography (IVP). The other half of their cases were associated with graft complications including thrombosis, false aneurysm, graft-enteric fistula, and infection.[5, 6] Thus, patients who present with ureteral complications should be investigated for associated graft complications, and conversely, patients who present with aortic graft complications should have a full urologic work-up because 5 per cent will be found to have an abnormality.

Diagnosis

Sant and colleagues[2] reported that 13 per cent of patients with obstructive uropathy were asymptomatic, 31 per cent had nonurologic symptoms (anorexia, hypertension, nephrotic syndrome), and 56 per cent had urologic symptoms (flank pain, anuria, frequency). Investigations are oriented toward four specific areas: (1) The presence of hydronephrosis may be detected by IVP, ultrasound, or CT scan. (2) The diagnosis of ureteral obstruction and assessment of the site of involvement are determined by retrograde pyelography. (3) Renal function is assessed by isotope renography, measuring creatinine clearance by inserting a percutaneous nephrostomy in the affected kidney, or evaluating the improvement in renal function after temporary decompression. (4) The position of the ureter relative to the graft is determined by a simultaneous retrograde pyelogram and angiogram.

Management

Ureteral dilatation in the early postoperative period is usually the result of edema from operative trauma but rarely may be due to ischemia from local interruption of the ureter's blood supply. Conservative treatment is usually successful, but surgery may be indicated if progressive hydronephrosis, renal deterioration, or recurrent pyelonephritis develops.

Chronic ureteral obstruction with symptoms, evidence of impaired renal function, or recurrent infection requires surgery. However, in poor-risk patients, if the cause is fibrosis, the use of a permanent ureteral stent can be considered. Although stents are associated with risk of infection and may be occluded by debris, this approach is relatively noninvasive and can be used on a long-term basis.

If the *ureter lies anterior to the graft,* ureterolysis is performed and subsequent fibrosis minimized by omental wrapping and possibly steroid administration. A severely scarred and narrowed segment of ureter may have to be excised and continuity reestablished by primary anastomosis, usually over a stent and protected by a proximal diversion and omental wrapping. Other procedures used to reestablish ureteral continuity include ureteroneocystotomy with or without a bladder flap or anastomosis to the contralateral ureter through a retroperitoneal tunnel.

If the *ureter lies posterior to the graft,* the graft can be divided and reanastomosed posteriorly to the ureter, or perfusion can be reestablished by an extra-anatomic bypass, such as a femoral crossover graft. The ureter is freed by ureterolysis. Alternatively, the ureter can be divided and reanastomosed anteriorly to the graft as described above.

There are no reports of the long-term results of ureteral repair.

References

1. Rutherford RB, Flanigan DP, Gupta SK, et al: Suggested standards for reports dealing with lower extremity ischemia. J Vasc Surg 4:80, 1986.
2. Sant G, Heaney JA, Parkhurst EC, Blaivas JG: Obstructive uropathy—Potentially serious complication of reconstructive vascular surgery. Urology 19:16, 1983.
3. Kaufman JE, Parsons CL, Gosink BB, Schmidt JD: Retrospective study of ureteral obstruction following vascular bypass surgery. Urology 19:278, 1982.
4. Goldenberg SL, Gordon PB, Cooperberg PL, McLoughlin MG: Early hydronephrosis following aortic bifurcation graft surgery: A prospective study. J Urol 140:1367, 1988.
5. Wright OJ, Ernst CB, Evans JR, et al: Ureteral complications and aortoiliac reconstruction. J Vasc Surg 11:29, 1990.
6. Schubart P, Fortner G, Cummings D, et al: The significance of hydronephrosis after aortofemoral reconstruction. Arch Surg 120:377, 1985.

31

Cardiac Complications

Bruce S. Cutler, M.D.

• • •

Complications of coronary artery disease (CAD) account for 70 per cent of the early and late morbidity and mortality following operations for peripheral arterial disease. This proportion has remained relatively constant since the early 1970s, during which time the overall safety of major vascular operations has undergone dramatic improvement. Because of the systemic nature of atherosclerosis, some degree of coronary occlusive disease coexists in nearly all patients with symptomatic peripheral arterial disease. Since the median age of the general population is gradually rising, vascular surgeons can expect to encounter older patients with more extensive coronary and peripheral arterial occlusive disease in the future. It is therefore important for the vascular specialist to be well acquainted with the current methods of cardiac evaluation and perioperative management of potential candidates for vascular reconstructive procedures.

PREVALENCE OF CORONARY ARTERY DISEASE

The true incidence of CAD in patients with symptomatic peripheral arterial disease is unknown. However, very useful data come from five studies in which patients underwent routine coronary angiography preoperatively prior to vascular reconstruction (Table 31–1). Such reports are inherently biased because only patients who were considered for operation were studied, and not all patients agreed to coronary angiography. The collected results from 1545 patients indicate that the incidence of hemodynamically important CAD involving at least one major vessel was 77 per cent and for three vessels, 44 per cent. Of equal significance was the observation that 40 per cent of patients with no history of CAD were found to have significant stenosis of at least one coronary artery. The high incidence of occult coronary disease is important because the risk of a postoperative cardiac complication has been shown to correlate with the severity of the CAD and to be independent of symptoms. Therefore, all patients, even those who lack symptoms of CAD, should be considered to be at risk for cardiac complications following a vascular operation.

PATHOPHYSIOLOGY OF CORONARY BLOOD FLOW

Normal homeostatic mechanisms adjust coronary artery blood flow to meet myocardial oxygen demands in response to changes in heart rate, wall tension, and contractility. Coronary vasodilatation is the primary mechanism by which coronary blood flow and oxygen delivery are increased. Coronary stenosis dramatically limits autoregulation of coronary blood flow and this may lead to ischemia if the demand for oxygen exceeds the supply.

The majority of coronary blood flow occurs during ventricular diastole when the pressure gradient across the coronary vascular bed is highest. Coronary perfusion pressure is determined by the difference between systemic arterial diastolic pressure and left ventricular end-diastolic pressure (LVEDP). Therefore, factors such as systemic hypotension or an increase in LVEDP due to ventricular failure, or both, can result in reduced coronary perfusion. Tachycardia is particularly insidious because it results in reduced coronary perfusion through a decrease in the duration of diastole and also causes an increase in myocardial oxygen consumption due to the accelerated heart rate. The oxygen-carrying capacity of the blood is determined by the hemoglobin concentration and oxygen saturation; consequently, anemia or reduced inspired oxygen fraction (FIO_2) may contribute to myocardial ischemia. Unfortunately, during the course of a vascular operation and subsequent con-

Table 31–1. Prevalence of Coronary Artery Disease Based on Routine Coronary Angiography Prior To Aortic Reconstruction

		Asymptomatic Coronary Artery Disease		Symptomatic Coronary Artery Disease	
Author	**No. Patients**	*≤ 1 Vessel (%)*	*3 Vessel (%)*	*≤ 1 Vessel (%)*	*3 Vessel (%)*
Tomatis et al,[1] 1972*	100	28	16	—	—
Hertzer et al,[2] 1984*	1000	37	15	78	44
Young et al,[3] 1986*	302	46	20	85	52
Blombery et al,[4] 1986†	84	48	9	44	22
Orecchia et al,[5] 1988*	59	64	29	84	36
Average	1545 (Total)	40	16	77	44

From Cutler BS: Assessment and importance of coronary artery disease in patients with aortoiliac occlusive and aneurysmal disease. In *Ernst CB, Stanley JC (eds): Current Therapy in Vascular Surgery, 2nd ed. Philadelphia, BC Decker, 1991, by permission of Mosby–Year Book, Inc.*

**Critical stenosis ≥ 70 per cent.*

†Critical stenosis ≥ 50 per cent.

valescence, many of the factors mentioned above conspire to cause an imbalance between myocardial oxygen supply and demand that may be poorly tolerated by the patient with coronary occlusive disease.[6].

PREOPERATIVE RISK ASSESSMENT

All vascular patients should undergo preoperative assessment of cardiac risk because of the prevalence of CAD. The evaluation should begin with careful questioning about risk factors associated with CAD, including hyperlipidemia, diabetes, smoking, angina pectoris, myocardial infarction, or a family history of atherosclerosis. It is widely understood that a recent myocardial infarction increases the risk of even a limited operative procedure. Although still true, during the last decade the risk of reinfarction following a vascular procedure within 3 months has dropped from 37 per cent[7] to only 5 per cent.[8–10] The risk of reinfarction following a myocardial infarction more than 3 months previously is 3 per cent. The risk of reinfarction is the same whether the initial event was transmural or subendocardial.[11]

Logistic regression analysis of clinical risk factors has identified those that are potentially useful in predicting perioperative cardiac complications. Scoring systems developed by Goldman and colleagues,[11, 12] Detsky and colleagues,[13] Yeager and associates,[14] Cooperman and coworkers[15] and Eagle and colleagues[16] have established the following as important preoperative risk factors for coronary artery disease: (1) myocardial infarction within 6 months, (2) history of congestive heart failure, (3) Q wave on electrocardiography (ECG), (4) angina, (5) diabetes, (6) ventricular arrhythmia, (7) age over 70, (8) emergency operation, and (9) recent cerebrovascular accident. Each of the scoring systems assigns a weight to each risk factor, which are then summed or incorporated into a formula to determine operative risk. The advantage of such a scheme is that it makes use of easily available clinical data and is applicable to all patients. Although individual risk factors undoubtedly have a strong association with underlying CAD, the risk factor indices have proved to be poor predictors of perioperative cardiac complications.[17–23] Detsky and colleagues[13] cautioned that multi-variant models are usually not transferable between institutions and may even vary from year to year. Last, risk factor analysis is of no benefit in detecting patients with asymptomatic CAD. Therefore, to identify all patients with hemodynamically significant CAD, an objective screening method should be applied preoperatively. A number of noninvasive and semi-invasive tests originally developed for evaluating patients after myocardial infarction have been adapted for preoperative testing of vascular patients.

The clinical utility of a screening test to predict cardiac events following vascular surgery can be statistically described by its sensitivity, specificity, and likelihood ratio. The likelihood ratio expresses the odds that a positive test result will occur in a patient with a cardiac complication. Ratios may be calculated for positive and negative test results. The ideal test should have a very high ratio (greater than 10) for a positive test result, and a value of less than 0.2 for a negative outcome. Likelihood ratios may be used to compare predictive values between different tests or to compare the same test performed in different institutions, or they can be chained together to evaluate the combined accuracy of two or more tests. Specificity, sensitivity, and likelihood ratios have been calculated to help the reader compare the clinical utility of the tests shown in Tables 31–2 to 31–5. (*Note*: To increase the validity of comparisons between studies, the original data have been recalculated using only fatal and nonfatal myocardial infarctions as endpoints.)

Electrocardiographically Monitored Exercise Test

The ECG-monitored exercise test was the first used to screen peripheral vascular patients preoperatively for CAD. The rationale for exercise testing was that the cardiac demand for oxygen during exercise may be analogous to the stress of a vascular operation and subsequent recovery. Therefore, the results of exercise testing could be used to predict the occurrence of perioperative cardiac complications.

Table 31–2. Exercise Testing to Predict Perioperative Myocardial Infarction

Author	Year	No. Patients	Pretest Probability (%)	Sensitivity	Specificity	Likelihood Ratio *Positive*	Likelihood Ratio *Negative*	Post-Test Probability (%)
Cutler[24]	1981	130	6.9	0.88	0.65	2.54	0.17	16
Von Knorring[25]	1985	105	2.9	0.67	0.76	2.79	0.43	8
McPhail[26]	1989	60	36*	0.23	0.89	2.09	0.87	54

**Includes pulmonary edema as an end-point.*

The results of several series of ECG monitored stress tests show that it has moderate sensitivity for detecting coronary artery disease but limited specificity in predicting adverse cardiac outcomes (Table 31–2). On the other hand, patients with a normal exercise test have a very low risk of having a cardiac complication. In fact, simply being able to achieve 85 per cent of the maximum predicted heart rate is a useful discriminant. In one study, the risk of a cardiac event was 7 per cent for patients who achieved their target heart rate compared to 24 per cent for those who could not.[27]

The major advantage of stress testing is its low cost, wide applicability, and potential for detecting occult CAD in asymptomatic patients. Most hospitals have exercise laboratories and personnel experienced in interpreting exercise electrocardiograms. The primary disadvantage of stress testing is the requirement for exercise. Nearly one third of all vascular patients are unable to exercise sufficiently to produce a meaningful test owing to claudication or other disease.[24] In addition, medications such as digitalis or diuretics and electrolyte abnormalities may produce resting ST-segment alterations that can yield false-positive results. Beta-adrenergic blocking medications may limit the heart rate response to exercise. Because of these drawbacks, stress testing has been largely replaced by other screening tests not requiring exercise.

Radionuclide Ventriculography

Radionuclide ventriculography is a widely available, noninvasive means of estimating residual left ventricular function after a myocardial infarction. Since the test does not require exercise and is minimally invasive, it is not surprising that it has been applied to the preoperative evaluation of cardiac risk in vascular patients. Several studies have compared preoperative ejection fraction determined by radionuclide ventriculography prior to aortic,[23, 28–30] lower extremity,[31, 32] and carotid[33] surgery to the incidence of postoperative cardiac events. Although some studies[28, 30, 32, 34] have shown a strong association between an ejection fraction of less than 0.35 and the incidence of postoperative myocardial infarction or congestive heart failure, others have not (Table 31–3).[23, 31, 35] Although the data are inconclusive, it is reasonable to assume in general that a patient with a very low left ventricular ejection fraction is at significantly greater risk for a perioperative cardiac event than his counterpart with normal function. However, even a normal ejection fraction is no assurance that the patient does not have significant underlying CAD. In one study, 44 per cent of patients with an ejection fraction of greater than 0.56 had at least one symptom of CAD, and 22 per cent had suffered a previous myocardial infarction.[31] Consequently, radionuclide ventriculography is of limited value as a preoperative screening test for CAD. Instead, it should be used selectively in patients in whom impaired left ventricular function is suspected or to complement another screening test such as dipyridamole thallium scintigraphy.

Continuous Electrocardiographic Monitoring

Continuous electrocardiographic monitoring permits detection of silent myocardial ischemia throughout the perioperative period. The majority of episodes of myocardial

Table 31–3. Radionuclide Ventriculography to Predict Perioperative Myocardial Infarction

Author	Year	No. Patients	Pretest Probability (%)	Sensitivity	Specificity	Likelihood Ratio *Positive*	Likelihood Ratio *Negative*	Post-Test Probability (%)
Pasternak[32] EF* < 0.35	1985	100	14.0	0.43	0.98	18.7	5.81	75
Mosley[28] EF < 0.30	1985	41	12.2	0.75	0.97	27.8	0.26	79
Kazmers[29] EF < 0.35	1988	60	6.6	0.25	0.84	1.56	0.89	9.9
Franco[31] EF < 0.35	1989	85	20.0	0.29	0.85	1.97	0.83	33
McPhail[36] EF < 0.5	1990	85	39.0†	0.27	0.85	1.75	0.86	53

**EF = Ejection fraction.*
†Includes pulmonary edema as an end-point.

Table 31–4. Preoperative Continuous ECG Monitoring to Predict Perioperative Myocardial Infarction

Author	Year	No. Patients	Pretest Probability (%)	Sensitivity	Specificity	Likelihood Ratio		Post-Test Probability (%)
						Positive	*Negative*	
Raby[45]	1989	176	2.8	0.80	0.84	5.0	0.24	13
Pasternak[39]	1989	120	5.0	1.00	0.63	2.70	0.	13
Fleisher[43]	1991	67	4.5	0.50	0.77	2.25	0.65	9.6

ischemia are unaccompanied by typical chest pain but carry the same adverse prognosis as those that produce angina.[37, 38] Holter monitors have been refined through the addition of microprocessors to generate a *real time* analysis of the electrocardiogram that can alert physicians to myocardial ischemia even when the perception of chest pain is impaired by anesthesia or sedative medication.

Silent myocardial ischemia occurs in 18 to 40 per cent of patients monitored for 18 to 48 hours preoperatively.[39–44] Several studies have compared the occurrence of preoperative ischemia with the incidence of adverse postoperative cardiac events and have come to conflicting conclusions (Table 31–4). In a study of 176 patients who were monitored for 24 to 48 hours prior to vascular surgery, 32 developed silent myocardial ischemia, and 12 went on to have a cardiac complication, half of which were fatal.[45] Statistical comparison to a variety of clinical risk factors showed that preoperative myocardial ischemia was the best predictor of cardiac events. In another study, preoperative myocardial ischemia increased the risk of a cardiac complication by 5.2 times.[39] Furthermore, those who developed myocardial infarction had a significantly greater number and duration of ischemic episodes than those who did not. Unfortunately, the most recent studies have not confirmed the utility of preoperative ischemia for predicting cardiac events.[42, 43] Fleisher and colleagues[43] found a positive predictive value of only 0.38 among 67 vascular patients. Mangano and associates[42] monitored 172 vascular and 302 general surgical patients throughout the perioperative period. Postoperative ischemia occurred in 41 per cent of patients, which was twice the incidence observed preoperatively. Postoperative ischemia increased the risk of an adverse cardiac outcome by 2.8 times, whereas preoperative ischemia was not predictive. McCann and Clements[41] monitored 50 patients throughout the perioperative period and also found that silent ischemia was most prominent in the postoperative period and was the best predictor of cardiac events. Although preoperative cardiac monitoring is a potentially attractive means of estimating cardiac risk because it is noninvasive and low in cost, it lacks sufficient sensitivity to be a useful screening test. Furthermore, 10 to 20 per cent of patients cannot be tested because of QRS or resting ST abnormalities that interfere with analysis including those commonly produced by digitalis therapy.[39–41] Until further data become available, preoperative ECG monitoring should not be used as the sole method for cardiac risk assessment.

Dipyridamole Thallium Scintigraphy

Dipyridamole thallium scintigraphy (DTS) is the most widely used method for preoperative stratification of cardiac risk in vascular surgery patients. It is therefore important that the vascular specialist be aware of the mode of action, clinical applications, and limitations of this method of testing.

The intravenous administration of dipyridamole causes intense coronary vasodilatation at least equal to that produced by exercise but with no significant increase in myocardial oxygen consumption.[46] Because dipyridamole is poorly absorbed from the gastrointestinal tract, significant coronary vasodilatation is not produced by the relatively small doses used to inhibit platelet aggregation. Dipyridamole produces coronary vasodilatation that is most marked in the small resistance vessels supplied by normal coronary arteries, and correspondingly less in areas supplied by stenotic vessels. Thus, dipyridamole maximizes the disparity in blood flow between normal and ischemic areas of the myocardium. Intravenous administration of aminophylline promptly reverses the effects of dipyridamole and thus is the ideal drug for treatment of side effects. From a practical standpoint, xanthine medications (e.g., aminophylline and caffeine), should be withheld for 48 hours prior to testing. DTS should not be performed in patients with severe bronchospastic conditions or in those who cannot safely stop aminophylline.[47, 48] In this group, an alternative coronary vasodilator may be substituted for dipyridamole. Exercise has been widely used as a vasodilating stimulus but is usually not feasible because of the lung disease.[49–54] An infusion of dobutamine produces coronary vasodilatation through an increase in heart rate and work, which, when combined with thallium, yields a scan of similar quality to that produced with dipyridamole.[55, 56] Alternatively, rapid atrial pacing[57] can increase heart rate and induce coronary vasodilatation. Although still experimental, these methods may be alternatives to the intravenous use of dipyridamole.

Thallium-201 is used as a marker for viable myocardium. The uptake of this isotope is proportional to blood flow except at very high flow rates. Following infusions of dipyridamole and thallium-201, scanning is performed in three planes at 15 minutes and again at 3 hours. The isotope is promptly absorbed by normal myocardium on the initial scan (Fig. 31–1). Infarcted, avascular tissue does not take up thallium and produces a ''fixed defect'' on the initial scan. Isotope absorption is delayed in ischemic areas owing to slower blood flow through stenotic or collateral vessels and produces an area of delayed uptake or ''redistribution.'' By comparing thallium uptake on the initial and 3-hour scans in three planes, infarcts and ischemic areas can be localized to the territory of each of the three major coronary arteries. For descriptive purposes, each of the three views is divided into three segments (Fig. 31–2).

Dipyridamole thallium scintigraphy was first used in 1985 by Boucher and colleagues[58] to stratify cardiac risk in vascular patients. They performed DTS in 48 patients prior

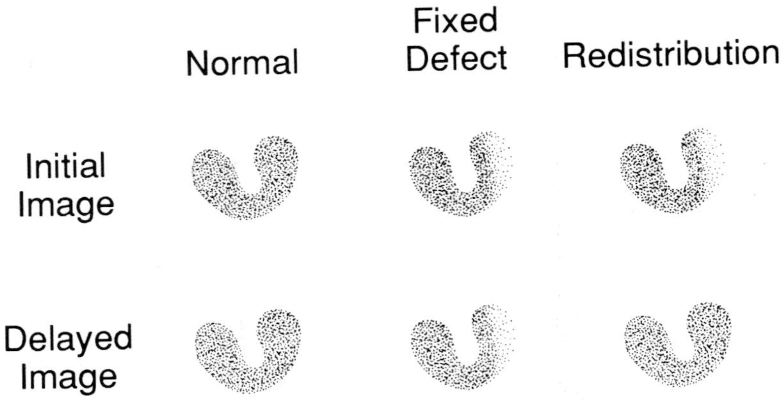

FIGURE 31–1. Dipyridamole thallium-201 scintigraphy. Thallium is promptly absorbed by normally perfused myocardium, and initial and delayed scans are identical. Thallium is not absorbed by infarcted myocardium, which produces a fixed defect on the initial and delayed scans. Delayed uptake of thallium-201, or redistribution, occurs in ischemic areas. (From Cutler BS: Cardiac evaluation prior to aortic surgery. *In* Bergan JJ, Yao JST [eds]: Arterial Surgery. New Diagnostic and Operative Techniques. Orlando, Fl, Grune & Stratton, 1988, p 248.)

to vascular surgery. Thallium redistribution was observed in 16 patients, of whom eight had postoperative cardiac complications. There were no events among 32 patients with normal scans or only fixed defects. Since this initial study, there have been a number of reports employing DTS as a means of screening preoperative patients for coronary artery disease (Table 31–5). Nearly all studies have demonstrated a high sensitivity but limited specificity in predicting postoperative cardiac morbidity. *Multi-variant comparison of DTS with a variety of clinical risk factors and risk factor indices has consistently shown thallium redistribution to be the best predictor of postoperative cardiac events.*[17, 19–21, 23, 61–64] It has also been found superior in direct comparisons with other screening methods such as exercise testing[26] and radionuclide ventriculography.[23] *Nevertheless, the clinical utility of DTS has been questioned because of its limited specificity: Up to 70 per cent of patients with a positive test will not have a postoperative cardiac event.*[65, 66] Various measures have been employed to improve specificity. A quantitative relationship has been demonstrated between the location and total area of thallium redistribution and the risk of a cardiac event. The positive predictive value increased from 13 per cent when redistribution involved only one segment to 43 per cent when two or three segments were involved. However, the increase in specificity resulted in a corresponding loss of sensitivity.[17] A similar approach involves the development of semi-quantitative scintigraphic indices that grade the extent and severity of

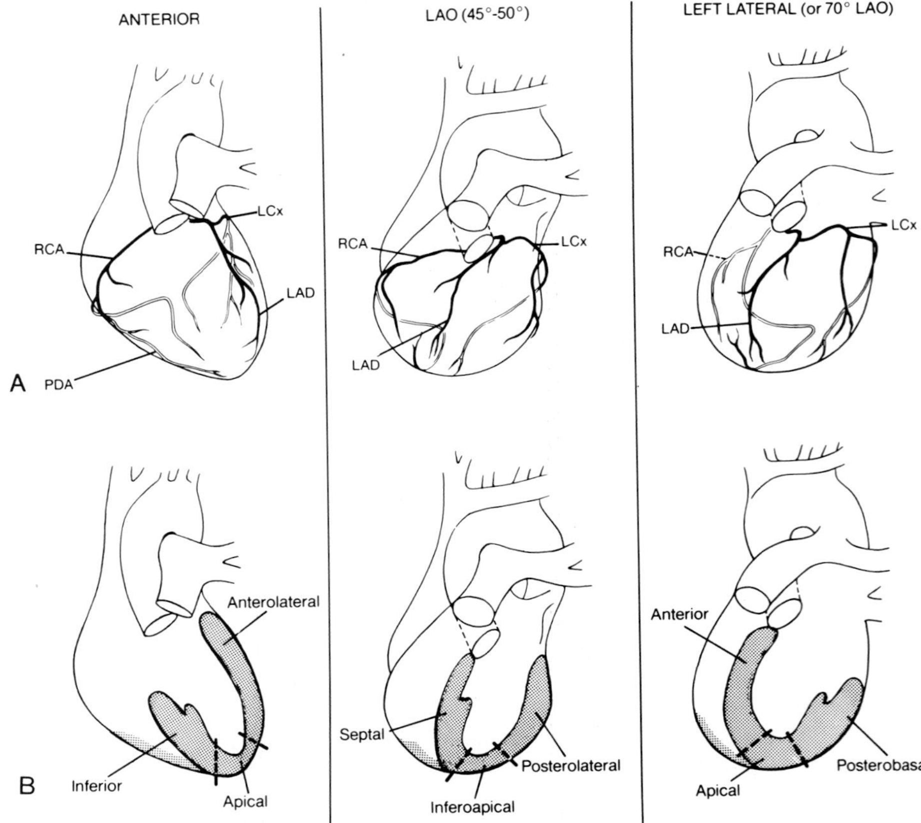

FIGURE 31–2. *A*, Coronary anatomy in standard projections. *B*, Schematic drawing of a normal thallium-201 scan subdivided into anatomic segments. LAO, left anterior oblique; RCA, right coronary artery; PDA, posterior descending artery; LAD, left anterior descending; LCx, left circumflex. (*A* and *B*, From Introduction to Nuclear Cardiology: A Technology Training Manual. 2nd ed. North Billerica, MA, EI du Pont de Nemours & Company, 1984.)

Table 31–5. Dipyridamole Thallium Scintigraphy to Predict Perioperative Myocardial Infarction

Author	Year	No. Patients	Pretest Probability (%)	Sensitivity	Specificity	Likelihood Ratio		Post-Test Probability (%)
						Positive	*Negative*	
Eagle[59]	1989	200	7.5	0.87	0.63	2.33	0.21	16
Lane[19]	1989	101	8.9	0.88	0.32	1.29	0.35	11
Younis[60]	1990	111	7.2	0.75	0.67	2.27	0.37	15
McPhail[36]	1990	85	38.8*	0.92	0.76	3.83	0.11	71
Cutler[61]	1992	262	8.8	0.87	0.53	1.85	0.25	15

**Includes pulmonary edema and ventricular arrhythmia as end-points.*

redistribution.[21] These indices may be used to stratify patients into an intermediate-risk group with a 5 per cent chance of a cardiac event, and a high-risk group with an 85 per cent chance. It therefore appears that the risk of cardiac morbidity is related not only to redistribution on DTS but also to the total number of segments involved and to the presence of thallium redistribution in the anatomic territories of multiple coronary arteries, particularly that of the left anterior descending artery.[20]

Two observations have suggested that some fixed defects on a 3-hour scan may represent viable but very ischemic areas of myocardium. First, some fixed defects were found to perfuse normally following successful coronary bypass surgery. Second, some patients with only fixed defects on a preoperative scan developed myocardial infarctions following vascular procedures.[23] Scanning delayed for 4 or more hours after a second thallium injection subsequently demonstrated that 31 to 49 per cent of fixed defects on the 3-hour scan showed delayed redistribution.[67, 68] Delayed imaging may therefore be another means of improving DTS specificity and should be performed in all patients with unexpected fixed defects.

Dipyridamole thallium scintigraphy may also be used to provide useful information about postoperative survival. Fixed defects on a preoperative scan are related to long-term survival, possibly because they reflect loss of ventricular function. In one study, the 5-year survival for patients with one or more fixed defects was 42 per cent compared to 82 per cent when the scan showed only redistribution and 96 per cent when the scan was normal.[61] Obviously, a patient's prognosis for long-term survival is an important factor to consider, together with perioperative risk, in making the initial decision on the method of treatment.

There are several potential sources of error in the interpretation of DTS with which the vascular specialist should be familiar. DTS interpretation relies on the differential uptake of thallium to identify ischemic areas of myocardium. Global ischemia caused by left main coronary artery stenosis may produce a uniformly poor uptake of thallium that may be mistaken for a normal test result. False-positive scans may also result from soft tissue attenuation from overlying breast tissue, left ventricular hypertrophy, or variations in coronary anatomy.

Despite the shortcomings of limited specificity, at present DTS is the most useful screening test for coronary artery disease in vascular patients because exercise is not necessary and it can detect asymptomatic coronary disease. It is cost-effective because only patients with a positive test result need further cardiac evaluation.

PREOPERATIVE MANAGEMENT OF CARDIAC RISK

Despite the widespread use of thallium scans, clinical judgment remains of paramount importance in the management of cardiac risk. The patient's cardiac history, the severity of associated diseases, and the urgency of a vascular operation must be thoughtfully evaluated together with the result of DTS to decide upon the best therapeutic alternative. *Frequently, an abnormal DTS test result simply confirms the suspicion that the patient has significant coronary artery disease but it is of little additional value in determining whether further cardiac evaluation and treatment are warranted.*

Which patients should undergo further cardiac evaluation? In general, patients with either chronic stable angina or a remote myocardial infarction who have only a single segment of redistribution or only fixed defects on DTS may undergo operation without further evaluation with an anticipated perioperative risk in the range of 2 per cent. Patients with a recent myocardial infarction, a history of congestive heart failure, or angina at rest or whose DTS test shows redistribution in the territories of multiple coronary arteries are clearly at increased risk and should be considered for further cardiac evaluation prior to a major operation.

The risk of a major vascular operation may be reduced by choosing an alternative surgical procedure or by instituting measures that will improve cardiac tolerance for a given procedure, or both. An alternative operative approach is most applicable in the treatment of aortoiliac occlusive disease. If the patient's only symptom is claudication, nonoperative management may be the safest choice. If the patient has ischemic tissue necrosis or rest pain and revascularization is therefore essential, angioplasty, atherectomy, or an extra-anatomic bypass graft are usually safer than an intra-abdominal procedure, although even extra-anatomic procedures have been reported to carry a cardiac morbidity of as much as 23 per cent when performed in high-risk patients.[61] In contrast, there is usually no acceptable alternative for treatment of a large or symptomatic abdominal aortic aneurysm or for limb-threatening ischemia due to femorotibial occlusive disease. *Recent evidence indicates that cardiac complications occur as frequently following infrainguinal procedures as they do after aortic operations.*[61, 69, 70] When there is no alternative to a major procedure, cardiac risk may be minimized through careful preoperative preparation and vigilant monitoring both intraoperatively and postoperatively or by improving cardiac tolerance for the proposed procedure through preliminary coronary revascularization.

Coronary Revascularization

Coronary revascularization prior to aortic or infrainguinal surgery may be a consideration in any patient with symptomatic CAD or multiple segments of thallium redistribution on DTS. The rationale for this approach is based on the observation that prior coronary artery bypass reduces the cardiac morbidity for a subsequent noncardiac operation.[71] However, the data from such retrospective studies are not directly applicable to patients with symptomatic peripheral vascular disease, who tend to be older, have more associated illnesses including diabetes, and have a higher mortality rate for aortocoronary surgery than the population of patients undergoing coronary revascularization for symptomatic CAD.[72, 73] Therefore, in assessing the potential benefit of preliminary coronary revascularization, the mortality of cardiac catheterization, coronary revascularization, and the vascular procedure *must be summed.* The risk for the coronary procedure may be as much as 10 per cent higher than that for an elective vascular operation, but the risk for the subsequent vascular procedure will be reduced by an undefined amount. The delay between the procedures is also an added risk to life for the patient with a large aortic aneurysm and a threat to the limb in patients with peripheral occlusive disease.

Coronary angiography usually demonstrates severe three-vessel involvement that is frequently not amenable to angioplasty or atherectomy. As much as one third of patients have disease that is so diffuse that coronary artery bypass grafting is not anatomically feasible or would not be expected to improve myocardial perfusion. Of the remaining patients, those with stenosis of the left main coronary artery or equivalent involvement of the three major vessels are clearly at high risk for a coronary event and should undergo preliminary coronary revascularization. Whether graftable patients without left main disease or its three-vessel equivalent will benefit from preliminary aortocoronary surgery remains controversial. The decision must be individualized, based on age, associated illnesses, urgency of the vascular disease, and the patient's willingness to undergo two procedures.

An occasional patient with a large or symptomatic abdominal aortic aneurysm who also has unstable angina or known stenosis of the left main coronary artery will require coronary revascularization and aneurysm resection at the same operation. Although no institution has had extensive experience with simultaneous procedures, reported mortality rates have ranged from 0 to 9 per cent.[71, 74, 75] When myocardial revascularization is not possible due to diffuse disease, poor ventricular function, or failed previous aortocoronary surgery and an intra-abdominal procedure is unavoidable, the cardiac risk may be reduced by the use of counterpulsation with an intra-aortic balloon pump.[76, 77]

Preoperative Treatment

Careful preoperative preparation can significantly reduce the intraoperative and postoperative cardiac risks of a major vascular operation. Control of hypertension is of particular importance because of its adverse effect on myocardial oxygen consumption. Antihypertensive agents should be continued up to the time of operation and resumed as promptly as feasible postoperatively. It is especially important to continue beta-antagonists and calcium channel blocking agents because their withdrawal has been associated with rebound tachycardia and hypertension. The intraoperative infusion of beta-antagonists may decrease the frequency of intraoperative myocardial ischemia.[78] The patient's state of hydration should be evaluated and corrected if necessary. Some degree of dehydration commonly occurs in vascular patients owing to the chronic use of diuretics, contrast-induced diuresis resulting from angiography, and from fasting for diagnostic procedures. Conversely, even mild congestive heart failure significantly increases the risk of myocardial injury and should be vigorously treated before operation. Preoperative determination of a Starling myocardial performance curve by plotting cardiac index against pulmonary capillary wedge pressure (PCWP) is an effective means of ensuring optimal hydration and reducing perioperative cardiac complications.[79, 80] Because this approach requires preoperative transfer to an intensive care unit, it is feasible only for selected patients. In practice, PCWP and cardiac output determinations are used to monitor volume administration and to develop a Starling curve intraoperatively.

INTRAOPERATIVE TREATMENT

Safe intraoperative treatment requires appropriate communication between the surgeon and the anesthesiologist, both of whom should be cognizant of those factors that increase myocardial oxygen requirements. For example, the surgeon should employ careful operative technique to minimize blood loss while the anesthesiologist titrates volume replacement to avoid hypotension or overtransfusion. Clamping of the aorta causes an abrupt rise in LVEDP, decreased coronary perfusion pressure, and reduced myocardial oxygen delivery. Conversely, unclamping of the aorta causes a drop in peripheral resistance, which may produce systolic and diastolic hypotension, which also decrease oxygen supply. Therefore, the surgeon should give the anesthesiologist ample warning before clamping and unclamping the aorta to minimize the hemodynamic consequences.

Intraoperative anesthetic management requires invasive hemodynamic monitoring of those parameters that reflect the myocardial oxygen balance. At the very least, this includes arterial pressure, a flow-directed pulmonary artery catheter, continuous ECG monitoring of limb and precordial leads, and core temperature. PCWP is a useful guide to volume replacement but is an unreliable measure of systolic and diastolic ventricular dysfunction.[81] Two-dimensional transesophageal echocardiography (TEE) is a recently developed means of monitoring ventricular wall motion abnormalities, which often precede electrocardiographic indications of myocardial ischemia. Intraoperative TEE has shown that ventricular hypokinesis occurs in nearly 50 per cent of patients during major vascular operations but is rarely associated with permanent myocardial injury.[82, 83] Consequently, the place of TEE monitoring in vascular surgery awaits further comparison with other standard monitoring methods.

The choice of anesthetic technique for the patient with CAD is not as important as the experience and expertise of the anesthesiologist. All inhalation anesthetics are myocardial depressants, which to a variable extent decrease heart rate, blood pressure, and myocardial oxygen consumption. These characteristics make these agents potentially useful in patients with coronary artery disease provided diastolic pressure is not permitted to drop to a level that would compromise coronary blood flow. Intravenous narcotic analgesics, such as fentanyl, are often used as an alternative to inhalation anesthetics because they produce minimal myocardial depression, a property that makes them especially useful for patients with impaired left ventricular function. However, large doses of narcotics may be necessary to avoid hypertension during intra-abdominal procedures and as a consequence may produce respiratory depression, necessitating controlled ventilation intraoperatively and postoperatively. Spinal or epidural anesthesia have no direct effect on the myocardium but may increase myocardial oxygen consumption because they may be associated with hypertension due to anxiety or hypotension and bradycardia resulting from sympathetic blockade. Prospective studies that have compared general and epidural anesthesia have found no advantage to either technique in reducing perioperative cardiac complications in patients undergoing aortic[84] or infrainguinal procedures.[85] However, epidural anesthesia may be associated with fewer pulmonary complications because the catheter may be left in place for postoperative pain control, obviating the need for intravenous narcotics.[86] Even local anesthesia is not completely safe because incomplete analgesia and anxiety can lead to catecholamine release, causing hypertension and tachycardia. In addition, lidocaine is absorbed from the subcutaneous tissue and is a myocardial depressant. Safe anesthesia for the patient with CAD requires skillful matching of the degree of anesthesia to the magnitude of the surgical stimulus combined with attentive monitoring and prompt treatment of electrical and hemodynamic indications of myocardial ischemia.

POSTOPERATIVE TREATMENT

Emergence from anesthesia is potentially stressful and may precipitate arrhythmias and myocardial ischemia. *Patients should not be awakened when hypothermic because shivering can increase tissue oxygen demands by as much as four to five times, causing an undesirable increase in cardiac output.* Intraoperative electrocardiographic and hemodynamic monitoring should be continued postoperatively in an intensive care unit. Atrial and ventricular dysrhythmias may signify, or left untreated, may produce myocardial ischemia. Continuous ECG monitoring has confirmed that silent myocardial ischemia is a frequent event in patients recovering from a major vascular operation and consequently, any indication of myocardial ischemia should be vigorously and promptly treated.[41, 42]

Careful pain management is critical to prevent catechol-induced hypertension and tachycardia. Fluids should be titrated to maintain optimal systolic and diastolic pressure and to avoid congestive heart failure. In this regard, PCWP is a particularly useful guide in patients with poor left ventricular function. Patients undergoing an intra-abdominal procedure usually begin to mobilize "third space" fluids 48 to 72 hours postoperatively, a time that coincides with the peak occurrence of myocardial infarction.[45, 88] Therefore, creatine phosphokinase isoenzymes and the ECG should be monitored for at least 2 to 3 days postoperatively. Intravenous beta-antagonists and antihypertensive medications should be promptly resumed to control hypertension. Prophylactic intravenous infusions of nitroglycerin may produce desirable coronary vasodilatation. *Many seemingly unrelated common postoperative problems such as atelectasis, fever, anxiety, and anemia have a cumulative deleterious effect on myocardial oxygen needs.* It has become clear that the recovery period following a major vascular procedure is at least as important as the operation itself in determining whether the patient will suffer a potentially fatal myocardial infarction. It is therefore essential that intensive care unit personnel promptly recognize and treat those physiologic alterations that contribute to myocardial ischemia before infarction ensues.

LONG-TERM TREATMENT

Myocardial infarction accounts for the majority of postoperative deaths and is also responsible for most of the mortality during the first 5 years after a vascular procedure.[61, 88, 89] Fatal myocardial infarctions occur more frequently in vascular surgery patients than in others with CAD of similar severity but without peripheral vascular disease.[73, 89, 90] Following a successful vascular reconstructive procedure, many patients who were minimally symptomatic, or even asymptomatic preoperatively, may increase their level of physical activity to the point where they develop angina. In others, the severity of CAD may have been appreciated for the first time as a consequence of the preoperative evaluation. Because of the risk of late cardiac morbidity, virtually all vascular patients should have close follow-up of their CAD, including strict control of risk factors, careful titration of medications, and angiographic or surgical revascularization, when appropriate, to derive the best chance for long-term survival following a major vascular operation.

References

1. Tomatis LA, Fierens EE, Verbrugge GP: Evaluation of surgical risk in peripheral vascular disease by coronary arteriography: A series of 100 cases. Surgery 71:429, 1971.
2. Hertzer NR, Beven EG, Young JR, et al: Coronary artery disease in peripheral vascular patients: A classification of 1000 coronary angiograms and results of surgical management. Ann Surg 199:223, 1984.
3. Young JR, Hertzer NR, Beven EG, et al: Coronary artery disease in patients with aortic aneurysm: A classification of 302 coronary angiograms and results of surgical management. Ann Vasc Surg 1:36, 1986.
4. Blombery PA, Ferguson IA, Rosengarten DS, et al: The role of coronary artery disease in complications of abdominal aortic aneurysm surgery. Surgery 101:150, 1987.
5. Orecchia PM, Berger PW, White CJ, et al: Coronary artery disease in aortic surgery. Ann Vasc Surg 2:28, 1988.
6. Nussmeier NA: Anesthetic management of the patient with ischemic heart disease. Lecture from the University of Southern California Review Course in Anesthesiology. March, 1987.
7. Wells PH, Kaplan JA: Optimal management of patients with ischemic heart disease for noncardiac surgery by complementary anesthesiologist and cardiologist interaction. Am Heart J 102:1029, 1981.

8. Shah KB, Kleinman BS, Sami H, et al: Reevaluation of perioperative myocardial infarction in patients with prior myocardial infarction undergoing noncardiac operations. Anesth Analg 71:231, 1990.
9. Rao TLK, Jacobs KH, El-Etr AA: Reinfarction following anesthesia in patients with myocardial infarction. Anesthesiology 59:499, 1983.
10. Rivers SP, Scher LA, Gupta SK, et al: Safety of peripheral vascular surgery after recent acute myocardial infarction. J Vasc Surg 11:70, 1990.
11. Goldman L: Cardiac risks and complications of noncardiac surgery. Ann Intern Med 98:504, 1983.
12. Goldman L, Caldera DL, Nussbuam SR, et al: Multifactorial index of cardiac risk of noncardiac surgical procedures. N Engl J Med 297:845, 1977.
13. Detsky AS, Abrams HB, McLaughlin JR, et al: Predicting cardiac complications in patients undergoing non-cardiac surgery. J Gen Intern Med 1:211, 1986.
14. Yeager RA, Weigel RM, Murphy ES, et al: Application of clinically valid cardiac risk factors to aortic aneurysm surgery. Arch Surg 121:278, 1986.
15. Cooperman M, Pflug B, Martin EW Jr, et al: Cardiovascular risk factors in patients with peripheral vascular disease. Surgery 84:505, 1978.
16. Eagle KA, Coley CM, Newell JB, et al: Combining clinical and thallium data optimizes preoperative assessment of cardiac risk before major vascular surgery. Ann Intern Med 110:859, 1989.
17. Lette J, Waters D, Lassonde J, et al: Multivariate clinical models and quantitative dipyridamole-thallium imaging to predict cardiac morbidity and death after vascular reconstruction. J Vasc Surg 14:160, 1991.
18. Lette J, Waters D, Lassonde J, et al: Postoperative myocardial infarction and cardiac death. Predictive value of dipyridamole-thallium imaging and five clinical scoring systems based on multifactorial analysis. Ann Surg 211:84, 1990.
19. Lane SE, Lewis SM, Pippin JJ, et al: Predictive value of quantitative dipyridamole-thallium scintigraphy in assessing cardiovascular risk after vascular surgery in diabetes mellitus. Am J Cardiol 64:1275, 1989.
20. Lette J, Waters D, Lapointe J, et al: Usefulness of the severity and extent of reversible perfusion defects during thallium-dipyridamole imaging for cardiac risk assessment before noncardiac surgery. Am J Cardiol 64:276, 1989.
21. Levinson JR, Boucher CA, Coley CM, et al: Usefulness of semiquantitative analysis of dipyridamole thallium-201 redistribution for improving risk stratification before vascular surgery. Am J Cardiol 66:406, 1990.
22. Reifsnyder T, Bandyk DF, Lanza D, et al: Use of stress thallium imaging to stratify cardiac risk in patients undergoing vascular surgery. J Surg Res 52:147, 1992.
23. McEnroe CS, O'Donnell TF Jr, Yeager A, et al: Comparison of ejection fraction and Goldman risk factor analysis to dipyridamole thallium-201 studies in the evaluation of cardiac morbidity after aortic aneurysm surgery. J Vasc Surg 11:497, 1990.
24. Cutler BS, Wheeler HB, Paraskos JA, et al: Applicability and interpretation of electrocardiographic stress testing in patients with peripheral vascular disease. Am J Surg 141:501, 1981.
25. Von Knorring J, Lepäntalo M: Prediction of perioperative cardiac complications by electrocardiographic monitoring during treadmill exercise testing before peripheral vascular surgery. Surgery 99:610, 1986.
26. McPhail NV, Ruddy TD, Calvin JE, et al: A comparison of dipyridamole-thallium imaging and exercise testing in the prediction of postoperative cardiac complications in patients requiring arterial reconstruction. J Vasc Surg 10:51, 1989.
27. McPhail N, Calvin JE, Shariatmadar A, et al: The use of preoperative exercise testing to predict cardiac complications after arterial reconstruction. J Vasc Surg 7:60, 1988.
28. Mosley JG, Clarke JMF, Ell PJ, et al: Assessment of myocardial function before aortic surgery by radionuclide angiocardiography. Br J Surg 72:886, 1985.
29. Kazmers A, Cerqueira MD, Zierler RE: The role of preoperative radionuclide ejection fraction in direct abdominal aortic aneurysm repair. J Vasc Surg 8:128, 1988.
30. Pasternack PF, Imparato AM, Bear G, et al: The value of radionuclide angiography as a predictor of perioperative myocardial infarction in patients undergoing abdominal aortic aneurysm resection. J Vasc Surg 1:320, 1984.
31. Franco CD, Goldsmith J, Veith FJ, et al: Resting gated pool ejection fraction: A poor predictor of perioperative myocardial infarction in patients undergoing vascular surgery for infrainguinal bypass grafting. J Vasc Surg 10:656, 1989.
32. Pasternack PF, Imparato AM, Riles TS, et al: The value of the radionuclide angiogram in the prediction of perioperative myocardial infarction in patients undergoing lower extremity revascularization procedures. Circulation 72(Suppl II):13, 1985.
33. Kazmers A, Cerqueira MD, Zierler RE: The role of preoperative radionuclide left ventricular ejection fraction for risk assessment in carotid surgery. Arch Surg 123:416, 1988.
34. Jones RH, Douglas JM Jr, Rerych SK, et al: Noninvasive radionuclide assessment of cardiac function in patients with peripheral vascular disease. Surgery 85:59, 1979.
35. McCann RL, Wolfe WG: Resection of abdominal aortic aneurysm in patients with low ejection fractions. J Vasc Surg 10:240, 1989.
36. McPhail NV, Ruddy TD, Calvin JE, et al: Comparison of left ventricular function and myocardial perfusion for evaluating perioperative cardiac risk of abdominal aortic surgery. Can J Surg 33:224, 1990.
37. Epstein SE, Quyyumi AA, Bonow RO: Myocardial ischemia—Silent or symptomatic. N Engl J Med 318:1038, 1988.
38. Gottlieb SO, Weisfeldt ML, Ouyang P, et al: Silent ischemia as a marker for early unfavorable outcomes in patients with unstable angina. N Engl J Med 314:1214, 1986.
39. Pasternack PF, Grossi EA, Baumann FG, et al: The value of silent myocardial ischemia monitoring in the prediction of perioperative myocardial infarction in patients undergoing peripheral vascular surgery. J Vasc Surg 10:617, 1989.
40. Ouyang P, Gerstenblith G, Furman WR, et al: Frequency and significance of early postoperative silent myocardial ischemia in patients having peripheral vascular surgery. Am J Cardiol 64:1113, 1989.
41. McCann RL, Clements FM: Silent myocardial ischemia in patients undergoing peripheral vascular surgery: Incidence and association with perioperative cardiac morbidity and mortality. J Vasc Surg 9:583, 1989.
42. Mangano DT, Browner WS, Hollenberg M, et al: Association of perioperative myocardial ischemia with cardiac morbidity and mortality in men undergoing noncardiac surgery. N Engl J Med 323:1781, 1990.
43. Fleisher LA, Rosenbaum SH, Nelson AH, et al: The predictive value of preoperative silent ischemia for postoperative ischemic cardiac events in vascular and nonvascular surgery patients. Am Heart J 122:980, 1991.
44. Muir AD, Reeder MK, Foëx P, et al: Preoperative silent myocardial ischaemia: Incidence and predictors in a general surgical population. Br J Anaesthesiol 67:373, 1991.
45. Raby KE, Goldman L, Creager MA, et al: Correlation between preoperative ischemia and major cardiac events after peripheral vascular surgery. N Engl J Med 321:1296, 1989.
46. Younis LT, Chaitman BR: Update on intravenous dipyridamole cardiac imaging in the assessment of ischemic heart disease. Clin Cardiol 13:3, 1990.
47. Beer SG, Heo J, Iskandrian AS: Dipyridamole thallium imaging. Am J Cardiol 67:18D, 1991.
48. Iskandrian AS, Heo J, Askenase A, et al: Dipyridamole cardiac imaging. Am Heart J 115:432, 1988.
49. Albro PC, Gould KL, Westcott RJ, et al: Noninvasive assessment of coronary stenoses by myocardial imaging during pharmacologic coronary vasodilatation. III. Clinical trial. Am J Cardiol 42:751, 1978.
50. Josephson MA, Brown BG, Hecht HS, et al: Noninvasive detection and localization of coronary stenoses in patients: Comparison of resting dipyridamole and exercise thallium-201 myocardial perfusion imaging. Am Heart J 103:1008, 1982.
51. Feldman RL, Nichols WW, Pepine CJ, et al: Acute effect of intravenous dipyridamole on regional coronary hemodynamics and metabolism. Circulation 64:333, 1981.
52. Leppo J, Boucher CA, Okada RD, et al: Serial thallium-201 myocardial imaging after dipyridamole infusion: diagnostic utility in detecting coronary stenoses and relationship to regional wall motion. Circulation 66:649, 1982.
53. Freeman MR, Chisholm RJ, Armstrong PW: Usefulness of exercise electrocardiography and thallium scintigraphy in unstable angina pectoris in predicting the extent and severity of coronary artery disease. Am J Cardiol 62:1164, 1988.
54. Kaul A, Finkelstein DM, Homma S, et al: Superiority of quantitative

exercise thallium-201 variables in determining long-term prognosis in ambulatory patients with chest pain: A comparison with cardiac catheterization. J Am Coll Cardiol 12:25, 1988.
55. Zellner JL, Elliott BM, Robison JG, et al: Preoperative evaluation of cardiac risk using dobutamine-thallium imaging in vascular surgery. Ann Vasc Surg 4:238, 1990.
56. Elliott BM, Robison JG, Zellner JL, et al: Dobutamine-^{201}Tl imaging. Assessing Cardiac risks associated with vascular surgery. Circulation 84(Suppl III):54, 1991.
57. Stratmann HG, Mark AL, Walter KE, et al: Preoperative evaluation of cardiac risk by means of atrial pacing and thallium 201 scintigraphy. J Vasc Surg 10:385, 1989.
58. Boucher CA, Brewster DC, Darling RC, et al: Determination of cardiac risk by dipyridamole-thallium imaging before peripheral vascular surgery. N Engl J Med 312:389, 1985.
59. Eagle KA, Coley CM, Newell JB, et al: Combining clinical and thallium data optimizes preoperative assessment of cardiac risk before major vascular surgery. Ann Intern Med 110:859, 1989.
60. Younis LT, Aguirre F, Byers S, et al: Perioperative and long-term prognostic value of intravenous dipyridamole thallium scintigraphy in patients with peripheral vascular disease. Am Heart J 119:1287, 1990.
61. Cutler BS, Hendel RC, Leppo JA: Dipyridamole-thallium scintigraphy predicts perioperative and long-term survival after major vascular surgery. J Vasc Surg 15:972, 1992.
62. Sachs RN, Tellier P, Larmignat P, et al: Assessment by dipyridamole-thallium-201 myocardial scintigraphy of coronary risk before peripheral vascular surgery. Surgery 103:584, 1988.
63. Cutler BS, Leppo JA: Dipyridamole thallium 201 scintigraphy to detect coronary artery disease before abdominal aortic surgery. J Vasc Surg 5:91, 1987.
64. Leppo JA, O'Brien J, Rothendler JA, et al: Dipyridamole-thallium-201 scintigraphy in the prediction of future cardiac events after acute myocardial infarction. N Engl J Med 310:1014, 1984.
65. Mangano DT, London MJ, Tubau JF, et al: Dipyridamole thallium-201 scintigraphy as a preoperative screening test. A reexamination of its predictive potential. Circulation 84:493, 1991.
66. Kazmers A, Kispert JF, Roitman L, et al: Thallium redistribution does not predict perioperative cardiac complications following vascular surgery. Kentucky Med J 89:279, 1991.
67. Dilsizian V, Rocco TP, Freedman NMT, et al: Enhanced detection of ischemic but viable myocardium by the reinjection of thallium after stress-redistribution imaging. N Engl J Med 323:141, 1990.
68. Rocco TP, Dilsizian V, McKusick KA, et al: Comparison of thallium redistribution with rest ''reinjection'' imaging for the detection of viable myocardium. Am J Cardiology 66:158, 1990.
69. Krupski WC, Layug EL, Reilly LM, et al: Comparison of cardiac morbidity between aortic and infrainguinal operations. J Vasc Surg 15:354, 1992.
70. Howell MA, Colgan MP, Seeger RW, et al: Relationship of severity of lower limb peripheral vascular disease to mortality and morbidity: A six-year follow-up study. J Vasc Surg 9:691, 1989.
71. Reul GJ Jr, Cooley DA, Duncan JM, et al: The effect of coronary bypass on the outcome of peripheral vascular operations in 1093 patients. J Vasc Surg 3:788, 1986.
72. Gersh BJ, Rihal CS, Rooke TW, et al: Evaluation and management of patients with both peripheral vascular and coronary artery disease. J Am Coll Cardiol 18:203, 1991.
73. Gersh BJ, Califf RM, Loop FD, et al: Coronary bypass surgery in chronic stable angina. Circulation 79(Suppl I):46, 1989.
74. Ruby ST, Whittemore AD, Couch NP, et al: Coronary artery disease in patients requiring abdominal aortic aneurysm repair. Ann Surg 201:758, 1985.
75. Carrell T, Niederhäuser U, Pasic M, et al: Simultaneous revascularization for critical coronary and peripheral vascular ischemia. Ann Thorac Surg 52:805, 1991.
76. Hollier LH, Spittell JA Jr, Puga FJ: Case reports. Intra-aortic balloon counterpulsation as adjunct to aneurysmectomy in high-risk patients. Mayo Clin Proc 56:565, 1981.
77. Bonchek LI, Olinger GN: Intra-aortic balloon counterpulsation for cardiac support during noncardiac operations. J Thorac Cardiovasc Surg 78:147, 1979.
78. Pasternack PF, Grossi EA, Baumann FG, et al: Beta blockade to decrease silent myocardial ischemia during peripheral vascular surgery. Am J Surg 158:113, 1989.
79. Whittemore AD, Clowes AW, Hechtman HB, et al: Aortic aneurysm repair. Reduced operative mortality associated with maintenance of optimal cardiac performance. Ann Surg 192:414, 1980.
80. Golden MA, Whittemore AD, Donaldson MC, et al: Selective evaluation and management of coronary artery disease in patients undergoing repair of abdominal aortic aneurysms. A 16-year experience. Ann Surg 212:415, 1990.
81. Kalman PG, Wellwood MR, Weisel RD, et al: Cardiac dysfunction during abdominal aortic operation: The limitations of pulmonary wedge pressures. J Vasc Surg 3:773, 1986.
82. Gewertz BL, Kremser PC, Zarins CK, et al: Transesophageal echocardiographic monitoring of myocardial ischemia during vascular surgery. J Vasc Surg 5:607, 1987.
83. London MJ, Tubau JF, Wong MG, et al: The ''natural history'' of segmental wall motion abnormalities in patients undergoing noncardiac surgery. Anesthesiology 73:644, 1990.
84. Baron J, Bertrand M, Barré E, et al: Combined epidural and general anesthesia versus general anesthesia for abdominal aortic surgery. Anesthesiology 75:611, 1991.
85. Rivers SP, Scher LA, Sheehan E, et al: Epidural versus general anesthesia for infrainguinal arterial reconstruction. J Vasc Surg 14:764, 1991.
86. Yeager MP, Glass DD, Neff RK, et al: Epidural anesthesia and analgesia in high-risk surgical patients. Anesthesiology 66:729, 1987.
87. Salem DN, Chuttani K, Isner JM: Assessment and management of cardiac disease in the surgical patient. Curr Probl Cardiol 14:167, 1989.
88. Hertzer NR: Basic data concerning associated coronary disease in peripheral vascular patients. Ann Vasc Surg 1:616, 1987.
89. Mullany CJ, Darling GE, Pluth JR, et al: Early and late results after isolated coronary artery bypass surgery in 159 patients aged 80 years and older. Circulation 82(Suppl IV):229, 1990.
90. Wong T, Detsky AS: Preoperative cardiac risk assessment for patients having peripheral vascular surgery. Ann Intern Med 116:743, 1992.

32

Respiratory Complications in Vascular Surgery

Gerald B. Zelenock, M.D., and Louis M. Messina, M.D.

• • •

Respiratory complications are common following surgical procedures, including vascular reconstruction. Fortunately, in normal clinical vascular surgery practice, most such complications are self-limited, and despite the near-universal presence of significant pulmonary risk factors, the average patient undergoes vascular reconstruction without the need for elaborate preoperative testing or unusual degrees of postoperative support. Nevertheless, such patients need a detailed and careful clinical assessment because they frequently experience minor pulmonary complications that, if unappreciated or undertreated, may rapidly progress to potentially catastrophic respiratory failure. The key to preventing this progression is the recognition of the potential for such complications, appropriate preemptory steps to minimize the frequency and severity of pulmonary complications, and aggressive and vigorous treatment when they do occur.

Patients undergoing elective vascular reconstruction are frequently elderly and frail and may be afflicted with a number of significant medical problems that compromise their overall vitality and restrict their ability to cough and deep breathe. The ravages of chronic obstructive pulmonary disease (COPD), bronchitis, emphysema, and asthma from years of smoking often become clinically manifest about the same time as their vascular disorder. Lengthy operations, upper abdominal and thoracic incisions, and the requisite need for anesthesia and analgesia place them at further risk of pulmonary complications. Patients requiring emergent operations have all of the same risk factors, but in addition, the urgency of the vascular procedure precludes a detailed assessment and preoperative preparation. Shock, sepsis, lower torso ischemia, or massive transfusion, as might occur with a ruptured aneurysm, may precipitate additional pulmonary complications including the adult respiratory distress syndrome (ARDS).

Numerous excellent and detailed treatises on mechanical ventilation, pulmonary function and dysfunction, and other critical care issues exist.[1–7] These topics will not be detailed here, but all vascular surgeons must be knowledgeable about such topics and expert in the application of the available technology to provide proper care for their patients. This discussion will briefly outline the preoperative assessment of risk factors and the diagnosis and treatment of pulmonary complications.

PREOPERATIVE ASSESSMENT OF RISK FOR PULMONARY COMPLICATIONS

The identification of patients who are at high risk for pulmonary complications is fundamental to minimizing the effect of these complications on postoperative outcome.[8–10] As a complement to the detailed vascular examination and assessment of cardiac risk, vascular patients require a skillful clinical appraisal of potential pulmonary risk. This assessment includes a careful general medical history and physical examination, a chest x-ray, and, when indicated, formal pulmonary function testing. Specific signs and symptoms are sought (Table 32–1). Extent of smoking, expressed in pack-years, exercise tolerance, dyspnea, sputum production, and cough are specifically queried. Patients with limited exercise tolerance secondary to severe intermittent claudication may be particularly difficult to assess with respect to exercise tolerance. Any history of steroid use for pulmonary indications, supplemental oxygen at home, or a prolonged period of ventilation following previous surgical procedures is noteworthy. Physical examination includes inspection to detect the presence of a barrel chest, kyphoscoliosis, clubbing of the fingers, cyanosis, and the use of accessory muscles to breathe. Tobacco-stained fingers and teeth, significant obesity, and any thoracic deformity limiting respiratory excursions are readily apparent. Auscultation and percussion will detect wheezing, rales, rhonchi, and a low-lying flattened diaphragm with poor respiratory excursion. Observation of the patient as he or she moves about the office or examining room may reveal signs of exertional dyspnea. Walking for a block or two in the hospital or clinic corridors or up a flight of stairs is usually a satisfactory pulmonary stress test in patients without limiting lower extremity vascular complaints.

If the planned procedure requires an upper abdominal, thoracic, or thoracoabdominal incision, the patient is older than 40 to 45 years, or there are any positive historical or physical findings, a chest x-ray and room air arterial blood gas determination are obtained. The latter may identify carbon dioxide (CO_2) retention ($Pa_{CO_2} \geq 45$ mmHg) or hypoxemia ($Pa_{O_2} \leq 70$ mmHg) but are of greatest value in providing a baseline for the postoperative management period.

Table 32–1. Clinical Signs and Symptoms of Respiratory Disorders

	Comments
Dyspnea	
With exertion	Patients able to tolerate walking two flights of stairs are usually fit for operation
At rest	Indicates severe impairment
Tachypnea/tachycardia	Resting tachypnea (>20 beats/min) or tachycardia (>100 beats/min) should mandate formal testing
Cyanosis	Cyanosis implies unsaturated hemoglobin ≥ 5 gm/dl
Cough	Irritation of respiratory tract epithelium
Hemoptysis	Irritation and loss of structural integrity of the respiratory mucosa
Stridor	Upper airway stenosis
Altered level of consciousness	Most common respiratory cause is hypoxia
Hypotension	Nonspecific and late sign
Hypertension	Nonspecific and late sign
Use of accessory muscle	
Gasping and pursing of lips	Signs of advanced respiratory distress
Suprasternal and intercostal muscle retraction	
Hypoxia	
Systemic	Three main causes (right-to-left shunt, inadequate provision, diffusion block)
Mixed venous	Imbalance between supply and delivery
CO_2 retention	Inadequate ventilation
Pulmonary hypertension	May markedly impair respiratory and cardiac function

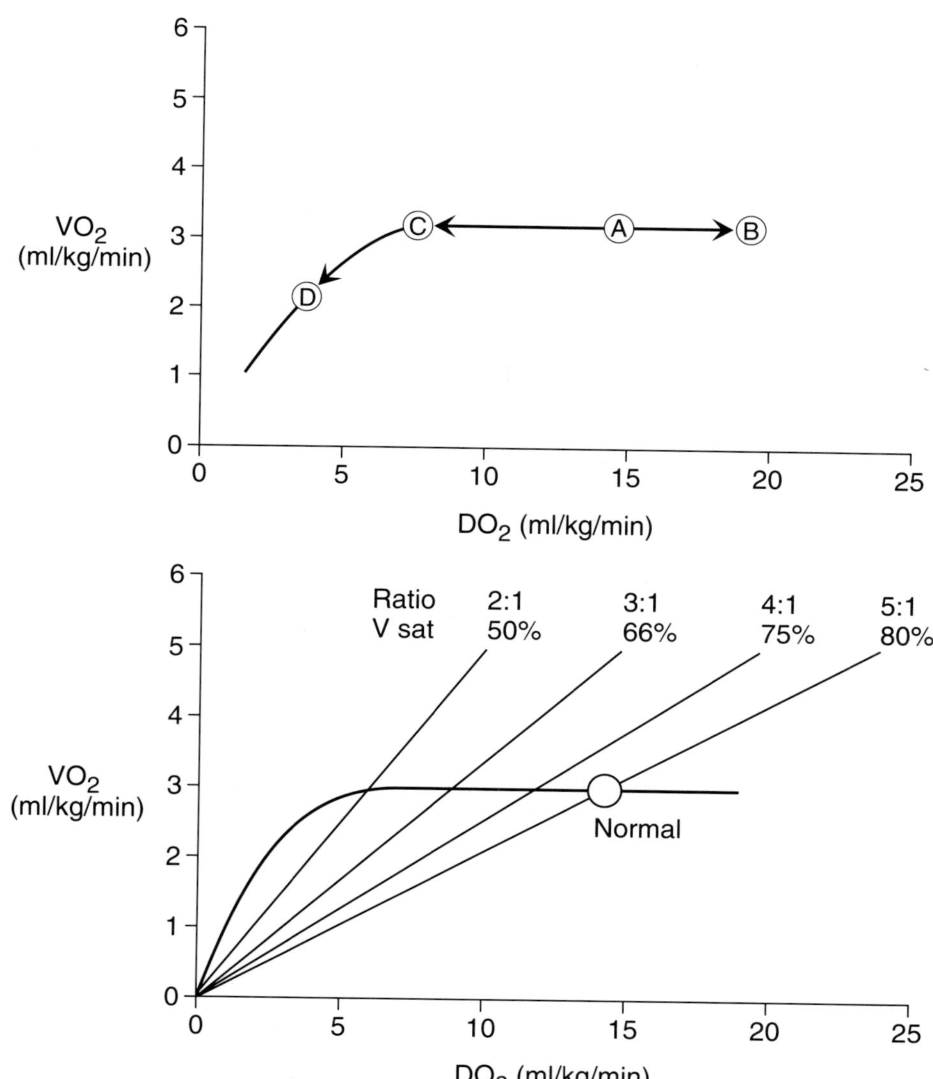

FIGURE 32–1. *Top*, Mixed venous oxygen saturation ($S\bar{v}O_2$) is a sensitive indicator of the relationship between oxygen delivery (DO_2) and consumption (VO_2). Normally (point A), about 20 per cent of the delivered oxygen is consumed (DO_2 : VO_2 is 5 : 1). Over a wide range (point B to point C), oxygen consumption is relatively independent of delivery. Oxygen delivery can be increased to meet increased metabolic demand (point A to point B). Below point C, consumption becomes dependent on delivery. The metabolic rate is unchanged unless the ratio is less than 2 : 1 (point D). *Bottom*, A pulmonary artery catheter with a fiberoptic oximeter (Oximetrix, Abbott Critical Care, Chicago) can be used to determine mixed venous oxygen saturation (V sat). Normal mixed venous saturation (80 per cent) implies consumption of 20 per cent of the available oxygen (DO_2 : VO_2 is 5 : 1). A progressive decrease in venous saturation reflects significant changes in the DO_2 : VO_2 ratio. At a mixed venous saturation of 50 per cent, a ratio of 2 : 1 exists and indicates supply-side dependency. (*Top* and *bottom*, Modified from Bartlett RH, Anderson HL: Multiorgan failure. *In* Zelenock GB, et al [eds]: Clinical Ischemic Syndromes: Mechanisms and Consequences of Tissue Injury. St. Louis, CV Mosby, 1989, pp 565–572.)

In patients undergoing a major vascular reconstruction, any positive finding in the general history or physical examination should be cause for a more detailed assessment. Bedside spirometry measures tidal volumes (VT), inspiratory capacity, vital capacity (VC), and maximal voluntary ventilation (MVV). Significant abnormalities detected by history or physical examination or simple bedside spirometry mandate formal pulmonary function testing and should trigger preoperative referral to the anesthesia service.[11] In select circumstances, a formal pulmonary medicine consultation should be considered. A brief trial to correct potentially reversible bronchospasm or infection is appropriate. Bronchodilators are the mainstay of treatment for bronchospasm; aerosolized, intravenous, or oral medications are all appropriate. Broad-spectrum antibiotics will often quickly effect a change in sputum color, consistency, or volume. Permanent cessation of smoking is desirable, but perioperative cessation of smoking is imperative. Detection and preoperative correction of deficits in hemoglobin and nutritional status as well as vigorous deep-breathing exercises, through instruction and short-term training with an incentive spirometer, will lessen potentially serious postoperative pulmonary complications.[12]

Highly individualized operative planning is essential to minimize risk in specific patients. The use of retroperitoneal versus transabdominal approaches, transverse rather than vertical incisions, and spinal or epidural anesthesia rather than general anesthesia are techniques suggested as beneficial in patients with respiratory compromise. Clearly, the operation itself and the technical requirements for access are the principal determinants of surgical approach, and secure control of the airway may obviate any perceived benefit from spinal or epidural anesthesia. Optimal outcomes depend on minimizing any and all adverse effects resulting from the planned surgical procedure, the necessary anesthesia, and perioperative analgesics.

PERIOPERATIVE MONITORING

Daily assessment of cardiac, pulmonary, hemodynamic, and renal function is a responsibility of the vascular surgeon and the essence of surgical critical care. Certain techniques have long been used and others have recently been developed to facilitate this assessment. For patients undergoing major vascular reconstruction, the use of an array of sophisticated monitoring devices is routine. Fortunately, standard cardiovascular monitoring is also state-of-the-art for critical pulmonary conditions that require maximal surveillance. It goes without saying that any patient requiring other than the most transient ventilatory support must be in an intensive care unit with continuous monitoring of heart rate and rhythm, systemic arterial blood pressure, and central pulmonary artery pressure. In most instances this requires an arterial line, a Swan-Ganz catheter, preferably an oximetric pulmonary artery catheter (Abbott Critical Care, Chicago), as well as a continuously displayed electrocardiogram (ECG) and a Foley catheter for bladder drainage.

Pulse oximeters that provide on-line percentage of O_2 saturation of hemoglobin and the use of end-tidal CO_2 measurements have reduced the need for repetitive arterial blood gas sampling. The oximetric Swan-Ganz catheter provides on-line assessment of mixed venous oxygen saturation, which reflects the adequacy of the balance between O_2 delivery (Do_2) and consumption (Vo_2) (Fig. 32–1). Although this technique has not yet acquired universal acceptance, we have found it to be very sensitive to the multiple factors that influence the balance between oxygen delivery and consumption.

RECOGNITION AND TREATMENT OF POSTOPERATIVE PULMONARY COMPLICATIONS

Prompt recognition of postoperative complications allows aggressive and specific treatment to avoid progression to overwhelming pulmonary dysfunction. The presenting signs and symptoms of postoperative pulmonary problems are essentially the same as those sought during the preoperative assessment (see Table 32–1). However, during this period, recovery from anesthesia, the use of analgesics, or an indwelling endotracheal tube may mask or prevent patients from expressing their symptoms, and the classic clinical signs may be obscured by bandages and mechanical ventilators. The additional physiologic data available in well-monitored postoperative patients may partially compensate for the difficulty of clinical evaluation.

CLINICAL CLASSIFICATION OF RESPIRATORY COMPLICATIONS

Nonpulmonary Causes

Nonpulmonary causes of respiratory compromise occur frequently, and it is important to recognize them, since in most instances they are readily treatable. Further, when prompt recognition and treatment do not occur, they are often rapidly lethal. Such nonpulmonary causes of respiratory compromise frequently affect the central nervous system (CNS), the upper airway, or the mechanical aspects of breathing (Table 32–2). Excessive anesthesia, sedation, or narcotic administration, provision of excess oxygen to patients with COPD or other advanced chronic lung disorder, or retention of CO_2 from any mechanical cause can lead to CNS-mediated respiratory arrest. In such circumstances, pharmacologic reversal or temporary ventilator support is usually adequate treatment. Mechanical problems such as malplaced oral or nasotracheal tubes, pneumothorax and hemothorax (and tension pneumothorax), gastrointestinal dilatation causing ventilatory compromise or aspiration, and abdominal tamponade from hemoperitoneum are usually readily recognized. Because these problems can occur unexpectedly and progress rapidly, constant awareness of their potential occurrence is mandatory. The airway is particularly vulnerable during transfers from the operating room to the recovery room, from the recovery room to the surgical intensive care unit, or when patients are en route to diagnostic studies. Observation for a properly secured airway, proper positioning of orotracheal tubes and chest wall motion, and the presence of bilateral breath sounds should suffice in most instances.

Table 32–2. Mechanisms of Respiratory Complications

Nonparenchymal, Nonpulmonary
Central Nervous System
Excess:
Anesthesia
Narcotics/sedatives
Muscle relaxants
O_2 in chronic obstructive pulmonary disease patients
CO_2
Diminished consciousness due to stroke, coma, or metabolic causes
Mechanical
Malplaced or displaced orotracheal or nasotracheal tubes
Tension pneumothorax or hemopneumothorax
Gastric, gastrointestinal distention
Abdominal tamponade (hemo-peritoneum, tense ascites)
Chest wall pain (thoracoabdominal incision) or instability
Ventilator malfunction
Upper Airway
Mucous plugs
Aspiration
Laryngeal edema/spasm
Laryngeal dysfunction (nerve injury)
Pulmonary, Parenchymal
Atelectasis
Pneumonia
Pulmonary edema, congestive heart failure, fluid overload
Adult respiratory distress syndrome
Pulmonary embolus

The frequent utilization of invasive monitoring devices placed through central venous routes and the need for mechanical ventilation in vascular surgery patients means that pneumothorax is a not uncommon problem. This potentially serious problem is fortunately readily treated in most instances. If the pneumothorax is small and stable and no immediate operation is planned, observation or simple aspiration will suffice. If the collapse is large or enlarging, or if the patient requires positive pressure ventilation, tube thoracostomy is required. A pneumothorax developing in the operating room or while the patient is in the intensive care unit (ICU) on a ventilator is often a tension pneumothorax. Classic findings of diminished breath sounds, a hyperresonant percussion note, distended neck veins, and deviation of mediastinal structures away from the tension pneumothorax may be difficult to detect owing to surgical drapes and dressings or obscured physical findings due to mechanical ventilation. It is noteworthy that the clinical presentation of tension pneumothorax is often hypotension. The fact that there are many causes of postoperative hypotension in vascular patients must not delay diagnosis because untreated tension pneumothorax promptly results in cardiac arrest. Prompt decompression of a suspected tension pneumothorax is essential. There is no need to wait for chest x-ray confirmation of the diagnosis; needle aspiration followed by tube thoracostomy may be life saving.

Pulmonary Parenchymal Causes

Complications involving the lung parenchyma itself are not peculiar to vascular patients but occur with regularity in this particular population. A brief discussion of the most common types is presented.

Atelectasis is the collapse of alveoli and produces hypoxia as a result of right-to-left shunting. Four types (obstructive, compressive, contraction, and patchy atelectasis) have been recognized and have many underlying causes[5] (Table 32–3). Untreated atelectasis may result in severe hypoxemia, fever, consolidation, and infection. Treatment depends upon the underlying cause and may require nasal tracheal suctioning or bronchoscopy to clear inspissated secretions or mucous plugs. Pleural drainage via thoracocentesis or placement of a chest tube relieves compressive atelectasis; in patients with abdominal tamponade, which causes airspace collapse by restricting diaphragmatic excursion, return to the operating room for decompression and control of bleeding is required. Contraction atelectasis improves with treatment of the underlying condition, which is often infectious or inflammatory in nature. Patchy atelectasis is very common in vascular surgical patients and nearly universal in patients with abdominal incisions. Fortunately, in its usual presentation, it is self-limited and with appropriate attention to pulmonary hygiene, tracheal suctioning, incentive spirometry, and other deep breathing maneuvers it will resolve in 24 to 48 hours. Aerosolized mucolytic agents and bronchodilators are considered helpful, whereas intermittent positive pressure breathing (IPPB) by itself is not.

Pneumonia is a frequently lethal complication of surgical procedures.[13] Well-treated postoperative pneumonia has a 10 per cent mortality; pneumonia superimposed on other lung injuries has a mortality of 50 to 60 per cent, but as part of the multi-organ failure syndrome (MOFS), the mortality approaches 80 to 90 per cent. Fever, tachypnea, tachycardia, purulent sputum production, and a dyspneic sensation due to progressive hypoxia are common. Cyanosis, rales, rhonchi, and either absent or bronchial breath sounds develop as consolidation occurs. Vigorous culture-specific antibiotic therapy, provision of supplemental oxygen and other respiratory support are the essentials of treatment. Bronchoscopy to remove inspissated secretions or to obtain good cultures may be required.

Aspiration of gastric contents causes a chemical injury

Table 32–3. Types and Causes of Atelectasis

Obstructive Atelectasis
Excess mucus
Airway edema
Infection
Impaired mucociliary clearance (due to smoking or anesthesia)
Bronchial neoplasms
Foreign bodies
Compressive Atelectasis
Pneumothorax
Hemothorax
Hydrothorax
Excessive elevation of diaphragm
Contraction Atelectasis
Local inflammation or fibrotic process
Abscess
Prior infection with scar formation
Patchy Atelectasis
Surfactant denaturation
ARDS

Modified from Demling RH: Decision Making in Surgical Critical Care. Philadelphia, BC Decker, 1988. By permission of Mosby–Year Book, Inc.

to the respiratory epithelium and sets the stage for bacterial infection. Gastric dilatation and gastrointestinal hypomotility are the usual precipitating factors and are preventable or treatable by decompression with a nasogastric tube. Unfortunately, nasogastric tubes, especially large-bore tubes, also allow reflux of gastric contents past the lower esophageal sphincter, particularly in supine patients. Prevention of aspiration is far more effective than treatment. Proper nasogastric decompression and elevation of the head of the bed by 30 degrees lessens the likelihood of significant aspiration. The clinical presentation of aspiration can be dramatic, with severe dyspnea, rhonchi, wheezes, profound cyanosis, and obvious acute respiratory distress. Aspiration of gastric contents from the airway confirms the diagnosis and is an essential step in treatment. Owing to direct injury from the acid aspirate, inflammatory and then infectious changes rapidly ensue. Despite their theoretical attractiveness and common usage, neither steroids (intratracheal instillation or parenteral administration) nor *prophylactic* antibiotics have been demonstrated to benefit the clinical outcome. Supplemental oxygen and ventilatory support are provided using standard indications, and antibiotics are indicated if bacterial infection is documented. Occasionally bronchoscopy to remove particulate matter is required. Recurrent bouts of aspiration that are less dramatic in their presentation may occur and can have an insidious effect on pulmonary function.

Pulmonary edema that results from marginal cardiac performance, with or without a superimposed fluid load, is termed "high pressure" or "cardiogenic" pulmonary edema. It is neither unusual nor particularly difficult to recognize in postoperative vascular surgery patients. Any patient with a cardiac history is at risk, and the addition of a significant operative stress or vigorous fluid resuscitation puts virtually all patients potentially at risk. Dyspnea, rales, rhonchi, wheezes, tachycardia, tachypnea, distended neck veins, and peripheral (or presacral) edema in a patient who is hypoxemic and has elevated pulmonary artery wedge pressure detected by Swan-Ganz catheter and a chest x-ray showing cardiomegaly, congested hila, apical redistribution of blood flow and bronchovascular cuffing, Kerley B lines, or pleural effusions establishes the diagnosis. Treatment is directed at elimination of the relative volume overload, augmentation of the performance of the heart as a pump, correction of any oncotic abnormality, and expert use of supplemental oxygen and mechanical ventilation. The last maneuver typically requires high inspired oxygen concentrations and positive end-expiratory pressure (PEEP).

Adult respiratory distress syndrome (ARDS) is a generic term that refers to a number of conditions that present as acute respiratory distress and resemble in some ways classic cardiogenic pulmonary edema. Distinguishing factors include the pulmonary wedge pressure, which is low or normal, and other important clinical and radiographic differences as well. The mechanism of this "low-pressure pulmonary edema" is an abnormally permeable capillary membrane precipitated by specific mediators. Although the list of predisposing clinical factors contributing to ARDS in general patient populations is long, certain of these commonly occur in vascular surgery patients (Table 32–4). Systemic shock, prolonged ischemia of the gut or skeletal muscle as might occur with a ruptured aneurysm, and the vigorous fluid resuscitation and multiple transfusions required by such patients are widely recognized as precipitating causes of ARDS.

Table 32–4. Factors Associated With ARDS in Vascular Patients

Factors
Shock
Prolonged ischemia
Multiple transfusions
Hypothermia
"Sepsis syndrome"
Aspiration of gastric contents
Narcotic overdose
Oxygen toxicity
Disseminated intravascular coagulation
Pancreatitis
Prolonged cardiopulmonary bypass
Viral pneumonitis
Bacterial pneumonia

Other causes of ARDS such as near-drowning, hyperthermia, burns, skeletal fractures, lung contusion, smoke inhalation, phosgene inhalation, ethchlorvynol overdose, salicylate overdose, tricyclic antidepressant overdose, paraquat toxicity, bleomycin toxicity, eclampsia, amniotic fluid embolus, miliary tuberculosis, and Pneumocystis carinii *pneumonia are relatively uncommon in vascular surgery patients.*

Even moderate lower torso ischemia such as that occurring during elective aortic reconstruction places patients at risk for permeable lung injury. In a series of experimental and clinical studies, Klausner and coworkers documented the presence of thromboxane A_2 (TXA_2) and white blood cell–mediated pulmonary injury with hind limb or lower torso ischemia.[14–16] In operations requiring infrarenal aortic clamping ranging from 76 ± 27 to 118 ± 25 minutes, they demonstrated noncardiogenic interstitial pulmonary edema on chest x-rays, an increase in physiologic shunting from 9 ± 2 per cent to 16 ± 2 per cent, and an increase in peak inspiratory pressure from 23 ± 2 to 33 ± 2 cm H_20. Correlated with these physiologic pulmonary changes was an increase in TXA_2 generation, which began with the application of the aortic clamp. The changes in pulmonary function were further explored in dog and sheep models and were found to be clearly white blood cell–dependent and mediated by thromboxane and leukotriene B_4 (LTB_4). Complement appeared not to be involved. Whether the same mediators are active in the ARDS seen in vascular surgery patients with intestinal ischemia, profound shock, prolonged aortic clamping, or massive blood transfusion has not been determined. It seems highly likely that additional mediators with adverse pulmonary effects will be identified.

Pulmonary embolism should be considered whenever pulmonary insufficiency is of sudden onset or is otherwise not readily explained. It may present as either a primary problem referred to the vascular surgeon or as a complication of vascular surgical procedures. With respect to the latter, most vascular patients fulfill the elements of Virchow's classic triad, with *stasis* due to immobility at the time of hospitalization and operation, *local injury* secondary to angiography and the surgical procedure, and, in 5 to 15 per cent of patients, a *hypercoagulable state.* This state has several clearly defined syndromes and is being increasingly recognized. A detailed description of the recognition and management of hypercoagulable states is provided in Chapter 17, and the recognition and clinical management of pulmonary embolism is covered in detail in Chapters 134 and 135.

Although pulmonary complications of vascular reconstructive procedures have not achieved the same recognition as cardiac and renal complications, they are extremely common. Fortunately, in most instances they are self-limited or respond rapidly to intervention. In some circumstances, despite optimal surveillance and treatment, they have the potential to prove rapidly fatal. New developments in monitoring and better definition of the role of advanced therapeutic devices such as the extracorporeal membrane oxygenator (ECMO) in adult patients should expand the surgeon's ability to recognize and treat pulmonary complications.[18]

References

1. Bartlett RH: Pulmonary insufficiency. *In* Wilmore DW, Brennan MF, Harken AH, et al (eds): Care of the Surgical Patient. New York, Scientific American, 1989.
2. Bartlett RH: Use of the mechanical ventilator. *In* Wilmore DW, Brennan MF, Harken AH, et al (eds): Care of the Surgical Patient. New York, Scientific American, 1989.
3. Bonner JT, Hall JR: Respiratory Intensive Care of the Adult Surgical Patient. St. Louis, CV Mosby, 1985.
4. Dantzker DR (ed): Cardiopulmonary Critical Care. 2nd ed. Philadelphia, WB Saunders, 1991.
5. Demling RH, Goodwin CW: Pulmonary dysfunction. *In* Wilmore DW, Brennan MF, Harken AH, et al (eds): Care of the Surgical Patient. New York, Scientific American, 1989.
6. Shoemaker WC, Ayres SM, Grenvik A, et al: Textbook of Critical Care. 2nd ed. Philadelphia, WB Saunders, 1989.
7. Stanley JC, Wakefield TW: Cardiopulmonary assessment for major reconstructive procedures. *In* Haimovici H, Callow AD, DePalma RG, et al (eds): Haimovici's Vascular Surgery. 3rd ed. Norwalk, CT, Appleton and Lange, 1989.
8. Bartlett RH, Brennan ML, Gazzaniga AB, Hanson EL: Studies on the pathogenesis and prevention of postoperative pulmonary complications. Surg Gynecol Obstet 137:925, 1973.
9. Brewster DC, Edwards JD: Cardiopulmonary complications related to vascular surgery. *In* Bernhard VM, Towne JB (eds): Complications in Vascular Surgery. 2nd ed. St. Louis, Quality Medical Publishing, 1991.
10. Garibaldi RA, Britt MR, Coleman ML, et al: Risk factors for postoperative pneumonia. Am J Med 70:677, 1981.
11. Lawrence VA, Page CP, Harris GD: Preoperative spirometry before abdominal operations: A critical appraisal of its predictive value. Arch Intern Med 149:280, 1989.
12. Celli BR, Rodriguez KS, Snider GL: A controlled trial of intermittent positive pressure breathing, incentive spirometry, and deep breathing exercises in preventing pulmonary complications after abdominal surgery. Am Rev Respir Dis 130:12, 1984.
13. Eickhoff TC: Pulmonary infections in surgical patients. Surg Clin North Am 60:175, 1980.
14. Klausner JM, Paterson IS, Valeri R, et al: Limb ischemia–induced increase in permeability is mediated by leukocytes and leukotrienes. Ann Surg 208:755, 1988.
15. Klausner JM, Anner H, Paterson IS, et al: Lower torso ischemia–induced lung injury is leukocyte-dependent. Ann Surg 208:761, 1988.
16. Klausner JM, Paterson IS, Kobizik L, et al: Leukotrienes but not complement mediate limb ischemia–induced lung injury. Ann Surg 209:462, 1989.
17. Carson JC, Kelley MA, Duff A, et al: The clinical course of pulmonary embolism. N Engl J Med 326:1240, 1992.
18. Bartlett RH: Critical care. *In* Greenfield LJ, Mulholland MW, Oldham KT, Zelenock GB (eds): Surgery: Scientific Principles and Practice. Philadelphia, JB Lippincott, 1992.

33

Renal Complications

Richard H. Dean, M.D., B.A., and David L. Robaczewski, M.D., B.S.

• • •

The factors affecting fluid shifts and renal function have interested scientists and physicians for 300 years. Nevertheless, our understanding remains fragmentary, and therapeutic regimens for prevention or correction of renal dysfunction are imperfect. Examination of the nomenclature used for the description of renal dysfunction underscores the relative simplicity with which the medical community views renal injury and its management. For instance, acute tubular necrosis (ATN) is commonly used by clinicians as the only term to describe the kidney's response to injury. The implication that an insult to renal function must produce tubular cell death in order to be considered clinically important is too simplistic.

To address the potential renal insults associated with vascular surgery, one must first understand normal renal physiology. From this reference point, a better appreciation of the spectrum of aberrations in renal function that can be induced by the stress of major vascular surgery can be achieved.

NORMAL RENAL FUNCTION

A complete discussion of normal renal physiology is beyond the scope of this text; excellent reviews of normal anatomy and physiology are available for the reader in standard surgical texts.[2, 3] However, an understanding of certain components of intrarenal and excretory renal function is germane to comprehending the effects of insults on such function.

The kidney serves as the dominant site for maintenance of normal intravascular volume and solute constituency. Under normovolemic baseline states, the kidneys receive approximately 25 per cent of the cardiac output. Based on a 5 L/min cardiac output, this means that the kidneys receive 900 L/day of plasma flow. Given the fact that the glomeruli filter 20 per cent of the renal plasma flow into the tubular space within Bowman's capsule and that the normal 24-hour urinary output for a 70-kg man is less than 1.8 L, the kidneys must reabsorb more than 99 per cent of the 180 L/day of filtered water to maintain homeostasis. Similarly, the initial composition of the tubular fluid is essentially an ultrafiltrate of plasma with a concentration of electrolytes and other solutes similar to that in plasma. Therefore, electrolytes and other solutes such as glucose must also be almost totally reabsorbed. For the purposes of this review, the mechanisms of sodium, potassium, and water reabsorption are reviewed primarily.

Reabsorption of electrolytes from the tubular fluid occurs both by active transport and by passive back-diffusion. The sodium ion is reabsorbed in the early proximal tubule by its cotransportation with organic solutes, bicarbonate, and divalent cations through an active transport mechanism. Similarly, sodium is actively transported in the late proximal tubule in linkage with chloride transport. Since water freely follows this movement of solutes and ions, the tubular fluid is isosmotic to plasma as it enters the loop of Henle (Fig. 33–1).

The tubular cells of the loop of Henle vary in their permeability depending on their location in the loop. This establishes a hypotonic tubular fluid and medullary osmotic gradient. Whereas the descending loop of Henle is permeable to water but relatively impermeable to sodium and chloride, the ascending loop of Henle is impermeable to water but actively transports the chloride ion, with sodium passively following. The resulting countercurrent mechanism produces a medullary osmotic gradient that regulates urine osmolarity from 50 to 1200 mOsm.[4] Distal tubular reabsorption of sodium is also active. In the distal tubule and in the proximal collecting ducts, sodium is actively and almost completely reabsorbed under the control of aldosterone. Of the approximately 25,000 mEq of sodium filtered daily, only 50 to 200 mEq is ultimately excreted through urination (less than 1 per cent).

Filtered potassium is almost totally reabsorbed in the proximal tubule and the loop of Henle. However, influenced by the electronegativity of the tubular fluid and the intracellular concentration of potassium, potassium is also passively secreted by the distal tubules and early collecting ducts into the tubular lumen. Essentially all of the potassium in the urine is transported there through this process.

Neuroendocrine Modulators of Renal Function

Intravascular volume is regulated primarily by a series of stretch or baroreceptors located in systemic and renal arteries and the atria. Since these receptors not only sense pressure or volume changes (atrial receptors) but also monitor their rates of change during the cardiac cycle, they predominately sense what might be called the effective

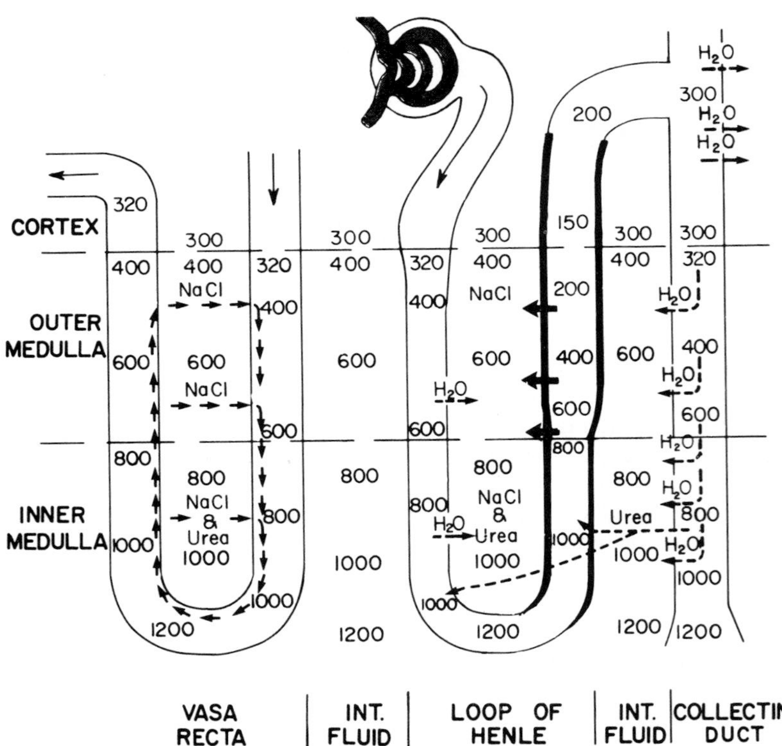

FIGURE 33–1. Depiction of the loop of Henle demonstrating the development of the countercurrent mechanism. Int., interstitial.

circulating volume. Factors that decrease cardiac performance will alter the intravascular volume perceived by these receptors and thereby also alter the renal function to retain water and increase the effective circulating volume. Similarly, when the concentration of circulating plasma proteins is reduced, there is a net diffusion of intravascular water into the extracellular space secondary to the decreased intravascular oncotic pressure. This net decrease in circulating volume is sensed by these same receptors. The neuroendocrine regulators of urinary output inhibit excretion of water to correct the perceived deficiency.

When the baroreceptors perceive a reduction in circulating volume, their afferent signals are reduced, which decreases their tonic inhibition over the neuroendocrine system. This leads to increased secretion of vasopressin, beta-endorphins, growth hormone, and adrenocorticotropic hormone through the central nervous system (CNS) and to an increase in release of epinephrine. Likewise, when baroreceptors within the juxtaglomerular apparatus of the kidney perceive a decrease in intravascular pressure they are stimulated to increase the release of renin.

Other monitors and regulators of intravascular volume include the macula densa of the juxtaglomerular apparatus, the osmoreceptors located near the hypothalamic ventricles of the CNS and in the liver, and sensors of plasma potassium concentration in the adrenal cortex.

The primary hormonal regulators of fluid and electrolyte balance are aldosterone, cortisol, vasopressin, and angiotensin. However, the interactions between insulin, epinephrine, plasma glucose concentration, acid-base balance of the plasma, and other factors play a vital role in modulating the release of these hormones and directly affect the renal tubular management of water and the respective filtered solutes. Further discussion of their interactions and impact on renal function and fluid shifts will be limited to the effects of major vascular surgery. More detailed descriptions of their respective roles and integrated functions are provided elsewhere.[3,4]

FLUID SHIFTS ASSOCIATED WITH AORTIC SURGERY

Intra-abdominal arterial reconstructive surgery can be appropriately considered a major injury. To appreciate the response to such an insult and its impact on the fluid balance in the respective fluid compartments of the body, one must examine the factors influencing transcapillary and transcellular movement of fluid.

Normally, water and its respective solutes move from the plasma into the interstitial space at the precapillary level because of the net hydrostatic pressure at that level. Reentry into the intravascular space in the distal capillary bed is predominantly governed by the net intravascular oncotic pressure produced by plasma proteins. Among these proteins, albumin is the most plentiful and important. Normally, approximately 7 per cent of intravascular albumin arriving at the capillary level crosses the capillary membrane into the interstitial space. This is a unidirectional flow of albumin, and it ultimately returns to the intravascular pool by transport through the lymphatic system.

Following trauma to tissue and as a result of multiple complex hemodynamic mechanisms induced by any major insult, capillary membrane permeability to albumin is dramatically enhanced. This net egress of albumin into the interstitial space is further enhanced by interruption or alteration of poorly understood complex mechanisms governing the lymphatic transport of albumin following systemic or local trauma.[5–7] Therefore, the increased amount of albumin transported across the capillary membranes stays in the interstitial space longer. The effect of the increased migration of albumin into the interstitial fluid space is a decrease in distal capillary oncotic pressure and a resultant decrease in the reabsorption of water into the intravascular compartment. This in turn decreases intravascular volume and enhances the neuroendocrine mechanisms that decrease renal excretion of sodium and free water.

The normal homeostatic method of contending with a decreased circulating intravascular volume is to mobilize the extracellular (third-space) interstitial fluid. Indeed, the extracellular fluid space is expanded as a consequence of the aforementioned response to the stress of major intra-abdominal surgery. Unfortunately, this excess extracellular third space fluid might be conceptually described as "entrapped" by its greater oncotic pressure, and the functional reserve of fluid available for return to the plasma for expansion of the contracted intravascular volume is severely reduced. When one considers the additive impact of temporary ischemia to tissue beds during major vascular surgery, the ensuing shift in acid-base balance in the involved tissue beds, the adverse impact of unreplaced blood loss, the potential reductions in cardiac performance during aortic cross-clamping, and the stimulation of stress response neuroendocrine mechanisms, one can easily visualize the vicious cycle of events leading to a shifting of total body water out of the functional circulating blood volume into the third space.[8,9]

This obligatory loss of circulating free water and its associated solutes following major surgery has only recently been appreciated. The impact of such knowledge, however has been of dramatic benefit to the intraoperative and early postoperative fluid management of patients undergoing major vascular surgery. Recognition of increased obligatory losses of intravascular volume associated with major surgery has led to the current use of balanced salt solutions for replenishment.[10] Although formulas for calculation of required intraoperative and postoperative fluid administration are available,[11] of greatest importance is the appreciation that hourly parenteral fluid replacement requirements during surgery are severalfold those required during a resting state and may vary from 100 to 500 ml/hr. Even this range of additional replacement fluids is inadequate during and after acute blood loss. These increased fluid replacement requirements continue in the immediate postoperative period owing to continued sequestration of fluid into the areas of the operative site.

Mobilization of the sequestered third-space fluid is delayed for a variable period of days depending on the magnitude of ongoing postoperative stress, cardiac performance, and intravascular oncotic pressure. Reabsorption of this third space fluid usually begins on the second or third postoperative day. If not managed with appropriate reduction in maintenance parenteral fluid administration or addition of diuretic therapy, this mobilization phase of third-space fluid can lead to intravascular volume overload and acute congestive heart failure.

RENAL DYSFUNCTION AFTER VASCULAR SURGERY

The severity of renal dysfuncton following vascular surgery may range from minor inappropriate loss of sodium in the urine to anuric acute renal failure. Similarly, its causes span a wide range of prerenal, postrenal, and parenchymal causes (Table 33–1). Fortunately, the incidence of clinically severe acute renal failure after major surgery has dramatically decreased during the last 50 years as knowledge of the factors affecting fluid and electrolyte balance has increased and as early intervention to abort underlying causes has been implemented. Nevertheless, mortality due to postoperative acute renal failure remains high and varies from 10 to 80 per cent depending on the associated presence of multi-organ system failure.

Prerenal Causes

Prerenal causes are the most frequent source of acute renal dysfunction in the early postoperative period. Usually, renal failure from a prerenal cause is a direct result of a contracted intravascular volume secondary to inadequate fluid replacement following intraoperative and immediate postoperative fluid losses or fluid sequestration into the third space. Less commonly, it is secondary to reduced cardiac performance, which likewise triggers the neurohormonal reflexes to increase intravascular volume by increasing tubular reabsorption of sodium and water. In their pure forms, these two causes of reduced renal function are easily discernible. Whereas hypovolemia is associated with flat neck veins, dry mucous membranes, reduced central venous pressure, and reduced pulmonary artery wedge pressure, renal dysfunction secondary to poor cardiac performance is associated with distended neck veins, apparent fluid overload (evident when the lungs are ausculated), elevated central venous pressure, and elevated pulmonary artery wedge pressure. Obviously, the therapy for hypovolemic prerenal azotemia is to increase intravascular volume by administering a balanced salt solution and red blood cells as needed. Conversely, therapy for renal dysfunction of cardiogenic origin is directed at improving myocardial performance by administering afterload-reducing agents and inotropic agents and instituting diuretic therapy as needed to diminish preloading of the failing myocardium.

Unfortunately, the diffusely atherosclerotic patient who is undergoing major vascular surgery frequently has associated coronary artery disease and impaired myocardial function. Distinction between the two causes of renal dysfunction (hypovolemic vs. cardiogenic) can be problematic. In this circumstance, preexisting heart disease may raise the euvolemic level for an individual to higher central filling pressures, and apparently normal or low-normal cardiac filling pressures may in fact reflect hypovolemia. In this clinical situation, the authors maintain a constant infusion of afterload-reducing agents (e.g., nitroprusside or nitroglycerine) and inotropic agents (e.g., dobutamine) and cautiously administer sequential boluses of balanced salt solutions while monitoring cardiac output and left atrial filling pressure (pulmonary artery wedge pressure). If no urinary response is noted once filling pressures begin to rise, we then begin diuretic therapy as an added measure to treat the cardiac origin of the reduced urinary output.

The final prerenal cause is occlusive disease of the renal arteries. Because occlusive disease is initially a diagnosis made by exclusion of other causes, one should first evaluate the patient for other sources of renal failure. If other causes have been excluded, the authors' initial study to determine whether there is occlusive disease of the renal arteries is a technetium-99m pertechnetate perfusion scan of the kidneys. Because intense interstitial swelling from parenchymal causes of ATN may dramatically increase renal parenchymal resistance, a slow renal perfusion as determined by isotope renography may be misleading. In all instances in which correction of a renovascular occlusion may be contemplated, the authors perform contrast arteriography to clarify the presence of the occlusion and to plan its correction.

Postrenal Causes

Although an uncommon cause of postoperative oliguria and apparent renal failure, postrenal obstruction to urine flow may be the easiest to overcome and can be quite embarrassing when not excluded. Kinking or obstruction of the indwelling urinary catheter may produce sudden cessation of urinary flow. For this reason, the catheter should be irrigated as the first maneuver in diagnostic evaluation and potential therapy. Obstruction by clotted blood in the bladder can follow a traumatic catheter insertion. Therefore, one should be especially sensitive to this cause following a difficult bladder catheterization.

Table 33–1. Sites and Causes of Acute Renal Failure

Prerenal	Parenchymal	Postrenal
Low cardiac output/cardiogenic shock	Nephrotoxic drugs	Catheter kinking
Increased vascular space	Radiologic contrast	Catheter clot
Septic shock	Myoglobinuria	Bladder clot
Hypovolemia	Acute tubular necrosis	Ureteral obstruction
Blood loss	Other cause	Renal pelvic obstruction
Dehydration		
Third-space sequestration		

Ureteral or renal pelvic obstructions also can cause postrenal oliguria. If other causes of oliguria have been excluded, preliminary diagnosis of the cause can be obtained with isotope renography, but definitive diagnosis requires retrograde urography. When identified, placement of a ureteral stent can frequently relieve such an obstruction.

Renal Parenchymal Causes

Parenchymal causes of acute renal dysfunction cover a wide range and pose the greatest potential for permanent compromise of renal function. The pathophysiology of the dysfunction is dependent on the specific etiology.

Ischemic Injury

Caused by either temporary periods of interruption of perfusion to the kidney or periods of shock during or after major vascular procedures, the pathophysiology of ischemic injury is twofold. First, as a consequence of the magnitude and duration of ischemia, tubular cell swelling occurs following reperfusion. This in turn can cause tubular obstruction, leading to further reduction or cessation of glomerular filtration in the nephron. Second, tubular cells can either lose their basement membrane attachment secondary to the interstitial edema that develops after reperfusion or undergo cell death during ischemia, subsequently being sloughed into the tubule. The finding of tubular cells in the urinary sediment is the genesis of the term acute tubular necrosis. Although it is a poor pathologic description of this form of injury, ATN is commonly used to describe all renal parenchymal causes of acute renal failure. The medullary thick ascending loop of Henle and the pars recta of the proximal tubule appear to be the segments of the tubular epithelium that are most sensitive to ischemia.[12, 13] Following loss of the tubular cell, a backleak of glomerular filtrate into the renal parenchyma then develops.[14]

Toxic Injury

Chemical injury to the kidney can result from many sources. The most common compounds responsible for such injury in the postoperative period are aminoglycosides, but myoglobin and radiologic contrast media have also been implicated. Aminoglycosides appear to exert their toxicity primarily on the tubular cell in relation to their trough level of plasma concentration.[15] Because of this relationship and the frequent history of reduced renal function in postoperative vascular surgery patients requiring the administration of aminoglycosides, it is important to monitor the peak and trough levels of the antibiotic to establish appropriate dosage levels.

Myoglobinuria is an important cause of renal failure in patients submitted to revascularization of limbs with prolonged extreme ischemia. Circulating as a breakdown product of muscle death, myoglobin is freely filtered by the glomerulus. Myoglobin exerts its toxicity through direct tubular cell injury and through precipitation and obstruction of the tubule.[16, 17] Therefore, prevention of injury to the kidney is directed toward maximizing the urine flow rate by administering intravenous crystalloid infusion and diuretics and by alkalinizing the urine.

Although there are a multitude of other parenchymal causes of acute renal failure, most are infrequent in surgical patients. Causes that are peculiar to vascular surgery and vascular contrast imaging have special pertinence and are discussed separately.

Renal Failure Associated With Aortic Surgery

Acute renal failure following aortic surgery continues to be a complication that is associated with an extremely high mortality. Although it is reported to have an incidence ranging from 1 to 13 per cent in elective aortic surgery,[18–25] its occurrence depends on the clinical circumstances of the operation, intraoperative and postoperative events, and the overall prior health status of the patient. The incidence of acute renal failure following elective surgery for abdominal aortic aneurysm and bypass for aortoiliac occlusive disease and operations performed for ruptured abdominal aortic aneurysms in several reported series is summarized in Tables 33–2 and 33–3. The mortality rate associated with postoperative renal failure has remained formidable. Nevertheless, recognition of the clinical syndrome of multiorgan system failure has shed some light on factors that increase this mortality. In patients with postoperative renal failure as an isolated system failure, the associated mortality

Table 33–2. Acute Renal Dysfunction or Failure After Elective Infrarenal Aortic Surgery

Series	No. Patients	Type of Procedure	Severity of Dysfunction	Incidence (%)
Gardner et al[18] (1970)	56	AAA	Dialysis	1
David et al[25] (1974)	69	AAA	Dialysis	13
Thompson et al[20] (1975)	108	AAA	Not requiring dialysis	8
Volpetti et al[21] (1976)	585	AAA	Dialysis	4
McCombs and Roberts[23] (1979)	361	AAA	Dialysis	2
Diehl et al[24] (1983)	350	AAA	Not requiring dialysis	6
	173	AIO		5
Bergqvist et al[22] (1983)	205	AIO	Not requiring dialysis	8
Breckwoldt et al[30] (1992)	221	AAA	Not requiring dialysis	2
Johnson et al[62] (1989)	666	AAA	Not requiring dialysis	3–39*

Key: *AAA, abdominal aortic aneurysm; AIO, aortoiliac occlusion.*
**Varied depending on preoperative creatinine and ligation of left renal vein.*

Table 33–3. Acute Renal Failure in Surgery for Ruptured Aneurysm

Series	No. Patients	Incidence (%)	Severity of Dysfunction	Mortality (%)
Tilney et al[29] (1973)	18	100	Dialysis	95
Hicks et al[26] (1975)	56	18	Dialysis	70
Sink et al[27] (1976)	28	46	Not requiring dialysis	69
McCombs and Roberts[23] (1979)	38	21	Dialysis	50
Gornick and Kjellstrond[28] (1983)	30	—	Dialysis	64

is low. In contrast, when renal failure is only one of several system failures, mortality is extremely high.[29] It might be surmised that one simply needs to prevent or provide improved treatment of multi-organ system failure to improve the probabilty of survival in the group with renal failure. To date, however, the prevention of multi-organ system failure has been an unachieved goal of allied research and clinical care.

Pathophysiology of Postaortic Surgery Renal Failure

The development of acute renal failure following procedures involving the juxtarenal aorta seldom parallels pure pathophysiologic models but rather stems from a mixture of underlying causes. However, for the sake of clarity, the respective causes are addressed here as independent sources of acute renal failure on the understanding that all of these mechanisms may be active in the production of postoperative renal failure in an individual patient.

A temporary isolated period of renal ischemia caused by suprarenal aortic cross-clamping, temporary renal artery occlusion, a single episode of hypovolemic shock, declamping hypotension, or cardiogenic shock in the perioperative period is the most common cause of acute renal dysfunction and renal failure associated with aortic surgery. Through observations of patients and use of investigative models, Myers and associates[31–34] have postulated that a pathophysiologic cascade of events following temporary renal ischemia leads to acute renal failure. The observation that renal biopsies and autopsy studies in patients with postischemic acute renal failure showed minimal if any disturbance in glomerular architecture yet demonstrated profound disruption of tubular morphology led Oliver and colleagues[35] to conclude that this form of acute renal failure was initiated through tubular luminal obstruction caused by sloughed tubular cells. The resultant tubular obstruction is postulated first to cause a transtubular backleak of glomerular filtrate. Since obstruction of tubular flow also leads to an increase in the tubular luminal hydrostatic pressure above the obstruction, less hydrostatic pressure differential exists between the glomerular capillary lumen and the tubular space within Bowman's capsule. This reduced hydrostatic pressure differential leads to a reduction in glomerular filtration. Then, because of the increased permeability of the tubular lining and the resultant increased interstitial oncotic pressure, further backdiffusion of filtered water occurs. This increased backdiffusion of glomerular filtrate causes further progression of oliguria. The final mechanism that leads to filtration failure and oliguria is the impact of an increased solute load presented to the macula densa as a consequence of the dramatic backdiffusion of fluid. This solute load is believed to stimulate the macula densa to activate the renin-angiotensin-aldosterone system. This mechanism triggers afferent or preglomerular arteriolar vasoconstriction, which decreases the glomerular capillary hydrostatic pressure and further encourages filtration failure. The magnitude and duration of the resulting ischemia are the predominant factors that determine the clinical severity and duration of this type of acute renal failure.

An alternative cause of acute renal failure in aortic surgery that might be considered a permanent form of ischemic insult is microscopic embolization of cholesterol-rich atheromatous debris into the renal vasculature during the act of cross-clamping or declamping of the juxtarenal aorta. Although this mechanism receives much less attention in the literature than the pathophysiologic consequences of temporary ischemia, we suspect that it is the dominant cause of acute renal failure in patients without prolonged renal ischemia, excessive blood loss and hypotension, or other recognized nephrotoxic insult to renal function. Obviously, the quantity of microembolization produced by clamping or declamping the aorta and by manipulating the juxtarenal aorta during dissection depends on the embologenic potential of the atheromatous debris and the operative techniques employed to prevent such an event. Furthermore, the clinical impact of such renal microembolization depends on the quantity of functioning renal parenchyma embolized and the presence of other causes of acute renal failure. In the absence of other causes of acute renal failure and a normal mass of functioning nephron units, relatively large amounts of atheromatous microemboli can occur without immediate impact on renal function. In contrast, if there is a minimal renal reserve, the added insult of even minor losses of nephron units by microembolization can lead to decompensation and acute renal failure.

Diagnosis of Renal Dysfunction

The patient with postoperative renal dysfunction or failure is usually identified by oliguria or increases in serum creatinine. Consideration of the many possible causes of postoperative renal dysfunction helps the clinician develop an organized plan of diagnosis and treatment. In the oliguric patient, our first step involves physical examination of the patient. Observation of the patient and his or her vital signs for evidence of intravascular volume depletion, hemodynamic instability, sepsis, and congestive heart failure allows us to focus our differential diagnosis on possible prerenal, renal, and postrenal causes of renal dysfunction. Nevertheless, the first step in any evaluation of oliguria should always be evaluation of the status of the Foley catheter. As mentioned, prerenal causes are the most frequent source of acute renal dysfunction in the early postoperative period. An evaluation of the patient's intravascular volume status and cardiac performance is then carried out. In the patient with signs of volume depletion such as flat neck veins, dry mucous membranes, and reduced filling pressures, we proceed with replenishment of intravascular volume with saline. In light of the possibility of renal failure, we initially avoid infusing potassium-containing solutions and blood products. If examination reveals that diminished cardiac performance is responsible for the oliguria as suggested by findings of distended neck veins, S_3 gallop, pulmonary edema, acute electrocardiographic changes, dysrhythmias, decreased cardiac output, and elevated central venous pressure, we proceed with ruling out a possible myocardial infarction and provide judicious inotropic support while monitoring the patient closely with Swan-Ganz catheter measurements of cardiac performance. If correction of filling pressures or myocardial performance fails to improve urinary output, we obtain samples of urine and blood and begin diuretic therapy. Serum electrolytes, blood counts, and urine studies allow evaluation of other possible sources of oliguria and renal failure such as ATN or myoglobinuria. Urine studies include urinalysis, urine sodium, urea and creatinine concentrations, urine osmolality, and fractional excretion of sodium. An abdominal plain film is useful at this point to rule out obstructive nephrolithiasis. When these sources of renal dysfunction are ruled out, we entertain the possibility of renal artery occlusive disease. Our approach to evaluating this was mentioned earlier. In general, we screen for this possibility with a technetium-99m pertechnetate scan of the kidneys. We proceed with this scan only if we are prepared to follow the scan with angiographic confirmation and surgical intervention.

Protection of Renal Function

Several fundamental concepts for protection of renal function during aortic surgery are widely understood and practiced. These include limiting the period of warm renal ischemia, providing adequate circulating blood volume prior to operation by means of preoperative intravenous fluid hydration and adequate blood volume replacement during and immediately after surgery, avoiding repetitive or prolonged renal ischemia, and maintaining maximal parameters of cardiac performance. Additional modalities include the use of mannitol and other diuretics, renal hypothermia, renal vasodilating drugs, and other, more investigational, techniques.[36–41] Conceptually, all of these modalities are directed toward reduction of the severity or duration of renal tubular ischemia, reduction of renal tubular metabolic needs during periods of ischemia, or prevention of tubular obstruction by sloughed tubular cells. No single modality or combination of modalities prevents the insult of aortic surgery on renal function, but by using these preventive measures, one can lessen the severity and duration of renal dysfunction.

Careful attention should be given to limiting the period of warm renal ischemia. For the normally perfused kidney, anything less than 45 minutes of warm ischemia is generally safe. For the chronically ischemic kidney, the duration of safe warm ischemic time is extended for an unknown period depending upon the amount of collateral flow that has been developed. Meticulous preoperative evaluation, planning, and intraoperative set-up can help to reduce the necessary cross-clamp time and diminish the chances of time-consuming intraoperative complications.

Intravenous administration of mannitol, 12.5 to 25 gm, before aortic cross-clamping is widely practiced as a routine measure to prevent acute renal failure. Extensive investigation of its actions suggests that mannitol not only acts as an osmotic diuretic to increase urine flow rate but may also attenuate the reduction in cortical blood flow that occurs during and immediately after aortic cross-clamping; mannitol also acts as a free radical scavenger.[36]

Regional renal hypothermia has been used sporadically for many years to protect renal function during periods of ischemia. Its use is based on the valid premise that even modest decreases in core temperature significantly reduce metabolic needs. These unmet metabolic needs during ischemia lead to the cascade of events that produce acute renal failure. The technique usually employs the infusion of 500 ml to 1 L of cold (4 to 5° C) crystalloid solution with or without other additives into the isolated segment of the aorta containing the renal arteries or directly into the renal artery ostia using a handheld cannula or infusion balloon catheters. The protective effect of minimal changes in core temperature has recently been evaluated in rats. Postoperative serum creatinine levels and renal tubular morphology data revealed that a protective effect occurred with a minimal, sustained decrease in core temperature to 35°C.[42] It would be interesting to see whether a similar well-controlled study in humans would reveal like findings.

Finally, one cannot overstate the importance of operative technique in preventing microembolization of atheromatous debris during juxtarenal aortic manipulation or clamping. Because the embologenic potential of the debris cannot be judged definitively until after the aorta is opened, one should assume the worst until it is proved otherwise. For this reason, we temporarily occlude renal artery flow immediately before the application of the aortic clamp whenever the aortogram suggests the presence of succulent atheromatous debris. This applies both to cross-clamping immediately below the renal arteries and to suprarenal aortic cross-clamping. For infrarenal cross-clamping, we "flash unclamp" the proximal aortic clamp after opening the aorta to flush out any loose debris. Then we reapply the aortic clamp, remove any renal artery–occluding device, and reestablish renal perfusion. Although we can provide only anecdotal support for this maneuver, we believe it has been an important adjunct in minimizing the incidence of postoperative acute renal failure among our patients.

Renal Failure Associated With Arteriography

Contrast arteriography is the gold standard of diagnostic studies used in the evaluation of vascular disease. Conventional contrast agents have iodine incorporated into their structure to absorb x-ray photons, thereby achieving visualization of the vasculature. The nephrotoxicity of such iodinated contrast agents has been recognized for many years.[43] The ionization and high osmolarity of these agents may contribute to their nephrotoxicity. Nonionic contrast agents (e.g., iopamidol) are now available that provide comparable absorption of x-ray photons yet are significantly less charged than traditional agents. It was hoped that this reduction in ionization would decrease their nephrotoxicity,[44] but significant alterations in incidence of complications have not been achieved.[45]

The incidence of acute renal dysfunction following contrast arteriography varies from 0 to 92 percent[46–48] and is dependent on several factors: the quantity of contrast material injected, the patient population, and the prearteriographic preparation of the patient. A number of factors have been identified that increase the risk of contrast-induced acute renal failure (Table 33–4). Among these, diabetes and preexisting renal insufficiency are of the greatest concern because they are common in vascular surgery patients. Risk factors such as dehydration, volume depletion, volume of contrast used, and simultaneous exposure to other nephrotoxins are common but should be avoidable through proper patient preparation. Other risk factors such as multiple myeloma and severe proteinuria are uncommon and may be lesser risk factors in the absence of secondary renal insufficiency.

The impact of diabetes on the risk of acute renal failure following arteriography appears to be dependent on the type of diabetes and the magnitude of secondary diabetic nephropathy. Type I diabetics appear to be more susceptible to contrast-induced acute renal failure than type II diabetics.[49–50] Harkonen and Kjellstrand[49] found that 22 of 26 patients (76 per cent) with a prestudy serum creatinine level of greater than 2 mg/dl who underwent excretory urography developed acute renal failure. Weinrauch and associates[48] reported that acute renal failure following coronary arteriography developed in 12 of 13 patients (92 per cent) with juvenile-onset diabetes and severe diabetic nephropathy. The cause of chronic renal insufficiency also appears to affect the permanency of contrast-induced acute renal failure. Whereas both diabetic and nondiabetic patients with renal insufficiency are at increased risk for contrast-induced acute renal failure, diabetic patients appear to recover less often and are at much greater risk of permanent dependence on dialysis as a consequence of contrast-induced acute renal failure.

The cause of acute renal failure following angiography is probably multifactorial. In contrast to the widely known potential for the nephrotoxicity of contrast agents, there are relatively little experimental data confirming the pathogenesis. This is partially explained by the difficulty of creating animal models that mimic the human conditions known to predispose to the injury. Factors considered important in the pathogenesis include the osmolality of the contrast material,[51] the presence of proteinuria,[52] tubular obstruction,[53] allergic reactions,[54] enzymuria,[55] direct toxicity of the agent,[56] and altered glomerular permeability.[57] Although the newer nonionic contrast materials have been developed to address some of these potential causes (e.g., osmolality and magnitude of ionic change), they are significantly more expensive. They appear to diminish the pain experienced by the patient immediately following injection, yet prospective and controlled trials have not demonstrated a significant reduction in risk of acute renal failure with their use.[45, 58]

Table 33–4. Factors Implicated in Arteriography-Induced Renal Failure

Advanced age	Exposure to other nephrotoxins
Renal insufficiency	Repeated exposure to radiocontrast material
Diabetes mellitus	Excessive volume of contrast material
Multiple myeloma	Intra-arterial vs. intravenous administration of contrast material
Anemia	Cardiovascular disease
Proteinuria	Hypertension
Abnormal liver function	Renal transplantation
Dehydration	
Hyperuricemia	

Prevention of Contrast-Induced Renal Failure

Specific measures used to minimize the risk of contrast-induced acute renal failure remain controversial and lack controlled studies to confirm their efficacy. Nevertheless, experimental parallels and understanding of factors that increase the risk of this complication have led to generally accepted tenets of prevention. The basic relationship between the use of contrast material and the risk of causing acute renal failure for any of the currently used agents in any high-risk patient population appears to be related to the amount of time the kidney is exposed to a given concentration of contrast material. For this reason, maximizing urine flow rate during and immediately after arteriography and limiting the quantity of agent used during an arteriographic session are important considerations. Maximal urine flow rate should be achieved by preliminary intravenous hydration of the patient and the use of diuretic therapy. We routinely admit any patient with recognized risk factors for 12 hours before arteriography to administer intravenous hydration and infuse 5 per cent dextrose in 25 per cent normal saline at 1.5 ml/kg/hr during this period. Immediately before arteriography the patient usually receives a bolus of intravenous fluid (3 to 5 ml/kg). In addition, 12.5 gm of mannitol or 20 to 40 mg of furosemide are given intravenously at the time of arteriography. Finally, intravenous hydration is continued for 4 to 6 hours after completion of the study.

Though attempts to calculate a safe upper limit of contrast material have met with some success, no definitive formula currently exists.[59] Even small doses (30 to 60 ml) may induce renal failure in patients with extreme renal insufficiency (glomerular filtration rate less than or equal to 15 ml/min). In contrast, more than 300 ml of contrast material may be safely administered to other patients with no risk of acute renal failure. Our practice is to limit the quantity of nonionized contrast agent to less than 50 to 75 ml in patients with a significant reduction in glomerular filtration rate (less than 20 to 30 ml/min). If additional contrast material is required to evaluate other areas of the vasculature, we postpone such studies and approach the total evaluation in a sequential manner after confirming that no adverse effect from the prior study has occurred. The introduction of digital substraction techniques has been useful in limiting the quantity of contrast material used in patients with renal insufficiency. Digital subtraction techniques are especially useful when the areas to be viewed would require multiple injections if conventional radiologic techniques were employed. Nevertheless, we have found that a single midstream aortic injection, using 30 ml of nonionic contrast material and standard radiologic techniques, is just as safe as digital substraction techniques. We believe that it provides superior visualization of the renal vasculature and related aortic anatomy in patients with renal insufficiency in whom the presence of ischemic nephropathy is being evaluated.

Finally, we believe that future advancements in the safe visualization of the vasculature will not come from further modification of the chemical composition of the contrast agents. Rather, we believe that the greatest innovations and progress will be made in the application of noncontrast agent studies. The reported use of carbon dioxide is generally overlooked but may be a viable alternative to the use of standard contrast agents for limited studies.[60] Most important, however, is the development of nuclear magnetic imaging of the vasculature.[61] Through further technological modification, this field holds the greatest promise for providing excellent visualization of the vascular anatomy without the risks induced by injection of any noxious agents.

References

1. Harvey W: Exercitatio Anatomica de Motu Cordis et Sanguinis, 1628. *Cited in* Harvey W: The Works of William Harvey. London, Syndenham Society, 1847.
2. Shires TG, Canizaro PC, Shires TC III, Lowry SF: Fluid, electrolyte, and nutritional management of the surgical patient. *In* Schwartz SI: Principles of Surgery, 5th ed, vol. 1. New York, McGraw-Hill, 1989, pp 68–104.
3. Gann DS, Amaral JF: Preoperative electrolyte management. *In* Sabiston DC Jr (ed): Sabiston's Essentials of Surgery. Philadelphia, WB Saunders, 1987, pp 29–61.
4. Valtin H: Renal function: Mechanisms preserving fluid and solute balance in health. *In* Renal Dysfunction: Mechanisms Involved in Fluid and Solute Imbalance. Boston, Little, Brown, 1983.
5. Carey LD, Lowery BD, Cloutier CT. Hemorrhagic shock. Curr Prob Surg 8:1048, 1971.
6. Granger H, Dhar J, Chen HI: Structure and function of the interstitium. *In* Squoris JT, Rene A (eds): Proceedings of the Workshop on Albumin. Bethesda, MD, National Institutes of Health, 1976, pp 114–123.
7. Taylor AE, Granger DN: A model of protein and fluid exchange between plasma and interstitium. *In* Squoris JT, Rene A (eds): Proceedings of the Workshop on Albumin. Bethesda, MD, National Institute of Health, 1976, pp 93–113.
8. Lucas CE, Ledgerwood AM: The fluid problem in the critically ill. Surg Clin North Am 63(2):439, 1983.
9. Dawson CW, Lucas CE, Ledgerwood AM: Altered interstitial fluid space dynamics and post-resuscitation hypertension. Arch Surg 116:657, 1981.
10. Baxter CA: Balanced salt solutions as renal prophylaxis. *In* Brown BR Jr (ed): Fluid and Blood Therapy in Anesthesia. Philadelphia, FA Davis, 1983, pp 137–150.
11. Thorén L, Wiklund L: Intraoperative fluid therapy. University Hospital, Uppsala, Sweden. World J Surg 7:581, 1983.
12. Glaumann B, Glaumann H, Trump BF: Studies of cellular recovery from ischemia: III. Ultrastructural studies on the recovery of the pars recta of the proximal tubule (P_1 segment) of the rat kidney from temporary ischemia. Virchows Arch B 25:281, 1977.
13. Brezis M, Rosen S, Silva P, et al: Renal ischemia: A new perspective. Kidney Int 26:275, 1984.
14. Jones DB: Ultrastructure of human acute renal failure. Lab Invest 46:254, 1982.
15. Matzke GR, Lucarotti RL, Shapiro HS: Controlled comparison of gentamicin and tobramycin nephrotoxicity. Am J Nephrol 3:11, 1983.
16. Eneas JF, Schoenfeld PY, Humphreys MH: The effect of infusion of mannitol–sodium bicarbonate on the clinical course of myoglobinuria. Arch Intern Med 139:801, 1979.
17. Braun SR, Weiss FR, Keller AL, et al: Evaluation of the renal toxicity of hemoproteins and their derivatives: A role in the genesis of acute tubular necrosis. J Exp Med 131:443, 1979.
18. Gardner RJ, Lancaster JR, Tarney TJ, et al: Five year history of surgically treated abdominal aortic aneurysms. Surg Gynecol Obstet 130:981, 1970.
19. O'Donnell D, Clarke G, Hurst P: Acute renal failure following surgery for abdominal aortic aneurysm. Aust NZ J Surg 59:405, 1989.
20. Thompson JE, Hollier JH, Patman RD, et al: Surgical management of abdominal aortic aneurysms: Factors influencing mortality and morbidity—A 20-year experience. Ann Surg 181:654, 1975.
21. Volpetti B, Barker CJ, Berkowitz H, et al: A twenty-two year review of elective resection of abdominal aortic aneurysms. Surg Gynecol Obstet 142:321, 1976.
22. Bergqvist D, Olsson P-O, Takolander R, et al: Renal failure as a complication to aortoiliac and iliac reconstructive surgery. Acta Chir Scand 149:37, 1983.
23. McCombs PR, Roberts B: Acute renal failure following resection of abdominal aortic aneurysm. Surg Gynecol Obstet 148:175, 1979.
24. Diehl JT, Cali RF, Hertzer NR, Beven EG: Complications of abdominal aortic reconstruction, An analysis of perioperative risk factors in 557 patients. Ann Surg 197(1):49, 1983.
25. David JP, Marks C, Bonneval M: A ten-year institutional experience with abdominal aneurysms. Surg Gynecol Obstet 138:591, 1974.
26. Hicks GL, Eastland MW, DeWeese JA, et al: Survival improvement following aortic aneurysm resection. Ann Surg 181:863, 1975.
27. Sink JD, Myers RT, James PM: Ruptured abdominal aortic aneurysms: Review of 33 cases treated surgically and discussion of prognostic indicators. Am Surg 42:303, 1976.
28. Gornick CC Jr, Kjellstrand CM: Acute renal failure complicating aortic aneurysm surgery. Nephron 35:145, 1983.
29. Tilney NL, Bailey GL, Morgan AP: Sequential system failure after rupture of abdominal aortic aneurysms: An unsolved problem in postoperative care. Ann Surg 178:117, 1973.
30. Breckwoldt WI, Mackay WC, Belkin M, et al: The effect of suprarenal cross-clamping on abdominal aortic aneurysm repair. Arch Surg 127:510, 1992.
31. Myers BD, Moran SM: Hemodynamically mediated acute renal failure. N Engl J Med 314:97, 1986.
32. Myers BD, Miller DC, Mehigan JT, et al: Nature of the renal injury following total renal ischemia in man. J Clin Invest 73:329, 1984.
33. Moran SM, Myers BD: Course of acute renal failure studied by a model of creatinine kinetics. Kidney Int 27:928, 1985.
34. Hilberman M, Myers BD, Carrie G, et al: Acute renal failure following cardiac surgery. J Thorac Cardiovasc Surg 77:880, 1979.
35. Oliver J, MacDowell M, Tracy A: Pathogenesis of acute renal failure associated with traumatic and toxic injury. Renal ischemia, nephrotoxic damage, and the ischemuric episode. J Clin Invest 30:1305, 1951.
36. Miller DC, Myers BD: Pathophysiology and prevention of acute renal failure associated with thoracoabdominal or abdominal aortic surgery. J Vasc Surg 5(3):518, 1987.
37. Abbott WM, Abel RM, Beck CH: The reversal of renal cortical ischemia during aortic occlusion by mannitol. J Surg Res 16:482, 1974.
38. Hanley MJ, Davidson K: Prior mannitol and furosemide infusion in a model of ischemic acute renal failure. Am J Physiol 241:F556, 1981.
39. Ochsner JL, Mills NL, Gardner PA: A technique for renal preservation during suprarenal abdominal aortic operations. Surg Gynecol Obstet 159:388, 1984.
40. Hilberman M, Maseda J, Stinson EB, et al: The diuretic properties of dopamine in patients following open heart operations. Anesthesiology 61:489, 1984.
41. Lindner A, Cutler RE, Bell AJ: Attenuation of nephrotoxic acute renal failure in the dog with angiotensin-converting enzyme inhibitor (SQ-20, 881). Circ Res 51:216, 1982.
42. Pelkay TJ, Frank RS, Stanley JJ, et al: Minimal physiologic temperature variations during renal ischemia alter functional and morphologic outcome. J Vasc Surg 15:619, 1992.
43. Ansell G: Adverse reaction to contrast agents: Scope of problem. Invest Radiol 5:374, 1979.

44. Evans JR, Cutler RE, Pettis JL: Low-osmolar radiocontrast agents and nephrotoxicity. Dialysis Transplant 16:504, 1987.
45. Davidson CJ, Hlatky M, Schwab SJ, et al: Nephrotoxicity and nephrotic risk factors: A prospective trial of nonionic contrast media. Ann Intern Med 110(2):119, 1989.
46. Miller DL, Chang R, Wells WT, et al: Intravascular contrast media: Effect of dose on renal function. Radiology 167:607, 1988.
47. Martin-Paredero V, Dixon SM, Baker JD, et al: Risk of renal failure after major angiography. Arch Surg 118:1417, 1983.
48. Weinrauch LA, Healy RW, Leland OS, et al: Coronary angiography and acute renal failure in diabetic azotemic nephropathy. Ann Intern Med 86:56, 1977.
49. Harkonen S, Kjellstrand CM: Exacerbation of diabetic renal failure following intravenous pyelography. Am J Med 63:939, 1977.
50. Shieh SD, Hirsch SR, Boshell BR, et al: Low risk of contrast media induced acute renal failure in nonazotemic type 2 diabetes mellitus. Kidney Int 21:739, 1982.
51. Morris TW, Katzberg RW, Fisher HW: A comparison of the hemodynamic responses to metrizamide and meglumine/sodium diatrizoate in canine renal angiography. Invest Radiol 13:74, 1978.
52. Tejler L, Almen T, Holtas S: Proteinuria following nephroangiography. Acta Radiol (Diagn) 18:634, 1977.
53. Rees ED, Waugh WH: Factors in renal failure in multiple myeloma. Arch Intern Med 116:400, 1965.
54. Light JA, Hill GS: Acute tubular necrosis in a renal transplant recipient: Complication from drip-infusion excretory urography. JAMA 232:1267, 1975.
55. Goldstein EJ, Feinfeld DA, Fleischner GM, Elkin M: Enzymatic evidence of renal tubular damage following renal angiography. Radiology 121:617, 1976.
56. Humes HD, Hunt DA, White MD: Direct toxic effect of the radiocontrast agent diatrizoate on renal proximal tubule cells. Am J Physiol 252:F246, 1987.
57. Vari RC, Natarajan LA, Whitescarver SA, et al: Induction, prevention and mechanisms of contrast media–induced acute renal failure. Kidney Int 33:699, 1988.
58. Parfrey PS, Griffiths SM, Barrett BJ, et al: Contrast material–induced renal failure in patients with diabetes mellitus, renal insufficiency, or both: A prospective controlled study. N Engl J Med 320:143, 1989.
59. Cigarroa RG, Lang RA, Williams RH, Hillis LD: Dosing of contrast material to prevent contrast nephropathy in patients with renal disease. Am J Med 86:649, 1989.
60. Weaver FA, Pentecost MJ, Yellin AE: Carbon dioxide digital subtraction arteriography: A pilot study. Ann Vasc Surg 4(5):437, 1990.
61. Kim D, Edelman RR, Kent KC, et al: Abdominal aorta and renal artery stenosis: Evaluation with MR angiography. Radiology 174:727, 1990.
62. Johnston KW: Multicenter prospective study of nonruptured abdominal aortic aneurysms: II. Variables predicting morbidity and mortality. J Vasc Surg 9:437, 1989.

34

Perioperative Hemorrhage

Michael F. X. Glynn, M.D., D.Phil.(Oxon.), F.R.C.P.(C.) London, and K. Wayne Johnston, M.D., F.R.C.S.(C.)

• • •

Hemorrhage is one of the most serious complications faced by the vascular surgeon and is serious enough to necessitate reoperation in 1 to 3 per cent of cases.[1, 3, 5, 6] It may result from technical factors, vascular pathology (e.g., collagen vascular diseases), or a coagulopathy. This chapter outlines the prevention and management of bleeding in the preoperative, operative, and postoperative periods.

MECHANISM OF HEMOSTASIS

A simple model of hemostasis, the sine wave, is used to describe hemostasis and relate bleeding and its treatment to pathophysiology. Vascular injury triggers the most fundamental reactions of blood vessels: retraction and spasm. This stops blood loss but at the cost of reducing the blood flow beyond the site of injury and potentially jeopardizing the viability of tissues downstream. This ''physiologic ligature'' fatigues and is succeeded by hemostasis, an orderly sequence of reactions and counter-reactions that direct hemostasis away from bleeding but toward thrombosis then back toward bleeding again before finally regaining hemostatic equilibrium: This is the sine wave of hemostasis (Fig. 34–1). The sine curve emphasizes the continuity of successive hemostatic events as well as the logic of treatment. There are three stages in the response of hemostasis to injury that compose the sine wave: initiation turns hemostasis away from bleeding; amplification turns hemostasis toward thrombosis; and finally, restraints deflect hemostasis back toward bleeding until equilibrium is reached. A brief account of each of these stages is given here and is shown in Figure 34–2.

Initiation of Hemostasis

Platelets recognize and adhere to exposed subendothelium, collagen, and damaged endothelium but not to healthy endothelium. Normally, blood flows in a column composed of a central axis of erythrocytes and a peripheral surrounding annulus of plasma. Near the wall, convection and radial diffusion currents of plasma transport platelets, which are smaller and lighter than erythrocytes, to the vessel wall. If the platelets encounter normal endothelium, they stick only briefly. Receptors—specialized glycoproteins traversing the platelet membrane—are structured at the platelet surface to

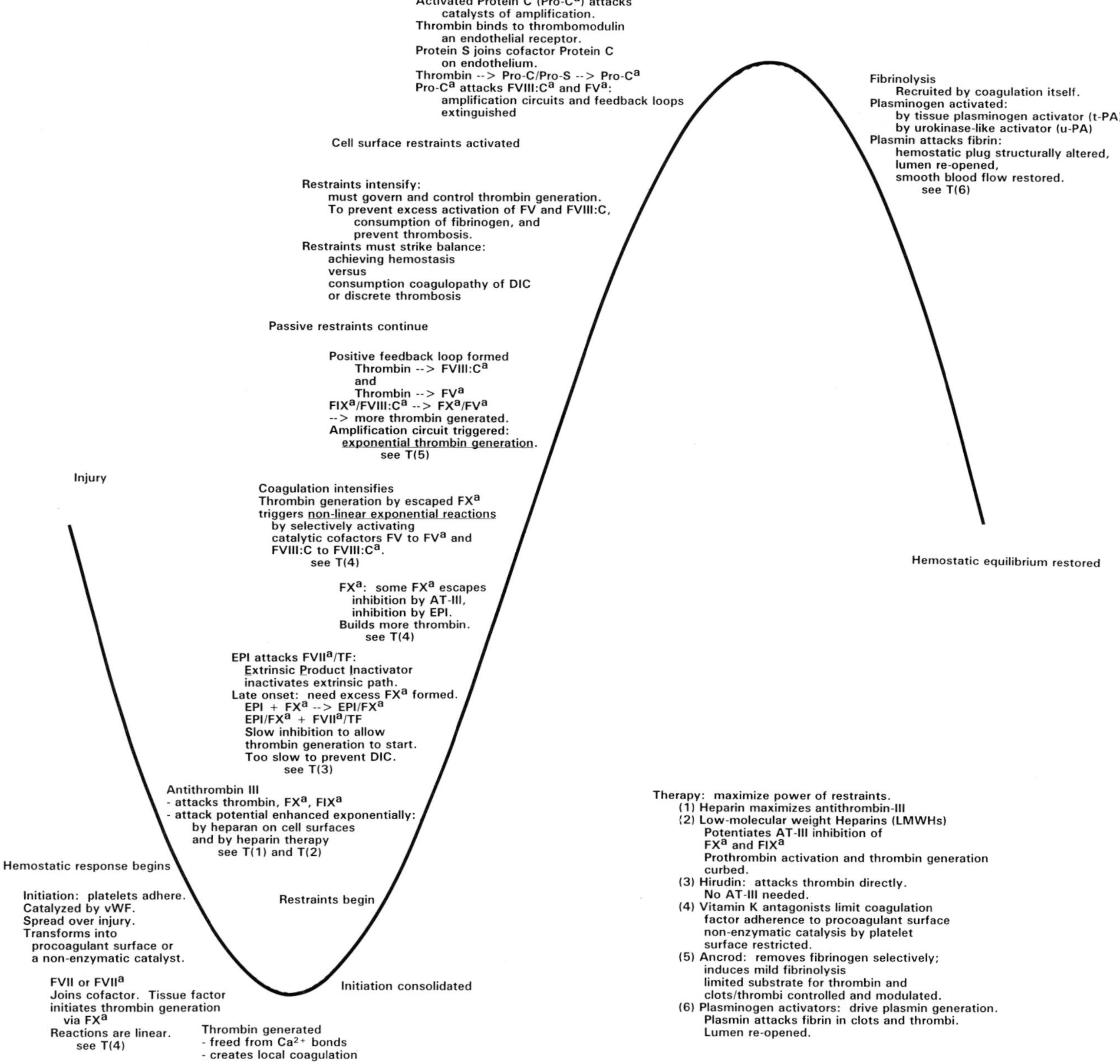
Injury
Hemostatic response begins
Initiation: platelets adhere.
Catalyzed by vWF.
Spread over injury.
Transforms into
procoagulant surface or
a non-enzymatic catalyst.
FVII or FVII^a
Joins cofactor. Tissue factor
initiates thrombin generation
via FX^a
Reactions are linear.
see T(4)
Thrombin generated
- freed from Ca^{2+} bonds
- creates local coagulation
Bleeding
Initiation consolidated
Restraints begin
Antithrombin III
- attacks thrombin, FX^a, FIX^a
- attack potential enhanced exponentially:
by heparan on cell surfaces
and by heparin therapy
see T(1) and T(2)
EPI attacks FVII^a/TF:
Extrinsic Product Inactivator
inactivates extrinsic path.
Late onset: need excess FX^a formed.
EPI + FX^a --> EPI/FX^a
EPI/FX^a + FVII^a/TF
Slow inhibition to allow
thrombin generation to start.
Too slow to prevent DIC.
see T(3)
FX^a: some FX^a escapes
inhibition by AT-III,
inhibition by EPI.
Builds more thrombin.
see T(4)
Coagulation intensifies
Thrombin generation by escaped FX^a
triggers non-linear exponential reactions
by selectively activating
catalytic cofactors FV to FV^a and
FVIII:C to FVIII:C^a.
see T(4)
Positive feedback loop formed
Thrombin --> FVIII:C^a
and
Thrombin --> FV^a
FIX^a/FVIII:C^a --> FX^a/FV^a
--> more thrombin generated.
Amplification circuit triggered:
exponential thrombin generation.
see T(5)
Passive restraints continue
Restraints intensify:
must govern and control thrombin generation.
To prevent excess activation of FV and FVIII:C,
consumption of fibrinogen, and
prevent thrombosis.
Restraints must strike balance:
achieving hemostasis
versus
consumption coagulopathy of DIC
or discrete thrombosis
Cell surface restraints activated
Activated Protein C (Pro-C^a) attacks
catalysts of amplification.
Thrombin binds to thrombomodulin
an endothelial receptor.
Protein S joins cofactor Protein C
on endothelium.
Thrombin --> Pro-C/Pro-S --> Pro-C^a
Pro-C^a attacks FVIII:C^a and FV^a:
amplification circuits and feedback loops
extinguished
Fibrinolysis
Recruited by coagulation itself.
Plasminogen activated:
by tissue plasminogen activator (t-PA)
by urokinase-like activator (u-PA)
Plasmin attacks fibrin:
hemostatic plug structurally altered,
lumen re-opened,
smooth blood flow restored.
see T(6)
Hemostatic equilibrium restored
Therapy: maximize power of restraints.
(1) Heparin maximizes antithrombin-III
(2) Low-molecular weight Heparins (LMWHs)
Potentiates AT-III inhibition of
FX^a and FIX^a
Prothrombin activation and thrombin generation
curbed.
(3) Hirudin: attacks thrombin directly.
No AT-III needed.
(4) Vitamin K antagonists limit coagulation
factor adherence to procoagulant surface
non-enzymatic catalysis by platelet
surface restricted.
(5) Ancrod: removes fibrinogen selectively;
induces mild fibrinolysis
limited substrate for thrombin and
clots/thrombi controlled and modulated.
(6) Plasminogen activators: drive plasmin generation.
Plasmin attacks fibrin in clots and thrombi.
Lumen re-opened.

FIGURE 34–1. The sine wave of normal hemostasis. AT-III, antithrombin III; DIC, disseminated intravascular coagulation; F, factor; T, therapy; vWF, von Willebrand's factor.

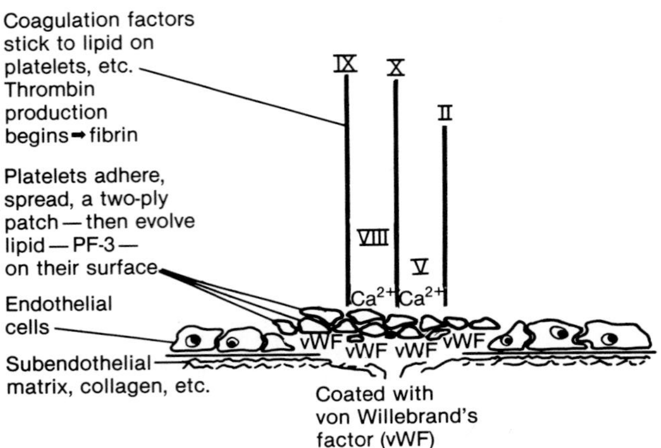

FIGURE 34–2. The development of hemostasis. (1) Injury exposes the subendothelial matrix. (2) von Willebrand's factor secreted by endothelial cells coats collagen. (3) Platelets adhere to the subendothelial matrix, spread, and evolve phospholipid (platelet factor 3 [PF-3]) on the surface. (4) Coagulation factors II, X, and IX (and VII) adhere to the phospholipid surface by calcium bonds and by special groups such as gamma-carboxyglutamic acid placed onto factors by vitamin K. (Co) factors VIII and V mediate the reaction. (5) Coagulation is amplified by thrombin acting on cofactors. Platelet response is amplified by thrombin and the release of platelet contents, both of which recruit and activate more platelets. The restraints of coagulation are not shown. Antithrombin inactivates thrombin and prevents amplification. Proteins S and C are activated by thrombin and then rapidly destroy factors VIII and V. Fibrinolysis is activated. Pharmacologically, heparin activates antithrombin. Warfarin (Coumadin) prevents vitamin K from providing gamma-carboxyglutamic acid, so the factors are unable to adhere.

recognize and bind only to subendothelium and damaged endothelium. These receptors do not recognize or bind with normal endothelium, so the platelets do not adhere and are dislodged easily back into the circulation. This encounter with healthy endothelium is repeated throughout the vascular tree but at the cost of structural damage to the platelet membrane during each encounter, so that eventually the spleen clears those platelets that have become damaged beyond a critical threshold. If the platelets make contact with damaged endothelium or subendothelium, the receptors recognize and bind to the injured tissue, fastening the platelet in place. These adherent platelets are much less easily displaced.

After the receptor recognizes and binds with its programmed target, its next function is to signal intracellular messengers to trigger platelet activation: the exposure of different sets of receptors and cytoskeletal changes. Adherence and activation initiate hemostasis.

The initial adherence by these primary platelet receptors eventually results in hemostasis, especially if it is augmented by local pressure, but normally hemostasis is greatly facilitated by the emergence of another set of platelet receptors that recognize fibrinogen. But more important, at this stage they recognize and react with the adhesive protein, von Willebrand's factor (vWF). vWF is secreted by endothelial cells along their undersurface coating the subendothelium. Binding of the platelet receptors to vWF enables the platelet to adhere more firmly and the cytoskeletal apparatus to spread the platelet over the injury. Where platelet meets platelet, these same receptors induce cohesion between them by linking with fibrinogen to construct a primary platelet layer one to two cells thick.

Securing Initiation. Fibrin is needed to bind and secure the initial platelet adhesion. A procoagulant surface to initiate and foster thrombin generation must be formed but localized to the zone of injury. Thrombin and fibrin are needed to reinforce and secure adhesion of the initial platelets. What is needed is a procoagulant surface to initiate and foster thrombin generation but only at the site of injury. Normally, the heparin-like, carbohydrate-rich surface of endothelium and the glycoprotein coating of circulating blood cells are not procoagulant but are actively anticoagulant. The receptors and cytoskeletal maneuvers of the platelets provide the needed focus for coagulation.

Adherent activated platelets evolve the required procoagulant surface by transforming their normally anticoagulant surface membrane. As the platelets spread to cover the injury, negatively charged phospholipid molecules rich in phosphatidylserine are "flip-flopped" from the inside to the outer layer of the platelet membrane, creating a procoagulant surface. The four vitamin K–dependent coagulation proenzymes are able to form calcium bonds with the negatively charged phospholipids now composing the platelet surface and covering the injury. Gamma carboxyglutamic acid (gamma-gla) groups are unique chemical groups, structured on the coagulation factors by vitamin K–mediated induced carboxylation. These gamma-gla groups bind the attached factor to the platelet by calcium bonding with the negatively charged phospholipids. In patients with vitamin K deficiency or in the presence of vitamin K antagonists such as warfarin, vitamin K cannot construct the groups, so there is no localization and coagulation, and hemostasis fails.

Factor V, the essential procoagulant catalytic cofactor for factor Xa, is stored in the platelet granules. During platelet activation it is released from the granules and inserted into the surface of the platelet along with the phospholipid molecules. The procoagulant transformation of the platelet membrane and the exposure of factor V direct the anchoring of the four coagulation factors onto the procoagulant surface as well as the changes in the conformation of the adherent factors. The result is a group of procoagulant enzymes concentrated in a stereochemically optimal configuration for amplifying thrombin generation.

Factor Xa/factor Va is called prothrombinase because factor Xa complexed with its cofactor, factor Va, is the principal activator of prothrombin to thrombin. Factor VIIa and its cofactor, tissue factor (TF), initiate factor Xa activation and thrombin formation. TF is present as a constituent on the surface membrane of many cells, and after perturbation of endothelium and circulating monocytes, it can appear transiently in their plasma membranes in the circulation. Factor VII or factor VIIa complexed with TF undergoes self-activation to factor VIIa TF, catalyzed by the factor Xa generated by the factor VII or factor VII/TF complex. Neither factor VII nor factor VIIa has inhibitors in the blood, so both are able to circulate for hours, providing an ongoing, ready trigger for hemostasis; they can also induce thrombosis under circumstances of injury to the vessels themselves. All factors VII and VIIa need to fulfill this potential is to encounter and complex with TF, the cofactor needed by factor VIIa to activate factor Xa.

TF can appear in the plasma membranes of endothelium and circulating monocytes and is present on the surface membrane of many other cells, usually after perturbation and cell injury. Factor VIIa joins with TF on these cells to form the reactive complex factor VIIa/TF, whereas the complex of factor VII/TF likely activates itself to the reactive complex factor VIIa/TF. This self-activation is the first in a series of positive feedback or amplification reactions that generate thrombin.

The primary platelet-fibrin hemostatic patch constructed by thrombin initiation can stop bleeding from superficial cuts and mucosal lining and prevent most superficial bruising. It is not able to withstand even moderately severe trauma and cannot overcome bleeding that occurs deep into muscle, joints, and other closed cavities. This is the characteristic picture of hemophilia.

Amplification

Factor IX and its cofactor factor VIII:C meet on the platelet surface to become activated and form factor IXa/factor VIII:C, the key complex in the amplification of thrombin generation.

Relation Between Platelets and Amplification. The transformed platelet surface, with its phosphatidylserine-rich negatively charged phospholipids, is collectively referred to as platelet factor 3. This is the procoagulant surface for the vitamin K–dependent factors. The platelet provides factor V, factor VIII:C, and TF, the catalytic cofactors for factor Xa, factor IXa, and factor VIIa, respectively. Factor V is set into the platelet membrane as it transforms. TF is created after injury. Factor IX is actively bound by calcium bonds, but factor VIII:C, its cofactor, does not have the gamma-gla groups needed for binding to the platelet. Instead, vWF, carrying and sheltering factor VIII:C in the circulation, binds to specific receptors on the surface of the platelet membrane. This binding positions factor VIII:C exactly where it is needed for factor IX to be able to react with prothrombin and generate thrombin.

The transformed platelet membrane with factor V studded throughout its surface not only directs proper conformational changes by the factors but also shelters them from circulating and fixed cell surface inactivators or inhibitors. Concentrating the factors on the platelet membrane in the ideal stereochemical configuration for optimal thrombin generation is the key to forming the positive amplification circuits and feedback loops for the exponential generation of thrombin. If not bound to such a catalytic surface, it would take 2 weeks for the factors, fully activated and complexed with their activated cofactors, to generate as much thrombin as they could have generated in 1 minute if they had been anchored in place.

The negatively charged, phosphatidylserine-rich phospholipids, the factor V inserted from granules, and the receptors evolved to bind vWF/factor VIII:C all lend unique properties of a catalytic nature to the transformed platelet membrane. For this reason, it is called a nonenzymatic catalytic cofactor for coagulation.

Amplification—The Reactions. The factor VIIa/TF complex responsible for triggering the initial, *linear* formation of thrombin via factor Xa also sets the scene for the *exponential* generation of thrombin by activating factor IXa. Unlike the enzyme cofactor complexes, thrombin loses its anchor once it is activated and spreads both upstream and downstream by blood flow convection and radial diffusion, creating a zone of intense activation and autogeneration. Thrombin then triggers the exponential generation of more thrombin. First, thrombin takes over as principal activator of factor IXa, compensating for the inhibition of factor VIIa/TF/factor Xa by the extrinsic product inhibitor. Second, thrombin activates the two catalytic cofactors, factor Va, the cofactor of factor Xa and factor VIIIa, and the cofactor of factor IXa. These two activated catalytic cofactors drive thrombin generation exponentially. Furthermore, as fresh prothrombin is bound and quickly activated to free thrombin, it moves to activate even more of the catalytic cofactors factor Va and factor VIIIa. Thus, a positive feedback loop or amplification circuit is created. Once activated by thrombin, the two activated catalytic cofactors in turn generate even more molecules of thrombin, thus widening the zone of activation. Furthermore, thrombin autoactivates prothrombin to thrombin in a limited positive feedback loop to further amplify its production. Finally, thrombin amplifies the platelet response by activating platelets passing through its zone of activation and augmenting convection and radial diffusion. These interactions, catalyzed by the contents of activated adherent platelets, create the platelet-rich hemostatic plug.

Amplification—The Outcome. In contrast to the zero, first-, and even second-order linear reactions of initiation, amplification evolves second-, third-, and higher-order nonlinear exponential reactions, all with positive feedback loops and amplification circuits. Amplification can have one of the two general outcomes of any positive feedback system. The system can exhaust itself and collapse, or it can be brought under control by built-in governors and regulators of thrombin generation. The first outcome, exhaustion, comes about when pathologic stimuli to hemostasis have driven amplification to the point where all the catalytic cofactors and fibrinogen are consumed, culminating in disseminated intravascular coagulation (DIC) or have driven the activation of plasmin to excess. Both DIC and excessive activation of plasminogen create circulating plasma proteolysis with the consumption and destruction of the catalytic cofactors and fibrinogen. The second outcome is the outcome of normal hemostasis. Governors and regulators restrain amplification and limit thrombin generation to what is needed for hemostasis, while complementary enzyme systems actively lyse excess hemostatic plugs and fibrin.

Restraint

Restraints control amplification and restore hemostasis to baseline equilibrium. Clearly, the initial generation of thrombin must be amplified to provide an adequate hemostatic plug to withstand the disruption of blood flow, protect against circulation inhibitors, and repair the damage of significant trauma. Also, the amplification must itself be restrained, lest it create hemostasis to excess (i.e., thrombosis). For this reason, although the completely activated enzyme-cofactor complexes react to form a positive feedback loop or amplification circuit of thrombin production, the component reactions are nonetheless tightly regulated during normal hemostasis. The governors of hemostasis can be pharmacologically enhanced to reassert their control over the component reactions and amplification loops in the presence of excessive thrombin generation during its exponential amplification.

Natural circulating anticoagulants, principally antithrombin III, actively attack the thrombin in the zone of activation. The inactivation potential of antithrombin III can be enhanced exponentially by heparin to overcome amplified thrombin generation. The pharmacologic advantage of heparin is used during the physiologic inactivation of thrombin. Heparin sulfate and other similar glycosaminoglycans from cell membranes also enhance the ability of antithrombin III to limit thrombin generation at cell surfaces. Extrinsic pathway inhibitor (EPI) also attacks factor Xa by forming a complex, EPI/factor Xa. This complex in turn adjoins the initiating tissue enzyme complex, factor VIIa/TF, bringing this reaction sequence, the extrinsic or tissue pathway, under control.

Circulating and endothelial cell surface–bound anticoagulants are mobilized to deal with the thrombin forming the zone of activation. The most significant of these is the activation by thrombin itself of the protein C–protein S complex formed on endothelial cells within and surrounding the zone of activation created by thrombin. Once activated, protein Ca then diffuses throughout the zone of activation, reaching the sites of thrombin generation, where it attacks and inactivates the procoagulant catalytic cofactors, factor Va and factor VIIIa. Once the catalysts are inactivated, the factors are no longer able to drive thrombin generation, and the amplification circuits and feedback loops are quenched.

Equally important, blood flow rapidly removes activated coagulation factors that are not firmly bound, especially thrombin, and carries them to the liver and other organs of the reticular endothelial system (RES) or macrophage phagocytic system (MPS), where they are cleared and inactivated.

Finally, fibrinolysis is triggered. Plasminogen within hemostatic plugs and on the surface of plugs is activated, enabling plasmin to attack and modify the physical architecture of the fibrin hemostatic structure. The end result is a smooth endothelial surface.

Note that even in the restraints, the capacity for hemorrhage is possible. Excess fibrinolysis can dismantle hemostasis, regardless of how rapidly thrombin is generated, and bleeding may result.

PREOPERATIVE PREVENTION

Prevention of hemorrhage begins in the preoperative period with (1) the detection of preexisting coagulation abnormalities and (2) specific treatment of preoperative coagulopathies.

Preoperative Detection of Coagulopathy

Prior to any vascular surgery procedure, the integrity of the hemostatic system should be evaluated by an appropriate clinical history and laboratory tests. Of these, a thorough directed history is the more important.

History should include specific questions designed to detect easy bruising, bleeding, or petechiae that occur spontaneously or that followed previous operations, trauma, pregnancy or menstrual cycles and to determine whether or not a positive family history of hemostatic abnormalities exists. Table 34–1 shows the important questions in the preoperative evaluation of a patient's hemostatic system.

Screening tests to evaluate hemostasis include (1) platelet count and bleeding time, (2) prothrombin time (PT), (3) activated partial thromboplastin time (APTT) and (4) thrombin time (TT) and will detect most significant coagulation abnormalities. Figures 34–3 to 34–5 detail the interpretation of the results of these tests and outline other investigations that may be necessary if an abnormality is detected.

Screening tests of hemostasis are helpful, but unfortunately their limitations are not generally appreciated. First, they are relatively insensitive. Only 30 to 35 per cent of a particular coagulant activity is needed to give results for screening tests in the normal range. Yet the same patients are at risk of bleeding during surgery or after trauma. Second, screening tests are seldom unexpectedly abnormal and generally confirm the historical data.

Unexpected positive test results call for repeating the tests, taking a more thorough history, and searching for a disorder early in its development—e.g., thrombocytopenia without bleeding reflects the onset of immune thrombocytopenia (ITP). A history of bruising or bleeding nearly always precedes laboratory findings of thrombocytopenia, prolonged bleeding time, or a delayed coagulation time. The data from a thorough history, supplemented by any abnormal blood test results will provide sufficient information to direct more specific investigations and precautions.

Specific Treatment of Coagulopathies

Resources for Replacement or Substitution Therapy to Correct Bleeding From a Deficiency of Clotting Activity

Fresh frozen plasma contains the clotting activity of all of the coagulation factors. *Stored plasma* contains the clotting activities of all the factors except that of factor V and factor VIII:C, the two catalytic cofactors for factor Xa and factor IXa. Without these two cofactors, factor X and factor IX are virtually inert, seriously impeding thrombin generation and hemostasis. Fresh plasma can be subjected to different physical or chemical treatments to isolate distinct fractions of plasma that have specific clotting activities. For example, *cryoprecipitate* is simply the cold precipitate of fresh plasma. In a volume of 10 ml, cryoprecipitate contains 80 per cent of both factor VIII:C and vWF as factor VIII complex as well as upward of 80 per cent of the

Table 34–1. Important Questions to Ask in Evaluating the Hemostatic System

Bruising

Have you any tendency to bruise easily? How much force or trauma is needed to elicit bruises? Any spontaneous bruising? If yes to any of these, ask:
Where are your bruises most often located—shins, thighs, forearms, trunk?
Any bruises around face, especially in areas of pressure by glasses or other areas of wear and tear?
What color are the bruises? Deep dark blue, reddish-purple, or bright red?
When the bruises are fading, are they multicolored orange-yellow, or do they turn from red directly to brown?
Have you ever bruised around an injection site—for example, where you had an injection for pain or for immunization?
Have you ever bruised along scratches?
Can you feel a tenderness or sensation of pain or itching before the bruise actually appears?
Can you feel a knot or lump in the center of the bruise?
Have you ever had a bruise that covered your whole arm, leg, abdomen, or one side of your back?

Bleeding

Have you had nose bleeds? Have the nose bleeds continued in adulthood? Is the bleeding enough to soak tissues?
Have you bled for more than 1 hour after a slight, superficial cut or laceration?
Have you bled for more than 1 day after tooth extraction or after a laceration that required closure with sutures?
Have you experienced cuts that began to rebleed hours or even a day or so after it had been stopped with pressure, bandage, or stitches?
Have you bled during or directly after childbirth?
Have you passed clots at any time during menstrual flow?
Have you ever passed blood in your urine?
Have you ever bled into a joint?
Have you ever coughed up, vomited, or passed blood from the rectum?
Have you ever bled into your nervous system (i.e., had a stroke)?
Has a surgeon or your doctor ever said you were a "bleeder" or advised you to have investigations for a bleeding tendency or treatment for bleeding?
Have you ever needed a transfusion for bleeding after surgery or for any reason?
Have you ever had to return to surgery after an operation because of bleeding?
Has any member of your family, even a distant relative, had any of the problems cited previously? Were the affected relatives male or female?
Have you experienced a bleeding difficulty for as long as you can remember or has it only recently come to your attention?

Petechiae

Do you ever have tiny pinhead-sized bruises beneath a tight belt, strap, etc?
Do you experience bruises on the skin of the forearm, periorbital area, beneath eyeglasses, or at other wear-and-tear areas?

Comment. The answers given to the directed questions guide the choice of laboratory investigations. Simple algorithms of the screening test and their application are set out in Figures 34–3 to 34–5.

Answers to questions about bleeding after tooth extraction or any oropharyngeal surgery, persistent heavy nose bleeds, and heavy menstrual flow are especially important. The mucosa in these areas is especially rich in tissue-type plasminogen activator (t-PA). A hemostatic plug that is in any way defective—poorly initiated or poorly amplified—will be lysed easily and the defect made apparent by bleeding. Large ecchymoses, often after only trivial trauma, suggest that fibrinolytic activity has been generated and spread at the site of vascular injury, likely by the abnormal circulating blood cells or perivascular cells of patients with polycythemia vera. Patients who have had arterial surgery often generate primary fibrinolysis from the large reservoir of fibrinolytic potential within the vessels and in perivascular tissue.

plasma fibrinogen. When infused, large amounts of the factor VIII complex and fibrinogen can be administered without challenging intravascular volume. The plasma remaining after cryoprecipitate is removed can be treated with sequences of physical-chemical manipulations to isolate specific fractions of plasma, each containing other *specific clotting activities.* A specific fraction of plasma enriched in factors VII, IX, X, and II, the vitamin K–dependent factors, is easily isolated. It is useful to correct specific deficiencies of clotting activity as well as to overcome the effects of warfarin.

The advantages of using fractions of plasma enriched in specific clotting activities are offset by the possibility of transmitting blood-borne diseases, especially hepatitis, cytomegalovirus inclusion disease, and human immunodeficiency virus (HIV). Only a single donor contributing to the pool of plasma need have one of these diseases to contaminate the entire plasma pool in each fraction. The load of antigen transfused during repeated infusions of plasma and concentrates of specific clotting activity modulates the recipient's immune system so that the immune response is impaired even without HIV infection. Plasma and its derivatives contain antibodies to blood groups and can provoke a hemolytic anemia in a recipient who has a blood group complementary to the antibodies. Some of these preparations contain activated coagulation factors to allow them to better overcome the inhibitor. The potential for causing thrombosis is especially great with the activated concentrate but is present with any plasma isolate of clotting activity containing the vitamin K–dependent factors. Patients with liver disease are at special risk.

Replacement of sufficient coagulation factor V to

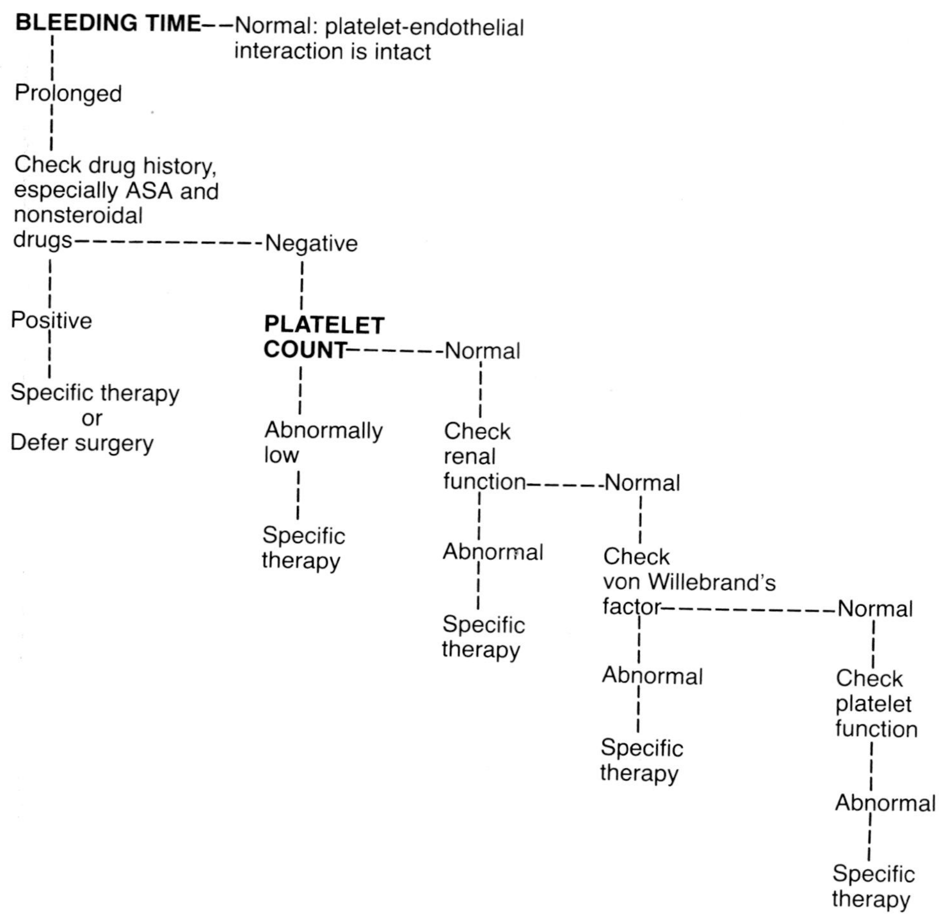

FIGURE 34–3. Interpretation of results of bleeding time and platelet count determinations. ASA, acetylsalicylic acid.

overcome an acquired or genetically related deficiency can be problematic because neither fresh frozen plasma nor cryoprecipitate contains much coagulation factor V activity. On the other hand, platelets contain at least one third of the total plasma factor V activity and, hence, should be infused when factor V is reduced (e.g., in primary fibrinolysis, severe liver disease) despite a seemingly adequate number of platelets.

The use of *platelet transfusions* is discussed later.

The following sections describe specific treatments for the abnormalities detected by the screening tests shown in Figures 34–3 to 34–5.

Reversal of Anticoagulant Effect of Heparin

The specific antidote to heparin is protamine, available as protamine sulfate in North America. Protamine sulfate must be injected intravenously and infused slowly to prevent cardiac depression and hypotension.

Urgent Reversal of Heparin Anticoagulation. For neutralization of heparin anticoagulation in a patient who develops life-threatening bleeding or has a need for immediate surgery, 10 mg of protamine sulfate dissolved in 50 ml of normal saline is infused intravenously over 10 minutes, followed by 20 mg of protamine dissolved in 50 ml of normal saline infused intravenously over 30 minutes. This amount of protamine sulfate should be adequate to reverse the anticoagulation achieved by therapeutic doses of heparin and restore hemostasis to normal. Protamine in excess should not be given. Thrombus formation can be initiated if protamine, in the absence of heparin, contacts injured arteriolar endothelium.

Nonurgent Reversal of Heparin Anticoagulation. The half-life of heparin in the circulation is about 90 minutes. Stopping heparin 3 hours before surgery means that only about 25 per cent of the original anticoagulant effect remains. This intensity of effect is sufficiently low for nearly all surgery to be undertaken safely. If complete reversal is necessary because of the nature of the procedure, e.g., neurologic or ophthalmic surgery, heparin should be stopped 6 hours preoperatively.

Reversal of Warfarin Anticoagulant Effect

The specific antidote to warfarin, sintrom, or any vitamin K antagonist is vitamin K_1. Vitamin K menadione is no longer available for oral use. Vitamin K_1, 5 to 10 mg in 50 to 100 ml of 5 per cent dextrose in water or normal saline infused over 30 to 60 minutes or up to 5 mg injected subcutaneously should counteract the therapeutic anticoag-

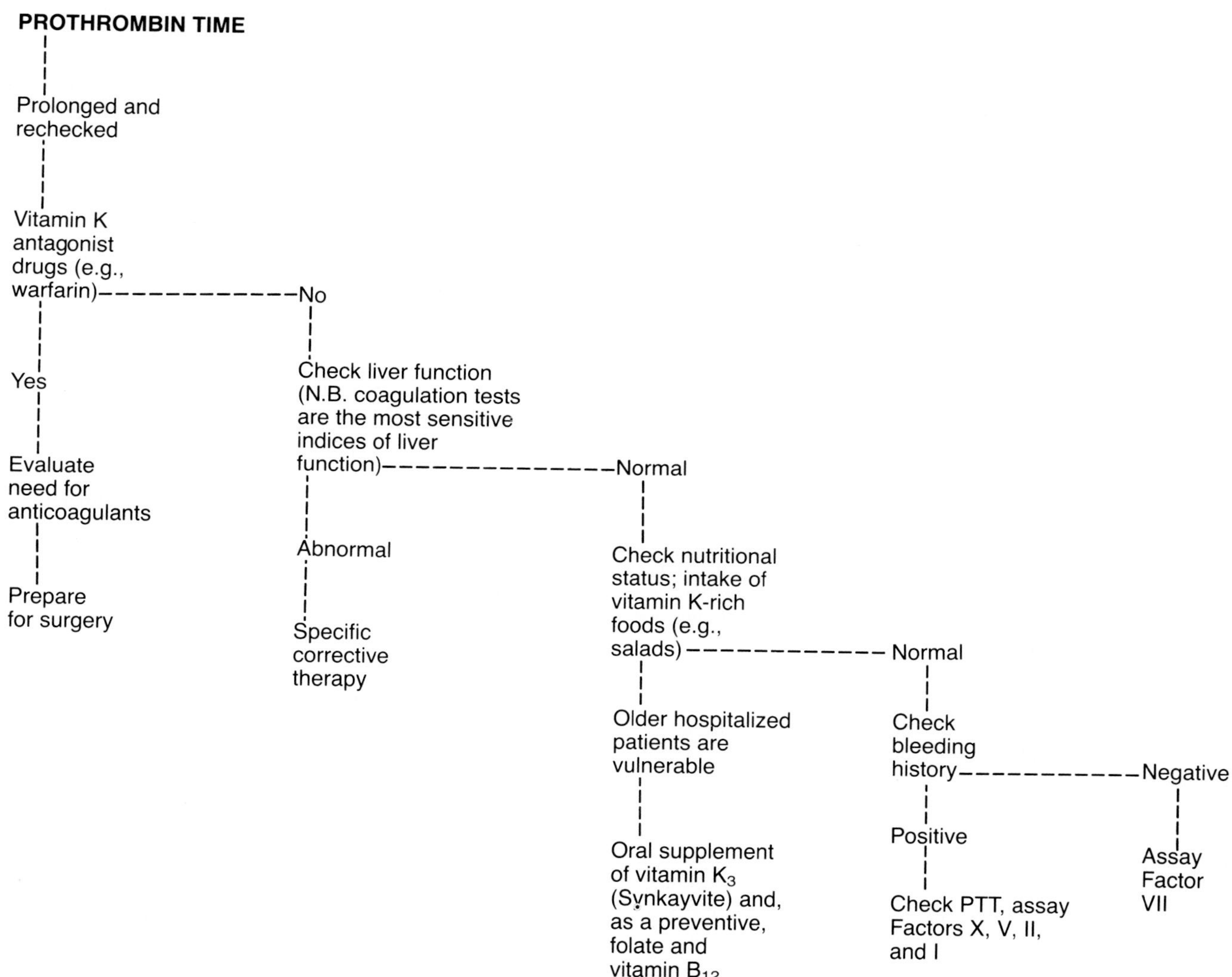

FIGURE 34–4. Interpretation of results of prothrombin time determination. *Note*: A deficiency of factor XIII (the fibrin-stabilizing factor) can cause serious bleeding without prolonging the prothrombin time (PT) or the partial thromboplastin time (PTT). A specific assay can be performed simply and should be done whenever a bleeding diathesis is suspected.

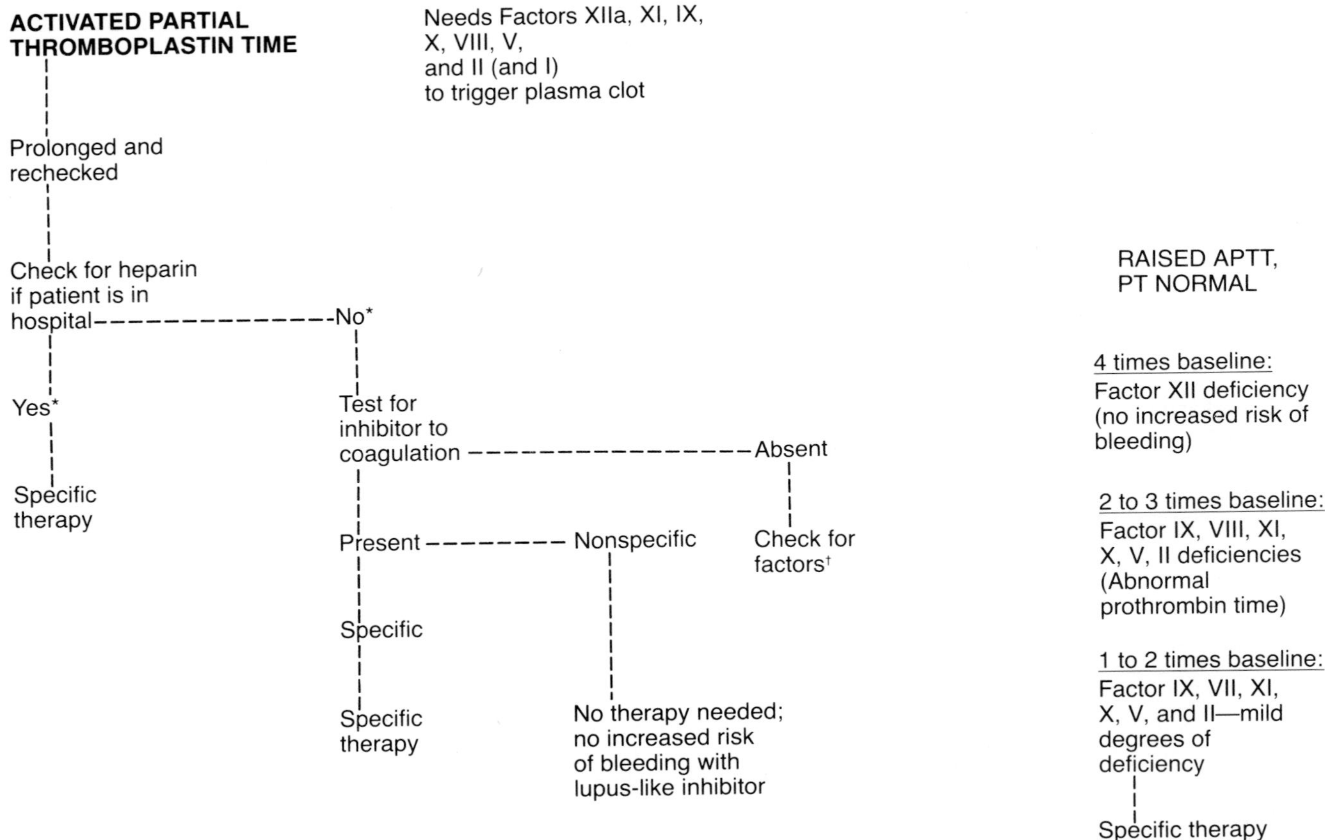

FIGURE 34–5. Interpretation of results of activated partial thromboplastin time (APTT) determination. Other tests, such as thrombin time with protamine or toluidine blue and reptilase time, are useful *(asterisks)*. Heparin inhibitor can prolong APTT to any degree *(dagger)*. *Note*: A deficiency of factor XIII (the fibrin-stabilizing factor) can cause serious bleeding without prolonging the PT or the PTT. A specific assay can be performed simply and should be done whenever a bleeding diathesis is suspected.

ulation effect of warfarin. Vitamin K_1 has caused severe allergic reactions and even anaphylaxis; hence, slow infusion of a dilute solution of vitamin K_1 is prudent. Vitamin K_1 begins to implement gamma carboxylation of synthesized factors stored in hepatic cells, and they are released in about 6 hours. Significant correction of the PT toward normal is seen in 18 to 24 hours. The time needed to achieve complete normalization depends on the amount of warfarin present, the intensity of the anticoagulation, and the affinity of hepatic receptors to warfarin.

Alternatively, plasma may be infused to replenish the four vitamin K_1–dependent factors that are depleted by warfarin (i.e., factors VII, IX, X, and II [prothrombin]), or commercially available concentrates of coagulation factors (''prothrombin complex'') can be administered. Plasma (250 ml) should be infused over 30 to 60 minutes. Surgery can be started after about 100 ml have been given. There is no need to wait for results of a PT. Infusion of plasma seldom, if ever, completely normalizes the coagulation test reading. Note that both plasma and the concentrations of coagulation factors made from plasma pooled from many donors can potentially transmit blood-borne diseases.

In the event of *life-threatening bleeding* (e.g., ruptured aneurysm, central nervous system or intraocular bleeding, multiple trauma, massive hemoptysis, or other urgent situations), recommended treatment is as follows. Infuse at least 4 units of fresh frozen or stored plasma, or alternatively, give prothrombin complex concentrate to 3000 units of clotting activity for each of the vitamin K–dependent factors (factors VII, X, IX, and II [prothrombin]) and infuse 5 to 10 mg of vitamin K_1 over 30 to 60 minutes. After the acute episode subsides, resume anticoagulation with heparin to provide anticoagulation protection if the patient is at high risk for thrombosis. Heparin anticoagulation lends flexibility in therapy to deal quickly with another bleed or to prepare the patient for surgery.

In the event of significant but *not life-threatening bleeding,* infuse 2 units of stored or fresh frozen plasma. Vitamin K_1 should also be given if the clinical situation warrants.

If the *patient is not bleeding but the international normalized ratio (INR) is high,* exceeding 5.0, or the PT is more than three to four times control, appropriately small doses of vitamin K_1 should be administered to avert bleeding. The exact amount of vitamin K_1 depends on the degree of INR or PT prolongation and the clinical situation itself.

If *elective surgery* is to be undertaken in patients taking warfarin, the management of anticoagulation must reflect the competing risks of bleeding and thrombosis or thromboembolism. Two criteria especially demand evaluation. First, what is the condition for which the patient is being anticoagulated and what is the risk of thromboembolism if anticoagulants are discontinued, even temporarily? Second, what is the risk of bleeding associated with the procedure and to what degree would this risk be increased if the anticoagulant therapy is continued?

Note that impaired coagulation or pharmacologic anticoagulation producing an INR of less than 1.4 should not impair hemostasis unduly. If the INR is greater than 1.4, some modification of anticoagulation will be needed (e.g., vitamin K_1, with or without plasma, depending on the competing risks of thromboembolism versus bleeding). If the surgery is straightforward and the wound accessible, direct pressure and local coagulants may be sufficient to secure hemostasis. If the site of surgery is not easily accessible or the operation is complicated, control of systemic anticoagulation is required to minimize the risk of bleeding without undue risk of thrombosis.

In *patients with a relatively high risk of thromboembolism (e.g., mechanical heart valve or established history of thromboembolism),* one of two options is appropriate. The first option is to admit the patient 2 to 3 days before surgery, start an infusion of heparin in a concentration sufficient to achieve therapeutic anticoagulation and discontinue warfarin on admission, and wait for the therapeutic effects of warfarin to wane. The heparin should be discontinued 3 hours before surgery. Since its half-life is about 90 minutes, after 3 hours about 25 per cent of heparin remains in the circulation, providing adequate protection against thrombosis without an undue risk of bleeding during surgery. The heparin infusion may be resumed 12 hours after hemostasis is judged to be intact. During surgery, no heparin is given unless there is a high risk (e.g., clot in a ventricle) or anticoagulants are required for the surgical procedure. A second option is to admit the patient the day before surgery, discontinue warfarin, start heparin to achieve therapeutic anticoagulation, and infuse vitamin K_1 intravenously. Subsequent anticoagulation may be implemented as in the first option.

In *patients with a moderate to low risk of thromboembolism,* three options are available. (1) Discontinue warfarin 3 days before surgery, and admit the patient to hospital 1 day before surgery. On admission, begin prophylaxis against thrombosis. Usually, 5000 units of heparin injected subcutaneously the night before surgery and every 6 to 12 hours thereafter should provide adequate protection against thrombosis, but the heparin therapy can be intensified if the risk of thrombosis is sufficiently great. Adjusted-dose heparin therapy has been successful. The dose of the subcutaneous injection is altered until a blood sample taken at the mid-point in time between successive injections attains an APTT of about 1.5 times normal baseline. (2) Discontinue the usual dose of warfarin 5 days before surgery, and instead prescribe warfarin 1 mg/day for prophylaxis. This program is still under study. In any of the options, warfarin may be resumed once the patient can tolerate oral feeding. Whether or not to use heparin while anticoagulation with warfarin is being reestablished depends on the patient's risk of thromboembolism. (3) For patients who are undergoing invasive investigations only (e.g., angiography, colonoscopy with biopsy) or minor superficial surgery, infuse 2 units of plasma, each over 30 to 45 minutes, starting the first unit 10 minutes before the procedure begins. The fully formed, competent coagulation factors maintain hemostasis long enough for short procedures to be undertaken safely. Hemostatic competence is only transient, lasting at best 3 to 4 hours, depending on the patient's hemostatic reserves.

Note that in any option that requires the administration of blood products, the risk of transmission of blood-borne diseases must be fully explained to the patient and informed consent obtained.

Bleeding During Thrombolytic Therapy: Pharmacologically Activated Plasminogen

The following paragraphs provide guidelines for the reversal of thrombolytic therapy if bleeding occurs or if it is necessary to undertake immediate surgery. Local bleeding from accessible sites can often be dealt with by pressure and the plasminogen activator infusion can be continued; however, when bleeding occurs from inaccessible sites (e.g., respiratory, gastrointestinal, or genitourinary tracts), usually the plasminogen activator infusion must be stopped. Bleeding into the central nervous system—or even a suspicion of bleeding owing to development of an unexplained headache—requires suspension and generally termination of treatment.

If it is necessary to terminate treatment with streptokinase, urokinase, or any of the plasminogen activators because of bleeding or because surgery is imperative, the targets of plasmin—fibrinogen (factor I), factor V, and, to a lesser extent, factor VIII—must be replaced. Plasma (2 to 3 units) or cryoprecipitate (12 units) suffices to replace the substrates of plasmin. Platelet infusions may be necessary because not only are they a rich source of factor V, but also the surface membrane of the platelet and the receptors essential to platelet function can be attacked and destroyed by plasmin generated on the surface of the platelet itself or by circulating plasmin.

Drugs designed to protect hemostatic plugs from plasmin attack or to inhibit the enzymatic action of plasma should be administered. The drugs include epsilon-aminocaproic acid (EACA, Amicar), tranexamic acid (Cyklokapron), and aprotinin (Trasylol). EACA and tranexamic acid prevent the destruction of hemostatic plugs by blocking the action of plasmin. Both EACA and tranexamic acid compete for lysine binding sites on plasmin or plasminogen by which the enzyme or its precursor binds to its substrates. The drugs displace fibrinogen or fibrin and occupy the lysine binding sites. This prevents activation of plasminogen built into hemostatic plugs as well as any attack by plasmin on its substrates. Although some enzymatic inhibition is claimed for EACA and tranexamic acid, the principal inhibitor of plasmin in clinical use is aprotinin. Aprotinin inhibits kallikrein generation and plasmin and interferes with the inflammatory response.

The dose of all these drugs is empirical. EACA 5 gm is infused in 60 ml of 0.9 per cent normal saline over 1 hour, and 5-gm doses are given over 2 and then 3 hours. If bleeding continues, 5 gm is infused over 15 hours. Tranexamic acid 10 gm may be given in 50 ml of 0.9 per cent normal saline over 1 hour. Case reports have documented occasional accounts of thrombosis, DIC, or other adverse effects, but these are few in number and do not clearly implicate the fibrinolytic drugs as the cause. The only contraindication to these drugs is bleeding from the kidney. The kidney is absolutely dependent on urokinase generated locally to maintain fluidity of the small amount of blood that normally escapes from the glomerulus into the urine. Fibrinolytic inhibitors would prevent the lysis of any blood excreted or pathologic bleeding from tissue damage, which could then clot in the renal pelvis, obstruct urinary outflow, and lead to hydronephrosis.

Finally, if the improvement in vessel patency from successful thrombolytic therapy is to be maintained, anticoagulation with heparin or ancrod must be undertaken as soon as bleeding is under control. If surgery is to be undertaken, a lower intensity of anticoagulation, (e.g., 100 units of heparin infused intravenously each hour) might well preserve the gains of fibrinolysis while not interfering with surgical hemostasis.

The biologic half-life of all plasminogen activators is short—minutes to hours—but the effects in terms of substrate depletion of fibrin monomer concentrations can last for many hours; hence, careful attention to adequate replacement must be continued for at least 24 hours.

Reversal of Bleeding in Patients Taking Ancrod

Ancrod (Arvin) is a thrombin-like enzyme derived from the venom of the Malayan pit viper. Ancrod achieves its anticoagulation effect by selectively depleting the plasma of fibrinogen. A mild systemic fibrinolysis is also induced. If bleeding occurs in these patients, hemostasis can be regained by infusing 1 unit of plasma each hour for about 3 to 4 hours or 2 units of cryoprecipitate each hour for 3 to 4 hours. A specific antidote is available, but it is a foreign protein and its complications generally exceed the risks of bleeding; also, the time needed to establish that the patient is not sensitive may be longer than the time of bleeding. Nevertheless, if bleeding appears to be life-threatening, administration of the antidote may be life-saving.

Treatment of Thrombocytopenia and Abnormal Platelet Function

Platelet transfusion may be required because of thrombocytopenia or an acquired or inborn functional abnormality of platelet function. Since concentrations of blood platelets less than 50×10^9/L, even if they are functionally intact, may not be able to support hemostasis—especially the hemostatic challenge imposed by surgery—it is prudent to transfuse platelets to patients with a low platelet concentration. A single platelet pack contains 6×10^{10} platelets concentrated in about 50 ml of plasma. Consequently, infusion of a single pack should increase the platelet count by about 5×10^9/L whole blood, measured 1 hour after the platelets have been infused. In general, platelets are transfused not as a single pack but as a six pack, and a corresponding rise in platelet count should be observed. Platelet transfusions may also be needed if the patient's platelets are functionally abnormal.

It is preferable to give platelets from ABO, Rhesus (Rh) identical blood donors. Although the ABO antigens are expressed only weakly on platelet membranes and the Rh antigens not at all, platelet preparations invariably contain residual erythrocytes. A 50-ml pack of platelet concentrate can contain 1 ml of packed erythrocytes, enough to sensitize the patient and cause a reaction. However, if the clinical situation is urgent, as with erythrocytes, one should not hesitate to use other ABO and Rh-group platelets. If platelets from an Rh-positive donor are given to an Rh-negative female who may yet conceive and bear children, Rh immunoglobulin should be administered within 72 hours.

Platelet transfusions should be given *just as the scalpel cuts the skin* and not before. If transfused earlier, they may be consumed or sequestered in the reticuloendothelial system before they can perform their hemostatic function. Empirically, we have found that the infusion of a six pack of platelet concentrate as surgery begins is adequate to support most vascular procedures. Occasionally a second pack is required to ensure that hemostasis remains adequate, and this may be given as the surgery ends.

Abnormalities of Platelet Function. Disorders of platelet function compromise initiation. The platelets may not be able to interact with endothelium or subendothelium because of abnormalities of the plasma as in uremia; lack of adhesive proteins such as a deficiency of the large, hemostatically active multimers of vWF in the different forms of von Willebrand's disease (vWD); lack of fibrinogen; inherited afibrinogenemia; or abnormalities of the subendothelium or collagen. These disorders are separate from abnormalities of platelet function per se.

Platelets that are unable to adhere and thus unable to initiate endothelial interaction may have no receptors for collagen (Bernard-Soulier syndrome) or for fibrinogen, fibronectin, or vWF itself (Glanzman's thrombasthenia), or their membranes may be altered by drugs (e.g., acetylated membranes altered by acetylsalicylic acid [ASA]). Other platelet disorders imply a disjunction of receptor to messenger or an inability to translate biochemical energy (e.g., adenosine triphosphate [ATP]) into mechanical energy so that the platelets have difficulty in responding to activation, transforming membranes, or amplifying their response. Alternatively, the platelets have poor internal contents that prevent them from furnishing a procoagulant nonenzymatic catalytic surface, recruiting other platelets, or amplifying the platelet response by inducing coherence and aggregation. An easy way to remember these is that the platelet is either impotent or sterile and that, regardless of which is true, the bleeding time is prolonged despite a numerically adequate platelet population.

In the acute situation, the only treatment for intrinsic platelet disorders is immediate platelet transfusion. Treatment of abnormalities of plasma, vWD, and similar disorders are discussed in other sections. Diagnosis of the exact platelet disorder can be made later. Providing functionally adequate platelets in excess of 50×10^9/L will *prevent* bleeding, but platelets amounting to 100×10^9/L or more may be needed to *restore* hemostasis.

Treatment of Coagulopathy Associated With Abnormal Renal Function

The hemostatic defect in azotemia centers at the platelet-endothelial interface: interaction is poor. Specific platelet and plasma abnormalities are ill defined, so treatment is directed toward vigorous improvement of the azotemia while the treatment to improve hemostasis remains empirical. The alternatives for managing a patient with a coagulopathy associated with azotemia are summarized here.

Transfusion. Enough functionally intact platelets must be continually driven onto the endothelium and vessel wall by the central axial column of erythrocytes to initiate hemostasis. Patients with renal insufficiency are anemic because insufficient erythropoietin, the humoral stimulus to erythropoiesis, is secreted by the damaged kidneys. In smaller arteries and arterioles, where cellular and humoral hemostasis is paramount, erythrocytes, platelets, and leukocytes are not equally distributed in the column of flowing blood. Instead, the large, dense erythrocytes and leukocytes flow in a central or axial core, with plasma displaced to a peripheral annulus that is contiguous with the arterial wall. Because platelets are lighter and less dense than erythrocytes or leukocytes, they are forced centrifugally into the outer plasma annulus along the wall. Flow in this region is slow, and the relatively long residence time gives platelets more time to interact with the endothelium. In patients with anemia, the central axial column of erythrocytes is smaller, and below a hematocrit of 30, the platelets flow in a much thicker layer of plasma, encountering the vessel wall much less frequently and with much less force. Hemostasis can be improved by a transfusion of erythrocytes to a hematocrit of 30. This enlarges the central axial cylinder of erythrocytes enough that it is able to drive the platelets more effectively and frequently onto the endothelium, augmenting convection and radial diffusion of plasma and platelets.

Erythropoietin is now available for treatment and is produced by human recombinant cell cultures employing the human erythropoietin gene. The administration of erythropoietin corrects the anemia of renal failure and shortens the bleeding time. Doubtless this therapy will be utilized more in the future.

Conjugated estrogens[4] (Premarin 0.6 mg/kg/day for 5 consecutive days) are useful for the prevention and treatment of bleeding associated with renal failure. The mechanism of action is unknown, but treatment protects the patient from disorders of hemostasis and provides a long duration of action, maximal effect being observed between days 5 and 7. Unfortunately, onset of the effect is delayed from 6 to 24 hours. The course of estrogens can be repeated.

DDAVP (1-deamino-(8-D-argenine)-vasopressin; desmopressin) is a synthetic analogue of the antidiuretic hormone, L-arginine-vasopressin, but unlike the natural hormone, it has little effect on the V_1 vasopressin receptors of smooth muscle. Accordingly, it produces little or no vasoconstriction, no increase in blood pressure, and no contraction of the uterus or the small intestine. The standard dose of 0.2 μg/kg exerts three principal hemostatic effects. First, it induces endothelial cells to secrete high-molecular-weight vWF into the plasma. These vWF multimers are especially active as adhesive proteins. Second, tissue plasminogen activator is released from endothelial cells, but not to a great extent. It can lead to increased fibrinolysis; however, this is seldom of consequence and can be overcome by a simultaneous infusion of tranexamic acid or epsilon-aminocaproic acid. Third, and most important in the context of renal disease, desmopressin promotes elevated concentrations of noradrenaline in the circulating plasma approximately 1 to 4 hours after the infusion. Small increases in the concentration of noradrenaline improve platelet endothelial interactions, probably by sensitizing or activating the alpha-adrenergic receptors of platelets. This effect of producing a tide of noradrenaline is independent of the the effects of releasing high-molecular-weight, hemostatically active factor VIII/vWF from the endothelial cells. Nonetheless, the combination of the high multimeric forms of factor VIII/vWF released from the endothelial cells and the increased noradrenaline concentration may act synergistically to improve initiation and primary hemostasis enough to overcome the impediment to initiation in patients with renal failure.

Infusion of 10 units of cryoprecipitate to patients with azotemia results in immediate and nearly complete hemostatic competence that lasts 4 to 12 hours. The unique value of cryoprecipitate is that it contains nearly all of the hemostatically active high-molecular-weight vWF that is valuable for correction of classic vWD and helpful for restoring hemostasis in patients with mild hemophilia by stimulating factor VIII:C production or release and then carrying it as the factor VIII complex, vWF/factor VIII:C, to the site of active hemostasis. Nonetheless, the exact mechanism by which it restores hemostasis in patients with azotemia remains incompletely understood. The mechanism of hemostatic improvement by cryoprecipitate might well be different from that brought about by desmopressin. The high-molecular-weight, large-multimer type vWF probably becomes insolubilized onto damaged subendothelium. The insolubilization, altered structural configuration, and intense local concentration lend vWF enhanced potential for interacting with platelets and initiating hemostasis. As with the administration of any blood product, there is risk of exposure to viruses and other infectious agents. An infusion of 10 bags of cryoprecipitate immediately before surgery should secure hemostasis, even for a prolonged and complex vascular procedure, and is indicated when the patient proves refractory to treatment with DDAVP or conjugated estrogens. Infusion may be repeated after 24 hours or even earlier if hemostasis is endangered. Tachyphylaxis does not develop with repeated infusions of cryoprecipitate.

Dialysis. Hemodialysis should improve platelet function and reduce the risk of bleeding but is seldom successful in completely restoring hemostasis. The exposure of blood to heparin and to the artificial surfaces of the membrane and its circuits can compromise platelet function and even cause thrombocytopenia. System heparinization can be minimized if heparin is confined to the extracorporeal circuit, but dialysis still causes hemostatic problems with cell absorption activation and rupture.

Platelet Transfusions. Platelet transfusions are not helpful. They achieve only a temporary or transient improvement in hemostasis before the uremia compromises them also.

Treatment of von Willebrand's Disease and Hemophilia

The most frequently encountered inherited disorders of blood coagulation are vWD, classic hemophilia (deficiency of factor VIII:C), and rarely, hemophilia B (deficiency of factor IX activity). The clinical manifestations of vWD are the result of difficulties in initiating hemostasis. Patients with vWD have the symptoms and signs of failure of initiation of hemostasis: easy bruising, mucosal bleeding, and prolonged bleeding after superficial cuts. The bleeding stops if pressure is applied, and cuts seldom, if ever, rebleed once hemostasis is achieved. The clinical manifestations of hemophilia are the result of a failure to amplify the initiation of hemostasis: deep bruises into muscle, bleeding into joints, often spontaneously, and frequent rebleeding from deep cuts well after hemostasis has been secured even with primary closure. Hemophiliacs do not bleed or bruise after superficial cuts and trauma and bleed from mucosal surfaces only when there is significant trauma to the surface or an underlying lesion such as a tumor or ulcer. The ability to initiate hemostasis is intact in patients with hemophilia, and this explains why patients with only mild to moderate hemophilia can escape detection well into middle age or until significant trauma or bleeding during surgery uncovers the defect in the amplification of hemostasis.

Von Willebrand's Disease

If bleeding at surgery is excessive but can be controlled by local pressure and blood platelets are normal in number, the patient may have vWD. vWD results from a quantitative or qualitative deficiency of the adhesive protein, vWF. vWF is responsible for facilitating the initiation of platelet-endothelial interaction. Of the three inherited defects of coagulation frequently encountered, only vWD is transmitted on an autosomal chromosome. Thus, if the patient is a female whose bleeding can be stopped with pressure and has a normal platelet count, it is even more likely that vWD is responsible for the excessive bleeding.

The key screening test to identify any disorder of the initiation of hemostasis is the bleeding time. The bleeding time is abnormal in vWD, but the definitive diagnosis of vWD rests upon the results of more specific tests to evaluate the function of a patient's vWF. A helpful test that can be performed rapidly to establish the diagnosis of vWD is to measure the aggregation response of the patient's platelets after the exhibition of ristocetin in vitro. Other screening tests are generally not helpful in making the diagnosis of vWD, although in these patients the APTT is often at or slightly above the upper limit of normal.

Differential Diagnosis. Disorders of platelet function are described elsewhere in this chapter and must be distinguished from vWD. Patients with either vWD or dysfunctional platelets have an adequate number of platelets and a prolonged bleeding time. Clinically, patients with platelet disorders frequently exhibit petechiae, whereas patients with vWD seldom have petechiae. Laboratory evidence of platelet dysfunction versus definitive tests for vWD decide the issue.

Treatment. If decisive laboratory tests cannot be undertaken, desmopressin or DDAVP should be infused intravenously. DDAVP will improve the condition of patients with vWD by releasing hemostatically active vWF. DDAVP will also improve any acquired or inherited disorder of platelet function, probably by inducing a tide of norepinephrine secretion such that the alpha-receptors of the platelets are sensitized, and hemostatic competence is restored, at least in part.

Hemophilia and Other Disorders of Amplification of Hemostasis

When local pressure fails to achieve hemostasis and previously secured wounds begin to rebleed, a disorder of amplification of thrombin production and hemostasis is possible. The following approach to diagnosis and treatment is suggested.

Anticoagulant effects, either from pharmacologic treatment or natural anticoagulants, or the presence of a plasma proteolytic state (e.g., DIC or primary fibrinolysis [PF]) must be excluded. The key screening tests are the PT and the TT. A prolonged PT suggests the effects of vitamin K antagonist anticoagulation (warfarin or coumadin), vitamin K deficiency, or liver disease compromising the ability to utilize vitamin K for gamma carboxylation. A prolonged thrombin time identifies the presence of heparin and can distinguish the anticoagulant effect of heparin from that of DIC or PF. Protamine sulfate is added to a fresh sample of plasma, and the thrombin time is repeated. If the thrombin time was prolonged by heparin, the addition of protamine sulfate to the plasma will neutralize the heparin, and the thrombin time performed on this sample will be normal. The plasminemia secondarily generated by DIC or the primary plasminemia of PF creates circulating products of fibrin and fibrinogen digestion. The larger fragments, termed X and Y, act as antithrombins and prolong the thrombin time. Protamine sulfate precipitates some but not all of these fragments, so that the thrombin time performed on the sample with protamine added will show some shortening but will always remain prolonged.

If the screening tests exclude heparin as well as a plasma proteolytic state, the APTT and bleeding time should be reviewed. If the APTT is prolonged but the bleeding time is normal, fresh frozen plasma, 2 to 4 units, should be infused. This will help correct either type of hemophilia as well as vWD. If hemophilia itself is suspected from the patient's history or the history of his relatives but the type of hemophilia cannot be determined, then intensive treatment with substitution or replacement therapy should be directed initially toward correcting a deficiency of factor VIII:C because this type of hemophilia is 10 times as prevalent as factor IX–deficient hemophilia. Cryoprecipitate, 8 to 12 units, and DDAVP should also be infused. Cryoprecipitate contains vWF and an abundance of factor VIII:C. DDAVP causes endothelial cells to release stored vWF into the circulation. The vWF complexes with factor VIII:C and shelters it in the circulation. Platelet and endothelial receptors for vWF are exposed in activated platelets and perturbed endothelium. The vWF complexed to factor VIII:C binds to these receptors, the site of active thrombin generation. Neither cryoprecipitate nor DDAVP will help to correct the defect in amplification resulting from a deficiency of factor IX clotting activity. Cryoprecipitate contains little or no factor IX, and the vWF released from the endothelial cells by DDAVP does not transport or shelter factor IX in the circulation. Hence, if factor IX–deficient hemophilia is suspected, 4 to 6 units of fresh frozen plasma or a specific concentrate of factor IX activity should be infused.

Treatment of Coagulopathy Associated With Ingestion of Acetylsalicylic Acid or Other Nonsteroidal Anti-Inflammatory Drugs

ASA damages the platelet membrane and reduces platelet adhesiveness. This abnormality is manifested by a prolonged bleeding time and a tendency to "ooze" at surgery. Since the damage to individual platelets is permanent and their average life span is 7 to 10 days, waiting 2 to 3 days after stopping ASA administration allows time for production of enough fresh, unaffected platelets to sustain hemostasis at surgery. Other nonsteroidal anti-inflammatory drugs act similarly, but since their effect on the platelets is dissipated within 4 to 6 hours, they seldom if ever pose a problem. Bleeding due to the abnormalities of platelet function caused by drugs can be overcome by prolonged local pressure. The characteristic of being able to restore hemostasis with local pressure is a feature of platelet endothelial abnormalities and is in contrast to a coagulopathy, in which bleeding cannot be similarly controlled.

Treatment of Coagulopathy Associated With Liver Disease

All coagulation factors are synthesized entirely or in part by the liver. In mild hepatic insufficiency it is possible to replace the coagulation factors by an infusion of plasma or plasma products. However, in frank liver failure this is rarely possible, especially if there is ongoing consumption, because 8 L of plasma would be required each day to compensate for lack of synthesis and consumption. Often, hepatic insufficiency is also associated with compromised renal function, which limits the fluid volumes that can be infused. For patients with hepatic insufficiency who must undergo vascular surgery, an infusion of plasma is begun 2 to 3 hours before the procedure. With severe liver disease, it is preferable to use fresh frozen plasma rather than stored plasma. The main and probably only significant difference between stored plasma and frozen plasma is that frozen plasma contains all the coagulation factors, including the labile factors V and VIII and complement, as well as cold insoluble globulin. In most patients, the constraints of volume expansion, cardiac reserve, and renal excretion limit the total infusion to 3 to 4 units—enough for at least transient hemostasis.

In patients with liver disease, the normal activators and inhibitors of the fibrinolytic system may become unbalanced, and systemic fibrinolysis can occur, jeopardizing hemostasis by attacking functionally adequate hemostatic plugs. Epsilon-aminocaproic acid or tranexamic acid can preserve the hemostatic plug by competing with plasminogen for lysyl binding sites. A 24-hour infusion of epsilon-aminocaproic acid or tranexamic acid, beginning just before surgery and continuing during and after surgery, may help to preserve hemostasis.

Treating Bleeding From Inhibitors of Coagulation

Catastrophic bleeding can result if surgery is undertaken in a patient who has a circulating inhibitor to a specific coagulation factor. These inhibitors arise in about 6 to 10 per cent of hemophiliacs. It is for this reason that surgery is not begun in hemophiliacs or other individuals who lack specific clotting activities until the laboratory confirms that the substitution or replacement therapy given before operation is adequate to support surgical hemostasis.

Inactivating or inhibiting antibodies to the coagulant activity of factor VIII are by far the most frequent inhibitors encountered; inhibitors to factor IX activity are much less frequent. Even more unexpectedly, these inhibitors can arise rapidly in patients with no history of hemostatic problems, for example, women early in the postpartum period; at any time during the course of autoimmune or rheumatic connective tissue disease; as part of systemic hypersensitivity, particularly a reaction to the drug penicillin; in patients with malignancies, especially lymphomas; and in elderly patients without any obvious disease.

The pathogenesis of these nonspecific inhibitors is not known. In hemophiliacs, the most severely affected and hence more commonly transfused patients acquire these antibodies more frequently, suggesting that the immune system is producing alloantibodies in response to the transfused antigens. Other studies demonstrating concordance of incidence in twins who are only mildly affected implicate a genetic predisposition to produce these antibodies.

These inhibitors are antibodies directed against a specific coagulation factor. Interaction of these antibodies with the target coagulation factor neutralizes the clotting action of the specific factor. In contrast to a simple deficiency of clotting activity, inhibitors prevent further enzyme activation in the enzyme sequence, and a barrier to activation of subsequent coagulation factors is created at the site of inhibition. The degree of inhibition and the impediment to hemostasis depend upon the kinetics of the reaction between the antibody and its target coagulation factor antigen. Usually, the degree of hemostatic jeopardy is determined by the titer of antibody in relation to the amount of coagulation factor or clotting activity.

Fortunately, these inhibitors occur rarely and are always accompanied by abnormal coagulation test results. Often the clotting time is prolonged over 5 minutes, but because there is usually no history of bleeding at previous surgery and no history of bruising, a detailed history directed toward eliciting subtle recent changes in hemostasis may not have been taken, and screening tests may not have been performed. Thus the bleeding can be an unanticipated surprise.

Treatment. If hemostasis collapses during surgery, especially early, when other factors such as consumption are not yet operative, a complete blood count with a platelet count, PT, and PTT should be performed at once. If the initial tests suggest the effects of an inactivating inhibitor but the specific target factor has not yet been identified, an infusion of cryoprecipitate (8 to 24 units) should be started immediately. Cryoprecipitate is rich in factor VIII, and by far the majority of circulating inhibitors are directed against factor VIII. If cryoprecipitate or factor VIII concentrates are not available, fresh frozen plasma can be infused because it contains all of the clotting factors. The replacement should be continued until hemostasis is brought back under control.

Once the specific target factor is identified, massive amounts of the specific factor should be infused until some clotting activity persists long enough to participate in thrombin generation, fibrin formation, and hemostasis. Local mechanical and topical hemostasis can be life-saving in these situations.

If only tenuous hemostasis can be achieved, clotting activity can be supplemented by exchange transfusion with normal fresh frozen plasma, accomplished most easily if plasmapheresis is available. Alternatively, preparations of procoagulant activities isolated and concentrated from the plasma of many donors pooled together can be infused. These are designed to bypass the inhibited activity and trigger the sequence of clotting enzyme reactions beyond the inhibited activity, thus generating thrombin. For example, if factor VIII coagulant activity is inhibited, concentrates of the prothrombin complex isolated from plasma (factors II [prothrombin], VII, IX, and X) can be infused in an attempt to bypass the barrier of factor VIII inhibition.

Restoring hemostasis is the first priority in patients with inhibitors of activity. The second priority is eradicating the clone of immunologically competent cells that is producing the circulating inhibitor. Immunosuppression coupled with intense substitution therapy is generally employed by immunohematologists.

Nonspecific Lupus-Like Anticoagulant. The specific inhibiting antibodies described above must be distinguished from global, nonspecific inhibitors. Both specific and nonspecific global inhibitors prolong the APTT even after reference plasma is added in sufficient amounts to replace any missing but not inhibited clotting activity in the patient's plasma. Nevertheless, only specific, inactivating, or inhibiting antibodies targeted toward a specific clotting factor jeopardize hemostasis. As said earlier, the degree to which hemostasis is endangered depends upon the degree of inhibition of the clotting activity of the target factor. This in turn depends on the combining affinities of the specific inactivating inhibitor with the target coagulation factor and on the relative amounts of competent coagulation factor and titer of specific inactivating or inhibiting antibody.

Nonspecific global inhibitors do not inhibit the clotting activity of a specific or target coagulation factor and do not delay thrombin generation even though they may prolong the APTT by many minutes. At worst, analysis of the clotting activities of all the coagulation factors shows a variable lessening of clotting activity by factors XII, XI, and occasionally IX. The decrease in activity is rarely if ever complete, and usually 30 to 50 per cent of the clotting activities of the factors XII, XI, and IX remain. Regardless of how much the clotting activity is decreased, thrombin generation is not impaired. These nonspecific global inhibitors are probably directed against the procoagulant phospholipid on transformed platelets and other cells such as monocytes and endothelium. The effect of this interference is to prevent the factors from interacting with one another, at least in vitro, but not to inhibit any specific clotting activity. Hemostasis with its intense procoagulant focus overrides this interference, and as a result, the nonspecific global inhibitors have seldom been implicated as the cause of bleeding.

The importance of the nonspecific global circulating inhibitors of anticoagulants lies in the clinical context in which they arise. Indeed, these global circulating inhibitors or anticoagulants are seen so often in systemic lupus erythematosus that they have been given the name lupus-like anticoagulant. The presence of the lupus anticoagulant can antedate the clinical manifestations of systemic lupus erythematosus by months or years. Also, lupus-like anticoagulants are seen in patients taking drugs known to induce clinical lupus erythematosus as well as in individuals with cancer.

It may be that the lupus anticoagulant or the global nonspecific inhibitor is a response to phospholipid, in particular the phospholipid generated to excess in clotting and thrombus formation. Studies have repeatedly suggested that lupus and lupus-like inhibitors or anticoagulants are associated with venous thromboembolism rather than jeopardizing hemostasis and causing bleeding. Thus, surveillance of patients who manifest the lupus-like anticoagulant is an absolute necessity but more because of its associations with the underlying disease and the development of thrombosis.

INTRAOPERATIVE PREVENTION

In the operative period, the risk of hemorrhage can be prevented by (1) paying attention to the important details of operative technique, and (2) preventing of intraoperative coagulopathy.

Attention to Technical Details

Certain technical details are important in preventing perioperative hemorrhage. Excellent hemostasis is provided if *blended electrocautery* is used for tissue dissection and coagulation. *Minimal dissection* of the inflow and outflow arteries reduces the risk of inadvertently damaging surrounding vessels and opening large tissue planes. For the average patient, 5000 units of *heparin* is adequate to prevent thrombosis during the vascular procedure; larger doses may be associated with excessive blood loss. Aortic aneurysmorraphy can be performed without heparinization, and the risk of graft thrombosis, atheromatous embolization, and amputation is not increased.[3]

Selection of the *appropriate graft* will minimize blood loss. Woven grafts are generally selected for thoracic aortic replacement. Knitted grafts are more porous and are usually used to bypass aortoiliac arterial occlusive disease because of their improved handling characteristics. Coated knitted grafts provide better hemostasis, but the cost is higher and their greater thrombogenicity requires attention to technique in order to prevent graft limb thrombosis. Knitted grafts can be *preclotted* by soaking or irrigating them with fresh arterial or venous blood. Excessive irrigation predisposes to clot lysis by activating the fibrinolytic system, and this prolongs the preclotting process. During the preclotting stage, the graft should be under tension so that interstices are maximally clotted. Grafts used in the thoracic aorta, especially those that are used while the patient is undergoing cardiopulmonary bypass, can be preclotted using cryoprecipitate.[2]

In suturing anastomoses, *deep bites* should be taken except at the apex and base of an end-to-side anastomosis; in these areas the sutures must be smaller and closer together in order to prevent lumen constriction. *Tension* on the anastomosis should not be excessive.

In aortic surgery, after completion of the proximal anastomosis, the aortic clamp is released in order to *evaluate hemostasis* of the anastomosis and to determine if the graft has been adequately preclotted. In applying *clamps to the graft,* care must be taken not to disrupt the fabric and cause bleeding. After completion of the bypass, optimal hemostasis is obtained if the *heparin is reversed* with a slow infusion of 25 to 50 mg of protamine sulfate over 10 to 15 minutes. In selected cases with large dissection planes and incomplete hemostasis, *closed suction drains* may be useful in obliterating any tissue dead space and preventing accumulation of hematoma. These drains should be removed as soon as possible.

Intraoperative Prevention of Coagulopathy

If large amounts of packed erythrocytes are required during surgery, specific blood components should also be administered. In general, if 4 to 6 units of packed erythrocytes and a corresponding amount of crystalloid or colloid have been transfused, 1 or 2 units of *fresh frozen plasma* should also be given. This will ensure that concentrations of the stable and labile factors of coagulation (factors V and VIII) are present in amounts adequate to support continuing hemostasis. After the infusion of 6 to 8 units of blood and crystalloid or colloid, *platelets* should be infused. A standard pack consisting of all the platelets harvested from 6 units of fresh plasma is adequate. Precautions relating to ABO and Rh compatibility have been set out earlier.

Autotransfusion devices have an important role in the management of selected patients, but they must be used with care to prevent development of coagulopathy. Disseminated intravascular coagulation can result if tissue fluid or clotted blood is salvaged and readministered. Because this salvaged blood is washed and platelets and plasma are removed, platelet transfusions and fresh frozen plasma are necessary if large volumes are reinfused. Although heparin is added by the autotransfusion system, it is usually removed when the blood is washed by the cell saver. However, because heparin may remain bound to the red cells and be released later, it may be wise to administer 25 mg of protamine sulfate slowly, over 15 minutes, after the cell-saved blood is retransfused.

MANAGEMENT OF BLEEDING

Anastomotic Bleeding

Anastomotic bleeding is controlled by technical methods, local application of hemostatic agents, or both.

Technical Factors

Anastomotic bleeding usually stops spontaneously with local pressure or a simple suture. If additional suturing is required, only small bites are necessary; deeper bites may distort the anastomosis and not control bleeding. If a suture has torn out of the artery, a horizontal mattress suture with a Dacron felt pledget or a small pledget fashioned from an extra piece of graft will suffice. It is best to resuture the vessel with the inflow clamped to reduce the tension and risk of tearing while the suture is tied. In some cases, if the aorta has been completely divided, bleeding from an end-to-end anastomosis can be controlled by sliding a sleeve, cut from the remaining body of the aortic graft, over the anastomosis.

Local Hemostatic Agents

Bleeding from needle holes, suture lines, or tissue planes can be controlled by the topical application of absorbable gelatin sponge (Gelfoam), oxidized cellulose (Surgicel), microfibrillar collagen (Avitene), thrombin, cryoprecipitate, or epsilon-aminocaproic acid (Amicar).

Gelfoam. Gelfoam sponge is prepared from a purified gelatin solution. Its method of action in hemostasis is related to its ability to draw up, by capillary action, many times its weight of whole blood and to trigger coagulation. It is reabsorbed in 4 to 6 weeks without producing significant scar tissue formation.

Surgicel. Surgicel is a knitted fabric of oxidized cellulose that appears to aid clotting by the mechanical effect of swelling into a gelatinous mass after it has been saturated with blood. It should be applied loosely against the bleeding surfaces and in small amounts to facilitate subsequent reabsorption and minimize the possibility of a foreign body reaction.

Tisseel. Tisseel is a fibrin sealant that is formed when a mixture of fibrinogen : factor XIII, which causes the fibrin to cross-link; and aprotinin, which inhibits fibrinolysis, is sprayed onto the bleeding surface with a mixture of activators, including thrombin and calcium chloride. It is useful for controlling graft bleeding from needle holes or significant suture line bleeding.

Avitene. Avitene is made from purified bovine collagen. It is an adjunct to hemostasis because it provides a surface that promotes the adhesion of platelets. They adhere to the fibrils of Avitene and undergo a release reaction that triggers aggregation of nearby platelets into thrombi. Although it is more expensive than other hemostatic agents and can be more difficult to apply, since it must be kept dry, nonetheless, it readily conforms to irregular bleeding surfaces, including anastomoses, and can be used in a heparinized patient.

Topical Thrombin. Dressings soaked with topical thrombin and placed directly on the wound are useful to arrest bleeding from suture holes and tissue cavities. The topical thrombin reacts with the patient's own fibrinogen and any other coagulation factors to achieve a fibrin-rich hemostatic plug. Because the thrombin is provided, the patient may remain anticoagulated systemically by drugs or by an inborn or acquired hemostatic defect. The patient need only provide fibrinogen in his or her blood.

Topical thrombin, usually of bovine origin, is provided as a lyophilized powder. Ordinarily, the powder is dissolved in saline, and the reconstituted mixture has an activity of 1000 biologic thrombin units/ml. However, for local application, the powder does not need to be reconstituted with saline. Rather, it is applied onto an absorbable or nonabsorbable dressing and then placed directly on the wound. Pressure is maintained on the dressing for as long as needed, usually 5 to 10 minutes.

Topical Cryoprecipitate and Thrombin. Dressings soaked with cryoprecipitate and then sprayed with thrombin are useful in stopping bleeding from deep wounds or large bleeding surfaces. This technique is especially helpful in patients who are systemically anticoagulated, either pharmacologically or naturally, and also in those who have undergone extensive tissue dissection. Topical cryoprecipitate is reconstituted as for intravenous injection, except that double the volume of reconstituting fluid is used. It is poured into a sterile basin on the operating table and absorbable or nonabsorbable dressings are placed in the basin, to be impregnated with cryoprecipitate. While the dressings are soaking, a vial of thrombin (1000 units/ml reconstituted with 10 ml saline) and 10 ml of calcium chloride (1 gm/10 ml) are drawn up in a 20-ml syringe. The impregnated dressings are applied directly to the bleeding surfaces, and the topical thrombin is then sprayed over the dressings. A fibrin-rich coagulum results, as the fibrinogen polymerizes over the wound. Alternatively, the cryoprecipitate can be drawn up in a separate syringe and sprayed over the bleeding surface. Immediately thereafter the surface is sprayed with the syringe containing the thrombin. The use of cryoprecipitate is associated with a risk of blood-borne infections.

Topical Epsilon-Aminocaproic Acid. Clotting normally triggers fibrinolysis, which helps prevent excessive clot formation and thrombosis. Intense thrombolytic activity can be triggered by tissue damage, including extensive dissection or inflammation of any vascular tissue. The resultant fibrinolytic activity is often so intense that if there is even a mild deficiency in the patient's ability to generate thrombin, a less than optimal hemostatic plug results, and the lytic activity can disperse the hemostatic plugs and cause bleeding. Enhanced fibrinolysis generated by tissue damage and inflammation can be counteracted by the local administration of epsilon-aminocaproic acid (EACA, Amicar), tranexamic acid (Cyklokapron), or soybean trypsin inhibitor (aprotinin). Dressings impregnated with these agents may be placed directly on the wound or, more usefully, added to the cryoprecipitate and either sprayed on the wound or impregnated into dressings, followed in each instance by thrombin spray. Specifically, one vial (20 gm) of epsilon-aminocaproic acid or equivalent quantities of another antifibrinolytic agent is diluted with saline to 100 ml. Dressings are soaked in epsilon-aminocaproic acid, applied directly to the wound, and sprayed with cryoprecipitate and thrombin. Alternatively, 1.0 ml (5 gm) of the epsilon-aminocaproic acid solution can be added to the syringe containing cryoprecipitate and this mixture sprayed on the wound, followed by the thrombin spray.

Bleeding From the Graft

Diffuse hemorrhage from the graft is usually the result of a consumptive coagulopathy and is managed as described farther on. However, on occasion, the graft may be inadequately preclotted. Reclamping the inflow and waiting a few minutes usually permits the bleeding to stop spontaneously. In difficult cases, it may rarely be necessary to reclamp the graft and apply a dry sponge or one of the local hemostatic agents described earlier to control bleeding. As a final alternative, the graft may have to be replaced with a woven or coated prosthesis.

Disseminated Intravascular Coagulation and Primary Fibrinolysis: Plasma Proteolytic States

Although DIC and primary fibrinolysis (PF) are distinctly different in terms of etiology and pathogenesis, whichever occurs first provokes the other as a compensatory mechanism, and both result in plasma proteolysis. Normally, shortly after hemostasis reacts to injury and thrombin generation is amplified, the onset of fibrin monomer formation triggers fibrinolysis. In this respect, fibrinolysis is a restraint to hemostasis. It lyses the intravascular fibrin thrombi that have lodged throughout the body as a result of unrestricted thrombin generation. Fibrinolysis is a necessary response if vessels are to remain patent and blood flow to continue. In PF, plasminogen activation is driven to exceed the set of restraints and inhibitors, especially plasminogen activator inhibitor 1 (PAI-1). Plasmin generation then saturates its inhibitors, especially alpha$_2$-antiplasmin, so that plasmin in the circulation attacks fibrinogen, factor V, and even factor VIII. Plasmin generated on the surface of platelets and endothelial cells, as well as within hemostatic plugs, attacks the cell membranes and their receptors and inappropriately lyses hemostatic plugs. The cellular and vascular injury initiates coagulation. Thrombin generation is quickly amplified, and platelets are recruited in an effort to restore endothelial competence and hemostasis in the face of ongoing plasma proteolysis.

Some of the conditions capable of driving hemostasis to DIC are sepsis (especially gram-negative sepsis), trauma (especially burn trauma), necrotic tissue and severe infection through activating leukocyte cytokines and cachectin, or tumor necrosis factor, intravascular antibody-antigen and immune reactions, obstetric disorders (dead fetus, retention of placenta), toxins or venoms, intravascular prosthetic devices by destroying circulation blood cells, and hematologic and other malignancies by releasing procoagulant material, often during active treatment and tumor cell lysis.

Although disorders that initiate DIC inevitably result in plasma proteolysis as a compensatory mechanism, PF itself is usually caused by liver failure, associated with deficient synthesis of competent PAI-1 and other barriers to plasminogen activation or with pathologically intense stimuli to plasminogen activation as in vascular surgery involving the great vessels of the thorax and abdomen, especially from their perivascular tissue, or as in the rapid synthesis and release of activators by kidney neoplasms.

Disseminated Intravascular Coagulation

The elements of the cytokine cascade, in particular interleukin-1 and tissue necrosis factor, in some way direct and amplify the pathologic stimuli from the inciting events to drive hemostasis beyond its restraints. Thrombocytopenia usually precedes the triggering of the coagulation cascades. During infection and sepsis and in some of the other etiologic circumstances, platelets are consumed peripherally at the site of infection or tissue damage. Platelets can also be coated with IgG as well as specific antibodies. The consequent membrane damage and partial or complete activation signals the spleen and other organs of the reticuloendothelial system (RES) and macrophage phagocytic system (MPS) to clear them from the blood.

The damage to circulating blood cells and endothelium as well as other fixed tissue cells causes their membranes to either transform into procoagulant surfaces as in hemostasis or at least evolve TF (tissue factor, the cofactor of factor VIIa) on their surfaces. In particular, TF, the activating cofactor of coagulation factor VII, is expressed on the luminal surfaces of endothelial cells and platelets. The widespread activation of factor VII, with the formation of tissue factor/factor VIIa complex and the formation of factor Xa, follows. Widespread generation of factor Xa triggers an intense exponential generation of thrombin. Ordinarily, the RES and MPS are able to deal with these circulating activated complexes along with the natural inhibitors directed toward factor VIIa, but the underlying pathology may also have damaged the major organs of the RES and MPS. If there is significant damage to the inhibitory or clearing capacity of the fixed and circulating elements of the RES and MPS, then factor VIIa may trigger amplification by directly activating factor IXa. Thus, thrombin may be produced at a rate that exceeds the natural constraints intended to contain hemostasis and may preliminarize fibrinogen to circulating fibrin monomers and higher polymers.

Should thrombin generation and fibrin accumulation continue to be amplified, fibrin microthrombi can be laid down throughout the circulation. The intravascular microthrombi lodge throughout the microcirculation but especially in the vascular beds of the kidney, brain, lung, adrenal gland, and skin. The polymerization of fibrin monomers initiates compensatory fibrinolysis. The degree of organ damage from occlusion of the microcirculation by these fibrin-rich microthrombi depends upon the balance between their formation and lysis by plasmin. If the original pathologic stimuli are sustained, the reserves of coagulation factors are exhausted, and the production of fresh coagulation factors is finally outstripped by consumption. Although all the activated clotting factors are subject to inhibition, their activation while on procoagulant surfaces is usually protected. Moreover, thrombin diffuses to create larger and larger zones of activation, upstream and downstream, to further amplify its production. The nonenzymatic coagulation factors—fibrinogen (factor I), factor V, and factor VIII complex—finally become exhausted. Paradoxically, fibrinolysis activated to restrain hemostasis and lyse intravascular fibrin thrombi results in further damage to hemostasis. The products of fibrinolysis, especially the larger fibrin degradation products, such as X and Y, further compromise normal hemostasis by acting as antithrombins and interfering with fibrinogen polymerization. Excessive activation of plasminogen can outstrip its restraints and inhibitors to result in plasminemia, plasma proteolysis, and further attack of intravascular coagulation factors. The progressive consumption of fibrinogen, factor V, and factor VIII by unrestricted hemostasis and their destruction by plasmin as part of plasma proteolysis worsens the hemostasis potential, and the clinical picture relentlessly progresses from trivial oozing to hemorrhage.

Clinical and Laboratory Findings and Treatment. The sequence of clinical and laboratory events making up DIC, plasma fibrinolysis, or primary fibrinolysis is best described with reference to the changes taking place in the normal sine wave of hemostasis caused by DIC. The mechanism begins with thrombosis and culminates in the picture of the hemostatic collapse with consumption of coagulation factors.

The first clinical indications that amplification of coagulation has escaped its restraints and is generating circulating fibrin are that hemostasis becomes more difficult and then impossible to achieve: cautery is effective but only transiently; ligatures hold, but there is bleeding around them; suture holes begin to ooze, and areas previously hemostatically intact break down. The first laboratory clue that unrestrained amplification may be ongoing is the presence of circulating fibrin monomers and soluble fibrin. In DIC, these arise from thrombin generation and fibrin polymerization in the circulation as well as intravascular fibrinolysis recruited and stimulated by thrombin and the deposition of fibrin thrombi.

The most important aspect of treatment is elimination of the original stimulus driving hemostasis and coagulation in DIC. This may require immediate surgery to remove a neoplasm or drain an abscess. During the initial stage of intravascular coagulation, when thrombosis is occurring, heparin and other forms of anticoagulation and antithrombotic therapy are appropriate. In the later stages of DIC, as fibrinogen and the catalytic procoagulant cofactors Va and VIII:C are consumed, the immediate problem is insufficiency of coagulation substrates in the face of the continuing stimulus to coagulation, fibrin formation, and fibrinolysis. Replacement of coagulation factors, plasma restraints, and cellular hemostatic elements is vital. Replacement of the factors consumed during coagulation (factors I, VIII, and V) is best accomplished with cryoprecipitate and blood platelets, the latter being rich in factor V. Once hemostatic measurements begin to return to normal, anticoagulation at low intensity (heparin 100 u/hr) is started. Gradually, replacement therapy is decreased while anticoagulation is increased to regain control over coagulation.

The conflict between those advocating the use of heparin and those advocating the use of replacement therapy alone can be seen as one of timing. Heparin and the other approaches to anticoagulation may be used to counter the effects of ongoing activation. Eventually, in unchecked DIC, hypercoagulability and thrombosis decay into hypocoagulability and bleeding, which makes replacement therapy necessary. The hemostatic vector first climbs above the baseline during thrombosis and then falls below the baseline hemostasis when the coagulation system becomes incompetent. Replacement deflects the hemostatic vector upward, back toward normal hemostatic equilibrium. Anticoagulant treatment is started only when the vector begins to deflect upward, indicating that replacement is supplying adequate substrates for hemostasis. Eliminating the drive to excess hemostasis with anticoagulants prevents an overshoot to thrombosis or a continual oscillation between thrombosis and bleeding.

Primary Fibrinolysis

In PF, the activation of plasmin from plasminogen exceeds restraints to plasminogen activation such that the concentration of plasmin in turn exceeds that of circulating plasma inhibitors, principally alpha$_2$-antiplasmin. This means that plasmin can attack its preferred substrates fibrin and fibrinogen as well as secondary substrates of coagulation factor V and factor VIII complex, especially factor VIII:C. Platelets are also attacked but are rendered poorly functional rather than destroyed completely. In PF, the fibrin monomers and fibrin degradation products arise from the attack of unrestrained plasmin on fibrinogen and fibrin. In both DIC and PF, decompensation takes place when the RES and MPS are saturated and are no longer able to clear the circulation. The result is the same for PF as for DIC—consumption of factor V and factor VIII:C as well as fibrinogen—to the point of hemostasis collapse.

Clinical and Laboratory Diagnosis and Treatment. The clinical picture of PF resembles that of DIC, but the clinical setting of PF is usually different from that of DIC. In PF, patients have liver impairment with decreased synthesis of restraints to plasminogen activation and to plasma itself. Tissue plasminogen activator synthesis and release carry on and can be stimulated by cytokines. If the resultant imbalance becomes excessive, the excess plasminogen can trigger PF. PF is present to a limited degree in patients with polycythemia vera. tPA is released sporadically resulting in large ecchymoses, or systemically from neoplastic cells in patients with promyelocytic leukemia. The therapy of PF is different from DIC, and thus laboratory diagnosis is crucial. In PF, thrombocytopenia is seldom profound because the inciting disorders do not necessarily cause platelet destruction. The concentration of fibrinogen is disproportionately lower than that of factor V, and that of factor V is lower than that of factor VIII:C. Fibrin degradation products are increased in both DIC and PF, but in the latter, products of fibrinogen degradation are attacked by plasma whereas in DIC these are not present.

The treatment of PF requires replacement therapy and the use of fibrinolytic inhibitors. The target substrates of plasmin—fibrinogen (factor I), factor V, and, to a lesser extent, factor VIII—must be replaced. Platelet infusions may be necessary to supply factor V and to replace the platelets that are damaged since their surface shares with endothelium specific receptors for plasminogen. In PF, replacement therapy cannot be limited to one treatment because the disorder causing excess plasminogen activation must be treated. The use of fibrinolytic inhibitors, such as EACA, tranexamic acid, or aprotinin may be necessary. The first two displace plasmin from substrates and bind it. The last is a direct inhibitor of plasmin, kallikrein, and so on. Antifibrinolytic agents are contraindicated in DIC. The fibrinolytic response seen in DIC is secondary to the fibrin thrombi and must not be interfered with lest fibrinolysis fail to clear the thrombi and permanent organ damage result.

Summary: Treatment of the Plasma Proteolytic States

The treatment of DIC and PF, the two disease syndromes that most frequently cause plasma proteolysis, has evolved as the relationship between them has become more clearly appreciated and the pathogenesis more clearly understood. The initial therapy must be directed toward inhibiting and controlling the primary enzyme that causes the hematologic disturbance. Replacement of the targets of the enzyme must be undertaken carefully to provide *minimal* resources to regain homeostasis until the body itself can provide resources for ongoing needs and reserves. Then therapy for the secondary or respondent enzyme activity can be considered.

In DIC, the primary enzyme that threatens hemostasis is unrestrained thrombin production. Primary therapy is anticoagulation with heparin, which is directed towards inhibiting and controlling thrombin. Replacement is provided only to enable primary hemostasis; excessive replacement could cause intravascular thrombus formation. The secondary or respondent enzyme in DIC is plasmin, provoked by intravascular clotting. Drugs to displace or inhibit fibrinolysis can only be given cautiously and not until thrombin generation is extinguished and well under control with heparin. Fibrinolysis is needed to dismantle intravascular microthrombi and restore vascular continuity and blood flow.

In PF, the primary abnormality is uncontrolled plasmin generation and indiscriminate plasmin attack. The main potential for tissue damage is direct attack by plasmin at cell membrane surfaces, whereas the main danger to hemostasis is the attack and destruction of hemostatic structures (plugs, platelet patches, etc.) and endothelium, especially at sites of hemostasis. Circulating factor I, fibrinogen, factor V, and factor VIII are attacked during plasmin action. The secondary consequence is unrestrained thrombin production. The destruction of hemostatic plugs and damage to endothelium provides an overriding demand for hemostasis and eventually an exaggerated generation of thrombin. The thrombin in turn acts synergistically with the plasmin destruction of coagulation substrates to deplete hemostatic reserves even further. Treatment is first directed toward displacing the plasmin enzyme from fibrin, especially on stabilized hemostatic plugs, with tranexamic acid (Cyklokapron) or inhibiting plasmin's enzyme action with aprotinin (Trasylol). Depleted reserves are replenished *only* if necessary to recover hemostasis: factor I, fibrinogen, and factor VIII complex are replaced with cryoprecipitate, 4 to 8 units (bags), and factor V activity is restored with platelet infusion because platelet granules carry factor V. Once replacement is underway, heparin therapy should be considered to moderate the thrombin generated secondarily in response to the attack on hemostasis by unrestrained plasmin.

Postoperative Bleeding

Patients with postoperative bleeding who exhibit signs of hypovolemia require reoperation. The principles for managing anastomotic and graft bleeding and systemic coagulopathy are the same as those described earlier. A wound hematoma is best evacuated under sterile conditions in the operating room to reduce the risk of infection and the possibility of a false aneurysm and to speed wound healing.

SUMMARY

Perioperative bleeding is one of the most common of the serious complications of vascular surgery. All vascular surgery patients should be screened by history, physical examination, and coagulation studies in order to detect primary and secondary coagulation abnormalities. Coagulopathies should be corrected before surgery. Bleeding is prevented in the operating room by careful attention to technical details. If large volumes of blood are administered, blood component therapy is necessary to prevent a coagulopathy.

References

1. Bergqvist D. Ljungstrom K-G: Hemorrhagic complications resulting in reoperation after peripheral vascular surgery: A fourteen-year experience. J Vasc Surg 6:134, 1987.
2. Glynn MFX, Williams WG: A technique for preclotting vascular graft. Ann Thorac Surg 29:182, 1980.
3. Johnston KW, Scobie TK: Multicenter prospective study of nonruptured abdominal aortic aneurysms. I. Population and operative management. J Vasc Surg 7:69, 1988.
4. Livio M, Mannucci PM, Vigano G, et al: Conjugated estrogens for the management of bleeding associated with renal failure. N Engl J Med 315:731, 1986.
5. Mulherin JL. Allen TR, Edwards WH, et al: Management of early postoperative complications of arterial repairs. Arch Surg 112:1371, 1977.
6. Sproul G, Pinto JM, Trummer MJ, et al: Reoperation for early complications of arterial surgery. Arch Surg 104:814, 1972.

35

Graft Thrombosis and Thromboembolic Complications

Anthony J. Comerota, M.D., F.A.C.S., and Robert B. Rutherford, M.D.

• • •

The vascular surgeon constantly tries to avoid the two extreme complications of vascular surgery, bleeding and thrombosis. This chapter considers the thromboembolic complications of arterial reconstruction with an emphasis on graft thrombosis.

The responsibility of the vascular surgeon is not limited to the performance of a technically satisfactory bypass. The timing and appropriateness of the procedure must be put into the context of the patient's symptoms and disability, the natural history of the disease, and the durability and complications of the planned procedure. All treatment alternatives must be considered, including noninterventional care. If a bypass is chosen, not only are the proper location of the bypass and graft selection important, but the subsequent management (i.e., graft surveillance and the treatment of the failing and failed graft) can have a significant effect on long-term patency. The latter is a major focus of this chapter.

After a discussion of the causes, prevention, and management of graft thrombosis, the thromboembolic complications of arterial reconstruction are reviewed, with a focus on intravascular thrombosis at or distal to the site of reconstruction and the embolic events that may occur during the dissection or at the time flow is restored.

GRAFT THROMBOSIS

In the minds of most vascular surgeons, graft thrombosis is the ultimate complication of arterial reconstruction. Although other complications, such as graft sepsis or distal thromboembolic complications, may have more dire consequences, thrombosis is the most tangible measure of graft failure. Indeed, the success of a bypass procedure is traditionally measured by graft patency rates.

Incidence

Early graft thrombosis probably occurs more frequently than is generally appreciated because of the practice of excluding from life table calculations of graft patency occlusions occurring in the first days after surgery in which patency can be successfully restored. The reported incidence of early graft thrombosis varies widely, from less than 2 per cent in large-diameter or high-flow grafts (e.g., aortobifemoral or aortorenal bypasses) to 20 per cent for difficult distal bypasses.[1] Furthermore, late occlusion rates are rarely less than 10 per cent in 5 years, even for the best-performing bypass grafts, and they may exceed 80 per cent for some infrainguinal bypasses performed for limb salvage. When prosthetic bypasses are carried to the infrapopliteal arteries, less than 25 per cent are still patent by 5 years. Similar dismal results are experienced after some extra-anatomic bypasses, such as an axillofemoral bypass, when performed in the presence of superficial femoral artery occlusion.[2] Because of the relative frequency of this complication, it has a major bearing on the overall results of arterial reconstruction, and its prevention and management must be considered integral parts of the successful operative approach to limb salvage. The discussion that follows focuses on infrainguinal bypass procedures because the problem is greatest here and more critical investigation has been carried out with grafts in this location.

Etiology

Understanding the fate of bypass grafts and the likely causes of graft failure at different intervals after implantation will help direct appropriate preventive measures and substantially influence the management of these graft occlusions. This background information may materially influence the initial choice of procedures and the graft material used. The likely etiology of graft thrombosis changes as the time from implantation increases (Fig. 35–1). Occlusion within 1 week of operation and particularly within 2 to 3 days is generally attributed to technical error or to poor patient selection. Occlusions occurring after the first few days but within 1 month may well be due to more subtle technical imperfections, persistent underlying disease, or surface thrombogenicity of the graft that exceeds its thrombotic threshold. Sauvage and coworkers suggested that there is a *critical threshold velocity* for sustaining early graft patency.[3] This not only varies with graft material but also changes with time for the same graft material. Thus, although early graft thrombosis must be assumed, for all

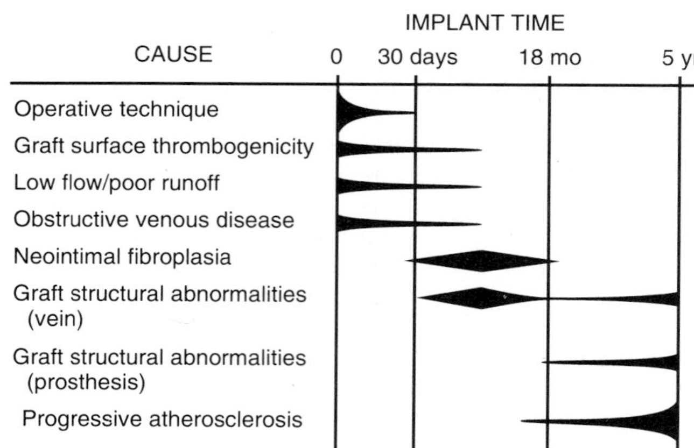

FIGURE 35–1. The factors contributing to graft occlusion with time. (Modified from Rutherford RB: The prevention and management of graft thrombosis. *In* Kempczinski RF [ed]: The Ischemic Leg. Chicago, Year Book Medical Publishers, 1985.)

practical purposes, to be due to technical error, graft surface thrombogenicity must be accepted as a bonafide cause of early graft thrombosis, particularly in distal bypasses in which small-caliber grafts are placed into a low-flow, high-resistance circulation.

All vascular surgeons have observed instances of early graft thrombosis corrected by simple thrombectomy in which subsequent long-term patency was achieved. This is particularly true with prosthetic grafts. Properly harvested autologous veins slough their endothelial surface for only a brief period, so that their increased surface thrombogenicity is rather transient. In contrast, the surfaces of prosthetic and modified heterologous grafts reduce their thrombogenicity after a period of weeks or months, but unfortunately they never reduce their thrombogenicity comparably to that of autologous veins. Abnormal platelet consumption on prosthetic bypass grafts often does not subside until 6 months after implantation and may never return to normal.[4] In humans, such grafts do not undergo significant endothelialization but are lined with a layer of compacted fibrin. Although this has a negative charge and is much less thrombogenic than the initial prosthetic surface, it does not compare with a healthy endothelial layer in resisting thrombosis. Although the length and the diameter of bypass grafts can also be shown to correlate with patency, the lack of an endothelial surface and graft compliance are the two major contributors to the failure of today's arterial substitutes, and of the two, the lack of surface endothelium appears to be the more important. Current research into endothelial seeding and sodding and other means of endothelializing graft surfaces may change this outlook (see Chapter 26).

Although more patients with graft thrombosis are suspected of harboring predisposing clotting abnormalities than are documented, hypercoagulability must be considered among the important causes of graft occlusion. Towne and associates implicated low levels of antithrombin III in patients with repeated graft failure.[5] Even patients with normal preoperative coagulation profiles have significant increases in clotting factors (Factor VIII) and platelet reactivity, as well as reductions in antithrombin III levels in the early period after lower extremity bypass.[6] Furthermore, hypotension, hypothermia, and acidosis are common features after major transabdominal aortic reconstruction, and all can contribute to periods of abnormal coagulability during the perioperative period. Thus, coagulation disturbances probably play a greater role in producing graft thrombosis than is generally realized. Whittemore and colleagues studied 60 patients who had had acute graft thrombosis and found that the presence of a circulating lupus anticoagulant was the most frequent hypercoagulable abnormality, followed by protein C deficiency and heparin-induced platelet aggregation.[7] As the sophistication of routine coagulation laboratories continues to improve, greater numbers of hypercoagulable states undoubtedly will be identified and appropriately treated. In turn, pharmacologic manipulation can be expected to play an increasingly important role in maintaining graft patency and improving limb salvage.

Occlusive disease in the vessels beyond the reconstructed segment, known as *poor runoff,* can play a role in determining early graft patency. Runoff is commonly graded from arteriographic patterns of occlusive disease in vessels beyond the distal anastomosis;[8] however, this method is crude and allows only gross correlation with patency. When good- and poor-runoff groups are compared, the slopes of projected patency rates for femoropopliteal bypasses run roughly parallel courses after an initial period of more rapid dropoff in the poor-runoff group. The degree of separation primarily represents significantly different rates of early postoperative thrombosis.[9, 10] LiCalzi and Stansel combined a number of factors (runoff, graft length, and graft diameter) to create a *closure index*, which achieves better correlation with graft patency.[11] Although impractical for routine clinical use, flow measurements obtained with electromagnetic flow probes have proved to be of prognostic value in distal reconstructions. Both basal flow levels and the response to drug-induced hyperemia have correlated with graft patency.[12, 13] Grafts with flow rates lower than 100 ml/min have been shown to have a lower patency than those with higher flow rates. Resistance measurements have also been correlated with graft patency.[14] Graft diameter plays a role in determining graft flow only in extreme situations.[15] Given a flow rate that is fixed over a large range by the peripheral resistance in the runoff vessels, increasing diameter *decreases* flow velocity. At the other extreme, a graft that is too small may serve as an impediment to flow, and the layering of fibrin on its inner surface may cause it to become significantly more narrow. For example, a 1-mm circumferential fibrin lining results in more than a 50 per cent reduction in the cross-sectional area of a graft that is 6 mm in diameter.

Venous obstruction, both acute and chronic, can increase arterial outflow resistance and is an underappreciated factor that adversely affects graft patency. Patients with symptomatic obliterative arterial disease can develop rapidly progressive ischemic symptoms following the onset of acute proximal deep vein thrombosis. Unrecognized acute deep vein thrombosis can lead to early graft failure due to high outflow resistance. Similar observations have been made in patients with chronic venous obstruction, as demonstrated by Filippone and coworkers when they analyzed the results of femoropopliteal bypass for limb salvage in patients with grade III chronic venous disease.[16] Seven of the nine grafts were prosthetic, and two were saphenous vein. There were five early failures (30 days), resulting in a 1-month patency rate of 45 per cent. All five of the early failures occurred in prosthetic grafts. Of the remaining four patients, three had thrombosis by 6 months and one required a below-knee amputation for uncontrolled infection. Therefore, increased venous resistance on the other side of the capillary bed increases arterial runoff resistance, resulting in early graft failure. Although the availability of saphenous veins may be limited if these patients require a bypass for limb salvage, it is particularly important that autogenous material be used. The surgeon must seriously question performing a bypass for intermittent claudication in these patients because the likelihood of failure is so high.

Graft length has been shown to correlate adversely with graft patency, but this factor probably has an impact later,[17] as does graft compliance. Both may contribute to graft occlusion during the intermediate postoperative period (1 to 18 months). Most graft occlusions occurring during this period have been blamed on the development of *neointimal fibroplasia,* to which these two factors may contribute. The understanding and control of neointimal fibroplasia play such an important role in the success of revascularization procedures that it has been given independent coverage elsewhere in this text (see Chapter 14).

After 12 to 18 months, most occlusions are caused by either local recurrence or progressive atherosclerosis of the proximal or distal vessels. Szilagyi and coworkers' classic study of autologous vein femoropopliteal grafts showed that approximately 33 per cent developed some structural abnormalities during the 10-year follow-up.[18] There was an 8 per cent incidence of intimal thickening and a 4 per cent incidence of fibrous stenosis in the intermediate period. Identical incidences of atheromatous narrowing and aneurysm formation (8 and 4 per cent, respectively) were observed, with the latter occurring much later (mean onset, at 45 and 28 months, respectively). Structural abnormalities occur less frequently in prosthetic grafts, although *fabric failure* has been reported for most grafts,[19] particularly the porous, ultralightweight grafts popular in the early 1980s.[20] One survey revealed approximately a 4 per cent rate of such fabric failures, with aneurysm formation and, occasionally, rupture or local extravasation. Such dilatated prostheses can also develop considerable mural thrombus, as seen in natural aneurysms, and this can eventually lead to graft thrombosis or distal embolism. Bovine (carotid artery) heterografts and modified human umbilical vein grafts have been observed to undergo aneurysmal changes.[21–23] However, these degenerative changes have not led to significant graft occlusion, because most studies have shown that disease progression at or beyond the distal anastomosis is the most common cause of late graft failure.[14, 24–26]

In situ saphenous vein bypasses have grown in popularity, especially for revascularizing infrapopliteal vessels. Donaldson and associates reviewed 455 consecutive patients to evaluate the primary cause of failure in the 92 grafts that occluded during follow-up.[27] Among the likely causes of graft failure, 60 per cent (55 of 92) were intrinsic to the graft. These causes included (in order of decreasing frequency) perianastomotic stenosis, vein stricture, focal stenosis, valvulotome injury, kink, retained valve leaflet, intimal flap, and residual arteriovenous fistula. Of these intrinsic causes, 36 per cent (20 of 55) were directly related to the in situ technique. Thirty-seven per cent of the failures were extrinsic to the graft and included (in order of decreasing frequency) compromised outflow, hypercoagulability, systemic hypotension, compromised inflow, and graft sepsis. The authors hypothesized that improvements in operative technique, patient selection, and perioperative management might have prevented 44 per cent of the primary in situ graft failures.

Diagnosis

Early recognition of graft thrombosis is extremely important. Even if graft thrombosis does not immediately threaten limb viability, the success of management (i.e., thrombectomy or thrombolysis) decreases as the time between graft thrombosis and treatment increases. Evaluation of graft status by physical examination alone may be difficult even for the experienced observer, particularly when peripheral pulses are not palpable postoperatively because of residual occlusive disease in the distal arterial tree. Assessment of a peripheral pulse by nurses or inexperienced house officers is clearly unreliable. However, frequent monitoring of Doppler velocity signals over pedal arteries, with determination of ankle systolic pressure, overcomes much of this uncertainty and is now accepted as standard care for early postoperative monitoring after lower extremity arterial reconstruction. Doppler monitoring of flow through the graft itself may be instructive if the clinician is familiar with the significance of qualitative differences in the audible Doppler signals or their analog tracings. However, polytetrafluoroethylene grafts frequently cannot be directly insonated with Doppler monitoring during the early postoperative period because of the air trapped in the interstices of the graft, which transmits ultrasound waves poorly.

Late monitoring of graft patency by periodic examination of ankle pressures, direct graft surveillance by duplex imaging, and observation of the patient's response to treadmill exercise or some other means of induced hyperemia may detect impending graft failure. This close surveillance has been demonstrated to add significantly to graft patency after femoropopliteal bypasses when an impending lesion is identified and corrected before thrombosis.[28, 29] Patients with subcutaneously placed bypasses or easily palpable pulses should be taught to monitor their grafts frequently; if claudication symptoms, weakness, numbness, or changes in temperature or color develop abruptly, they should seek attention. If patients are taught the signs and symptoms of graft failure, with an emphasis on the importance of immediate presentation for treatment, prompt intervention may result in improved secondary patency rates.

Prevention

Preventing operative and postoperative graft thrombosis begins with a careful preoperative anatomic and hemodynamic evaluation of the patient. Thorough angiographic study, a thorough search with duplex imaging for all potential sources of autogenous vein grafts, and attention to detail (i.e., resisting short cuts) all help to avoid intraoperative pitfalls and prevent early graft failure. Obviously, the vascular surgeon's approach to prevention should be based on an understanding of the etiologic factors discussed earlier and should use measures designed to avoid or minimize them. Technical errors are avoided with experience and continued attention to detail. The best available arterial substitute for the proposed bypass should always be chosen. Beyond this, some method of intraoperative detection of technical flaws should be part of the operative routine. The most practical method of evaluating the bypass intraoperatively is completion arteriography. Narrowing at the site of controlling clamps or vessel loops; the presence of intimal flaps, a suture line, or mural or intramural thrombus; axial twisting or extrinsic compression of the graft; and other unexpected problems can be readily detected when proper angiographic technique is used.[30] Stept and colleagues demonstrated that 15 per cent of early graft failures were due to technical problems, and another 10 per cent were due to undetected emboli (Fig. 35–2);[31] therefore, 25 per cent (or more) of early graft failures were potentially detectable with good completion arteriography.

Listening over the graft and vessels adjacent to the

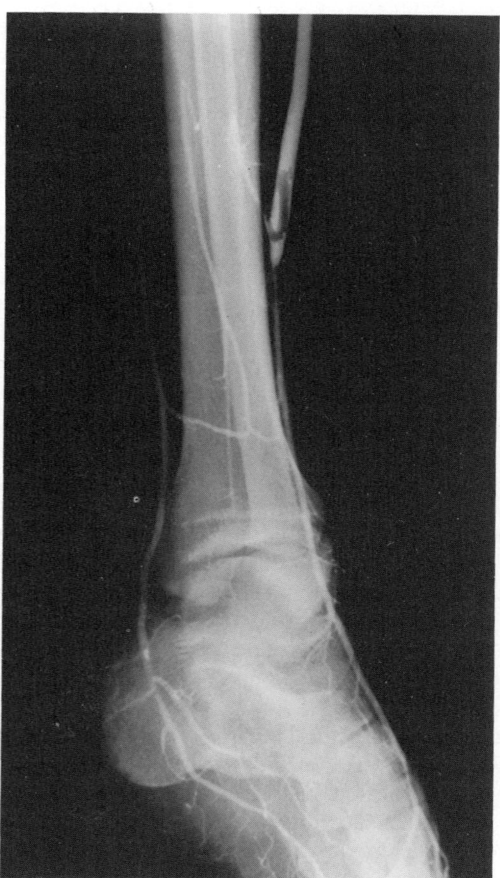

FIGURE 35–2. Completion arteriogram obtained after a femoral–anterior tibial bypass demonstrates an unsuspected distal embolus. This demonstrates the value of completion arteriography for identifying the problem and the value of sequential release of the vascular clamps. Through the restoration of perfusion to the least important outflow bed first (the proximal anterior tibial artery), the embolus was directed proximally, protecting the important distal outflow tract.

anastomoses with a Doppler probe,[32] imaging them with a B-mode or duplex ultrasound scanner,[33] and looking at them from within with a fiberoptic angioscope[34] all have merit. In most centers, these new techniques have yet to match the confidence and accuracy of good-quality completion arteriography. The completion arteriogram is far more accurate than clinical assessment and has provided invaluable information during the follow-up period; in selected instances, it has also identified patients in whom numerous reoperations for graft occlusion could be avoided. In a prospective study, Gilbertson and coworkers intraoperatively evaluated in situ bypasses with angiography, angioscopy, and duplex scanning.[35] Grafts were evaluated for anastomotic stenosis, residual valve cusps, and patent vein side branches. Angioscopy was significantly more sensitive than either duplex scanning or angiography in detecting residual valve cusps. No anastomotic stenosis was confirmed; however, the false-positive rates for stenosis detection were 20 per cent for angiography, 10 per cent for duplex scanning, and 0 per cent for angioscopy. Therefore, for the intraoperative evaluation of the in situ graft itself and the sites of anastomosis, angioscopy may be preferable. A thorough discussion of the methods of assessing the technical adequacy of bypass grafts is presented in Chapter 24.

Avoidance of hypotension by hemodynamic monitoring is part of basic patient care and underlines the role of low flow in causing early postoperative thrombosis. Increasing flow velocity by constructing an arteriovenous fistula at or near the distal anastomosis has been advocated to improve the patency of difficult distal bypasses, with varying results.[36–38] Until more convincing evidence exists, most surgeons are unwilling to add this additional technical maneuver to an already difficult procedure.

Sympathectomy increases the flow primarily through the opening of arteriovenous communications; for this reason, it has been used as an adjunctive procedure. Experimentally, it has been shown to enhance the early patency of small vascular anastomoses[39] and injured arteries.[40] In at least one clinical series, it has been suggested to enhance the patency of femoropopliteal bypasses.[9] Unfortunately, in the proximal reconstructions that would readily permit concomitant sympathectomy, it is not needed, whereas in distal bypasses, a second, anatomically separate operation would be required. Better proof of efficacy is required for its recommendation. Pharmacologic methods have demonstrated sufficient efficacy to make an operation unnecessary for sympathetic ablation.[41, 42]

Pharmacotherapy is the most commonly used adjunctive method of preserving graft patency. The goals of pharmacologic intervention are to (1) decrease platelet deposition on the bypass graft or endarterectomy site, (2) minimize thrombus formation, (3) prevent the development of neointimal fibroplasia, and (4) prevent disease progression. Use of each method must be balanced by an awareness of its efficacy and its potential for complications.

Although heparin is used routinely to prevent thrombosis intraoperatively during periods of arterial occlusion, heparin use carries a significant risk of hemorrhagic complications of the wound when it is continued postoperatively. Such risk is ordinarily accepted only after graft thrombectomy or thrombolysis or in patients undergoing reconstructive procedures associated with a high risk of failure. Low-molecular-weight heparin appears to provide greater protection against thrombosis relative to the risk of bleeding,[43, 44] and when approved, it may offer a reasonable compromise in the future. Warfarin compounds are not of much value in the immediate postoperative period unless they are started preoperatively. Most vascular surgeons do not begin patients on warfarin compounds preoperatively; therefore, these compounds require 3 to 4 days to achieve a therapeutic effect and their action cannot be rapidly adjusted. Many surgeons use warfarin compounds to enhance intermediate patency. Although one study has shown this practice to be ineffective,[45] others have demonstrated a significantly better 30-month patency rate in patients who received femoropopliteal bypasses for limb salvage[46] and in those who have prosthetic bypasses to the tibial vessels.[47] Warfarin compounds are commonly given to patients undergoing secondary reconstructions and to those with axillofemoral or axillobifemoral bypass grafts. Warfarin's ability to elevate depressed antithrombin III levels,[48] even at low dosages, has encouraged its use in this setting, even though this specific cause of graft failure has been implicated in no more than 20 per cent of patients.[49] Because the perioperative period may be associated with physiologically diminished antithrombin III levels, these compounds may offer greater advantage than previously recognized. Warfarin is also the drug of choice in most other hypercoagulable states (e.g., protein C and protein S deficiencies, hyperfibrinogenemia, and lupus-like anticoagulant).

Platelet inhibitors (e.g., aspirin) are the pharmacologic agents most frequently used to prolong patency of bypass grafts. They have also been demonstrated to reduce cardiovascular complications of atherosclerosis significantly. Perhaps most important is the confidence physicians have in their safety. In experimental canine studies, platelet inhibitors have improved low-caliber graft patency, primarily because a significant number of dogs' platelets are hyperaggregable. This factor has been shown to be of greater importance than the graft alternatives under comparison in some experimental studies.[50] An important basis for the use of platelet inhibitors in humans undergoing arterial reconstruction comes from the demonstration that for months after surgery, there is increased platelet utilization on endarterectomy and prosthetic surfaces. In a prospective, randomized study, Goldman and associates showed in humans that compared with a placebo, aspirin and dipyridamole significantly reduced platelet deposition on prosthetic femoropopliteal bypasses.[51] No difference in platelet deposition at 1 week was noted in patients in whom an autogenous vein was used; this result was due to the naturally low platelet deposition on veins in the control group. Long-term patency of coronary artery bypass grafts has been demonstrated with the use of platelet inhibitors. This was conclusively shown by a prospective, randomized, double-blind trial performed by Chesebro and coworkers.[52, 53] Significantly better angiographically proven patency was found in patients receiving aspirin (325 mg) plus dipyridamole (75 mg three times daily) than in those receiving a placebo. To achieve this benefit, however, patients should be given the drugs preoperatively. Additionally, mural thrombus formation after carotid endarterectomy was shown to be diminished in patients who received perioperative platelet inhibition.[54] Green and coworkers showed significantly better patency of above-knee femoropopliteal bypasses in patients taking aspirin and dipyridamole than in controls.[55]

Although not uniformly successful in preventing neointimal hyperplasia, platelet inhibition is commonly used for this purpose, and selected studies have demonstrated benefit. In carefully performed animal studies, McCann and associates demonstrated a significant decrease in intimal hyperplasia in experimental vein grafts in animals receiving aspirin and dipyridamole.[56] Metke and colleagues likewise demonstrated a reduction in intimal thickening in canine coronary bypass vein grafts with the use of dipyridamole and aspirin.[57] These experimental observations parallel the clinical benefit observed in patients, as reported by Chesebro and coworkers.[53]

Neointimal thickening is a complex phenomenon resulting from many factors[58–62] (see also Chapter 14). *Pure neointimal fibroplasia* refers to the proliferation of smooth muscle cells that gain access to the lumen through damage to the endothelium and continue to proliferate and transform into secretory cells, synthesizing the extracellular matrix that contributes to this lesion. The process is initiated by endothelial damage, which is followed by the interaction of platelets with the vessel wall, which is followed by the release of growth factors. Inflammatory cells that are involved release cytokines and other substances, which further stimulate migration and proliferation. It has also been demonstrated that organized luminal thrombus in an advanced state demonstrates both gross and microscopic features of the thickened mural fibroplastic tissue, which is difficult to differentiate from primary, smooth muscle neointimal fibroplasia.[63] Therefore, any pharmacologic agent that reduces thrombus formation at suture lines, endarterectomy surfaces, angioplasty sites, or prosthetic surfaces may reduce the clinical development of neointimal fibroplasia. It is imperative, however, that these agents be pharmacologically active and have sustained effect at the time of vessel injury and thrombus formation.

Dextran 40 is a drug that improves blood flow and decreases coagulability. The former depends on volume expansion; the latter, on decreased platelet adhesiveness[64] and reduction of factor VIII activity.[65] This agent is also believed to have a coating effect on endothelial surfaces, to decrease electronegativity, and to increase clot lysability.[66] Hemodilution also occurs, which reduces blood viscosity. Rutherford and associates reported on a randomized, multicenter trial in which dextran 40 decreased the early postoperative occlusion rate of "difficult" distal bypasses more than threefold.[1] The 4-day regimen was particularly effective in femorotibial bypasses and in any femorodistal bypass in which a prosthetic was used. It consisted of five 500-ml units of dextran 40, the first unit with induction of anesthesia at 100 ml/hr, the second unit on the day of the operation at 75 ml/hr, and additional units on each of the first 3 postoperative days, all at 75 ml/hr. This is the most efficacious method of preventing early postoperative thrombosis in patients undergoing distal bypasses. The volume administered may need to be modified in patients with a history of congestive heart failure and in those with compromised myocardium. If increased flow is not needed (e.g., in patients undergoing carotid endarterectomy or during reactive hyperemia following distal bypass) or if increased volume will not be well tolerated, a single 500-ml unit daily at 20 to 25 ml/hr will suffice. However, because dextran 40's effect is short-lived, its benefit may need to be consolidated by combining it with other agents, such as platelet inhibitors or warfarin.

Newer antithrombotic agents and platelet inhibitors show promise in improving efficacy and reducing complication rates. Low-molecular-weight heparin,[43, 44, 66] hirudin,[67–70] specific platelet receptor glycoprotein blockade,[71] and saralasin[72] all have been demonstrated to be beneficial in animal models, either in reducing thrombus formation, in decreasing platelet aggregation, or by inhibiting the development of intimal fibroplasia.

Graft Surveillance

Bypass graft surveillance and intervention for the failing graft will avert a significant number of graft occlusions. As alluded to earlier, careful attention to signs and symptoms of impending graft failure, such as recurrent or progressive intermittent claudication, a decreasing ankle pressure or pulse waveform, or diminished flow velocity with routine arterial duplex surveillance can identify lesions. Correction of these lesions before graft thrombosis will significantly improve long-term patency. Whittemore and colleagues clearly demonstrated this when they reported the results of secondary femoropopliteal reconstruction.[73] Frequent postoperative follow-up examinations allowed recognition of a failing graft, and correction of the lesion before graft thrombosis yielded an 85 per cent 5-year patency rate. If graft failure was not appreciated before graft thrombosis and correction followed graft thrombectomy, a significantly lower patency rate at 5 years (19 per cent) was observed ($p = .008$). New autogenous vein grafts resulted in a 37 per cent 5-year patency rate, in contrast to prosthetic grafts, none of which was patent at 5 years. These observations were supported by Berkowitz and Greenstein when they reported an 80 per cent 4-year patency rate after correction of a graft stenosis before thrombosis, compared with a 13 per cent 1-year patency rate and a 0 per cent 4-year patency rate after a thrombosed graft was reopened.[29] Bandyk and coworkers extended these observations to in situ grafts, with careful surveillance and correction of developing lesions.[28] Graft velocities of less than 40 cm/sec identified grafts at risk and generated a careful search to identify and correct a causative lesion. This approach improved the patency of femoropopliteal bypasses from 48 per cent to 89 per cent at 4 years ($p < .0001$) and that of femorotibial bypasses from 58 per cent to 80 per cent at 4 years ($p < .005$). Careful graft surveillance should improve overall graft patency rates by 15 to 20 per cent.

Management

Appropriate management of a graft occlusion depends on numerous considerations:

1. Likely cause of occlusion
2. Degree of ischemia
3. Patient's ability to tolerate reoperation
4. Graft type
5. Original indications for operation

6. Current indications for revascularization
7. Condition of proximal and distal arteries
8. Likelihood of success (and complications) of intervention

The approach to the failed bypass graft depends on the time of failure: graft failure is divided into early graft thrombosis and late graft occlusion.

Early Graft Thrombosis

Most of the considerations mentioned earlier apply to late graft failures. With early graft failure, the original indications for surgery still apply, and either the status of the inflow and the outflow vessels is unchanged or they can be restored to their preoperative status by thrombectomy and intraoperative thrombolysis. Therefore, if thrombosis is recognized early, at a stage of reversible ischemia and without a substantial change in the patient's general condition, immediate reoperation with thrombectomy, intraoperative intra-arterial infusion of thrombolytic agents, intraoperative arteriography, and correction of any technical errors must be considered the accepted means of management.

Exceptions to this policy require justification. The decision not to operate could be justified if the patient has suffered an acute myocardial infarction or some other life-threatening complication after the original operation, forcing the surgeon to observe the priority of life over limb. Occasionally, uncorrectable difficulties, such as a very poor vein graft or severity of disease in the recipient vessels unrecognized at the original operation, may convince the surgeon to accept graft thrombosis rather than pursue attempts to postpone the inevitable. However, such a decision should be made at the time of the original operation, not at the time of occlusion. More objective means of making this latter decision are desirable, such as the approach described by Ascer and associates of measuring the outflow resistance in the distal arterial bed.[14]

Late Graft Occlusion

For the purpose of this discussion, *late graft occlusion* refers to graft failure that occurs more than 30 days after implantation. With these patients, the clinician has several options:

1. No intervention
2. Catheter-directed thrombolysis with identification and correction of the underlying stenosis
3. Operative thrombectomy and revision
4. New bypass

In patients who present late with advanced and irreversible ischemic change or in patients who have no reasonable options following occlusion (e.g., bypass to small, distal arteries with compromised outflow and no autologous vein available), primary amputation should be considered. A suggested management plan is outlined in Figure 35–3. The

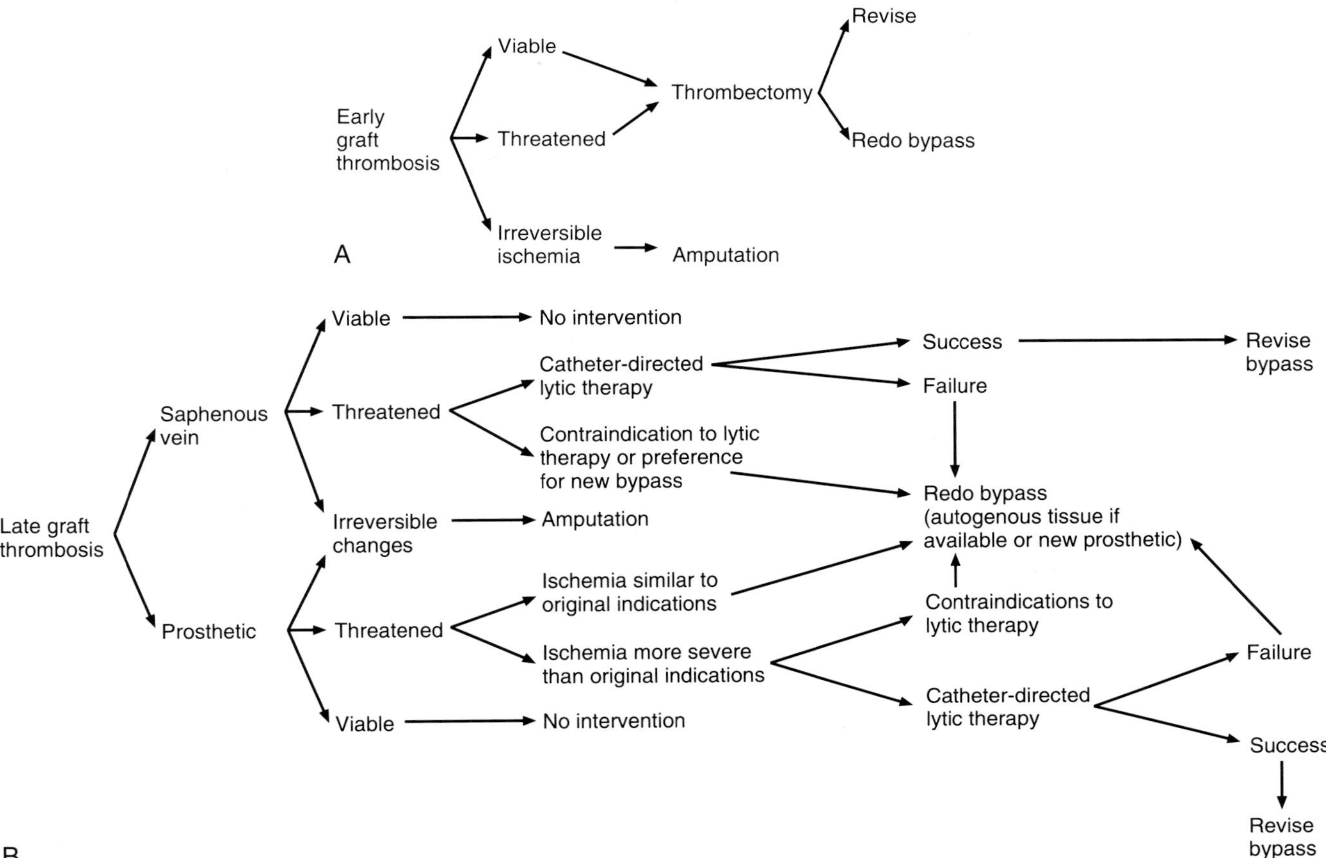

FIGURE 35–3. Algorithm outlining the management of early graft thrombosis *(A)* and late graft thrombosis *(B)*.

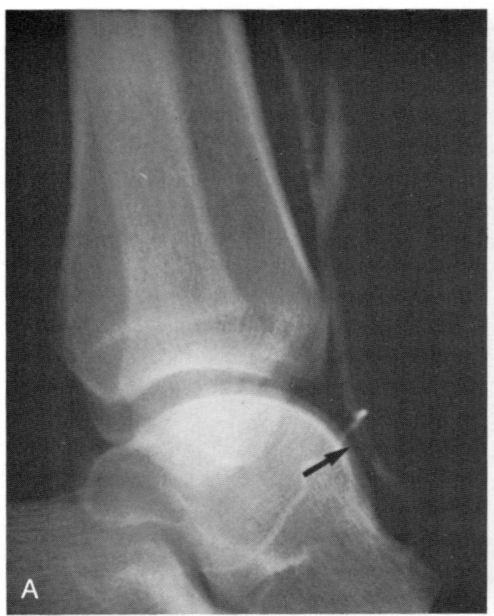

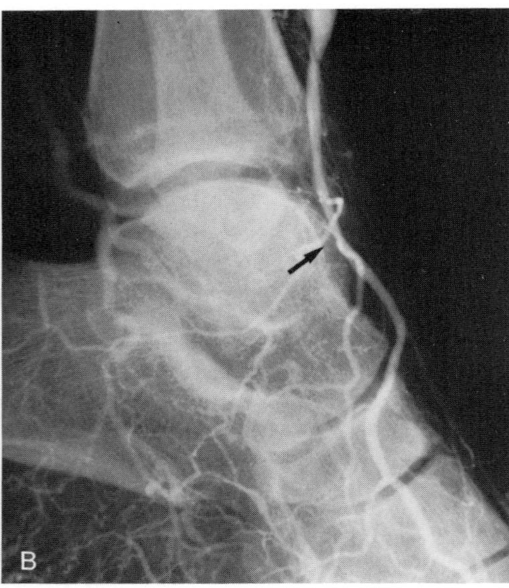

FIGURE 35–4. *A*, Completion arteriogram obtained after a femoral–distal anterior tibial in situ bypass in a patient with a circulating lupus anticoagulant and gangrene of the tip of the great toe. A thrombus formed in the dorsalis pedis artery during the procedure, or an embolus occurred after reperfusion *(arrow)*. The patient's heparin was supplemented intraoperatively, the graft was clamped, and 250,000 units of urokinase (UK) was infused over 30 minutes. The vascular clamps were removed, and Doppler signals sounded normal. *B*, The angiogram obtained after UK infusion demonstrates lysis of the thrombus in the dorsalis pedis artery, with return of the foot vasculature to its preoperative condition *(arrow)*.

first consideration in this decision tree is limb viability. Irreversible ischemia leaves primary amputation as the only option. At the other extreme, patients presenting with a viable extremity after some delay following graft occlusion may require no treatment if the original indication for reconstruction no longer applies. This is most likely in patients with claudication, but it can also occur following bypass for limb salvage if an ischemic ulcer or open foot wound has healed and the limb is no longer at risk. This is attested to by the fact that limb salvage rates are higher than patency rates following distal bypass for this indication. The threatened but reversibly ischemic extremity must be promptly evaluated because it needs immediate reperfusion, with treatment planned accordingly. In patients with severe motor and sensory dysfunction, immediate thrombectomy with operative arteriography is indicated, with the need for further revision being determined by the findings on the operative arteriogram. Patients with less severe ischemia may be candidates for catheter-directed thrombolytic therapy. Whereas thrombectomy is the procedure of choice for early graft thrombosis, it gives disappointing results with late graft occlusions,[73] particularly if patients present after some delay.

Thrombolytic therapy has several advantages and in many centers has become the preferred means of managing late graft occlusion. Graor and colleagues demonstrated better patency and limb salvage rates in patients who had lytic therapy and graft revision than in those who had operative thrombectomy and revision.[74] When the follow-up was extended to 500 days, the majority of patients in both treatment groups had rethrombosis of their grafts; however, patients in the thrombolysis group continued to show better patency and limb salvage rates. Although the initial experience with catheter-directed thrombolysis was encouraging, longer-term follow-up reported from many centers was disappointing, and these results appeared no better than those with operative thrombectomy.[75, 76] As experience with catheter-directed thrombolysis has expanded[77] and more critical analyses have been performed, a number of observations have been made that might assist in the selection of patients who are likely to gain the greatest benefit. The authors' experience indicates that although thrombosis of prosthetic grafts can be successfully treated with catheter-directed thrombolysis, long-term results appear better for saphenous vein grafts, especially saphenous vein grafts that thrombose more than 1 year after implantation (Fig. 35–4).

Sullivan and associates evaluated multiple factors influencing the initial outcome and long-term results of thrombolysis for failed infrainguinal bypass grafts.[78] They found that complete lysis could be achieved in 88 per cent, whereas only 74 per cent received clinical benefit. This common observation identifies the hemodynamic graft failure that may be associated with extensive and unreconstructable pathology. Although initial lysis occurred more frequently with prosthetic grafts than with vein grafts, once secondary patency was restored, vein grafts had significantly better long-term patency at 30 months than prosthetic grafts (69.3 per cent vs 28.6 per cent, respectively). When an underlying lesion was identified and corrected, patency at 2 years was 79 per cent, compared with 10 per cent when a lesion was not identified or corrected ($p = .01$) (Fig. 35–5). Bleeding complications occurred in 9 per cent, and in all but one case, bleeding occurred locally. Thrombolysis for thrombosed grafts less than 1 month of age resulted in a 33 per cent bleeding complication rate, compared with a rate of 3 per cent for grafts more than 1 month old.

Patients likely to have initially successful lysis can be identified by passage of a guidewire through the soft thrombus of the occluded bypass graft. Guidewire passage indicates that with proper catheter position, thrombolysis will probably be successful and patency most likely will be restored. If the guidewire cannot be passed through the occluded graft, the authors abandon attempts at thrombolysis and consider the best operative alternative. A prospective, randomized study comparing surgical procedures with thrombolysis is underway. Patients are stratified according to native arterial or bypass graft occlusion and are treated with urokinase, recombinant tissue plasminogen activator, or the best operative procedure. The results of the Surgery Versus Thrombolysis for the Ischemic Lower Extremity

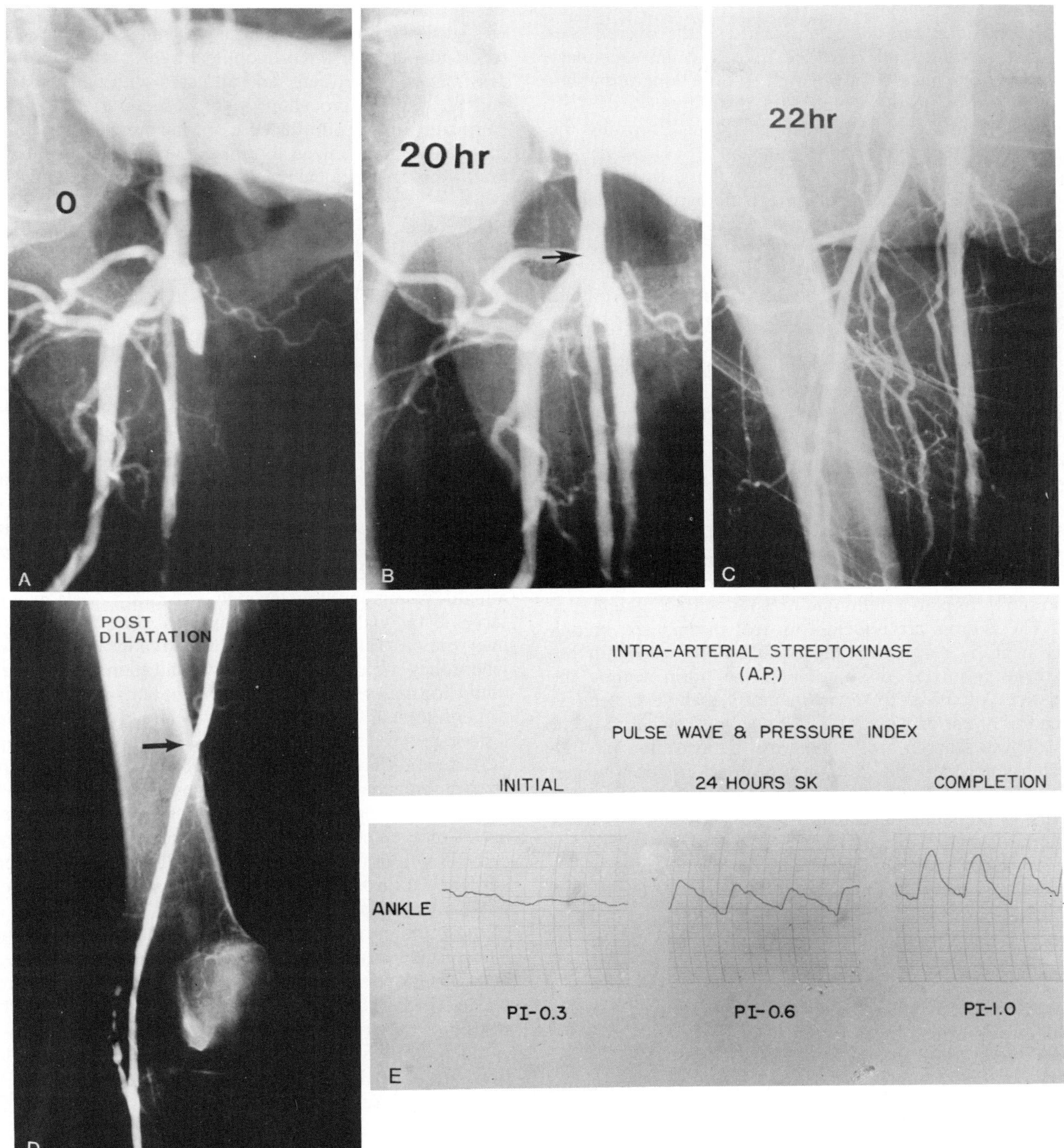

FIGURE 35–5. *A*, Arteriogram of a patient presenting 3 to 4 days after acute thrombosis of a femoropopliteal reversed saphenous vein graft placed 3 years earlier for ischemic rest pain. The arteriogram demonstrates a patent profunda with the femoropopliteal bypass occluded immediately distal to the proximal anastomosis. *B*, The catheter was positioned above the proximal anastomosis near the origin of the profunda. After 20 hours of streptokinase (SK) infusion, only 3 inches of the proximal thrombus had lysed, despite the fact that the patient had been systemically lytic for at least 16 hours. The catheter was then advanced into the saphenous vein graft and positioned with the tip *(arrow)* in the thrombus. *C*, After an additional 2 hours of infusion, significant lysis occurred. *D*, With continuation of the infusion, the entire thrombus lysed and the graft regained patency. The distal graft fibrosis responded well to percutaneous balloon dilatation. The sclerotic venous valve *(arrow)* did not dilate; however, it was excised and a small autogenous vein patch angioplasty was performed. *E*, The patient initially had flat pulse waveforms with an ankle brachial index (PI) of 0.3. Following lysis but before correction of the underlying lesions, she regained a pulsatile (but abnormal) pulse waveform and her ankle brachial index improved to 0.6. After operative correction of the sclerotic vein valve, her pulse waveform returned to normal, with an ankle index of 1.0. The patient's graft remained patent for the next 3½ years, after which she suffered a fatal myocardial infarction.

(STILE) study should offer insight into the proper selection of patients for therapy.

Reoperation can add significantly to the overall success rate in these patients. Late revisions and secondary reconstructions have been reported to offer long-term success rates of 50 to 60 per cent for distal bypasses.[73, 79, 80] The best results are those achieved by reperforming the bypass with autogenous saphenous vein.[81, 82] However, secondary vascular procedures with prosthetic bypasses are also reasonable,[24, 82] and a new prosthetic bypass appears to function better than a thrombectomized prosthetic bypass.[24]

The aforementioned comments refer primarily to occlusions of infrainguinal bypass grafts, which are, of course, far more common than occlusions with proximal reconstructions. Except in the case of rare technical errors, such as the inadvertent kinking or twisting of the limb of the graft, proximal bypasses rarely thrombose early unless the superficial femoral artery is occluded, concomitant profundaplasty has not been performed, or adequate profunda-geniculate pathways into a patent popliteal artery do not exist. At the time of arteriography for proximal graft failure, if the guidewire can be passed into the occluded limb and the patient has no contraindication to lytic therapy, catheter-directed thrombolysis can be offered. Elimination of the thrombus should offer a good look at the specific etiology leading to failure and should allow the surgeon the opportunity to plan a definitive revision with confidence.

The authors are reluctant to treat thrombosed knitted Dacron grafts because of the likelihood of transgraft hemorrhage following dissolution of the fibrin sealing the interstices of the graft, even in grafts that have been in place for 1 year or more.[83, 84] This does not appear to occur with woven Dacron grafts. Contrast extravasation through polytetrafluoroethylene grafts has been observed; however, this is likely to be similar to the serous "weeping" that occurs at implantation and is not indicative of transgraft hemorrhage.

If the patient is not a candidate for thrombolysis, either because of contraindications to lytic therapy or because of the inability to pass a guidewire or to position the catheter properly, operative reconstruction should be offered. A balloon catheter thrombectomy can usually restore perfusion; however, if this procedure fails to disobliterate the occluded graft limb satisfactorily, the balloon catheter ring stripper technique described by Ernst and Daugherty can be used.[85] Hyde and colleagues showed that removal of a hard proximal plug is frequently the critical maneuver in restoring good inflow in late graft occlusions.[86] If attempts at disobliteration continue to be unsuccessful, a femorofemoral bypass can be performed, although good inflow can be obtained from the proximal stump of the graft approached extraperitoneally. If these options are unsuitable, the ipsilateral axillary artery may also be used as an inflow source. The best means of establishing good outflow depends on the condition of the deep femoral artery and its collateral branches, because the superficial femoral artery is almost always occluded in these instances. A generous profundaplasty should be performed if it was not done during the original operation. However, unless a satisfactory outflow is achieved via the profunda, a femoropopliteal bypass should be performed with the proximal anastomosis attached to the graft limb. LeGrand and associates achieved an overall success rate of 78 per cent in dealing with occlusions of aortobifemoral graft limbs.[87] Thrombectomy alone was successful in 62 per cent; adding an outflow procedure (profundaplasty or femoropopliteal bypass) raised this success rate to 79 per cent, and all cases with both an inflow and an outflow procedure were successful. Fogarty and Hermann[110] have introduced a special wire-spring catheter for removing organized thrombus from occluded proximal graft limbs, but clinical results are not available at this time.

THROMBOEMBOLIC COMPLICATIONS

The thromboembolic complications of arterial reconstruction are much less frequent than graft thrombosis and are primarily an intraoperative event. Late thromboembolic complications are rare but can occur as a result of sloughing of the graft pseudointima or as distal emboli from aneurysmal degeneration or pseudoaneurysm formation.

Thromboembolic complications are more common with reconstruction for aneurysmal disease than with that for occlusive disease and are more frequent with proximal than with distal reconstructions. The opposite is true with graft thrombosis, in which the distal arterial tree commonly remains patent and flow through collateral vessels may preserve distal viability or at least buy time for corrective intervention. Emboli may occlude smaller distal vessels, where they are difficult to retrieve and there is less opportunity for major collateral reentry. Embolism may be more difficult to deal with in patients who already have occlusive lesions in the distal arterial tree. For example, if the superficial femoral artery is occluded, clots may enter profunda femoris branches, where removal by a Fogarty catheter is difficult, or if the posterior tibial artery is occluded distally, a clot may enter the anterior tibial artery but the Fogarty catheter will not. The consequences of acute limb ischemia and arterial thromboembolism are discussed in more detail in Chapters 42 and 43. In general, they depend on the size of the embolus and the site of occlusion. Obviously, embolism to vital circulation, such as the brain, kidney, or gut, is more serious than that to pelvic branches or to an extremity, in which either tissues tolerate ischemia better or arborization of the arterial tree provides a better opportunity for compensatory collateral flow. Although embolic complications are more difficult to diagnose and treat, they are fortunately more readily prevented.

Incidence

The incidence of thromboembolic complications varies widely, depending on the indications for operation, the procedure performed, and whether the procedure was elective or an emergency. The incidence of lower limb ischemia following reconstruction for abdominal aortic aneurysm ranged from as high as 25 per cent to 7 per cent in a series reviewed by Imparato.[88] In 100 consecutive cases from the Cleveland Clinic, it occurred in 7 per cent, but early postoperative deaths were excluded and systemic heparinization was not routinely used.[89] Acute peripheral ischemia was seen in 4.4 per cent of elective aneurysm repairs reported on by Ruberti and associates.[90] Thrombectomy was performed in fewer than one third, but amputation was required in more than one third. In the Baylor experience, reported on by Starr and colleagues, thromboembolic complications occurred in 4.6 per cent of emergency aneurysm repairs, compared with only 0.23 per cent of elective reconstructions.[91] Scobie and coworkers found thrombosis in 1.6 per cent and embolism in 2.1 per cent, with little difference between results in elective and emergency repairs.[92] In a more recent review by Strom and associates of the Milwaukee experience with aortoiliac reconstruction, acute ischemia occurred postoperatively in 10.3 per cent: in 9.5 per cent in the aneurysm group, in 8 per cent in the occlusive disease group, and in 17 per cent in the combined group.[93] The ischemia was due to embolism in 4.7 per cent of the aneurysm group, 2.4 per cent of the occlusive disease group, and 9.4 per cent of the combined group (total, 4.0 per cent). Every major complication was several times more frequent in those who developed ischemic complications.

In an analysis of a large series of patients who had repair of nonruptured abdominal arterial aneurysms, Johnston reported that intraoperative limb ischemia occurred in 3.5 per cent.[109] There was a strong association of intraoperative ischemia and aortoiliac or femoropopliteal occlusive disease. Intraoperative anticoagulation did not reduce the risk of ischemic complications. Graft thrombosis occurred in only 0.9 per cent, and as would be expected, it was associated with femoropopliteal occlusive disease and the need to perform a femoral anastomosis. Minor amputations were required in 0.8 per cent, and major amputations (above-knee or below-knee) in 0.4 per cent.

Causes of Intraoperative Thromboembolism

Thrombus may form intraoperatively or may already be present on or adjacent to the arterial segment being revascularized. Preexisting thrombus or atheromatous material capable of being dislodged results in greater difficulties in diagnosis, prevention, and management because it is firmer and more organized and is usually unrecognized. Manipulation of that segment during the initial dissection required for exposure and control of the inflow and outflow vessels may dislodge thrombus or atheromatous debris from an ulcerated surface or mural thrombus from the inner wall of an aneurysm. Clot is often dislodged by the very manipulations designed to remove it, as in graft thrombectomy or thrombolysis. When vascular clamps are applied, underlying plaque or unrecognized mural thrombus may be fragmented and loosened, only to be swept downstream when flow is restored. Unless specific measures (discussed later) are taken, intravascular thrombus formation will occur during prolonged interruption of flow in the static segments above or below the points of interruption or in the sluggish distal circulation.[91] The other two elements of Virchow's triad are less important here, but some patients may be innately hypercoagulable or become so because of hypotension (e.g., a ruptured aneurysm), whereas in others endothelial injury may be inflicted by surgical manipulation (e.g., repeated Fogarty catheter passages).

Prevention

Although there are routine measures for the prevention of thromboembolic complications with which all vascular surgeons must be familiar, it is helpful to be aware of certain patients who are at increased risk for these complications. Preoperative coagulation profiles of patients with a previous history of thromboembolic complications may identify those likely to develop intraoperative events. Additionally, careful evaluation of the preoperative arteriogram may reveal luminal irregularities that represent mural thrombus, shagbark aorta, or ulcerated plaques, all of which might require special prophylactic measures. Routine operative measures to prevent thromboembolic complications include

1. Gently handling and minimally manipulating arterial segments that contain thrombus, have ulcerated surfaces, or are aneurysmal.
2. Using adequate systemic anticoagulation with heparin during the entire period of flow interruption. The heparin should be given at least 5 minutes or more before cross-clamping, and during longer operations, the adequacy of heparinization should be monitored by serial testing, using the activated clotting time.[94]
3. Gently palpating the inflow and the outflow segments to detect the presence of plaque and other abnormalities in vessel wall or contents and to help determine the safest sites and orientation for clamp application.
4. Using the most atraumatic occluding devices available (see Chapter 21), with enough pressure applied to control luminal bleeding with a single application. Release plus reapplication of the vascular clamp is to be avoided.
5. Avoiding stagnation of blood in prosthetic grafts during anastomosis by aspirating it beforehand and flushing (filling) the graft with heparinized saline.
6. Releasing the occluding devices to flush out the thrombotic and other debris before the completion of each arteriotomy closure or anastomosis, and if flow is less than expected, exploring the vessel with Fogarty balloon catheters and removing any luminal thrombus.
7. Releasing occluding devices in sequence, with that to the least vital outflow released first (e.g., the external before the internal carotid, the hypogastric before the external iliac, and the profunda femoris before the superficial femoral artery.

These procedures do not prevent all embolic complications but minimize them and direct emboli to where they do the least harm (see Fig. 35–2). The sequential release offers the additional advantage of mitigating declamping shock, which might also contribute to intravascular thrombosis.

Diagnosis

The final precaution recommended for inclusion in this stepwise routine is not preventative but diagnostic: the clinician should check to be sure that the foregoing measures have been successful in preventing thromboembolism. Methods routinely used to assess the technical adequacy of the reconstruction (described earlier) are also valuable here, but they are useful in detecting thromboembolic events only to the extent that they evaluate the status of the distal arterial tree (see Chapter 24). That is, a duplex image will not normally visualize the lumen beyond the reconstructed segment, and even a completion arteriogram may be focused more proximally and cut off the distal vessels. A fiberoptic angioscope may visualize some distal clot but does not explore the most distal vessels. From a practical viewpoint, most thromboembolic complications following lower extremity revascularization are best detected by evaluation of the pedal circulation at the end of the procedure. Pallor, mottled cyanosis, collapsed veins, poor capillary filling, and absent or attenuated pulses and Doppler signals over pedal arteries indicate inadequate distal flow, and if the graft or the reconstructed segment has been shown to be widely patent proximally, the problem must lie distally. Experienced judgment is required before the findings can be ascribed to cooling and vasospasm or poor runoff, even though these factors can contribute to poor reflow, especially after transabdominal reconstruction performed in the presence of superficial femoral artery occlusion.[95] Appreciation of the degree of occlusive disease distal to the lowest anastomosis gleaned from adequate pre- or intraoperative arteriograms is helpful in this appraisal. It may allow the surgeon to accept reduced but audible signals in the pedal arteries on Doppler examination and be rewarded by steadily increasing ankle pressures postoperatively. As a rule, however, the absence of Doppler signals over distal arteries is unacceptable, and the burden of proof lies heavily on any surgeon who accepts a degree of reflow that is less than expected from preoperative or intraoperative arteriographic views of the distal arterial tree. At this point, thorough arteriographic visualization of the distal tree is indicated and is clearly preferable to continued observation and the possibility of returning the patient to the operating room after an extended period of ischemia. The vascular surgeon can be grateful for the opportunities and options available for intervening in thromboembolic complications of lower extremity arterial reconstruction; as difficult as these decisions can be, the surgeon at least has the time and opportunity for proper assessment and appropriate response. Intraoperative embolism to the brain, kidney, or gut does not allow these opportunities.

Management

General Measures

Removal of the distal thrombus or embolus by passage of a Fogarty balloon catheter according to the techniques described in Chapter 21 is the treatment of choice for this complication. Unfortunately, this procedure is often not as effective as it is for emboli from the heart, which frequently lodge in larger vessels. It is difficult to remove the clot from the infrapopliteal arteries or branches of the profunda femoris or hypogastric arteries. Soft clots that form intraoperatively may gradually break up or lyse; however, they are most appropriately treated by the intraoperative infusion of thrombolytic agents (see the next section). Older, organized clot that characterizes most small, fragmented distal emboli will not readily lyse. If the degree of ischemia created by small vessel emboli threatens significant tissue loss, the balloon embolectomy catheter and thrombolytic agents introduced from above generally fail to relieve the situation, and exploration of the distal vessels is mandatory. Repeating these maneuvers through an arteriotomy in the distal popliteal artery, placed close enough to the anterior tibial orifice that it and the posterior tibial and peroneal arteries can each be entered individually, may succeed when proximal attempts have failed. Because vascular surgeons today are familiar with handling of small vessels, attempts to disobliterate distal vessels at the level of the ankle can be pursued if necessary.[96] However, it must be understood that significant tissue loss will probably occur if this approach is not successful. Furthermore, balloon catheter embolectomy of small arteries raises great concern because of the extensive endothelial damage and the subsequent risk of neointimal fibroplasia in the thrombectomized vessels. In such situations, especially when acute thrombus is present, intraoperative thrombolysis is preferable.

Intraoperative Intra-Arterial Thrombolytic Therapy

The infusion of thrombolytic agents intraoperatively into the artery or graft containing residual thrombi offers valuable adjunctive therapy to thrombectomy and bypass procedures[96–100] (Fig. 35–6). Intraoperative thrombolysis is particularly useful in clearing a thrombosed graft or the distal arterial circulation of residual thrombi after thrombectomy for acute arterial or graft occlusion. New thrombotic (or embolic) events occurring intraoperatively can also be treated in this manner. Patients likely to benefit are those who have thrombotic occlusion or fragments of thrombi that have embolized to the distal circulation. Atherosclerotic debris is of course not susceptible to fibrinolytic agents, although superimposed secondary thrombus is.

A recent operation has been (and continues to be) a strong relative contraindication to the use of systemic fibrinolytic therapy. For this reason, most vascular surgeons were initially reluctant to infuse lytic agents intra-arterially in the operating room: it appeared to contradict the clear contraindications traditionally accepted. Since the early 1980s, numerous instances have been recorded in which patients demonstrated rapid lysis of acutely occluded arteries or bypass grafts (in 1 to 3 hours).[101] Many patients who responded within a short period failed to show any evidence of bleeding or a coagulopathy.

These observations were welcome in light of the recognition that residual intra-arterial thrombi remained following clinical and experimental balloon catheter thromboembolectomy for acute arterial occlusion. Greep and colleagues showed that almost all patients treated with standard balloon catheter techniques had additional thrombus removed with a modified wire basket catheter retrieval system.[102] Plecha and Pories performed an angiographic study and showed that 36 per cent of patients had residual thrombus after the best attempts at balloon thromboembolectomy for acute arterial occlusion.[103] These data were corroborated by Quinones-Baldrich and associates in an experimental study in which they demonstrated that 85 per cent of dogs

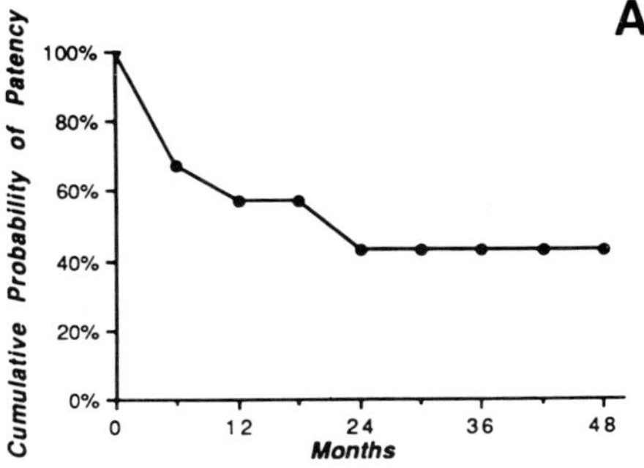

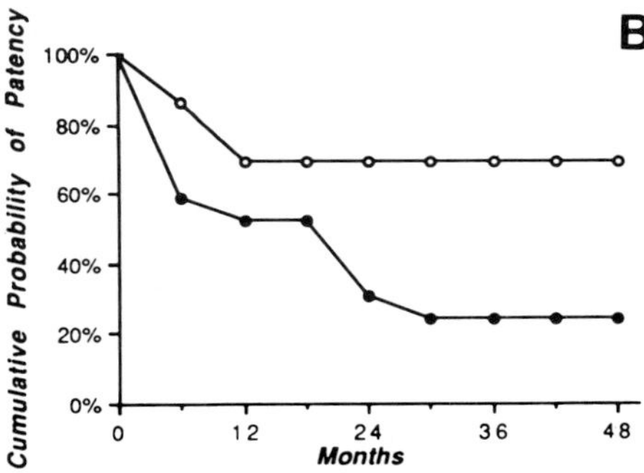

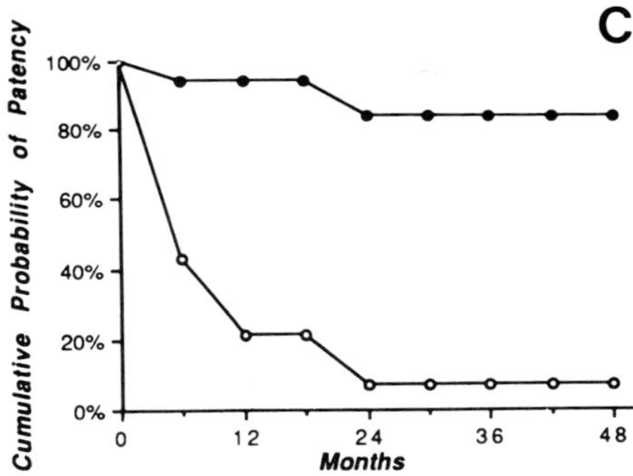

FIGURE 35–6. Life table results of catheter-directed thrombolysis for occluded bypass grafts. *A*, Cumulative patency of all grafts successfully treated with catheter-directed thrombolysis (n = 43) by means of Kaplan-Meier survival per period. *B*, Comparison of the cumulative patencies of vein *(closed circles)* and prosthetic *(open circles)* grafts by means of Kaplan-Meier survival curves. *C*, Kaplan-Meier survival curves comparing the cumulative patencies of grafts with *(open circles)* and those without *(closed circles)* identification and correction of the underlying lesion. (*A–C*, from Sullivan KL, Gardiner GA, Kandarpa K, et al: Efficacy of thrombolysis in infrainguinal bypass grafts. Circulation 83[Suppl 1]:1–99, 1991. Reproduced with permission. Copyright 1991 American Heart Association.)

had angiographically demonstrable residual thrombi following balloon catheter thromboembolectomy.[104] Intraoperative thrombolysis after balloon catheter thrombectomy produced significantly improved angiographic results and a trend toward increased blood flow compared with that in controls.

Laboratory studies have shown that experimental hindlimb ischemia produces arteriolar thrombosis after 6 hours of complete inflow occlusion.[105] It is not usually possible to perform mechanical thrombectomy of branch vessels from main arteries, and it is never possible to remove thrombi mechanically from the primary arterioles. Belkin and colleagues showed, in an isolated ischemic muscle preparation, that the group with urokinase (UK) infusion had more ischemic muscle salvaged and less reperfusion edema than did the control group.[106] Therefore, laboratory data confirm the clinical observations that balloon catheter thromboembolectomy frequently leaves residual thrombus. The data also demonstrate that arteriolar perfusion can be restored, tissue can be salvaged, and reperfusion injury can be reduced with the judicious use of intra-arterial infusion of lytic agents. The rationale for the intraoperative use of lytic agents is further supported by their short half-life, which minimizes the likelihood of a lytic effect persisting after wound closure.

An earlier report on the use of intraoperative streptokinase (SK) dampened the enthusiasm of many surgeons for intraoperative thrombolysis. Cohen and coworkers reported a 42 per cent mortality and a 42 per cent major bleeding complication rate with the use of an intraoperative SK infusion.[107] However, the doses ranged from 25,000 to 250,000 units, using a repeated bolus technique with 30 to 100 minutes of inflow occlusion. It is likely that patient selection, the choice of lytic agent, and the method of infusion significantly contributed to the high complication rate. Other investigators have reported marked clearing of thrombi with intraoperative infusion, without complications.[96, 99] An alternative clinical benefit from intraoperative thrombolysis is the ease with which residual thrombus can be retrieved with subsequent attempts at balloon catheter thrombectomy 30 minutes after the infusion of SK or UK.[97, 98]

Parent and associates treated 28 patients who had acute ischemia and residual thrombus after balloon catheter thrombectomy.[99] Seventeen patients had operative angiograms showing the residual thrombi. Of these 17, 15 had successful lysis when they were treated with intraoperative thrombolytic therapy. Both SK and UK were used and were shown to be equally effective; however, hypofibrinogenemia and bleeding complications were significantly more frequent in patients treated with SK than in those treated with UK.

At Temple University Hospital, 62 patients who had impending limb loss and occlusions of their runoff vessels were treated with intraoperative intra-arterial lytic therapy from 1982 to 1993. Included were patients with extensive distal thrombosis in whom complete thrombectomy was difficult or impossible, many of whom suffered graft thrombosis. It was believed by the attending surgeon that tissue loss was imminent. SK, UK, or recombinant tissue plasminogen activator was infused into the most distal vessel containing the thrombus with a short-duration infusion (usually with either a single- or a double-bolus technique). Up to 50,000 IU of SK, up to 250,000 IU of UK, and up to 10 mg of recombinant tissue plasminogen activator were given for routine intraoperative use (excluding patients having the isolated limb perfusion technique). Inflow was restored to the site of infusion in each instance by thrombectomy or bypass, whichever was necessary. Limb salvage was achieved in 71 per cent. In 73 per cent of the limbs salvaged, success was directly attributable to lysis. In 27 per cent, it was difficult to determine whether the limb would have been saved without intraoperative thrombolysis because thrombectomy and bypass procedures were also performed on these patients. Twenty-nine per cent of the patients ultimately underwent major amputation. Although there was an 8 per cent mortality rate, none of the deaths was thought to be due to use of the lytic agent. Two major bleeding complications occurred, one on the 3rd and one on the 4th postoperative day; they were thought to be due to systemic anticoagulation.

A prospective, randomized, blinded, and controlled study of intraoperative intra-arterial UK infusion in patients undergoing routine lower extremity revascularization has been completed.[108] The study was performed to evaluate the regional (leg) and systemic (body) effects of three doses of UK infused intraoperatively into the distal arterial tree during routine infrainguinal revascularization procedures. Blood samples were drawn simultaneously from the femoral vein and the arm before UK infusion, immediately before reperfusion, and shortly after the bypass graft was open. Regional and systemic fibrinolysis were simultaneously evaluated, as was the breakdown of cross-linked fibrin in the distal arterial tree. Plasminogen activation occurred in a stepwise fashion with increasing doses of UK. The breakdown of cross-linked fibrin in the distal circulation increased as the dose of UK increased from 125,000 to 500,000 units (250,000 to 500,000 IU). Although there was a progressively greater decrease in fibrinogen, absolute differences were small and values were not significantly different from those obtained with placebo (Fig. 35–7).

An important new technique is *high-dose isolated limb perfusion* (Fig. 35–8).[96] This procedure can be applied to patients with multi-vessel occlusion in whom a single- or double-bolus infusion will not be effective or to patients in whom any degree of systemic fibrinolysis, however transient, will pose significant risk. The technique includes full anticoagulation, exsanguination of venous blood from the limb with a rubber bandage, application of a tourniquet to achieve complete arterial and venous occlusion, direct arterial infusion into the affected vessels with a high dose of UK (1 million units or more) or recombinant tissue plas-

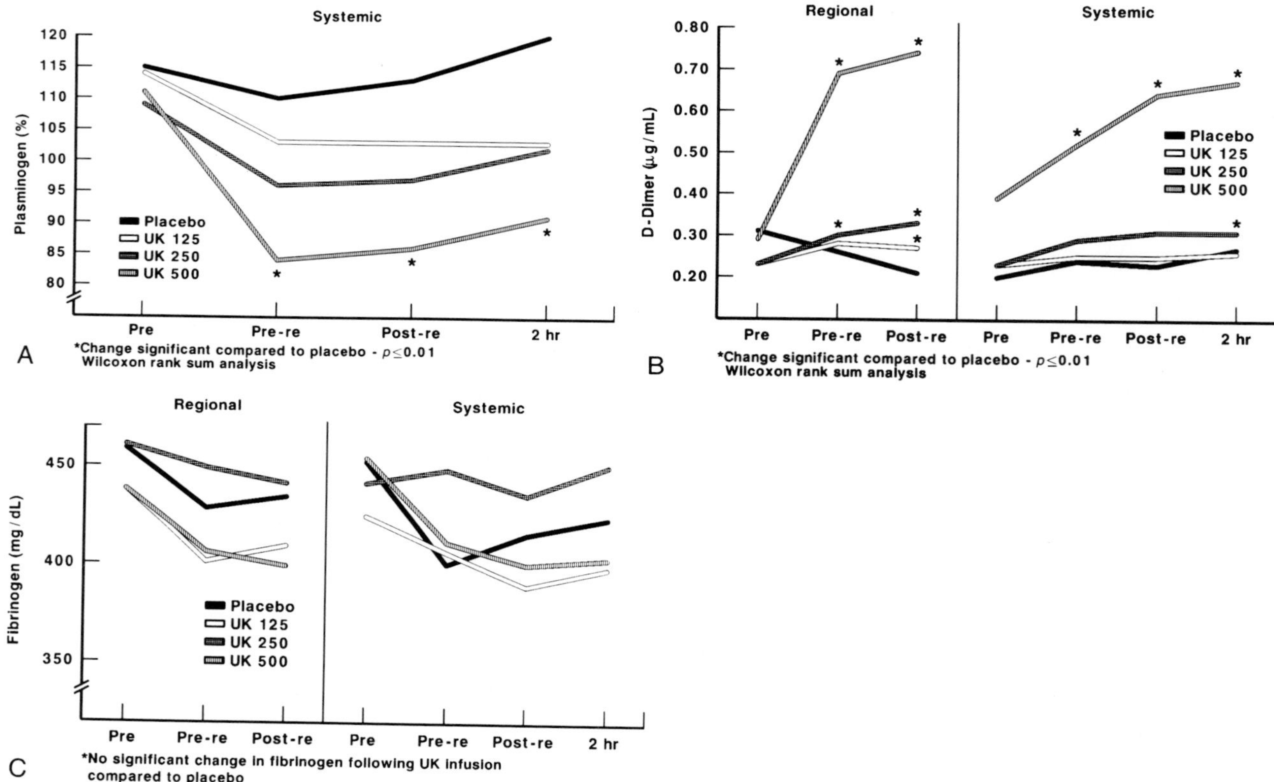

FIGURE 35–7. Results of a prospective, randomized, placebo-controlled trial of intraoperative UK infusion. In these graphs of the mean assay values of plasma factors by time period and dosage level of UK, regional samples are femoral vein blood and systemic samples are arm blood. The regional and systemic samples were drawn simultaneously for each time period. Blood samples were drawn: immediately before the infusion of intraoperative UK into the distal circulation at the time that the distal anastomosis was being performed for infrainguinal revascularization (Pre); after all anastomoses were completed but before perfusion was restored (Pre-re); and approximately 1 minute after reperfusion (Post-re). The last blood sample was obtained systemically 2 hr after infusion (frequently this was in the recovery room). The p values were calculated by the Wilcoxon rank sum analysis because of the nonparametric distribution of data. A significant change compared with placebo is considered to be $p \leq .01$. *A*, Mean assay values of systemic plasminogen by time period and dosage level. There is dose-related activation of plasminogen, which becomes significant at a dose of 500,000 units (UK 500) ($p < .001$). *B*, Mean assay values of D-dimer by region, time period, and dosage level. Note the significant and dose-related elevations for all doses of UK, both regionally and systemically. *C*, Mean assay values of fibrinogen by region, time period, and dosage level. There was no significant drop in fibrinogen for any of the UK treatment groups compared with the placebo group. (*A–C*, From Comerota AJ, Rao AK, Throm RC, et al: A prospective randomized, blinded and placebo-controlled trial of intraoperative, intra-arterial urokinase infusion during lower extremity revascularization: Regional and systemic effects. Ann Surg 218:534, 1993.)

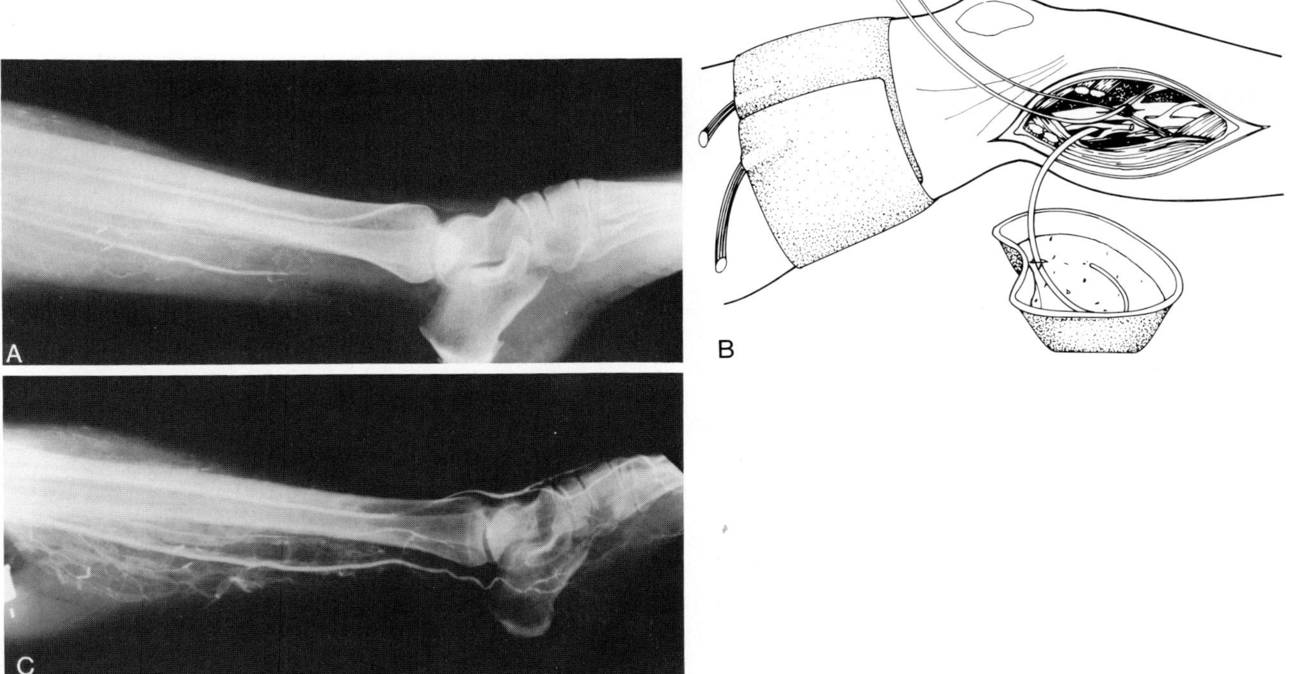

FIGURE 35–8. Technique of high-dose isolated limb perfusion of a fibrinolytic agent. This technique is useful in patients who cannot tolerate any degree of systemic fibrinolysis and who have multi-vessel distal occlusion that is unlikely to resolve with a single dose of a fibrinolytic agent. *A*, Intraoperative arteriogram after balloon catheter thrombectomy of the popliteal and the tibial vessels, following acute embolic or thrombotic occlusion. Additional thrombus could not be mechanically removed with a balloon catheter. Infusion catheters were placed into the origin of the posterior tibial and anterior tibial arteries, and arteriography was performed with a selective injection technique. There is no evidence of contrast material entering the foot. Because no additional thrombus could be retrieved, it was apparent that the patient was facing major amputation. *B*, The limb was elevated and the venous blood exsanguinated with a rubber bandage. A sterile blood pressure cuff (tourniquet) was placed on the distal thigh and inflated to 350 mmHg. The popliteal vein was cannulated with a red rubber catheter and drained into a basin. One million units of UK was infused into the lower leg in a volume of 1 L of saline (500,000 units each in the anterior tibial and posterior tibial arteries). After the UK infusion, the limb was flushed with heparinized saline. The venotomy was closed primarily, and the arteriotomy was closed with a patch. *C*, A postinfusion arteriogram documents significant improvement of perfusion to the foot. The patient had a palpable dorsalis pedis pulse and a pink foot following wound closure.

minogen activator (40 mg or more), and drainage of the venous effluent. Exposure of a direct-acting lytic agent to the thrombus for 45 to 60 minutes has yielded impressive results in a small number of patients suffering from acute multi-vessel distal thrombi or emboli. If distal vessel occlusion is due to atheromatous emboli or well-formed thrombus, treatment has not been successful.

CONCLUSIONS

Vascular surgeons have pushed back the frontiers of lower extremity revascularization by bypassing to branches of the pedal arteries. Intraoperative lytic therapy can maximize outflow in some patients by dissolving acute thrombotic (or embolic) occlusion in the runoff bed before a revascularization procedure. Ongoing interest in treating the ischemic limb will continue to improve outcome by addressing the important issues of minimizing reperfusion injury and sustaining patency. It is the responsibility of the vascular surgeon to be familiar with all available techniques of restoring and maintaining perfusion in the severely ischemic limb, because vascular surgeons are the last hope for limb salvage for most of these patients.

References

1. Rutherford RB, Jones DN, Bergentz S, et al: The efficacy of dextran 40 in preventing early postoperative thrombosis following difficult lower extremity bypass. J Vasc Surg 1:765, 1984.
2. Rutherford RB, Patt A, Pearce WH: Extra-anatomic bypass: A closer view. J Vasc Surg 6:437, 1987.
3. Sauvage LR, Berger KE, Mansfield PB, et al: Future directions in development of arterial prostheses for small and medium caliber arteries. Surg Clin North Am 54:213, 1974.
4. Harker LA, Slichter SJ, Sauvage LR: Platelet consumption by arterial prostheses. Ann Surg 186:594, 1977.
5. Towne JB, Bernhard VM, Husssey C, et al: Antithrombin III deficiency: A cause of unexplained thrombosis in vascular surgery. Surgery 89:735, 1981.
6. McDaniel MD, Pearce WH, Yao JST, et al: Sequential changes in coagulation and platelet function following femorotibial bypass. J Vasc Surg 1:261, 1984.
7. Whittemore AD, Donaldson MC, Mannick JA: Detection and treatment of hypercoagulable states: Can they improve infrainguinal bypass results? Presented at the Symposium on Current Critical Problems and New Horizons in Vascular Surgery, New York, November 16–18, 1990.
8. Morton DL, Ehrenfeld WK, Wylie EJ: Significance of outflow obstruction after femoropopliteal endarterectomy. Arch Surg 94:592, 1967.
9. Cutler BS, Thompson JE, Kleinsasser LB, et al: Autologous saphenous vein femoropopliteal bypass: Analysis of 298 cases. Surgery 79:325, 1976.

10. Linton RR, Darling RC: Autogenous saphenous vein bypass in femoropopliteal obliterative arterial disease. Surgery 51:62, 1962.
11. LiCalzi LK, Stansel HC: The closure index: Prediction of long term patency of femoropopliteal vein grafts. Surgery 91:413, 1982.
12. Barner HB, Judd DR, Kaiser GC, et al: Blood flow in femoropopliteal bypass vein grafts. Arch Surg 96:619, 1968.
13. Sumner DS: Objective diagnostic techniques: Role of the vascular laboratory. *In* Rutherford RB (ed): Vascular Surgery. 3rd ed. Philadelphia, WB Saunders, 1989, pp 41–60.
14. Ascer E, Veith F, Morin L, et al: Quantitation of outflow resistance in lower extremity arterial reconstruction. J Surg Res 37:8, 1984.
15. Sanders RJ, Kempczinski RF, Hammon W, et al: The significance of graft diameter. Surgery 88:856, 1980.
16. Filippone ND, Shah DM, Welch HF, Powers SR: Chronic venous obstruction as a factor in the early failure of bypass grafts in the leg. Am J Surg 140:671, 1980.
17. DeWeese JA, Rob CG: Autogenous venous bypass grafts five years later. Ann Surg 174:348, 1971.
18. Szilagyi DE, Elliott JP, Hageman JH, et al: Biologic fate of autogenous vein implants as arterial substitutes. Ann Surg 178:232, 1973.
19. Campbell CD, Brooks DH, Webster MW, et al: Aneurysmal formation in expanded polytetrafluoroethylene prostheses. Surgery 79:491, 1976.
20. Ottinger LW, Darling RC, Wirthlin LS, et al: Failure of ultralightweight knitted Dacron grafts in arterial reconstruction. Arch Surg 111:146, 1976.
21. Dardik H, Miller N, Dardik I, et al: A decade of experience with the glutaraldehyde-tanned human umbilical cord vein graft for revascularization of the lower limb. J Vasc Surg 7:336, 1988.
22. Karkow WS, Cranley JJ, Cranley RD, et al: Extended study of aneurysm formation in umbilical vein grafts. J Vasc Surg 4:486, 1986.
23. Miyata T, Tada Y, et al: A clinicopathologic study of aneurysm formation of glutaraldehyde-tanned human umbilical vein grafts. J Vasc Surg 10:605, 1989.
24. Ascer E, Collier P, Gupta SK, et al: Reoperation for polytetrafluoroethylene bypass failure: The importance of distal outflow site and operative technique in determining outcome. J Vasc Surg 5:298, 1987.
25. Mozersky DJ, Sumner DS, Strandness DE: Disease progression after femoropopliteal surgical procedures. Surg Gynecol Obstet 135:700, 1972.
26. Mozersky DJ, Sumner DS, Strandness DE: Long term results of reconstructive aortoiliac surgery. Am J Surg 123:503, 1972.
27. Donaldson MC, Mannick JA, Whittemore AD: Causes of primary graft failure after in situ saphenous vein bypass grafting. J Vasc Surg 15:113, 1992.
28. Bandyk DF, Schmitt DD, Seabrook GR, et al: Monitoring functional patency of in situ saphenous vein bypasses: The impact of a surveillance protocol and elective revision. J Vasc Surg 9:286, 1989.
29. Berkowitz HD, Greenstein SM: Improved patency in reversed femoral-infrapopliteal autogenous vein grafts by early detection and treatment of the failing graft. J Vasc Surg 5:755, 1987.
30. Maddison FE, Rutherford RB, Kumpe DA, Redmond PL: Contrast arteriography. *In* Rutherford RB (ed): Vascular Surgery. 3rd ed. Philadelphia, WB Saunders, 1989, pp 157–177.
31. Stept LL, Flinn WR, McCarthy WJ III, et al: Technical defects as a cause of early graft failure after femorodistal bypass. Arch Surg 122:599, 1987.
32. Sumner DS: Perioperative assessment of patient revascularization: Intraoperative assessment by Doppler ultrasound. *In* Bergan JJ, Yao JST (eds): Gangrene and Severe Ischemia of the Lower Extremities. New York, Grune & Stratton, 1978.
33. Sigel B, Coelho JCU, Flanigan DP, et al: Ultrasonic imaging during vascular surgery. Arch Surg 117:764, 1982.
34. Towne JB, Bernhard VM: Vascular endoscopy: An adjunct to carotid surgery. Stroke 8:569, 1977.
35. Gilbertson JJ, Walsh DB, Zwolak RM, et al: A blinded comparison of angiography, angioscopy, and duplex scanning in the intraoperative evaluation of in situ saphenous vein bypass grafts. J Vasc Surg 15:121, 1992.
36. Dardik H, Sussman B, Ibrahim IM, et al: Distal arteriovenous fistula as an adjunct to maintaining arterial and graft patency for limb salvage. Surgery 94:478, 1983.
37. Paty PSK, Shah DM, Saiki J, et al: Remote distal arteriovenous fistula to improve infrapopliteal bypass patency. J Vasc Surg 11:171, 1990.
38. Snyder SO, Gregory RT, Wheeler JR, et al: Failure of arteriovenous fistulas at distal tibial bypass anastomotic sites. Presented at the XVI World Congress of the International Society for Cardiovascular Surgery, Rio de Janeiro, September 19, 1983.
39. Casten DF, Sadley AH, Foreman D: An experimental study of sympathectomy on patency of small vessel anastomoses. Surg Gynecol Obstet 114:462, 1962.
40. Williams GD, Crumpler JB, Campbell GS: Effects of sympathectomy on the severely traumatized artery. Arch Surg 101:704, 1970.
41. Boas RA, Hatangdi VS, Richards EG: Lumbar sympathectomy—A percutaneous chemical technique. Adv Pain Res Ther 1:685, 1976.
42. Cousins MJ, Reeve TS, Glynn CJ, et al: Neurolytic lumbar sympathetic blockade: Duration of denervation and relief of rest pain. Anaesth Intensive Care 7(2):121, 1979.
43. Bergqvist D, Burmark US, Frisell J, et al: Low molecular weight heparin once daily compared with conventional low dose heparin twice daily. A prospective double-blind multicenter trial on prevention of postoperative thrombosis. Br J Surg 73:204, 1986.
44. Bergqvist D, Matzsch T, Burmark US, et al: Low molecular weight heparin given the evening before surgery compared with conventional low dose heparin in prevention of postoperative thrombosis. Br J Surg 75:888, 1989.
45. Ware JA, Lewis JL, Salzman EW: Antithrombic therapy. *In* Rutherford RB (ed): Vascular Surgery. 3rd ed. Philadelphia, WB Saunders, 1989, pp 287–299.
46. Kretschmer G, Wenzl E, Piza F, et al: The influence of anticoagulant treatment on the probability of function in femoropopliteal vein bypass surgery: Analysis of a clinical series (1970 to 1985) and interim evaluation of a controlled clinical trial. Surgery 102(3):453, 1987.
47. Flinn WR, Rohrer MJ, Yao JST, et al: Improved long-term patency of infragenicular polytetrafluoroethylene grafts. J Vasc Surg 7:685, 1988.
48. Thaler E, Niessner H, Kleimberger G, et al: Antithrombin IV replacement therapy in patients with congenital and acquired antithrombin III deficiency. Thromb Haemost 42:324, 1979.
49. Pearce WH: In discussion of McDaniel MD, Pearce WH, Yao JST, et al: Sequential changes in coagulation and platelet function following femorotibial bypass. J Vasc Surg 1:261, 1984.
50. Freeman MB, Sicard GA, Allen BT, et al: Endogenous canine thrombogenicity is equally important in vascular graft patency as platelet inhibition. Surg Forum 37:453, 1986.
51. Goldman MD, Simpson D, Hawker RJ, et al: Aspirin and dipyridamole reduce platelet deposition on prosthetic femoropopliteal grafts in man. Ann Surg 198(6): 713, 1983.
52. Chesebro JH, Clements IP, Furter V, et al: A platelet inhibitor drug trial in coronary arterial bypass operations. N Engl J Med 307:73, 1982.
53. Chesebro JH, Fuster V, Elverback LR, et al: Effect of dipyridamole and aspirin on late vein-graft patency after coronary bypass operations. N Engl J Med 310:209, 1984.
54. Findlay JM, Lougheed WM, Gentili F, et al: Effect of perioperative platelet inhibition on postcarotid endarterectomy mural thrombus formation. Results of a prospective randomized controlled trial using aspirin and dipyridamole in humans. J Neurosurg 63:693, 1985.
55. Green RM, Roedersheimer LB, DeWeese JA: Effects of aspirin and dipyridamole on expanded polytetrafluoroethylene patency. Surgery 92:1016, 1982.
56. McCann RL, Hagen PO, Fuchs JCA: Aspirin and dipyridamole decrease intimal hyperplasia in experimental vein grafts. Ann Surg 191(2):238, 1980.
57. Metke MP, Lie JT, Fuster V, et al: Reduction of intimal thickening in canine coronary bypass vein grafts with dipyridamole and aspirin. Am J Cardiol 43:1144, 1979.
58. Abbot W, Megerman J: Does compliance mismatch alone cause neointimal hyperplasia? [Letter to the editor]. J Vasc Surg 9:507, 1989.
59. Bulkley BH, Hutchins GM: Accelerated ''atherosclerosis'': A morphologic study of 97 saphenous vein coronary artery bypass grafts. Circulation 55:163, 1977.
60. DeWeese JA, Green RM: Control of anastomotic neointimal fibrous hyperplasia in vascular grafts. *In* Stanley JC (ed): Biological and Synthetic Vascular Prostheses. New York, Grune & Stratton, 1982, pp 653–659.

61. Haudenschild CC: Morphology of intimal hyperplasia [Special communication]. J Vasc Surg 10:591, 1989.
62. Bassiouny HS, White S, Glagov S, et al: Anastomotic intimal hyperplasia: Mechanical injury or flow induced. J Vasc Surg 15:708, 1992.
63. Kuwano H, Hashizume M, Yang Y, et al: Patterns of pannus growth of the expanded polytetrafluoroethylene vascular graft with special attention to the intimal hyperplasia formation. Am Surg 52:663, 1986.
64. Cronberg S, Robertson B, Nilsson IM, et al: Suppressive effect of dextran on platelet adhesiveness. Thromb Diath Haemorr 16:384, 1966.
65. Aberg M, Hedner U, Bergentz SE: Effect of dextran on factor VIII (antihemophilic factor) and platelet function. Ann Surg 189:243, 1979.
66. Ooasta GM, Gardner WT, Beeler DL, Rosenberg RD: Multiple functional domains of the heparin molecule. Proc Natl Acad Sci USA 78:829, 1981.
67. Chesebro J: Hirudin: A specific thrombin inhibitor [Special communication]. J Vasc Surg 12:201, 1990.
68. Glusa E, Urban U: Studies in platelet functions in hirudin plasma. Folia Haematol (Leipz) 115:88, 1988.
69. Hoffman A, Markwardt F: Inhibition of the thrombin-platelet reaction by hirudin. Haemostasis 14:164, 1984.
70. Donayre CE, Ouriel K, Rhee RY, Shortell CK: Future alternatives to heparin: Low-molecular-weight heparin and hirudin. J Vasc Surg 15:675, 1992.
71. Rubin BG, McGraw DJ, Sicard GA, Santoro SA: New RGD analogue inhibits human platelet adhesion and aggregation and eliminates platelet deposition on canine vascular grafts. J Vasc Surg 15:683, 1992.
72. Pan XM, Nelken N, Colyvas N, Rapp JH: Inhibition of injury induced intimal hyperplasia by saralasin in rats. J Vasc Surg 15:693, 1992.
73. Whittemore AD, Clowes AW, Counch NP, et al: Secondary femoral-popliteal reconstruction. Ann Surg 143:35, 1981.
74. Graor RA, Risius B, Young JR, et al: Thrombolysis of peripheral arterial bypass grafts: Surgical thrombectomy compared with thrombolysis. J Vasc Surg 7:347, 1988.
75. Belkin M, Donaldson MC, Whittemore AD, et al: Observations on the use of thrombolytic agents for thrombotic occlusion of infrainguinal vein grafts. J Vasc Surg 11:289, 1990.
76. Wolfson RH, Kumpe DA, Rutherford RB: Role of intra-arterial streptokinase in treatment of arterial thromboembolism. Arch Surg 19:697, 1984.
77. McNamara TO, Fischer JR: Thrombolysis of peripheral arterial and graft occlusions: Improved results using high-dose urokinase. AJR 144:769, 1985.
78. Sullivan KL, Gardiner GA, Kandarpa K, et al: Efficacy of thrombolysis in infrainguinal bypass grafts. Circulation 83(Suppl 1):1–99, 1991.
79. Bartlett ST, Olinde AJ, Flinn WR, et al: The reoperative potential of infrainguinal bypass: Long term limb and patient survival. J Vasc Surg 5:170, 1987.
80. Veith FJ, Gupta S, Daly V: Management of early and late thrombosis of expanded polytetrafluoroethylene femoropopliteal bypass grafts: Favorable prognosis with appropriate reoperation. Surgery 87:581, 1980.
81. Edwards JE, Taylor LM, Porter JM: Treatment of failed lower extremity bypass grafts with new autogenous vein bypass grafting. J Vasc Surg 11:136, 1990.
82. Dennis JW, Littooy FN, Greisler HP, et al: Secondary vascular procedures with polytetrafluoroethylene grafts for lower extremity ischemia in a male veteran population. J Vasc Surg 8:137, 1988.
83. Comerota AJ: Complications of thrombolytic therapy. *In* Comerota AJ (ed): Thrombolytic Therapy. Orlando, FL, Grune & Stratton, 1988, pp 255–281.
84. Rabe FE, Beck GJ, Richmond BD, et al: Contrast extravasation through Dacron grafts: A sequela of low dose streptokinase therapy. AJR 138:917, 1982.
85. Ernst CG, Daugherty ME: Removal of a thrombotic plug from an occluded limb of an aortofemoral graft. Arch Surg 113:301, 1978.
86. Hyde GL, McCready RA, Schwartz RW, et al: Durability of thrombectomy of occluded aortofemoral graft limbs. Surgery 94:748, 1983.
87. LeGrand DR, Vermillion BD, Hayes JP, et al: Management of the occluded aortofemoral graft limb. Surgery 93:818, 1983.
88. Imparato AM: Abdominal aortic surgery: Prevention of lower limb ischemia. Surgery 93:112, 1983.
89. Tchirkow G, Beven EG: Leg ischemia following surgery for abdominal aortic aneurysm. Ann Surg 188:166, 1978.
90. Ruberti U, Scorza R, Biasi GM, et al: Nineteen year experience on the treatment of aneurysms of the abdominal aorta: A survey of 832 consecutive cases. J Cardiovasc Surg 26:547, 1985.
91. Starr DS, Lawrie GM, Morris GC: Prevention of distal embolism during arterial reconstruction. Am J Surg 138:764, 1979.
92. Scobie K, McPhail N, Hubbard C: Early and late results of resection of abdominal aortic aneurysms. Can Med Assoc J 117:147, 1977.
93. Strom JA, Bernhard VM, Towne JB: Acute limb ischemia following aortic reconstruction. Arch Surg 119:470, 1984.
94. Effency DJ, Goldstone J, Chin D, et al: Intraoperative autocoagulation in cardiovascular surgery. Surgery 90:1065, 1981.
95. Brewster DC, O'Hara PJ, Darling RC, et al: The value of intraoperative monitoring using the pulse volume recorder during peripheral vascular reconstructive operations. Surg Gynecol Obstet 152:275, 1981.
96. Comerota AJ, White JV, Grosh JD: Intraoperative, intra-arterial thrombolytic therapy for salvage of limbs in patients with distal arterial thrombosis. Surg Gynecol Obstet 169:283, 1989.
97. Garcia R, Saroyan RM, Senkowsky J, et al: Intraoperative intra-arterial urokinase infusion as an adjunct to Fogarty catheter embolectomy in acute arterial occlusion. Surg Gynecol Obstet 171:201, 1990.
98. Norem RF, Short DH, Kerstein MD: Role of intraoperative fibrinolytic therapy in acute arterial occlusion. Surg Gynecol Obstet 167:87, 1988.
99. Parent NE, Bernhard VM, Pabst TS, et al: Fibrinolytic treatment of residual thrombus after catheter embolectomy for severe lower limb ischemia. J Vasc Surg 9:153, 1989.
100. Quinones-Baldrich WJ, Zierler RE, Hiatt JC: Intraoperative fibrinolytic therapy: An adjunct to catheter thromboembolectomy. J Vasc Surg 2:319, 1985.
101. Comerota AJ, Rubin R, Tyson R, et al: Intra-arterial thrombolytic therapy in peripheral vascular disease. Surg Gynecol Obstet 165:1, 1987.
102. Greep JM, Allman PJ, Janet F, et al: A combined technique for peripheral arterial embolectomy. Arch Surg 105:869, 1972.
103. Plecha FR, Pories WJ: Intraoperative angiography in the immediate assessment of arterial reconstruction. Arch Surg 105:902, 1972.
104. Quinones-Baldrich WJ, Ziomek S, Henderson TC, et al: Intraoperative fibrinolytic therapy: Experimental evaluation. J Vasc Surg 4:229, 1986.
105. Dunnant JR, Edwards WS: Small vessel occlusion in the extremity after periods of arterial obstruction: An experimental study. Surgery 75:240, 1973.
106. Belkin M, Valeri R, Hobson RW: Intra-arterial urokinase increases skeletal muscle viability after acute ischemia. J Vasc Surg 9:161, 1989.
107. Cohen LJ, Kaplan M, Bernhard VM: Intraoperative fibrinolytic therapy: An adjunct to catheter thromboembolectomy. J Vasc Surg 2:319, 1985.
108. Comerota AJ, Rao AK, Throm RC, et al: A prospective randomized, blinded and placebo-controlled trial of intraoperative, intra-arterial urokinase infusion during lower extremity revascularization: Regional and systemic effects. Ann Surg 218:534, 1993.
109. Johnston KW: Multicenter prospective study of nonruptured abdominal aortic aneurysms. II. Variables predicting morbidity and mortality. J Vasc Surg 9:437, 1989.
110. Fogarty TJ, Hermann GD: New techniques for clot extraction and managing acute thromboembolic limb ischemia. *In* Veith FJ (ed): Current clinical problems in vascular surgery. St. Louis, Quality Medical Publishing, 1991, vol. 3, pp 197–203.

36

Infection in Prosthetic Vascular Grafts

Dennis F. Bandyk, M.D., and Thomas M. Bergamini, M.D.

• • •

The fabrication of biomaterials as arterial substitutes was a seminal technical advance of vascular surgery that revolutionized the management of arterial disease. In the peripheral circulation, prosthetic grafts have proved to be durable conduits with acceptable patency for the treatment of both aneurysmal and occlusive disease. The use of prosthetic grafts has permitted palliation of otherwise fatal or disabling vascular conditions, with a graft-related morbidity due to biomaterial degeneration (dilatation or rupture), allergic foreign body reactions, or anastomotic false aneurysm formation of less than 5 per cent. Infection remains the most serious complication of prosthetic grafting because it dramatically alters patient outcome. Even when treatment of an established graft infection is successful, patient morbidity is often worse than the natural history of the vascular disease process that led to implantation.

The reported incidence of graft infection varies with the indication for implantation and the site of the graft (Table 36–1). The true incidence may be higher because many graft infections do not present until years after graft implantation. Early postoperative graft infection rates of less than 2 per cent have been reported without antibiotic prophylaxis. Graft infection is more common after emergency procedures (e.g., for ruptured abdominal aortic aneurysm) and when the prosthesis is anastomosed to the femoral artery or placed in a subcutaneous tunnel (e.g., with axillofemoral or femorofemoral bypass).

Table 36–1. Incidence of Prosthetic Vascular Graft Infections

Graft Site	Reference	Incidence (%)
Thoracic aorta	Hargrove and Edmunds, 1984[46]	1.9
	Coselli et al, 1990[28]	3.0
Aortoiliac	Szilagyi et al, 1972[90]	0.7
	Goldstone and Moore, 1974[44]	1.2
	Yashar et al, 1978[105]	1.3
	Lorentzen et al, 1985[59]	0.0
	O'Hara et al, 1986[66]	0.4
Aortofemoral	Szilagyi et al, 1972[90]	1.6
	Goldstone and Moore, 1974[44]	3.0
	Yashar et al, 1978[105]	2.4
	Lorentzen et al, 1985[59]	3.0
	O'Hara et al, 1986[66]	1.3
Femoropopliteal	Szilagyi et al, 1972[90]	3.0
	Goldstone and Moore, 1974[44]	2.3
	Yashar et al, 1978[105]	4.6
	Lorentzen et al, 1985[59]	3.5
	Durham et al, 1986[34]	0.9
Femorotibial	Durham et al, 1986[34]	3.4
Axillofemoral	Goldstone and Moore, 1974[44]	5.3
Carotid-subclavian	Criado, 1982[30]	1.5
Axilloaxillary	Criado, 1982[30]	4.1

Despite aggressive antibiotic administration and surgical treatment, the mortality (10 to 50 per cent) and amputation (15 to 60 per cent) rates associated with infections of vascular prostheses remain high, with the greatest morbidity occurring when sepsis or anastomotic bleeding is a presenting sign. Successful management of this uncommon and dreaded clinical condition requires an understanding of the pathogenesis, the microbiology, and the surgical principles required to eradicate a biomaterial-associated vascular infection. This chapter reviews these facets and emphasizes patient risk factors and operative techniques important in the prevention of prosthetic graft infection.

PATHOGENESIS

Etiologic Factors

Any mechanism that exposes the vascular prosthesis to microorganisms (bacteria or fungi) can result in colonization of the biomaterial and subsequent clinical infection. Microorganisms can contact graft surfaces via a *direct route* during the implantation procedure, through the surgical wound in the event of a healing complication, or via *hematogenous* or *lymphatic routes* from remote sites of infection or colonization (e.g., urinary tract infection, tinea pedis, pneumonia, venous or arterial catheter sepsis, endocarditis, and ischemic foot ulcer). Important potential sources of direct graft contamination include breaks in aseptic technique by the operative team, contact with the patient's endogenous flora harbored within sweat glands, lymph nodes, diseased artery walls (e.g., atherosclerotic plaque or aneurysm thrombus), disrupted lymphatics, or fluid that accumulates within a bowel bag during aortic surgery. If the surgical wound does not develop a fibrin seal or heal promptly following operation, the underlying vascular prosthesis is susceptible to colonization from initially trivial superficial wound problems (e.g., erythema, dermal necrosis, and lymphocele). With persistent wound drainage, a septic focus can develop in ischemic or injured tissues and progress by deep extension to involve the prosthesis.[10] Diseased artery walls are a frequent unrecognized source of bacteria, especially coagulase-negative staphylococci, as are reoperative wounds. Patients requiring graft revision for failed vascular reconstructions commonly harbor bacteria within scar tissue and lymphoceles and on the surfaces of previously implanted prosthetic vascular grafts and suture material. In explanted graft material, microorganisms were cultured from 90 per cent of grafts associated with anastomotic aneurysm and from 69 per cent of thrombosed grafts.[4]

Bacterial seeding of the prosthesis via a hematogenous route is an uncommon but potentially important mechanism of graft infection. Experimentally, intravenous infusion of 10^7 colony-forming units of *Staphylococcus aureus* will produce a clinical graft infection in nearly 100 per cent of animals during the immediate postimplantation period. Bacteremia from sources such as intravascular catheters, an infected urinary tract, or remote tissue infection (e.g., pneumonia or an infected foot ulcer) is common in elderly vascular patients, particularly during the postoperative period. In high-risk, leukopenic, or septic patients, it is best to avoid the use of prosthetics, if possible. Experimentally, parenteral antibiotic therapy significantly decreased the risk of graft colonization from bacteremia and is the basis for culture-specific antibiotic therapy in patients with known remote sites of infection. The prosthesis becomes less susceptible to colonization as the luminal pseudointimal lining develops and matures over time, but vulnerability to infection from bacteremia has been documented beyond 1 year after implantation. Transient bacteremia, in combination with altered immune status, may account for graft infections occurring years after the original operation. Clinicians should consider this mechanism of infection rather than assuming that the virulent bacteria have remained dormant since graft implantation.

The most common cause of graft infection is *microorganism contamination* of the graft during implantation or in the immediate postoperative period. The pathogenesis of biomaterial-associated infection involves several fundamental steps: (1) bacterial adhesion to biomaterial surfaces, (2) microcolony formation within a bacterial biofilm, (3) activation of host defenses, and (4) an inflammatory response involving perigraft tissues and the graft-artery anastomoses (Fig. 36–1). Bacterial adherence to the prosthesis depends on cell wall and growth characteristics of the bacteria species, as well as on physical and chemical properties of the vascular biomaterial. The prevalence of staphylococcal biomaterial infections can be explained in part by the relatively increased adherence of gram-positive bacteria to biomaterials. Under experimental conditions, *Staphylococcus* species adhere in greater numbers (10 to 1000 times) to vascular graft materials (Dacron or polytetrafluoroethylene) than do gram-negative bacteria.[11] The differential adherence of staphylococci is postulated to be due to specific capsular adhesions that mediate microorganism attachment and colonization. Antibodies to these specific cell surface glycoproteins have been developed, and adherence to biomaterials of adhesin-producing strains has been inhibited.

Vascular biomaterials and bacteria act together, producing coinflammatory stimuli to activate the immune system. This results in an inflammatory process that attempts to localize the infection, but with tissue-damaging effects. Activation is via humeral and cellular defenses, with secretion of cytokines and recruitment of polymorphonuclear granulocytes. Importantly, biomaterials invoke an immune foreign body reaction that produces an acidic, ischemic microenvironment conducive to bacterial biofilm formation and proliferation. Unlike autogenous grafts, implanted prosthetic grafts do not develop rich vascular connections with surrounding tissue. This prevents host immune defenses and antibiotics from exerting maximal effect on infecting organisms. The extent of perigraft inflammation and tissue injury depends on the virulence of the infecting organism, but the ultimate manifestations of graft infection, regardless of location, are tissue autolysis, vessel wall or anastomotic disruption, and hemorrhage. Perigraft tissue destruction

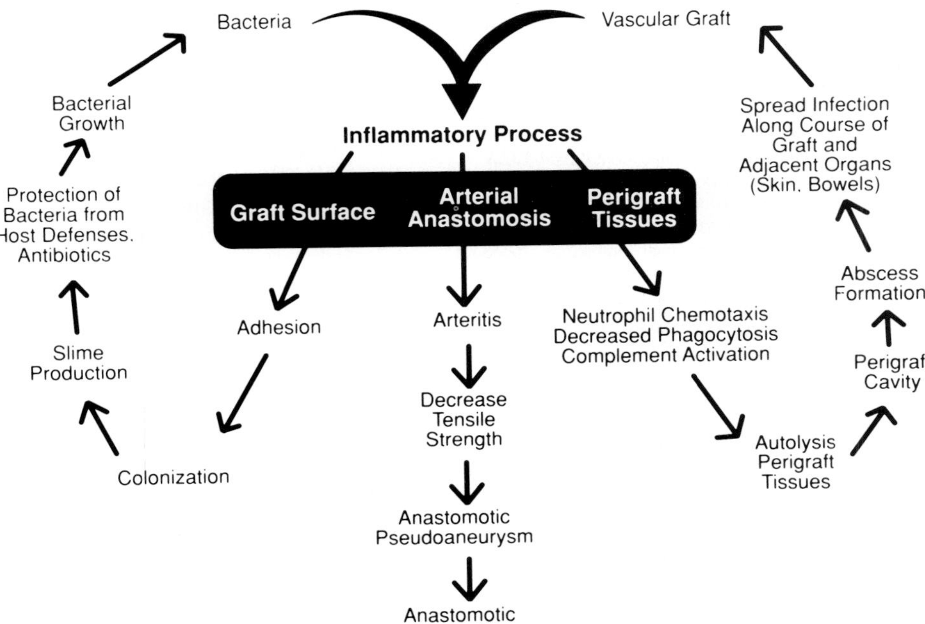

FIGURE 36–1. Pathogenesis of vascular biomaterial–associated infections.

leads to the formation of a perigraft cavity or abscess, spread of the infectious process along the length of the graft, and involvement of adjacent structures such as the adjacent artery, skin, or bowel. The pathobiology of graft infection can manifest clinically as a spectrum of presenting signs including graft sepsis, localized perigraft abscess, anastomotic pseudoaneurysm, graft cutaneous sinus tract, or graft-enteric erosion or fistula (aortoduodenal fistula).

Predisposing Factors

Graft infections are commonly associated with operative events leading to bacterial contamination of the graft or with patient risk factors that predispose to infection due to impaired host defenses (Table 36–2). The skin is an important reservoir of bacteria. Some graft infections originate from a break in sterile surgical technique with graft colonization from the patient's endogenous flora rather than the operating room environment or surgical team. A number of factors accentuate this mechanism, including a prolonged preoperative in-hospital stay with skin colonization by more resistant organisms, emergency procedures, long operative procedures (greater than 4 hours), and reoperation for hematoma or graft thrombosis.[57] The increased risk of infection following reoperative vascular procedures is due to a higher frequency of arterial wall and wound colonization, as well as to increased wound complications (e.g., hematoma, lymphocele, and dermal necrosis). Concomitant biliary (e.g., cholecystectomy), bowel (e.g., colon resection), and urologic (e.g., ureter repair) procedures also increase the risk of graft colonization by bacteria during the procedure, but more commonly, colonization results from a postoperative complication (e.g., bile fistula or anastomosis breakdown).

Most patients (more than 90 per cent) have one or more risk factors for the development of graft infection. Early graft infections are usually the result of wound sepsis, reoperation for hematoma, concomitant remote infection, and impaired immunocompetence. Patients with late-appearing graft infections often have a history of multiple operations for graft thrombosis or false aneurysm.

Table 36–2. Risk Factors Predisposing to Graft Infection

Bacterial Contamination of the Graft
Faulty sterile technique
Prolonged preoperative hospital stay
Emergency surgery
Extended operating time
Reoperative vascular procedure
Simultaneous gastrointestinal procedure
Remote infection
Postoperative superficial wound infection
Altered Host Defenses
Local factors
Biomaterial
Slime production
Systemic factors
Malnutrition
Leukopenia
Malignancy
Corticosteroid administration
Chemotherapy
Diabetes mellitus
Chronic renal failure
Autoimmune disease

Immune factors associated with the biomaterial itself (foreign body reaction) or products of bacterial growth on graft surfaces can impair neutrophil chemotaxis and bactericidal function and result in an indolent, low-grade perigraft infection. The architectural features of the graft material may permit bacteria to grow within the interstices of the biomaterial (e.g., in woven and knitted Dacron prostheses). Products of the bacteria, such as the extracellular glycocalyx called slime, protect the bacteria from both host defense mechanisms and antibiotics.[10] Slime production is an indicator of virulence and pathogenicity of both gram-positive and gram-negative bacteria. Body surface culture results indicate that most patients undergoing prosthetic implant procedures are colonized with pathogenic (i.e., slime-producing) strains of coagulase-negative staphylococci.[57] Coagulase-negative staphylococci are primary opportunists, infecting foreign bodies, injured tissues, or patients with profound leukopenia. The altered immune function associated with malignancy, lymphoproliferative disorders, or drug administration (e.g., steroids or chemotherapy) can predispose patients to graft infection with low numbers of contaminating bacteria.

PREVENTION

Prevention of graft infection is an important concept, and every surgeon must be cognizant of preoperative, operative, and postoperative prophylactic measures. A prolonged preoperative hospital stay should be avoided to minimize the development of skin flora resistant to commonly used antibiotics (i.e., hospital-acquired strains). Prophylactic antibiotic administration is standard with the implantation of a vascular prosthesis and has been shown to decrease the occurrence of wound infections that potentially lead to graft infection.[4] The antibiotic should be administered systemically before incision of the skin and at regular intervals during the procedure in order to maintain tissue levels above the minimal bactericidal concentration for expected pathogens. Alterations in the antibiotic regimen may be needed during the operation based on the elimination and volume of distribution of the antibiotic, with higher or more frequent doses necessary in patients with excessive changes in blood volume, fluid administration, or renal blood flow during the procedure. Cefazolin sodium, 1 gm given intravenously 1 hour before surgery and then 1 gm given every 2 to 3 hours during surgery, will achieve excellent tissue levels in the majority of patients undergoing prosthetic graft implantation. In patients with allergies to penicillin or the cephalosporins, parenteral vancomycin (1 gm) plus gentamicin (1.5 mg/kg), administered 1 hour before surgery and then repeated every 8 to 12 hours for three additional doses, is also an appropriate prophylactic antibiotic regimen. Culture-specific antibiotics should be prescribed for patients undergoing vascular graft implantation who have coexisting infections of the leg or at other remote sites. At some vascular centers, prophylactic antibiotics are continued for 3 to 5 days in patients deemed to be at high risk for transient bacteremia, or until all central intravascular catheters are removed. However, there are no solid data to support continuing prophylactic antibiotics for more than two to three postoperative doses (i.e., 24 hours of antibiotic administration).

Attention to meticulous sterile technique is imperative to avoid bacterial contamination of the graft, especially during emergency procedures and prolonged reconstructive procedures. The graft should be protected from contact with any potentially contaminating sources, especially the exposed skin adjacent to the operative field, by the use of iodine-impregnated plastic drapes or antibiotic-soaked towels or cotton pads. Simultaneous gastrointestinal procedures should be avoided during grafting procedures to prevent graft contamination with enteric organisms. The performance of an enterotomy during celiotomy should preclude graft implantation; the patient's incision should be closed and the arterial reconstruction scheduled for a second operative setting a few days later. A possible exception to the admonition against simultaneous gastrointestinal procedures is with cholecystectomy for asymptomatic cholelithiasis, which can be performed safely in patients undergoing aortic graft implantation. An 18 per cent incidence of postoperative acute cholecystitis in the face of cholelithiasis following elective aneurysm repair without cholecystectomy has been reported.[18] In addition, an increased risk of graft infection has not been demonstrated when cholecystectomy is performed at the same time as aortic graft implantation. Cholecystectomy should be performed only after the aortic graft has been implanted and the retroperitoneum has been totally closed.

After prosthetic graft implantation, patients should be fully informed of the potential risk of late graft colonization and infection via bacteremia, especially following interventional procedures such as dental work, colonoscopy, and cystoscopy. Antibiotic prophylaxis is recommended in these instances.

Early recognition and aggressive treatment of postoperative wound infections is an absolute necessity if extension that involves the underlying graft is to be avoided. Careful handling of the tissues, meticulous hemostasis to prevent hematoma formation, and closure of the groin incisions in multiple layers to eliminate dead space are important technical caveats for decreasing the likelihood of wound healing problems and subsequent infection. The use of topical antibiotics may also be of benefit before wound closure in order to achieve a high antibiotic concentration adjacent to the prosthetic graft.

BACTERIOLOGY

Although virtually any microorganism can infect a vascular prosthesis, *Staphylococcus aureus* is the most prevalent pathogen (Table 36–3). Since the early 1970s, graft infections due to *Staphylococcus epidermidis* and other gram-negative bacteria have increased in frequency. Surgeons have also become cognizant of the possibility of microbiologic sampling error when low numbers of bacteria are present, despite clinical and anatomic signs of perigraft infection.[56] Late-appearing graft infections caused by *S. epidermidis* and other coagulase-negative staphylococci are typically associated with negative results in cultures of perigraft fluid or tissue.[11] Infections due to gram-negative bacteria such as *Escherichia coli* and *Pseudomonas, Klebsiella, Enterobacter,* and *Proteus* species are particularly virulent. The incidence of anastomotic dehiscence and artery rupture is high and is due to the organisms' ability to produce destructive endotoxins (e.g., elastase and alkaline protease) that act to compromise vessel wall structural integrity.[19, 20] Fungal infections of grafts (e.g., with *Candida, Mycobacterium,* and *Aspergillus* species) are rare, and most patients who develop them are either severely immunosuppressed or have an established fungal infection elsewhere.

Graft infections that occur within 4 months of graft implantation are associated with virulent pathogens, with *S. aureus* predominating. Coagulase-positive strains produce hemolysis and toxins to leukocytes that provoke an intense local and systemic host response and permit early recogni-

Table 36–3. Bacteriology of Prosthetic Vascular Graft Infections: Incidence From Collected Cases (n = 1258)

	Incidence (%)					
Microorganism	***AEF***	***AI***	***AF***	***FD***	***TA***	***ICS***
Staphylococcus aureus	4	3	27	28	22	50
Staphylococcus epidermidis	2	3	26	11	25	20
Streptococcus species	19	3	10	11	2	—
Escherichia coli	18	30	12	7	2	—
Pseudomonas species	3	7	6	16	14	—
Klebsiella species	5	10	5	2	2	10
Enterobacter species	5	13	2	2	—	—
Enterococcus species	8	10	2	7	4	—
Bacteroides species	8	3	3	2	—	—
Proteus species	4	—	4	7	2	—
Candida species	3	—	1	1	4	—
Serratia species	1	—	1	2	—	—
Other species	3	2	4	6	0	—
No growth culture	18	13	2	2	16	20

AEF, aortoenteric fistula or erosion (n = 397); AI, aortoiliac or aortic tube graft (n = 39); AF, aortobifemoral or iliofemoral graft (n = 460); FD, femoropopliteal, femorotibial, axillofemoral, or femorofemoral graft (n = 251); TA, thoracic aorta graft (n = 55); ICS, innominate, carotid, or subclavian bypass graft or carotid patch following endarterectomy (n = 56).

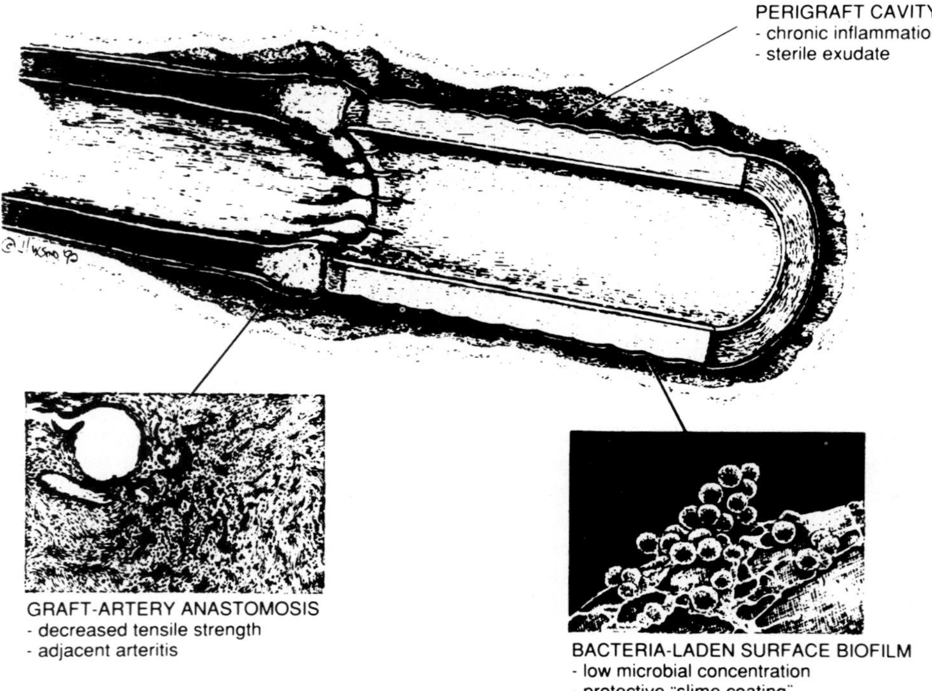

FIGURE 36–2. Anatomic characteristics of prosthetic graft infection caused by a bacterial biofilm. (Courtesy of Medical College of Wisconsin.)

tion of the infectious complications. Gram-negative organisms such as *Proteus, Pseudomonas, Klebsiella,* and *Enterobacter* species can also be involved in early postoperative graft infections, with anastomotic bleeding most commonly associated with a *Pseudomonas aeruginosa* infection. Graft healing complications, such as graft-enteric erosion or fistula, typically involve infection with gram-negative enteric bacteria and can develop in both the early and the late postoperative periods.

Late-appearing graft infections (i.e., those occurring more than 4 months after graft implantation) are commonly associated with less virulent bacteria. *S. epidermidis* and other coagulase-negative staphylococci are common pathogens for graft infections occurring months to years after implantation. These organisms are a component of normal skin flora but have the ability to adhere to and colonize biomaterials and to grow within a biofilm adherent to the prosthetic surfaces, resulting in an indolent infection. The bacterial biofilm is eventually recognized by host defense mechanisms, leading to inflammation of the perigraft tissue and adjacent artery and to the subsequent clinical manifestations of a late graft infection (Fig. 36–2).

DIAGNOSIS

Prompt diagnosis and treatment of prosthetic graft infections are essential to avoid complications (e.g., sepsis and hemorrhage) and death. Clinical manifestations are varied and may be subtle, particularly for grafts confined to the abdomen or thorax. Operative exploration is the most accurate method of excluding infection of a vascular prosthesis and may be required when clinical suspicion of graft-enteric erosion exists. In equivocal cases, the vascular surgeon has the onus to prove a graft infection is not present. The majority of graft infections are diagnosed more than 4 months after graft implantation,[6, 7, 66, 75] and fewer than 20 per cent are detected in the early postoperative period. Diagnosis of vascular prosthesis infection is based on clinical signs, characteristic abnormalities on vascular imaging, and microbiologic analysis of the graft.

Clinical Manifestations

History. Because graft infections are often subtle in presentation, the vascular surgeon must develop a low threshold for diagnostic testing based on any symptom or sign suggestive of graft infection. Infection of grafts confined to the abdomen can present as unexplained sepsis, prolonged postoperative ileus, or abdominal distention and tenderness as the only clinical signs. If the infection involves a superficial graft segment (i.e., in leg, groin, or neck incisions), local signs of graft infection are usually apparent by findings of an inflammatory perigraft mass, cellulitis, a drainage sinus tract, or a palpable anastomotic pseudoaneurysm. Patients with an aortic graft infection and graft-enteric fistula often present with an upper or lower gastrointestinal herald bleed. Any patient with gastrointestinal bleeding and an aortic graft should be considered to have graft infection and graft-enteric fistula or erosion until another source of bleeding is conclusively identified or no graft-bowel communication is verified at operation.[6, 66, 75, 103] In patients with vague symptoms suggestive of a low-grade graft infection, careful review of the operative history and surgical notes may furnish clues that further support the diagnosis of graft infection and provide the rationale for more detailed and invasive diagnostic testing. The patient should also be queried about recent medical illnesses that could have resulted in hematogenous or lymphatic seeding of the graft with bacteria. Early graft infections due to *S. aureus* or other gram-negative bacteria typically present within weeks of the procedure as fever, leukocytosis, and obvious perigraft purulence. Bacteremia is a late sign and is associated with artery wall or mural thrombus infection or with secondary endocarditis. Patients with a graft infection due to *S. epidermidis* present months to years after graft implantation with graft healing complications (e.g., anastomotic aneurysm, perigraft cavity with fluid, or graft cutaneous sinus tract) but no systemic signs of sepsis (e.g., fever, leukocytosis, and bacteremia). The preoperative diagnosis of a vascular prosthesis infection due to *S. epidermidis* is based on the clinical presentation, physical signs, and a high index of suspicion.

Physical Examination. In the physical examination, the clinician should closely scrutinize the site or sites of graft implantation for signs of inflammation. Surgical incisions should be carefully inspected for healing complications or draining sinuses. Masses in juxtaposition to anastomotic sites can represent perigraft abscesses or anastomotic pseudoaneurysms. The extremities should be examined for signs of septic embolization manifesting as a cluster of petechiae downstream from the infected graft. Other sources of infection, such as infected foot lesions, osteomyelitis, and infected urinary calculi, should be sought because these conditions can predispose to hematogenous bacterial seeding and graft colonization.

Laboratory Studies. An elevated white blood cell count (15,000 to 18,000 cells/ml) with left-shifted differential and an increased erythrocyte sedimentation rate (greater than 20 mm/min) are common but nonspecific findings in patients with graft infection and fever. Routine laboratory testing should also include urinalysis, blood cultures, and cultures of any other potential sources of infection, such as foot and surgical wound drainage. A stool guaiac test for blood is indicated in patients with suspected graft-enteric fistula or erosion, but findings are positive in only approximately two thirds of patients with documented lesions. All laboratory test results may be normal in patients with late-appearing perigraft infections due to *S. epidermidis*.

Vascular Imaging

Various vascular imaging modalities are currently used to diagnose graft infection. Anatomic signs of graft infection, such as perigraft abscess or anastomotic aneurysm, can be identified by ultrasonography, computed tomography (CT), magnetic resonance imaging (MRI), arteriography, and contrast sinography. Functional radionuclide imaging can confirm the presence of a clinically suspected graft infection when anatomic signs of perigraft abscess are equivocal. The combination of anatomic and functional vascular imaging techniques is highly accurate for confirming the presence of infection, planning management, and assessing operative sites for residual or recurrent infection. Arteriography is particularly useful in the development of a treatment strategy and should be routine. Anatomic definition of the infectious process identifies safe locations for vascular clamp placement and minimizes the likelihood of vascular injury or organ ischemia secondary to anatomic anomalies or concomitant arterial occlusive disease.

Contrast-Enhanced CT. Contrast-enhanced CT is the preferred initial imaging technique for patients with suspected infection of aortofemoral, abdominal aorta, or thoracic aorta grafts. Diagnostic criteria suggestive of infection include the loss of normal tissue planes of the retroperitoneal structures, indicative of inflammation; abnormal collections of fluid or gas around the graft; false aneurysm formation; hydronephrosis; adjacent vertebral osteomyelitis; and juxta-aortic retroperitoneal abscess (Fig. 36–3). The presence of fluid and air surrounding a vascular prosthesis is normal in the early postoperative period, and this limits the diagnostic accuracy of CT. However, any gas in the periprosthetic tissues on CT scans should be judged as abnormal beyond 6 to 7 weeks after implantation. CT should be performed with intravenous and oral contrast to better identify the lumen of the graft, delineate periprosthetic abscess, and define the relationship of the duodenum and small bowel to the aortic prosthesis. Scanning can be performed with sufficient speed to be useful in evaluating symptomatic but hemodynamically stable patients with suspected graft-enteric fistula or erosion.

Ultrasonography. Ultrasonography is a readily available imaging technique that is suited for portable examination of patients with suspected graft infection. Color duplex scanning can reliably differentiate perigraft fluid collection from anastomotic pseudoaneurysm or hematoma and is thus useful in the evaluation of pulsatile masses. Diagnostic accuracy depends on the skill of the examiner and the ability to adequately image the graft, which can be obscured by abdominal distention due to large amounts of intestinal gas or obesity. Duplex scanning is the most useful initial imaging technique for verifying vessel or graft patency and assessing pulsatile masses adjacent to grafts in the groin and limbs.

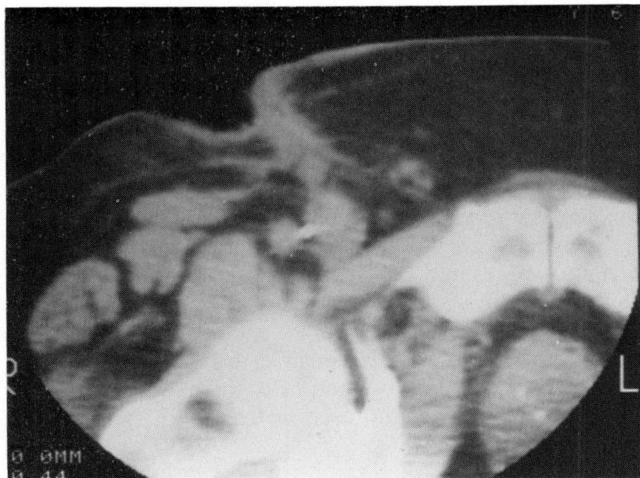

FIGURE 36–3. Computed tomographic scan of an infected aortofemoral graft limb showing perigraft inflammation extending to the skin. The patient presented with groin sinus tract. Graft culture isolated *Staphylococcus epidermidis*.

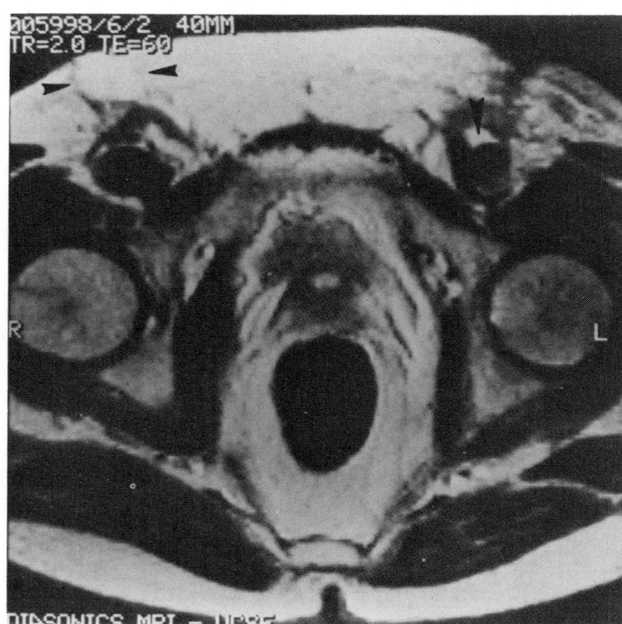

FIGURE 36–4. Magnetic resonance image of prosthetic graft infection. Soft tissue inflammation delineated by *arrowheads.* (From Olofsson PA, Auffermann W, Higgins CB, et al: Diagnosis of prosthetic aortic graft infection by magnetic resonance imaging. J Vasc Surg 8:99, 1988.)

MRI. MRI is a newer modality for determining the presence of graft infection (Fig. 36–4). It may become the preferred method because of its superior imaging, compared with CT, of the soft tissues surrounding the graft. MRI is useful in differentiating between perigraft fluid collection and inflammation of the perigraft tissues. In a review by Olofsson and colleagues, MRI clearly identified perigraft fluid collection and inflammation in 11 of 14 patients with aortic graft infection at operation. In contrast, CT was correct in only 4 of 10 patients with verified graft infection.[67] MRI and CT, however, share the limitation of not being able to differentiate a perigraft abscess from sterile perigraft fluid.

Contrast Sinography. Percutaneous localization of the perigraft fluid and performance of a contrast study can demonstrate the extent of the perigraft cavity along the graft limb. This study, however, is not routinely recommended because of the risks of contaminating the sterile graft. In addition, the contrast material in the perigraft space does not necessarily give the full extent of the graft infection.

Gram's stain and culture of fluid aspirated from the perigraft space may identify the causative organism or organisms. Gram's stain of tissue or perigraft fluid showing no organisms is not sufficient to exclude the presence of infection. It is not uncommon with a late-appearing graft infection for only white blood cells to be seen on Gram's stain and for no bacteria to be isolated by a swab culture plated on agar media.[6, 11]

White Blood Cell Scanning. Gallium-67 scanning, indium-111 labeling of white blood cells, and polyclonal human IgG scanning are useful radionuclide imaging techniques for demonstrating sites of leukocyte accumulation and for diagnosing graft infection. These functional imaging techniques are not useful during the early postoperative course because of nonspecific radionuclide take-up in the perigraft tissues. False-negative scan findings are unusual, so exclusion of early graft infection is possible, but normal findings have been reported in late-appearing aortic graft infection complicated by graft-enteric erosion. Three to 4 months after graft implantation, the accuracy of the functional imaging scans, especially indium-111–labeled white blood cell scans, approaches 90 per cent in the detection of graft infection. Positive scan findings are associated with a positive predictive value of 80 per cent. IgG scans are preferred over leukocyte scans because of the ease of preparation, the lack of staff exposure to the patient's blood, the absence of concomitant red blood cell and platelet imaging, and the long shelf-life. Functional imaging studies can be used with MRI and CT to delineate accurately the extent of graft involvement.

Endoscopy. Endoscopy is an important diagnostic modality in patients with suspected secondary aortoenteric fistula or erosion (Fig. 36–5). It is essential that the entire upper gastrointestinal tract be inspected, including the third and fourth portions of the duodenum, which are the most common sites of graft-enteric fistula. Patients with recent massive gastrointestinal hemorrhage should be examined *in the operating room,* with preparation for operation should exsanguination from the fistula be induced.[54] Endoscopy can sometimes visualize the graft eroded through the bowel mucosa or the clot at the bleeding site, but its main purpose is to rule out other sources of bleeding, such as gastritis or ulcer disease. Negative examination findings do *not* exclude the possibility of an aortoduodenal fistula.

Arteriography. Although arteriography cannot be used to make the diagnosis of graft infection, it can accurately identify infection-associated complications, such as graft rupture and anastomotic aneurysm. Biplanar angiography should be performed on all patients with confirmed or suspected aortic graft infection to assess the patency of the involved vessels and graft and to evaluate the status of the

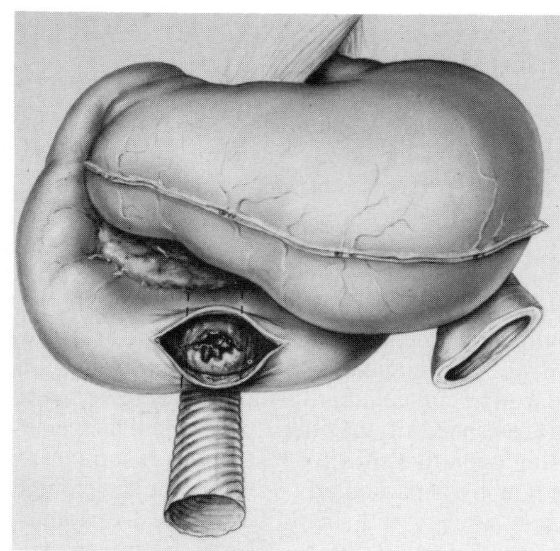

FIGURE 36–5. Graft enteric fistula.

proximal and distal vessels as potential sites for extra-anatomic bypass grafts.

Microbiologic Methods

Identification of the bacteria causing the graft infection is necessary to confirm the diagnosis and to select appropriate antibiotic therapy. Routine techniques for culture of graft surfaces and perigraft fluid are usually adequate in patients who have graft infections associated with fever, leukocytosis, and perigraft abscess with cellulitis. Virulent organisms, such as *S. aureus*, streptococci, and gram-negative bacteria, result in systemic signs of graft sepsis by invading the perigraft tissues and blood and are readily identified. However, routine microbiologic techniques will *not* recover less virulent pathogens that do not result in invasion of the perigraft tissues. More sensitive microbiologic techniques should be employed to identify the causative organism when organisms are not seen on Gram's stain of the perigraft fluid or tissues and when patients show no signs of graft sepsis (no fever or leukocytosis), especially when they present more than 4 four months postoperatively (Fig. 36–6). Mechanical disruption of the bacteria from the graft surface, either by tissue grinding or by ultrasonic disruption, and culture in broth media increase the identification of the bacteria, compared with routine culture methods.[11] Culture of the graft material with mechanical disruption and broth media identified the bacteria in more than 80 per cent of cases, despite negative findings on Gram's stain and culture of the perigraft tissue and fluid. Disruption of the bacteria from the surface of the graft disperses the bacteria into the culture media for growth. Even though broth and agar have the same biochemical composition, placement of the graft in broth is believed to maximize bacterial growth and recovery because the liquid medium allows submersion of the graft and optimal exposure of the bacteria to the nutrient medium. The use of mechanical disruption and broth cultures is particularly useful for confirming graft infections with *S. epidermidis*. These techniques overcome the sampling errors of routine culturing methods in isolating slowly growing microorganisms that reside in low numbers on the vascular biomaterial surfaces. Culture results may also be influenced by concomitant antibiotic administration, the degree of tissue invasion, and the adequacy of host defenses.

Operative Findings

The definitive diagnostic test for patients with suspected graft infection is operative exploration. Operation permits the surgeon to inspect the graft and surrounding tissues for signs of infection, including graft incorporation, the presence of perigraft fluid, anastomotic integrity, and graft-enteric fistulae. Exploration, graft excision, and culture of the graft material are often the only reliable methods of identifying the causative bacteria.[6, 11] Operation is also an essential diagnostic test in patients with prior aortic surgery and gastrointestinal bleeding in whom all other sources of bleeding have been excluded. Fewer than one half of patients with graft-enteric fistula are diagnosed with certainty using the preoperative testing methods described previously.[66, 75] Thorough mobilization and exploration of the duodenum, the small bowel, and the aortic graft and proximal anastomoses will identify an infection in this situation in more than 80 per cent of cases. Successful treatment can be expected if the diagnosis is established before the development of life-threatening complications, such as hypotension and sepsis.

MANAGEMENT OF GRAFT INFECTIONS

General Principles

Preparing the Patient for Surgery. Patients who present in septic shock or hypovolemia due to anastomotic

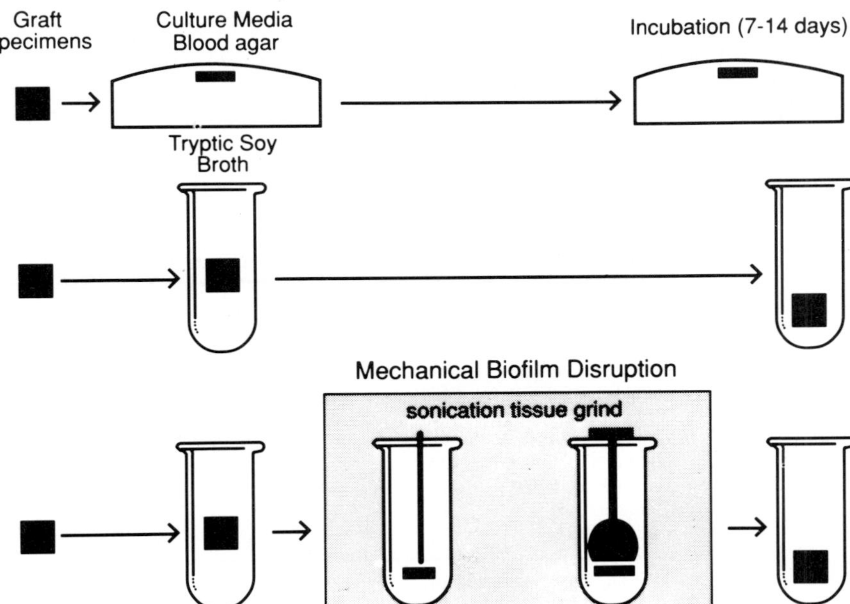

FIGURE 36–6. Culture techniques for recovery of bacteria from prosthetic vascular grafts.

bleeding secondary to a graft infection allow little time for preparation. Adequate resuscitation with blood and fluid volume, perioperative cardiopulmonary monitoring, administration of broad-spectrum high-dose antibiotics, and careful planning of the surgical approach form the essential elements of urgent preoperative treatment of these critically ill patients.

Fortunately, the majority of patients with graft infection allow time for adequate preoperative preparation, identification of the infecting pathogen, and determination of the extent of graft infection. Patients should be prepared physiologically and psychologically for the most extensive operation that may be required. Cardiac function should be determined, and the cardiac index and peripheral vascular resistance should be optimized with the administration of nitrates, antiarrhythmia medications, beta-blockers, and alpha-antagonists. The patient's pulmonary status should be evaluated and augmented with bronchodilators and respiratory therapy as needed. Baseline renal function should be established and renal perfusion improved by hydration or low-dose dopamine (3 to 5 μg/kg/min). Patients who have depleted nutritional reserves or are anergic to a battery of standard skin tests should be given enteral or parenteral nutrition, if time permits. Glucose levels should be closely monitored and controlled in patients with diabetes. The bowels should be cleansed with mechanical and antibiotic preparations in patients who have an intra-abdominal graft infection. Arterial circulation to the upper and lower extremities should be assessed by Doppler-derived pressure measurements and arteriography for adequate determination of appropriate revascularization alternatives to maintain limb perfusion after graft excision. Systemic antibiotics should be selected according to isolated or suspected pathogens. Other sites of infection, such as the urinary tract, lung, or foot, should be appropriately evaluated and treated.

Determining the Extent of Graft Infection. Persistent infection of a nonexcised graft segment or in the arterial graft bed is the major reason for treatment failure and the cause of morbidity and death.[75] Local control of infection is more successful when there is no gross purulence and when culture results are negative or *S. epidermidis* is recovered. CT, MRI, and white blood cell radionuclide scans are helpful in localizing the infected portion of the graft, but surgical exploration remains the most reliable method of determining the extent of graft infection.

Removing the Graft. Removal of the entire infected graft is absolutely essential for eradicating the infectious process in patients who are septic, present with anastomotic bleeding, or have complete involvement of the graft. Attempts at graft preservation with antibiotics and drainage have been reported, but the persistence of infection is common and patients remain at risk for exsanguination from anastomotic or arterial rupture during the period of observation.

For patients with infection localized to only a portion of an aortic graft, the surgeon should develop an individualized treatment plan because no single approach is applicable to all patients. Excision of the entire graft and extra-anatomic bypass are associated with amputation and mortality rates of 11 to 27 per cent (Table 36–4). Morbidity continues to be high due to persistent infection of the aortic stump (10 per cent incidence), recurrent infection of the extra-anatomic bypass (5 to 10 per cent incidence), and multiple secondary procedures for treatment of the failed extra-anatomic bypass (25 to 50 per cent incidence). In highly selected cases, amputation and mortality rates may be decreased by excising only the infected portion of the graft, with distal revascularization via remote bypass through tissues not involved with infection. At the site of graft retention, culture specimens should be obtained and topical antibiotics instilled via wound irrigation systems to cleanse perigraft tissues. The quantity and the virulence of the pathogens, the adequacy of local and systemic host defenses, and the extent of the infection are critical factors that influence decision making and treatment outcomes.

Débridement of the Arterial Wall and Perigraft Tissues, and Drainage. After graft excision, débridement of all inflamed tissues and drainage of the graft bed are important principles for avoiding persistence of the infectious process. The artery wall adjacent to the infected graft is a potential reservoir of bacteria, and positive artery wall culture findings increase the risk of aorta stump or artery disruption.[5, 7] The artery wall and perigraft tissues should be débrided back to normal-appearing tissues, especially in the presence of purulence or false aneurysm. Adequate débridement of the aorta should be confirmed by histologic examination, and if positive wall culture results are obtained, patients should be treated with long-term antibiotic therapy.[5] It is essential to use monofilament permanent sutures to close the artery. Closed suction drainage should be

Table 36–4. Results of Treatment of Aortic Graft Infections

Reference	No. of Cases	Mortality Rate (%)	Early Amputation (%)	Stump Blowout (%)	Survival > 1 Year (%)	Infection of EAB (%)
Bandyk et al, 1984[6]	18	11	11	0	66	17
O'Hara et al, 1986[66]	84	18	27	22	58	25
Reilly et al, 1987[75]	92	14	25	13	73	20
Schmitt et al, 1990[82]	20	15	5	6	75	6
Yeager et al, 1990[106]	38	14	21	4	76	22
Quinones-Baldrich et al, 1991[73]	45	24	11	0	63	20

EAB, extra-anatomic bypass.

positioned in the infected graft bed when gross purulence is present. Coverage of the arterial closures with viable, noninfected tissue, such as an omental pedicle or rotational muscle flaps, lessens the risk of stump blowout and separates the arterial closures from adjacent organs, the graft bed, and drains.

Antibiotic Therapy. If the pathogen or pathogens can be identified before operation, bactericidal antibiotics in large doses should be administered pre- and perioperatively. If the infecting organism has not been identified, broad-spectrum antibiotics, such as an aminoglycoside plus semisynthetic penicillin, a second-generation cephalosporin, or ampicillin plus sulbactam should be given. If *S. aureus* or *S. epidermidis* is suspected, an intravenous first- or second-generation cephalosporin and vancomycin would be appropriate. It is essential that antibiotics be administered preoperatively and that adequate tissue levels be maintained throughout the operation. Before closure of the incision, topical antibiotics (kanamycin and bacitracin) should be used in combination with a wound pulsed-irrigation system to cleanse tissues and remove debris. Once the graft infection has been treated and the operative cultures have isolated the bacteria, antibiotic coverage should be modified according to antibiotic susceptibility testing of the recovered strains. The duration of antibiotic administration after treatment by graft excision is unclear. Reilly and associates recommended at least 2 weeks of systemic antibiotics.[75] Patients who received long-term antibiotics (parenteral antibiotics for 6 weeks, followed by oral antibiotics for 6 months) had significantly better results than patients treated with short-term therapy (10 to 14 days). The incidences of recurrent infection and aortic stump blowout may be decreased with long-term antibiotic administration, especially in patients with positive arterial wall culture findings.[5] In patients with negative arterial wall culture findings, parenteral antibiotics should be administered for 2 to 4 weeks, followed by 3 months of oral therapy specific to the infecting pathogen or pathogens.

Revascularization of Organs and Limbs. Rarely can graft excision alone, without revascularization, be performed for the treatment of a patent, infected prosthetic graft. Occluded grafts and grafts implanted to alleviate symptoms of claudication may be treated by total graft excision without revascularization or in combination with endovascular angioplasty. An end-to-side anastomotic configuration permits reconstruction of the native arteries via autogenous patch angioplasty alone or in combination with endarterectomy. If a phasic Doppler arterial signal is present at the ankle after graft excision or if arterial systolic pressure is greater than 40 mmHg, delayed reconstruction is an option because sufficient collaterals have been preserved. In the presence of critical limb ischemia (i.e., if there is no audible Doppler signal at the ankle), arterial revascularization should not be delayed because of the associated increased morbidity and limb loss.

It is preferable to perform limb revascularization before the infected graft is removed, but in the presence of anastomotic bleeding and shock, control of hemorrhage takes precedence. Autogenous tissue grafts (greater saphenous vein or endarterectomized iliac or superficial femoral artery), if available, are the conduits of choice for limb or organ revascularization. If a prosthetic graft is used for an ex situ bypass, polytetrafluoroethylene (PTFE) conduits are preferred to Dacron grafts, although antibiotic-impregnated grafts may eventually be the conduits of choice for the treatment of established graft infections by either in situ replacement or extra-anatomic bypass grafting. Trout and coworkers[99] and Reilly and associates[75] showed a trend toward decreased morbidity and mortality with staged or sequential treatment as compared with traditional treatment (i.e., total graft excision followed by immediate extra-anatomic bypass). Preliminary revascularization can be performed without increasing the risk of death, amputation, or new graft infection, and with staged treatment (i.e., revascularization followed in 1 to 2 days by total graft excision), the physiologic stress on the patient may be reduced. Sequential treatment (i.e., preliminary revascularization followed by graft excision) prevents lower limb ischemia and avoids the necessity of keeping the patient heparinized during total graft excision and artery or aorta stump closure.

Selective graft preservation and in situ replacement should be applied only in carefully selected patients. When infection involves the thoracic aorta, in situ replacement may be the only practical approach. The perigraft infectious process should be low-grade and not associated with anastomotic hemorrhage, and cultures should be sterile or the anatomic and microbiologic characteristics of the graft infection should suggest infection with *S. epidermidis.* In situ replacement has been used successfully to treat secondary aortoduodenal fistula, with an operative mortality rate as low as 19 per cent. Patients with graft-enteric erosion and minimal retroperitoneal infection fared best. In situ replacement appears to be a safe option for patients with graft infections secondary to *S. epidermidis.* From 1987 to 1993, the authors treated 20 patients presenting with groin false aneurysm (n = 10), inflammatory mass (n = 6), or groin sinus tract (n = 4). No deaths or early graft failures occurred, and during follow-up, all replacement grafts remained patent and without signs of infection. Two patients required an additional graft replacement for infection that developed proximal to the in situ replacement graft. In situ treatment of bacterial biofilm graft infections is effective treatment for localized graft healing problems, but because of the indolent nature of this type of biomaterial infection, subsequent infection of previously uninvolved graft segments may be expected.

Treatment for Specific Infected Graft Sites

Aortoiliac or Aortic Interposition Graft Infections. Aortoiliac or aortic interposition graft infections are best treated by preliminary (right-sided) axillobifemoral bypass grafting through clean, uninfected tissues, followed during the same operation by total graft excision of the infected aortic graft (sequential treatment). Preliminary remote bypass is safe and is associated with lower morbidity than is traditional treatment.[66, 75, 99] Extra-anatomic bypass grafting should be performed without entry into the contaminated abdomen or retroperitoneum. Because the aortic graft is confined to the abdomen, the distal axillofemoral anastomoses can usually be performed to the common femoral arteries bilaterally. After completion of the extra-anatomic bypass grafting, all wounds should be closed and covered with sterile protective dressings. The patient is then reprepared and draped for excision of the infected aortic graft. Heparinization should be used during the revascularization procedure but can be reversed during excision of the infected graft. In cases with proximal and distal end-to-side anastomoses, in situ autogenous reconstruction should be considered an option. However, this scenario is uncommon because the majority of aortic interposition and aortoiliac grafts were implanted to treat aneurysmal disease rather than atherosclerotic occlusive disease.

The entire infected abdominal aortic graft should be excised. Achieving proximal control at the supraceliac aorta before approaching the proximal anastomosis is of value, especially in patients who have a proximal anastomotic aneurysm or juxtarenal anastomosis. Meticulous care is necessary to dissect adherent viscera and duodenum from the graft capsule. If graft-enteric erosion or fistula is present, débridement of all necrotic or inflamed bowel wall is imperative, and primary end-to-end anastomosis of the bowel is preferred. Further details of the diagnosis and treatment of aortoenteric fistula are provided in Chapter 38. The iliac arteries distal to the graft should also be mobilized for distal control before excision of the graft. Culture of explanted graft material should be performed with standard broth and biofilm culture techniques.

The aorta should be débrided back to normal-appearing wall and closed with interlocking monofilament sutures. A pedicle of omentum should be passed through the transverse mesocolon and carefully positioned around the aortic stump and into the bed of the excised aorta and graft. If necessary, the aorta can be excised to above the level of the renal arteries, with renal revascularization achieved via bypasses originating from the splenic or hepatic arteries.[63] Fortunately, infection involving the juxtarenal aorta is rare. Closed suction drains should be placed in the infected graft bed and brought out the flank opposite from the axillofemoral graft limb.

The distal aorta or iliac arteries should also be closed with monofilament suture. The ureter should be located and protected from injury throughout the procedure. Preoperative placement of ureteral stents can be helpful; however, they are usually not necessary unless hydronephrosis is present. The site and the method of iliac artery ligation should be chosen to maintain perfusion to the colon, the pelvis, and the buttock musculature. With infrarenal aorta ligation, pelvic circulation can be adequately maintained via retrograde blood flow from the extra-anatomic femoral bypass through the external and internal iliac arteries. With excision of an infected aorta–external iliac graft, salvage of perfusion to one iliac artery via autogenous reconstruction should be considered. Inflow to a single internal iliac artery is usually sufficient to maintain adequate pelvic perfusion because of abundant collateral flow via the visceral and deep femoral arteries.

Aortobifemoral Graft Infections. Aortobifemoral graft infections are more difficult to treat because involvement of the groin complicates lower limb revascularization and mandates distal anastomoses of the ex situ bypass to the deep femoral, superficial femoral, or popliteal arteries. Preoperative vascular imaging studies can identify patients with localized aortofemoral graft limb infection, thus permitting partial graft excision, typically of the distal groin segment. Patients should have no anatomic evidence of infection involving the proximal aorta and an intact aorta-graft anastomosis. If the graft infection is localized to the femoral region only and the distal anastomosis is not involved, local treatment by drainage of the perigraft abscess without graft excision, radical débridement of the perigraft tissues, and topical povidone-iodine irrigation has been successful.[56] Muscle flap coverage of the exposed graft facilitates graft coverage and wound healing.[73] Treatment without graft excision is appropriate only in carefully selected patients and is not recommended when patients are septic, the prosthetic graft is occluded, anatomic signs of arterial infection are present, and the infecting organism is a *Pseudomonas* species.[19, 20] Patients treated by graft preservation should be monitored in the intensive care unit, and persistence of perigraft purulence or systemic signs of infection should prompt the surgeon to recommend total graft excision.

Patients whose infection is localized to the femoral region of a single aortofemoral graft limb but who demonstrate sepsis or anastomotic involvement (e.g., femoral pseudoaneurysm or bleeding) are best treated by graft excision. If vascular imaging studies indicate that the graft infection is limited to the groin, a retroperitoneal approach through an oblique, suprainguinal incision is recommended to confirm that the retroperitoneal aortic graft limb is not involved and to obtain proximal control (Fig. 36–7). If the graft limb is well incorporated and culture of the excised graft shows negative results, removal of the graft limb, with retention of the remainder of the graft, is appropriate treatment. After division of the graft limb through the retroperitoneal approach, adjacent tissue should be interposed between the oversewn proximal and distal ends of the graft. The retroperitoneal incision should then be closed, and the infected femoral graft limb should be excised through an inguinal incision. The entire graft-artery anastomosis to the femoral artery should be excised, the adjacent artery wall débrided, and autogenous patch closure attempted if possible. Local endarterectomy may be required to facilitate closure. Salvage of the common femoral artery is important in maintaining retrograde flow into the pelvis. If the superficial femoral artery is open, an alternative method is to anastomose the superficial femoral artery to the deep femoral artery end to end in order to maintain pelvic flow via collaterals from the deep femoral system (Fig. 36–8). After graft excision, all arterial ligation sites or anastomoses should be covered with viable tissue. A rotational sartorius muscle flap is particularly useful for groin infections. The groin wound should be left open and treated with topical 0.1 per cent povidone-iodine or antibiotic dressings. Revascularization of the limb should be performed as necessary to maintain limb viability. Alternatives to revascularization depend on the patency of the distal circulation and can be performed to the deep femoral artery, the superficial femoral artery, or the popliteal artery. Revascularization should be accomplished via noninfected tissue planes using crossover femorofemoral grafts with medial tunneling or tunneling in the retropubic or suprapubic space, obturator bypass

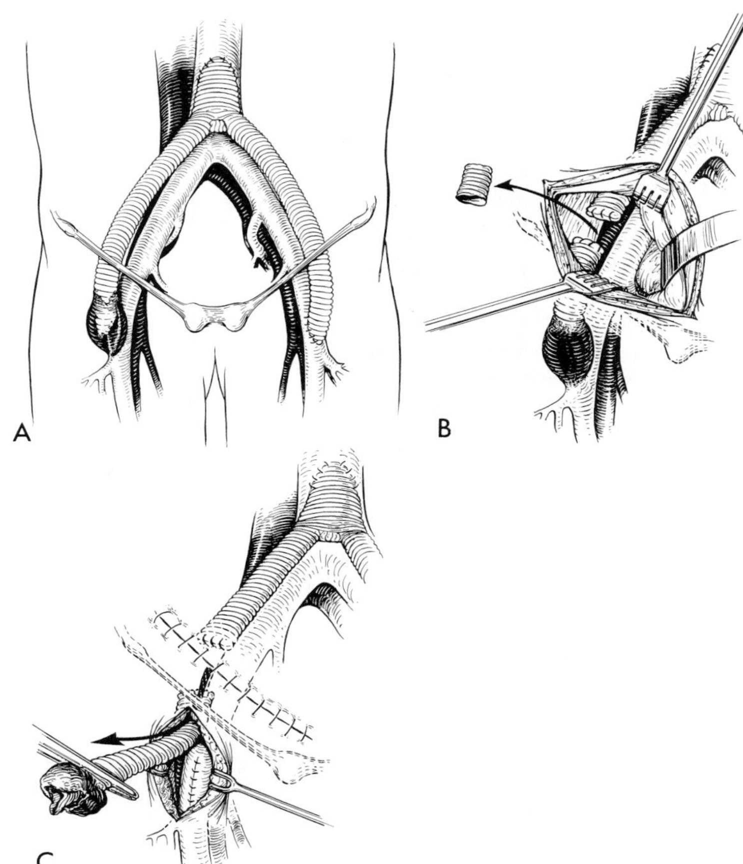

FIGURE 36–7. Excision of an infected femoral graft. *A*, Localized groin infection. *B*, Retroperitoneal exposure of noninfected graft segment. *C*, Excision of infected graft segment. (See text for details.)

via the obturator canal, or lateral tunneling through the psoas tunnel to course diagonally distal to the distal outflow artery. These bypasses are usually performed with PTFE or saphenous vein if it is of adequate caliber (5 mm in diameter or greater).

Highly selected cases of femoral graft limb infection that are localized only to the groin region, occur late in the postoperative course, and are secondary to *S. epidermidis* may be treated by graft excision and in situ replacement. Perioperative and postoperative use of antibiotics, both systemic and topical, is imperative in treatment with graft excision and in situ replacement. Wide débridement of all inflamed perigraft tissues, including the inflamed adjacent artery wall, is essential. In situ replacement with a PTFE prosthesis is recommended because it does have the best early graft healing after in situ replacement, both experimentally and clinically.[7, 10] It is recommended that patients continue intravenous antibiotics for 2 to 4 weeks and then receive oral antibiotics for 3 months after treatment.

Results of Treatment of Aortic Graft Infections. In some series, treatment of aortic graft infections with extra-anatomic bypass and excision of the entire graft has resulted in high operative mortality rates and early amputation rates (see Table 36–4). The persistence of sepsis and aortic stump blowout are the major causes of early and late mortality. Reilly and associates reported that 43 per cent of the early deaths and 71 per cent of the late deaths were due to aortic stump blowout. Lower extremity amputation and recurrent infection of the extra-anatomic bypass are major causes of late morbidity. The risk of major amputation of the extremity and of failure of extra-anatomic bypass grafts is higher for aortic grafts with groin infections than for infected aortoiliac grafts.[91] A subsequent infection of an axillofemoral graft is also associated with a significantly higher amputation rate than with no infection of the extra-anatomic bypass graft but failure due to thrombosis.[106]

As discussed earlier, the morbidity and mortality of extra-anatomic bypass grafting and total graft excision, combined with the high rate of late infection or failure of extra-anatomic bypass resulting in late lower extremity amputation, have resulted in investigations into alternative methods of treatment in highly selected patients. Infected aortobifemoral prostheses that have infection limited to the groin, no sepsis, a patent graft, and an intact distal anastomosis can be treated with local operative débridement, antibiotic use, and muscle flap coverage, as reported in several small series with good results.[62, 70] Calligaro and associates achieved complete graft preservation and wound healing in 16 of 22 cases (73 per cent) of graft infection due to gram-negative bacteria and in 23 of 33 cases (70 per cent) of graft infection due to gram-positive bacteria.[20] However, the potential for treatment failure exists, and patients must be carefully monitored. All four deaths (10 per cent mortality) in this series were due to graft sepsis; nine patients ultimately required total graft excision, and in seven patients, surgical wounds never healed. *Pseudomonas* was a particularly virulent pathogen and was associated with non-

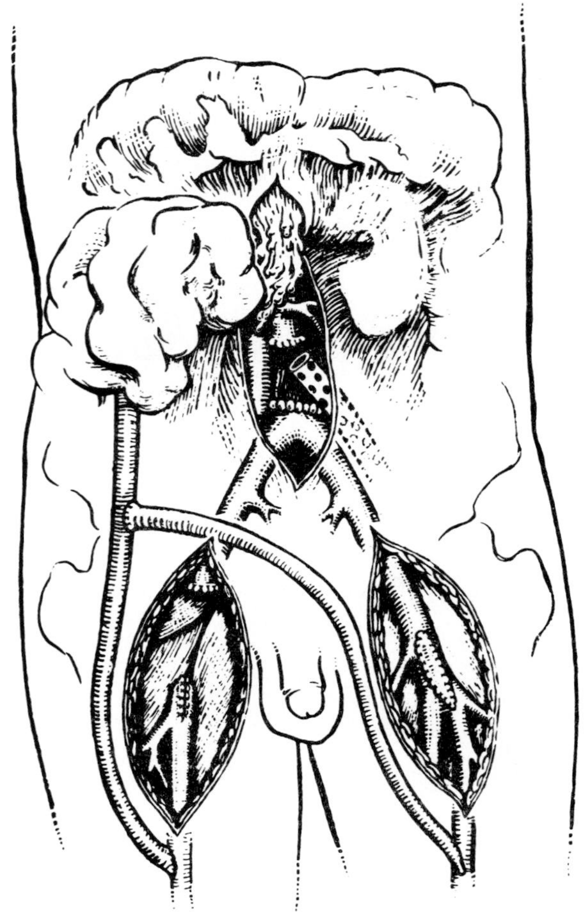

FIGURE 36–8. Excision of an infected aortobifemoral graft with extra-anatomic bypass.

healing wounds, anastomotic disruption, and arterial bed hemorrhage. Selective graft preservation carries a small but definite risk of hemorrhage due to destruction of an anastomosis by the septic process. One study indicated preservation of exposed or infected Dacron grafts was less successful than that of PTFE grafts.[19]

In situ replacement following prosthetic graft infections has been reported sporadically, with initial reports describing high (greater than 50 per cent) mortality rate in patients with graft-enteric fistula. More recent reports by Jacobs and coworkers[50] and Robinson and Johansen[78] indicated a mortality rate of less than 20 per cent, and long-term survival in 70 per cent of patients when this procedure was applied for low-grade infections. Treatment of bacterial biofilm graft infections by in situ replacement was uniformly successful in one report, but confirmation from additional vascular centers is warranted.[7]

Femoral, Popliteal, and Tibial Graft Infections. Once the diagnosis of infrainguinal prosthetic bypass graft infection is made, excision of the entire graft is recommended in patients who have anastomotic disruption or graft sepsis. The same principles that apply to aortic graft infection should be followed, including removal of the entire graft; radical débridement of infected perigraft tissues; débridement of the artery wall back to noninfected, uninflamed tissue; closure of the arteriotomies with monofilament suture; and the administration of systemic and topical antibiotics. The treatment of peripheral graft infections is associated with a low mortality rate but a high amputation rate as compared with the treatment of aortic graft infections (Table 36–5). Heparin should be administered intravenously to patients in whom limb viability is jeopardized by graft excision. Patients who had prosthetic grafts inserted for claudication may be treated with graft excision alone. Patients with limb-threatening ischemia resulting from excision of the infected bypass should have revascularization, preferably with autogenous tissue. Autogenous tissue, however, is frequently not available, and reconstruction with prosthetic graft via remote, noninfected planes should be performed.

The local treatment of infrainguinal graft infections by aggressive perigraft tissue débridement, antibiotic use, and muscle flap coverage, without graft excision, has been successful in patients without graft sepsis or anastomotic disruption. Multiple small series[20, 59, 62] have shown that this alternative treatment method can result in healing in approximately 70 per cent of cases and may not be harmful to the patient as long as early aggressive management by graft excision is undertaken if sepsis or anastomotic disruption or bleeding occurs.[70] If local treatment is successful, it may result in a decreased rate of limb amputation due to infrainguinal graft infection; however, there is no conclusive evidence to support this treatment in favor of the more conventional therapy of total graft excision and remote revascularization as needed.

Thoracic Aortic Graft Infections. Thoracic aortic graft infection is a very grave complication (Table 36–6). The principles of graft excision and extra-anatomic bypass are not applicable to most cases of prosthetic aortic valve or ascending or transverse aortic arch graft infection.[28, 46] The principle of in situ maintenance of circulation must be followed. The operative approach to this severe infection should be wide débridement of the infected tissues, graft excision and replacement if anastomotic areas are involved or disrupted because of the infection, and coverage of the

Table 36–5. Results of Treatment of Femoropopliteal or Tibial Prosthetic Graft Infections

Reference	No. of Cases	Mortality Rate (%)	Amputation Rate (%)
Szilagyi et al, 1972[90]	10	0	50
Liekweg and Greenfield, 1977[58]	55	9	33
Yashar et al, 1978[105]	3	0	67
Durham et al, 1986[34]	3	0	67

Table 36–6. Collected Series Results of Treatment of Thoracic, Innominate, Carotid, or Subclavian Prosthetic Graft Infections

Graft Site	No of Cases	Operative Deaths	Perioperative Strokes*	Survival > 1 Year†
Thoracic	50	6	0	42
Innominate, carotid, or subclavian bypass graft	33	9	3	14
Carotid patch	11	3	2	5

Data from Kieffer et al, 1986; Ehrenfeld et al, 1979; and Bergamini et al, 1993.

**All patients with strokes were treated by carotid ligation without reconstruction, which resulted in 4 operative deaths and 1 late death.*

†Late follow-up was not reported for 13 patients with an innominate, a carotid, or a subclavian bypass graft and for 1 patient with a carotid patch.

graft with viable, noninfected tissues. Pericardial fat pads; adjacent muscle, including the pectoralis major, the rectus abdominis, and the latissimus dorsi; and the greater omentum pedicle have been used for graft coverage. These principles of treatment were used by Coselli and colleagues in 40 patients. There were five operative deaths due to coagulopathy and hemorrhage (n = 2) or to cardiopulmonary and renal complications (n = 3).[28] Twenty-eight patients (70 per cent) were alive and without any evidence of recurrent graft infection at 4 months to 6.5 years.

Infections involving prosthetic grafts in the descending thoracic aorta may be amenable to graft excision and revascularization through clean, uninfected planes. A remote bypass graft can be placed through a median sternotomy from the ascending aorta to the abdominal aorta, tunneling through the diaphragm through clean, uninfected tissue. This graft should be placed before excision of the descending thoracic graft. After placement of this graft, the patient should undergo graft excision via a left thoracotomy.[46] The aortic closure should be covered with viable tissue transferred locally.

Innominate, Subclavian, and Carotid Graft Infections. Management of infection of a bypass or patch graft of the innominate, subclavian, or carotid arteries should be based on the same principles used for lower extremity graft infections. The risks of treatment of prosthetic infections at this location include not only persistent sepsis and death but also stroke (see Table 36–6). The surgical approach to a patient with prosthetic infection of a transthoracic bypass graft often requires a median sternotomy and preparation for cardiopulmonary bypass and total circulatory arrest, if needed for proximal control.[52] Treatment should include total graft excision, administration of parenteral and topical antibiotics, and remote bypass, preferably with autogenous tissue, if needed. There have been reports of successful treatment of infected prostheses with local irrigation, but this is not recommended because graft excision and remote revascularization are usually possible.

An infected transthoracic or extrathoracic bypass graft for upper extremity ischemia can often be removed without the need for immediate revascularization. Ligation of the proximal innominate or subclavian arteries, unlike ligation of the iliac or common femoral arteries, is often tolerated without the onset of extremity ischemia. A subsequent bypass, if needed, can be performed after the infection is cleared. Only one case of upper extremity amputation following removal of a subclavian bypass graft for infection has been reported.[52] If upper extremity ischemia results from graft excision, bypass with autogenous tissue through remote planes is preferred. Patients with transthoracic bypass grafts to the innominate and subclavian arteries often have multi-vessel disease of the aortic arch, necessitating that remote bypasses use the femoral artery, the descending thoracic aorta, or the supraceliac abdominal aorta as the inflow vessel. Remote bypass following excision of an infected carotid-subclavian bypass can be performed with a carotid-carotid bypass using saphenous vein or an axilloaxillary bypass using vein or PTFE (Fig. 36–9). Blood flow after excision of an infected axilloaxillary graft can be successfully reestablished with a supraclavicular subclavian-subclavian bypass, a carotid-carotid bypass, or a femoroaxillary bypass.

Patients with prosthetic infections of bypasses to the carotid arteries or with prosthetic patch infection of a carotid artery endarterectomy frequently do not tolerate simple ligation. In review of the reported cases of the treatment of carotid prosthetic infections, all five perioperative strokes occurred in patients treated by ligation without reconstruction. Simple ligation of the common or internal carotid

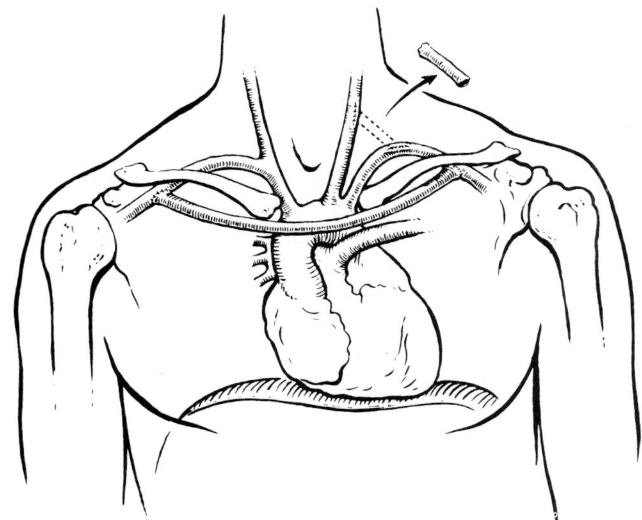

FIGURE 36–9. Excision of an infected carotid-subclavian graft with axilloaxillary bypass.

artery may be safely performed in patients with stump pressures of higher than 70 mmHg, but reconstruction of the artery to maintain cerebral blood flow and prevent stroke should be performed if possible. After graft excision, revascularization is preferably done with autogenous tissue. The anatomy of the extracranial carotid artery often does not permit remote bypass through noninfected, uninflamed tissues, and it often requires autogenous bypass in infected areas. Coverage of the bypass with muscle can be of value in this situation in preventing the recurrence of infection. Autogenous bypasses with saphenous vein or internal iliac artery are successful alternatives.[35] Treatment of carotid prosthetic patch infections is usually best achieved by excision of the patch and reconstruction with vein. Carotid shunts have been successfully and safely used to maintain cerebral perfusion during these difficult, challenging procedures. Stroke, recurrent infection, and carotid pseudoaneurysm formation are late complications in 12 per cent of cases.[12]

FUTURE DIRECTIONS

Dissatisfaction with the morbidity and mortality of treating graft infections, regardless of location, by total graft excision and remote bypass has been an impetus to the investigation of selective graft retention or in situ reconstruction. Selection criteria for these less aggressive treatment options have not been clinically verified, but experimental models have shown that treatment outcome depends on the virulence of the infecting organism, the extent of graft-artery infection, and the immune status of the patient. Appropriately designed and executed clinical trials are required to determine the patient group likely to benefit from these alternative treatments.

Studies are also warranted to investigate infection-resistant arterial conduits further. Cadaveric venous homografts and aortic allografts are being studied as replacement grafts following the excision of an infected prosthetic vascular graft.[40, 51] The development of and indications for the use of antibiotic-impregnated grafts are on the clinical horizon. Experimentally, antibiotic bonding to vascular biomaterials is now possible, and efficacy has been demonstrated under a variety of conditions (i.e., bacteremia, direct graft inoculation, and treatment of an established graft infection). Antibiotic-bonded grafts will probably be of most clinical benefit in patients at high risk for graft infection or of value to treat established infection by in situ replacement. The role of omental or muscle coverage of infected or replacement bypass grafts is also undergoing study. Future investigations of the pathogenesis, microbiology, anatomy, clinical presentation, and treatment of graft infections would be advantageous for all surgical specialties using biomaterials.

References

1. Aarnio P, Hannukainen J: Aortic graft—Enteric fistula. Ann Chir Gynaecol 78:329, 1989.
2. Arnold PG, Pairolero PC: Intrathoracic muscle flaps in the surgical management of life-threatening hemorrhage from the heart and great vessels. Plast Reconstr Surg 81:831, 1988.
3. Bakker-deWekker P, Alfieri O, Vermeulin F, et al: Surgical treatment of infected pseudoaneurysms after replacement of the ascending aorta. J Thorac Cardiovasc Surg 88:447, 1984.
4. Bandyk DF: Vascular graft infections: Epidemiology, microbiology, pathogenesis and prevention. *In* Bernhard VM, Towne JB (eds): Complications in Vascular Surgery. St. Louis, Quality Medical Publishing, 1991, pp 223–234.
5. Bandyk DF: Aortic graft infection. Semin Vasc Surg 3:122, 1990.
6. Bandyk DF, Berni GA, Thiele BL, et al: Aortofemoral graft infection due to *Staphylococcus epidermidis*. Arch Surg 119:102, 1984.
7. Bandyk DF, Bergamini TM, Kinney EV, et al: In situ replacement of vascular prostheses infected by bacterial biofilms. J Vasc Surg 13:575, 1991.
8. Becker RM, Blundell PE: Infected aortic bifurcation grafts: Experience with fourteen patients. Surgery 80:544, 1976.
9. Bennion RS, Hiatt JR, Williams RA, et al: Surgical management of unilateral groin infection after aortofemoral bypass. Surg Gynecol Obstet 156:724, 1983.
10. Bergamini TM: Vascular prostheses infection caused by bacterial biofilms. Semin Vasc Surg 3:101, 1990.
11. Bergamini TM, Bandyk DF, Govostis D, et al: Identification of *Staphylococcus epidermidis* vascular graft infections: A comparison of culture techniques. J Vasc Surg 9:665, 1989.
12. Bergamini TM, Seabrook GR, Bandyk DF, et al: Symptomatic recurrent carotid stenosis and aneurysmal degeneration following endarterectomy. Surgery 113:580, 1993.
13. Blaisdell FW, DeMattei GA, Gauder PJ: Extraperitoneal thoracic aorta to femoral bypass graft as replacement for an infected aortic bifurcation prosthesis. Am J Surg 102:583, 1961.
14. Branchereau A, Magnan PE: Results of vertebral artery reconstruction. J Cardiovasc Surg 31:320, 1990.
15. Brenner WI, Richman H, Reed GE: Roof patch repair of an aortoduodenal fistula resulting from suture line failure in an aortic prosthesis. Am J Surg 127:762, 1974.
16. Buchbinder D, Leather R, Shah D, et al: Pathologic interactions between prosthetic aortic grafts and the gastrointestinal tract. Am J Surg 140:192, 1980.
17. Busuttil RW, Rees W, Baker JD, et al: Pathogenesis of aortoduodenal fistula: Experimental and clinical correlates. Surgery 85:1, 1979.
18. Calligaro KE, Veith FJ: Surgery of the infected aortic graft. *In* Bergan JJ, Yao JST (eds): Aortic Surgery. Philadelphia, WB Saunders, 1989, pp 485–496.
19. Calligaro KD, Westcott CJ, Buckley RM, et al: Infrainguinal anastomotic arterial graft infections treated by selective graft preservation. Ann Surg 216:74, 1993.
20. Calligaro KD, Veith FJ, Gupta SK, et al: A modified method of management of prosthetic graft infections involving an anastomosis to the common femoral artery. J Vasc Surg 11:485, 1990.
21. Carter SC, Cohen A, Whelan TJ: Clinical experience with management of the infected Dacron graft. Ann Surg 158:249, 1963.
22. Champion MC, Sullivan SN, Coles JC, et al: Aortoenteric fistula. Incidence, presentation, recognition, and management. Ann Surg 3:314, 1982.
23. Cherry KJ, Roland CF, Pairolero PC, et al: Infected femorodistal bypass: Is graft removal mandatory? J Vasc Surg 15:295, 1992.
24. Cohn R, Angell WW: Late complications from plastic replacement of aortic abdominal aneurysms. Arch Surg 87:696, 1968.
25. Conn JH, Hardy JD, Chavez CM: Infected arterial grafts: Experience in 22 cases with emphasis on unusual bacteria and techniques. Ann Surg 171:704, 1970.
26. Connelly JE, Kwaan JHM, McCart PM, et al: Aortoenteric fistula. Ann Surg 4:402, 1981.
27. Conte CC, Ellison LH: Management of extracranial carotid artery aneurysms. Conn Med 50:501, 1986.
28. Coselli JS, Crawford ES, Williams TW, et al: Treatment of postoperative infection of ascending aorta and transverse aortic arch, including use of viable omentum and muscle flaps. Ann Thorac Surg 50:868, 1990.
29. Crawford ES, DeBakey ME, Morris GC Jr, et al: Evaluation of late failures after reconstructive operations for occlusive lesions of the aorta and iliac, femoral, and popliteal arteries. Surgery 17:79, 1960.
30. Criado FJ: Extrathoracic management of aortic arch syndrome. Br J Surg 69(Suppl):S45, 1982.
31. Dean RH, Allen TR, Foster JH, et al: Aortoduodenal fistula: An uncommon but correctable cause of upper gastrointestinal bleeding. Am Surg 44:37, 1978.

32. DeBakey ME, Crawford ES, Morris GC Jr, et al: Patch graft angioplasty in vascular surgery. J Cardiovasc Surg 3:106, 1962.
33. Diethrich EB, Noon GP, Liddicoat JE, et al: Treatment of infected aortofemoral arterial prosthesis. Surgery 68:1044, 1970.
34. Durham JR, Rubin JR, Malone JM: Management of infected infrainguinal bypass grafts. *In* Bergan JJ, Yao JST (eds): Reoperative Arterial Surgery. Orlando, FL, Grune & Stratton, 1986, pp 359–373.
35. Ehrenfeld WK, Wilbur BG, Olcott CN, et al: Autogenous tissue reconstruction in the management of infected prosthetic grafts. Surgery 85:82, 1979.
36. Elliott JP, Smith RF, Szilagyi DE: Aortoenteric and paraprosthetic-enteric fistulas. Arch Surg 108:479, 1974.
37. Ferris EJ, Koltay MRS, Koltay OP, et al: Abdominal aortic and iliac graft fistulae—Unusual roentgenographic findings. Surgery 94:416, 1965.
38. Flye MW, Thompson WM: Aortic graft-enteric and paraprosthetic-enteric fistulas. Am J Surg 146:183, 1983.
39. Fry WJ, Lindenauer SM: Infection complicating the use of plastic arterial implants. Arch Surg 94:600, 1966.
40. Fujitani RM, Bassiouny HS, Gewertz BL, et al: Cryopreserved saphenous vein allogenic homografts: An alternative conduit in lower extremity arterial reconstruction in infected fields. J Vasc Surg 15:519, 1992.
41. Fulenwider JT, Smith RB, Johnson RW, et al: Reoperative abdominal arterial surgery—A ten-year experience. Surgery 93:20, 1983.
42. Garrett HE, Beall AC, Jordan GL Jr, et al: Surgical considerations of massive gastrointestinal tract hemorrhage caused by aortoduodenal fistula. Am J Surg 105:6, 1963.
43. Geary KJ, Tomkiewicz ZM, Harrison HN, et al: Differential effects of a gram-negative and a gram-positive infection on autogenous and prosthetic grafts. J Vasc Surg 11:339, 1990.
44. Goldstone J, Moore WS: Infection in vascular prostheses. Clinical manifestations and surgical management. Am J Surg 128:225, 1974.
45. Graver JM, Mulcare RJ: Pseudoaneurysm after carotid endarterectomy. J Cardiovasc Surg 27:294, 1986.
46. Hargrove WC III, Edmunds H Jr: Management of infected thoracic aortic prosthetic grafts. Ann Thorac Surg 37:72, 1984.
47. Hoffert PW, Gensler S, Haimovici H: Infection complicating arterial grafts. Arch Surg 90:427, 1965.
48. Humphries AW, Young JR, deWolfe VG, et al: Complications of abdominal aortic surgery. Arch Surg 86:43, 1963.
49. Jamieson GG, DeWeese JA, Rob CG: Infected arterial grafts. Ann Surg 181:850, 1975.
50. Jacobs MJHM, Reul GJ, Gregoric I, et al: In situ replacement and extra-anatomic bypass for the treatment of infected abdominal aortic grafts. Eur J Vasc Surg 5:83, 1991.
51. Kieffer E, Bahnini A, Koskas F, et al: In situ allograft replacement of infected infrarenal aortic prosthetic grafts: Results in 43 patients. J Vasc Surg 17:349, 1993.
52. Kieffer E, Petitjean C, Bahnini A: Surgery for failed brachycephalic reconstruction. *In* Bergan JJ, Yao JST (eds): Reoperative Arterial Surgery. Orlando, FL, Grune & Stratton, 1986, pp 581–607.
53. Kitka MJ, Goodson SF, Rishara RA, et al: Mortality and limb loss with infected infrainguinal bypass grafts. J Vasc Surg 5:566, 1987.
54. Kleinman LH, Towne JB, Bernhard VM: A diagnostic and therapeutic approach to aortoenteric fistulas: Clinical experience with twenty patients. Surgery 86:868, 1979.
55. Kozol RA, Bredenberg CE: Alternatives in the management of atherosclerotic occlusive disease of aortic arch branches. Arch Surg 116:1457, 1981.
56. Kwaan JHM, Connolly JE: Successful management of prosthetic graft infection with continuous povidone-iodine irrigation. Arch Surg 116:716, 1981.
57. Levy MF, Schmitt DD, Edmiston CE, et al: Sequential analysis of staphylococcal colonization of body surfaces of patients undergoing vascular surgery. J Clin Microbiol 28:664, 1990.
58. Liekweg WG Jr, Greenfield LJ: Vascular prosthetic infections: Collected experience and results of treatment. Surgery 81:335, 1977.
59. Lorentzen JE, Nielsen OM, Arendrup H, et al: Vascular graft infection: An analysis of sixty-two graft infections in 2411 consecutively implanted synthetic vascular grafts. Surgery 98:81, 1985.
60. Martinez NS: Extracranial carotid aneurysm—A complication of carotid endarterectomy. Illinois Med J 150:583, 1976.
61. McCollum CH, Wheeler WG, Noon GP, et al: Aneurysms of the extracranial carotid artery. Am J Surg 137:196, 1979.
62. Mixter RC, Turnipseed WD, Smith DJ Jr, et al: Rotational muscle flaps: A new technique for covering infected vascular grafts. J Vasc Surg 9:472, 1989.
63. Moncure AC, Brewster DC, Darling RC, et al: Use of the splenic and hepatic arteries for renal revascularization. J Vasc Surg 3:196, 1986.
64. Najafi H, Javid H, Dye WS, et al: Management of infected arterial implants. Surgery 65:539, 1969.
65. Ochsner JL, Mills NL: Profound hypothermia and circulatory arrest in control and repair of infected aortic prostheses. J Cardiovasc Surg 20:1, 1979.
66. O'Hara PJ, Hertzer NR, Beven EG, et al: Surgical management of infected abdominal aortic grafts: Review of a 25-year experience. J Vasc Surg 3:725, 1986.
67. Olofsson PA, Auffermann W, Higgins CB, et al: Diagnosis of prosthetic aortic graft infection by magnetic resonance imaging. J Vasc Surg 8:99, 1988.
68. O'Mara CS, Williams GM, Ernst CB: Secondary aortoenteric fistula. Am J Surg 142:203, 1981.
69. Pinkerton JA: Aortoduodenal fistula. JAMA 225:1196, 1973.
70. Piotrowski JJ, Bernhard VM: Management of vascular graft infections. *In* Bernhard VM, Towne JB (eds): Complications in Vascular Surgery. St. Louis, Quality Medical Publishing, 1991, pp 235–258.
71. Popovsky J, Singer S: Infected prosthetic grafts. Arch Surg 115:203, 1980.
72. Proctor CD, Rice KL, Lucas MR: Comparison of ankle-brachial indexes and magnetic resonance flowmetry in predicting outcome in diabetic foot lesions [Abstract]. J Vasc Surg 15:242, 1992.
73. Quinones-Baldrich WJ, Hernandez JJ, Moore WS: Long-term results following surgical management of aortic graft infection. Arch Surg 126:507, 1991.
74. Raskind R, Doria A: Wound complications following carotid endarterectomy: Report of two cases. J Vasc Surg 1:127, 1967.
75. Reilly LM, Stoney RJ, Goldstone J, et al: Improved management of aortic graft infection: The influence of operation sequence and staging. J Vasc Surg 5:421, 1987.
76. Reilly LM, Altman H, Lusby RJ, et al: Late results following surgical management of vascular graft infection. J Vasc Surg 1:36, 1984.
77. Reul GJ Jr, Cooley DA: False aneurysms of the carotid artery. *In* Bergan JJ, Yao JST (eds): Reoperative Arterial Surgery. Orlando, FL, Grune & Stratton, 1986, pp 537–553.
78. Robinson JA, Johansen K: Aortic sepsis: Is there a role for in situ graft reconstruction? J Vasc Surg 13:677, 1991.
79. Rosato FE, Barker C, Roberts B: Aorto-intestinal fistula. J Thorac Cardiovasc Surg 53:511, 1967.
80. Samson RH, Veith FJ, Janko GS, et al: A modified classification and approach to the management of infections involving peripheral arterial prosthetic grafts. J Vasc Surg 8:147, 1988.
81. Santschi DR, Frahm CJ, Pascale LR, et al: The subclavian steal syndrome. Clinical and angiographic considerations in 74 cases in adults. J Thorac Cardiovasc Surg 51:103, 1966.
82. Schmitt DD, Seabrook GR, Bandyk DF, et al: Graft excision and extra-anatomic revascularization: The treatment of choice for the septic aortic prosthesis. J Cardiovasc Surg 31:327, 1990.
83. Schroeder T, Hansen HJH: Arterial reconstruction of the brachycephalic trunk and the subclavian arteries. Acta Chir Scand 502:122, 1980.
84. Shaw RS, Baue AE: Management of sepsis complicating arterial reconstructive surgery. Surgery 53:75, 1963.
85. Seeger JM, Wheeler JR, Gregory RT, et al: Autogenous graft replacement of infected prosthetic grafts in the femoral position. Surgery 93:39, 1983.
86. Smith RB III, Lowry K, Perdue GD: Management of the infected arterial prosthesis in the lower extremity. Am Surg 33:711, 1967.
87. Snyder SO, Wheeler JR, Gregory RT, et al: Freshly harvested cadaveric venous homografts as arterial conduits in infected fields. Surgery 101:283, 1987.
88. Spanos PK, Gilsdorf RB, Sako Y, et al: The management of infected abdominal aortic grafts and graft-enteric fistulas. Ann Surg 183:397, 1976.
89. Sproul G: Rupture of an infected aortic graft into jejunum: Resection and survival. JAMA 182:1118, 1962.
90. Szilagyi DE, Smith RF, Elliott JP, et al: Infection in arterial reconstruction with synthetic grafts. Ann Surg 176:321, 1972.

91. Taylor SM, Mills JL, Fujitani RM, et al: The influence of groin sepsis on extra-anatomic bypass patency in patients with prosthetic graft infection. Ann Vasc Surg 6:80, 1992.
92. Thompson JE: Complications of carotid endarterectomy and their prevention. World J Surg 3:155, 1979.
93. Thistlethwaite JR, Hughes RK, Smyth NPD, et al: Spontaneous arteriovenous fistula between the abdominal aorta and vena cava. Arch Surg 81:79, 1960.
94. Thomas WEG, Baird RN: Secondary aorto-enteric fistulae: Towards a more conservative approach. Br J Surg 73:875, 1986.
95. Thompson BW, Read RC, Campbell GS: Operative correction of obstructed subclavian or innominate arteries. South Med J 71:1366, 1978.
96. Thompson BW, Read RC, Campbell GS: Operative correction of proximal blocks of the subclavian or innominate arteries. J Cardiovasc Surg 21:125, 1980.
97. Thompson JE, Kartchner MM, Auston DJ, et al: Carotid endarterectomy for cerebrovascular insufficiency (stroke): Follow up of 359 cases. Ann Surg 163:751, 1966.
98. Tobias JA, Daicoff GR: Aortogastric and aortoileal fistulas repaired by direct suture. Arch Surg 107:909, 1973.
99. Trout HH, Kozloff L, Giordano JM: Priority of revascularization in patients with graft enteric fistulas, infected arteries, or infected arterial prostheses. Ann Surg 199:669, 1984.
100. Turnipseed WD, Berkoff HA, Detmer DE, et al: Arterial graft infections. Delayed v. immediate vascular reconstruction. Arch Surg 118:410, 1983.
101. Van De Water JM, Gaal PG: Management of patients with infected vascular prostheses. Am Surg 31:651, 1965.
102. Veith FJ, Hartsuck JM, Crane C: Management of aortoiliac reconstruction complicated by sepsis and hemorrhage. N Engl J Med 270:1389, 1964.
103. Walker WE, Cooley DA, Duncan JM, et al: The management of aortoduodenal fistula by in situ replacement of the infected abdominal aortic graft. Ann Surg 205:727, 1987.
104. Welling RE, Cranley JJ, Krause RJ, et al: Obliterative arterial disease of the upper extremity. Arch Surg 116:1593, 1981.
105. Yashar JJ, Weyman AK, Burnard RJ, et al: Survival and limb salvage in patients with infected arterial prostheses. Am J Surg 135:499, 1978.
106. Yeager RA, Moneta GL, Taylor LM, et al: Improving survival and limb salvage in patients with aortic graft infection. Am J Surg 159:466, 1990.

37

Anastomotic Aneurysms

Wesley S. Moore, M.D.

• • •

An anastomotic aneurysm results from partial or total separation of the anastomosis between an artery and a vascular prosthesis. The fibrous tissue capsule surrounding the graft and host artery maintains vascular continuity; however, because the capsule lacks inherent strength, it can stretch and become aneurysmal. An anastomotic aneurysm differs from a true aneurysm in that the wall consists of fibrous tissue, whereas a true aneurysm contains the anatomic layers of an artery, including intima, media, and adventitia. Incidence is estimated to be between 1 and 4 per cent.[27] Aneurysms created by dilatation or disruption of graft material itself are addressed in relation to the particular prosthetic substances (see Chapter 29).

PATHOGENESIS

Suture Failure

Because primary healing between a prosthetic graft and a host artery does not occur, the ultimate strength of the anastomosis depends on the integrity of the suture line. During the early experience with prosthetic grafts, anastomotic aneurysms were often a direct result of the failure of silk suture. Silk is a biologic material, not a permanent suture; it is slowly absorbed and usually disappears within 4 years. Once the continuity of the suture is interrupted by absorption and phagocytosis, the graft begins to separate from the artery. Vascular continuity is maintained only by the fibrous tissue capsule that surrounds the graft and the host artery.[9, 11, 15–17, 21, 24] This capsule expands and becomes the wall of an anastomotic false aneurysm (Fig. 37–1).

Use of any suture material that is absorbable or easily broken can lead to this complication. Polyethylene was one example of a suture that fragmented with age and stress. Polypropylene (Prolene) suture had been viewed with caution, but there is no evidence to incriminate it in anastomotic aneurysm formation. Care must be taken not to grasp polypropylene suture with forceps or clamps because it may disrupt and later break, leading to pseudoaneurysm formation. The use of braided Dacron has been effective in virtually eliminating suture failure as a cause of anastomotic aneurysms. However, as with polypropylene, careless handling of braided suture may weaken it and result in late failure.

Graft Material

Studies have shown that polytetrafluoroethylene grafts may result in a better fibrous attachment between artery and

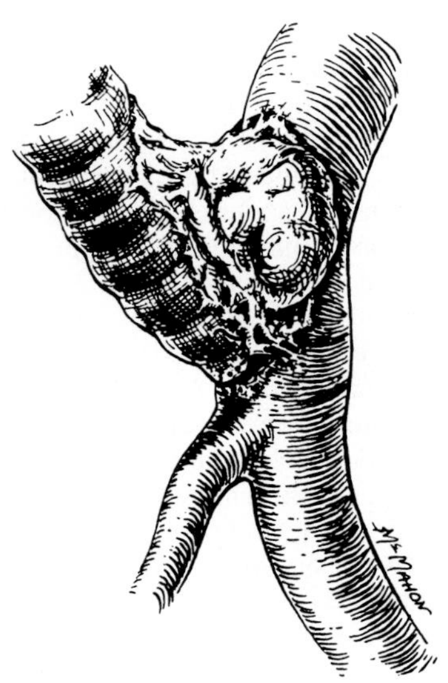

FIGURE 37–1. Separation of a graft-artery anastomosis, with associated aneurysmal dilatation of the bridging fibrous tissue capsule. Note the disruption of the suture line caused by absorption.

graft than Dacron grafts. Furthermore, the bond between the graft-graft anastomosis is stronger.[19] This tensile strength has not been demonstrated with other types of grafts.

Graft Infection

If a graft infection develops adjacent to a suture line, the necrotizing effect of the septic process may destroy the adjacent artery, allow the sutures to pull free, and lead to an anastomotic aneurysm. As this may occur over a prolonged time, infection should be considered as a prime etiologic factor, no matter what the time interval between graft placement and pseudoaneurysm formation. Most commonly, *Staphylococcus aureus* is cultured from pseudoaneurysms associated with infection.[22] *Staphylococcus epidermidis* is now emerging as a more common organism in graft infections, and infection with this organism may be an important etiologic factor in anastomotic aneurysm formation. The most common site for an infected pseudoaneurysm is the femoral anastomosis.[8]

Hematoma Communicating With Fresh Anastomosis

Following wound closure, a leak from the suture line may produce a hematoma that communicates with the arterial stream through a small suture line separation. The outer portion of the hematoma becomes organized, but the central part remains liquid and communicates with the arterial lumen through the defect in the anastomosis. This results in a saccular anastomotic aneurysm that will continue to enlarge.

Inadequate Suture Purchase

If sutures are placed too close to the edge of the arteriotomy and incorporate an inadequate amount of arterial wall, one or more of the suture loops may pull through the edge of the artery, leaving a gap that can lead to anastomotic aneurysm formation (Fig. 37–2). This is probably the most common mechanism of anastomotic aneurysm formation today.

Stress on the Anastomosis

Extraneous stress on the anastomosis line may increase the tendency of an inadequately placed suture to pull free from the arterial wall. Such stress includes the distraction force produced by joint motion when the anastomosis is located in the femoral or popliteal positions.[12–14, 25] In addition, the motion associated with normal pulsatile flow can result in shearing forces at the interface between areas of different compliance that exist at the junction between prosthetic graft and host artery.

One subtle but possibly important cause of anastomotic stress is the tension placed on the graft during anastomosis. Crimped fabric prostheses are often fully stretched during the distal anastomosis. The elastic force tending to return the graft to a crimped configuration is a cause of anastomotic stress. This is best illustrated angiographically in axillofemoral bypass grafts by the downward displacement of the axillary artery at the site of anastomosis. This factor may also account for the reduced tendency for polytetrafluoroethylene graft anastomoses to result in anastomotic aneurysms. Because the polytetrafluoroethylene graft is uncrimped, no force is exerted to stretch it for anastomosis. Therefore, the anastomosis is not subjected to the force of elastic recoil.

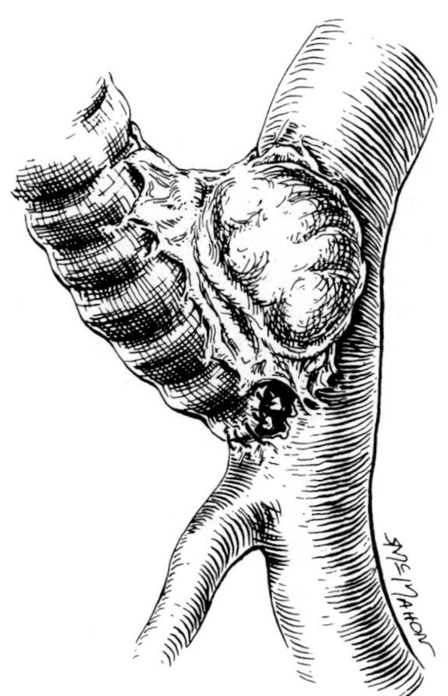

FIGURE 37–2. Anastomotic aneurysm developing because suture loops pulled out from the edge of the arterial wall.

Degeneration of the Arterial Wall

Degeneration of the arterial wall has also been implicated in suture line disruption. In instances of true degeneration, infection with low-virulence bacteria is the most likely etiologic factor. Other cases, sometimes blamed on arterial degeneration, more likely result from sutures placed at an inadequate depth that have pulled free from the edge of the arterial wall.

Previous Endarterectomy

Construction of an anastomosis to an arterial segment following intimectomy or endarterectomy can lead to an anastomotic aneurysm. After local removal of an atherosclerotic plaque, the tensile strength of the arterial segment is lower than that of the original diseased artery, and the sutures may pull out. Following such procedures, sutures must be placed deeper in the arterial wall in order to prevent suture line disruption and anastomotic aneurysm formation.

The etiologic factors described earlier are reflected in the published statistics relative to the incidence of anastomotic aneurysm.[27] Stepwise decreases in incidence can be related to the abandonment of silk sutures and, more recently, to the use of the more compliant knitted Dacron grafts and prophylactic antibiotics. The significantly higher incidence in the femoral region (even allowing for its greater frequency as an anastomotic site) is due to the greater shearing forces produced by joint flexing, the more frequent occurrence of perigraft hematoma and wound infection, and the placement of end-to-side anastomoses in the commonly thinned anterior arterial wall.

INCIDENCE

It is difficult to identify the true contemporary incidence of anastomotic false aneurysm in patients undergoing vascular grafting. The difficulty occurs in the identification of a false aneurysm by physical examination. For example, an anastomotic aneurysm at an aortic or iliac anastomosis may not be detected until the aneurysm increases to a relatively large size. Attempts to screen patients after aortoiliac and aortofemoral graft operations have provided some insight into both the true and the relative incidences of anastomotic aneurysm at various sites. Satiani, in a collective review of 444 anastomotic aneurysms, noted that 79 per cent were located at prosthetic graft–femoral artery anastomoses.[33] Although this may be a disproportionately high percentage because of the difficulty in correctly identifying anastomotic aneurysms at the aortoiliac position, it clearly represents a repeated observation that the femoral artery location is more vulnerable to anastomotic aneurysm formation.

Several authors reported their experience with a routine survey of patients undergoing aortoiliac and aortofemoral grafting operations. Sieswerda and colleagues reported their experience with 303 patients undergoing aortic reconstruction during a 4-year interval from 1977 to 1980.[34] At the time of final analysis, 122 patients had been assessed by physical examination, ultrasonography, and intravenous digital subtraction angiography and had complete data for analysis. A total of 36 patients developed 52 anastomotic aneurysms, for an incidence of 29.5 per cent of the patient population. The sites of aneurysm formation included 3 of 115 aortic anastomoses (incidence, 2.6 per cent), 18 of 146 iliac artery anastomoses (incidence, 12.3 per cent), and 31 of 70 femoral anastomoses (incidence, 44.3 per cent).

Edwards and colleagues used abdominal sonography to monitor 138 patients over a 33-month interval.[31] One hundred eleven patients were available for analysis. A total of seven anastomotic aneurysms were identified, for an incidence of 6.3 per cent. The authors determined the appearance of anastomotic aneurysm to be a function of the time interval between original operation and identification. They noted that the incidence was only 1 per cent at 8 years but rose to 20 per cent at 15 years. The mean time for development of an anastomotic aneurysm was 180 months ± 97 months. Although their principal interest was in the appearance of intra-abdominal anastomotic aneurysm, they also noted that 64 of the 111 patients had femoral artery anastomoses. Fifteen of 64 femoral anastomoses (23 per cent) were found to have anastomotic aneurysm.

Ernst, in a discussion of the paper by Edwards and colleagues, related a 30-year experience at the Henry Ford Hospital.[32] He had the opportunity to review 6090 aortoiliac anastomoses. He found 15 aortic anastomotic aneurysms, for an overall incidence of 0.25 per cent, and 21 iliac artery anastomotic aneurysms, for an incidence of 0.34 per cent. He noted that the average interval between operation and anastomotic appearance was 9.1 years.

CLINICAL MANIFESTATIONS

Clinical findings depend on the location of the anastomotic aneurysm. Most often, the aneurysm presents as a palpable pulsatile mass. In the femoral region, it enlarges and is noted by the patient. Rupture of an anastomotic aneurysm may be contained, or bleeding may occur into the adjacent soft tissues or hollow viscera. As with any aneurysm, mural thrombus may be the source of distal emboli. Finally, the aneurysm may thrombose, resulting in concomitant thrombosis of the graft.

An anastomotic aneurysm located within the abdomen may remain obscure for some time, only to be discovered on a subsequent arteriogram; at the time of an unrelated abdominal exploration; or as the result of rupture, gastrointestinal bleeding, or distal embolization.

Anastomotic aneurysms can occur in any anatomic position in which there is a junction of prosthetic graft and host artery.[20] An analysis of the clinical manifestations associated with the most commonly reported locations, in order of frequency, follows.

Femoral Artery

Patients with an anastomotic aneurysm in the femoral artery position usually become aware of an enlarging pulsatile mass beneath the scar. Because this is in a relatively superficial site, patients tend to observe these changes

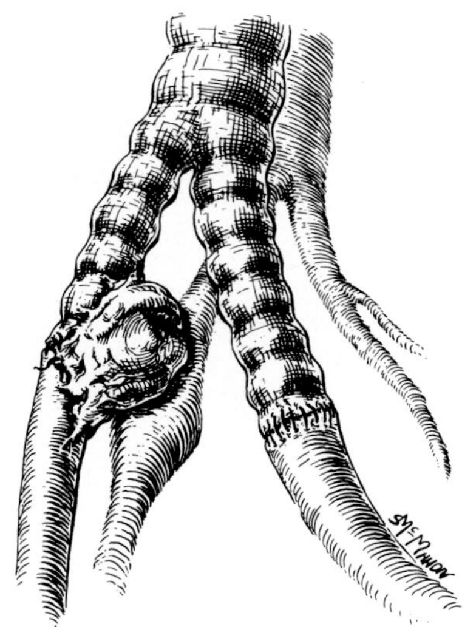

FIGURE 37–3. An anastomotic aneurysm at the junction of a graft and the right common iliac artery. Enlargement causes compression of the adjacent iliac vein, leading to stasis and possible thrombosis.

early and seek treatment before other complications ensue. Less commonly, patients may present with symptoms of rupture or acute ischemic changes of the lower extremity secondary to thrombosis or embolization of mural thrombus.[2–5, 10, 23, 26, 28, 29]

Abdominal Aorta

Anastomotic aneurysms of the abdominal aorta may occur as a complication of either replacement grafting or bypass grafting of the aortoiliac system.[6, 18] These aneurysms may remain undetected unless arteriography is performed because of clinical suspicion or for an unrelated cause. The aneurysm may occasionally erode into the overlying duodenum, resulting in an aortoduodenal fistula with gastrointestinal bleeding. In this instance, the fistula is due to erosion into the duodenum by the expanding false aneurysm or infection combined with anastomotic degeneration. Any anastomotic aneurysm that reaches sufficient size and is not encased by fibrous tissue can rupture. The clinical manifestations of rupture include hemorrhagic shock combined with abdominal distention, tenderness, and signs of a pulsatile mass.

Iliac Arteries

Anastomotic aneurysms of the iliac artery present very much like those of the abdominal aorta. However, if intestinal fistulization occurs, the jejunum, ileum, or sigmoid colon will be involved, rather than the duodenum. Enlargement of an iliac anastomotic aneurysm may produce iliac vein compression, with concomitant iliofemoral venous thrombosis (Fig. 37–3). If the ureter becomes incorporated into the surrounding fibrous tissue, ureteral obstruction and hydronephrosis with possible urinary tract infection may also occur as the aneurysm expands.

Popliteal Artery

Aneurysms in the popliteal artery occur following femoropopliteal bypass grafting and usually present as enlarging pulsatile masses in the popliteal fossa. A popliteal anastomotic aneurysm may also compress and cause thrombosis of the reconstruction or cause symptoms by compression of adjacent nerves and veins. These pseudoaneurysms are usually noted early by the patient because of their superficial location.

Carotid Artery

Although saphenous vein patches can also dilate over time and become quite aneurysmal, anastomotic aneurysms of the carotid artery occur most commonly when a carotid arteriotomy is closed with a prosthetic patch in which a nonpermanent suture material such as silk is used.[1] Aneurysm formation is not an inevitable consequence because the patch is relatively small and tends to be adequately held in place by the surrounding fibrous tissue capsule, even after the sutures have been absorbed. If the patch begins to separate, the patient may notice a pulsatile mass in the neck. An anastomotic aneurysm may also present as recurrent hemispheric transient ischemic attacks secondary to intermittent embolization of platelet aggregate material or thrombus from the lining of the aneurysm wall (Fig. 37–4).

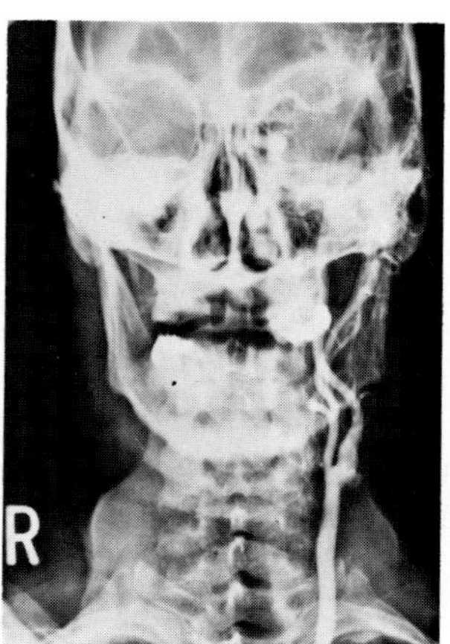

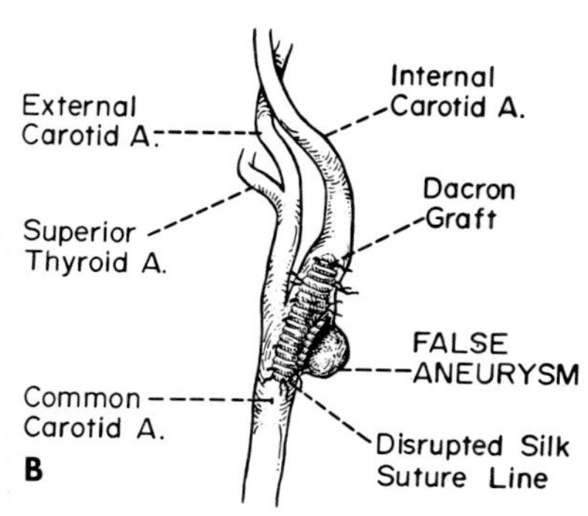

FIGURE 37–4. *A*, Left carotid arteriogram showing a false aneurysm at the lower lateral margin of the carotid bulb. *B*, Operative findings of false aneurysm that occurred when silk suture disruption permitted separation of a Dacron patch from the carotid artery.

DIAGNOSIS

History

The patient usually becomes aware of an anastomotic aneurysm in the femoral or popliteal region because of an enlarging pulsatile mass. Intra-abdominal anastomotic aneurysms tend to be silent until they enlarge and produce back pain, rupture, or erode into adjacent small bowel and produce intestinal bleeding. The clinician should be alert to the possibility of anastomotic degeneration and aneurysm formation in the following situations: whenever an operative note describes the use of a nonpermanent suture material, such as silk or polyethylene for an anastomosis; whenever the surgeon uses tiny sutures of host artery tissue, especially if an endarterectomy was performed at the graft site; and whenever a wound hematoma was documented following the original operation.[7, 8]

Physical Examination

The principal finding on physical examination is an aneurysm at the anastomotic site. When the site is superficial, as in the femoral region, the diagnosis is quite obvious. However, femoral anastomotic aneurysms can be mistaken for hernias, abscesses, or lymphoceles by the untrained examiner. Small intra-abdominal anastomotic aneurysms may not be palpable. Further diagnostic study is warranted if an aneurysm is suspected, particularly if any of the predisposing factors occurred during the operation.

An aortic anastomotic aneurysm can be misdiagnosed if the bypass graft is anastomosed in an end-to-side fashion. The enlarged pulsatile mass produced by the summation of native abdominal aortic and graft pulsations may alarm an examiner who is not familiar with this surgical technique.

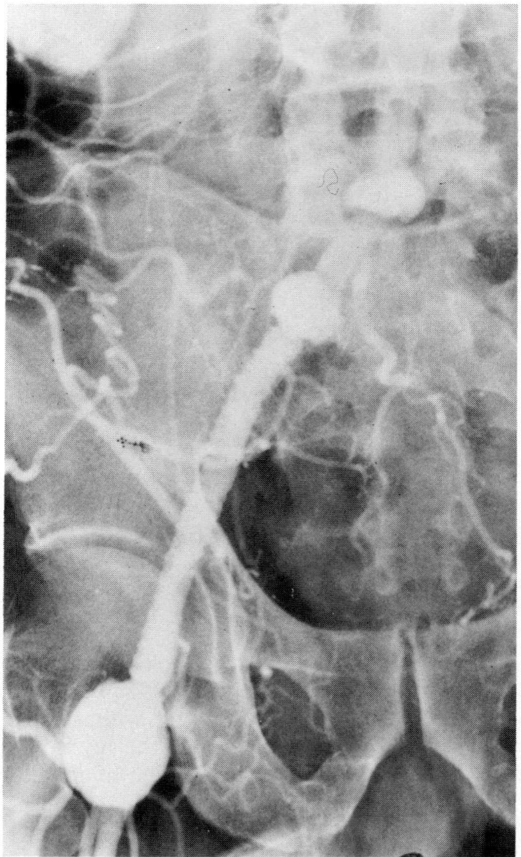

FIGURE 37–5. Aortogram demonstrating anastomotic aneurysms at the distal aorta, right iliac, and common femoral anastomoses. At the time of repair, no trace of silk suture used for the original operation could be found.

Special Studies

Ultrasonography can confirm the diagnosis of a femoral or popliteal false aneurysm and may help to identify an occult intra-abdominal anastomotic aneurysm. Computed tomography has been particularly helpful in identifying occult anastomotic aneurysms, especially when they are intra-abdominal. The definitive diagnosis is usually made by angiography (Fig. 37–5). Because of the graft's position in relation to the host artery, oblique projections that place the aneurysm in profile may be necessary. Computed tomography may be superior to angiography when the aneurysm is lined with thrombus and thus may be missed.

MANAGEMENT

Once the diagnosis of anastomotic aneurysm is made, surgical repair is indicated. Conservative management is not generally warranted. The natural history of anastomotic aneurysm has not been documented; thus, it is not possible to estimate the risk of rupture relative to size. Nevertheless, it is logical to assume that any false aneurysm, lacking as it does the strength-giving structural elements of the original arterial wall, will inexorably enlarge at a more rapid rate than most true aneurysms. Ernst reported on the conservative management of 15 poor-risk patients with intra-abdominal anastomotic aneurysms.[32] Three patients (20 per cent) died of aneurysm rupture. Treiman and colleagues reported their experience with 22 intra-abdominal anastomotic aneurysms in 18 patients.[35] Six of 22 (27 per cent) presented with rupture. As soon as the anastomosis begins to separate and the surrounding fibrous tissue capsule becomes aneurysmal, the lateral wall forces will increase as the diameter of the anastomotic aneurysm increases. The rate of enlargement accelerates because of the action of these physical forces.

General Principles of Operative Management

1. Obtain control of the vessels proximal and distal to the site of the anastomotic aneurysm. Because the aneurysm wall consists only of fibrous tissue, a plane of dissection about the aneurysm may not exist. Inadvertent entry into the lumen during dissection is quite likely if extensive dissection is attempted (Fig. 37–6).

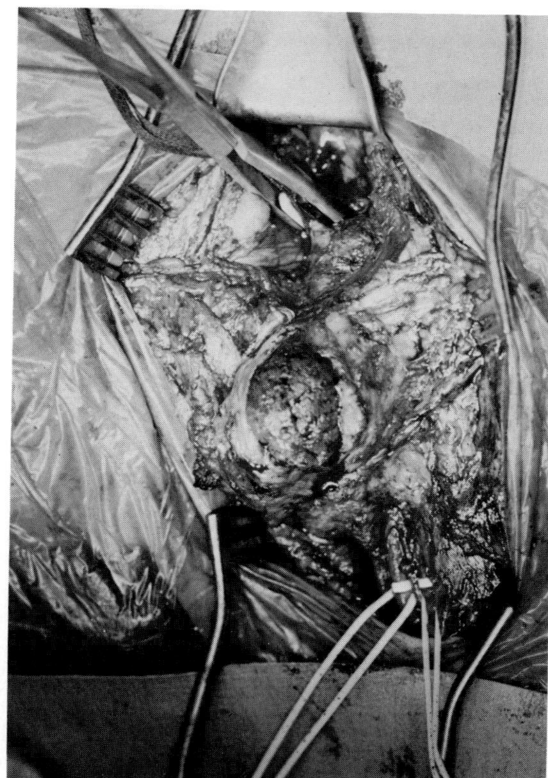

FIGURE 37–6. Intraoperative photograph of a femoral anastomotic aneurysm demonstrating proximal and distal control before resection and repair.

2. Identify the cause of the anastomotic aneurysm. Because the majority of aneurysms are caused by suture line failure, carefully observe the suture line for signs of suture fragmentation, absorption, or pulling out from the arterial wall. Also examine the arterial wall for defects.

3. Rule out graft infection as a cause of anastomotic degeneration. A Gram stain for bacteria should be performed on fluid from the space between the fibrous tissue capsule and the prosthetic graft, and a small piece of distal graft should be sent for culture. If no organisms are identified, the surgeon can assume that the anastomotic aneurysm is primary rather than secondary to infection and should repair the vessel. However, if culture results are positive, management should proceed as in the case of an infected graft.

4. Carefully detach the fibrous tissue aneurysmal capsule and residual graft before constructing a new anastomosis.

Technique of Operative Repair

The principal techniques employed for repair of anastomotic aneurysms are similar and are illustrated in the following description of the surgical repair of a femoral aneurysm.

Reopen the femoral incision and carry it proximally over the inguinal ligament. Deepen the incision proximal to the palpable aneurysm so as to expose and gain control of the prosthetic graft. If the original anastomosis was end-to-side, expose the proximal common femoral artery, if it is patent, in order to obtain complete proximal control. Continue soft tissue dissection distal to the aneurysm and expose the superficial femoral and deep femoral arteries in order to obtain distal control (Fig. 37–7). If the mass and the fibrous tissue reaction to the aneurysm are too extensive, distal control can also be obtained intraluminally by inserting occlusive balloon catheters of appropriate size into the lumina of the runoff vessels.

Administer 5000 units of aqueous heparin intravenously. Once the patient is heparinized, clamp the inflow and outflow. Make an incision directly over the anterior surface of the aneurysm in order to gain access to the anastomosis. Do not try to excise a large femoral false aneurysm because injury to the adjacent femoral vein or nerve is likely to occur.

Carefully search for the cause of the anastomotic failure. If the graft is not completely separated, detach the remaining portion and trim the aneurysm sac away from the edges of the arteriotomy (Fig. 37–8). Use a new segment of prosthetic graft, appropriately beveled, to reconstruct the distal anastomosis (Fig. 37–9). Do not attempt a simple repair by resuturing the original graft to the anastomosis. Clarke and coworkers reported recurrence of 5 of 14 (36 per cent) femoral anastomotic aneurysms that had simple repair.[30] In contrast, there were no recurrences among 17 femoral anastomotic aneurysms repaired by interposing a new graft segment. This may be further evidence to support the theory that anastomotic stress due to recoil of a stretched, crimped graft may be important in the contemporary etiology of anastomotic aneurysm formation. The new anastomosis should be performed with a permanent-type braided Dacron suture or a polypropylene suture. The new segment of graft can be used to bridge the gap created by excising a portion of the old graft and the native artery. A simple graft-graft anastomosis is carried out, and the reconstruction is completed (Fig. 37–10). Flow is then re-

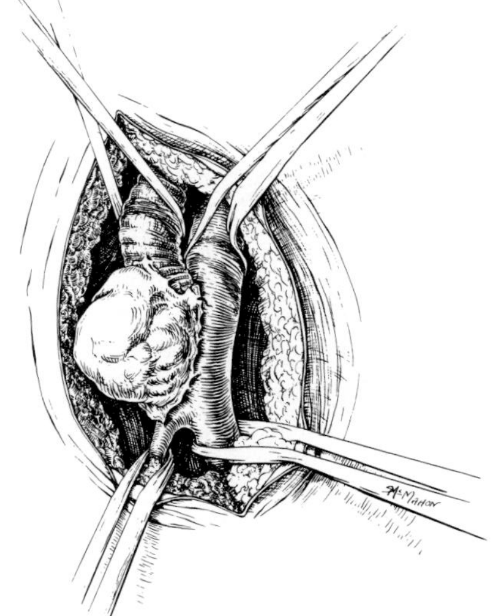

FIGURE 37–7. Proximal and distal control of the anastomotic aneurysm is complete with tapes placed around the graft and around the common femoral, superficial femoral, and profunda femoris arteries.

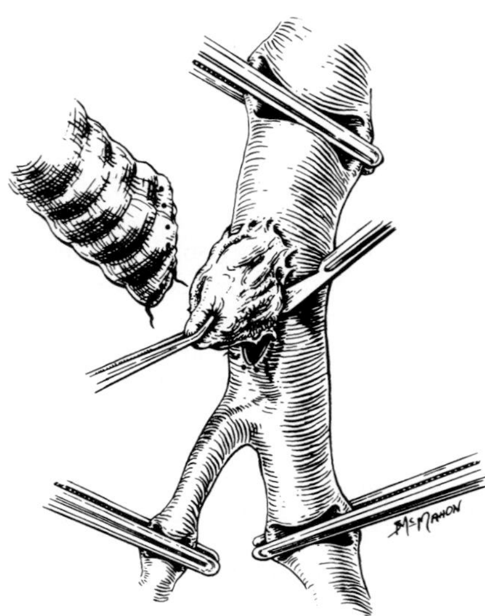

FIGURE 37–8. The aneurysm sac is trimmed away from the edge of the artery to ensure that the new anastomosis will be to arterial tissue.

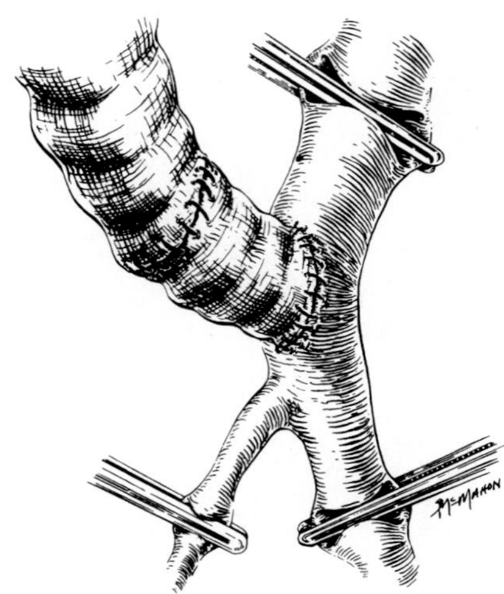

FIGURE 37–10. The new graft segment allows adequate length to bridge the gap left after excision of the false aneurysm.

stored, the wound is appropriately irrigated, and the aneurysm wall is incorporated as part of the soft tissue closure.

PREVENTION

1. Use permanent synthetic sutures. Because historically a major cause of anastomotic aneurysm was suture failure, this etiology can be eliminated by the use of braided synthetic sutures that will not fracture or be absorbed or by the use of polypropylene suture.

2. Use relatively large suture bites of the artery receiving a prosthetic graft. Sutures that pull out of the host artery are now the most common cause of anastomotic aneurysms. When performing an end-to-side anastomosis, take small bites at the base and at the apex in order to avoid compromise of the arterial inflow and outflow. Large bites can, however, be taken in the mid-portion of the anastomosis without compromising the lumen, because the bevel of the graft serves as a patch of host artery and provides ample margin to ensure a generous cross-sectional area for the anastomosis.

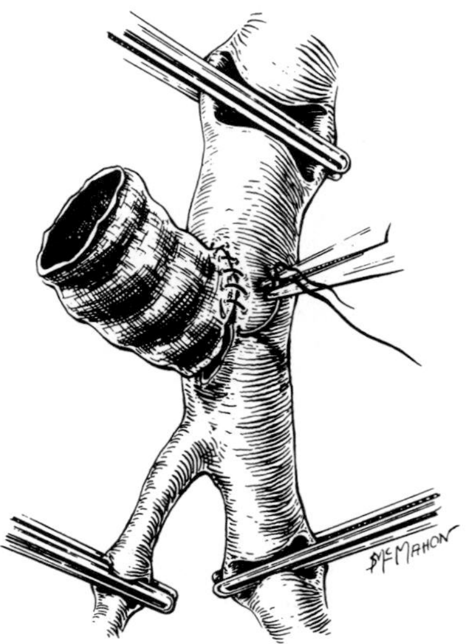

FIGURE 37–9. A new segment of prosthetic graft is used to facilitate the anastomosis.

3. Prevent wound hematomas. Careful attention to wound and anastomotic hemostasis, combined with a wound closure designed to eliminate dead space, should prevent the majority of hematomas, which are the third most frequent cause of sterile anastomotic aneurysms. If a hematoma occurs in the early postoperative period, the patient should be returned to the operating room for sterile evacuation and reclosure of the incision. Do not try to treat the hematoma conservatively.

4. Do not suture the distal anastomosis under stress. Pull the graft limb down to correct redundancy, then allow recoil of the crimped segment to take place before cutting the graft limb to conform to the distal arteriotomy.

5. Prevent graft infection. Use prophylactic antibiotics and pay careful attention to sterile techniques.

References

1. Buscaglia LC, Moore WS, Hall AD: False aneurysm after carotid endarterectomy. JAMA 209:1529, 1969.
2. Chavez CM: False aneurysms of the femoral artery: A challenge in management. Ann Surg 183:694, 1976.
3. Christensen RD, Bernatz PE: Anastomotic aneurysms involving the femoral artery. Mayo Clin Proc 47:313, 1972.
4. Crawford ES, Manning LG, Kelly TF: "Redo" surgery after operations for aneurysm and occlusion of the abdominal aorta. Surgery 81:41, 1977.
5. Dennis JW, Littooy FN, Greisler HP, et al: Anastomotic pseudoaneurysms—A continuing late complication of vascular reconstructive procedures. Arch Surg 121:314, 1986.
6. Drury JK, Leiberman DP, Gilmour DG, et al: Operation for late complications of aortic grafts. Surg Gynecol Obstet 163:251, 1986.
7. Edwards WS, Dalton D Jr, Quattlebaum R: Anastomoses between synthetic graft and artery. Arch Surg 86:477, 1963.
8. Gardner TJ, Brawley RK, Gott VL: Anastomotic false aneurysms. Surgery 72:474, 1972.

9. Hohf RP: Tensile strength of the arterial-prosthesis anastomosis during healing. Ann Surg 156:805, 1962.
10. Hollier LH, Batson RC, Cohn I Jr: Femoral anastomotic aneurysms. Ann Surg 191:715, 1980.
11. Kottmeier CA, Wheat MW Jr: Strength of anastomoses in aortic prosthetic grafts. Am Surg 31:128, 1965.
12. Knox GW: Peripheral vascular anastomotic aneurysms. Ann Surg 183:120, 1976.
13. Millili JJ, Lanes JS, Nemir P Jr: A study of anastomotic aneurysms following aortofemoral prosthetic bypass. Ann Surg 192:69, 1980.
14. Moore WS, Cafferata HT, Hall AD, et al: In defense of grafts across the inguinal ligament: An evaluation of early and late results of aortofemoral bypass grafts. Ann Surg 168:207, 1968.
15. Moore WS, Hall AD: Late suture failure in the pathogenesis of anastomotic false aneurysms. Ann Surg 172:1064, 1970.
16. Moore WS, Hall AD, Allen RE: Tensile strength of arterial prosthetic anastomoses. J Surg Res 13:209, 1972.
17. Nichols WK, Stanton M, Silver D, et al: Anastomotic aneurysms following lower extremity revascularization. Surgery 88:366, 1980.
18. Olsen WR, DeWeese MS, Fry WJ: False aneurysm of abdominal aorta. A late complication of aortic aneurysmectomy. Arch Surg 92:123, 1966.
19. Quiñones-Baldrich WJ, Ziomek S, Henderson T, et al: Primary anastomotic bonding in polytetrafluoroethylene grafts? J Vasc Surg 5:311, 1987.
20. Richardson JV, McDowell HA Jr: Anastomotic aneurysms following arterial grafting: A 10-year experience. Am Surg 184:179, 1976.
21. Sauvage LR, Berger KE, Wood SJ, et al: Interspecies healing of porous arterial prostheses. Arch Surg 169:698, 1974.
22. Sawyer JL, Jacobs K, Sutton JP: Peripheral anastomotic aneurysms. Development following arterial reconstruction with prosthetic grafts. Arch Surg 95:802, 1967.
23. Spratt EM, Doran ML, Baird RJ: False aneurysms in the lower extremity. Surg Gynecol Obstet 124:562, 1967.
24. Starr DS, Weatherford SC, Lawrie GM, et al: Suture material as a factor in the occurrence of anastomotic false aneurysms. Arch Surg 114:412, 1979.
25. Stoney RJ, Albo RS, Wylie EJ: False aneurysms occurring after arterial grafting operations. Am J Surg 110:153, 1965.
26. Sumner DS, Strandness DE Jr: False aneurysms occurring in association with thrombosed prosthetic grafts. Arch Surg 94:360, 1967.
27. Szilagyi DE, Smith RF, Elliott JP, et al: Anastomotic aneurysms after vascular reconstruction: Problems of incidence, etiology and treatment. Surgery 78:800, 1975.
28. West JP, Lattes C, Knox WG: Anastomotic false aneurysms. Arch Surg 103:348, 1971.
29. Youkey JR, Clagett GP, Rich NM, et al: Femoral anastomotic false aneurysms: An 11-year experience with a case control study. Ann Surg 199:703, 1984.
30. Clarke AM, Poskitt KR, Baird RN, Horrocks M: Anastomotic aneurysms of the femoral artery: Aetiology and treatment. Br J Surg 76:1014, 1989.
31. Edwards JM, Teefey SA, Zierler E, Kohler TR: Intraabdominal paraanastomotic aneurysms after aortic bypass grafting. J Vasc Surg 15:344, 1992.
32. Ernst C: In discussion of Edwards JM, Teefey SA, Zierler E, Kohler TR: Intraabdominal paraanastomotic aneurysms after aortic bypass grafting. J Vasc Surg 15:344, 1992.
33. Satiani B: False aneurysms following arterial reconstruction. Surg Gynecol Obstet 152:357, 1981.
34. Sieswerda C, Skotnicki SH, Berentsz JO, Heystraten FMJ: Anastomotic aneurysms—An underdiagnosed complication after aortoiliac reconstructions. Eur J Vasc Surg 3:233, 1989.
35. Treiman GS, Weaver FA, Cossman DV, et al: Anastomotic false aneurysms of the abdominal aorta and the iliac arteries. J Vasc Surg 8:268, 1988.

38

Aortoenteric Fistulae

Victor M. Bernhard, M.D.

• • •

Direct communication between the aorta and the intestinal lumen is a very infrequent complication of aortoiliac reconstructive surgery and a very rare consequence of untreated abdominal aortic aneurysm. The inevitable outcome is death from hemorrhage or sepsis, unless the diagnosis is promptly established and appropriate surgical therapy employed.

Primary aortoenteric fistulae (AEFs) are usually due to erosion of an aortic aneurysm into the intestine, generally at the level of the duodenum.[9, 11, 18, 20, 22, 37, 44, 45] This has become less frequent because of aggressive operative treatment of abdominal aortic aneurysms. The most common etiology currently is *secondary* to aortoiliac reconstruction for aneurysm or occlusive disease, with erosion of a prosthesis or vascular suture line into an adjacent loop of bowel.[7–9, 14, 17, 24, 26, 34, 41, 43] This complication usually appears months to years after the original operation, with a reported incidence of 0.4 to 4 per cent.[9, 17, 26, 34, 38]

PATHOGENESIS AND CLINICAL PRESENTATION

The segments of intestine most frequently involved in AEF are the third and fourth portions of the duodenum and the duodenojejunal flexure because of their anatomic location draped over the anterior bulge of an aneurysm or the proximal anastomosis and upper portion of an aortic prosthesis (Fig. 38–1*A* and *B*).[7, 9, 10, 11, 26, 34, 39] The distal ileum, the cecum, the sigmoid colon, and the appendix are occasionally the sites of fistula formation because of their proximity to right and left iliac anastomoses (Fig. 38–1*B* and *F*).[1, 17, 39]

The pathogenesis is usually based on direct adhesion of a segment of the gastrointestinal tract to an aortoiliac aneurysm, an anastomotic aneurysm, or a vascular prosthesis, usually at an anastomosis, followed by progressive erosion through the bowel wall and secondary contamination by intestinal flora (Fig. 38–1*A* to *C*).[3, 9, 10, 12, 17, 24] The ensuing infection further contributes to necrosis of the adjacent aortic wall or aortoprosthetic suture line, with gastrointestinal hemorrhage as a consequence of necrosis.

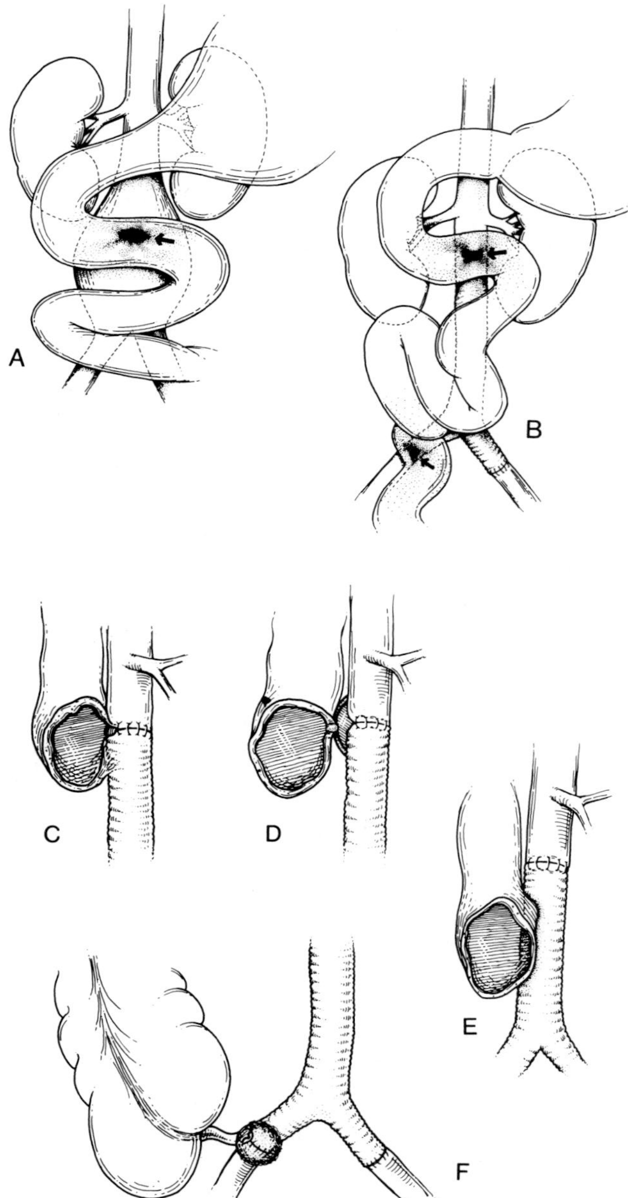

FIGURE 38–1. Pathogenesis of aortoenteric fistula (AEF). *A*, Primary AEF due to an abdominal aortic aneurysm (*arrow*). *B*, Secondary AEF due to graft anastomotic erosion into the distal duodenum or occasionally into the ileum at the graft-iliac anastomoses (*arrow*). *C*, Direct AEF. *D*, AEF due to anastomotic aneurysm erosion into an overlying loop of bowel. *E*, Erosion of graft directly into the bowel not involving anastomosis (aortoenteric erosion [AEE]). *F*, Appendiceal enteric fistula associated with an anastomotic false aneurysm.

The most important factor predisposing to secondary fistula formation is failure to separate the prosthesis and anastomoses from adjacent bowel with an adequate layer of retroperitoneal tissue and peritoneum at the time of the initial aortic surgery.[14, 17, 26] Contributing factors include false aneurysm at a suture line (as shown in Fig. 77–1*D*), kinking or redundancy of a retroperitoneal graft (Fig. 38–2; see also Fig. 38–5), reoperation for graft complications, endarterectomy, and primary graft infection.[9, 10, 17, 24, 26, 30, 41, 43]

The initial bleeding episode is usually modest and self-limited owing to the formation of thrombus, which can temporarily plug the fistula when it is small.[18, 24, 26] Bouts of bleeding recur over a period of hours, days, or weeks, eventually culminating in massive hemorrhage.

Occasionally, a graft that lies in direct contact with a loop of bowel may erode into the bowel lumen at some distance from a suture line, producing a paraprosthetic aortoenteric erosion (AEE) (see Figs. 38–1*E* and 38–2).[17, 26, 33] Although adherence of the bowel wall to the graft prevents leakage of intestinal contents, digestion of the fibrous tissue encasing the prosthesis permits blood to seep through its interstices into the intestine, or bleeding may arise from the ulcerated edges of the bowel, producing anemia and guaiac-positive stools without evidence of gross hemorrhage. This process may be accompanied by sepsis manifested by fever, back pain, and leukocytosis.[26, 33] Ultimately, infection may extend along the graft to involve a suture line, producing anastomotic necrosis with recurrent episodes of gross hemorrhage similar to the clinical presentation of a direct anastomotic enteric fistula.[26]

Gastrointestinal bleeding is not invariably present, although it is by far the most common and characteristic manifestation of the disease process. Reilly and associates[39] noted the absence of clinical evidence of gastrointestinal bleeding in 1 of 15 direct anastomotic fistulae and in 50 per cent of aortoenteric graft erosions. On the other hand, some form of gastrointestinal bleeding, from a variety of causes, is frequently encountered at various times after aortic surgery; however, AEF is infrequently the etiology. In a series of 253 patients who had received their primary operative procedure at the author's institution, there were 74 episodes of gastrointestinal bleeding in 52 patients during an average follow-up of 46 months, but only 1 of these was due to an aortoenteric communication.[35] Yeager and coworkers found AEF in only 5 of 19 patients with gastrointestinal bleeding after prosthetic aortic repair.[48]

DIAGNOSIS

Regardless of the nature of clinical presentation, AEF should always be placed high on the list of possible diagnoses in any patient with gastrointestinal bleeding following recent or remote aortic surgery or in the presence of an abdominal aortic aneurysm.[9, 17, 23, 24, 26, 28] Moreover, this diagnosis should not be discarded until there is clear proof that this pathologic process is not the cause.[26, 28, 35] A history of previous aortic surgery and the presence of an abdominal aortic aneurysm are the important clues that raise the clini-

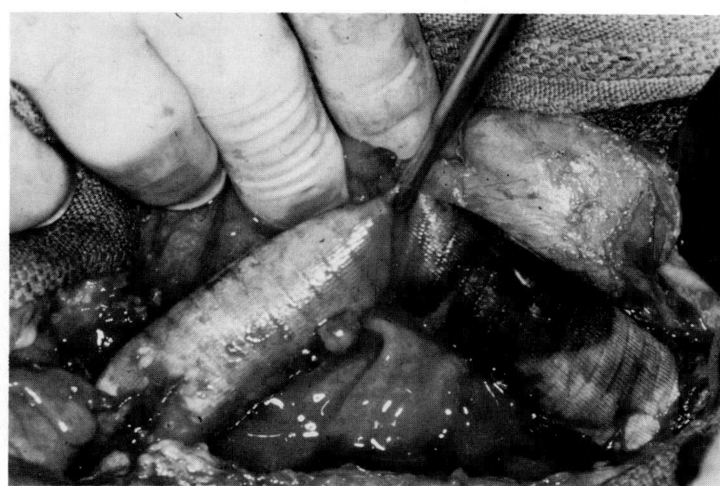

FIGURE 38–2. Erosion of a redundant mid-section of an aortic graft into the adjacent duodenum. The prosthetic wall is darkly bile stained.

cian's suspicions for a diagnosis of AEF or AEE.[26, 35] A pulsatile abdominal mass is the only physical finding that may be helpful in the differential diagnosis.[34, 37] Although this is frequently encountered in fistulae associated with untreated abdominal aneurysms, it is rarely present with secondary fistula formation unless an anastomotic false aneurysm is present and large enough to be palpable.[26, 34, 37, 48]

The diagnosis of AEF is often difficult to establish owing to the usual site of erosion into the distal duodenum or the bowel at or beyond the ligament of Treitz. Immediate laparotomy is required only when the patient is hemodynamically unstable because of continuing or massive hemorrhage.[3, 16, 34] Usually, the initial episodes of melena or hematemesis stop spontaneously, and the characteristic picture is that of intermittent "herald" bleeding, which tends to recur over periods of hours or days before the final exsanguinating hemorrhage.[24, 26, 46] Appropriate investigation to establish the diagnosis or to rule out other causes of gastrointestinal bleeding can be performed during this interval.[26]

Computed tomography (CT) with contrast should be the primary diagnostic maneuver whenever AEF or AEE is suspected. Findings that strongly support the diagnosis are perigraft fluid or gas more than 2 to 3 months after aortic surgery, an increase in perigraft soft tissue, pseudoaneurysm formation, loss of continuity of the aneurysmal wrap around the graft, and thickening of adjacent bowel wall or prosthetic erosion into the lumen (Fig. 38–3).[2, 9, 25, 29, 31] Although normal CT findings suggest that an undefined clinical picture of gastrointestinal bleeding and sepsis is due to some cause other than AEF or graft infection,[29] this is not invariably true.[21] Magnetic resonance imaging is also highly reliable for demonstrating perigraft infection, although experience with this technique is not as precisely defined as that with CT.

Fiberoptic endoscopy should be performed promptly in all hemodynamically stable patients, unless the diagnosis has been firmly established by CT.[9, 26, 39] If possible, the examination should be carried down through the terminal portion of the duodenum in order to visualize the mucosal defect associated with the fistula.[26, 32] An operating room should be available for immediate laparotomy in the event that endoscopic manipulation precipitates active hemorrhage. Even though the fistula may not be directly visualized, the absence of an actively bleeding lesion in the esophagus, stomach, or proximal duodenum rules out these more common sources and, by exclusion, supports the diagnosis of fistula.[26, 34, 35] Demonstration of an ulcer or varices without active bleeding, however, does not clearly rule out an aortoenteric communication. On the other hand, bleeding arising from a point distal to the second portion of the duodenum in the absence of a proximal lesion strongly suggests this diagnosis. In the author's experience, endoscopy was helpful in seven of eight cases in which this technique was employed: it directly demonstrated the lesion in two patients and showed the absence of any other source of bleeding in five.[26]

Aortography may demonstrate a false aneurysm at the proximal anastomosis,[26, 38] as shown in Figure 38–4, or an abdominal aortic aneurysm that was not palpated on physical examination. These findings suggest the presence of an AEF; however, extravasation of dye into the intestinal lumen is rarely seen (Fig. 38–5).[26] Furthermore, aortography before surgical intervention provides important information for subsequent surgical management of graft excision and lower extremity revascularization.

CT, endoscopy, and aortography can be accomplished within a few hours after admission, while preparations are being made for laparotomy.

Barium contrast investigation of the upper gastrointestinal tract[19] is usually not helpful and frequently confuses the picture.[9, 26, 34, 39] The finding of varices or gastric or duodenal ulceration does not identify these lesions as the source of bleeding. A deformity in the third or fourth portion of the duodenum, such as that shown in Figure 38–6, strongly suggests an aortoduodenal fistula. Extraluminal extravasation of contrast or outlining of the vascular prosthesis establishes the diagnosis.[19, 34] Unfortunately, these findings are infrequently present.[26] Upper gastrointestinal roentgenography should not precede aortography because residual barium will obscure angiographic details. Colonoscopy and barium enema should be employed whenever the clinical presentation suggests distal gastrointestinal bleeding on the basis of anemia, guaiac-positive stools, or hematochezia.[26] Fistulization of a graft or aneurysm into the colon is extremely rare, and the most likely source of bleed-

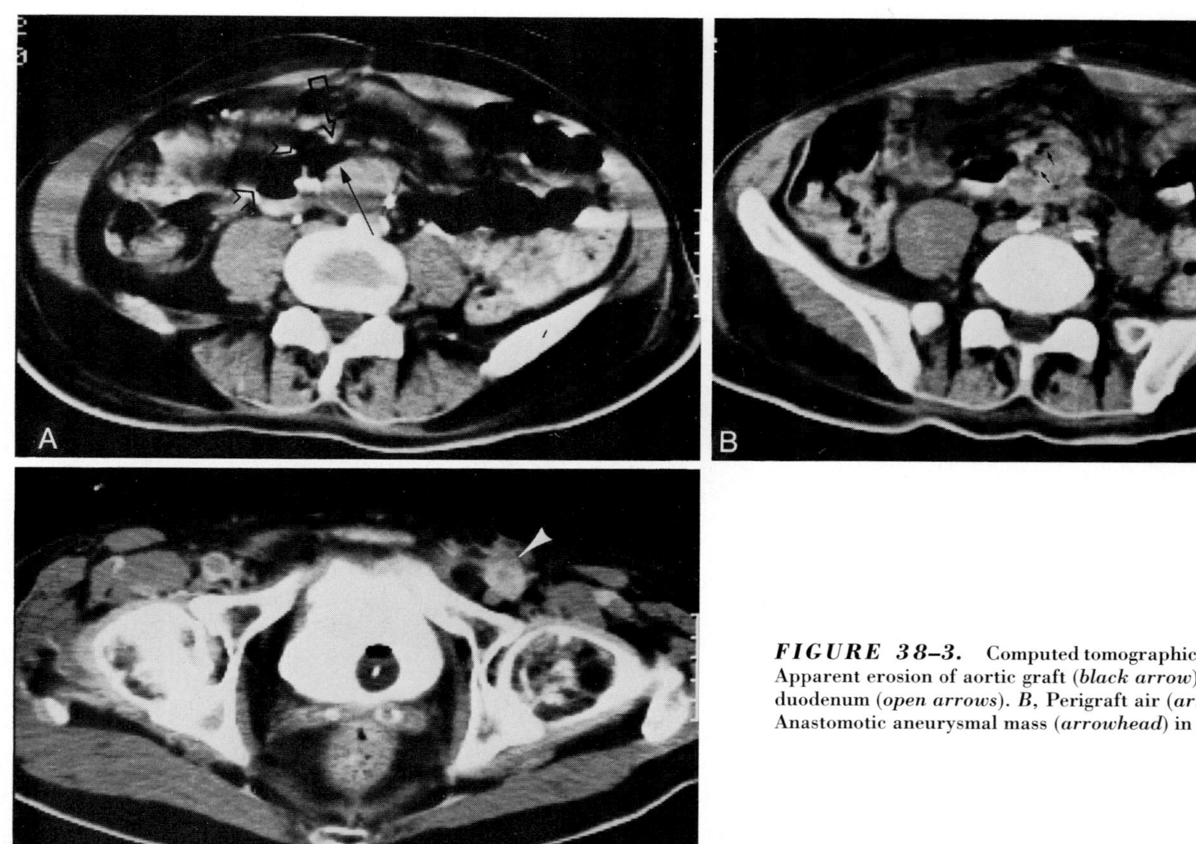

FIGURE 38–3. Computed tomographic scans of AEE. *A*, Apparent erosion of aortic graft (*black arrow*) into the overlying duodenum (*open arrows*). *B*, Perigraft air (*arrows*). *C*, Anastomotic aneurysmal mass (*arrowhead*) in the left groin.

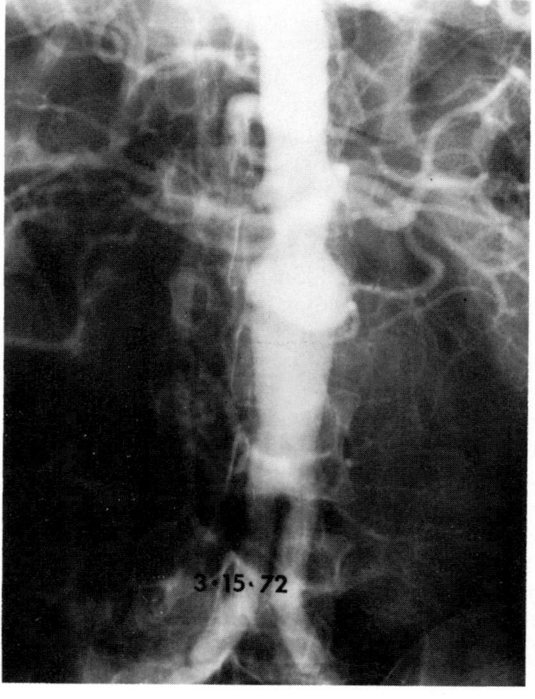

FIGURE 38–4. A false aneurysm at the proximal aortoprosthetic suture line is identified by arteriography. The patient had an 18-hour history of intermittent hematemesis and melena due to an aortoduodenal fistula.

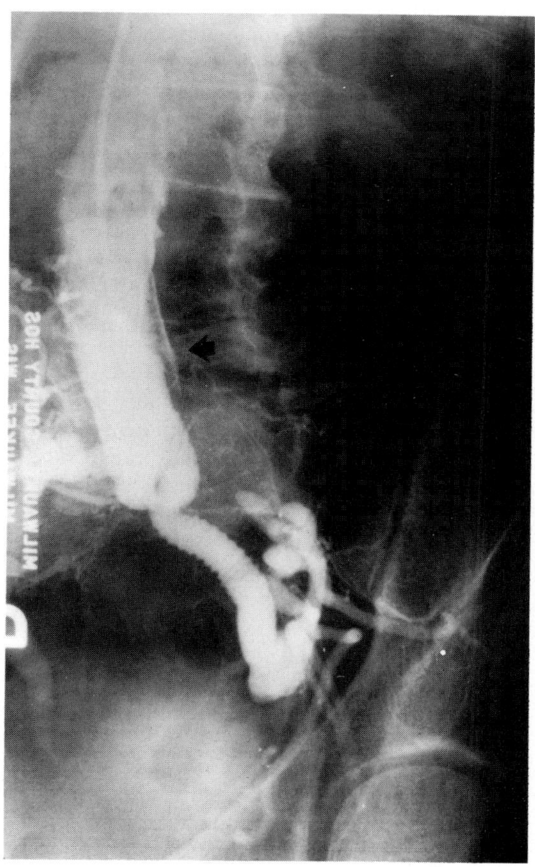

FIGURE 38–5. Aortogram reveals the graft erosion into the duodenum shown in Figure 38–2. Extravasation of dye through the interstices of the prosthesis (*arrow*) demonstrates the mechanism of chronic blood loss that had produced severe anemia.

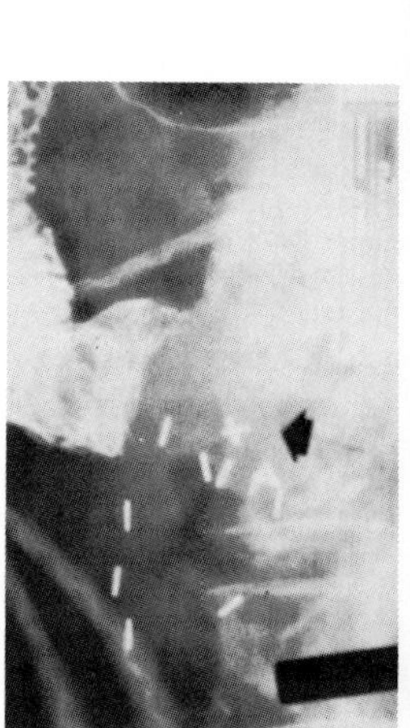

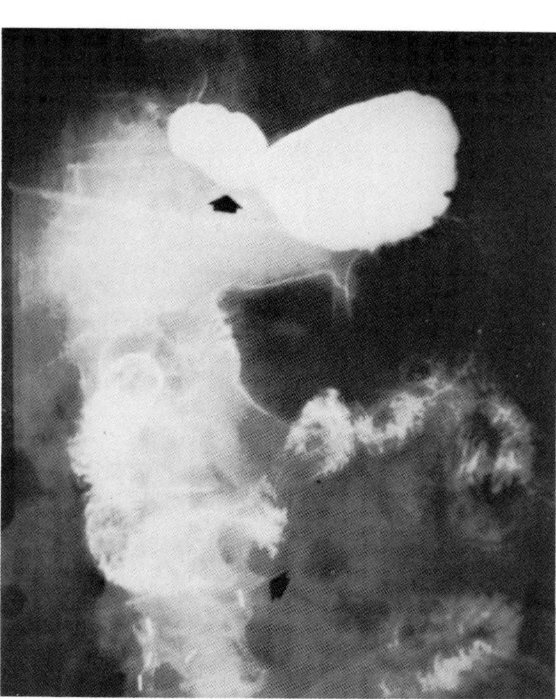

FIGURE 38–6. Upper gastrointestinal barium study demonstrating an external compression deformity in the third portion of the duodenum (*arrows, left and lower right*). A hiatus hernia (*upper arrow, right*) is also present and may confuse the picture.

ing under these circumstances is an intrinsic bowel lesion, which requires specific preparation for surgery.[20]

Radionuclide scanning with indium-111–labeled leukocytes or human immunoglobulin will detect perigraft inflammation associated with fistula formation and is useful when the results of other investigations are equivocal or negative.[27, 28] Tagged red blood cell studies during a bleeding episode may define the presence and location of a fistula and was helpful for diagnosing an aortoappendiceal fistula when the results of all other investigations were negative.[1]

OPERATIVE MANAGEMENT

Laparotomy to confirm the diagnosis and prevent further hemorrhage is the mandatory first step when bleeding is massive or ongoing.[3] This should be performed with continuous cardiopulmonary monitoring and multiple large-bore venous access ports for rapid transfusion. Broad-spectrum antibiotic coverage is begun before surgery and is continued throughout the postoperative period, with appropriate changes as indicated by bacterial sensitivities determined from operative cultures.[3]

A mid-line incision from the xiphoid to a point 2 inches above the pubis provides rapid entry and full access to any fistula site and does not interfere with subsequent placement of extra-anatomic bypass grafts along the lateral abdominal wall or across the pubis (Fig. 38–7*A*). Initially, the aorta should be exposed above the celiac trunk by incising the gastrohepatic omentum and dividing the fibers of the overlying diaphragmatic crura so that temporary proximal aortic control can be readily achieved if necessary (Fig. 38–7*B*).[3] Thereafter, the infrarenal aorta proximal to the presumed site of the fistula is mobilized for control, if possible, before the fistula is entered. The duodenojejunal flexure is then completely separated from the underlying graft or aneurysm, and the fistula site is disconnected. Bleeding from the aortic defect is controlled by direct finger pressure if the bleeding point is small or by temporarily clamping the aorta at the diaphragm until infrarenal control can be established if the defect is large or associated with the fragile wall of an anastomotic false aneurysm (Fig. 38–7*B*). Stasis thrombosis in the lower extremities is avoided by local injection of heparin into the distal graft or iliac vessels as soon as possible after proximal vascular control has been achieved (Fig. 38–7*C*). Clamps are then applied to the graft below the fistula or to the iliac arteries distal to an aortoiliac aneurysm.

Maneuvers to identify other bleeding sources should not be performed until an AEF has been clearly ruled out. If the fistula is actively bleeding, exsanguination may occur during the time consumed by such activity.[26]

The duodenal or jejunal defect is closed transversely with standard intestinal suture techniques. If extensive destruction of the intestinal wall has taken place, segmental resection with end-to-end anastomosis is preferred,[16, 26, 34] or the proximal end of the third portion of the duodenum may be closed and intestinal continuity restored by anastomosing the jejunum to the side of the second portion of the duodenum.[3]

The vascular side of the fistula poses a more hazardous problem because of infection extending to a variable degree into the aortic wall and the presence of, or need for, a foreign body prosthesis in a septic or at least contaminated area. The abdominal aortic aneurysm associated with a primary fistula can usually be managed in the standard fashion by direct insertion of a prosthesis in the aortic bed after thorough débridement of the infected and necrotic tissue in the aneurysm wall. The graft is covered or wrapped with a vascularized pedicle of omentum to separate it from bowel and the contaminated area.[13, 42] Unless the aneurysm is mycotic or the fistula is accompanied by extensive local sepsis, secondary infection of the graft is unlikely because contamination from the duodenum is minimal. In the collected experience presented by Daugherty and associates[13] and updated by Sweeney and Godacz,[42] simple closure of the duodenal defect and replacement of the aneurysm with a

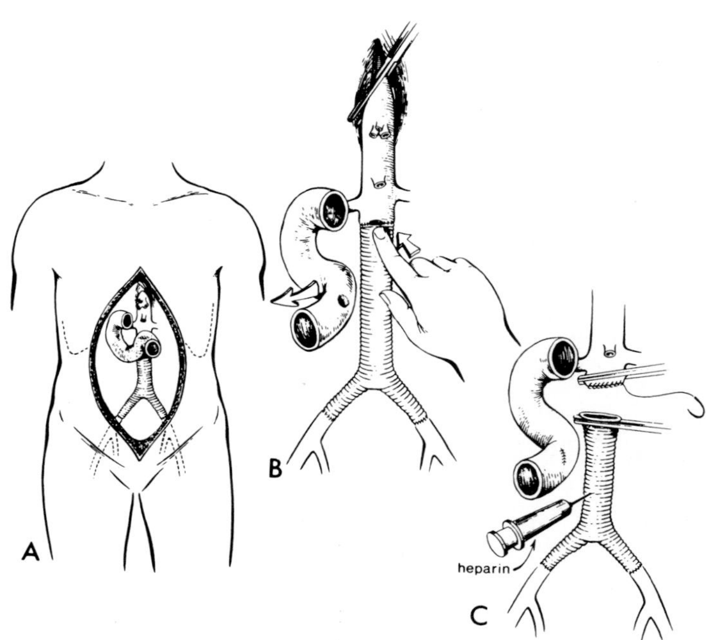

FIGURE 38–7. *A*, Exposure of AEF through a mid-line incision. *B*, The diaphragm over the aorta above the celiac axis is incised prior to takedown of the fistula to facilitate application of a clamp. The aortic side of the fistula is frequently small enough to permit temporary finger control. *C*, Transverse closure of the duodenal defect and suture of the infrarenal aortic stump after takedown of the proximal anastomosis. Heparin is injected into the graft to prevent distal thrombosis. (*A–C*, From Bergan JJ, Yao JST [eds]: Operative Techniques in Vascular Surgery. New York, Grune & Stratton, 1980, p 196.)

graft resulted in long-term recovery in 17 of 18 patients with primary AEFs.[42]

By contrast, successful eradication of a secondary fistula and prevention of further vascular infection usually require complete removal of all foreign material and the surrounding infected necrotic tissue.[3, 8, 9, 15, 26, 34, 36]

Extra-anatomic bypass, therefore, is generally considered to be the most reliable method for restoring lower extremity circulation. Although attempts to retain the original prosthesis, insert a new graft in the same bed, or patch the vascular defect have been advocated,[4, 6, 17, 24, 41] the incidence of necrosis of the aortic suture line, hemorrhage, or recurrent aortoduodenal fistulization has been very high whenever vascular prosthetic materials have been allowed to remain in the retroperitoneum. Nevertheless, reports have suggested that in situ revascularization with a new prosthesis may be safely performed with lower morbidity and mortality if thorough débridement back to healthy uninfected tissue can be accomplished with complete removal of the old prosthesis.[40, 47] However, guidelines for this approach are not clear, and wider experience will be required to determine its appropriate application.

When complete removal of the old graft is performed in the presence of an end-to-side anastomosis, the aortic defect after graft removal may be closed by simple monofilament suture; this allows some flow to the extremities through the patient's remaining native circulation if the aortic lumen is not completely obliterated.[38] The aorta must be transected, however, when the original proximal anastomosis was end-to-end. In a high percentage of cases, the remaining infrarenal aortic stump has been prone to disruption or at least delayed aneurysmal dilatation (Fig. 38–8).[3, 7, 17] To prevent this, the aortic stump may be buttressed by the application of a flap of anterior spinal ligament[23] or a vascularized pedicle derived from an isolated segment of jejunum after removal of the mucosa.[7] However, studies have indicated that stump disruption is probably caused by residual infection in the aortic wall; therefore, adequate débridement to remove all infected aortic tissue is necessary to prevent disruption.[30, 38] Adequate débridement may require sacrifice of one or both renal orifices, which then necessitates renal revascularization by splenorenal anastomosis, vein graft from the hepatic artery, or both.[38] In addition, long-term culture-specific antibiotics should be administered if the results of culture of the arterial wall proximal to the area of débridement are positive.[30] A tongue of omentum or other adjacent healthy soft tissue should be sutured in place around the aortic closure to prevent bowel loops from readhering to this area. Continuous antibiotic irrigation and suction drainage of the retroperitoneal space have also been recommended.[17]

After the abdomen has been closed, the lower extremities are inspected to determine the adequacy of collateral circulation. This may be sufficient if one or both limbs of the graft have been chronically occluded or if the legs have been previously amputated.[3, 26] Doppler ultrasound and ankle pressure measurements may help the surgeon evaluate limb perfusion in marginal cases. Pulsatile Doppler arterial flow and a measurable ankle pressure usually indicate that circulation is sufficient to maintain viable limbs,[3] so that revascularization can be deferred until the patient is better able to tolerate further surgery and the potential for contamination of the new graft is minimal. However, if limb viability is clearly threatened or in doubt, circulation must be restored immediately to preserve the extremities and also to restore hypogastric perfusion, because infarction of the colon frequently accompanies gangrene of the extremities under these circumstances.[3]

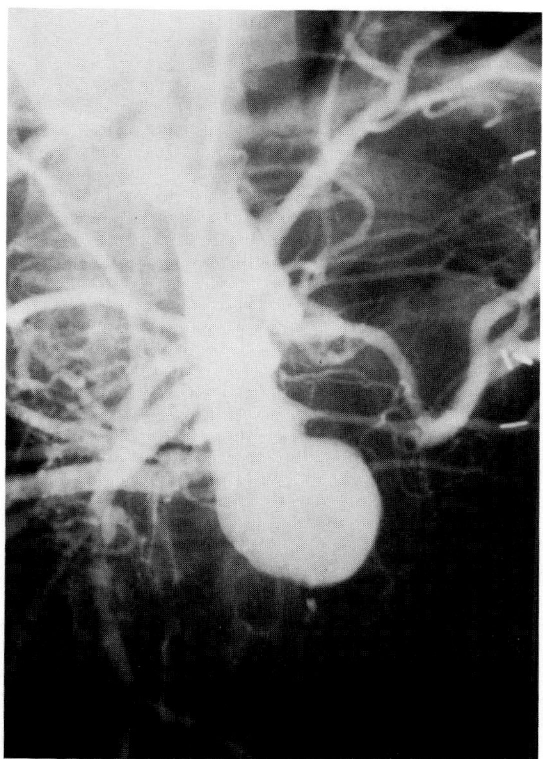

FIGURE 38–8. Aortic stump aneurysm following excision of an aortic graft for AEF.

Axillobifemoral bypass is currently considered to be the most practical and reliable method for restoring limb circulation in the presence of sepsis from AEF or AEE (Fig. 38–9*A*).[3, 5, 9, 15, 26, 34, 38] If a fistula develops in association with an aortobifemoral graft, this procedure must be modified to prevent secondary infection in the new extra-anatomic bypass because the groins may be infected or are likely to be contaminated during removal of the original prosthesis. A variety of techniques have been devised for extending grafts through clean tissues away from previous groin incisions to the popliteal or distal deep femoral vessels. Autogenous vein or endarterectomized artery may be used in contaminated fields to meet specific circumstances.[16] Some of the solutions to this difficult problem are diagrammed in Figure 38–9*B*. Regardless of the method chosen, revascularization must be performed in a freshly prepared field, with new gowns, drapes, and instruments, after all wounds associated with excision of the infected prosthesis have been closed and sealed.

When the diagnosis of fistula is unequivocal and the patient is not threatened by immediate hemorrhage, it may be preferable to stage surgical management.[38] Axillofemoral bypass is performed as the initial procedure, and repair of the fistula with removal of the old prosthesis is delayed for a few days in order to avoid excessive operative trauma and prolonged anesthesia in these debilitated patients.

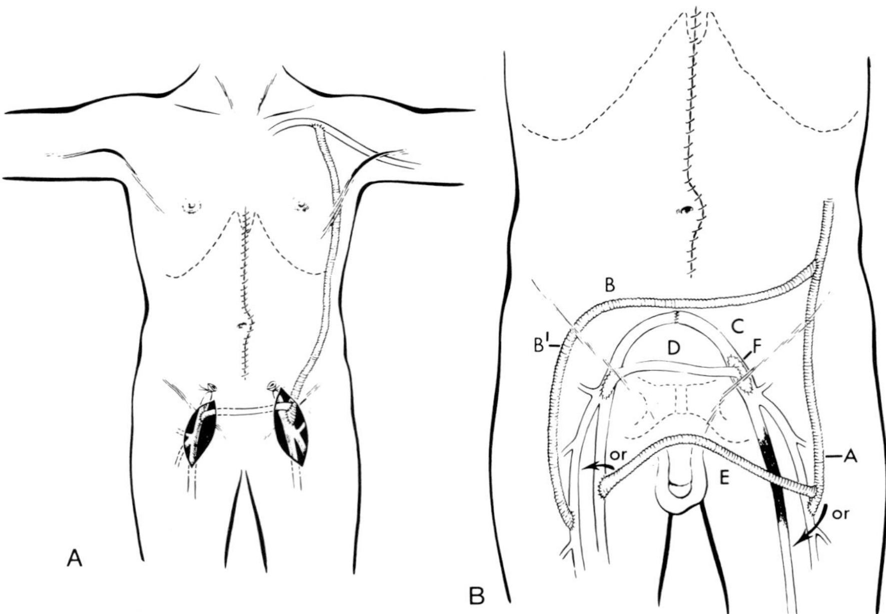

FIGURE 38–9. *A*, Axillobifemoral bypass can be performed in the standard fashion when the aortic prosthesis is confined entirely to the abdomen. In order to prevent contamination, the abdominal incision is closed and sealed with plastic drapes before the extra-anatomic bypass is carried out. *B*, Variations of the axillobifemoral technique to avoid contamination from the groin wounds required to excise an infected aortofemoral graft include lateral placement of the axillofemoral limb just medial and deep to the anterior superior iliac spine with anastomosis to the mid-profunda femoris or distal femoropopliteal segment (A); high takeoff of the femorofemoral limb tunneled between the distal end of the abdominal incision and the pubis but sufficiently proximal to the old femoral incisions to remain in fresh uncontaminated tissue (B); the descending limb placed laterally (B'); iliac arteries anastomosed to each other to provide transpelvic crossover (C); autogenous saphenous vein femorofemoral bypass through contaminated groin wounds (this graft is not inserted until the wounds for the lateral axillofemoral graft have been closed) (D); femorofemoral graft tunneled through clean tissue medial and distal to the groin wounds and crossing over to the opposite thigh below the pubic prominence (E); and vein-patch closure of the common femoral defect after excision of an aortofemoral graft limb (F).

AEF is invariably fatal unless treated aggressively by surgery.[9, 17, 26, 34, 38] Despite appropriate intervention, morbidity and mortality rates are high owing to the immediate consequences of hemorrhage and sepsis and the frequent occurrence of cardiac, pulmonary, and renal failure. A survival rate of 26 per cent was reported by Elliott and coworkers[17] in a series of 19 fistulae, whereas Garrett and associates[24] recorded a 64 per cent survival rate in their series of 14 cases. In an experience with 20 secondary fistulae reported by Kleinman and colleagues,[26] the overall survival rate was 35 per cent. However, when the diagnosis was made preoperatively and the surgical principles of graft excision and judicious extra-anatomic limb revascularization were employed, a 78 per cent survival rate was achieved. This experience has been confirmed by Perdue and associates,[36] who reported a 93 per cent long-term survival rate without limb loss, and by Bunt[9] in his collective review of AEFs and AEEs.

References

1. Alfrey EJ, Stanton C, Dunnington G, et al: Graft appendiceal fistulas. J Vasc Surg 7:814, 1988.
2. Auffermann W, Olofsson PA, Rabahie GN, et al: Incorporation versus infection of retroperitoneal aortic grafts. Radiology 172:359, 1989.
3. Bernhard VM: Reoperation for graft complications: Aortoenteric fistulas. *In* Bergan JJ, Yao JST (eds): Operative Techniques in Vascular Surgery. New York, Grune & Stratton, 1980, pp 193–202.
4. Billingham GT, Bessen HA: Aortoenteric fistula in a 21-year-old. J Emerg Med 9:343, 1991.
5. Blaisdell FW, Hall AD: Axillary-femoral artery bypass for lower extremity ischemia. Surgery 54:563, 1963.
6. Brenner WI, Richman H, Reed GE: Roof patch repair of an aortoduodenal fistula resulting from suture line failure in an aortic prosthesis. Am J Surg 127:762, 1974.
7. Brock RC: Aortic homografting. Guy's Hosp Rep 102:204, 1953.
8. Buchbinder D, Leather R, Shah D, Karmody A: Pathologic interactions between prosthetic aortic grafts and the gastrointestinal tract: Clinical problems and a new experimental approach. Am J Surg 140:192, 1980.
9. Bunt TJ: Synthetic vascular graft infections. Secondary graft enteric erosions and graft enteric fistulas. Surgery 94:1, 1983.
10. Busuttil RW, Rees W, Baker JD, et al: Pathogenesis of aortoduodenal fistula: Experimental and clinical correlates. Surgery 85:1, 1979.
11. Cooper A: The Lectures of Sir Astley Cooper on the Principles and Practice of Surgery With Additional Notes and Cases by Tyrell F. 5th ed. Philadelphia, Haswell, Barrington, and Haswell, 1939.
12. Cordell AR, Wright RH, Johnston FR: Gastrointestinal hemorrhage after aortic operations. Surgery 48:997, 1960.
13. Daugherty M, Shearer GR, Ernst CB: Primary aortoduodenal fistula: Extra-anatomic vascular reconstruction not required for successful management. Surgery 86:399, 1979.
14. DeWeese MS, Fry WJ: Small-bowel erosion following aortic resection. JAMA 179:882, 1962.
15. Ehrenfeld WK, Lord RSA, Stoney RJ, et al: Subcutaneous arterial bypass grafts in the management of fistulae between the bowel and plastic arterial prostheses. Ann Surg 168:19, 1968.

16. Ehrenfeld WK, Wilbur BG, Olcott CN, et al: Autogenous tissue reconstruction in the management of infected prosthetic grafts. Surgery 85:82, 1979.
17. Elliot JP Jr, Smith RF, Szilagyi DE: Aortoenteric and paraprosthetic-enteric fistulas. Problems of diagnosis and management. Arch Surg 108:479, 1974.
18. Evans DM, Webster JHH: Spontaneous aortoduodenal fistula. Br J Surg 59:368, 1972.
19. Ferris EJ, Koltay MRS, Koltay OP, et al: Abdominal aortic and iliac graft fistulae: Unusual roentgenographic findings. AJR 94:416, 1965.
20. Foster JH, Vetto RM: Aortic intra-aneurysmal abscess caused by sigmoid-aortic fistula. Am J Surg 104:850, 1962.
21. Freimanis IE, Kozak B, Taylor LM Jr, et al: Failure of CT scanning to diagnose aortic graft infection [Letters to the editors]. J Vasc Surg 5:531, 1987.
22. Frosch HL, Horowitz W: Rupture of abdominal aorta into duodenum (through a sinus tract created by a tuberculous mesenteric lymphadenitis). Ann Intern Med 21:481, 1944.
23. Fry WJ, Lindenauer SM: Infection complicating the use of plastic arterial implants. Arch Surg 94:600, 1967.
24. Garrett HE, Beall AC Jr, Jordan GL Jr, et al: Surgical considerations of massive gastrointestinal tract hemorrhage caused by aortoduodenal fistula. Am J Surg 105:6, 1963.
25. Harris KA, Kozak R, Carrol SF, et al: Confirmation of infection of an aortic graft. J Cardiovasc Surg 30:230, 1989.
26. Kleinman LH, Towne JB, Bernhard VM: A diagnostic and therapeutic approach to aortoenteric fistulas: Clinical experience with twenty patients. Surgery 86:868, 1979.
27. La Muraglia GM, Fischman AJ, Strauss HW, et al: Utility of the indium^{111}-labeled human immunoglobulin G scan for the detection of focal vascular graft infection. J Vasc Surg 10:20, 1989.
28. Lawrence PF, Dries DJ, Alazraki N, et al: Indium^{111}-labeled leukocyte scanning for detection of prosthetic graft infection. J Vasc Surg 2:165, 1985.
29. Low RN, Wall SD, Jeffrey RB Jr, et al: Aortoenteric fistula and perigraft infection: Evaluation with CT. Radiology 175:157, 1990.
30. Malone JM, Lalka SG, McIntyre KE, et al: The necessity for long-term antibiotic therapy with positive arterial wall cultures. J Vasc Surg 8:262, 1988.
31. Mark AS, Moss AA, McCarthy S, et al: CT of aortoenteric fistulas. Invest Radiol 20:272, 1985.
32. Mir-Madjlessi SH, Sullivan BH, Farmer RG, et al: Endoscopic diagnosis of aortoduodenal fistula. Gastrointest Endosc 19:187, 1973.
33. O'Mara CS, Imbembo AL: Paraprosthetic-enteric fistula. Surgery 81:556, 1977.
34. O'Mara CS, Williams GM, Ernst CB: Secondary aortoenteric fistula. A 20 year experience. Am J Surg 142:203, 1981.
35. Pabst TS III, Bernhard VM, McIntyre KE, et al: Gastrointestinal bleeding following aortic surgery. The place of laparotomy to rule out aortoenteric fistula. J Vasc Surg 8:280, 1988.
36. Perdue GD Jr, Smith RB III, Amsley JD, et al: Impending aortoenteric hemorrhage: The effect of early recognition on improved outcome. Ann Surg 192:237, 1980.
37. Reckless JPD, McColl I, Taylor GW: Aortoenteric fistulae: An uncommon complication of abdominal aortic aneurysms. Br J Surg 59:458, 1972.
38. Reilly LM, Altman H, Lusby RJ, et al: Late results following surgical management of vascular graft infection. J Vasc Surg 1:36, 1984.
39. Reilly LM, Ehrenfeld WK, Goldstone J, et al: Gastrointestinal tract involvement of prosthetic graft infection. The significance of gastrointestinal hemorrhage. Ann Surg 202:342, 1985.
40. Robinson JA, Johansen K: Aortic sepsis: Is there a role for in situ graft reconstruction? J Vasc Surg 13:677, 1991.
41. Sproul G: Rupture of an infected aortic graft into jejunum: Resection and survival. JAMA 182:1118, 1962.
42. Sweeney MS, Godacz TR: Primary aortoduodenal fistula: Manifestations, diagnosis, and treatment. Surgery 96:492, 1984.
43. Syme RG, Doobay BS, Gregor P, Franchetto A: Aortoenteric fistula 24 years after aortic endarterectomy. Can J Surg 3:100, 1992.
44. TenEyck FW, Wellman WE: Salmonellosis associated with abdominal aortic aneurysm and edema of lower extremities. Case report. Postgrad Med 26:334, 1954.
45. Thompson WM, Jackson DC, Johnsrude IE: Aortoenteric and paraprosthetic-enteric fistulae. Radiologic findings. AJR 127:235, 1976.
46. Voyles WR, Moretz WH: Rupture of aortic aneurysms into gastrointestinal tract. Surgery 43:666, 1958.
47. Walker WE, Cooley DA, Duncan JM, et al: The management of aortoduodenal fistula by in situ replacement of the infected abdominal aortic graft. Ann Surg 205:727, 1987.
48. Yeager RA, Sasaki TM, McConnell DB: Clinical spectrum of patients with infrarenal aortic grafts and gastrointestinal bleeding. Am J Surg 153:459, 1987.

39

Ischemic Neuropathy

J. Jean E. Turley, M.D., F.R.C.P.(C.), and K. Wayne Johnston, M.D., F.R.C.S.(C.)

• • •

Ischemic neuropathy is a term used to describe any injury of peripheral nerve caused by a reduction in blood supply. These disorders may be associated with diseases of large or small arteries. Large artery lesions may be acute (e.g., those due to arterial embolism, thrombosis, or injury) or chronic (e.g., those due to atherosclerosis). Small endoneurial arteries may be involved in periarteritis nodosa, rheumatoid vasculitis, Churg-Strauss syndrome, and Wegener's granulomatosis. Capillary disease may be significant in diabetic neuropathy. For the surgeon, ischemic disorders of nerve resulting from large artery disease are important.

ANATOMY AND PHYSIOLOGY OF PERIPHERAL NERVE

Peripheral nerves are composed of fascicles of nerve fibers. The fascicles are made up of nerve fibers, Schwann's cells, collagen, small vessels, and endoneurial fluid. Nerve fibers are bathed in endoneurial fluid that is maintained within narrow metabolic limits by blood-nerve and perineurial barriers.

Structural proteins and macromolecules are produced in the nerve cell body and transported in the axon. Axon transport is energy dependent and requires oxygen and glucose, which are supplied locally to the endoneurial fluid by endoneurial vessels. Transmission of nerve impulses is accomplished by transient depolarization of limited portions of the axonal membrane, during which time sodium and potassium diffuse across the membrane and are then restored to resting levels. This flow uses stored energy that is replenished by glycolysis in the Krebs cycle through aerobic metabolism. Although the nerve continually uses energy to maintain resting ionic gradients, the oxygen requirement of mammalian nerve is small, and even when this requirement is increased by activity, it is less than that of other tissues.[1] As a result, peripheral nerves are relatively resistant to ischemia.

BLOOD SUPPLY OF PERIPHERAL NERVE

The metabolic needs of large nerves are met by intraneural blood vessels, the vasa nervorum, whereas those of small nerves are met by diffusion from surrounding tissues. The vasa nervorum arise from nearby major arteries and enter nerve trunks at multiple levels, frequently near joints. The epineural arteries branch, and then arteriolar and precapillary branches penetrate the perineurium to perfuse the endoneurium. There is a complete terminal network of capillaries through the perineurium that supplies blood to nerve at some distance from the nutrient arteries.[1–4] The abundant collateral circulation pattern of peripheral nerve explains why it is difficult to injure a peripheral nerve by occlusion of one or even several nutrient arteries. Regional nutrient arteries have been ligated over considerable lengths of a nerve trunk without disturbing blood supply to nerve or adversely affecting the structure and function of nerve fibers.[5] Extensive studies of the microvasculature of peripheral nerve have demonstrated that the organization of vasa nervorum is such that a total interruption of circulation in nerves is very unlikely unless drastic interference with the blood supply is produced.[6]

The pattern of epineural vessels varies in different nerves, and some nerves may be more susceptible than others to ischemia.[5] In some cases, a single nutrient artery provides the major blood supply to a considerable length of nerve, and this may predispose to ischemic damage to the nerve trunk. At its upper end, the human sciatic nerve receives an arterial branch from the inferior gluteal artery. As the sciatic nerve enters the popliteal fossa, its blood supply is taken over by the popliteal artery and its branches. The tibial nerve is intimately related to the posterior tibial artery, which supplies a large number of direct nutrient arteries. The peroneal nerve, on the other hand, diverges from the main vessels and is supplied in the region of the fibular head by small adjacent arteries. At the neck of the fibula, the major intraneural vessels occupy a superficial position that may expose them to damage from pressure. In the calf, the posterior tibial and peroneal nerves receive branches from the anterior and posterior tibial arteries. The intraneural arterial pattern in the buttock and thigh contains several arterial channels of fairly large caliber, whereas below the knee, one major vessel usually dominates. The peroneal nerve at the knee and perhaps the more distal portions of the peroneal and posterior tibial nerves may therefore be more liable to ischemic damage.[5]

Sympathetic nerve fibers innervate vessels in the epineurium and perineurium. High sympathetic drive may significantly reduce intraneural circulation. Sympathetically mediated vasoconstriction may be important in the pathogenesis of reflex sympathetic dystrophy and chronic pain.[3]

PATHOPHYSIOLOGY OF ISCHEMIC NERVE

Many studies have been carried out to determine the effect of anoxia on nerve function. A short period of experimental ischemia results in disturbed function of nerve, which can recover if circulation is restored. Severe acute ischemia appears to result in decreased or abolished conduction of impulses. Thus, if ischemia is of short duration or is mild, function in peripheral nerve can be impaired in a transient manner.[7] The slight metabolic needs of nerve and the diffusion of nutrients from surrounding tissues enable it to survive. However, if ischemia is prolonged or severe, damage may be permanent.[5, 8]

Exactly how these functional changes of nerve occur is unknown. Obviously, ischemia impairs the metabolic processes that maintain the ionic gradient necessary for impulse transmission. Fast axoplasmic transport also depends on an adequate blood supply. The transport of material in the axon is impaired by ischemia at the same time that conduction is impaired, suggesting that both depend on the same sources of energy.[9] The block of fast axoplasmic transport becomes irreversible after 6 to 8 hours of ischemia. The permeability of endoneurial vessels during ischemia is impaired after 8 to 10 hours.[11] Metabolic factors including anoxia, hypercapnia, hyperkalemia, and acidosis are probably important. Potassium accumulation in the extracellular space during anoxia may cause irreversible depolarization of cell membrane.[2, 10]

There is controversy about the relative vulnerabilities of nerve and muscle to ischemia. The idea is entrenched in the literature that muscle is more sensitive, and Dyck, in a review of hypoxic neuropathy, still considers skeletal muscle to be more vulnerable to ischemic injury than nerve.[11] Korthals and coworkers ligated the abdominal aorta and femoral artery in cats and found necrotic changes in muscle at 2 to 3 hours, whereas no nerve lesions appeared until 5 hours of ischemia.[12] However, a study by Chervu and associates of the relative sensitivities of skeletal muscle and peripheral nerve function to ischemia and reperfusion suggests that peripheral nerve is more susceptible to ischemia than skeletal muscle.[13]

PATHOLOGIC CHANGES IN ISCHEMIC NERVE

Pathologic studies have been performed of peripheral nerves in ischemic limbs. Farinon and colleagues, examining muscle and nerve biopsy specimens from patients with chronic arterial insufficiency, found a combination of segmental demyelination and axonal degeneration. They believed that large fibers and small fibers were equally affected, and further noted that the severity of the nerve pathology did not correlate well with the severity of vascular disease.[14] Eames and Lange described the pathologic changes in sural nerve biopsy specimens from eight patients with vascular disease: they found evidence of segmental demyelination and remyelination, axonal degeneration and regeneration, and an increase in endoneurial collagen.[16] The unmyelinated fibers were essentially normal. Rodriguez-Sánchez and associates examined morphologic alterations in the sural nerve from patients with chronic atherosclerotic disease. Both axonal degeneration and regeneration, and demyelination and remyelination were seen.[15] In cases of atherosclerotic disease of large vessels, the lumina of the epineurial and endoneurial vasa nervorum in the sural nerves have been found to be markedly narrowed and the walls thickened.[16]

Many experimental studies have examined the morphology of animal nerve after ischemic injury.[17–21] In general, large myelinated fibers, particularly in the center of nerves, seem to undergo axonal degeneration.

ISCHEMIC POLYNEUROPATHY ASSOCIATED WITH CHRONIC ARTERIAL INSUFFICIENCY

In humans, the effects of chronic ischemia on the structure and function of nerves are not well defined, nor is the limit of tolerance of peripheral nerve to ischemia.

The incidence of neurologic deficits in patients with chronic peripheral vascular disease has not been ascertained. Peripheral nerve involvement in atherosclerosis is probably underestimated because neuropathic symptoms—pain, sensory changes, and even weakness—may be confused with claudication or rest pain. A number of series have reported symptoms such as painful burning and signs varying from sensory impairment to reflex loss, muscle wasting, and weakness in patients with peripheral arterial occlusive disease. Hutchison and Liversedge found peripheral nerve dysfunction, as manifested by sensory deficits and absent reflexes, in 50 per cent of their patients with peripheral vascular disease.[22] They believed that the presence of neuropathy was related to the severity of the vascular disease. Eames and Lange found impaired sensation in 88 per cent of their 32 atherosclerotic patients, muscle weakness in 50 per cent, and decreased or absent reflexes in 41 per cent.[16] Again, the extent of the deficit was proportional to the degree of ischemia. All patients with claudication at less than 100 yards had a neurologic abnormality. Twenty patients had a superficial femoral artery occlusion, and the remainder had proximal vascular disease. Hunter and colleagues found neurologic deficits in 22 per cent of ischemic limbs.[23] Miglietta found decreased ankle jerks and decreased vibration sense in 54 per cent of his patients with atherosclerosis.[24]

When electrophysiologic studies are added to the clinical evaluation, neurologic abnormalities are uncovered in an even greater number of individuals who have no apparent clinical symptoms or signs. Miglietta and Lowenthal found slowing of motor conduction velocity in peroneal nerves in nearly all patients with severe vascular disease and no neurologic signs, but many patients were diabetic.[25] Hunter and colleagues found abnormal peroneal nerve compound muscle action potential amplitudes in 86 per cent and abnormal conduction velocities in the lower extremities in 36 per cent of atherosclerotic patients, whereas only 22 per cent had clinical neurologic abnormalities.[23]

Therefore, it seems that some patients with chronic occlusive vascular disease develop peripheral neuropathy. The precise location and the severity of the requisite arterial lesion have not been defined, nor has the precise incidence. Nevertheless, there is considerable clinical importance in detecting the presence of neuropathy before surgery. If some of the patient's symptoms are neuropathic in origin, it is to be expected that improvement of vascular supply to the limb may not immediately relieve all of the symptoms, even if adequate revascularization is achieved.

ISCHEMIC POLYNEUROPATHY FOLLOWING ACUTE ARTERIAL INSUFFICIENCY

Incidence

Acute arterial occlusion due to embolism, thrombosis, or arterial injury is often associated with acute neural dysfunction. The motor and sensory deficit usually has a distal limb distribution, but selective peroneal palsy has been described.[26] The frequency of clear neurologic signs in the acutely ischemic limb has seldom been carefully analyzed. Haimovici reported that 22 per cent of his patients presented with sensory symptoms, but no data are presented on physical signs.[27] A number of other reports have documented neurologic deficits with motor signs in about 20 per cent and sensory deficits in 50 per cent.[1] After acute arterial occlusion, if flow is not reestablished within several hours (and this time limit has not been clearly defined), symptoms and signs of neurologic dysfunction may persist when circulation is restored, and the neurologic deficit may be permanent.

Clinical Features

The clinical features of ischemic neuropathy following trauma to major blood vessels were summarized by Sunderland.[5] He reported that sensory loss is distal and of a stocking-and-glove type, is associated with distal muscle wasting and weakness, and is sometimes accompanied by late fibrosis and contracture. Wilbourn and coworkers subsequently described 14 cases of ischemic monomelic neuropathy in a single limb,[28] with pain, paresthesia, and paralysis following the restoration of blood flow after acute occlusion of a proximal limb artery.

The precise incidence of ischemic neuropathy and the various factors that predispose to the development of neuropathy in an ischemic limb have not as yet been characterized by the publication of a large series or by a prospective study. However, after an episode of severe ischemia, it is not unusual for patients with a satisfactorily revascularized leg to continue to complain of pain that is due to neuropathy. The neuropathic pain is burning and paresthetic in nature, is frequently worse with rest and at night, and is unaffected or relieved by walking, in marked contrast to the pain of claudication. The patient perceives the foot to be cold, although it is in fact warm. The patient may remark on loss of mobility of the toes.

Examination no longer reveals signs of significant ischemia. Instead, the small muscles of the affected foot are wasted compared with those of the normal side, and they are weak. There may be slight ankle weakness, and the ankle reflex may be depressed compared with that of the normal side. There is a unilateral stocking sensory loss, particularly to vibration sense. Unlike the findings in neuropathies caused by diabetes, uremia, drug intoxication, or alcoholism, the findings in ischemic neuropathy are very asymmetric, with sensory and motor findings exclusively or prominently in the limb that was afflicted by severe ischemia.

Diagnosis

Vascular Assessment. The severity of ischemia can be assessed clinically or may be determined more objectively by noninvasive methods, including the measurement of ankle and toe pressures and Doppler waveform recordings. If the ankle pressure is greater than 50 to 60 mmHg or the toe pressure is greater than 30 mmHg, ischemic rest pain is unlikely and the diagnosis of ischemic neuropathy should be suspected. Flat or monophasic Doppler waveforms confirm that the arterial disease is severe. If clinical examination and noninvasive assessment confirm that the peripheral circulation is adequate, the pain is probably not due to ischemia. If the perfusion is inadequate, the pain may be due to ischemia, neuropathy, or both, and treatment should be directed first toward improvement of the limb blood flow.

Electrophysiologic Studies. Careful electrophysiologic studies can establish the diagnosis of ischemic neuropathy and define its severity. Typically, a unilateral axonal neuropathy involving distal nerves is present.

Motor nerve conduction studies show a decrease in or an absence of the compound *muscle action potential* amplitude from the extensor digitorum brevis muscle when the peroneal nerve is stimulated and from the flexor hallucis brevis muscle when the posterior tibial nerve is stimulated in the affected foot. Frequently, the distal posterior tibial nerve is more involved than the distal peroneal nerve. The abnormality is always most severe in the distal nerves. The distal latency, if one can be recorded, and the velocity of conduction in the calf portion of the peroneal and posterior tibial nerves are relatively well preserved. These findings are in sharp contrast to those in diabetic and uremic neuropathies, in which distal latencies and conduction velocities tend to be symmetrically reduced well below normal velocities at an early stage in *both* lower limbs.

Sensory nerve conduction studies show decreased or absent sensory potential amplitudes from sural, superficial peroneal, and plantar nerves, whereas sensory conduction velocity, when recordable, is normal.

Needle electrode examination reveals the changes of muscle denervation in the small muscles of the affected foot, particularly in the sole of the foot, with fibrillation potentials at rest and large motor units of long duration in much reduced numbers. Lesser denervation changes are seen in the muscles of the calf if the ischemia has been severe.

Treatment. Once a diagnosis of ischemic neuropathy has been made by clinical and electrophysiologic investigations, what treatment can be offered? If peripheral blood flow is significantly reduced, vascular reconstructive surgery is justified. However, if perfusion is adequate, conservative treatment is indicated. Wilbourn and coworkers suggest that phenytoin, tricyclic antidepressants, and analgesics are ineffective but that carbamazepine produces partial relief.[28] Three of their patients had sympathectomy, and two reported pain relief. Persistent pain that is uncontrolled by such drugs, if dramatically relieved by sympathetic blocks, may well deserve sympathectomy, particularly if the passage of time does not indicate spontaneous regression is taking place. Many clinicians believe that tricyclic antidepressants, sometimes in combination with small amounts of phenothiazine, are quite effective.

Prognosis. The prognosis is uncertain. After other types of axonal nerve injury, peripheral nerves show a considerable capacity to regenerate, and regeneration has been seen in animal models after ischemia. Therefore, particularly in the absence of any other causes of neuropathy, such as diabetes, uremia, blood dyscrasias, or carcinoma, axon repair might be expected to occur slowly, with relief of symptoms.

ISCHEMIC MONONEUROPATHY ASSOCIATED WITH ATHEROSCLEROTIC DISEASE OF LARGE ARTERIES

Ischemic mononeuropathy is a frequent occurrence in diseases of small vessels associated with vasculitis and diabetes. Ischemic mononeuropathies that seem distinct from compressive neuropathies have occasionally been documented in the literature in association with atherosclerotic disease of large vessels.

Peroneal Neuropathy

Ferguson and Liversedge reported seven cases of peroneal palsy with vascular disease: three resulted from cardiac emboli, and four were associated with atherosclerosis.

The precise location of the arterial occlusions was not documented angiographically.[26] As described earlier, the nature of the vascular supply to the peroneal nerve at the fibular head certainly predisposes to ischemic damage, although the nerve is also prone to compression in the same area.

Peroneal neuropathy presents as weakness of dorsiflexion and eversion of the ankle, with preservation of inversion and plantar flexion, which are functions of the posterior calf muscles. The sensory deficit is confined to the dorsum of the foot and perhaps to the lateral calf, and the ankle jerk is preserved. It is possible to confirm the diagnosis with nerve conduction studies, which will demonstrate abnormality in peroneal function while all other nerve conduction is intact. It is usually possible to distinguish a compressive peroneal neuropathy, which produces a local area of conduction slowing and block at the fibular head, from an ischemic lesion, which is primarily axonal in nature and produces a uniform conduction velocity throughout the length of the nerve and a reduction in the motor and sensory potential amplitudes.

Femoral Neuropathy

Whether a femoral neuropathy occurs with vascular occlusion in the absence of compression, traction, or hemorrhage is unclear. Chopra and Hurwitz reported slight wasting and weakness of the quadriceps muscle in 1 of 29 patients with atherosclerosis and claudication symptoms,[29] and Archie reported a femoral neuropathy due to common iliac artery occlusion in a nondiabetic.[30] D'Amour and associates reported two cases of femoral neuropathy, one following surgery for abdominal aortic aneurysm with aortobifemoral bypass grafting and one following placement of an intra-aortic balloon pump.[31]

The main trunk of the femoral artery receives nutrient arteries from the iliac branch of the iliolumbar artery, from the deep circumflex iliac artery in the iliac fossa, and from the lateral circumflex femoral artery in the femoral triangle.[5]

A femoral nerve lesion results in flaccid paralysis of the quadriceps muscle, an absent knee jerk, and loss of sensation over the anterior and medial thigh and the inner aspect of the calf down to the level of the medial malleolus. Electrophysiologic studies show decreased or absent motor evoked response from the quadriceps muscle when the femoral nerve is stimulated in the groin and an absent saphenous sensory potential at the ankle, together with fibrillation potentials and motor unit loss, on needle electrode examination of the quadriceps muscle. Other nerves in the limb will be normal. Femoral neuropathy is a frequent complication of diabetes and is presumably due to abnormalities of the vasa nervorum. The prognosis for recovery in both traumatic and diabetic femoral neuropathy is excellent. The incidence of and prognosis for ischemic femoral neuropathy await further reports.

Lumbosacral Plexus Lesions

Whether lumbosacral plexus lesions rather than lower cord or cauda equina lesions result from occlusive vascular disease is also not well documented.

The lumbosacral plexus really has two parts: a lumbar plexus arising from the second, third, and fourth lumbar roots and forming the femoral and obturator nerves, and a sacral plexus arising from the fourth and fifth lumbar roots and the first three sacral roots and forming the superior and inferior gluteal nerves and the sciatic nerve. Blood supply to the lumbosacral plexus is through five lumbar arteries from each side of the abdominal aorta, the deep circumflex iliac artery, a branch of the external iliac artery, and the iliolumbar and gluteal branches of the internal iliac artery.[5]

Usubiaga and colleagues described a lumbosacral plexus lesion after resection of an abdominal aortic aneurysm and aortobifemoral grafting.[32] At autopsy, the plexus was totally infarcted. Voulters and Bolton reported lumbosacral plexus damage following aortofemoral bypass grafting for repair of an abdominal aortic aneurysm.[33] D'Amour and associates described a number of cases, one following aortofemoral bypass grafting for stenosis of the common and external iliac arteries; one following acute occlusion of an aortobifemoral graft; one following aortofemoral bypass and femoropopliteal thrombectomy for occlusion of the common iliac, internal iliac, and superficial femoral arteries; and one following occlusion of the common iliac and femoral arteries.[31] In these cases, the sciatic nerve seemed to be mainly involved. In two cases, neurologic symptoms appeared following vascular occlusion before surgery. Partial slow recoveries were reported. Gloviczki and coworkers reported on a non–insulin-dependent diabetic patient who had bilateral leg weakness following aorta–profunda femoris bypass grafting for internal iliac disease.[34] The patient experienced slow partial recovery.

Clinical evaluation of the patient with unilateral lower limb dysfunction can often distinguish a lesion of the lumbosacral plexus from one affecting the spinal cord or a major peripheral nerve. When the abnormality resides in the plexus, motor and sensory loss affect more than one peripheral nerve and dermatomal segment. Weakness involves proximal muscles (the iliopsoas, hip adductors and abductors, or glutei) as well as distal muscles. The limb is flaccid and areflexic, with no response to plantar stimulation. This is in contrast to spinal lesions, which produce a spastic, hyper-reflexic limb with extensor plantar response and dissociated sensory loss. Electromyography is usually essential to confirm the diagnosis. Localization to the lumbosacral plexus depends on the unilateral absence of sensory potentials (these are preserved in cauda equina and proximal root lesions), the absence of paraspinal denervation, and the presence of denervation changes in muscles innervated by multiple nerves and roots.

It is important to attempt to distinguish the precise level of the lesion when severe unilateral limb dysfunction occurs. Whereas lesions of the lower spinal cord or cauda equina have a very poor prognosis, there is some hope of recovery if the damage has occurred to part of the lumbosacral plexus.

CONCLUSIONS

Nerve injury due to ischemia has been discussed. Although there has been an enormous amount of publication of experimental animal studies, the association of atherosclerotic disease with clinical neuropathic lesions in humans has not been as clearly reported. Occlusive vascular disease, both acute and chronic, seems capable of producing a painful unilateral axonal polyneuropathy, and major vascular occlusion may occasionally cause a mononeuropathy or lumbosacral plexus lesion. In the clinical setting, attempts should be made to diagnose the location and severity of the neurologic lesion precisely so that clearer therapeutic and prognostic guidelines can be established. In general, if significant ischemia is present, revascularization is indicated; however, if perfusion is adequate, a conservative approach is justified.

Acknowledgment: *The authors wish to thank Ms. P. Purdy for her assistance in the preparation of the manuscript.*

References

1. Daube JR, Dyck PJ: Neuropathy due to peripheral vascular diseases. *In* Dyck PJ, Thomas PK, Lambert EH, et al (eds): Diseases of the Peripheral Nervous System. Philadelphia, WB Saunders, 1984, pp 1458–1478.
2. Olsson Y: The involvement of vasa nervorum in diseases of peripheral nerves. *In* Vinken PJ, Bruyn GW (eds): Handbook of Clinical Neurology. Amsterdam, North Harvard Publishing, 1972, vol. 12, pp 644–664.
3. Lundborg G: Intraneural microcirculation. Orthop Clin North Am 19:1, 1988.
4. Lundborg G: The intrinsic vascularization of human peripheral nerves—Structural and functional aspects. J Hand Surg 4:34, 1979.
5. Sunderland S: Nerve and Nerve Injuries. Edinburgh, Churchill Livingstone, 1978.
6. Lundborg G: Ischemic nerve injury. Experimental studies on intraneural microvascular pathophysiology and nerve function in a limb subjected to temporary circulatory arrest. Scand J Plast Reconstr Surg Suppl 6:3, 1970.
7. Parry GJ, Linn DJ: Transient focal conduction block following experimental occlusion of the vasa nervorum muscle and nerve. Muscle Nerve 9:345, 1986.
8. Schmetzer JD, Zochodne E, Low PA: Ischemic and reperfusion injury of rat peripheral nerve. Proc Natl Acad Sci USA 86:16, 1989.
9. Leone J, Ochs S: Anoxic block and recovery of axoplasmic transport and electrical excitability of nerve. J Neurobiol 9:229, 1978.
10. Fox JL, Kenmore PI: The effect of ischemia on nerve conduction. Exp Neurol 17:403, 1967.
11. Dyck PJ: Hypoxic neuropathy: Does hypoxia play a role in diabetic neuropathy? The 1988 Robert Wartenberg Lecture. Neurology 39:111, 1989.
12. Korthals JK, Maki T, Gieron MA: Nerve and muscle vulnerability to ischemia. J Neurol Sci 71:283, 1985.
13. Chervu A, Moore WS, Homsher E, et al: Differential recovery of skeletal muscle and peripheral nerve function after ischemia and reperfusion. J Surg Res 47:12, 1989.
14. Farinon AM, Marbini A, Gemignani F, et al: Skeletal muscle and peripheral nerve changes caused by chronic arterial insufficiency—Significance and clinical correlations—Histological, histochemical and ultrastructural study. Clin Neurol 3:240, 1984.
15. Rodriguez-Sánchez C, Medina Sánchez M, Malik RA, et al: Morphological abnormalities in the sural nerve from patients with peripheral vascular disease. Histol Histopathol 6:63, 1991.
16. Eames RA, Lange LS: Clinical and pathological study of ischemic neuropathy. J Neurol Neurosurg Psychiatry 30:215, 1967.
17. Benstead TJ, Dyck PJ, Sangalang V: Inner perineurial cell vulnerability in ischemia. Brain Res 489:177, 1989.
18. Korthals JK, Korthals MA, Wisniewski HM: Peripheral nerve ischemia. 2. Accumulation of organelles. Ann Neurol 4:487, 1978.
19. Parry GJ, Brown MJ: Selective fiber vulnerability in acute ischemic neuropathy. Ann Neurol 11:147, 1981.
20. Nukada H, Dyck PJ: Acute ischemia causes axonal stasis, swelling, attenuation, and secondary demyelination. Ann Neurol 22:311, 1987.
21. McManis PG, Low PA: Factors affecting the relative viability of centrifascicular and subperineurial axons in acute peripheral nerve ischemia. Exp Neurol 99:84, 1988.
22. Hutchison EC, Liversedge LA: Neuropathy in peripheral vascular disease. Its bearing on diabetic neuropathy. Q J Med 25:267, 1956.
23. Hunter GC, Song GW, Nayak NN, et al: Peripheral nerve conduction abnormalities in lower extremity ischemia: The effects of revascularization. J Surg Res 45:96, 1988.
24. Miglietta O: Electrophysiologic studies in chronic occlusive peripheral vascular disease. Arch Phys Med Rehabil 48:89, 1967.
25. Miglietta O, Lowenthal M: Nerve conduction velocity and refractory period in peripheral vascular disease. J Appl Physiol 17:837, 1962.
26. Ferguson FR, Liversedge LA: Ischemic lateral popliteal nerve palsy. Br Med J 2:333, 1954.
27. Haimovici H: Peripheral arterial embolism. Angiology 1:20, 1950.
28. Wilbourn AJ, Furlan AJ, Hulley W, et al: Ischemic monomelic neuropathy. Neurology 33:447, 1983.
29. Chopra JS, Hurwitz LJ: Femoral nerve conduction in diabetes and chronic occlusive vascular disease. J Neurol Neurosurg Psychiatry 31:28, 1968.
30. Archie JP Jr: Femoral neuropathy due to common iliac artery occlusion. South Med J 76:1073, 1983.
31. D'Amour ML, Lebrun LH, Rabbat A, et al: Peripheral neurological complications of aortoiliac vascular disease. Can J Neurol Sci 14:127, 1987.
32. Usubiaga JE, Kolodny J, Usubiaga LE: Neurologic complications of prevertebral surgery under regional anaesthesia. Surgery 68:304, 1970.
33. Voulters L, Bolton C: Acute lumbosacral plexus neuropathy following vascular surgery. Can J Neurol Sci 10:153, 1983.
34. Gloviczki P, Cross SA, Stanson AW, et al: Ischemic injury to the spinal cord or lumbosacral plexus after aorto-iliac reconstruction. Am J Surg 162:131, 1991.

40

Lymphatic Complications of Vascular Surgery

Peter Gloviczki, M.D., and Robert C. Lowell, M.D.

• • •

Injury to the lymphatic system during vascular reconstructions may be unavoidable. Lymph vessels usually run parallel to corresponding arteries and veins, and major groups of lymph nodes are close to major vessels. However, the ability of transected or ligated lymphatics to regenerate and reestablish normal lymphatic transport is remarkable. Lymphatic injury frequently heals spontaneously and causes minimal or no morbidity. Injury to the lymphatics is, however, a major factor responsible for the development of edema of the lower extremity after infrainguinal reconstructions.[1–11] Interruption of lymphatic vessels during surgical dissection may also cause a lymphatic fistula[12–17] or lymphocele.[17–27] Rarely, injury to the para-aortic or mesenteric lymphatics may result in chylous ascites,[22, 28–46] and thoracic duct injury during thoracic or thoracoabdominal aortic reconstruction[31, 47–56] or after high translumbar aortography[57] may result in chylothorax. This chapter reviews the pathophysiology, diagnosis, and management of the most frequent lymphatic complications following vascular reconstructions and suggests guidelines for prevention.

POSTBYPASS EDEMA

Lower extremity edema occurs in 50 to 100 per cent of patients who undergo successful infrainguinal arterial reconstruction for chronic ischemia.[2, 7] Leg swelling after femoropopliteal or femorotibial bypass becomes evident with dependency, usually when the patient resumes ambulation. Pitting edema usually subsides within 2 to 3 months after reconstruction. During this period, normal ambulation may be impaired and wound healing delayed. In some patients, the edema may become chronic and cause persistent functional disability, despite the successful arterial reconstruction.

Etiology and Pathogenesis

Lymphedema develops if the rate of production of protein-rich interstitial fluid exceeds the ability of the lymphatic system to remove the increased volume of lymph. Insufficiency of the lymphatic transport plays the most important role in the development of postbypass edema.[58] Lymphatic insufficiency has two main causes (Fig. 40–1). First, increased production of interstitial fluid after successful revascularization results in a significant increase in the lymphatic load. Second, the transport capacity of the lymphatic system is reduced because of lymphatic injury and the obstruction of deep and superficial lymph channels during dissection in the popliteal space, along the greater saphenous vein and at the groin.

Increased capillary filtration results from elevated arterial pressure after revascularization, alterations in the regulation of the microcirculatory flow, and probable endothelial and smooth muscle injury from chronic ischemia.[1, 7] Decreased arterial and arteriolar smooth muscle tone as a cause of hyperemia following revascularization was first proposed by Simeone and Husni in 1959.[59] Experiments by Eickhoff,[8] however, demonstrated that abnormalities in local blood flow regulation normalized within about 1 week after reconstruction, whereas edema persisted much longer in these patients. Although derangement of the microcirculation contributes to postbypass edema to some degree, Eickhoff's experiments support the theory that lymphatic obstruction due to surgical injury is the most important cause of postbypass edema.

If the number of functioning major lymph channels decreases to a critical level, lymphedema will develop. In one study, in which patients underwent lymphangiography after infrainguinal bypass, the average number of patent visualized superficial lymph vessels was reduced to 1.7 per patient, as compared with the normal average of 9.5.[1] In a similar series of 37 patients, edema was not significant when more than three intact superficial lymph vessels were visualized on the postoperative lymphangiogram.[4]

AbuRahma and colleagues examined the involvement of the lymphatic system in the pathophysiology of edema formation in patients undergoing femoropopliteal bypass grafting.[9] Twenty-nine of the 72 patients (40 per cent) developed edema. Leg swelling occurred in 85 per cent of the patients (17 of 20) who had conventional dissection of the femoropopliteal arteries. If careful dissection was performed that preserved the lymphatics, edema developed in only 2 of 20 patients (10 per cent). Postoperative lymphangiography showed normal anatomy in 6 of the 8 patients without edema, but the anatomy was markedly abnormal in all 8 patients with edema who underwent lymphangiography. Persson and coworkers found less edema in those patients who needed less dissection during surgery.[10] Sig-

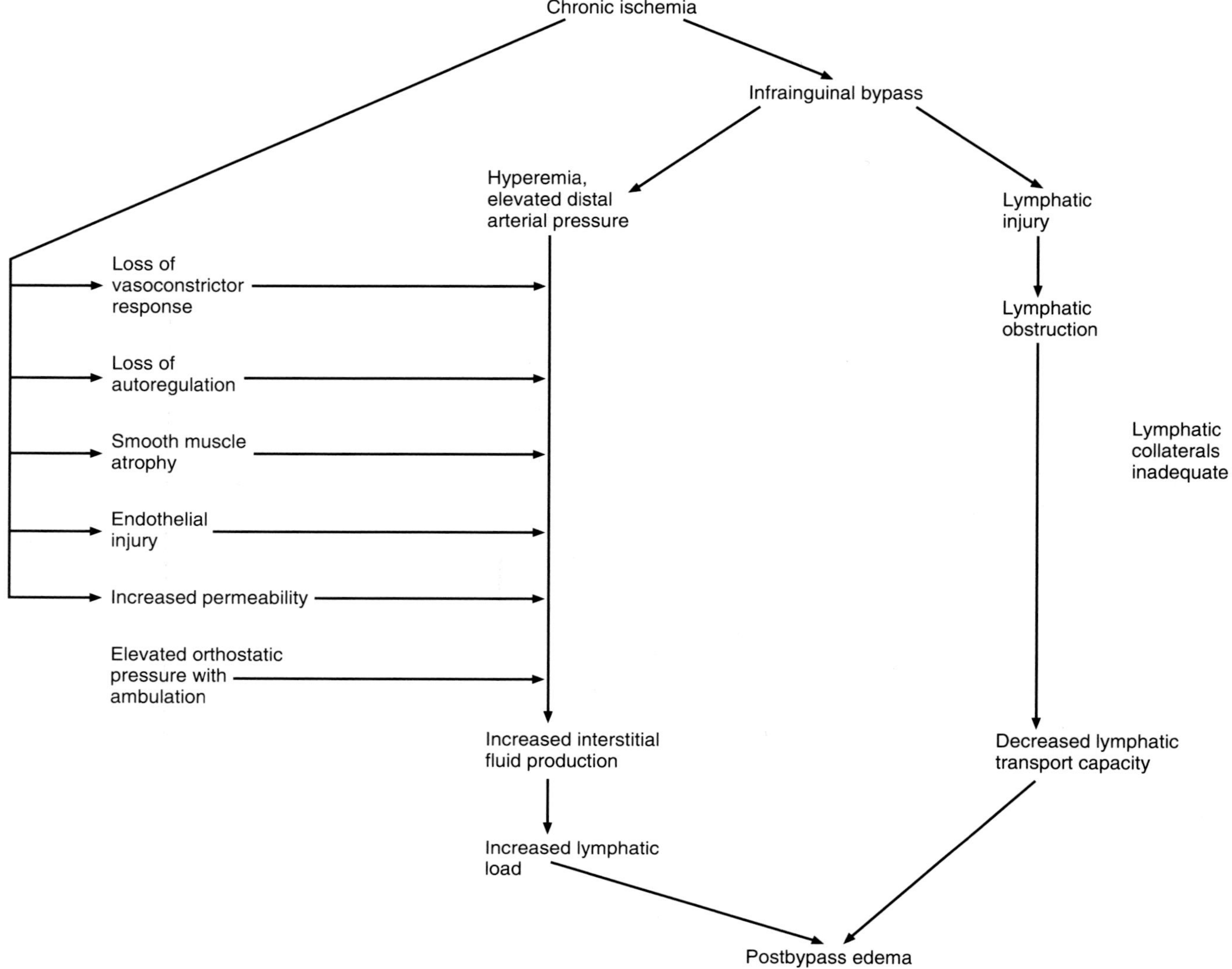

FIGURE 40–1. Mechanism of postbypass edema. (Adapted from Gloviczki P, Bergman RT: Lymphatic problems and revascularization edema. *In* Bernhard VM, Towne JB [eds]: Complications in Vascular Surgery. 2nd ed. St. Louis, Quality Medical Publishing, 1991, p 366.)

nificantly less swelling was found in patients with prosthetic grafts than in those with vein grafts. Less edema was also found in patients with above-knee grafts than in those with below-knee bypasses.[10]

Studies using albumin clearance in patients with postrevascularization edema also support the idea that edema is mainly lymphatic in origin. A reduction in plasma albumin level with a concomitant increase in the extremity albumin content was noted after femoropopliteal bypass.[60] The increase in albumin content was three times higher in limbs revascularized with femoropopliteal bypass than in those with aortoiliac grafts. These data correspond to the clinical observation that edema rarely develops after aortofemoral revascularization.

Although venous thrombosis has been proposed as a cause of postoperative leg edema,[61, 62] studies have demonstrated a low incidence of deep venous thrombosis in patients with postbypass edema.[63, 64] In one series, normal venous hemodynamics and morphology were confirmed in 41 of 45 patients with leg edema after arterial bypass.[65] The incidence of deep venous thrombosis following femoropopliteal bypass was found to be similar in patients with edema (7 per cent) and in those without edema (10 per cent).[9] Deep venous thrombosis, therefore, seems to play a minor role in postbypass edema in most patients.[7, 58, 66]

Diagnosis

Mild, partially pitting ankle edema appears on the 2nd or 3rd postoperative day and almost completely resolves with leg elevation and bed rest. Deep venous thrombosis as a cause of postoperative edema should be excluded if there is excessive postoperative swelling, cyanosis, muscle tenderness, or unusual pain. Duplex scanning of the deep veins is the test of choice for excluding deep venous thrombosis. If the cause of the edema is still in question, lymphoscintigraphy will confirm lymphedema (Fig. 40–2).

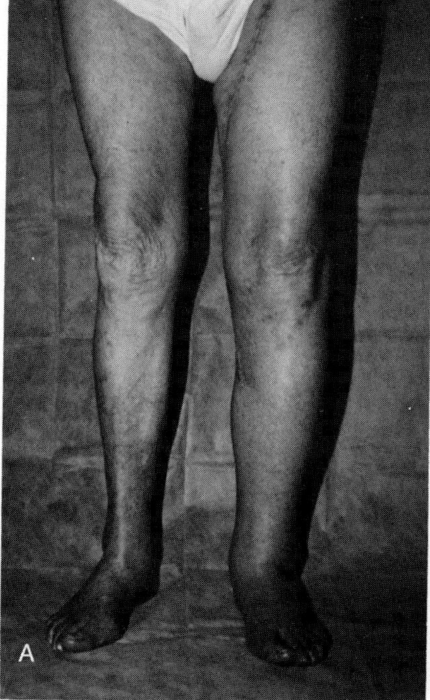

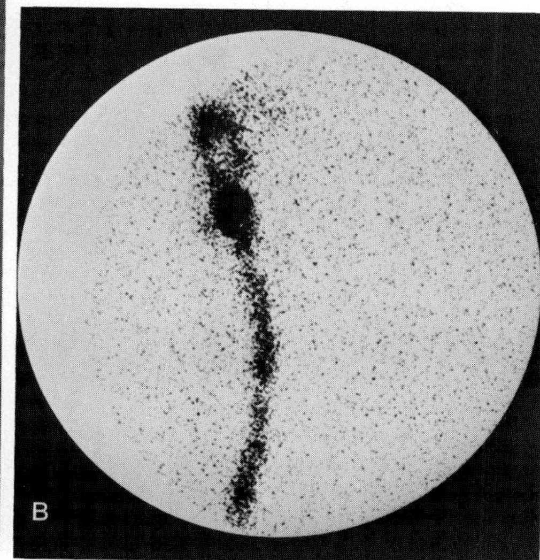

FIGURE 40–2. *A*, Edema of the left lower extremity in an 88-year-old man 4 weeks after left femoropopliteal saphenous vein bypass performed for severe chronic ischemia. *B*, Lymphoscintigraphy confirmed the severe lymphedema of the left leg with no visualization of the lymph vessels or inguinal lymph nodes. The lymphatic transport was normal on the right.

Management

Postoperatively, mild edema of the extremity should be treated with frequent elevation of the limb and some restriction of ambulation. Cardiac failure should be promptly treated to help preserve the normal pressure gradient and to allow venous return and lymphatic flow toward the heart. Moderate to severe postbypass edema is treated with compression stockings. In general, the authors prescribe calf-length therapeutic elastic stockings with a compression of 30 to 40 mmHg at the ankle level. In patients with a below-knee in situ bypass or any bypass to the distal tibial or pedal arteries, management is individualized to avoid direct compression of a subcutaneous vein graft. Attempts to prevent or limit postbypass edema pharmacologically with steroids, mannitol, terbutaline, or furosemide have not been proved to be effective[10] and are not recommended.

Prevention

Meticulous, lymphatic-preserving surgical dissection is needed to minimize postbypass edema.[9, 58] For infrainguinal bypass, a vertical groin incision slightly lateral to the femoral pulse should be made in an attempt to preserve the patency of lymph vessels and the integrity of lymph nodes. The inguinal lymphatics should be retracted medially, and a vertical incision should be made in the femoral sheath to dissect the femoral arteries. The use of loupe magnification facilitates the identification of lymph nodes and lymph vessels. The lymphatics should be carefully preserved, or if they have to be divided, they should be ligated or cauterized to avoid lymphatic leakage. Attempts should be made to preserve as much lymphatic tissue between the saphenofemoral junction and the femoral artery as possible. A skin bridge should be left between the groin incision and the incision made in the thigh to dissect the more distal saphenous vein. Multiple short skin incisions to dissect the saphenous vein will disrupt fewer superficial lymphatics.[9]

Dissection around the popliteal artery should be performed with the same care as previously described. The vascular sheath should be opened longitudinally without dissection of the popliteal vein or the posterior tibial nerve in the neurovascular bundle. Fibroadipose tissue, which contains the deep lymphatics in the popliteal fossa, should be left intact.

LYMPHATIC FISTULA

Because of the rich lymphatic network of the femoral triangle, lymphatic fistula following vascular reconstructions occurs most often at the groin. In 4000 vascular operations, Kalman and associates observed lymphatic fistula in 45 patients (incidence, 1.1 per cent).[16] In other series, the incidence of this complication was similar, ranging from 0.8 to 6.4 per cent.[13, 67, 68]

Etiology

Important factors contributing to lymphatic leakage are a failure to ligate or cauterize divided lymphatics and a failure to approximate well the tissue layers at closure. Lymphatic leakage occurs more frequently in elderly diabetic patients with poor wound healing. Excessive early limb motion, infection of the operated leg or foot, reoperation, and the placement of a prosthetic graft to the groin are additional possible causes.[16]

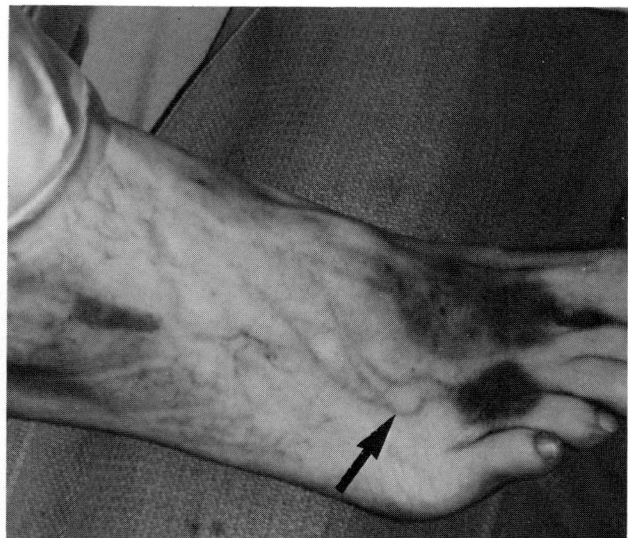

FIGURE 40–3. Injection of isosulfan blue (Lymphazurin) dye into the first and third interdigital spaces of the foot immediately visualizes the foot lymphatics (*arrow*) and during surgery helps to identify the site of lymphatic injury at the groin.

Diagnosis

Persistent leakage of clear yellow fluid from a groin incision establishes the diagnosis. Lymphoscintigraphy to confirm that the fluid is lymphatic in origin is seldom needed if the fistula develops within days or a few weeks after the operation. If lymphatic leakage occurs several months or years after vascular reconstruction, lymphoscintigraphy is helpful. However, in these patients, computed tomography, white blood cell scanning, and sometimes fistulography must be performed to exclude infection of an underlying vascular graft. Computed tomography is also valuable for diagnosing concomitant retroperitoneal lymphatic injury because retroperitoneal lymphocele or chylous ascites may present with lymphatic fistula at the groin.[58]

Management

Early diagnosis and management of lymphatic fistula are important to prevent prolonged hospitalization and delayed wound healing. Although in one study of 35 patients with lymphatic leakage, infection of an underlying vascular graft was not noted,[14] most studies have reported a small but definite risk of deep wound infection from persistent lymphatic leakage.[13, 16] In the first few days, conservative management is indicated in these patients. It should include local wound care, administration of systemic antibiotics, and bed rest with leg elevation to reduce lymph flow. Like other authors,[13, 16] the authors of this chapter favor surgical closure in the operating room if the fistula has persistent high volume despite several days of conservative management. First, 5 ml of isosulfan blue (Lymphazurin dye) is injected subcutaneously into the first and third interdigital spaces in the foot (Fig. 40–3).[15, 58] The groin incision is then opened, and the site of the lymphatic injury is readily apparent by the leakage of blue fluid droplets. The area is oversewn, and the wound is closed in multiple layers over a small polyethylene drain. In cases in which it is impossible to oversew the damaged lymphatic, injection of ''tissue glue'' may be useful.

THORACIC DUCT FISTULA

Injury to the thoracic duct may occur after dissection of the proximal left common carotid artery or after left subclavian or vertebral artery dissection.[22, 74] Neglected cases of thoracic duct cutaneous fistula may lead to malnutrition, lymphocytopenia, anemia, or infection of an underlying prosthetic graft. Early operation with lateral closure using 7–0 or 8–0 nonabsorbable monofilament sutures is the optimal treatment. If lateral closure is not possible, ligation of the thoracic duct at the neck is an accepted alternative because the collateral lymphatic circulation is usually adequate. The incision is closed over a subcutaneous drain, which is left in place for a short period postoperatively.

LYMPHOCELE

A lymphocele is a localized collection of lymph fluid. Early after injury to the lymphatic pathways, the lymph collects between tissue planes. Unless it reabsorbs spontaneously or drains through a cutaneous fistula, a pseudocapsule will develop. In contrast to a seroma, a lymphocele usually has a well-localized connection with one or more of the lymphatic channels. For this reason, lymphoscintigraphy can readily demonstrate a lymphocele (Fig. 40–4).

Groin Lymphocele

As is the case with lymphatic fistula, the most frequent location of lymphocele after vascular reconstructions is the

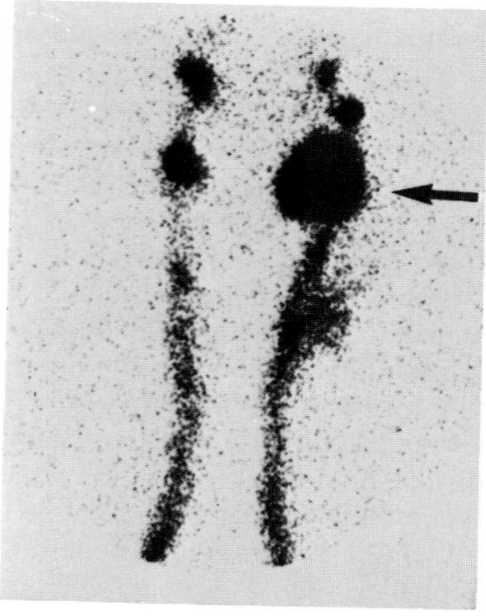

FIGURE 40–4. Bilateral lower extremity lymphoscintigraphy demonstrates a large left groin lymphocele (*arrow*) and extravasation of the colloid in the left thigh.

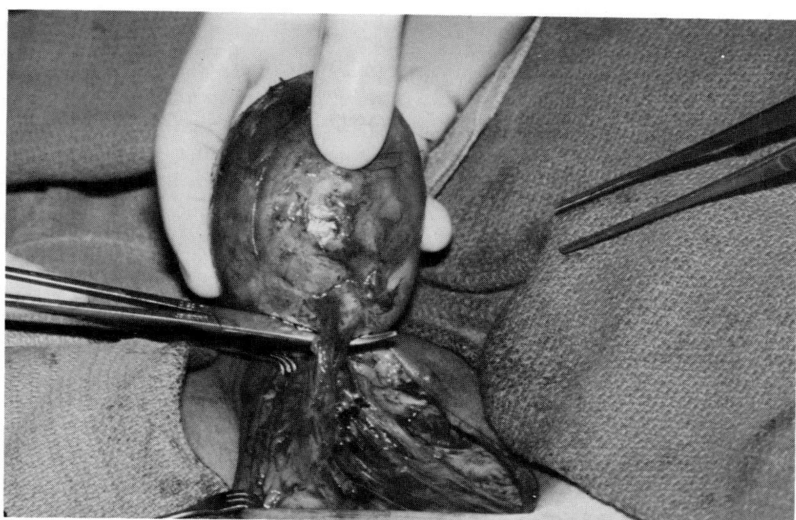

FIGURE 40–5. Intraoperative photograph of a dissected left groin lymphocele with an easily identifiable lymphatic pedicle. The pedicle was ligated and the lymphocele was removed.

groin. Most lymphoceles develop in the early postoperative period, but may appear later in follow-up. Large lymphoceles cause local discomfort, pain, and leg swelling. Hematoma, seroma, and wound infection should be considered in the differential diagnosis. The presence of a soft, fluid-filled cyst and intermittent drainage of clear lymph through a fistula confirm the diagnosis of lymphocele. Ultrasound is helpful in distinguishing a solid, dense hematoma from a cystic lymphocele. Computed tomography is performed if lymphocele develops several weeks to months after the operation. This test is helpful for excluding graft infection or for identifying retroperitoneal lymphocele with extension to the groin.

Small lymphoceles can be observed safely because they may reabsorb spontaneously. In patients who have enlarging or symptomatic lymphoceles or in those whose lymphoceles are in close proximity to a prosthetic graft, the authors advocate early surgery to reduce the risk of graft infection. Injection of isosulfan blue into the foot is helpful for identifying the lymphatic channels supplying the lymphocele. The lymphocele is excised, and the lymphatic pedicle is ligated or oversewn (Fig. 40–5). The wound is closed in multiple layers over a small subcutaneous drain.

Retroperitoneal Lymphocele

Symptomatic retroperitoneal lymphoceles are rare. In a review of more than 4000 aortic reconstructions, an incidence of 0.1 per cent was reported by Garrett and colleagues.[25] In reviewing the literature, the authors of this chapter found 11 well-documented cases of this complication following aortic reconstruction.[18, 19, 21–23, 25, 58] The number of unreported and asymptomatic cases is undoubtedly higher. Retroperitoneal lymphoceles have been reported more frequently after renal transplantation, with an incidence of 0.6 to 18 per cent.[26, 69–73] In these patients, however, lymphocele develops not only because of injury to the recipient pelvic lymphatics but also because of increased lymph production and lymph leakage from the donor kidney.[26]

Diagnosis

The most common symptoms of retroperitoneal lymphocele are abdominal distention, nausea, and abdominal pain, and the most frequent finding is an abdominal or a flank mass. Although signs or symptoms may develop early, in almost half of the patients the lymphocele is discovered 1 or several years after the operation.[58] In patients who present with signs or symptoms of a retroperitoneal lymphocele, computed tomography should be performed (Fig. 40–6). In 5 of 11 published cases of retroperitoneal lymphocele, a groin mass was also present.[58] Evaluation of these patients showed a communication of the groin lymphocele with a retroperitoneal lymphocele. This observation illustrates the importance of performing computed tomography if a groin mass develops after aortofemoral reconstruction. If infection is suspected, white blood cell scanning should also be performed, unless computed tomography has already confirmed graft infection. Lymphoscintigraphy will be diagnostic of a retroperitoneal lymphocele and should differentiate it from a perigraft seroma. However, lymphoscintigraphic findings positive for lymphocele do not exclude graft infection.

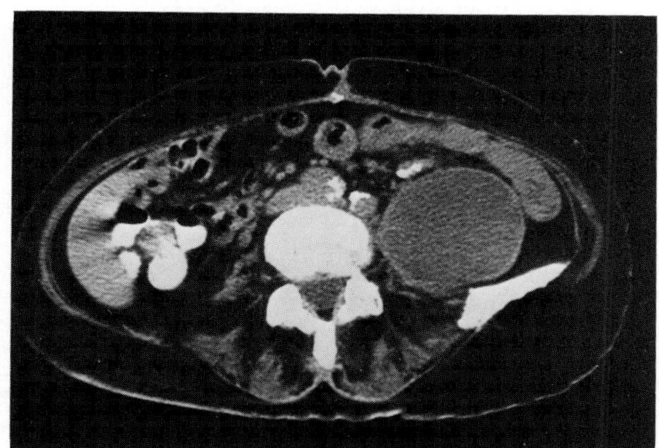

FIGURE 40–6. Computed tomographic scan of a 70-year-old woman reveals a large left retroperitoneal lymphocele 9 months after repair of a thoracoabdominal aortic aneurysm.

Management

In patients with a small asymptomatic retroperitoneal lymphocele, observation with serial ultrasound or computed tomography is warranted. If the lymphocele is increasing in size or causes local compression to adjacent structures, needle aspiration under computed tomographic or ultrasound guidance is performed. This maneuver is both diagnostic and therapeutic. In 4 of 11 patients, aspiration alone was used with success.[58] Placement of an indwelling irrigation-drainage system may be associated with a high risk of infection. Garrett and colleagues reported on two patients who developed prosthetic graft infection after placement of an irrigation-drainage system for retroperitoneal lymphocele.[25] Therefore, if repeated aspiration is unsuccessful, operative repair should be considered.

Abdominal exploration is performed after injection of 5 ml of isosulfan blue into the ipsilateral foot, using the technique detailed previously. The lymphocele is unroofed, and the site of the lymphatic injury is oversewn, ligated, or both. If the prosthetic graft is exposed, it is covered by retroperitoneal tissue or omentum. If preoperative aspiration confirms the presence of chyle in the cyst, 24 ounces of cream is given to the patient through a nasogastric tube 4 hours before exploration. Absorption of the cream helps to identify the site of lymphatic leakage in the mesenteric lymphatics around the left renal vein or at the cisterna chyli (Fig. 40–7). Whereas the mesenteric lymphatic trunks should be ligated or oversewn, lateral closure of the cisterna should be attempted first, using loupe magnification.

For post-transplant lymphocele, peritoneal fenestration has been advocated for treatment.[69, 70] With the advent of surgical laparoscopy, however, several reports have described aspiration and peritoneal fenestration under laparoscopic control.[72, 73] A tongue of omentum is brought down and placed through the peritoneal window to prevent premature closure and recurrence of the cyst. Laparoscopic transperitoneal drainage may become a useful addition to the vascular surgeon's armamentarium for the occasional treatment of lymphoceles following vascular reconstruction.

CHYLOUS ASCITES

The development of chylous ascites after abdominal aortic reconstructions is rare, but morbidity and mortality related to this complication can be significant. In reviewing the literature, the authors found 23 patients who were reported to have chylous ascites following aortic reconstruction.[22, 28–46, 73] Eighteen patients (78 per cent) underwent repair of an abdominal aortic aneurysm, and 5 (22 per cent) had surgery for occlusive disease. Ascites developed in the first 6 weeks after surgery in all but 1 patient.

Diagnosis

Symptoms of chylous ascites include progressive abdominal pain, dyspnea, and nausea. Abdominal distention can be significant, and the loss of proteins and fat may result in malnourishment. Lymphopenia and anemia can also develop, frequently resulting in poor immune function. Ascites can usually be detected by physical examination and confirmed by ultrasonography or computed tomography. Paracentesis is necessary to verify the presence of chyle in the ascitic fluid. Chyle is an odorless, sterile alkaline fluid that is milky in appearance. It has a specific gravity that is greater than 1012 gm/dl. Its protein content is usually above 3 gm/dl, and its fat content ranges from

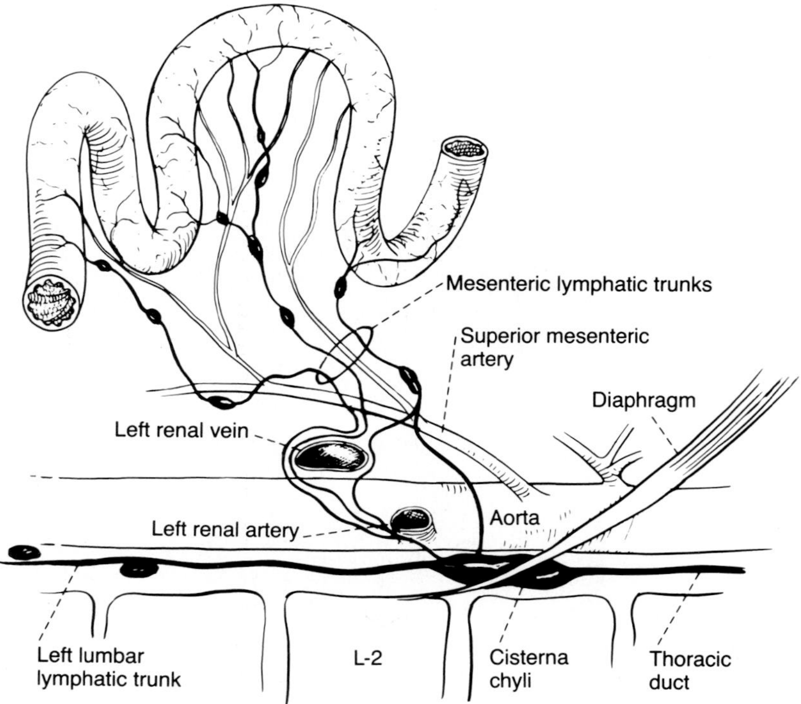

FIGURE 40–7. The anatomy of the mesenteric and ascending lumbar lymphatic trunks and the cisterna chyli. (From Gloviczki P, Bergman RT: Lymphatic problems and revascularization edema. *In* Bernhard VM, Towne JB [eds]: Complications in Vascular Surgery. 2nd ed. St. Louis, Quality Medical Publishing, 1991, p 366.)

0.4 to 4 gm/dl. The fat in the fluid stains positively with Sudan stain.

Management

Although the presence of chylous ascites in patients with abdominal malignancies carries an ominous prognosis, the outcome in patients who developed chylous ascites after aortic surgery has been somewhat better. Still, following aortic surgery, 4 of 23 patients with this complication died, a mortality rate of 17 per cent.[22, 31, 47, 73] The causes of death were sepsis in 2 patients and pulmonary embolus and malnutrition in 1 patient each.[22, 31, 42, 73]

Most patients with chylous ascites after aortic surgery can be successfully treated nonoperatively. The mainstay of treatment in patients with mild to moderate ascites is a medium-chain triglyceride diet to decrease chyle formation. In severe cases, however, complete bowel rest and total parenteral nutrition must be introduced. Repeated paracentesis results in resolution of the symptoms in most patients. Placement of a peritoneovenous shunt was reported in five patients, but sepsis caused death in one.[73] If repeated paracentesis is unsuccessful, exploration and closure of the site of the lymphatic injury should be carried out. Larger mesenteric or para-aortic lymphatic channels should be ligated or oversewn, but lateral closure of the injured cisterna chyli can be attempted with fine monofilament sutures, as mentioned earlier. Of the six patients who had exploration and surgical closure of the fistula, all recovered without recurrence.[28, 34, 39, 41, 44, 45]

Prevention

Injury to the retroperitoneal and mesenteric lymphatics during aortic dissection should be carefully avoided. The cisterna chyli is formed by the right and left lumbar and the mesenteric lymphatic trunks, and it is usually located at the level of the second lumbar vertebra, between the inferior vena cava and the abdominal aorta.[58] In half of patients, a well-developed cisterna chyli is absent. Several large mesenteric lymph vessels are located on the anteroinferior aspect of the left renal vein (see Fig. 40–7). Injury to these vessels will result in leakage of chyle. Failure to close the divided lymphatics may lead to the development of chylous ascites or retroperitoneal lymphocele. All large lumbar, para-aortic, and mesenteric lymph vessels should be ligated or clipped if division is necessary during aortic dissection. Lateral closure of the injured cisterna chyli with 7–0 monofilament sutures should be attempted.

CHYLOTHORAX

Effusion of chyle into the pleural cavity after vascular procedures is uncommon: it occurs in 0.2 to 1 per cent of cases following cardiothoracic surgery.[55] It is more frequent in neonates and small children operated on for congenital vascular anomalies, most frequently for aortic coarctation.[51–56] Chylothorax following repair of thoracic aortic aneurysm has been reported,[47–50] and in one patient it occurred after repair of an abdominal aortic aneurysm.[31] Chy-

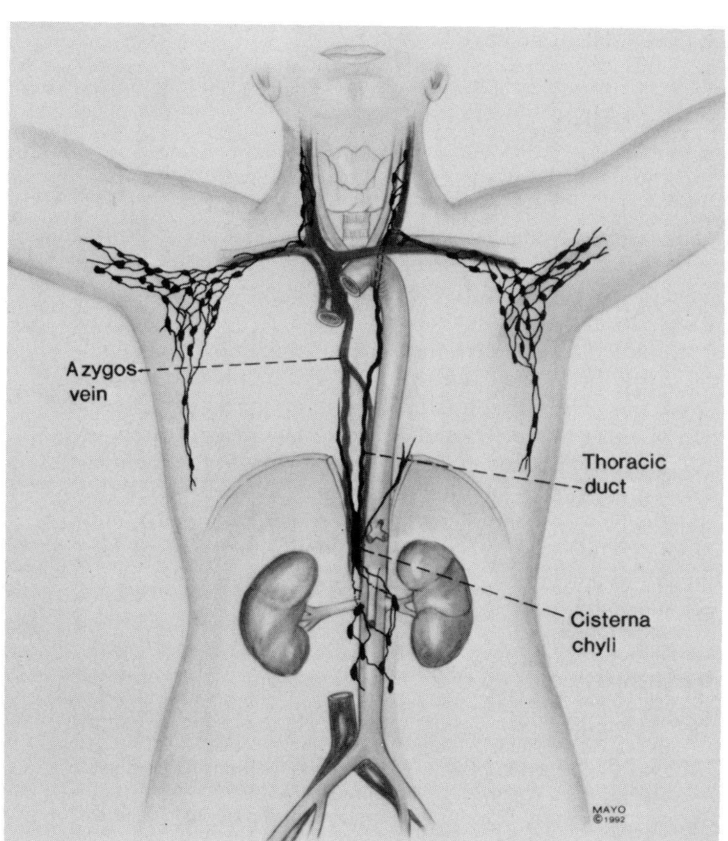

FIGURE 40–8. The anatomy of the thoracic duct. (By permission of Mayo Foundation.)

lothorax may develop as a complication of transthoracic dorsal sympathectomy[48, 74] or following high translumbar aortography.[57]

Diagnosis

Pleural effusion is confirmed on chest x-ray studies or computed tomographic scans. Analysis of the fluid obtained through thoracentesis or through the thoracostomy tube will confirm the diagnosis. Laboratory analysis of the milky or serous fluid is similar to that described for chylous ascites.

Management

Because respiratory embarrassment is frequent, drainage of the chylous fluid through a thoracostomy tube is usually necessary. The principles of treatment for decreasing chyle formation are the same as those discussed for chylous ascites. Conservative management, consisting of closed drainage through a thoracostomy tube and nutritional support, has been effective in the majority of cases. If a low-fat, high-protein diet with medium-chain triglyceride supplementation is not successful, intravenous hyperalimentation is started. Rarely, surgical closure of the site of the leak by oversewing or ligating the thoracic duct must be performed. Pleurodesis facilitates closure of the pleural space and decreases the potential for recurrence. Of the six patients who developed chylothorax after aortic aneurysm repair, only one needed thoracotomy to treat a large chylous pseudocyst.[47] However, one patient treated conservatively died after a long postoperative course complicated by both chylous ascites and chylothorax.[31]

Prevention

Injury to the thoracic duct during thoracic aortic dissection should be carefully avoided. The thoracic duct extends upward from the cisterna chyli and enters the posterior mediastinum through the aortic hiatus, slightly to the right of the aorta and to the left of the azygos vein (Fig. 40–8). In the posterior mediastinum, it is mostly a right-sided structure. It enters the superior mediastinum behind the aortic arch and subclavian artery, to the left of the esophagus. Therefore, it is exposed to injury during dissection of either the proximal thoracic aorta, the aortic arch, or the proximal subclavian artery. Once injury to the thoracic duct is recognized, an attempt at lateral closure should be made with 7–0 monofilament sutures, using loupe magnification. If this is not successful, ligation of the thoracic duct should be performed. Adequate collateral lymphatic circulation usually develops.

References

1. Vaughan BF, Slavotinek AH, Jepson RP: Edema of the lower limb after vascular operations. Surg Gynecol Obstet 133:282, 1970.
2. Porter JM, Lindell TD, Lakin PC: Leg edema following femoropopliteal autogenous vein bypass. Arch Surg 105:883, 1972.
3. Storen EJ, Myhre HO, Stiris G: Lymphangiographic findings in patients with leg oedema after arterial reconstructions. Acta Chir Scand 140:385, 1974.
4. Schmidt KR, Welter H, Pfeifer KJ, et al: Lymphographic investigations of oedema of the extremities following reconstructive vascular surgery in the femoropopliteal territory. ROEFO 128:194, 1978.
5. Stillman RM, Fitzgerald JF, Varughese G, et al: Edema following femoropopliteal bypass: Etiology and prevention. Vasc Surg 18:354, 1983.
6. Stranden E: Edema in the lower limb following arterial reconstruction for atherosclerosis: A study of pathogenetic mechanisms. J Oslo City Hosp 34:3, 1984.
7. Schubart PJ, Porter JM: Leg edema following femorodistal bypass. *In* Bergan JJ, Yao JST (eds): Reoperative Arterial Surgery. Orlando, FL, Grune & Stratton, 1986, p 311.
8. Eickhoff JH: Local regulation of subcutaneous blood flow and capillary filtration in limbs with occlusive arterial disease: Studies before and after arterial reconstruction. Dan Med Bull 33:111, 1986.
9. AbuRahma AF, Woodruff BA, Lucente FC: Edema after femoropopliteal bypass surgery: Lymphatic and venous theories of causation. J Vasc Surg 11:461, 1990.
10. Persson NH, Takolander R, Bergqvist D: Edema after lower limb arterial reconstruction: Influence of background factors, surgical technique and potentially prophylactic methods. Vasa 20:57, 1991.
11. Esato K, Ohara M, Seyama A, et al: ^{99m}Tc-HSA lymphoscintigraphy and leg edema following arterial reconstruction. J Cardiovasc Surg 32:741, 1991.
12. Stolzenberg J: Detection of lymphaticocutaneous fistula by radionuclide lymphangiography. Arch Surg 113:306, 1978.
13. Kwaan JHM, Berstein JM, Connolly JE: Management of lymph fistulae in the groin after arterial reconstruction. Arch Surg 114:1416, 1979.
14. Murphy JL, Cole WC, White PM, et al: Lymphatic fistula after vascular reconstruction: A case control study. Can J Surg 34(1):76, 1991.
15. Weaver FA, Yellin AE: Management of postoperative lymphatic leaks by use of isosulphan blue [Letter]. J Vasc Surg 14(4):566, 1991.
16. Kalman PG, Walker PM, Johnston KW: Consequences of groin lymphatic fistulae after vascular reconstruction. Vasc Surg 25:210, 1991.
17. Khauli RB, Mosenthal AC, Caushaj PF: Treatment of lymphocele and lymphatic fistula following renal transplantation by laparoscopic peritoneal window. J Urol 147(5):1353, 1992.
18. Dillon ML, Postlethwait RW: The management of an abdominal mass recurring after resection of abdominal aortic aneurysm. Surg Clin North Am 50:1021, 1970.
19. Fitzer PM, Sallade RL, Graham WH: Computed tomography and the diagnosis of giant abdominal lymphocele. Va Med Q 107:448, 1980.
20. Patel BR, Burkhalter JL, Patel TB, et al: Interstitial lymphoscintigraphy for diagnosis of lymphocele. Clin Nucl Med 10:175, 1985.
21. Puyau FA, Adinolfi MF, Kerstein MD: Lymphocele around aortic femoral grafts simulating a false aneurysm. Cardiovasc Intervent Radiol 8:195, 1985.
22. Jensen SR, Voegeli DR, McDermott JC, et al: Lymphatic disruption following abdominal aortic surgery. Cardiovasc Intervent Radiol 9:199, 1986.
23. Pardy BJ, Harris P, Mourad K, et al: Case reports: Upper abdominal lymphocele following urgent aortorenal bypass grafting. J R Soc Med 79:674, 1986.
24. Scott AR: A report on the management of a lymphocyst after vascular surgery. Aust N Z J Surg 57:205, 1987.
25. Garrett HE Jr, Richardson JW, Howard HS, et al: Retroperitoneal lymphocele after abdominal aortic surgery. J Vasc Surg 10:245, 1989.
26. Malovrh M, Kandus A, Buturovic-Ponikvar J, et al: Frequency and clinical influence of lymphoceles after kidney transplantation. Transplant Proc 22:1423, 1990.
27. Velanovich V, Mallory P, Collins PS: Lower extremity lymphocele development after saphenous vein harvesting. Mil Med 156:149, 1991.
28. Bradham RR, Gregorie HB, Wilson R: Chylous ascites following resection of an abdominal aortic aneurysm. Am Surg 36:238, 1970.
29. Klippel AP, Hardy DA: Postoperative chylous ascites. Mo Med 68:253, 1971.
30. DeBartolo TF, Etzkorn JR: Conservative management of chylous ascites after abdominal aortic aneurysm repair: Case report. Mo Med 73:611, 1976.
31. Lopez-Enriquez E, Gonzalez A, Johnson CD, et al: Chylothorax and chyloperitoneum: A case report. Bol Asoc Med P R 71:54, 1979.

32. Meinke AH III, Estes NC, Ernst CB: Chylous ascites following abdominal aortic aneurysmectomy: Management with total parenteral hyperalimentation. Ann Surg 190:631, 1979.
33. Stubbe LTHFL, Terpstra JL: Chylous ascites after resection of an abdominal aortic aneurysm. Arch Chir Neerlandicum 31:111, 1979.
34. McKenna R, Stevick CA: Chylous ascites following aortic reconstruction. Vasc Surg 17:143, 1983.
35. Savrin RA, High JR: Chylous ascites after abdominal aortic surgery. Surgery 98:866, 1985.
36. Sarazin WG, Sauter KE: Chylous ascites following resection of a ruptured abdominal aneurysm. Arch Surg 121:246, 1986.
37. Fleisher HL III, Oren JW, Sumner DS: Chylous ascites after abdominal aortic aneurysmectomy: Successful management with a peritoneovenous shunt. J Vasc Surg 6:403, 1987.
38. Schwein M, Dawes PD, Hatchuel D, et al: Postoperative chylous ascites after resection of an abdominal aortic aneurysm: A case report. S Afr J Surg 25:39, 1987.
39. Williamson C, Provan JL: Chylous ascites following aortic surgery. Br J Surg 74:71, 1987.
40. Boyd WD, McPhail NV, Barber GC: Case report: Chylous ascites following abdominal aortic aneurysmectomy: Surgical management with a peritoneovenous shunt. J Cardiovasc Surg 30:627, 1989.
41. Heyl A, Veen HF: Iatrogenic chylous ascites: Operative or conservative approach. Neth J Surg 41:5, 1989.
42. Ablan CJ, Littooy FN, Freeark RJ: Postoperative chylous ascites: Diagnosis and treatment. Arch Surg 125:270, 1990.
43. Bahner DR Jr, Townsend R: Chylous ascites after ruptured abdominal aortic aneurysm. Contemp Surg 36:37, 1990.
44. Sultan S, Pauwels A, Poupon R, et al: Ascites chyleuses de l'adulte aspects étiologigues, thérapeutiques et évolutifs: A propos de 35 cas. Ann Gastroenterol Hepatol (Paris) 26:187, 1990.
45. Williams RA, Vetto J, Quinones-Baldrich W, et al: Chylous ascites following abdominal aortic surgery. Ann Vasc Surg 5:247, 1991.
46. Sanger R, Wilmshurst CC, Clyne CA: Chylous ascites following aneurysm surgery: Case report. Eur J Vasc Surg 5:689, 1991.
47. Mack JW, Heydorn WH, Pauling FW, et al: Postoperative chylous pseudocyst. J Thorac Cardiovasc Surg 77:773, 1979.
48. Kostiainen S, Meurala H, Mattila S, et al: Chylothorax: Clinical experience in nine cases. Scand J Thorac Cardiovasc Surg 17:79, 1983.
49. Okabayashi H, Tamura N, Hirose N, et al: Aortic aneurysm associated with coarctation of the aorta [in Japanese]. Kyobu Geka 42(12):1032, 1989.
50. Sachs PB, Zelch MG, Rice TG, et al: Diagnosis and localization of laceration of the thoracic duct: Usefulness of lymphangiography and CT. AJR 157:703, 1991.
51. Hallman GL, Bloodwell RD, Cooley DA: Coarctation of the thoracic aorta. Surg Clin North Am 46(4):893, 1966.
52. Bortolotti U, Faggian G, Livi U, et al: Postoperative chylothorax following repair of coarctation of the aorta. Report of a case with unusual clinical manifestation. Thorac Cardiovasc Surg 30:319, 1982.
53. Fairfax AJ, McNabb WR, Spiro SG: Chylothorax: A review of 18 cases. Thorax 41:880, 1986.
54. Baudet E, Al-Qudah A: Late results of the subclavian flap repair of coarctation in infancy. J Cardiovasc Surg 30:445, 1989.
55. Cooper P, Paes ML: Bilateral chylothorax. Br J Anaesth 66:387, 1991.
56. Chun K, Colombani PM, Dudgeon DL: Diagnosis and management of congenital vascular rings: A 22 year experience. Ann Thorac Surg 53:597; discussion 602, 1992.
57. Negroni CC, Ortiz VN: Chylothorax following high translumbar aortography: A case report and review of the literature. Bol Asoc Med P R 80:201, 1988.
58. Gloviczki P, Bergman RT: Lymphatic problems and revascularization edema. *In* Bernhard VM, Towne JB (eds): Complications in Vascular Surgery. 2nd ed. St. Louis, Quality Medical Publishing, 1991, p 366.
59. Simeone FA, Husni EA: The hyperemia of reconstructive arterial surgery. Ann Surg 150:575, 1959.
60. Campbell H, Harris PL: Albumin kinetics and oedema following reconstructive arterial surgery of the lower limb. J Cardiovasc Surg 26:110, 1985.
61. Taylor GW: Arterial grafting for gangrene. Ann R Coll Surg Engl 31:168, 1962.
62. Hamer JD: Investigation of oedema of the lower limb following successful femoropopliteal by-pass surgery: The role of phlebography in demonstrating venous thrombosis. Br J Surg 59:979, 1972.
63. Myhre HO, Dedichen H: Haemodynamic factors in the oedema of arterial reconstructions. Scand J Thorac Cardiovasc Surg 6:323, 1972.
64. Myhre HO, Storen EJ, Ongre A: The incidence of deep venous thrombosis in patients with leg oedema after arterial reconstruction. Scand J Thorac Cardiovasc Surg 8:73, 1974.
65. Husni EA: The edema of arterial reconstruction. Circulation 35(Suppl):I169, 1967.
66. Cass AJ, Jennings SA, Greenhalgh RM: Leg swelling after aortic surgery. Int Angiol 5(3):207, 1986.
67. Skudder PA, Geary J: Lymphatic drainage from the groin following surgery of the femoral artery. J Cardiovasc Surg (Torino) 28:460, 1987.
68. Johnston KW: Multicenter prospective study of nonruptured abdominal aortic aneurysm. II. Variables predicting morbidity and mortality. J Vasc Surg 9:437, 1989.
69. Howard RJ, Simmons RL, Najarian JS: Prevention of lymphoceles following renal transplantation. Ann Surg 18:166, 1976.
70. Greenberg BM, Perloff LJ, Grossman RA, et al: Treatment of lymphocoele in renal allograft recipients. Arch Surg 120:501, 1985.
71. Längle F, Schurawitzki H, Mühlbacher R: Treatment of lymphoceles following renal transplantation. Transplant Proc 22(4):1420, 1990.
72. Clayman RV, So SSK, Jendrisak MD, et al: Laparoscopic drainage of a posttransplant lymphocele. Transplantation 51:725, 1991.
73. Ancona E, Rigotti P, Zaninotto G, et al: Treatment of lymphocele following renal transplantation by laparoscopic surgery. Int Surg 76:261, 1991.
74. Servelle M, Nogues CL, Soulie J, et al: Spontaneous, postoperative and traumatic chylothorax. J Cardiovasc Surg (Torino) 21:475, 1980.

41

Postoperative Sexual Dysfunction Following Aortoiliac Revascularization

D. Preston Flanigan, M.D.

• • •

The relationship between altered male sexual function and arterial occlusive disease in the aortoiliac system is now established. Also well known is the complication of postoperative sexual dysfunction in male patients undergoing aortoiliac reconstructive surgery. In 1923, Leriche first pointed out the association between aortic occlusion and impotence.[1] The classic Leriche syndrome consists of weariness of the thighs, impotence, and terminal aortic occlusion.[2] Historically, surgery on the aortoiliac vessels carries a high risk of iatrogenic sexual dysfunction, but it also has the possible benefit of reversing preoperative impotence. Numerous investigators have demonstrated that approximately 25 per cent of patients with preoperative sexual dysfunction will regain normal sexual function after aortoiliac revascularization.[3–11] Although sexual improvement following aortoiliac revascularization was presumed to be secondary to an improvement in pelvic circulation, not until the application of Doppler technology to the measurement of penile blood pressure could the actual relationship between sexual function and penile circulation be established. Using Doppler-derived penile blood pressure measurements preoperatively and postoperatively, Queral and coworkers conclusively demonstrated the relationship between improved or worsened sexual function after aortoiliac revascularization and improved or worsened penile perfusion.[12]

The significant interconnections between the sympathetic and the parasympathetic nerves at the levels of the para-aortic and superior hypogastric plexuses have been demonstrated.[13] Both erection and ejaculation may be impaired after injury to these nerve plexuses. Sparing these nerve plexuses during aortoiliac surgery has been shown to decrease the incidence of postoperative sexual dysfunction.[3, 4, 7] Thus, it is important for vascular surgeons to maintain or improve pelvic circulation *and* to avoid injury to autonomic nerve plexuses during aortoiliac revascularization if the incidence of postoperative sexual dysfunction is to be lessened.

Women do not seem to be susceptible to iatrogenic sexual dysfunction following aortoiliac surgery, probably because of the lush pelvic collateral circulation to the female sex organs and because of the fact that female sexual sensation depends locally on intact pudendal somatic nerve fibers.[14] The pudendal nerve is covered by a thick layer of endopelvic fascia and is unlikely to incur surgical injury.

Although the previously mentioned considerations are important, they are not the only factors that may affect sexual function in vascular patients. These patients may have other preoperative and postoperative risk factors for sexual dysfunction, including neurogenic, psychogenic, and pharmacologic causes (Table 41–1). It is important for vascular surgeons to be well versed in the anatomy and physiology of male sexual function, the various etiologies of sexual dysfunction, the diagnostic methods used in the evaluation of sexual dysfunction, the methods of preventing iatrogenic sexual dysfunction during revascularization, and the treatment of postoperative sexual dysfunction.

ANATOMY

The blood supply to the penis is through the aortoiliac segment. Flow to the penis is via the dorsal artery of the penis, the deep penile artery, and the urethral artery. These arteries are the terminal arteries of the internal pudendal artery, which is a branch of the anterior division of the internal iliac artery (the hypogastric artery). Arterial obstruction anywhere in this arterial axis has been shown to be associated with sexual dysfunction.

At the penile level, there are two paired corpora cavernosa and a single corpus spongiosum. Each corpus cavernosum is surrounded by a thick fibrous sheath that encases multiple interconnected lacunar spaces lined by vascular endothelium. The arterial circulation to the corpora cavernosa is from paired cavernosal arteries. Numerous muscular corkscrew-shaped and helicine arteries lead from the cavernosal arteries directly to the lacunar spaces. Venous drainage from the corpora is through subtunical venules, which coalesce to form larger emissary veins that pierce the tunica albuginea. Drainage proceeds through the deep dorsal vein and the cavernosal and crural veins.

Table 41–1. Etiology of Impotence

Psychogenic
Neurogenic
Vasculogenic
Pharmacologic
Iatrogenic
Developmental
Endocrinologic
Traumatic

Innervation of the vessels of the penis is by sympathetic nerves arising from the 11th thoracic through the 2nd lumbar segments, whereas parasympathetic innervation and somatic innervation arise from the 2nd through the 4th lumbar segments. Somatic innervation is via the pudendal nerves. Erectile function is thought to be controlled primarily by parasympathetic innervation, whereas ejaculation is primarily a sympathetically mediated function;[15] however, numerous interconnections between the two systems have been demonstrated in the para-aortic plexus and the superior hypogastric plexus.[13] These plexuses are particularly susceptible to injury during infrarenal aortic dissection (Fig. 41–1).

PHYSIOLOGY

Erection occurs as a result of local genital stimulation or through central psychogenic stimuli. Genital stimulation is mediated by a spinal reflex pathway. Several areas of the brain have been implicated in psychogenic erection, including the thalamic nuclei, the rhinencephalon, and the limbic structures. Hypothalamic projections to the spinal cord have been identified; they probably control thoracolumbar sympathetic and sacral parasympathetic outflow to the penis.

Erection is the result of penile arterial smooth muscle relaxation. Cavernosal and helicine artery dilatation leads to filling of the lacunar spaces, which become dilated, thus causing penile engorgement. Increased pressure within the tunica albuginea compresses subtunical venules, resulting in restriction of venous outflow from the lacunar spaces, which maintains tumescence.

Loss of erection is the result of penile arterial smooth muscle vasoconstriction, which reduces arterial inflow and causes collapse of the lacunar spaces and decreased venous outflow resistance.[16]

Control of penile arterial smooth muscle is through adrenergic nerves, cholinergic nerves, and nerves immunoreactive to vasoactive intestinal peptide. Adrenergic nerves cause smooth muscle constriction through norepinephrine release, whereas smooth muscle relaxation is via cholinergic neurotransmitters. The latter work through effects on other neuroeffector systems. Vascular endothelium can also influence underlying smooth muscle tone, possibly through the release of endothelium-derived relaxing factor, endothelium-derived hyperpolarizing factor, prostaglandins, and the peptide endothelin.[16]

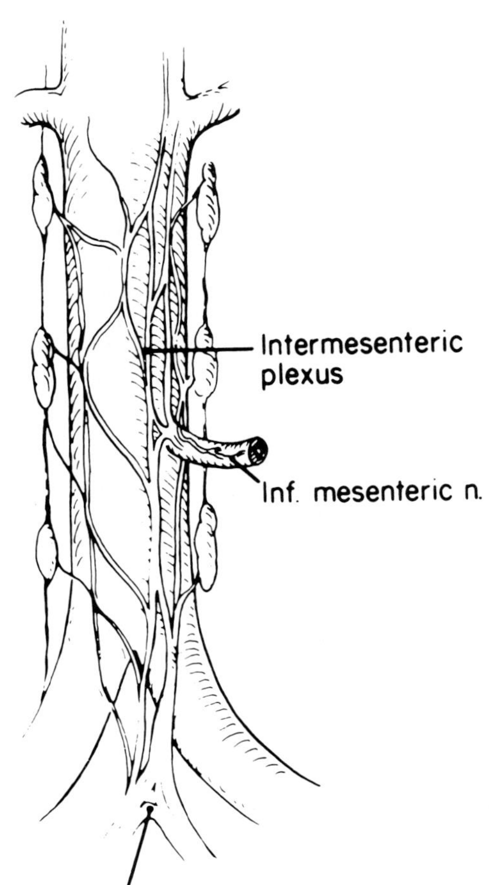

FIGURE 41–1. Anatomy of the autonomic nerve plexuses at the level of the infrarenal aorta and the proximal iliac arteries. The nerves are predominantly on the left side of the aorta and cross the proximal left common iliac artery as they course distally. (From Weinstein MH, Machleder HI: Sexual function after aortoiliac surgery. Ann Surg 181:787, 1975.)

INCIDENCE AND ETIOLOGY

The incidence of male sexual dysfunction has not been accurately assessed. Pertinent to vascular surgery, however, is the incidence of preoperative sexual dysfunction in patients being considered for aortoiliac revascularization. Flanigan and coworkers showed this incidence to be 27 per cent in 110 patients, an incidence similar to that reported in other surgical series.[4] The etiology of impotence in vascular patients is not always circulatory. Multiple etiologic factors such as diabetes mellitus, drug therapy, psychogenic factors, and previous surgery are often present. Impotence in diabetic patients has been reported to be as high as 50 per cent.[17]

There are numerous causes of impotence that must be considered (see Table 41–1). Psychogenic impotence is thought to be the most common form. Although this is usually not a major postoperative consideration, there may be a perception of change in body image and decreased masculinity that follows major abdominal surgery. Neurogenic sexual dysfunction can be secondary to nerve injury or diabetic neuropathy. Vasculogenic impotence is usually the result of decreased pelvic blood supply due to either arterial occlusive disease or surgery. Malfunction of the venous occlusive mechanism can also cause vasculogenic impotence.[18] Pharmacologic sexual dysfunction most commonly results from antihypertensive medications, but numerous other agents have been implicated (Table 41–2). For an exhaustive list of drugs associated with male sexual dysfunction, the reader is referred to *The Medical Letter*, vol. 29 (issue 744), July 17, 1987. Iatrogenic impotence is usually the result of urologic or vascular surgery. Developmental causes, including hypospadias, are rare. Except for diabetes mellitus, endocrinologic causes are also unusual; they include such states as eunuchoidism, hypopituitarism,

Table 41–2. Drugs Associated With Impotence

Antihypertensive agents
Thiazide diuretics
Guanadrel
Clonidine
Methyldopa
Propranolol
Angiotensin-converting enzyme inhibitors
Calcium channel blockers
Hydralazine
H_2 receptor antagonists
Cimetidine
Ranitidine
Antipsychotics
Tricyclic antidepressants
Central nervous system depressants
Anticancer drugs

hypothyroidism, Cushing's syndrome, and prolactin disorders. It has been postulated that sexual dysfunction secondary to circulatory impairment might, at least in part, be due to decreased production of testosterone secondary to testicular hypoperfusion.[19] Traumatic sexual dysfunction usually follows spinal or pelvic trauma and is mostly neurogenic in nature.

Detailed discussion of the etiology, diagnosis, and management of sexual dysfunction, and specifically vasculogenic impotence, is beyond the scope of this chapter; however, a knowledge of causes other than iatrogenic ones is important for the vascular surgeon in both the preoperative and the postoperative evaluation of men with sexual dysfunction. For a more comprehensive coverage of vasculogenic impotence, the reader is referred to Chapter 63. Documentation of the presence and cause of sexual dysfunction before elective aortoiliac revascularization is obviously important for medicolegal reasons and for informing the patient about the possibilities for postoperative improvement.

DIAGNOSIS OF SEXUAL DYSFUNCTION

The etiology of impotence can often be determined by history taking and physical examination alone. Recent psychological trauma or marital problems may be associated with the onset of impotence. A careful medication history may detect the use of agents associated with sexual dysfunction. Developmental and traumatic problems should be easily discovered. Known endocrine pathology may be associated with impotence. A history of the onset of impotence following surgery should be sought.

Of primary importance in the diagnosis of sexual dysfunction is differentiating psychogenic from organic etiologies. Organic impotence is nonsituational. Psychogenic impotence may be intermittent, partner specific, and absent during masturbation. Psychological impotence can probably best be differentiated from organic impotence through the use of nocturnal penile tumescence studies. It has been well documented that all males from 3 to 79 years of age have nocturnal penile tumescence during normal sleep, with the amount being a function of age.[20] Monitoring during sleep for nocturnal penile tumescence has been shown to be approximately 80 per cent accurate in differentiating psychogenic from organic impotence.[19]

If organic impotence is suspected based on the history, the physical examination findings, and the results of nocturnal penile tumescence studies, penile blood pressure measurement and penile duplex ultrasonography with penile papaverine injection are reliable diagnostic tests for detecting the presence of vasculogenic impotence. If this testing indicates that arterial inflow obstruction is probably present, arteriography with selective pelvic catheterization is indicated as a guide to the type of therapy that should be considered.

If the results of vascular studies are normal and if developmental, traumatic, surgical, and pharmacologic etiologies have been ruled out, neurogenic or endocrinologic causes are most likely. Neurogenic impotence may be associated with an absent bulbocavernosus reflex, abnormal findings on perineal electromyographic studies, and abnormal cystometrographic findings. These abnormal study results are often seen in diabetics with sexual dysfunction. The diagnosis of endocrine dysfunction is usually made through the measurement of hormone levels.

PREVENTION

Analysis of the major surgical series addressing the problem of sexual function changes associated with aortoiliac revascularization indicates that approximately one fourth of patients are impotent preoperatively.[3–11] Postoperatively, roughly one fourth of these patients will regain normal sexual function, and one fourth of patients with normal preoperative sexual function will develop impotence following surgery.[21] Both erectile dysfunction and ejaculatory dysfunction can follow aortoiliac revascularization, and collected surgical series published before 1975 demonstrated an average 43 per cent incidence of postoperative retrograde ejaculation.[21] The authors of these series postulated that postoperative sexual dysfunction was secondary to reduction of pelvic blood supply, and they demonstrated that injury to the para-aortic and hypogastric nerve plexuses could cause both impotence and retrograde ejaculation. The association between postoperative impotence and postoperative decreases in penile perfusion pressure has now been well documented.[12] Thus, prevention of iatrogenically induced sexual dysfunction following aortoiliac revascularization requires preservation of pelvic circulation and avoidance of injury to the para-aortic and hypogastric autonomic nerve plexuses.

Preservation of pelvic blood flow requires careful evaluation of arteriographic findings and consideration of the type of proximal aortic anastomosis. End-to-side anastomoses do not divert pelvic blood flow but may not be desirable for other reasons. End-to-side aortic anastomoses may carry a greater risk of atheroembolization, may preclude routine retroperitoneal coverage of the graft, and may create a competitive flow situation with the native iliac arteries. It has been suggested that end-to-side anastomoses may have a lower patency rate than end-to-end anastomoses.[22] When end-to-end anastomoses are used, pelvic flow may be diverted if there is not adequate retrograde flow up

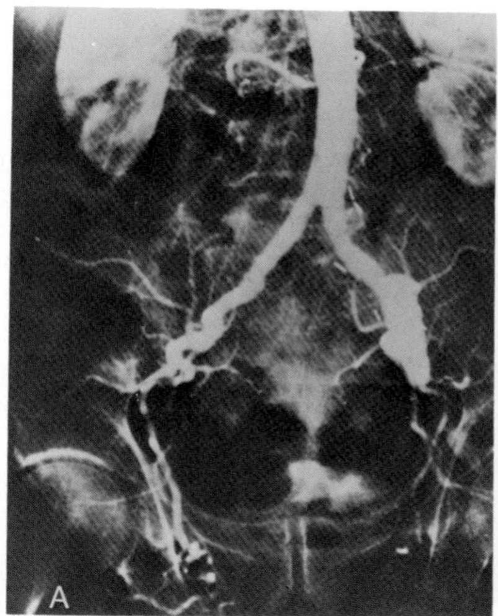
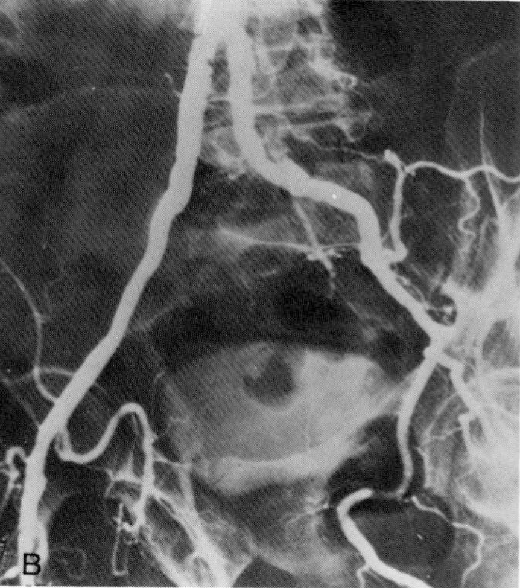
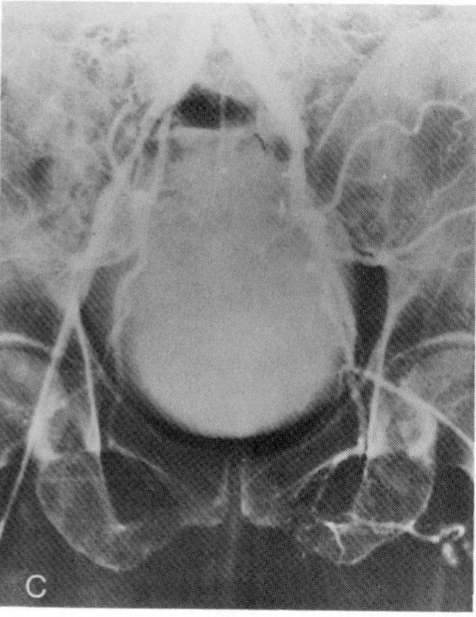

FIGURE 41–2. Examples of disease distribution in which end-to-end aortic anastomoses should be avoided if possible. *A*, Bilateral external iliac artery occlusion. *B*, Unilateral external iliac artery occlusion and contralateral internal iliac artery occlusion. *C*, Unilateral external iliac artery occlusion and contralateral external iliac artery stenosis. (*A–C*, From Flanigan DP, Schuler JJ, Keifer T, et al: Elimination of iatrogenic impotence and improvement of sexual dysfunction after aortoiliac revascularization. Arch Surg 117:544, 1982. Copyright 1982, American Medical Association.)

the external iliac arteries postoperatively. Examples of disease distributions that probably should not be treated with end-to-end anastomoses are shown in Figure 41–2. The requirement for retrograde external iliac artery flow is probably important even if there is occlusion of the hypogastric arteries.

Bilateral hypogastric occlusion or ligation is thought to be associated with a high risk of pelvic ischemia. Although it is commonly believed that hypogastric flow is necessary for normal sexual function, several studies have indicated that this may not always be the case. Kawai showed that branches of the femoral artery may provide significant collateral circulation to the penis in the face of hypogastric artery occlusion.[23] Iliopoulos and associates showed that in the presence of acute hypogastric artery ligation, hypogastric collateral flow is more dependent on the ipsilateral external iliac artery than it is on the contralateral hypogastric artery, although in the chronic state, lush collateralization between the left and the right internal iliac arteries is common (Fig. 41–3).[24] Ohshiro and Kosaki suggested that preservation of the hypogastric nerve plexus is more important than preservation of hypogastric blood flow and showed that little correlation exists between postoperative sexual dysfunction and hypogastric circulation.[25] Of 26 patients with bilateral hypogastric atherosclerotic occlusion or bilateral hypogastric artery ligation at the time of surgery who were studied by Flanigan and coworkers, 17 had normal sexual function postoperatively.[4]

Although hypogastric artery patency may not be necessary for normal sexual function in all patients, in many patients it is necessary[12] not only for sexual function but also for preventing colon or buttock ischemia.[26]

The important role of the hypogastric circulation in sexual function is further supported by evidence of im-

FIGURE 41–3. Selective right internal iliac artery arteriogram demonstrating lush pelvic collaterals filling the contralateral left internal iliac artery circulatory bed. (From Flanigan DP, Schuler JJ: Sexual function and aortic surgery. *In* Bergan JJ, Yao JST [eds]: Aortic Surgery. Philadelphia, WB Saunders, 1989, pp 547–560.)

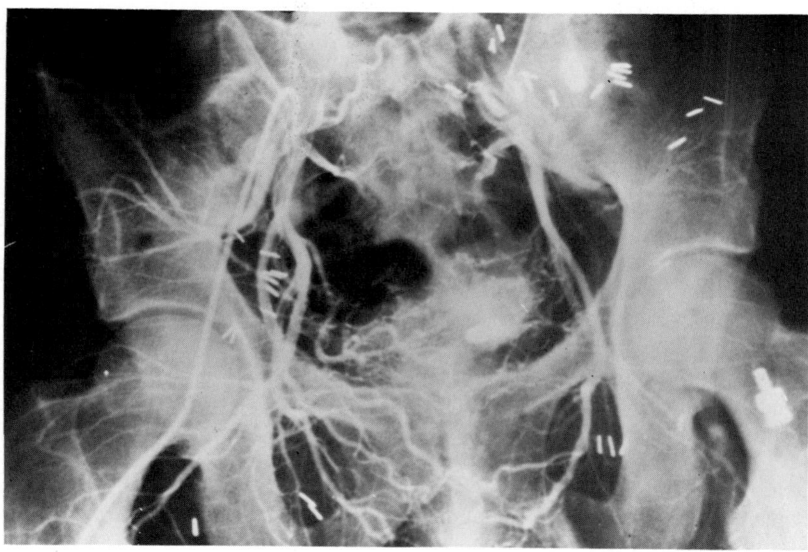

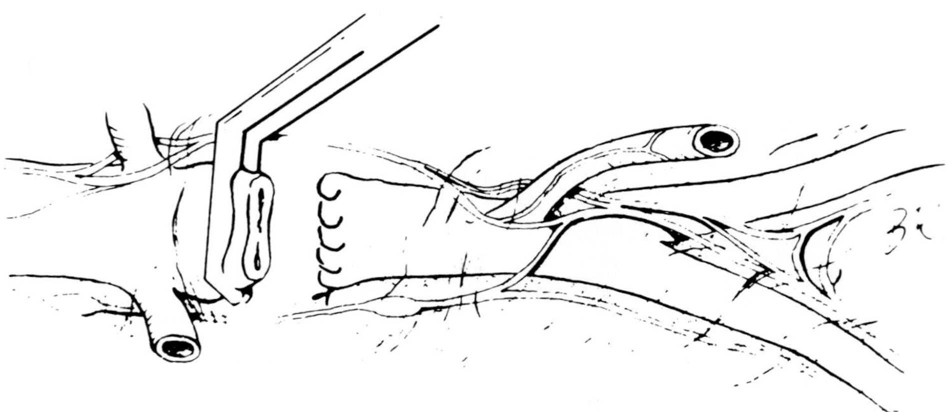

FIGURE 41–4. Suggested approach to aortic dissection and clamping: a right lateral approach to the aorta just below the renal arteries lessens possible injury to the para-aortic and superior hypogastric plexuses. (From DePalma RG, Levine SB, Feldman S: Preservation of erectile function after aorto-iliac reconstruction. Arch Surg 113:958, 1978. Copyright 1978, American Medical Association.)

provement in sexual function after internal iliac revascularization. Flanigan and associates demonstrated that revascularization of the internal iliac artery at the time of aortoiliac revascularization reversed vasculogenic impotence in five of five men.[27] Subsequently, Gossetti and colleagues studied 148 patients with vasculogenic impotence who were undergoing aortoiliac revascularization and found that 14 of 18 patients (77 per cent) who had concomitant hypogastric revascularization had normal postoperative sexual function.[28]

Caution would dictate that at least unilateral hypogastric flow be maintained whenever possible during aortoiliac revascularization. Nevertheless, bilateral hypogastric artery ligation or exclusion may be unavoidable in some patients. No clear criteria have emerged that indicate the need for direct hypogastric revascularization in such patients. Iwai and coworkers used transanal Doppler monitoring as a guide, but more experience will be needed to establish clear guidelines for revascularization.[29] When there is uncertainty regarding the adequacy of pelvic circulation, hypogastric revascularization should probably be performed. This may take the form of internal iliac endarterectomy, side-to-side anastomosis between a bifurcation graft limb and an iliac vessel, or a graft between a bifurcation graft limb and a hypogastric artery.[4, 28, 30]

The incidence of iatrogenic neurogenic sexual dysfunction is lessened through nerve-sparing dissections of the aortoiliac segment. This is best achieved through a right lateral aortic approach just below the renal arteries (Fig. 41–4). Tissues over the anterior aorta are reflected rather than transected. Tunnels are created posterior to the ureters and superior hypogastric plexus. When iliac anastomoses are required, dissection over the iliac arteries is carried out in the longitudinal plane, with meticulous care taken not to transect the autonomic nerves. The wall of aortic aneurysms should not be resected, and inferior mesenteric artery control should be achieved from within the aneurysm cavity. When iliac aneurysms are present, graft limbs can often be tunneled through the iliac aneurysm to avoid dissection and incision of the iliac aneurysm and damage to the overlying autonomic plexus (Fig. 41–5).

Another approach for avoiding iatrogenic impotence is the use of revascularization procedures that do not require dissection of the aortoiliac segment. Axillofemoral bypass, femorofemoral bypass, and aortoiliac transluminal balloon angioplasty all achieve this purpose. In addition, like aortoiliofemoral bypass, these procedures have been shown to reverse vasculogenic impotence in selected patients.[4, 31–36] It is important to inform prospective patients for aortoiliac revascularization of the risk of iatrogenic sexual dysfunc-

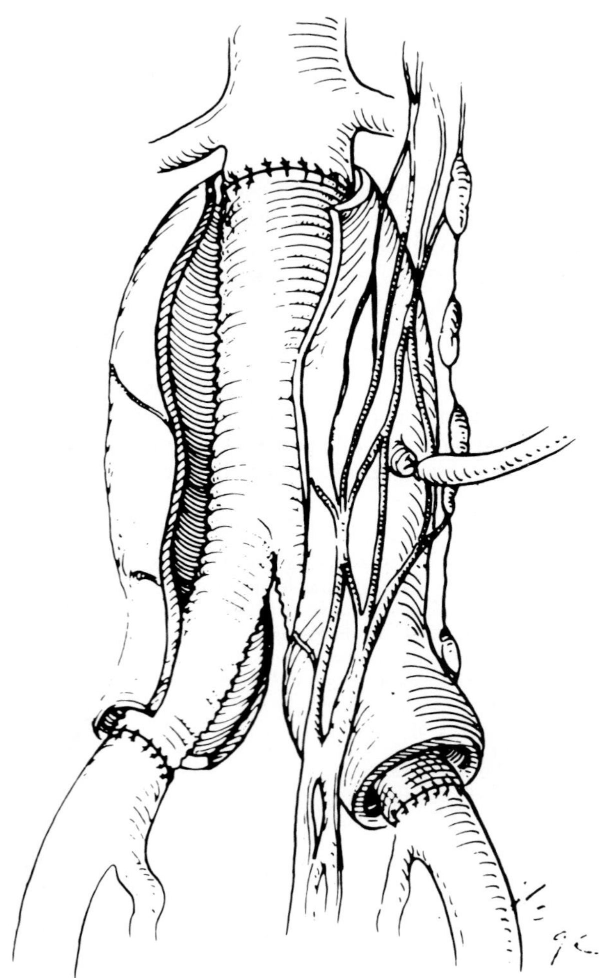

FIGURE 41–5. Bifurcation graft limbs may often be tunneled through iliac aneurysms, thus avoiding transection of the overlying hypogastric nerve plexus. (From Weinstein MH, Machleder HI: Sexual function after aortoiliac surgery. Ann Surg 181:787, 1975.)

tion and of the availability of alternative indirect methods of revascularization that essentially eliminate this risk but may provide less satisfactory revascularization.

Flanigan and coworkers demonstrated that when careful operative planning is undertaken to avoid diversion of pelvic blood flow, nerve-sparing aortoiliac dissections are carried out, and indirect methods of aortoiliac revascularization are employed, iatrogenic impotence can be eliminated and many patients can regain normal sexual function postoperatively.[4] In a series of 110 patients undergoing direct and indirect aortoiliac revascularization, 45 per cent of patients with preoperative vasculogenic impotence regained normal sexual function postoperatively, no patients with normal preoperative sexual function were rendered impotent, and only 2 patients developed retrograde ejaculation.[4] Despite the use of these techniques, however, patients requiring iliac dissections and those with ruptured aneurysms remain susceptible to iatrogenic sexual dysfunction, especially retrograde ejaculation secondary to nerve injury.

TREATMENT

The treatment of postoperative sexual dysfunction depends on an accurate assessment of the etiology. This fact emphasizes the need for a careful preoperative assessment of the cause of sexual dysfunction in patients being considered for aortoiliac revascularization. Before treatment of postoperative impotence, a complete diagnostic work-up may be required as described earlier, especially if no preoperative work-up was performed. If sexual dysfunction is determined to be iatrogenic in origin, then it is due to either reduced pelvic blood flow and penile ischemia or nerve injury.

Penile ischemia can be corrected by penile revascularization when possible. This may take the form of angioplasty, endarterectomy, or bypass to the hypogastric vessels. Direct penile revascularization has also been attempted, with mixed results. Currently, direct revascularization of the penis is accomplished by inferior epigastric artery anastomosis to the dorsal penile[37] or cavernosal[38] arteries. Alternatively, a vein graft can be used.[39] Good results have been reported in 31 to 80 percent of patients.[37, 40] Older men with diffuse atherosclerosis have poorer results, and vein grafts may, in some cases, provide excess flow resulting in priapism.[3]

Treatment of neurogenic impotence requires the placement of a penile prosthesis. This may also be useful in patients with vasculogenic impotence in whom revascularization is not possible or is unsuccessful. Several models of penile prostheses are now available, and about 25,000 prostheses are implanted yearly in the United States.[16] Approximately 90 per cent of patients report satisfactory results.[41, 42] Infection rates vary from 1 to 9 per cent, and reoperation because of mechanical failure is necessary in 14 to 44 per cent of patients.[43–47]

Vacuum constriction devices are also available. These devices suck blood into the penis, causing tumescence, and maintain erection through constriction of the venous outflow at the base of the penis.[48] With these devices, patients may have ejaculatory restriction (12 per cent), initial pain (41 per cent),[49] and penile ecchymosis or petechiae (10 to 27 per cent), although satisfactory use is generally achieved.[50]

Clearly, the best approach to the problem of iatrogenic sexual dysfunction is prevention through the use of appropriate preoperative evaluation, the use of nerve-sparing aortoiliac dissections or indirect methods of aortoiliac revascularization, and intraoperative attention to the maintenance of pelvic blood flow through the use of proper graft configurations and selective hypogastric revascularization.

References

1. Leriche R: Des obliterations arterielles hautes (obliteration de la terminaison de l'aorte) comme causes des insuffisances circulatoires des members inferieurs. Bull Mem Soc Chir 49:1404, 1923.
2. Leriche R, Morel A: The syndrome of thrombotic obliteration of the aortic bifurcation. Ann Surg 127:193, 1948.
3. DePalma RG, Levine SB, Feldman S: Preservation of erectile function after aorto-iliac reconstruction. Arch Surg 113:958, 1978.
4. Flanigan DP, Schuler JJ, Keifer T, et al: Elimination of iatrogenic impotence and improvement of sexual dysfunction after aortoiliac revascularization. Arch Surg 117:544, 1982.
5. Spiro M, Cotton LT: Aorto-iliac thrombo-endarterectomy. Br J Surg 57:161, 1979.
6. Hallbrook T, Holmquist B: Sexual disturbances following dissection of the aorta and the common iliac arteries. J Cardiovasc Surg 11:255, 1970.
7. Sabri S, Cotton LT: Sexual function following aortoiliac reconstruction. Lancet 2:1218, 1971.
8. Weinstein MH, Machleder HI: Sexual function after aortoiliac surgery. Ann Surg 181:787, 1975.
9. Harris JD, Jepson RP: Aorto-iliac stenosis: A comparison of two procedures. Aust J Surg 34:211, 1965.
10. May AG, DeWeese JA, Rob CG: Changes in sexual function following operation on the abdominal aorta. Surgery 65:41, 1969.
11. Miles JR, Miles DG: Aortoiliac operations and sexual dysfunction. Arch Surg 117:1177, 1982.
12. Queral LA, Whitehouse WM, Flinn WR: Pelvic hemodynamics after aortoiliac reconstruction. Surgery 36:799, 1979.
13. Pick J: Anatomy of the Autonomic Nervous System. Philadelphia, JB Lippincott, 1979, pp 439–441.
14. Queral LA, Flinn WR, Bergan JJ, et al: Sexual function and aortic surgery. *In* Bergan JJ, Yao JST (eds): Surgery of the Aorta and Its Body Branches. New York, Grune & Stratton, 1979, pp 263–276.
15. Whitelaw GP, Smithwick RH: Some secondary effects of sympathectomy. N Engl J Med 245:121, 1951.
16. Krane RJ, Goldstein I, De Tejada IS: Impotence. N Engl J Med 321:1648, 1989.
17. McCulloch DK, Campbell IW, Wu FC, et al: The prevalence of diabetic impotence. Diabetologia 18:279, 1980.
18. Ebbehoj J, Wagner G: Abnormal drainage of the corpora cavernosa causing erectile dysfunction. *In* Zorgniotti AW, Rossi G (eds): Vasculogenic Impotence. Springfield, IL, Charles C Thomas, 1980, pp 309.
19. Foresta C, Ruzza G, Mioni R, et al: Male hypogonadism in aorto-iliac arteriopathies. Arch Androl 9:297, 1982.
20. Wasserman MD, Pollak CP, Spielman AJ, et al: The differential diagnosis of impotence. JAMA 243:2038, 1980.
21. Flanigan DP, Schuler JJ: Sexual function and aortic surgery. *In* Bergan JJ, Yao JST (eds): Aortic Surgery. Philadelphia, WB Saunders, 1989, pp 547–560.
22. Pierce GE, Turrentine M, Stringfield S, et al: Evaluation of end-to-side v end-to-end proximal anastomosis in aortobifemoral bypass. Arch Surg 117:1580, 1982.
23. Kawai M: Pelvic hemodynamics before and after aortoiliac vascular reconstruction: The significance of penile blood pressure. Jpn J Surg 18:514, 1988.
24. Iliopoulos JI, Hermreck AS, Thomas JH, et al: Hemodynamics of the hypogastric arterial circulation. J Vasc Surg 9:637, 1989.

25. Ohshiro T, Kosaki G: Sexual function after aorto-iliac vascular reconstruction. Which is more important, the internal iliac artery or hypogastric nerve? J Cardiovasc Surg (Torino) 25:47, 1984.
26. Iliopoulos JI, Horwanitz PE, Pierce GE, et al: The critical hypogastric circulation. Am J Surg 154:671, 1987.
27. Flanigan DP, Sobinsky KR, Schuler JJ, et al: Internal iliac artery revascularization in the treatment of vasculogenic impotence. Arch Surg 120:271, 1985.
28. Gossetti B, Gattuso R, Irace L, et al: Aorto-iliac/femoral reconstructions in patients with vasculogenic impotence. Eur J Vasc Surg 5:425, 1991.
29. Iwai T, Sakurazawa K, Sato S, et al: Intra-operative monitoring of the pelvic circulation using a transanal Doppler probe. Eur J Vasc Surg 5:71, 1991.
30. Cronenwett JL, Gooch JB, Garrett HE: Internal iliac artery revascularization during aortofemoral bypass. Arch Surg 117:838, 1982.
31. Blaisdell FW, Hall AD: Axillary-femoral artery bypass for lower extremity ischemia. Surgery 54:563, 1963.
32. Schuler JJ, Gray B, Flanigan DP, et al: Increased penile perfusion and reversal of vasculogenic impotence following femorofemoral bypass. Br J Surg 69(Suppl):S6, 1982.
33. Merchant RF, DePalma RG: Effects of femorofemoral grafts on postoperative sexual function: Correlation with penile pulse volume recordings. Surgery 90:962, 1981.
34. Dewar ML, Blundell PE, Lidstone, et al: Effects of abdominal aneurysmectomy, aortoiliac bypass grafting and angioplasty on male sexual potency: A prospective study. Can J Surg 28:154, 1985.
35. Ravimandalam K, Rao VR, Kumar S, et al: Obstruction of the infrarenal portion of the abdominal aorta: Results of treatment with balloon angioplasty. Am J Roentgenol 156:1257, 1991.
36. Castaneda-Zuniga WR, Smith A, Kaye K, et al: Transluminal angioplasty for treatment of vasculogenic impotence. AJR 139:371, 1982.
37. Goldstein I: Overview of types and results of vascular surgical procedures for impotence. Cardiovasc Intervent Radiol 11:240, 1988.
38. McDougal WS, Jeffery RF: Microscopic penile revascularization. J Urol 129:517, 1983.
39. Krotovsky GS, Turpitko SA, Gerasimov VB, et al: Surgical treatment and prevention of vasculopathic impotence in conjunction with revascularization of the lower extremities in Leriche's syndrome. J Cardiovasc Surg (Torino) 32:340, 1991.
40. Sharlip ID: Treatment of iatrogenic impotence by penile revascularization. *In* Proceedings of the Sixth Biennial International Symposium for Corpus Cavernosum Revascularization and Third Biennial World Meeting on Impotence, Boston, October 6, 1988, p 135.
41. Gregory GJ, Purcell MH: Scott's inflatable penile prosthesis: Evaluation of mechanical survival in the series 700 model. J Urol 137:676, 1987.
42. Malloy TR, Wein AJ, Carpeniello VL: Reliability of AMS M700 inflatable penile prosthesis. Urology 28:385, 1986.
43. Thomalla JV, Thompson ST, Rowland RG, et al: Infectious complications of penile prosthetic implants. J Urol 138:65, 1987.
44. Carson CC: Infections in genitourinary prostheses. Urol Clin North Am 16:139, 1989.
45. Kaufman JJ, Linder A, Raz S: Complications of penile prothesis surgery for impotence. J Urol 128:1192, 1982.
46. Kessler R: Surgical experience with the inflatable penile prosthesis. J Urol 124:611, 1980.
47. Furlow WL, Goldwasser B, Gundian JC: Implantation of model AMS 700 penile prosthesis: Long term results. J Urol 139:741, 1988.
48. Witherington R: Vacuum constriction device for management of erectile impotence. J Urol 141:320, 1989.
49. Witherington R: Suction device therapy in the management of erectile impotence. Urol Clin North Am 15:123, 1988.
50. Nadig PW, Ware JC, Blumoff R: Noninvasive device to produce and maintain an erection-like state. J Urol 27:126, 1986.

SECTION VII

Acute Ischemia and Its Sequelae

Edited by Malcolm O. Perry, M.D.

42

Acute Limb Ischemia

Malcolm O. Perry, M.D.

• • •

ETIOLOGY

Acute arterial insufficiency most often is the result of *intrinsic* obstruction of major arteries by clot, and emboli originating in the heart frequently are the cause of such obstructions. Patients who have had myocardial infarcts or who have mitral stenosis or atrial fibrillation have the greatest risk of developing intracardiac clots that are potential emboli. Such emboli usually lodge where vessels taper or branch and consequently are seen most commonly in the lower extremities, particularly in the iliac, femoral, and popliteal arteries. In the upper extremities, the most common site for an embolus to lodge is in the brachial artery, but emboli also may occlude the subclavian or axillary vessels. Unfortunately, some emboli of cardiac origin enter the cerebral circulation and produce serious neurologic deficits. Embolic episodes tend to be recurrent, and if the predisposing factors cannot be corrected, the prognosis for recovery is poor.

In patients with arterial aneurysms or disseminated atherosclerosis, arterioarterial embolization may produce occlusion of smaller distal vessels and subsequent tissue necrosis. In these instances, the discharge of atheromatous debris from proximal arterial lesions results in intermittent and repetitive occlusion of small vessels, usually in the feet or hands. This increasingly recognized phenomenon is commonly called atheroembolism, although the term "blue toe syndrome" has also been applied (see Chapter 44). Such ulcerative plaques also may occur in the brachiocephalic vessels, and fibrin or platelet aggregates may embolize to the cerebral circulation and produce transient episodes of cerebral ischemia or cerebral infarction.

In patients with preexisting atherosclerosis and significant narrowing of major arteries, thrombosis may occur, producing acute intrinsic arterial obstruction. Such a complication is most likely to occur in areas where the vessels are severely stenotic and particularly in association with other predisposing factors such as congestive heart failure, hypovolemia, polycythemia, and trauma. This is the most common cause of acute arterial insufficiency, but because the stenotic lesion may have stimulated the development of collateral circulation, the final occlusive events may not produce the severe degree of arterial insufficiency seen in other forms. In fact, the patient may not seek medical attention, and as a result, the incidence of this form of acute arterial occlusion is commonly underestimated.

Intrinsic arterial obstruction may be caused by insertion of a catheter or medical device. Modern techniques employed in monitoring patients (e.g., arterial pressure monitoring and blood gas analysis), attempts to alleviate arterial occlusive lesions (transluminal angioplasty), administration of intra-arterial infusions (chemical agents, vasopressin, streptokinase), cardiac assist devices (intra-aortic balloon pumping) all require extended catheterization of arteries, and this encourages the formation of local clots that may result in occlusion at the site of catheterization or may produce distal emboli. Similarly, occlusion of small vessels may be the result of drug abuse associated with the intentional or inadvertent injection of foreign materials into peripheral arteries. In many cases these reactions are particularly violent, and the ensuing necrotizing arteritis causes extensive tissue loss (see Chapter 45). Occasionally, migration of foreign bodies inserted into the heart may produce intrinsic arterial obstruction. Rare cases have been reported of secondary migration of instruments, bullets, and other foreign bodies acting as arterial emboli.

Direct arterial injury by blunt and penetrating injuries is the most common cause of *extrinsic* arterial obstruction. Because of associated wounds, penetrating arterial injuries usually are an obvious cause of acute vascular insufficiency. Laceration and transection are seen most often, but in some cases mural contusion and severe spasm may produce acute arterial obstruction. Secondary thrombosis is commonly seen with arterial injuries, particularly when significant periods of hypotension occur. In a substantial number of cases, however, such arterial injuries are not associated with severe distal ischemia. In fact, some patients with proven arterial injuries have few or no immediate clinical signs of significant arterial damage, and 10 to 15 per cent may have normal distal pulses on admission.

Arterial injury or obstruction resulting from fractures of the long bones or dislocations of major joints may be very difficult to assess because of associated soft tissue swelling and osseous deformity. External compression of the artery may be the initial injury, but this may be complicated by subsequent thrombosis distal to the site of occlusion. In other cases, angulation and kinking may be associated with contusion, laceration, or even transection. The arteries are most vulnerable where they are relatively fixed by the muscles and fascia, and thus supracondylar dislocations or fractures of the humerus or femur are likely to injure or obstruct the axillary, brachial, and popliteal arteries. Less commonly, fractures of the clavicle may produce injuries of the subclavian artery, and tibial plateau fractures have been associated with damage of the popliteal and tibial arteries.

On rare occasions, extrinsic neoplastic masses or abscesses produce arterial compression and vascular insufficiency. In some instances, massive soft tissue swelling associated with extensive trauma may interfere with arterial supply. This is seen most frequently in the lower leg, and because of its relatively rigid fascial sheath, the anterior compartment is most vulnerable to this type of vascular compression. Such compartment syndromes may be seen as a complication of other types of vascular obstruction or may follow repair of direct arterial injuries (see Chapter 48).

Another infrequent cause of acute vascular insufficiency is venous outflow blockade, as seen in phlegmasia cerulea dolens, the more massive form of ileofemoral venous thrombosis. In this serious venous disease, extensive obstruction of the venous outflow from the leg interferes with arterial inflow and can pose a threat to the viability of the extremity and the life of the patient.

Low-flow states may occur in patients with cardiac disease, endotoxemia, and debilitating diseases associated with extensive neoplasia. In these patients, arterial obstruction may supervene and cause ischemia sufficient to produce gangrene, often seen symmetrically in the extremities. Several drugs, including digitalis, corticosteroids, and phenothiazines, are thought to increase the risk of nonobstructive arterial occlusion in some instances. The exact mechanisms causing these changes are unknown, but low cardiac output and splanchnic vasoactivity have been incriminated in the production of nonocclusive mesenteric vascular insufficiency (see Chapter 96). Digitalis, for example, produces significant splanchnic vasoconstriction. Presumably, similar mechanisms associated with other drugs can explain many instances of acute arterial insufficiency observed in debilitated patients undergoing intensive multidrug therapy.

PATHOPHYSIOLOGY

Tolerance of the extremities to ischemia may be difficult to assess because some cells are more susceptible to anoxia than others. Presumably, these differences reflect the oxygen requirements for that particular type of cell, and it is interesting to compare the respiratory rates of tissues. There is, for example, a fourfold difference between the respiratory rate of the skin and that of the retina. It also is widely held that the brain is especially vulnerable to hypoxia because of its oxygen requirements. Previous studies have shown that peripheral nerves and muscles have relatively less resistance to ischemia than skin. Other investigators have indicated that irreversible changes in the skeletal muscle and peripheral nerves occur after 4 to 6 hours of ischemia. Because of differences in susceptibility to hypoxia, it is apparent that the skin and subcutaneous tissue may survive periods of hypoxia that would not be tolerated by skeletal muscle and peripheral nerves.

There is much evidence to suggest that the outcome following a period of ischemia depends not only on the specific tissue tolerance to hypoxia and the duration of the period of circulatory interruption but also on local changes that impair restoration of normal flow after the initial cause has been removed or corrected. This has been called, among other things, the impaired reflow phenomenon.

Ames and his coworkers state that this phenomenon is the result of narrowing of the vascular lumen secondary to compression by swollen cells.[1] Other investigators subsequently confirmed that perivascular glial cell swelling does occur in such experiments.[2] They also showed a secondary type of capillary narrowing associated with the formation of intravascular blebs of injured capillary endothelium. Further studies by Fischer and Ames,[2] and Merrill[4] suggest that, despite adequate perfusion pressure, vascular trapping of red cells in these narrowed capillaries contributes to impaired reflow and extends the hypoxic interval. Capillary occlusion by leukocyte plugs has been observed in skeletal muscle and in the lungs during hemorrhagic shock. This phenomenon has also been seen in cardiac muscle capillaries following coronary artery occlusion.[3, 5] The importance of this hypothesis is strengthened by demonstration of the beneficial effect of acute hemodilution. Fischer and Ames,[2] Jameson,[6] and Sheehan and Davis[7] have reported similar findings in the ischemic kidney. Flores and his colleagues examined renal tissue by both light and electron microscopy and demonstrated swelling of different cells in the ischemic kidney.[8]

Similar studies of skeletal and cardiac muscle suggest that cellular swelling may follow hypoxia and may also play an important role in irreversibility. Volkmann's contracture has been attributed to obstruction of arterial flow to the extremity, with subsequent fibrosis and contracture of the skeletal muscles. In 1948, Harman, using rabbits, produced temporary complete ischemia of the hind leg with a tourniquet and subsequently injected bromphenol blue to examine the rate of penetration into and elimination of this vital dye from ischemic muscle.[9] He noted that bromphenol blue stained normal and mildly ischemic muscle as soon as the tourniquet was released and concluded that the arteries did not remain occluded. When ischemia was extended beyond 3 hours, however, there was considerable retention of dye within the muscle, and if the ischemia lasted as long as 6 hours, the dye did not enter the muscle for at least 30 minutes. His findings suggested that the circulation was stagnant, and this was confirmed by the histologic picture;

capillaries were dilated and engorged with red blood cells, and yet no thrombi were seen. The probable cause of the reduced flow through the damaged muscle was obstruction of the small vessels. Generalized swelling of the tissue was documented by demonstration of a gain in weight of the ischemic limb, and this increased with the duration of ischemia.

Similar studies of myocardium by Krug and his colleagues suggested that cellular edema occurred because of failure of the sodium pump, and thus the period of myocardial ischemia was increased.[10] Subsequent studies by Willerson and associates demonstrated that these changes could be reduced by pretreatment with a mannitol infusion, suggesting that this agent acted to reduce cell swelling and thus to restore capillary patency.[11] More recent studies have shown that mannitol is a scavenger of the oxygen-derived toxic hydroxyl radical. This free radical can cause lipid peroxidation of the cell membrane, and its neutralization may prevent cellular damage that contributes to changes in permeability leading to cell swelling.[12]

If there is a disturbance in the maintenance of normal intracellular volume, tissue swelling may occur. Studies by Stern and his group indicate that the maintenance of normal cell volume is dependent on tissue respiration and that in the absence of oxygen, tissues gain weight because of an increase in water content.[13] The final duration of ischemic insult may be much greater than is apparent because the impaired reflow phenomenon may extend the ischemic interval.

Merrill has shown that blood is a non-Newtonian fluid with increased viscosity during low-flow states.[4] The "yield stress," the pressure required to reinstitute flow from a state of rest inertia, is a function of the third power of packed red cell volume and the square of the plasma fibrinogen concentration. Thus, the increased viscosity of blood trapped during the ischemic period may present another barrier to reestablishment of blood flow.

Because of resident tone in the circular muscle fibers in the arterial wall, a critical intraluminal pressure must be present to maintain patency.[14] At very low arterial blood pressures, small muscular arteries close, and flow ceases. In accordance with the physical laws governing the relationship between vessel diameter and lateral pressure, reopening of the artery requires a finite pressure increase, and this may be especially difficult in the face of increased blood viscosity and cellular swelling. Such a combination of events may prolong ischemia; adenosine triphosphate levels fall, and cell membrane function continues to deteriorate, finally culminating in cell death.[15] Although it is apparent that the exact mechanisms responsible for this impaired reflow phenomenon have not been established, the phenomenon itself is real and, when the interruption of circulation has been prolonged, it may play an important role in determining the survival or death of the affected tissue.

Recent clinical and experimental evidence suggests that even short periods of ischemia can cause cell damage that may not be apparent if only the overall function of the organ is examined. Eklof and associates reported that temporary aortic occlusion in patients undergoing vascular surgery caused metabolic changes in the muscles of the legs that lasted for at least 16 hours.[16] Two experimental studies in dogs showed that 3 hours of partial ischemia (mean arterial pressure of 50 mmHg) resulted in longer lasting cell membrane dysfunction than 3 hours of tourniquet ischemia.[17, 18] Walker and coworkers, in a series of dog experiments, found that the skeletal muscle necrosis following 5 hours of total ischemia could be reduced by controlling oxygen delivery in the reperfusion period.[15] The salutary effect of hemodilution was increased when free radical scavengers were given. In a rat model of temporary infrarenal aortic occlusion, Perry and Fantini found that superoxide dismutase prevented progressive cell membrane dysfunction as reflected by changes in transmembrane electrical potential.[18] These studies suggest that skeletal muscle is susceptible to injury by oxygen-derived free radicals (as has been shown in the intestine, kidney, and heart). Furthermore, it appears that partial ischemia, which is the type most often encountered in clinical practice, is capable of causing cell damage.[19] Prevention of reperfusion tissue injury by scavengers of free radicals may occupy an important position in the treatment of acute vascular insufficiency.

CLINICAL MANIFESTATIONS AND DIAGNOSIS

Acute arterial insufficiency often occurs abruptly and without warning, and early diagnosis is essential. Emboli most commonly lodge at the points where the major arteries branch, and atherosclerosis tends to be more severe in these same areas. Either embolus or in situ thrombosis, therefore, is likely to compromise more than one vessel, limiting the ability to establish adequate collateral flow immediately. With the sluggish flow distal to the arterial obstruction and the hypercoagulability frequently attending the thrombotic episode, distal extension of the thrombus is likely if definitive therapy is delayed.

If the collateral circulation is not well developed, muscle necrosis and irreversible changes may appear as early as 4 to 6 hours after onset. If specific therapy can be initiated early in the course of the illness, a successful outcome can be expected. Revascularization is considerably less effective after 8 to 12 hours of ischemia.

The urgent need for surgical revascularization usually is obvious in patients presenting with acute vascular insufficiency, but this is not always the case. During the early stages of the disease, the severity of the ischemia may not be readily apparent. It is clear that because of intervening collateral beds, obstruction of major arteries may occur without early symptoms, but as the thrombotic process extends, or as fragmentation and distal embolization supervene, signs of peripheral ischemia develop or increase. Occlusion of a brachial artery, for example, usually does not produce the acute dramatic picture of severe ischemia seen after abrupt occlusion of the common femoral or popliteal artery. If the collateral circulation is disrupted by injury or extension of the occlusive process, acute ischemia supervenes. Because of these characteristics, it probably is not reasonable to assume that a period of "safe" ischemia exists. Although severe ischemia usually can be reversed successfully if adequately treated in the first 4 to 6 hours after its inception, this cannot always be accomplished.[20]

Five cardinal features of arterial insufficiency have been described and are frequently referred to as the five Ps: pain, paralysis, paresthesia, pallor, and pulselessness. In more than three quarters of the patients, pain occurs suddenly and is well localized to the afflicted extremity. It usually is quite severe, but may not be prominent in patients with relatively good collateral circulation. In some patients, the onset of ischemia is so severe and dramatic that paralysis and anesthesia appear early and pain is not a persistent symptom. Paresis and paresthesia are very important symptoms in assessing viability of an ischemic extremity. It is important to separate perception of light touch from that of pressure, pain, and temperature, because the larger fibers serving these latter functions are relatively less susceptible to hypoxia. Thus, a patient may maintain sensation to pinprick and yet be unable to perceive light touch. Similarly, proprioception may be lost relatively early. Subtle degrees of weakness of the small muscles of the feet or hands may be hard to detect and must be carefully separated from the function of the long muscles that, lying more proximally, are better perfused, but whose distal tendinous insertions greatly affect digital movement. It is clear that a paralyzed, anesthetic extremity is not viable, and if revascularization is not possible, irreversible changes appear in 6 to 8 hours. These are important findings in the evaluation of the severity of the ischemia, and they present compelling indications for immediate treatment.

Distal pulses usually are absent in patients with acute arterial insufficiency, but in some instances, significant disturbances in nutritive flow occur even when distal pulses are detectable. In most cases, however, there are no pulses distal to the level of obstruction. Thus, the site of occlusion may be localized on examination. In some patients, detection of distal pulses may be difficult because of swelling of the extremity associated with soft tissue or bony injury, and arteriography may be required. Detection of distal pulses by palpation or demonstration of flow by noninvasive methods does not preclude the presence of significant ischemia. If disturbances in sensation and motor function can be demonstrated, a more extensive evaluation is urgently required.

An acutely ischemic extremity is often pale and cool, with almost empty veins. Evaluation of skin temperature may reveal a definite line of change that is somewhat below the true level of occlusion, usually one joint distal to the site of the arterial obstruction. Careful palpation along the course of the involved artery may detect the characteristic tenderness overlying an acute embolus and will confirm the absence of pulses distal to this site. Pulsations immediately proximal to the arterial obstruction may be abnormally strong. These signs are easily elicited along the brachial artery and proximal portion of the superficial femoral arteries and are of practical aid in directing the surgical approach to these obstructions.

Evaluation of the consistency of skeletal muscle tissue is an important part of the assessment of the severity of the ischemia. With increasing ischemia, cellular swelling occurs, and the muscles no longer feel soft but thick and inelastic. As ischemic edema progresses, the muscles become quite stiff and firm; this is clear evidence of early necrosis and carries an ominous prognosis. In this group of patients, surgical revascularization is likely to fail, and although the extremity may be partly salvageable, extensive muscle débridement almost certainly will be required.

Associated diseases in certain patients may aid in the diagnosis of arterial occlusion. Some patients have obvious preexisting cardiac disease that predisposes to embolization and have no evidence of disseminated peripheral vascular disease. In contrast are those patients who give a history of intermittent claudication, have other signs of segmental atherosclerosis, and then suddenly develop acute ischemia. In this group, physical examination will often reveal the stigmata of diffuse arterial disease, and a diagnosis of in situ thrombosis complicating a preexisting stenosis is likely. Since the surgical management of these two groups of patients is quite different, separation of these problems is important in planning operative management (see Chapter 43).

Adjunctive Diagnostic Studies

In many cases, the cause of acute arterial insufficiency is readily apparent. An arterial embolus to a superficial artery often is easily detectable on physical examination, and the exact location may be determined by simple palpation of the artery. A femoral or brachial embolus may be quickly identified, and if severe ischemia is present, adjunctive diagnostic studies may be deferred. In some cases, even more proximal emboli may easily be diagnosed. The saddle embolus in the terminal aorta often is associated with clear signs of peripheral ischemia in both lower extremities, and in the absence of clinical involvement of the intestines or the urinary tract, other angiographic studies may not be required. It is apparent, therefore, that in cases of severe ischemia when the diagnosis is firm and solid indications for surgical intervention exist, a delay for arteriography may be unwise.

In contrast are those instances in which modest ischemia of the extremities is present and doubt exists about the exact nature of the arterial obstruction. Occasionally, it may be difficult on physical examination to separate those patients with emboli from those who have in situ thrombosis complicating preexisting arterial disease. Since the operative management of the patient with a simple embolus and a relatively normal artery differs drastically from that required in the person with preexisting arterial disease, arteriography is valuable if not essential in planning the operation, even when the diagnosis of arterial obstruction is relatively secure. During the period of preoperative evaluation and resuscitation, arteriograms may be obtained and a more definite plan of operative management formulated. Simple, abbreviated arteriographic studies are indicated in these patients, and they usually can be obtained satisfactorily by direct needle puncture proximal to the suspected area of obstruction. Delayed arteriograms of the distal circulation are helpful because the success of the operation often depends on patency of the distal vascular tree. Many patients also require immediate postoperative arteriography because patency of the distal circulation is not always confirmed on preoperative evaluation.

Concomitant venous thrombosis, although infrequent, may complicate acute arterial obstruction. This is especially likely in patients in whom revascularization is delayed. The diagnosis of concurrent venous obstruction often can be made by clinical evaluation with the aid of a Doppler probe. Since venous autografts may be required in patients with severe preexisting arterial disease, preoperative duplex studies may be of value in identifying suitable veins. Exploration along the course of the greater saphenous or other major superficial vein using a Doppler probe and proximal and distal compressive maneuvers is helpful, although it will not give information regarding the adequacy of the prospective donor vein. Such adjunctive procedures are preferable to prolonged and repeated attempts at local exploration of potential vein grafts.

Other ancillary diagnostic methods as described in Section II may be helpful in the clinical and operative evaluation of these patients. Of all the adjunctive methods, ultrasonic detection of flow provides the most practical information and offers reliable evidence about the patency of major vessels. Because of the well-described disparity between pressure and flow in the major vessels and nutritive flow to the tissues, these measurements cannot be the only criteria used in evaluating viability. Nevertheless, they may be useful when combined with a careful clinical evaluation and selective use of angiography.

Since the heart is usually the source of arterial emboli, careful examination of cardiopulmonary function is mandatory. The ultimate success of the treatment of emboli depends largely on the ability to control their source. Similarly, patients with arterial thrombosis as a complication of arteriosclerosis must be examined in the context of possibly requiring major vascular reconstruction. It is desirable to defer these procedures (echocardiography, proximal arteriography) until the emergency is over, but this may not be feasible. Failure to manage predisposing causes often results in recurrent thrombosis, which may not be susceptible to repair.

MANAGEMENT

Protective Measures

Protection of the vascular bed distal to a proximal obstruction is very important and often can be accomplished by immediate systemic anticoagulation with intravenous heparin. Systemic heparinization offers protection against the propagation of distal thrombosis and usually does not cause significant problems during the operative procedure. Patients with severe associated injuries or other systemic diseases that tend to be complicated by bleeding may not tolerate systemic anticoagulation, but local irrigation with a dilute heparin solution may be useful during surgery.

Some rheologic benefits have been claimed for the administration of hypertonic solutions of mannitol. The studies of Jameson and others suggest that it may reduce cellular swelling and thus to some extent ameliorate the impaired reflow phenomenon.[6] Osmotic diuresis also will result and may be of value after hypovolemia has been corrected. Severe muscle ischemia may cause myoglobinuria, and mannitol is considered by some to be the drug of choice in this situation. When such a pigment load may further compromise renal function, diuresis and alkalinization of the urine are important therapeutic measures.

Potassium may be released whenever cell membrane integrity is compromised by ischemia. The resultant hyperkalemia often responds to the judicious administration of glucose and insulin, reestablishment of adequate volume, and, in severe cases, administration of an ion-exchange resin. In rare instances of severe peripheral ischemia, peritoneal dialysis or hemodialysis may be required to control rapidly rising levels of serum potassium (see Chapter 43).

Low-flow states, whether the result of central or peripheral factors, may induce lactic acidemia, and the increased hydrogen ion concentration may interfere with cardiac function. It is apparent from the studies of McClelland and associates that the major requirement for correction of these compositional abnormalities is restoration of adequate tissue flow.[21] This is best accomplished preoperatively by repairing volume deficits and improving cardiac output, thus removing the primary cause of acidosis.[22] The judicious administration of sodium bicarbonate may be useful after this stage of treatment.

Protection of the ischemic extremity is important because a severe reduction in arterial flow renders it more vulnerable to external forces. The application of heat to an ischemic extremity may produce significant thermal damage to the skin and subcutaneous tissues and should be avoided. Because the primary problem is lack of arterial flow, it is unlikely that external heat will change core temperature, but it may increase the metabolic rate beyond the ability of a limited blood flow to supply the required oxygen and nutrients, causing further cellular damage and extending the ischemic injury. The primary function of the subcutaneous veins is mainly thermoregulation, and external heat may produce superficial venous vasodilatation, thus diverting blood flow through physiologic arteriovenous fistulae. Focal points of extrinsic pressure, particularly over the malleoli and heels, may exceed the local perfusion pressure and may produce focal necrosis in areas that might otherwise have survived. Therefore, ischemic extremities should be protected from extremes of heat and cold and guarded from undue pressure.

Preoperative Preparation

Even during the brief preoperative period, many supportive measures can be accomplished satisfactorily. Complete resuscitation may not always be possible, but administration of sufficient intravenous fluids to stabilize cardiopulmonary function is essential. Central venous pressure monitoring is a useful guide in these efforts, but in some cases, placement of a flow-directed, balloon-tipped (Swan-Ganz) catheter for the direct measurement of pulmonary artery pressure may be required. Since the intravenous administration of fluids and drugs may be important throughout the perioperative period, secure catheters in large veins are needed. Indwelling venous catheters, one of which is committed to the restoration of blood volume only, should be placed in two extremities prior to the administration of anesthesia.

Those patients who have associated fractures causing arterial obstruction often need external stabilization or reduction. In certain cases, reduction of dislocations of the femur and humerus or fractures of other long bones may restore adequate flow and reduce the period of ischemia.

Perioperative Management

In the operating room, the patient usually is placed in the supine position to allow access to all four extremities. When certain injuries are present, different positioning may be necessary. For example, in patients with suspected injuries or thrombosis of the left subclavian artery, anterolateral thoracotomy may be required.

In most cases, placing the patient supine with the arms extended will offer satisfactory exposure to the majority of vessels in the extremities. This positioning also allows easy access to autogenous vein grafts if they are required for vascular reconstruction. The most useful veins for interposition grafts are the greater saphenous and the cephalic veins. Since vascular reconstructive procedures may require exposure of the proximal arterial and venous system, access to the thorax and abdomen should be provided for at the time of preparation and draping of the surgical field.

Although many peripheral emboli and thrombi can be handled quite satisfactorily under local anesthesia, general anesthesia should be employed when extensive vascular reconstruction is necessary. In addition, even when local anesthesia is adequate, cardiorespiratory monitoring and the management of intraoperative blood loss require close attention and support, especially in patients with cardiopulmonary disease. The maintenance of normal blood pressure is important in patients who are dependent upon collateral beds for tissue viability. Therefore, anesthetic techniques that cause minimal hemodynamic disturbance should be chosen.

Since they may be extended easily in either direction, vertical incisions are most useful in exposing major vessels in the extremities; these may be modified in order not to compromise function. In certain cases, when the location of the occlusion is firmly established, small incisions along natural skin lines may be satisfactory, as in patients with emboli in the common femoral artery or the brachial artery. Proximal and distal control of the major vessels and important adjacent collaterals should be obtained before the artery is opened. Atraumatic occlusion is important, because atheromata tend to be deposited preferentially at areas of injury. It usually is not necessary to apply vascular clamps until the vessel has been cleared of local thrombi. Control of hemorrhage often can be accomplished by digital pressure at appropriate points, by gently encircling the vessels with double-looped Silastic strands or umbilical tapes and applying a Rummel tourniquet, or by carefully applying soft, atraumatic vascular clamps. Intraluminal tamponade also may be obtained with plain or balloon-tipped catheters, causing minimal trauma to the arterial wall. Every effort should be made to avoid disruption of the arterial wall, a complication particularly likely to occur in patients with preexisting arteriosclerosis. In many cases in which embolectomy or thrombectomy is the only procedure necessary, a transverse arteriotomy is preferable. Care should be taken to avoid fragmenting and disseminating intraluminal clots.

Once the artery has been cleared, distal flow must be assessed. Arterial backflow may be misleading because intervening collateral beds may produce a relatively vigorous backflow, even with remote distal obstruction. The procedure should not be terminated until distal flow is ensured, either by return of normal distal pulses or, as is frequently required, by operative arteriography. The patency of associated major veins should be confirmed prior to wound closure because secondary venous thrombosis may accompany arterial occlusion. If this is the case, the veins should be cleared of thrombus and flow restored prior to reestablishing arterial flow. In patients in whom severe ischemia has been prolonged, it may be desirable to open the major accompanying vein temporarily to drain the initial venous effluent externally. Venous blood from a severely ischemic extremity may contain thrombotic debris and large amounts of potassium and hydrogen ions. Removal of these components usually is more effective than an attempt to neutralize them by giving buffers and other medications.[23]

Postoperative Management

In the immediate postoperative period, arterial and venous flow should be carefully monitored by checking pulses, skin temperature, capillary and venous filling, and segmental limb systolic pressures. If any deterioration occurs, immediate arteriography is required. The evaluation of neuromuscular function of the extremity must also be repeated frequently. Although major arterial flow may be restored, nutritive flow to the tissues may remain impaired, particularly in those patients who have had prolonged ischemia, shock, and associated soft tissue and bony injuries. In these cases, the evaluation of motor function and perception of touch and proprioception is an integral part of the postoperative care because early treatment of ischemia is necessary if viability of the extremity is to be ensured.

References

1. Ames A, Wright RL, Kowada M, et al: Cerebral ischemia—The no-reflow phenomenon. Am J Pathol 52:437, 1968.
2. Fischer EG, Ames A: Studies on mechanisms of impairment of cerebral circulation following ischemia: Effect of hemodilution and perfusion pressure. Stroke 3:538, 1972.
3. Bagge U, Amundson B, Lauritzen C: White blood cell deformability and plugging of skeletal muscle capillaries in hemorrhagic shock. Acta Physiol Scand 108:159, 1980.
4. Merrill EW: Rheology of blood. Physiol Rev 49:863, 1969.
5. Ernst E, Hammerschmidt DE, Bagge U, et al: Leukocytes and the risk of ischemic diseases. JAMA 257:2318, 1987.
6. Jameson RL: The role of cellular swelling in the pathogenesis of organ ischemia. West J Med 3:205, 1974.
7. Sheehan HL, Davis JC: Renal ischemia with failed reflow. J Pathol Bacteriol 78:105, 1959.
8. Flores J, DiBona DR, Beck CH, et al: The role of cell swelling in ischemic renal damage and the protective effect of hypertonic solution. J Clin Invest 51:118, 1972.
9. Harman JW: The significance of local vascular phenomena in the production of ischemic necrosis in skeletal muscle. Am J Pathol 24:625, 1948.
10. Krug S, de Rochemont W, Korb G: Blood supply of the myocardium after temporary coronary occlusion. Clin Res 19:57, 1966.
11. Willerson JT, Powell WJ, Guiny TE: Improvement in myocardial function and coronary blood flow in ischemic myocardium after mannitol. J Clin Invest 11:2981, 1972.
12. McCord JM: Oxygen-derived free radicals in post-ischemic tissue injury. N Engl J Med 313:159, 1985.

13. Stern JR, Eggleston LV, Herns R, et al: Accumulation of glutamic acid in isolated brain tissue. Biochem J 44:410, 1949.
14. Burton AC: On the physical equilibrium of small blood vessels. Am J Physiol 164:319, 1951.
15. Walker PM, Lindsay TF, Labbe R, et al: Salvage of skeletal muscle with free radical scavengers. J Vasc Surg 5:68, 1987.
16. Eklof B, Neglan P, Thompson D: Temporary incomplete ischemia of the legs induced by aortic clamping in man. Ann Surg 93:89, 1980.
17. Perry MO, Shires GT III, Albert SA: Cellular changes with graded limb ischemia and reperfusion. J Vasc Surg 1:536, 1984.
18. Perry MO, Fantini G: Ischemia: Profile of an enemy. J Vasc Surg 6:231, 1987.
19. Roberts JP, Perry MO, Hariri RJ, et al: Incomplete recovery of muscle cell function following partial but not complete ischemia. Circ Shock 17:253, 1985.
20. Malan E, Tattoni G: Physio- and anatopathology of acute ischemia of the extremities. J Cardiovasc Surg 4:2, 1963.
21. McClelland RN, Shires GT, Perry MO: Balanced salt solution in the treatment of hemorrhagic shock. JAMA 199:830, 1967.
22. Canizaro PC, Prager MD, Shires GT: The infusion of Ringer's lactate solution during shock: Changes in lactate, excess lactate and pH. Am J Surg 122:494, 1971.
23. Anderson MN, Mouritzen C: Effect of acute respiratory and metabolic acidosis on cardiac output and peripheral resistance. Ann Surg 163:161, 1966.

43

Arterial Thromboembolism

David C. Brewster, M.D., Albert K. Chin, M.D., George D. Hermann, B.S., and Thomas J. Fogarty, M.D.

• • •

Despite significant advances in the management of cardiovascular diseases, arterial embolism remains a common and important cause of limb-threatening ischemia and loss of vital organ function. Although innovative improvements have greatly simplified the surgical approach, the morbidity and mortality associated with embolic events continue to be substantial and remain a challenge to the vascular surgeon.

The overall incidence of arterial embolic disease appears to be increasing. A report from the Henry Ford Hospital revealed that admissions for arterial embolism increased from 23.1 per 100,000 hospital admissions during the period 1950 to 1964 to 50.4 per 100,000 admissions between 1960 and 1979.[1] This may, in part, be due to better diagnosis and recognition, but there is little doubt that a substantial increase in the number of elderly patients, longer survival of patients with advanced cardiac disease, and more frequent use of cardiac and vascular prosthetic devices and invasive diagnostic techniques all contribute to the rising incidence of thromboembolic problems.[2, 3]

The term embolus, derived from the Greek ''embolos'' meaning plug or stopper, was first introduced by Virchow in 1854. By definition, an embolus is a blood clot or other foreign body that is formed in, or gains access to, the vascular system in one location and is then carried by blood flow to another site where it produces vascular obstruction. Following the first successful reports of surgical removal of an embolus in the early parts of this century,[4] operative management slowly gained increasing acceptance over the next 50 years, with recognition of the necessity for early operation to avoid irreversible intimal damage and secondary thrombosis distal to the point of embolic occlusion.[5–7] A significant advance in clinical management was achieved with the introduction of heparin for use both during and after surgery.[8]

Complete removal of the embolus, particularly associated secondary propagated thrombus, continued to be problematic, however. A variety of methods, including retrograde ''milking'' or arterial flushing,[9, 10] use of suction catheters,[11] or even wire corkscrew-like devices,[12] were employed for this purpose. In 1963, the most notable advance in the surgical treatment of thromboembolic disease was achieved with introduction of the balloon catheter by Fogarty and associates.[13]

Changing Patient Population

Although introduction of the Fogarty catheter greatly simplified and improved the technique of embolectomy and has led to a substantial increase in limb salvage, it is somewhat surprising that the mortality associated with arterial emboli has remained high, ranging from 10 to 25 per cent in even more recently reported series.[14–27] This persistently high death rate reflects the serious underlying disease, principally cardiac, present in patients with an arterial embolus. In fact, analysis of the patient population with arterial emboli reveals a gradual but definite increase in clinical risk factors in the typical patient with an embolus. Increased age, severity of associated medical problems, and the presence of coexisting chronic arterial occlusive disease appear to have largely offset the technical advances in surgical treatment and improvements in supportive care that promised dramatic decreases in morbidity and mortality rates and limb salvage.

Table 43–1. Arterial Emboli—Clinical Trends, Massachusetts General Hospital Experience*

	1937–1953[29,30]	1954–1963[28]	1964–1980[14]
Average patient age	52	63	70
Source of embolus			
Arteriosclerotic heart disease	38%	51%	66%
	84%	87%	86%
Rheumatic heart disease	46%	36%	20%
Noncardiac	3%	6%	9%
Unknown	13%	7%	5%

**773 patients, 974 embolic events; cerebral emboli excluded.*

Such trends in the clinical characteristics of patients with arterial emboli have been clearly documented in a series of reports over a period of four and one-half decades from the Massachusetts General Hospital.[14, 28–30] As shown in Table 43–1, in earlier years patients with an embolus were most often in the 40- to 50-year age group, with rheumatic heart disease the most common cause. In contrast, the average patient age is currently 70 years, and arteriosclerotic heart disease and its complications are by far the most frequent causes. Many patients are currently in or beyond their eighth decade of life, with widespread coronary artery, cerebrovascular, and peripheral occlusive disease all contributing significantly to the persistently high mortality and risk of limb loss in patients with embolic disease. Similar changes in the patient population have been recognized by other investigators as well.[31, 32]

ETIOLOGY AND SOURCES OF EMBOLI

Cardiac Sources

Arterial emboli are largely a reflection of cardiac disease (Fig. 43–1). The heart is by far the predominant source of arterial emboli, cited as the site of origin in 80 to 90 per cent of cases in all reported series. As noted in Table 43–1, at the Massachusetts General Hospital approximately 85 per cent of arterial emboli originate in the heart, a rate that has remained remarkably constant over the last half century. The type of heart disease responsible for the embolus has changed substantially, however, with arteriosclerotic heart disease and its related complications currently implicated in 60 to 70 per cent in recent reviews.[1, 14, 15, 19, 33] Rheumatic heart disease, predominantly mitral valvular stenosis with atrial fibrillation, has been declining steadily as a cause of arterial emboli but is still seen on occasion. Fifty per cent of patients with unrepaired rheumatic mitral stenosis experience peripheral embolism.[34] This is due to the high incidence of concomitant atrial fibrillation and mitral valve disease. In isolated aortic valvular disease, clinically detectable thromboembolism is rare owing to the infrequency of atrial fibrillation.[35]

Regardless of its cause, atrial fibrillation is associated with two thirds to three quarters of peripheral thromboembolic cases.[14, 23, 33] Clot formation is especially prominent in the left atrial appendage secondary to stasis in the noncontractile atrium. In this location, standard echocardiographic detection is often difficult and unreliable.[36–38] Therefore, the absence of intracardiac thrombus on echocardiography does not rule out the heart as a source of peripheral embolism in a patient with atrial fibrillation. Indeed, this cardiac arrhythmia is usually a reliable indicator of an embolic cause of acute arterial ischemia.

Myocardial infarction is the next most frequent cause of peripheral arterial embolism. In Panetta and colleagues' recent review of a 34-year experience with 400 patients from Baylor Medical Center in Dallas, recent myocardial infarction was believed to be the cause of an arterial embolus in nearly 20 per cent of cases.[22] Left ventricular thrombus is common in transmural anterior infarction and is generally situated at the left ventricular apex. It is less common for ventricular thrombus formation to occur in subendocardial or inferior myocardial infarction. Mural thrombus was found at autopsy in 44 per cent of patients with fatal myocardial infarctions.[39] Although left ventricular thrombus is present in approximately 30 per cent of patients suffering acute transmural anterior myocardial infarction, the incidence of arterial thromboembolism is less than 5 per cent in all patients following myocardial infarction.[40, 41] Nonetheless, the sheer magnitude of coronary artery disease and myocardial infarction makes this a relatively common cause of arterial embolism. In Darling and associates' report from the Massachusetts General Hospital, an acute myocardial infarction was the source of the arterial embolus in

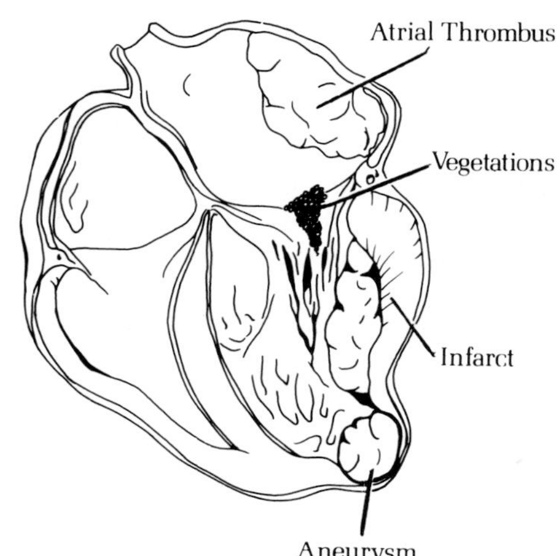

FIGURE 43–1. **Cardiac sources of arterial emboli.**

more than half of patients presenting without atrial fibrillation. Myocardial infarction had occurred from 3 to 28 days prior to the embolic episode, with an average of 14 days.[28] This is similar to findings in other reports of emboli following acute myocardial infarction.[42, 43] Because an arterial embolus may be the initial manifestation of a "silent" myocardial infarction, careful evaluation of the electrocardiogram and determination of serial cardiac enzymes are essential in patients presenting with an acute embolus, especially if they are not in atrial fibrillation.

Myocardial infarction may also be the cause of an embolus after longer intervals, usually due to areas of hypokinesia or ventricular aneurysm formation after infarction. Thrombus is present within the aneurysm in 50 per cent of cases, and peripheral embolism is found in approximately 5 per cent.[44] When embolism occurs, it is usually within 6 weeks following the infarction, but much longer intervals may be noted.[45]

Valves and other prostheses are another cardiac source of arterial emboli. Thrombus formation may occur around the sewing ring in a caged-ball or caged-disc valve.[46] Tilting disc valves predispose to thrombus formation at the hinge points, which correspond to sites of low-velocity blood flow. Rarely, mechanical stresses may lead to embolization of parts of the prosthetic devices themselves.[47] Anticoagulation is required with prosthetic mechanical valves, and embolic complications are particularly common when postimplantation anticoagulation is inadequate or discontinued. With bioprosthetic valves, such as the porcine xenograft, anticoagulation is not required in most cases.[48]

Although rare, intracardiac tumors such as atrial myxoma may give rise to tumor emboli sufficiently large to occlude major vessels.[28, 49] Similarly, vegetation from mitral or aortic valve leaflets or prosthetic valve devices in patients with bacterial or fungal endocarditis may cause recognizable arterial embolic events. The incidence of bacterial endocarditis has increased in recent years owing to more widespread intravenous drug abuse, and this is a potentially important cause of an embolus in a young patient without other discernible risk factors.[50–52] For these reasons, careful examination of embolic material removed at embolectomy by both gross and microscopic pathologic methods as well as bacteriologically is important and will occasionally provide unexpected diagnostic dividends.

Noncardiac Sources

An identifiable noncardiac source of an embolus is found in 5 to 10 per cent of patients. At the Massachusetts General Hospital (see Table 43–1), such noncardiac sources were believed to be responsible for approximately 9 per cent of emboli in the most recent era reviewed.[14] This percentage has steadily risen, and the frequency of undetermined causes has decreased, as diagnostic methods have improved.

In most instances, diseased proximal large vessels are the site of thrombus formation (Fig. 43–2). Most common is downstream embolization of mural thrombus from aneurysms of the aortoiliac, femoral, or popliteal arteries.[53] In the upper extremity, small unsuspected subclavian aneurysms, often due to thoracic outlet compression, may cause distal embolic events in the arm, hand, or fingers. Proximal ulcerated arteriosclerotic plaques may also be a site of thrombus formation and subsequent embolization.[54–57] Although these often involve only the terminal digital arteries as microemboli (see Chapter 44), on occasion surprisingly large emboli may obstruct major vessels and may be clini-

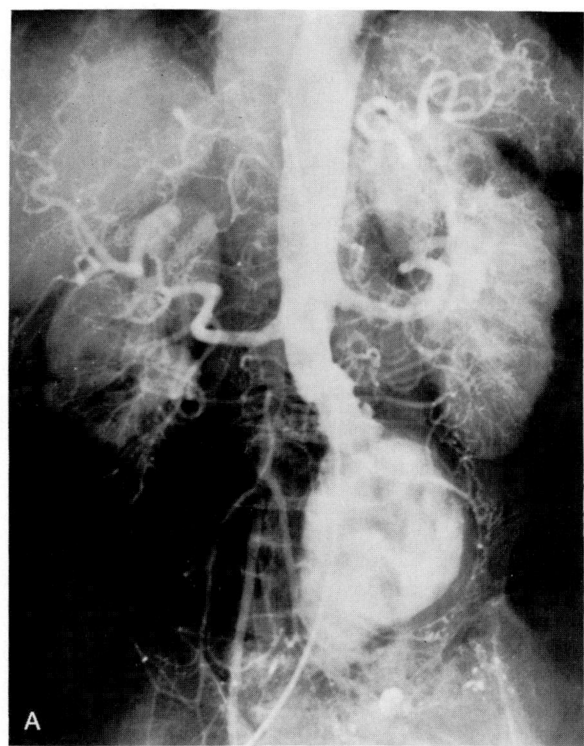

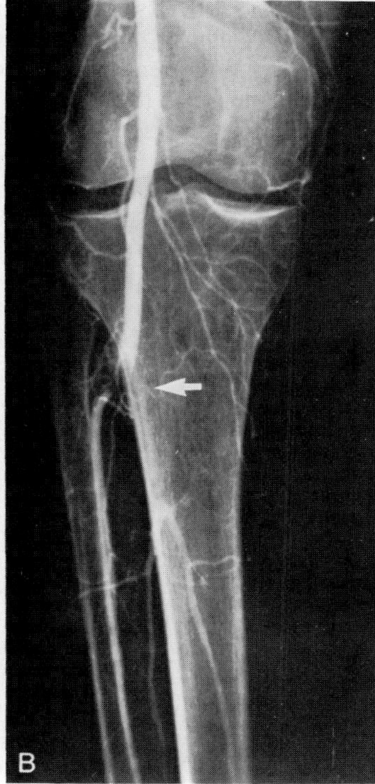

FIGURE 43–2. *A*, Large abdominal aortic aneurysm, the source of the popliteal embolus shown in *B*. Aneurysmal or occlusive lesions in proximal vessels are the most common noncardiac sources of emboli.

cally indistinguishable from emboli of cardiac origin. Thrombus or bits of poorly adherent fibrin from the pseudointimal lining of previously implanted prosthetic grafts are increasingly a source of peripheral embolus. Similarly, vessel injuries due to trauma or the growing use of invasive diagnostic or therapeutic intravascular catheters, balloons, and other devices may lead to intramural clots or dislodgment of plaque which may embolize and cause distal vascular obstruction.[58–60]

Rarely, noncardiac tumors or other foreign bodies may gain access to the arterial circulation and form arterial emboli. Such tumors are usually primary or metastatic lung neoplasms that invade the pulmonary vasculature or heart, but occasionally direct arterial invasion has been reported.[61, 62] Bullet emboli have also been recognized.[63, 64] ''Paradoxical'' embolization occurs when a thrombus arising in the venous system or right heart passes through an intracardiac communication, most often a patent foramen ovale, to become a systemic arterial embolus. These are rare but should be considered in any patient with coexisting systemic arterial thromboembolism and deep venous thrombosis or pulmonary embolism, especially if another source of embolus is not evident. A complete diagnostic work-up should include lung scan to determine the presence of pulmonary emboli, peripheral venography, and cardiac catheterization with angiography to establish the presence of a right-to-left intracardiac shunt secondary to increased right-sided pressure, allowing venous emboli to cross to the left side of the heart.[65–67]

Unknown Source

In the remaining 5 to 10 per cent of cases, the specific source of an embolus cannot be determined clinically or even at autopsy.[1, 14, 19, 22, 28, 32, 68] The incidence of such ''cryptogenic'' emboli has decreased as diagnostic modalities have improved and recognition of noncardiac sources of embolic events has increased (see Table 43–1). More frequent use of arteriography and other imaging techniques has contributed to identification of likely proximal arterial sites of origin of peripheral emboli. In addition, a recent diagnostic technique, transesophageal echocardiography, permits more thorough and accurate evaluation of possible cardiac sources of emboli and identification of potentially important lesions in the proximal thoracic aorta.[69–71] Unlike the more commonly performed standard transthoracic echocardiography, in the transesophageal approach an ultrasound transducer is passed orally into the mid-thoracic esophagus. From a vantage point directly behind the left atrium, this technique offers good visualization of the entire heart and most of the thoracic aorta, with improved diagnostic evaluation of left atrial appendage thrombi, cardiac valvular vegetations, or thoracic aortic atheromas or lesions, all of which are potentially important sources of peripheral arterial emboli.[37, 38, 69–72]

In some instances of presumed cryptogenic emboli, confusion with local thrombosis in situ may be responsible. Possible hypercoagulable states should be suspected and appropriately evaluated, particularly in younger patients with no history of antecedent occlusive disease who present with sudden arterial occlusions, or in patients with malignant disease.[73]

SITES OF EMBOLISM

Approximately 20 per cent of arterial emboli involve the carotid vessels or their intracranial branches, and about 10 per cent involve the visceral arteries.[28] Emboli to both of these locations may be underdiagnosed. Acute strokes secondary to cerebrovascular embolic events may be attributed to other pathologic causes. Many visceral emboli may go undetected; if small, little physiologic disturbance may result to indicate their occurrence, whereas if large they may prove rapidly fatal and may frequently be confused with other causes of sudden death such as myocardial infarction, pulmonary embolus, or other intra-abdominal catastrophes. Carotid and visceral emboli will not be considered further in this chapter.

The axial limb vessels are involved in 70 to 80 per cent of embolic episodes in most series of arterial emboli,[1, 22, 28] and this is indeed fortunate because such locations are most readily approached surgically. As shown in Figure 43–3, the lower extremity vessels are involved approximately five times as frequently as those of the upper extremity. Because vessel diameters change most abruptly at points of arterial branching, sites of embolic occlusion are most often related to major arterial bifurcations. However, with the advancing age of patients with emboli and the

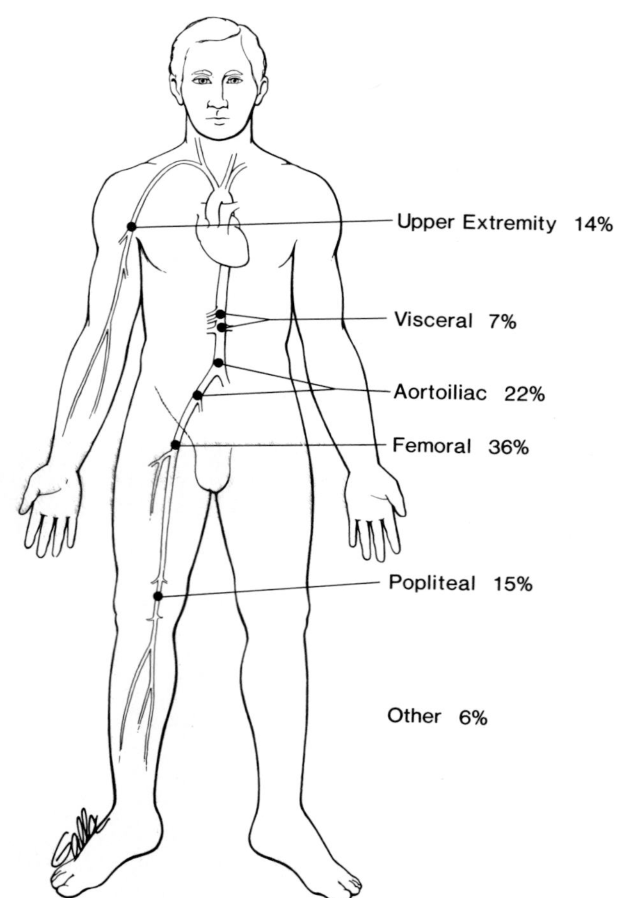

FIGURE 43–3. Incidence of embolic occlusion at different sites. Compiled from 1303 embolic events at Massachusetts General Hospital[14] and Stanford University.[33]

increased incidence of associated occlusive disease, the frequency of acute embolic occlusion in already stenotic portions of vessels unrelated to points of bifurcation appears to be increasing.

In all series, the common femoral bifurcation is the most frequent site of embolic occlusion, usually noted in 35 to 50 per cent of instances.[1, 16, 22, 28, 31–33, 68] Together, the femoral and popliteal arteries are involved more than twice as often as the aorta and iliac vessels, probably reflecting the simple mechanical fact that only a thrombus of considerable size will have any effect at the aortic or iliac bifurcation unless it is narrowed by preexisting occlusive disease.

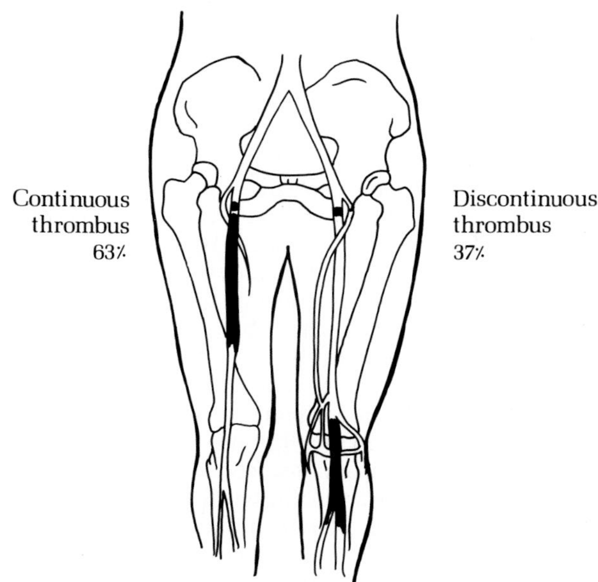

FIGURE 43–5. Continuous and discontinuous clot propagation following embolism. Discontinuous thrombus occurs in approximately 37 per cent of cases.

PATHOPHYSIOLOGY

In general, the clinical outcome of any embolic event depends upon the size of the vessel involved, the degree of obstruction, and, most important, the amount of collateral circulation available. The adequacy of collateral blood flow around the site of acute embolic occlusion is the chief determinant of severity and outcome.

If an acute embolus obstructs a previously normal artery, severe distal ischemia may result owing to the paucity of collateral pathways. Or even a small embolic event may have serious impact in a limb with marginal vascular status, in which both the artery and collateral circulation have already been appreciably narrowed by chronic occlusive disease. In contrast, it is well known that sudden occlusion imposed upon a severely stenotic vessel with a well-formed collateral system may produce only mild clinical symptoms. The latter is most characteristic of acute arterial thrombosis, of course.

Formerly, much emphasis was placed upon the necessity to intervene therapeutically within a 4- to 6-hour period, the so-called golden period, which was felt to represent the maximal length of tolerable ischemia. Although this may be true in some instances, it is now well recognized that no arbitrary time limit can be applied to all cases. The physiologic state of the limb, determined mainly by the balance between supply and metabolic demand rather than simply elapsed time from onset of occlusion, best determines operability and the likelihood of limb salvage. In many instances, enough collateral circulation may be present to allow survival of the ischemic limb or organ, although its function may be severely impaired. Obviously, different tissues vary significantly in their susceptibility to ischemia, depending largely on their individual metabolic activity and hence their demand for nutrient blood flow.

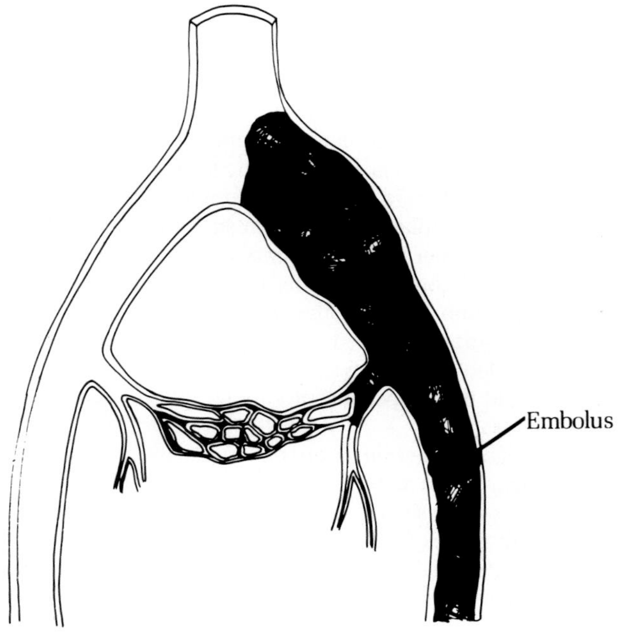

FIGURE 43–4. Proximal and distal propagation of clot following the lodging of an embolus.

Following initial obstruction of an arterial bifurcation by an embolus, three possible events may occur to aggravate ischemia. Of primary importance is proximal and distal thrombus propagation (Fig. 43–4), as recognized by Linton.[74] Impairment of collateral circulation by propagation of clot, which tends to be most serious distal to the site of embolic occlusion, is the major secondary factor leading to worsening of ischemia following an embolus. Prevention of such secondary clotting is the principal reason why immediate therapy with full-dose heparin is so important. In addition, effective surgical therapy requires complete removal of such propagated thrombus, one of the main advantages of the balloon embolectomy catheter. Secondary thrombus may occur in both a continuous and discontinuous fashion (Fig. 43–5). The possibility of such distal discontinuous clot makes cannulation of the distal vasculature necessary at the time of embolectomy. The presence of backbleeding at the site of embolectomy is an unreliable guide to the patency of the distal circulation because it may occur from intervening arterial branches proximal to distal clot.

A second event that may aggravate distal ischemia is

fragmentation of an embolus, with subsequent migration to distal vessels beyond collateral sources. Occasionally, however, partial clot lysis and fragmentation may be the mechanism for the spontaneous clinical resolution of an embolic episode that is noted in some patients.

Finally, associated venous thrombosis may occur with prolonged severe arterial ischemia, presumably due to a combination of sluggish flow and ischemic injury to the intima of veins in the involved area. With advanced ischemia, development of venous thrombosis may further reduce arterial blood flow or worsen edema following revascularization. Pulmonary embolus has been a significant cause of death in advanced cases of arterial thromboembolism.[28, 75]

Patients with sudden severe ischemia resulting from acute embolic occlusion are prone to several other severe systemic and metabolic complications. The most grave of these is the myonephropathic-metabolic syndrome, emphasized by Haimovici, who estimated that one third of the deaths from peripheral arterial thromboembolism are the result of such disastrous metabolic complications following revascularization.[76] Recognition of the potentially severe metabolic derangements due to such an "ischemia-reperfusion syndrome" has also led Blaisdell and associates to recommend treatment with heparin alone in patients with advanced ischemia, with early primary amputation as necessary, in an effort to reduce mortality associated with surgical embolectomy.[75]

The content of venous blood in the severely ischemic limb has been studied by Fischer and colleagues[77] and reflects the metabolic consequences of severe hypoxia in a predominantly muscular organ. High concentrations of potassium, lactic acid, myoglobin, and cellular enzymes such as creatinine phosphokinase, lactate dehydrogenase, and serum glutamic-oxaloacetic transaminase (SGOT) and a significant fall in blood pH result from anaerobic metabolism, paralysis of the sodium-potassium cellular pump, and rhabdomyolysis. The mean venous effluent pH was 6.80 and the serum potassium was 7.2 mEq/L 5 minutes after restoration of arterial continuity.[77] With revascularization, the sudden release of these accumulated products in the venous effluent may have profound consequences. Hyperkalemia, metabolic acidosis, and myoglobinuria (red urine, clear plasma) are the key features of the syndrome. Renal tubular necrosis may occur when myoglobin is precipitated in the renal tubules under acidotic conditions.

Significant edema may also follow revascularization of the acutely ischemic limb. The integrity of capillary walls may be disrupted owing not only to the ischemic insult but also to arterial reperfusion itself.[78] With reperfusion, large quantities of oxygen-free radicals may overwhelm the intracellular scavenger system and cause damage to the phospholipid cell membrane and intracellular organelles. Damaged cells and cell membranes allow transudation and subsequent edema to occur, potentially reducing local perfusion further ("no-reflow phenomenon") and aggravating skeletal muscle injury. This edema is particularly prominent in patients with profound limb ischemia. When edema occurs in fixed spaces of an extremity, a compartment syndrome may develop, perhaps perpetuating ischemia and leading to arterial reocclusion; this occurs most often in the anterior compartment of the lower extremity. Fasciotomy may be required to correct this situation.[79–81]

The specific mechanisms of reperfusion injury, acting in concert with the initial ischemic insult itself, remain an area of intense laboratory investigation currently. It is hoped that further elucidation of the cellular components involved (leukocytes, endothelial cells, etc.), the cellular receptors that mediate responses, and the biochemical consequences of ischemia-reperfusion will someday enable specific pharmacologic measures to be employed in addition to surgical revascularization to improve the outcome of treatment of acute ischemia.

DIAGNOSIS

Clinical Manifestations

Most frequently, an arterial embolus is associated with sudden onset of acute arterial ischemia. The cardinal signs and symptoms are denoted by the mnemonic five Ps: pulselessness, pain, pallor, paresthesia, and paralysis. Although a useful axiom in general, it is important to stress that none of these characteristics, either singly or together, definitely establishes the diagnosis of acute limb ischemia, nor do they lend themselves to grading or quantification. Furthermore, considerable clinical acumen is required to assess them in combination to gauge the severity of ischemia reliably.[82]

Sudden loss of a previously present pulse is the hallmark of an embolic occlusion. Recognition is easiest when a known pulse existed at a particular site, and obviously more difficult if the prior pulse status of the limb is unknown or abnormal due to associated arteriosclerotic occlusive disease. It is also important to emphasize that a normal or even bounding pulse may often be felt initially at the actual site of embolic impaction, representing transmitted pulsations through the fresh clot (Fig. 43–6). Occasionally, tenderness can be noted over a deep vessel with acute embolic occlusion, clearly defining the point of obstruction.

Pain and pallor are well-known classic symptoms of acute arterial insufficiency. The pain is characteristically a severe and steady ache, involving major muscle groups, below the level of obstruction and usually becoming progressively worse at locations increasingly distal to the point of occlusion. Occasionally, however, sensory disturbances secondary to ischemic neuropathy predominate and may mask primary complaints of pain. In such instances, seen in perhaps 10 to 20 per cent of patients with an acute embolus, the patient may complain primarily of numbness or paresthesias. The limb distal to the occlusion is initially white and waxy—often termed "cadaveric." Subsequently, blotchy mottled areas of cyanosis may appear with eventual blistering and the deeper discoloration typical of early gangrene.

Advanced ischemia is characterized by clinically detectable neurologic deficits, manifested by diminished to absent motor and sensory function, reflecting ischemia to muscles and nerves (or both) distal to the arterial occlusion. The extent of anesthesia and motor paralysis of a limb is a good index of the degree of tissue anoxia and correlates well with the ultimate prognosis. Preservation of sensitivity to light touch is often the best guide to viability and should be compared with that in the uninvolved extremity. Its

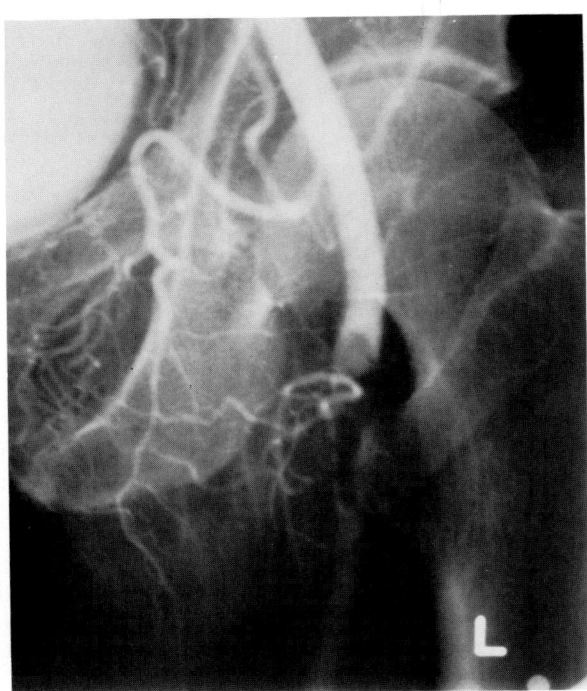

FIGURE 43–6. Femoral embolus obstructing femoral bifurcation, with extension into proximal superficial femoral artery. A bounding femoral pulse was present.

absence demands surgical intervention if at all possible. Paralysis is a similarly grave sign, a late symptom signaling impending gangrene. It represents a combination of severe neural and skeletal muscle ischemia with potential irreversibility. When paralysis proceeds to rigor, the woody hardness associated with involuntary muscle contracture, irreversible ischemia has often developed. Although the limb may still be salvaged by surgical intervention, ultimate function is often permanently compromised, and the metabolic effects of revascularization may be profound and sometimes lethal.

Determination of the site of occlusion is often possible by careful physical examination. In addition to the site of pulse disappearance, a point of temperature demarcation can usually be noted approximately "one joint" distal to the point of occlusion; that is, temperature change just above the ankle often denotes occlusion at the popliteal bifurcation, whereas such a finding at or just above the knee suggests blockage at the femoral bifurcation. Similarly, changes in the upper thigh on one side suggest an iliac embolus, and involvement of both thighs to the groin, lower abdomen, or buttocks suggests an aortic bifurcation *saddle embolus.* In the latter case, one must also be aware of possible associated renal, visceral, or spinal cord ischemia.

Use of a Doppler probe by the examining physician can also provide useful data for stratifying acutely ischemic limbs for therapeutic purposes.[82] The combination of a careful clinical evaluation and assessment of distal arterial and venous Doppler signals allows limbs to be categorized into clinically relevant groupings: viable, threatened, and irreversibly ischemic, as suggested by the Society for Vascular Surgery/International Society for Cardiovascular Surgery (SVS/ISCVS) committee on reporting standards.[83] These are summarized below and shown in Table 43–2.

1. *Viable.* Not immediately threatened; there is no ischemic pain, no neurologic deficit, adequate skin capillary circulation, and clearly audible Doppler pulsatile flow signal in pedal arteries or ankle pressure above 30 mmHg.

2. *Threatened viability.* Implies reversible ischemia and a limb salvageable without major amputation if arterial obstruction is promptly relieved. Ischemic pain or mild and incomplete neurologic deficit is present (e.g., sensory loss involves only vibration, touch, position, or weakness of toe or foot dorsiflexion). "Pulsatile flow" in pedal arteries is *not* audible with Doppler instrument but venous patency is demonstrable.

3. *Major, irreversible ischemic change.* Requires major amputation regardless of therapy. Profound sensory loss and muscle paralysis, absent capillary skin flow or evidence of more advanced ischemia (e.g., muscle rigor or skin marbling) are characteristic; neither arterial nor venous flow signals are audible distally.

Differential Diagnosis

Acute Arterial Thrombosis. Acute arterial occlusion due to an embolus is often difficult to distinguish clinically from in situ thrombosis of a diseased and stenotic artery involved with occlusive disease. Sudden thrombosis may also occasionally occur in a vessel with preexisting aneurysmal disease. Nevertheless, differentiation is of signifi-

Table 43–2. Clinical Categories of Acute Limb Ischemia

					Doppler Signals	
Category	**Description**	**Capillary Return**	**Muscle Weakness**	**Sensory Loss**	***Arterial***	***Venous***
Viable	Not immediately threatened	Intact	None	None	Audible (AP >30 mmHg)	Audible
Threatened	Salvageable if promptly treated	Intact, slow	Mild, partial	Mild, incomplete	Inaudible	Audible
Irreversible	Major tissue loss, amputation regardless of treatment	Absent (marbling)	Profound, paralysis (rigor)	Profound, anesthetic	Inaudible	Inaudible

AP, ankle pressure.
From Rutherford RB, Flanigan DP, Gupta SK, et al: Suggested standards for reports dealing with lower extremity ischemia. J Vasc Surg 64:80, 1986.

Table 43–3. Differentiation of Embolus From Thrombosis

	Embolus	Thrombosis
Identifiable source for embolus	Usual, particularly atrial fibrillation	Less common
History of claudication	Rare	Common
Physical findings suggestive of occlusive disease	Few; proximal and contralateral limb pulses normal	Often present; proximal or contralateral limb pulses diminished or absent
Arteriography	Minimal atherosclerosis; sharp cutoff; few collaterals	Diffuse atherosclerosis; tapered, irregular cutoff; well-developed collaterals

cance in planning treatment.[16, 84] Whereas embolectomy is often successful and the surgical procedure usually limited, attempts at thrombectomy for thrombosis in situ often fail and sometimes even aggravate ischemia, requiring major arterial reconstruction on an emergency basis in a poorly prepared patient.[85, 86] For these reasons, most vascular surgeons prefer to manage acute arterial thrombosis nonoperatively in its initial stages, if feasible.[16, 49, 75, 84–87]

As indicated in Table 43–3, several clues may be obtained from a careful history and physical examination. Typically, patients with an embolus have a sudden onset of symptoms and usually have a recognizable source for an embolus, most often cardiac disease with atrial fibrillation. In Cambria and Abbott's report of acutely ischemic limbs, atrial fibrillation was found in 74 per cent of patients with embolic occlusion, as opposed to only 4 per cent who were thought to have acute thrombotic occlusion.[87] As many as one third of patients with an embolus have had a prior embolic episode. A history of claudication is usually absent in the patient with an embolus, and no evidence of occlusive disease is present in the contralateral limb on pulse examination. The level of temperature change is often quite sharply demarcated in embolic occlusion, in contrast to the patient with preexisting occlusive disease, who has better developed collateral networks.

Angiography. Angiography may also be extremely helpful. In the patient with an embolus, a sharp cutoff, sometimes with a convex filling defect, or ''reversed meniscus,'' in an otherwise fairly normal vessel is seen (Figs. 43–6 and 43–7). Other arteriographic features of embolic occlusion include scant, poorly developed collateral vessels in the region of occlusion and an absence of associated atherosclerotic disease in adjacent arterial segments or the vessels of the contralateral limb. In contrast, patients with acute thrombosis have more obvious and diffuse atheromatous changes and better developed collaterals, with an irregular tapering and end-point at the site of vascular occlusion.

Several other angiographic features may help in differentiation. Obviously, the finding of multiple filling defects within several different arterial beds is almost certain to suggest an embolic etiology. The location of occlusion in an artery may also be helpful. For instance, occlusion noted in the mid to distal superficial femoral artery, centered on the adductor canal, would be typical of acute thrombotic occlusion, whereas an embolus typically lodges at arterial bifurcations. These findings may be obscured, however, by subsequent propagation of clot. For example, an acute popliteal embolus occluding the popliteal bifurcation may develop secondary retrograde thrombus up to the superficial femoral artery at a level of a large geniculate vessel, making determination of the exact point of initial occlusion less certain.

The use of angiography in the evaluation and management of patients with an acutely ischemic extremity remains controversial. In general, most surgeons feel that preoperative angiography for patients with a history and physical findings typical of embolic occlusion is rarely necessary or helpful. Indeed, the additional time taken often only prolongs the ischemia and increases the possibility of a poor outcome. In acute emboli, the distal outflow tract is often not visualized, and little useful information is gained. If distinction between an acute embolus and thrombotic occlusion is difficult, however, angiography may be extremely valuable and is generally advisable in all patients with acute

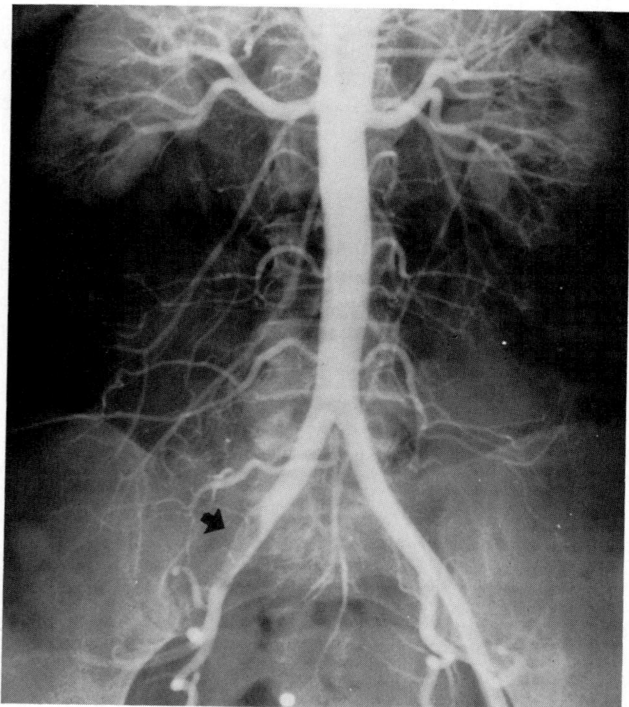

FIGURE 43–7. Acute iliac bifurcation embolus is shown occluding the external iliac artery. Typical reversed meniscus (*arrow*) is seen in the distal common iliac artery, and other vessels are relatively free of atherosclerotic disease.

ischemia as long as the clinical status of the acutely threatened ischemic limb will allow the time (generally 1 to 3 hours) required to obtain such studies. Careful clinical judgment remains of paramount importance in such management decisions.

Aortic Dissection. Acute aortic dissections may sometimes cause sudden limb or organ ischemia with abrupt loss of pulses and other signs of acute ischemia.[88] However, it can usually be differentiated from an acute embolic occlusion by the presence of hypertension and chest or intrascapular back pain radiating downward. A murmur of aortic insufficiency may be present or a difference in the strength and character of right- and left-sided carotid or upper extremity pulses may be detected. Widening of the mediastinum may be noted on chest x-ray. The diagnosis is usually confirmed by aortography, computed tomography (CT) scan, magnetic resonance imaging (MRI), or transesophageal echocardiography. Sometimes limb or visceral ischemia may be transient if spontaneous reentry of the aortic dissection occurs. In some instances, the actual pathologic problem may not be appreciated until embolectomy is attempted,[89] when the surgeon notes that a Fogarty balloon catheter will either not pass beyond the point of occlusion, or if it does, no clot is retrieved nor is blood flow restored. In such instances, the possibility of aortic dissection must be immediately suspected and pursued by further diagnostic evaluation or surgical exploration (see also Chapter 78).

Phlegmasia Cerulea Dolens. Several other conditions are occasionally confused with lower extremity emboli. Phlegmasia cerulea dolens due to massive iliofemoral deep venous thrombosis may present with a suddenly painful leg. Indeed, swelling often makes pulses difficult to feel, and in its late stages secondary arterial insufficiency may in fact develop. However, it is usually differentiated initially by the sudden acute swelling of the limb always present at the onset, an atypical initial presentation for acute arterial occlusion. In addition, the intense cyanotic congestion of the limb with deep venous thrombosis and phlegmasia is in distinct contrast to the typical pallor and collapsed superficial veins seen with acute arterial insufficiency.

Neurologic Disorders. In some patients, neurologic manifestations of acute ischemia may predominate and cause confusion with primary neurologic disorders. This is most common in patients with limb numbness as the presenting sign of an acute embolus. On occasion, aortic saddle emboli may present primarily with the sudden onset of bilateral lower extremity weakness and sensory loss, progressing rapidly to a paraplegic-like state. Care must be taken to avoid initial confusion with acute neurologic problems, leading to time-consuming and misdirected therapeutic efforts.[90]

Low Output States. Hypovolemia and diminished cardiac output, particularly in a patient with longstanding absent distal pulses, may occasionally be confused with acute limb ischemia due to emboli. Sepsis, myocardial infarction, pulmonary embolus, dehydration, and acute intra-abdominal catastrophes are among the disease states sometimes confused with an acute arterial occlusion. Swan-Ganz catheter insertion with determination of cardiac output and systemic vascular resistance usually permits differentiation of these disorders. Recognition of the primary underlying disease also facilitates differentiation from primary acute arterial insufficiency. Nevertheless, a major aortic saddle embolus in a patient with a massive acute myocardial infarction may present in precisely this manner.

SURGICAL TREATMENT

Today, optimal therapy in the great majority of cases of arterial embolism is prompt surgical removal by embolectomy. This requires an expeditious diagnosis of acute arterial ischemia followed by recognition of a probable embolic etiology based on the clinical features already outlined. With the availability of anticoagulants, improved vascular surgical techniques, and particularly simplification of the operative procedure by use of the Fogarty embolectomy catheter, there has been a dramatic trend toward surgical management over the past three decades; whereas only 23 per cent of arterial emboli were treated by embolectomy in the years 1937 to 1946 at the Massachusetts General Hospital, 88 per cent underwent surgical treatment between 1964 and 1980, the most recent era reviewed.[14]

Full doses of intravenous heparin should be administered as soon as the diagnosis of acute arterial ischemia is made. This is intended to prevent clot propagation and stabilize the patient long enough to allow consideration of diagnostic possibilities and, most important, evaluation and initial treatment of the cardiac abnormalities present in the great percentage of patients with embolic disease. Overt or subtle cardiac failure, myocardial ischemia, arrhythmias, electrolyte disturbances, and similar problems are managed by judicious use of cardiac glycosides, antiarrhythmic agents, diuretics, and other appropriate maneuvers.

Preoperative preparation should otherwise be minimal so that operation is delayed as little as possible. Laboratory studies include complete blood count, serum electrolyte, blood urea nitrogen (BUN) and creatinine determinations, baseline cardiac enzymes, coagulation parameters, and blood typing and cross-matching. A chest film and electrocardiogram are obtained to detect and evaluate cardiac disease. Doppler studies may be performed in both extremities as an aid in assessing and stratifying the severity of ischemia and to serve as a baseline for postoperative comparison. A central venous catheter is inserted via the subclavian or internal jugular vein to diagnose and treat hypovolemia. If necessary in an unstable patient, a thermodilution Swan-Ganz catheter may be placed to facilitate cardiac monitoring. A radial artery line may be indicated when large fluid- or acid-based shifts are likely, as for example in patients with a suspected aortic saddle embolus.

Except in unusual circumstances, the operation is performed employing local anesthesia and limited incisions, both helpful in the generally high-risk group of patients with an arterial embolus. Close monitoring by an anesthesiologist is generally advisable; however, wide prepping and draping are recommended in case modification of the operative approach is required.

Iliac and Femoral Emboli

Most lower extremity emboli can be successfully managed via a groin incision and femoral arteriotomy. Under local anesthesia, the common, superficial, and deep femoral arteries are gently exposed and controlled with Silastic loops. Either a transverse or a vertical arteriotomy may be utilized; if the femoral artery is diseased, a vertical arteriotomy may be preferable because it generally affords better access to branches for catheter manipulation and is more appropriate in case local endarterectomy, profundaplasty, or bypass grafting becomes necessary. A vertical arteriotomy may be closed with a patch if primary closure of the diseased vessel appears likely to compromise the lumen.

The technique of catheter embolectomy is familiar to all vascular surgeons (see Chapter 21), although several recent modifications of catheter design and adjunctive maneuvers have been developed to improve the management of acute thromboembolic arterial occlusions.[9] An appropriately sized embolectomy balloon catheter is inserted proximally or distally past the occlusive clot and carefully withdrawn in the inflated position (Fig. 43–8). Generally, No. 2 and No. 3 balloon catheters are used for embolectomy of the profunda femoris, popliteal, and tibial arteries, No. 3 and No. 4 catheters are used for common and superficial artery embolectomies, and a No. 4 or No. 5 catheter is used in the proximal aortoiliac system. Passage down the profunda femoris should not exceed 25 to 30 cm. Several passes are made until no further thrombus is extracted, and forceful, pulsatile inflow is obtained. It is important that one surgeon inflate and withdraw the catheter to determine the appropriate amount of traction and inflation pressure to be used, thereby minimizing the chance of vessel trauma or dislodgment of arteriosclerotic plaques in a diseased vessel. Inability to pass the balloon catheter distally is more commonly due to occlusive disease or vessel angulation than to blockage by the embolic clot, which is usually readily passed with the embolectomy catheter. Overly forceful attempts to pass the catheter should be avoided, lest arterial injury produce hemorrhage, false aneurysm, arteriovenous fistula formation, dissection, or thrombosis. Maneuvers that are helpful if vessel angulation or tortuosity hampers distal passage of the catheter include simultaneous insertion of several catheters, varying the angle of the knee joint, or preforming an angle in the tip of the catheter followed by rotation of the catheter tip during introduction. If fluoroscopy is available, passing two catheters with contrast used to inflate the balloon so that its location can be noted may be helpful, particularly if the fluoroscopic equipment has roadmapping capabilities. Use of intraoperative angioscopy may similarly help in guiding the direction of an embolectomy catheter into specific distal vessels. Partial inflation of the balloon at the site of obstruction may recenter the catheter in a diseased vessel, and deflation and gentle advancement may then allow the catheter to pass. After satisfactory exploration of the distal vasculature, dilute heparinized saline solution (1000 units in 50 ml saline) is flushed distally, and the vessels are occluded with gentle vascular clamps.

After good inflow has been restored and all distal clot removed, the arteriotomy is closed primarily or with a patch, the clamps are removed, and flow is restored. It is essential for the surgeon to then assess the adequacy of revascularization. Failure to recover any additional distal thrombus and the presence of backbleeding are no assurance that distal patency and adequate revascularization have been achieved. Indeed, when arteriography is employed routinely following embolectomy, as many as 35 to 40 per cent of embolectomies are found to be incomplete with residual thrombus being noted.[92] Assessment may be made by clinical examination of the distal limb and palpation of distal pulses, but these criteria are frequently difficult to evaluate immediately after revascularization. Associated occlusive disease, vasospasm, and related problems may cause uncertainty about the adequacy of clot removal. Doppler pressure measurements or pulse volume recordings may supplement clinical evaluation.[93] In many instances, however, completion intraoperative arteriography remains the best means of ensuring the completeness of the embolectomy procedure. If available, angioscopy may also be very useful in assessing the completeness of embolectomy.[91] However, overall evaluation of the adequacy of distal runoff by this means may be difficult. Regardless of the method used, it is vital for the surgeon to document in some fashion the effectiveness of revascularization.

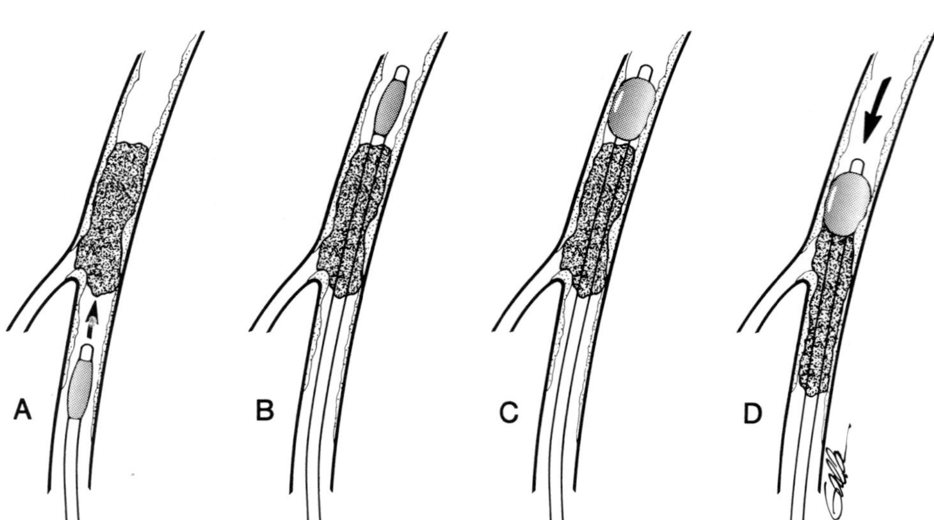

FIGURE 43–8. Extraction of an embolus by balloon-tipped embolectomy catheter. *A* and *B*, The deflated catheter is passed beyond the thromboembolus, the balloon is inflated (*C*) and then gently withdrawn (*D*), carrying thromboembolic material with it.

New Catheters for Adherent Thrombus

If intraoperative evaluation by any of these described methods suggests incomplete clot removal, additional steps must be taken. Recent modifications of the conventional balloon embolectomy catheter may be helpful in this regard. Although the standard balloon catheter is quite effective in removing soft, fresh clot, older and more organized and adherent thrombus, particularly in areas of atherosclerotic disease or within synthetic grafts, may be much more difficult to retrieve completely from a remote access site. The Fogarty adherent clot catheter (Fig. 43–9) has a retrieval end that is composed of a latex-covered spiral coil instead of an inflatable balloon. The diameter may be manually adjusted from 2 to 10 mm. It is passed in the low profile configuration so that the retrieval portion of the catheter is positioned within the region of the adherent material. To effect removal of the thrombus, the pitch of the spiral corkscrew balloon is adjusted according to feel via a control knob on the handle of the catheter. This engages the adherent material within the spiral coils of the device. Although the technique of insertion, inflation, and withdrawal is quite similar to that of the standard balloon catheter, the mechanism of thrombus entrapment and removal is quite different and is more effective in removing tenacious organized and adherent thrombus.[91] A related catheter, the graft thrombectomy catheter, is quite similar in design except that the spiral retrieval wire elements are shorter and stiffer and have no latex covering (Fig. 43–10). This design enables the surgeon to exert additional traction on the wall of the lumen, a feature that is particularly useful for removing the mature adherent pannus or pseudointima often found in occluded synthetic grafts or arteriovenous fistulae. It is meant for more aggressive thrombectomy in occluded prostheses and consists of a variable diameter ring stripper that allows the surgeon to vary the force and amount of traction exerted on the wall of Dacron or polytetrafluoroethylene (PTFE) grafts.

As an alternative to further attempts at catheter thromboembolectomy, the surgeon may attempt to remove residual thrombus under direct visualization with the angioscope, using various grabbing or biopsy tools that are commonly available in this era of increasing endoscopic surgical procedures. Or intraoperative lytic therapy (discussed later) may be considered for removal of residual distal thrombus.

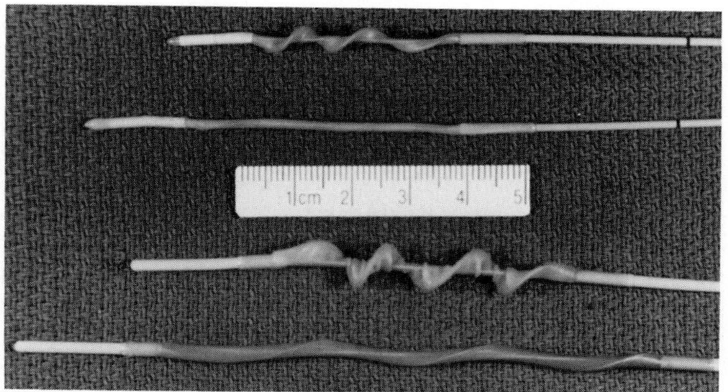

FIGURE 43–9. Adherent clot catheter in low profile and partially expanded configuration. Note corkscrew-type configuration of retrieval element in 4 Fr and 6 Fr sizes.

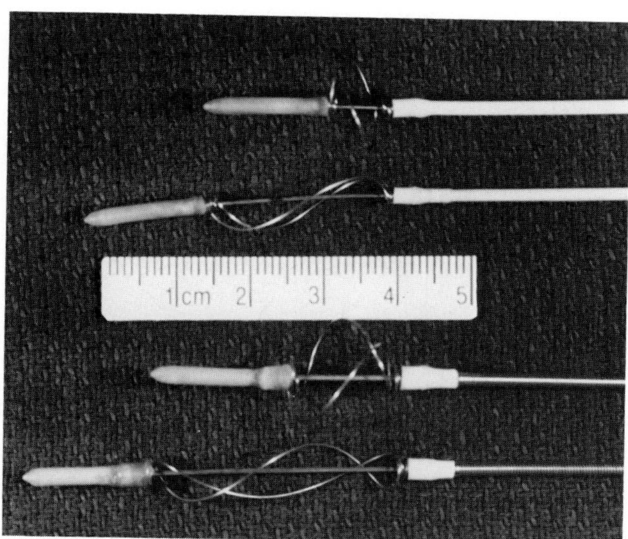

FIGURE 43–10. Graft thrombectomy catheter in low-profile and partially expanded configurations in 5 Fr *(above)* and 6 Fr *(below)* sizes. Wire elements of varying diameter retrieve adherent thrombus from the walls of synthetic grafts.

Aortic Saddle Emboli

In most instances of embolic occlusion of the terminal aorta, a transfemoral approach will still be feasible.[94] This obviously is a major advantage of the balloon catheter. As shown in Figure 43–11, both femoral arteries are exposed and opened, with passage of embolectomy catheters up both sides to prevent dislodgment of thrombus down the other side. Larger embolectomy catheters are required. Blood loss associated with the flushing required with a bilateral femoral approach may be substantial, and careful assessment of the volume status may require transfusion.

If good inflow cannot be restored, usually due to preexisting occlusive disease at the aortic bifurcation, or if concern exists about concomitant mesenteric or renal artery embolic compromise, which may coexist in up to 20 per cent of aortic saddle emboli,[28] a direct transperitoneal or retroperitoneal approach is indicated, obviously requiring induction of general anesthesia.

Popliteal Emboli

Most surgeons still prefer to approach lower limb emboli via a groin incision and distal passage of the embolectomy catheter through a femoral arteriotomy. In many instances, a popliteal embolus can be successfully removed in this fashion, and adequate clot retrieval can be documented by completion arteriography. In some cases, however, residual clot cannot be adequately extracted; this is particularly true if clot extension down the tibial vessels is present (Fig. 43–12). Since anatomic studies have shown

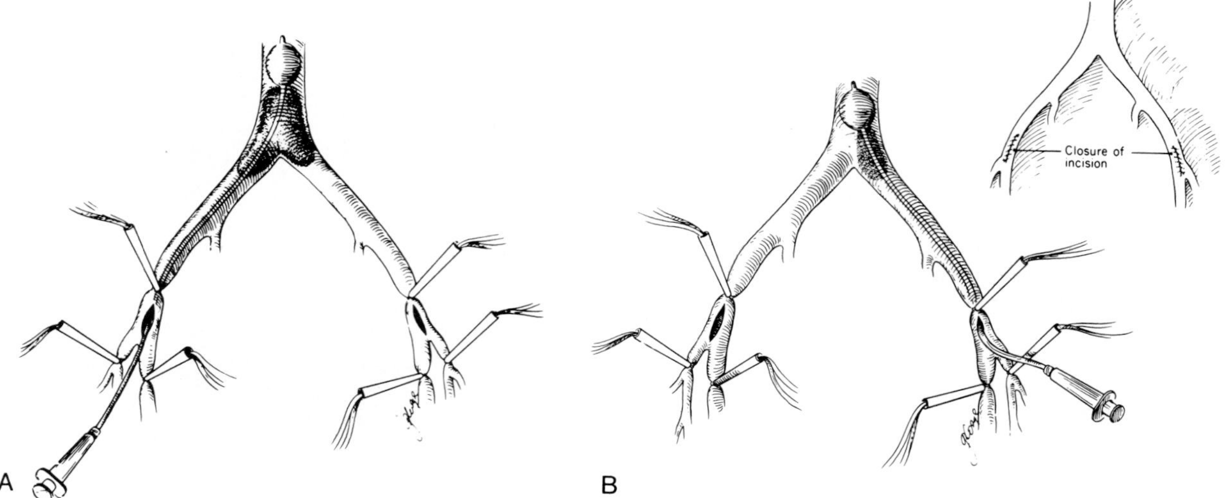

FIGURE 43–11. Transfemoral extraction of aortic saddle embolus. *A*, A No. 5 or 6 Fogarty catheter is passed from a femoral arteriotomy after exposure and control of both femoral arteries in the groin have been obtained. This is then withdrawn, extracting the bulk of the embolus. Contralateral femoral vessel is occluded simultaneously to prevent distal thromboemboli. *B*, Remaining thrombus is removed by passing a catheter from the other side, followed by closure of arteriotomies. (*A* and *B*, From Busuttil RW, Keehn G, Milliken J, et al: Aortic saddle embolus: A twenty-year experience. Ann Surg 197:698, 1983.)

that a catheter passed from above will go down the peroneal artery in nearly 90 per cent of patients,[95] clot in the anterior or posterior tibial vessels that branch from the popliteal artery at varying angles may be impossible to remove via a proximal femoral approach. Insertion of additional catheters, with angulation of the knee, can sometimes achieve cannulation of other tibial vessels, or some of the other maneuvers previously described using adjunctive fluoroscopy, guidewires, or angioscopy, may be successful.[9]

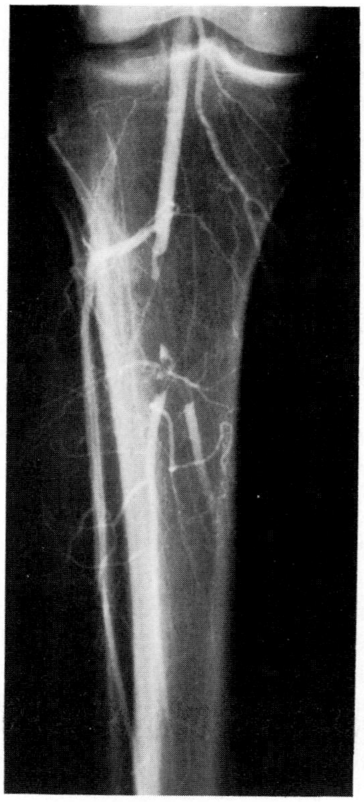

FIGURE 43–12. Distal popliteal embolus with extension into posterior tibial and peroneal branches.

If an initial transfemoral approach is used, the extracted thrombus should be examined: a smooth taper suggests adequate clot removal; a sharp cutoff implies retained clot. An arteriogram is then performed. If it reveals residual thrombus that cannot be extracted from above, direct exploration of the below-knee popliteal artery is required. Although this can sometimes be accomplished under local anesthesia, regional or general anesthesia is frequently necessary for adequate exposure and patient comfort. The distal popliteal artery is exposed, the soleal muscle insertion taken down, and the anterior tibial vein ligated and divided to expose the anterior tibial artery origin and tibioperoneal trunk (Fig. 43–13). Upon exposure of the distal popliteal artery and its tibial branches, the embolectomy catheter can be advanced from above and guided into the individual branches by external compression of the other branches with vascular forceps. Or a distal popliteal arteriotomy may be performed, and each tibial vessel selectively catheterized under direct vision with a No. 2 catheter. In this fashion, the ability to completely remove distal clot is maximized.[96, 97]

In Abbott and colleagues' report from the Massachusetts General Hospital, a transfemoral approach for popliteal emboli was successful in only 49 per cent of instances without direct popliteal artery exposure.[96] It is recommended that the appropriate surgical approach to patients with popliteal embolism be based upon the presence or absence of a popliteal pulse. If the pulse is absent, the initial attempt at embolectomy may be made via the transfemoral route using a Fogarty balloon-tipped catheter. However, if a popliteal pulse is present, presumably the embolus is at or distal to the popliteal artery bifurcation, and the popliteal artery below the knee is exposed as the initial step. In either case, completion arteriography is an essential feature of a

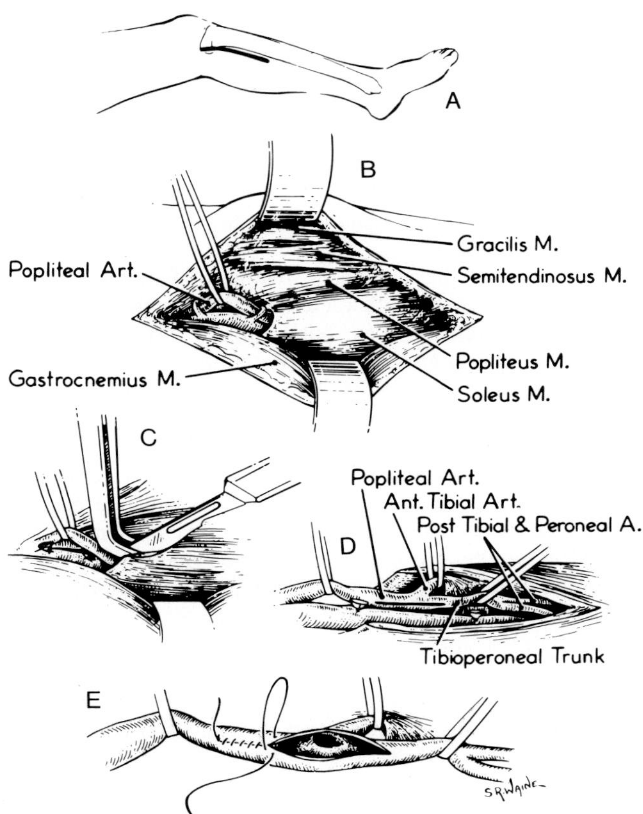

FIGURE 43–13. *A*, Incision for exposure of the distal part of the popliteal artery. *B*, Exposure of the vascular bundle after incision of the deep fascia and retraction of gastrocnemius muscle medially and posteriorly. *C*, Division of overlying soleus muscle fibers. *D*, Mobilized distal popliteal artery, anterior tibial artery, and tibioperoneal trunk and position of longitudinal incision in the artery. *E*, Ostia of anterior tibial artery as seen through the arteriotomy, and closure of the arteriotomy with fine vascular sutures without producing any stenosis. (*A–E*, From Gupta SK, Samson RH, Veith FJ, et al: Embolectomy of the distal part of the popliteal artery. Surg Gynecol Obstet 153:255, 1981. By permission of *Surgery, Gynecology & Obstetrics*.)

properly conducted popliteal embolectomy and should always be done at the termination of the procedure.

Distal Tibial Embolectomy

Occasionally, thromboembolic material will remain in the distal tibial vessels despite a direct approach through the distal popliteal artery and selective catheterization of the tibial vessels from this level. This is particularly likely if substantial delay in operative intervention has occurred, making propagation of clot in distal vessels and greater inflammatory organization and adherence of the thromboembolic material more likely. In such circumstances, direct exploration of the distal tibial vessels at the ankle may be required.[33, 98] Each vessel is approached through a longitudinal incision just proximal to the ankle joint. The posterior tibial artery is located deep to the flexor retinaculum midway between the medial malleolus and calcaneus tendon. The anterior tibial artery is located deep to the extensor retinaculum between the tendons of the extensor hallucis longus and the extensor digitorum longus. By direct manipulation of the vessels with gentle simultaneous probing of the catheter from the popliteal arteriotomy, it may be possible to pass the catheter beyond the point of obstruction and remove the embolic material. If not, a small transverse arteriotomy is made, and a No. 2 Fogarty catheter is passed retrograde and antegrade to extract distal thrombus. The arteriotomies are closed with 7–0 monofilament sutures under magnification. Although infrequently required, such maneuvers may occasionally be necessary for limb salvage.

Intraoperative Thrombolytic Therapy

An alternative method for dealing with retained distal tibial and small vessel thromboembolic material that cannot be adequately managed with conventional catheter techniques is the intraoperative adjunctive use of fibrinolytic agents. Although recent surgical procedures are generally accepted as a strong relative contraindication to systemic thrombolytic therapy owing to the high incidence of bleeding complications, accumulating clinical experience has suggested that more localized direct distal infusion of lytic agents during standard surgical procedures is safe and often beneficial.[99–103]

Experimental work has suggested that blood flow is improved and salvage of ischemic muscle is accomplished with less reperfusion edema and ischemic muscle injury when lytic agents are infused.[104–106] This result, which is presumably due to restoration of perfusion in the small arteriolar branches of larger axial vessels, is not possible with mechanical catheter thromboembolectomy.

The specific lytic agent employed, the dosage, and the method of infusion vary considerably among different investigators. At present, urokinase appears to be faster and safer than streptokinase and is just as effective as the more expensive and less easily available recombinant tissue plasminogen activator. From 250,000 to 350,000 units of urokinase are infused through a small catheter into the most distal vessel containing thrombus, either as a bolus or as a dripping infusion over approximately 30 minutes, and a distal arteriogram is then repeated. In Comerota and White's experience with 53 patients with persistent ischemia and impending limb loss due to extensive distal thrombosis despite maximal standard efforts with catheter thromboembolectomy, use of adjunctive regional intraoperative lytic therapy resulted in limb salvage in 70 per cent of patients. In 47 per cent, limb salvage was judged to be directly attributable to lysis, and only one patient (2 per cent) had a major bleeding complication.[100] Although it is always difficult in such reports to determine precisely whether the ultimate outcome was due to the initial surgical procedure or to the lytic therapy itself, growing evidence suggests that adjunctive lytic therapy should be considered whenever arteriography or angioscopy demonstrates residual small vessel distal clot beyond the reach of the embolectomy catheter, or whenever persistent pedal or digital ischemia follows standard surgical efforts at revascularization. As an extension of this concept in truly desperate situations with extensive multi-vessel distal occlusions and severely ischemic extremities, investigation of a technique of "high-dose isolated limb perfusion" is being undertaken.[99, 100] This technique involves exsanguination of blood from the limb with a rubber bandage, application of a thigh tourniquet to achieve complete arterial and venous occlusion, and direct arterial infusion of a high dose (1 million units or more) of urokinase into the affected vessels. The venous effluent is drained by a catheter placed in the popliteal vein, and lytic perfusion of the isolated distal limb segment is continued over a 45- to 60-minute period. Although this technique appears promising in difficult clinical situations, lytic agents are ineffective in patients with a "trash foot" due to cholesterol-atheromatous embolic debris or highly organized thrombus, and this remains a significant clinical problem.[100]

Upper Extremity Emboli

Embolic occlusion of upper extremity vessels is the most common cause of acute ischemia of the arm or hand. In the review by Ricotta and associates, 57 per cent of cases of acute upper extremity ischemia were due to emboli that originated in the heart.[107] Twenty-five per cent had arm ischemia as a result of upper extremity catheterization for angiographic study or hemodynamic monitoring, and the remaining 18 per cent had ischemia resulting from proximal arterial disease of diverse types. In a significant percentage of this latter group, the acute event developed from embolization from the proximal arterial site, however. Examples of proximal arterial abnormalities that may be a source of upper extremity emboli include atherosclerotic plaques or aneurysms of the great vessels, problems related to thoracic outlet compression, arteritis or postradiation changes, traumatic aneurysms, and prior axillofemoral grafts.

The great majority of upper extremity emboli lodge at or just below the brachial artery and are most commonly approached by a brachial arteriotomy under local anesthesia in the antecubital fossa. Although more abundant collateral circulation makes limb loss less likely than with lower extremity embolic events, the relative ease, safety, and excellent results of transbrachial embolectomy warrant a surgical approach in all but a few patients. Only patients expected to die from their underlying disease or in whom the embolus is so peripheral that there is insignificant ischemia should be denied the potential benefits of embolectomy. The relatively unusual proximal subclavian and axillary emboli also nearly always can be successfully managed by a retrograde transbrachial approach.

If a noncardiac proximal source of an embolus is suspected from the history, physical findings, or lack of evident heart disease, preoperative arteriography is of utmost importance to avoid overlooking such a source. Direct surgical repair of the proximal cause is required in addition to embolectomy.

Delayed Embolectomy

It has been traditionally taught that arterial embolism must be recognized and treated early, and many series have documented that early operation improves survival and limb salvage rates. Nonetheless, it has been well established that there is a significant group of patients who may present days or weeks after an embolic event with a viable but compromised extremity.[108–110] The absence of muscle necrosis in these patients indicates that propagated thrombus has not extended into inaccessible branch vessels and suggests that effective collateral channels and a patent distal arterial tree exist.

In some of these patients, recognition of an embolic cause may be based on characteristic features of the history and clinical circumstances, but in many instances of delayed presentation arteriography is required. The diagnosis of an embolic cause may be suggested by the lack of well-formed collaterals, abrupt termination of the dye column, or an atypical location of the occlusion. In many such instances, balloon catheter embolectomy can successfully restore arterial patency. In some patients with late presentation, retrieval of an embolus by a balloon catheter inserted through a remote arteriotomy may be unsuccessful because an embolic clot that has been present in an artery for a prolonged period may well have engendered a localized inflammatory response and become adherent to the vessel wall. In such circumstances, a direct approach to the site of occlusion, with arteriotomy directly over the involved vessel is required (Fig. 43–14). Removal of such chronic organized adherent emboli often requires sharp dissection off the vessel wall with an endarterectomy spatula or similar instrument. It is nearly always possible to establish an appropriate plane of dissection between the thromboembolus and the vessel wall; dissection in a true endarterectomy plane within the vessel wall media is avoided to prevent jeopardy to the patency of outflow tract vessels.[108] Following thromboembolectomy, closure with a patch may be elected. In a few instances, bypass grafting, profundaplasty, or similar reconstructive techniques may be required. It should be emphasized that late embolectomy should not be attempted in the limb with advanced, probably irreversible, ischemia; the metabolic dangers of revascularization are very real and outweigh the small likelihood of salvaging a functional limb.[75]

Perioperative Management

Because of the potential for severe adverse systemic effects of revascularization of acute severely ischemic extremities due to the ischemia-reperfusion syndrome previously described, steps should be taken in the operating room at the time of embolectomy to minimize the consequences of reperfusion. Anticipation of possible sudden acidosis or hyperkalemia requires administration of sodium bicarbonate or glucose and insulin if necessary. Induction of diuresis with mannitol and alkalinization of the urine will help to avoid precipitation of myoglobin in the renal collecting tubules and will lessen the chances of acute renal failure following revascularization. Mannitol may have other beneficial effects by acting as a scavenger of oxygen-derived free radicals, which appear to be an important intermediary in ischemia-reperfusion injury.[111–113] Active investigation of numerous other pharmacologic agents or other methods of ameliorating reperfusion injury are underway in

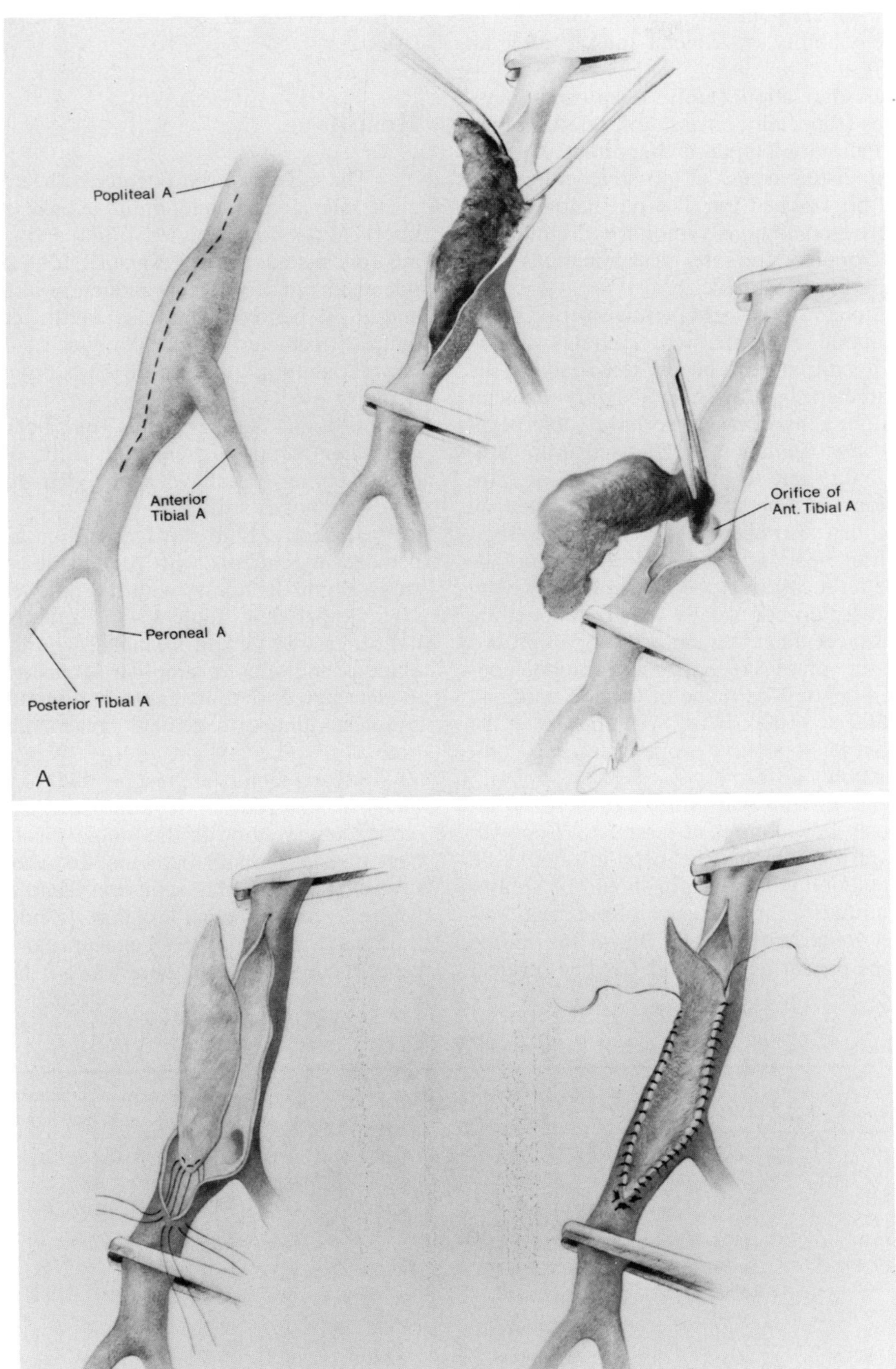

FIGURE 43–14. *A*, Direct exposure of popliteal artery allowing longitudinal arteriotomy, embolectomy assisted by endarterectomy spatula, and direct visualization of orifice of anterior tibial artery. *B*, Closure of arteriotomy with saphenous vein patch using interrupted mattress technique at distal end of arteriotomy. (*A* and *B*, From Cambria RP, Ridge BA, Brewster DC, et al: Delayed presentation and treatment of popliteal artery embolism. Ann Surg 214:50, 1991.)

many laboratories.[114] Although none is currently in standard clinical use, it is hoped that further experimental work may yield agents or strategies that can be used by the surgeon during the period of standard operative revascularization to further increase the viability of skeletal muscle after an ischemic episode.

Following revascularization, careful monitoring of vital signs, electrolytes (especially potassium), arterial blood gases and pH, and urinary output is important. Cardiac ischemia or rhythm disturbances, or possible congestive heart failure should be watched for. The circulatory status of the limb should be continuously monitored clinically, supplemented by Doppler pressure determinations and pulse volume recordings as available.

Heparin is continued in the perioperative period, both to reduce the likelihood of a recurrent embolus and to minimize chances of arterial reocclusion secondary to the intimal damage inflicted by the embolectomy catheter itself.[115, 116] In addition, heparin may also have some properties other than its anticoagulation capability that are beneficial in lessening injury due to muscle ischemia-reperfusion.[114] Continuation of heparin in the immediate postoperative period can also decrease the risks of associated deep venous thrombosis or pulmonary embolism. Although there will be an increase in the incidence of wound hematomas,[28, 31, 117] these do not usually require reoperation and appear to be an acceptable "trade-off" for improved patency and reduction of early recurrent thromboembolism.[1, 115, 118] Use of a continuous mode of heparin administration, generally 500 to 1000 U/hr, will minimize the chances of significant postoperative wound bleeding compared to intermittent bolus doses.[119]

Oral anticoagulation with warfarin (Coumadin) is instituted simultaneously but requires at least 5 to 7 days to become effective, during which time heparin should be continued. Anticoagulation with warfarin should be continued indefinitely to minimize the incidence of recurrent emboli (see later under Recurrent Emboli), unless the source of the embolus can be primarily corrected. Cardiac surgical repair, successful cardioversion of atrial fibrillation, and resection and grafting of proximal aneurysmal lesions are some examples of correctable sources of emboli, repair of which may obviate the necessity for long-term anticoagulation.

Results

The advent of the Fogarty catheter has simplified surgical management and improved the results of operative intervention in most series. Elliott and colleagues cited a 75 per cent increase in good results, a 66 per cent decrease in fair results, a 35 per cent reduction in the amputation rate, and a 50 per cent decrease in the death rate since the balloon catheter was introduced. The improvements brought about by the use of the balloon catheter were particularly evident in their series of patients with aortoiliac embolization.[1] Similar trends have been noted in other series when results of treatment in the pre- and postballoon embolectomy eras have been compared, although differences are not as striking.[14, 22, 31, 32]

Currently, limb salvage may be achieved in 85 to 95 per cent of patients with peripheral emboli who undergo surgical embolectomy, with mortality rates in the range of 10 to 20 per cent (Table 43–4). Differences among individual series are often attributable to variations in patient populations and sites of embolic occlusion. Nonetheless, it is evident that despite its apparent simplicity, arterial embolization continues to present considerable risk to life and limb.

Several factors are responsible for this substantial morbidity and mortality. Most surgeons agree that prompt operative intervention is the single most important determinant of a successful outcome. In Abbott and colleagues' review from the Massachusetts General Hospital, patients whose treatment began less than 12 hours after onset had a limb salvage rate of 93 per cent and mortality of 19 per cent. In contrast, when there was a delay of greater than 12

Table 43–4. Results of Surgical Treatment of Arterial Emboli

Year of Report	Author	No. Patients	No. Emboli	Mortality (%)	Limb Salvage (%)
1967	Darling[28]	260	426	23	91
1970	Thompson[68]	163	203	15	93
1971	Fogarty[33]	300	330	16	95
1975	Green[31]	228	247	23	84
1976	Hight[32]	124	152	30	78
1978	Satiani[18]	122	135	11	81
1980	Elliott[1]	225	260	4	84
1980	Silvers[20]	106	156	22	87
1981	Kendrick[17]	90	121	28	71
1982	Abbott[14]	313	349	20	86
1982	Sheiner[19]	134	148	20	87
1984	Connett[15]	111	130	14	95
1984	Dale[16]	65	71	11	73
1985	Tawes[21]	739	739	12	95
1985	Galbraith[23]	120	129	20	87
1986	Panetta[22]	326	400	11	91
1987	Degrelid[24]	202	202	26	82
1987	Englund[25]	253	269	16	92
1988	Baxter-Smith[26]	221	248	22	83
1992	Varty[27]	84	84	39	89

hours, only 78 per cent had limb salvage and 31 per cent died.[14] Elliott and coworkers found that within a range of 8 hours to 7 days, the effect of delayed treatment had a linear relationship to severity of ischemic changes and unfavorable results.[1]

Other factors that continue to exert a negative influence on the outcome of arterial embolectomy are the severity of underlying cardiac problems responsible for the embolus, the increasing incidence of associated arteriosclerotic peripheral vascular occlusive disease, which hampers limb salvage, and the systemic metabolic complications associated with increasingly aggressive attempts at limb salvage.[120] As patients with emboli get older and the incidence of arteriosclerotic heart disease increases, risks of operation largely offset the gains of a simplified technique and better postoperative care. When data are broken down into arteriosclerotic and nonarteriosclerotic causes of emboli, the marked differences in risk are apparent. In Freund and coworkers' report, the mortality rate for arteriosclerotic cases was 52 per cent compared to 18 per cent in those without arteriosclerotic heart disease, whereas Haimovici and associates noted a rate of 46 per cent versus 7.7 per cent.[120, 121] Advancing age is also a significant risk factor. Jarrett and Detmer reported a 6.8 per cent mortality rate for patients less than 70 years of age, whereas older patients had a mortality rate of 22 per cent.[122]

Complications

Complications associated with embolectomy can be categorized as those related to use of the balloon catheter itself and those related to the condition of advanced ischemia.

Arterial Injuries. Acute complications directly related to catheter application occur in approximately 0.5 to 1.0 per cent of cases.[123, 124] The true frequency of arterial injury is unknown because manifestations are often delayed, angiographic follow-up after catheter embolectomy is relatively uncommon, and minor injuries may be overlooked or attributed to the underlying disease process itself. Arterial perforation is most common, but arterial rupture, pseudoaneurysm formation, intimal dissection, arteriovenous fistula formation, and even catheter-tipped separation with fragment embolization have been reported.[125–128] With retrograde passage of larger-sized balloon catheters from a femoral arteriotomy, care should be taken to limit the length of catheter insertion to 30 to 35 cm to avoid possible damage to renal or visceral vessels.[129] In addition to such immediate problems, later adverse effects of catheter-related trauma to the endothelial flow surface and vessel wall may result in myointimal hyperplasia or accelerated atherosclerosis and marked narrowing of such vessels, which is noted on subsequent arteriography.[130–133]

These problems underscore the fact that despite its simplicity, catheter embolectomy must be carried out gently, with awareness that diseased vessels are frequently encountered in patients with arterial emboli. Repeated and forceful probing is responsible for many such injuries. Little force is required to generate high lateral wall pressures (500 to 1200 mmHg or more) with the mechanical advantage of a small-bore syringe. The smallest balloon size sufficient for clot removal should be used, overdistention of the balloon and excessive traction during balloon withdrawal should be avoided, and the number of catheter passages should be kept as few as possible.[128]

Arterial Reocclusion. Recurrent arterial ischemia may occur in the early postoperative period following embolectomy. Although recurrent emboli to the same site are occasionally responsible, thrombosis secondary to areas of intimal injury or incomplete removal of the thromboembolic material is more likely. It is well recognized that the process of balloon catheter embolectomy often denudes the endothelium, rendering the arterial surface thrombogenic.[116, 130] Increasing use of catheters in vessels already compromised by associated arteriosclerosis also increases the likelihood of rethrombosis. The importance of diligent clinical observation of the embolectomized limb and the value of peri- and postoperative use of anticoagulants are underscored by such observations.

If recurrent ischemia is noted, prompt reoperation is generally indicated. In many instances secondary arterial reconstructive procedures may be necessary to achieve limb salvage.[134] In the large experience reported by Tawes, Fogarty, and associates, 21 per cent of surviving patients undergoing balloon embolectomy required early secondary surgical procedures to ensure a favorable long-term result.[21] Such secondary procedures included repeat thromboembolectomy, endarterectomy, profundaplasty, patch angioplasty, bypass procedures, and sympathectomy.

Compartment Syndrome. Following revascularization, significant limb swelling may occur, leading to compartmental compression, particularly in the anterior compartment. Concomitant venous thrombosis may exacerbate the situation. Such compartmental swelling may lead to neurologic compromise or impairment of distal blood flow. If prolonged severe ischemia has existed prior to embolectomy, the surgeon may elect to perform fasciotomy empirically in conjunction with embolectomy.[79–81] Alternatively, because fasciotomy can usually be easily performed subsequently, the limb can be watched carefully after revascularization and fasciotomy carried out as a delayed procedure if necessary. Although some authorities have advocated use of compartmental pressure measurements as a more objective indication of the need for fasciotomy,[135, 136] most surgeons have found them difficult and of uncertain reliability. Most often, decisions regarding fasciotomy in the management of acute embolic ischemia are based upon individual preferences, prior clinical experience, and empiricism.

The major risk of fasciotomy is infection. Necrotic muscle, which often atrophies and resorbs if left alone, is exposed to possible infection after fasciotomy, with limb- or even life-threatening consequences. The decision to perform fasciotomy should therefore be weighed carefully against these risks.[75, 137]

Metabolic Complications. As discussed previously, serious systemic complications can follow revascularization of a severely ischemic limb. Acidosis, hyperkalemia, renal failure secondary to myoglobinuria, and pulmonary insufficiency secondary to washout of platelet aggregates and thrombotic debris in the venous effluent of the revascularized limb can result.[75, 76] Indeed, the likelihood of such potentially devastating complications has led some authorities such as Blaisdell to advocate avoidance of embolectomy in patients with advanced ischemia (see later section, Nonoperative Management).

As noted earlier under Perioperative Management, it is important for the surgeon and anesthesiologist to anticipate the possible development of such systemic problems. Use of bicarbonate to offset acidosis and correction of hyperkalemia by use of intravenous insulin and glucose, oral or rectal administration of exchange resins, or even hemodialysis are essential. Establishment of a brisk diuresis by means of vigorous hydration, use of an osmotic diuretic such as mannitol, and alkalinization of the urine are employed to reduce the risk of renal failure. Phlebotomy of the involved limb following reestablishment of arterial flow, with removal of the first 300 to 500 ml of venous blood flow, may be advisable to prevent the toxic venous effluent from entering the systemic circulation.[21] If available, autotransfusion devices can salvage this blood and return the packed cells to the patient after washing.

Recurrent Emboli. The incidence of recurrent embolic events is significant, particularly if postoperative anticoagulation is not carried out or is inadequate. The reported incidence of recurrent emboli has ranged from 6 to 45 per cent in various series.[1, 20, 28, 32, 118] The importance of anticoagulation was shown by Green and associates, who found a 9 per cent incidence of in-hospital recurrent emboli in patients who were appropriately anticoagulated postoperatively, in contrast to a rate of 31 per cent in those not receiving such treatment.[31] In the 102 patients reentering the hospital with recurrent emboli in Darling and associates' series, only 22 were appropriately anticoagulated.[28] The effectiveness of anticoagulation in prevention of recurrent emboli is shown graphically in Figure 43–15 from Elliott's data.[1]

The mortality rate and limb loss secondary to recurrent emboli are significantly greater than those associated with an initial embolic event.[17, 20, 28] Associated cerebral and visceral arterial emboli, often fatal and untreatable, are more common. Such experience reemphasizes the value of long-term, carefully monitored anticoagulant treatment in patients with arterial emboli, unless the embolic source can be corrected or eliminated.

NONOPERATIVE MANAGEMENT

High-Dose Heparin Therapy Alone. Noting the persistently high mortality and limb loss rates associated with emergency surgical treatment of acute ischemia, Blaisdell and associates in 1978 first advocated avoidance of an initial surgical approach and reliance on primary therapy with high-dose anticoagulation therapy alone.[75] In their view, the high mortality rate is not due to failure to reestablish circulation because the mortality rate appears to be higher in successful than in unsuccessful procedures; rather, the systemic consequences of revascularization in the high-risk patient typically presenting with acute ischemia are responsible.

In the opinion of Blaisdell and associates, embolectomy is indicated only in low-risk patients with ischemia of less than 8 hours' duration. Emergency operation on patients with ischemia of longer duration is avoided because it is thought that if the ischemic insult is severe enough to result in muscle necrosis, the necrosis will already be established within 8 hours. Revascularization after this period of time will save no more muscle than that salvaged by anticoagulation, a treatment associated with lower mortality. Primary amputation is recommended for nonviable limbs.

Employing such selective criteria and high-dose heparin therapy (20,000 units initial bolus followed by 2000 to 4000 U/hr), Blaisdell and associates found a mortality rate of 7.5 per cent and a limb salvage rate of 67 per cent.[75] The authors compared their results with those reported in a compilation of 3350 cases of acute ischemia treated with thromboembolectomy in surgical series published between 1963 and 1978, which had a cumulative mortality rate of 27 per cent and a limb salvage rate of 61 per cent in the survivors. They concluded that such selective management was successful in lowering mortality without leading to a corresponding increase in limb loss compared to such pre-

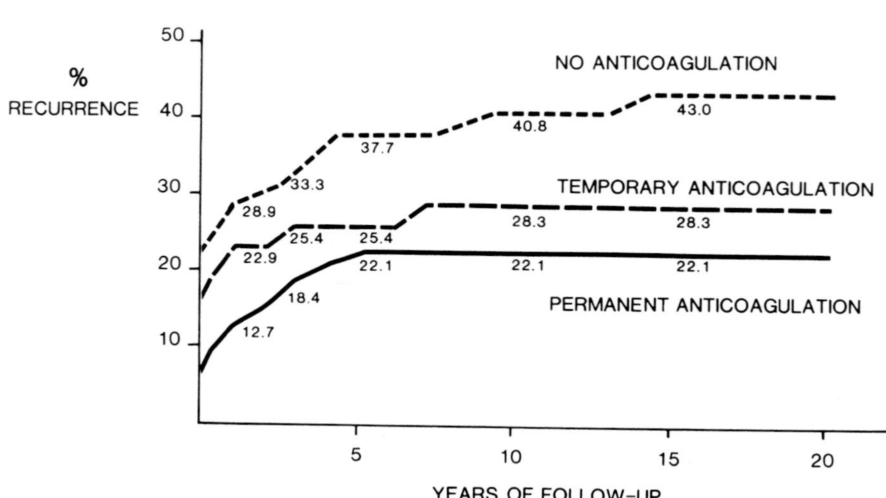

FIGURE 43–15. Cumulative rate of recurrence of embolization in 215 survivors of initial embolic episode with permanent anticoagulation (n = 97), temporary anticoagulation (n = 19), and no anticoagulation (n = 69). (From Elliott JP Jr, Hageman JH, Szilagyi DE, et al: Arterial embolization: Problems of source, multiplicity, recurrence, and delayed treatment. Surgery 88:833, 1980.)

viously published historical controls, and recommended high-dose heparin therapy as the initial management in all cases of acute arterial ischemia.

This remains a controversial recommendation. Many surgeons believe that more recent results of surgical embolectomy are much improved over those of older reports. Further, there was no attempt to differentiate between embolic and thrombotic etiologies of acute ischemia in Blaisdell and associates' series. Although his recommendations fit nicely into the management scheme for patients with acute arterial thrombosis who have viable limbs, most surgeons continue to favor prompt embolectomy for those patients with an acute arterial embolus. Certainly, however, high-dose heparin alone or immediate amputation may be best for patients with truly advanced, probably irreversible ischemia, in whom ill-advised revascularization presents almost no hope of salvage and may be associated with devastating and frequently fatal complications.

Thrombolytic Therapy. In recent years, thrombolytic therapy has occasionally been employed as the primary treatment for acute embolic arterial occlusions.[138–141] Two primary agents have been utilized for this mode of therapy; streptokinase and urokinase. Selective intra-arterial infusion has the advantage of delivering a higher concentration of the agent directly to the region of clot, allowing a lower total infusion dose and potentially fewer side effects.

At present, the exact role of this type of therapy has yet to be fully delineated.[142, 143] Several shortcomings have been identified. First, the duration of the procedure can be quite lengthy and unpredictable and its efficacy uncertain. In general, an embolus is much more easily and effectively treated by expeditious operation. Since thrombolytic therapy often requires from 24 to 72 hours to achieve clot lysis, it is not appropriate for many patients with significant acute ischemia that requires immediate revascularization to preserve limb viability. In addition, some have suggested that the organized older clot typical of an embolus may be more resistant to thrombolysis than a recent thrombosis.[140] The time requirements, complexity of patient care, need for multiple arteriographic studies to monitor progress, and the expense of lytic agents themselves are substantial, and all detract from the cost-effectiveness of lytic therapy.[144]

It is also important to recognize that thrombolytic therapy carries complications of its own in a significant number of patients.[145, 146] Most prominent is severe bleeding secondary to systemic effects of the lytic drugs. Distal migration of thrombotic material as partial clot dissolution occurs is well recognized and may aggravate ischemia. In addition, the potential exists for partial clot lysis at the source of an embolus, such as mural clot in a ventricular aneurysm or abdominal aortic aneurysm, possibly causing multiple recurrent embolic events.[145] The significant number of both minor and major complications of thrombolytic therapy noted in many series reemphasizes the point that nonoperative therapy is not necessarily better or safer than surgery.[142, 143, 147]

Nonetheless, consideration of thrombolytic therapy may be appropriate in selected circumstances of acute limb ischemia as an alternative to surgical thromboembolectomy.[148] This is particularly true if the embolus is difficult to approach surgically, or if the surgical approach carries a truly excessive risk.[140, 142] An example might be an unstable patient with recent myocardial infarction and an acute popliteal embolus. As previously described, adjunctive intraoperative use of thrombolytic agents following balloon catheter embolectomy may potentially improve surgical results when distal small vessel clots are inaccessible to the embolectomy catheter.[99–103] Finally, initial lytic therapy may be advantageous in acutely ischemic limbs that are viable but in which the differentiation between embolic and thrombotic causes of occlusion cannot be clearly established.[148]

Percutaneous Aspiration Thromboembolectomy (PAT). Percutaneous aspiration of thrombotic material from the vascular system was first utilized by Greenfield and associates for treatment of pulmonary embolism in 1968.[149] Application of intra-arterial catheter aspiration was initially associated with management of iatrogenic embolism coincident with balloon angioplasty. Turnipseed and associates expanded the use of PAT for selective treatment of acute arterial occlusions caused by primary as well as iatrogenic thromboembolism.[150] PAT is performed following standard angiography and is best limited to occlusions distal to the femoral artery. The authors reported use of PAT in 42 patients with acute limb-threatening ischemia. Seventy-five per cent had distal arterial occlusion resulting from acute embolic events. Successful clot retrieval and limb salvage were achieved in 40 of the 42 patients.

Although it is possible to use catheter aspiration in concert with surgical embolectomy, the limiting factor for use of aspiration embolectomy in the operating room is adequate fluoroscopy. Overall, experience is currently far too limited with this technique to evaluate its utility in the management of embolic disease.

SUMMARY

Arterial emboli remain an important cause of acute arterial ischemia. Despite simplification of operative techniques, the substantial morbidity and mortality still associated with an acute embolus remain a challenge to the vascular surgeon.

An embolus originates from the heart in over 80 per cent of cases. Most patients are 70 years of age or older, and arteriosclerotic heart disease and its complications are the underlying cause of the embolic event. Noncardiac arterial sources of emboli are being recognized more frequently. An acute arterial embolus must be differentiated from other causes of ischemia, most commonly acute arterial thrombosis due to preexisting occlusive disease. Preoperative arteriography is sometimes required to make the proper diagnosis and guide therapeutic intervention.

Prompt balloon catheter embolectomy performed under local anesthesia is a safe, simple, and effective method of treatment and the preferred mode of management in the great majority of patients. Concomitant anticoagulation with heparin is of great associated importance in the perioperative period to improve results. Long-term anticoagulation with oral agents is also vital to decrease the incidence of recurrent emboli, unless the source of an embolus can be corrected or eliminated.

Nonoperative management with thrombolytic agents or high-dose heparin therapy alone is occasionally indicated in highly selected patients. Patients too ill to tolerate any efforts to revascularize the limb or with evidence of irreversible ischemia should be treated with primary amputation.

References

1. Elliott JP Jr, Hageman JH, Szilagyi DE, et al: Arterial embolization: Problems of source, multiplicity, recurrence, and delayed treatment. Surgery 88:833, 1980.
2. Brewster DC: Acute peripheral arterial occlusion. Cardiol Clin 9:497, 1991.
3. Brewster DC: Arterial embolism: Diagnosis and management. *In* Coodley E (ed): Geriatric Heart Disease. Littleton, MA, PSG Publishing Co, 1985, pp 239–247.
4. Moynihan BGA: An operation for embolus. Br Med J 2:826, 1907.
5. Key E: Embolectomy in the treatment of circulatory disturbances in the extremities. Surg Gynecol Obstet 36:309, 1923.
6. Key E: Embolectomy on the vessels of the extremities. Br J Surg 24:350, 1936.
7. Lerman J, Miller FR, Lund CC: Arterial embolism and embolectomy. JAMA 94:1128, 1930.
8. Murray DWG, Best CH: The use of heparin in thrombosis. Ann Surg 108:163, 1938.
9. Crawford ES, DeBakey ME: The retrograde flush procedure in embolectomy and thrombectomy. Surgery 40:737, 1956.
10. Keeley JL, Rooney JA: Retrograde milking: An adjunct in technic of embolectomy. Ann Surg 134:1022, 1951.
11. Dale WA: Endovascular suction catheters: For thrombectomy and embolectomy. J Thorac Cardiovasc Surg 44:557, 1962.
12. Shaw RS: A method for the removal of the adherent distal thrombus. Surg Gynecol Obstet 110:255, 1960.
13. Fogarty TJ, Cranley JJ, Krause RJ, et al: A method for extraction of arterial emboli and thrombi. Surg Gynecol Obstet 116:241, 1963.
14. Abbott WM, Maloney RD, McCabe CC, et al: Arterial embolism: A 44 year perspective. Am J Surg 143:460, 1982.
15. Connett MC, Murray DH Jr, Wenneker WW: Peripheral arterial emboli. Am J Surg 148:14, 1984.
16. Dale WA: Differential management of acute peripheral arterial ischemia. J Vasc Surg 1:269, 1984.
17. Kendrick J, Thompson BW, Read RC, et al: Arterial embolectomy in the leg: Results in a referral hospital. Am J Surg 142:739, 1981.
18. Satiani B, Gross WS, Evans WE: Improved limb salvage after arterial embolectomy. Ann Surg 188:153, 1978.
19. Sheiner NM, Zeltzer J, MacIntosh E: Arterial embolectomy in the modern era. Can J Surg 25:373, 1982.
20. Silvers LW, Royster TS, Mulcare RJ: Peripheral arterial emboli and factors in their recurrence rate. Ann Surg 192:232, 1980.
21. Tawes RL Jr, Harris EJ, Brown WH, et al: Arterial thromboembolism: A 20-year perspective. Arch Surg 120:595, 1985.
22. Panetta T, Thompson JE, Talkington CM, et al: Arterial embolectomy: A 34-year experience with 400 cases. Surg Clin North Am 66:339, 1986.
23. Galbraith K, Collin J, Morris PJ, et al: Recent experience with arterial embolism of the limbs in a vascular unit. Ann R Coll Surg Engl 67:30, 1985.
24. Dregelid EB, Strangeland LB, Eide GE, et al: Patient survival and limb prognosis after embolectomy. Eur J Vasc Surg 1:263, 1987.
25. Englund R, Magee HR: Peripheral arterial embolism: 1961–1985. Aust NZ J Surg 57:27, 1987.
26. Baxter-Smith D, Ashton F, Slaney G, et al: Peripheral arterial embolism. A 20 year review. J Cardiovasc Surg 29:453, 1988.
27. Varty K, St. Johnston JA, Beets G, et al: Arterial embolectomy: A long-term perspective. J Cardiovasc Surg 33:79, 1992.
28. Darling RC, Austen WG, Linton RR: Arterial embolism. Surg Gynecol Obstet 124:106, 1967.
29. Warren R, Linton RR: The treatment of arterial embolism. N Engl J Med 238:421, 1948.
30. Warren R, Linton RR, Scannell JG: Arterial embolism: Recent progress. Ann Surg 140:311, 1954.
31. Green RM, DeWeese JA, Rob CG: Arterial embolectomy before and after the Fogarty catheter. Surgery 77:24, 1975.
32. Hight DW, Tilney NL, Couch NP: Changing clinical trends in patients with peripheral arterial emboli. Surgery 79:172, 1976.
33. Fogarty TJ, Daily PO, Shumway NE, et al: Experience with balloon catheter technic for arterial embolectomy. Am J Surg 122:231, 1971.
34. Hinton RC, Kistler JP, Fallon JT, et al: Influence of etiology of atrial fibrillation on incidence of systemic embolism. Am J Cardiol 40:509, 1977.
35. Levine JH, Pauker SG, Salzman EW: Antithrombotic therapy in valvular heart disease. Chest 89:36S, 1986.
36. Shrestha NK, Moreno FL, Narcisco FV, et al: Two-dimensional echocardiographic diagnosis of left-atrial thrombus in rheumatic heart disease. A clinicopathologic study. Circulation 67:341, 1983.
37. Schweizer P, Bardos F, Erbel R: Detection of left atrial thrombi by echocardiography. Br Heart J 45:148, 1981.
38. Aschenberg W, Schluter M, Krenner P, et al: Transesophageal two-dimensional echocardiography for the detection of left atrial appendage thrombus. J Am Coll Cardiol 7:163, 1986.
39. Hellerstein HK, Martin JW: Incidence of thromboembolic lesions accompanying myocardial infarction. Am Heart J 33:443, 1947.
40. Asinger RW, Mikell FL, Elsperger J, et al: Incidence of left ventricular thrombosis after acute transmural myocardial infarction. Serial evaluation by two-dimensional echocardiography. N Engl J Med 305:297, 1981.
41. Keating EC, Gross SA, Schlamowitz RA: Mural thrombi in myocardial infarctions. Am J Med 74:989, 1983.
42. Satiani B, Evans WE: Immediate prognosis and five year survival after arterial embolectomy following myocardial infarction. Surg Gynecol Obstet 150:41, 1980.
43. Thompson JE, Weston AS, Sigler L, et al: Arterial embolectomy after acute myocardial infarction: A study of 31 patients. Ann Surg 171:979, 1970.
44. Loop FD, Effler DB, Navia JA, et al: Aneurysms of the left ventricle: Survival and results of a ten-year surgical experience. Ann Surg 178:399, 1973.
45. Lapeyre AC III, Steele PM, Kazmier FJ, et al: Systemic embolism in chronic left ventricular aneurysm: Incidence and the role of anticoagulation. J Am Coll Cardiol 6:534, 1985.
46. Perier P, Bessou JP, Swanson JS, et al: Comparative evaluation of aortic valve replacement with Starr, Bjork, and porcine valve prostheses. Circulation 72:II140, 1985.
47. Schwarcz TH, Coffin LH, Pilcher DB: Renal failure after embolization of a prosthetic mitral valve disc and review of systemic disc embolization. J Vasc Surg 2:697, 1985.
48. Pipkin RD, Buch WS, Fogarty TJ: Evaluation of aortic valve replacement with a porcine xenograft without long-term anticoagulation. J Thorac Cardiovasc Surg 71:179, 1976.
49. Brewster DC: How can you best identify and treat arterial embolism? J Cardiovasc Med 7:354, 1982.
50. Vo NM, Russell JC, Becker DR: Mycotic emboli of the peripheral vessels: Analysis of forty-four cases. Surgery 90:541, 1981.
51. Kitts D, Bongard FS, Klein SR: Septic embolism complicating infective endocarditis. J Vasc Surg 14:480, 1991.
52. Freischlag JA, Asbun HA, Sedwitz MM, et al: Septic peripheral embolization from bacterial and fungal endocarditis. Ann Vasc Surg 3:318, 1989.
53. Lord JW Jr, Rossi G, Daliana M, et al: Unsuspected abdominal aortic aneurysm as the cause of peripheral arterial occlusive disease. Ann Surg 177:767, 1973.
54. Kempczinski RF: Lower-extremity arterial emboli from ulcerating atherosclerotic plaques. JAMA 241:807, 1979.
55. Kwaan JHM, Vander Molen R, Stemmer EA, et al: Peripheral embolism resulting from unsuspected atheromatous aortic plaques. Surgery 78:583, 1975.
56. Machleder HI, Takiff H, Lois JF, et al: Aortic mural thrombus: An occult source of arterial thromboembolism. J Vasc Surg 4:473, 1986.
57. Williams GM, Harrington D, Burdick J, et al: Mural thrombus of the aorta: An important, frequently neglected cause of large peripheral emboli. Ann Surg 194:737, 1981.
58. Johnston KW, Sniderman KW: Complications of percutaneous transluminal angioplasty of peripheral arterial occlusive disease. *In* Bernhard VM, Towne JB (eds): Complications in Vascular Surgery. St. Louis, Quality Medical Publishing, 1991, pp 409–419.

59. Gardiner GA Jr, Meyerovitz MF, Stokes KR, et al: Complications of transluminal angioplasty. Radiology 159:201, 1986.
60. White RA: Complications associated with intravascular instrumentation: Endoscopy, atherectomy, lasers, and dilatation devices. *In* Bernhard VM, Towne JB (eds): Complications in Vascular Surgery. St. Louis, Quality Medical Publishing, 1991, pp 420–431.
61. Harris RW, Andros G, Dulawa LB, et al: Malignant melanoma embolus as a cause of acute aortic occlusion: Report of a case. J Vasc Surg 3:550, 1986.
62. Prioleau PG, Katzenstein AA: Major peripheral arterial occlusion due to malignant tumor embolism: Histologic recognition and surgical management. Cancer 42:2009, 1978.
63. Symbas PN, Harlaftis N: Bullet emboli in the pulmonary and systemic arteries. Ann Surg 185:318, 1977.
64. Shannon JJ, Nghia MV, Stanton PE Jr, et al: Peripheral arterial missile embolization: A case report and 22-year literature review. J Vasc Surg 5:773, 1987.
65. Gazzaniga AB, Dalen JE: Paradoxical embolism: Its pathophysiology and clinical recognition. Ann Surg 171:137, 1970.
66. Laughlin RA, Mandel SR: Paradoxical embolization: Case report and review of the literature. Arch Surg 112:648, 1977.
67. Katz S, Andros G, Kohl R, et al: Arterial emboli of venous origin. Surg Gynecol Obstet 174:17, 1992.
68. Thompson JE, Sigler L, Raut PS, et al: Arterial embolectomy: A 20 year experience. Surgery 67:212, 1970.
69. Tunick PA, Perez JL, Kronzon I: Protruding atheromas in the thoracic aorta and systemic embolization. Ann Intern Med 115:423, 1991.
70. Rubin BG, Barzilai B, Allen BT, et al: Detection of the source of arterial emboli by transesophageal echocardiography: A case report. J Vasc Surg 15:573, 1992.
71. Seward JB, Khandheria BK, Oh JE, et al: Transesophageal echocardiography: Technique, anatomic correlations, implementation, and clinical applications. Mayo Clin Proc 63:649, 1988.
72. Kuecherer HF, Lee E, Schiller NB: Role of transesophageal echocardiography in diagnosis and management of cardiovascular disease. Cardiol Clin 2:377, 1990.
73. Eason JD, Mills JL, Beckett WC: Hypercoagulable states in arterial thromboembolism. Surg Gynecol Obstet 174:211, 1992.
74. Linton RR: Peripheral arterial embolism: A discussion of the postembolic vascular changes and their relation to the restoration of circulation in peripheral embolism. N Engl J Med 224:189, 1941.
75. Blaisdell FW, Steele M, Allen RE: Management of acute lower extremity arterial ischemia due to embolism and thrombosis. Surgery 84:822, 1978.
76. Haimovici H: Muscular, renal and metabolic complications of acute arterial occlusions. Myonephropathic-metabolic syndrome. Surgery 85:461, 1979.
77. Fischer RD, Fogarty TJ, Morrow AG: Clinical and biochemical observations of the effect of transient femoral artery occlusion in man. Surgery 68:323, 1970.
78. Walker PM: Pathophysiology of acute arterial occlusion. Can J Surg 29:340, 1986.
79. Patman RD, Thompson JE: Fasciotomy in peripheral vascular surgery: Report of 164 patients. Arch Surg 101:663, 1970.
80. Perry MO: Compartment syndromes and reperfusion injury. Surg Clin North Am 68:853, 1988.
81. Padberg FT, Hobson RW II: Fasciotomy in acute limb ischemia. Semin Vasc Surg 5:52, 1992.
82. Rutherford RB: Acute limb ischemia: Clinical assessment and standards for reporting. Semin Vasc Surg 5:4, 1992.
83. Rutherford RB, Flanigan DP, Gupta SK, et al: Suggested standards for reports dealing with lower extremity ischemia. J Vasc Surg 64:80, 1986.
84. Meier GH, Brewster DC: Acute arterial thrombosis. *In* Bergan JJ, Yao JST (eds): Vascular Surgical Emergencies. Orlando, FL, Grune and Stratton, 1987, pp 499–515.
85. McPhail NV, Fratesi SJ, Barber GG, et al: Management of acute thromboembolic limb ischemia. Surgery 93:381, 1983.
86. Jivegard L, Holm J, Schersten T: The outcome in arterial thrombosis misdiagnosed as arterial embolism. Acta Chir Scand 152:251, 1986.
87. Cambria RP, Abbott WM: Acute arterial thrombosis of the lower extremity. Arch Surg 119:784, 1984.
88. Cambria RP, Brewster DC, Gertler JP, et al: Vascular complications associated with spontaneous aortic dissection. J Vasc Surg 7:199, 1988.
89. Brewster DC, Cambria RP: Role of the vascular surgeon in the management of dissecting aortic aneurysms. *In* Veith FJ (ed): Current Critical Problems in Vascular Surgery. St. Louis, Quality Medical Publishing, 1989, pp 291–302.
90. Meagher AP, Lord RSA, Graham AR, et al: Acute aortic occlusion presenting with lower limb paralysis. J Cardiovasc Surg 32:643, 1991.
91. Fogarty TJ, Hermann GD: New techniques for clot extraction and managing acute thromboembolic limb ischemia. *In* Veith FJ (ed): Current Critical Problems in Vascular Surgery. St. Louis: Quality Medical Publishing, 1991, vol. 3, pp 197–203.
92. Pleacha FR, Pories WJ: Intraoperative angiography in the immediate assessment of arterial reconstruction. Arch Surg 105:902, 1972.
93. O'Hara PJ, Brewster DC, Darling RC, et al: The value of intraoperative monitoring using the pulse volume recorder during peripheral vascular reconstructive operations. Surg Gynecol Obstet 152:275, 1981.
94. Busuttil RW, Keehn G, Milliken J, et al: Aortic saddle embolus: A twenty-year experience. Ann Surg 197:698, 1983.
95. Short D, Vaughn GD III, Jachimczyk J, et al: The anatomic basis for the occasional failure of transfemoral balloon catheter thromboembolectomy. Ann Surg 190:555, 1979.
96. Abbott WM, McCabe CC, Maloney RD, et al: Embolism of the popliteal artery. Surg Gynecol Obstet 159:533, 1984.
97. Gupta SK, Samson RH, Veith FJ: Embolectomy of the distal part of the popliteal artery. Surg Gynecol Obstet 153:255, 1981.
98. Youkey JR, Clagett GP, Cabellon S Jr, et al: Thromboembolectomy of arteries explored at the ankle. Ann Surg 199:367, 1984.
99. Comerota AJ, White JV, Grosh JD: Intraoperative intraarterial thrombolytic therapy for salvage of limbs in patients with distal arterial thrombosis. Surg Gynecol Obstet 169:283, 1989.
100. Comerota AJ, White JV: Intraoperative, intra-arterial thrombolytic therapy as an adjunct to revascularization in patients with residual and distal arterial thrombus. Semin Vasc Surg 5:110, 1992.
101. Norem RS, Short DH, Kerstein MD: Role of intraoperative fibrinolytic therapy in acute arterial occlusion. Surg Gynecol Obstet 167:87, 1988.
102. Parent NE, Bernhard VM, Pabst TS, et al: Fibrinolytic treatment of residual thrombus after catheter embolectomy for severe lower limb ischemia. J Vasc Surg 9:153, 1989.
103. Quinones-Baldrich WJ, Baker JD, Busuttil RW, et al: Intraoperative infusion of lytic drugs for thrombotic complications of revascularization. J Vasc Surg 10:408, 1989.
104. Dunnant JR, Edwards WS: Small vessel occlusion in the extremity after periods of arterial obstruction: An experimental study. Surgery 75:240, 1973.
105. Quinones-Baldrich WJ, Ziomek S, Henderson TC, et al: Intraoperative fibrinolytic therapy: Experimental evaluation. J Vasc Surg 4:229, 1986.
106. Belkin M, Valeri R, Hobson RW: Intra-arterial urokinase increases skeletal muscle viability after acute ischemia. J Vasc Surg 9:161, 1989.
107. Ricotta JJ, Scudder PA, McAndrew JA, et al: Management of acute ischemia of the upper extremity. Am J Surg 145:661, 1983.
108. Cambria RP, Ridge BA, Brewster DC, et al: Delayed presentation and treatment of popliteal artery embolism. Ann Surg 214:50, 1991.
109. Jarrett F, Dacumos GC, Crummy AB, et al: Late appearance of arterial emboli: Diagnosis and management. Surgery 86:898, 1979.
110. Levin BH, Giordano JM: Delayed arterial embolectomy. Surg Gynecol Obstet 155:549, 1985.
111. McCord JM: Oxygen derived free radicals in postischemic tissue injury. N Engl J Med 312:159, 1985.
112. Perry MO, Fantini G: Ischemia: Profile of an enemy. Reperfusion injury of skeletal muscle. J Vasc Surg 6:231, 1987.
113. Rubin BB, Walker PM: Pathophysiology of acute skeletal muscle injury: Adenine nucleotide metabolism in ischemic reperfused muscle. Semin Vasc Surg 5:11, 1992.
114. Wright JG: Pharmacological and non-pharmacological methods for preservation of skeletal muscle viability: Mechanisms and potential clinical applications. Semin Vasc Surg 5:28, 1992.
115. Campbell HC, Hubbard SG, Ernst CB: Continuous heparin anticoagulation in patients with arteriosclerosis and arterial emboli. Surg Gynecol Obstet 150:54, 1980.

116. Jorgensen RA, Dolbrin PB: Balloon embolectomy catheters in small arteries. IV. Correlation of sheer forces with histological injury. Surgery 93:798, 1983.
117. Hammarsten J, Holm J, Schersten T: Positive and negative effects of anticoagulant treatment during and after arterial embolectomy. J Cardiovasc Surg 19:373, 1978.
118. Tawes RL Jr, Beare JP, Scribner RG, et al: Value of postoperative heparin therapy in peripheral arterial thromboembolism. Am J Surg 146:213, 1983.
119. Salzman EW, Deykin D, Shapiro RM: Management of heparin therapy. N Engl J Med 292:1046, 1975.
120. Haimovici H, Moss CM, Veith FJ: Arterial embolectomy revisited. Surgery 78:409, 1975.
121. Freund U, Romanoff H, Floman Y: Mortality rate following lower limb arterial embolectomy: Causative factors. Surgery 77:201, 1975.
122. Jarrett F, Detmer E: Arterial thromboemboli: Factors affecting mortality and morbidity. J Cardiovasc Surg 22:454, 1981.
123. Albrechtsson U, Einarsson E, Tylen U: Complications secondary to thrombectomy with the Fogarty balloon catheter. Cardiovasc Intervent Radiol 4:14, 1981.
124. Dainko EA: Complications of the use of the Fogarty balloon catheter. Arch Surg 105:79, 1972.
125. Foster JH, Carter JW, Graham CP Jr, et al: Arterial injuries secondary to the use of the Fogarty catheter. Ann Surg 171:971, 1970.
126. Schweitzer DL, Aguam AS, Wilder JR: Complications encountered during arterial embolectomy with the Fogarty balloon catheter. Report of a case and review of the literature. Vasc Surg 10:144, 1976.
127. Cronenwett JL, Walsh DB, Garrett HE: Tibial artery pseudoaneurysms: Delayed complication of balloon catheter embolectomy. J Vasc Surg 8:483, 1988.
128. Dobrin PB: Mechanisms and prevention of arterial injuries caused by balloon embolectomy. Surgery 106:457, 1989.
129. Charlesworth PM, Brewster DC, Darling RC: Renal artery injury from a Fogarty balloon catheter. J Vasc Surg 4:573, 1984.
130. Chidi CC, DePalma RG: Atherogenic potential of the embolectomy catheter. Surgery 83:549, 1978.
131. Schwarcz TH, Dobrin PB, Mrkvicka R, et al: Early myointimal hyperplasia after balloon catheter embolectomy: Effect of shear forces and multiple withdrawals. J Vasc Surg 7:495, 1988.
132. Bowles CR, Olcott C, Pakter RL, et al: Diffuse arterial narrowing as a result of intimal proliferation. J Vasc Surg 7:487, 1988.
133. McGurrin MA, Driscoll JL, Seifert KB, et al: Myointimal hyperplasia as a result of balloon-catheter thromboembolectomy. Arch Surg 126:786, 1991.
134. Field T, Littooy FN, Baker WH: Immediate and long-term outcome of acute arterial occlusion of the extremities: The effect of added vascular reconstruction. Arch Surg 117:1156, 1982.
135. Matsen FA, Winquist RA, Krugmire RB: Diagnosis and management of compartment syndromes. J Bone Joint Surg [Am] 62:286, 1980.
136. Whitesides TE, Haney TC, Harada H, et al: A simple method of tissue pressure determination. Arch Surg 110:1311, 1975.
137. Rush DS, Frame SB, Bell RM, et al: Does open fasciotomy contribute to morbidity and mortality after acute lower extremity ischemia and revascularization? J Vasc Surg 10:343, 1989.
138. Berni GA, Bandyk DF, Zierler RE, et al: Streptokinase treatment of acute arterial occlusion. Ann Surg 198:185, 1983.
139. Katzen BT, Edwards KC, Albert AS, et al: Low-dose direct fibrinolysis in peripheral vascular disease. J Vasc Surg 1:718, 1984.
140. Taylor LM Jr, Porter JM, Baur GM, et al: Intraarterial streptokinase infusion for acute popliteal and tibial artery occlusion. Am J Surg 147:583, 1984.
141. McNamara TO, Bomberger RA, Merchant RF. Intraarterial urokinase as the initial therapy for acute ischemic lower limbs. Circulation 83(Suppl I):106, 1991.
142. Porter JM, Taylor LM Jr: Current status of thrombolytic therapy. J Vasc Surg 2:239, 1985.
143. Ricotta JJ, Green RM, DeWeese JA. Use and limitations of thrombolytic therapy in the treatment of peripheral arterial ischemia: Results of a multi-institutional questionnaire. J Vasc Surg 6:45, 1987.
144. Dacey LJ, Dow RW, McDaniel MD, et al: Cost effectiveness of intraarterial thrombolytic therapy. Arch Surg 123:1218, 1988.
145. Comerota AJ, Rubin RN, Tyson RR, et al: Intra-arterial thrombolytic therapy in peripheral vascular disease. Surg Gynecol Obstet 165:1, 1987.
146. Sicard GA, Schier JJ, Totty WG, et al: Thrombolytic therapy for acute arterial occlusion. J Vasc Surg 2:65, 1985.
147. Yeager RA, Moneta GL, Taylor LM Jr, et al: Surgical management of severe acute lower extremity ischemia. J Vasc Surg 15:385, 1992.
148. McNamara TO: Thrombolysis as an alternative initial therapy for the acutely ischemic lower limb. Semin Vasc Surg 5:89, 1992.
149. Greenfield LJ, Kimmell GO, McCurdy WC III: Transvenous removal of pulmonary emboli by vacuum-cup catheter technic. J Surg Res 9:347, 1969.
150. Turnipseed WD, Starck EE, McDermott JC, et al: Percutaneous aspiration thromboembolectomy (PAT): An alternative to surgical balloon techniques for clot retrieval. J Vasc Surg 3:437, 1986.

44

Atheroembolism and Microthromboembolic Syndromes (Blue Toe Syndrome and Disseminated Atheroembolism)

Jeffrey L. Kaufman, M.D., Dhiraj M. Shah, M.D., and Robert P. Leather, M.D.

• • •

The observation that some arterial emboli arise from fragmentation of atheromatous plaques or from thrombotic material adherent to these plaques was first documented over a century ago. Since the mid-1940s,[18] the pathology of plaque degeneration has come to the attention of clinicians as a unifying mechanism for the production of profound cerebrovascular, visceral, cardiac, and limb ischemia. Microembolization of platelet aggregates and cholesterol-laden debris into end-arteries has been documented in every part of the human body.[8, 25, 42, 49] The production of stroke or cerebrovascular insufficiency by this mechanism is discussed in Section XVI. Upper extremity microembolic phenomena are discussed in Section IX and in Chapter 80. Coronary artery microembolization is a significant factor in the pathogenesis of myocardial ischemia and is discussed elsewhere.[19] This chapter deals with embolization to the lower extremities and viscera.

Aside from the Hollenhorst plaque in a retinal artery, evidence of atheroembolism is visible to the clinician only in the extremities, most often in the feet, rarely in the fingers. In its classic presentation, the "blue toe syndrome" is marked by a toe that is suddenly cool, painful, and cyanotic in the presence of palpable distal pulses (Fig. 44–1).[26] In its more subtle manifestation, the syndrome may occur in patients without palpable pulses at the ankle: These patients have sufficiently adequate peripheral collateral circulation by vascular laboratory criteria, so that impending gangrene of a toe is not expected.

The term atheroembolism is employed here as a generic term for cholesterol or atherothrombotic microembolism. Numerous misleading labels have been applied to this condition, including vasospasm, cold injury, localized Raynaud's phenomenon, and idiopathic digital artery thrombosis.[22] Connective tissue and autoimmune disorders such as vasculitis, polyarteritis, and polymyositis have also been implicated.[5, 10, 44] The source of this confusion is obvious because these disorders share the pathophysiology of end-arterial occlusion. Despite the longstanding recognition that atheroemboli arise from severely degenerative atherosclerotic plaques in the proximal circulation, there remain many questions to be answered about the pathophysiology and natural history of this disorder. This inattention to atheroembolism is likely related in part to the lack of understanding and concern about problems of the feet in the medical community at large. The threat to the survival of a single toe may not appear to be of great consequence, but repeated untreated episodes of atheroembolism with continued destruction of the collateral circulation may portend disaster for the leg or life-threatening visceral damage.[8] Diagnostic efforts should be promptly concentrated on the location, stabilization, and, preferably, eradication of the source of such microemboli.

PATHOPHYSIOLOGY

Atheroembolism may originate from a variety of lesions, and virtually any artery may degenerate to produce microemboli.[20] Lesions located in the arterial tree from the infrarenal aorta to the distal popliteal arteries account for the majority of emboli to the lower extremities. Aneurysms have long been recognized as a source of microemboli, particularly popliteal aneurysms, as discussed in Chapter 79. Microembolic showers have been noted coincident to occlusion of polytetrafluoroethylene grafts. Nevertheless, the most important sources of emboli are degenerative, stenotic, hemorrhagic, irregular, and ulcerative plaques (Fig. 44–2). Although these lesions have been documented in the suprarenal aorta, the distribution of infrarenal arterial

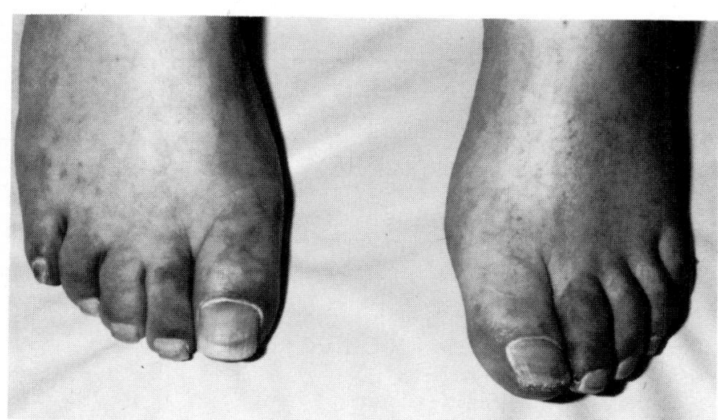

FIGURE 44–1. Typical appearance of the toes after bilateral atheroembolism.

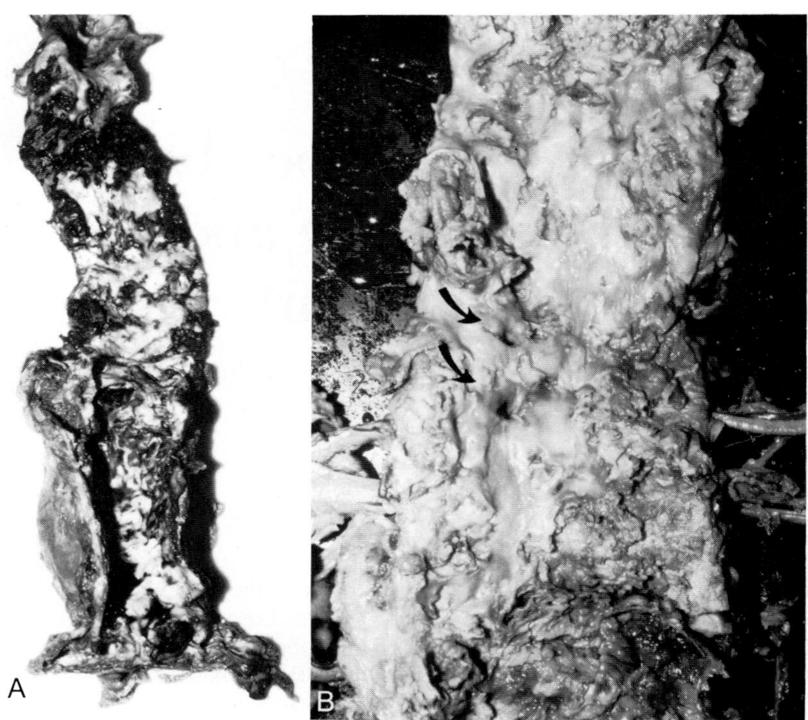

FIGURE 44–2. Two patients with extensive degenerative atherosclerosis and disseminated atheroembolism. *A*, Total aortic degeneration extending from the ligamentum arteriosum to the iliac arteries. The aorta is diffusely aneurysmal but without the thick laminated thrombus that typically lines infrarenal aneurysms. *B*, View of a visceral aortic segment, showing the friable atheromatous plaques and visceral ostial occlusive disease (*arrows*).

sources is approximately equal in the aortoiliac and femoropopliteal segments (Table 44–1). Widespread degeneration has been frequently noted, and in these cases it is difficult to locate precisely the specific anatomic area responsible for the production of microemboli. In general, bilateral atheroembolism signifies a proximal or aortic source, whereas unilateral emboli usually arise distal to the aortic bifurcation (Fig. 44–3).[46]

Fragmentation of atheromatous plaques may occur as they undergo central necrosis, with development of virtual liquefaction of cholesterol and calcium debris as well as hemorrhage.[6, 11, 19, 26, 30] With ulceration of the fragile intima overlying this material, debris may be released into the bloodstream, leading to distal embolization. Intact plaques with stenosis or irregularities may have regions of turbulent blood flow with flow stagnation, analogous to the "coral reef" plaque described in the upper abdominal aorta.[50] Mural thrombi formed in such regions have been observed to embolize into distal arteries (Fig. 44–4). Interestingly, the authors have observed repeated unilateral distal embolization from aortic sources, which implies that pulsatile flow in the distal aorta is sufficiently laminar to carry microemboli in a repetitive flow pattern. In the case of aneurysmal sources, emboli may be dislodged from the laminated thrombus that lines the vascular channel. Considerable friability of atheromatous plaques is a common surgical finding, and it is not unusual to find shaggy, frond-like clumps of fibrinoplatelet debris at the site of a high-grade arterial stenosis as a preocclusive phenomenon. The fact that atheroembolic events occur with arterial catheterization for angiography and with cross-clamping of the ascending aorta has provided additional evidence of the fragility of degenerative plaques.[21, 41, 43] Less often, large fragments of cholesterol debris or crystals have been noted to dislodge

Table 44–1. Sources of Recurrent Microembolism

		Embolic Sources		
Author	**No. Cases**	***Abdominal Aortic Aneurysm***	***Aorta/Iliac***	***Femoral/Popliteal***
Karmody et al[26]	31	6	2	23
Kwaan and Connolly[31]	15	15		
Schechter[47]	17	3	9	2
Crane[11]	3		2	1
Carvajal et al[8]	4	4		
Branowitz and Edwards[6]	4		4	
Kempczinski[30]	10		8	
Mehigan and Stoney[36]	12		5	7
Jenkins and Newton[24]	15		8	6
McFarland et al[34]	42		14	28

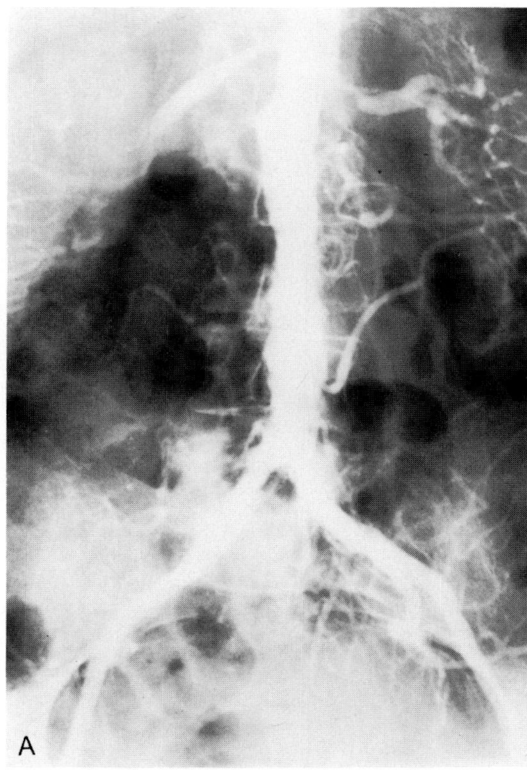

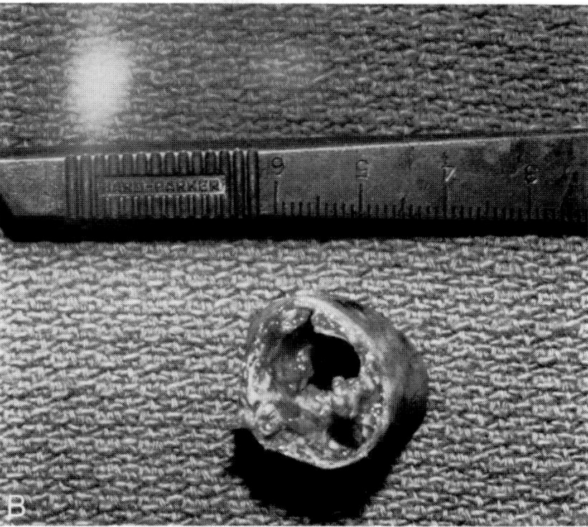

FIGURE 44–3. Same patient as in Figure 44–1. *A*, The angiogram shows severe diffuse irregularity of the aortic wall and stenoses of the inferior mesenteric and left renal arteries. *B*, Cross-sectional appearance of the aorta, a segment removed at the time of aortobifemoral reconstruction. The friability of the "toothpaste"-like atheromatous debris is apparent.

from severely degenerative plaques.[52] Atheromatous gravel has been observed in the tibial arteries where it becomes firmly impacted, leading to distal propagation of additional thrombus.[17] It is therefore difficult to determine the exact nature of the atheromatous debris and microthrombotic material that may be involved in the clinical picture of atheroembolism. Although cholesterol emboli tend to be diffuse and lodge in arteries 100 to 200 μm in size,[30] small crystals have been observed in capillaries in the end-arterial circulation. The authors have observed similar cholesterol crystal emboli in the pulmonary capillary circulation. It appears that the smallest elements of this debris may pass through peripheral arteriolar-capillary shunts and thereby return in the venous circulation to lodge in the lung. This phenomenon has been confirmed for the 10- to 20 μm atheromatous debris produced by transcatheter high-speed burr atherectomy.[1] Obviously, digital arteries are most often involved in this embolic phenomenon, but larger emboli have been recovered from the tibial, popliteal, and superficial femoral arteries (Fig. 44–5). Emboli may occlude the circulation in a cumulative manner, thereby leading to more proximal thromboses. Larger emboli of atheromatous debris appear generally to arise from the aorta and iliac arteries, in which severe atheromatous degeneration may occur.

Pathologists have long noted the autopsy finding of clinically silent extensive degeneration of the whole aorta.[20, 29, 28] Nevertheless, patients with a defined blue toe syndrome remain unusual, and practitioners treating vascular disease exclusively will find patients with atheroembolism a minority within their clinical experience. In a recent series, atheroembolism constituted a significant clinical problem in 0.03 per cent of hospitalized patients.[24] Fully disseminated atheroembolism has an autopsy prevalence of 0.79 per cent.[29]

Indeed, it is remarkable that this debris may remain stable and clinically silent in many patients for years. This has been confirmed at autopsy.[9, 18] In more recent studies, the presence of such silent degeneration has been documented by intraoperative ultrasonography in the ascending aorta in approximately 20 to 25 per cent of patients undergoing coronary bypass.[43] The reasons why atheroembolism remains a generally silent phenomenon are still unclear.[3] The onset of symptoms does not appear to be directly related to the cumulative burden of debris showering an extremity because some patients with relatively minor plaques have severe symptoms at their first episode, whereas others seemingly tolerate severe arterial degeneration for years. The fact that antiplatelet drugs are useful in treatment (see later discussion) implies a role for platelet-derived humoral factors in the pathogenesis of symptoms and signs.[19, 32]

The type of emboli causing the blue toe syndrome cannot be differentiated on clinical grounds. From aneurysms, the material is usually fragmented laminated clot. Friable granular amorphous thrombus (with the consistency of oatmeal) has been observed to embolize from mural aortic plaques or from isolated iliac or superficial femoral artery stenoses. When cholesterol crystals are found in histologic sections of infarcted tissue, the source is usually the aorta or the common iliac arteries. Atheroembolism is a clinical diagnosis: It is remarkably difficult to find the site of microembolic lodgment or cholesterol debris in periph-

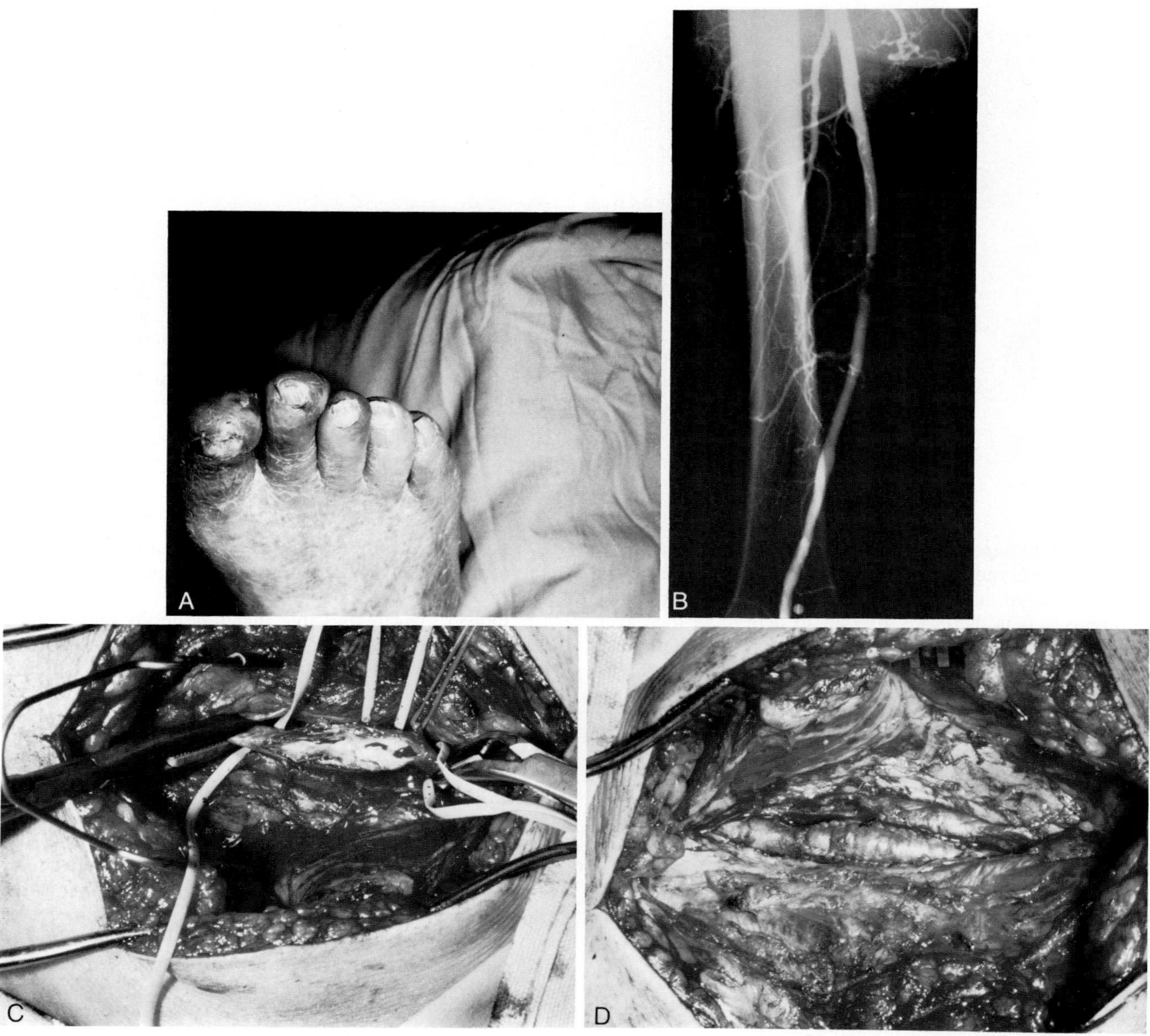

FIGURE 44–4. *A*, Unilateral "blue toe" syndrome. Angiograms demonstrated a high-grade superficial femoral artery stenosis (*B*), on which friable fresh thrombus was found at the time of reconstruction (*C*). A limited endarterectomy and vein patch angioplasty were performed (*D*).

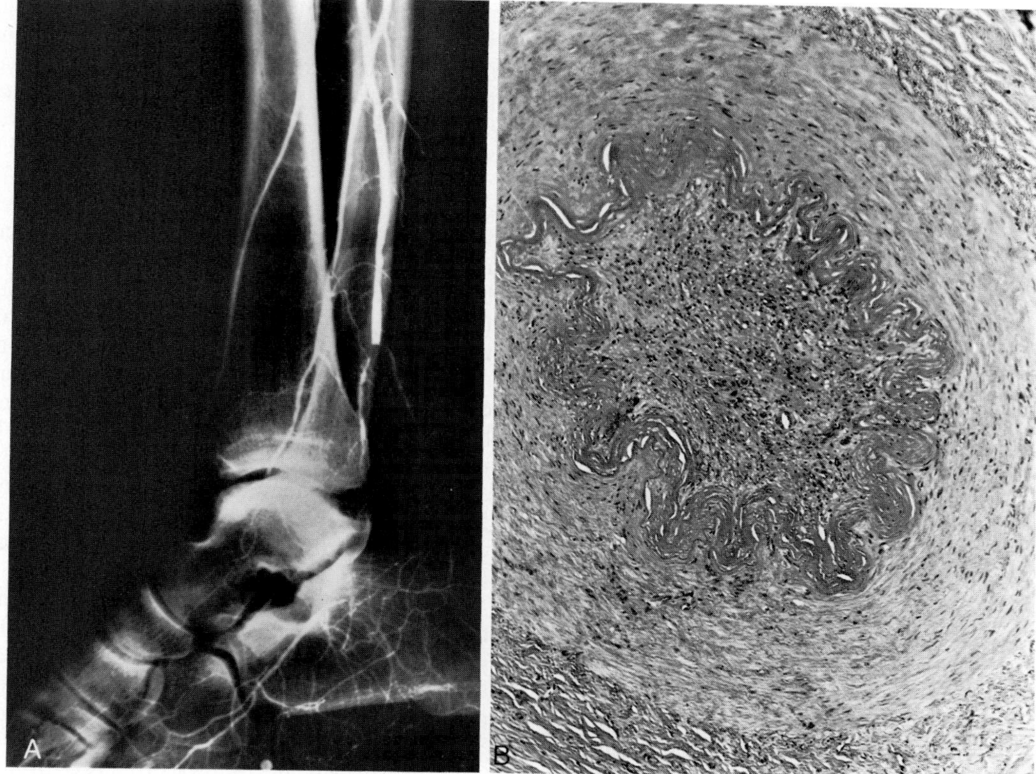

FIGURE 44–5. Atheroembolism from a friable common iliac lesion. Angiography demonstrated a sharp cutoff of the posterior tibial artery (*A*) and multiple intraluminal defects in the peroneal and pedal vessels. After 9 months, a below-knee amputation was performed. The posterior tibial artery contains organized atheromatous debris (*B*).

eral tissues that are infarcted or debrided, even when a pathologist takes care to search for these findings in multiple tissue sections.

Finally, it must be noted that the sequence of clinical events in microembolization of the lower extremity is analogous to that occurring in the carotid circulation, a problem that has achieved far greater clinical recognition. Obviously, this is due to the dramatic nature of stroke and transient ischemic attack symptoms and to the fact that Hollenhorst plaques may be seen in retinal arteries. Many of the issues pertaining to the diagnosis and treatment of peripheral atheroembolism are thus similar to those related to carotid disease.

Physicians must avoid the false sense of security that may occur after discomfort subsides from the first embolic episode. Since the symptoms of atheroembolism may be evanescent, a careful history is required to reveal the typical features of the syndrome, in particular the fact that more than one episode has occurred. If neglected, recurrent microembolization carries the unfortunate consequence of extensive tissue infarction.[6, 47] A significant feature of atheroembolism is the appearance of lesions in crops, as if intermittent showers of debris occur.[36, 47] Collateral circulation in the affected beds is either undeveloped in the presence of this acute shower or destroyed by the emboli, accounting for the progressive nature of the symptoms.

CLINICAL DIAGNOSIS

The typical presentation of microembolism to the lower extremity is the sudden appearance of a painful small area on the foot, typically a toe, which is mottled blue in color, has sluggish capillary return, and is tender to touch.[15, 26, 39] The discoloration may be patchy, and comparison of both feet shows that the distribution is usually not symmetric. If the presentation is late (1 or more weeks after the onset), there may be early ulceration of the toe tip or formation of an eschar. There is no history or sign of recent trauma or local infection. Accessory lesions may be present on the lateral and posterior aspects of the heels, which later may develop linear fissures with skin edge gangrene and a dark necrotic base. Severe atheroembolism from a proximal source may be accompanied by livedo reticularis of the knees, thighs, and buttocks.

The symptoms may last only a few minutes and may cause little noticeable disability. More commonly, the initial insult causes discomfort for several days, long enough to prompt a visit to the patient's local physician or a vascular surgery consultation. If the pain is minor, the lesions generally heal without tissue loss. Occasionally, the presentation of an embolic shower is marked by severe pain, which requires hospitalization and parenteral narcotics for control. These patients often have lesions that progress to gangrene, and, on careful questioning, a history consistent with previous showers is elicited. The outcome is determined by the presence of collateral circulation to the involved skin, and this circulation is dependent on the size of the emboli and the effects of previous or unrecognized embolic episodes. It is important to note that diabetic patients with neuropathy may suffer totally silent atheroembolism resulting in gangrene.

The clinical examination should include assessment of all peripheral arteries, including an examination for aneurysms. In its classic form, microembolism occurs with palpable pedal pulses. A bruit may be present over the affected artery, particularly if the source of microembolism is a highly stenotic common or superficial femoral artery. Duplex ultrasonography may be useful to determine the location of such high-grade stenotic lesions. The ankle blood pressures, the ankle-brachial indices, and pulse volume studies should be obtained because they are important in determining the prognosis for healing skin lesions. A Doppler stethoscope is also used to perform mapping of the digital arteries, which may demonstrate abrupt occlusion sounds (a ''tap'' or ''thunk'' without forward systolic or diastolic flow) or absence of flow at the ankle, in the midfoot, or in affected toes. Since microemboli can traverse relatively large collateral channels, it is possible for a proximal arterial source to lead to the signs and symptoms of atheroembolism even in the presence of chronic occlusive disease. Patients with stable occlusions as documented by vascular laboratory studies over time may heal without a proximal reconstruction, provided that laboratory results are within a range in which healing is expected. The authors have found that atheroembolic lesions usually heal if the ankle pressure exceeds 100 mmHg as measured in compressible arteries or if the metatarsal pulse volume tracings have a standard amplitude of 5 mm (see Chapter 5). In the clinical examination it is of vital importance to differentiate this chronic disease state from an acute thrombosis (usually at the adductor canal) that involves ''trashing'' of the distal circulation, a situation that often requires reconstruction for limb salvage.

Patients with evidence of atheroembolism should also be studied with duplex ultrasonography to determine the presence of aneurysms, particularly in the abdominal aorta and femoral popliteal segments. In thin patients, the iliac arteries can be adequately studied with this technique. Not uncommonly, diffuse aneurysmal disease is present throughout the arterial tree, with development of a fusiform dilatation of the aorta extending from the thoracic level to the iliac arteries. Ultrasound studies may define calcified irregular plaques, and the aneurysm may be notable for the absence of laminated thrombus. Computed tomography may also be helpful, particularly to define iliac aneurysms. With duplex scanning, friable thrombi or fungating plaques in the femoral and popliteal arteries may be documented.

There are no blood or laboratory tests specific to atheroembolism. Eosinophilia has been noted on blood smears and in urine.[53] Renal function is often checked in patients with bilateral lesions. A deterioration in renal function may indicate a suprarenal source of emboli. Muscle biopsy has received prominent attention in the literature pertaining to atheroembolism, and gastrocnemius muscle biopsies have confirmed atheroembolism in patients with suspicious clinical findings.[2, 4, 8, 48] However, this method has not found widespread use, and the overall accuracy of muscle biopsy has never been determined. The authors have been impressed that the symptoms are usually far more prominent than would be suspected from the degree of vascular occlusion evident in histologic sections of affected tissue.

At present, biplane angiography is the most accurate diagnostic method for determining the source of emboli. Ideally, this examination should define arteries from the infrarenal aorta to the toes. If the patient has evidence of bilateral embolization, the angiogram should include the lower thoracic aorta. Arterial irregularities may be present in many areas, and a complete examination is therefore necessary to determine the most likely arterial source of emboli. Intra-arterial digital subtraction angiography is helpful in avoiding excessive contrast loads because these patients are frequently seriously ill. Digital subtraction is also helpful in obtaining good anterior and posterior angiograms of the pedal arches of the foot, where abrupt cutoffs due to impacted atheroemboli may occasionally be visualized.

It should be stressed that the classic manifestation of atheroembolism is the development of ischemic skin in the presence of a continuous anatomic arterial channel between the source and the foot. Nevertheless, it is still possible for cholesterol debris to move through collateral channels. Therefore, it may be difficult to differentiate lesions due to occlusive disease in the foot or caused by local trauma to chronically ischemic or diabetic toes from lesions due to atheroembolism. A patient may ultimately need to undergo treatment for both entities in the course of the disease.

DIFFERENTIAL DIAGNOSIS

The manifestations of microemboli are frequently confused with those of other states of abnormal perfusion to the distal lower extremity. While the foot is dangling, a generalized bluish discoloration of the whole forefoot or a discoloration that involves all toe tips equally denotes rubor if it disappears into pallor with elevation of the leg. This implies severe proximal occlusive disease, and the pattern of pain may mimic that of atheroembolism if gangrene is impending. Acrocyanosis is associated with abnormal cardiopulmonary function, usually has a symmetric and constant distribution through all parts of the extremity, and may be associated with similar cutaneous discoloration in the hands, nose, helices of the ear, and lips. Confirmation of low cardiac output and abnormal oxygenation may be necessary to make this differentiation. Patients who receive beta-blocking medications may develop sluggish distal circulation, also symmetric in pattern, but it occurs in the presence of otherwise normal cardiac function. These lesions are not painful, although the sensation of a cool foot may be bothersome. Previous frostbite or exposure injury may leave an extremity sensitive to cold, with early development of bluish discoloration. Connective tissue disorders and microthrombotic episodes due to cryoglobulinemia may also mimic atheroembolism. These are usually more symmetric in nature but may be difficult to differentiate unless specific blood tests are performed. A severe atheroembolic shower may lead to livedo reticularis over the thighs and knees, a finding shared with connective tissue disorders, cold intolerance, and low cardiac output states. Repeated microthromboembolism or acute thrombosis distal to chronic occlusive disease has been documented in hypercoagulable states, such as protein S or protein C deficiency, antithrombin III deficiency, or occult carcinomatosis.[14] The foot affected by causalgia (reflex sympathetic dystrophy, see Chapter 49) is cool, clammy, and painful, and markedly different in appearance from the mottled, patchy, localized lesions of atheroembolism. The purpuric lesions of intravascular coagulopathy may mimic the early lesions of microemboli, but are differentiated by the signs and symptoms of systemic sepsis. Nevertheless, a patient may harbor occult endocarditis or a proximal septic arteritis (mycotic aneurysm) as a source of similar lesions in the toes. Localized injury to a diabetic foot may lead to patchy skin discoloration. A careful history and examination of the patient's footwear will assist in substantiating this diagnosis. Finally, the most important entity to be differentiated from atheroembolism is common impending gangrene of a toe due to critical lower extremity ischemia. The appearance of the ischemic foot may be identical to that of a repeatedly embolized extremity, and differentiation of these two entities may depend on angiography or histologic examination of the tissue. Therefore, because early or subsequent episodes of microembolism may be short-lived and cause few symptoms, the most important aspect of diagnosis is a careful history. Frequently, details of sudden attacks of pain in the calf muscles or previous episodes of skin discoloration are best confirmed by a family member rather than the patient.

MANAGEMENT

The primary treatment of lower extremity atheroembolism is, first and foremost, removal of the embolic source. Secondarily, if the source is associated with hemodynamically significant proximal occlusive disease, arterial reconstruction may be needed to guarantee healing through improved end-arterial bed perfusion. The long-term therapeutic goals also include palliation of severe pain due to atheroembolism and local care of the damaged skin envelope to minimize the potential for amputation. If an aneurysm is associated with microembolism, conventional operative repair is the best choice. Limited occlusive lesions in the aorta or iliac arteries may be approached by either local endarterectomy or bypass, and conventional anatomic aortofemoral or aortoiliac bypass grafts may be necessary to exclude more extensive diseased segments (see Fig. 44–3).[16, 31, 36, 46] If the source of embolization is a highly stenotic lesion in the femoral or popliteal segments, localized endarterectomy with vein patch angioplasty has proved satisfactory (see Fig. 44–4).[23, 26] If the degree of infrainguinal occlusive disease is extensive, conventional femoropopliteal bypass is indicated, with exclusion of the offending segment from the distal arterial circulation. Severe plaque degeneration is frequently a generalized phenomenon, and the surgeon should be alert to the possibility of plaque disruption following any manipulation of arteries, particularly with repeated clamping, passage of catheters for angiography,[21, 41] or transluminal balloon angioplasty. Prevention of intraoperative microembolization (''trashing'' of the outflow circulation) is particularly important during aortic procedures.[45] For these, it is usually best to clamp the outflow vessels before clamping or performing major manipulation of the aorta to prevent dislodgment of friable material. The graft and proximal arterial cuff should be flushed (''blown out'') just prior to completing the distal or outflow anastomosis, and initial blood flow for aortofemoral procedures should be directed retrograde into the external iliac arteries before flow is released into the legs. Care must be taken in reclamping after testing the proximal aortic suture line for hemostasis: Reclamping repeatedly may lead to dislodgment of debris into the renal arteries.

Sympathectomy has received attention as a measure for palliation of atheroembolic lesions.[33, 36] Not only is it an adjunct to direct surgical treatment of the offending arterial segment, but also it may be useful to control the pain of severe atheroembolic toe lesions in patients who otherwise cannot undergo direct reconstruction of the embolic source or when correction does not improve distal perfusion. Sympathectomy is easily performed during aortic procedures, or it can be achieved postoperatively through lumbar sympathetic blocks.

In some instances, the exact identification of the embologenic area can be quite difficult. The authors have observed occlusion of infrainguinal bypasses by dislodgment of sizable emboli from the proximal arteries.[17] This is both a frustrating and puzzling phenomenon because the occlusion is associated with a technically adequate reconstruction. When this occurrence is noted, treatment of the proximal circulation with either bypass or endarterectomy may be necessary to remove the offending lesion.

The degree of damage to the lower extremities by atheroemboli may be impressive. After extirpation of the embolic source, extensive healing may ensue. If dry gangrene of toes is noted after reconstruction, near autoamputation should be allowed before revision or closure. As long as these digits do not become infected, this course will preserve the greatest amount of tissue in the foot. Dry dressings are used for protection, and the injured areas are painted twice daily with povidone iodine liquid. In diabetic patients the lesions can heal with these measures, but careful home management and frequent office visits are necessary to prevent wet gangrene and disastrous necrotizing infection. Atheroembolism results in a permanent microvascular insult to the skin, not unlike that occurring with frostbite or exposure injury. Major forefoot injury is treated with conventional transmetatarsal amputation after demarcation has occurred. Amputation through damaged skin may fail to heal properly. Skin flaps must be fashioned and handled with meticulous atraumatic technique and tension-free closure.

Like the controversy associated with the ''medical'' management of cerebrovascular microembolism leading to a transient ischemic attack or stroke, disagreement exists about the nonsurgical treatment of lower extremity atheroembolism. Prior to initial surgical evaluation, episodes of microembolization are frequently treated by nonsurgical practitioners with a variety of medications, typically aspirin, dipyridamole, warfarin, or steroids.[13] Only one study has examined the efficacy of aspirin for the treatment of atheroembolism, and clinical improvement occurred in over

50 per cent of patients so managed.[37] Because plaque hemorrhage and surface disruption are notable pathologic findings, these medications may actually lead to paradoxical accentuation of atheroembolism by decreasing the stability of the diseased flow surface.[7] After a minor initial embolic event, it is reasonable to treat some patients with long-term antiplatelet therapy, which appears to carry little morbidity. This decision should be based on the best information about the state of the circulation, using vascular laboratory studies and appropriate angiography. Patients treated in this manner must be followed closely to determine whether treatment failure has occurred.

The bilateral occurrence of lower extremity atheroembolism is important because it generally indicates a source proximal to the aortic bifurcation.[28, 46] Because the suprarenal aorta or aortic arch may be degenerative (see Fig. 44–2), it is necessary initially to document the patient's renal function and to determine, by history, whether the patient has had symptoms consistent with intestinal atheroembolism (pain, diarrhea, hematochezia, loss of appetite). In the most flagrant form of disseminated atheroembolism, in which the source is in the thoracic aorta and embolization occurs to multiple organ systems, the patient is usually found to have pronounced cardiopulmonary disease, frequently with repeated episodes of congestive heart failure.[8, 12, 28, 40, 49] Renal dysfunction due to multiple episodes of atheroembolism is difficult to treat medically because there is poor response to either antiplatelet medication or steroids. Atheroembolism to the intestinal tract may be confused with diverticular disease, ischemic colitis, pancreatitis, or gastritis.[4, 12, 28] The definitive diagnosis of this syndrome is based on appropriate clinical findings, including weight loss, malaise, bilateral lower extremity lesions, cardiac disease, and recent, rapid deterioration of renal function. Angiograms demonstrate the severe degenerative atherosclerosis of the suprarenal aorta. Renal, prostatic or rectal biopsy may provide confirmatory evidence of cholesterol embolization to the viscera.[38, 51] If the patient has good cardiopulmonary function, the theoretical treatment of choice is aortic replacement to remove the offending source, commencing with repair of the aorta proximal to or including the visceral and renal ostia. However, the majority of these patients are seriously ill at presentation, with marked asthenia, and the prognosis has been early death in 64 to 89 per cent of all cases.[12, 28, 40] Occasionally, patients with this syndrome develop progressive embolization to the feet, with severe associated pain and impending gangrene. In such cases, an axillobifemoral bypass with exclusion ligation of the external iliac arteries may be the only viable alternative.[27] This procedure allows healing of the feet by creation of a new proximal inflow source from an uninvolved subclavian artery and results in gratifying relief of pain. Lumbar sympathetic blocks may be a useful adjunct to this operation. Short of primary reconstruction of the aorta, there is no satisfactory treatment for documented atheroembolism to the gut or pancreas. Unfortunately, the majority of these patients are diagnosed only after an abdominal catastrophe has occurred or at autopsy. Likewise, there is little that can be done to treat spontaneous atheroembolism to the kidneys if the patient's condition does not permit direct aortic reconstruction. Renal failure in these patients usually develops rapidly during a period when new cutaneous lesions are noted. Because of the friable nature of the involved aorta in these patients, care must be taken in performing any angiographic studies to prevent further embolization, which may affect adjacent soft tissue structures and the spinal cord. Renal failure after atheroembolism has a poor prognosis, and early provision of access for hemodialysis or peritoneal dialysis is indicated.

SUMMARY

Atheroembolism and microembolic phenomena are common complications of severe atherosclerosis, most often from limited lesions in the aortoiliac and femoropopliteal segments. The most common clinically apparent manifestation is the blue toe syndrome, but atheroembolism may affect any organ, most significantly the central nervous system as a cause of transient ischemic attacks and stroke. At the occurrence of atheroembolism, diagnostic measures should be aimed at determining the location and character of the source of microemboli and the perfusion state of the involved extremity. Minor single atheroembolic events affecting the feet can be treated with antiplatelet drugs, if the source is diffuse degenerative disease as typically found in the infrarenal aorta. However, these patients must have close follow-up because the efficacy of nonsurgical therapy is not well demonstrated, and some patients suffer recurrent events, especially after the administration of anticoagulants. Because repeated episodes of atheroembolism may result in limb loss, surgical therapy should be focused on removal of the embolic source from the proximal circulation, either by local endarterectomy or bypass procedures. Disseminated atheroembolism, with associated damage to the viscera and kidneys, has a poor prognosis. If the primary aortic source cannot be replaced in these patients, surgical attention should be focused on providing access for hemodialysis or peritoneal dialysis and on performing exclusion bypass to prevent further embolization to the feet.

References

1. Ahn SS, Auth D, Marcus DR, Moore WS: Removal of focal atheromatous lesions by angioscopically guided high-speed rotary atherectomy: Preliminary experimental observations. J Vasc Surg 7:292, 1988.
2. Adamson AS, Pittman MR, Karke SG: Atheroembolism presenting as selective muscle embolisation. J Cardiovasc Surg 32:705, 1991.
3. Amarenco P, Duyckaerts C, Tzourio C, et al: The prevalence of ulcerated plaques in the aortic arch in patients with stroke. N Engl J Med 326:221, 1992.
4. Anderson WR: Necrotizing angiitis associated with embolization of cholesterol: Case report with emphasis on the use of the muscle biopsy as a diagnostic aid. Am J Clin Pathol 43:65, 1965.
5. Berkman M, Berkman N, Favre M, et al: Les embolies de cholesterol: Confrontation clinique, ophthalmoscopique et anatomique, a l'occasion de trois observations. Nouv Presse Med 1:795, 1972.
6. Branowitz JB, Edwards WS: The management of atheromatous emboli to the lower extremities. Surg Gynecol Obstet 143:941, 1976.
7. Bruns FJ, Segel DP, Adler S: Control of cholesterol embolization by discontinuation of anticoagulant therapy. Am J Med Sci 275:105, 1978.
8. Carvajal JA, Anderson WR, Weiss L, et al: Atheroembolism: An etiologic factor in renal insufficiency, gastrointestinal hemorrhages and peripheral vascular diseases. Arch Intern Med 119:593, 1967.
9. Case records of the Massachusetts General Hospital 50-1977. N Engl J Med 297:1337, 1977.

10. Case records of the Massachusetts General Hospital 30-1986. N Engl J Med 315:308, 1986
11. Crane C: Atherothrombotic embolism to lower extremities in arteriosclerosis. Arch Surg 94:96, 1967.
12. Dahlberg PJ, Frecentese DF, Cogbill TH: Cholesterol embolism: Experience with 22 histologically proven cases. Surgery 105:737, 1989.
13. Darsee JR: Cholesterol embolism: The great masquerader. South Med J 72:174, 1979.
14. Eason JD, Mills JL, Beckett WC: Hypercoagulable states in arterial thromboembolism. Surg Gynecol Obstet 174:211, 1992.
15. Falanga V, Fine MJ, Kapoor WN: The cutaneous manifestations of cholesterol crystal embolization. Arch Derm 122:1194, 1986
16. Fisher DF, Clagett GP, Brigham RA, et al: Dilemmas in dealing with the blue toe syndrome: Aortic versus peripheral source. Am J Surg 148:836, 1984.
17. Flinn WR, Harris JP, Rudo ND, et al: Atheroembolism as a cause of graft failure in femoral distal reconstruction. Surgery 90:698, 1981.
18. Flory CM: Arterial occlusions produced by emboli from eroded aortic atheromatous plaques. Am J Pathol 21:549, 1945.
19. Fuster V, Badimon L, Badimon JJ, Chesebro JH: The pathogenesis of coronary artery disease and the acute coronary syndromes. N Engl J Med 326:310, 1992.
20. Gore L, Collins DP: Spontaneous atheromatous embolization: Review of the literature and a report of 16 additional cases. Am J Clin Pathol 33:416, 1960.
21. Harrington JT, Sommers SC, Kassirer JP: Atheromatous emboli with progressive renal failure: Renal arteriography as the probable inciting factor. Ann Intern Med 68:152, 1968.
22. Haygood TA, Fessel WJ, Strange DA: Atheromatous microembolism simulating polymyositis. JAMA 203:423, 1968.
23. Inahara T, Scott CM: Endarterectomy for segmental occlusive disease of the superficial femoral artery. Arch Surg 116:1547, 1981.
24. Jenkins DM, Newton WD: Atheroembolism. Am Surg 57:588, 1991.
25. Karmody AM, Jordan FR, Zaman SM: Left colon gangrene after acute inferior mesenteric artery occlusion. Arch Surg 111:972, 1976.
26. Karmody AM, Powers SR, Monaco VJ, et al: ''Blue toe'' syndrome: An indication for limb salvage surgery. Arch Surg 111:1263, 1976.
27. Kaufman JL, Saifi J, Chang BB, et al: The role of extraanatomic exclusion bypass in the treatment of disseminated atheroembolism syndrome. Ann Vasc Surg 4:260, 1990.
28. Kaufman JL, Stark K, Brolin RE: Disseminated atheroembolism from extensive degenerative atherosclerosis of the aorta. Surgery 102:63, 1987.
29. Kealy WF: Atheroembolism. J Clin Pathol 31:984, 1978.
30. Kempczinski RF: Lower-extremity arterial emboli from ulcerating atherosclerotic plaques. JAMA 241:807, 1979.
31. Kwaan JHM, Connolly JE: Peripheral atheroembolism: An enigma. Arch Surg 112:987, 1977.
32. Labs JD, Merillat JC, Williams GM: Analysis of solid phase debris from laser angioplasty: Potential risks of atheroembolism. J Vasc Surg 7:326, 1988.
33. Lee BY, Brancato RF, Thoden WR, et al: Blue digit syndrome: Urgent indication for digital salvage. Am J Surg 147:418, 1984.
34. McFarland RJ, Taylow RS, Woodyer AB, Eastwood JB: The femoropopliteal segment as a source of peripheral atheroembolism. J Cardiovasc Surg 30:597, 1989.
35. McLean NR, Irvine BH, Calvert MH: Peripheral embolic phenomena from proximal arterial disease. J R Coll Surg Edinb 29:205, 1984.
36. Mehigan JT, Stoney RJ: Lower extremity atheromatous embolization. Am J Surg 132:163, 1976.
37. Morris-Jones W, Preston FE, Greaney M, Chatterjee DK: Gangrene of the toes with palpable peripheral pulses: Response to platelet suppressive therapy. Ann Surg 193:462, 1981.
38. O'Briain DS, Jeffers M, Kay EW, Hourihane DO: Bleeding due to colorectal atheroembolism. Diagnosis by biopsy of adenomatous polyps or of ischemic ulcer. Am J Surg Pathol 15:1078, 1991.
39. Perdue GD, Smith RB: Atheromatous microemboli. Ann Surg 169:954, 1969.
40. Pizzolitto S, Rocco M, Antonucci F, Antoci B: Atheroembolism: A form of systemic vascular disease. Pathologica 83:147, 1991.
41. Ramirez G, O'Neill WM, Lambert R, et al: Cholesterol embolization: A complication of angiography. Arch Intern Med 138:1430, 1978.
42. Retan JW, Miller RE: Microembolic complications of atherosclerosis. Arch Intern Med 118:534, 1966.
43. Ribakove GH, Katz ES, Galloway AC, et al: Surgical implications of transesophageal echocardiography to grade the atheromatous aortic arch. Ann Thorac Surg 53:758, 1992.
44. Richards AM, Eliot RS, Kanjuh VI, et al: Cholesterol embolism: A multiple-system disease masquerading as polyarteritis nodosa. Am J Cardiol 15:696, 1965.
45. Robicsek F: Prevention of cholesterol embolism (trash foot) during aorto-iliac reconstruction using a blood filtering device. J Cardiovasc Surg (Torino) 27:63, 1987.
46. Rosenberg MW, Shah DP: Bilateral blue toe syndrome: A case report. JAMA 243:365, 1980.
47. Schechter DC: Atheromatous embolization to lower limbs. NY State Med J 79:1180, 1979.
48. Schipper H, Gordon M, Berris B: Atheromatous embolic disease. Can Med Assoc J 113:640, 1975.
49. Smith MC, Ghose MK, Henry AR: The clinical spectrum of renal cholesterol embolization. Am J Med 71:174, 1981.
50. Stoney RJ, Skioldebrand CG, Ovarfordt PG, et al: Juxtarenal aortic atherosclerosis: Surgical experience and functional result. Ann Surg 200:345, 1984.
51. Sussman B, Stahl R, Ibrahim IM, et al: Atheroemboli to the lower urinary tract: A marker of atherosclerotic vascular disease—a case report. J Vasc Surg 12:655, 1990.
52. Williams GM, Harrington D, Burdick J, et al: Mural thrombus of the aorta: An important, frequently neglected cause of large peripheral emboli. Ann Surg 194:737, 1981.
53. Wilson DM, Salazer TL, Faroukh ME: Eosinophiluria in atheroembolic renal disease. Am J Med 91:186, 1991.

45

Acute Vascular Insufficiency due to Drug Injection

William W. Turner, Jr., M.D., R. James Valentine, M.D., and Creighton B. Wright, M.D.

• • •

Substance abuse is a worldwide social concern. Of the many problems associated with drug addiction, acute vascular insufficiency is the most common disorder for which the vascular surgeon is consulted. The modern addict is skilled at achieving intravenous access. The lack of precise anatomic knowledge and inexperience with sterile technique frequently lead to acute complications involving both arterial and venous systems. The more common complications of drug-induced vascular insufficiency are listed in Table 45–1.

ARTERIAL INJURIES

The first report of an accidental intra-arterial drug injection with resulting gangrene appeared 50 years ago.[1] Subsequently, a number of instances of barbiturate-induced vascular insufficiency have been described.[2–8] In earlier years, these problems were due primarily to unintentional intra-arterial injections by physicians or nurses. The complications of intra-arterial injections are now most often associated with illicit drug use. There are numerous reports of extremity gangrene following intra-arterial injections of a variety of drugs, and a number of authors have attempted to delineate the mechanisms of the injuries.[2–4, 6, 7, 9–15]

Clinical Presentation

There is no way to calculate accurately the incidence of arterial injections associated with drug abuse or to describe fully the variety of resulting vascular insufficiency syndromes. Only the worst complications of intra-arterial drug injections come to medical attention, and it is possible that many inadvertent intra-arterial injections go unnoticed. Several large centers have reported their experiences.[9, 16–25] Complicating the clinical presentation are the multiple and variable manifestations. One report noted hand ischemia secondary to intra-arterial drug injections in five patients who denied any history of substance abuse.[26]

Drug users, depending on ''self-taught'' skills, may directly inject a superficial artery, or they may accidentally enter an artery while attempting to gain access to any vessel deep in the antecubital fossa or femoral triangle. Only with the production of a ''hand trip'' does the addict recognize the error of intra-arterial injection.[5] The result has been described as a burning discomfort extending from the point of injection to the tips of the fingers, followed by blanching, severe pain, and subsequent swelling and cyanosis. The exact timing of these events, particularly the development of gangrene, remains unclear. Delay in seeking medical attention is frequent. It is common for digital or even total extremity gangrene to be the presenting complaint (Fig. 45–1).

Before, during, and after administration of a drug, a number of additional factors can play roles in the development of gangrene. In the quest for vascular access, an individual may use a variety of tourniquets, and the sedative effects of the drug may lead to prolonged tourniquet compression with the induction of venous or arterial thrombo-

Table 45–1. Complications of Drug-Induced Vascular Insufficiency

Infections
Cellulitis
Abscesses
Osteomyelitis
Septic arthritis
Endocarditis
Lymphatic complications
Puffy hand
Vascular complications
Compartment syndrome
Rhabdomyolysis
Vasospasm
Direct arterial injury
Intimal disruption
Thrombosis
Embolism
Mycotic aneurysm
Skin ulcers
Thrombophlebitis
Venous aneurysm
Neurologic complications
Direct nerve injury
Polyneuritis
Ischemic neuritis
Acute transverse myelitis

Modified from Ritland D, Butterfield W: Extremity complications of drug abuse. Am J Surg 126:639, 1973.

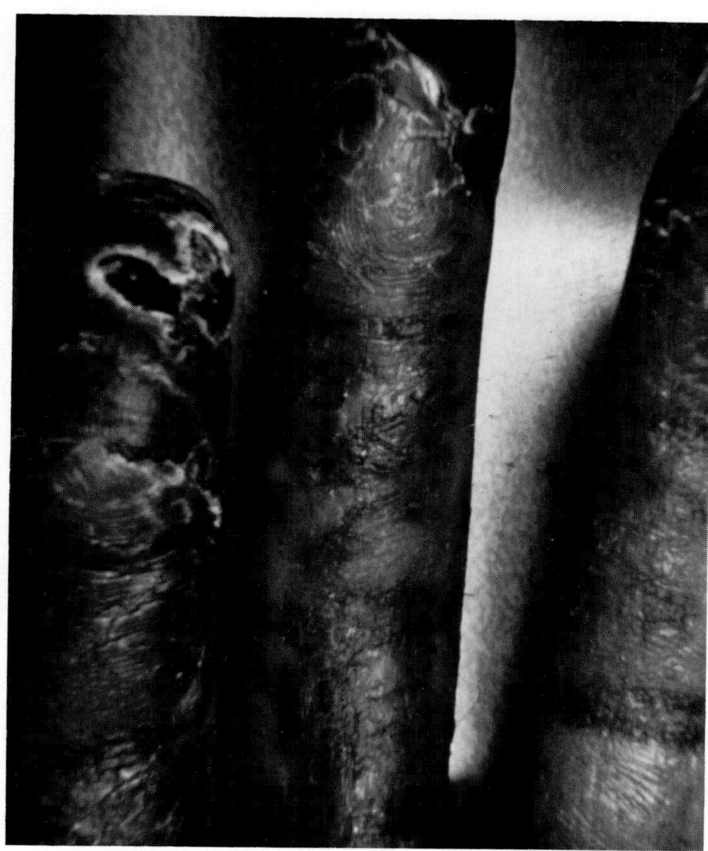

FIGURE 45–1. Distal digital gangrene following intra-arterial administration of heroin.

sis. The intra-arterially injected drug may remain in sustained contact with the vessel intima prior to release of the tourniquet. Abnormal posturing with arm or thigh flexion or with the extremity compressed under the full weight of the obtunded person may add to circulatory compromise. Experimental studies using catheters placed in normal volunteers have documented marked elevations of intramuscular pressures sufficient to cause muscle and capillary ischemia and local obstruction of the circulation when the extremities are placed in postures similar to those of overdosed, sedated, stuporous individuals.[27]

Local injury is a problem associated with arterial access, even when it is performed by skilled clinicians.[28] Arterial injections by the less adept addict may lead to a variety of vessel injuries that cause thrombosis at injection sites. These include intimal flaps, perivascular hematomas, and perivascular inflammation. Certain drugs are also more likely to damage the intima directly.[3, 29] Severe damage to arteries at injection sites can cause pseudoaneurysms. These may develop at any site as a result of a through-and-through puncture or from ineffectual tamponade of a puncture site after removal of a needle. Superimposed infection is common. Mycotic aneurysms are being reported more frequently both at sites of injections and at distant locations, including cerebral, aortic, splenic, coronary, and pulmonary arteries. Additional unusual sites of mycotic aneurysms are the inferior mesenteric, carotid, and superior mesenteric arteries.[24, 30–34] The more superficial pseudoaneurysms of the brachial, femoral, and radial arteries are often used by drug addicts for vascular access because they are more easily palpable than peripheral veins (Fig. 45–2).

Upper Extremity

The brachial artery is the most common site of accidental injections in the upper extremity.[35] Pseudoaneurysm is the most common sequela. Patients with pseudoaneurysms frequently present with cellulitis and pain associated with infection or distal ischemia. Severe ischemia accompanies such lesions in approximately 30 per cent of cases. Fortunately, systemic sepsis is usually not a major problem. In a series of 32 patients with upper extremity lesions only 12 per cent had positive blood cultures.[35] Mycotic aneurysms associated with intra-arterial injections are treated by ligation and excision, and immediate distal revascularization is generally not required. This form of treatment has been associated with few complications. Severely involved gangrenous digits may require amputation.

Lower Extremity

Approximately three fourths of all admissions for accidental intra-arterial drug injections involve the lower extremities.[35] Pseudoaneurysm is the most common arterial abnormality, with arteriovenous fistula being second in frequency. The major presenting symptom is a painful, pulsatile mass, often associated with cellulitis. Examination often reveals a bruit over the involved area. Local infections are

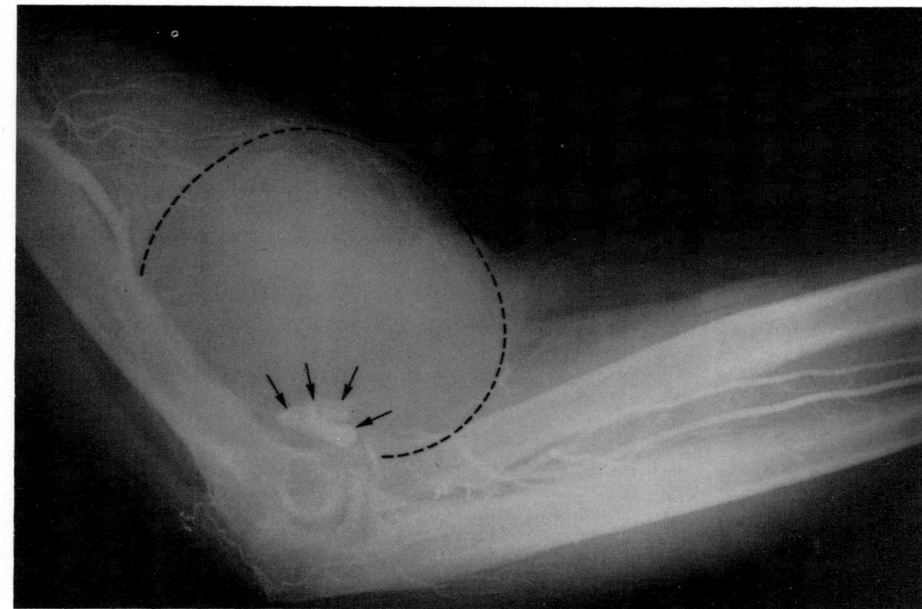

FIGURE 45–2. Operative arteriogram of an expanding brachial artery false aneurysm. The small false aneurysm (*arrows*) had been used for drug injections. It ruptured suddenly into the soft tissues (*outlined*), resulting in overlying skin necrosis and neural compression. Patch angioplasty (autogenous vein) was used for arterial repair.

common, and there is a higher incidence of positive blood cultures than with mycotic aneurysms of the upper extremities.

In a review of 54 infected femoral artery pseudoaneurysms in drug addicts, 11 per cent of patients required amputation.[36] There was a 33 per cent risk of amputation when the common femoral bifurcation was involved and required excision. Twenty-eight aneurysms were reconstructed using either prosthetic grafts or autologous saphenous veins. All synthetic grafts eventually developed septic complications, and graft removals were required. Of 18 patients who were treated by ligations without vascular reconstructions, one third required amputation. This study supports the conclusion that if a pseudoaneurysm involves only a single artery, ligation and excision is the treatment of choice. When the common femoral bifurcation is involved, immediate autogenous reconstruction should be considered. Obturator artery bypasses have been utilized successfully for the treatment of mycotic aneurysms in drug addicts.[37] Such extra-anatomic bypass techniques may be excellent alternatives to direct revascularization through contaminated tissues.

Head and Neck

The head and neck are the least common sites of vascular insufficiency secondary to drug abuse. This is perhaps due to the infrequent use of these highly visible areas and to addicts' desires to keep their injection sites hidden. In a review of 172 consecutive patients admitted to the hospital for vascular injuries from drug abuse, approximately 2 per cent of patients presented with head and neck lesions; 19 per cent presented with upper extremity lesions; and 79 per cent presented with lower extremity complications.[35] Of the head and neck lesions studied, the carotid artery was the vessel most commonly involved. There were two carotid pseudoaneurysms, one carotid-jugular arteriovenous fistula, and one arterial wall necrosis. The most common presenting complaint was a pulsatile mass with associated induration and cellulitis. All of the patients were treated with ligations of the common carotid artery and no neurologic sequelae resulted from this treatment.

Deep abscesses may be associated with arterial lesions in the neck. Various abused drugs have been implicated, but methylphenidate (Ritalin) has been associated with more than 50 per cent of the deep neck abscesses in some series.[38] Since the majority of these abscesses are acquired outside the hospital setting, it is not surprising that most cultures reveal staphylococci and streptococci. A less common organism, *Eikenella corrodens*, has been implicated as a synergistic pathogen with streptococci in association with Ritalin-induced abscesses. Oral flora are the most likely source of organisms that contaminate the head and neck.

Lung

Multiple mycotic pulmonary artery aneurysms have been reported secondary to intravenous drug abuse.[39–41] Patients frequently present with dyspnea, cyanosis, and hemoptysis. Physical examination sometimes reveals a harsh systolic murmur in the left second interspace. Right ventricular hypertrophy with right axis deviation is common.[42] These lesions are difficult to manage because they are frequently multiple and often central in location. Bilaterality occurs, which precludes surgical treatment by resection and ligation in some cases. To date fewer than 70 cases have been collected in the world literature. As intravenous drug abuse increases, it is possible that mycotic aneurysms of the pulmonary arteries will be diagnosed more frequently.

Pulmonary hypertension associated with talc granulomas can occur when drugs intended for oral use are injected intravenously. Pulmonary hypertension and, in extreme cases, cor pulmonale result from small vessel occlusions due to excipients.[43, 44]

Mechanisms of Injury

Numerous mechanisms for producing ischemia have been proposed: vessel obstruction by inert particles (excipients) or drug crystals, endarteritis, hemolysis, platelet aggregation, vasospasm, and venous thrombosis.[7, 18, 19, 23, 45–49] Most of these factors lead to thrombosis of the arterial supply to digits as the final common pathway leading to extremity gangrene. The addict may obtain pure parenteral drugs, but more commonly the drugs have been ''cut'' by the addition of other materials, either by the producer or by the distributor. Oral preparations are often diluted or suspended and injected along with debris from the tablet (Table 45–2)[24, 50, 51] Each of these additives can compound the vascular injury produced by the specific drug. Excipients may also have systemic effects. Oral suspensions of methylphenidate hydrochloride (Ritalin) containing talc and cornstarch have been injected intravenously. Excipients have been identified in the retinal fundi and choroid, producing transient blindness and decreased visual acuity as well as neovascularization.[50, 52–57] The microvasculature of the digits may, like the eye, be particularly sensitive to excipient collections. Such effects may result from both intravenous and intra-arterial injections.

Crystalline emboli, like excipients, can play roles in producing arterial injuries. A series of experiments studied in vitro crystallization of thiopental sodium in freshly drawn blood at room and body temperatures.[58] Concentrations of 5, 2.5, and 1.25 per cent thiopental were evaluated to show the amount of precipitated thiopental in mixtures with blood. The obstructing capacity of these mixtures was demonstrated by perfusing them through a No. 20 hypodermic needle and, in addition, by postmortem perfusion of a human arm. Crystals formed in 5 per cent and 10 per cent thiopental solutions but occurred less frequently in solutions of lower concentrations.

Crystal formation does not account for all instances of arterial gangrene. Direct endothelial damage is another effect associated with injection of some agents. A series of experiments in dogs produced gangrene with dextroamphetamine sulfate (Dexedrine), promazine hydrochloride (Sparine), ether, and sulfobromophthalein sodium (Bromsulphalein). Temporary occlusion of the femoral artery proximal to the site of injection was necessary to produce gangrene. Biopsies and vascular casts of the necrotic tissue demonstrated severe necrosis of the small artery walls, with pronounced edema and congestion with thrombi in some of the larger vessels. The vascular casts demonstrated complete occlusion of larger arterioles and small arteries corresponding to the areas of gangrene. It was concluded that these drugs are transported in undiluted forms as boluses of highly irritating solutions to induce the subsequent gangrene.

Table 45–2. Common Excipients

Caffeine	Starch
Lactose	Stearic acid
Procaine	Talcum powder
Quinine	

Table 45–3. Drugs Associated With Hypersensitivity Vasculitis

Allopurinol	Isoniazid
Ampicillin	Levamisole
Bromide	Methylthiouracil
Carbamazepine	Oxyphenbutazone
Chloramphenicol	Phenylbutazone
Chlorpropamide	Phenytoin
Chlortetracycline	Potassium iodide
Chlorthalidone	Procainamide
Cromolyn sodium	Propylthiouracil
Colchicine	Quinidine
Dextran	Spironolactone
Diazepam	Sulfonamides
Diphenhydramine	Tetracycline
Griseofulvin	Trimethadione
Indomethacin	

From McAllister HA Jr, Mullick FG: The cardiovascular system. In *Riddel RH (ed): Pathology of Drug-Induced and Toxic Disease. Churchill Livingstone, New York, 1982.*

Many drugs have been associated with a hypersensitivity vasculitis syndrome. Some of these substances are listed in Table 45–3. Additionally, several drugs have been associated with toxic vasculitis (Table 45–4). A lupus-like syndrome occurring after injection of certain substances has also been reported (Table 45–5).

A study of 10 barbiturate solutions at varying concentrations demonstrated that in addition to crystal formation, hemolysis and platelet aggregation occur with barbiturates.[45] Following these reports, thiopental has been supplied in the reduced concentration (2.5 per cent), and reports of problems with this drug have become much less frequent.

Vasospasm secondary to drug acidity, alkalinity, vascular trauma, and norepinephrine or epinephrine release has been studied. The contribution of arterial constriction to the sequelae of intra-arterial drug injection remains controversial. Contraction of aortic strips and ear arteries was produced in rabbits by thiopental.[59] This may have been due to local norepinephrine release or to direct chemical effects.[46] Vasospasm may also result from local trauma or irritation by particulate matter.[60] Most clinical studies that have implicated vasospasm have lacked arteriographic data.[16, 19, 23, 51]

In one experiment investigators employed micrometer measurements of rabbit femoral arteries before, during, and after injections of 5 per cent thiopental or a buffer of equal pH.[6] Transient (30-second) vasoconstriction was followed by prompt vasodilatation in response to thiopental, and no effect was noted from the buffer. In subsequent experiments, tissue necrosis developed after injections of 0.2 ml

Table 45–4. Drugs Associated With Toxic Vasculitis

Organic arsenicals	Methamphetamine
Gold salts	DDT
Mercurials	Serum
Bismuth	Sulfonamides
Amphetamine	Penicillin

From McAllister HA Jr, Mullick FG: The cardiovascular system. In *Riddel RH (ed): Pathology of Drug-Induced and Toxic Disease. Churchill Livingstone, New York, 1982.*

Table 45–5. Drugs That Induce Lupus-Like Syndrome

Hydralazine	Sulfonamides
Procainamide	Tetracycline
Isoniazid	Propylthiouracil
Aminosalicylic acid	Methylthiouracil
Phenytoin	Methyldopa
Mephenytoin	Barbiturates
Primidone	Griseofulvin
Trimethadione	Streptomycin
Ethosuximide	Quinidine
Methsuximide	Phenylbutazone
Reserpine	Chlorpromazine
Penicillin	Methotrimeprazine
Penicillamine	Perphenazine
	Promazine

From McAllister HA Jr, Mullick FG: The cardiovascular system. In *Riddel RH (ed): Pathology of Drug-Induced and Toxic Disease. Churchill Livingstone, New York, 1982.*

of 10 per cent thiopental into the central artery of the rabbit ear followed by application of an intestinal clamp across the base of the ear for 15 minutes. It required prolonged observation for 3 to 4 weeks before a standard amount of necrosis was seen. In this model, sympathetic denervation by cervical ganglionectomy significantly decreased the area of gangrene, as did administration of 2500 units of heparin every 8 hours. When a decreased concentration of thiopental (2.5 per cent) was substituted for the 10 per cent thiopental solution the incidence of tissue loss was very low. If procaine or tolazoline was administered following thiopental, no significant reduction in the area of gangrene occurred. The authors concluded that prolonged arterial spasm was not the cause of ischemia after intra-arterial injection of thiopental because the area of injury could be diminished by lowering the thiopental concentration, by sympathectomy, or by heparinization but not by vasodilator drugs.

A recent study in the rabbit ear intra-arterial thiopental model also suggested that vasospasm might have only a limited effect on the clinical events following intra-arterial drug injections. Vasodilators administered after the injection of thiopental had no effect on the course of tissue necrosis.[61] This study did not employ arteriography to assess the degree of vasospasm, and the conclusion that vasospasm played a minor role in the development of gangrene was drawn indirectly from evidence of the ineffectiveness of vasodilators in preventing gangrene. The results of these animal experiments differ from anecdotal cases in humans in which intra-arterial injection of the vasodilator reserpine resulted immediately in improved distal perfusion in patients who had injected crushed pentazocine tablets into their brachial arteries.[62]

Although arterial constriction may occupy a debatable position in the etiology of drug-related extremity ischemia, venospasm may play an indirect but significant role. Concentrated drugs can cause venostasis. Repetitive angiography was used to study the effects of 0.4 ml of 10 per cent thiopental on the central arteries and veins of rabbit ears.[12] The study demonstrated dramatic changes in the venous circulation, including marked venospasm along with segmental thrombosis, which probably contributed to the development of ischemia and gangrene. Acute outflow obstruction with transudation into interstitial spaces leading to persistent arterial stasis with thrombosis may have been the mechanism underlying the ischemic necrosis.[63] An absence of superficial veins may further contribute to flow reduction and ischemia.[3, 13, 58, 64, 65]

Therapeutic Considerations

Therapy should include immediate measures to relieve pain, prevent local limb and systemic hypothermia, and improve venous drainage by patient positioning. Long-term efforts should be directed toward encouraging discontinuance of drug abuse and cessation of smoking. Arteriography should be performed early with a catheter positioned proximal to the suspected site of drug injection. An arteriogram will define local arterial injuries such as an intimal flap, a pseudoaneurysm, an arteriovenous fistula, or thrombosis, as well as distal vasospasm or thrombosis. The arteriogram catheter may be left in place for subsequent intraluminal therapy.

Vasodilators

Vasodilators can play a role in the treatment of acute arterial ischemia secondary to drugs of abuse.[23, 58, 61, 66–68] Tolazoline (Priscoline) in doses of 25 to 50 mg has been used successfully by injection into the proximal artery.[69] Tolazoline competitively blocks arterial wall alpha-adrenergic receptors, dilates precapillary arterioles, and opens precapillary arteriovenous shunts in the skin. Other vasodilators that have been used in patients following intra-arterial drug injections include verapamil and phentolamine.[70, 71] If vasospasm is not a major component of the process, vasodilator therapy will not directly alter the response to the drug, although it may serve to maintain collateral circulation.

Anticoagulation

Animal studies have demonstrated a benefit of heparin in reducing gangrene following intra-arterial injections of thiopental.[6, 72] Beneficial reports in humans have included several anecdotal reports and a noteworthy description of a patient in whom an occluded palmar arch was reconstituted; the patient also experienced improved digital flow in the hand after the administration of intra-arterial heparin.[9, 18, 23, 69] Evidence suggests that treatment for at least 4 days may be beneficial.[6]

Thrombolysis

Persistent vessel occlusion and poor response to vasodilators may indicate a need for thrombolysis. Low dose intra-arterial streptokinase has been used successfully in patients with palmar arterial thromboses secondary to causes *other* than intra-arterial drug injections.[73, 74] A patient with hand ischemia after forearm arterial drug injection experienced improved hand perfusion within 24 hours of receiving intra-arterial streptokinase (Fig. 45–3).[69] This patient received an initial intra-arterial dose of 25,000 units of streptokinase followed by 3000 u/hr for 24 hours. Traditionally, the infusion catheter has been placed within the

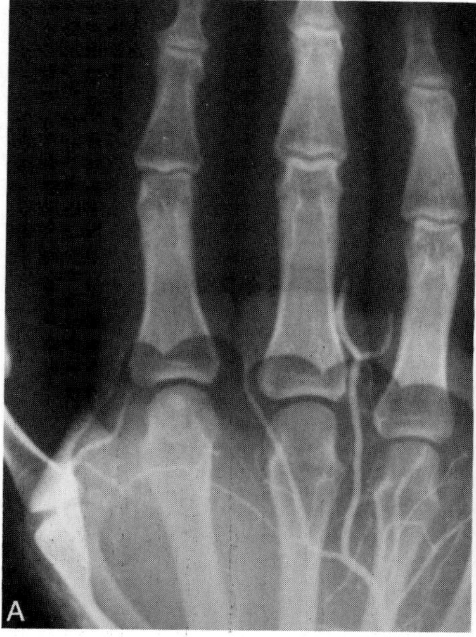

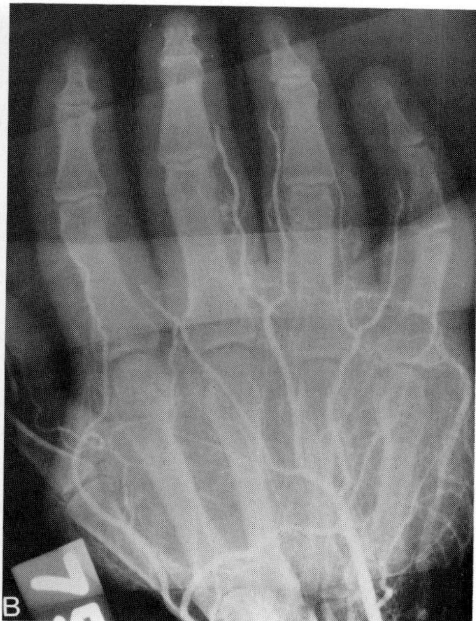

FIGURE 45–3. *A*, Initial arteriogram of the left hand demonstrates absent visualization of the digital arteries. *B*, Arteriogram after intra-arterial streptokinase infusion demonstrates improved flow to all digits of the left hand. (*A* and *B*, From Silverman SH, Turner WW Jr: Intra-arterial drug abuse: New treatment options. J Vasc Surg 14:111, 1991.)

thrombus to produce a high local concentration of the drug and to reduce perfusion of collaterals with the drug. This technique may limit the success of thrombolytic therapy in patients with distal thrombi, which are frequently seen secondary to intra-arterial drug injections. Urokinase may have the advantage of producing fewer allergic reactions; however, it is more expensive.

Tissue plasminogen activator (t-PA) is used increasingly in the treatment of intra-arterial thrombosis.[73, 75, 76] The ready availability of recombinant DNA-produced t-PA has facilitated widespread use. Thrombolysis may be achieved more rapidly with t-PA than with streptokinase, and it is theoretically safer than streptokinase or urokinase because of its affinity for fibrin.[77, 78] A report comparing the success of low-dose streptokinase with t-PA noted comparable fibrinolytic effects, shorter duration of therapy required with t-PA, and lower t-PA doses than were traditionally reported with the drug.[78] The investigators advocated intra-arterial infusions of t-PA at 0.5 mg/h; the median time needed to achieve reperfusion was 22 hours.

Infusions of thrombolytic agents, even those administered intra-arterially, may cause systemic thrombolysis if they are used for prolonged periods (more than 48 hours). Although monitoring of plasma fibrinogen levels and other clotting profiles is advocated, the evidence indicates no reduction in bleeding complications with these measurements.[73]

Steroids

Chemical endarteritis following intra-arterial drug injections has in some studies been ameliorated by intra-arterial dexamethasone sodium phosphate (Decadron).[46, 67, 79] Dexamethasone administered in doses ranging from 40 to 70 mg followed by 40 mg every 6 hours (orally or intravenously) decreases progressive tissue necrosis.[18, 46] A precautionary note should be made of a case report of digital ischemia resulting from intra-arterial injection of methylprednisolone acetate (Depo-Medrone, Depo-Medrol).[80] The latter response may have been due to distal small arterial obstruction by the relatively water insoluble methylprednisolone acetate compared with dexamethasone.

Operative Therapy

Fasciotomy is indicated in selected cases associated with massive edema and compartment syndrome. Clinical findings may be subtle, and compartment pressure measurements may be useful.[3, 48, 81] If drug injections are subfascial, necrotizing fasciitis can develop, necessitating débridement of necrotic tissue and decompression.[19] Local vessel problems may indicate embolectomy, primary repair, resection, or ligation. Najjar and colleagues observed improvement in a patient with microscopic emboli of the digits who was treated with vasodilator therapy, open arteriotomy, and thorough irrigation of the limb with heparinized saline.[82] It is possible that microscopic debris was irrigated from the vessel. Unfortunately, no follow-up angiogram was obtained to document the effectiveness of the procedure.

VENOUS INJURIES

Habitual use of superficial hand veins as drug injection sites eventually results in venous thrombosis. When combined with lymphatic obstruction secondary to recurrent infection and uptake of injected particulate debris, the result is often the puffy hand syndrome (Fig. 45–4).[19, 83] Other than treatment of acute compartment syndrome, operative management of the puffy hand syndrome is usually not required. Along with elevation, antibiotics and anticoagulation may be indicated. Intractable edema may require management with fitted or pneumatic compression devices.

The appearance of erythema or tenderness over a superficial vein may indicate suppurative thrombophlebitis. Diagnosis is confirmed by needle aspiration, Gram stain,

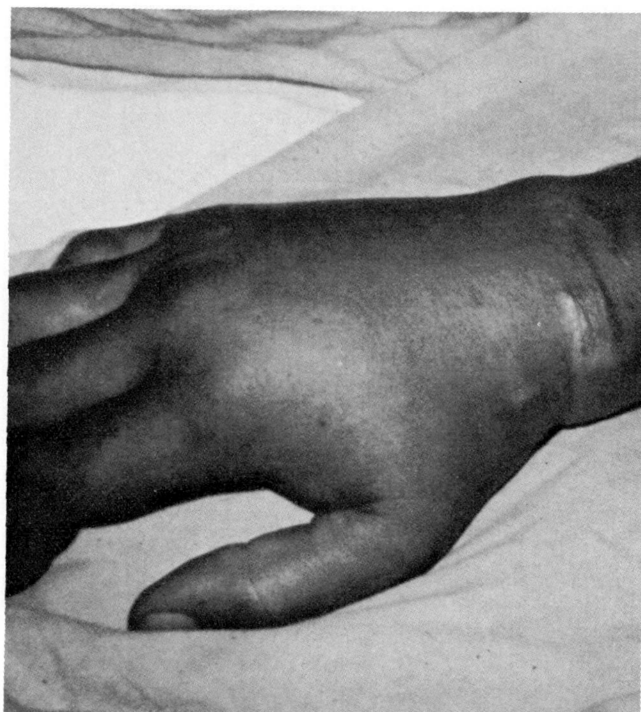

FIGURE 45–4. Puffy hand in an addict secondary to superficial venous and chronic lymphatic obstruction. (From Gellhoed GW, Joseph WL: Surgical sequelae of drug abuse. Surg Gynecol Obstet 139:749, 1974. By permission of Surgery, Gynecology & Obstetrics.)

and culture. If suppuration is found, or if elevation and antibiotics do not resolve the infection, operative intervention is indicated. This may include incision or excision of the entire involved superficial vein. Infections with a variety of organisms occur in drug abusers who have suppurative thrombophlebitis.[84] Contributing factors are needle sharing, immune system incompetence, and drug injection rituals (''needle licking'').[85]

Progressive loss of superficial venous access in chronic drug abusers leads inevitably to deep injections into major venous tributaries. Mechanisms similar to those causing injuries after arterial injections lead to deep venous thrombosis. Absence of venous collaterals due to preexisting superficial venous thrombosis may exacerbate the venous hypertension that occurs with deep venous thrombosis. The resulting presentation can be that of catastrophic venous obstruction. Management includes elevation, anticoagulation, and, under conditions of impending gangrene, fasciotomy and venous thrombectomy.

Venous aneurysms may be the consequence of repeated injections into the same area. Because of the close proximity of the femoral vein to the skin, venocutaneous fistula may occur.[35, 86] Venous pseudoaneurysms may also present as infected groin masses. Treatment consists of draining the soft tissue abscess, excising the involved venous segment, and ligating the vein proximally and distally.

Poor compliance with prescribed treatment in drug abusers often mandates inpatient treatment with long-term antibiotics and anticoagulants. Long-term central venous catheterization for outpatient antibiotic administration is rarely indicated.

In summary, acute vascular insufficiency following drug abuse is common in this era of increased use and abuse of a variety of pharmacologic agents. Resultant gangrene and other extremity complications as well as systemic, cerebral, and pulmonary complications are frequent. Treatment should be aggressive. Success has been greatest when a selective, multimodal approach has been used, including elevation, anticoagulation, vasodilators, thrombolysis, fasciotomy, and operative control of sepsis and gangrene.

References

1. Van der Post CWH: A case of mistaken injection of pentothal sodium into an aberrant ulnar artery. S Afr Med J 16:182, 1942.
2. Burn JH: Why thiopentone injected into an artery may cause gangrene. Br Med J 2:414, 1960.
3. Cohen SM: Accidental intra-arterial injection of drugs. Lancet 2:361, 1948.
4. Davies DD: Local complications of thiopentone injection. Br J Anaesthesiol 38:530, 1966.
5. Gay GR: Intra-arterial injection of secobarbital sodium into the brachial artery: Sequelae of a ''hand trip.'' Anesth Analg 50:979, 1971.
6. Kinmonth JB, Shepherd RC: Accidental injection of thiopentone into arteries. Br Med J 2:914, 1959.
7. Klatte EC, Brooks AL, Rhamy RK: Toxicity of intra-arterial barbiturates and tranquilizing drugs. Radiology 92:700, 1969.
8. Stone HH, Donnelly CC: Accidental intra-arterial injection of thiopental. Anesthesiology 22:995, 1961.
9. Albo D, Cheung L, Ruth L, et al: Effect of intra-arterial injections of barbiturates. Am J Surg 120:676, 1970.
10. Alix EC, Bogumill GP, Wright CB: Intra-arterial injection of abused drugs. Cardiovasc Res 9:266, 1975.
11. Blackwell SJ, Huang TT, Lewis SR: Intra-arterial drug abuse. Tex Med 74:64, 1978.
12. Ellerston DG, Lazarus HM, Auerbach R: Patterns of acute vascular injury after intra-arterial barbiturate injection. Am J Surg 126:813, 1973.
13. Hewitt JC, Hamilton RC, O'Donnell JF, et al: Clinical studies of induction agents. XIV. A comparative study of venous complications following thiopentone, methohexitone, and propanidid. Br J Anaesth 38:115, 1966.
14. Rumbaugh CL, Fang HCH, Higgins, RE, et al: Cerebral microvascular injury in experimental drug abuse. Invest Radiol 11:282, 1976.
15. Tasker FL, DeBoer B: Vascular changes during oxy- and thiobarbiturate perfusion modified by reserpine and iproniazid. Arch Intern Pharmacodyn 160:223, 1966.
16. Beebe HG, Keats NM: Surgical patients and drug abuse syndrome. Am Surg 38:88, 1973.
17. Daniel DM: The acutely swollen hand in the drug user. Arch Surg 107:548, 1973.
18. Gaspar MR, Hare RR: Gangrene due to intra-arterial injection of drugs by drug addicts. Surgery 72:573, 1972.
19. Geelhoed GW, Joseph WL: Surgical sequelae of drug abuse. Surg Gynecol Obstet 139:749, 1974.
20. Hager DL, Wilson JN: Gangrene of the hand following intra-arterial injection. Arch Surg 94:86, 1967.
21. Hawkins LG, Lisher CG, Sweeney M: The main line accidental intra-arterial drug injection: A review of seven cases. Clin Orthop 94:268, 1973.
22. Joseph WL, Fletcher HS, Giordano JM, et al: Pulmonary and cardiovascular implications of drug addiction. Ann Thorac Surg 15:263, 1973.
23. Maxwell TM, Olcott C, Blaisdell FW: Vascular complications of drug abuse. Arch Surg 105:875, 1972.
24. Sternbach G, Moran J, Eliastam M: Heroin addiction: Acute presentation of medical complications. Ann Emerg Med 9:161, 1980.
25. Wilson SE, Van Wagenen P, Passaro E Jr: Arterial infection. Curr Probl Surg 15:1, 1978.

26. Charney MA, Stern PJ: Digital ischemia in clandestine intravenous drug users. J Hand Surg 16A:308, 1991.
27. Owen CA, Mubarak SJ, Hargens AR, et al: Intramuscular pressures with limb compression: Clarification of the pathogenesis of the drug-induced muscle-compartment syndrome. N Engl J Med 300:1169, 1979.
28. Rich NM, Hobson RW, Fedde CW: Vascular trauma secondary to diagnostic and therapeutic procedures. Am J Surg 126:639, 1973.
29. Citron BP, Halpern M, McCarron M, et al: Necrotizing angiitis associated with drug abuse. N Engl J Med 283:1003, 1970.
30. Espiritu MB, Medina JE: Complications of heroin injections of the neck. Laryngoscope 90:1111, 1980.
31. Ho K, Rassekh ZS: Mycotic aneurysms of the right subclavian artery: A complication of heroin addiction. Chest 74:116, 1978.
32. Lau J, Mattox KL, DeBakey ME: Mycotic aneurysm of the inferior mesenteric artery. Am J Surg 138:443, 1979.
33. Ledgerwood M, Lucas CE: Mycotic aneurysm of the carotid artery. Arch Surg 109:496, 1974.
34. Yellin AE: Ruptured mycotic aneurysm: A complication of parenteral drug abuse. Arch Surg 112:981, 1977.
35. Berguer R, Benitez P: Surgical emergencies from intravascular injection of drugs. *In* Bergan JJ, Yao JST (eds): Vascular Surgical Emergencies. Orlando, FL, Grune & Stratton, 1987, pp 309–318.
36. Reddy DJ, Smith RD, Elliott JP Jr, et al: Infected femoral artery false aneurysms in drug addicts: Evolution of selective vascular reconstruction. J Vasc Surg 3:718, 1986.
37. Fromm SH, Lucas CE: Obturator bypass for mycotic aneurysm in the drug addict. Arch Surg 100:82, 1970.
38. Zemlenyi J, Colman MF: Deep neck abscesses secondary to methylphenidate (Ritalin) abuse. Head Neck Surg 6:858, 1984.
39. Morgan JM, Morgan AD, Bradley GW, et al: Fatal hemorrhage from mycotic aneurysms of the pulmonary artery. Thorax 41:70, 1986.
40. Navarro C, Dickinson PCT, Kondlapoodi P, et al: Mycotic aneurysms of the pulmonary arteries in intravenous drug addicts: Report of three cases and review of the literature. Am J Med 76:1124, 1984.
41. SanDretto MA, Scanlon GT: Multiple mycotic pulmonary artery aneurysms secondary to intravenous drug abuse. AJR 142:89, 1984.
42. Boyd LJ, McGavack TH: Aneurysm of the pulmonary artery: Review of the literature and report of two cases. Am Heart J 18:562, 1939.
43. Robertson CH Jr, Reynolds RC, Wilson JE III: Pulmonary hypertension and foreign body granulomas in intravenous drug abusers: Documentation by cardiac catheterization and lung biopsy. Am J Med 61:657, 1976.
44. Waller BF, Brownlee WJ, Roberts WC: Self-induced pulmonary granulomatosis: A consequence of intravenous injection of drugs intended for oral use. Chest 78:90, 1980.
45. Brown SS, Lyons SM, Dundee JW: Intra-arterial barbiturates: A study of some factors leading to intravascular thrombosis. Br J Anaesthesiol 40:13, 1968.
46. Buckspan GS, Franklin JD, Novak GR, et al: Intraarterial drug injury: Studies of etiology and potential treatment. J Surg Res 24:294, 1978.
47. Goldberg I, Bahar A, Yosipovitch Z: Gangrene of the upper extremity following intra-arterial injection of drugs. Clin Orthop 188:223, 1984.
48. Pearlman HS, Wollowick BS, Alvarez EV: Intra-arterial injection of propoxyphene into brachial artery. JAMA 214:2055, 1970.
49. Williams AW, Montgomery GL: Chemical injury of arteries. J Pathol Bact 77:63, 1959.
50. Atlee WE Jr: Talc and cornstarch emboli in eyes of drug abusers. JAMA 219:49, 1972.
51. Lindell TD, Porter JM, Langston JC: Intra-arterial injections of oral medications. A complication of drug addiction. N Engl J Med 287:1132, 1972.
52. Appen RE, Wray SH, Cogan DG: Central retinal artery occlusion. Am J Ophthalmol 79:374, 1975.
53. Brucker AJ: Disk and peripheral retinal neovascularization secondary to talc and cornstarch emboli. Am J Ophthalmol 88:864, 1979.
54. Friberg TR, Gragoudas ES, Regan CDJ: Talc emboli and macular ischemia in intravenous drug abuse. Arch Ophthalmol 97:1089, 1979.
55. Kresca. LJ, Goldberg MF, Jampol LM: Talc emboli and retinal neovascularization in a drug abuser. Am J Ophthalmol 87:334, 1979.
56. Lee J, Sapira JD: Retinal and cerebral microembolization of talc in a drug abuser. Am J Med Sci 265:75, 1973.
57. Schatz H, Drake M: Self-injected retinal emboli. Ophthalmologica 86:468, 1979.
58. Waters DJ: Intra-arterial thiopentone. Anaesthesia 21:346, 1966.
59. Burn JH, Jobbs R: Mechanism of arterial spasm following intra-arterial injection of thiopentone. Lancet 1:1112, 1969.
60. Begg EJ, McGrath MA, Wade DN: Inadvertent intra-arterial injection: A problem of drug abuse. Med J Aust 2:561, 1980.
61. Crawford CR, Terranova WA: The role of intraarterial vasodilators in the treatment of inadvertent intraarterial injection injuries. Ann Plast Surg 25:279, 1990.
62. Stueber K: The treatment of intra-arterial pentazocine injection injuries with intraarterial reserpine. Ann Plast Surg 18:41, 1987.
63. Wright, CB, Hobson, RW, Swan KG, et al: Extremity venous ligation: Clinical and hemodynamic correlation. Am Surg 41:203, 1975.
64. Myers MB, Cherry G: Necrosis due to venous inadequacy: An experimental model in the skin of rabbits. Surg Forum 18:513, 1967.
65. Wright CB, Swan KG: The hemodynamics of venous occlusion in the canine hindlimb. Surgery 73:141, 1973.
66. Corser G, Masey S, Jacob G, et al: Ischaemia following self-administered intra-arterial injection of methylphenidate and diamorphine: A case report of treatment with intra-arterial urokinase and review. Anaesthesia 40:51, 1985.
67. Enloe G, Sylvester M, Morris LE: Hazards of intra-arterial injection of hydroxyzine. Can Anaesth Soc J 16:425, 1969.
68. Lloyd WK, Porter JM, Lindell TD, et al: Accidental intraarterial injection in drug abuse. Am J Roentgenol 117:892, 1973.
69. Silverman SH, Turner WW Jr: Intraarterial drug abuse: New treatment options. J Vasc Surg 14:111, 1991.
70. Gallacher BP: Intra-arterial verapamil to reverse acute ischemia of the hand after radial artery cannulation. Can Anaesth 38:138, 1991.
71. Roberts JR, Krisanda TJ: Accidental intra-arterial injection of epinephrine treated with phentolamine. Ann Emerg Med 18:424, 1989.
72. Lazarus HM, Hutto BS, Ellertson DG: Therapeutic prevention of ischemia following intraarterial barbiturate injection. J Surg Res 22:46, 1977.
73. Earnshaw JJ: Thrombolytic therapy in the management of acute limb ischaemia. Br J Surg 78:261, 1991.
74. Kartchner MM, Wilcox WC: Thrombolysis of palmar and digital arterial thrombosis by intra-arterial thrombolysin. J Hand Surg 1:67, 1976.
75. Buckenham TM, Darby M: Thrombolysis with t-PA. Br J Hosp Med 46:269, 1991.
76. Juhan C, Haupert S, Miltgen G, et al: A new intra arterial rt-PA dosage regimen in peripheral arterial occlusion: Bolus followed by continuous infusion. Thromb Haemost 65:635, 1991.
77. Dawson KJ, Reddy K, Platts AD, et al: Results of a recently instituted programme of thrombolytic therapy in acute lower limb ischaemia. Br J Surg 78:409, 1991.
78. Earnshaw JJ, Westby JC, Gregson RHS, et al: Local thrombolytic therapy of acute peripheral arterial ischaemia with tissue plasminogen activator: A dose-ranging study. Br J Surg 75:1196, 1988.
79. Treiman GS, Yellin AE, Weaver FA: An effective treatment protocol for intraarterial drug injection. J Vasc Surg 12:456, 1990.
80. Taweepoke P, Frame JD: Acute ischaemia of the hand following accidental radial artery infusion of Depo-Medrone. Hand Surg 15:118, 1990.
81. Gall WE, Burr JW, Wright CBV: Noninvasive evaluation and correlation of hemodynamics in ''compartment syndrome.'' Surg Forum 29:222, 1978.
82. Najjar FB, Bridi G, Rizk G: Management of micro-emboli of the digital arteries. J Med Liban 27:467, 1974.
83. Neviaser RJ, Butterfield WC, Wieche DR: The puffy hand of drug addiction: A study of the pathogenesis. J Bone Joint Surg 54-A:629, 1972.
84. Tuazon CU, Hill R, Sheagren JN: Microbiologic study of street heroin and injection paraphernalia. J Infect Dis 129:327, 1974.
85. Moustoukas NM, Nichols RL, Smith JW, et al: Contaminated street heroin: Relationship to clinical infections. Arch Surg 118:746, 1983.
86. Yeager RA, Hobson RW II, Padberg FT, et al: Vascular complications related to drug abuse. J Trauma 27:305, 1987.

46

Thoracic and Abdominal Vascular Trauma

Fred Bongard, M.D.

• • •

THORACIC VASCULAR TRAUMA

The term thoracic vascular trauma typically refers to injuries of the aorta and arch vessels, the pulmonary arteries and veins, the superior and inferior vena cava, the intercostal vessels, and the internal mammary vessels. These injuries, although life threatening, constitute only a minority of patients with vascular trauma treated at a metropolitan center. In a review of our experience, only 9 per cent of all vascular injuries over a 10-year period were in the chest.[1]

Interest in the diagnosis and treatment of these relatively uncommon injuries stems from the fact that patients may harbor a rapidly lethal injury with minimal or no signs and symptoms. Although penetrating mechanisms predominate, the number of patients with aortic dissection due to blunt trauma has continued to increase.[2] Nearly 10 to 15 per cent of those who die from automobile accidents sustain an aortic rupture. Greendyke reported a 27 per cent incidence of rupture in those who were ejected from a vehicle and only a 12 per cent incidence in those who were not.[3] The majority of such ruptures occur in patients aged 20 to 30, with very few at the extremes of life. Males predominate in a 9:1 sex ratio. Since the first report of a successful repair in 1958, advances in diagnostic and surgical technique have improved the overall results of management, although morbidity and mortality still remain high.[4] Approximately 10 to 20 per cent of those with acute thoracic disruptions survive the initial trauma. Of these, nearly 30 per cent die within 6 hours, 40 per cent within 24 hours, 72 per cent within the first week, and over 90 per cent within 10 weeks if no treatment is instituted.[5,6]

Pathophysiology

The combinations of forces that contribute to traumatic rupture of the thoracic aorta and its branch vessels vary depending on the location and direction of the force applied.[7,8] Theories advanced to explain the predominance of disruption at the aortic isthmus (between the left subclavian artery and the ligamentum arteriosum) are based upon the observation that during a deceleration injury, the heart, the ascending aorta, and the transverse arch continue to move forward, while the motion of the isthmus and descending aorta is limited by their posterior attachments. There is additional evidence that the isthmus is inherently weaker than other parts of the thoracic aorta.[9] Lundevall, using isolated strips of aorta free of adventitia, reported that the isthmus was only two thirds as strong as the ascending aorta. The descending aorta was of intermediate strength.[10] Injuries most commonly become manifest as transverse tears beginning at the intima and progressing outward. The adventitia typically remains intact because of its tough collagenous nature. Rapid increases in intraluminal pressure may also rupture the aorta.[11] The pressure required may be as low as 580 mmHg or as high as 2500 mmHG.[8,11]

The forces responsible for rupture at the isthmus include:

1. Vertically directed deceleration following an impact that produces transient stretching of the aorta. Falls that caudally displace the thoracoabdominal aorta are common examples.
2. Compression that follows a frontal impact.
3. Horizontal deceleration with or without chest compression (motor vehicle collision).
4. Crush injury.

The mechanical factors thought to contribute to injury at the isthmus include shearing stress, bending stress, and torsion stress. Shearing stress is created by the different rates of deceleration between the mobile aortic arch and the immobile descending aorta. Shear stress leads to rupture opposite the site of fixation and accounts for the *anterior* location of proximal descending ruptures at the isthmus. Bending stress is created when the heart is displaced caudally and produces flexion of the aortic arch around a "fulcrum" created by the hilar structures of the left lung. Anteroposterior compression with displacement of the heart to the left produces a pressure wave referred to as torsion stress. Torsion stress is also responsible for tears of the *ascending* aorta that occur with the vertical deceleration that accompanies falls from heights. The rapid downward displacement of the heart results in an acute lengthening of the aorta. The pressure wave thus created produces a water-hammer effect that exerts its greatest influence in the ascending aorta.

Compression and tension forces may combine to produce tears of the subclavian and innominate arteries. Reporting on the first successful repair of an innominate artery avulsion in 1962, Binet and colleagues theorized that a compressive force would shorten the distance between the sternum and the vertebral column.[12] The decrease in volume would push the heart and the ascending aorta posteriorly and to the left. The curvature of the aortic arch would be accentuated creating tension on its convex surface at the points of insertion of the brachiocephalic vessels. Binet and colleagues also noted that patients tend to rotate the head to one side to protect against facial injury, and in doing so place the opposite carotid artery under tension in the longitudinal axis. The tearing force thus created may avulse the carotid artery from the aortic arch. When first rib fractures occur, injuries to the subclavian arteries may also result from being stretched over the rib margin.

An alternative theory advanced by Voigt and Wifert implicates the cranially directed impact of the sternum following contact with a dashboard. When the sternum is fractured, the lower portion is displaced upward and backward. The mediastinum and ascending aorta are forced (shoveled) superiorly by the sternal fragment. The cranial displacement puts tensile stretch on the proximal descending aorta, which ruptures in proximity to its fixed point at the ligamentum arteriosum.[13] Crass and coworkers advanced the theory that aortic isthmus lacerations result from a "pinch" of the aorta between the spine and the anterior bony thorax (manubrium, clavicle, and first ribs) during chest compression caused by abrupt deceleration.[14]

Other thoracic vascular injuries resulting from blunt trauma include *distal* descending aortic tears and disruption of intercostal vessels. The descending aorta is most likely ruptured by fracture-dislocations of the lower thoracic spine, whereas inter-costal vessels are often associated with rib fractures.

Penetrating injuries include complete transection, partial transection, and arteriovenous fistulae. Because the vessels involved are large, the mechanism of muscular retraction usually fails to control hemorrhage, and rapid blood loss may result.

Diagnosis

A high index of suspicion is the most important factor in initiating a search for thoracic aortic disruption in trauma victims. Because the forces imparted on the aorta are directly related to the energy absorbed, falls from more than three stories or motor vehicle accidents at speeds in excess of 40 miles per hour should arouse suspicion of thoracic vascular injury, even in the absence of physical findings (Fig. 46–1). Circumstances surrounding the incident such as the death of other automobile occupants or the use of harness seat belts (associated with innominate and subclavian injuries) are also helpful.[16]

THE TRAUMA EPIDEMIC

Total Impact Velocity and Injury Risk

IMPACT VELOCITY (miles/hr.)	INJURY RISK (%) morbidity	INJURY RISK (%) mortality	EQUIVALENT FREE FALL MPH	EQUIVALENT FREE FALL Feet
1–10	2.5	.1	10 →	5
11–20	6	1.0	20 →	13
21–30	25	3.0	30 →	28
≥40	70	40.0	40 →	54
			50 →	84
			60 →	121

FIGURE 46–1. A comparison of automobile deceleration injuries and equivalent free falls.

Table 46–1. Clinical Findings Associated With Traumatic Rupture of the Thoracic Aorta

History of high-speed deceleration injury
Multiple rib fractures or flail chest
Fractured first or second rib
Fractured sternum
Pulse deficits
Upper extremity hypertension
Interscapular systolic murmur
Blood in the carotid or subclavian sheaths
Hoarseness or voice change without laryngeal injury
Superior vena cava syndrome

Modified from Wilson RF: Thoracic vascular trauma. In *Bongard F, Wilson SE, Perry MO (eds): Vascular Injuries in Surgical Practice. Norwalk, CT, Appleton & Lange, 1991, p 107.*

Symptoms on admission are often related to associated injuries. Wilson noted that retrosternal or interscapular pain may result from "stretching" or dissection of the aortic adventitia.[7] A detailed review of the English language literature by Duhaylongsod and colleagues summarized 1188 patients in whom the most frequent presenting symptoms were chest pain (76 per cent) and dyspnea (56 per cent).[17] Loss of consciousness or coma (36.8 per cent) and hypotension (25.9 per cent) were other common complaints.

Only one third of those with blunt aortic trauma have physical evidence of thoracic injury on presentation.[8] No single physical finding or combination of findings is diagnostic of acute thoracic aortic rupture. The "acute coarctation syndrome," first reported by Symbas and associates, is characterized by hypertension in the arms and a difference in pulse amplitude between the upper and lower extremities.[18] The syndrome may be caused either by intimal dissection and flap, or by compression of the aortic lumen by hematoma. Another cause of the hypertension may be the stretching or stimulation of receptors in or near the aortic isthmus. A systolic murmur over the precordium or posterior interscapular area may accompany the coarctation syndrome and is due to the turbulence created as blood flows past the intimal flap. In our experience, the acute coarctation syndrome is uncommon.

Physical findings are summarized in Table 46–1. The frequency of these findings varies significantly between authors and series. Clark and coworkers found that a hemothorax of more than 500 cc, pseudocoarctation, or neck hematoma were present in patients at "high risk."[20] Duhaylongsod and colleagues reported that physical findings usually considered "highly suggestive" such as mid-scapular back pain, differences in pulse amplitude, and generalized hypertension were not commonly observed.[17] However, preoperative paresis or paraplegia or indeterminate findings on physical examination were present in one third of patients.[17]

Associated injuries are common and frequently obscure the underlying thoracic aortic injury. The most commonly reported associated injuries include fractures (both local and remote), pulmonary contusion, closed head injury, intra-abdominal solid organ injury (spleen, kidney, liver), and maxillofacial injuries.[17]

Radiographic imaging remains pivotal in the diagnostic algorithm. The commonly cited findings on plain chest x-ray suggestive of rupture of the aorta or brachiocephalic vessels after blunt trauma are summarized in Table 46–2.[21] Recent reports have evaluated the importance of individual findings that suggest the diagnosis.[22–24] Of greatest utility are signs with sufficient sensitivity to include all true positive aortic injuries but with adequate specificity to minimize the number of unnecessary angiograms (Fig. 46–2). Supine chest x-rays may enlarge the mediastinal structures because of magnification obtained at short focal film distances. Ayella and others suggested that erect chest radiographs be performed to compensate for this artifact.[25, 26] Mirvis and coworkers found that although the supine chest radiograph was more sensitive for detecting signs of mediastinal hemorrhage than the erect view, it was less specific for aortic rupture than an erect film.[26] However, a subsequent study found that an erect view was normal in 6 per cent of patients with proven blunt aortic or brachiocephalic arterial rupture.[27] Therefore, the reduced sensitivity of the erect chest radiograph for signs of mediastinal hemorrhage will result in a reduction in the number of negative aortograms performed but will do so at the expense of increasing the number of missed aortic or brachiocephalic arterial injuries.

In an effort to quantitate mediastinal enlargement, Marsh and Sturm reported that a superior mediastinal transverse width (just above the aortic arch) of greater than 8 cm on supine chest x-ray was abnormal.[28] However, a subsequent report by the same group found that the aortic arch may exceed 8 cm in up to 81 per cent of normal patients.[29]

Table 46–2. Radiographic Findings Associated With Traumatic Rupture of the Thoracic Aorta

Deviation of esophagus to the right at T4 (>1.0 to 2.0 cm)
Superior mediastinal widening
Obscuration of the aortic knob
Obliteration of the outline of descending aorta
Tracheal deviation to the right
Apical cap
Depression of left main stem bronchus (>40 degrees)
Obliteration of the aortopulmonary window
Obscuration of medial aspect of left upper lobe
Widened paravertebral stripe
Thickened or deviated paratracheal stripe
Fracture of first or second rib
Fractured sternum

Modified from Wilson RF: Thoracic vascular trauma. In *Bongard F, Wilson SE, Perry MO (eds): Vascular Injuries in Surgical Practice. Norwalk, CT, Appleton & Lange, 1991, p 107.*

Seltzer and coworkers described the mediastinal width–to–chest width (M/C), which is calculated by dividing the width of the mediastinum at the aortic arch (M) by the internal diameter of the chest at the same level (C).[30] The initial critical value of 0.25 was later found to allow too many false-positive results, whereas a higher ratio potentially discounted patients with true rupture.[30] Failure of objective measures to predict reliably which patients require aortography has led the author and others to rely upon the observer's experience and knowledge of mediastinal anatomy to determine the need for aortography.[31] Interobserver variability for mediastinal widening is low, and agreement can usually be reached.[32] It must be noted, however, that the width of the mediastinum in the supine position progressively increases with age, probably due to atherosclerosis. Thus, the presence of mediastinal widening may be less important in those over 65 years of age.

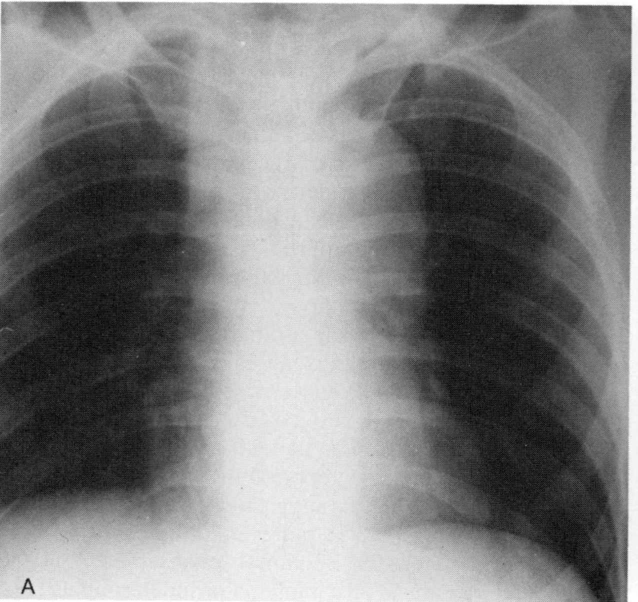

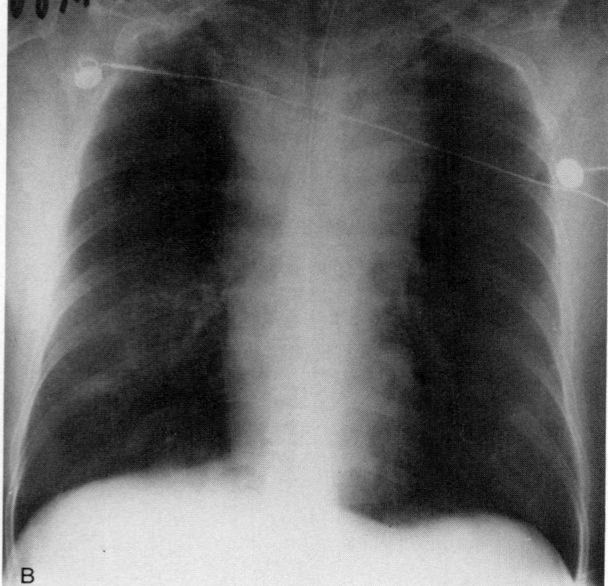

FIGURE 46–2. *A*, The classic appearance of a widened mediastinum on supine chest radiography. *B*, This abnormal chest x-ray occurred after a malpositioned resuscitation line infused fluid into a patient's mediastinum. Aortography was normal.

Adjunctive findings on chest x-ray such as hemothorax, first rib fracture (unilateral and bilateral), pneumothorax, apical cap, depression of the left mainstem bronchus to more than 40 degrees from the horizontal, deviation of the nasogastric tube to the right, and widening of the right paratracheal stripe have also been evaluated for their utility in predicting the need for aortography.[26] Extension of a mediastinal hematoma typically displaces the esophagus to the right. In two series reported by Ayella and Gerlock and associates, no patient with esophageal deviation of less than 1.0 cm from the midline had aortic injury, whereas deviation of more than 2 cm to the right was highly suggestive.[33, 34] When an innominate injury is present, the superior mediastinal hematoma tends to have a pointed appearance and actually displaces the nasogastric tube to the left. It must be remembered, however, that none of these findings, alone or in combination, is absolutely reliable for the diagnosis of aortic or arch vessel injury. Subjective evaluation of the mediastinum by an experienced observer remains the most valuable tool.

Computed tomography (CT) and transesophageal echo (TEE) have been used for the diagnosis of aortic rupture (Fig. 46–3). Because of limited experience, neither modality can be recommended for establishing aortic injury or for determining the need for angiography. The considerations of sensitivity and specificity previously discussed for plain chest radiographs apply to these modalities as well. Concerns about CT imaging primarily relate to the fact that it may not be sufficiently sensitive to detect small aortic branch injuries. Further, the usual 8 to 10-mm sections may make satisfactory evaluation of the aorticopulmonary window difficult because of partial volume averaging. Morgan and coworkers addressed these concerns by obtaining 5-mm contrast-enhanced CT scans in patients who had sustained deceleration injuries with a low-to-moderate probability of having an aortic disruption.[35] Twenty-eight patients had abnormal chest x-rays on admission and underwent thin-section CT scanning. Of the 22 with normal CT scans, 19 were treated without angiography; there were no adverse outcomes. Six patients with mediastinal hematomas on CT scan underwent angiography; one was found to have an aortic injury. The authors concluded that 5-mm contrast-enhanced CT scans can reduce the number of angiograms needed in a select group of patients.[35] A similar study by Raptopoulos and coworkers found that CT scans offered a significant improvement over plain radiographs in specificity, accuracy, and predictive value of positive results.[36] By their criteria, 79 per cent of patients with normal scans had false-positive chest radiographs, whereas none of the patients with normal CT scans had evidence of aortic disruption.

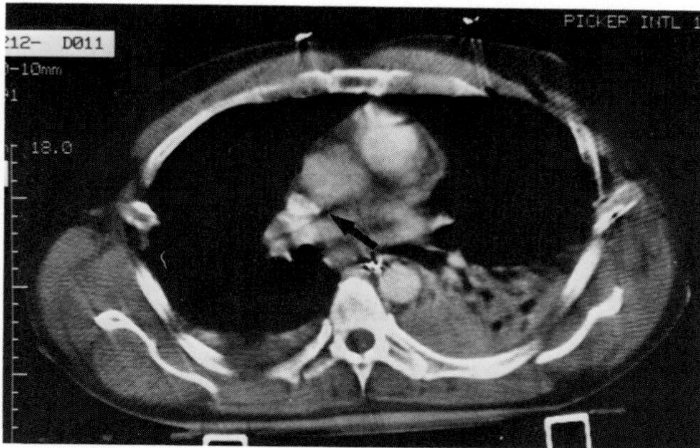

FIGURE 46–3. Computed tomographic study of a patient after a motor vehicle accident. *Arrow* indicates the widened mediastinum and evidence of hematoma around the proximal descending aorta.

Transesophageal echo has been used as a relatively noninvasive means of detecting thoracic aortic disruption.[37–39] The majority of reports are isolated incidents, with no carefully controlled series using angiography for comparison. One of the major disadvantages of the technique is that it is highly operator dependent and requires specialized equipment and technicians that may not be available when trauma patients arrive.

The author's decision to obtain thoracic angiograms continues to revolve around the mechanism of injury and the results of plain chest radiographs. In stable patients who are victims of high-speed vehicular accidents or falls from more than three stories, angiographs are usually obtained. Whenever the mediastinum is widened or the severity of associated injuries warrants it, angiographs are obtained provided that the patient remains stable.

The author approaches thoracic angiography via the femoral artery, with retrograde introduction of the guidewire and catheter to the ascending arch. When unequal lower extremity pulses are present or when pelvic injuries preclude the use of a femoral artery, the axillary or brachial arteries may be cannulated. If blunt injury to the innominate artery is suspected by the location of hematoma on plain film, the right axillary artery should not be used.[40] A small amount of obliquity (15 to 20 degrees left anterior oblique) aids in evaluating the ascending aorta by rotating it away from the thoracic spine (Fig. 46–4). The most common positive finding is that of a contained disruption located on the anterior face of the aorta just opposite the ligamentum arteriosum. We have occasionally seen intimal defects and extravasation. When injury to the innominate or subclavian artery has occurred, an oval-shaped widening at the orifice of the vessels is seen (Fig. 46–5).[41] In the rare patient with multiple lesions, the need for cardiopulmonary bypass can be appreciated and the appropriate personnel notified.

Preoperative Management

Initial management of blunt or penetrating injuries to the thoracic vasculature depends upon rapid resuscitation. A secure airway is the first priority. When deceleration was responsible, associated cervical spine injuries may be present, and hyperextension of the neck must be avoided. In these circumstances, intubation with a fiberoptic bronchoscope or cricothyroidotomy is preferable. After the airway has been secured, adequate gas exchange usually necessitates mechanical ventilation. Patients who have sustained penetrating injuries or blunt trauma with rib fractures are at high risk for developing tension pneumothoraces when positive pressure ventilation is applied. Bilateral tube thoracostomies may be required, and particular care should be ex-

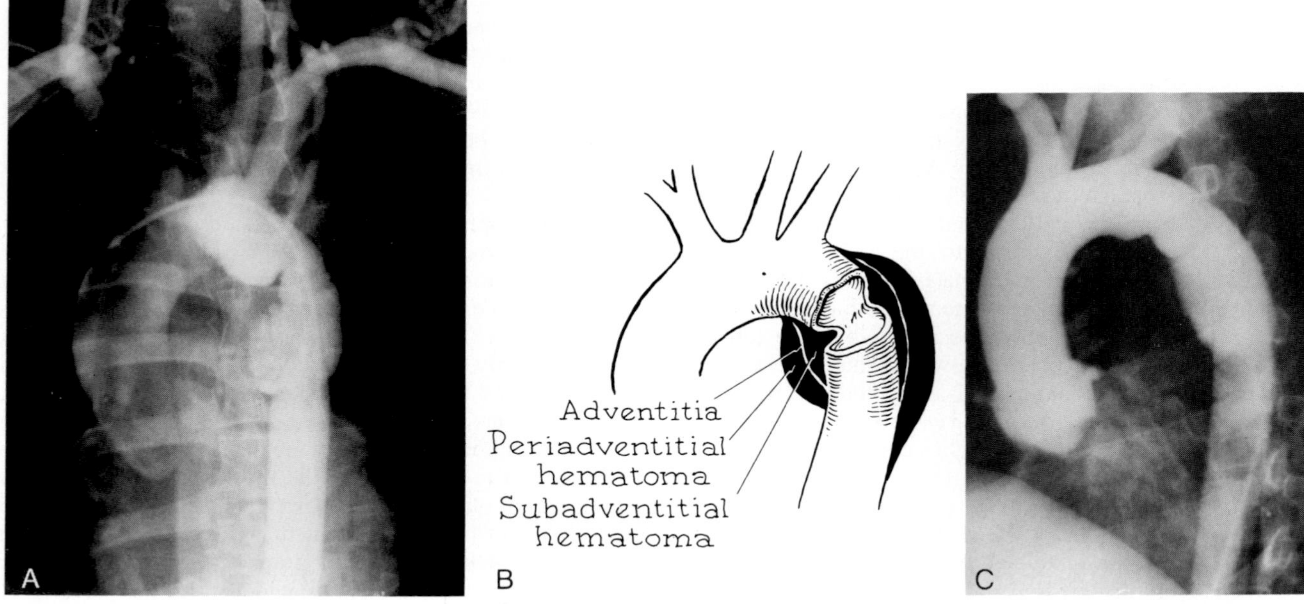

FIGURE 46–4. *A*, An anteroposterior aortogram shows disruption of the aorta at the isthmus with proximal extension. *B*, Schematic representation of injury in *A*. *C*, A similar aortogram shot from an oblique angle "opens" the aortic arch and provides a better view of the injury and great vessels. (*B*, From Wilson RF: Thoracic vascular trauma. *In* Bongard FS, Wilson SE, Perry MO [eds]: Vascular Injuries in Surgical Practice. Norwalk, CT, Appleton & Lange, 1991, p 119.)

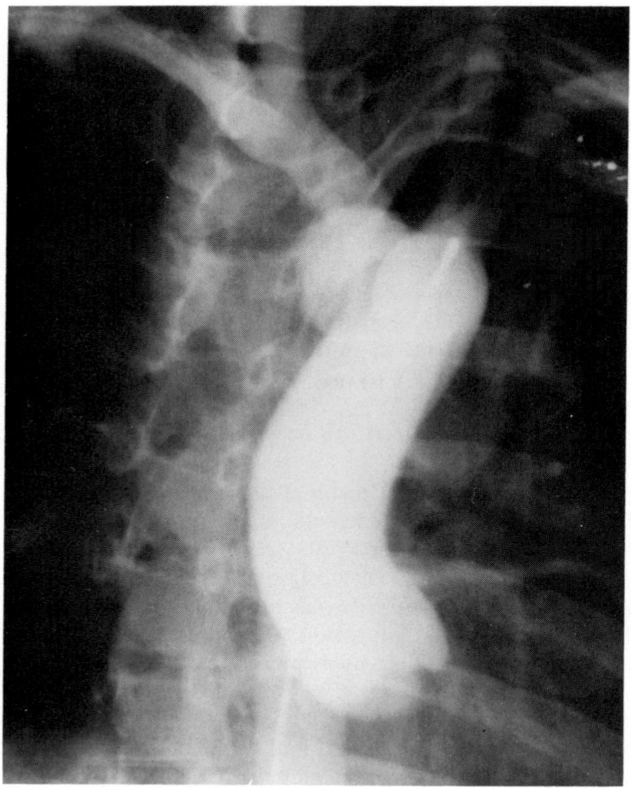

FIGURE 46–5. A gunshot wound to the chest caused a pseudoaneurysm of the innominate artery at its origin from the aorta. Note the oval appearance of the injury.

ercised during their placement to prevent disturbing a tamponading periaortic hematoma. The need for secure and reliable venous access cannot be overstated. When penetrating injuries of the thoracic inlet are present, ipsilateral upper extremity access sites are undesirable. In these situations, lower extremity venous catheterization is preferable. In patients with associated abdominal trauma, iliac or vena cava lacerations may be present, and upper extremity sites should be used. In any case, catheters of sufficiently large caliber to infuse fluids rapidly are an absolute requirement.

Air emboli may occur during resuscitation. Although most common following penetrating injuries, they may also be problematic after blunt trauma accompanied by rib fractures. Venous air emboli require 100 to 200 ml of air before airlock of the right ventricle occurs.[42] The patient should be placed in the left decubitus position with the legs elevated. This will displace air into the apex of the heart and open the outflow tract. Paradoxical air emboli may occur when a patent foramen ovale is present. In contrast to venous air emboli, systemic emboli require less than 1 cc of air to produce devastating effects. Until proved otherwise, any dysrhythmia or sudden drop in blood pressure occurring soon after the application of positive pressure ventilation should be considered to be due to systemic air emboli. In this event, the head should be lowered and a thoracotomy performed to clamp the lung proximal to the injured area.[7]

Hypotension following penetrating injury may require emergency thoracotomy to facilitate resuscitation. On the other hand, resuscitative thoracotomy following blunt injury is seldom successful. Because the thoracic great vessels are located in the superior mediastinum, thoracic inlet, and supraclavicular areas, the approach used should be higher than that used for penetrating cardiac injuries. The author prefers to gain access through a third or fourth space anterolateral thoracotomy. When a penetrating wound is present on the right, a left thoracotomy is still required to provide adequate exposure to clamp the descending thoracic aorta.

Once adequate exposure has been achieved, the first priority is localization and identification of the bleeding site. Intercostal vessels are frequently lacerated by rib fractures following blunt injury. The internal mammary may be disrupted following a stab wound or during a hastily performed thoracotomy. Pulmonary hilar vessels are also potential bleeding sites. Wide exposure is the key to success. Frequently a unilateral thoracotomy must be extended across the sternum to provide bilateral exposure. A longitudinal incision of the pericardium parallel to the course of the phrenic nerve will permit open cardiac massage. Further dissection to the opposite phrenic nerve will permit exposure of the intrapericardial portion of the great vessels. When injury of the ascending aorta is present, control can usually be accomplished with a partially occluding Satinsky or Wylie-J clamp placed so as to isolate the defect. Bleeding from the pulmonary hilum can be secured by applying an aortic vascular clamp across all hilar structures until the patient can be moved to the operating room.

Operative Strategy

The operative repair of thoracic injuries requires a preplanned and coordinated approach to optimize the outcome. Upon arrival in the operating room, the following equipment should be available: rib spreaders, saws, aortic cross-clamps, shunts or cardiopulmonary bypass pump tubing (as preferred), and woven grafts of various sizes. The author stores this equipment on the trauma resuscitation ''crash'' cart kept outside the main trauma surgery suite. Following injury, extrication, transport, and emergency room resuscitation, patients with aortic injuries are frequently profoundly hypothermic. Because of its undesirable effects on myocardial function and the clotting cascade, hypothermia must be prevented. Useful measures in the operating suite include (1) a warming pad placed under the patient, (2) a silver thermal blanket (Thermadrape) placed over the patient to retain body heat, (3) warming of all blood products and fluids used, and (4) use of a heated gas mixture from the anesthesia ventilator.

Patients are positioned on the operating table to facilitate the repair anticipated. In general, exposure and skin preparation should include the anterior neck, thorax, abdomen, and a lower extremity. When a subclavian injury is suspected, the ipsilateral arm should be prepared and draped in such a fashion that free mobility of the shoulder is maintained to aid in operative dissection and exposure. The posterolateral thoracotomy provides excellent exposure to virtually all portions of the hemithorax. The contralateral decubitus position brings the affected side into view. The incision extends from behind the medial border of the scapula below its tip and then anteriorly to the anterior axillary line. The chest can be entered through the fourth to seventh intercostal spaces. Particular care must be exercised in positioning hypotensive patients for this incision because the decubitus position interferes with venous return and may aggravate the condition. Blood and bronchial contents also may flow to the uninjured dependent lung, causing profound respiratory embarrassment. Use of a split-lumen endotracheal tube allows selective collapse of the left lung to facilitate exposure.

When severe shock or hemoptysis precludes the decubitus position, an anterior thoracotomy may be used instead. This is also the incision of choice for rapid access to the mediastinum for open cardiac massage. The incision should start 2 cm lateral to the sternum to avoid injury to the internal mammary artery. It then follows a gentle curve laterally to the axilla. Overzealous use of rib spreaders usually results in posterior rib fractures, which create the possibility of intercostal vessel disruption. When additional exposure is required, the anterior thoracotomy may be extended across the midline as a ''clamshell'' incision. Large shears should be used to transect the sternum to avoid splintering. Both internal mammary arteries will be divided during this approach and require ligation.

A median sternotomy is preferred for injuries of the ascending aorta, innominate, or proximal carotid arteries. Extension into the neck along the anterior border of the right sternocleidomastoid muscle allows access to the proximal right subclavian artery and the origin of the right common carotid artery as well as the right vertebral artery. Although the author does not prefer leftward extension for exposure of the proximal left subclavian, some have noted that if the shoulders are thrown back by placing a vertical roll between the scapulae, the origin of the left subclavian is accessible.[43]

Controversy continues about the optimal technique for aortic control and repair because of concern about spinal cord ischemia and the potential for lower extremity paralysis. Safe time and pressure limits are not well defined. Several methods for indirect assessment of perfusion are available and have received mixed reviews. Intraoperative evaluation of evoked somatosensory potential, monitoring of lumbar spinal fluid pressure, and measurement of distal aortic pressure have all been employed.[45, 46] Because such modalities are awkward in emergent situations, extensive experience in trauma cases is lacking. The author prefers to perform the operation as expeditiously as possible without these techniques.

Methods of control and repair include partial or complete bypass via an external pump with systemic anticoagulation, external heparin-bonded (triclodecylmethylammonium chloride) shunts from the ascending aorta to the descending aorta or femoral artery, and simple clamp and repair. The need for systemic anticoagulation with heparin in a patient with multi-system trauma makes widespred hemorrhage a possibility. For this reason, partial or complete cardiopulmonary bypass has largely fallen into disfavor. Patients with thoracic aortic injuries at multiple levels who require extensive repairs are notable exceptions. The torroidal centrifugal pump, which is connected between the left atrium and a femoral artery, can be used with little or no heparin because an oxygenator is not required. It offers the following advantages over complete cardiopulmonary bypass: (1) It does not require systemic anticoagulation, (2) it automatically deprimes itself if air enters, effectively reducing the risk of systemic embolization, (3) it is flow dependent and will decrease flow if inflow is obstructed, and (4) it is resistance dependent and will stop pumping if excessively high pressures in the outflow are present.[47–50]

Clamp and repair, either by simple suture, prosthetic graft, or sutureless graft, is the most direct method. Its advantages are that it requires no additional equipment, dissection in another area, systemic anticoagulation, or vessel cannulation. Many centers prefer this technique to the more complex bypass or shunt methods.[51–53] There is general agreement that operating times of 30 minutes or less reduce the risk of paralysis.

The customary operative technique for clamp and repair begins by positioning the patient in a right decubitus position, followed by creation of a left posterolateral thoracotomy in the fourth intercostal space. After retraction of the lung, the area of injury is identified. Vascular tapes are placed sequentially around (1) the aortic arch between the left common carotid and subclavian arteries, (2) the subclavian artery just beyond its origin, and (3) the descending aorta just below the injury (Fig. 46–6). Dissection proceeds from distal to proximal, so that the inferior aortic clamp can be moved as close to the site of injury as possible.

Once vascular isolation has been achieved, options for repair include simple repair, graft insertion, or a sutureless graft. When a partial laceration is present or the disruption is small, some prefer mobilization, resection of the injured segment, and simple suture repair. Caution is required to ensure adequate mobilization because tension on the anastomosis will increase further after inflow is restored. It is generally believed that only 20 per cent of aortic tears can be repaired in this fashion.[54] Its advantages include the speed with which it can be performed, the absence of a prosthetic graft, and the decreased risk of a prosthetic infection.[55]

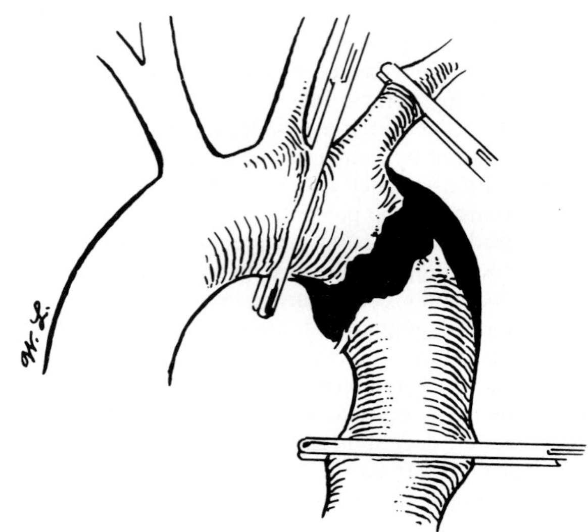

FIGURE 46–6. **Control of injuries at the isthmus can be achieved by placing clamps between the left common carotid artery and the left subclavian artery, beyond the origin of the left subclavian and distal to the injury. (From Wilson RF: Thoracic vascular trauma. *In* Bongard FS, Wilson SE, Perry MO [eds]: Vascular Injuries in Surgical Practice. Norwalk, CT, Appleton & Lange, 1991, p 122.)**

Prosthetic graft insertion is the customary method of repair. It is an absolute requirement when more than 2 cm of vessel is injured. Although knitted grafts are more flexible and handle more easily, woven grafts are preferable because they can be inserted without preclotting. If the segment of damaged aorta is relatively short, a sleeve patch may be used to bridge the gap. Antunes described the use of a polytetrafluoroethylene (PTFE) graft (18 to 20 mm in diameter) that is opened into a sleeve patch.[52] Although two suture lines are still required, the open rather than tubular graft facilitates sewing.

Sutureless grafts are made of woven Dacron with support rings at each end. The graft is placed through a longitudinal aortotomy with the rings on either side of the defect. The graft is fixed in place with sutures or external rings. Although this graft can theoretically reduce cross-clamp time, familiarity with its handling and placement are prerequisites. The utility of intraluminal stents in this setting also requires further study.

Clamp and repair times vary depending on a number of factors including location, associated injuries, and the skill and experience of the surgeon. The decreased distal blood flow during clamp application and the need to control proximal blood pressure with antihypertensives such as nitroprusside compromise spinal cord perfusion. For this reason, many surgeons have opted for extracorporeal shunting with a heparin-bonded (triclodecylmethylammonium chloride heparin) shunt. Because of its special surface, clotting is inhibited, and the need for systemic anticoagulation is eliminated. After filling the shunt with heparinized saline, the distal end is clamped. The proximal end is inserted through a pursestring into either the ascending aorta or the aortic arch. The distal end can be inserted into either the descending thoracic aorta or the femoral artery. Although femoral insertion is preferable to avoid clutter in the field, studies have shown that flow is reduced by as much as 50 per cent compared with thoracic aorta insertion.[56] Flow also depends on the size of the shunt; a 7.5-mm cannula can provide 1500 to 2000 ml/min, whereas a 9.0-mm cannula can provide 3000 to 4000 ml/min. The presence of a functioning shunt does not provide absolute protection against paraplegia. In the study by Duhaylongsod and colleagues, 3 of 41 patients (7 per cent) still developed paraplegia despite being shunted.[17] This result may be related in part to the distal aortic pressure. Cunningham and coworkers commented that a pressure of 60 mmHg or greater beyond the shunt is required to prevent paralysis.[57] Shunt use may be complicated by vessel laceration at the time of placement, bleeding, and pseudoaneurysm formation at the insertion site.

In most cases, immediate repair of thoracic aortic injuries is indicated, although delayed repair in selected cases has received recent attention. Soots and coworkers reported on four patients who underwent delayed repair (after 5 to 43 days) because of severe associated injuries.[58] They commented that major brain injury or pulmonary contusions are indications for delay in hemodynamically stable patients. Fisher and colleagues described three patients with thoracic aortic injuries who were observed because of either trivial findings on angiography or severe associated injuries. On prolonged follow-up, the lesions resolved in one, diminished in another, and remained unchanged in the third. The author believes that unless the patient has multiple and severe associated injuries that are likely to be rapidly fatal, immediate repair is warranted. Minimal vascular injuries in this location have received insufficient study to advocate a "wait and see" policy.

INJURIES OF THE INTRATHORACIC GREAT VESSELS

Blunt trauma is responsible for the majority of injuries to the great vessels of the chest, with the innominate artery being affected most commonly. A survey of 36 cases of blunt injury to the aortic arch branch vessels found 22 cases of innominate trauma (61 per cent), 7 of the right subclavian artery, and 7 of the left subclavian artery. Eleven patients had associated injuries of the aortic arch proper.[59] Penetrating injuries of the innominate or subclavian arteries typically occur with gunshot wounds or with inferiorly directed stab wounds.

As with aortic injuries, patients with branch vessel trauma may present with stable vital signs or in profound shock. The initial diagnostic impression may be that of an aortic arch injury. The most common findings among those sustaining blunt trauma are decreased ipsilateral extremity pulses, physical evidence of chest wall trauma, and hypotension.[60] Associated injuries are common and include head injuries, tracheal or bronchial injuries, facial injuries, brachial plexus injuries, and abdominal trauma. Penetrating injuries may present with an arteriovenous fistula and palpable distal pulses. Profound shock may be present owing to bleeding into the hemithorax. Occasionally, these patients present with a supraclavicular hematoma that expands into the neck. When penetration has extended caudally to the mediastinum, pericardial tamponade may occur.[61]

Subclavian artery injuries are largely due to penetrating mechanisms, although improperly worn shoulder harnesses are a common cause of blunt trauma. The most important sign of a subclavian artery occlusion is absence of the radial pulse. An occasional patient may develop the subclavian steal syndrome when the injury causes stenosis proximal to the origin of the vertebral artery. Associated brachial plexus injuries are common.

Plain chest x-rays typically reveal widening of the superior aspect of the mediastinal silhouette (Fig. 46–7). The widened mediastinum noted with an innominate artery injury is usually more superior than that seen with an aortic injury. With penetrating injuries, a large hemithorax may also be present. When the film is taken with the patient supine, only a diffuse haziness may be apparent over the involved hemithorax.[7] Angiography remains the definitive modality for the demonstration of branch vessel injuries. (Figs. 46–8 to 46–11). Femoral or contralateral axillary approaches are preferred. Penetrating injury to the subclavian vessels may be diagnosed by a retrograde ipsilateral axillary or brachial arteriogram performed in the emergency department.[41] A blood pressure cuff is placed distal to the injury and inflated to 300 mmHg. The action of the blood pressure cuff forces contrast, injected into either the axillary or brachial artery, backward toward the aortic arch to demonstrate the injury.

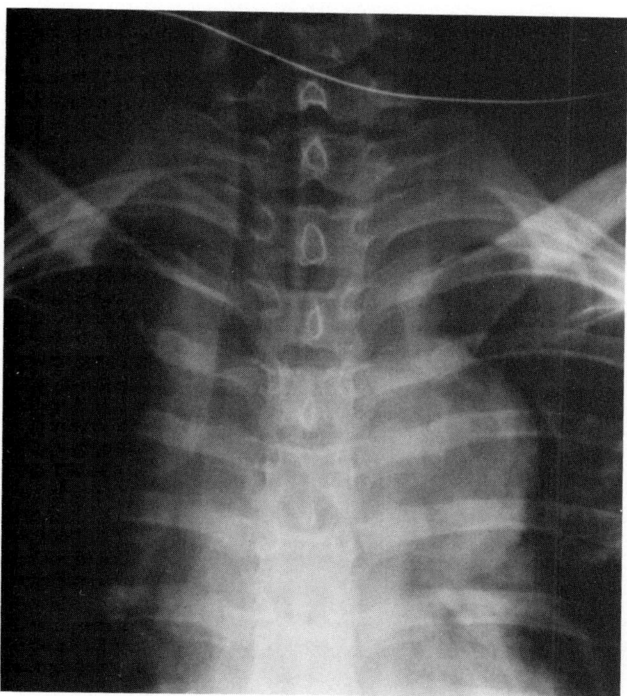

FIGURE 46–7. The mediastinal widening associated with this left subclavian arterial injury is somewhat higher and more displaced than that occurring with an injury at the aortic isthmus.

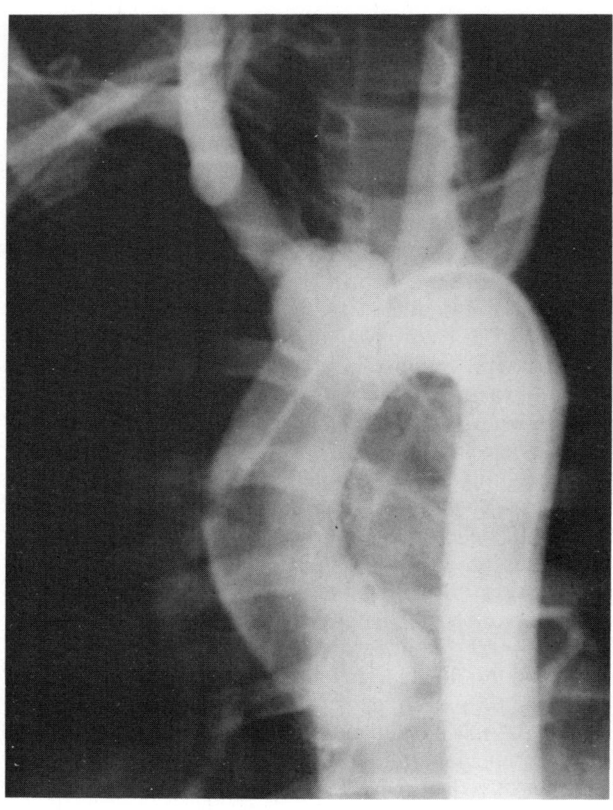

FIGURE 46–8. Blunt injury at the origin of the innominate artery.

FIGURE 46–9. Occlusion of the proximal left subclavian artery.

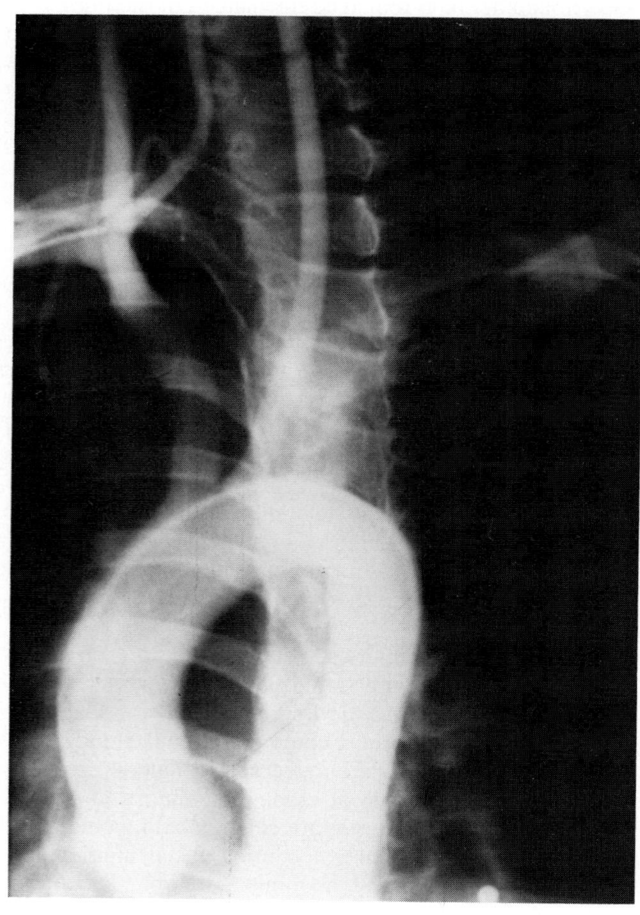

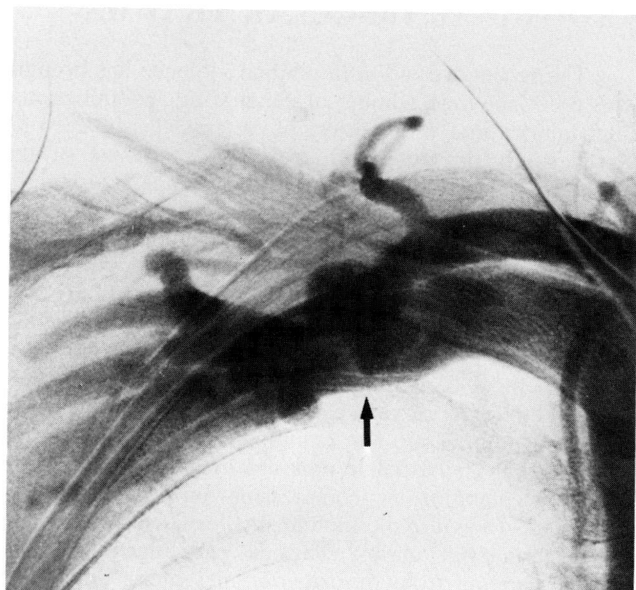

FIGURE 46–10. A subtraction angiogram shows a midsubclavian arteriovenous fistula that occurred after the patient sustained an inferiorly directed knife wound of the supraclavicular fossa.

Preoperative Management

Prior to diagnostic angiography or transport to the operating room, patients must be resuscitated and stabilized using the strategies outlined for injuries of the aorta. Because of the possibility of concomitant venous trauma, lower extremity venous access sites are preferred.

A penetrating wound of the subclavian artery or vein may result in rapid intrapleural hemorrhage unless it is controlled. When moribund patients have a right-sided injury, an emergent high right anterolateral thoracotomy may be performed to allow packing and manual compression of the bleeding site from within the chest.[62] Manual pressure may also be applied to the right supraclavicular fossa to aid in control. When the injury is to the left subclavian artery, an anterolateral thoracotomy is required to gain control of the vessel's proximal intrapleural position. If satisfactory hemostasis is not achieved, digital pressure in the supraclavicular fossa may help.

Operative Strategy

Injuries of the Innominate Artery. Access to the innominate artery is best obtained through a median sternotomy. If the proximal right subclavian artery is involved, the incision can be extended into the right neck as needed. In the absence of profound intraoperative hypotension or an extensive injury that requires simultaneous occlusion of both the innominate and the left common carotid artery, cardiopulmonary bypass or common carotid artery shunting is not required. When the repair is likely to be lengthy, or if there are concerns about blood pressure, some have used ''stump pressures'' to ensure adequate cerebral perfusion.[60] When a carotid shunt is used, it should be placed so that it extends from the proximal ascending aorta to the distal common carotid artery. When injuries involve the aortic arch as well, partial occluding clamps are used to gain control. We have found that cardiopulmonary bypass is seldom required. Vosloo and Reichart reported inflow occlusion as an alternative to cardiopulmonary bypass.[63] In their patient with partial transection of the innominate artery, clamps were placed on the superior and inferior vena cava for 1.5 minutes, during which time the repair was completed.

Blunt injuries typically involve the origin of the innominate artery. Proximal control is obtained with a curved instrument such as a Wylie-J clamp. Distal control of the innominate artery is obtained proximal to its bifurcation. When the innominate vein obscures the field, it can be either retracted or divided. An 8 to 12-mm Dacron graft should be placed end-to-side to the proximal ascending aorta away from the pseudoaneurysm and then connected to the innominate artery just proximal to its bifurcation. The final step is oversewing of the innominate stump.

Penetrating injuries in the distal portion of the innominate artery are best approached through a median sternotomy extended into the right neck. Removal of the middle portion of the clavicle facilitates exposure and distal control, although this is seldom necessary. Repair of the vessel can usually be performed by lateral arteriorrhaphy, although bypass grafting from the ascending aorta is occasionally required.

Injuries of the Left Common Carotid. Access to the left common carotid artery is obtained with a median sternotomy extended upward along the anterior border of the left sternocleidomastoid muscle. Proximal control can be achieved at the origin of the vessel from the aortic arch, with distal control obtained cephalad to the injury. Concern

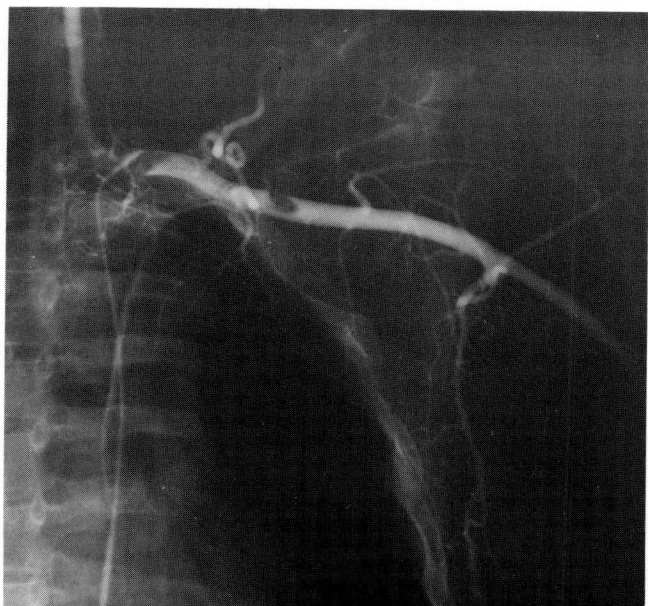

FIGURE 46–11. Traumatic occlusion of the proximal left subclavian artery caused this vertebral steal. The lucency just beyond the vertebral origin is a balloon at the tip of the angiography catheter. Note the second defect in the mid-subclavian artery.

about the patient's neurologic status dictates the type of repair performed. Liekweg and Greenfield reported on 233 injuries of the common and internal carotid arteries and found that reconstruction was beneficial in all patients except those in severe coma.[64] Some surgeons believe that if the patient is seen shortly after injury, repair is warranted because prolonged ischemia may be the more significant threat.[65] Shunts should be used only when intraoperative hypotension is a concern, or when both the innominate and the left common carotid arteries must be occluded simultaneously.

Injuries of the Subclavian Vessels. Optimal exposure for repair of the proximal right subclavian artery is obtained by a median sternotomy with extension into the right neck. Removal of the middle third of the clavicle provides exposure of all three portions of the artery. Injuries to the more distal portions of either subclavian artery can be exposed by supraclavicular incision with removal of the clavicle. Caution must be exercised because the artery is extremely fragile and can be damaged easily by overzealous dissection.

Because of its intrapleural location, the proximal left subclavian artery is best approached through an anterolateral thoracotomy. Although this incision facilitates proximal control, the more distal extrapleural portions cannot be reached. A supraclavicular incision is added for this purpose. Although many authors speak of the "open book" created when a median sternotomy connects an anterolateral thoracotomy to a supraclavicular incision, the author has found that the approach does not open easily and typically results in multiple posterior rib fractures.

Subclavian artery repairs following penetrating injury can usually be performed by débridement and primary anastomosis.[66] When a defect is present, we have used reversed saphenous grafts with success. Associated subclavian vein injuries are common and merit repair if possible. For simple lacerations, lateral venorrhaphy is usually adequate. When larger defects are present, a paneled repair may be required to prevent narrowing of the lumen. Although the subclavian artery and vein can be ligated, blunt trauma may disrupt the collateral supply around the shoulder and produce effort fatigue of the arm and ischemia of the hand.

Results

The outcome of acute thoracic aortic injury depends not only on the aortic lesion but also on the severity of associated trauma. A study from Duke University examined 108 patients who had sustained blunt trauma.[17] Of the 86 per cent who survived initial resuscitation, 71 per cent survived their injuries. Significantly, only 11 of 42 deaths (26 per cent) were directly attributable to the thoracic aortic injury. Postoperative paraplegia developed in 6.8 per cent of patients.

Survival after injuries of the innominate vessels was reported to be 86 per cent in a series by Graham and coworkers.[67] Injuries of the individual common carotid arteries have survival rates near 80 per cent.[68] The mortality of isolated acute subclavian artery injuries is less than 15 per cent.

ABDOMINAL VASCULAR TRAUMA

The recent escalation in civilian violence has brought with it an increased number of penetrating abdominal vascular injuries in a wide variety of patterns. Tissue destruction depends on the speed, trajectory, and size of the wounding object. If vessel transection occurs, free hemorrhage into the abdominal cavity may result. Occasionally, injury may be partially or completely contained within the retroperitoneum. Rarely, a tangential injury produces thrombosis with ischemia of the respective mesenteric or peripheral bed. Slow-speed penetrating injuries may cause arteriovenous fistulae between adjacent vessels. This type of injury most commonly occurs between the infrarenal aorta and the inferior vena cava.

Blunt injuries are less common than their penetrating counterparts. The usual lesions are avulsions and thromboses. Deceleration or compression produces sufficient shear stress to avulse the mobile smaller vessels from their fixed mesenteric origins. This is particularly true for branches arising from the superior mesenteric artery and from the portal vein. These patients present in shock due to intraperitoneal hemorrhage when sufficient energy has been absorbed. In other instances, stretching during deceleration may cause intimal tears that lead to vessel thrombosis. Occlusion by an intimal flap is thought to be responsible for the "seat belt aorta" and for occlusions of the proximal renal arteries (Fig. 46–12).

Diagnosis

Patients with intra-abdominal vascular injuries who survive the initial insult commonly present with hypoten-

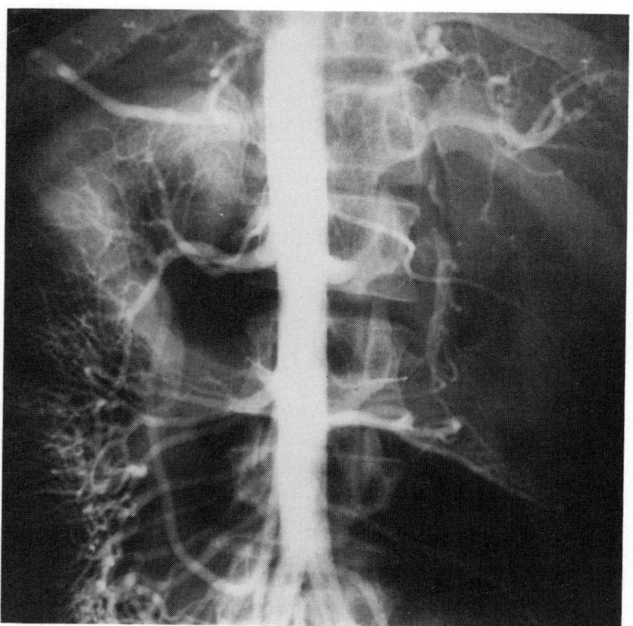

FIGURE 46–12. High-speed motor vehicle accidents may cause intimal stretching and flaps that result in thrombosis. This patient sustained occlusion of the left renal artery after a motorcycle accident.

sion or frank shock. It has been estimated that only 15 per cent of patients with penetrating injuries of the abdominal aorta survive long enough to reach the hospital. Because trauma to the lower thorax may also involve the abdominal aorta, all patients with penetrating injuries between the nipples and the groin should be suspected of harboring an abdominal vascular injury. Retroperitoneal location, a contained hematoma, and hypotension may all be protective, and exsanguination may be prevented by peritoneal tamponade and decreased pulsatile pressure.[69] As volume resuscitation is instituted, increased cardiac output and blood pressure expand the hematoma and lead to free hemorrhage. The key to diagnosis is a history of moderate hypotension prior to arrival and failure to maintain a stable blood pressure after fluid resuscitation.[62]

Rapid and aggressive fluid resuscitation is paramount. Because of the possibility of associated venous injury, the author uses only upper extremity intravenous access sites in these patients. If the patient's condition deteriorates or if he or she has a cardiac arrest, open cardiac massage and cross-clamping of the thoracic aorta are required. These maneuvers will decrease intra-abdominal blood loss and may substantially improve the critical coronary and cerebral circulations.[70]

While resuscitation is proceeding, physical assessment and radiographic studies are performed. Physical findings of significance include a rapidly expanding abdomen, an audible bruit, or asymmetric lower extremity pulses. An asymmetric femoral arterial pulse is evidence of a common or external iliac artery injury. All patients should have an indwelling urinary bladder catheter placed to monitor resuscitation and provide information about possible renal injury. The author obtains both a chest x-ray and a *one-shot* intravenous pyelogram (IVP). The chest x-ray helps to eliminate associated pathology such as pneumothorax or thoracic vascular injury. Additionally, it may reveal a missile embolism in patients with venous injuries. The one-shot IVP is obtained by infusing 50 ml of Renografin contrast along with the resuscitation fluids. A flat plate view of the abdomen is taken 5 to 10 minutes later and provides information about the kidneys and ureters. Optimally, bilateral renal function and ureteral continuity will be present. This information is critical for subsequent intraoperative decision-making if a perinephric hematoma is found.

Blunt injuries of the abdominal vasculature are more difficult to diagnose. If an artery is completely avulsed, hemorrhage into the peritoneal cavity may produce profound hypotension and signs of peritoneal irritation.[62] If the abdominal examination is equivocal, a diagnostic peritoneal lavage or CT scan may be helpful.[62]

Diagnostic evaluation of renal vascular injury begins with a urinalysis. Although 25 to 50 per cent of patients with renal artery injuries have neither gross nor microscopic hematuria, the presence of either should be interpreted with caution.[71–73] A prospective study of 1146 consecutive patients by Mee and colleagues found no significant renal injuries among blunt trauma patients who had microscopic hematuria *without* shock. The author has adopted their recommendations that all patients with penetrating trauma to the flank or abdomen, and those with blunt trauma who have either gross or microscopic hematuria and are in shock, should undergo radiographic evaluation.[74] The one-shot IVP seems a reasonable tool in patients who are unstable and require rapid evaluation of renal function. Unfortunately, the IVP may have a 30 per cent false-negative rate and may be uninterpretable in those who are hypotensive.[73] In stable patients who require evaluation for intra-abdominal injury by CT scan, the author routinely includes intravenous contrast injection to examine bilateral renal function. Absence of renal enhancement and excretion, or the presence of a cortical rim sign, is evidence of thrombosis of the renal artery. If a kidney is present but not functioning, the author proceeds with angiography to identify the location and nature of the lesion. Although it has been suggested that CT can substitute for angiography, the author and others believe that angiography remains the modality of choice.[75, 76] Once the diagnosis of renal artery injury has been made, repair must proceed expeditiously because ischemic time is inversely related to the chances of functional repair.

Operative Management

An operative team familiar with aortic surgery is mandatory. Equipment requirements include an aortic compression device or balloon occluders, cardiovascular instruments, and a selection of straight and bifurcated grafts.

Aortic Injuries. The abdominal aorta is divided into three surgical regions:

1. The diaphragmatic aorta: the aorta at or above the celiac axis.
2. The suprarenal aorta: the portion extending from the celiac axis to the level of the renal arteries.
3. The infrarenal aorta: the portion extending from below the renal arteries to the bifurcation into the common iliac arteries (L4).

After the patient is positioned supine on the operating table, he or she is prepared and draped from the mid-thorax (nipples) to the knees *prior to the induction of anesthesia.* Muscle relaxants used during induction relax the abdominal wall and may relieve the tamponade, resulting in sudden and profound hypotension.

Several incisions have been described for this procedure including (1) extended midline laparotomy, (2) thoracoabdominal, and (3) left thoracotomy with laparotomy. The advantage of the added left thoracotomy is that it provides access for immediate control of the descending thoracic aorta if the abdominal injury is so high that subdiaphragmatic control is not possible. The thoracoabdominal approach offers the added advantage of additional exposure in the left upper quadrant. The author prefers the traditional extended midline laparotomy incision and obtains subdiaphragmatic control just below the aortic hiatus. This is done by bluntly dissecting the lesser omentum with the forefinger to gain entry to the lesser sac. This provides access to the posterior peritoneum, which overlies the pancreas and the crura of the diaphragm. The posterior peritoneum is divided, and the muscle fibers of the crura are separated, exposing the periadventitial tissue along the supraceliac aorta.[77] The anterior, left, and right walls of the aorta are dissected bluntly for about 1 inch, enabling placement of a slightly curved aortic clamp along the course of the surgeon's fingers. If the aorta is not well dissected prior to placing the clamp, it may slip off the dense periaortic tissue. Associated venous injuries, such as aortocaval fistulae, must also be addressed quickly. Because the veins are fragile, the author prefers to control venous hemorrhage with sponge sticks rather than attempt clamp control. By progressively reducing the length of vein between the sponges, the area of hemorrhage can usually be controlled sufficiently to permit suture repair. When the area of injury contains an avulsion, the proximal and distal ends are controlled with sponges until clamps can be placed accurately around the segments. Blood loss during these maneuvers is often considerable, and it is imperative that once preliminary hemostasis has been achieved, the surgeon pause long enough to allow the anesthesiologist to replace shed volume, correct metabolic acidosis, and restore platelets as needed.

After hemorrhage has been controlled, a survey should determine whether bowel injuries are present. For small isolated rents, a few single-layer closures can be performed while the anesthesiologist is correcting metabolic and hematologic abnormalities. When large segments of intestine have been damaged, noncrushing clamps are used to isolate the injured segments. Affected bowel should be packed out of the field until the vascular repair has been completed and protected by soft tissue coverage.

Diaphragmatic (Supraceliac) Injuries. Supraceliac injuries traditionally have a high mortality rate owing to exsanguination.[78] Upon entering the abdomen, active supramesocolic hemorrhage or an expanding central hematoma signals an aortic injury. Direct pressure controls bleeding until dissection through the lesser omentum allows proximal control. When a large active hematoma and tissue destruction are present, aortic occluders, transaortic balloon catheters, or transthoracic aortic occlusion may be required. The author has recently employed a balloon catheter inserted through a femoral artery in difficult situations. The disadvantage of this method is that an assistant must isolate the femoral artery and introduce the device, taking him or her away from the operative field.

Optimal exposure of the supraceliac aorta is obtained via a left lateral retroperitoneal incision with medial rotation of the intestines (Fig. 46–13).[78, 79] The dissection is begun inferiorly along the fusion plane between the left colon and the posterior peritoneum. Further medial mobilization is accomplished by performing blunt dissection of the entire left colon, splenic flexure, spleen, and tail of the pancreas.[77] The left kidney may remain in place or can be rotated medially along with the viscera. Dissection is carried out proximally in the plane of the preaortic fascia to the level of entry of the aorta into the abdomen. In the unlikely event that more proximal exposure is required, a transthoracic extension can be accomplished by extending the midline wound as a median sternotomy or by making a radial incision in the diaphragm to expose the thoracic aorta. This approach exposes the aorta from T9 to the bifurcation. Potential complications include injury to the spleen, left renal artery, and lumbar arteries.[80]

A right-sided approach may also be used. A wide Kocher maneuver is performed, and the duodenum and head of the pancreas are rotated medially. This produces excellent exposure of the vena cava and aorta at the level of the celiac axis and superior mesenteric artery.

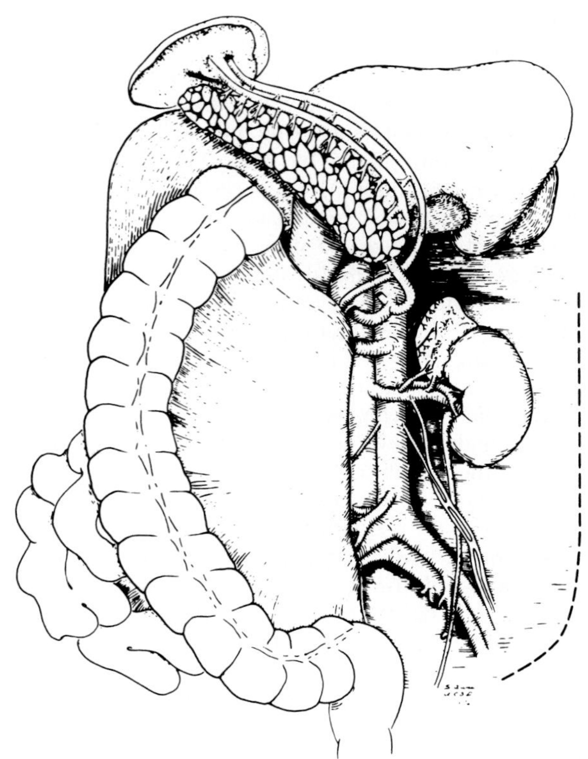

FIGURE 46–13. **Incision along the left lateral fusion plane with rotation of the viscera to the midline provides excellent exposure of the aorta and mesenteric vessels. The left kidney may be reflected with the intestines or left in place, as shown here. (From Shackford SR, Sise JR: Renal and mesenteric vascular trauma. *In* Bongard FS, Wilson SE, Perry MO [eds]: Vascular Injuries in Surgical Practice. Norwalk, CT, Appleton & Lange, 1991, p 178.)**

The supraceliac aorta is typically repaired using a lateral suture of 3–0 polypropylene. If extensive tissue destruction is present near the head of the pancreas along the course of the gastroduodenal arteries, celiac ligation must not be performed because collateral pathways may have been destroyed. If the aortic defect is sufficiently large to require a patch, we prefer autogenous tissue. Hypogastric artery is usually readily available and can be opened and trimmed to suitable size. This avoids the need to dissect and excise a segment of saphenous vein. Although others have reported routine use of prosthetic materials such as PTFE or Dacron in this location, we avoid their use whenever possible, particularly in the presence of gastrointestinal contamination.[81]

Suprarenal Injuries. Injuries to the segment between the origin of the renal arteries and the celiac axis have the highest mortality rate. Because dense periaortic neural tissue surrounds the celiac axis, the superior mesenteric artery, and the pancreas, this segment is best exposed by medial rotation of the viscera in the same manner as that described for the supraceliac aorta. When an injury of the inferior vena cava is suspected as well, a right rather than a left gutter incision is preferable. With this technique, the right colon, hepatic flexure, and duodenum are mobilized to the left.

Suprarenal aortic injuries are usually repaired with 3–0 monofilament polypropylene via a lateral arteriorrhaphy. When two lacerations closely approximate each other, they can be connected and repaired transversely as a single defect using a horizontal mattress suture.

Infrarenal Injuries. Injuries of the infrarenal aorta generally have the best outcome because of their accessibility. Upon entering the abdomen, a large retroperitoneal hematoma extending into the flanks is the first finding. The initial approach requires cephalad traction on the transverse colon mesentery, accompanied by evisceration of the small bowel to the right. The retroperitoneum is then opened in the midline superiorly near the transverse colon mesentery. This permits identification of the left renal vein, which serves as a marker for the renal arteries. For most infrarenal injuries, proximal control can be obtained at this level. The left renal vein is usually very mobile and can be retracted superiorly after minimal dissection to expose the renal arteries. When this is not possible, the left renal vein can be ligated medially as it passes over the aorta. If a supraceliac or thoracic aortic cross-clamp has been placed, it can be repositioned below the renal arteries. We prefer to obtain distal control with a gently curved Crafoord clamp placed tangentially to simultaneously control the aorta and the posteriorly arising lumbar arteries. When the injury extends inferiorly toward the bifurcation, the iliac arteries may need to be controlled individually. Particular care must be exercised to prevent injury to the left iliac vein as it passes under the right iliac artery.

When the injury is less than 1 cm in length, gentle dissection may provide enough mobility to allow resection and repair. Great care must be exercised to ligate and divide lumbar arteries with clips or suture before mobilization is attempted. Repair is performed with 3–0 monofilament polypropylene suture. Careful closure of the peritoneum over the aorta is imperative.

When a large segment of aorta is damaged, in-line bypass, or ligation of the proximal and distal ends with extra-anatomic bypass, may be performed. Because young trauma victims have relatively small aortas, the maximum size of graft usable is typically 12 to 14 mm. Feliciano and coworkers summarized the results in 33 patients from eight studies and found only 1 reported graft infection.[82] If the surgeon chooses to use a prosthetic graft, the repair must be meticulously covered with soft tissue and peritoneum before intestinal injuries are repaired. Careful postoperative monitoring is required to detect the earliest evidence of graft infection.

Blunt Aortic Injuries. Blunt trauma to the aorta most commonly occurs following motor vehicle accidents or falls. Downward traction produces intimal disruption, particularly in the infrarenal aorta.[83] Bowel injuries are present in 100 per cent of cases when seat belts are the causative agent.[83] Typical acute findings include diminished lower extremity pulses in the presence of a normal upper extremity examination. Transaxillary angiography will locate the injury and demonstrate its length. Treatment depends on the extent of the injury and associated findings. Simple intimal disruption with limited dissection can be repaired by simple suture, whereas lengthy dissections may require endarterectomy beyond the end-point. Vessel replacement is required when injury is extensive or presentation has been delayed.

Iliac Vessels. Iliac injuries most commonly occur after penetrating trauma and are often accompanied by cecal, sigmoid colon, ureteral, or urinary bladder injuries. Blunt injuries that produce trauma to the common or external iliac vessels are unusual. Hemorrhage is usually due to disruption of branches of the hypogastric artery or vein. A falling hematocrit after pelvic fracture without evidence of other injuries is best managed by external fracture stabilization and angiography for therapeutic embolization.[84] Operative ligation of bleeding vessels in this location is usually not required.

When laparotomy is performed for penetrating trauma, injuries of the iliac vessels often present as pulsatile and expanding hematomas in the inferior quadrants. Exposure of the right common iliac artery is best obtained by elevating the cecum and terminal ileum toward the left. The left common iliac artery can be exposed by reflecting the sigmoid and left colon toward the right. Exposure of the left iliac vein may require division and reanastomosis of the right common iliac artery.[85] Proximal and distal control are mandatory before entering the hematoma. Sponge sticks placed on either side of the injury provide rapid hemostasis and permit more careful dissection in a relatively blood-free field.

Repair of external iliac arterial injuries can usually be performed via lateral arteriorrhaphy with 4–0 or 5–0 polypropylene.[86] Resection with mobilization of cut ends provides a tension-free anastomosis for injuries less than 2 cm in length. The internal iliac artery makes an excellent autologous graft for short segments. Injuries that extend proximally to include the aortic bifurcation may be repaired by performing an aortoiliac anastomosis on one side, followed by an end-to-side anastomosis of the iliac artery to the contralateral reconstruction. This repositioned ''aortic bifurcation'' has the advantage of placing the anastomosis out of direct contact with other injured tissue. Reconstructions should be covered by viable retroperitoneal tissue and replaced in the pelvis. In the presence of significant enteric contamination, the author prefers to ligate the injured artery and perform femoral crossover grafting rather than use prosthetic grafts in the field. If repair or extra-anatomic reconstruction is not possible, a four-compartment calf fasciotomy should be performed because of the high incidence of compartment syndrome.[82]

Iliac venous injuries are exposed using the same methods described for their arterial counterparts. Control is achieved by applying direct pressure or by using sponge sticks. These injuries are usually fairly simple to repair via lateral venorrhaphy, although care must be exercised to prevent narrowing of the vein, which will lead to subsequent thrombosis. Ligation of an iliac vein in a young patient is usually well tolerated but should be avoided if possible.

Mesenteric and Portal Vessels. Injuries of the mesenteric and portal vessels are often accompanied by overlying intestinal trauma, creating difficulty with isolation and repair. Exposure of the origin of the celiac and superior mesenteric arteries is best obtained through lateral mobilization and rightward rotation of the viscera as outlined for suprarenal aortic injuries. Associated mesenteric venous injuries are common and should be repaired first to prevent venous engorgement of the bowel.[87]

Isolated injuries of the celiac axis are extremely uncommon and can usually be ligated. The common hepatic artery tends to be the largest branch of the celiac artery and can occasionally be repaired with an end-to-end anastomosis or saphenous vein graft if the patient's overall condition warrants. Ligation of the common hepatic artery, when necessary, should be done proximal to the origin of the gastroduodenal artery because this constitutes a large collateral from the superior mesenteric artery. Several anatomic variants of the celiac axis exist including a common origin with the superior mesenteric. For this reason, the pertinent anatomy must be clearly identified before any vessels are sacrificed.[69]

The superior mesenteric artery (SMA) can be divided into four segments based on their location and the presence of collateral blood flow: (1) at its origin behind the pancreas proximal to the takeoff of the pancreaticoduodenal artery, (2) in the base of the transverse mesocolon between the pancreaticoduodenal and middle colic branches, (3) beyond the middle colic branch, and (4) at the level of the mesenteric arcades.[88] At its origin, exposure of the SMA is difficult but can be obtained by rightward rotation of the viscera or by transection of the pancreas. When the aorta and SMA are sufficiently damaged to preclude direct repair, the splenic artery can be turned down and an end-to-end anastomosis to the stump of the artery performed. A splenectomy is usually included. Alternatively, a graft can be placed from the anterior surface of the aorta to the stump of the mesenteric vessel. Care must be exercised when pancreatic injuries are present to shield the anastomosis from the potentially disruptive effect of pancreatic enzymes. Ligation of the proximal SMA, if required, is usually tolerated because of collateral flow from the pancreaticoduodenal artery, although associated injuries and vasospasm make midgut viability problematic. Beyond the middle colic branch, repair is mandatory to prevent midgut ischemia.

The superior mesenteric vein lies just to the right of the artery as they cross over the uncinate process of the pancreas and third portion of the duodenum. Presumed injuries of the artery frequently involve the vein or prove to be the vein on exposure. Repair of the superior mesenteric vein is preferred to ligation, although this may be difficult, especially in the segment that exits from beneath the pancreas. Pancreatic division may be necessary to obtain access and control for repair. Collaterals must be ligated before visualization of posterior perforations is possible. Control is obtained with sponge sticks or finger pressure. Repair can be performed with 5–0 or 6–0 polypropylene fashioned to prevent narrowing of the lumen. Methods of repair include saphenous vein interposition, anastomosis to the splenic vein, and ligation. Splenic vein injuries that cannot be repaired simply should be managed by ligation and splenectomy. Ligation of the splenic vein may lead to gastric varices if the spleen is not removed. When the superior mesenteric vein requires ligation, postoperative fluid balance must be monitored carefully because the resultant splanchnic hypervolemia leads to peripheral hypovolemia for 72 hours after ligation.

Inferior mesenteric artery injuries are best treated by ligation as long as SMA and hypogastric collaterals are patent. Assessment of bowel viability is mandatory and is best accomplished by reexploration at 48 to 72 hours, or sooner if indicated.

Repair of portal venous injuries is preferred to ligation when possible. In the hypovolemic and hypotensive patient, portal vein ligation may lead to hepatic necrosis. Portacaval shunting is difficult in this situation and has a high complication rate.[89] Exposure of the portal vein and the confluence of the mesenteric and splenic veins is achieved by mobilizing the hepatic flexure and colon (Fig. 46–14). A Kocher maneuver also facilities exposure. Injuries of the porta hepatis require dissection of the common bile duct and cystic duct, which are then mobilized and displaced. Trauma in this area may also include hepatic artery injuries and may be accompanied by profuse hemorrhage. Placement of a noncrushing clamp across the common bile duct, portal vein, and hepatic artery (Pringle's maneuver) may be required. Injuries of the portal vein and hepatic artery to a liver segment will result in hepatic ischemia and, if ligated, will require segmental hepatectomy. Anterior and left lateral portal vein exposure may require division of the pancreas, which is best accomplished by clamping the head of the pancreas with two straight intestinal clamps and opening between them. Lateral venorrhaphy or end-to-end anastomosis should be performed, although panel grafts may be required when significant disruption has occurred. When the patient is unstable or when a coagulopathy is present, portal venous ligation is required. As in the situation following superior mesenteric venous ligation, this produces systemic hypovolemia and requires aggressive fluid resuscitation during the first few days after surgery.

Renovascular Injuries. At the time of laparotomy, previously unsuspected renovascular injuries are indicated

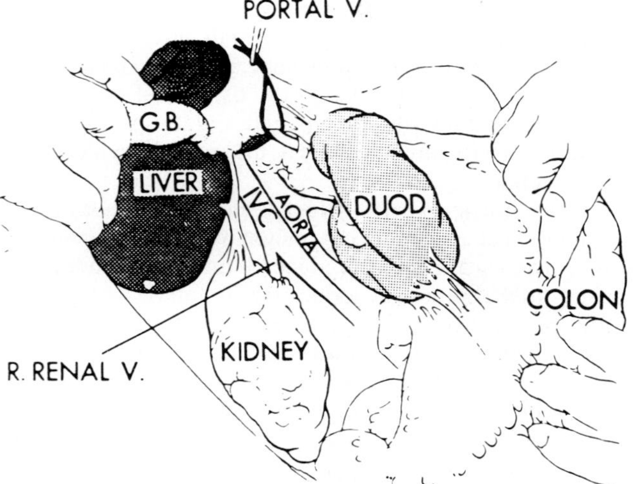

FIGURE 46–14. Exposure of the portal vein is best achieved by incision of viscera along the right fusion line with medial rotation. (From Petersen SR, Sheldon GF, Lim RC: Management of portal vein injuries. J Trauma 19[8]:616–620, © Williams & Wilkins, 1979.)

by the presence of a central hematoma or by a pulsatile and expanding lateral perirenal hematoma. Wilson and Zeigler commented that up to 10 per cent of patients with unexplored perirenal hematomas developed complications that might have been avoided.[73]

The renal vasculature must be controlled prior to exploring a perirenal hematoma. The proximal renal artery can be exposed either through an incision in the retroperitoneum over the aorta, or by mobilizing the viscera from lateral to medial. Mobility of the left renal vein can be achieved by dividing the distal branches, although this maneuver eliminates the possibility of ligating the vein subsequently. Control of the distal left renal artery is achieved by dissecting along the course of the vessel until the hilum is identified. Leftward retraction of the inferior vena cava will permit isolation of the right renal pedicle. Care must be exercised to ensure that the right renal vein is not avulsed from the inferior vena cava or that small posterior lumbar veins are not damaged. Ligation of the right renal vein will require ipsilateral nephrectomy. Very proximal right renal artery injuries may also be controlled by this maneuver, although mobilization of the ascending colon and a Kocher maneuver are usually required for enough exposure to permit repair.

Strategy regarding repair or ligation of the injured vessel depends upon (1) the overall condition of the patient, (2) the extent of injury to the renal artery, (3) the condition of the ipsilateral kidney, and (4) the condition of the contralateral kidney.[69] Additionally, the duration of renal ischemia is important. Renal function is severely impaired after 6 hours of warm partial ischemia and after 3 hours of total ischemia.[90] Although successful repairs have been reported after extended periods, it does not seem prudent to attempt revascularization of a unilateral injury after more than 6 hours. However, if there is only one kidney, or if there are bilateral renal vascular injuries, a more aggressive approach is warranted if the patient's condition permits.

After the decision to revascularize has been made, proximal and distal control must be ensured. Lacerations of the distal vessel may be controlled with a sponge stick or with an occluding balloon inserted through the proximal vessel. Simple lacerations should be débrided and repaired end-to-end to prevent narrowing of the lumen. If insufficient length is present, interposition grafting with saphenous vein is preferred. Occasionally the graft must be connected proximally to the aorta. Moving the splenic artery down to replace the left renal artery or the hepatic artery to replace the right renal artery may be necessary in a stable patient without contralateral renal function. Following any type of renal vascular repair, follow-up assessment of renal function by excretion scanning is mandatory. Repairs thought to be successful at the time of completion may subsequently cause hypertension and require medication or late nephrectomy to correct.[91]

Injuries of the Inferior Vena Cava. Injuries of the inferior vena cava occur in two regions: (1) the infrarenal vena cava, which extends from the junction of the left and right common iliac veins at the level of the fifth lumbar vertebrae to L2, where it receives the left and right renal veins, and (2) the suprarenal and retrohepatic vena cava, which extends cephalad until it enters the right atrium inside the pericardial sac.

Infrarenal Vena Cava. One third to one half of inferior vena caval injuries occur in this segment. Exposure requires mobilizing the right colon, hepatic flexure, duodenum, and pancreas to the left. Initial hemostasis is best achieved by placing sponge sticks to isolate the injury. A drop in blood pressure may occur if the patient has not had adequate fluid resuscitation. Subdiaphragmatic aortic occlusion may help to restore blood pressure and prevent pooling in the lower extremities. When posterior injuries are present, some hemorrhage may persist because of collateral and lumbar veins. The author usually does not completely mobilize the vena cava because such maneuvers can tear the posterior collaterals. For anterior injuries, a side-biting Satinsky clamp will control the injury while permitting some continued venous return. Once controlled, the posterior wall should be inspected carefully for injury. If present, small posterior lacerations can be repaired from within the vessel. Suture lines should be kept as short as possible to avoid unnecessary thrombogenesis.

The majority of injuries can be repaired by lateral venorrhaphy, provided that the diameter is not narrowed to less than 50 per cent.[92] For large anterior defects, an opened segment of saphenous vein or a panel graft may be required. When an entire segment of vena cava is damaged, replacement or ligation is necessary. Although the creation of spiral vein grafts from a segment of saphenous vein has been described, these patients are usually not able to withstand the operative time required to create such a graft.[89] A number of graft materials and techniques including creation of distal femorosaphenous fistulae to improve flow through the graft have been described. The time, potential blood loss, and likelihood of eventual thrombosis make such efforts inadvisable.[93, 94] The author prefers infrarenal caval ligation to prosthetic repair for complex injuries. Postoperatively, these patients require volume expansion and prevention of lower extremity venous pooling. The use of venous pumps, elastic wraps, and leg elevation should be maintained for at least 1 week after surgery.

If a small and stable hematoma is present on laparotomy, an isolated posterior defect may be responsible. Recently, several authors have advocated management without repair.[95, 96] Experience with this approach has been limited but may be reasonable under carefully defined and controlled circumstances.[97] Animal studies have confirmed the general absence of sequelae in experimental models.[96]

Suprarenal and Retrohepatic Vena Cava. Injuries of the suprarenal and retrohepatic vena cava carry a mortality of between 33 and 67 per cent because of extensive blood loss, difficulty in repair, and associated trauma. When the injury is at the confluence of the renal veins and the inferior vena cava, compression at the site of injury will limit hemorrhage until suprarenal and infrarenal sponge sticks or loops can be placed. Once this is done, the left renal vein is looped or ligated medially, and the vena cava is gently mobilized medially until the right renal vein is visualized and controlled. If the rent is large, a 30-ml Foley catheter can be inserted into the defect and inflated. Particular care is required to prevent excessively rapid inflation, which results in complete disruption of the injury.

Exposure of extrahepatic suprarenal injuries can be achieved by use of a Kocher maneuver that mobilizes the duodenum and ascending colon toward the midline. Initial hemostasis can be achieved with sponge sticks, finger pressure, or balloon occlusion. Repair is performed in the manner described for infrarenal injuries. Ligation in this position carries a high mortality rate.

The retrohepatic portion of the inferior vena cava is the most difficult to expose and control. This segment receives the hepatic veins, which are short and extremely fragile. When initial mobilization of the liver is met with increased hemorrhage, the author packs the area and places downward pressure on the liver to achieve immediate hemostasis. The injury is exposed by division of the triangular and anterior and posterior coronary ligaments of the overlying hepatic lobe. This limited dissection is occasionally adequate to permit direct repair of the lacerated hepatic veins and vena cava. Pachter and associates have suggested that the hepatic laceration can be extended along the injury tract until exposure of the hepatic venous or vena caval injury is obtained.[98] On occasion, extension of the laparotomy to a median sternotomy with radial incision of the diaphragm to the vena caval hiatus is required. Inflow to the area of injury is achieved by aortic occlusion and a clamp applied across the afferent portal and arterial supplies of the liver (Pringle's maneuver).

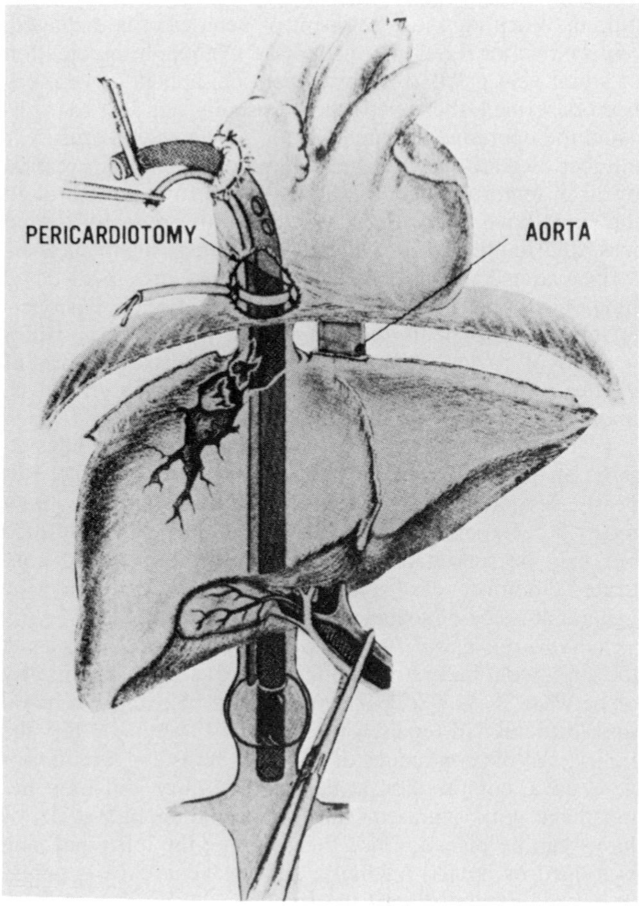

FIGURE 46–15. An endotracheal tube is used to bypass a retrohepatic caval injury. The balloon at the end of the tube eliminates the need for a tourniquet above the renal veins. (From Yellin AE, Chaffee CB, Donovan AJ: Vascular isolation in treatment of juxtahepatic venous injuries. Arch Surg 102:566–573, 1972. Copyright 1971, American Medical Association.)

Vascular isolation of the liver has received great attention but not much use. Indeed, Nance has commented, "Somewhat like a chicken whose neck has been wrung and still survives, the caval shunt still persists."[99] Multiple techniques and modifications have been described, although the majority of surgeons have had little experience with any of them.[100] The author has found the endotracheal tube technique effective and relatively easy to learn and apply (Fig. 46–15). A sterile 7-mm cuffed endotracheal tube is used. A pursestring suture is placed in the right atrial appendage of sufficient size to accept the endotracheal tube. The intrapericardial inferior vena cava is dissected, and a Rumel tourniquet is placed around it. The proximal end of the endotracheal tube is clamped and the balloon tipped end is advanced distally. A finger palpates for the tip of the tube until it lies just below the renal veins. The tube is withdrawn from the atrium for several centimeters while side holes are cut with rongeurs so that they will lie within the right atrium when the tube is repositioned. The shunt is advanced until the tip lies just *above* the renal veins. The balloon is inflated to secure the shunt in place while the pursestring suture is secured. Care must be taken while the shunt is being advanced to prevent laceration of tributary veins. Hemostasis in the area is greatly reduced, although some residual hemorrhage continues because of small tributaries that enter between the renal veins and the hepatic veins. When the shunt is ready to be removed, the balloon is deflated, and the shunt withdrawn through the pursestring. Fluid resuscitation through the exposed portion of the shunt is possible; however, the author prefers not to do this because air embolization will occur if the connectors become dislodged.[101]

Results

Survival following injury of the abdominal aorta depends largely upon the number of associated injuries and on the location of aortic injury. Results following infrarenal injuries are best and carry a reported 44 to 58 per cent survival.[79, 102] With suprarenal injuries, the survival rate is slightly lower, ranging from 28 to 46 per cent, although some small studies have reported better results.[79, 102–104] Function is generally good; however, a recent report of follow-up on 11 survivors of abdominal repair found decreased ankle-brachial indices in 5. Pathologic calcifications were noted in the area of repair on examination by CT scanning.[105] Iliac arterial injuries have a somewhat higher average survival rate, but function of the ipsilateral lower extremity may be suboptimal. Typical survival rates for iliac artery injuries range from 48 to 71 per cent, and for iliac venous injury the rates range from 69 to 82 per cent.[106, 107]

Isolated injuries of the mesenteric vessels are uncommon, so survival rates of patients with these injuries need to be evaluated in the context of associated trauma. Superior mesenteric artery injuries have a survival rate ranging from 32 to 67 per cent.[102, 107] Most series are small, and the results are not necessarily comparable. Portal vein injuries are also typically found in the polytrauma patient and carry a mortality near 50 per cent.[82]

Infrarenal vena caval injuries, especially when due to penetrating trauma, typically have good outcomes. Survival rates are better than 70 per cent. Suprarenal and retrohepatic injuries have lower survival rates, however, and average about 40 to 50 per cent.[108]

References

1. Bongard F, Dubrow T, Klein SR: Vascular injuries in the urban battleground. Experience at a metropolitan trauma center. Ann Vasc Surg 4:415, 1990.
2. Feliciano DV, Bitondo CG, Mattox KL, et al: Civilian trauma in the 1980s. A 1-year experience with 456 vascular and cardiac injuries. Ann Surg 199:717, 1984.
3. Greendyke RM: Traumatic rupture of the aorta. Special references to automobile accidents. JAMA 195:527, 1966.
4. Passaro E, Pace WG: Traumatic rupture of the aorta. Surgery 46:787, 1959.
5. DelRossi AJ, Cernaianu AC, Madden LD, et al: Traumatic disruptions of the thoracic aorta: Treatment and outcome. Surgery 108:864, 1990.
6. Avery JE, Hall DP, Adams JE: Traumatic rupture of the thoracic aorta. South Med J 75:653, 1979.
7. Wilson RF: Thoracic vascular trauma. *In* Bongard F, Wilson SE, Perry MO (eds): Vascular Injuries in Surgical Practice. Norwalk, CT, Appleton & Lange, 1991, p 107.
8. Kirsh MM, Sloan H: Blunt Chest Trauma. Boston, Little, Brown, 1977.
9. Sevitt S: The mechanisms of traumatic rupture of the thoracic aorta. Br J Surg 64: 166, 1977.
10. Lundevall J: The mechanism of traumatic rupture of the aorta. Acta Pathol Microbiol Scand 62: 34, 1964.
11. Besson A, Saegesser F: Chest Trauma and Associated Injuries. Oradell, NJ, Medical Economics, 1983, p 2.
12. Binet JP, Langlois J, Cormier JM, et al: A case of recent traumatic avulsion of the innominate artery at its origin from the aortic arch. J Thorac Cardiovasc Surg 43: 670, 1962.
13. Voigt GE, Wifert K: Mechanisms of injuries to unrestrained drivers in head-on collisions. *In* Proceedings of the Thirteenth Stapp Car Crash Conference, New York. Society of Automotive Engineers, pp 295–313.
14. Crass JC, Cohen AM, Motta AO, et al: A proposed new mechanism of traumatic aortic rupture: The osseous pinch. Radiology 176:645, 1990.
15. Harrington DP, Barth KH, White RI Jr, et al: Traumatic pseudoaneurysm of the thoracic aorta in close proximity to the anterior spinal artery: A therapeutic dilemma. Surgery 87:153, 1980.
16. Wexler L, Silverman J: Traumatic rupture of the innominate artery—A seat-belt injury. N Engl J Med 282:1186, 1970.
17. Duhaylongsod FG, Glower DD, Wolfe WG: Acute traumatic aortic aneurysm: The Duke experience from 1970 to 1990. J Vasc Surg 15:331, 1992.
18. Symbas PN, Tyras DH, Ware RE, et al: Rupture of the aorta—a diagnostic triad. Ann Thor Surg 15:405, 1973.
19. Fox S, Pierce WS, Waldhausen JA: Acute hypertension: Its significance in traumatic aortic rupture. J Thorac Cardiovasc Surg 75:622, 1973.
20. Clark DE, Zeiger MA, Wallace KL, et al: Blunt aortic trauma: Signs of high risk. J Trauma 30:701, 1990.
21. Fisher RG, Hadlock F, Ben-Menachem Y: Laceration of the thoracic aorta and brachiocephalic arteries by blunt trauma. Report of 54 cases and review of the literature. Radiol Clin North Am 19:91, 1981.
22. Gundry SR, Williams S, Burney RE, et al: Indications for aortography in blunt thoracic trauma: A reassessment. J Trauma 22:664, 1982.
23. Woodring JH: The normal mediastinum in blunt traumatic rupture of the thoracic aorta and brachiocephalic arteries. J Emerg Med 8:467, 1990.
24. Mirvis SE, Bidwell JK, Buddemeyer EU, et al: Value of chest radiography in excluding traumatic aortic rupture. Radiology 163:487, 1987.
25. Ayella RJ, Hankins JR, Turney SZ, et al: Ruptured thoracic aorta due to blunt trauma. J Trauma 17:199, 1977.
26. Mirvis SE, Bidwell JK, Buddemeyer EU: Value of chest radiography in excluding aortic rupture. Radiology 163:487, 1982.
27. Woodring JH, King JG: The potential effects of radiographic criteria to exclude aortography in patients with blunt chest trauma. J Thorac Cardiovasc Surg 97:456, 1989.
28. Marsh DG, Sturm JT: Traumatic aortic rupture: Roentgenographic indications for angiography. Ann Thorac Surg 21:337, 1976.
29. Sturm JT, Olson FR, Cicero JJ: Chest roentgenographic findings in 26 patients with traumatic rupture of the thoracic aorta. Ann Emerg Med 12:598, 1983.
30. Seltzer SE, D'Orsi C, Kirshner R, et al: Traumatic aortic rupture: Plain radiographic findings. AJR 137:1011, 1981.
31. Williams S, Burney RE, MacKenzie J, Cho K: Indications for aortography. Radiography after blunt chest trauma: A reassessment of the radiographic findings associated with traumatic rupture of the aorta. Invest Radiol 18:230, 1983.
32. Burney RE, Gundry SR, Mackenzie JR, et al: Chest roentgenograms in diagnosis of traumatic rupture of the aorta: Observer variation in interpretation. Chest 85:605, 1984.
33. Ayella RJ: Radiologic Management of the Massively Traumatized Patient. Baltimore, Williams & Wilkins, 1978.
34. Gerlock AJ, Muhletaler CA, Coulam CM, et al: Traumatic aortic aneurysm: Validity of esophageal tube displacement sign. Am J Radiol 135:713, 1980.
35. Morgan PW, Goodman LR, Aprahamian C, et al: Evaluation of traumatic aortic injury: Does dynamic contrast-induced CT play a role? Radiology 182:661, 1992.
36. Raptopoulos V, Sheiman RG, Phillips DA, et al: Traumatic aortic tear: Screening with chest CT. Radiology 182:667, 1982.
37. Erbel R, Mohr-Kahaly S, Rennollet H, et al: Diagnosis of aortic dissection: The value of transesophageal echocardiography. Thorac Cardiovasc Surg 35:126, 1987.
38. Taams MA, Gussenhoven WJ, Schippers LA, et al: The value of transesophageal echocardiography for diagnosis of thoracic aorta pathology. Eur Heart J 9:1308, 1988.
39. Brooks SW, Cmolik BI, Young JC, et al: Transesophageal echocardiographic examination of a patient with traumatic aortic transection from blunt chest trauma: A case report. J Trauma 31:841, 1991.
40. Graham JM, Feliciano DV, Mattox KL, et al: Innominate vascular injury. J Trauma 22: 647, 1982.
41. O'Gorman RB, Feliciano DV: Arteriography performed in the emergency center. Am J Surg 152:323, 1986.
42. Oppenheimer MJ, Durant TM, Lynch P: Body position in relation to venous air embolism and the associated cardiovascular-respiratory changes. Am J Med Sci 252:362, 1953.
43. Robbs JV, Baker LW, Human RR, et al: Cervicomediastinal injuries. Arch Surg 116:663, 1981.
44. Marvisti MA, Meyer JA, Ford BE, et al: Spinal cord ischemia following operation for aortic transection. Ann Thorac Surg 42:425, 1986.
45. Laschinger JC, Cunningham JN Jr, Nathan IM, et al: Experimental and clinical assessment of the adequacy of partial bypass in maintenance of spinal cord blood flow during operations on the thoracic aorta. Ann Thorac Surg 36:417, 1983.
46. Kewalramani LS, Katta RSR: Atraumatic ischemic myelopathy. Paraplegia 19:352, 1981.
47. Olivier HF, Maher TD, Liebler GA, et al: Use of the BioMedicus centrifugal pump in traumatic tears of the thoracic aorta. Ann Vasc Surg 38:586, 1984.
48. Von Oppell UO, Thierfelder CF, Beningfield SJ, et al: Traumatic rupture of the descending thoracic aorta. S Afr Med J 19:595, 1991.
49. McCroskey BL, Moore EE, Moore FA, et al: A unified approach to the torn thoracic aorta. Am J Surg 162:473, 1991.
50. Hess PJ, Howe HR, Robicsek FR, et al: Traumatic tears of the thoracic aorta: Improved results using the Bio-Medicus pump. Ann Thorac Surg 48:6, 1989.
51. DelRossi AJ, Cernaianu AC, Madden LD, et al: Traumatic disruptions of the thoracic aorta: Treatment and outcome. Surgery 108:864, 1990.
52. Antunes MJ: Acute traumatic rupture of the aorta: Repair by simple aortic cross-clamping. Ann Thorac Surg 44:257, 1987.

53. Mattox KL, Holtzman M, Pickard LR, et al: Clamp repair: A safe technique for treatment of blunt injury to the descending thoracic aorta. Ann Thorac Surg 40:456, 1985.
54. Orringer MB, Kirsh MM: Primary repair of acute traumatic aortic disruption. Ann Thorac Surg 35:672, 1982.
55. McBride LR, Tidik S, Stothert JC, et al: Primary repair of traumatic aortic disruption. Ann Thorac Surg 43:65, 1987.
56. Kouchoukos NT, Lell WA: Hemodynamic effects of aortic clamping and decompression with a temporary shunt for resection of the descending thoracic aorta. Surgery 25:58, 1983.
57. Cunningham JN, Lanschinger JC, Merking HA, et al: Measurement of spinal cord ischemia during operations upon the thoracic aorta: Initial clinical experience. Ann Surg 185:196, 1982.
58. Soots G, Warembourg H, Prat A, et al: Acute traumatic rupture of the thoracic aorta: Place of delayed surgical rupture. J Cardiovasc Surg 30:173, 1989.
59. Castagna J, Nelson RJ: Blunt injuries to branches of the aortic arch. J Thorac Cardiovasc Surg 69:521, 1975.
60. Rosenberg JM, Bredenberg CE, Marvast MA, et al: Blunt injuries to the aortic arch vessels. Ann Thorac Surg 48:508, 1989.
61. Knott-Craig CJ, Przybojewski JZ, Barbard PM: Penetrating wounds of the heart and great vessels—A new therapeutic approach. S Afr Med J, 62:316, 1982.
62. Feliciano DV, Burch JM, Graham JM: Vascular injuries of the chest and abdomen. *In* Rutherford R (ed): Vascular Surgery. Philadelphia, WB Saunders, 1989, p 588.
63. Vosloo SM, Reichart BA: Inflow occlusion in the surgical management of a penetrating aortic arch injury: Case report. J Trauma 30:514, 1990.
64. Liekweg WG, Greenfield LJ: Management of penetrating carotid arterial injury. Ann Surg 188:587, 1978.
65. Brown MF, Graham JM, Feliciano DV, et al: Carotid artery injuries. Am J Surg 144:748, 1982.
66. Parmley LF, Mattingly TW, Manion WC: Penetrating wounds of the heart and aorta. Circulation 17:953, 1958.
67. Graham JM, Feliciano DV, Mattox KL, et al: Innominate vascular injury. J Trauma 22:647, 1982.
68. Brown MF, Graham JM, Feliciano DV, et al: Carotid artery injuries. Am J Surg 144:748, 1982.
69. Shackford SR, Sise MJ: Renal and mesenteric vascular trauma. *In* Bongard F, Wilson SE, Perry MO (eds): Vascular Injuries in Surgical Practice. Norwalk, CT, Appleton & Lange, 1991, p 173.
70. Lim RC, Miller SE: Management of acute civilian vascular injuries. Surg Clin North Am 62:113, 1982.
71. Holcroft JW: Abdominal arterial trauma. *In* Blaisdell FW, Trunkey DT (eds): Trauma Management, vol. I. Abdominal Trauma. New York, Thieme-Stratton, 1982, p 253.
72. Cass AS, Bubrisk M, Luxenberg M, et al: Renal pedicle injury in patients with multiple injuries. J Trauma 25:892, 1985.
73. Wilson RF, Zeigler DW: Diagnostic and treatment problems in renal injuries. Am Surg 53:399, 1987.
74. Mee SL, McAninch JW, Robinson AL, et al: Radiographic assessment of renal trauma: A 10 year prospective study of patient selection. J Urol 141:1095, 1989.
75. Steinberg DL, Jeffrey RB, Federle MP, et al: The computerized tomography appearance of renal pedicle injury. J Urol 132:1163, 1984.
76. Lang EK, Sullivan J, Frentz G: Renal trauma: Radiologic studies. Radiology 15: 1, 1985.
77. Talhouk AS, Lim RC, Bongard FS: Abdominal aortic injuries. *In* Bongard F, Wilson SE, Perry MO (eds): Vascular Injuries in Surgical Practice. Norwalk, CT, Appleton & Lange, 1991, p 165.
78. Accola KD, Feliciano DV, Mattox KL, et al: Management of injuries to the suprarenal aorta. Am J Surg 154:613, 1987.
79. Brinton M, Miller SE, Lim RC, et al: Acute abdominal aortic injuries. J Trauma 22:481, 1982.
80. Mattox KL, McCollum WB, Beall AC, et al: Management of penetrating injuries of the suprarenal aorta. J Trauma 15:808, 1975.
81. Feliciano DV, Burch JM, Graham JM, et al: Abdominal vascular injury. *In* Mattox KL, Moore EE, Feliciano DV (eds): Trauma. Norwalk, CT, Appleton-Century-Crofts, 1987, p 519.
82. Feliciano DV, Burch JM, Graham JM: Abdominal vascular injury. *In* Moore EE, Mattox KL, Feliciano DV (eds): Trauma. 2nd ed. Norwalk, CT, Appleton & Lange, 1991, p 523.
83. Lassonde J, Laurendeau F: Blunt injury of the abdominal aorta. Ann Surg 194:745, 1981.
84. Klein SR, Mehringer CM, Bongard FS: Endovascular occlusive intervention in the management of trauma. Ann Vasc Surg 4:424, 1990.
85. Salam AA, Stewart MT: New approach to wounds of the aortic bifurcation and inferior vena cava. Surgery 98:105, 1985.
86. Burch JM, Richardson RJ, Martin RR, et al: Penetrating iliac vascular injuries: Recent experience with 233 consecutive patients. J Trauma 30:1450, 1989.
87. Courcy PA, Brotman S, Oster-Granite NL, et al: Superior mesenteric vein injuries from blunt abdominal trauma. J Trauma 18: 419, 1978.
88. Fullen WD, Hunt J, Altemeier WA: The clinical spectrum of penetrating injury to the superior mesenteric arterial circulation. J Trauma 12:656, 1978.
89. Conti S: Abdominal venous trauma. *In* Blaisdell FW, Trunkey DD (eds): Trauma Management, vol I. Abdominal Trauma. New York, Thieme-Stratton, 1982, p 253.
90. Lohse JR, Shore RM, Belzer FO: Acute renal artery occlusion. Arch Surg 117:801, 1982.
91. Maggio AJ, Brosman S: Renal artery trauma. Urology 1978 II:125, 1978.
92. State DL, Bongard FS: Abdominal venous injuries. *In* Bongard FS, Wilson SE, Perry MO (eds): Vascular Injuries in Surgical Practice. Norwalk, CT, Appleton & Lange, 1991, p 185.
93. Lau JM, Mattox KL, Beall AC, et al: Use of substitute conduits in traumatic vascular surgery. J Trauma 23:207, 1983.
94. Johnson V, Eiseman B: Evaluation of arteriovenous shunt to obtain patency of venous autografts. Am J Surg 118:915, 1969.
95. Stewart MT, Stone HH: Injuries of the inferior vena cava. Am Surgeon 52:9, 1988.
96. Posner MC, Moore EE, Greenholz SL, et al: Natural history of untreated inferior vena cava injury and assessment of venous access. J Trauma 26:698, 1986.
97. Burch JM, Feliciano DV, Mattox KL, et al: Injuries of the inferior vena cava. Am J Surg 158: 548, 1988.
98. Pachter HL, Spencer FC, Hofstetter S, et al: The management of juxtahepatic venous injuries without an atriocaval shunt: Preliminary clinical observations. Surgery 99:569, 1986.
99. Nance F: Comments in Wieneck RG, Wilson RF: Inferior vena cava injuries—the challenge continues. Am Surg 54: 423, 1988.
100. Beall SL, Wards RE: Successful atrial caval shunting in the management of retrohepatic venous injuries. Am J Surg 158:409, 1988.
101. Mattox KL: Abdominal venous injuries. Surgery 91:497, 1982.
102. Kashuk JL, Moore EE, Millikan JS, et al: Major abdominal vascular trauma—A unified approach. J Trauma 22:672, 1978.
103. Millikan JS, Moore EE: Critical factors in determining mortality from abdominal aortic trauma. Surg Gynecol Obstet 160:313, 1985.
104. Buchness MP, LoGerfo FW, Mason GR: Gunshot wounds of the suprarenal abdominal aorta. Ann Surg 42: 1, 1976.
105. Soldano SL, Rich NM, Collins GJ, et al: Long-term follow-up of penetrating abdominal aortic injuries after 15 years. J Trauma 28:1358, 1988.
106. Millikan JS, Moore EE, Van Way CW III, et al: Vascular trauma in the groin: Contrast between iliac and femoral injuries. Am J Surg 142:695, 1981.
107. Sirinek KR, Gaskill HV III, Root HD, et al: Truncal vascular injury—Factors influencing survival. J Trauma 23:372, 1983.
108. Kudsk KA, Bongard F, Lim RC Jr: Determinants of survival after vena caval injury: Analysis of a 14-year experience. Arch Surg 119:1009, 1984.

47

Injuries of the Brachiocephalic Vessels

Malcolm O. Perry, M.D.

• • •

INITIAL EVALUATION

In this author's view, management of penetrating trauma to the neck is straightforward: Wounds that pierce the platysma muscle and enter the anterior triangles require surgical exploration. Selective observation is gaining popularity but requires reliance on multiple diagnostic studies and close monitoring.

It is useful to divide penetrating wounds of the neck into three zones as suggested by Monson and associates.[1] Although the exact levels vary according to the authorities who have suggested them, the division described below is simple. Zone I extends from the head of the clavicle inferiorly to include the thoracic outlet; zone II extends from the clavicle to the angle of the mandible; and zone III extends from the angle of the mandible to the base of the skull. By clinical examination it may be difficult to determine if injuries in zone I and zone III include damage to major vascular structures. In these situations, if the patients are hemodynamically stable, preoperative biplane arteriography is extremely useful. In selected patients with penetrating wounds in zone II, it may be acceptable to proceed with surgery without preoperative arteriograms, although even in this group of patients, such studies can be helpful.

CAROTID ARTERY TRAUMA

Most wounds of the cervical vessels are caused by penetrating trauma, and the common carotid artery is usually involved (Table 47–1).[2, 3] The left carotid is injured slightly more often than the right, perhaps because most assailants are right-handed. Reviews by Thal and coworkers, Bradley, Yamada and associates, and Liekweg and Greenfield have emphasized the special problems encountered in these patients.[2–5] In addition to the vascular injury, major neurologic deficits may exist. Also, there may be associated wounds of the larynx, esophagus, and trachea, thus increasing the likelihood of bacterial contamination.

In the series reported by Thal and coworkers, the patients were divided into three groups in order to better evaluate treatment (Table 47–2).[3] The first and largest group contained patients with common or internal carotid artery wounds but no neurologic deficits. The second group included those with mild deficits, and the third, patients with a severe deficit. Experience in the management of patients with occlusive extracranial arterial disease has clearly underscored the risks of vascular reconstruction in people with acute strokes, especially if there are alterations in consciousness or coma. When vascular reconstructions are attempted in these patients, mortality rates of 40 per cent and higher are found.

This high death rate was thought to be mainly the result of conversion of an anemic cerebral infarct into a hemorrhagic infarct, with subsequent extension of the stroke. It was believed that restoration of normal arterial pressure and blood flow to the damaged brain was followed by bleeding into the softened tissue. Recent investigations suggest that microhemorrhage is a part of many cerebral infarctions and that extensive intracerebral bleeding may supervene even without restoration of normal arterial pressure. In fact, it is believed that some lacunar microinfarcts commonly are hemorrhagic. These observations suggest that other factors may be involved in the sudden neurologic deterioration seen when vascular reconstruction is performed in patients with acute severe strokes.[4, 6, 7] The precise role that hypertension, heparinization, anesthesia, and surgery play is uncertain at present, but it seems clear that patients with severe strokes caused by complete occlusion of the carotid artery are poor candidates for vascular reconstruction. Almost all studies report high mortality rates in this group of patients.[2, 5, 8]

Accurate preoperative assessment is essential for the successful management of the patient with carotid injuries because it appears that the eventual outcome depends on the extent of the initial preoperative neurologic deficit. Moreover, a significant number of these patients have other injuries; closed head trauma, especially, can distort the diagnostic picture. Such combined problems are particularly confusing when the indications for surgery are being considered. A precise neurologic evaluation is mandatory before extensive vascular repairs are begun in these patients.

The results of several studies strongly support surgical repair of all carotid injuries in patients who have either no neurologic deficit or only a mild deficit.[3, 4, 8] This decision is easier when the arterial injury is bleeding actively than when there is complete carotid artery occlusion and no neurologic symptoms. In this situation, technical problems encountered during surgery could conceivably produce brain damage, although in the reported experience this has been rare. The risk exists, however, and careful neurologic and arteriographic studies are needed before operation is undertaken in order to accurately assess the danger and formulate the sequence of treatment.

Even the artery that appears completely blocked on arteriography may at operation be patent; the slow flow of

Table 47–1. Distribution of Cervical Arterial Injuries

	Number
Common carotid	58
Internal carotid	17
External carotid	19
Vertebral	7

blood through a small channel may not be visible even with good arteriograms. Left untreated, this lesion is likely to progress to complete occlusion, with occasional extension into the cerebral arteries, thus causing a stroke. Thromboembolic events may also supervene, and middle cerebral artery emboli have been observed in such situations. Although some arterial wounds heal spontaneously, this is not predictable, and delayed development of a false aneurysm is possible, although such lesions are uncommon. For these reasons, many surgeons believe that practically all carotid wounds should be repaired if the patients do not have a complete occlusion complicated by an acute severe stroke.[1, 4]

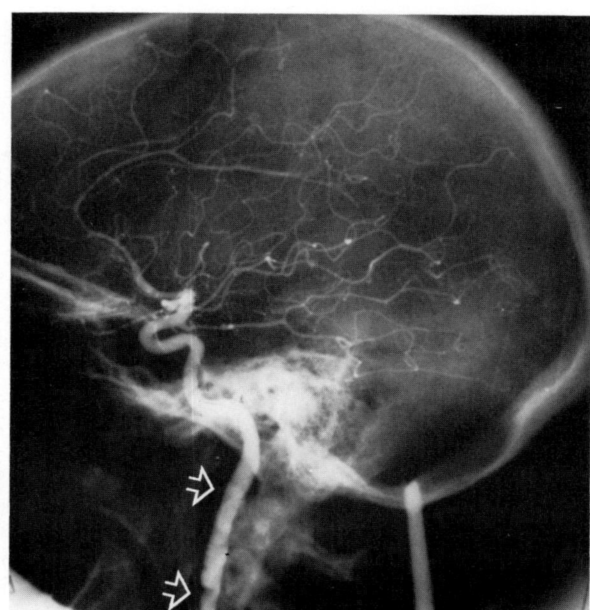

FIGURE 47–1. **Hyperextension injury of the internal carotid artery. There are multiple intimal and mural defects (*arrows*).**

Diagnosis

Carotid wounds from blunt trauma may be more difficult to detect and evaluate (Fig. 47–1).[9] Such trauma is not invariably accompanied by telltale bruises and cuts; in fact, about half of the patients have no superficial evidence of trauma. Clinical features suggesting the presence of blunt trauma to the carotid artery include Horner's syndrome, transient attacks of cerebral ischemia, lucid interval after injury, and limb paresis in an alert patient.[10] In some patients there may be no neurologic symptoms even in the presence of severe carotid damage. Hyperextension injuries of the neck are particularly likely to produce contusion and intimal damage in the distal internal carotid artery; the artery at this level is fixed by its entry into the skull, and it can be forcibly stretched over the cervical vertebra by hyperextension. This type of stretch injury, or even direct contusion, predisposes to a special sequence of events.[7] Initially there may be no sign of injury and no neurologic symptoms, but as thrombosis of the vessel or intramural hemorrhage occurs, stroke becomes evident. This can be delayed for several hours but is almost always apparent within the first 24 hours. By this time there usually is complete occlusion of the artery, often with extension of the clot into the head and occasionally even distal embolization. If an initial neurologic problem is suspected, it is often thought to be caused by direct brain damage (i.e., a subdural or epidural hematoma), resulting in delayed diagnosis.

Table 47–2. Carotid Injuries: Neurologic Status on Admission

Classification	Number
Group 1 (no neurologic deficit)	54
Group 2 (mild neurologic deficit)	8
Group 3 (severe neurologic deficit)	15

Most of these arterial wounds will eventually cause specific symptoms, but unfortunately by then they may not be reversible. Also, the delay between injury and the emergence of neurologic symptoms can be protracted. Crissey and Bernstein report a case in which 15 years elapsed before the injury was diagnosed, having by then caused a severe carotid stenosis.[11] One patient in the author's series also developed common carotid stenosis and transient attacks of cerebral ischemia more than a year after the carotid contusion occurred (Fig. 47–2).[7]

Diagnostic Tests

Although the noninvasive vascular tests can be useful in the chronic, stable case, they are not particularly helpful in the acute evaluation. Arteriography is the definitive test, and when properly employed, it is quite reliable in diagnosing or excluding carotid artery injuries.[12] Moreover, knowing the type and location of the wound preoperatively assists materially in planning the operation. Because complete exposure of the internal carotid artery requires an extensive surgical dissection, and some blunt injuries may not be easily detected by examining the exterior of the vessel, angiography is very helpful.[7, 12] For example, the identification of an acute fistula between the internal carotid artery and the jugular vein permits the surgeon to prepare special techniques for management. If a graft is needed to replace a damaged artery, it is best to know this in advance and have it ready and thus reduce the carotid occlusion time. If the patient is stable, preoperative cerebral arteriography is recommended, particularly if there are neurologic problems; if for other reasons this cannot be done, an angiogram can be obtained in the operating room. Most penetrating wounds of the mid-cervical region can be managed adequately without arteriograms, but distal clots or other injuries near the base of the skull may pose serious problems, and operative arteriography can be very helpful.

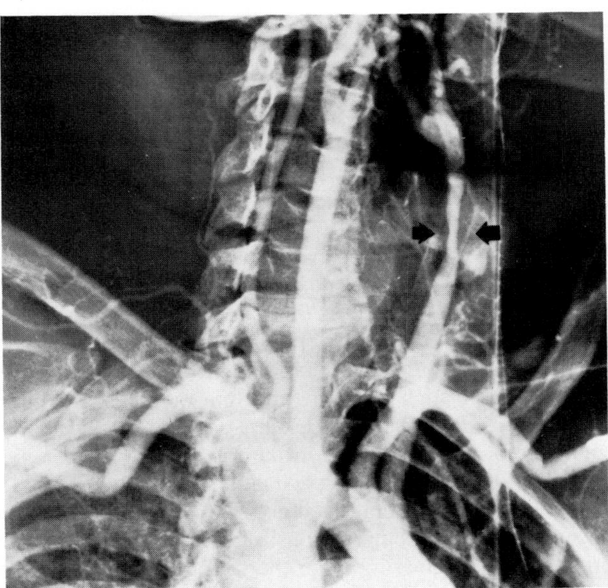

FIGURE 47–2. A contusion of the common carotid artery during an assault led to this stenosis (*arrows*), discovered 2 years later. A graft was needed to restore continuity.

Treatment

Preoperative Preparation

With isolated carotid wounds, extensive monitoring is not usually required, but a radial arterial line is helpful for measurement of arterial blood pressure and blood-gas tension. General anesthesia, hypercapnia, and some neurologic wounds interfere with cerebral autoregulation, and cerebral blood flow then will respond directly to changes in systemic arterial pressure. The maintenance of normal blood pressure is an important aspect of the management of these situations.

As in almost all cases of cervical trauma, the induction of anesthesia must be accomplished gently to prevent the dislodgment of tamponading clots, which might cause recurrence of bleeding or embolize into the intracranial circulation.[3] Endotracheal intubation is required in these patients, and preoperative knowledge of laryngeal nerve function is essential. If this information is not known before the patient reaches the operating room, the vocal cords can be inspected directly during tracheal intubation.

Operative Technique

Because the investing fascia and the deep cervical fascia are relatively strong structures, bleeding may be contained deeply within the neck, and the external evidence of blood accumulation may be modest, although a hematoma is often seen. If the wound has not been accurately identified, wide exposure will be needed for further surgical exploration. The neurovascular structures are approached through the usual carotid incision made along the anterior border of the sternocleidomastoid muscle. Proximal control of the carotid artery is obtained before the area of suspected injury is exposed. Even with a laceration of the artery, gentle digital pressure will usually control bleeding and thus minimize the time of carotid occlusion. If the injury is in the external carotid, it is controlled with vascular clamps and either repaired or ligated, as indicated. Unless there is evidence that the external carotid artery is functioning as a major cerebral collateral, it is usually not grafted or shunted.

More often, the common or internal carotid arteries are damaged and should be repaired. Once control of bleeding is obtained, internal carotid artery backflow is assessed. Brisk, pulsatile backflow is usually satisfactory evidence of adequate cerebral perfusion, but measurements of carotid stump pressure may be helpful. Pressures greater than 60 or 70 mmHg are believed to indicate adequate cerebral perfusion.[13] If shunts are needed because of low pressure or scanty backflow, a variety of instruments and techniques can be used. The simple inlying No. 10 Fr size tube shunt advocated by Thompson is usually satisfactory.[14] Most surgeons use systemic heparin when shunts are in place, and anticoagulants are not contraindicated, although it seems more important to heparinize the patient if the distal carotid artery is filled with a stagnant pool of blood. Most studies of shunting and heparinization during operations on carotid injuries have failed to document clearly the need for and results of these maneuvers.[3]

Standard vascular techniques are used, but because of the size of the carotid and the importance of securing a smooth intimal surface, resection and anastomosis are preferred. This is especially important with blunt trauma because the mural damage is likely to be extensive. After resection, a repair without tension is required or graft interposition will be necessary.

Several special maneuvers are helpful in these cases. Substitution of the external carotid for the internal carotid or use of the external as a patch for the internal carotid may simplify the repair (Fig. 47–3). If grafts are needed and a shunt is to be used, it can be placed through the graft prior to insertion and then removed prior to completion of the final anastomosis (Fig. 47–4).

Injuries at the base of the skull are difficult to expose and repair. Division of the digastric muscle and excision of the styloid process may aid the exposure. Subluxation of the mandible can be of assistance in obtaining adequate exposure of the distal internal carotid artery. This maneuver usually requires preoperative placement of dental wires and appliances and must be performed with care to prevent compression of the opposite carotid or other structures.[7]

The following method of control and shunting can be very helpful. Through a small proximal transverse incision in the common carotid artery a No. 4 Fogarty catheter with an attached three-way stopcock is prepared by threading a straight carotid shunt over it. (A Pruitt-Inahara shunt is also useful.) The catheter is then inserted and advanced beyond the area of injury. Precise expansion of the balloon will control carotid backflow. If needed, the shunt can be guided beyond the laceration into the distal carotid and then the balloon deflated and prograde cerebral perfusion restored. The arterial injury can be repaired accurately and without haste; then the catheters are removed and a completion arteriogram performed prior to closure of the small access arteriotomy. In this manner the shunt not only allows a deliberate and disciplined repair but also acts as a stent and reduces the chances of narrowing the artery.

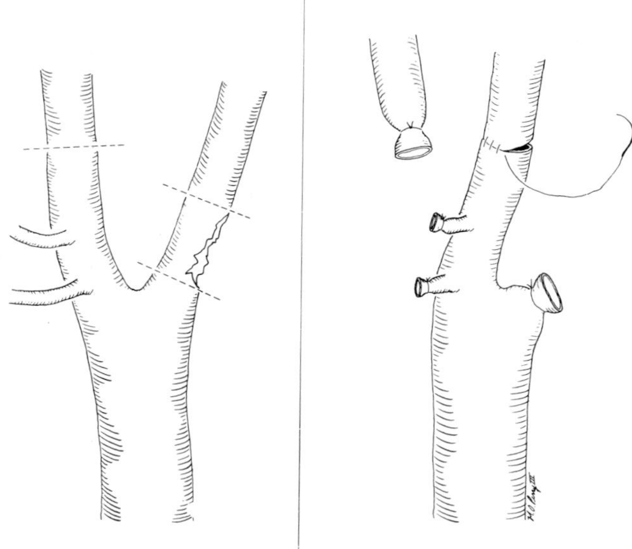

FIGURE 47–3. Severe wounds of the internal carotid artery can be repaired by using the external carotid artery.

Some of these maneuvers are useful in controlling and repairing acute arterial venous fistulae. If these lesions are known to exist before exploration, the balloon-tipped catheter can be inserted from a remote area and advanced to the fistula and then inflated to assist in controlling bleeding.

If resection is required and direct anastomosis is impossible, a saphenous vein graft is preferred to restore continuity. The vein taken from the groin is preferred; if it is unavailable, the cephalic vein is satisfactory. Local cervical veins may be too fragile for this purpose. Plastic grafts may be needed in the common carotid, especially in large or hypertensive patients. Whatever the need for repair, it must be met, and all injured and devitalized artery débrided. If damaged intima is left behind, local thromboembolic events can cause a delayed stroke. This is particularly a danger in blunt injuries in which the artery may sustain extensive damage, and in this situation a graft will almost certainly be needed.

When concomitant injuries of the trachea, the esophagus, or the pharynx are present and drains are needed, these should be routed away from the repaired artery and all fascial layers closed between wounds. There is little room for changing the path of the arteries, and local protection will be needed. In a few cases when heavy contamination is expected to cross the operating field, it might be necessary to redirect the carotid artery through the posterior triangles of the neck and interpose other tissues. This has not been required in the author's experience, however.[3, 7]

With the advent of combined extracranial and intracranial vascular procedures for treating occlusive arterial disease, difficult intracranial injuries of the cerebral arteries may be repaired. Injuries of the carotid in the petrous bone or the cavernous canal are surgically inaccessible and may require proximal and distal ligation to control bleeding. Alternatively, it may be possible to construct bypasses from the cervical carotid to the intracranial vessels, and thus perhaps improve cerebral perfusion.[15] Although these are formidable procedures, in special circumstances they may prevent serious neurologic problems caused by carotid ligation.

With the advent of better methods of diagnosis, patient selection, and vascular repair, ligation of the carotid artery is rarely indicated.[4] In a few patients in whom arterial damage is so extensive that repair cannot be done, ligation may be necessary. If distal backflow and blood pressure are high, carotid occlusion probably will be safe. This is not always true, however, because distal thrombosis of the intracranial carotid artery may lead to a stroke. Heparin has been used to control the extent of thrombosis in the distal carotid following proximal ligation. A lower stroke rate was found in a few such patients, and this therapeutic adjunct may prove useful in selected trauma cases also.[13] It must be remembered, however, that stroke rates up to 50 per cent are to be expected following acute carotid ligation.

If there is sufficient distal artery available for pressure measurements, a vascular reconstruction can often be done, perhaps even originating from the subclavian or the opposite carotid artery, if the ipsilateral common carotid cannot be used. Also, the extracranial to intracranial techniques may improve perfusion in selected cases.

It now appears that carotid ligation is needed in only a very small group: patients with complete internal carotid occlusion and severe neurologic deficits, including coma.[4, 6] Revascularization, with repair of all the damaged artery and complete removal of all clots, is seldom possible in a patient who has a carotid artery that is totally occluded as a result of blunt trauma. If total repair is attempted but not completed, the results often are progressive neurologic deterioration and death.[5, 7] Obviously, restoration of flow through the carotid without clearing the distal artery is dangerous and contraindicated. In these patients, carotid

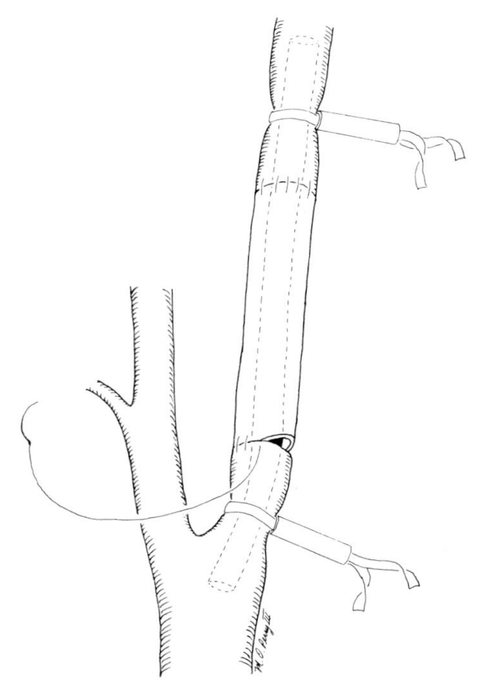

FIGURE 47–4. If an intraluminal shunt is needed, it is inserted into the saphenous vein graft and then the repair is completed.

ligation is probably best, especially because it appears that the neurologic damage caused by the occlusion will have already occurred, and it is unlikely that delayed disobliteration will reverse fixed deficits.

Many surgeons believe that completion arteriography should be routine after repair of the carotid artery, particularly the internal carotid artery (ICA). If any question exists about the adequacy of the repair, or if there is a possibility of distal embolism, an arteriogram is needed. This can be done easily by placing the x-ray film in a lateral position to permit an across-the-table study. Ten milliliters of a 60 per cent contrast medium is injected via an 18-gauge Cournand needle inserted into the common carotid artery, and the film is exposed as the final milliliter goes in. A single film will usually show the entire ICA, cervical and intracranial, and the major branches. The information obtained from this study is of particular value if postoperative problems appear.

Postoperative Care

Although any vascular repair can bleed, this is unusual unless the patient has multiple injuries or coagulation defects. Drains are not usually employed in treating isolated vascular wounds, but in selected patients they may be used for 12 to 24 hours to prevent the accumulation of blood, a technique commonly used in elective carotid surgery.[14] Even with the low incidence of bleeding, this complication should be kept in mind because the relatively strong cervical fascia can contain blood under pressure, causing acute respiratory difficulties. Elevation of the head and upper body to reduce venous engorgement, adequate hemostasis, selective drainage, and careful observation in the postoperative period will usually prevent these problems.

Thromboembolic events are also unusual, but when they do occur serious neurologic problems are likely to ensue. Early identification and treatment are essential if irreversible brain damage is to be avoided. Adequate fluid resuscitation and maintenance of normal systemic blood pressure are important, and therefore drugs likely to produce hypotension as a side effect should be avoided. Frequent evaluation of the hemodynamic and neurologic status of these patients is mandatory. In the early postoperative period, this should be performed every hour, at least for several hours, and then every 4 hours for the first 2 days. Any aberration in the findings is a clear indication for more exact studies. If a buildup of thrombus in the artery is suspected, noninvasive tests may be helpful.[11, 12] Oculoplethysmography, for example, may expose this complication before complete carotid occlusion supervenes, thus allowing time to return the patient to surgery for thrombectomy and repair. The test may be falsely positive, however. Other noninvasive studies using ultrasound (duplex Doppler) can be used to assess patency, although some problems exist in evaluating cervical vessels under a fresh surgical wound.

High-grade arterial stenosis can be diagnosed in this manner, and similarly, patency can be confirmed. If doubt exists about the interpretation of the findings, repeat arteriography is indicated. Intracranial views are needed to ascertain whether cerebral arterial embolization has occurred. In some cases, intracranial emboli have been extracted successfully with complete recovery, but these are difficult cases and require close cooperation among vascular surgeons, neurosurgeons, and vascular radiologists. If postoperative carotid thrombosis does occur, immediate carotid disobliteration is indicated and is likely to be successful. Correction of the cause of failure may require a thorough surgical exploration and operative arteriography, but these are obviously essential to success. Such problems are unusual but do happen, and they should be treated aggressively in a postoperative patient who appears to be developing a stroke. If the patient has a frank stroke, it is probably best not to wait for confirmatory arteriograms but to return the patient to the operating room for exploration and restore cerebral perfusion as rapidly as possible. The problem is likely to be clot at the site of repair, which can be treated successfully if cerebral infarction has not occurred.

Results

The long-term results of repair of carotid injuries are quite good (Table 47–3). In fact, in the absence of infection and problems generated by other injuries, most of these patients do very well.

False aneurysms and arteriovenous fistulae, a result of untreated arterial wounds, are rare when the vessels are repaired. False aneurysm as a complication of infection of the repaired artery is seen on rare occasions and presents a formidable problem. Although not supported by unequivocal data, it is widely held that this problem is more likely when plastic prosthetic material has been used in the vascular repair, either as a graft or as patch material. The diagnosis is usually easily, although reluctantly, established. Local signs of infection, a draining sinus, bleeding, sepsis, and a mass are seen. Arteriography confirms the diagnosis, and operative therapy is indicated. Although a few isolated cases of successful cure of infection without removal of plastic grafts have been reported, most infected grafts must be removed. Reconstruction with autogenous tissue or rerouting of the vessel through clean tissue planes is generally satisfactory treatment if the patient has no neurologic deficits.

VERTEBRAL ARTERY INJURIES

Wounds of the vertebral arteries are rare—the vessels enter the bony canal at the C6 level and exit at C2 and apparently are protected from many injuries. In the past, without preoperative arteriograms, vertebral artery damage usually was undetected unless it was discovered because of bleeding during exploration. Treatment consisted of proxi-

Table 47–3. Results of Repair of Carotid Injuries

Classification	No. Died
Group 1 (no neurologic deficit)	0
Group 2 (mild neurologic deficit)	1
Group 3 (severe neurologic deficit)	5
Total	6 (7.8%)

mal ligation, packing, and on rare occasions, direct exposure and suture ligation.

Since preoperative arteriography is now employed more frequently to assess the damage accurately and evaluate the collateral circulation, more vertebral artery wounds will probably be discovered.[16] Direct repair, even in the bony canal, is possible with modern vascular techniques.[17] A penetrating injury to a dominant or single vertebral artery should be considered for repair. Continued bleeding or the late development of a false aneurysm or arteriovenous fistula is a serious complication of such wounds. A penetrating vertebral artery wound must be controlled in some fashion. If the arteriograms reveal an intact circle of Willis and the opposite vertebral artery is normal, ligation of the injured vessel is acceptable.

Bleeding from the vertebral canal can be profuse and difficult to control, especially when the injury is caused by a gunshot wound that also shatters a cervical vertebra. Some of the bleeding can be from the multiple vertebral veins that traverse the canal with the artery; these are attached to the periosteum and thus tend to remain open when they are torn. Proximal exposure and control of the artery below C6, where it enters the canal, are often needed in these cases. Backbleeding usually remains fairly brisk because of the extensive collateral circulation, some vessels even reaching the artery in the canal itself. Direct pressure, packing, application of bone wax, proximal ligation, and even distal exposure up to C1 may be needed in rare cases. Balloon catheter control as described in the preceding section can be very helpful in recalcitrant cases.

Although the artery can be repaired, even in the bony canal, ligation has been used more often than not.[16] The vertebral arteries usually are paired and join to form the basilar artery, but this is not invariable, and occasionally one vertebral artery may be hypoplastic or perhaps terminate as the posterior inferior cerebellar artery. If the extracranial cerebral architecture is known in advance in a given patient, the repairs can be planned with more accuracy and unusual problems better managed. Arteriography, therefore, may be as important as surgical technique in handling patients with vertebral artery injuries.

VASCULAR INJURIES IN THE THORACIC OUTLET

Injuries of the intrathoracic aorta and great vessels have the highest mortality rate of all arterial wounds, often ending in early exsanguination and death.[18, 19] In several studies, many patients were dead on arrival in the emergency room or were in profound hemorrhagic shock when initially seen.[20] As pointed out by Hewitt and associates, these injuries present special problems because of the difficulty in making a specific diagnosis and the wide surgical exposure required to obtain control of bleeding.[19] In the report by Flint and his associates, 40 per cent of 146 patients were in shock when first seen, and Reul and coworkers observed that almost half of their patients were hypotensive and more than 40 per cent had other serious wounds.[18, 19] Such combined injuries appear to be a major reason for the lethality of penetrating injuries of the upper chest and root of the neck.

Etiology

Most major vascular wounds in this area are caused by bullets or stabbing (97 per cent of the cases of Flint and associates), but blunt trauma may also be causative (Table 47–4). Multiple injuries are more likely to be caused by gunshot wounds, especially when the wound tract is in an oblique or lateral plane, thus passing through several vessels. Major venous injuries are also common and can seriously compromise efforts at control.[18] With venous injuries in this area, bleeding is not the only risk, because with resuscitation and operative manipulation air embolism can occur.

Certain types of blunt trauma are particularly likely to result in vascular injury: Steering wheel injuries, deceleration forces, falls, and crushing blows to the chest and root of the neck often involve serious vascular wounds. Posterior fractures of the first and second ribs, for example, are an indication that the chest has been subjected to tremendous forces, and the likelihood of associated serious vascular damage is increased.

Evaluation

The diagnosis of vascular injury is obvious in the presence of specific findings such as bleeding, large or expanding hematomas, weak or absent distal pulses, and continued intrathoracic hemorrhage, but in one large series a third of the patients had no diagnostic signs.[18] Injuries of nearby nerves occur with more frequency with penetrating trauma here than in other areas, a feature explained by the close anatomic relation of the vessels to the brachial plexus, phrenic nerve, vagus nerves, and even the spinal cord.[19, 21]

Most of the patients with serious vascular injuries have large hematomas at the base of the neck, a widened mediastinum (more than 8 cm in the second interspace on an upright chest radiograph), continued intrathoracic bleeding, or massive hemothorax. Unfortunately, persistent bleeding in the chest may not be apparent until after a period of observation and even greater blood loss. Also, a number of patients may experience cardiac tamponade or cardiac arrest soon after injury, especially when there are multiple injuries. In a few cases, the only early symptom of internal bleeding is refractory hypotension, but when a chest tube is inserted, massive bleeding becomes apparent.

Table 47–4. Distribution of 206 Vascular Injuries in the Root of the Neck

Vessel	Number
Arterial	
Common carotid	36
Subclavian	37
Innominate	7
Vertebral	6
Venous	
Internal jugular	53
Subclavian	50
Innominate	17

Arteriography

If the injured patient is stable, arteriography may be of great help in defining the extent and location of the injuries. High-quality biplane angiography can be reliable, but it is also clear that it is not infallible, particularly with vascular wounds in this area. Several surgeons have observed false-negative studies, perhaps reflecting the difficulty in obtaining the multiple views needed for precise evaluation.[18, 19, 22] When preoperative arteriograms can be obtained safely, they may offer information that can materially assist in the conduct of surgery, particularly if special preoperative maneuvers are needed (shunts, cardiac bypass pump, remote catheter control techniques, and so forth). It has been emphasized by several workers that a delay in required surgery may be dangerous in unstable patients, and if firm indications for immediate operation exist, it is best not to hesitate. If arteriograms are necessary they can be obtained in the operating room; then if sudden collapse ensues, immediate exploration can be begun.

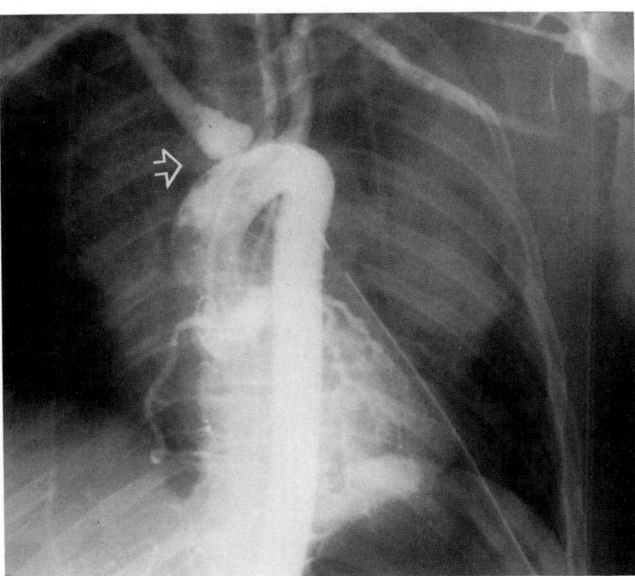

FIGURE 47–5. Blunt trauma from a steering wheel injury in an automobile accident nearly avulsed the innominate artery (*arrow*). An 8-mm graft from the ascending aorta to the transected normal distal innominate completed the repair. The innominate artery origin was oversewn with monofilament sutures.

Treatment

Incisions

The decision regarding surgical exposure is often complex; whether to approach the wound through a thoracotomy or via an extrathoracic route is an important aspect of management. The proximity and number of vital structures in this area are well known, and the danger of combined injuries of the large arteries and veins is apparent. If exsanguination is to be avoided, early operation and vascular control are essential, and several experienced trauma surgeons recommend initial thoracotomy when dealing with suspected vascular wounds in the root of the neck. Some even suggest a median sternal splitting incision for all penetrating wounds below the cricoid cartilage or below C7.[20] Others suggest a more moderate approach, but all support the view that if major vascular wounds are strongly suspected, early thoracotomy is needed.[18] Unnecessary thoracotomy may introduce an additional risk, and therefore most surgeons recommend that specific plans be formulated and followed, and this is easier if the number and location of the vascular injuries are known.

The data reported by Flint and associates, Hewitt and associates, and others suggest that when firm signs of major vascular wounds of the root of the neck and upper mediastinum are present, control through a midline sternal splitting incision is best.[18, 19] This approach affords access to the heart, major veins, and the great vessels of the arch, except for the origin of the left subclavian artery (Fig. 47–5). This incision can be opened quickly, is usually well tolerated, and is easily closed. It may be extended into the supraclavicular area or into the anterior triangle along the sternocleidomastoid muscle to reach the common carotid artery. For exposure of the intrathoracic portion of the left subclavian artery, many surgeons prefer a separate anterolateral fourth or fifth interspace thoracotomy. In most trauma centers, the sternal splitting incision is generally used because it is simple, fast, familiar to most surgeons, and affords ready access to the most vulnerable and commonly injured vessels. A limited median sternotomy can be enlarged quickly by extending the original incision or by adding an intercostal incision.

Extrathoracic incisions for managing vascular injuries of the subclavian and common carotid arteries are also useful. In stable patients with isolated, well-defined penetrating injuries, exposure and repair of these vessels can be easily managed with this approach (Fig. 47–6). In selected cases, especially on the left side, injuries of the second and third portion of the subclavian artery may require resection of the medial half of the clavicle for adequate exposure. In patients with penetrating wounds suspected of causing only subclavian injury, the extrathoracic approach is satisfactory and causes little late morbidity. Venous repairs can be performed through these same incisions.

When exploration is undertaken with a firm clinical diagnosis or after a positive arteriogram, exposure of the injury is usually straightforward, but in some cases the damage may not be apparent. If bleeding or large hematomas are absent, a thorough exploration is still required. Hematoma in the carotid sheath or in the adventitia of the proximal portion of the vessel is an indication for wider exposure. A rather extensive wound can be present in this situation, being effectively tamponaded by the surrounding fascia and the neurovascular sheath, which may have more substance in this region than in some others.

Operative Technique

Direct control of bleeding can be accomplished by the usual techniques in most situations; digital pressure is used most often. In some cases, in fact, small lateral wounds of the large vessels can be controlled with direct pressure and repaired by simply passing the vascular sutures under the occluding finger. Packing may offer temporary assistance

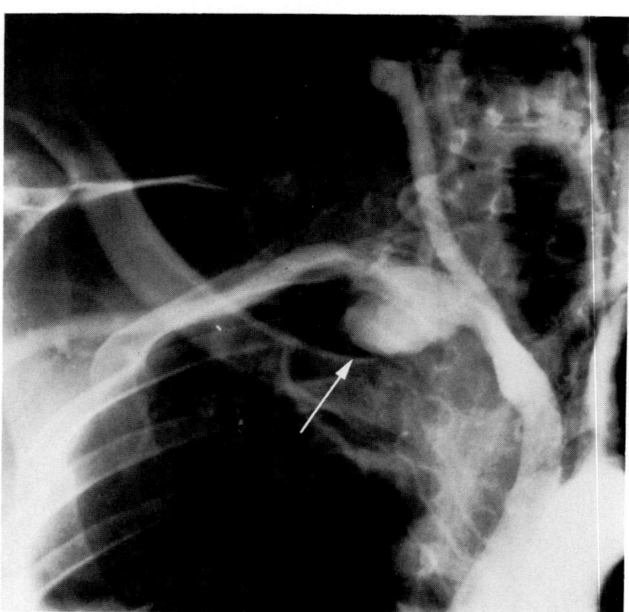

FIGURE 47–6. This false aneurysm of the subclavian artery (*arrow*) occurred as a result of an automobile accident. It was discovered after the man experienced microembolization to his right hand. Repair was accomplished with an interposition saphenous vein graft.

while incisions are widened or additional ones opened, but it cannot be recommended for prolonged use. Lack of complete control and pressure occlusion of other vascular structures are hazards that can contribute to blood loss and perhaps to ischemic complications.

Once vascular clamps have been applied, standard vascular techniques of repair are satisfactory. With large vessels, lateral repair can be used more often, but if the wound cannot be closed without narrowing the artery, patch graft angioplasty is indicated. With more extensive wounds of the great vessels, resection and anastomosis will be required, and if the closure cannot be accomplished without tension, an interposition graft is needed. Most surgeons use plastic grafts for repair of these large vessels, although a few recommend vein grafts, especially if the gastrointestinal or respiratory tract is also injured. Remote bypass techniques may be needed to avoid placing a graft into a field heavily contaminated with bacteria. Subclavian-carotid, axillary-axillary, and carotid-carotid bypasses have been used successfully in a number of cases. Such precautionary procedures may be particularly important when infection is extremely likely, as when the wound has been caused by erosion from a tracheostomy tube, for example.

Shunting

Temporary shunt procedures to maintain cerebral blood flow while the innominate or common carotid arteries are being repaired are used infrequently. Several reports allude to these maneuvers, but none describes the indications or documents the basis for their use.[18, 19, 22] No statistically valid study has been conducted to clarify this problem, but many trauma surgeons suggest that if there is scanty backflow or low back pressures in the distal arteries (less than 70 mmHg), insertion of a temporary shunt may be indicated.[13] A variety of techniques have been used, including inlying tube shunts, combined external and internal shunts, and external shunts.

VENOUS INJURIES

Major venous wounds in this area are quite dangerous, as described by several authors.[18] Multiple injuries are often seen and control of bleeding is difficult. Although repair of the superior vena cava is an accepted procedure, other veins are sometimes simply ligated. This is particularly common when there are multiple wounds, especially of other major arteries, whose repair often takes precedence.

Although there have been sporadic reports of long-term disability after subclavian vein ligation, the true incidence of the problem has not been widely appreciated. Several recent reports concerned with vascular injuries in this region note some late venous problems after subclavian vein ligation, whereas others have observed little disability. It is not possible from published data to clearly state the indications, risks, outcome, and desirability of venous repair, but several related studies are of interest. Adams and coworkers and Tilney and his colleagues have described a progressive increase in the incidence and severity of venous insufficiency after subclavian vein thrombosis with each passing year of follow-up.[23, 24] Up to 60 per cent of their patients ultimately had significant symptoms. Although these patients are not strictly comparable to the trauma patient, several reports concerned with injured patients describe similar problems, but they have not been observed in all cases. No actual study of this type has been reported, but inferentially one might suggest that venous repair is indicated if it does not introduce additional risks. In Rich's study of popliteal vein trauma, postphlebitic and thromboembolic events were seen less often after vein repairs than after ligation.[25] These same features may be important in the upper extremity in selected cases, but at present only a general statement supporting venous repair is appropriate. If obvious venous hypertension is present, if there has been destruction of collateral vessels, and if concomitant major arterial injuries exist, venous repair rather than ligation appears to be indicated.

References

1. Monson DU, Saletta JD, Freeark RJ: Carotid vertebral trauma. J Trauma 9:987, 1969.
2. Bradley EL: Management of penetrating carotid injuries: an alternative approach. J Trauma 13:248, 1973.
3. Thal ER, Snyder WH, Hays RJ, et al: Management of carotid artery injuries. Surgery 76:955, 1974.
4. Liekweg WG, Greenfield LJ: Management of penetrating carotid arterial injury. Ann Surg 188:587, 1978.
5. Yamada S, Kindt GW, Youmans JR. Carotid injuries due to nonpenetrating injury. J Trauma 7:333, 1967.
6. Ledgewood AM, Mullins RJ, Lucas CE: Primary repair vs ligation for carotid artery injuries. Arch Surg 115:488, 1980.
7. Perry MO, Snyder WH, Thal ER: Carotid artery injuries caused by blunt trauma. Ann Surg 192:74, 1980.
8. Unger SW, Tucker WS, Mudeza MA, et al: Carotid arterial trauma. Surgery 87:477, 1980.

9. Krajewski LP, Hertzer NR: Blunt carotid trauma. Ann Surg 191:341, 1980.
10. Jernigan WR, Gardner WC: Carotid artery injuries due to closed cervical trauma. J Trauma 11:429, 1971.
11. Crissey MM, Bernstein EF: Delayed presentation of carotid intimal tear following blunt craniocervical trauma. Surgery 75:543, 1974.
12. Fry WJ, Fry RE: Management of carotid artery injury. *In* Bergan JJ, Yao JST (eds): Vascular Surgical Emergencies. Orlando, Grune & Stratton, 1986, pp 153–162.
13. Ehrenfeld WK, Stoney RJ, Wylie EJ: Relation of carotid stump pressure to safety of carotid artery ligation. Surgery 93:299, 1983.
14. Thompson JE, Talkington CM: Carotid endarterectomy. Ann Surg 184:1, 1976.
15. Gewertz B, Samson D, Ditmore QM, et al: Management of penetrating injuries of the internal carotid artery at the base of the skull utilizing extracranial-intracranial bypass. J Trauma 20(5):365, 1980.
16. Meier DE, Brink BE, Fry WJ: Vertebral artery trauma. Arch Surg 116:236, 1981.
17. Brink BJ, Meier D, Fry WJ: Operative exposure and management of lesions in the vertebral artery. J Cardiovasc Surg 20:435, 1979.
18. Flint LM, Snyder WH, Perry MO, et al: Management of major vascular injuries in the base of the neck. Arch Surg 106:407, 1973.
19. Hewitt RL, Smith AD, Becker ML, et al: Penetrating vascular injuries of the thoracic outlet. Surgery 76:715, 1974.
20. Reul GJ, Beall AC, Jordon GL, et al: The early operative management of injuries to the great vessels. Surgery 74:862, 1973.
21. Smith RF, Elliott JP, Hagaman JH, et al: Acute penetrating arterial injuries of the neck and limbs. Arch Surg 109:198, 1974.
22. Lim LT, Saletta JD, Flanigan DP: Subclavian and innominate artery trauma. Surgery 86:890, 1979.
23. Adams JT, McEvoy RK, DeWeese JA: Primary deep venous thrombosis of upper extremity. Arch Surg 91:29, 1965.
24. Tilney NL, Griffiths HJG, Edwards EA: Natural history of major venous thrombosis of the upper extremity. Arch Surg 101:792, 1970.
25. Rich NM, Hobson RW, Collins GJ, et al: The effect of acute popliteal venous interruption. Ann Surg 183:365, 1979.

48

Vascular Injuries of the Extremities

Erwin R. Thal, M.D., William H. Snyder III, M.D., and Malcolm O. Perry, M.D.

• • •

The diagnosis and management of vascular trauma continues to undergo scrutiny and change. The pendulum has swung from a policy of mandatory exploration for all suspected and potential vascular injuries to one of selective evaluation and nonoperative treatment of ''minimal injuries.'' Studies now in progress ideally will identify injuries that can safely be classified as ''minimal.'' Adequate long-term studies of these injuries have not yet been done, and their natural history is unclear.

The diagnosis and repair of vascular injuries are crucial in the management of traumatized extremities. Although upper extremity wounds account for more than one third of peripheral vascular injuries, most of the difficult clinical problems occur with lower extremity injuries. Survival is infrequently threatened by extremity wounds; amputation or the retention of a painful, functionless limb is the most serious untoward result of severe injury or inadequate treatment. The amputation rate following major arterial injuries in the extremities approached 50 per cent in World War II,[16, 102] fell to 13 per cent in the Korean conflict,[92] and has been reported to be 1.5 per cent in civilian series.[68] Prompt and effective diagnosis, resuscitation, and revascularization are the necessary ingredients for successful results.

Complications of vascular trauma such as thrombosis, delayed bleeding, arteriovenous fistulae, and false aneurysms are more likely to occur and are more difficult to manage if the injury is not treated promptly.[6, 21, 26, 56, 62, 93, 127] Such lesions may be evident immediately or may produce delayed symptoms hours to decades after the injury.[46] The initial arterial repair of such wounds is simple in comparison with the problems presented by well-developed false aneurysms or arteriovenous fistulae.[26, 93] The risk of these delayed complications underscores the importance of early recognition and repair.

Although the management of vascular injuries of the extremities has progressively improved, some clinical problems and controversial issues remain. These include (1) the indications for immediate amputation without attempted vascular reconstruction; (2) the appropriate use of diagnostic arteriography; (3) the management of injuries that are arteriographically ''minor'' or involve nonessential vessels; (4) the optimal sequence of operative repair of multiple injuries (artery, vein, and bone); (5) the operative management of injured veins; and (6) the choice of interposition graft when primary repair is not possible.

TYPES OF TRAUMA

In urban America, vascular wounds of the extremities most commonly result from penetrating trauma. Single, low-velocity bullets and sharp instruments are the usual causes, and gunshot wounds predominate. Penetrating vascular wounds are produced by direct trauma or, in the case of high-velocity missiles, blast injury. In rural populations, blunt vascular injuries are more common and are caused by compression forces, traction from fracture displacement, or direct wounds from bone fragments. Bishara and associates have documented an incidence of vascular injuries of 6.5 per cent of hospitalized patients with orthopedic injuries.[5] The highest incidence was in patients with knee dislocations and those with combined fractures of the bones of the leg or of the forearm. Adjacent tissue damage commonly accompanies vascular injuries, especially with blunt trauma and high-velocity bullet wounds. Failure to recognize and effectively treat these associated injuries can lead to complications that jeopardize vascular repair and increase the mortality rate. Vessel spasm is common with adjacent tissue injury or minimal arterial damage. It rarely results in arterial insufficiency but suggests that a vascular injury is present and a thorough examination is needed.

The risk of limb loss is greatest following blunt trauma and injuries from high-velocity missiles or close-range shotgun wounds.[55, 105, 109] This is largely related to the extent of associated tissue damage from these mechanisms. Wounds from sharp instruments and single, low-velocity missiles seldom result in amputations. Injury sites most prone to limb loss are the popliteal and proximal shank vessels. In Shah and associates' series, no amputations resulted from 151 arterial injuries due to low-velocity, single-missile gunshot wounds or sharp instruments; 10 amputations followed 35 injuries from blunt or shotgun wounds ($p < .001$).[107] The effect of adjacent fractures, probably reflecting the magnitude of trauma, was an amputation rate of 26 per cent in 33 patients with fractures or dislocations and a rate of 0.6 per cent in extremities without skeletal injuries ($p < .001$). In these patients the amputation rate was not significantly influenced by associated venous injuries.

PATIENT SELECTION AND EVALUATION

Initial Management of Potential Vascular Injuries

Peripheral vascular injuries do not compete with those that are immediately life threatening but take priority over most other injuries. Once the initial resuscitation is underway, bleeding controlled, and the airway secure, the extent and nature of the vascular injuries are fully assessed. Vessel wounds causing distal ischemia require urgent operative restoration of flow; the repair is delayed only for hemodynamic stabilization and treatment of other life-threatening problems. Additional resuscitation or further diagnostic evaluation (such as arteriography) can be accomplished in the operating room, if indicated.

Probes and fingers are not inserted into wounds that potentially harbor vascular injuries because of the danger of dislodging a clot and causing recurrent hemorrhage. Bleeding is best controlled by direct pressure. Tourniquets should be avoided, since they can occlude collateral inflow and lead to further circulatory compromise and greater ischemic damage. Vascular clamps should not be applied in the depths of the wound without adequate exposure; accurate clamping usually requires operating room facilities. Attempts to place clamps blindly can damage adjacent structures and extend the arterial injury, further complicating reconstruction.

All arterial injuries should be repaired as soon as they are recognized unless other wounds or illnesses require priority attention. The treatment of venous injuries is more controversial, but injured veins may cause massive hemorrhage, requiring early control. Those major venous injuries associated with arterial wounds require operative repair. The appropriate management of isolated asymptomatic venous injuries has not been defined, and the importance of extensive diagnostic maneuvers is, therefore, unknown.

Diagnosis and Indications for Operation

History and Physical Examination

Impressive advances in diagnostic techniques have been made in recent years, but the history and physical examination remain the basis for diagnosing vascular injury. Careful questioning about the mechanism of injury, the amount and location of blood loss, and the symptoms of circulatory, sensory, or motor impairment often lead to the correct diagnosis. A meticulous physical examination is essential and should include a careful record of baseline observations with which changes can be compared. The adequacy of arterial perfusion distal to an injury is determined by evaluation of the presence and volume of pulses, the filling of peripheral veins, the speed of capillary refill, and the color, temperature, and neurologic function of the extremity. Signs of arterial injury without occlusion include hematoma formation, arterial bleeding, evidence of adjacent nerve injury, and thrills or bruits caused by turbulent flow. Careful auscultation with a stethoscope distal to the area of injury usually is sufficient to detect the murmur.

The signs suggesting arterial injury are listed in Table 48–1. The first four (hard signs) are almost pathognomonic of an underlying arterial injury. The last four are less specific, though suggestive, and are considered soft signs. Specific, or hard, signs of arterial injury mandate operative exploration. The urgency depends on the number and severity of associated injuries, the presence of hemorrhage or distal ischemia, and the site of injury. Equivocal, or soft, signs suggest the presence of arterial injury, and arteriography or operative exploration may be necessary to exclude or confirm this possibility. Some arterial injuries may be difficult to detect, even with a careful history and examina-

Table 48–1. Signs of Arterial Injury

Hard signs
Distal circulatory deficit
Ischemia
Pulses diminished or absent
Bruit
Expanding or pulsatile hematoma
Arterial bleeding
Soft signs
Small or moderate-size stable hematoma
Adjacent nerve injury
Shock (unexplained by other injuries)
Proximity of penetrating wound to a major vascular structure

tion. Certain overt physical manifestations reliably indicate the presence of an arterial injury, but their absence does not preclude one.

Diminished distal pulse volume may be caused by hypotension, and the diagnostic validity of this finding as a sign of arterial injury depends on comparison with the pulse volume in the contralateral extremity. Pulses may be palpable distal to an arterial injury because the vessel may not be occluded or because pressure waves can be transmitted through soft clots or because flow may be maintained through collateral channels (Fig. 48–1). The important observation, documented by numerous clinical reports, is that the presence of a pulse does not ensure the absence of a proximal arterial injury.[42] Physical findings, confirmed by exploration or arteriography, were falsely positive in 42 per cent and falsely negative in 20 per cent of 91 patients reported by McCormick and Burch.[65]

The major factors responsible for misleading physical findings associated with an arterial injury are the extent of damage to the vessel wall and the location of the injury. Saletta and Freeark reported finding palpable pulses in 61 per cent of patients with *partially* severed arteries (almost half of whom had normal pulses).[103] The effect of a rich collateral arterial system is illustrated by comparison of the distal pulses in subclavian arterial injuries with those in popliteal arterial injuries. In two series, normal pulses were present distal to 56 per cent of the subclavian injuries but only 16 per cent of the popliteal arterial injuries.[115]

The lack of specific physical findings caused by some arterial injuries and the morbidity from missed injuries have led some authorities in the past to recommend exploration of all wounds in proximity to major vessels.[20, 87, 112] This approach was the diagnostic standard with which other techniques were compared. Routine exploration will generally prevent vascular injuries from being missed; however, it will also result in unnecessary explorations, some morbidity, and, rarely, a patient's death. Even the accuracy of operative exploration has been questioned by data collected by Richardson and associates.[97] Long-term clinical follow-up demonstrated six missed injuries in 72 patients (8 per cent) undergoing operative exploration. The yield and risk of routine operative exploration for suspected vascular injuries is documented in a report by Sirinek and associates.[112] Sixty-four per cent of 390 explorations failed to demonstrate injuries and were associated with morbidity in 5 per cent, and 0.4 per cent of the patients died.

Noninvasive Studies

More recently, there has been a tendency to withhold operative intervention in a select subgroup of patients thought to have minimal injury.[17] With this in mind, perhaps more reliance is now placed upon the history and physical examination than was common in the past. Frykberg and coauthors reported their experience in a prospective study of 310 patients with 366 injuries in whom physical examination was the sole method of evaluation in penetrating extremity trauma.[29] They reported 2 false-negative diagnoses (0.7 per cent), which included transected popliteal and radial arteries but no morbidity or mortality. Their positive predictive value was 100 per cent.

Reliance on Doppler studies and arterial pressure indices (APIs) as part of the physical examination has added to its accuracy; however, minimal injuries such as intimal defects and small pseudoaneurysms may still not be detected. Johansen and colleagues reported a series of patients in which the negative predictive value for an API of more than 0.90 was 99 per cent and the sensitivity and specificity were 95 per cent and 97 per cent, respectively, for major arterial injury if the API was less than 0.90.[49] In their evaluation of 100 injured limbs in 96 patients, 16 of 17 patients with an API of less than 0.90 had positive findings, with 7 requiring arterial reconstruction. Only 5 minor injuries (4 pseudoaneurysms, none of which required surgery, and 1 arteriovenous fistula, which was repaired 1 year later) were seen in the 83 limbs with an API of more than 0.90. The authors acknowledged that it is difficult to evaluate minor vessels, lesions that do not reduce flow, or venous injuries with the Doppler technique. Nevertheless, they concluded that noninvasive tests can reliably exclude major occult arterial damage and that arteriography should be limited to patients with an API of less than 0.90. This enthusiasm for Doppler studies is not necessarily shared by all surgeons treating these injuries. Late complications from missed or untreated arterial injuries continue to occur.

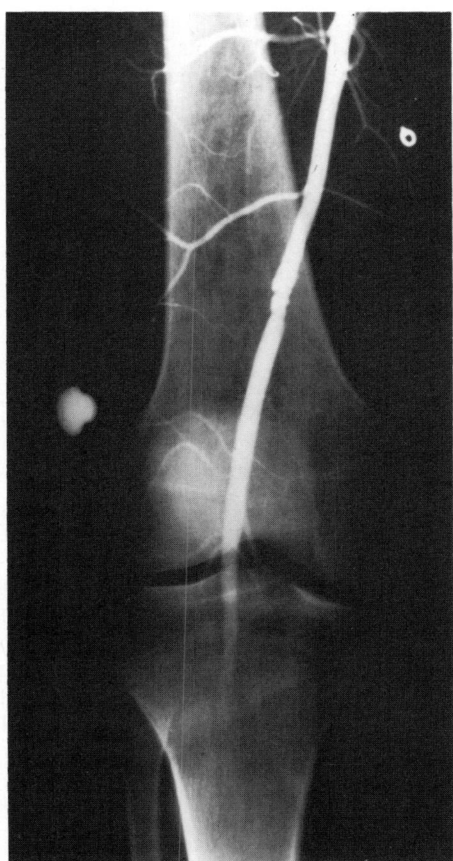

FIGURE 48–1. Arteriogram shows injured but patent artery with continued flow, demonstrating why pulses are often maintained.

Another noninvasive study that may have a role in the diagnosis of vascular injury is duplex ultrasonography. Not only can it detect injuries, it may also become an excellent study with which to follow selected patients who are managed nonoperatively. Meissner and colleagues reported their experience with 89 patients who sustained 93 injuries.[66] Four of 60 scans performed solely for reasons of proximity were positive for injury. There were 4 false-negative studies; however, no major injuries were missed. There were no false-positive studies. The authors warn that the study is operator-dependent and that there is indeed a ''learning curve'' that governs its reliability. This study is cost-effective and may serve as a reliable substitute for contrast angiography if occult injury is suspected.

Arteriography

Arteriography is the single most accurate diagnostic procedure for detecting an arterial injury. The validity of normal arteriography in arterial trauma was addressed in a prospective study reported in 1978 in which 177 patients with 183 penetrating extremity wounds underwent arteriography followed by operative vessel explorations.[114] Most of those patients had equivocal physical findings for arterial injuries. Surgical exploration revealed that 36 arteriograms were true positives, 132 were true negatives, 14 were false positives, and 1 was a false negative. It was concluded that arteriography was sufficiently sensitive to exclude the presence of arterial injuries in patients with equivocal clinical signs.

The indications for preoperative arteriography in arterial trauma fall into two categories: establishing the diagnosis and planning the operation. Precise injury location may be especially helpful in blunt or multiple missile trauma, which often requires extensive dissection. Such studies also aid in planning the sequence of operative procedures in patients with trauma of more than one system.

Although arteriography is accurate in identifying the presence or absence of injury, it may be less precise than once thought in predicting the actual type of injury. Reid and coworkers, in a review of vertebral artery injuries, noted that 50 per cent of the injuries found at operation were different from those predicted by the angiogram.[90] Francis and coauthors also noted that less than half of a small series of extremity injuries were the same as those seen on arteriography.[27]

Since it may be necessary to delay the operation to obtain high-quality arteriograms, arteriography should be reserved for patients in whom the findings may eliminate the need for surgery or simplify the performance of an operation. Patients with unequivocal signs of arterial injury that are adequately localized by physical examination or plain radiographs are best served by early operation. Urgent operation is mandatory in patients with ischemia because delay may prevent a successful revascularization. A single-film arteriogram can be obtained rapidly in the operating room if additional information is required.

Table 48–2. Arteriographic Findings in Trauma*

Obstruction (see Fig. 48–2)
Extravasation (see Fig. 48–3)
Early venous filling/arteriovenous fistula (see Fig. 48–4)
Wall irregularity/filling defect (see Fig. 48–1)
False aneurysm

**Any abnormality makes a study positive*

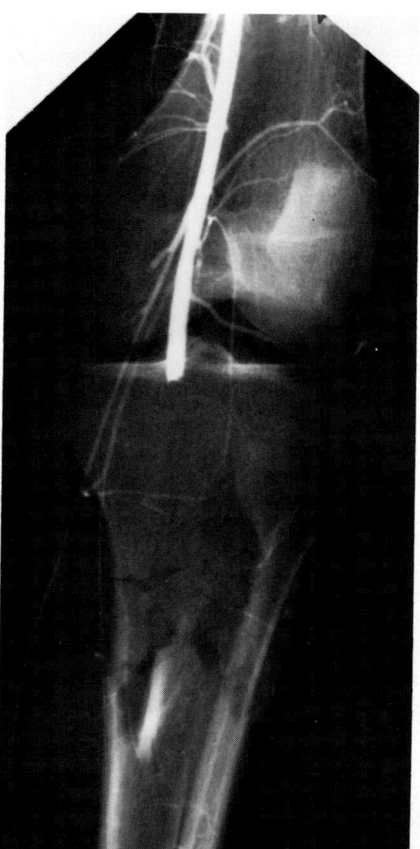

FIGURE 48–2. Arteriogram demonstrates obstruction of flow.

Exclusion arteriography should be limited to patients with equivocal signs of arterial injury in whom no other operative procedure (débridement or internal fracture fixation) is required. Equivocal (soft) signs of arterial injury include the last four signs listed in Table 48–1. Experienced personnel and special angiographic facilities must be available, day or night, if high-quality arteriograms are to be obtained.

Specific arteriographic findings of arterial injuries are listed in Table 48–2. Arteriographic features seen in various types of trauma are illustrated in Figures 48–1 through 48–4. Though these findings are usually obvious, extensive injury may produce only minor radiographic changes. Some arteriographic findings have been labeled soft signs and are used to identify a select subgroup of patients with arterial injury that are occasionally managed nonoperatively. These signs include vessel narrowing, intimal defect, injury in noncritical arteries, and intimal flaps that are adherent or downstream. Other findings such as small false aneurysms, small arteriovenous fistulae, and spasm are more controversial, but spontaneous cure of post-traumatic false aneurysms and anteriovenous fistulae is unusual. More often, these lesions are progressive in extent and complexity. Any abnormality is strongly suggestive of a vascular injury.

Reliable arteriographic evaluation of arterial trauma requires strict attention to the details of performance and

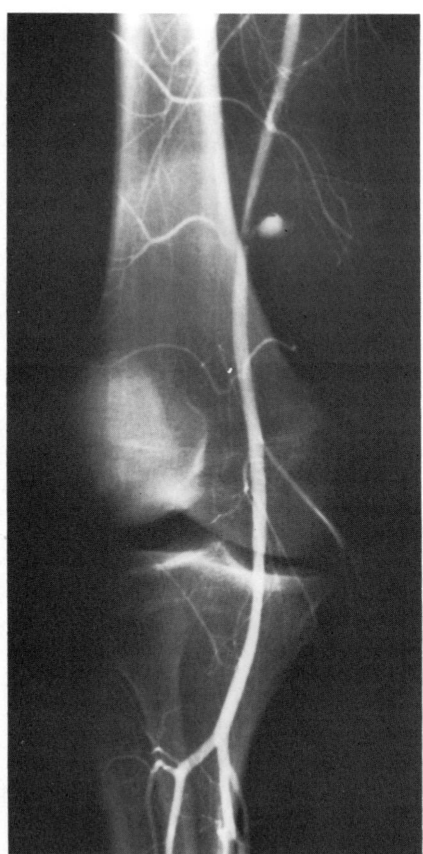

FIGURE 48–3. Arteriogram demonstrating extravasation.

interpretation. This is especially true if the study is performed to exclude arterial injury. The complete contrast column must be clearly seen in two projections and throughout the entire region of potential injury. Subtraction techniques may be useful to suppress surrounding densities, and not infrequently, this will accentuate a minor defect that might otherwise be missed. The two findings that may be subtle and demand excellent technique and close scrutiny are early venous filling and wall irregularities or filling defects. Incorrectly timed single-film studies may easily miss the former, and single-projection examinations may miss the latter. Guidelines for accurate arteriography in trauma patients are listed in Table 48–3. The importance of precise technique is emphasized in a study by Richardson and associates in which long-term clinical follow-up uncovered missed injuries in 8 of 133 patients (6 per cent) undergoing exclusion arteriography.[97]

Table 48–3. Technical Considerations in Arteriography in Trauma

Use opaque markers on entrance and exit sites
Inject a distance from suspected injury
Include 15 cm on both sides of potential injury
Obtain sequential films for "early" venous filling
Obtain at least two different projections
Surgeon must review films before removal of catheter or needle to judge adequacy of study
Any abnormality equals a positive study
Repeat inconclusive studies or explore operatively

The need for venography in vascular trauma is much less well defined than that for arteriography. Preoperative venograms define venous anatomy, which may be helpful for intraoperative decision making. For instance, paired veins may mean that the surgeon can safely ligate one of the pair—a consideration of particular importance in the popliteal region. The demonstration of a venous thrombus indicates the need for thrombectomy.[34] In patients with arterial injuries but without ischemia, venography can be obtained in conjunction with preoperative arteriograms.

Another approach to the arteriographic evaluation of extremities potentially harboring arterial wounds was described by O'Gorman and associates.[81] This procedure is performed in the emergency department and consists of single-film, hand-injected arteriograms. The authors reported 515 arteriograms performed on 488 patients; studies were abnormal in 130 patients (25 per cent), and 102 (20 per cent) required operations. The examinations included axillary injections for subclavian (retrograde), axillary, and brachial injuries, brachial injections for radial and ulnar injuries, and femoral injections for lower extremity injuries. One false normal and four false abnormal studies were documented. Although this appears to be a simple, rapid, and cost-effective technique, normal examinations were validated only by limited clinical follow-up. A concern about missed injuries, as discussed previously, suggests caution in recommending the widespread use of this technique to exclude arterial injuries. However, it is probably the preferred technique for patients requiring operations in whom additional preoperative information would be beneficial.

Several reports have described the use of digital subtraction arteriographic techniques for the evaluation of po-

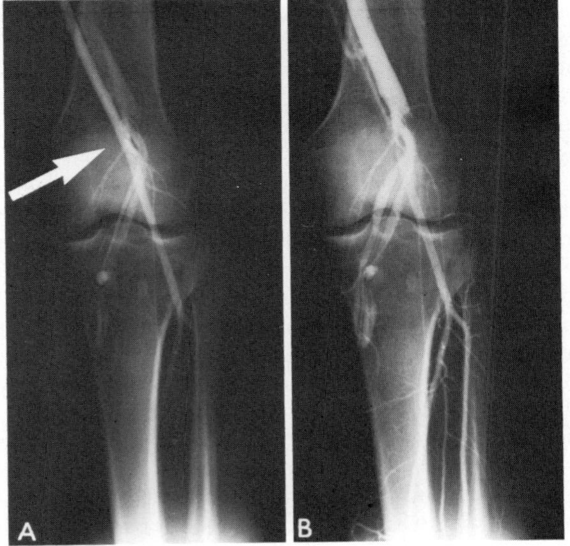

FIGURE 48–4. *A* and *B*, Arteriogram demonstrates early venous filling in acute arteriovenous fistula with tibial fracture (*arrow* in *A*). (*A* and *B*, From Perry MO: The Management of Acute Vascular Injuries, p. 126, ©1981, The Williams & Wilkins Co., Baltimore.)

tential arterial injuries. Both intravenous and arterial injections have been studied.[22, 37, 110] Two studies prospectively compared digital techniques with conventional arteriography.[22, 110] The advantages of the digital studies are reductions in contrast media, time required, and patient discomfort. The disadvantages are the degree of patient cooperation required and the limited area that can be studied with a single injection. Accuracy has been similar to that achieved with conventional studies except in the detection of intimal abnormalities. This additional limitation has led to the recommendation that digital studies not be used for the evaluation of wounds from high-velocity missiles, shotgun pellets, or blunt trauma. It is worth stressing that diagnostic accuracy requires arterial catheterizations for selective injections and a motionless subject, a difficulty for most trauma patients.

Angioscopy is a potentially useful technique for evaluating arterial injury. It can be performed in conjunction with arteriography or under local anesthesia, or may complement an equivocal angiogram. It is still under investigation for trauma situations and is not recommended for routine use at this time.

Evaluation of Patients With Minimal Signs

Validation of the superior accuracy of arteriography has spawned an enormous increase in its use for the evaluation of patients with minimal signs of arterial injury. As with all screening techniques, a judgment must be made regarding the risk : benefit ratio. In studies of patients in whom the only indication for arteriography was the proximity of wounds to a major vessel, the frequency of arterial injuries varied between 4 and 16 per cent.[27, 68, 69, 81, 90, 111, 114, 116] One report suggests that exclusion arteriography in patients with such "proximity" as the only indication seldom uncovers an arterial injury and is not indicated for this purpose.[36] A prospective study of 143 extremities with penetrating trauma in which the only indication for exploration was proximity of the wound to a major vessel found 12 arterial injuries (8 per cent).[114] In O'Gorman and associates' study of emergency center arteriography, proximity was the sole indication for study in 352 extremities, and 45 of these patients (13 per cent) required operations for arterial injuries.[81]

Whereas proximity of an injury to a major vessel used to be an indication for operative exploration, the large number of nontherapeutic procedures led most surgeons to rely on arteriography to rule out an injury. Recent interest has focused on the incidence of injury that requires repair when proximity is the sole indication in an otherwise *completely asymptomatic* patient. Several studies have addressed this issue, and most conclude that proximity is no longer an indication for arteriography. Reid and colleagues, in a retrospective series of over 500 patients, found an incidence of injury of 3.6 per cent, and only half of those patients required a repair.[90] The complication rate associated with the arteriogram was 3.2 per cent in those patients in whom no injury was detected. Francis and coauthors reported a similar incidence of injury of only 4.4 per cent in a prospective study of 134 patients.[27] They concluded that proximity as a sole indication was no longer a valid reason to obtain an arteriogram in a totally asymptomatic patient with an extremity injury. The patient should have a complete clinical evaluation including a Doppler examination before a decision is made not to obtain the angiogram. It is important to stress that this concept applies to extremity injuries only and not to cervical or thoracic outlet injuries as has been recommended by some authors.

One must acknowledge that occasional injuries will be missed if this policy of not obtaining arteriograms for proximity is adopted. Authors recommending this policy state that neither life nor limb will be put in jeopardy and that it is an acceptable trade-off for the cost-effectiveness and preservation of resources that will be gained.

The judgment that a penetrating injury traverses the course of a major artery requires anatomic knowledge of the course of the vessel in relation to superficial landmarks and to radiographic findings such as the missile or metallic fragments in bone. However, if all penetrating wounds of extremities are studied arteriographically, the yield of arterial injuries will be extremely low. The yield from operative exploration or arteriography of penetrating extremity trauma without specific signs of arterial injury is proportional to the anatomic knowledge and experience of the examiner.

Nonoperative Management

There is still a consensus that patients with evidence of injury to major vascular structures warrant early and aggressive operative treatment. However, the development of new and less invasive diagnostic studies coupled with a better understanding of the natural history of untreated vascular injuries has allowed identification of a subset of patients who may be safely observed.

In an attempt to better elicit the natural history of minimal lesions Frykberg and coauthors reported a prospective study of 20 injuries in 19 patients with angiographically proven lesions.[30] Sixty-five per cent had intimal flaps, 30 per cent demonstrated focal narrowing, and one (5 per cent) had a false aneurysm. Their follow-up consisted of 95 per cent of the patients, and 15 of the 19 patients (79 per cent) had angiographic follow-up. The authors stated that 53 per cent of the lesions resolved, 16 per cent improved, and 26 per cent remained unchanged. One false aneurysm enlarged at 10 weeks and was repaired without sequelae.

Another report by Frykberg and associates detailed their experience with nonoperative management in a prospective study of 50 occult injuries in 47 patients, of whom 43 were observed nonoperatively.[28] One patient died of an unrelated injury, and three were operated on after the initial arteriogram was obtained. The patients in the study had arteriographically documented injuries to major arteries with either absent or equivocal clinical signs of vascular injury but intact and distally patent vessels. There were 22 intimal flaps, 21 cases of segmental narrowing, 6 pseudoaneurysms, and 1 arteriovenous fistula. Follow-up averaged 3.1 months, and 39 of the patients (85 per cent) had a subsequent arteriogram, whereas 7 were reevaluated only by clinical examination. Complete resolution was documented for 29 (63 per cent) of the injuries, whereas 3 were improved, 9 remained unchanged, and 3 became worse. The three injuries that failed to improve were all pseudoaneurysms, and all three patients were operated on without subsequent morbidity. The authors concluded that because 89 per cent of the followed injuries did not require surgery, nonoperative observation was a safe and effective management option for clinically occult arterial injuries.

Although other authors share this philosophy, a word of caution must be given.[118] As better understanding of the natural history of occult vascular injuries begins to evolve, there appears to be a select group of patients who will do well with nonoperative treatment. These are patients who are essentially asymptomatic, have arteriographic evidence of minimal injury, and are amenable to close follow-up. We still do not know how long these injuries are at risk for developing complications, but past experience indicates it is longer than has been recently reported. Until more data are available, this form of treatment should be limited to injured vessels that will not cause significant morbidity and certainly no mortality if an injury progresses or an occasional injury is missed on initial evaluation.

Indications for Primary Amputation

Immediate amputation of a severely traumatized limb is a difficult but critical decision that presents itself early in the care of patients with such injuries. This decision relates to the projected likelihood that a functional and durable extremity can result and does not apply to isolated vascular injuries. The attitude that vascular reconstruction is always indicated is inappropriate and may result in serious morbidity. It is basically a matter of judgment of the magnitude of the extremity trauma, the most important components of which are the nerve and skeletal injuries. An anesthetic and paralyzed extremity is usually best treated by immediate amputation. However, operative confirmation of nerve destruction, rather than contusion or ischemia, as the basis of the functional loss is important. Another factor that portends a poor functional result is the loss of bone continuity of more than 6 cm. The importance of soft tissue injury is relative, and in the absence of other unrepairable injuries, reconstruction is usually attempted. Extensive remote trauma that deserves prior attention for the preservation of life is a relative factor in the decision for immediate amputation. The vascular injury itself is almost never the deciding factor. The final decision about primary amputation should usually be made under ideal circumstances, as are found when exploring an anesthetized patient in the operating room.

Little has been written about the decision regarding primary amputation, and until fairly recently, no objective data have been brought to bear on it. Gregory and associates reported a group of patients with massively injured extremities and devised a scoring system to describe the effect of multi-system extremity trauma and to define the boundary between salvageable and unsalvageable extremities.[39] Multi-system extremity injuries were defined as those involving at least three of the four organ systems (integument, nerve, artery, and bone). Sixty consecutive patients with severely injured extremities were reviewed, and 17 met the definition of the "mangled extremity syndrome." Injuries were retrospectively scored to quantitate the extent of extremity injury and also to include components characterizing the extent of remote injury, age, and preexisting illness. Ten of the 17 extremities eventually required amputations, and all could have been prospectively identified using the scoring system. The authors concluded that (1) a multi-disciplinary approach is essential, including specialists in vascular, orthopedic, and reconstructive surgery; (2) the final decision about limb salvage should be made under ideal circumstances, i.e., in the operating room; and (3) extensive injury to a single tissue system may negate the importance of the total score.

PREPARATION FOR SURGERY

Hemodynamic stabilization should be started immediately and, if possible, accomplished before operation. Fluid resuscitation is begun with balanced salt solution, and when it is anticipated that operative blood loss may be excessive, appropriate quantities of blood are typed and crossmatched. Because small vessel thrombosis and myonecrosis may occur in ischemic limbs, systemic anticoagulation with heparin may be beneficial in patients with profound or prolonged ischemia secondary to isolated vascular injuries. On the other hand, patients with associated abdominal, ophthalmic, central nervous system, or extensive soft tissue and skeletal injuries should *not* be given full-dose heparin. Parenteral antibiotic administration is begun as soon after injury as possible, and always before operation. Injuries of the extremities require an agent effective against gram-positive skin organisms, such as staphylococci. Short-term administration (usually less than 48 hours) is sufficient to combat contaminating organisms, and this regimen avoids the complications of prolonged treatment.

TECHNICAL CONSIDERATIONS

General anesthesia is preferable to regional techniques in treating major injuries, although local or regional anesthesia may occasionally be used for patients with distal minor vascular injuries. Regardless of the type of anesthesia used, an experienced anesthesiologist is required to monitor vital signs and regulate fluid therapy because intraoperative blood loss may be substantial.

Positioning of the patient and preparation of the sterile field require consideration not only of extended operative exposure but also of the possible need to "harvest" venous autografts. Normally, the entire involved extremity is included in the sterile field; distal access is important for palpation of pulses or intraoperative Doppler examination and occasionally for retrograde thrombectomy. With proximal injuries, access to the abdomen or chest may be required to obtain vascular control.[25] An uninjured lower extremity should also be prepared for harvest of a segment of saphenous vein if this is needed for reconstruction.

Longitudinal incisions are made over the vessels to be explored to allow proximal and distal extensions, if required. If possible, the initial dissection exposes the vessels outside the hematoma and away from the suspected site of vascular injury. Control is accomplished by encircling the vessel with umbilical tapes or latex loops proximal and distal to the injury. In the event of hemorrhage during exposure, bleeding is controlled with digital pressure until vascular clamps can be applied. Following isolation of the injured arterial segment, the extent of damage is evaluated and nearby veins, nerves, and other structures are examined. Vessel wall contusions may, on superficial inspection, appear to be innocuous. When there is no bleeding from the artery, suggesting that the vessel wall is only contused, a serious injury may escape detection. If the gross external appearance of the vessel is not consistent with preoperative information suggesting an arterial injury, intraoperative arteriography or arteriotomy should be considered. Dissecting or false aneurysms can occur when the vessel wall is only partially disrupted and intimal injuries are thrombogenic and may lead to later occlusion.

If the collateral circulation is adequate, the vessel may safely be occluded during repair. If impaired backflow suggests that collateral blood flow is inadequate and a delay of more than an hour or two is anticipated before revascularization is completed, *an indwelling shunt* may be useful.[48, 54, 80, 122]

Intraluminal thrombus is often present, especially with injuries that cause vessel occlusion. *Proximal and distal balloon catheter thrombectomy* of injured arteries and veins is carried out before flow is restored by shunt or reconstruction. Thrombectomy of adjacent segments may enhance collateral flow if the vessel needs to be clamped during the dissection and repair and is essential to ensure shunt patency. If collateral flow is inadequate, the distal vessels are irrigated with copious amounts of *cold* balanced salt solution containing a 1:10 dilution of heparin. An approach that has been used with some success at the authors' institution in patients with distal ischemia and combined arterial and venous injuries is to flush the distal arterial tree with a solution of 1000 units of heparin and 12.5 gm of mannitol in a liter of lactated Ringer's until the venous effluent is clear. Heparin affords some protection to the occluded segment by retarding intravascular thrombosis, the irrigation removes thrombotic debris, and mannitol may decrease muscle edema and the need for subsequent fasciotomy. Regional heparin will remain effective only in blind segments of vessels containing stagnant blood—it is rapidly removed from other areas. Balloon catheter thrombectomy and flushing are repeated just prior to completion of the repair and restoration of flow.

Adequate débridement of injured vessels is as important as for other tissues. There is a natural reluctance to débride vessels widely, since this may preclude primary anastomosis, but leaving a transmural injury in continuity may result in the development of a false aneurysm. Moreover, damaged intima promotes platelet aggregation and may increase the risk of occlusion. Débridement is particularly important in gunshot wounds and blunt trauma because there is often blast damage and contusion beyond the visible limits of injury. This usually requires resection of 4 to 5 mm of vessel beyond the visible limits of injury in low-velocity missile wounds and 1 cm in high-velocity missile wounds and blunt injuries. Additional vessel length for primary anastomosis can often be obtained by proximal and distal mobilization, dividing small branches.

Adequate débridement of vessel injuries from blunt trauma or high-velocity missiles often precludes primary anastomosis, and autogenous grafts should be used preferentially in the repair of these injuries. At some point during the repair, the extremity should be placed in an unflexed position to ensure that the reconstituted vessel will be of proper length when the limb is fully extended. Undue tension at the anastomosis should be avoided.

Sequence of Procedures

The appropriate sequence for arterial and venous reconstruction and the repair of skeletal injuries is important. If distal flow is maintained, the sequence of repair is a matter of personal preference. Arterial injuries causing distal ischemia or venous injuries causing venous hypertension require immediate restoration of blood flow. Flow can be temporarily restored by indwelling shunts if a delay in reconstruction is required for attention to adjacent or remote injuries or harvesting of a graft.[48, 54, 80, 122] Venous reconstruction usually precedes arterial repair if the injured vein is the major or sole source of venous return. This provides better outflow and may enhance the success of arterial repair.[92, 96]

Controversy continues regarding the need to stabilize fractures before reconstructing arteries. Initial bone stabilization protects the vascular repair from movement at the fracture site. The disadvantages of this sequence include delay in restoration of flow to ischemic tissue and possible interference with the vascular repair by the fixation device, which may not only block access to the injury but also obscure the completed reconstruction on arteriography (Fig. 48–5). Repair of vascular injuries first is recommended, especially in patients with significant ischemia. This ap-

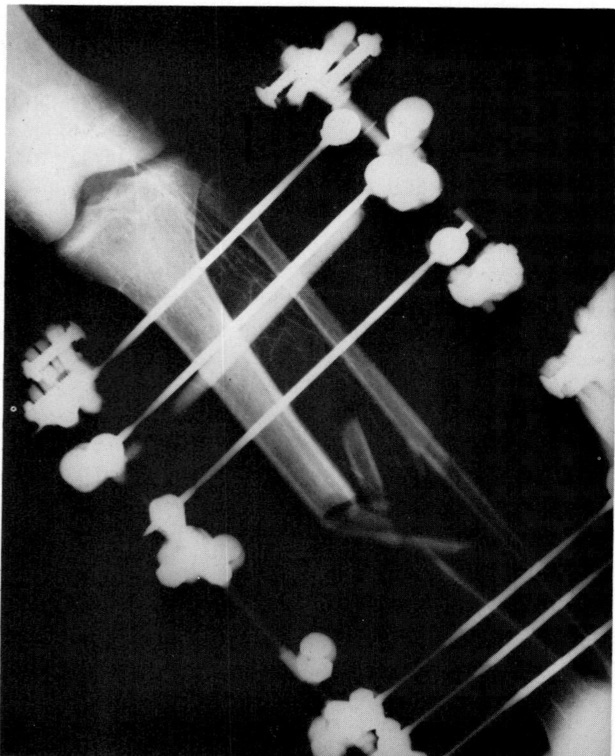

FIGURE 48–5. External fixation device (Roger-Anderson).

proach requires that the vascular surgeon remain in attendance during the orthopedic manipulation to ensure that the vascular repair is not exposed to excessive movement. Managed in this way, orthopedic manipulations disturbed fewer than 10 per cent of vascular repairs in a series of patients with popliteal artery injuries.[115] With the vascular surgeon in attendance, such complications are readily detected and corrected. Occasionally, an extremity is so shortened or a fracture so unstable that initial stabilization is mandatory. This situation is limited almost entirely to upper extremity injuries.

Thorough débridement of nonviable soft tissue and bone is extremely important. Infection commonly occurs in wounds with extensive soft tissue trauma, and this risk is best minimized by aggressive initial débridement. Fragments of clothing and other foreign material must be completely removed, and this is enhanced by copious irrigation with balanced salt solution. In the upper extremity, considerable lengths of bone and vessels can be sacrificed without impairing function, but this cannot be done with impunity in the lower extremity.[100]

Methods of Repair

The type of vessel injury and the extent of débridement required will determine which method of repair is best. Lateral repair is often satisfactory for minor lacerations and puncture wounds in large vessels. Autogenous patch angioplasty is chosen for minor injuries if lateral repair would compromise the lumen and if resection would necessitate an interposition graft. A small patch can often be obtained from an adjacent nonessential vein, thus avoiding interruption of the saphenous system. Most of today's violent injuries (i.e., gunshot wounds) require segmental arterial resection. After resection for low-velocity missile injury, an end-to-end vascular anastomosis is often feasible, but any difficulty in approximating the vessel ends without tension indicates the need for an interposition graft. The lumen size of the injured vessel usually dictates the choice of graft material—autogenous saphenous or cephalic vein is recommended by most authorities if the diameter of the injured vessel allows this choice although a few surgeons prefer prosthetic material.[59, 95, 125]

The vein is best taken from the side opposite the injury to preserve superficial venous flow on the injured side. The ipsilateral vein may be used if there is clearly no injury or disease in the deep venous system or if the distal vein is a satisfactory graft. The saphenous vein near the ankle is an excellent donor site if the lumen is sufficiently large. This site should be considered for patch grafts or for interposition grafts of the brachial, popliteal, and more distal arteries, preserving the proximal saphenous vein for whatever future needs might arise. The proximal vein is necessary for most major venous reconstructions. If a vein of suitable diameter is not available, and autogenous vein is essential, a panel or spiral graft may be constructed from the saphenous vein. The lumen size can be increased by 50 per cent by incising the vein vertically, dividing it in half transversely, and sewing the two pieces together. A catheter similar in diameter to the host vessel is used as a stent over which the graft is constructed, which makes the longitudinal anastomosis easier. A luminal diameter greater than twice the size of the saphenous can be obtained by spiral construction, as described by Chiu and coworkers.[13]

Interposition saphenous vein grafts are being used with increasing frequency in the reconstruction of vascular injuries. In reports from Cook County Hospital, this method was used in 62 per cent of 139 penetrating arterial injuries, including 81 per cent of popliteal wounds.[83] In the same institution, saphenous vein was used to reconstruct arterial injuries in 78 per cent with associated fractures and 90 per cent of those from shotgun wounds.[5, 70]

Mitchell and Thal reviewed an experience with 180 patients with saphenous vein graft reconstruction of 181 arterial injuries.[72] There were 22 graft-related complications (12 per cent), including 16 thromboses (9 per cent) and 7 graft infections (4 per cent). All infected grafts eventually ruptured, and this risk is one of the reasons why some surgeons recommend prosthetic grafts.

Prosthetic grafts have been proposed for reconstruction of arterial injuries in patients with inadequate venous autografts, to eliminate the time required to harvest saphenous vein and because of clinical experience and experimental data suggesting an increased resistance to infection. Before the late 1970s, prosthetic conduits were used infrequently in vascular trauma because of the fear of subsequent infection. Rich and Hughes reported complications in 20 of 26 injuries in which prosthetic material was used to repair contaminated vascular wounds.[95] Infection and thrombosis predominated, each occurring in nine patients. In most of these patients, infection progressed to anastomotic disruption and massive hemorrhage. A conflicting experience involving 122 interposition grafts equally divided between Dacron and autogenous vein was subsequently reported from Houston.[59] Perigraft infections developed in about 10 per cent of repairs with either type of material, but the autogenous vein grafts more frequently progressed to disruption and massive hemorrhage. These authors recommended using Dacron grafts in trauma patients because of data suggesting a lesser tendency for anastomotic disruption *if* infection occurs. Occasionally, large vessel grafts are required, and Dacron has been used successfully in this situation. Graft infections are uncommon but occur sufficiently often to suggest caution in using Dacron in contaminated areas.

Several experimental studies have demonstrated enhanced resistance to infection of polytetrafluoroethylene (PTFE) grafts.[106, 119] In studying animals contaminated with *Staphylococcus aureus* and not treated with antibiotics, Stone and coworkers found disruption in 86 per cent of veins and in only 28 per cent of PTFE grafts. Disruption occurred in the body of the vein graft but at the suture line in the PTFE grafts because of necrosis of the adjacent arterial wall. All animals treated with antibiotics had intact grafts when sacrificed 6 weeks postoperatively.[119]

PTFE was used for reconstruction of twenty arterial and five venous wounds by Shah and associates.[108] Most of the injuries were blunt but were open and potentially contaminated. One patient died and all but one of the arterial and one of the venous grafts were patent on clinical examination at up to 2 years follow-up. The authors emphasize the importance of placing the suture lines in healthy vascular tissue and covering them with viable muscle.

A large series of patients in whom PTFE was used to reconstruct arterial and venous wounds has been reported from Houston.[24] Two hundred and six arterial and 30 venous injuries were reconstructed with PTFE in 206 patients. Thirty-eight patients (18 per cent) had follow-up for an average of 25 months. The authors concluded that (1) PTFE is an acceptable prosthesis for arterial wounds, but long-term patency is less than with saphenous vein grafts. (2) Many occlusions occurred with 4-mm PTFE grafts inserted in brachial arteries, and this size graft is consequently not recommended. (3) Peripheral PTFE graft infection did not occur in the absence of exposure of the graft or of osteomyelitis. (4) Exposed PTFE grafts are easier to manage than exposed autogenous vein grafts, but delay in coverage will inevitably lead to occlusion, infection, or disruption of the graft-artery suture line. (5) PTFE grafts in proximal extremity veins usually occlude in the early postoperative period but are good temporary conduits that decrease hemorrhage in blast cavities and fasciotomy sites.

Autogenous vein continues to be the preferred conduit for the reconstruction of vascular injuries. PTFE is an acceptable substitute in patients with inadequate saphenous veins, those with severe or multiple injuries in whom the time needed to harvest autogenous vein may compromise results, and those with bilateral injuries in whom deep venous patency is in question.

The choice of suture material and anastomotic technique for repairing injured vessels is based on the same standards established for elective vascular surgery. The suture used is the smallest that will provide adequate tensile strength, and monofilament material such as polypropylene is less reactive and more hemostatic. To ensure intimal coaptation, a simple over-and-over suture technique is used, and normal vessel diameter is restored. Patency of vessels with diameters of 5 mm or less is enhanced by spatulation of the anastomosis as shown in Figure 48–6. Interrupted sutures are recommended in small vessels (less than 5 mm in diameter) and continuous techniques in larger vessels.

Removal of all intravascular thrombi before completion of the anastomosis reduces the incidence of early occlusion. A Fogarty catheter is gently passed proximally and distally through the nearly completed anastomosis to remove thrombus. Palpation of the balloon tip at the ankle or wrist, along with perception of a gentle pressure pulse when the distal segment is irrigated, serves as a "poor man's arteriogram." Routine arteriography on completion (*completion arteriography*) is ideal, although not always convenient, but it is especially important in managing injuries in which failure carries the greatest risk of amputation (e.g., injuries of the popliteal artery).

There are times when ligation rather than repair of injured arteries and veins is indicated. If the injured vessel is minor and expendable, ligation is preferable. A more important consideration, however, is the surgeon's assessment of the patient's overall condition relative to other injuries. Thus, it is sometimes advisable to ligate even a major vessel in a severely injured or deteriorating patient, accepting tissue loss in exchange for survival.[92]

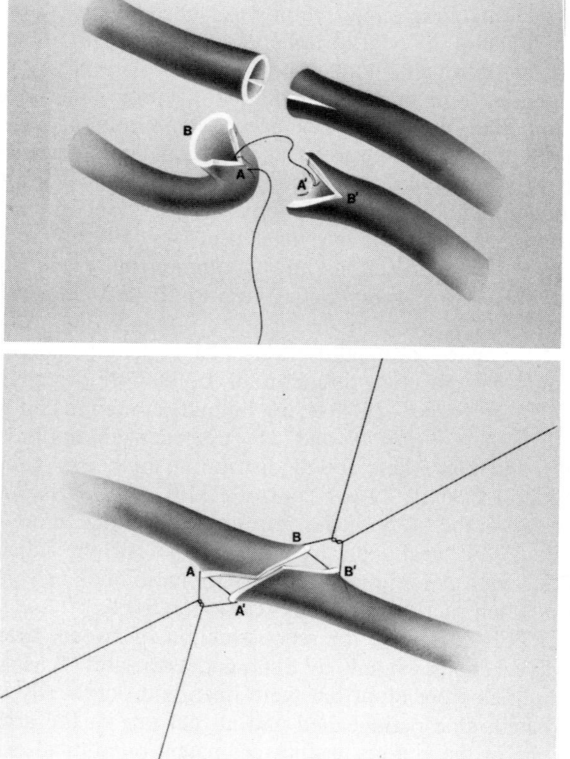

FIGURE 48–6. Spatulation technique for small-vessel anastomoses. The vessel ends are slit longitudinally and fashioned into a cobrahead shape.

Vein Injuries

Whether venous injuries are best treated by repair or by ligation remains controversial. Most authorities agree that simple venorrhaphies are indicated for injured, unpaired major veins. The controversy relates to complex venous reconstruction, especially in seriously injured patients who require extensive procedures for other injuries. The suggested benefits of repairing major venous injuries are (1) the successful repair of a concomitant arterial injury is enhanced by better outflow; (2) the likelihood of postoperative venous insufficiency is reduced; and (3) even transient patency of the venous repair may allow time for the development of collateral circulation.[84, 91, 96, 102] The crux of the problem is whether the patency of complex reconstructions is sufficiently frequent and prolonged to have an important effect on chronic venous insufficiency and whether this effect is worth a longer and more complicated procedure. Available data offer a partial answer, but the issue remains unsettled. It is axiomatic, however, that patient survival and repair of an adjacent arterial injury take precedence over any venous reconstruction.

Associated arterial injury is usually an indication for venous repair: venous ligation may impede outflow and compromise the patency of the arterial repair. Animal studies have demonstrated a transient (72 hours) reduction in arterial flow following venous ligation.[43] Clinical series suggest improved limb salvage after combined arterial and venous injuries of the lower extremity in those patients undergoing venous reconstruction.[89, 113, 120]

A reduction in lower extremity morbidity after repair

of venous injuries was demonstrated in Rich and associates' review of 110 patients with isolated popliteal vein injuries.[94] Operative treatment was almost equally divided between repairs and ligations; postoperative edema occurred in 51 per cent of ligated injuries but in only 13 per cent of those repaired. In long-term follow-up, chronic edema was present in 9 of 14 patients undergoing ligations but in only 3 of the 15 whose injuries were repaired. The long-term patency of repairs was documented by venography in 11 of the 12 patients studied.[94] Additional support for venous repair is provided by Agarwal and associates, who found postoperative edema in 50 per cent of patients with infrailiac venous injuries treated by ligations as compared with 7 per cent in those undergoing reconstructions.[3] Other authors have reported large series of patients in whom the incidence of lower extremity edema was similar whether the venous injuries were ligated or repaired.[40, 123] Such conflicting data have stimulated objective studies of the results of venous reconstructions for trauma.

Several reports provide data concerning the patency rate of venous repairs and the relationship of patency to symptomatic venous insufficiency. Meyer and associates prospectively studied 36 patients with venous injuries of the extremities who underwent repair and had postoperative studies to determine patency.[71] The patency of repair was evaluated by clinical examination, impedence plethysmography, Doppler ultrasonography, and contrast venography. No amputations were required. Venography, performed on the 7th postoperative day, demonstrated venous repairs to be patent in 22 (61 per cent) and occluded in 14 extremities. Local venous repair, including lateral venorrhaphy, end-to-end anastomosis, and patch venoplasty, had a significantly higher patency rate (79 per cent) than interposition vein grafts (41 per cent) ($p < .03$). Compared with venography, accuracy in the assessment of venous patency was 67 per cent by clinical evaluation and 53 per cent by noninvasive studies. At 3-month follow-up, mild lower extremity edema was present in 2 of 14 patients with occluded repairs, compared with no edema in the 22 patients whose repairs were initially patent ($p > .05$).

Borman and associates reviewed 82 infrailiac venous injuries; 38 were treated with simple repair, 36 required complex reconstructions, and 7 required ligation.[7] Venography was performed postoperatively in 41 patients with repaired injuries; 26 had patent repairs (63 per cent), and 15 were occluded. Seventy-four per cent of the simple repairs were patent, compared with 54 per cent of the complex reconstructions. Outpatient follow-up was available for 36 patients whose repairs were documented by venography, including 23 patients with patent repairs and 13 with occlusions. Asymptomatic extremities were more frequent in patients with patent repairs (74 per cent) than in those whose repairs had occluded (38 per cent). Edema or postphlebitic changes were present during late follow-up in 13 per cent of extremities with patent repairs, 23 per cent with occluded repairs, and 40 per cent of those treated by ligations.

The repair of lower extremity venous injuries from blunt trauma is especially important, according to Ross and associates' experience with 22 patients.[101] Postoperative edema did not occur in the 5 patients with patent venous repairs. In contrast, 6 of 7 patients having ligations or whose repairs were occluded had postoperative vascular compromise or edema. Venous repair and early complete fasciotomies are recommended in patients with such injuries because of the associated soft tissue injury and occlusion of lymphatic and venous collateral pathways.

The potential for long-term patency and continued normal valvular function in injured veins undergoing repair has been infrequently documented. Such data are available for five patients with reconstructions of six venous injuries, between 6 and 20 years postoperatively.[88] Patency was documented by venography in five of the six repairs, including two lateral venorrhaphies, two saphenous vein interposition grafts, and one end-to-end anastomosis. Normal valvular function was demonstrated by exercise venography in all five patent reconstructions. The only occluded repair was a Teflon graft of an injured common femoral vein inserted 20 years previously. All five patients with patent repairs had intact and asymptomatic extremities, but postphlebitic changes were present in the limb with the occluded repair.

The reviewed data support the value of repair of venous injuries, including complex reconstructions, in selected patients with major injuries, especially of the lower extremity. The incidence of postoperative thrombophlebitis and pulmonary embolism is not increased by the repair of venous injuries. Limb salvage after combined arterial and venous injuries is not influenced by occlusion of venous reconstruction. Documentation of the patency of venous repairs requires contrast venography. Early postoperative patency is present in about 75 per cent of local venous repairs, but in only one half of more complex reconstructions.[7, 71] The sequelae of venous insufficiency appear to be reduced by even short-term patency. Although few patients with venous repairs have undergone late venography, continued patency and normal valvular function have been shown to be possible.

The morbidity from venous ligation is due to muscle edema resulting from acute venous hypertension and from the late development of venous insufficiency. The extent of venous hypertension following ligation is dependent upon the amount of collateral venous flow. Stahl suggests that a pressure of 35 cm or less of saline distal to an occluded superficial femoral vein indicates adequate collateral flow and acute venous hypertension will not occur.[117]

Ligation of a major extremity vein may cause a rapid increase in muscle compartment pressure that further compromises venous and arterial flow. Early fasciotomy is an important adjunct in reducing the acute morbidity of venous ligation. In a report of infrailiac venous injuries, compartment syndromes developed in 37 per cent of patients with combined proximal venous and arterial injuries compared with 5 per cent of those with isolated arterial injuries.[3] For this reason, fasciotomies are recommended in most patients with combined arterial and venous injuries of the femoral and popliteal vessels.

Veins are less forgiving than arteries in regard to technical precision of repair. Thrombosis can be expected unless vein repairs are virtually perfect and lumen size is preserved. Intimal coaptation is particularly important, and special care is necessary to ensure that no adventitial tissue intrudes into the lumen. Vessel manipulation and clamp occlusion must be performed gently because endothelial damage predisposes to delayed thrombosis.[57] Encircling the vessel with latex loops to control bleeding during repair may cause less endothelial damage than vascular clamps. The importance of balloon catheter thrombectomy and intraoperative venography during the repair of venous injuries is suggested by data presented in a study by Borman and associates. Postoperative venograms demonstrated intraluminal thrombi, separate from the site of repair, in 25 per cent of patients undergoing venous repairs.[7]

Late morbidity from venous stasis after venous ligation may be decreased by prolonged postoperative elevation to reduce edema formation. In Mullins and coworkers' report, persistent edema requiring external support occurred in only 4 of 21 patients after ligations of injured femoral veins.[77] Additional measures that may reduce venous stasis morbidity after venous ligation or repair include intermittent pneumatic calf compression and low-molecular-weight dextran.[44] Although it is reasonable to assume that postoperative anticoagulation might enhance the patency of venous repair and promote collateral flow, there are no data supporting this contention.

The surgeon's first objective in treating venous injuries is to prevent exsanguination. The choice between ligation and repair is based on the severity of associated injuries and the general condition of the patient, the technical complexity of reconstruction, and the potential for collateral venous return in the area involved. The indications for complex venous reconstructions remain controversial. Patients in whom venous injury or its ligation has resulted in obvious venous hypertension and stable patients whose arterial reconstructions have not been especially prolonged or complicated usually are candidates for these procedures. Further studies are needed to define optimal treatment methods for venous injuries, and these should include measurements of venous and compartmental pressures as well as phlebographic documentation of results.[7, 34, 71]

The appropriate management of isolated asymptomatic venous injuries has likewise not been delineated. If an extremity requires exploration for other reasons and such an injury is found, the previously described principles pertain. However, until more is known about the long-term effects of untreated isolated venous injuries that are asymptomatic, it does not seem reasonable to recommend routine diagnostic venography and subsequent operative repair.

Adjunctive Measures

Vasodilatation

Spasm is rarely the sole cause of severe ischemia in patients with vascular trauma: it should never be accepted as the explanation for a circulatory deficit from trauma unless an occlusion has been excluded. Spasm of muscular vessels does occur after arterial injury and operative repair. This is the result of sustained smooth muscle contraction, unrelated to the autonomic nervous system, and is not affected by pharmacologic or operative sympatholysis. Spasm is best overcome by direct gentle dilatation by means of intraluminal injections of balanced salt solution against the resistance of compression applied distal to the spasm. Alternatively, graded dilators or balloon-tipped catheters may be used. The direct application of pharmacologic agents has been advocated, but most appear to be ineffective. Topical application of a 20 per cent solution of magnesium sulfate or a 2.5 per cent solution of papavarine has occasionally been considered successful.[1, 85]

Intra-arterial infusion of tolazoline (Priscoline) has been used by angiographers to increase peripheral vasodilatation. This drug is an alpha-adrenergic blocker; it has a direct relaxant effect on smooth muscle and opens precapillary arteriovenous shunts. It acts by competitively blocking the vasoconstrictive receptors in the arterial wall, which results in vasodilatation. This effect is of no nutritional benefit but increases flow and thereby lessens stasis and thrombosis. Selective intra-arterial infusion has been successfully used to improve distal flow in traumatized ischemic extremities after large-vessel reconstruction and fracture reduction.[18] Before tolazoline is infused, vascular patency should be confirmed arteriographically and compartmental hypertension excluded as the cause of diminished arterial flow.

Peck and coworkers have reported 15 patients with extremity ischemia related to severe distal arterial injuries that persisted after angiographically patent arterial reconstructions.[86] A catheter was inserted intraoperatively through a small branch of the common femoral artery and tolazoline solution (500 mg tolazoline with 1000 units of heparin in 1 liter of normal saline) delivered by constant infusion pump. Distal vascular perfusion was restored in 13 patients (87 per cent), and 10 limbs (67 per cent) were salvaged.

Soft Tissue Coverage

At the conclusion of the vascular repair, it is important that the soft tissue be closed over the vessel. This may be difficult to achieve in patients with widespread soft tissue damage, but the vessel *must be covered* with muscle or skin. Musculocutaneous flaps are occasionally needed, and operative planning should include preservation of muscle groups with intact neurovascular supply for use in covering the repair. Porcine heterograft and homograft skin are suggested alternatives for covering the vascular repair when adjacent soft tissue is inadequate.[60] It is often difficult to predict the extent of muscle necrosis at the initial operation, and an early "second look" in the operating room after 24 to 48 hours is often useful.[58] In extensive or severely contaminated wounds, an extra-anatomic bypass, routed through clean tissue planes, may circumvent problems with soft tissue coverage.

Fasciotomy

Increased compartmental pressure from muscle edema frequently complicates vascular injuries, especially in the lower extremity, and may threaten tissue viability or impede successful vascular reconstruction. The edema may be caused by direct trauma, by proximal venous occlusion, or by the reperfusion of ischemic muscle. Operative decompression of the fascial compartments effectively reverses this process, if performed before myoneural necrosis has occurred. The clinical problems of compartmental hypertension accompanying vascular injuries of the extremities are delayed diagnosis and incomplete operative decompression of all four compartments.

Pain is an important symptom of compartmental hypertension, but it is often present in the trauma patient as a result of other causes. Pain on stretching of uninjured muscles is strongly suggestive. The physical findings of reversible compartmental hypertension are often subtle and may be overlooked without careful and repeated examinations. The loss of palpable pulses, capillary refill, and Doppler flow signals are late findings, usually indicating irreversible damage. Earlier signs include the loss of light touch, hypoesthesia on the dorsum of the first interdigital cleft of the foot, decreased motor function, and swelling or increased tissue tension on palpation. A measured increase in intracompartmental pressure may be helpful, especially in unreliable or unresponsive patients or those with a nerve deficit from another cause.[74]

The early recognition of compartmental hypertension may be difficult in patients with severely injured extremities. In patients with obvious arterial injuries causing ischemia, in whom the distal extremity is swollen and tense preoperatively, immediate fascial decompression is indicated before beginning the vascular exploration. Relieving the acutely elevated intracompartmental pressure may improve collateral blood flow and improve tissue viability until main channel flow can be reestablished by vascular reconstruction. However, most patients with arterial injuries of the extremities do not have initial evidence of compartmental hypertension. Many of them develop the problem intraoperatively after the restoration of flow or in the early postoperative period. To obviate the difficult diagnosis of reversible compartmental hypertension and avoid the risk of compromising vascular repairs, criteria have evolved to select, for "early" or prophylactic fasciotomies, patients most likely to develop compartmental hypertension. These criteria include prolonged hypotension, an extended period of compromised flow (4 to 6 hours) between injury and repair, combined arterial and venous injuries, severe distal soft tissue trauma, and distal limb swelling.[87]

Methods to prevent compartmental hypertension may be useful in patients with arterial injuries. Experimental studies have suggested that infusing hypertonic mannitol decreases the edema resulting from the reperfusion of ischemic muscle and reduces the incidence of compartmental hypertension.[10] The clinical efficacy of this technique has been demonstrated in a series of 30 patients with blunt popliteal vascular injuries.[109] Fasciotomies were required in 9 of 14 patients not receiving mannitol, but were necessary in only 2 of 16 patients in whom hypertonic mannitol was infused before flow was restored. One hundred milliliters of 20 per cent mannitol was given as an intravenous bolus immediately before flow was restored, and this was followed by a constant infusion of 10 gm of mannitol an hour for 6 to 24 hours.[10]

If fasciotomy is not performed "early" as a part of the initial procedure, the extremity must be carefully observed for evidence of increasing compartment pressure and circulatory compromise.[87] Monitoring compartmental pressures during the operation and in the early postoperative period may be useful in reaching a decision to perform fasciotomy.[77] Mubarak and coworkers have demonstrated the efficacy of the wick technique for monitoring intracompartmental pressures and suggest that a pressure greater than 30 cm of water indicates the need for fasciotomy.[74, 76] These methods appear to be valid if proper technique is followed and only normal pressures are accepted. In the authors' opinion, liberal indications for fasciotomies during the initial operation are appropriate because the morbidity resulting from the failure to perform a needed fasciotomy is greater than that caused by the procedure itself.

The subtlety of the diagnostic signs of intracompartmental hypertension demand that the emphasis of operative technique should be on complete decompression of all compartments. There are several alternative procedures for lower extremity fasciotomy, all of which provide good decompression if performed properly. The three techniques most frequently described are combined lateral and medial incisions, a lateral incision with perifibular release, and a lateral incision combined with fibulectomy.[75, 78, 99] Although some civilian injuries may be adequately decompressed through limited skin incisions, complete and dependable four-quadrant fasciotomy requires full skin incisions.

The four compartments of the leg—anterior, lateral, superficial posterior, and deep posterior—at about the level of the mid-calf, are illustrated in Figure 48–7. The anterior compartment contains the anterior tibial nerve and vessels and is the one most prone to damage from muscle edema. The lateral compartment contains the superficial peroneal nerve and is bounded by anterior and posterior intermuscular or crural septa. The superficial posterior compartment contains the gastrocnemius and soleus muscles. The deep posterior compartment is dorsal to the interosseous membrane, contains the posterior tibial nerve and vessels and the peroneal vessels, and is the one most often missed or incompletely decompressed.

In the technique most commonly used, bilateral skin incisions are made to gain entrance into the four compartments (Fig. 48–7).[75] The anterior and lateral compartments are decompressed through a 20- to 25-cm incision midway between the fibula and tibial crest (this is approximately over the anterior intermuscular septum, which separates the anterior and lateral compartments). The anterior compartment fascia is incised longitudinally. By making a transverse incision in the anterior septum, the adjacent superficial peroneal nerve can be identified as it courses distally in the lateral compartment, penetrating the deep fascia between the peroneus longus and brevis muscles, assuming a subcutaneous position. Injury of the nerve should be avoided when making the incision in the investing fascia of the lateral compartment.

The superficial and deep posterior compartments are then approached through a medial incision of similar length, placed 2 cm posterior to the tibial margin to avoid injuring the saphenous vein. Once the fascia is reached, the subcutaneous tissue is reflected anteriorally, protecting the saphenous vein to the posterior tibial margin. The deep posterior compartment is entered and incised through the attachment of the soleus muscle, immediately behind the tibial border. The fascia of the superficial posterior compartment is then incised, posterior and parallel to the incision in the deep compartment.

Another technique is the perifibular fasciotomy, which is performed through a single anterolateral incision, similar to that described for the bilateral incision technique.[78, 99] The lateral compartment is initially decompressed as previously described. The peroneus muscles are then retracted

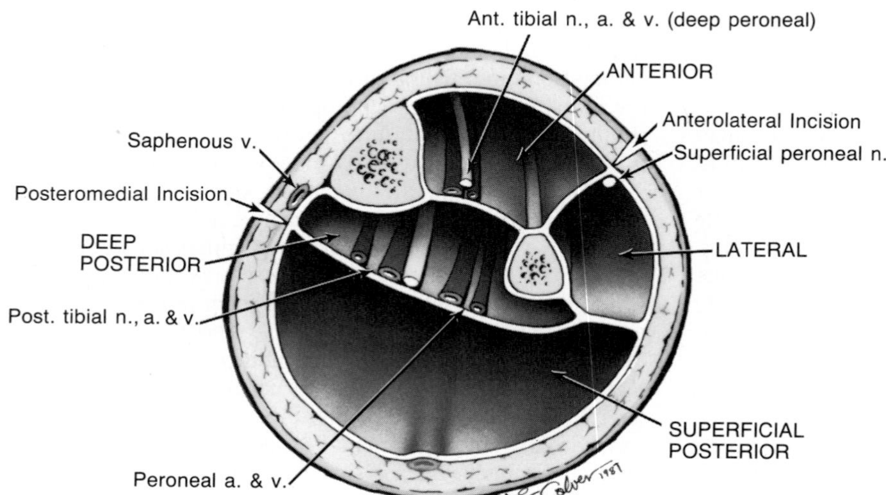

FIGURE 48–7. Fascial compartments of the leg.

anteriorally and the fascia overlying the soleus and gastrocnemius muscles (posterior intermuscular septum) is incised vertically to open the superficial posterior compartment.

A skin and subcutaneous tissue flap is then raised anteromedially, and the anterior compartmental fascia is opened. The deep posterior compartment can be approached ventrally by medially reflecting the muscles of the anterior compartment and incising the fibular attachment of the interosseus membrane, or dorsally by incising the fibular attachment of the soleus and reflecting the soleus and gastrocnemius posteriorally. If the dorsal approach is used, the intermuscular septum between the superficial and deep compartments is incised longitudinally. With either route, care is required to avoid injuring the peroneal vessels on the posteromedial aspect of the fibula.

Forearm compartmental hypertension is decompressed through a skin incision beginning proximal to the antecubital fossa and extending into the palm. Important areas of fascial release in the volar forearm include the lacertus fibrosus, the proximal edges of the pronator teres and the superficial flexor muscles, and the carpal tunnel. The fascial envelopes of the radial and dorsal extensor muscles are longitudinally opened through the volar skin incision by undermining the subcutaneous tissue on the radial aspect of the forearm.[74]

Once the swelling has subsided, the skin incisions can frequently be closed in a delayed primary fashion, or it may be necessary to apply a split-thickness skin graft. Avoidance of a skin graft for closure is not a justification for a limited skin incision.

Anticoagulants

Distal small vessel thrombosis may prevent the successful reconstruction of injured arteries, especially in areas without good collateral blood flow. Early administration of systemic anticoagulants may reduce distal thrombosis and should be considered in peripheral injuries with diminished distal circulation. Anticoagulants are contraindicated in patients with neurologic and ophthalmic injuries and in those with multiple wounds and major fractures. When appropriate, heparin is administered intravenously as soon as occlusion is suspected in isolated peripheral vascular injuries. Because of the short half-life of heparin (90 minutes), its effect is not reversed with protamine at the completion of the procedure unless there is diffuse bleeding. Local or regional heparin infusion may be useful in injured patients with poor collateral flow in whom systemic anticoagulation is contraindicated. A 1:10 solution of heparin and saline cooled to 4°C is intermittently infused into the distal arterial tree during the vascular reconstruction.

Anticoagulation is not used postoperatively after repair of arterial injuries. If arterial reconstruction is technically competent, there is no need for postoperative anticoagulation; if the repair is technically imprecise, no amount of heparin will sustain patency. The role of anticoagulation in venous reconstruction for trauma is controversial, but, based primarily on experience with deep venous thrombosis, anticoagulants are often used for 6 weeks after repair of venous injuries. If extracellular volume has been replaced with blood and electrolyte solutions, there is usually no need for other rheologic agents.[87, 122]

POSTOPERATIVE COMPLICATIONS

Patients with peripheral vascular injuries must be observed closely in the postoperative period. Thrombotic occlusion and bleeding are the two most common early complications—both require immediate reoperation. Patients are best monitored postoperatively by physical and Doppler ultrasound examinations. Arteriography is performed only for specific indications. Postoperative swelling may compromise the circulation, especially if fasciotomy has not been performed. Perception of light touch and normal motor function are good indicators of adequate perfusion, but extremity skin temperature and color may be misleading. Because of the greater blood flow requirements of muscle and nerves, it is possible to have an envelope of viable skin surrounding a necrotic muscle mass. Unexplained fever, tachycardia, or distal sensory or motor deficits may be caused by nerve or muscle ischemia. To exclude this possibility, it may be necessary to incise the skin and fascia and directly inspect the underlying muscle.

Infection is a serious threat to the patient with a vascular injury and often suggests residual necrotic tissue. The aggressive management of infection, with early drainage of pus, débridement, and appropriate antibiotic therapy, is mandatory. Inability to control the septic process may endanger both the vascular repair and the patient's life. Exsanguinating hemorrhage can occur if an infected anastomosis becomes disrupted.

False aneurysm, arteriovenous fistula, hemorrhage, and occlusion may occur as late complications of vascular injuries. These are best managed by operative intervention, which usually requires resection and either a primary repair or an interposition bypass graft.[93] They are discussed in detail in Chapters 83 and 88.

MANAGEMENT OF SPECIFIC INJURIES

Upper Extremity Vascular Injuries

The vascular injuries of the upper extremity discussed here are those distal to the lateral border of the first rib and include the axillary, brachial, radial, and ulnar arteries and adjacent veins.[8, 16, 20, 52, 82, 87] Brachiocephalic vascular injuries are discussed in Chapter 47.

Upper extremity injuries constitute 30 to 40 per cent of peripheral vascular injuries. Penetrating trauma is the predominant cause, although blunt trauma with adjacent skeletal injury occasionally produces axillary or brachial arterial injuries. Complications of arterial catheterizations for diagnostic studies are the most common cause of distal brachial artery injuries.

The reported incidence of limb loss from upper extremity arterial injuries has varied from 0 to 40 per cent, depending on the vessel involved, the type of injury, and the mode of treatment.[2, 8, 16, 82, 87] Sequelae of associated neurologic injuries account for most of the late morbidity. The anatomic characteristics that influence upper extremity arterial injuries and their treatment are the relative lack of protection from overlying bone or muscle, the high frequency of adjacent nerve and skeletal trauma, the extensive collateral blood supply, and the infrequency of significant sequelae from venous ligation. The superficial course of most of the upper extremity arterial tree makes the diagnosis of injury and the operative exposure for control and repair less complicated than for lower extremity injuries. Hemorrhage can usually be readily controlled with external pressure. The rich collateral circulation frequently maintains limb viability despite arterial occlusion; distal pulses are preserved in at least 20 per cent of upper extremity arterial wounds. In a civilian series comprising 269 injuries, definite signs of arterial trauma were present preoperatively in almost 90 per cent of brachial, radial, and ulnar arteries, but in only two thirds of axillary injuries.[8] Isolated arterial injuries were uncommon (18 per cent); associated injuries involved adjacent nerves, bones, veins, or soft tissue in 73 per cent. Amputations were required in 1.5 per cent of injured extremities and serious neurologic deficits persisted in 27 per cent.

The operative techniques used for upper extremity vascular injuries are essentially the same as those used for other injured vessels. The prepared operative field should include the major arterial trunk proximal to the suspected site of injury, to allow vascular control and the injection of contrast material, and the entire extremity distally for evaluation of pulses and for changing position to improve exposure. For proximal injuries, the supraclavicular area and chest are included in the prepared field, although thoracotomy is infrequently required.[8]

Axillary Vessels

Most axillary arterial injuries are due to penetrating trauma, although repeated damage from improper use of crutches and proximal humeral fractures or dislocations are occasional causes. The axillary artery is a continuation of the subclavian artery, extending from the lateral border of the first rib to the inferior margin of the teres major muscle, where it becomes the brachial artery. Its 6-inch length is divided into three segments by the pectoralis minor muscle. The cords of the brachial plexus surround the axillary artery, explaining the frequently associated peripheral nerve injuries. The amputation rate after ligation of injured axillary arteries varied from 8.8 per cent in Makins' World War I report to 43.2 per cent in World War II injuries.[16] Amputations followed 3 per cent of civilian injuries in one series.[8]

Diagnosis and Initial Management. The physical signs suggesting axillary artery injury are listed in Table 48–1. Distal perfusion and palpable pulses are often maintained because of the rich collateral network about the shoulder. Arteriography requires special attention to the details of performance and interpretation. The spatial relationships of the course of the axillary artery and the overlying bone can interfere with arteriographic visualization, and minor defects can be obscured by the numerous overlying branches. Arteriography is indicated in any patient with a skeletal injury near the shoulder in whom a distal circulatory deficit is observed initially despite the return of adequate perfusion after orthopedic manipulation. It should be remembered that patients with injuries from a single traumatic event or from repeated low-grade damage from improperly used crutches may present subsequently with a palpable axillary aneurysm, distal emboli, or thrombosis.

The initial management of axillary artery injuries does not differ significantly from the principles previously outlined for other peripheral arterial injuries. Hemorrhage can usually be controlled by external pressure; wounds should not be locally explored with fingers or instruments. Blind application of clamps to stop hemorrhage is particularly dangerous in axillary artery wounds because of the risk of damaging adjacent nerves.

Operative Technique. Repair of axillary vascular injuries is indicated because it minimizes the risk of ischemia and provides optimal late extremity function. If concomitant problems mandate arterial ligation, it is most safely performed immediately proximal to a major patent branch in order to maintain collateral flow and avoid an adjacent cul-de-sac. Venous ligation infrequently results in serious problems, but repair is preferable.

Axillary vessel injuries are best approached with the arm abducted 90 degrees and externally rotated; hyperabduction may stretch and injure the brachial plexus and should be avoided. The incision is made along the lower border of the clavicle, beginning at its mid-portion and extending over the pectoralis major insertion to the anteromedial upper arm. The mid-portion of the incision is curved laterally to avoid crossing the axillary fold. The axillary fascia is incised, and the pectoralis major and minor muscles are divided near their insertions, the tendon of the pectoralis major being carefully preserved for reapproximation.[4, 12, 98] Abundant collateral flow often prevents complete control of axillary artery injuries by proximal and distal clamping; a direct approach to the injury is usually more expedient. However, when the need for more proximal exposure is anticipated, horizontal extension of the incision with medial resection of the clavicle is carried out, allowing the distal subclavian artery to be controlled. Distal control can be obtained by first exposing the proximal brachial artery before the pectoralis muscles are transected. Exposure is completed by dividing the coracoid attachment of the pectoralis minor and the humeral insertion of the pectoralis major muscles.

The principles of vascular reconstruction for trauma have already been described and do not differ for the axillary vessels. Muscular compartmental hypertension is infrequently a problem in the upper extremity, but fasciotomies may be needed in patients with prolonged ischemia and combined arterial and venous wounds. If venous ligation is necessary, postoperative elevation of the extremity is important to decrease edema.

Brachial Vessels

Owing in part to frequent iatrogenic trauma, the brachial artery is the most commonly injured artery and accounts for 20 to 30 per cent of peripheral arterial injuries.[87] Most brachial artery injuries are from penetrating trauma; many follow catheterizations for diagnostic studies. Injuries are occasionally seen with supracondylar fractures of the humerus and with posterior elbow dislocations.[35]

The brachial artery begins as a continuation of the axillary artery at the lateral margin of the teres major muscle and terminates by dividing into the radial and ulnar arteries about an inch distal to the antecubital skin crease. The deep brachial and the superior and inferior ulnar collateral arteries are the three major branches of the brachial artery in the arm. These vessels provide collateral flow to the distal extremity through a network about the elbow, much as the deep femoral artery functions in the thigh. The contribution of the deep brachial artery to distal collateral flow is reflected in a doubling of the amputation rate after ligation above compared with ligation below its origin. The amputation rate was 42.9 per cent following ligation and 4.7 per cent after repair of brachial artery injuries in Vietnam.[92] This high amputation rate reflects the influence of extensive soft tissue injuries and the destruction of collateral channels in this area. In contrast, one amputation was required in a civilian series of 142 brachial artery injuries.[8]

Operative Technique. Exposure is gained through an incision along the medial aspect of the arm in the groove between the biceps and triceps muscles. If the wound is conveniently located, it can be extended and incorporated into the incision. Once the neurovascular sheath is entered, care is taken to protect the median nerve crossing the brachial artery from lateral to medial.[4, 12, 98] Exposure near the elbow is best obtained through a vertical incision that briefly traverses the crease in the antecubital space horizontally before continuing again vertically down the forearm across the brachial artery bifurcation.

Proximal and distal vascular control is obtained first, the injury is identified, and the adjacent vessel is dissected free. If the extremity is ischemic, thrombus is extracted with a balloon-tipped catheter. An intraluminal shunt can be inserted if remote injuries require priority treatment or an unstable humeral fracture exists. Unstable upper extremity fractures often require reduction and fixation *before* the vascular reconstruction because of the lack of muscle bulk to assist stabilization and the substantial shortening that often exists.

Sufficient mobilization to perform end-to-end anastomoses is often possible, but if it is not, the cephalic vein or saphenous vein near the ankle provides appropriate interposition grafts. The brachial vein is often paired, in which case ligation of one injured vein is appropriate. Repair is recommended for injured single veins if it can be accomplished simply. Upper extremity collateral venous flow is usually adequate and symptomatic venous stasis is uncommon.

Complications of Brachial Artery Catheterization. Brachial artery catheterization for arteriography and cardiac studies frequently is the cause of arterial trauma. The reported incidence of these complications varies from less than 1 per cent to more than 30 per cent, but most institutions report a 2 to 3 per cent complication rate.[124] Factors contributing to brachial artery complications are repeat catheterizations, prolonged procedures, catheter change, brachial artery atherosclerosis, improper arteriotomy closure, inexperienced cardiologist, female patient, and failure to use heparin.[64] Usually there is an immediate loss of wrist pulses, but the pulses may disappear several hours after the procedure. The obstruction often results from a thrombotic occlusion secondary to intimal damage, but it may also result from adherent clot that was stripped off the catheter during its removal.[9]

The intimal damage is usually on the posterior arterial wall at or near (0.5 to 15 mm proximal) the puncture or arteriotomy site.[9, 50] The natural history of these lesions has been well described, and if they are treated nonoperatively, tissue loss is unusual, but late effort-related symptoms occur in 20 to 40 per cent of patients.[67, 79, 124] Because delayed symptoms are frequent, operative treatment is recommended for all patients in whom repair does not present a prohibitive risk.[79]

The operation usually can be performed with local anesthesia and consists of catheter thrombectomy and excision of damaged intima. The site of intimal damage should be diligently sought, focusing on the frequent site of catheter-related damage on the posterior wall at or just proximal to the entry site.[50] Resection and end-to-end anastomosis are often required and are usually successful. The extent of intimal damage necessitated resection in two-thirds of patients in one large series, one-third of whom required saphenous vein interposition grafts for reconstruction.[64] Vein grafts are necessary in most patients undergoing delayed reconstructions for *late* ischemic symptoms.

Radial and Ulnar Arterial Injuries

Injuries of the radial and ulnar arteries constitute 15 to 20 per cent of civilian peripheral vascular trauma, and in one large series of upper extremity arterial wounds, they accounted for more than 40 per cent of the injuries.[8] Almost all are penetrating injuries. Inadvertent intra-arterial injection of drugs has become more common, and this can cause a diffuse necrosis of the distal artery that is not amenable to operative treatment (see Chapter 45).

Borman and colleagues reported one amputation in 17 patients (6 per cent) with combined radial and ulnar artery injuries; the overall amputation rate for radial or ulnar artery injuries was less than 1 per cent.[8]

The management of injuries of the arteries of the forearm is based on knowledge of the unique anatomy and physiology of this region. Because of the rich collateral arterial flow through the palmar arches, both wrist pulses are often present after wounds of a single artery in the forearm, and acute ischemia is very uncommon. Typically, the superficial arch is a continuation of the ulnar artery, and the deep and dorsal arches are formed by the radial artery. The superficial and deep arches are complete in 80 and 97 per cent of hands, respectively.[14]

Diagnosis and Initial Management. Both wrist pulses are often palpable, and ischemia is uncommon after wounds of either the radial or ulnar arteries. Injuries causing obstruction can be confirmed by demonstrating a pulse deficit with digital occlusion of the opposite vessel. A modification of this so-called Allen test can be performed with a directional Doppler. Normally flow is antegrade and is augmented by collateral artery compression. If the artery is obstructed proximally, flow will be retrograde and diminished by compression of the companion artery (see Chapter 5). Nonobstructing injuries may only be suspected because of a penetrating forearm wound. The need to submit all such patients to exclusion arteriography has not been substantiated. In patients with normal distal flow, the main concern is the later manifestations of false aneurysms or arteriovenous fistulae. However, the small caliber and superficial position of the forearm arteries reduce the morbid consequences of these late complications. For these reasons, the selective management of asymptomatic penetrating wounds of the forearm requires individualization based on the severity of the wound, associated adjacent or remote injuries, and available facilities.

Operative Treatment. Radial or ulnar arterial injuries that cause acute ischemia require immediate reconstruction. Continued bleeding, arteriovenous fistulae, or false aneurysms also require prompt operation. Ligation is only permissible for isolated radial or ulnar injuries with evident good collateral flow. Ischemic risk is increased by incomplete palmar arches and anatomic anomalies, which are found in 9 per cent of extremities.[31] The safety of forearm artery ligation should be confirmed by some form of Allen test or may be evident from arteriography. The management of isolated asymptomatic forearm arterial injuries with good collateral flow presents a dilemma. Unrepaired injuries cause identifiable alterations in hand vascularity, but signs of ischemia or cold intolerance are infrequent.[32] If palmar arch patency is unknown, restitution of flow is advisable.[33] If there is good collateral circulation through the palmar arches, it is usually safe to ligate either the radial or ulnar arteries,[87] but if other injuries do not require priority treatment, primary revascularization is appropriate. This may prevent ischemic symptoms in some patients, and in the event of later injury or the need for hemodialysis, two patent wrist vessels are helpful.

The proximal radial artery is exposed through an antecubital incision that crosses the fossa transversely and extends distally along the radial aspect of the forearm. The mid and distal radial artery is exposed through an incision along the medial border of the brachioradialis muscle. The proximal ulnar artery can be exposed through the sigmoid-shaped antecubital incision. The distal two thirds is exposed through an incision that begins four finger-breadths distal to the medial epicondyle and follows the lateral border of the flexor carpi ulnaris to the pisiform. The ulnar neurovascular bundle is exposed between the superficial flexor muscles and the flexor carpi ulnaris.

The technique of repair of these small vessels is more demanding than that required for larger vessels. Loupes providing two to three times magnification, vessel dilatation, interrupted fine suture technique, and spatulation of the anastomoses are important principles.

An additional, though uncommon, problem with penetrating forearm injuries is continued bleeding, which may result in compartmental hypertension and Volkmann's ischemic contracture. If not explored, these injuries require careful observation for signs of neurovascular compression.[121]

Lower Extremity Vascular Injuries

The injuries described here lie distal to the inguinal ligament and include the femoral, popliteal, and tibioperoneal arteries and adjacent veins. (More proximal injuries are discussed in Chapter 46.) They account for approximately two-thirds of arterial wounds on the battlefield and one-third of civilian injuries. Most lower extremity vascular trauma is penetrating, although at least 15 to 20 per cent of civilian wounds distal to the common femoral artery result from blunt trauma. Distal ischemia is the predominant problem—hemorrhage can usually be controlled with external pressure. The possibility of a penetrating arterial injury is suggested by a wound in proximity to a major vessel and further supported by the signs listed in Table 48–1. However, diagnostic persistence is necessary to avoid overlooking blunt arterial injuries as well as those involving the profunda femoris and the tibioperoneal vessels from any cause. Preoperative arteriography is beneficial in the management of these injuries, especially those arising from blunt trauma, and is usually essential in order to diagnose profunda femoral and tibioperoneal arterial wounds. In addition, when time and facilities permit, venography may be helpful because of the morbid potential of lower extremity venous injuries and their thromboembolic sequelae.[8, 34]

The reconstruction of most injured lower extremity arteries is strongly recommended. As discussed above, some authors suggest nonoperative management of minor injuries in selected patients. The detection and repair of venous injuries is more important in the lower extremity than in other sites. Venous hypertension resulting from ligation or thrombotic occlusion may adversely affect the success of arterial reconstruction, and the late morbidity from venous stasis is substantial.[94, 96] Timely and complete fasciotomy also is more important for limb salvage in the lower extremity than in the upper.

Groin and Thigh Wounds

Common femoral arterial injuries constitute less than 5 per cent, superficial femoral 15 to 20 per cent, and deep femoral about 2 per cent of peripheral arterial wounds.[16, 87, 92] Most injuries of the common femoral artery are caused by penetrating trauma, but, depending on the population studied, 15 per cent or more of superficial femoral injuries are blunt in origin. The incidence and causes of profunda femoris injuries are incompletely documented because these injuries were not often detected before arteriography was commonly used.

Amputations were not required in *any* of the 63 surviving patients with common and superficial femoral arterial injuries in a large civilian series.[87] Traumatic occlusion of the profunda femoris artery does not normally result in distal ischemia if the superficial femoral is patent. The effect of such trauma in patients with atherosclerotic occlusion of the superficial femoral artery or in those subsequently developing such an occlusion is not well documented.

Diagnosis and Initial Management. The general principles of trauma care apply to the initial management of patients with arterial injuries of the groin and thigh. Hemorrhage can usually be controlled by external pressure. Common and superficial femoral arterial injuries can generally be diagnosed by the typical signs of arterial injury, but profunda femoris injury is usually only diagnosed arteriographically because overt signs are rare. Signs of distal ischemia indicate the need for operation without delay for arteriography. In patients with femoral shaft fractures and inadequate distal circulation, arteriography is indicated despite improvement after orthopedic manipulation.[100]

Operative Technique. The entire lower extremity is included in the operative field to allow access to distal vessels and for fasciotomies. In addition, part or all of the contralateral extremity should be prepared in the event that a saphenous vein autograft is required. Femoral vein injuries accompany almost half the common and superficial femoral artery wounds, and in this circumstance, interruption of the ipsilateral saphenous vein is not advisable.[92] Proximal and distal arterial and venous control should be obtained before entering the hematoma. It may be necessary to incise the inguinal ligament to gain proximal control of common femoral or proximal superficial femoral injuries. Before making the vertical groin incision, the external iliac artery can be controlled through a proximal extraperitoneal approach if there is a large, obscuring hematoma. The internal oblique muscle is detached from the inguinal ligament, the transversalis fascia is incised, and the peritoneum is bluntly swept superiorly. The external iliac artery and vein are easily and rapidly exposed in this manner. The common femoral and most of the superficial femoral arteries are exposed through a vertical incision along the anterior border of the sartorius muscle. As the artery is approached in the mid-thigh, care is required to avoid injury to the saphenous nerve as it crosses in front of the artery and distally at the adductor canal as it leaves to join the more superficial saphenous vein.[4, 12, 98]

The profunda femoris artery lies dorsal and somewhat lateral to the superficial femoral vessels and can be exposed, though with more difficulty, through the anteromedial vertical incision. It is separated from the superficial vessels by the adductor longus muscle, which must be detached from the femur to expose the distal portion of the artery. Branches of the profunda femoris vein pass ventral to the artery and must be carefully divided.

Once control has been obtained, the hematoma is entered and both the artery and vein are carefully examined because concomitant venous injuries can easily be missed. Reconstruction of injured common and superficial femoral arteries is essential. If an inter-position vein graft is required for the former, it may be necessary to construct a panel or spiral graft because of size discrepancy. Proximal profunda femoris arterial injuries require operative treatment, despite the absence of acute ischemia, because of the risk of late complications such as arteriovenous fistulae and false aneurysms.[104] For injuries of the proximal several centimeters of the profunda femoris, reconstruction is preferable to ligation. Atherosclerotic occlusive disease may later involve the superficial femoral artery, leaving the deep artery as the major source of flow to the lower extremity.

Reconstruction of injured common and superficial femoral veins is indicated to enhance patency of an arterial repair and lessen the likelihood of chronic venous insufficiency. Even complex repairs, including interposition grafts, are used to reduce the incidence of acute venous occlusion, unless hemodynamic instability or injuries of greater priority dictate otherwise. Vascular reconstruction usually should precede the operative treatment of femoral fractures. Flaps of sartorius or other adjacent muscles are mobilized to cover the vascular repair if soft tissue damage is extensive.

Wounds in the Region of the Knee

Popliteal artery injuries constitute 20 per cent of battlefield arterial injuries and 5 to 10 per cent of civilian wounds.[16, 23, 52, 87, 92] Penetrating trauma is the most common cause, but depending on the patient source, 25 to 50 per cent of these injuries are due to blunt trauma.[15, 115] Popliteal artery trauma results in amputation more often than any other arterial injury. An amputation rate of 12.7 per cent was documented in a civilian series of 110 popliteal arterial injuries treated in one institution during a 14-year period.[113] The amputation rate for penetrating injuries was 9 per cent compared with 24 per cent for blunt injuries.

In a smaller series, reported by Lim and associates

from the Cook County Hospital, 31 consecutive popliteal artery injuries were treated *without a single amputation.*[61] These are remarkable results, and some of the concepts outlined below are borrowed from their experience.

The major deterrents to limb salvage after injury of the popliteal artery are extensive adjacent tissue injuries and delayed treatment resulting in distal small vessel thrombosis and muscle necrosis.[19, 47, 63]. The anatomy of the popliteal artery predisposes to ischemia after acute traumatic occlusion. The collateral arterial network around the knee is abundant but frail. No large vessels run parallel to the popliteal artery, and some of the geniculate collaterals may be involved in the segmental occlusion. These delicate vessels maintain some distal perfusion after occlusion of the untraumatized popliteal artery, but, in the trauma setting, they are easily obliterated by swelling of the surrounding soft tissues. This partially explains why fewer limbs are salvaged after diffuse injury than after sharp penetrating injury. The paucity of resilient, high-flow arterial channels about the knee increases the risk of distal small vessel thrombosis. This outcome is most effectively prevented by early diagnosis and expedient revascularization.

Diagnosis and Initial Management. Extravascular injuries of such magnitude as to preclude a functional extremity are best treated by primary amputation. Criteria upon which to base this decision are not clearly defined. However, as a general rule, primary amputation is appropriate in the anesthetic extremity in which nerve destruction is documented and when there is substantial bone loss. The final decision is best made in the operating room and in consultation with orthopedic and plastic surgeons.

Popliteal arterial injury can usually be diagnosed early if the initial examiner appreciates certain signs and the implications of certain types of injury Snyder and colleagues reported that 70 per cent of such patients presented with pulseless extremities, and most also had other signs of ischemia.[113] Such findings usually lead to rapid diagnosis and immediate operation. However, 30 per cent presented with less obvious signs, and half of these had wounds in close proximity to the popliteal vessels as the only sign of arterial injury. Most penetrating popliteal injuries can be promptly identified by arteriography or operation. The diagnosis of blunt injury often is less obvious and explains most treatment delays. Thirty-two per cent of patients with knee dislocations have arterial injuries; the amputation rate has been reported to be as high as 86 per cent in those limbs not revascularized within 8 hours.[38] Other types of trauma around the knee, though less precisely defined, are also frequently associated with arterial injury.[58]

On the basis of these considerations, arteriography is recommended to identify or exclude blunt arterial injury in patients with (1) knee dislocation; (2) knee instability after acute blunt trauma; (3) displaced fractures near the knee with circulatory deficits that resolve after reduction; (4) compression injuries from automobile bumpers; and (5) fractures near the knee requiring operation, particularly if a tourniquet is to be used.

Urgent operation, without delay for arteriography, is indicated in patients with popliteal injuries and signs of distal ischemia. Unless contraindications exist, these patients are immediately given heparin to limit distal small-vessel thrombosis. Arteriography is used selectively in patients with overt injury but without signs of ischemia. Multi-plane arteriographic catheter studies may be performed in the radiology department, single exposure femoral angiograms may be made in the operating room, or preoperative arteriography may be omitted entirely. The appropriate choice is based on the urgency of revascularization and obvious localization of the arterial injury by the external wound.

The initial management of patients with major knee trauma is most effectively based on the state of the distal circulation at the time of presentation. These concepts are summarized in Table 48–4.

Operative Technique. The prepared operative field should include the entire injured limb and the contralateral extremity as a potential saphenous vein donor site. The medial approach to the popliteal vessels is favored for most trauma explorations because it can be easily extended for access to the superficial femoral proximally or the tibioperoneal trunk distally. In addition, saphenous vein autografts are more easily obtained with the patient supine. The extremity is supported at the knee in slight flexion with the hip abducted and externally rotated. If there is evidence of compartmental hypertension in the ischemic extremity, fasciotomy should precede vascular reconstruction. This can be completed in a few minutes and, as Lim and coworkers have demonstrated, collateral flow is enhanced during the time required for definitive reconstruction.[61] The incision for upper popliteal exploration is made along the medial aspect of the lower thigh, parallel to and just behind the tendon of the adductor magnus. Depending on the level of exploration, the sartorius muscle is divided or retracted anteriorly or posteriorly to provide maximum exposure. Careful dissection is required to avoid injury to the adjacent saphenous vein and nerve. The artery is found by displacing the semimembranosus muscle posteriorly and dissecting the space between it and the adductor magnus tendon. Through this approach, the artery is the most superficial of the neurovascular structures, the vein and nerve lying subjacent, laterally and posteriorly. More distal exposure may be obtained by dividing the medial head of the gastrocnemius and the tendons of the semimembranosus, semitendinosus, and gracilis muscles.[4, 12, 98]

After proximal and distal control is obtained, the hematoma is entered, the artery and vein carefully dissected, and the extent of injury defined. Restoration of both arterial

Table 48–4. Early Management of Knee Trauma

- Ischemic limb (pulseless, cool, or both)
  - Systemic heparin unless contraindicated
  - Urgent operation
    - Consider initial fasciotomy
    - Consider intraoperative femoral arteriography
    - Priority revascularization or shunt
- Nonischemic limb
  - Arteriography of suspicious lesions
    - Penetration in proximity to vascular structures
    - Dislocation, instability, "bumper" injury
    - Limbs needing urgent operative reduction and fixation
  - Expedient operative revascularization

and venous flow is essential for successful limb salvage. This is best accomplished by prompt reconstruction, but an indwelling shunt may be inserted to maintain flow if more urgent injuries require treatment or if extensive fractures must first be reduced. Proximal and distal balloon catheter thrombectomy is performed before reconstruction or shunt insertion. Arterial resection is often required, and adequate margins are particularly important in blunt and high-velocity missile injuries to avoid leaving a residual thrombogenic arterial wall. End-to-end anastomosis may be possible, but vein grafts should be willingly used to avoid inadequate resection or anastomotic tension. Autogenous vein interposition or by-pass grafts were used for reconstruction in more than 80 per cent of popliteal arterial injuries in several series.[83, 126] Completion arteriography is recommended to detect technical defects at the anastomosis, missed additional injuries, and residual thrombus (see also Chapter 8). It is important to obtain patency of at least two of the three infrapopliteal branches.

Restoration of venous flow is perhaps more important in the popliteal area than elsewhere, to enhance patency of arterial anastomoses and lessen the likelihood of late venous stasis.[94, 96, 113] Extensive venous injuries may require interposition grafts; these are recommended unless the additional time imposes substantial risks. Venous thrombectomy also may be needed to clear the system. Completion venography should be considered to ensure the patency of venous reconstructions and exclude intraluminal thrombus. Complete, four-compartment fasciotomies often are necessary to restore and preserve adequate distal flow and are performed in more than half of the patients with popliteal artery injuries.[115]

Management of Adjacent Injuries. Some of the most difficult problems associated with popliteal artery trauma are concomitant vein, bone, nerve, and soft tissue injuries. They are common, and their management requires careful attention for successful limb salvage and functional rehabilitation. Vein injuries accompany more than half of the arterial wounds. In a series of 110 popliteal artery injuries, 49 of 58 injured veins (84 per cent) were repaired and five of these limbs (10 per cent) required amputation.[113] In contrast, four of the nine limbs (44 per cent) in which the veins were ligated were ultimately amputated. These data support venous repair. Venous reconstruction is considered an important aspect of limb salvage, especially with popliteal artery trauma.

In the same series of 110 patients, 37 of the 52 adjacent fractures were unstable and required operative fixation.[113] In 29 of these 37, the vascular injuries were repaired before fracture reduction and fixation, and the vascular surgeon stayed in the operating room during the orthopedic manipulation to monitor continued arterial flow and prevent excessive movement of the repaired vessels. Of the 29 patients, 2 lost flow during fracture reduction, but this was rapidly detected and easily corrected. Therefore, revascularization is given priority unless the associated fracture is so unstable or bone length so reduced that initial reduction and fixation are mandatory. In the latter circumstances, catheter thrombectomies are performed and indwelling shunts are inserted to maintain flow during the orthopedic procedure.

Extensive soft tissue trauma is a serious impediment to limb salvage despite an appropriately managed vascular injury. Residual nonviable soft tissue promotes subsequent infection and contributes to late failure. Thorough débridement is an important aspect of the operative treatment of these injuries and should not be limited in order to avoid a soft tissue defect. The use of musculocutaneous flaps may improve outcome in limbs with massive soft tissue trauma. This adjunct is most effectively applied when the plastic surgeon participates in the initial operation. The reconstruction can then be planned before muscles or their vascular supplies are tampered with.

Important concepts that may improve overall limb salvage were derived from demonstration of repeated technical or judgmental errors or identification of maneuvers that appeared to improve or simplify patient management. These recommendations are proposed in the foregoing discussion and summarized in Table 48–5.

Lower Leg Injuries

Vascular injuries of the leg are defined as those distal to the popliteal artery, including the tibioperoneal trunk and the anterior and posterior tibial and peroneal arteries. These injuries constitute 15 to 20 per cent of battlefield arterial trauma but less than 5 per cent of reported civilian injuries.[16, 52, 87, 92] Before arteriography was commonly used in extremity trauma, many tibial and peroneal arterial injuries were probably missed because exploration was recommended only for overt signs of vascular injury.[87] Blunt trauma causes about one-third of civilian injuries, and severe soft tissue trauma is common. Amputations were required in 13 of 88 patients (15 per cent) in civilian series of patients with infrapopliteal arterial injuries.[41, 45, 51, 53]

The termination of the popliteal artery is frequently referred to as a trifurcation giving rise to the anterior and posterior tibial and peroneal arteries. This pattern is unusual, however, because the popliteal artery most often terminates as a bifurcation forming the anterior tibial artery and tibioperoneal trunk, which then divides into the posterior tibial and peroneal arteries, usually 2 to 5 inches farther distal than the anterior tibial artery.[73] The malleolar vessels form a rich collateral network around the ankle that may maintain distal pulses after occlusion of one of these major inflow arteries.

Table 48–5. Management Principles for Popliteal Injuries

Avoidance of lower extremity "reimplantation"
Expeditious diagnosis
Despite intact pulses or capillary filling
Arteriography of suspicious injuries
Avoid undue attention to skeletal injury
Early systemic anticoagulation (unless contraindicated)
Urgent and complete revascularization
"Routine" balloon catheter thrombectomy
Vessel repair before bone reduction
Adequate débridement of injured vessel
Liberal use of autogenous vein grafts
Repair of venous injuries
"Routine" completion arteriography
Liberal, though selective, fasciotomy
Thorough débridement of nonviable soft tissue
Appropriate use of myocutaneous flaps

Diagnosis and Initial Management. The indications for exploration and repair of injured leg arteries have not been completely defined. Signs of impaired distal circulation, arteriovenous fistula, or false aneurysm clearly require operative treatment. The potential for limb loss from these distal injuries is not commonly appreciated, as evidenced by an average preoperative delay of 7 hours in one civilian series of 51 patients.[51] In this series, amputations were most often required following blunt trauma (23 per cent) and shotgun wounds (33 per cent) and in those with injuries of all three infrapopliteal vessels (60 per cent) or the tibioperoneal trunk (50 per cent). These data emphasize the need for expedient evaluation and operation in patients with major wounds below the knee.

The indications for arteriography or operative exploration of lower leg wounds in which there are no signs of arterial injury are less clear. The frequency of late complications from initially undiagnosed tibial and peroneal arterial wounds is not known. In one series, chronic false aneurysms and arteriovenous fistulae accounted for 90 per cent of the operations performed for tibial and peroneal injuries.[11] In addition, these problems represented 31 per cent of the late complications requiring operation in the 94 patients with peripheral arterial injuries. These data suggest that late problems may be more common than previously realized and underscore the need for more attention to early diagnosis.

The indications to reconstruct, rather than ligate, injured tibial and peroneal arteries are also not well clarified by available data. A logical rule of thumb is that patency should be maintained in at least two of the three distal vessels. Following this rule, all injuries of the tibioperoneal trunk should be repaired.[51]

The guidelines for managing leg wounds potentially harboring arterial injuries are as follows: (1) overt signs of arterial injury are an indication for operation and revascularization to ensure patency of at least two vessels; (2) arteriographic exclusion of arterial injury is indicated for penetrating wounds of the proximal third of the leg and more distal wounds in which two vessels may be injured, although this recommendation has recently been challenged in the *totally* asymptomatic patient; (3) operation or arteriographic exclusion is indicated for injuries causing intracompartmental bleeding; and (4) reconstruction is indicated for single-vessel transmural wounds detected operatively or arteriographically if time and conditions permit, failing which, ligation is indicated to prevent false aneurysms.

Operative Technique. The prepared operative field should include the entire involved extremity to provide proximal access for extension of original incisions or injection sites for arteriograms. In addition, a portion of the contralateral extremity should be included to make venous autografts available, if needed. Vertical incisions are used because extensions are often required for adequate vascular control and repair. For proximal lesions, the incision described for popliteal exploration is extended distally. Exposure of the mid-portion of all three vessels may be obtained through a proximally placed lateral incision with resection of part of the fibular shaft. The distal posterior tibial artery is easily located immediately beneath the muscular fascia, through a medial incision. Isolated anterior tibial injuries are approached through an anterolateral incision between the tibialis anterior and extensor hallucis longus muscles.

Success is enhanced by minivascular techniques, including optical magnification, spatulation, and interrupted fine sutures. Completion arteriography is recommended and is specifically indicated if the repair is being performed to relieve ischemia. Restoration of venous flow may be important for proximal injuries or those in which flow may be important for proximal injuries or those in which there is extensive soft tissue destruction and compromise of venous collateral flow. Fasciotomy should be considered and is particularly valuable in blunt injuries and those with extensive intracompartmental bleeding.

References

1. Ackard R: Prevention of thrombosis in microvascular surgery by the use of magnesium sulfate. Br J Plas Surg 25:292, 1972.
2. Adar R, Schramek A, Khodadadi J, et al: Arterial combat injuries of the upper extremity. J Trauma 20:297, 1980.
3. Agarwal N, Shah PM, Clauss RH, et al: Experience with 115 civilian venous injuries. J Trauma 22:827, 1982.
4. Anson BJ, McVay CB: Surgical Anatomy. Philadelphia, WB Saunders, 1971.
5. Bishara RA, Pasch AR, Lim LT, et al: Improved results in the treatment of civilian vascular injuries associated with fractures and dislocations. J Vasc Surg 3:707, 1986.
6. Bole PV, Munda R, Purdy RT, et al: Traumatic pseudoaneurysms: A review of 32 cases. J Trauma 16:63, 1976.
7. Borman KR, Jones GH, Snyder WH III: A decade of lower extremity venous trauma: Patency and outcome. Am J Surg. 154:608, 1987.
8. Borman KR, Snyder WH III, Weigelt JA: Civilian arterial trauma of the upper extremity: An 11 year experience in 267 patients. Am J Surg 148:796, 1984.
9. Brener BJ, Couch NP: Peripheral arterial complications of left heart catheterization and their management. Am J Surg 125:521, 1973.
10. Buchbinder D, Allastair MK, Leather RP, et al: Hypertonic mannitol. Arch Surg 116:414, 1981.
11. Burnett HF, Parnell CL, Williams GD, et al: Peripheral arterial injuries: A reassessment. Ann Surg 183: 701, 1976.
12. Cain A: The exposure of the blood-vessels of the extremities. *In* McNair TS (ed): Bailey's Emergency Surgery, 9th ed. Baltimore, Williams & Wilkins, 1972, Chap 80.
13. Chiu CJ, Terzis J, MacRae ML: Replacement of superior vena cava with the spiral composite vein graft. Ann Thorac Surg 17:555, 1974.
14. Coleman SS, Anson BJ: Arterial patterns in the hand based upon a study of 650 specimens. Surg Gynecol Obstet 113:409, 1961.
15. Conkle DM, Richie RE, Sawyers JL, et al: Surgical treatment of popliteal artery injuries. Arch Surg 110:1351, 1975.
16. DeBakey ME, Simeone FA: Battle injuries of the arteries in World War II. Ann Surg 123:534, 1946.
17. Dennis JW, Frykberg ER, Crump JW, et al: New perspectives on the management of penetrating trauma in proximity to major limb arteries. J Vasc Surg 11:85, 1990.
18. Dickerman RM, Gewertz BL, Foley DW, et al: Selective intra-arterial tolazoline infusion in peripheral arterial trauma. Surgery 81:605, 1977.
19. Downs AR, MacDonald P: Popliteal artery injuries: Civilian experience with sixty-three patients during a twenty-four year period (1960 through 1984). J Vasc Surg 4:55, 1986.
20. Drapanas T, Hewitt RL, Weichert RF, et al: Civilian vascular injuries: A critical appraisal of three decades of management. Ann Surg 172: 351, 1970.
21. Escobar GA, Escobar SC, Marquez L, et al: Vascular trauma: Late sequelae and treatment, J Cardiovasc Surg 27: 35, 1980.
22. Fabian TC, Reiter CB, Gold RE, et al: Digital venous angiography: A prospective evaluation in peripheral arterial trauma. Ann Surg 199: 710, 1984.
23. Fabian TC, Turkleson ML, Connelly TL, et al: Injury to the popliteal artery. Am J Surg 143: 225, 1982.

24. Feliciano DV, Mattox KL, Graham JM, et al: Five-year experience with PTFE grafts in vascular wounds. J Trauma 25: 71, 1985.
25. Flint LM, Snyder WH, Perry MO, et al: Management of major vascular injuries in the base of the neck: An 11 year experience with 146 cases. Arch Surg 106: 407, 1973.
26. Fomon JJ, Warren WD: Late complications of peripheral arterial injuries. Arch Surg 91: 610, 1965.
27. Francis H, Thal ER, Weigelt JA, et al: Vascular proximity: Is it a valid indication for arteriography in the asymptomatic patient? J Trauma 31:512, 1991.
28. Frykberg ER, Crump JM, Dennis JW, et al: Nonoperative observation of clinically occult arterial injuries: A prospective evaluation. Surgery 109: 85, 1991.
29. Frykberg ER, Dennis JW, Bishop K, et al: The reliability of physical examination in the evaluation of penetrating extremity trauma: Results at one year. J Trauma 31:502, 1991.
30. Frykberg ER, Vines FS, Alexander RH: The natural history of clinically occult arterial injuries: A prospective evaluation. J Trauma 29:577, 1989.
31. Gelberman RH, Blasingame JP: The timed Allen test. J Trauma 21: 477, 1981.
32. Gelberman RH, Blasingame JP, Fronek A, et al: Forearm arterial injuries. J Hand Surg 4: 401, 1979.
33. Gelberman RH, Nunley JA, Koman LA, et al: The results of radial and ulnar arterial repair in the forearm. J Bone Joint Surg 64A: 383, 1982.
34. Gerlock AJ, Thal ER, Snyder WH III: Venography in penetrating injuries of the extremities. Am J Roentgenol 126:1023, 1976.
35. Goldman MH, Kent S, Schaumburg E: Brachial artery injuries associated with posterior elbow dislocation. Surg Gynecol Obstet 164: 95, 1987.
36. Gomez GA, Kreis DJ Jr, Ratner L, et al: Suspected vascular trauma of the extremities: The role of arteriography in proximity injuries. J Trauma 26: 1005, 1986.
37. Goodman PC, Jeffrey RB Jr, Brant-Zawadzki M: Digital subtraction angiography in extremity trauma. Radiology 153: 61, 1984.
38. Green NE, Allen BL: Vascular injuries associated with dislocation of the knee. J Bone Joint Surg 59A: 236, 1977.
39. Gregory RT, Gould RJ, Peclet M, et al: The mangled extremity syndrome (M.E.S.): A severity grading system for multisystem injury of the extremity, J Trauma 25: 1147, 1985.
40. Hardin WD, Adinolfi MF, O'Connell RC, et al: Management of traumatic peripheral vein injuries: Primary repair or vein ligation? Am J Surg 144: 235, 1982.
41. Hartsuck JM, Moreland HJ, Williams GR: Surgical management of vascular trauma distal to the popliteal artery. Arch Surg 105: 937, 1972.
42. Hewitt RL, Smith AD, Becker M, et al: Penetrating vascular injuries of the thoracic outlet. Surgery 76: 715, 1974.
43. Hobson RW, Howard EW, Wright CB, et al: Hemodynamics of canine femoral venous ligation: Significance in combined arterial and venous injuries. Surgery 74: 824, 1973.
44. Hobson RW II, Yeager RA, Lynch TG, et al: Femoral venous trauma: Techniques for surgical management and early results. Am J Surg 146: 220, 1983.
45. Holleman JH Jr, Killebrew LH: Tibial artery injuries. Am J Surg 144: 362, 1982.
46. Hunt JL, Snyder WH III: Late false aneurysm of the carotid artery: Repair with extra-intracranial arterial bypass. J Trauma 19:198, 1979.
47. Jaggers RC, Feliciano DV, Mattox KL, et al: Injury to popliteal vessels. Arch Surg 117:657, 1982.
48. Johansen K, Bandyk D, Thiele B, et al: Temporary intraluminal shunts: Resolution of a management dilemma in complex vascular injuries. J Trauma 22: 395, 1982.
49. Johansen K, Lynch K, Paun M, et al: Non-invasive vascular tests reliably exclude occult arterial trauma in injured extremities. J Trauma 31:515, 1991.
50. Karmody AM, Zaman SN, Mirza RA, et al: The surgical management of catheter injuries of the brachial artery. J Thorac Cardiovasc Surg 73: 149, 1977.
51. Keeley SB, Snyder WH III, Weigelt JA: Arterial injuries below the knee: Fifty-one patients with 82 injuries. J Trauma 23: 285, 1983.
52. Kelly G, Eiseman B: Civilian vascular injuries. J Trauma 15: 507, 1975.
53. Kelly G, Eiseman B: Management of small arterial injuries: Clinical and experimental studies. J Trauma 16: 681, 1976.
54. Khalil IM, Livingston DH: Intravascular shunts in complex lower limb trauma. J Vasc Surg 4: 582, 1986.
55. Koivunen D, Nichols WK, Silver D: Vascular trauma in a rural population. Surgery 91: 723, 1982.
56. Kollmeyer KR, Hunt JL, Ellman BA, et al: Acute and chronic traumatic arteriovenous fistulae in civilians. Arch Surg 116: 697, 1981.
57. Krupski W, Thal ER, Gewertz BL, et al: Endothelial response to venous injury. Arch Surg 114: 1240, 1979.
58. Lange RH, Bach AW, Hansen ST Jr, et al: Open tibial fractures with associated vascular injuries: Prognosis for limb salvage. J Trauma 25: 203, 1985.
59. Lau JM, Mattox KL, Beall AC Jr, et al: Use of substitute conduits in traumatic vascular injury. J Trauma 17: 541, 1977.
60. Ledgerwood AM, Lucas CE: Biological dressings for exposed vascular grafts: A reasonable alternative. J Trauma 15: 567, 1975.
61. Lim LT, Michuda MS, Flanigan DP, et al: Popliteal artery trauma: 31 consecutive cases without amputation. Arch Surg 115:1307, 1980.
62. Lindenauer SM, Thompson NW, Kraft RO, et al: Late complications of traumatic arteriovenous fistulas. Surg Gynecol Obstet 129: 525, 1969.
63. McCabe CJ, Ferguson CM, Ottinger LW: Improved limb salvage in popliteal artery injuries. J Trauma 23: 982, 1983.
64. McCollum CH, Mavor E: Brachial artery injury after cardiac catheterization. J Vasc Surg 4: 355, 1986.
65. McCormick TM, Burch BH: Routine angiographic evaluation of neck and extremity injuries. J Trauma 19: 384, 1979.
66. Meissner M, Paun M, Johansen K: Duplex scanning for arterial trauma. Am J Surg 161:552, 1991.
67. Menzoian JO, Corson JD, Bush HL Jr, et al: Management of the upper extremity with absent pulses after cardiac catheterization. Am J Surg 135: 484, 1978.
68. Menzoian JO, Doyle JE, Cantelmo NL, et al: A comprehensive approach to extremity vascular trauma. Arch Surg 120: 801, 1985.
69. Menzoian JO, Doyle JE, LoGerfo FW, et al: Evaluation and management of vascular injuries of the extremities. Arch Surg 118: 93, 1983.
70. Meyer JP, Lim LT, Schuler JJ, et al: Peripheral vascular trauma from close-range shotgun injuries. Arch Surg 120: 1126, 1985.
71. Meyer J, Walsh J, Schuler J, et al: The early fate of venous repair after civilian vascular trauma: A clinical, hemodynamic, and venographic assessment. Ann Surg 206: 458, 1987.
72. Mitchell FL III, Thal ER: Results of venous interposition grafts in arterial injuries. J Trauma 25: 703, 1985.
73. Morris GC Jr, Beall AC Jr, Berry WB, et al: Anatomical studies of the distal popliteal artery and its branches. Surg Forum 10: 498, 1959.
74. Mubarak SJ, Hargens AR: Acute compartment syndromes. Surg Clin North Am 63: 539, 1983.
75. Mubarak SJ, Owen CA: Double-incision fasciotomy of the leg for decompression in compartment syndromes. J Bone Joint Surg 59A: 184, 1977.
76. Mubarak SJ, Owen CA, Hargeas AR, et al: Acute compartment syndromes: Diagnosis and treatment with the aid of the wick catheter. J Bone Joint Surg 60A: 1091, 1978.
77. Mullins RJ, Lucas CE, Ledgerwood AM: The natural history following venous ligation for civilian injuries. J Trauma 20: 737, 1980.
78. Nghiem DD, Boland JP: Four-compartment fasciotomy of the lower extremity without fibulectomy: A new approach. Am Surgeon 46: 414, 1980.
79. Nicholas GG, DeMuth WE: Long-term results of brachial thrombectomy following cardiac catheterization. Ann Surg 183: 436, 1976.
80. Nichols JG, Svoboda JA, Parks SN: Use of temporary intraluminal shunts in selected peripheral arterial injuries. J Trauma 26: 1094, 1986.
81. O'Gorman RB, Feliciano DV, Bitondo CG, et al: Emergency center arteriography in the evaluation of suspected peripheral vascular injuries. Arch Surg 119: 568, 1984.
82. Orcutt MB, Levine BA, Gaskill HV, et al: Civilian vascular trauma of the upper extremity. J Trauma 26: 63, 1986.
83. Pasch AR, Bishara RA, Lim LT, et al: Optimal limb salvage in penetrating civilian vascular trauma. J Vasc Surg 3: 189, 1986.
84. Pasch AR, Bishara RA, Schuler JJ, et al: Results of venous reconstruction after civilian vascular trauma. Arch Surg 121: 607, 1986.

85. Patman RD, Poulos E, Shires GT: The management of civilian arterial injuries. Surg Gynecol Obstet 118: 725, 1964.
86. Peck JJ, Fitzgibbons TJ, Gaspar MR: Devastating distal arterial trauma and continuous intraarterial infusion of tolazoline. Am J Surg 145: 562, 1983.
87. Perry MO, Thal ER, Shires GT: Management of arterial injuries. Ann Surg 173: 403, 1971.
88. Phifer TJ, Gerlock AJ Jr, Rich NM, et al: Long-term patency of venous repairs demonstrated by venography. J Trauma 25:342, 1985.
89. Phifer TJ, Gerlock AJ Jr, Vekovius WA, et al: Amputation risk factors in concomitant superficial femoral artery and vein injuries. Ann Surg 199: 241, 1984.
90. Reid JDS, Weigelt JA, Thal ER, et al: Assessment of proximity of a wound to major vascular structures as an indication for arteriography. Arch Surg 123:942, 1988.
91. Rich NM: Principles and indications for primary venous repair. Surgery 91: 492, 1982.
92. Rich NM, Baugh JH, Hughes CW: Acute arterial injuries in Vietnam: 1000 cases. J Trauma 10: 359, 1970.
93. Rich NM, Hobson RW II, Collins GJ: Traumatic arteriovenous fistulas and false aneurysms: A review of 558 lesions. Surgery 78: 817, 1975.
94. Rich NM, Hobson RW II, Collins GJ Jr, et al: The effect of acute popliteal venous interruption. Ann Surg 183: 365, 1976.
95. Rich NM, Hughes CW: The fate of prosthetic material used to repair vascular injuries in contaminated wounds. J Trauma 12: 459, 1972.
96. Rich NM, Hughes CW, Baugh JH: Management of venous injuries. Arch Surg 171: 724, 1970.
97. Richardson JD, Vitale GC, Flint LM Jr: Penetrating arterial trauma. Arch Surg 122: 678, 1987.
98. Rob C, Smith R (eds): Operative Surgery. Vol. 3, Vascular Surgery. Philadelphia, JB Lippincott, 1968.
99. Rollins DL, Bernhard VM, Towne JB: Fasciotomy: An appraisal of controversial issues. Arch Surg 116: 1474, 1981.
100. Rosenthal JJ, Gaspar MR, Gjerbrum TC, et al: Vascular injuries associated with fractures of the femur. Arch Surg 110: 494, 1975.
101. Ross SE, Ransom KJ, Shatney CH: The management of venous injuries in blunt extremity trauma. J Trauma 25: 150, 1985.
102. Rutherford RB, Kelly GL: Peripheral vascular injuries. *In* Zuidema GD, Rutherford RB, Ballinger WF (eds): The Management of Trauma. 3rd ed. Philadelphia, WB Saunders, 1979.
103. Saletta JD, Freeark RJ: The partially severed artery. Arch Surg 97: 198, 1968.
104. Saletta JD, Freeark RJ: Injuries to the profunda femoris artery. J Trauma 12: 778, 1972.
105. Seller JG III, Richardson JD: Amputation after extremity injury. Am J Surg 152: 260, 1986.
106. Shah PM, Ito K, Clauss RH, et al: Expanded microporous polytetrafluoroethylene (PTFE) grafts in contaminated wounds: Experimental and clinical study. J Trauma 23: 1030, 1983.
107. Shah PM, Ivatury RR, Babu SC, et al: Is limb loss avoidable in civilian vascular injuries? Am J Surg 154: 202, 1987.
108. Shah DM, Leather RP, Corson JD, et al: Polytetrafluoroethylene grafts in the rapid reconstruction of acute contaminated peripheral vascular injuries. Am J Surg 148: 229, 1984.
109. Shah DM, Naraynsingh V, Leather RP, et al: Advances in the management of acute popliteal vascular blunt injuries. J Trauma 25: 793, 1985.
110. Sibbitt RR, Palmaz JC, Garcia F, et al: Trauma of the extremities: Prospective comparison of digital and conventional angiography. Radiology 160: 179, 1986.
111. Sirinek KR, Gaskill HV, Dittman WI, et al: Exclusion angiography for patients with possible vascular injuries of the extremities—A better use of trauma center resources. Surgery 94: 598, 1983.
112. Sirinek KR, Levine BA, Gaskill HV, et al: Reassessment of the role of routine operative exploration in vascular trauma. J Trauma 21: 339, 1981.
113. Snyder WH III: Vascular injuries near the knee: An updated series and overview of the problem. Surgery 91: 502, 1982.
114. Snyder WH III, Thal ER, Bridges RA, et al: The validity of normal arteriography in penetrating trauma. Arch Surg 113: 424, 1978.
115. Snyder WH III, Watkins WL, Whiddon LL, et al: Civilian popliteal artery trauma: An eleven year experience with 83 injuries. Surgery 85: 101, 1979.
116. Spencer AD: The reliability of signs of peripheral vascular injury. Surg Gynecol Obstet 114: 490, 1962.
117. Stahl WM: Discussion of paper by Mullins RJ, et al. J Trauma 20: 743, 1980.
118. Stain SC, Yellin AE, Weaver FA, et al: Selective management of non-occlusive arterial injuries. Arch Surg 124:1136, 1989.
119. Stone KS, Walshaw R, Sugiyama GT, et al: Polytetrafluoroethylene versus autogenous vein grafts for vascular reconstruction in contaminated wounds. Curr Surg 41: 267, 1984.
120. Sullivan WG, Thornton FH, Baker LH, et al: Early influence of popliteal vein repair in the treatment of popliteal vessel injuries. Am J Surg 122: 528, 1971.
121. Symonds FC, Garnes AL, Porter V, et al: Pitfalls in the management of penetrating injuries of the forearm. J Trauma 11: 47, 1971.
122. Thal ER, Snyder WH III, Hayes R, et al: Management of carotid artery injuries. Surgery 76: 955, 1974.
123. Timberlake GA, O'Connell RC, Kerstein MD: Venous injury: To repair or ligate, the dilemma. J Vasc Surg 4: 553, 1986.
124. Tuzzeo S, Saad SA, Hastings OM, et al: Management of brachial artery injuries. Surg Gynecol Obstet 146: 21, 1978.
125. Vaughan GD, Mattox KL, Feliciano DV, et al: Surgical experience with expanded polytetrafluoroethylene (PTFE) as a replacement graft for traumatized vessels. J Trauma 19: 403, 1979.
126. Weimann S, Nicolo MS, Sandbichler P, et al: Civilian popliteal artery trauma. J Cardiovasc Surg 28: 145, 1987.
127. Winegarner FG, Baker AG Jr, Bascom JF, et al: Delayed vascular complications in Vietnam casualties. J Trauma 10: 867, 1970.

49

Causalgia and Post-Traumatic Pain Syndromes

Robert B. Rutherford, M.D.

• • •

Post-traumatic pain syndromes, most often called causalgia or reflex sympathetic dystrophy, remain one of the most poorly understood and frequently misdiagnosed entities encountered in clinical practice. These painful afflictions can develop following irritation or damage to peripheral nerves in a variety of settings, and in the susceptible patient the initiating event may be relatively insignificant, even obscure. Although a discussion of the management of all types of post-traumatic pain is beyond the scope of this chapter, the management of causalgic-like pain is relevant to the vascular surgeon for the following reasons. First, one form of causalgic pain is caused by ischemic damage to nerves following delayed revascularization, and, of course, the vascular surgeon may inadvertently injure peripheral nerves during revascularization procedures, so that he or she may encounter it in patients as a postoperative complication. Second, the vasomotor phenomena associated with causalgic pain often cause such patients to be referred to a vascular surgeon. The associated vascular signs often convince the referring physician that he or she is dealing primarily with a painful vascular condition. This may be fortuitous because, although sympathectomy is now rarely used for vascular disease (as discussed in Chapter 59), it is the vascular surgeon who has perfected and made safe this procedure, and it is sympathectomy that provides the most dramatic and lasting relief from causalgic pain.

TERMINOLOGY

The term causalgia is derived from the Greek words "causos," meaning heat, and "algos," meaning pain, i.e., it means burning pain.[14] Although described in detail by Mitchell in 1864, it was probably Paré in the 16th century who reported the first case.[14, 16] These early reports described incomplete peripheral nerve injury secondary to penetrating trauma (e.g., partial rather than complete transection) with subsequent burning pain, autonomic dysfunction, and "limb atrophy." With time, however, symptoms of similar severity were noted to occur with trauma of a less serious nature and even without obvious injury to a peripheral nerve. In 1973, Patman consolidated the numerous terms that had appeared in the literature to describe a variety of pain syndromes similar to causalgia, but of different etiologies, under the name mimocausalgia.[17] This term is also derived from the Greek and means imitating causalgia. Previously, it had been popular to refer to these syndromes as minor causalgia, in contrast to the full-blown symptom complex seen with incomplete nerve injuries, referred to as major causalgia. Table 49–1 includes over 30 different terms in the literature that describe similar symptom complexes, with minor variations from the classic triad of burning pain, sympathetic dysfunction, and limb atrophy.

PATHOGENESIS

Numerous theories have been proposed to explain causalgia, but none have been universally accepted. Most of these were developed to explain the causalgic pain associated with nerve injury. The most popular theory is probably that of "artificial synapses" occurring at the site of a nerve injury, as first proposed by Doupe and associates.[5] According to this theory, a "short circuit" occurs at the point of partial nerve interruption or demyelinization, which allows *efferent sympathetic impulses to be relayed back along afferent somatic fibers.* Such an artificial synapse has been demonstrated experimentally in crushed nerves,[2] and the interruption of sympathetic efferent impulses may explain the warm, red, and dry extremity seen *initially* in cases of *major* causalgia. It has also been demonstrated that stimuli to a sensory nerve along its course make the nerve more

Table 49–1. Terms Used to Describe Causalgia and Minor Causalgia

Major causalgia	Post-traumatic spreading neuralgia
Minor causalgia	Chronic segmental arterial spasm
Post-traumatic sympathetic dystrophy	Post-traumatic sympathetic dysfunction
Reflex sympathetic dystrophy	Reflex dystrophy of the extremities
Sudeck's atrophy	Post-traumatic painful osteoporosis
Post-traumatic dystrophy	Traumatic neuralgia
Shoulder-hand syndrome	Mitchell's causalgia
Traumatic edema	Homans' minor causalgia
Reflex dystrophy	Sympathalgia
Post-traumatic pain syndromes	Acute atrophy of bones
Sympathetic neurovascular dystrophy	Traumatic angiospasm
	Chronic traumatic edema
Causalgia-like states	Peripheral trophoneurosis
Post-traumatic vasomotor disorders	Reflex nervous dystrophy
Painful osteoporosis	Sudeck's syndrome
Steinerocher's shoulder-hand syndrome	

sensitive to the usual types of sensory stimulus.[18] The work of Walker and Nielsen in humans suggests the presence of this artificial synapse.[26] Stimulation of the postganglionic sympathetics after upper thoracic preganglionic sympathectomy reproduced the causalgic pain for which the surgery was performed. No such pain was produced, however, in patients in whom the sympathectomy was performed for conditions other than causalgia. These findings have been confirmed by White and Sweet.[27]

One piece of evidence weighing against this theory was the demonstration that nerve block beyond the site of nerve injury and presumably beyond this artificial synapse not infrequently afforded relief.[2] However, proponents of this theory have countered that the efferent sympathetic impulses that are ''short circuited'' at the site of injury may not always be strong enough by themselves to cause a retrograde propagation of impulses, and summation of these impulses together with other afferent somatic impulses may be necessary. It has also been suggested by Barnes[1] that impulses at sympathetic-sensory fiber short circuits may travel both proximally and distally. Impulses traveling proximally would then cause pain, and those traveling distally would release ''antidromic'' substances demonstrated by Chapman and coworkers.[4] Release of these antidromic substances has been shown to lower the threshold for sensory stimuli, thus further increasing the sensory input.

Although these explanations are plausible enough in cases with demonstrable nerve injuries, obvious difficulties arise in extending them to explain the similar pain experienced in minor causalgia. They do not explain the sympathetic overactivity often seen in the latter stages of this condition, the relief of pain associated with intra-arterial injections of a peripheral adrenergic blocking agent, such as tolazoline hydrochloride, or the fact that, in early cases, the relief of causalgic pain not infrequently lasts beyond the duration of a sympathetic block by anesthetic agents. The appropriate hypothesis for the mechanism of minor causalgia must also explain the modification of pain by emotional and sensory stimuli and the relief of pain by contralateral sympathectomy after failure of an apparently adequate ipsilateral sympathectomy.[19] The hypothesis must also be compatible with the relief of pain by spinal anesthesia *below* the sympathetic-lumbar outlet and before sympathetic blockade response,[10] and finally, it must explain the failure of sympathectomy in some long-standing cases.

In the late 1930s, Livingston[10] proposed that in causalgia, there was a ''vicious cycle of reflexes'' consisting of three components: (1) chronic irritation of a peripheral sensory nerve with increasingly frequent afferent impulses; (2) abnormal (heightened) activity in the ''internuncial pool'' in the anterior horn of the spinal cord; and (3) increase in efferent (sympathetic) activity. This theory was supported experimentally by Toennie's demonstration that individual stimulation of over one third of the afferent fibers of a cat's saphenous nerve resulted not only in related impulses cephalad from the spinal center but also in impulses back down efferent fibers, including sympathetics.[24] This theory, therefore, explains a number of characteristics of minor causalgia that cannot be explained by the artificial synapse theory of Doupe and colleagues.[5] In particular, it explains the high incidence of ''sympathetic overactivity'' in these patients, and the effect of emotional or sensory stimuli, all of which could exert their influence by heightening the background activity of this internuncial pool. It was suggested that anything that broke this vicious cycle, whether it be interruption of sympathetic efferents by spinal anesthesia or interruption of somatic nerve conduction, would relieve pain.

However, this latter theory enjoyed only a brief wave of enthusiasm, probably because it did not conform to the classic concepts of sensory perception, as originally proposed by von Frey.[25] According to von Frey, individual receptors existed for pain, touch, warmth, and cold, and these sensations involved simple transmission of a sensory impulse up a modality-specific peripheral nerve fiber, followed by relay from the spinal center to the brain via the spinothalamic tract.[25]

However, modern neurophysiology has come a long way from the attractive but simplistic views of von Frey, and, although it has not supported a return to Livingstone's concepts, it has shown that the responsible mechanisms are indeed complex. Further understanding has spawned the ''gate control'' theory of pain mediation.[23] In the substantia gelatinosa of the dorsal horns of the spinal cord, the synapses between the peripheral nerves and those that relay their impulses up the long tracts to the brain are played upon or modulated by sympathetic input. Simplified for the sake of explanation, it is as if a gate existed at this point of relay and transmission that controlled the relationship between the number or frequency of incoming peripheral impulses and the number or frequency of outgoing pulses reaching the brain. High-frequency stimulation of the latter pathways in awake patients is reported as burning pain. Thus if the gate is open, an effect of increased sympathetic activity, sensations of, for example, touch or pressure, which would normally result in lower frequency impulses being relayed up to the brain, might be perceived as burning pain because of the higher frequency of impulses getting through the ''open gate.'' This theory is still under study and will obviously undergo modification and definition with time, but it does offer an explanation, not only for causalgia and the role of sympathetic tone (the susceptible patient, the associated peripheral sympathetic activity, and relief by sympathectomy, which ''closes the gate''), but also for other heretofore unexplained observations (e.g., variations in ''pain threshold,'' relief by transcutaneous stimulators, and even acupuncture in ''receptive'' individuals).

CLINICAL PRESENTATION AND DIAGNOSIS

The natural history of causalgia has been divided by Drucker into three clinical stages.[6]

1. Acute. At this stage the clinical course is reversible and is characterized by warmth, erythema, burning, edema, hyperalgesia, hyperhidrosis, and, after a few months, patchy osteoporosis. At this stage, a good result can be expected with a Bier block or chemical sympathectomy, often lasting beyond the normal duration of the block. Spontaneous resolution may occur in this stage, particularly with therapeutic support (see later section, Treatment).

2. Dystrophic. The clinical course is marked by a

fixed duration, but still good response to sympathetic block, and patients rarely experience spontaneous resolution. Characteristics include coolness; mottling of the skin; cyanosis; brawny edema; dry, brittle nails; continuous pain; and diffuse osteoporosis. At this stage, not only is a bone scan positive but usually changes in the bone structure are seen on plain films.

3. Atrophic. Pain beyond the area of injury is common, and fixed, trophic changes occur, including atrophy of the skin and its appendages and fixed joint contractures. Radiographs show severe demineralization and ankylosis.

Although these stages may be oversimplified, they do provide a framework for diagnosis, treatment, and prognosis in the patient with causalgia or mimocausalgia. For example, among patients who are in stage 1 or 2, prompt treatment may eventually result in permanent relief of their pain, and sympathectomy may not even be required in the former group. However, for patients in stage 3, the likelihood of a poor result is increased and even sympathectomy may not give lasting relief.

The diagnosis of causalgia is certain when the clinical presentation includes superficial burning pain in the distribution of a single somatic sensory nerve, hyperesthesia, vasomotor abnormalities, radiographic evidence of osteoporosis, and a good response to sympathetic blockade. However, this classic picture can be reliably expected only in major causalgia. In minor or mimocausalgia, certain of these clinical features may be minimal or absent, though the response to sympathetic block may still be reliable. In fact, the ultimate relief obtained by surgical sympathectomy is predictable by careful documentation of the response to sympathetic blockade.

In the differential diagnosis of causalgia, one of the most important diagnoses to consider is that of nerve entrapment. Causalgic-like pain may also occur if a nerve is caught in a suture, entrapped by scar, or compressed by surrounding structures. The former obviously must be considered in causalgic pain appearing immediately postoperatively, but since nerve irritation or injury can occur by any compressing or pinching mechanism, there may be a causalgic component to the pain associated with any nerve compression. This is important because relief of the compression may only partially relieve the pain, and the causalgic component may persist. This is discussed below in relation to residual pain following operations to relieve a herniated disc. If peripheral nerve entrapment is suspected, there will often be a ''trigger point'' where the focal application of pressure will cause sharp pain. The pain will be relieved by the infiltration of a small amount of local anesthetic at this point.

Patients presenting with signs and symptoms characteristic of Drucker's stage 2 may be thought to have Raynaud's syndrome. However, in the latter, the symptoms are intermittent, primarily related to cold exposure, and relieved by warmth. Furthermore, hyperesthesia is rare, and the pain is not usually severe or burning in character.

The pain of peripheral neuritis is often burning and associated with hyperesthesia and vasomotor phenomena. In fact, the pathogenetic mechanisms for the two may be quite similar. However, the process here is more diffuse in location and gradual in onset, without a history of trauma or some other discrete precipitating event.

As stated earlier, the clinical diagnosis of major or minor causalgia is greatly strengthened by a positive response to sympathetic blockade. Patients should be encouraged to quantitate the degree of relief obtained by expressing the percentage of pain relief experienced, e.g., 100 per cent relief, 50 per cent relief, and so on. The degree of pain relief a patient enjoys with such a block is an excellent predictor of the degree of relief that can be expected postoperatively should sympathectomy be undertaken.[29] Some caution should be exercised here, however, because sympathectomy can give some degree of nonspecific relief of almost any pain, including ischemic pain.[3, 11] However, causalgic pain is usually dramatically relieved by sympathetic blockade (e.g. 75 to 100 per cent relief), whereas other pain usually receives only mild to moderate (25 to 50 per cent) relief.

The diagnosis of major versus minor causalgia is based on the history of injury, the degree and characteristics of the pain and associated findings, and the response to treatment. Patients with major causalgia have a clear-cut history of nerve injury, present earlier with a full-blown classic picture, and have a better response to treatment. Patients with minor causalgia usually present later, because their initiating event is more obscure, and their clinical features may be less obvious. Treatment response may be less dramatic and less long-lasting, but this may be due, at least in part, to delay in presentation or recognition, and therefore, to treatment.

TREATMENT

Once the diagnosis has been confirmed by sympathetic blockade, the question of whether to try to achieve this degree of relief more permanently by sympathectomy usually promptly arises. The answer depends on the clinical stage of development, severity of symptoms, and the degree and duration of relief by sympathetic block.

For example, in a patient with recent onset of pain with relief from sympathetic blockade lasting well beyond the known duration of the anesthetic agent used, one should persist with nonoperative measures. Patients in whom the condition has persisted for several months, whose pain is disabling, and who receive near total relief from sympathetic block, but only for the duration of the anesthetic, may be considered immediate candidates for surgical sympathectomy. Patients with symptoms of long duration, those with associated trophic changes, or those with less classic and less severe symptoms and who receive only mild to moderate relief from sympathetic block should be told that the long-term results are likely to be disappointing. The reader will note the similarity of these examples with Drucker's three stages. This is deliberate because sympathectomy is, for the most part, applied in stage 2, before progression to stage 3, and after progression from stage 1, despite nonoperative therapy.

Nonoperative therapy, particularly as it applies to stage 1 or early stage 2 patients, consists of drug therapy, intermittent sympathetic blocks, and physiotherapy. Drug therapy may require nonspecific analgesics, but these should be superimposed, only if necessary, on a background of medication designed to attenuate the symptoms by direct effect. Of these, phenytoin, amitriptyline, carbamazepine, and baclofen may be used effectively, usually in that order, because of increasing side effects. Nonsteroidal anti-inflammatory agents may be useful not only in relieving joint swelling but also, in combination with the agents just listed, in allowing reduced dosage and fewer side effects. The methods previously discussed are appropriate in stage 1 because the condition at this stage may be reversible, and complete remission can be achieved, particularly in patients with long-lasting relief from sympathetic blocks, which allow the vicious cycle to be broken and aggressive physiotherapy to be applied. However, when relief is of short duration, persisting with repeated blocks is counterproductive and expensive.

Injections of alcohol and phenol have been used rather than sympathectomy in an attempt to produce lasting sympathetic denervation. However, there is a significant incidence of incomplete or transient sympathetic block with this approach. Its risks include painful neuralgias and inflammation with scarring, all of which make subsequent surgery more difficult.[19]

Radiofrequency ablation has been advocated as a more precise method of achieving percutaneous sympathetic denervation.[30] Admittedly, it represents an advance over phenol or alcohol blocks, but its effect is still not as complete or durable as sympathectomy, and its local reaction would seriously interfere with subsequent sympathectomy. Furthermore, it requires a general anesthetic.

Such methods have been justified primarily because of the morbidity of sympathectomy, particularly transthoracic sympathectomy, which may cause significant post-thoracotomy discomfort, but this objection is no longer valid now that the procedure can be safely and precisely done through a thoracoscope[31–33] and the patient discharged the following day. Through the modern thoracoscope, with its view enlarged on videoscreen, and using instruments such as those developed for laparoscopic cholecystectomy, removal of T2 and T3 and division of the rami to the lower part of the stellate ganglion can be performed with precision and safety, but only in the absence of inflammation and scarring. In view of this development and the fact that lumbar sympathectomy is so well tolerated, any percutaneous method that does not produce a complete and lasting sympathectomy cannot be condoned because it precludes safe sympathectomy later. As will be seen below, if sympathectomy is limited to those obtaining excellent relief from a sympathetic block produced by local anesthetic, it produces long-term relief in nearly 90 per cent of patients.[15, 29]

Results of Sympathectomy

The techniques of dorsal and lumbar sympathectomy and their effectiveness for many indications are well described in Chapters 72 and 59, respectively. This discussion reviews the results of sympathectomy for causalgia, including our own experience.[15]

The first reports of surgical sympathectomy for causalgia were probably those of Spurling in 1930[22] and Kwan in 1935.[9] Both described trauma to an extremity complicated by causalgia and relieved by sympathectomy. Clinical series from World War II helped to clearly define a role for sympathectomy in causalgia.[7, 12, 21] In 1951, Mayfield reported on 75 patients with causalgia treated and followed for 5 years; 73 of the 75 patients had significant early pain relief, and in 63 per cent this was sustained for 5 years. In the other 37 per cent the pain relief was significantly improved but not completely gone at 5 years. In Thompson's 1979 series of 147 patients, 27 patients with causalgia were treated with sympathectomy, and among 120 patients with minor causalgia, 55 were treated with sympathectomy and 65 with medical management; 82 per cent of the patients had excellent pain relief, 11 per cent had good pain relief, and 7 per cent had a poor result. Residual symptoms, however, largely secondary to associated injuries, were present in 31 per cent.[23] The author has twice published his experience with causalgia and sympathectomy. The first series was from Johns Hopkins and included 27 patients.[28] Immediate pain relief was achieved in 24 patients (all of whom received a trial block), and in 15 patients followed for 2 to 17 years, pain relief was sustained in 13. The second series, from the University of Colorado, included 31 patients.[15] All patients in this series were evaluated preoperatively with sympathetic block, and 97 per cent of the patients obtained a satisfactory level of immediate pain relief. In extended follow-up, this level of pain relief was sustained in 94 per cent. In a similar, more recent series of 28 patients, AbuRahma and colleagues reported 95 per cent long-term success in patients reporting an excellent response to a trial block.[29] Olcott and associates also reported 91 per cent good to excellent results in 35 patients.[34]

An interesting subgroup of patients was identified in the last two reports.[15, 29] In the first series,[15] patients with causalgic pain persisting after disc surgery formed a subgroup of 12 patients for whom sympathectomy offered a therapeutic benefit equal to that in other patients. These cases constituted more than half of those in whom lumbar sympathectomy was performed; this relates both to a high index of suspicion and indoctrination of local neurosurgeons. In the second series,[29] 10 patients (36 per cent of the total) had had lumbar discectomy and they too reported uniformly excellent results. Neither the true frequency of this condition nor its nature is known. Once called "arachnoiditis" and thought to be due to inflammation and nerve sheath irritation following disc surgery, it probably relates to residual nerve damage that occurs before nerve root compression is relieved by removal of the herniated nucleus pulposis. Clearly, the recognition of causalgia as a potential component of lumbar disc pain, its persistence after discectomy, and its potential relief by sympathectomy has not been well recognized in the English literature.

Complications

Failure to recognize promptly and appropriately treat causalgic pain is one of the most tragic complications because it often results in a complicated clinical course with irreversible changes, including wasting of the skin and muscles, fixed joint contractures, and severe demineralization of bone, as well as a missed opportunity for relief by sympathectomy. The complications of sympathectomy itself have been described in depth by the author[20] and are also discussed in Chapter 59. In general, the complications of sympathectomy can be classified by origin: preoperative, i.e., failure to achieve the anticipated benefit because of improper patient selection; intraoperative, i.e., related to improper technique; or postoperative, i.e., those encountered after an appropriate and properly executed sympathectomy. Preoperative complications can be minimized by the use of nerve blocks, sham saline blocks in questionable cases, and careful psychiatric evaluation. Intraoperative complications can be avoided by meticulous attention to the anatomic relationships and normal variations of anatomy among the most frequently injured structures—the genitofemoral nerve, ureter, lumbar veins, aorta, and inferior vena cava. The most frequent postoperative complication is postsympathectomy neuralgia, which, though frequent, almost always resolves spontaneously.[1, 15] In summary, when selectively applied for causalgia, sympathectomy gives excellent symptomatic relief, far superior to its other indications. Although it used to carry a significant mortality and morbidity when performed on elderly patients with advanced arteriosclerosis, current technique results in negligible mortality with very few permanent adverse sequelae in the characteristically younger, healthier patients with causalgia.

References

1. Barnes R: The role of sympathectomy in the treatment of causalgia. J Bone Joint Surg 35B:172, 1953.
2. Bergan JJ, Con J: Sympathectomy for pain relief. Med Clin North Am 52:147, 1968.
3. Bobin A, Anderson WP: Influence of sympathectomy in α-2 adrenoreceptor binding sites in canine blood vessels. Life Sci 33:331, 1983.
4. Chapman LF, Ramos AV, Goodell H, et al: Neurohumoral features of afferent fibers in man. Arch Neurol 4:617, 1961.
5. Doupe J, Cullen CH, Chance GQ: Post-traumatic pain and the causalgic syndrome. J Neurol Psychiat 7:33, 1944.
6. Drucker WR, Hubay CA, Holden WD, et al: Pathogenesis of post-traumatic sympathetic dystrophy. Am J Surg 97:454, 1959.
7. Kirklin JW, Chenoweth AE, Murphy F: Causalgia: a review of its characteristics, diagnosis and treatment. Surgery 21:321, 1947.
8. Kleiman A: Causalgia. Am J Surg 87:839, 1954.
9. Kwan ST: The treatment of causalgia by thoracic sympathetic ganglionectomy. Ann Surg 101:222, 1935.
10. Livingston WK: Pain Mechanisms: A Physiological Interpretation of Causalgia and its Related States. New York, Macmillan, 1943, pp 83–113.
11. Lon L, Nathan PW: Painful peripheral states and sympathetic blocks. J Neurol Neurosurg Psychiat 41:664, 1978.
12. Mayfield FH: Causalgia. Springfield IL, Charles C Thomas, 1951.
13. Melzack R, Wall PD: Gate control theory of pain. *In* Soulairoc A, Cahn J, Charpentier J (eds): Pain. New York, Academic Press, 1968, pp 11–31.
14. Mitchell SW, Morehouse GR, Keen WW: Gunshot Wounds and Other Injuries of Nerves. Philadelphia, JB Lippincott, 1964, p 164.
15. Mockus MB, Rutherford RB, Rosales C, et al: Sympathectomy for causalgia: patient selection and long-term results. Arch Surg 122:668, 1987.
16. Paré A: Les Oeuvres D'Ambroise Pare, Paris, Gabriel Bron. Historie de defunct. Roy Charles 10th book, 1598, p 401.
17. Patman RD, Thompson JE, Persson AV: Management of post-traumatic pain syndromes: Report of 113 cases. Ann Surg 177(6):780, 1973.
18. Porter EL, Taylor AN: Facilitation of flexion reflex in relation to pain after nerve injuries (causalgia). J Neurophysiol 8:289, 1945.
19. Ramos M, Almazan A, Lozano F, et al: Phenol lumbar sympathectomy in severe arterial disease of the lower limb: A hemodynamic study. Int Surg 68:127, 1983.
20. Rutherford RB: Complications of sympathectomy. *In* Bernhard VM, Towne JB (eds): Complications in Vascular Surgery. New York, Grune & Stratton, 1980.
21. Shumaker HB Jr, Abramson DI: Post-traumatic vasomotor disorders. Surg Gynecol Obstet 88:417, 1949.
22. Spurling RG: Causalgia of the upper extremity: treatment by dorsal sympathetic ganglionectomy. Arch Neurol Psychiat (Chir) 23:704, 1930.
23. Thompson JE: The diagnosis and management of post-traumatic pain syndromes (causalgia). Aust NZ J Surg 49(3):299, 1979.
24. Toennie JF: Reflex discharges from the spinal cord over the dorsal roots. J Neurophysiol 1:370, 1938.
25. von Frey R: Cited in White JC, Sweet WH: Other varieties of peripheral neuralgia. *In* White JC (ed): Pain and the Neurosurgeon. Springfield, IL, Charles C Thomas, 1969, pp 87–109.
26. Walker AE, Nielsen S: Electrical stimulation of the upper thoracic portion of the sympathetic chain in man. Arch Neurol Psychiat 59:559, 1947.
27. White JC, Sweet WH: Other varieties of peripheral neuralgia. *In* White JC (ed): Pain and the Neurosurgeon. Springfield, IL, Charles C Thomas, 1969, pp 87–109.
28. Wirth FP, Rutherford RB: A civilian experience with causalgia. Arch Surg 100:633, 1970.
29. AbuRahma AF, Robinson PA, Dowel M, et al: Sympathectomy for reflex sympathetic dystrophy: Factors affecting outcome. Presented at the 40th Scientific Meeting of the International Society for Cardiovascular Surgery, North American Chapter, Chicago, June 9–10, 1992.
30. Noe CE, Haynsworth RF Jr: Lumbar radiofrequency sympatholysis. J Vasc Surg 17:801, 1993.
31. Appleby TC, Edwards WH Jr: Thoracoscopic dorsal sympathectomy for hyperhidrosis: Technique of choice. J Vasc Surg 16:121, 1992.
32. Horgan K, O'Flanagan S, Duignan PJ, et al: Palmar and axillary hyperhidrosis treated by sympathectomy by transthoracic endoscopic electrocoagulation. Br J Surg 71:1002, 1984.
33. Malone PS, Cameron ALP, Rennie JA: Endoscopic thoracoscopic sympathectomy in the treatment of upper limb hyperhidrosis. Ann Coll Surg Engl 68:93, 1986.
34. Olcott C, Eltherington LG, Wilcosky BR, et al: Reflex sympathetic dystrophy—The surgeon's role in management. Presented at the Western Vascular Society meeting, January 15, 1991.

SECTION VIII

Management of Chronic Ischemia of the Lower Extremities

Edited by Richard F. Kempczinski, M.D.

50

Introduction and General Considerations

Richard F. Kempczinski, M.D., and Victor M. Bernhard, M.D.

Since the 1950s, numerous technical and clinical developments have revolutionized the management of chronic ischemia of the lower extremities. The vascular surgeon is now armed with a bewildering array of diagnostic and therapeutic options for the management of arterial occlusive disease. Refinements in traditional angiographic techniques and the introduction of digitized vascular imaging have made detailed visualization of the lower extremity arterial tree feasible, and noninvasive methods of hemodynamic testing have provided objective documentation of each patient's physiologic derangement. In addition to a wide variety of traditional bypass and disobliterative (i.e., endarterectomy) techniques, an ingenious modification of the angiographer's catheter made percutaneous dilatation of arterial stenoses practical. An extensive selection of artificial vascular substitutes has been developed and promises to provide durable vascular prostheses for virtually every clinical situation. The resurgence of interest in the in situ autogenous saphenous vein for lower extremity bypasses promises to increase the availability of this nearly ideal conduit and to improve long-term patency. Modifications in amputation techniques and prosthetic design have enhanced the rehabilitation of the dysvascular amputee. The indications for lumbar sympathectomy have been defined more clearly. Finally, careful clinical studies and retrospective analyses have clarified the natural history of lower extremity arterial insufficiency and the prognosis for survival and limb loss in patients afflicted with this disease.

This introductory chapter reviews the principles underlying the current understanding of atherosclerosis and the pathophysiology of chronic lower extremity ischemia. The impact of gradual arterial occlusion and the development of collateral circulation on lower extremity perfusion is discussed, as are the associated diseases that influence its development and progression and the general principles that govern vascular reconstruction of the chronically ischemic lower extremity. Subsequent chapters deal with the nonoperative management of the ischemic limb, give detailed descriptions of the indications for and the techniques and results of the various reconstructive procedures, and discuss some of the rarer conditions that may produce lower extremity ischemia.

ETIOLOGY AND PREDISPOSING FACTORS

A thorough understanding of the arterial obliterative process and its natural history is essential for the proper selection of candidates for operation and the appropriate surgical procedures to achieve limb revascularization. Atherosclerosis is the underlying cause of chronic limb ischemia in the vast majority of patients. Although its etiology remains unclear, its incidence and progression are clearly accelerated by the coexistence of diabetes mellitus, hypertension, lipoprotein abnormalities, and most importantly, chronic addiction to the use of tobacco.[11, 19, 20, 25, 31, 47, 55, 58, 60, 63] The already diminished flow through atherosclerotic vessels and the high-resistance collateral channels that have opened to carry blood around them is further compromised by the increased viscosity of the blood in patients with polycythemia and by the reduced cardiac output from associated heart disease.[32, 47, 73, 75] Alterations in fibrinogen, fibrinolytic activity, and platelet adhesiveness or aggregation may also contribute to the progression of atherosclerosis or promote thrombosis of already diseased vessels.[23, 46, 47, 50]

Although it is a more common problem in the Middle East and the Far East, thromboangiitis obliterans, or Buerger's disease, is a very infrequent cause of lower limb ischemia in the United States (see Chapter 11).[40] Despite challenges by some investigators to its very existence, there can no longer be any doubt that it is a distinct pathologic entity.[12, 40, 45, 74] Many cases that in the past would have been classified on clinical grounds as Buerger's disease are now correctly identified, on the basis of more precise angiographic and clinical scrutiny, as peripherally distributed premature atherosclerosis.[12] Occasionally, the two diseases may coexist in the same patient.[45] Pathologically, thromboangiitis obliterans presents as a severe, chronic inflammatory process that involves the entire neurovascular bundle of the small vessels of the hands and feet and leads to arterial and venous thrombosis and fibrosis.[12, 40] Its inflammatory nature and distal localization generally preclude direct surgical reconstruction. Typically, it occurs in individuals during the 3rd and 4th decades of life and is invariably associated with heavy use of tobacco.[40] If the patient can be persuaded to stop smoking, progression of the disease process will be halted.

Other types of vasculitis may involve the small arteries and arterioles and result in lower extremity ischemia. Proper treatment depends on recognition and management of the underlying disease process and is rarely the direct concern of the vascular surgeon.

Ischemia that is due to arterial trauma is usually an acute problem. Nonocclusive arterial trauma occasionally may be overlooked during the initial evaluation or may be obscured by the patient's more pressing, life-threatening associated injuries. Subsequently, as the patient recovers and resumes ambulation, the arterial injury may become apparent.

Popliteal artery entrapment and cystic adventitial disease of the popliteal artery are rare causes of chronic arterial ischemia that generally affect young, otherwise healthy, active individuals.* Although these diseases can produce severe disability if they are unrecognized and left untreated, normal circulation can usually be restored in the majority of these patients.

PATHOLOGY OF ATHEROSCLEROSIS

Atherosclerosis is primarily a disease of the arterial intima that extends into the media but usually spares the outer media and adventitia[11] (see Chapter 10). The pathogenesis of its sentinel lesion, the fatty intimal streak, remains the subject of continuing debate.[23, 47, 71] It may begin as a platelet and fibrin thrombus sealing a break in the intima that has exposed subintimal collagen, or increased permeability of the damaged intima to low-density lipoproteins may lead to focal accumulations of this material and cholesterol, particularly in association with proteoglycan, in the vessel wall.† Further accumulation of thrombus with the development of fibrosis then leads to plaque formation and progressive luminal encroachment.[11, 23] Continuing lipid accumulation, hemorrhage into the plaque, or deposition of mural thrombus may progressively narrow the lumen until occlusion eventually occurs.[23] Nonocclusive but ulcerated plaques may be the source of peripheral emboli.[27, 51] These can lodge in the smaller, more distal arteries and further aggravate limb ischemia by reducing the runoff bed.

Although atherosclerosis is a generalized disease, it is remarkably segmental in its distribution.[22, 33, 39] It develops at major arterial bifurcations and in areas of posterior fixation or acute angulation.[68] Disruption of laminar flow in these areas creates eddy currents that traumatize the intima and are responsible in part for the increase in atheroma formation at these points.[73] In addition, the marked change in the direction of blood flow at arterial bifurcations and pronounced curves induces a relatively negative force on the intima along the convex inner wall of the curvature (the air foil effect), which further promotes plaque formation in these areas.[68]

The arterial segment that lies in Hunter's canal and represents the transition between the distal superficial femoral and the popliteal arteries is the lower extremity site most commonly involved with atherosclerosis.[22, 33, 39] It is not only a point of arterial fixation and oblique passage through the adductor magnus tendon but also the site of origin of the large superior genicular branch. Atheromata occur with nearly equal frequency on the posterior wall of the common femoral artery and extend into the proximal superficial femoral and profunda femoris arteries. The infrarenal abdominal aorta commonly has atherosclerotic involvement, which is especially prominent immediately distal to the origin of the inferior mesenteric artery, where it becomes confluent with the plaque arising at the aortic bifurcation. This heavily diseased segment often contains an irregular, ulcerated intima covered by friable, exuberant thrombus that may embolize spontaneously or at the time of surgical manipulation[27] (see Chapter 44).

The true extent of atherosclerotic involvement of the posterior arterial wall may be difficult to appreciate on routine arteriograms taken in a single anteroposterior projection.[42, 61] However, careful palpation at the time of surgery usually reveals the magnitude of the problem and permits appropriate modification or extension of the proposed reconstructive procedure.

Other sites for which atherosclerosis exhibits a predilection include the common iliac bifurcation; the mid-popliteal artery opposite the knee joint; and the popliteal trifurcation, including the proximal portions of the tibial vessels.[33, 39] The experienced clinician who is cognizant of atherosclerosis's remarkable propensity for segmental localization can usually predict the sites of arterial involvement on the basis of a careful history and physical examination, occasionally supplemented by noninvasive hemodynamic measurements, without the need for arteriography.

HEMODYNAMIC CONSIDERATIONS IN THE ISCHEMIC LEG

A complete discussion of circulatory physiology is presented in Section II. Some of the principles, however,

*See references: entrapment, 34; cystic adventitial disease, 21.
†See references: thrombus sealing a break, 46; increased permeability to lipoproteins, 29.

deserve reemphasis in order to provide the foundation for a rational approach to lower limb revascularization.

Blood Flow

Blood flow is directly proportional to arterial pressure and inversely related to peripheral resistance.[73] *Arterial pressure* is determined by cardiac output, peripheral resistance, and circulating blood volume. *Peripheral resistance* in the normal limb is a function of the precapillary arterioles, blood viscosity, tissue pressure, and venous pressure. A hemodynamically significant obstruction within a major limb artery results in a drop in perfusion pressure distal to the obstruction and an increase in total peripheral resistance that reduces limb blood flow.

Within certain limitations, arterial blood flow is governed by the Poiseuille equation:[73]

$$P_1 - P_2 = \overline{V} \cdot \frac{8L\eta}{r^2} = Q \cdot \frac{8L\eta}{\pi r^4}$$

where

$$\begin{aligned} Q &= \text{Flow} \\ P_1 - P_2 &= \text{Pressure differential} \\ \eta &= \text{Viscosity} \\ r &= \text{Radius} \\ L &= \text{Length} \\ \overline{V} &= \text{Mean flow velocity} \end{aligned}$$

Therefore, the flow through a stenotic major artery or through narrow collateral vessels is largely governed by the radius of the arterial lumen and by the length of the stenotic segment.

When a main limb artery is occluded, the total resistance to flow that results is the sum of the parallel resistances imposed by the collateral vessels that bypass that segment and is expressed by the formula:[73]

$$\frac{1}{r_{total}} = \frac{1}{r_1} + \frac{1}{r_2} + \text{- - -} \frac{1}{r_n}$$

As the vessels dilate over time, this resistance diminishes and flow improves. If a second segment of the same artery becomes occluded, adding a resistance *in series,* the total resistance is expressed by the formula:

$$r_{total} = r_1 + r_2 + \text{- - -} r_n$$

Thus, the impact of resistance in series is additive and further diminishes the capacity of the arterial tree to meet the functional demands imposed by exercise, infection, or the dissipation of external heat. Finally, even the minimal flow needed to sustain viability is compromised, and tissue necrosis ensues.[67]

Collateral Circulation

Collateral vessels develop from the distributing branches of large and medium-sized arteries.[66] Anatomically, as well as functionally, it is convenient to divide the collateral bed into stem arteries, mid-zone collaterals, and reentry arteries. These vessels are generally preexisting pathways that enlarge when a stenosis or an occlusion develops in a main artery of supply and do not represent neovascularization. Although the precise mechanism that stimulates their development remains unknown, it appears that the pressure differential that develops across the collateral bed as a result of the arterial occlusion causes a reversal of flow in the distal mid-zone collateral channels and increases the velocity of flow through them as they dilate in response to this stimulus (Fig. 50–1). Exercise further enhances this effect by producing relative tissue hypoxia and acidosis, which reduce peripheral resistance, thus magnifying the pressure gradient across the obstruction.[3]

Collateral channels that form in response to a chronic, unisegmental occlusion can usually provide adequate blood flow to meet the resting needs of the limb and sufficient

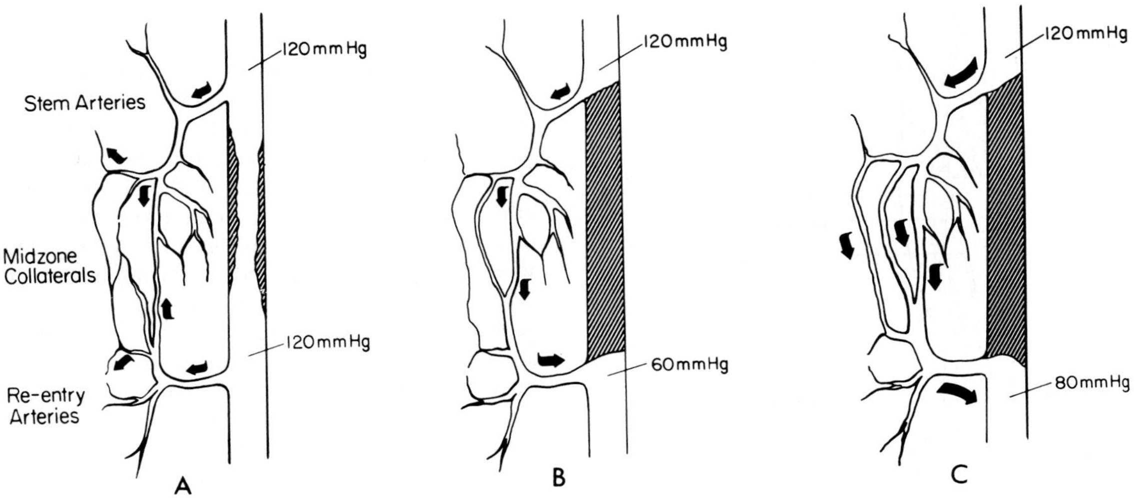

FIGURE 50–1. Hemodynamic theory of collateral formation. *A,* Developing stenosis in main vessel without drop in pressure across it; *arrows* indicate direction and volume of blood flow in side branches. *B,* Lesion has progressed to acute thrombosis with 60 mmHg pressure drop and reversal of flow in reentry below occlusion. *C,* Over several weeks, collateral flow increases in response to the pressure differential, and the gradient across the lesion decreases.

additional flow to sustain moderate exercise.[39] However, sudden occlusion of a previously normal vessel, as might occur with an arterial embolus, may not allow sufficient time for the collateral circulation to compensate for the acute ischemia and may result in tissue necrosis or frank gangrene.[66, 67] On the other hand, if the collateral development around an arterial stenosis keeps pace with any progression of the disease, there may be little change in the patient's symptoms or the patient may experience a transient period of severe limb ischemia that gradually relents over the next few weeks as the collateral circulation expands to its ultimate potential (see Fig. 50–1*C*).

Although atherosclerosis usually spares the mid-zone collateral vessels, progressive intimal disease or extension of the main vessel thrombosis may occlude the stem or reentry vessels, thus compromising the effectiveness of the entire collateral network. In the absence of mechanical occlusion, the collateral blood flow may be reduced by decreased cardiac output, increased blood viscosity,[53] hyperfibrinogenemia,[50] or dehydration.

Several well-recognized anatomic patterns of collateral development are illustrated in Figure 50–2. Occlusion of the distal abdominal aorta recruits stem collaterals from the intercostal and lumbar arteries to connect with reentry collaterals of the iliolumbar, gluteal, deep circumflex iliac, and epigastric arteries.[66] A secondary visceral pathway arises from the left colic branch of the superior mesenteric artery, continues through the meandering mesenteric artery, and finally reenters the hypogastric artery via the hemorrhoidal plexus.[18] For external iliac or common femoral artery occlusions, collateral supply develops by way of the hypogastric artery and its gluteal branches with the femoral circumflex branches of the deep femoral artery. This important collateral pathway is known as the *cruciate anastomosis.* The relationship between aortoiliac collateral vessels and the visceral circulation explains how occlusive disease involving both systems may predispose the patient to bowel ischemia and necrosis if these channels are disrupted at surgery or if flow through them is altered after aortofemoral bypass.[18, 49, 62, 69]

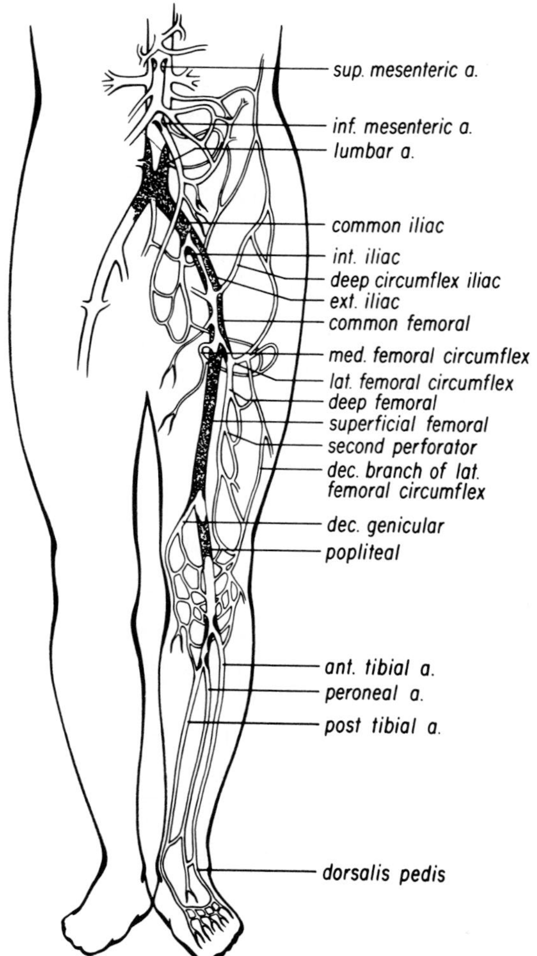

FIGURE 50–2. Diagram of the arterial circulation to the lower extremity, indicating the characteristic segments of obstruction by atherosclerosis *(shaded areas)* and the compensatory collateral network.

The interconnection of the perforating branches of the profunda femoris artery and the genicular branches of the popliteal readily compensates for occlusion of the superficial femoral artery. This network in the upper leg depends largely on the profunda femoris artery as a critical link between the cruciate and genicular networks and emphasizes the importance of a patent popliteal artery that serves as the reentry vessel for this vital collateral pathway. In similar fashion, the genicular arteries, via their tibial connections, bypass popliteal obstructions.[66] Occlusion of the anterior and posterior tibial arteries is often compensated for by the peroneal artery, which sends large collateral branches to the patent distal segments of the tibial arteries at the ankle.[4] Figure 50–2 graphically illustrates the paucity of collaterals in the lower leg and helps to explain why even unisegmental occlusion of the distal popliteal and proximal tibial arteries may result in such severe ischemia of the distal lower extremity.

CLASSIFICATION OF LIMB ISCHEMIA

Limb ischemia is classified as "functional" or "critical." *Functional ischemia* occurs when blood flow is normal in the resting extremity but cannot be increased in response to exercise. Clinically, this is manifested as *claudication.* The term is derived from the Latin verb meaning "to limp" and indicates one of the best-defined entities in clinical medicine. It is the single most important symptom of arterial occlusive disease in an extremity and develops whenever blood flow to the exercising muscle mass is unable to meet the requirements of this increased metabolic activity. It consists of three essential features: the pain is always experienced in a functional muscle unit; it is reproducibly precipitated by a consistent amount of exercise; and it is promptly relieved by merely stopping the exercise. Although a number of syndromes are regularly confused with claudication, careful attention to these features will facilitate accurate diagnosis.[26]

Chronic critical limb ischemia is defined by either of the following two criteria: (1) recurring ischemic rest pain that persists for more than 2 weeks and requires regular analgesics, with an ankle systolic pressure of 50 mmHg or less, a toe systolic pressure of 30 mmHg or less, or both, or (2) ulceration or gangrene of the foot or toes, with similar hemodynamic parameters.[77]

Unlike claudication, *ischemic rest pain* is experienced not in a muscle group but rather in the foot, specifically the toes and metatarsal heads. It should not be confused with *night cramps,* which are common in patients with atherosclerosis and occur as painful cramps of the calf muscle that usually begin after the patient has fallen asleep and are relieved by massaging the muscle. In its earliest manifestations, rest pain may be experienced as dysesthesias in the foot after it has been elevated for some time. At this stage, the pain is usually relieved by dangling the affected extremity over the side of the bed or, paradoxically, by getting up and walking around. Because this typically occurs at night, some clinicians call it *night pain* to distinguish it from the more severe rest pain that is constant and present even with dependency. Ischemic rest pain implies a reduction of blood flow in the extremity to a level below that required for normal resting tissue metabolism. If left untreated, it almost invariably results in tissue necrosis. Such limbs are relatively useless or frankly incapacitated by the constant pain, the paresthesias, and the muscle paresis. Because the patients typically keep such limbs dependent, there is often a considerable amount of edema, which further compromises tissue perfusion. Angiography in such extremities invariably demonstrates at least two, and often three or more, serial obstructions of the arterial tree. By contrast, patients with claudication usually have only one or, at most, two segments involved.

Although the pathophysiology of *critical limb ischemia* (CLI) is not firmly established, the following hypothesis attempts to incorporate much of the new information on this entity.[77] Arteriolar vasodilatation, probably mediated by local hypotension and the release of vasoactive metabolites, is a microvascular compensation that tends to maintain nutritive flow in the presence of proximal arterial occlusion.[78] Paradoxically, some patients with CLI have increased *total* skin blood flow in the ischemic foot, probably because of maximal vasodilatation in the neighboring ischemic tissue.[79] Therefore, the ultimate cause of CLI is presumably maldistribution of skin microcirculation in addition to reduced total blood flow. The importance of the microcirculation in CLI is emphasized by the wide overlap in ankle or toe systolic blood pressures when patients who have CLI are compared with patients who have peripheral arterial disease without CLI.

The ultimate sequence of events leading to decreased capillary perfusion in CLI is not established. However, the potential mechanisms probably include collapse of precapillary arterioles because of low transmural pressure; arteriolar vasospasm; abnormal vasomotion; microthrombosis; collapse of capillaries caused by interstitial edema; capillary occlusion by endothelial cell swelling, platelet aggregates, rigid adhesive leukocytes, rigid red blood cells, or blood cell–platelet aggregates; and local activation of the immune system.[80] Figure 50–3 attempts to summarize the changes in CLI at different levels of the circulation. Regardless of the precise pathophysiologic mechanisms that are operational, the net result is an inhomogeneous perfusion of the skin microvessels.

Certainly, a clear distinction between the two categories (i.e., functional ischemia and CLI) is not always possible, and a certain amount of overlap is to be expected because they represent merely two points on the spectrum of the same disease. Patients with severe claudication may develop CLI without any actual change in limb perfusion if they sustain an injury to the ischemic limb or develop an infection in it. Because there is no functional arterial reserve to meet the increased demands required for healing, the stage is set for progressive necrosis and spreading infection.

The diagnosis of ischemic rest pain may be particularly difficult in the patient with diabetes mellitus. Because atherosclerosis with loss of peripheral pulses is more common in such patients and is often associated with a peripheral neuropathy that can mimic rest pain, the noninvasive vascular laboratory can be very helpful in correctly identifying them.[37] The use of such physiologic testing as well as angiography to define the extent, severity, and operability of the occlusive lesions is discussed in greater detail in Chapters 2 and 4 to 8.

ASSOCIATED DISEASES

Because the underlying condition (i.e., atherosclerosis) cannot be treated directly, it is important for the clinician to identify any of the associated diseases that are known to influence its course and to direct his or her therapeutic efforts against them. This approach is outlined more completely in Chapter 51, but it should include abstinence from all tobacco products; control of hypertension, diabetes mellitus, and hyperlipoproteinemia; weight reduction when necessary; and treatment of congestive heart failure or azotemia.[11, 19, 55, 63] The presence and severity of these problems not only may influence the course of the disease but also may determine whether surgical correction is feasible and the type of reconstruction that will be most suitable. The importance of meticulous foot care and avoidance of trauma in the ischemic limb cannot be overemphasized.

Diabetes and Arteriosclerosis Obliterans

Because of the unique and important role that diabetes mellitus plays in the pathogenesis of atherosclerosis, it is extensively discussed in Chapter 62. For the present, the authors only highlight some of the more relevant considerations. Although atherosclerosis is not qualitatively different in the diabetic patient, it appears at an earlier age and progresses more rapidly.[20] Furthermore, its distribution differs significantly.[22, 31, 65] The popliteal, tibial, and profunda femoris arteries are more severely and diffusely involved, whereas the aorta and the iliac arteries may remain largely undiseased.[22, 66]

Although the term *small vessel disease* is frequently used in discussing diabetic patients, no anatomically distinct lesion can be identified in their extremity vessels. The degenerative changes seen in the media of the small arterioles and the basement membrane thickening so often iden-

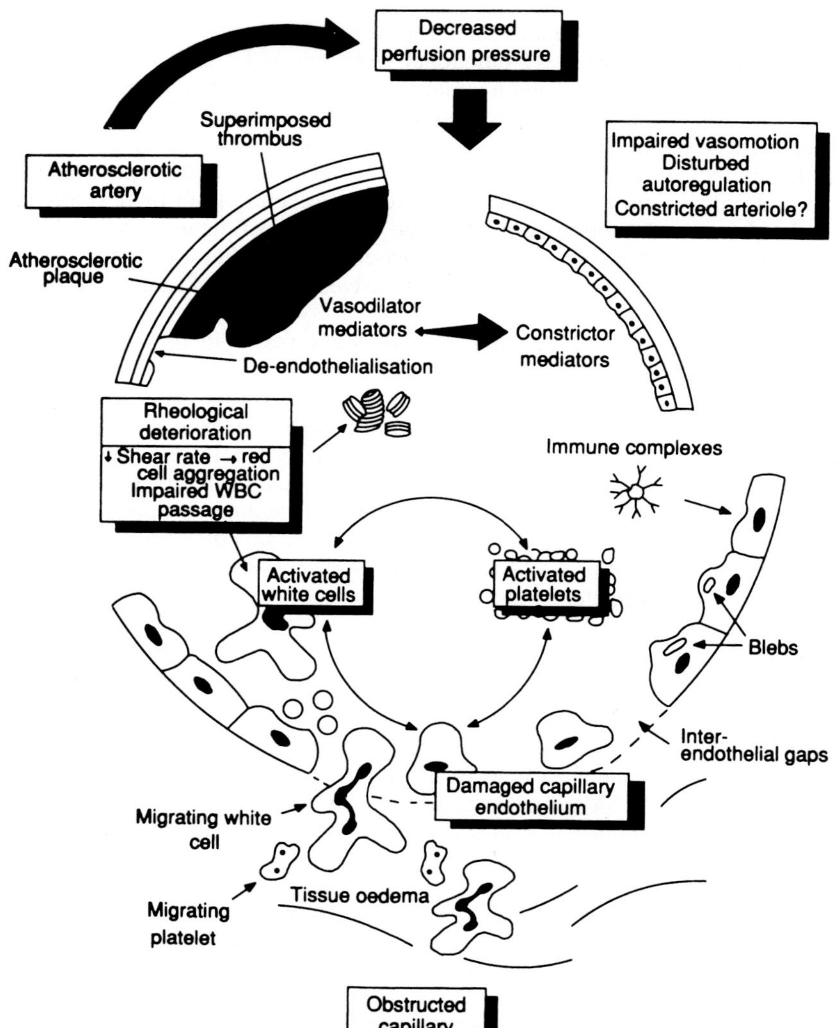

FIGURE 50–3. Summary of suggested pathophysiologic changes in critical leg ischemia at different levels of the circulation. WBC, white blood cell. (From Dormandy J, Verstraete M, Andreani D, et al: Second European consensus document on chronic critical leg ischemia. Circulation 84[Suppl 4]:1, 1991.)

tified in most diabetics are, unfortunately, not unique and can be found in nondiabetic patients with advanced atherosclerosis.[76] These lesions are believed to result in impaired tissue perfusion and nutrition.[2, 5] They may also play a role in the peripheral neuropathy that frequently accompanies diabetes.[31] Because the vascular lesions in both diabetic and nondiabetic persons are qualitatively similar and differ primarily in frequency of occurrence, severity, and distribution, the pathogenetic mechanisms involved are probably comparable but are accelerated in the diabetic.

The combination of neuropathy and peripherally distributed atherosclerosis makes diabetics especially vulnerable to foot lesions. It also greatly complicates the evaluation of their frequent complaints of foot pain. In association with the absence of pedal pulses, such pain might be considered ischemic in origin. Attempts to quantitate perfusion noninvasively are frequently confounded by the presence of *calcific medial sclerosis,* which renders the vessels virtually incompressible and makes ankle pressure measurements meaningless. More distal determinations, such as toe pressures, may be needed to help resolve the question.[8] Even in the absence of demonstrable vascular occlusive disease, diabetic neuropathy and its resulting hypesthesia render the diabetic's foot insensitive to repeated minor trauma, which may lead to the development of ulcers over pressure points or provide a portal of entry for bacteria that can spread rapidly and establish extensive deep-seated infection with remarkably few clinical signs (see Chapter 62). Finally, diabetic neuropathy may also involve the sympathetic nervous system and produce a lower extremity autosympathectomy.[31] This helps to explain the frequent failure of empirically performed surgical sympathectomy to improve skin perfusion in the diabetic patient (see Chapter 59).

Although impaired resistance to infection is frequently invoked to explain the virulence of septic complications in diabetic patients, this concept remains unproved. Nevertheless, they appear less able to contain the spread of infection once it becomes established. It is this triumvirate of peripherally distributed atherosclerosis obliterans, neuropathy, and a reduced ability to contain infection that underlies the frequent foot lesions seen in the diabetic person and ultimately results in a significantly greater rate of limb loss.

NATURAL HISTORY OF THE ATHEROSCLEROTIC LIMB

The development of mild to moderate intermittent claudication poses little threat of limb loss to the nondiabetic patient. Approximately three fourths of such patients will remain symptomatically stable or actually show some improvement 2 to 5 years after onset of their symptoms, and only 5 to 7 per cent will ultimately need extremity amputation.[9, 24] This is in striking contrast to patients who present with ischemic ulceration or rest pain and face an immediate amputation in 19.6 per cent of cases.[25]

The presence and control of coexistent risk factors significantly influence the natural history of atherosclerosis. One study showed that 11.4 per cent of those who continued to smoke required amputation of a limb, whereas none of those who abstained did so.[25] Similarly, the presence of diabetes mellitus adversely affects the course of atherosclerosis. Amputations were required in 8 per cent of nondiabetic and 34 per cent of diabetic patients.[60] Unfortunately, these risk factors are additive, and the prognosis is worst in diabetics who continue to smoke.

The impact of atherosclerosis on the patient's life expectancy is more important than the risk of amputation. The overall survival rate for patients with intermittent claudication is only 72 per cent at 5 years and approximately 50 per cent at 10 years.[25] This is in contrast to an expected 90 per cent 5-year survival rate for age-adjusted control subjects. Evidence of atherosclerosis in other locations further reduces survival. Thus, only 61 per cent of patients with associated cerebrovascular disease and 59 per cent of those with symptomatic coronary artery disease lived for 5 years. Three quarters of these deaths were due to coronary artery disease.[25] Hypertension had a slightly adverse effect on survival, but hypercholesterolemia had no significant effect at the 5-year level.

Serial angiographic studies indicate that progression of atherosclerosis occurs primarily in the arteries proximal to the initial lesion and suggest that it may exert some type of protective influence on the distal vessels.[15, 33, 44, 72] Following successful bypass of the obstruction, this protection is lost.[72]

In summary, the majority of nondiabetic persons with intermittent claudication can expect their symptoms to remain stable, especially if they abstain from tobacco use. On the other hand, those with ischemic rest pain, ulcers, or gangrene are at high risk for both limb loss and premature death. They deserve an aggressive approach to limb salvage when feasible. However, because all patients with symptomatic atherosclerosis are at increased risk for early death, the overall goals of therapy should be to relieve pain and preserve bipedal gait without further jeopardizing the patient's already limited life expectancy.

INDICATIONS FOR SURGERY

It is important to decide which patients are candidates for surgery because only these individuals should undergo arteriography. The mere documentation of symptomatic lower extremity atherosclerosis is not an absolute indication for surgical intervention. This decision is facilitated by first assigning patients to one of two categories: those with functional ischemia and those with CLI.

As already discussed, patients with functional ischemia face little risk of limb loss, especially if they are able to abstain from tobacco use, engage in a program of regular exercise, and control associated medical diseases. Often, merely reassuring such patients that they are not facing impending gangrene will produce a dramatic improvement in their subjective response to their disease. However, if claudication precludes gainful employment or imposes an unacceptable alteration in lifestyle, surgical revascularization should be considered. This decision can be facilitated by physiologic testing of such patients (see Chapter 5). Stress testing, such as treadmill exercise, can reproduce patients' symptoms under controlled conditions, objectively document the degree of disability, and exclude more limiting medical conditions such as coronary artery disease or chronic obstructive pulmonary disease. A further benefit of such testing stems from its ability to localize the arterial lesions with reasonable precision and thus indirectly define the type of arterial repair that would be required to improve the circulation. For example, if a patient with mild to moderate claudication were shown to need a revascularization procedure that entailed a significant risk of limb loss should it fail, it would be foolish to proceed with arteriography. Such risks can be justified only when there is already a serious risk of amputation if the procedure is not performed.

Because the determination of disability resulting from functional limb ischemia is relative, it is the patient's prerogative to request revascularization, provided he or she understands the risks involved and the anticipated benefits of the more conservative, nonoperative approach. As the severity of claudication increases, the surgeon is under less constraint to recommend revascularization. It is now incumbent on the surgeon to select the procedure that will improve circulation most effectively, taking into consideration the patient's risk status and the pattern of the vascular disease.

Critical limb ischemia constitutes a definite indication for arterial reconstruction if the patient's disease is sufficiently localized to permit endarterectomy or bypass grafting with a reasonable likelihood of success and if he or she is able to tolerate the proposed procedure. Even if a patient presents with the recent onset of rest pain or even localized gangrene, amputation or surgical revascularization is not inevitable. Provided that the limb is viable, the conditions of approximately 25 to 30 per cent of such patients can be expected to improve, in time, to intermittent claudication alone as collateral circulation develops. As a result of advances in anesthetic and postoperative management and the development of a variety of percutaneous endovascular techniques for surgical revascularization, currently reported operative mortality rates for most vascular surgical procedures, in the hands of an experienced surgeon, are actually lower that those for amputation of an extremity.[17] Furthermore, even temporary graft patency may be sufficient to permit healing of an ischemic ulcer or toe amputation. Subsequent failure of the vascular repair will not inevitably jeopardize survival of the limb. Patients whose grafts become occluded 6 months to 1 year postoperatively frequently maintain a remarkably comfortable foot at rest and enjoy better rehabilitation than would have been possible with amputation and a prosthesis.[4, 48, 67] Such encouraging exceptions should not, however, delude the vascular surgeon into attempting arterial reconstruction in all patients with critical limb ischemia on the grounds that "they have little to lose." Although several reports have suggested that a failed vascular reconstruction does not appear to affect the level of subsequent amputation adversely, the mortality and morbidity rates for successive, futile attempts at limb salvage are cumulative, and the emotional and physical toll on these often elderly patients with a limited life expectancy is considerable. Furthermore, other experienced vascular surgeons contend that failed distal bypass, especially femoropopliteal, may indeed precipitate an above-knee amputation when a below-knee amputation might have succeeded had the salvage procedure not been attempted.[16, 28, 59] Refinements in amputation techniques that often make it possible to preserve the knee joint and modern limb prostheses can preserve bipedal gait even in elderly patients and restore them to a remarkably normal existence. Heroic surgery in hopeless situations does these patients a disservice and is to be condemned.

On the other hand, in the presence of severe multilevel occlusive disease, blood flow to such extremities can be so poor that preoperative arteriograms may fail to visualize patent distal vessels that would be suitable for bypass. If Doppler insonation of these vessels reveals audible flow signals and if tissue loss can be confined to the toe or distal metatarsal level, popliteal or tibial artery exploration with intraoperative direct arteriography is a reasonable alternative approach to empiric major amputation.[57] However, owing to the increased availability of computer-enhanced digital arteriograms to supplement traditional angiograms, this step is rarely necessary.

GENERAL PRINCIPLES GOVERNING VASCULAR RECONSTRUCTION

Like success in so many areas of medicine, success in vascular surgery is dependent on judicious patient selection, meticulous attention to technical details, and a knowledgeable choice of operative procedure based on certain important principles. Paramount among these is the assurance of a relatively unobstructed inflow and a patent distal runoff if both early and long-term patency are to be achieved. For example, if a femoropopliteal bypass is being planned, it is essential that there be no significant obstruction in the aorta or the iliac arteries and that a patent segment of popliteal artery with sufficient runoff to sustain a graft be present. The auscultation of a femoral bruit or diminution of the femoral pulse, especially after exercise, suggests the presence of significant aortoiliac disease. In some patients, however, this may be difficult to appreciate on the basis of the physical examination alone, and the results of angiography, especially if it is uniplanar, may be confusing.[42, 61] Noninvasive techniques such as analysis of Doppler velocity waveforms from the femoral artery (see Chapter 4) or segmental plethysmography of the thigh may be helpful. If these measures fail to resolve the issue, direct femoral artery pressures can be obtained at the time of angiography or at the time of surgery (see Chapter 5).[10] By first recording aortic pressure and then pulling the catheter back into the femoral artery, the clinician can identify the presence of any pressure gradients at rest. A differential of 15 mmHg is considered significant. Because some lesions might not produce a 15-mmHg gradient at rest, reactive hyperemia should be produced by using cuff-induced ischemia or the intra-arterial injection of a vasodilator in those patients in whom no initial gradient is seen. The importance of ensuring adequate inflow cannot be overemphasized. In an experimental canine model, graft occlusion regularly occurred when an inflow stenosis was induced, but the graft remained patent despite an equivalent degree of outflow stenosis.[30]

The effectiveness of runoff vessels distal to an obstruction may be difficult to assess. Although a patent common femoral artery with disease-free superficial and deep femoral arteries or a patent popliteal artery with an intact crural runoff is ideal, the profunda femoris artery can be a perfectly adequate recipient for the entire inflow into the lower extremity.[1, 65] Excellent long-term patency and function can be expected from grafts carried into this vessel despite superficial femoral artery occlusion.[38, 43] Occasionally, an extensive angioplasty of the profunda femoris artery may be necessary before the anastomosis is fashioned (see Chapter 55).

Similarly, extensive disease in the popliteal artery or the tibial vessels does not preclude revascularization in limb-threatening situations. Bypass into a patent popliteal artery without direct runoff into the tibial arteries can be performed, with results comparable to those of conventional femoropopliteal grafting.[36] Distal perfusion relies on the geniculate collateral vessels arising from this so-called isolated popliteal segment to carry blood flow to the more distal vessels of the leg and foot. This approach is particularly suitable for the treatment of rest pain or superficial focal gangrene. When the gangrene is more extensive, higher perfusion pressures are needed to achieve healing, and direct bypass into the tibial arteries is usually required.[4, 48, 52] The technical failure rate for these demanding small vessel anastomoses is higher than that for femoropopliteal bypass, and only 50 to 60 per cent of them will still be patent 2 years after implantation. Limb salvage rates, however, are higher, averaging 75 per cent over the same period for the reasons already given. Some authors have suggested that these results can be improved by performing multiple sequential distal anastomoses to increase the available runoff bed, to augment the flow through the graft, and to improve long-term patency.[13] Although the sequential bypass technique has great theoretical appeal, sufficient long-term data are not yet available to confirm its effectiveness (see Chapter 53). Yet another approach for bypass to the infrapopliteal vessels is the use of the autogenous saphenous vein in situ (see Chapter 28). Although a technically more demanding and time-consuming procedure than conventional vein bypass, it offers a better size-match between the small distal vein and the tibial artery, increased utilization of the vein, and the possibility of improved long-term patency.

Most patients selected for vascular reconstruction have arterial obstructions at two or more levels in the same arterial system because chronic unisegmental lesions rarely produce disability serious enough to warrant revascularization. The general principles that govern the choice of operation in these cases are (1) if all lesions are of equal severity, correct the most proximal lesion first and (2) if the lesions are of greatly differing severity, correct the more severe occlusion first. However, if the more proximal lesion is hemodynamically significant, even if it is less severe than the distal lesion, failure to correct it will often lead to premature graft occlusion or failure to relieve the patient's symptoms. The importance of correcting "inflow" disease first is worth reemphasizing. Restoration of pulsatile arterial flow through or around the proximal obstruction will augment circulation through the distal collateral beds sufficiently to ensure limb salvage in most cases and will significantly improve exercise tolerance.[5, 35, 43, 67] The simultaneous addition of a distal bypass is rarely required. The most common example of this problem is the patient with significant aortoiliac stenosis and an ipsilateral occlusion of the superficial femoral artery. Aortofemoral bypass into a widely patent profunda femoris artery will heal ischemic lesions of the foot, relieve rest pain, and markedly reduce claudication, especially if the distal profunda femoris artery is disease-free and the popliteal artery and its tibial branches are patent.[41] In some instances, even pedal pulses may be restored through these collateral channels (see Chapter 52).[43]

Management of less severe degrees of proximal disease has been a particularly perplexing problem. Surgeons were unwilling to recommend repair of a lesion that was unlikely to improve the patient's arterial hemodynamics, but at the same time, they were aware that if left untreated, such lesions would progress with time and jeopardize the distal bypass. The development of percutaneous transluminal angioplasty has now provided surgeons with an acceptable alternative (see Chapter 59). Before the proposed distal bypass is undertaken, the proximal lesion can be corrected with angioplasty and the hemodynamic improvement of this procedure can be assessed by means of noninvasive tests. If the distal bypass appears to be still necessary, the surgeon can proceed with the assurance that good inflow has now been provided. Because of the ease and apparent simplicity of percutaneous transluminal angioplasty, some surgeons have extended its indications to cases in which the symptoms are so mild that surgical revascularization would never have been considered. Unfortunately, failure of the angioplasty may precipitate the need for urgent surgical intervention; angioplasty should therefore be considered only in those cases in which there are acceptable surgical indications. Conversely, some patients with critical limb ischemia have such severe associated diseases that standard surgical revascularization may be out of the question. Transluminal angioplasty in such patients may spell the difference between major amputation and a comfortable, viable extremity.

Another alternative available to the vascular surgeon in the management of such cases is so-called extra-anatomic bypass (see Chapter 54). Although not as durable as more conventional bypass grafts, these procedures can be performed under local anesthesia and provide the patient with adequate long-term blood flow to the extremity.

The role of lumbar sympathectomy in the treatment of chronic lower extremity arterial insufficiency continues to be hotly debated. Although it offers little objective benefit to the patient with functional ischemia, it may relieve mild rest pain or help heal limited areas of superficial gangrene of the pedal skin in some patients who do not have a surgically correctable arterial lesion. The advisability of adding it to an arterial reconstruction remains controversial. Conclusive evidence for either point of view is lacking. Theoretically, the augmented graft flow, which undeniably occurs in such circumstances, helps to prevent graft occlusion during the early postoperative period when the pseudointima is forming and thrombosis is most likely. This consideration may be important in poor runoff situations or in bypasses to small tibial arteries. This entire subject is discussed in greater detail in Chapter 59.

Because no vascular operation alters or arrests the underlying atherosclerotic process, the patient remains vulnerable to progression of the disease in the vessels contiguous to the bypass or in sites remote from the primary operation. The responsible surgeon thus must accept the obligation to perform continuous long-term follow-up of all patients with symptomatic arterial occlusive disease. The surgeon must be vigilant to detect the earliest signs of new occlusive lesions that might threaten the continued patency of the reconstruction and be alert to possible late deterioration or complications of the bypass graft itself. He or she must also remain cognizant of the risk to patients' survival posed by other other manifestations of their primary disease and take appropriate steps to control these whenever possible.

CONCLUSION

Many ischemic extremities that would certainly have been amputated just a few years ago can now be salvaged by a variety of ingenious techniques available to the trained vascular surgeon. Patients should be carefully selected for elective revascularization, and appropriate reconstructive procedures should be chosen that will ensure the maximal improvement in limb perfusion with the least risk to the patient. The surgeon is assisted in making these decisions by a wide range of new tests capable of assessing the physiologic impact of the patient's disease and by significant improvements in angiography that demonstrate the anatomy of the occlusive process with increased clarity. Proper selection of the most appropriate course of management from the bewildering array of alternatives now available requires a considerable degree of training and clinical experience. Only through extensive and ongoing involvement in the management of these clinical problems can the vascular surgeon maintain the judgment and technical skill required to achieve optimal results.

References

1. Baddeley RM, Ashton F, Slaney G, et al: Late results of autogenous vein bypass grafts in femoropopliteal arterial occlusion. Br Med J 1:653, 1970.
2. Barner HB, Kaiser GC, Willman VL: Blood flow in the diabetic leg. Circulation 43:391, 1971.
3. Barner HB, Kaiser GC, Willman VL, et al: Intermittent claudication with pedal pulses. JAMA 204:100, 1968.

4. Bernhard VM, Ashmore CS, Evans WE, et al: Bypass grafting to distal arteries for limb salvage. Surg Gynecol Obstet 135:219, 1972.
5. Bernhard VM, Militello JM, Geringer AM: Repair of the profunda femoris artery. Am J Surg 127:676, 1974.
6. Bernhard VM, Ashmore CS, Rodgers RE, et al: Operative blood flow in femoral-popliteal and femoral-tibial grafts for lower extremity ischemia. Arch Surg 103:595, 1971.
7. Blaisdell FW, Hall AD: Axillary-femoral artery bypass for lower extremity ischemia. Surgery 54:563, 1963.
8. Bone GE, Pomajzl MJ: Toe blood pressure by photoplethysmography: An index of healing in forefoot amputation. Surgery 89:569, 1981.
9. Boyd AM: Natural course of arteriosclerosis of lower extremities. Proc R Soc Med 53:591, 1962.
10. Brener BJ, Brief DK, Alpert J: The usefulness of intra-arterial pressure measurements in occlusive arterial disease. 1. Vasc Diagn Ther 3:37, 1982.
11. Brown AL, Juergens JL: Arteriosclerosis and atherosclerosis. *In* Fairbairns JF, Juergens JL, Spittel JA (eds): Peripheral Vascular Disease. Philadelphia, WB Saunders, 1972.
12. Brown H, Sellwood RA, Harrison CV, et al: Thromboangitis obliterans. Br J Surg 56:59, 1969.
13. Burdick JF, O'Mara C, Ricotta J, et al: The multiple sequential distal bypass graft: Improving nature's alternatives. Surgery 89:536, 1981.
14. Burgess EM, Marsden FW: Major lower extremity amputation following arterial reconstruction. Arch Surg 108:655, 1974.
15. Coran AG, Warren R: Arteriographic changes in femoropopliteal arteriosclerosis obliterans. N Engl J Med 274:643, 1966.
16. Dardik H, Kahn M, Dardik I, et al: Influence of failed vascular bypass procedures on conversion of below-knee to above-knee amputation levels. Surgery 91:64, 1982.
17. DeWeese JA, Blaisdell FW, Foster JH: Optimal resources for vascular surgery. Arch Surg 105:948, 1972.
18. Gonzalez LI, Jaffe MS: Mesenteric arterial insufficiency following abdominal aortic resection. Arch Surg 93:10, 1966.
19. Gordon T, Kannel WB: Predisposition to atherosclerosis in the head, heart and legs. The Framingham study. JAMA 221:661, 1972.
20. Guggenheim W, Koch G, Adams AP, et al: Femoral and popliteal occlusive vascular disease. A report on 143 diabetic patients. Diabetes 18:428, 1969.
21. Haid SP, Conn J Jr, Bergan JJ: Cystic adventitial disease of the popliteal artery. Arch Surg 101:765, 1970.
22. Haimovici H: Patterns of arteriosclerotic lesions of the lower extremity. Arch Surg 95:918, 1967.
23. Haust MD, More RH: Development of modern theories on the pathogenesis of atherosclerosis. *In* Wissler RW, Geer JC (eds): The Pathogenesis of Atherosclerosis. Baltimore, Williams & Wilkins, 1972, pp 1–19.
24. Imparato AM, Kim GE, Davidson T, et al: Intermittent claudication: Its natural course. Surgery 78:795, 1975.
25. Juergens JC, Barker NW, Hines EA: Arteriosclerosis obliterans. Review of 520 cases with special reference to pathogenic and prognostic factors. Circulation 21:188, 1960.
26. Kempczinski RF: The differential diagnosis of intermittent claudication. Pract Cardiol 7:53, 1981.
27. Kempczinski RF: Peripheral arterial atheroembolism. *In* Miller DC, Roon AJ (eds): Diagnosis and Management of Peripheral Vascular Disease. Menlo Park, CA, Addison-Wesley Publishing Company, 1982.
28. Kihn RB, Warren R, Beebe GW: The ''geriatric'' amputee. Ann Surg 176:305, 1972.
29. Kinlough-Rathbone RL, Mustard JF: Atherosclerosis. Current concepts. Am J Surg 141:638, 1981.
30. Kirkpatrick JR, Miller DR: Effects of decreased arterial inflow and runoff on vein graft patency. Surgery 69:870, 1971.
31. Levin ME, O'Neal LW: The Diabetic Foot. St. Louis, CV Mosby, 1973.
32. Levy MN, Share L: The influence of erythrocyte concentration upon the pressure flow relationships in the dog's hind limb. Circ Res 1:247, 1953.
33. Lindbom A: Arteriosclerosis and arterial thrombosis in the lower limb. A roentgenological study. Acta Radiol Suppl 80:1, 1950.
34. Love JW, Whelan TJ: Popliteal artery entrapment syndrome. Am J Surg 109:620, 1965.
35. Malone JM, Moore WS, Goldstone J: The natural history of bilateral aortofemoral bypass-grafts for ischemia of the lower extremities. Arch Surg 110:1300, 1975.
36. Mannick JA, Jackson BT, Coffman JD, et al: Success of bypass vein grafts in patients with isolated popliteal artery segments. Surgery 61:17, 1967.
37. Marinelli MR, Beach KW, Glass MJ, et al: Noninvasive testing vs. clinical evaluation of arterial disease. A prospective study. JAMA 241:2031, 1979.
38. Martin P, Frawley JE, Barabas AP, et al: On the surgery of atherosclerosis of the profunda femoris artery. Surgery 71:182, 1972.
39. Mavor GE: The pattern of occlusion in atheroma of the lower limb arteries. The correlation of clinical and arteriographic findings. Br J Surg 43(180):352, 1956.
40. McKusick VA, Harris WS, Ottesen OE, et al: Buerger's disease: A distinct clinical and pathologic entity. JAMA 181:93, 1962.
41. Mitchell RA, Bone GE, Bridges R, et al: Patient selection for isolated profundaplasty. Arteriographic correlates of operative results. Am J Surg 138:912, 1979.
42. Moore WS, Hall AD: Unrecognized aortoiliac stenosis. Arch Surg 103:633, 1971.
43. Morris GC Jr, Wheeler CG, Crawford ES, et al: Restorative vascular surgery in the presence of impending and overt gangrene of the extremities. Surgery 51:50, 1962.
44. Mozersky DJ, Sumner DS, Strandness DE Jr: Disease progression after femoropopliteal surgical procedures. Surg Gynecol Obstet 135:700, 1972.
45. Mozes M, Cahansky G, Doitsch V, et al: The association of atherosclerosis and Buerger's disease: A clinical and radiological study. J Cardiovasc Surg 11:52, 1970.
46. Mustard JF: Recent advances in molecular pathology: A review. Platelet aggregation, vascular injury and atherosclerosis. Exp Mol Pathol 7:366, 1967.
47. Newman EV, et al: Report by the National Heart and Lung Institute Task Force on Arteriosclerosis. 1971, vol. II. DHEW Publication (NIH) 72–219. Bethesda, MD, National Institutes of Health.
48. Noon GP, Diethrich EB, Richardson WP, et al: Distal tibial artery bypass. Arch Surg 99:770, 1969.
49. Ottinger LW, Darling RC, Nathan MJ, et al: Left colon ischemia complicating aortoiliac reconstruction. Arch Surg 105:841, 1972.
50. Pelgeram LO: Relation of plasma fibrinogen concentration changes to human arteriosclerosis. J Appl Physiol 16:660, 1961.
51. Perdue GD Jr, Smith RB: Atheromatous microemboli. Ann Surg 169:954, 1969.
52. Reichle FA, Tyson RR: Comparison of long-term results of 364 femoropopliteal or femorotibial bypasses for revascularization of severely ischemic lower extremities. Ann Surg 182:449, 1975.
53. Replogle RL, Muselman HJ, Merrell EW: Clinical implication of blood rheology studies. Circulation 36:148, 1967.
54. Roberts B, Gertner MH, Ring EJ: Balloon-catheter dilation as an adjunct to arterial surgery. Arch Surg 116:809, 1981.
55. Rosen AJ, DePalma RG: Risk factors in peripheral atherosclerosis. Arch Surg 107:303, 1973.
56. Samson RH, Gupta SK, Scher LA, et al: Level of amputation after failure of limb salvage procedures. Surg Gynecol Obstet 154:56, 1982.
57. Scarpato R, Gembarowicz R, Farber S, et al: Intraoperative prereconstruction arteriography. Arch Surg 116:1053, 1981.
58. Schadt DC, Hines EA Jr, Juergens JL, et al: Chronic atherosclerotic occlusion of the femoral artery. JAMA 175:937, 1961.
59. Schenker JD, Wolkoff JS: Major amputations after femoropopliteal bypass procedures. Am J Surg 129:495, 1975.
60. Silbert S, Zazeela H: Prognosis in arteriosclerotic peripheral vascular disease. JAMA 166:1816, 1958.
61. Slot HB, Strijbosch L, Greep JM: Interobserver variability in single-plane aortography. Surgery 90:497, 1981.
62. Smith RF, Szilagyi DE: Ischemia of the colon as a complication in the surgery of the abdominal aorta. Arch Surg 80:806, 1960.
63. Stamler J, Berkson DM, Lindberg HA: Risk factors: Their role in the etiology and pathogenesis of the atherosclerotic diseases. *In* Wissler RW, Geer JC (eds): The Pathogenesis of Atherosclerosis. Baltimore, Williams & Wilkins, 1972, pp 41–119.
64. Stary HC: Disease of small blood vessels in diabetes mellitus. Am J Med Sci 252:357, 1966.

65. Stoney RJ, James DR, Wylie EJ: Surgery for femoropopliteal atherosclerosis. A reappraisal. Arch Surg 103:548, 1971.
66. Strandness DF: Collateral Circulation in Clinical Surgery. Philadelphia, WB Saunders, 1969.
67. Taylor GW: Limb salvage arterial surgery for gangrene. Postgrad Med J 47:251, 1971.
68. Texon M, Imparato AM, Helpern M: The role of vascular dynamics in the development of atherosclerosis. JAMA 194:168, 1965.
69. Trippel OH, Jurayj MN, Medell AL: The aorto-iliac steal: A review of this syndrome and a report of one additional case. Ann Surg 175:454, 1972.
70. Vetto RM: The treatment of unilateral iliac artery obstruction with a transabdominal, subcutaneous, femorofemoral graft. Surgery 52:342, 1962.
71. Walton KW: Pathogenetic mechanisms in atherosclerosis. Am J Cardiol 35:542, 1975.
72. Warren R, Gomez RL, Marston JAP, et al: Femoropopliteal arteriosclerosis obliterans—Arteriographic patterns and rates of progression. Surgery 55:135, 1964.
73. Weale FE: An Introduction to Surgical Haemodynamics. Chicago, Year Book Medical Publishers, 1967.
74. Wessler S, Ming S, Gurewich V, et al: A critical evaluation of thromboangiitis obliterans. The case against Buerger's disease. N Engl J Med 161:1149, 1960.
75. Whittaker SRF, Winton FR: Apparent viscosity of blood in isolated hind limb of dog and its variation with corpuscular concentration. J Physiol 78:339, 1933.
76. Williamson JR, Kilo C, Crespin SR: Vascular disease. *In* Levin ME, O'Neil LW (eds): The Diabetic Foot. St. Louis, CV Mosby, 1977.
77. Dormandy J, Verstraete M, Andreani D, et al: Second European consensus document on chronic critical leg ischemia. Circulation 84(Suppl 4):1, 1991.
78. Bollinger A, Barras JP, Mahler F: Measurement of foot artery blood pressure by micromanometry in normal subjects and in patients with arterial occlusive disease. Circulation 53:506, 1976.
79. McEwan AJ, Ledingham IM: Blood flow characteristics and tissue nutrition in apparently ischaemic feet. Br Med J 3:220, 1971.
80. Lowe GD: Pathophysiology of critical limb ischaemia. *In* Dormandy J, Stock G (eds): Critical Leg Ischaemia: Its Pathophysiology and Management. Berlin, Springer-Verlag, 1990, pp 17–38.

51

Natural History and Nonoperative Treatment of Chronic Lower Extremity Ischemia

Lloyd M. Taylor, Jr., M.D., and John M. Porter, M.D.

• • •

Vascular surgery in North America occupies an unusual position in the organization of medical specialities. In contrast to the situation of most other surgical disciplines, no widely represented branch of internal medicine is primarily concerned with the diagnosis and treatment of peripheral vascular disorders. Thus, no internal medicine specialists have the same relationship to vascular surgeons as do cardiologists to cardiac surgeons, gastroenterologists to general surgeons, endocrinologists to endocrine surgeons, and so forth. This means that the vascular surgeon is placed regularly in the role of diagnostician, primary care provider, and nonoperative therapist for patients, without participation of an appropriately trained and knowledgeable internal medicine colleague. This situation is changing at present. Vascular medicine, long a recognized subspecialty in a few academic centers, is becoming a topic of interest and considerable national funding support. New departments and training programs are being formed, and the next decade will witness the arrival of a small but increasing number of trained specialists in vascular medicine. For the foreseeable future, however, the impact of these welcome colleagues on the scope of care of patients with vascular disease will remain small. Thus, vascular surgeons must become as knowledgeable in the nonoperative as in the operative treatment of vascular disease.

The requirement for such detailed knowledge is nowhere more evident than in dealing with patients who have chronic lower extremity ischemia. Lower extremity claudication caused by atherosclerotic occlusive disease[30, 76] affects an estimated 10 per cent of the US population over age 70 and 1 to 2 per cent of individuals aged 37 to 69. In view of the rapidly aging profile of the US population, it is clear that many more patients will be affected in the next several decades[79] (Fig. 51–1). At present, only about 100,000 operations for treatment of lower extremity ischemia are performed annually in the United States.[88] Clearly, a large majority of persons with lower extremity ischemia are currently treated nonoperatively. The modern practice of vascular surgery obviously requires a detailed knowledge of the natural history and nonoperative treatment of lower extremity ischemia.

A description of the authors' approach to the nonoperative treatment of lower extremity ischemia forms the basis for this chapter. The subjects discussed include the natural history of chronic lower extremity ischemia, the use of objective diagnostic tests to detect the severity and loca-

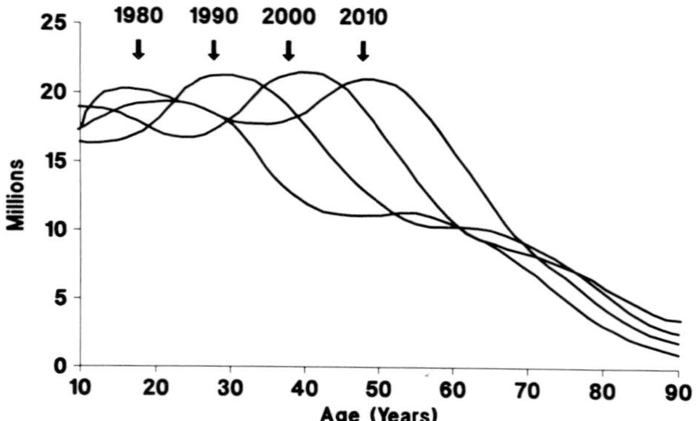

FIGURE 51–1. Age profile of United States population in each decade, 1980 to 2010. Note rapid increase in mean age of largest population group. (From Johnson G Jr: The second-generation vascular surgeon. J Vasc Surg 5:213, 1987.)

tion of occlusive lesions and to evaluate their physiologic significance, the therapeutic roles of exercise therapy and cessation of tobacco use, and finally, several proposed therapeutic approaches currently considered unconventional or of unproven benefit in the treatment of lower extremity ischemia.

NATURAL HISTORY OF LOWER EXTREMITY ISCHEMIA

Operative treatment of lower extremity arterial occlusive disease has been widely performed since the late 1950s. Although it may be thought that a large body of data concerning the natural history of unoperated lower extremity occlusive disease would have been collected before this era, such is not the case. As has often been true in the history of surgery, acquisition of accurate knowledge about the natural history of a condition unmodified by surgery appears to have been prompted by the evolution of a surgical treatment proposed as a superior alternative to the presumed natural history. Thus, well-documented studies of the natural history of untreated lower extremity ischemia date from the same historical period as the development of surgical treatment methods.

Patients with lower extremity ischemia have been traditionally divided into two distinct groups based on presumed markedly different natural histories: those with intermittent claudication and those with limb-threatening ischemia. Each of these is considered in detail in this chapter.

Claudication

Intermittent claudication is defined as a clinical condition of lower extremity muscle pain induced by exercise and relieved by short periods of rest. It is caused by fixed arterial obstruction at sites proximal to the affected muscle bed such that the normal exercise-induced increase in muscle blood flow cannot occur to a degree sufficient to meet the metabolic demands of exercising muscle. Interestingly, the perceived significance of claudication varies widely among affected individuals. Fully 50 to 90 per cent of patients with definite intermittent claudication do not complain of this symptom to their physicians.[52, 83] They appear to accept increasing difficulty in walking as a normal consequence of aging. In one well-documented prospective study, two thirds of patients with arteriographically proven lower extremity arterial occlusions denied claudication on an initial questionnaire, and one third steadfastly maintained that they were without symptoms even after a detailed interview.[104] Similar results noted by other investigators illustrate the relative nature of the claudication symptom: that is, the patient must both possess a sufficiently significant arterial stenosis and exercise sufficiently to induce relative muscle ischemia.[18] These observations are important because they emphasize that studies of the natural history of claudication are for the most part descriptive of the outcome of a symptom complex rather than a disease process. Indeed, the natural history of asymptomatic patients with arterial lesions morphologically identical to those found in claudicators is largely unknown.

The most feared consequence of lower extremity claudication is progression to severe ischemia, with an ultimate need for amputation. Almost all historical studies of large patient groups with claudication have convincingly demonstrated that this progression is an unusual event. Boyd prospectively followed up 1440 patients with intermittent claudication and found that after 10 years, only 12.2 per cent required amputation.[10] In the Framingham study, only 1.6 per cent of claudicators followed up for 8.3 years required amputation.[59] The results of multiple historical studies regarding the natural history of claudication are summarized in Table 51–1.

The risk factors associated with increased likelihood of worsening of claudication have been described by multiple authors. Continued cigarette smoking has repeatedly been identified as the most consistent adverse risk factor associated with progression of lower extremity ischemia in claudicators. Another important risk factor for disease progression is the severity of the initial arterial occlusive disease process, as assessed by symptoms, angiography,[55] or noninvasive segmental pressure measurements.[19, 56] Diabetics have been identified as having a higher likelihood of progression to gangrene and limb loss in some studies[52, 76] but not in others.[49, 56]

The low long-term likelihood of limb loss in claudicators demonstrated by multiple historical studies must be viewed with some skepticism. Clearly, many patients with leg pain on walking do not have occlusive arterial disease, and this obviously may have biased many long-term studies that admitted patients by history only, without objective documentation of arterial occlusion. An objective method that clearly identifies the claudicating patient and allows quantitation of the severity of the symptoms is readily available. Measurement of the ankle-brachial pressure index before and after treadmill walking is a simple noninvasive method that fulfills these requirements. Interestingly, modern studies in which abnormal findings on a noninvasive lower extremity arterial examination were an entrance requirement have demonstrated a more morbid prognosis than that outlined by historical studies that relied on patient history or on angiographic demonstration of arterial disease

Table 51–1. Historical Studies of the Natural History of Claudication Progression to Severe Limb Ischemia

Study	No. of Patients	Mean Follow-Up (yr)	Stable or Improved (%)	Worse (%)	Amputated (%)
Boyd, 1960[10]	1440	10.0	—	—	12.2
McAllister, 1976[72]	100	6.0	78	22	7
Imparato et al, 1975[55]	104	2.5	79	21	5.8
Peabody et al, 1974[76]	162	8.3	—	—	4.3

without further quantitation of severity. Table 51–2 lists the results of more recent studies of the natural history of claudication in which objective demonstration of lower extremity arterial occlusive disease was required for entry into the study. Importantly, in each of these studies, the *severity of the arterial obstruction as determined objectively at the time of initial patient encounter* was the most important factor in predicting the subsequent patient outcome. This objective information is important because it is readily obtained (the ankle-brachial systolic pressure index is easily measured in any physician's office) and allows stratification of patients into high- and low-risk groups. The information in Table 51–2 clearly indicates that by no means all patients with claudication have a benign prognosis and that prediction of a benign prognosis on the basis of symptoms alone may not represent the current state of the art. The published recommended standards for reporting the results of studies of lower extremity ischemia represent a proper first step in improving the validity of future information by insisting on objective characterization of the severity of ischemia in addition to a description of symptoms.[2]

The systemic nature of the atherosclerotic disease process producing claudication is emphasized by the incidence and severity of associated cerebral and coronary vascular disease found in claudicators. Until fairly recently, accurate assessment of the incidence of coronary and cerebral atherosclerosis in claudicators was limited by the lack of suitable diagnostic studies. However, several recent studies have contributed important new information in these areas. The first of these is the remarkable patient series accumulated at the Cleveland Clinic under the direction of Hertzer and colleagues, following a policy decision to perform coronary arteriography in 1000 consecutive patients before elective vascular surgery without regard to the presence of symptoms of coronary disease. Angiographically identifiable coronary atherosclerosis was detected in 90 per cent of all patients scheduled for operation to treat claudication (381 of the 1000 patients).[48] The same group of investigators detected only a 47 per cent incidence of coronary disease in similar patients when the clinical history and resting electrocardiographic findings were used for screening,[49] emphasizing the asymptomatic nature of a considerable portion of the coronary disease identified angiographically. An important finding from this study was the demonstration of severe surgically correctable coronary disease in 14 per cent of asymptomatic patients with no historical or electrocardiographic evidence of disease. These important data are seen in Table 51–3. The reader should remember that these data are derived from a population of patients being considered for surgical treatment of lower extremity ischemia, whose conditions thus represent the most severe portions of the clinical spectrum of lower extremity occlusive disease. It is reasonable to assume that the spectrum of coronary artery disease found in these patients is more severe than that found in the entire group of claudicators, most of whom are insufficiently symptomatic to prompt surgical intervention.

The availability of duplex scanning of the carotid bifurcation, a test that detects the presence of cervical carotid artery disease with accuracy comparable to that achieved with angiography, has made it possible to screen large numbers of claudicators for carotid artery atherosclerosis. In one study of preoperative patients, 52 per cent were found to have detectable carotid artery disease.[99] In the authors' experience, 40 per cent of patients examined by duplex scanning before surgery for correction of claudication had demonstrable cervical carotid artery disease. In the majority of these patients, the carotid stenosis was asymptomatic. Interestingly, one fourth of the claudicators with carotid disease, or 10 per cent of all claudicators, had carotid artery stenoses in excess of 60 per cent diameter reduction, emphasizing the severity of the generalized atherosclerotic process.[66]

A study by Ahn and coworkers used duplex scanning to examine the carotid arteries of 78 patients with lower extremity vascular disease who had no clinical evidence of

Table 51–2. Natural History of Claudication as Determined by Objective Studies

Study	No. of Patients	Mean Follow-Up (yr)	Stable (%)	Worse (%)	Amputated (%)
Cronenwett et al, 1984[19]	91	2.5	40	60	—
Rosenbloom et al, 1988[117]	195	8	59	41	—
Jonason and Ringqvist, 1985[118]	224	6	78	22	—
Walsh et al, 1991[119]*	38	3	72	28	—

**Evaluated superficial femoral stenoses only.*

Table 51–3. Incidence of Coronary Artery Disease in 1000 Consecutive Peripheral Disease Patients Screened by Coronary Angiography

	Clinical Assessment of Coronary Disease			
	No Indications of Coronary Disease		*Suspected Coronary Disease*	
	No. of Patients	Per Cent	No. of Patients	Per Cent
Normal coronary arteries	64	14	21	4
Mild to moderate CAD	218	49	99	18
Advanced but compensated CAD	97	22	192	34
Severe correctable CAD	63	14	188	34
Severe inoperable CAD	4	1	54	10

From Hertzer NR, Beven EG, Young JR, et al: Coronary artery disease in peripheral vascular patients: A classification of 1000 coronary angiograms and results of surgical management. Ann Surg 199:223, 1984.

CAD, coronary artery disease.

Table 51–4. Survival of Patients with Claudication Followed Up Without Operation

Study	No. of Patients	Mean Follow-Up (yr)	5-Year Survival (%)	10-Year Survival (%)	15-Year Survival (%)	Age
Bloor, 1961[8]	1476	7.0	79.0	54	—	45–54
			72.0	35	—	55–64
			60.0	20	—	65–74
Silbert and Zazeela, 1958[92]	1198	12.0	94.7	71	52	
Kallero, 1981[58]	193	9.7	—	52	—	
Schadt et al, 1961[90]*	362	9.0	76.0	59	—	
			54.0	38		
Lefevre et al, 1959[64]	500	5.0	57.0	—	—	

**The top line reflects data for nondiabetics; the bottom line is data for diabetics.*

Table 51–5. Survival of Patients with Claudication Treated by Operation

Study	No. of Patients	Follow-Up (yr)	5-Year Survival (%)	10-Year Survival (%)	15-Year Survival (%)
Szilagyi et al, 1979[96]	531	0–15	44	25	6
Hansteen et al, 1975[45]	307	8–16	70	50	37
Crawford et al, 1981[17]	949	0–25	74	50	30
Szilagyi et al, 1986[97]	1648	0–30	70	64	25
Hertzer, 1981[49]	256	6–11	80	60	—
Malone et al, 1977[67]	180	0–15	80	43	26

carotid artery disease (carotid bruit, abnormal carotid pulses, or neurologic symptoms).[105] They found 16 to 50 per cent stenosis of the internal carotid artery in 33 per cent of the patients, greater than 50 per cent stenosis in 14 per cent of the patients, and greater than 75 per cent stenosis in 5 per cent of the patients.

From these data, one may accurately predict lower long-term survival rates in claudicators than in age-matched controls. All investigations have found that the presence of claudication identifies a patient group with significantly shortened survival when compared with age-matched controls. Table 51–4 shows the results of several long-term studies of survival of unoperated claudicators. Table 51–5 gives similar data for patients operated on for claudication. Combining these data permits construction of an approximate life table survival curve allowing comparison with the anticipated survival of an age-matched control group. As shown in Figure 51–2, this indicates that the predicted mortality rates for patients with claudication at 5, 10, and 15 years' follow-up are approximately 30, 50, and 70 per cent, respectively, mortality rates significantly in excess of those observed in control groups.

As is evident from Tables 51–4 and 51–5, the anticipated long-term survival of patients with lower extremity ischemia appears to be related to the severity of ischemia. This stratification of survival risk also applies to patients with more severe degrees of ischemia. Thus, 5-year patient survival rates range from 87 per cent in a series of patients with claudication who were treated nonoperatively[106] to 80 per cent in a series of patients with claudication who were treated by operation,[67] to 48 per cent in a series of patients with limb-threatening ischemia who were treated by operation,[107] to 12 per cent in a series of patients requiring reoperative surgery for limb-threatening ischemia.[108]

The overwhelming cause of death in claudicators, as predicted from the preceding data, is arteriosclerotic vascular disease and its attendant complications. As seen in Figure 51–3, coronary deaths account for approximately 60 per cent of the deaths in claudicators, with cerebrovascular disease causing mortality in another 10 to 15 per cent. Other

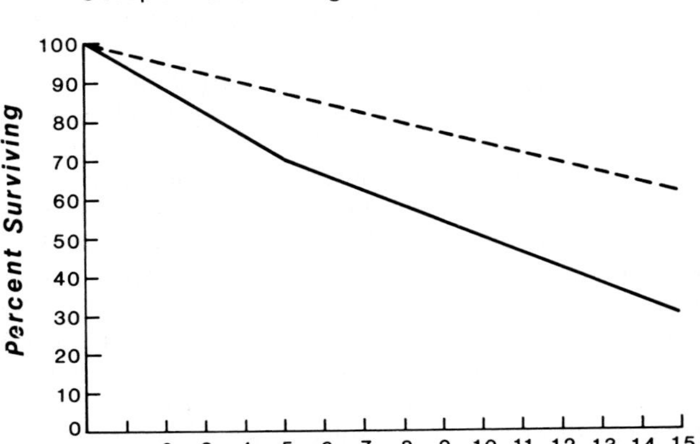

FIGURE 51–2. Survival of patients with claudication compared with controls. (Source: Composite of figures from references in Tables 51–4 and 51–5.)

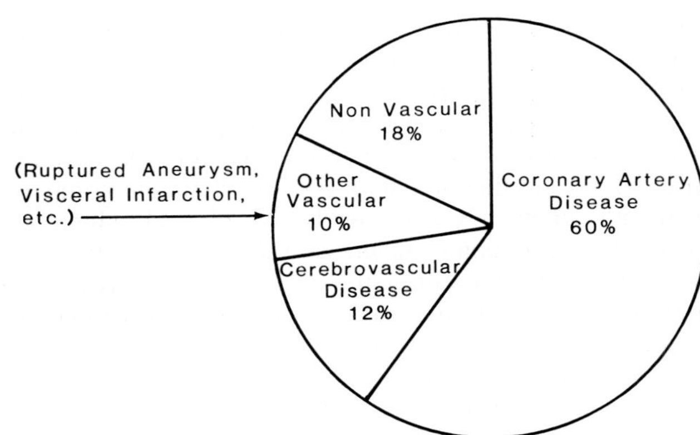

FIGURE 51–3. Causes of death in patients with claudication. (Source: Composite of figures from references in Tables 51–4 and 51–5.)

vascular events such as visceral infarction and ruptured aneurysm account for another 10 per cent. The remainder are due to non-vascular causes. Continued cigarette smoking, diabetes, and the presence of symptomatic coronary and cerebrovascular disease have been identified as independent risk factors associated with an increased risk of mortality exceeding that predicted for the entire group of claudicators.

Limb-Threatening Ischemia

Limb-threatening ischemia occurs when resting blood flow is insufficient to meet the maintenance metabolic requirements for nonexercising tissue. The clinical manifestations of limb-threatening ischemia include rest pain, ulceration, and gangrene. Ischemic rest pain is typically described as a burning, dysesthetic pain that is usually worse in the forefoot and toes and is frequently worse at night when the patient is recumbent. The pain is typically lessened or relieved by placing the foot dependent, with the consequent increase in arterial pressure resulting from gravity. Ischemic ulceration occurs when minor traumatic lesions fail to heal because of inadequate blood supply. Gangrene occurs when arterial perfusion is so inadequate that spontaneous necrosis occurs in the most poorly perfused areas.

Progressive gangrene with an ultimate need for amputation is believed by most vascular surgeons to be the inevitable outcome in patients with unrelieved limb-threatening ischemia. Although it is conceded that ischemic rest pain and ulceration may resolve in the occasional patient, in association with the development of collaterals, this is thought to be a rare event. An exception is recognized when limb-threatening ischemia occurs after an acute thrombotic event, such as closure of a previously stenotic superficial femoral artery. Such patients may experience a period of days to a few weeks of ischemic rest pain, after which the development of collateral circulation results in stabilization of symptoms at the level of claudication only.

Available data indicate that the true prognosis for limb loss in patients with presumed limb-threatening ischemia is not known with certainty. Progressive gangrenous changes and continuous ischemic rest pain unrelieved by dependency are unstable conditions associated with rapid progression to limb loss. In contrast, a number of patients with advanced ischemia describe occasional episodes of typical nocturnal ischemic rest pain that is easily relieved by limb dependency, and they maintain a stable symptom complex for months or even years. Clearly, the clinical symptoms and findings commonly included in the category of limb-threatening ischemia represent a spectrum of severity. In a single patient, the decrease in nutritive blood flow caused by progressive atherosclerosis in primary inflow vessels may be balanced by the development of collaterals such that symptoms remain stable for prolonged periods.

Chronic severe ischemia obviously renders the affected extremity vulnerable to such adverse influences as the need for increased blood flow to heal traumatic lesions or to dissipate external heat. In such patients, minor alterations in capillary flow induced by the improvement in cardiac output resulting from the treatment of congestive heart failure or by specific hemorrheologic drugs may be sufficient to prevent progressive ischemia leading to limb loss.[109] An important report documenting long-term improvement in a number of limbs with advanced ischemia without specific therapy[85] emphasizes that the prognosis for patients with severe limb ischemia is not necessarily the early development of gangrene. This clearly emphasizes the critical need for a control population in any study purporting to show a therapeutic benefit from a specific treatment method in patients with ischemic rest pain.

The few studies in which such a control group has been included have been most interesting. The results of these studies may be surprising to surgeons accustomed to equating the existence of rest pain or ischemic ulceration with inevitable limb loss. A 1982 Scandinavian trial randomized 22 patients with arterial ischemic ulcers to placebo or prostaglandin treatment and found a 40 per cent rate of ulcer healing in the placebo group.[35] A similar study in the United States of 120 patients reported a 49 per cent incidence of ulcer healing and greater than 80 per cent improvement in rest pain in the placebo group.[91] Similar findings have been noted in placebo groups from other studies of patients with ischemic rest pain and gangrenous ulcers, with overall improvement in 25 per cent to greater than 50 per cent of patients.[5, 20] These data obviously indicate that the prognosis for limb loss in patients grouped solely according to *symptoms* of severe lower extremity ischemia is uncertain. Clearly, objective quantitative information to permit better classification of patient groups is essential. There are at least some data of this type, indicating a grim prognosis for the group of patients characterized by the complete absence of pedal Doppler signals.[38]

Scandinavian investigators have identified alterations in the microcirculatory control mechanisms of ischemic limbs, which may in the future permit more precise identification of patients with actual threatened limb loss. In normal persons, the increased lower leg and foot venous pressure that results from the dependent position produces a reflex arteriolar constriction leading to a decrease in arteriolar flow with dependency, counteracting the expected increase in flow that should result from the gravitational increase in arterial pressure. The response is commonly known as the venoarterial reflex.[46] Henriksen,[47] Eickhoff,[34] and others have demonstrated that this normal reflex is absent in chronically ischemic limbs, thus allowing passive increases in arterial flow with dependency. In the future, this loss of venoarterial reflex may prove to be a sensitive physiologic marker of severe limb ischemia, with greater prognostic significance than that associated with patient symptoms or simple ankle pressure measurements. Clearly, more work in this important area is needed to allow early, accurate identification of patients with true threatened limb loss and no hope for improvement without revascularization.

The prognosis for survival of patients with severe limb ischemia is more clearly defined than the prospects of limb loss. All authorities agree that patients with ischemic rest pain and gangrene as a group are more elderly and have more advanced coronary and cerebrovascular disease than do patients with claudication. The decreased life expectancy of patients operated on for limb-threatening ischemia as compared with those operated on for claudication is clearly demonstrated in Figure 51–4. The causes of death in these patients are typically vascular and are quite similar in distribution to those outlined in Figure 51–3.

Chronic Lower Extremity Ischemia in Young Persons

Arteriosclerosis is generally a disease of later life. Symptomatic peripheral occlusive disease occurring in younger persons is often associated with the presence of identifiable risk factors such as hyperlipidemia, hypercoagulable states, Buerger's disease, or inborn errors of metabolism. As might be expected from the early age of onset, progression of disease in these patients has been found to be especially rapid, with a corresponding high incidence of amputation reported by most investigators.[24, 74] Most authorities have recommended that arterial reconstruction be avoided except in cases with clearly threatened limb loss because of a high anticipated failure rate of the arterial repair in these severely afflicted patients. Several studies have emphasized that a systematic approach to diagnosis should allow assignment of a cause in most patients and that the results of vascular treatment are more favorable when this treatment is combined with vigorous treatment of the associated risk factors.[44, 75]

Physicians must be wary of attributing a vascular cause to all typical leg pain syndromes, especially in young persons. Several unusual syndromes may produce exercise-induced leg pain, which by history alone cannot be reliably differentiated from claudication. *Chronic compartment syndrome* is a condition in which muscle exercise results in acute increases in compartment pressures to a level at which pain and neuromuscular compromise may occur.[110] This syndrome is most often seen in athletes and most frequently involves the anterior and lateral compartments of the calf. Treatment is by fascial incision or limited excision. *Neurogenic claudication* is a syndrome in which lower extremity pain induced by walking is caused by stenosis of the spinal canal from any of a number of causes.[111] Both direct nerve root compression and compression of the local neural blood supply have been implicated in this syndrome,[112] which

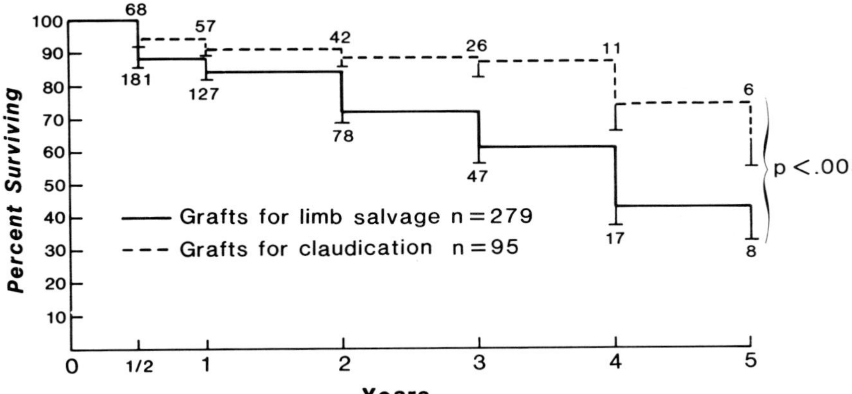

FIGURE 51–4. Survival of patients operated on for limb salvage compared with patients operated on for claudication. (From Taylor LM Jr, Porter JM: Current status of the reversed saphenous vein graft. *In* Bergan JJ, Yao J [eds]: Arterial Surgery: New Diagnostic and Operative Techniques. New York, Grune & Stratton, 1987, p 494.)

may be historically quite similar to claudication caused by large artery obstruction.

The key to diagnosis of these conditions is insistence on objective confirmation of the diagnosis of vascular occlusive disease in suspected claudication with the use of the noninvasive vascular laboratory, as described in the sections that follow and in Chapters 4 and 5. All patients with arterial vascular claudication have abnormal noninvasive test findings, although some patients with mild symptoms may have apparently normal test results at rest. Absence of a vascular abnormality after dynamic testing (treadmill walking or reactive hyperemia) should lead to a search for an alternative explanation for the patient's lower extremity symptoms.

Summary of Natural History

Patients with chronic lower extremity ischemia may present clinically with symptoms ranging from minor claudication to extensive gangrene. The arbitrary division of these patients into two distinct groups, those with claudication and those with threatened limb loss, on the assumption of markedly different natural histories, although a serviceable approach in the past, is probably no longer optimal. Great progress has been made in quantitating the degree of ischemia with a variety of noninvasive vascular laboratory methods. Evidence is emerging that the prognosis for patients with chronic lower extremity ischemia is more closely related to these objective findings than to patients' descriptions of symptomatic severity. The missing element in the current method of categorizing patients with chronic lower extremity ischemia is a consistent, objective method of quantitating the rate of progression of the occlusive process. Until this information can be added to the objective description of the current severity of ischemia, the ability of vascular surgeons to prognosticate remains imperfect at best.

Clearly, it is as inappropriate to predict a uniformly satisfactory clinical outcome solely on the basis of a history of claudication as it is to predict the inevitable occurrence of early limb loss in a patient with intermittent ischemic rest pain. Similarly, in the authors' opinion, it is as inappropriate to consistently refuse operation in patients with claudication only as it is to always insist on arterial reconstruction in patients with the recent development of an ischemic ulcer that, as noted previously, may heal spontaneously. Careful consideration of the objective findings pertinent to each patient and individualization of therapy on the basis of these findings will result in a more favorable clinical outcome than algorithmic assignment of treatment methods to symptom complexes as if each represented a uniquely distinctive disease process with a predictable clinical outcome.

NONOPERATIVE TREATMENT

Initial Evaluation

The foundation of the initial clinical patient evaluation remains an unhurried and detailed patient history taking and physical examination, the details of which with respect to vascular disease are fully discussed in Chapter 1 and are not repeated here. Lower extremity ischemia is a clinical condition especially suited to objective noninvasive vascular laboratory evaluation, which may be thought of as an extension of the physical examination. The authors perform complete lower extremity non-invasive laboratory examinations on all patients with chronic lower extremity ischemia as an integral part of the initial patient evaluation. The testing routinely performed consists of palpation of peripheral pulses and recording of Doppler waveforms over the femoral, popliteal, and pedal arteries. Segmental pressure indices at the upper thigh, above-knee, below-knee, ankle, and great toe levels are also determined. Patients with incompressible vessels are examined with plethysmographic recordings and toe reactive hyperemia testing. Toe photoplethysmography is used to detect significant obstructive disease below the ankle, as is frequently present in diabetic patients. Patients with claudication are examined with treadmill walking followed by measurement of ankle pressure recovery times. The authors' preference is to use a rather slow treadmill speed of 1.5 mph with a 0 per cent

Peripheral Arterial Exam

Resting Segmental Blood Pressures:

	RIGHT		LEFT	
	Pressure	Leg/Arm Ratio	Pressure	Leg/Arm Ratio
Arm	168		168	
Upper thigh	124	.74	127	.76
Above knee	99	.59	115	.68
Below knee	88	.52	100	.59
Ankle D.P.	82	.48	80	.48
P.T.	82	.48	74	.44
Toe .	60	.36	66	.39

Common femoral

Popliteal

Posterior Tibial

Dorsal Pedal

Treadmill: 1.5 mph at 0% grade.

Stopped arbitrarily; no discomfort at 5:00 (202 meters)

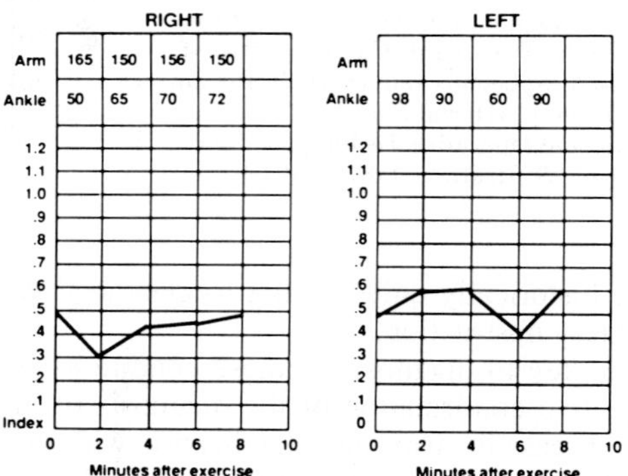

FIGURE 51–5. Information obtained from standard noninvasive peripheral arterial examination provides complete assessment of lower extremity circulation.

grade to duplicate normal ambulation and minimize the cardiopulmonary stress associated with exercise testing.

The clinical and vascular laboratory data obtained at the initial evaluation, an example of which is seen in Figure 51–5, provide the objective information required to form the first impression of the etiology and severity of the patient's symptoms. In addition, the vascular laboratory data serve as a baseline against which to judge progression of disease as well as to evaluate future changes in symptoms or response to therapy objectively.

The initial evaluation of patients with chronic lower extremity ischemia should include the identification of risk factors known to influence the natural history of the disease, including cigarette smoking, diabetes, and hyperlipidemia. Historical details suggesting coronary artery disease should be specifically sought, and objective information relative to coronary disease, including electrocardiograms, records of previous coronary bypass, and dipyridamole thallium or multi-gated acquisition scanning, should be reviewed if available.

Armed with this large body of information, the surgeon can decide whether to recommend operative or nonoperative treatment. It is important that both patient and surgeon understand that the decision for surgery always requires a careful consideration of whether the anticipated improvement outweighs the associated risk, discomfort, and expense of operative treatment. Patients should be clearly informed when appropriate nonoperative alternatives exist. A discussion of specific nonoperative measures that may be undertaken in the treatment of chronic lower extremity ischemia and the anticipated results of these measures forms the basis for the remainder of this chapter.

Cessation of Smoking

It is estimated that 325,000 to 350,000 deaths directly related to cigarette smoking occur yearly in the United States.[78] The direct relationship between tobacco use and lower extremity ischemia is well known. Smokers are nine times more likely than nonsmokers to develop claudication.[52] Smokers compose as many as 98 to 99 per cent of all patients who complain of intermittent claudication[32, 65] and an equally high percentage of patients undergoing lower extremity amputation for ischemia.[57] Interestingly, the pathophysiologic mechanisms through which smoking exerts its adverse effects on arteries are not known with certainty. This is in part due to the chemical complexity of cigarette smoke, which has been demonstrated to contain more than 3000 different substances.[104] Multiple individual components of tobacco smoke have been demonstrated to affect each of the important components of the atherosclerotic process adversely, as outlined in Table 51–6.

Tobacco smoke produces marked alterations in vascular endothelium, prostaglandin metabolism, lipid metabolism, blood viscosity, platelet function, and coagulation function, among other things.[43, 69] Smokers frequently demonstrate chronic vasoconstriction and hypertension, probably as a result of the nicotine in tobacco smoke. In addition to having adverse influences on atherogenesis, the carbon monoxide component of tobacco smoke has a demonstrably adverse effect on claudication. Aronow and associates demonstrated an immediate, significant decrease in treadmill walking in claudicators who breathed air containing 50 ppm of carbon monoxide.[3] For more detailed information on the pathophysiologic and epidemiologic association of cigarette

Table 51–6. Adverse Effects of Tobacco Smoking on Components of Atherogenesis

1. Endothelial effects
   a. Increased endothelial denudation[38]
   b. Increased endothelial cell turnover[39]
   c. Decreased endothelial cell prostacyclin production[42]
2. Platelet effects
   a. Increased platelet count[40]
   b. Increased platelet aggregation[39]
   c. Increased platelet adhesiveness[44]
   d. Increased thromboxane A_2 production[42]
3. Lipid effects
   a. Decreased high-density lipoprotein levels[44]
4. Coagulation effects
   a. Decreased fibrinolytic activity[45]
   b. Increased blood viscosity[46]
   c. Increased fibrinogen level[45]
5. Whole vessel effects
   a. Vasoconstriction
   b. Hypertension

smoking with lower extremity ischemia, the reader is referred to excellent reviews.[16, 39]

The overwhelming association between smoking and lower extremity ischemia emphasizes that cessation of all tobacco use is an essential first step in the nonoperative treatment of chronic lower extremity ischemia. The initial effort on the part of the vascular surgeon must be to identify clearly the patient's smoking addiction as an important component of the ischemic state. When the surgeon is taking the patient's history, questions such as "Do you still smoke?" or "How much do you smoke?" more effectively convey to the patient the impression that smoking is part of the problem than does the more neutral (and more typically asked) "Do you smoke?" Although almost all smokers are aware of an adverse health influence, most associate tobacco use with pulmonary disease, specifically lung cancer. The increased risks of myocardial infarction and stroke[1, 100] are less well recognized. The strong association with lower extremity ischemia was understood by only 37 per cent of smokers with peripheral vascular disease in the study by Clyne and colleagues.[14] The surgeon must therefore clearly and unequivocally inform the patient that smoking is the most important correctable cause of the patient's disease. An unwavering recommendation that patients with chronic lower extremity ischemia totally cease tobacco use in all forms must be an important part of the initial encounter with the patient and should be repeated at every subsequent encounter. In a study by Kirk and associates, strong and repeated advice by physicians to cease smoking resulted in abstinence by 37 per cent of smokers with arterial disease.[61]

However, it is important for vascular surgeons to remember that for most smokers, tobacco use represents a powerful chemical addiction, which has been defined by Pollin as the "inability to discontinue smoking despite awareness of the medical consequences."[78] The portion of the patient population able to cease smoking on being informed of the importance of this step may be thought of as the population of unaddicted users. How best to approach the problem of those addicted patients remains unsolved.

In the authors' opinion, it is important that the approach to vascular patients who are smokers be positive, nonjudgmental, and oriented toward the future. Poorly chosen statements may imply that the physician is condemning the patient rather than the smoking habit. An admonition to cease smoking accompanied by the threat of refusal to continue treatment if the patient cannot comply is inappropriate in the authors' opinion and indicates a lack of understanding by the physician of the nature of addiction. It is both appropriate and desirable for the vascular surgeon to indicate carefully and in detail to the patient that cessation of smoking not only removes a strong negative influence but also is associated with tangible positive benefits.

Abundant evidence indicates that abstinence from tobacco use improves the prognosis in patients with chronic lower extremity ischemia. When one is evaluating studies comparing smokers with nonsmokers or ex-smokers, the denial and deception common in addicted persons must be recalled. It is desirable that any study of smoking behavior and the consequences of it be controlled by objective measurements of smoking markers, such as blood thiocyanate or carboxyhemoglobin levels. Studies that rely only on patient history are likely to be skewed by the inclusion of smokers who claim to be abstainers within the group of ex-smokers. It is important to note that this inaccuracy reduces the detected benefit associated with cessation of tobacco use, and studies that demonstrate benefit based on patient history, although probably valid, most likely underestimate the magnitude of the benefit.

Patients with intermittent claudication who stopped smoking (by history) were found by Quick and Cotton to have significant improvement in both ankle pressure and treadmill walking when compared with continued smokers.[81] Mean walking distance improved from 214 to 300 m. In the authors' practice, claudicators who stop smoking usually experience prompt improvement in walking distance, which averages a doubling of the initial distance.

The prognosis for continued patency of lower extremity arterial repairs has been related to smoking by multiple authors. Using carboxyhemoglobin blood levels to indicate continued smoking, Greenhalgh and colleagues found that patients with failed grafts had carboxyhemoglobin levels that averaged 2.5 times those found in patients with patent grafts.[42] Provan and colleagues found significantly improved patency at 5 years in aortofemoral grafts in nonsmokers (71 per cent) and in patients who stopped smoking (77 per cent) compared with continued smokers (42 per cent). This favorable effect could not be confirmed for femoropopliteal grafts in this study, which relied on patient history for smoking information.[80] The study of Myers and associates, which also relied on patient history of smoking, demonstrated significantly improved patency of aortofemoral grafts (90 vs 79 per cent at 4 years) and femoropopliteal grafts (80 vs 61 per cent) for patients who smoked fewer than five cigarettes per day.[73] Similar findings were noted by Robicsek and coworkers in patients with aortoiliac disease.[86]

An improved prognosis for prevention of limb loss in patients with chronic lower extremity ischemia who stop smoking has been described by multiple authors. In the study by Jurgens and coworkers,[57] no patients who stopped smoking required amputation, whereas 11.4 per cent of those who continued smoking required amputation. Birkenstock and coworkers found that 85 per cent of persons who stopped smoking experienced improvement in symptoms of lower extremity ischemia, whereas only 20 per cent of continuing smokers had improvement.[6] This difference was maintained even in the subgroup of patients with severe ischemia manifested by ischemic rest pain, gangrene, or both, in which 86 per cent of 64 patients who stopped smoking had improvement and did not require amputation, whereas only 10 per cent of smokers had a similar favorable outcome.

In addition to giving the tobacco-addicted patient the information described, the vascular surgeon should provide a plan of action to achieve the goal of elimination of the addiction. The surgeon must be willing to recognize the limitations of his or her own expertise and to refer addicted patients to colleagues who specialize in substance abuse and addiction. Initial failure or relapse should not be regarded negatively: multiple attempts are common in the histories of successful abstinence and should be regarded as a necessary part of the process, which for most who successfully quit requires from 2 to 5 *years* and includes an average of six cycles of abstinence and relapse.[95] Continuing positively expressed encouragement to stop smoking by physicians, family members, and others is identified by many ex-smokers as the most important influence leading to success. The prescription of nicotine gum as an aid to ease the transition from tobacco use to abstinence is appropriate. Although the adverse effects of nicotine are well known, studies show that fewer than 5 per cent of successful ex-smokers among those using the gum continue its use on a long-term basis.[51]

More than any other factor, current changes in social norms regarding the acceptability of smoking may greatly aid the physician's efforts to influence patients to cease tobacco use. Prohibition of smoking in the workplace and in public places and an increasing awareness of the real health risk posed by passive smoking have led to increasing restrictions being placed on smokers. The authors have been impressed with how well their own hospital inpatients, essentially all of whom are smokers, have accepted almost with relief the recent decision of the authors' hospital administration to ban smoking from all areas of the hospital.

Exercise

Patients with chronic lower extremity ischemia and intermittent claudication typically greatly reduce their daily walking because of the inevitable discomfort. In addition, many claudicators assume that the occurrence of muscle discomfort, which is the hallmark of claudication, indicates tissue damage and should be avoided by voluntary reduction of activity. In fact, the opposite is true. It has long been known that a regular program of walking exercise results in a measurable improvement in walking distance in a large majority of claudicators. The improvement produced by exercise programs has ranged from an 80 per cent increase in walking distance in one British study of 21 patients[13] to a 234 per cent increase in a study of 148 patients from Sweden.[36] All studies have consistently demonstrated similar benefit and form a firm foundation for a recommendation for regular walking exercise as a basic principle of the initial therapy for intermittent claudication.[40, 87, 93]

The mechanism responsible for improved walking tolerance in claudicators following an exercise program is not fully understood. The frequent assumption that exercise results in an improvement in the number of collateral vessels, the size of collateral vessels, or both, with a resulting increase in exercise-induced blood flow, is not supported by available data. Using a variety of techniques, numerous investigators have shown that neither ankle blood pressure nor calf muscle blood flow improves in claudicators with improved walking tolerance after an exercise program.[13, 21, 36, 89, 94] Current opinion indicates that the improved muscle performance caused by exercise training is at least in part a result of adaptive changes in muscle enzymes leading to a more efficient oxygen extraction from blood.[11] Evidence in support of this mechanism was found when popliteal venous blood from exercising claudicators was examined for oxygen content. The extraction of oxygen was significantly increased following regular physical training. In addition, popliteal venous lactate levels were not increased, emphasizing that the increased muscle exercise capacity was aerobic in nature.[94]

Although this mechanism of increased exercise tolerance following a regular exercise program seems to be well established, other mechanisms may also be important. At least one study has observed improved hemorrheologic behavior of erythrocytes after regular exercise.[87] Others have speculated that improved mechanical efficiency of muscles, improved fatty acid metabolism, and increased muscle fiber : capillary ratios may all play a role.

The improvement in claudication following a program of regular walking exercise occurs with sufficient predictability that the surgeon can prescribe such a program with confidence. In the authors' practice, sedentary claudicators have generally experienced at least a doubling of their walking distance by following an exercise program. Interval treadmill examinations in the vascular laboratory may demonstrate incremental increases in walking distance to skeptical patients before they can be clinically appreciated and thus increase compliance during early phases of regular exercise. A sedentary lifestyle is a recognized risk factor for the development of atherosclerotic disease, and most patients with claudication fit this description. It is important for the physician to be aware of the major change in activities represented by the assumption of a regular exercise program and to prescribe a regimen that falls within the range of possibility.

Obviously, exercise programs should be individualized, but for the majority of their patients, the authors have found a recommendation of 1 hour of walking at a comfortable pace each day to be well accepted. The patient should be instructed to walk until claudication occurs, then rest until it subsides, then repeat the cycle for 1 hour each day. The indoor shopping malls in suburban locations across the United States provide a nearly ideal place for walking exercise during inclement weather, free from automobile traffic and often with conveniently spaced benches for periods of rest.

A study by Creasy and coworkers randomized patients with intermittent claudication to treatment by balloon angioplasty or to an exercise therapy program.[113] As expected, the initial improvement in leg circulation, as assessed by the ankle-brachial pressure index, was greater in the angioplasty group. Despite this, after 1 year of follow-up, the patients in the exercise group could walk farther, both on the treadmill in the laboratory and as assessed by questionnaire, and there was no longer a significant difference in the ankle pressure index. This study demonstrates again the important benefits associated with exercise therapy. In addition, it questions the superiority of invasive therapy, presumed by many, and indicates that most future studies of claudication treatment should contain a control group that is treated by a regular exercise program rather than not treated at all.

Summary of Data on Cessation of Smoking and Exercise

An overwhelming body of data clearly indicates that cessation of smoking and assumption of a regular exercise program favorably influence the natural history of chronic lower extremity ischemia. It is important for physicians to understand that patients' compliance with these recommendations frequently requires profound change of lifelong habits. Physicians recommending basic lifestyle changes must be prepared to deal with a high incidence of noncompliance and reversion to noncompliance after initial success. In the past, some investigators recommended that vascular surgeons refuse to treat patients who fail to exercise or stop smoking. In the authors' opinion, this is a counterproductive attitude that fails to recognize the difficulty of the recommended tasks and abandons the basic attitude of acceptance of the patient, which is the foundation of a professional physician-patient relationship. These considerations aside, however, one must be aware that most smokers who successfully quit do so after several initial failures, and most persons who develop the habit of regular exercise do so after a similar series of starts and stops. A disapproving attitude conveyed by the physician may abort this natural process, whereas repeated positive encouragements, based on the very real anticipated benefits outlined previously, may retain in the patient the growing desire for change that ultimately results in success.

In contrast to past times, when physicians may have been the only persons encouraging patients to exercise regularly and stop smoking, current societal fashion and public opinion now form strong allies for the medical profession. Family, church, and citizens groups now commonly join in general condemnation of smoking and offer programs to aid those wishing to quit. Health clubs abound, fitness is "in," and almost all communities have organized exercise classes and programs specifically intended for the sedentary and infirm wishing to make a change. The vascular surgeon should be aware of such resources in the community and recommend them as appropriate to patients.

It is the summation of influences suggesting change to the patient that ultimately produces favorable change in lifestyle. In addition to being aware of the importance of their own contribution to this summation, vascular surgeons must recognize their limitations and assist in applying other available community and family resources to the patient.

Pharmacologic Therapy

More recent years have witnessed the development of multiple new pharmacologic agents potentially useful in the treatment of chronic lower extremity ischemia, including hemorrheologic agents, prostaglandins, calcium channel blockers, and others. Use of these agents is described in detail in Chapter 18 and with the exception of hemorrheologic interventions is not discussed here.

Hemorrheology. The viscosity of blood has an important influence on blood flow, as is evident from Poiseuille's equation. Active current interest is focused on therapeutic interventions that may improve the flow characteristics of blood in the microcirculation primarily through drug-induced decreases in blood viscosity, an area termed hemorrheology. The pharmacologic approaches to this problem are discussed in Chapter 18.

The straightforward approach to a reduction in blood viscosity by simple hemodilution has been evaluated in a blinded, controlled fashion. Ernst and coworkers treated 24 patients with stable claudication and found significant improvement in resting blood flow and pain-free walking distance after hemodilution, changes that did not occur in control patients.[37] This study obviously indicates further investigation of this relatively simple approach to therapy, especially in patients with abnormally high blood viscosity.

Foot Care

For many patients with stable chronic lower extremity ischemia, the occurrence of minor injuries to the feet may initiate a relentless train of unmet increased demands for flow, chronic wounds, infection, further ischemia, gangrene, and ultimate limb loss. An unfortunately common scenario is that which follows the ill-advised application of external heat (e.g., with a "hot pack" or heating pad) to an ischemic foot. It is obvious that the only mechanism by which the extremity can dissipate excess heat is through vasodilatation and increased blood flow. In the setting in which blood flow is fixed by proximal obstructive lesions, the excess heat cannot be dissipated and full-thickness burns may (and frequently do) result from the application of heating pads set at temperatures that would not injure feet with normal arterial supply. Similarly, surgical operations designed to correct common foot problems may have disastrous consequences if performed in persons with chronic lower extremity ischemia whose blood supply is insufficient to achieve wound healing.

The desirability of preventing these unfortunate events is obvious. Patients with chronic lower extremity ischemia should be specifically instructed in the importance of foot care and the possibility of limb loss resulting from such seemingly inconsequential acts as careless nail or callus trimming, and so forth. *Any* procedure on the foot should be regarded as a major undertaking and be preceded by the clear demonstration of palpable pedal pulses, and in their absence a noninvasive vascular laboratory examination to assess the potential for healing. The risk inherent in the

Table 51–7. Guidelines for Patients With Poor Circulation to the Feet

1. It is essential that you not use tobacco in any form.
2. Set aside 1 hour each day for walking exercises. Walk at a comfortable pace until your legs hurt, then stop and rest. When the pain is gone, walk again until they hurt and then rest. Repeat this cycle until an hour has passed.
3. You should take one aspirin tablet every day.
4. Care of your feet is extremely important.
   a. Your feet must be inspected daily for abrasions, ulcerations, or infections.
   b. Clean your feet daily with soap and water, and dry them well.
   c. Dry skin can be treated with any common hand cream.
   d. You should avoid ill-fitting or worn-out shoes.
   e. You should see us before cutting your toenails, trimming any calluses, or performing any other such procedures on your feet.
   f. You should not apply external heat (e.g., heating pad or "hot pack") to your feet, and you should not soak your feet in hot water.
   g. You should avoid trauma to your feet. Do not walk barefoot.
5. Contact us immediately if you develop any problems with your feet.

application of external heat should be described carefully and in detail. Each patient with chronic lower extremity ischemia should be encouraged to report to the physician immediately the detection of any foot lesion, no matter how apparently minor. Patient instruction sheets are particularly useful in reinforcing the important points of such physician-patient discussions; the one the authors distribute to patients with chronic lower extremity ischemia is shown in Table 51–7.

INFLUENCE OF COEXISTING MEDICAL CONDITIONS AND THEIR TREATMENT ON CHRONIC LOWER EXTREMITY ISCHEMIA

Given the age range, smoking habits, and degree of infirmity of most patients with chronic lower extremity ischemia, multi-system disease is the rule rather than the exception. In general, the improvement in cardiac, pulmonary, or renal function and hypertension following careful medical management of each of these conditions beneficially affects patients' chronic lower extremity ischemia as well. However, a few treatment interactions may produce undesirable results and may not be familiar to internists making primary treatment decisions.

Cardiac function is obviously central to peripheral perfusion, and the adverse influence of lower extremity arterial obstructive lesions may be magnified by significant decreases in cardiac output. All vascular surgeons are familiar with patients with well-compensated chronic lower extremity ischemia who develop rest pain and even ischemic ulcerations during periods of decreased cardiac output caused by exacerbation of congestive heart failure. Likewise, patients with mild, previously unrecognized lower extremity occlusive disease may develop impressive findings of peripheral mottling and cyanosis during episodes of decreased cardiac output as, for example, may accompany myocardial infarction. The potential in this situation for mistaken diagnosis of acute arterial occlusion that may lead to the performance of an unnecessary and hazardous operation to revascularize the affected extremity is obvious. In the authors' experience, the true chronic nature of the occlusive process can best be recognized in such patients by the use of objective measurements such as the ankle-arm pressure index. The finding of a severely ischemic foot but an ankle-brachial index of greater than 0.4 in a nondiabetic with normally compressible arteries should immediately focus attention on decreased cardiac output as the acute cause of poor distal extremity perfusion.

Treatment of systolic hypertension rarely, in the authors' experience, produces worsening in symptoms of chronic lower ischemia related to blood pressure reduction alone. However, beta-adrenergic blocking agents are commonly used to treat hypertension or angina pectoris. Exacerbation of the symptoms of chronic lower extremity ischemia, including claudication, rest pain, gangrene, and Raynaud's symptoms, has been well described with the use of these agents.[41, 68, 82, 101] Although blockade of normal beta-adrenergic peripheral vasodilating influence is part of the involved mechanism, increased sensitivity of peripheral alpha-adrenergic receptors also occurs following beta-blockade.[102] In the study by Marshall and colleagues, Raynaud's symptoms occurred in 50 per cent of patients taking beta-blockers for hypertension but in only 5 per cent of patients achieving similar blood pressure control using methyldopa, emphasizing that the effect is drug specific and is not caused by decreased systemic blood pressure.[68] Fortunately, hypertension and angina pectoris can be treated with multiple alternative drug regimens. Patients with chronic lower extremity ischemia need not be maintained on beta-adrenergic blockers, and conversion to other agents may be associated with sufficient symptomatic improvement to avoid contemplated operative therapy.

NONCONVENTIONAL TREATMENT

The considerable expense, risk, and discomfort of surgical treatment, combined with the progressive nature of the underlying disease process, continue to provide both patients and physicians with a strong impetus to seek alternative methods of therapy for chronic lower extremity ischemia. The proven approaches to non-operative treatment described in the preceding section of this chapter involve primary changes in lifestyle and personal habits that for many patients prove difficult. Thus, new forms of therapy evolve that invariably require less effort by the patient. Unfortunately, appreciation of the variable natural history of chronic lower extremity ischemia is not widespread among patients, physicians, or, sadly, even many investigators. This is particularly true with regard to the natural history of ischemic rest pain and ischemic ulceration, which in the minds of many are symptoms associated with an inevitable progression to gangrene and limb loss. This belief leads to the erroneous attribution of therapeutic benefit to treatment modalities associated with improvement in chronic lower extremity ischemic symptoms in the absence of placebo-controlled patient groups. None of the treatment modalities described in the following section has been proved to be of benefit in the treatment of chronic lower extremity ischemia. The results of treatment reported with all of these methods fall within the range described in previous sections of this chapter for the natural history of the conditions being treated.

Epidural Electrical Stimulation

Epidural electrical stimulation was reported to be of benefit in healing skin ulcers, some of which were believed to be ischemic, by Cook and coworkers in 1976.[15] More recently, Tallis and associates reported improvement in claudication walking distance and exercise tolerance following spinal cord stimulation in 6 of 10 patients with arterial disease. The study was without controls.[98] A still more recent report by Augustinsson and colleagues described the treatment of 34 patients, 27 of whom had occlusive arterial disease and the remainder of whom had vasospastic disorders. Electrodes were implanted in the epidural space and were connected to a subcutaneous radio receiver. Stimulation was controlled by the patients using a hand-held transmitter. Pain relief was described as "adequate" or "complete" in 94 per cent of patients. Ten of the 27 patients with occlusive disease (37 per cent) required amputation at a mean interval of 5.4 months of therapy. This result was believed to be improved when compared with a historical group of "similar" but otherwise undescribed control patients, who had a 90 per cent amputation rate.[4] A similar study was reported by Jacobs and associates, who found that ischemic ulcers healed in 12 of 20 patients after treatment with epidural stimulation.[114] After 2 years of follow-up, 56 per cent of the limbs in this uncontrolled study had not been lost.

The mechanism of action of spinal cord stimulation is unknown. Pain relief may occur by inhibition of transmission of noxious stimuli, as postulated in the gate control theory of Melzack and Wall,[71] or by stimulation of local endorphin release.[22] Improvement in local blood flow is thought to result from vasodilatation, possibly by an effect on resting sympathetic tone.

The appropriate place of this form of therapy remains to be determined. Although spinal cord stimulation is an established form of pain control, regardless of the cause of the pain, no evidence thus far presented indicates any benefit with regard to limb salvage, ulcer healing, or limitation of localized gangrene when compared with the natural history expected for these symptoms.[115] To date, there have been no controlled studies demonstrating benefit from electrical epidural stimulation in chronic lower extremity ischemia.

Chelation Therapy

The basis for this unorthodox and unproven treatment for lower extremity ischemia lies in the administration of ethylenediaminetetra-acetic acid (EDTA) in the hopes that the calcium present in arteriosclerotic plaque will be extracted, solubilized by this chelating agent, and subsequently excreted, with a consequent reduction in the severity of arterial stenoses. Chelation therapy has been recommended by unorthodox practitioners since the 1950s.[12] In its most common form, EDTA is administered intravenously by infusion over several hours, on a near-daily basis for a treatment course of weeks or months. The therapy is most often prescribed as part of an overall approach to the treatment of arteriosclerosis that invariably includes sound recommendations such as cessation of tobacco use, exercise, weight reduction, and so forth. To date, no evidence has demonstrated effectiveness of this form of therapy for the treatment of arteriosclerosis of any site in a controlled trial setting. The results of numerous clinical reports of effectiveness fall within the expected range for the natural history of the conditions being considered.[12, 60, 62, 63] The reasoning behind this approach to therapy is obviously flawed because authorities generally agree that the important events in the generation of atherosclerotic plaques are related to the proliferation of smooth muscle cells and the subsequent deposition by them of collagen, proteoglycans, and elastic fibers, as well as the accumulation of large amounts of lipid. Calcification is a tertiary event, and many significantly occlusive arteriosclerotic plaques contain little or no calcium.

In contrast to many questionably effective therapies that at least involve little or no patient risk, chelation therapy with EDTA carries the potential for significant and even fatal complications. Nephrotoxicity that may produce renal failure is a recognized complication of EDTA therapy.[31] In addition, rapid infusion of EDTA may produce severe hypocalcemia, with resultant tetany and cardiac arrhythmias.[70] A possible role for this drug in the production of serious autoimmune reactions has been suggested.[77]

On the basis of these considerations, statements have been issued by the Medical Letter,[33] The American Medical Association, the American Heart Association, the American College of Physicians, the American Academy of Family Physicians, the American Society for Clinical Pharmacology and Therapeutics, the American College of Cardiology, and the American Osteopathic Association indicating that currently no basis exists for the use of chelation therapy in the treatment of arteriosclerotic disease.[25] A definitive randomized, controlled trial commissioned by the government of Denmark has conclusively shown no benefit associated with chelation therapy.[116]

Externally Applied Devices: The Circulator Boot

The lay public maintains a well-recognized fascination with the application of various external devices and contraptions aimed at relief or cure of diseases of the internal organs. This is particularly true of diseases that may manifest themselves with recalcitrant skin ulcerations, as is often true of chronic lower extremity ischemia. A currently available device purported to be of benefit in the treatment of lower extremity ischemia is the Circulator Boot, which encloses the extremity within a gas-filled inflatable bag. Pressure (50 to 70 mmHg) is applied to the leg by inflation during diastole. In theory, blood flow to the ischemic extremity is thus improved by augmentation of cardiac output, increased venous and lymphatic flow, and improved arterial collateral flow, as well as by enhanced fibrinolysis.[26] The treatments are applied for periods of up to 1 hour, from one to four times each day. The principal proponent of this form of therapy has demonstrated statistically significant increases in the ankle-arm pressure index and in subcutaneous Po_2 in patients who have had compression boot therapy.[27] These findings have never been independently confirmed, and the described increases in the ankle-arm blood pressure index seem to be minimally clinically significant (mean, 8 per cent).

Although the benefits of external compression therapy for venous and lymphatic disease are well known, application of this technology to the treatment of arterial insufficiency must be viewed with skepticism. No direct evidence of improved blood flow to ischemic tissue after Circulator Boot therapy has been provided. No controlled patient trials have been reported. The results of anecdotal uncontrolled patient studies reported to date fall within the range anticipated for the natural history of the conditions described.[26-28] In addition, it is difficult to hypothesize the mechanism by which a physical treatment method applied for 1 to 4 hours per day can improve arterial insufficiency that is present constantly. The placebo effect of such devices is sufficiently obvious that physicians must insist on controlled trials as proof of their efficacy, as with any other new or unproven therapeutic method.

SUMMARY

A clear knowledge of the natural history of chronic lower extremity ischemia forms the foundation on which all decisions related to therapy for this condition are based. In the authors' opinion, the classically described benign natural history of claudication and the morbid outcome associated with ischemic rest pain or ulceration are probably too simplistic and are based on questionable data. More accurate assessment of the prognosis for chronic lower extremity ischemia will be based on objective noninvasive vascular laboratory evaluation of the severity of ischemia.

A marked improvement in symptoms of chronic lower extremity ischemia may follow a regular program of exercise and cessation of tobacco use, both in claudicators and in some patients with limb-threatening ischemia. Although not discussed in this chapter, the appropriate use of pharmacologic agents as described in Chapter 18 obviously forms an important part of the nonoperative approach to treatment in occasional patients.

The nonconventional therapies described in the final section of this chapter are included because of the need for physicians undertaking the care of patients with chronic lower extremity ischemia to answer frequent patient inquiries regarding such treatment. Familiarity with the natural history of lower extremity ischemia as outlined in this chapter is critical to the accurate evaluation of treatment results attributed to these various therapies.

References

1. Abbott RD, Yin Y, Reed DM, et al: Risk of stroke in male cigarette smokers. N Engl J Med 315:717, 1986.
2. Ad Hoc Committee on Reporting Standards, Society for Vascular Surgery, North American Chapter, International Society for Cardiovascular Surgery: Standards for reports dealing with lower extremity ischemia. J Vasc Surg 4:80, 1986.
3. Aronow WS, Stemmer EA, Isbell MW: Effect of carbon monoxide exposure on intermittent claudication. Circulation 49:415, 1974.
4. Augustinsson LE, Carlsson CA, Holm J, et al: Epidural electrical stimulation in severe limb ischemia. Ann Surg 202:104, 1985.
5. Belch JJF, McArdle B, Pollack JG, et al: Epoprostenol (prostacyclin) and severe arterial disease: A double-blind trial. Lancet 1:315, 1983.
6. Birkenstock WE, Louw JHY, Terblanche J, et al: Smoking and other factors affecting the conservative management of peripheral vascular disease. S Afr Med J 49:1129, 1975.
7. Birnstingl MA, Brinson K, Chakrabarti BK: The effect of short-term exposure to carbon monoxide on platelet stickiness. Br J Surg 58:837, 1971.
8. Bloor K: Natural history of arteriosclerosis of the lower extremities. Ann R Coll Surg Engl 28:36, 1961.
9. Boobis LH, Bell PRF: Can drugs help patients with lower limb ischemia? Br J Surg 69(Suppl):517, 1982.
10. Boyd AM: The natural course of arteriosclerosis of the lower extremities. Angiology 11:10, 1960.
11. Bylund AC, Hammersten J, Holm J, et al: Enzyme activities in skeletal muscles from patients with peripheral arterial insufficiency. Eur J Clin Invest 6:425, 1976.
12. Clarke NE, Clarke CN, Mosher RE: The in vivo dissolution of metastatic calcium on approach to atherosclerosis. Am J Med Sci 229:142, 1955.
13. Clifford PC, Davies PW, Hayne JA, et al: Intermittent claudication: Is a supervised exercise class worthwhile? Br Med J 280:1503, 1980.
14. Clyne CA, Arch PJ, Carpenter D, et al: Smoking, ignorance, and peripheral vascular disease. Arch Surg 117:1062, 1982.
15. Cook AW, Oygar A, Baggenstos P, et al: Vascular disease of extremities: Electrical stimulation of spinal cord and posterior roots. NY State J Med 76:366, 1976.
16. Couch NP: On the arterial consequences of smoking. J Vasc Surg 3:807, 1986.
17. Crawford ES, Bomberger RA, Glaeser DH, et al: Aortoiliac occlusive disease: Factors influencing survival and function following reconstructive operation over a twenty-five year period. Surgery 90:1055, 1981.
18. Crigui MH, Fronck A, Klauber MR, et al: The sensitivity, specificity and predictive value of traditional clinical evaluation of peripheral arterial disease: Results from noninvasive testing in a defined population. Circulation 71:516, 1985.
19. Cronenwett JL, Warner KG, Zelenock GB, et al: Intermittent claudication: Current results of nonoperative management. Arch Surg 119:430, 1984.
20. Cronenwett JL, Zelenock GB, Whitehouse WM Jr, et al: Prostacyclin treatment of ischemic ulcers and rest pain in unreconstructible peripheral arterial occlusive disease. Surgery 100:369, 1986.
21. Dahllöf AG, Holm J, Sclersten T, et al: Peripheral arterial insufficiency. Effect of physical training on walking tolerance, calf blood flow and blood flow resistance. Scand J Rehabil Med 8:19, 1976.
22. Dahn I, Ekman CA, Lassen NA, et al: On the conservative treatment of severe ischemia of the leg. J Clin Lab Invest 19(Suppl 99):160, 1967.
23. Davis JW, Shelton L, Eigenberg DA, et al: Effects of tobacco and non-tobacco cigarette smoking on endothelium and platelets. Clin Pharmacol Ther 37:527, 1985.
24. DeBakey ME, Crawford ES, Garrett E, et al: Occlusive disease of the lower extremities in patients 16 to 37 years of age. Ann Surg 159:873, 1964.
25. Diagnostic and Therapeutic Technology Assessment (DATTA): Chelation therapy. JAMA 250:672, 1983.
26. Dillon RS: Successful treatment of osteomyelitis and soft tissue infections in ischemic diabetic legs by local antibiotic injections and the end-diastolic pneumatic compression boot. Ann Surg 204:643, 1986.
27. Dillon RS: Effect of therapy with the pneumatic end-diastolic leg compression boot in peripheral vascular tests and on the clinical course of peripheral vascular disease. Angiology 31:614, 1980.
28. Dillon RS: Vascular disease successfully treated with end-diastolic pneumatic compression boot [Abstract]. Diabetes 104A(Suppl), 1983.
29. Dintenfass L: Elevation of blood viscosity, aggregation of red cells,

hematocrit values and fibrinogen levels in cigarette smokers. Med J Aust 1:617, 1975.
30. Droller H, Pemberton J: Cardiovascular disease in a random sample of elderly people. Br Heart J 15:199, 1953.
31. Dudley HR, Ritchie AC, Schilling A, et al: Pathologic changes associated with the use of sodium ethylene diamine tetraacetate in the treatment of hypercalcemia. N Engl J Med 255:331, 1955.
32. Eastcott HHG: Arterial Surgery. 2nd ed. London, Pitman Medical Publishers, 1973, p 3.
33. EDTA chelation therapy for arteriosclerotic heart disease. Med Lett Drugs Ther 23:51, 1981.
34. Eickhoff JH: Forefoot vasoconstrictor response to increased venous pressure in normal subjects and in arteriosclerotic patients. Acta Chir Scand 502:7, 1980.
35. Eklund AE, Eriksson G, Olsson AG: A controlled study showing significant short term effect of prostaglandin E1 in healing of ischemic ulcers of the lower limb in man. Prostaglandins Leukotrienes Med 8:265, 1982.
36. Ekroth R, Dahllöf AG, Gundevall B, et al: Physical training of patients with intermittent claudication: Indications, methods and results. Surgery 84:640, 1978.
37. Ernst E, Matrai A, Kollar L: Placebo controlled, double-blind study of hemodilution in peripheral arterial disease. Lancet 1:1449, 1987.
38. Felix WR Jr, Sigel B, Gunther L: The significance for morbidity and mortality of Doppler absent pedal pulses. J Vasc Surg 5:849, 1987.
39. Fielding JE: Smoking: Health effects and control. N Engl J Med 313:555, 1985.
40. Gallasch G, Diehm C, Dorter C, et al: The influence of physical training on blood flow properties in patients with intermittent claudication. Klin Wochenschr 63:554, 1985.
41. Gokal R, Dornan TL, Ledingham JG: Peripheral skin necrosis complicating beta-blockage. Br Med J 1:721, 1979.
42. Greenhalgh RM, Laing SP, Colap V, et al: Progressing atherosclerosis following re-vascularization. *In* Bernhard VM, Towne JB (eds): Complications in Vascular Surgery. New York, Grune & Stratton, 1980, p 39.
43. Hadovic J: Endothelial injury by nicotine and its prevention. Experientia 34:1585, 1978.
44. Hallet JW Jr, Greenwood LH, Robinson JG: Lower extremity arterial disease in young adults. Ann Surg 202:647, 1985.
45. Hansteen V, Lorentsen E, Sivertssen E, et al: Long term follow-up of patients with peripheral arterial obliterations treated with arterial surgery. Acta Clin Scand 141:725, 1975.
46. Henriksen O: Local sympathetic reflex mechanism in regulation of blood flow in human subcutaneous adipose tissue. Acta Physiol Scand 450(Suppl):7, 1977.
47. Henriksen O: Orthostatic changes of blood flow in subcutaneous tissue in patients with arterial insufficiency of the legs. Scand J Clin Lab Invest 34:103, 1974.
48. Hertzer NR, Beven EG, Young JR, et al: Coronary artery disease in peripheral vascular patients: A classification of 1000 coronary angiograms and results of surgical management. Ann Surg 199:223, 1984.
49. Hertzer NR: Fatal myocardial infarction following lower extremity revascularization: Two hundred and seventy-three patients followed six to eleven post-operative years. Ann Surg 193:492, 1981.
50. Hillis LD, Hirsh PD, Campbell WB, et al: Interactions of the arterial wall, plaque, and platelets in myocardial ischemia and infarction. Cardiovasc Clin 14:31, 1983.
51. Hjalmarson AIM: Effect of nicotine chewing gum in smoking cessation. JAMA 252:2835, 1984.
52. Hughson WG, Munn JI, Garrod A: Intermittent claudication: Prevalence and risk factors. Br Med J 1:1379, 1978.
53. Hully SB, Cohen R, Widdowson G: Plasma high-density lipoprotein cholesterol level. Influence of risk factor intervention. JAMA 238:2269, 1977.
54. Hurlow RA, Strachan CJL, George AJ, et al: Thrombosis tests in smokers and non-smokers and patients with peripheral vascular disease. *In* Greenhalgh RM (ed): Smoking and Arterial Disease. London, Pitman Medical Publishers, 1981.
55. Imparato AM, Kim GE, Davidson T, et al: Intermittent claudication: Its natural course. Surgery 78:795, 1975.
56. Jonason T, Ringqvist I: Factors of prognostic importance for subsequent rest pain in patients with intermittent claudication. Acta Med Scand 218:27, 1985.
57. Jurgens IL, Barker NW, Hines EA: Arteriosclerosis obliterans: A review of 520 cases with special reference to pathogenic and prognostic factors. Circulation 21:188, 1960.
58. Kallero KS: Mortality and morbidity in patients with intermittent claudication as defined by venous occlusion in plethysmography: A ten year follow-up. J Chron Dis 34:455, 1981.
59. Kannel WB, Skinner JJ, Schwarz MJ, et al: Intermittent claudication: Incidence in the Framingham study. Circulation 41:875, 1970.
60. Kitchell JR, Palmon F, Ayton N, et al: The treatment of coronary artery disease with disodium EDTA: A reappraisal. Am J Cardiol 11:501, 1963.
61. Kirk CJC, Lund VJ, Woolcock NE, et al: The effect of advice to stop smoking on arterial disease patients, assessed by serum thiocyanate levels. J Cardiovasc Surg 21:568, 1970.
62. Lamar CP: Chelation endarterectomy for occlusive atherosclerosis. J Am Geriatr Soc 14:272, 1966.
63. Lamar CP: Chelation therapy of occlusive arteriosclerosis in diabetic patients. Angiology 15:379, 1964.
64. Lefevre FA, Corbacioglu C, Humphries AW, et al: Management of arteriosclerosis obliterans of the extremities. JAMA 170:656, 1959.
65. Lithell H, Hedstrand H, Karlsson R: The smoking habits of men with intermittent claudication. Acta Med Scand 197:473, 1975.
66. Luscombe JA, Taylor LM Jr, Porter JM: Incidence of cervical carotid artery disease in patients undergoing lower extremity bypass surgery. Oregon Health Sciences University Noninvasive Vascular Laboratory. Unpublished data.
67. Malone JM, Moore WS, Goldstone J: Life expectancy following aortofemoral arterial grafting. Surgery 81:551, 1977.
68. Marshall AJ, Roberts CJC, Barritt DW: Raynaud's phenomenon as a side effect of beta-blockers in hypertension. Br Med J 1:1498, 1976.
69. Meade TW, Chakrabarti R, Haines AP, et al: Characteristics affecting fibrinolytic activity and plasma fibrinogen concentrations. Br Med J 1:153, 1979.
70. Meltzer LE, Kitchell JR, Palmon F Jr: The long term use, side effects and toxicity of EDTA. Am J Med Sci 242:51, 1961.
71. Melzack R, Wall PD: Pain mechanism: A new theory. Science 150:971, 1975.
72. McAllister FF: The fate of patients with intermittent claudication managed nonoperatively. Am J Surg 132:593, 1976.
73. Myers KA, King RB, Scott DF, et al: The effect of smoking on the late patency of arterial reconstructions in the legs. Br J Surg 65:267, 1978.
74. Nunn DB: Symptomatic peripheral arteriosclerosis of patients under age 40. Ann Surg 39:224, 1973.
75. Pairolero PC, Joyce JW, Skinner CR, et al: Lower limb ischemia in young adults: Prognostic implications. J Vasc Surg 1:459, 1984.
76. Peabody CN, Kannel WB, McNamara PM: Intermittent claudication: Surgical significance. Arch Surg 109:693, 1974.
77. Peterson GR: Adverse effects of chelation therapy [Letter]. JAMA 250:2926, 1983.
78. Pollin W: The role of the addictive process as a key step in causation of all tobacco related diseases. JAMA 252:2874, 1984.
79. Projections of the population of the United States by age, sex and race: 1983–2080. Current Population Reports, Population Estimates and Projections, US Dept of Commerce, 1984 (Bureau of the Census; Series P-25, No. 952).
80. Provan JL, Sojka SG, Murnaghan JJ, et al: The effect of cigarette smoking on the long term success rates of aortofemoral and femoropopliteal reconstructions. Surg Gynecol Obstet 165:49, 1987.
81. Quick CRG, Cotton LT: The measured effect of stopping smoking on intermittent claudication. Br J Surg 69(Suppl):524, 1982.
82. Rees PJ: Peripheral skin necrosis complicating beta-blockade. Br Med J 1:955, 1979.
83. Reid DD, Brett GZ, Hamilton PJ, et al: Cardiorespiratory disease and diabetes among middle aged male civil servants. Lancet 1:469, 1974.
84. Reinders JH, Brinkman HJM, Van Mourik JA, et al: Cigarette smoke impairs endothelial cell prostacyclin production. Arteriosclerosis 6:15, 1986.
85. Rivers SP, Veith FJ, Ascer E, et al: Successful conservative therapy of severe limb threatening ischemia: The value of nonsympathectomy. Surgery 99:759, 1986.
86. Robicsek F, Daugherty HK, Mullen DC, et al: The effect of continued cigarette smoking on the patency of synthetic vascular grafts in Lericle syndrome. J Thorac Cardiovasc Surg 70:107, 1975.

87. Ruell PA, Imperial ES, Bonor FJ, et al: Intermittent claudication. The effect of physical training on walking tolerance and venous lactate concentration. Eur J Appl Physiol 52:420, 1984.
88. Rutkow IM, Ernst CB: An analysis of vascular surgical manpower requirements and vascular surgical rates in the United States. J Vasc Surg 3:74, 1986.
89. Saltin B: Physical training in patients with intermittent claudication. *In* Cohen LS, Mock MB, Ringquist I (eds): Physical Conditioning and Cardiovascular Rehabilitation. New York, Wiley, 1981, p 181.
90. Schadt DC, Hines EA, Jeurgens JHLO, et al: Chronic atherosclerotic occlusion of the femoral artery. JAMA 175:937, 1961.
91. Schuler JJ, Flanigan DP, Holcroft JW, et al: Efficacy of prostaglandin E1 in the treatment of lower extremity ischemic ulcers secondary to peripheral vascular occlusive disease: Results of a prospective randomized, double-blind, multicenter clinical trial. J Vasc Surg 1:160, 1984.
92. Silbert S, Zazeela H: Prognosis in atherosclerotic peripheral vascular disease. JAMA 166:1816, 1958.
93. Skinner JS, Strandness DE Jr: Exercise and intermittent claudication. II. Effect of physical training. Circulation 36:23, 1967.
94. Sprlie D, Myhre K: Effects of physical training in intermittent claudication. Scand J Clin Lab Invest 38:217, 1978.
95. Stachnik T, Stoffelmayr B: Worksite smoking cessation programs: A potential for national impact. Am J Public Health 73:1395, 1983.
96. Szilagyi DE, Hageman JHY, Smith RF, et al: Autogenous vein grafting in femoropopliteal atherosclerosis: The limits of its effectiveness. Surgery 86:836, 1979.
97. Szilagyi DE, Elliott JP, Smith RF, et al: A thirty-year survey of the reconstructive surgical treatment of aortoiliac occlusive disease. J Vasc Surg 3:421, 1986.
98. Tallis RC, Illip LS, Sedgwich EM, et al: Spinal cord stimulation in peripheral vascular disease. J Neurol Neurosurg Psychiatry 46:478, 1983.
99. Turnipseed WD, Berkoff HA, Belzer FO: Postoperative stroke in cardiac and peripheral vascular disease. Ann Surg 192:365, 1980.
100. Ulietstra RE, Kronmal RA, Oberman A, et al: Effect of cigarette smoking on survival of patients with angiographically documented coronary artery disease. JAMA 255:1023, 1986.
101. Vale JA, Jefferys DB: Peripheral gangrene complicating beta-blockade [Letter]. Lancet 1:1216, 1978.
102. White CB, Udwadia BP: Beta-adrenoreceptors in the human dorsal hand vein and the effects of propranolol and practolol on venous sensitivity to noradrenaline. Br J Clin Pharmacol 2:99, 1975.
103. Widmer LK, Greensher A, Kannel WB: Occlusion of peripheral arteries: A study of 6400 working subjects. Circulation 30:836, 1964.
104. Wynder EL: Tobacco and health: A societal challenge. N Engl J Med 300:894, 1979.
105. Ahn SS, Baker JD, Walden K, Moore WS: Which asymptomatic patients should undergo routine screening carotid duplex scan? Am J Surg 162:180, 1991.
106. Renaunen A, Takkunen H, Aromaa A: Prevalence of intermittent claudication and its effect on mortality. Acta Med Scand 537(Suppl):8, 1972.
107. Veith FJ, Gupta SK, Samson RH, et al: Progress in limb salvage by reconstructive arterial surgery combined with new or improved adjunctive procedures. Ann Surg 194:386, 1981.
108. Edwards JM, Taylor LM Jr, Porter JM: Treatment of failed lower extremity bypass grafts with new autogenous vein bypass. J Vasc Surg 11:132, 1990.
109. Salmasi A-M, Nicolaides A, Al-Katoubi A, et al: Intermittent claudication as a manifestation of silent myocardial ischemia: A pilot study. J Vasc Surg 14:76, 1991.
110. Turnipseed W, Detmer DE, Girdley F: Chronic compartment syndrome: An unusual cause for claudication. Ann Surg 210:557, 1989.
111. Moreland LW, Lopez-Mendez A, Alarcon GS: Spinal stenosis: A comprehensive review of the literature. Semin Arthritis Rheum 19:127, 1989.
112. Andersson GBJ, McNeill TW: Definition and classification of lumbar spinal stenosis. *In* Andersson GBJ, McNeill TW (eds): Lumbar Spinal Stenosis. St. Louis, Mosby–Year Book, 1992.
113. Creasy TS, McMillan PJ, Fletcher EW, et al: Is percutaneous transluminal angioplasty better than exercise for claudication? Preliminary results from a prospective randomized trial. Eur J Vasc Surg 4:135, 1990.
114. Jacobs MJHM, Jorning PJG, Beckers RCY, et al: Foot salvage and improvement of microvascular blood flow as a result of epidural spinal cord electrical stimulation. J Vasc Surg 12:354, 1990.
115. LoGerfo FW: Epidural spinal cord electrical stimulation: An unproven methodology for management of lower extremity ischemia. J Vasc Surg 13:518, 1991.
116. Sloth-Nielsen J, Guldager B, Mouritzen C, et al: Arteriographic findings in EDTA chelation therapy on peripheral arteriosclerosis. Am J Surg 162:122, 1991.
117. Rosenbloom MS, Flanigan DP, Schuler JJ, et al: Risk factors affecting the natural history of claudication. Arch Surg 123:867, 1988.
118. Jonason T, Ringqvist I: Factors of prognostic importance for subsequent rest pain in patients with intermittent claudication. Acta Med Scand 218:27, 1985.
119. Walsh DB, Gilbertson JJ, Zwolak RM: The natural history of superficial femoral artery stenoses. J Vasc Surg 14:299, 1991.

52

Direct Reconstruction for Aortoiliac Occlusive Disease

David C. Brewster, M.D.

• • •

The infrarenal abdominal aorta and the iliac arteries are among the most common sites of chronic obliterative atherosclerosis in patients with symptomatic occlusive disease of the lower extremities.[1] Indeed, atherosclerotic narrowing or occlusion of these vessels, most commonly centered around the aortic bifurcation, occurs to various degrees in the majority of patients with symptoms of arterial insufficiency severe enough to require surgical revascularization. Because arteriosclerosis is frequently a generalized process, obliterative disease in the aortoiliac segment frequently coexists with disease below the inguinal ligament. Despite its generalized nature, however, the disease is usually segmental in distribution and is thereby amenable to effective surgical treatment. Even in patients with several levels of disease, successful correction of hemodynamic impairment in the aortoiliac inflow system frequently provides highly satisfactory clinical relief of ischemic symptoms. In addition, careful assessment of the adequacy of arterial inflow is important even in patients whose primary difficulty is located in the femoropopliteal or tibial outflow segment if good and durable results are to be obtained.

Since the introduction of the initial reconstructive methods of thromboendarterectomy and homograft replacement in the late 1940s and early 1950s, great progress has been achieved in the surgical management of aortoiliac occlusive disease. Currently, a variety of methods exist to evaluate the extent and physiologic severity of the disease process accurately, and improvements in preoperative assessment of patient risk have helped to clarify the decision about the optimal management in each individual patient. Advances in graft materials, surgical techniques, intraoperative management, and postoperative care have all contributed to a steady reduction in perioperative morbidity and mortality and to excellent long-term results. Indications for operation have become fairly well accepted and standardized, and various operative approaches and methods of revascularization are available for use in differing clinical circumstances. With proper patient selection and a carefully performed, appropriate operative procedure, a favorable outcome may be anticipated at low risk to the patient, making surgical management of aortoiliac occlusive disease one of the most rewarding areas of vascular surgical practice today.

CLINICAL MANIFESTATIONS

The symptoms and natural history of the occlusive process are significantly influenced by its distribution and extent (Fig. 52–1). Truly localized aortoiliac disease (type I), with occlusive lesions confined to the distal abdominal aorta and common iliac vessels, is seen infrequently (5 to 10 per cent of patients) and in the absence of more distally distributed disease rarely produces limb-threatening symptoms.[2] In such localized aortic obstruction, the potential for collateral blood flow around the aortoiliac arterial segment is great. Collateral pathways include both visceral and parietal routes, such as internal mammary artery to inferior epigastric artery, intercostal and lumbar arteries to circumflex iliac and hypogastric networks, hypogastric and gluteal branches to common femoral and profunda femoris branches, and superior mesenteric to inferior mesenteric and superior hemorrhoidal pathways via the marginal artery of Drummond (meandering mesenteric artery).

It should be emphasized that the relatively low incidence of localized aortoiliac disease is derived from results of angiography in patients with symptomatology sufficiently severe to merit serious consideration of direct surgical intervention. With the increasing use of percutaneous transluminal angioplasty and related interventional treatment modalities that may represent ''less invasive'' forms of management, more liberal application of arteriography earlier in the disease process, when less advanced symptoms are present, may well document a higher incidence of localized occlusive lesions in the aortoiliac segment.[3]

Patients with localized, segmental disease typically present with various degrees of claudication, most often involving the proximal musculature of the thigh, hip, or buttock areas. The symptoms may be equally severe in both limbs, although often one leg is more severely affected than the other. More advanced ischemic complaints are absent unless distal atheroembolic complications have occurred. In men, impotence is an often associated complaint, present in different degrees in at least 30 to 50 per cent of male patients with aortoiliac disease. Patients with a type I dis-

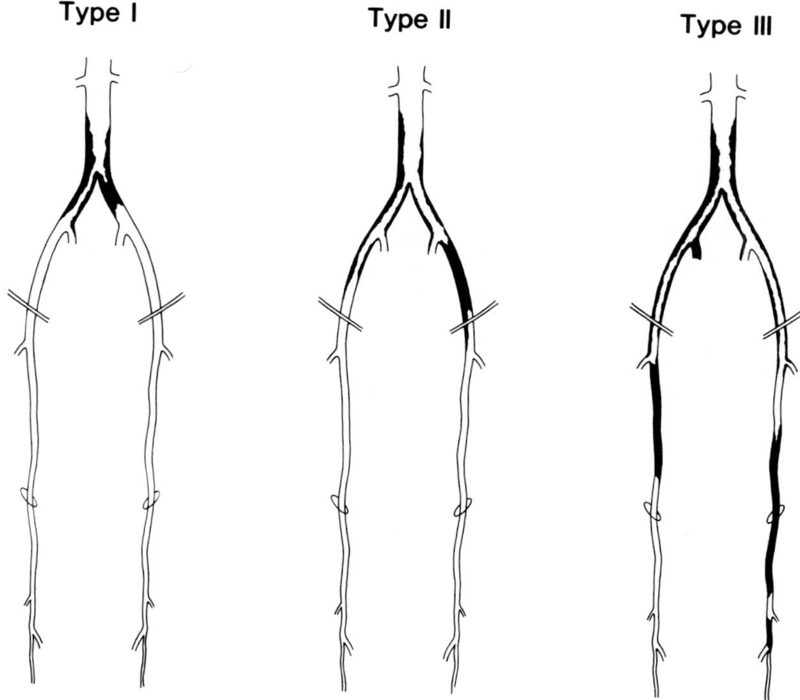

FIGURE 52–1. Patterns of aortoiliac occlusive disease. In type I, localized disease is confined to the distal abdominal aorta and common iliac arteries. In type II, more widespread intra-abdominal disease is present, whereas a type III pattern denotes multi-level disease with associated infrainguinal occlusive lesions.

ease pattern are characteristically younger, with a relatively low incidence of hypertension or diabetes but a significant frequency of abnormal blood lipid levels, particularly type IV hyperlipoproteinemia.[4, 5] In contrast to the usual male predominance in chronic peripheral vascular disease, almost one half of patients with localized aortoiliac lesions are women.[2] Indeed, the frequency of aortoiliac disease in women has been increasing substantially in recent years, coincident with the increased national incidence of cigarette smoking in women. Many female patients with localized aortoiliac disease exhibit a characteristic clinical picture often called the "hypoplastic aorta syndrome" (Fig. 52–2): typically a woman of about 50 years of age, invariably a heavy smoker, with angiographic findings of small aortic, iliac, and femoral vessels; a high aortic bifurcation; and occlusive disease often strikingly localized to the lower aorta or the aortic bifurcation.[5–8] Commonly, many such patients will have had an artificial menopause induced by hysterectomy or irradiation.

In more than 90 per cent of symptomatic patients, however, disease will be more diffuse. Approximately 25 per cent will have disease confined to the abdomen (type II), and approximately 65 per cent will have widespread occlusive disease above and below the inguinal ligament (type III).[2, 4] Patients in the latter group with such "combined-segment" or "multi-level" disease are typically older; more commonly male (about a 6 : 1 ratio); and much more likely to have diabetes, hypertension, and associated atherosclerotic disease involving cerebral, coronary, and visceral arteries. Progression of the occlusive process is also more likely in such patients than in patients with more localized aortoiliac disease.[8–10] For these reasons, the majority of patients with a type III pattern manifest symptoms of more advanced ischemia, such as ischemic pain at rest or various degrees of ischemic tissue necrosis, and they require revascularization more often for limb salvage than for relief of claudication alone. In addition, these characteristics not unexpectedly lead to a significant decrease in life expectancy of 10 or more years in patients with diffuse multisegment disease, whereas life expectancy may be nearly normal in patients with localized aortoiliac disease.[11]

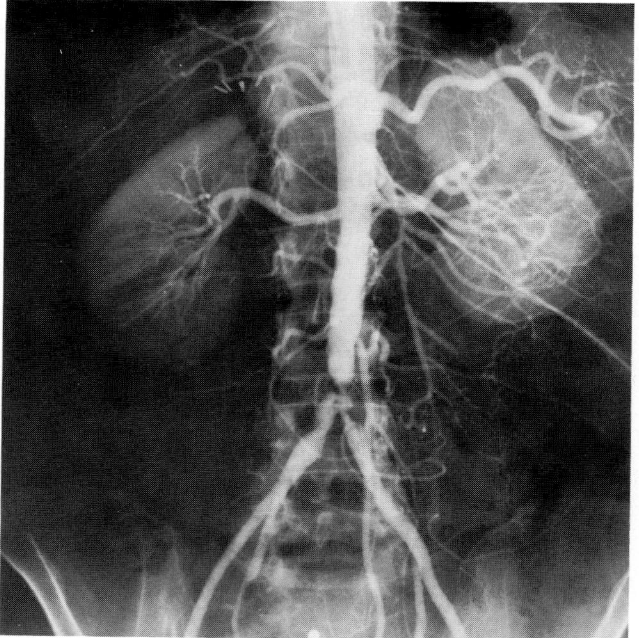

FIGURE 52–2. Translumbar aortogram of 50-year-old woman with localized type I aortoiliac disease.

DIAGNOSIS

In most instances, an accurate history and a carefully performed physical examination can unequivocally establish the diagnosis of aortoiliac disease. A reliable description of claudication in one or both legs, possible decreased sexual potency in the male patient, and diminished or absent femoral pulses define the characteristic triad often referred to as the Leriche syndrome. It should be remembered, however, that clinical grading of femoral pulses may sometimes be inaccurate, particularly in obese patients or in patients with scarred groins from prior operation.[12, 13] Although proximal claudication symptoms in the distribution of the thigh, hip, and buttock musculature are usually a reliable indicator of clinically important inflow disease, a significant number of patients with aortoiliac disease, particularly those with multi-level disease, will nonetheless complain only of calf claudication.[14, 15] Audible bruits may frequently be appreciated over the lower abdomen or the femoral vessels with a stethoscope, particularly after exercise. Elevation pallor, rubor on dependency, shiny atrophic skin in the distal limbs and feet, and possible areas of ulceration or of ischemic necrosis or gangrene may be noted, depending on the extent of atherosclerotic impairment. In some instances, however, the diagnosis of aortoiliac occlusive disease may not be readily apparent, and pitfalls may exist in terms of certain complaints that may cause diagnostic confusion. In some patients, pulse evaluation and appearance of the feet may be judged to be entirely normal at rest, despite the presence of proximal stenoses that are physiologically significant with exercise. This is often the case in patients presenting with distal microemboli secondary to atheroembolism, the so-called blue toe syndrome.[16, 17] In other instances, complaints of exercise-related pain in the leg, hip, buttock, or even low back may be mistaken for symptoms of degenerative hip or spine disease, nerve root irritation caused by lumbar disc herniation or spinal stenosis, diabetic neuropathy, or other neuromuscular problems. Many such patients may be distinguished from patients with true claudication by the fact that their discomfort is often relieved only by sitting or lying down, as opposed to simply stopping walking. In addition, the typical sciatic distribution of the pain and the fact that often the complaints are brought on by simply standing, as opposed to walking a certain distance, suggest nonvascular causes. However, in many such circumstances, the use of noninvasive vascular laboratory testing modalities, including treadmill exercise, may be extremely valuable.[18, 19]

Use of noninvasive studies (see Chapter 5) not only improves diagnostic accuracy but also allows physiologic quantification of the severity of the disease process. This may be of considerable clinical benefit, for instance in establishing the likelihood of lesion healing without revascularization or in differentiating neuropathic foot pain from true ischemic rest pain. Noninvasive studies may also serve as a reliable and objective baseline by which to follow a patient's disease course, and finally, they may often help in localization of the disease process. The author and his colleagues have found the use of segmental limb Doppler pressure measurements and pulse volume recordings to be most useful.[20]

ARTERIOGRAPHY

Purpose

If the patient's symptoms and clinical findings indicate sufficient disability or threat to limb survival, angiography is the next step. It should be emphasized that arteriography is rarely used in a truly diagnostic sense; the presence or absence of occlusive disease as a cause of the patient's symptoms can almost always be reliably established by clinical evaluation supplemented by pre- and postexercise noninvasive vascular laboratory studies. Instead, angiography is employed for the anatomic information it provides the surgeon in selecting and planning an operative procedure. On occasion, the angiogram may be the final bit of data involved in a decision whether or not to proceed with operation; in other instances, it may be employed to determine if occlusive disease is amenable to percutaneous transluminal balloon angioplasty. Neither of these uses is "diagnostic" in the usual sense of the word but is rather part of the therapeutic process.

In addition to noting the actual anatomic distribution of occlusive disease in the aortoiliac segment and distal vessels, the surgeon should examine the films for potentially important or critical anatomic variations or associated occlusive lesions in the renal, visceral, or runoff vessels. For example, an enlarged meandering left colic artery (Fig. 52–3) may often be an indicator of associated occlusive disease in the superior mesenteric artery, which can usually be appreciated only on a lateral view. Failure to recognize this may lead to catastrophic bowel infarction if the inferior mesenteric artery is ligated at the time of aortic reconstruction.[21]

Approach

The general preference of the author and his colleagues is for a retrograde transfemoral approach, which is feasible from the less involved side in most patients (see Chapter 8). In patients with severe bilateral occlusive disease or total aortic occlusion, a translumbar or transaxillary route may be employed, depending on the preferences of the angiographer or surgeon carrying out the study. A biplane study, providing oblique or lateral views, is highly desirable and often greatly enhances the ability to determine the clinical importance of visualized lesions.[12]

Extent of Study

For most patients, a full and complete arteriographic survey of the entire intra-abdominal aortoiliac segment and infrainguinal runoff vessels is advisable. Even if proximal operation alone is planned, knowledge of the anatomy of runoff disease is important because it helps the surgeon anticipate the probable outcome of proximal operation alone, aids in more effective management of possible technical misadventures, and is important for future planning. Only by such complete studies will unusual but highly important variations in the occlusive process, which may critically affect the conduct and outcome of operation, be detected. Some investigators believe that aortography is not necessary in patients with complete absence of both femoral pulses. Currently, however, most vascular surgeons believe that even in these cases angiographic study is important to define the exact anatomic distribution and extent of occlusive disease accurately and to facilitate selection of the appropriate arterial reconstruction.

In general, runoff views are obtained to at least the level of the mid-calf. In selected patients with advanced distal disease and threatened limbs, more distal views may be advisable, including views of the foot itself if the possibility of distal infrapopliteal bypass grafting is considered likely. In such instances, in which the amount of contrast material reaching these distal points may be significantly impaired by multi-level occlusive lesions, supplemental use of digital subtraction angiographic techniques may enhance adequate visualization and definition of anatomy.

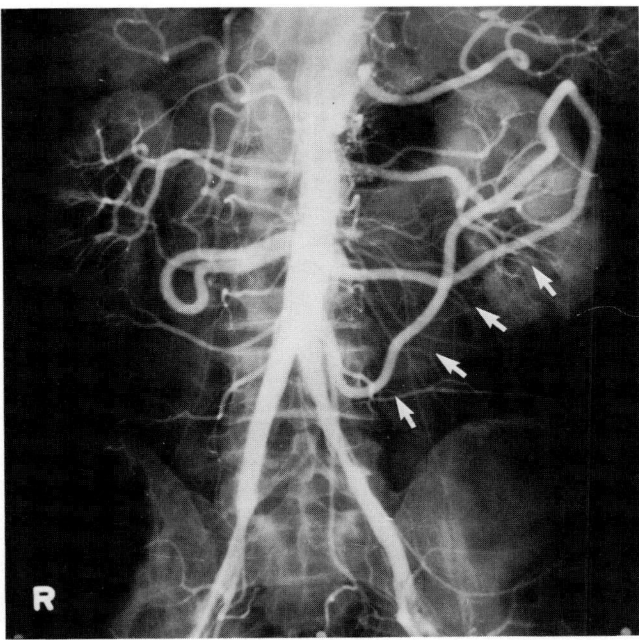

FIGURE 52–3. Aortogram demonstrating enlarged meandering inferior mesenteric and left colic arteries *(arrows)*, indicative of associated occlusive disease in the celiac and/or superior mesenteric arteries.

Renal Dysfunction After Angiography

Despite the relative lack of toxicity of contrast agents currently used for diagnostic arteriography, various degrees of deterioration of renal function may be noted following angiographic studies. Such dysfunction may be mild and transient or may lead to severe impairment requiring dialysis. Although the precise risk of acute renal dysfunction following aortic angiography is dependent on the definition of and criteria for functional impairment, the reported incidence varies between 0 and 10 per cent for low-risk patients and between 30 and 40 per cent for higher-risk patients.[22, 23] Renal deterioration appears to be related to contrast load and is clearly more likely to occur in patients with preexisting renal insufficiency and azotemia, dehydration, diabetes mellitus, increased age, or other predisposing factors.

Hydration of patients before angiography appears to be beneficial, and it should be liberally employed. The administration of mannitol to patients with preexisting renal disease at the time of angiography has also been recommended. In high-risk patients, digital subtraction angiography appears to be helpful, often providing diagnostic anatomic information with much lower volumes and dosages of contrast media. In general, contrast-induced renal failure usually resolves spontaneously within about 7 days. Because of its possible adverse effects, angiography should precede surgery by an interval of time sufficient to determine that the serum creatinine concentration has remained stable and that operation is not carried out at the time of developing renal failure.

FEMORAL ARTERY PRESSURE

Although an accurate assessment of occlusive disease is usually possible with traditional clinical evaluation and good-quality arteriography in most patients, difficulty may exist in patients with multi-level occlusive disease. Assessment of the hemodynamic significance of occlusive disease at each segmental level is obviously of critical importance in selecting an appropriate reconstructive procedure. It is well recognized that many atherosclerotic lesions may be of only morphologic significance on the arteriogram, with little or no actual hemodynamic importance. In such patients, proximal reconstruction alone may often fail to relieve the patient's symptoms adequately. Furthermore, if only moderate proximal disease is present in a patient with advanced distal disease, operative correction of both segmental levels may be required for limb salvage if severe ischemia is present in the foot.

Despite the availability of a wide array of noninvasive vascular laboratory testing methods, none is entirely accurate in establishing the hemodynamic importance of aortoiliac inflow lesions, particularly in the patient with multilevel disease. All appear to be influenced by the presence of infrainguinal occlusive disease, and abnormal results may not always be reliably attributable to the proximal lesions. Deficiencies of segmental limb Doppler pressures or pulse volume recordings are well recognized in this regard.[24–26] Analysis of femoral artery Doppler waveforms or calculation of a pulsatility index is also of questionable accuracy in the presence of multi-segment disease because they are affected by distal as well as proximal disease.[12, 27] Other, more complex modifications of Doppler waveform analysis have been devised, but their accuracy and value in combined-segment disease remain uncertain. Similarly, duplex scanning has been applied to the assessment of lower extremity occlusive disease,[28] but a threshold criterion for local increase of peak systolic velocity for hemodynamically significant iliac disease has not been conclusively established. Such examinations are also time consuming, require very experienced technicians, and may not visualize some arterial segments, all of which currently limit the applicability of duplex scanning for evaluating aortoiliac disease.

Reliance on the angiographic appearance of lesions also carries known hazards. It is now recognized that there is marked observer variability associated with the interpretation of the functional importance of arterial lesions visualized on arteriograms.[29] In addition, although the relationship of a simple arterial stenosis and hemodynamic impairment is well documented, the multiplicity and complexity of lesions occurring in the aortoiliac system make hemodynamic assessment based on morphology alone often inaccurate.[30] In such instances, actual measurement of femoral artery pressure (FAP) may be of considerable value.[12, 31–33] FAP measurements are usually obtainable in the arteriographic suite at the time of transfemoral catheter aortography. Separate arterial puncture by a relatively small caliber (19-gauge) needle may occasionally be required if pressure determinations are needed in the femoral artery contralateral to the angiographic catheter insertion site. As illustrated in Figure 52–4, peak systolic pressure in the femoral artery is compared with distal aortic or brachial systolic pressure. A resting systolic pressure difference of greater than 5 mmHg or a fall in FAP of greater than 15 per cent with reactive hyperemia induced pharmacologically or by inflation of an occluding thigh cuff for 3 to 5 minutes implies hemodynamically significant inflow disease. If revascularization is indicated in such patients, attention should first be directed at correction of the inflow lesions. With negative study findings, the surgeon may more confidently proceed directly with distal revascularization without fear of premature compromise or closure of the distal graft, and without subjecting the patient to an unnecessary inflow operation.[34]

Based on such criteria, selection of patients for an inflow procedure is greatly facilitated and benefit is accurately predicted. In the most recent review by the author's group, 96 per cent of patients with positive results of FAP studies had satisfactory clinical improvement in ischemic symptoms with proximal arterial reconstruction alone, despite uncorrected distal disease in the majority of patients. In contrast, 57 per cent of patients undergoing proximal operation despite a negative FAP result experienced unsatisfactory relief of symptoms and required subsequent distal procedures.[14] Similar results have been reported by other investigators using pressure determinations.[33, 35, 36]

INDICATIONS FOR OPERATION

Ischemic pain at rest or actual tissue necrosis, including ischemic ulcerations or frank digital gangrene, is well accepted as indicative of advanced ischemia and threatened limb loss. If untreated, most such patients will have disease progression and will require major amputation. Because of this, all surgeons agree that these symptoms are clear-cut

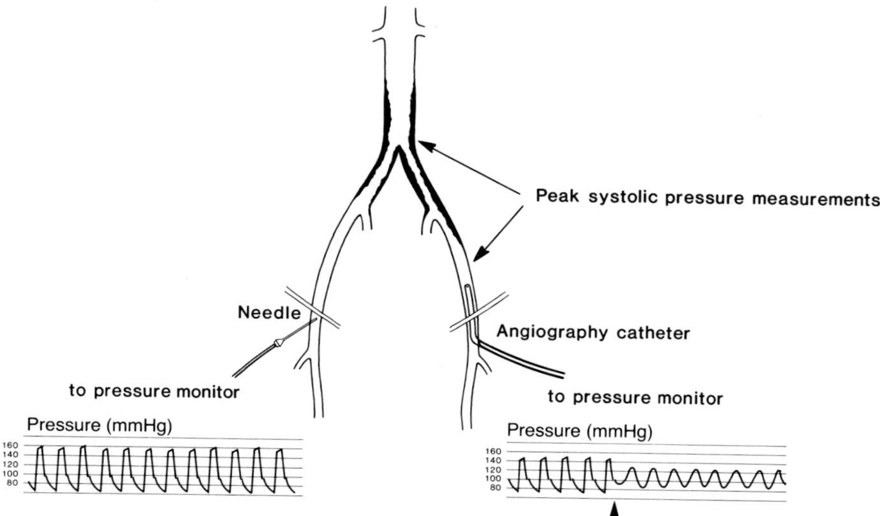

FIGURE 52–4. Femoral artery pressure (FAP) measurement. A significant fall in peak systolic pressure is noted on the left *(arrowhead)* as catheter is withdrawn down left iliac artery.

indications for arterial reconstruction, if anatomically feasible. Age per se is rarely an important consideration. Even elderly or frail patients or patients at high risk from multiple associated medical problems may generally be revascularized by alternative surgical methods if direct aortoiliac reconstruction is deemed inadvisable.

Some disagreement remains about the advisability of operation for claudication symptoms alone. Quite clearly, such decisions must be individualized, with each patient's age, associated medical disease, employment requirements, and lifestyle preferences taken into consideration. In general, claudication that jeopardizes the livelihood of a patient or significantly impairs the desired lifestyle of an otherwise low-risk patient may be considered to be a reasonable indication for surgical correction, assuming that a favorable anatomic situation for operation exists. It is usually advisable for the surgeon to have followed such a patient conservatively for a period of time and to have thoroughly discussed the merits and possible risks of any surgical procedure. The patient should have demonstrated his or her commitment to the therapeutic program by control of appropriate risk factors, most importantly elimination of cigarette smoking and appropriate weight reduction, when required, and by compliance with a low-fat, low-calorie diet. In general, most surgeons are more liberal in recommending surgical operation for patients with claudication alone if symptoms can be attributed to isolated proximal inflow disease, as opposed to more distal disease in the femoropopliteal arterial segment. This seems logical and appropriate because of the generally excellent and long-lasting results currently achieved with aortoiliac reconstruction, at low risk to the patient.

Another less frequent but well-recognized indication for aortoiliac reconstruction is peripheral atheromatous emboli from proximal ulcerated atherosclerotic plaques (see Chapter 44). The aortoiliac system has been recognized as a frequent source of spontaneous atheroembolization to more distal vessels. As already described, clinical evidence of occlusive disease in such patients may be minimal, with little or no history of claudication and fairly normal pulses at rest. However, if the clinical picture is consistent with a diagnosis of atheroembolization and aortography demonstrates shaggy or ulcerated atherosclerotic plaques in the aortoiliac system, aortofemoral grafting with total exclusion of the host aortoiliac system is frequently indicated to avoid repetitive episodes or even limb loss, even though the occlusive lesions may not be hemodynamically significant.

No truly effective medical treatment for aortoiliac occlusive disease is currently available. Nonoperative care is aimed at limiting disease progression, encouraging development of collateral circulation, and preventing local tissue trauma or infection in the foot. With such care, spontaneous improvement may be noted in a few patients, although in most instances slow progression of symptoms may be anticipated. Progression of the atheromatous process may, in some instances, be slowed by altering the patient's risk factors. Complete cessation of cigarette smoking is of paramount importance in this regard, and it cannot be overemphasized to the patient. Weight reduction, treatment of hypertension, correction of abnormal serum lipid levels, and regulation of diabetes all seem to be desirable and logical, although definite benefit in terms of stabilization or alleviation of occlusive symptoms is less well established. A regular exercise program, often involving no more than regular walking of a specific distance on a daily basis, seems to be the best stimulant to collateral circulation. Good local foot care is extremely important because trauma and digital infection are often the precipitating causes of gangrene and amputation, particularly in the diabetic patient. Although numerous vasodilator drugs exist, none are of established benefit in chronic occlusive disease.[37] None of these drugs have been shown to increase the exercising muscle blood flow in the claudicating extremity, the critical requirement for an effective agent in the treatment of claudication. A multi-institution double-blind, placebo-controlled trial of pentoxifylline (Trental) in the treatment of patients with claudication showed a significant increase in walking distance in patients who received this agent versus those treated with a placebo.[38] In the author's experience, perhaps 25 per cent of patients may find some alleviation of claudication symptoms. However, it is often difficult to know if this improvement is attributable to the drug. Although pentoxifylline may be used in patients with moderate claudication, it does not appear to have changed the eventual need for surgical revascularization in patients with severe claudication, resting ischemia, or more advanced symptoms.

The role of percutaneous transluminal angioplasty (PTA) is discussed more fully in Chapters 20 and 58. PTA may be a valuable treatment modality in some patients with aortoiliac occlusive disease. However, patient selection is of paramount importance. To be appropriate for PTA, the lesion should be relatively localized and preferably a stenosis rather than a total occlusion. A localized stenosis of the common iliac artery of less than 5 cm in length is the most favorable situation for PTA, with excellent early and late patency rates.[39, 40] Such a situation may exist in perhaps 10 to 15 per cent of patients with aortoiliac disease coming to arteriographic study.[41] PTA is generally not recommended for patients with diffuse iliac disease, unless they are extraordinarily poor surgical candidates, or for totally occluded iliac arteries because of the higher incidence of complications or recurrent occlusion.[42] Alternatives for revascularization in high-risk patients with such situations unfavorable to PTA almost always exist.

SURGICAL TREATMENT

Currently, methods of direct aortoiliac reconstruction offer the most definitive and durable means of surgical revascularization. A variety of inflow procedures are available to the surgeon. Most often, prosthetic bypass grafting is used, usually to the femoral arteries, although in a limited number of cases aortoiliac end-arterectomy may be feasible. Remote or "extra-anatomic" procedures are reserved for the relatively small group of truly high-risk patients unable to tolerate conventional anatomic reconstruction, or in circumstances of infection or other technical problems that may hamper standard direct operation. The proper choice of operation depends on the general condition of the patient, the extent and distribution of atherosclerotic disease, and the experience and training of the surgeon.

Preoperative Preparation

In addition to angiographic assessment, evaluation of associated cardiac, renal, and pulmonary disease is routinely performed. Any correctable deficiencies are best identified before operation and appropriately treated. For instance, patients with compromised pulmonary reserve may benefit from a period of preoperative chest physiotherapy, bronchodilator medication, appropriate antibiotic treatment, and so forth. Diminished renal function also requires evaluation, with correction of any prerenal component that is due to dehydration or treatment of other reversible deficiencies. Similarly, cardiac abnormalities demonstrated by clinical evaluation or 12-lead echocardiogram are evaluated and treated appropriately; in many instances, consultation with a cardiologist may be quite helpful. Without question, the most important and controversial aspect of the preoperative patient evaluation is the detection and subsequent management of associated coronary artery disease.[43, 44] Several studies have documented the existence of potentially important coronary artery disease in 40 to 50 per cent or more of patients requiring peripheral vascular reconstructive procedures, 10 to 20 per cent of whom may be relatively asymptomatic largely because of their inability to exercise.[45] Myocardial infarction is quite clearly responsible for the majority of both early and late postoperative deaths. However, most currently available screening methods suffer from a lack of sensitivity and specificity in predicting postoperative cardiac complications. In addition, many patients with vascular occlusive disease cannot achieve adequate exercise stress as a result of claudication or infirmity. Even with coronary angiography, it is difficult to relate anatomic findings to functional significance and hence surgical risk. In addition, coronary angiography is associated with its own inherent risks, and patients undergoing coronary artery bypass grafting or percutaneous transluminal coronary angioplasty before needed aortoiliac reconstructions are subjected to the risks and complications of both procedures.

In this regard, the author and his colleagues and others have found preoperative dipyridamole–thallium-201 imaging to be very valuable in identifying the subset of preoperative vascular patients who may indeed be at high risk for perioperative myocardial ischemic events and perhaps warrant more intensive preoperative evaluation.[46–49] This has allowed identification of a low-risk subset of patients in whom no further evaluation or intensive intraoperative monitoring appears to be warranted. Conversely, a subset of high-risk patients can be identified who often deserve preoperative coronary angiography, bypass surgery, or both or in whom operation may be deferred if more elective indications permit.[46–53] Good correlation with perioperative cardiac ischemic events and results of preoperative screening with continuous portable electrocardiographic monitoring to detect silent ischemia has also been reported.[54] Further experience with such monitoring, dipyridamole-thallium scanning, and other methods of preoperative evaluation of possible coronary artery disease will be of major importance to determine if they have a positive impact on the reduction of perioperative cardiac morbidity, which is currently low after elective operation in experienced centers.[55, 56]

Routine testing of coagulation parameters should be part of any preoperative evaluation. Baseline values should be obtained for hematocrit, complete blood count, platelet count, prothrombin time, and partial thromboplastin time. Any abnormalities of such screening studies will require further evaluation and correction of specific factor deficiencies. Patients taking aspirin, dipyridamole, or other drugs that may adversely affect platelet function or other aspects of the normal coagulation mechanisms should discontinue such medications approximately 1 week before operation.

On the day before surgery, only a liquid diet is given and a mechanical bowel preparation is ordered. Nonabsorbable oral antibiotics such as neomycin and erythromycin may be added if there is reason to believe that gastrointestinal trauma or ischemia may occur, but these are generally not used in the author's practice. Prophylactic parenteral antibiotics are routinely given, beginning 1 to 2 hours preoperatively and continuing for approximately 48 hours after arterial reconstruction. Several randomized studies have clearly established the value of such systemic prophylactic antibiotics in vascular surgery.[57–59]

Adequate preoperative hydration is ensured, often by administration of intravenous fluids during the evening preceding operation; occasionally, insertion of a central venous pressure catheter or Swan-Ganz catheter the day before surgery will be a helpful guide to the adequacy of intravascular volume. Such considerations are of additional importance if the patient has just undergone diagnostic angiography, with resultant osmotic diuresis. Careful attention to monitoring fluid intake and urinary output will reduce the likelihood of renal dysfunction following aortic operation.

Aortoiliac Endarterectomy

Aortoiliac endarterectomy may be considered in the group of approximately 5 to 10 per cent of patients with truly localized (type I) disease, and if properly performed in such circumstances, it may give excellent and durable results.[2, 60–62] Endarterectomy offers several theoretical advantages (see Chapter 21): no prosthetic material is inserted; the infection rate is practically nonexistent; and inflow to the hypogastric arteries, potentially improving sexual potency in the male patient, is perhaps somewhat better than with bypass procedures. Finally, because the procedure is totally autogenous and therefore more resistant to infection, it may be used in unusual circumstances in which reoperation in a contaminated or infected field requires innovative reconstructive methods.[63]

Proper selection of patients for endarterectomy is important: disease should terminate at or just beyond the common iliac bifurcation, allowing the surgeon to achieve a satisfactory end-point without extending more than 1 to 2 cm into the external iliac segment. Whether transverse or vertical arteriotomies are employed is of less importance than ensuring a proper plane of endarterectomy at the level of the external elastic lamina and achieving a secure end-point of endarterectomy, with or without the aid of tacking sutures. Primary closure of arteriotomies is generally feasible, although patch closure may occasionally be employed (Fig. 52–5).

Endarterectomy is definitely contraindicated in three circumstances. First, any evidence of aneurysmal change makes endarterectomy ill-advised because of possible continued aneurysmal degeneration of the endarterectomized segment in the future. Second, if total occlusion of the aorta exists to the level of the renal arteries, simple transection of the aorta several centimeters below the renal arteries with thrombectomy of the aortic cuff followed by graft insertion is technically easier and more expeditious. Finally, by far the most common consideration favoring bypass grafting will be extension of the disease process into the external iliac or distal vessels (types II and III). Difficulties with adequate endarterectomy of the external iliac artery as a result of its smaller size, greater length, somewhat more difficult exposure, and more muscular and adherent medial layer are well documented, with a higher incidence of both early thrombosis and late failure as a result of recurrent stenosis. For these reasons, extended aortoiliofemoral endarterectomy procedures have been generally abandoned and replaced by bypass grafting, which is simpler, faster, and associated with better late patency rates in such patients with more extensive disease.[2, 64, 65] In addition, aortoiliac

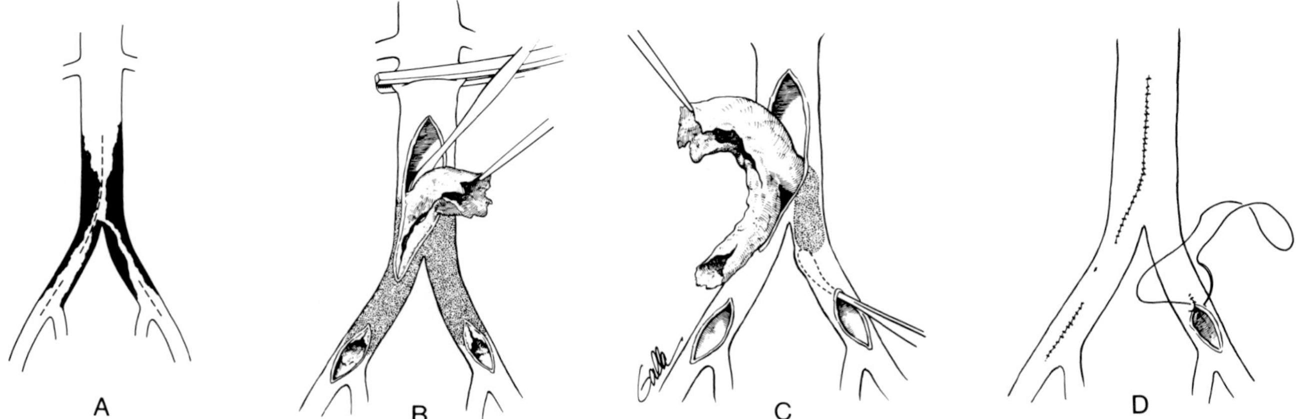

FIGURE 52–5. Aortoiliac endarterectomy. *A*, Endarterectomy may be considered if disease is localized to the distal abdominal aorta and common iliac arteries. *B*, A proper endarterectomy plane is established, and atheromatous disease is removed from the level of the aortic clamp proximally to the aortic bifurcation. *C*, Satisfactory end-point of endarterectomy at the iliac bifurcation is essential, with tacking sutures occasionally necessary. Atheromatous core is then mobilized proximally. *D*, Primary closure of the arteriotomies is usually feasible, with patch closure occasionally employed.

endarterectomy is generally acknowledged to be more demanding technically than bypass procedures. Therefore, bypass grafting may be preferable even for localized disease if the surgeon is not adequately trained in such alternative methods.

Bypass Grafting

Since the late 1960s, prosthetic graft insertion has become the standard method of direct surgical repair for aortoiliac occlusive disease, being used in more than 90 per cent of such patients by most vascular surgeons. Bypass grafts offer the most definitive, durable, and expeditious reconstruction currently available.[2, 9, 66–69] Although the technique of aortic graft insertion has been fairly well standardized, some differences in methods used do remain, and some are quite controversial. These are discussed in the following section.

PRINCIPLES OF AORTIC GRAFT INSERTION

Proximal Anastomosis

The proximal aortic anastomosis may be made either end-to-end or end-to-side. End-to-end anastomosis is clearly indicated in patients with coexisting aneurysmal disease or complete aortic occlusion extending up to the renal arteries. In addition, it is preferred by many vascular surgeons for routine use in most cases for several reasons. First, it appears to be more sound on a hemodynamic basis, with less turbulence, better flow characteristics, and less chance of competitive flow with still-patent host iliac vessels. Such considerations have led to better long-term patency and a lower incidence of aortic anastomotic aneurysms in grafts constructed with end-to-end proximal anastomosis in many reported series, although none have been randomized, prospective trials.[2, 4, 70–72] Other studies, however, have not demonstrated any differences in late patency rates between end-to-end and end-to-side grafts.[73–76] Second, application of partially occluding tangential clamps for construction of an end-to-side anastomosis may often carry a higher risk of dislodging intra-aortic thrombus or debris that may then be irretrievably carried to the pelvic circulation or lower extremities. Finally, resection of a small segment of host aorta and use of a short body of the prosthetic bifurcation graft for end-to-end anastomosis, as shown in Figure 52–6, allow the prosthesis to be placed in the anatomic aortic bed, greatly facilitating subsequent tissue coverage and reperitonealization and potentially reducing the late occurrence of aortoenteric fistula formation in subsequent years.[2, 4, 73]

End-to-side anastomosis appears to be potentially advantageous in certain anatomic patterns of disease (Fig. 52–7). For instance, if a large aberrant renal artery arises from the lower abdominal aorta or iliac arteries or if the surgeon wishes to avoid sacrifice of a large patent inferior mesenteric artery, end-to-side proximal anastomosis will presumably allow preservation of such vessels. Alternatively, they may be preserved and reimplanted into the body of the graft if end-to-end insertion is preferred. Most importantly, end-

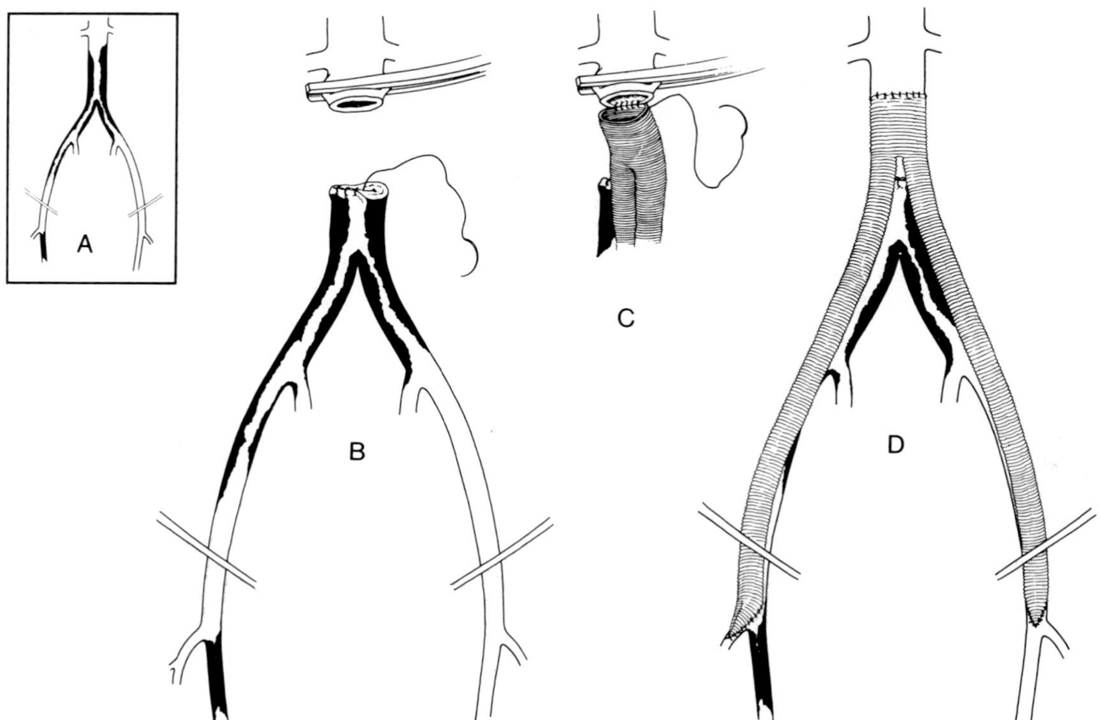

FIGURE 52–6. Aortofemoral graft. *A*, Schematic of preoperative aortogram. *B*, A segment of diseased aorta is resected, and the distal aortic stump is oversewn. *C*, End-to-end proximal anastomosis. *D*, Completed reconstruction.

to-side anastomosis appears to be advisable if the occlusive process is located principally in the external iliac vessels. In such instances, interruption of the infrarenal aorta for end-to-end bypass to the femoral level effectively devascularizes the pelvic region because no retrograde flow up the external iliac arteries to supply the hypogastric arterial beds can be anticipated. This may potentially increase the incidence of erectile impotence in the sexually potent male.[77, 78] Such hemodynamic consequences may also increase the incidence of postoperative colon ischemia, severe buttock ischemia, or even paraplegia secondary to spinal cord ischemia.[21, 79, 80] Troublesome hip claudication may also continue to plague the patient despite the presence of excellent femoral and distal pulses. Finally, if the limb of the graft occludes in later years, the resulting limb ischemia may be particularly severe and lead to difficulty with healing of even above-knee amputation if further revascularization proves to be infeasible. For these reasons, the surgeon may elect to use end-to-side proximal anastomosis in the anatomic circumstances described.

At present, one can only conclude that this area is controversial, and both methods have experienced and highly skilled vascular surgeons as advocates. Irrespective of the method of proximal anastomosis, the principle of placing the proximal anastomosis high in the infrarenal abdominal aorta, relatively close to the renal arteries in an area almost always less involved with the occlusive process, is of paramount importance to minimize later recurrent difficulties.

Distal Anastomosis

Although the distal anastomosis of the aortic graft may on occasion be accomplished at the level of the external iliac artery in the pelvis, it is almost always preferable in patients with occlusive disease to carry the graft to the femoral level, where exposure is generally better and anastomosis easier from a technical standpoint. With adequate personnel, both femoral anastomoses may often be performed simultaneously. Most importantly, anastomosis at the femoral level provides the surgeon with an opportunity to ensure adequate outflow into the profunda femoris artery. Experience has clearly demonstrated an increased late failure rate of aorta–external iliac grafts, with a higher incidence of subsequent ''downstream'' operations as a result of progressive disease at or just beyond the iliac anastomosis.[2, 64, 81] With meticulous surgical technique, proper skin preparation and draping, and use of a limited period of prophylactic antibiotic coverage, the anticipated higher incidence of infection if grafts were extended to the femoral level has not been borne out by extensive experience.[2, 9, 64–69] As a result, aortobifemoral grafting has become the procedure of choice for direct reconstruction in almost all patients with aortoiliac occlusive disease.

Profunda Runoff

Establishment of adequate graft outflow at the level of the femoral artery anastomosis, via the profunda femoris artery in patients with disease or occlusion of the superficial femoral artery, has been clearly documented to be of paramount importance in early and late graft results.[2, 67, 82–84] For these reasons, it is imperative that any lesion that might compromise profunda flow be carefully evaluated and corrected at the time of distal anastomosis. Preoperative arteriography should visualize the profunda orifice, particularly when occlusion of the superficial femoral artery is demonstrated. This is usually accomplished by oblique views of

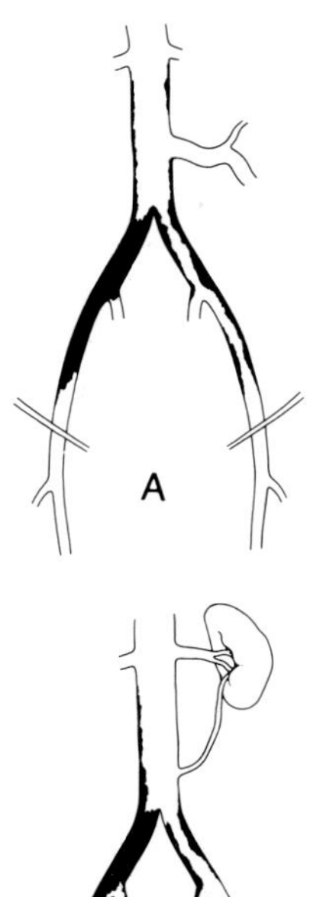

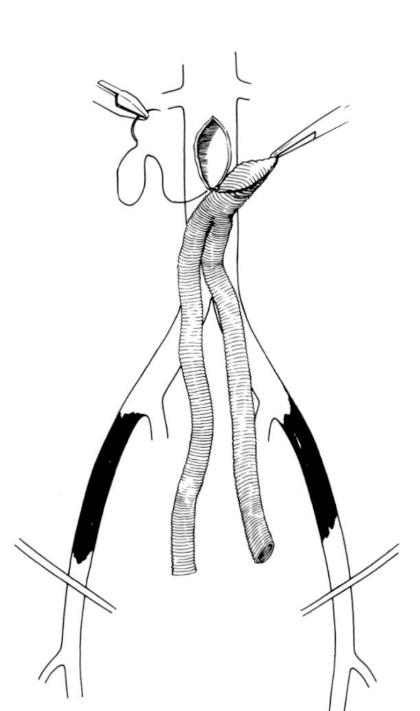

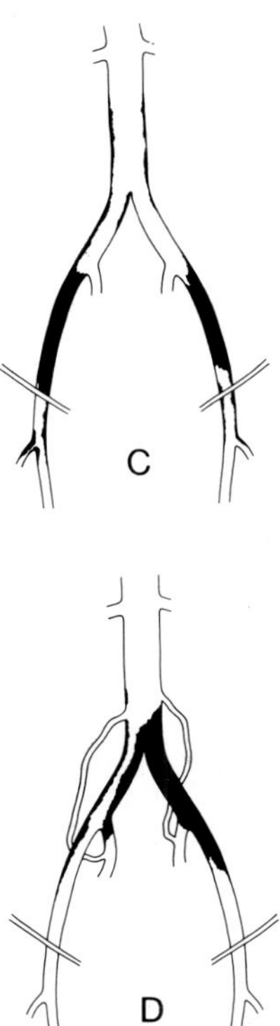

FIGURE 52–7. Anatomic findings or patterns of disease favoring end-to-side proximal anastomosis of aortofemoral graft. *A*, Patent and enlarged inferior mesenteric artery. *B*, Low-lying accessory renal artery arising from distal aorta or proximal iliac vessels. *C*, Occlusive lesions confined largely to the external iliac arteries, with aorta, common iliac, and internal iliac arteries fairly well preserved. This is the most common indication for end-to-side anastomosis in the author's experience. *D*, Reconstitution of pelvic circulation by collateral sources, which would be interrupted with end-to-end anastomosis. In all of these circumstances, end-to-side aortic anastomosis may be advantageous.

the groin. At operation, the surgeon must look for possible profunda-origin stenosis by palpation, gentle passage of vascular probes, or direct inspection. If any stenosis of the profunda origin exists, it should be corrected by endarterectomy or patch angioplasty techniques. The author's preference is for extension of the arteriotomy down the profunda beyond the orifice stenosis, with subsequent anastomosis of the beveled tip of the graft as a patch closure (Fig. 52–8). This achieves hemodynamic correction and is preferable to true endarterectomy, which may lead to a higher incidence of late false aneurysm formation when the prosthetic graft is sutured to the endarterectomized arterial wall. However, formal profunda endarterectomy will be required if the vessel is heavily diseased. Subsequent closure can still be achieved with the long, beveled tip of the graft hood. Other authors have preferred using autogenous arterial or saphenous vein patches for separate profundaplasty, then anastomosing the prosthesis to the common femoral artery above this.[83] In any case, it is imperative that the surgeon use precise anastomotic technique at the endpoint of the endarterectomy to ensure an adequate profunda outflow tract. In the hands of the author and his colleagues, this is usually best achieved by the use of three to five interrupted sutures at the distal end of the anastomosis (Fig. 52–8*C*), allowing excellent visualization, precise placement, and avoidance of any constricting effect of a running suture line at this critical outflow point.

Although some authors have suggested that the mere existence of an occluded superficial femoral artery in itself causes a ''functional'' stenosis despite the absence of orificial disease of the profunda,[85] most evidence suggests that ''routine'' profundaplasty in all such patients does not improve the hemodynamic result or late patency of the graft.[74]

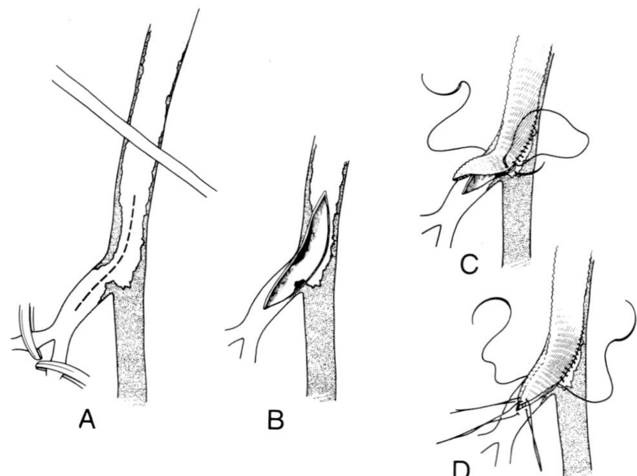

FIGURE 52–8. Femoral anastomosis in a patient with multilevel disease. *A*, With associated femoropopliteal occlusive disease, any disease at the orifice of the profunda femoris artery may limit graft limb runoff and subsequent patency. *B*, Extension of the common femoral arteriotomy into the proximal profunda femoris, distal to the origin stenosis. *C*, The heel of the long, beveled graft hood is anastomosed to the common femoral artery. *D*, Femoral anastomosis being completed with tip of the graft extended down the profunda, achieving a patch profundaplasty. Three to five interrupted sutures are first placed at the tip and not tied down, facilitating visualization and accurate placement, without constriction.

Graft Selection

Although standard fabric prosthetic grafts constructed from Dacron or Teflon and used during the initial era of aortofemoral reconstruction have generally performed well, in more recent years a wide variety of aortic prosthetic grafts have become available to the vascular surgeon. Numerous modifications in graft material (e.g., Dacron vs polytetrafluoroethylene [PTFE]), methods of fabrication (e.g., knitted vs woven, external velour vs double velour, and porosity differences), and addition of various biologic coatings (e.g., collagen or albumin) to the graft have been devised.

Such alterations have been proposed in the hope of improving the performance and characteristics of the graft, usually in terms of patency, durability, healing and incorporation within host tissue, resistance to infection, reduced blood loss through the graft, and improved handling qualities. Various claims concerning the benefits of one type over another have been made, although it is often difficult to discern science from salesmanship. Past studies performed to evaluate the differences frequently lacked adequate control to allow an accurate conclusion to be drawn. One attempt to help clarify this situation involved the use of ''half-and-half'' grafts of woven and knitted Dacron by Robicsek and associates.[86] Implanting a bifurcated Dacron graft constructed with one limb woven and the other knitted allowed them to compare patency of the two limbs directly. Although approximately half of their 158 patients underwent replacement for aneurysm, at an average of $5\frac{1}{2}$ years of follow-up, no significant difference was found in patency between the two limbs. In a related study, Robicsek and coworkers also reported no difference in platelet deposition in the two varieties of grafts and hence presumably no difference in the thrombogenicity of each graft.[87]

Many surgeons continue to prefer knitted Dacron grafts for aortofemoral grafting, mainly because of their flexibility and ease of handling and suturing, which is particularly helpful when a difficult profunda anastomosis is necessary. However, newer manufacturing techniques have begun to blur the former distinct differences in mechanical properties and characteristics between knitted and woven Dacron grafts and make such considerations less important in current practice. Whether internal or external velour surfaces or a combination of the two is beneficial remains unproven. Although porosity and incorporation by the host tissue remain desirable features, the successful use of PTFE grafts in other locations has made these considerations questionable. The bifurcated PTFE graft, introduced in 1982, has had too limited a use in the United States to allow meaningful evaluation of its long-term reliability. A study of PTFE use in the hypoplastic aorta syndrome by Burke and colleagues suggested better patency results than with Dacron grafts, but statistical significance was not achieved.[88] Similarly, the results of a comparison of PTFE bifurcated grafts and Dacron prostheses by Cintora and associates favored PTFE grafts: although cumulative patency at 4 years was not significantly different (97 vs 90 per cent, respectively), blood loss was less and late graft-related complications were less frequent with PTFE grafts.[89] High-porosity grafts sealed with protein matrix substances, fibrin glue, or other materials show promise for improvement in host tolerance and lower thrombogenicity but are too new to allow comment on long-term results. Clearly, both PTFE and biologically coated prosthetics do limit blood loss and facilitate the procedure by obviating the need for preclotting of the graft, but all such grafts are generally more expensive than conventional fabric prostheses and any improved performance is unproven. One may currently conclude in general that no single large-caliber graft is clearly superior and that long-term patency is more closely related to proper surgical methods of graft implantation and limitation of disease progression than to the specific graft employed.

Irrespective of the exact type of graft material and fabrication, the use of a proper-sized graft is important.[90, 91] Previously, many surgeons employed grafts that were too large in comparison with the size of outflow tract vessels, which tended to promote sluggish flow in graft limbs and deposition of excessive laminar pseudointima in the prosthesis. This in turn may often have a propensity to later fragmentation or dislodgment, leading to occlusion of one or both limbs of the graft. For occlusive disease, a 16 × 8-mm bifurcated graft is most often employed, with no hesitation to use a 14 × 7-mm or even smaller prosthesis when appropriate, as is frequently the case in some female patients. The limb size of such grafts will most closely approximate the femoral arteries of patients with occlusive disease, or more particularly the size of the profunda femoris, which often remains as the only outflow tract. In addition, it is now well recognized that many Dacron prosthetic grafts have a tendency to dilate 10 to 20 per cent when subjected to arterial pressure.[92] Selection of a smaller graft size will help compensate for this.

Intraoperative Evaluation of Revascularization

At the conclusion of the operative procedure, the surgeon must ensure the technical and hemodynamic integrity of the vascular reconstruction (see Chapter 24). This is traditionally done by visual inspection of the anastomoses and by palpation of satisfactory pulses at and just beyond the point of graft anastomosis. If feasible, some means of ensuring adequate distal flow intra-operatively is also advisable. Actual palpation of distal leg and pedal pulses is often cumbersome without contaminating the operative field. In addition, pulses are often difficult to appreciate immediately after reconstruction in the cold and vasoconstricted limb. Some surgeons prefer to prepare and drape the feet in transparent bags so as to allow visualization of their color and appearance, but this is often a rather subjective and uncertain method. It is the practice of the author and his colleagues to obtain pulse volume recordings following restoration of flow to evaluate hemodynamic adequacy of aortoiliac reconstruction more objectively.[93] Plethysmographic cuffs are placed at the calf or ankle level and are draped out of the operative field. Following graft insertion and release of clamps, postoperative pulse volume recordings are easily obtained by the circulating nurse and can be compared with preoperative tracings to assess the hemodynamic result of proximal revascularization. If more distal sterile draping is necessary, sterile intraoperative cuffs may be used for post-reconstructive determinations. Unless extensive uncorrected distal disease is present, such pulse volume recordings should show satisfactory or usually improved amplitude as compared with preoperative tracings. If extensive distal disease does complicate pulse volume recording monitoring, a sterile cuff may be applied to the distal thigh to ensure adequate profunda revascularization. Alternatively, some surgeons use postreconstructive determinations of distal ankle Doppler pressures or electromagnetic flow measurements through the open graft limb. Regardless of the method chosen, the importance of ensuring a satisfactory technical result before leaving the operating room cannot be overemphasized.

SPECIAL CONSIDERATIONS

Retroperitoneal Approach

Although a retroperitoneal approach to the infrarenal abdominal aorta was used by Rob and others during the early era of aortic reconstruction for occlusive or aneurysmal disease,[94] the traditional surgical approach for direct repair of infrarenal aortoiliac occlusive disease has been the transperitoneal route. Several reports have recommended a retroperitoneal approach as an alternative in patients with multiple prior intra-abdominal operations or in those high-risk patients with cardiac or significant pulmonary disease. In this latter group, possible advantages include less disturbance of pulmonary function, decreased postoperative ileus, and lessened third-space fluid losses. In other instances of occlusive disease extending close to the renal arteries or in patients with associated occlusive lesions of the visceral or renal arteries, a retroperitoneal approach may permit easier access, control, and repair.[95–97]

The patient is placed in a modified left thoracotomy position with the left shoulder and chest elevated to approximately a 45- to 60-degree angle, and the hips and pelvis are rotated posteriorly as far as possible to provide access to the femoral arteries. The mid-point between the left costal margin and the iliac crest is centered over the break in the table, and the table is flexed to widen the left flank. During the operative procedure, the operating table can be rotated either toward or away from the surgeon, who stands on the patient's left side. An oblique flank incision is made beginning at the left lateral border of the rectus muscle several inches below the umbilicus and extended superiorly to the tip of the 11th rib. Dissection is carried in a retroperitoneal plane either anterior to the kidney if standard infrarenal exposure is adequate, or the left kidney may be mobilized anteriorly if access to the supraceliac aorta is necessary. Further medial mobilization of the peritoneal envelope exposes the inferior mesenteric artery, which is divided and ligated close to the aorta, usually facilitating further exposure.

With such an approach, access to the right renal artery is often impossible, and control and repair of the right iliac artery are occasionally difficult. Similarly, tunneling to the right groin and right femoral anastomosis may sometimes be difficult, particularly in an obese patient. However, the approach may clearly be helpful for those patients with multiple prior intra-abdominal operations, prior aortic surgery, pararenal disease, or similar technical considerations. Whether or not it is advantageous for standard infrarenal aortic reconstruction, as compared with the conventional transperitoneal approach, remains uncertain; although several retrospective reviews[95, 98] have suggested that a retroperitoneal approach is less physiologically stressful, Cambria and coworkers found no differences between patients who underwent standard transperitoneal reconstruction and those who underwent retroperitoneal infrarenal aortic reconstruction in the only randomized, prospective study on this topic.[99]

Adjunctive Lumbar Sympathectomy

The use of a concomitant lumbar sympathectomy at the time of aortic reconstruction remains unsettled and controversial (see Chapter 59). Although it is well accepted that sympathectomy does increase skin and total limb blood flow, there are few objective data to document more favorable long-term graft patency or improved limb salvage results.[100, 101] However, available evidence does suggest that decreased pedal vasomotor tone and skin perfusion may be helpful as an adjunct to direct arterial revascularization, particularly in patients with multi-level disease and relatively minor superficial areas of pedal or digital ischemic lesions.[100, 102, 103] Therefore, limited (L2 to L3) sympathectomy in conjunction with direct aortic operation may be considered in such patients, particularly when it has been decided to limit operation to inflow reconstruction alone or when distal runoff is considered to be poor. This is easily and quickly accomplished, but it must be acknowledged that its benefit remains unproven.

The Totally Occluded Aorta

Approximately 8 per cent of the author's patients undergoing operation for aortoiliac occlusive disease have a chronic totally occluded aorta.[104] In about one half, the occlusion has extended retrograde to the level of the renal arteries (Fig. 52–9); in the rest, the occlusion has involved only the distal infrarenal aorta, with the proximal segment remaining open via runoff through a still-patent inferior mesenteric artery or lumbar vessels.

Surgical management of the latter group is straightforward and is similar to standard aortic graft insertion. However, with extension of the occluding thrombus to a juxtarenal level, the operative approach is more taxing and possible complications are more likely, particularly those complications involving disturbance of renal function.[104–106] Nevertheless, surgery may be advisable for such patients even if ischemic complaints are relatively mild and stable because of the potential for more proximal propagation of thrombus with compromise or occlusion of neighboring renal or visceral arteries. The actual threat of proximal propagation of untreated total aortic thrombosis remains controversial, however. Although some series have suggested that the danger is significant,[107, 108] other retrospective reviews have determined that subsequent compromise of renal or mesenteric circulation by further retrograde extension of clot is quite rare unless coexistent severe stenosis in renal or visceral arteries is also present.[109, 110]

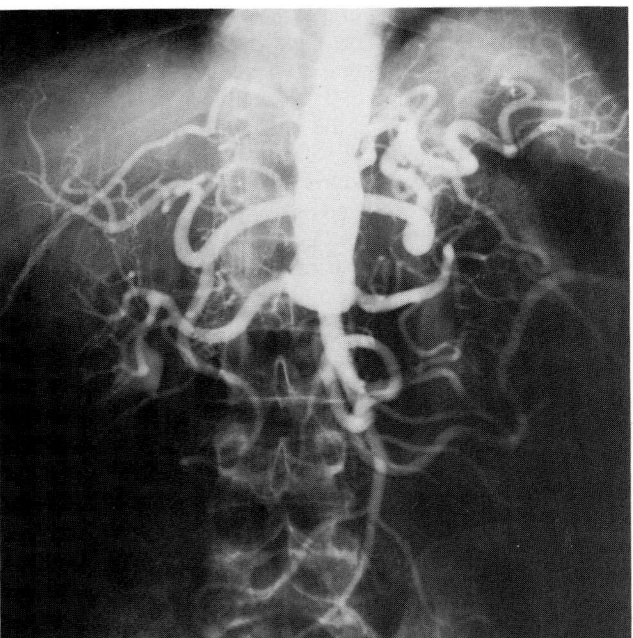

FIGURE 52–9. Transaxillary aortogram demonstrating total juxtarenal aortic occlusion.

In almost all patients with juxtarenal occlusion, the bulk of the actual occlusive disease lies in the distal aorta, with the proximal occlusive material composed largely of secondary thrombus. This proximal plug may almost always be removed by simple thrombectomy followed by routine graft insertion. Adequate dissection should be carried out to allow temporary control of the renal arteries to minimize chances of renal embolization at the time of juxtarenal thrombectomy. Division of the left renal vein may facilitate exposure and is a benign procedure if carried out correctly near the insertion of this vein into the vena cava, thereby preserving collateral venous drainage. This is generally unnecessary, however, and the mobilized left renal vein can usually be retracted cephalad or caudad as required for exposure and control of the juxtarenal aorta.[111] The completely occluded aorta should be opened through an arteriotomy placed several centimeters below the renal arteries. The infrarenal aorta should *not* be clamped at this juncture, to avoid compressing the apex of the thrombotic material and possibly dislodging it into the renal or mesenteric circulation. Indeed, infrarenal clamping is unnecessary at this stage because the thrombotic plug will prevent any bleeding. Thrombectomy of the aortic cuff to the level of the renal arteries is carried out with a blunt clamp. This is usually terminated by aortic pressure "blowing out" a typical organized cap of thrombus representing the apex of the thrombotic occlusion. The suprarenal aorta can then be controlled by manual pressure, or a suprarenal clamp can be temporarily applied. The aorta is then flushed, the renal artery bulldog clamps are removed, and an appropriate vascular clamp is applied to the now-patent infrarenal cuff. Graft insertion is then carried out in the routine fashion.

Formal endarterectomy is best avoided in most circumstances because this plane may be difficult to terminate without compromise of the renal artery origins. Simple thrombectomy at this level is preferred, and it is sufficient in almost all cases.

The Calcified Aorta

Occasionally, dense calcification of the infrarenal aorta appears to preclude successful insertion of an aortic graft and causes the surgeon to consider abandoning the procedure. This is particularly true of end-to-side anastomosis with the use of tangential, partially occluding clamps.

Reconstruction can always be accomplished with several possible alterations. First, a high end-to-end proximal anastomosis is preferred. By carrying dissection to or just above the left renal vein after its division or cephalad retraction, one often finds that the aorta immediately below the renal arteries is less involved and more manageable. Second, endarterectomy of a 1- to 2-cm cuff of totally transected aorta to the level of the infrarenal aortic clamp is usually possible and removes the calcification that always lies in the diseased intima and media. This greatly facilitates subsequent end-to-end graft anastomosis. Although the cuff of the endarterectomized aorta, which consists of aortic adventitia and external elastic lamina, always appears fragile, it invariably proves to be adequate for graft anastomosis without later difficulties with bleeding, suture line disruption, or false aneurysm formation. The surgeon must employ a tapered (not cutting-tip) needle, and the use of an interrupted mattress suture technique, with each suture backed with a pledget of Teflon felt (Fig. 52–10), is to be particularly recommended.

Clamping of such calcified vessels may also be problematic. This may usually be accomplished just below the renal arteries, where calcification is often less severe. Clamping in an anterior-to-posterior fashion, with the use of an arterial clamp applied from a lateral direction, may also be helpful. Finally, in truly difficult situations, the aorta may be clamped above the renal arteries at the level of the diaphragm, or intraluminal methods of vascular control employing balloon catheters may be used.

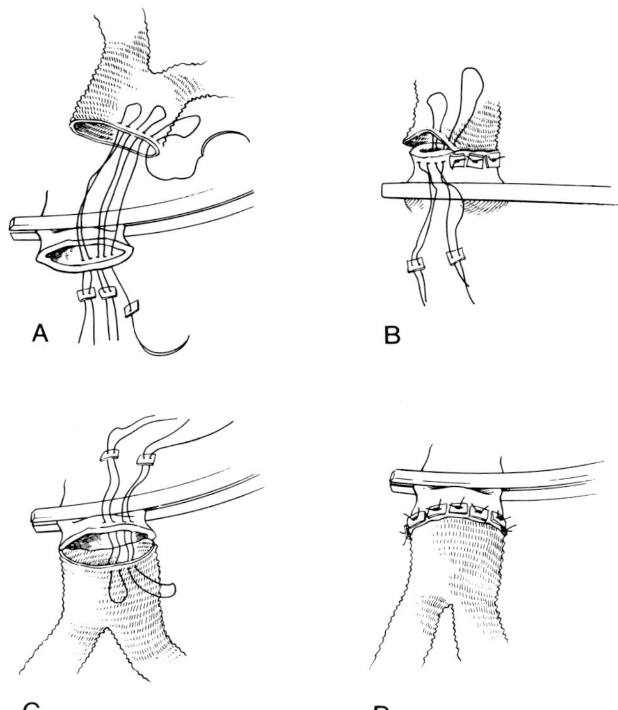

FIGURE 52–10. Interrupted mattress suture technique of aortic anastomosis. *A*, A posterior row of five mattress sutures is placed, with a double-armed suture passed through the posterior graft wall and then through the host aorta. *B*, Posterior row of sutures being tied down over pledgets of Teflon felt. *C*, The graft is turned inferiorly toward the patient's feet, and a similar anterior row of five mattress sutures is placed with pledgets. *D*, Completed interrupted suture line; extremely helpful for the small aorta or fragile, diseased vessel.

The Small Aorta

In approximately 5 to 10 per cent of patients, the infrarenal aorta and the iliac and femoral vessels will be small, which may make aortic reconstruction technically difficult. Actual anatomic definition of the small aorta is obviously arbitrary. Cronenwett and colleagues have defined the syndrome as characterized by infrarenal aortas measuring less than 13.2 mm just below the renal vessels or infrarenal aortas smaller than 10.3 mm just above the aortic bifurcation. Iliac and femoral vessels are typically correspondingly small, with the common femoral vessels often only about 5 mm in size.[5]

These patients appear to form a unique and distinct subgroup and are frequently characterized by the hypoplastic aorta syndrome.[6–8] Preferred surgical methods for reconstruction in patients with small vessels remain somewhat controversial; some authorities think the small size of the aorta and iliac vessels makes endarterectomy unsuitable, whereas others favoring bypass techniques advocate the use of end-to-side proximal aortic anastomosis to avoid size discrepancies with the usual prosthetic grafts.

Because the disease in such patients is frequently localized, aortoiliac endarterectomy may often be undertaken. Although the small size of the vessels demands greater care and occasionally requires the use of patch closures, endarterectomy in the hands of the author and his colleagues has worked well. If the disease is more diffuse, bypass grafting to the femoral vessels is preferred. Although end-to-side anastomosis is favored by many surgeons to overcome size differences between the graft and the host aorta, the author's group nonetheless still uses end-to-end techniques most often. A smaller prosthesis should be chosen to avoid the consequences of using inappropriately large grafts. In most cases, this will require the use of a 14 × 7-mm or even a 12 × 6-mm bifurcation graft. The limbs of such grafts, although small, will also be much more appropriate for the smaller femoral and outflow vessels of these individuals. Again, greater technical care must be exercised, but with attention to technical detail such grafts have not failed as a result of their small size; the author and his colleagues much prefer the insertion of such small grafts to the use of oversized prostheses. A study by Burke and colleagues suggested better patency rates when PTFE aortic bifurcation grafts were used for reconstruction in patients with a small abdominal aorta than when Dacron grafts were used, but statistical significance was not achieved.[88] Adjunctive lumbar sympathectomy is often carried out, particularly in women.

Simultaneous Distal Grafting

A frequent practical concern in patients with multi-level occlusive disease is whether or not an inflow operation alone will suffice. As already emphasized, such diffuse combined-segment disease (type III) is the most common pattern of occlusive disease, present in between one half and two thirds of the patients coming to surgery.[2, 65–69] Prior reports of patients with multi-level disease, treated in a generally accepted fashion by initial aortic reconstruction, have indicated that up to one third may fail to achieve satisfactory relief of ischemic symptoms with proximal operation alone.[10, 14, 67, 70, 74, 112–116] Although claudication symptoms are improved in more than 80 per cent of patients with multi-level disease who undergo aortofemoral grafting, only 35 per cent of patients in the author's series experienced total relief of claudication.[14] Many patients with unsatisfactory outcomes will require concurrent or subsequent distal bypass grafting. However, identification of patients likely to have insufficient relief of ischemic symptoms with an inflow procedure alone remains difficult.

In this regard, the author and his colleagues reviewed a 6-year experience with 181 patients with multi-level disease who underwent aortofemoral grafting.[14] A well-performed inflow procedure usually suffices if unequivocally severe proximal disease exists in the aortoiliac segment. Such clear-cut proximal disease is best identified by the findings of an absent or a clearly reduced femoral pulse and obvious severe aortic or iliac disease on angiography, and it is confirmed, if necessary, by positive findings on a femoral artery pressure study. Several intraoperative criteria may also be used. Restoration of an improved pulse volume recording at the calf or ankle, as compared with preoperative tracings, can give reassurance of satisfactory improvement in distal circulation. However, improvement in pulse volume recordings or Doppler ankle pressures may not be immediately apparent in the presence of significant distal disease, especially in the cold, vasoconstricted limb. Another useful intraoperative guide in predicting a good clinical response is assessment of the anatomic size of the profunda femoris vessel itself. If the proximal profunda accepts a 4-mm probe and if a No. 3 Fogarty embolectomy catheter can be passed for a distance of 20 cm or more, it is likely that the profunda femoris artery is well developed and will function satisfactorily as an outflow tract and collateral source.[4, 14, 117]

Possible benefits of simultaneous grafting include a more total correction of extremity ischemia and avoidance of the difficulties and potential complications associated with reoperation in the groin if later distal grafting proves to be necessary. Such advantages are usually outweighed by the greater magnitude of the synchronous two-level grafting and the fact that the majority of properly selected patients will be adequately benefited by proximal operation alone (76 per cent in the author's series). Distal bypass may be carried out in the future, if necessary; it was required in 17 per cent of the patients in the author's series followed up to 6 years.[14] Such a figure is in agreement with previously reported experience.[65, 66, 70, 81, 116]

In a small and carefully selected group of patients with multi-level disease and truly advanced limb-threatening ischemic problems in the foot, synchronous proximal and distal reconstruction seems appropriate.[118] This is particularly pertinent if only modest proximal occlusive disease is present because an inflow procedure will then be unlikely to improve blood flow to the foot markedly (Fig. 52–11). If the surgeon can reliably predict that a distal graft will almost certainly be necessary in the future for limb salvage, the author and his colleagues believe that simultaneous grafting is to be preferred because it offers the best chance of limb salvage and avoids a more demanding reoperation in the groin at a later time. Certainly, the use of two surgical teams can minimize the additional operative time required, and it is likely that synchronous grafting will become somewhat more common in the future.[119–124] Although some success has been claimed from preoperative noninvasive hemodynamic studies in selecting such patients,[14, 118, 122, 125] other investigators have found tests of this type to be unreliable indicators of the need for concomitant distal bypass.[74, 81, 113] Good clinical judgment remains extremely important, with reasoned and pragmatic decisions usually required.

Unilateral Iliac Disease

Not infrequently, proximal occlusive disease may appear unilaterally, with fairly normal pulses and no symptoms in the contralateral extremity. Truly unilateral iliac disease is relatively infrequent because aortoiliac disease is generally a more diffuse and eventually bilateral process. Progression of disease in the aorta or untreated contralateral iliac artery may necessitate later reoperation in a significant percentage of patients treated initially with unilateral operations for apparent one-sided disease,[64, 126] although the exact frequency of this occurrence remains controversial and several reports have suggested that it is relatively infrequent.[127–129] Thus, the most definitive and optimal long-term management for most patients is bilateral reconstruction with a bifurcated prosthetic graft.[130] For these reasons, almost all vascular surgeons have abandoned the use of unilateral aortofemoral grafts, except in unusual circumstances.[127] In the author's experience, whereas unilateral grafting was performed in 15 per cent of patients undergoing proximal operation from 1963 to 1969, only 4 per cent of patients had such procedures in the 1970 to 1978 era.[2] They are very rarely performed today.

In patients with a well-preserved aorta and contralateral iliac artery, the use of femorofemoral grafts has become increasingly important, owing to the ease of the procedure and the generally good long-term results.[131–134] In certain instances, however, the surgeon may wish to avoid the contralateral side and to confine reconstructive efforts to the symptomatic side (e.g., if the contralateral limb is asymptomatic but inflow in the proposed donor limb is of questionable reliability, and the patient is not a good risk for standard aortobifemoral grafting). In other instances, use of the contralateral groin may be relatively contraindi-

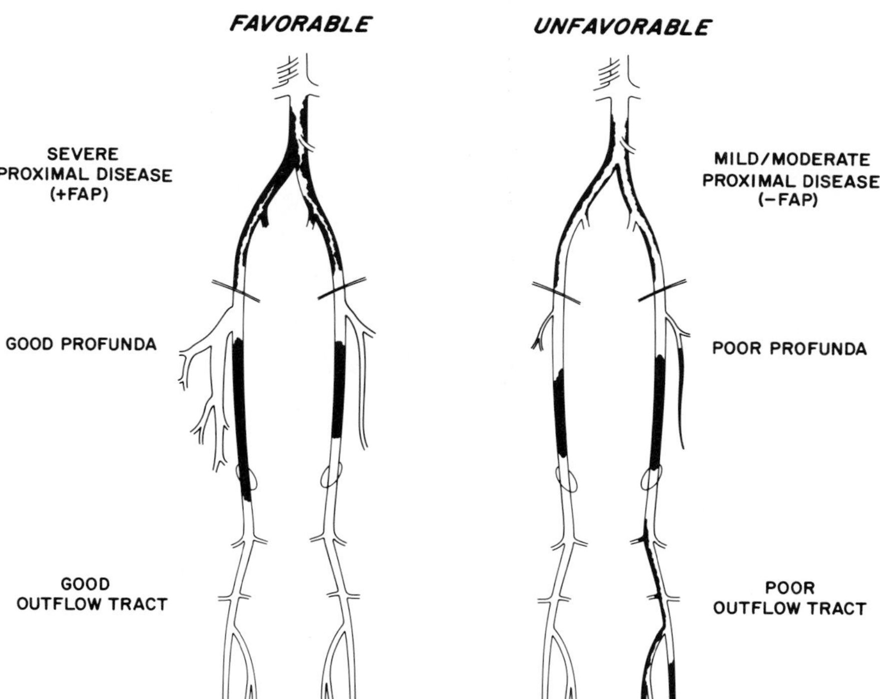

FIGURE 52–11. Clinical circumstances and disease patterns associated with favorable or unsatisfactory outcome of aortofemoral grafts alone in patients with multi-level disease.

cated as a result of heavy scarring from prior operative procedures, possible infection, and so forth. In these situations, occasional direct iliofemoral grafting may be used for disease that is largely unilateral at the time.[135–138] This procedure is used mainly for occlusive disease confined to the external iliac artery, because the ipsilateral common iliac must be relatively normal for the proximal graft anastomosis. A retroperitoneal approach through a separate lower quadrant incision (Fig. 52–12) usually provides good exposure and can be carried out with low patient morbidity. Whether femorofemoral bypass or iliofemoral grafting gives better results is currently debated, although several studies have demonstrated better long-term patency of direct ipsilateral iliofemoral bypass grafts.[139, 140] Nonetheless, femorofemoral grafting is a somewhat simpler procedure, has very low morbidity, and obviates any possibility of interfering with sexual function in the male patient.[141]

In similar situations, retroperitoneal iliac endarterectomy may be employed for relatively localized unilateral inflow lesions via a similar retroperitoneal approach,[128, 142, 143] although the established success of iliac PTA has replaced this approach in many patients. All methods of unilateral inflow revascularization may be readily combined with concomitant profundaplasty or simultaneous ipsilateral distal bypass and are therefore particularly helpful in patients with largely unilateral multi-level disease who may require extensive revascularization but in whom the surgeon wishes to limit the extent of the surgical procedure.[40, 118, 127, 142] Similarly, if proximal iliac disease is relatively localized and suitable for PTA, reestablishment of inflow by transluminal angioplasty may be combined with distal surgical procedures, with good long-term results.[40]

Associated Renal Artery or Visceral Artery Occlusive Lesions

Because of the diffuse nature of atherosclerotic occlusive disease in most patients, it is not surprising that individuals requiring aortic reconstruction for symptomatic lower extremity ischemia may be found to have associated occlusive lesions involving the renal or visceral arteries. Often these are unsuspected and detected only at the time of preoperative angiography. The dilemma of whether or not to attempt simultaneous correction of both abdominal aortic and visceral lesions is frequently encountered and difficult to resolve.[144, 145]

In these instances, each case must be considered individually and no general recommendations are feasible or appropriate. It is clear that extending aortic reconstruction to include visceral artery revascularization, although theoretically appealing, increases the complexity and magnitude of the operation and hence is associated almost invariably with some increased morbidity and mortality.[144, 146, 147] For these reasons, truly prophylactic revascularizations should generally be avoided. However, serial angiographic studies have demonstrated that renal occlusive disease is progressive in more than 50 per cent of patients and that approximately 10 per cent of high-grade lesions (80 per cent or more stenosis) go on to total occlusion, with resultant loss of function in that kidney.[144] Hence, if clinical evaluation suggests that the associated renal lesions are functionally important or preocclusive in severity, simultaneous correction is often appropriate.[144–150]

In the asymptomatic patient with visceral artery disease, careful evaluation of the anatomic pattern of disease

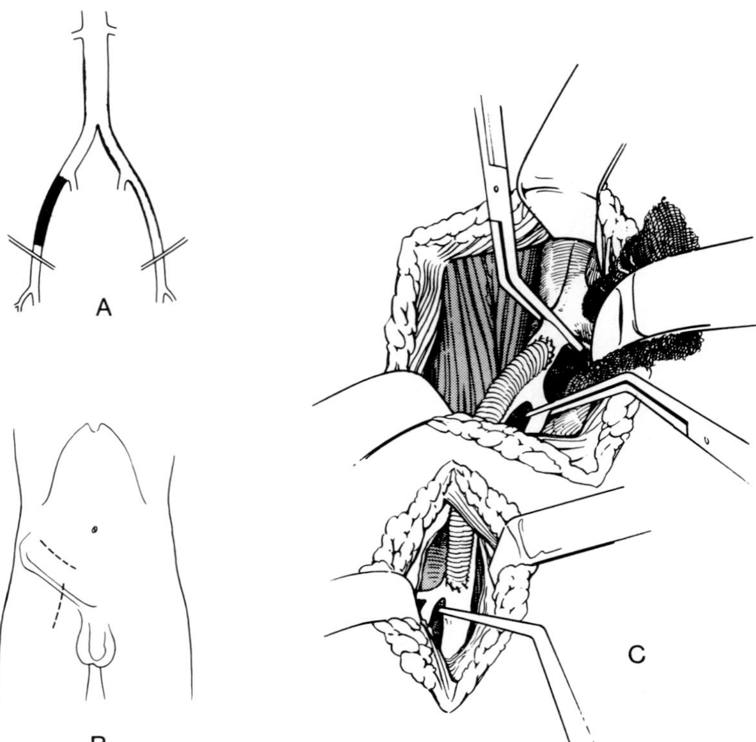

FIGURE 52–12. Unilateral iliofemoral bypass graft. *A*, Usual situation in which such a reconstruction may be considered, with occlusive disease confined largely to one external iliac artery. *B*, Positioning of skin incisions for retroperitoneal exposure of the iliac vessels and standard approach to the femoral arteries. *C*, Iliofemoral graft inserted.

on the preoperative arteriogram should indicate those patients at risk for postoperative intestinal ischemia if the visceral lesions are not dealt with. As emphasized by Ernst and others, avoidance of this catastrophic postoperative problem will require preservation of an important inferior mesenteric artery in those patients with celiac and superior mesenteric artery occlusive disease, or perhaps concomitant bypass grafting to the celiac or superior mesenteric artery itself.[21, 151] If associated renal artery disease is present, it is clear that combined reconstruction may improve associated hypertension or renal function in carefully selected patients.[146–148] Diminished renal function is rarely due to unilateral disease, and almost always significant bilateral disease (either intrarenal or extrarenal) must be present before overall renal function is adversely affected. Adding a unilateral renal bypass without first proving the functional significance of the renal lesion may unnecessarily risk further compromise of excretory function in a patient who may be azotemic predominantly on the basis of bilateral arteriolar nephrosclerosis. Therefore, it seems appropriate to assess the functional significance of such a unilateral renal artery lesion preoperatively and to proceed with correction only when study results are positive. If angiographically severe bilateral lesions are present and the patient has significant hypertension or diminished renal function, the addition of renal revascularization of at least one side to aortic reconstruction may well be the best course.

Because the morbidity and mortality of combined aortic operation and simultaneous bilateral renal artery revascularization are clearly substantially increased,[146, 147] the surgeon may elect to stage renal artery and aortic procedures, performing an isolated renal artery procedure either before or after the aortic procedure, which is combined with repair of only one renal artery. In such situations, the employment of extra-anatomic means of renal artery revascularization by use of the splenic or hepatic arteries may be particularly helpful in avoiding the necessity of operation in a previously dissected field.[152–154]

RESULTS OF DIRECT AORTOILIOFEMORAL RECONSTRUCTION

Currently, generally excellent early and late results of direct aortoiliofemoral reconstructions can be anticipated and are achievable at highly acceptable patient morbidity and mortality rates. A consensus of several large series in the modern era clearly supports this, indicating that it is reasonable to expect approximately 85 to 90 per cent graft patency at 5 years and 70 to 75 per cent at 10 years.[2, 66–69, 112, 155–158] Perioperative mortality rates well under 3 per cent are now commonplace in many centers. The mortality risk for direct reconstructions in patients with relatively localized aortoiliac disease can be expected to be extremely low, whereas those patients with multi-level disease and associated occlusive lesions in coronary, carotid, and visceral vessels will quite naturally have somewhat greater mortality risk. In this latter group of patients, it is hoped that continued improvement of screening methods for associated disease and continued refinements of anesthetic management, intraoperative monitoring, and postoperative intensive care can further reduce the risk of serious morbidity and mortality.

Long-term survival of these patients continues to be compromised, however. The cumulative long-term survival rate for patients undergoing aortoiliac reconstruction remains some 10 to 15 years less than that which might be anticipated for a normal age- and sex-matched population. Overall, approximately 25 to 30 per cent of patients will be dead at 5 years, and 50 to 60 per cent at 10 years.[11, 66, 68] Not unexpectedly, the majority of late deaths were attributable to atherosclerotic heart disease. Patients with more localized aortoiliac disease, who have a lesser incidence of coronary artery disease, distal occlusive disease, or diabetes, appear to have a much more favorable long-term prognosis, approaching that of a normal population at risk.[11, 112]

COMPLICATIONS AND THEIR PREVENTION

Early Complications

Hemorrhage

With current surgical methods and reliable prosthetic grafts and suture materials, early postoperative hemorrhage is a relatively unusual complication (1 to 2 per cent), most often the consequence of some technical oversight or abnormalities of the coagulation mechanism. Gentle surgical technique and proper methods of graft insertion are obviously of crucial importance in avoiding such difficulties. Routine screening for coagulation abnormalities preoperatively is essential.

Most currently applied reconstructive techniques emphasize minimal dissection, sufficient only to achieve adequate exposure for securing proper vascular control and graft insertion. Appropriate efforts at hemostasis during dissection are generally easier than localization and securing of bleeding points at the conclusion of the procedure. It is important that normal blood pressure be restored at the completion of the vascular reconstruction, to help avoid overlooking an insecure anastomotic suture line or improperly controlled bleeders. Leaks from vascular anastomoses, particularly those that are due to tearing of sutures in a fragile arterial wall, may acquire additional sutures, frequently with Teflon pledgets (see Fig. 52–10). Arterial inflow should be clamped briefly while such additional repair sutures are being placed and tied in order to avoid further tears. In many instances, operative bleeding may be due to injury of associated venous structures. Familiarity with the major venous anomalies is important to avoid such injuries.[159] If venous injury is present, bleeding is best controlled by gentle finger tamponade and fine vascular sutures rather than by application of clamps, which may only enlarge the size of the defect in the vein.

Adequate reversal of heparin after graft insertion is achieved by administration of protamine sulfate; however, considerable variations in individual responses to heparin exist, and monitoring of the activated clotting time before and after heparin administration may be helpful in determining the proper dose of intraoperative heparin and in judging the adequacy of its reversal before wound closure.[160] By far, the most common acquired coagulation deficiency leading to bleeding problems during aortic operations is dilutional coagulopathy. If blood loss intraoperatively is excessive and large amounts of avascular fluids and bank blood have been used during operation, administration of fresh frozen plasma and platelet concentrates is helpful and important and is often guided by serial testing of coagulation parameters. Finally, prompt recognition of ongoing volume requirements in the intensive care unit, with early appropriate reoperation as necessary, is essential.

Limb Ischemia

Acute limb ischemia occurring shortly after aortic operation for occlusive disease may be caused by either acute thrombosis of the reconstruction or more distal thromboembolic complications. Recognition of such difficulties is generally made by the failure of expected pulses to return after operation or the acute loss of previously present pulses and by ischemic deterioration of the involved extremity. Often this determination may be difficult in patients undergoing operation for multi-level disease, in whom reestablishment of peripheral pulses is not anticipated. In such patients, the use of Doppler signals, limb pressures, and distal pulse volume recordings may be quite helpful. In many patients, the perfusion of distal extremities should continue to improve during the early postoperative period, and a 4- to 6-hour interval of careful observation is often justified as long as the femoral pulse remains palpable. Careful clinical judgment is required, however.

If the diagnosis of acute limb ischemia is established, the patient should be returned promptly to the operating room. If aortoiliac endarterectomy has been performed, the usual causative factors are inadequacies in termination of the endarterectomy at the iliac bifurcation, leading to intimal flaps or constrictive closure of the arteriotomy at this point. In many instances, the basic underlying problem is inappropriate application of the endarterectomy procedure itself to patients with disease extending down the iliac vessels. In such circumstances, the abdominal incision must generally be reopened for direct inspection of the endarterectomized segments. If an aortoiliac bypass graft has been inserted, the surgeon may elect to first explore the groin and pass balloon embolectomy catheters, but often direct re-exploration is most appropriate. More commonly, an aortofemoral graft will have been extended below the inguinal ligament, and the distal anastomosis can be directly examined by reopening the groin incision. Acute thrombosis of an aortofemoral graft limb in the early perioperative period occurs in approximately 1 to 3 per cent of patients.[161] Kinking or twisting of the graft limb in the retroperitoneal tunnel may be responsible for acute graft occlusion, but most often technical anastomotic problems at the distal femoral artery are causative. Thrombectomy of the graft limb is easily carried out through a transverse opening in the distal graft hood, which also allows inspection of the interior of the anastomosis and passage of embolectomy catheters distally into the superficial and deep femoral systems. In the common clinical situation of associated superficial femoral occlusion, unobstructed runoff into the profunda femoris vessel must be ensured. If a small or diseased profunda exists and inadequate runoff is believed to be the reason for acute graft limb thrombosis, a distal bypass graft may be required to ensure adequate distal runoff.[161]

Thromboembolic mechanisms of acute limb ischemia may be more common than previously believed.[162, 163] Clot or atheromatous debris may be dislodged from proximal vessels by injudicious clamp application, or clot forming in the graft limb at the time of implantation may be inadequately flushed before flow is restored to the extremity. Thromboembolic occlusion may be best prevented by minimizing manipulation of the aorta, using full systemic heparinization during the procedure, carefully placing gentle vascular clamps on nondiseased portions of the vascular tree, and carefully flushing the reconstruction before restoration of flow. Thromboembolic occlusions of the graft limb or larger outflow vessels may generally be successfully corrected by passage of embolectomy catheters. However, more distal thromboembolic complications may be much more difficult to deal with surgically and are far better prevented if possible. A truly distal occlusion, involving tibial or digital arteries and colloquially referred to as "trash foot," is a well-recognized and frustrating problem to the surgeon. If pedal pulses are absent, it appears advisable to explore the distal popliteal artery, which allows passage of embolectomy catheters down each of the distal branches of the popliteal artery into the foot, enhancing the possibility of retrieving thrombotic material and improving perfusion. However, if the tibial vessels are patent and the occlusive debris is located in inaccessible foot and digital vessels, often little can be done. Systemic heparinization or the use of intravenous low-molecular-weight dextran is often recommended but of no proven benefit. More recently, the possible use of distally injected thrombolytic agents such as streptokinase or urokinase (see Chapters 19 and 35) has been suggested but also remains of uncertain benefit.[164, 165]

Renal Failure

In the absence of significant preoperative renal functional impairment, postoperative renal failure following elective aortic reconstruction for occlusive disease is currently an unusual event. In Diehl and associates' review of complications of abdominal aortic reconstruction in 557 patients at the Cleveland Clinic, 173 of whom underwent operation for aortoiliac occlusive disease, postoperative acute renal failure (ARF) developed in 4.6 per cent but was not fatal in any instance.[166] In other reports, the incidence of ARF after elective aortic surgery (both for aneurysm and for occlusive disease) varies from 1 to 8 per cent, with an overall mortality rate of 40 per cent. Emergency aortic surgery is associated with an increased incidence of ARF, with 50 to 90 per cent mortality.[167]

The most frequent cause is diminished renal perfusion secondary to a decrease in cardiac output and hypovolemia, which may occur during certain phases of aortic surgery, particularly at the time of declamping. Renal cortical vasospasm secondary to aortic clamping may also contribute by reducing glomerular filtration. Depending on the anatomy of occlusive disease and required repair, a period of suprarenal clamping may be necessary, or juxtarenal disease may result in intraoperative embolization of the renal circulation. Contrast-induced renal dysfunction following preoperative diagnostic arteriography may contribute, as may the use of potentially nephrotoxic antibiotics or other drugs. Finally, myoglobinuria may result from reperfusion of severely ischemic limbs and precipitate in renal tubules, resulting in ARF postoperatively.[167]

The current low rate of renal failure after elective aortic surgery is attributable to appreciation of the importance of maintaining appropriate intravascular volume by liberal use of intravenous fluids, careful monitoring of pulmonary capillary wedge pressure during operation, and avoidance of declamping hypotension.[167–169] Administration of intravenous mannitol, furosemide, or both to induce a brisk diuresis before aortic clamping is also used prophylactically by many surgeons, although the benefit of these agents in the prevention of renal failure is uncertain.

Milder forms of oliguric and nonoliguric renal dysfunction may be observed but rarely require dialysis support. Renal deterioration is much more common in patients with abnormal renal function before operation and in poorly prepared or dehydrated patients requiring emergency reconstruction for acute aortic thrombosis, and so forth. Most serious and probably irreversible are instances of renal failure secondary to embolization of thrombotic or atheromatous debris into the renal circulation. This can usually be prevented by avoiding excessive manipulation of the diseased aorta or by protecting the renal arteries by temporary clamping whenever extensive juxtarenal disease makes this advisable.

Intestinal Ischemia

Intestinal ischemia following aortic reconstruction may occur in approximately 2 per cent of cases;[21, 170] this almost always affects the colon, particularly the rectosigmoid region. The incidence of lesser degrees of ischemic colitis, involving only mucosal ischemia and resulting in less devastating consequences than transmural infarction or perforation, is undoubtedly more common, particularly if postoperative colonoscopy is used to identify patients with subclinical ischemic colitis. Small bowel ischemia following aortic operation is distinctly uncommon. Intestinal ischemia is more common after aneurysm repair than after reconstruction for occlusive disease, perhaps owing to a greater incidence of intraoperative hypotension and less well developed collateral networks.

The etiology of intestinal ischemia is often multifactorial, but it almost always involves a critical loss of blood flow to the involved intestinal segment by interruption of primary or collateral arterial flow to the bowel wall or by operative atheroembolization. Other predisposing causes may involve perioperative hypotension and hypoperfusion, manipulative trauma, or prior gastrointestinal tract surgery that may have interrupted vital collateral pathways. Recognition of anatomic situations more likely to result in intestinal ischemia following aortic operation is of vital importance. Hence, the surgeon must examine the preoperative arteriogram for associated occlusive lesions affecting the celiac axis, the superior mesenteric arteries, or both, and for a patent and enlarged inferior mesenteric artery, sacrifice of which would lead to likely colon ischemia. Identification of patients with such anatomic patterns of disease will allow preservation of the inferior mesenteric artery or concomitant revascularization of the superior mesenteric or celiac branches and, it is hoped, prevention of intestinal ischemia. The status of the hypogastric arteries should be ascertained on the aortogram, and the arterial reconstruction should be designed to maintain flow through at least one of these arteries by direct revascularization or retrograde perfusion from a femoral anastomosis if possible, especially if a patent inferior mesenteric artery must be ligated. If inferior mesenteric ligation is required, this should be carried out from within the aortic lumen or immediately adjacent to the aortic wall to avoid injury to its ascending and descending branches, which then assume increased importance as collateral pathways. Some authors have suggested reimplantation of all patent inferior mesenteric arteries during aortic reconstruction to minimize the risk of colon ischemia.[171] Although most surgeons do not believe that this is routinely necessary, careful evaluation and assessment are vital whenever a patent inferior mesenteric artery is interrupted because this is the most common identifiable factor in patients who do develop clinically significant postoperative colon ischemia, and reimplantation is advisable in selected circumstances.[170] Undue traction on the left colon mesentery must be avoided.

Recognition of intestinal ischemia intraoperatively may be difficult. Although various measures for detecting its presence intraoperatively have been reported, including use of a sterile Doppler probe, measurement of inferior mesenteric artery stump pressure, determination of intracolonic pH or transcolonic oxygen saturation, and injection of intravenous fluorescein, none have been found both practical and entirely reliable.[21, 170–172] If colon ischemia is recognized, maneuvers to increase colonic perfusion must be attempted, including revascularization of the inferior mesenteric artery by reimplantation or a short vein graft, superior mesenteric artery bypass, or hypogastric revascularization, depending on the individual circumstances and the anatomic distribution of disease.

Postoperatively, early diagnosis is the key to effective management. This often depends on a high degree of clinical suspicion and may be facilitated by prompt sigmoidoscopy or colonoscopy. Clinical manifestations in the immediate postoperative period are often masked by incisional discomfort and other problems common to the postoperative period. Findings that suggest the presence of intestinal ischemia include diarrhea, either liquid-brown or bloody; progressive abdominal distention; increasing signs of sepsis and peritonitis; and unexplained metabolic acidosis. Initial supportive care, gastrointestinal tract decompression, and intravenous antibiotic therapy may be used, with careful observation and frequent re-examination, but any evidence of clinical deterioration indicates the need for prompt operative intervention. Resection of nonviable bowel, end-sigmoid colostomy, and formation of a Hartmann pouch are generally necessary. Avoidance of graft exposure during such maneuvers, if feasible, is obviously crucial. Mortality rates for transmural colon infarction remain significant, approximating 50 to 75 per cent in many series.

Spinal Cord Ischemia

Spinal cord ischemia, resulting in paraplegia or paraparesis, is fortunately an unusual complication of aortoiliac surgery for occlusive disease. Szilagyi and associates reported an incidence of 0.25 per cent observed after 3164 operations involving temporary occlusion of the abdominal aorta, all of which were performed for aneurysmal disease. The incidence of spinal cord ischemia after intervention for ruptured aneurysms is 10 times higher than that after operations for unruptured aneurysmal lesions.[173] Although the etiology of paraplegia is multi-factorial, the usual cause of spinal cord ischemia is interruption of flow through the great radicular artery of Adamkiewicz, the major source of supply to the anterior spinal artery at the lower end of the cord. This vessel normally originates from one of the paired suprarenal intercostal arteries from T8 to T12, but it occasionally has a lower origin. In the latter situation, surgical interruption or thrombosis that is due to prolonged aortic occlusion or intraoperative embolization is believed to cause distal spinal cord ischemia. Because this anatomic variability is unpredictable, the occurrence of spinal cord ischemia is generally considered to be unavoidable. Preoperative or operative demonstration of the major blood supply to the lower spinal cord is difficult, impractical, and potentially dangerous. Several reports have also emphasized the importance of acute interruption of the pelvic circulation or atheroembolization through the pelvic arteries as another possible mechanism of ischemic neurologic injury.[79, 80, 174]

Currently, it is the consensus of almost all vascular surgeons that this tragic occurrence is essentially unpredictable and therefore not totally preventable in association with infrarenal aortic reconstruction. Monitoring of somatosensory evoked potentials during thoracic aortic surgery has been shown to correlate with cord ischemia. However, practical application of this technique to abdominal aortic reconstruction has not been established. Because of the potential importance of pelvic collateral circulation if the artery of Adamkiewicz is chronically stenosed or occluded, preservation of pelvic blood flow by revascularization of at least one hypogastric network or other technical modifications of the operative procedure is advisable, similar to the strategies for minimizing the occurrence of postoperative colon ischemia. When ischemic injury to the spinal cord does occur, treatment is confined to supportive care and rehabilitation.

Some authorities recommend the administration of high-dose intravenous steroids to decrease cord edema and hopefully improve perfusion, but the value of this is unproved and controversial.[80] The severity of paraplegia is often directly related to postoperative mortality. In the experience at the Henry Ford Hospital reported by Elliott and coworkers, 76 per cent of patients died when the neurologic deficit initially was complete; there were only two complete neurologic recoveries and one partial recovery. In contrast, when the initial loss was only partial motor and/or sensory loss, 24 per cent of patients died and some degree of recovery was noted in all but one case.[175]

Ureteral Injury

Because the ureter lies immediately adjacent to the operative field and crosses directly anterior to the iliac artery bifurcation, laceration, division, or ligature of the ureter must be constantly kept in mind and injury avoided during dissection, graft tunneling, and wound closure. This is particularly true of any reoperative surgery. A thorough knowledge of the anatomic relationship of the ureter at the level of the iliac bifurcation is essential. Direct injury to the ureter is best avoided by keeping dissection close to the arterial wall and elevating the ureter from the iliac vessels during retroperitoneal tunneling. This is particularly important during reoperative aortic surgery. Identification of the ureters during closure of the retroperitoneum, particularly the right ureter, is essential to avoid inclusion in the retroperitoneal closure.

Various degrees of hydronephrosis resulting from ureteral obstruction may also be seen in the late follow-up period, and this is probably an underdiagnosed entity. It may occur in up to 10 to 20 per cent of patients but is often asymptomatic and usually not detected unless intravenous pyelography, ultrasonography, or computed tomography (CT) scanning is carried out, often for other purposes.[176, 177] Such ureteral obstruction is most often mild and of no clinical consequence. This is occasionally attributable to placement of the graft limb anterior to the ureter, entrapping it between the graft and the native artery, but is most commonly due to compression by fibrotic changes caused by tissue reaction to the implanted graft. Occasionally, however, hydronephrosis may be a marker of graft complications such as pseudoaneurysm formation or graft infection.[178, 179] Such potential problems need to be carefully considered in patients presenting with severe or symptomatic ureteral obstruction, and the position of the ureters should be assessed before direct reoperative aortic surgery. Occasionally, preoperative placement of ureteral stents is helpful in this regard.

Late Complications

Despite the generally excellent long-term results of aortoiliofemoral reconstruction, late graft-related complications continue to occur throughout the follow-up period and detract from long-term effectiveness of the procedure. In the review of the late outcome of aortoiliac operation for occlusive disease by van der Akker and associates from Leiden, secondary operations for late complications such as reocclusion, false aneurysms, infection, and so forth were necessary in 21 per cent of 727 patients followed up over a 22-year period and contributed significantly (12.1 per cent) to the causes of late deaths.[180]

Graft Occlusion

The most frequent late complication of aortic operation for occlusive disease is graft thrombosis. Although the exact incidence of late graft occlusions varies from report to report, occlusion may be anticipated in 5 to 10 per cent of patients within the first 5 years after operation and in 15 to 30 per cent of patients if they are followed up 10 years or more postoperatively.[181–183] In the experience of the author and his colleagues, the average interval from original graft insertion to occlusion was 33.8 months.[181]

Most commonly, this will affect one limb of an aortofemoral graft, with the contralateral graft limb retaining patency. The resulting limb ischemia is often more severe than that prior to the primary procedure, and not infrequently urgent reoperation is required for limb salvage. Although thrombosis of an anastomotic aneurysm, compression that is due to fibrotic scarring, dilatation or degeneration of the graft, hypercoagulable states, or low-output syndromes may occasionally be responsible, the great majority of late graft failures are due to recurrent occlusive disease, usually occurring at or just beyond the distal anastomosis. If aortoiliac endarterectomy or aortoiliac bypass grafting has been performed, progressive occlusive disease in the external iliac artery is commonly responsible.[64, 81] In the most frequently encountered situation of occlusion of an aortofemoral graft limb, occlusive lesions interfering with profunda runoff are causative, because the majority of such patients have preexistent chronic occlusion of the superficial femoral artery.[83, 181–184] Recurrent disease compromising the proximal aortic anastomosis generally leads to failure of the entire reconstruction and is usually attributable to failure of the surgeon to carry the original procedure high enough in the infrarenal aorta.[90] Graft failure, particularly that due to recurrent or progressive inflow or outflow tract occlusive disease, is much more likely to occur in patients with ongoing risk factors for atherosclerosis, especially those who continue cigarette smoking postoperatively.[183, 185–189]

Reoperation for occlusion of the entire primary reconstruction almost always requires ''redo'' aortofemoral grafting, if the patient is an appropriate candidate.[64] Axillobifemoral grafting may be considered for the poor-risk patient. If various technical problems suggest that direct reoperation on the infrarenal abdominal aorta is ill-advised or unduly hazardous, the supraceliac aorta, descending thoracic aorta, or even ascending thoracic aorta may occasionally be used for the site of proximal anastomosis in reoperative bypass procedures.[190–194]

For unilateral limb failure of an aortoiliac procedure, direct reoperation, often employing a retroperitoneal approach, is generally feasible, with graft extension to the femoral level. Alternatively, femorofemoral transpubic grafting may be performed if the contralateral iliofemoral system is widely patent. For unilateral occlusion of one limb of an aortobifemoral graft, inflow can frequently be restored by thrombectomy of the graft limb using a balloon embolectomy catheter.[181, 184] A thromboendarterectomy stripper is often required to complete extraction of the adherent fibrinothrombotic plug.[184, 195] Or, the recently developed modification of the standard Fogarty balloon catheter, the Graft Thrombectomy catheter for adherent clot, appears to be quite useful in this situation. Once inflow has been reestablished, profunda revascularization by means of profundaplasty of varying extent or extension of a graft to the more distal profunda (Fig. 52–13) is used to reestablish reliable deep femoral outflow.[83, 181, 184, 196–198] In instances in which the profunda femoris is small or extensively diseased, addition of a femoropopliteal or femorotibial bypass may be required to provide adequate outflow and to maintain patency of the reoperated aortofemoral graft limb. Although this decision is often a difficult one, it was used in one third of such reoperations in the experience of the author and his colleagues[181] and has been advocated by other surgeons as well.[197, 199] In situations in which graft limb occlusion is more chronic and thrombectomy is not successful, a femorofemoral crossover graft from the patent contralateral graft limb is generally the most useful alter-

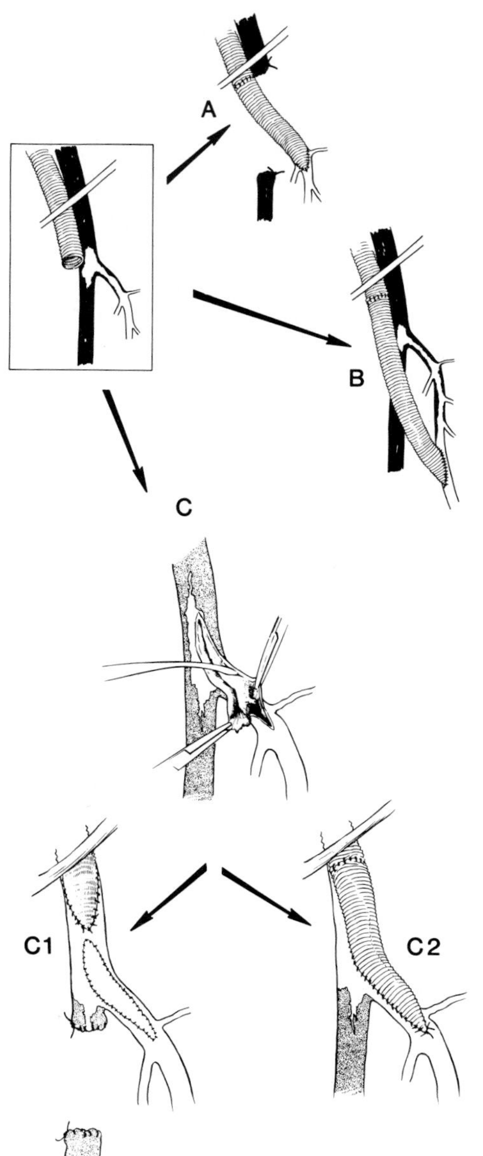

FIGURE 52–13. Options for outflow reconstruction during reoperation for aortofemoral graft limb occlusion. *A*, Addition of short extension of new prosthetic graft end-to-end to profunda below orificial profunda disease. *B*, If more extensive profunda disease is present, insertion of a longer new graft segment as a bypass to distal profunda is preferred. *C*, Most frequently, endarterectomy of the common femoral and profunda is performed, with separate patch closure employing autogenous or prosthetic material and graft reanastomosis above this *(C1)*, or closure with the long beveled tongue of new graft segment *(C2)*. *(A–C2*, From Brewster DC: Surgery of late aortic graft occlusion. *In* Bergan JJ, Yao JST [eds]: Aortic Surgery. Philadelphia, WB Saunders, 1989, p 533.)

native to reestablish inflow. Direct redo aortic surgery for unilateral aortofemoral graft limb occlusion, replacing either the entire graft or the involved graft limb, is generally unnecessary because proximal causes are infrequently responsible for unilateral failures and alternative methods of revascularizing the involved extremity are so often successful.[181, 182, 184]

Although such reoperative procedures are often difficult and may tax the skill and ingenuity of even the most experienced vascular surgeon, long-term results suggest that appropriate reoperation is indeed worthwhile, with highly satisfactory extension of long-term graft patency and associated limb salvage.[68, 181]

Anastomotic False Aneurysm

The incidence of anastomotic pseudoaneurysm formation varies between 1 and 5 per cent and is by far most common at the femoral anastomosis of an aortofemoral graft.[68] Although numerous factors may contribute to anastomotic aneurysm formation, degenerative changes within the host arterial wall leading to weakness and dehiscence of the intact suture line appear to be most common.[200] Predisposing factors include excessive tension on the anastomosis as a result of inadequate graft length, poor suture technique using inadequate bites of the arterial wall or excessive spacing between sutures, and a thin-walled artery. Many surgeons also believe that endarterectomy may weaken the arterial wall as a result of a reduction in tensile strength and lead to a higher incidence of subsequent pseudoaneurysm formation if anastomosis is done to such an arterial segment. Rarely, prosthetic suture materials may fracture, or degeneration may occur leading to late suture line disruption, such as was previously seen when silk sutures were used. Infection may be a contributing event and always needs to be considered as a possible etiologic factor when the surgeon is evaluating patients with even bland-appearing anastomotic aneurysms.[201]

Recognition of femoral anastomotic aneurysms is usually quite simple because a pulsatile mass, which is occasionally tender, is noted by both the patient and the surgeon. Retroperitoneal aortic or iliac anastomotic aneurysms are much less often noted until expansion or rupture produces pain, causes graft occlusion, or erodes into an abdominal hollow viscus. If these aneurysms are considered to be present, ultrasonography and computed tomography are reliable methods for evaluating intra-abdominal grafts and anastomoses. The true incidence of intra-abdominal anastomotic aneurysms may be much higher than previously thought after aortic surgery, with a study by Edwards and coworkers reporting a 10 per cent incidence at a mean interval of 12 years following initial operation.[202] This suggests that sonography or CT scans should be a routine part of the late follow-up of patients with aortic grafts. Diagnosis of a pseudoaneurysm is usually confirmed by angiography. Even if the diagnosis of a femoral anastomotic aneurysm is readily apparent, aortography is generally advisable to evaluate the proximal aortic anastomosis and to help plan the operative procedure. Indeed, the presence of a femoral anastomotic aneurysm may be a marker for other graft-related problems. In a report from Emory of 41 patients who had a femoral pseudoaneurysm after aortobifemoral grafting, 70 per cent had bilateral aneurysms and 17 per cent had proximal anastomotic aneurysms.[203]

An anastomotic aneurysm should generally be repaired as soon as it is identified. Even if the aneurysm is asymptomatic, the incidence of thrombosis or distal embolization warrants elective repair, which is usually easily and successfully carried out at the groin level by use of a short additional graft segment, with reanastomosis to a somewhat more distal arterial segment, often the profunda femoris artery itself. Cultures should always be obtained at the time of repair to detect unrecognized infection. Results of repair are generally highly successful, especially if repair is carried out electively rather than as an emergency.[204] Once they have been repaired, anastomotic aneurysms may recur in about 5 to 10 per cent of patients.[205] In such circumstances, occult infection must be seriously considered as a possible contributing cause.[206]

Impotence

Although a high percentage (50 to 80 per cent) of male patients presenting with aortoiliac occlusive disease significant enough to require surgical correction will have various degrees of sexual dysfunction when they are first seen, the incidence of iatrogenic impotence following aortic reconstruction may approach 25 per cent.[77, 207, 208] True impotence is the inability to achieve or maintain an erection sufficient for satisfactory coitus. Most often, such an occurrence following aortic operation implies inadequate preservation of hypogastric artery, and hence pelvic, circulation. Retrograde ejaculation, primarily a neurogenic disorder in which bladder neck closure does not occur and ejaculation occurs into the bladder, is also a frequent occurrence and is attributable to disturbance of autonomic nerve fibers that course along the left wall of the aorta and cross the proximal common iliac arteries.

Although the physiology of erection and ejaculation is complex and disturbances are not vasculogenic in all instances, it is clear that the surgeon should be aware of possible disturbance of sexual performance in the male patient and take steps to prevent or limit its incidence. As popularized by DePalma and others, a nerve-sparing approach to the infrarenal aorta emphasizing avoidance of autonomic nerve fibers along the left lateral wall of the aorta and minimal dissection in the region of the aortic bifurcation where such nerves usually cross the proximal common iliac arteries is helpful.[207–209] Preservation of hypogastric artery flow by a variety of techniques is also essential.[77, 78, 207, 210, 211] It remains controversial whether or not end-to-end proximal aortic anastomosis leads to a higher incidence of erectile dysfunction. With appropriate recognition and implementation of such considerations, it is hoped that the surgeon can minimize the incidence of postoperative sexual dysfunction and actually improve sexual function in some patients.[77]

Infection

Infection following aortic reconstruction remains the most feared complication, with formidable morbidity and mortality rates. Fortunately, with current reconstructive methods and the use of prophylactic antibiotics, this remains a rare occurrence, with an incidence of 1 per cent or less.[2, 68, 212–214] In most series, the highest incidence has been in the inguinal portion of an aortofemoral graft. Important contributing factors include (1) multiple vascular procedures; (2) postoperative wound problems such as hematoma, seroma, or lymph leakage, particularly in the groin; and (3) emergency operation. Infectious complications occur almost exclusively after prosthetic graft insertion, being exceedingly rare after autogenous operations such as endarterectomy. Although graft infection is often not clinically apparent for months to years, it is generally believed that graft contamination occurs most commonly at the time of primary graft implantation. This emphasizes the importance of meticulous sterile technique at the time of original operation, avoidance of skin contact with the prosthetic graft by use of adherent plastic drapes, careful attention to hemostasis and wound closure, and general avoidance of concomitant intra-abdominal operations that may increase the incidence of possible graft contamination. Several randomized series in the literature have now documented the efficacy of antibiotic prophylaxis in reducing the incidence of vascular graft infection,[57–59] and its perioperative use in vascular reconstruction is now well accepted. Late graft infection that is due to bacteremic implantation of organisms on the luminal surface of a functioning graft is uncommon but may occur; because current prostheses are rarely completely healed with a viable endothelial lining, antibiotic prophylaxis should probably be employed in patients with a previously implanted graft who are exposed to the risk of bacteremia in a manner similar to patients with rheumatic valvular disease or prosthetic heart valves.

Staphylococcus aureus remains the most common responsible organism, but more recent experience indicates that organisms such as *Staphylococcus albus* and gram-negative bacteria are of increasing importance.[213] In patients presenting with forefoot infection or wet gangrene, it is particularly important to use aggressive specific antibiotic treatment and débridement before placement of a vascular prosthesis. Several studies have implicated the importance of bacteria in lymph nodes in the groin as the mechanism of subsequent graft infection.[215]

Diagnosis and management of patients with infection following aortoiliofemoral reconstructive procedures are often complex and are discussed more fully in Chapter 36. Graft excision is usually required, and revascularization via remote uncontaminated routes or use of autogenous methods of anatomic revascularization is often necessary to maintain limb viability.[63, 216–221] If the patient's condition is stable and the diagnosis of graft infection is firmly established, extra-anatomic revascularization preceding graft excision appears to yield better outcome.[222, 223] If infection appears localized, as in a single groin, for example, local measures including antibiotic irrigation or débridement and soft tissue coverage without graft removal may sometimes be successful.[224–226]

Aortoenteric Fistula

Aortoenteric fistula and associated gastrointestinal hemorrhage are devastating complications, with a continued high incidence of death or limb loss despite efforts at their correction. Communication between the aortic prosthesis and a portion of the gastrointestinal tract invariably leads to massive gastrointestinal bleeding, although initial bleeding episodes may be limited and allow time for diagnosis and treatment. Such communications involve the third and fourth parts of the duodenum, which overlie the proximal aortic suture line in the majority of cases, but the small bowel or colon may be involved with an iliac anastomotic point in 10 to 20 per cent of cases. Such secondary aortoenteric fistulae must be differentiated from primary ones, which occur as a result of the rupture of unoperated aortic or iliac artery aneurysms into adjacent hollow organs.

Secondary aortoenteric fistula formation may occur as a result of several mechanisms. If the adjacent bowel is improperly separated from the prosthesis and suture line, fibrotic adherence and subsequent erosion may occur. In other instances, anastomotic aneurysm formation that is due to mechanical causes or infection may occur first, with subsequent erosion of the pseudoaneurysm into the gastrointestinal tract.

The diagnosis must be suspected whenever an episode of gastrointestinal hemorrhage occurs in a patient who has undergone previous aortic operation. Diagnosis is often elusive, but upper gastrointestinal series may show distortion or abnormality of the retroperitoneal duodenum, or endoscopy may actually visualize the site of hemorrhage or the prosthesis itself if the distal aspects of the duodenum are examined. Aortography is often nondiagnostic, but it may demonstrate a pseudoaneurysm involving an aortic or iliac anastomosis. Computed tomography is often helpful, demonstrating anastomotic or perigraft abnormalities.

As with all complications, such difficulties are far more easily prevented than treated. The incidence of aortoenteric fistula formation appears to be higher following end-to-side anastomosis, because it is much more difficult to cover such an anastomotic configuration with viable tissue and avoid contact with the bowel than with end-to-end proximal anastomosis.[2, 4, 73] In difficult situations, interposition of omentum between the graft and the duodenum is often helpful. Standard methods of treatment (see Chapter 38) generally require removal of all prosthetic material, closure of the infrarenal abdominal aorta, repair of the gastrointestinal tract, and revascularization by means of an extra-anatomic graft.[227–230] If local sepsis is minimal, some reports advocate excision of limited portions of the graft directly in contact with the bowel lumen and in situ repair with autogenous tissues, arterial homografts, or anatomic insertion of a new segment of prosthetic graft.[63, 231–236] However, further experience is necessary to determine the safety and wisdom of such an approach as compared with traditional removal of the graft and remote methods of revascularization. For more discussion, the reader is referred to Chapter 38. Despite advances in treatment, death or limb loss continues to occur in 50 per cent or more of patients, similar to the results of management of infected aortic grafts, to which aortoenteric fistulae are closely related in terms of mechanism of occurrence and subsequent management. Mortality is often due to continued sepsis, multi–organ system failure, or disruption of the proximal aortic stump closure.

SUMMARY

Arteriosclerotic aortoiliac occlusive disease is a common cause of lower extremity ischemic symptomatology. In the majority of patients, occlusive lesions will be multifocal in nature, involving the lower abdominal aorta, both iliac arteries, and frequently the infrainguinal arterial tree. Before proceeding with aortic reconstructive surgery, the surgeon must document the hemodynamic significance of inflow disease. This may often be accomplished by careful clinical examination, supplemented with vascular laboratory hemodynamic data and good arteriographic studies. If any doubt remains, however, direct measurement of femoral artery pressure is helpful. Because the results of surgical reconstruction in this anatomic area are so satisfactory, operation may be considered on carefully selected patients with limiting claudication as their only symptom. More advanced limb-threatening ischemia is a clear indication for aortic reconstructions in appropriate-risk patients. Aortoiliac endarterectomy may be used for a small group of patients, but in most instances aortofemoral grafting is the preferred procedure. The key features of aortofemoral grafting are high placement of the proximal anastomosis immediately distal to the renal arteries and careful techniques of distal anastomosis, with or without profundaplasty, to achieve adequate flow into the deep femoral artery.

Despite the presence of multi-level disease in the majority of patients, a properly performed inflow operation will achieve satisfactory improvement of ischemic symptoms in 70 to 80 per cent of patients. Approximately 10 to 15 per cent of patients with advanced distal ischemia may be best managed by simultaneous inflow and outflow reconstruction, but careful patient selection is important. In high-risk patients, a variety of alternative methods are available for inflow revascularization, including extra-anatomic grafting and unilateral extraperitoneal procedures. Modification of surgical methods will allow successful management of associated vascular lesions or other unusual situations.

Most complications of aortoiliofemoral reconstruction can be prevented, and those that do occur may generally be successfully managed by early recognition and appropriate methods of reoperation. Highly successful long-term patency and clinical function of aortic reconstructions for occlusive disease make this one of the most rewarding areas of vascular surgery today.

References

1. DeBakey ME, Lawrie GM, Glaeser DH: Patterns of atherosclerosis and their surgical significance. Ann Surg 201:115, 1985.
2. Brewster DC, Darling RC: Optimal methods of aortoiliac reconstruction. Surgery 84:739, 1978.
3. Brewster DC: Clinical and anatomic considerations for surgery in aortoiliac disease and results of surgical treatment. Circulation 83(Suppl I):I-42, 1991.
4. Darling RC, Brewster DC, Hallett JW Jr, et al: Aortoiliac reconstruction. Surg Clin North Am 59:565, 1979.
5. Cronenwett JL, Davis JT Jr, Gooch JB, et al: Aortoiliac occlusive disease in women. Surgery 88:775, 1980.
6. DeLaurentis DA, Friedmann P, Wolferth GC Jr, et al: Atherosclerosis and the hypoplastic aortoiliac system. Surgery 83:27, 1978.
7. Greenhalgh RM: Small aorta syndrome. *In* Bergan JJ, Yao JST (eds): Surgery of the Aorta and Its Body Branches. New York, Grune & Stratton, 1979, pp 183–190.
8. Staple TW: The solitary aortoiliac lesion. Surgery 64:569, 1968.
9. Moore WS, Cafferata HT, Hall AD, et al: In defense of grafts across the inguinal ligament. Ann Surg 168:207, 1968.
10. Mozersky DJ, Sumner DS, Strandness DE: Long-term results of reconstructive aortoiliac surgery. Am J Surg 123:503, 1972.
11. Malone JM, Moore WS, Goldstone J: Life expectancy following aortofemoral arterial grafting. Surgery 81:551, 1977.
12. Brewster DC, Waltman AC, O'Hara PJ, et al: Femoral artery pressure measurement during aortography. Circulation 60(Suppl I):120, 1979.

13. Sobinsky KR, Borozan PG, Gray B, et al: Is femoral pulse palpation accurate in assessing the hemodynamic significance of aortoiliac occlusive disease? Am J Surg 148:214, 1984.
14. Brewster DC, Perler BA, Robison JG, et al: Aortofemoral graft for multilevel occlusive disease: Predictors of success and need for distal bypass. Arch Surg 117:1593, 1982.
15. Johnston KW, Demorais D, Colapinto RI: Difficulty in assessing disease by clinical and arteriographic methods. Angiology 32:609, 1981.
16. Karmody AM, Powers FR, Monaco VJ, et al: "Blue toe" syndrome: An indication for limb salvage surgery. Arch Surg 111:1263, 1976.
17. Kempczinski RF: Lower extremity arterial emboli from ulcerating atherosclerotic plaques. JAMA 241:807, 1979.
18. Goodreau JJ, Creasy JK, Flanigan DP, et al: Rational approach to the differentiation of vascular and neurogenic claudication. Surgery 84:749, 1978.
19. Kempczinski RF: Clinical application of noninvasive testing in extremity arterial insufficiency. *In* Kempczinski RF, Yao JST (eds): Practical Noninvasive Vascular Diagnosis. Chicago, Year Book Medical Publishers, 1982, pp 343–365.
20. Raines JK, Darling RC, Buth J, et al: Vascular laboratory criteria for the management of peripheral vascular disease of the lower extremities. Surgery 79:21, 1976.
21. Ernst CB: Prevention of intestinal ischemia following abdominal aortic reconstruction. Surgery 93:102, 1983.
22. Martin-Paredero V, Dixon SM, Baker JD, et al: Risk of renal failure after major angiography. Arch Surg 118:1417, 1983.
23. Mason RA, Arbeit LA, Giron F: Renal dysfunction after arteriography. JAMA 253:1001, 1985.
24. Reidy NC, Walden R, Abbott WA, et al: Anatomic localization of atherosclerotic lesions by hemodynamic tests. Arch Surg 116:1041, 1981.
25. Lynch TG, Hobson RW, Wright CB, et al: Interpretations of Doppler segmental pressures in peripheral vascular occlusive disease. Arch Surg 119:465, 1984.
26. Rutherford RB, Lowenstein DH, Klein MF: Combining segmental systolic pressures and plethysmography to diagnose arterial occlusive disease of the legs. Am J Surg 138:211, 1979.
27. Thiele BL, Bandyk DF, Zierler RE, et al: A systematic approach to the assessment of aortoiliac disease. Arch Surg 118:477, 1983.
28. Kohler TR, Nance DR, Cramer MM, et al: Duplex scanning for diagnosis of aortoiliac and femoropopliteal disease: A prospective study. Circulation 76:1074, 1987.
29. Bruins Slot HB, Strijbosch L, Greep JM: Interobserver variability in single plane aortography. Surgery 90:497, 1981.
30. Flanigan DP, Tullis JP, Streeter VL: Multiple subcritical arterial stenosis: Effect on poststenotic pressure and flow. Ann Surg 186:663, 1977.
31. Brener BJ, Raines JK, Darling RC, et al: Measurement of systolic femoral artery pressure during reactive hyperemia: An estimate of aortoiliac disease. Circulation 49/50(Suppl II):259, 1974.
32. Flanigan DP, Williams LR, Schwartz JA, et al: Hemodynamic evaluation of the aortoiliac system based on pharmacologic vasodilatation. Surgery 93:709, 1983.
33. Moore WS, Hall AD: Unrecognized aortoiliac stenosis: A physiologic approach to the diagnosis. Arch Surg 103:633, 1971.
34. Kikta MJ, Flanigan DP, Bishara RA, et al: Long-term follow-up of patients having infrainguinal bypass performed below stenotic but hemodynamically normal aortoiliac vessels. J Vasc Surg 5:319, 1987.
35. Flanigan DP, Ryan TJ, Williams LR, et al: Aortofemoral or femoropopliteal revascularization? A prospective evaluation of the papaverine test. J Vasc Surg 1:215, 1984.
36. Verhagen PF, Van Vroonhaven TJMV: Criteria from intra-arterial femoral pressure measurements combined with reactive hyperemia to assess the aortoiliac segment: A prospective study. Br J Surg 71:706, 1984.
37. Coffman JD: Vasodilator drugs in peripheral vascular disease. N Engl J Med 300:713, 1979.
38. Porter JM, Cutler BS, Lee BY, et al: Pentoxifylline efficacy in the treatment of intermittent claudication: Multicenter controlled double-blind trial with objective assessment of chronic occlusive arterial disease patients. Am Heart J 104:66, 1982.
39. Johnston KW, Rae M, Hogg-Johnston SA, et al: Five-year results of a prospective study of percutaneous transluminal angioplasty. Ann Surg 206:403, 1987.
40. Brewster DC, Cambria RP, Darling RC, et al: Long-term results of combined iliac balloon angioplasty and distal surgical revascularization. Ann Surg 210:324, 1989.
41. Johnston KW, Colapinto RI, Baird RJ: Transluminal dilation: An alternative? Arch Surg 117:1604, 1982.
42. Morin JF, Johnston KW, Wasserman L, et al: Factors that determine the long-term results of percutaneous transluminal dilatation for peripheral arterial occlusive disease. J Vasc Surg 4:68, 1986.
43. Brewster DC, Edwards JP: Cardiopulmonary complications related to vascular surgery. *In* Bernhard VM, Towne JB (eds): Complications in Vascular Surgery. St. Louis, Quality Medical Publishing, 1991, pp 23–41.
44. Yeager RA, Moneta FL: Assessing cardiac risk in vascular surgical patients: Current status. Perspect Vasc Surg 2:18, 1989.
45. Hertzer NR, Beven EG, Young JR, et al: Coronary artery disease in peripheral vascular patients: A classification of 1000 coronary angiograms and results of surgical management. Ann Surg 199:223, 1984.
46. Boucher CA, Brewster DC, Darling RC, et al: Determination of cardiac risk by dipyridamole-thallium imaging before peripheral vascular surgery. N Engl J Med 312:389, 1985.
47. Brewster DC, Boucher CA, Okada RD, et al: Selection of patients for preoperative coronary angiography: Use of dipyridamole-stress thallium myocardial imaging. J Vasc Surg 2:504, 1985.
48. Cutler BS, Leppo JA: Dipyridamole thallium 201 scintigraphy to detect coronary artery disease before abdominal aortic surgery. J Vasc Surg 5:91, 1987.
49. Eagle KA, Coley CM, Newell JB, et al: Combining clinical and thallium data optimizes preoperative assessment of cardiac risk before major vascular surgery. Ann Intern Med 110:859, 1989.
50. Golden MA, Whittemore AD, Donaldson MC, et al: Selective evaluation and management of coronary artery disease in patients undergoing repair of abdominal aortic aneurysms: A 16-year experience. Ann Surg 212:415, 1990.
51. Cambria RP, Brewster DC, Abbott WM, et al: The impact of selective use of dipyridamole-thallium scans and surgical factors on the current morbidity of aortic surgery. J Vasc Surg 15:43, 1992.
52. Hollier LH: Cardiac evaluation in patients with vascular disease—Overview: A practical approach. J Vasc Surg 15:726, 1992.
53. Bunt TJ: The role of a defined protocol for cardiac risk assessment in decreasing perioperative myocardial infarction in vascular surgery. J Vasc Surg 15:626, 1992.
54. Raby KE, Goldman L, Creager MA, et al: Correlation between preoperative ischemia and major cardiac events after peripheral vascular surgery. N Engl J Med 321:1296, 1989.
55. Eagle KA, Boucher CA: Cardiac risk of non-cardiac surgery [Editorial]. N Engl J Med 321:1330, 1989.
56. Taylor LM, Yeager RA, Moneta GL, et al: The incidence of perioperative myocardial infarction in general vascular surgery. J Vasc Surg 151:52, 1992.
57. Kaiser AB, Clayson KR, Mulherin JL, et al: Antibiotic prophylaxis in vascular surgery. Ann Surg 188:283, 1978.
58. Pitt HA, Postier RH, MacGowan WL, et al: Prophylactic antibiotics in vascular surgery: Topical, systemic, or both? Ann Surg 192:356, 1980.
59. Hasselgren PO, Ivarsson L, Risberg B, et al: Effects of prophylactic antibiotics in vascular surgery: A prospective, randomized, double-blind study. Ann Surg 200:86, 1984.
60. Darling RC, Linton RR: Aortoiliofemoral endarterectomy for atherosclerotic occlusive disease. Surgery 55:184, 1964.
61. Inahara T: Evaluation of endarterectomy for aortoiliac and aortoiliofemoral occlusive disease. Arch Surg 110:1458, 1975.
62. van der Akker PJ, van Schilfgaarde R, Brand R, et al: Long-term results of prosthetic and non-prosthetic reconstruction for obstructive aorto-iliac disease. Eur J Vasc Surg 6:53, 1992.
63. Ehrenfeld WK, Wieber BC, Olcott CN, et al: Autogenous tissue reconstruction in the management of infected prosthetic grafts. Surgery 85:82, 1979.
64. Crawford ES, Manning LG, Kelly TF: "Redo" surgery after operations for aneurysm and occlusion of the abdominal aorta. Surgery 81:41, 1977.
65. Perdue GD, Long WD, Smith RB III: Perspective concerning aortofemoral arterial reconstruction. Ann Surg 173:940, 1971.
66. Crawford ES, Bomberger RA, Glaeser DH, et al: Aortoiliac occlusive disease: Factors influencing survival and function following reconstructive operation over a twenty-five year period. Surgery 90:1555, 1981.

67. Malone JM, Moore WS, Goldstone J: The natural history of bilateral aortofemoral bypass grafts for ischemia of the lower extremities. Arch Surg 110:1300, 1975.
68. Szilagyi DE, Hageman JH, Smith RF, et al: A thirty-year survey of the reconstructive surgical treatment of aortoiliac occlusive disease. J Vasc Surg 3:421, 1986.
69. Nevelsteen A, Wouters L, Suy R: Aortofemoral Dacron reconstruction for aorto-iliac occlusive disease: A 25-year survey. Eur J Vasc Surg 5:179, 1991.
70. Mulcare RJ, Royster TS, Lynn RA, et al: Long-term results of operative therapy for aortoiliac disease. Arch Surg 113:601, 1978.
71. Pierce HE, Turrentine M, Stringfield S, et al: Evaluation of end-to-side v. end-to-end proximal anastomosis in aortobifemoral bypass. Arch Surg 117:1580, 1982.
72. Mikati A, Marache P, Watel A, et al: End-to-side aortoprosthetic anastomoses: Long-term computed tomography assessment. Ann Vasc Surg 4:584, 1990.
73. Dunn DA, Downs AR, Lye CR: Aortoiliac reconstruction for occlusive disease: Comparison of end-to-end and end-to-side proximal anastomoses. Can J Surg 25:382, 1982.
74. Rutherford RB, Jones DN, Martin MS, et al: Serial hemodynamic assessment of aortobifemoral bypass. J Vasc Surg 4:428, 1986.
75. Ameli FM, Stein M, Aro L, et al: End-to-end versus end-to-side proximal anastomosis in aortobifemoral bypass surgery: Does it matter? Can Soc Vasc Surg 34:243, 1991.
76. Melliere D, Labastie J, Becquemin JP, et al: Proximal anastomosis in aortobifemoral bypass: End-to-end or end-to-side. J Cardiovasc Surg 31:77, 1990.
77. Flanigan DP, Schuler JJ, Keifer T, et al: Elimination of iatrogenic impotence and improvement of sexual function after aortoiliac revascularization. Arch Surg 117:544, 1982.
78. Queral LA, Whitehouse WM Jr, Flinn WR, et al: Pelvic hemodynamics after aortoiliac reconstruction. Surgery 86:799, 1979.
79. Picone AL, Green RM, Ricotta JR, et al: Spinal cord ischemia following operations on the abdominal aorta. J Vasc Surg 3:94, 1986.
80. Gloviczki P, Cross SA, Stanson AW, et al: Ischemic injury to the spinal cord or lumbosacral plexus after aorto-iliac reconstruction. Am J Surg 162:131, 1991.
81. Baird RJ, Feldman P, Miles JT, et al: Subsequent downstream repair after aorta-iliac and aorta-femoral bypass operations. Surgery 82:785, 1977.
82. Bernhard VM, Ray LI, Militello JP: The role of angioplasty of the profunda femoris artery in revascularization of the ischemic limb. Surg Gynecol Obstet 142:840, 1976.
83. Malone JM, Goldstone J, Moore WS: Autogenous profundaplasty: The key to long-term patency in secondary repair of aortofemoral graft occlusion. Ann Surg 188:817, 1978.
84. Morris GC, Edwards W, Cooley DA, et al: Surgical importance of profunda femoris artery: Analysis of 102 cases with combined aortoiliac and femoropopliteal occlusive disease treated by revascularization of deep femoral artery. Arch Surg 82:32, 1961.
85. Berguer R, Higgins RF, Colton LT: Geometry, blood flow, and reconstruction of the deep femoral artery. Am J Surg 130:68, 1975.
86. Robicsek F, Duncan GD, Daugherty HK, et al: "Half and half" woven and knitted Dacron grafts in the aortoiliac and aortofemoral positions: Seven and one-half years follow-up. Ann Vasc Surg 5:315, 1991.
87. Robicsek F, Duncan GD, Anderson CE, et al: Indium 111–labeled platelet deposition in woven and knitted Dacron bifurcated aortic grafts with the same patient as a clinical model. J Vasc Surg 5:833, 1987.
88. Burke PM, Herrmann JB, Cutler BS: Optimal grafting methods for the small abdominal aorta. J Cardiovasc Surg 28:420, 1987.
89. Cintora I, Pearce DE, Cannon JA: A clinical survey of aortobifemoral bypass using two inherently different graft types. Ann Surg 208:625, 1988.
90. Robbs JV, Wylie EJ: Factors contributing to recurrent limb ischemia following bypass surgery for aortoiliac occlusive disease, and their management. Arch Surg 193:346, 1981.
91. Sanders RJ, Kempczinski RF, Hammond W, et al: The significance of graft diameter. Surgery 88:856, 1980.
92. Nunn DB, Carter MM, Donohue MT, et al: Postoperative dilation of knitted Dacron aortic bifurcation graft. J Vasc Surg 12:291, 1990.
93. O'Hara PJ, Brewster DC, Darling RC, et al: The value of intraoperative monitoring using the pulse volume recorder during peripheral vascular surgery. Surg Gynecol Obstet 162:275, 1981.
94. Rob C: Extraperitoneal approach to the abdominal aorta. Surgery 53:87, 1963.
95. Sicard GA, Freeman MB, VanderWoude JC, et al: Comparison between the transabdominal and retroperitoneal approach for reconstruction of the infrarenal aorta. J Vasc Surg 5:19, 1987.
96. Williams GM, Ricotta J, Zinner M, et al: The extended retroperitoneal approach for treatment of extensive atherosclerosis of the aorta and renal vessels. Surgery 88:846, 1980.
97. Shepard AD, Tollefson DFJ, Reddy DJ, et al: Left flank retroperitoneal exposure: A technical aid to complex aortic reconstruction. J Vasc Surg 14:283, 1991.
98. Leather RP, Shah MS, Kaufman JL, et al: Comparative analysis of retroperitoneal and transperitoneal aortic replacement for aneurysm. Surg Gynecol Obstet 168:387, 1989.
99. Cambria RP, Brewster DC, Abbott WM, et al: Transperitoneal versus retroperitoneal approach for aortic reconstruction: A randomized prospective study. J Vasc Surg 11:314, 1990.
100. Barnes RW, Baker WH, Shanik G, et al: Value of concomitant sympathectomy in aortoiliac reconstruction: Results of a prospective randomized study. Arch Surg 112:1325, 1977.
101. Satiani B, Liapis CD, Hayes JP, et al: Prospective randomized study of concomitant lumbar sympathectomy in aortoiliac reconstruction. Am J Surg 143:755, 1982.
102. Imparato AM: Lumbar sympathectomy: Role in the treatment of occlusive arterial disease in the lower extremities. Surg Clin North Am 59:719, 1979.
103. Rutherford RB: The current role of sympathectomy in the management of limb ischemia. Semin Vasc Surg 4:195, 1991.
104. Corson JD, Brewster DC, Darling RC: The surgical management of infrarenal aortic occlusion. Surg Gynecol Obstet 155:369, 1982.
105. Liddicoat JE, Bekassy SM, Dang MH, et al: Complete occlusion of the infrarenal abdominal aorta: Management and results in 64 patients. Surgery 77:467, 1975.
106. Tapper SS, Jenkins JM, Edwards WH, et al: Juxtarenal aortic occlusion. Ann Surg 215:443, 1992.
107. Starrett RW, Stoney RJ: Juxta-renal aortic occlusion. Surgery 76:890, 1974.
108. Deriu GP, Ballotta E: Natural history of ascending thrombosis of the abdominal aorta. Am J Surg 145:652, 1983.
109. McCullough JL, Mackey WC, O'Donnell TF, et al: Infrarenal aortic occlusion: A reassessment of surgical indications. Am J Surg 146:178, 1983.
110. Reilly LM, Sauer L, Weinstein ES, et al: Infrarenal aortic occlusion: Does it threaten renal perfusion or function? J Vasc Surg 11:216, 1990.
111. Gupta SK, Veith FJ: Management of juxtarenal aortic occlusions: Technique for suprarenal clamp placement. Ann Vasc Surg 6:306, 1992.
112. Martinez BD, Hertzer NR, Beven EG: Influence of distal arterial occlusive disease on prognosis following aortobifemoral bypass. Surgery 88:795, 1980.
113. Sumner DS, Strandness DE Jr: Aortoiliac reconstruction in patients with combined iliac and superficial femoral arterial occlusion. Surgery 84:348, 1978.
114. Hill DA, McGrath MA, Lord RSA, et al: The effect of superficial femoral artery occlusion on the outcome of aortofemoral bypass for intermittent claudication. Surgery 87:133, 1980.
115. Galland RB, Hill DA, Gustave R, et al: The functional result of aortoiliac reconstruction. Br J Surg 67:344, 1980.
116. Jones AF, Kempczinski RF: Aortofemoral bypass grafting: A reappraisal. Arch Surg 116:301, 1981.
117. Brewster DC, Darling RC: Aortoiliofemoral bypass grafting. *In* Kempczinski RF (ed): The Ischemic Leg. Chicago, Year Book Medical Publishers, 1985, pp 305–326.
118. Brewster DC, Veith FJ: Combined aortoiliac and femoropopliteal occlusive disease. *In* Veith FJ, Hobson RW, Williams RA, et al (eds): Vascular Surgery: Principles and Practice, 2nd ed. New York, McGraw-Hill, 1994, pp 459–472.
119. Baird RJ: In discussion of Brewster DC, Perler BA, Robison JR, et al: Aortofemoral graft for multilevel occlusive disease. Arch Surg 117:1593, 1982.
120. Dardik H, Ibrahim IM, Jarrah M, et al: Synchronous aortofemoral or

iliofemoral bypass with revascularization of the lower extremity. Surg Gynecol Obstet 149:676, 1979.
121. Harris PL, Cave Bigley DJ, McSweeney L: Aortofemoral bypass and the role of concomitant femorodistal reconstruction. Br J Surg 72:317, 1985.
122. O'Donnell TF Jr, McBride KA, Callow AD, et al: Management of combined segment disease. Am J Surg 141:452, 1981.
123. Eidt J, Charlesworth D: Combined aortobifemoral and femoropopliteal bypass in the management of patients with extensive atherosclerosis. Ann Vasc Surg 1:453, 1986.
124. Dalman RL, Taylor LM Jr, Moneta GL, et al: Simultaneous operative repair of multilevel lower extremity occlusive disease. J Vasc Surg 13:211, 1991.
125. Garrett WV, Slaymaker EE, Heintz SE, et al: Intraoperative prediction of symptomatic result of aortofemoral bypass from changes in ankle pressure index. Surgery 82:504, 1977.
126. Levinson SA, Levinson HJ, Halloran LG, et al: Limited indications for unilateral aortofemoral or iliofemoral vascular grafts. Arch Surg 107:791, 1973.
127. Kram HB, Gupta SK, Veith FJ, et al: Unilateral aortofemoral bypass: A safe and effective option for the treatment of unilateral limb-threatening ischemia. Am J Surg 162:155, 1991.
128. van den Dungen JJAM, Boontje AH, Kropveld A: Unilateral iliofemoral occlusive disease: Long-term results of the semiclosed endarterectomy with the ringstripper. J Vasc Surg 14:673, 1991.
129. Ascer E, Veith FJ, Gupta SK, et al: Comparison of axillounifemoral and axillobifemoral bypass operations. Surgery 97:169, 1985.
130. Piotrowski JJ, Pearce WH, Jones DN, et al: Aortobifemoral bypass: The operation of choice for unilateral iliac occlusion? J Vasc Surg 8:211, 1988.
131. Brief DK, Brener BJ, Alpert J, et al: Crossover femorofemoral grafts followed up five years or more: An analysis. Arch Surg 110:1294, 1975.
132. Dick LS, Brief DK, Alpert J, et al: A twelve-year experience with femorofemoral crossover grafts. Arch Surg 115:1359, 1980.
133. Eugene J, Goldstone J, Moore WS: Fifteen-year experience with subcutaneous bypass grafts for lower extremity ischemia. Ann Surg 186:177, 1977.
134. Kalman PG, Hosang M, Johnston KW, et al: The current role for femorofemoral bypass. J Vasc Surg 6:71, 1987.
135. Couch NP, Clowes AW, Whittemore AD, et al: The iliac-origin arterial graft: A useful alternative for iliac occlusive disease. Surgery 97:83, 1985.
136. Kalman PG, Hosang M, Johnston KW, et al: Unilateral iliac disease: The role of iliofemoral graft. J Vasc Surg 6:139, 1987.
137. Cham C, Myers KA, Scott DF, et al: Extraperitoneal unilateral iliac artery bypass for chronic limb ischemia. Aust NZ J Surg 58:859, 1988.
138. Darling RC III, Leather RP, Chang BB, et al: Is the iliac artery a suitable inflow conduit for iliofemoral occlusive disease: An analysis of 514 aorto-iliac reconstructions. J Vasc Surg 17:15, 1993.
139. Perler BA, Burdick JF, Williams M: Femoro-femoral or ilio-femoral bypass for unilateral inflow reconstruction? Am J Surg 161:426, 1991.
140. Ricco J-B: Unilateral iliac artery occlusive disease: A randomized multicenter trial examining direct revascularization versus crossover bypass. Ann Vasc Surg 6:209, 1992.
141. Brener BJ, Eisenbud DE, Brief DK, et al: Utility of femorofemoral crossover grafts. *In* Bergan JJ, Yao JST (eds): Aortic Surgery. Philadelphia, WB Saunders, 1989, pp 423–438.
142. Taylor LM Jr, Freimanis IE, Edwards JM, et al: Extraperitoneal iliac endarterectomy in the treatment of multilevel lower extremity arterial occlusive disease. Am J Surg 152:34, 1986.
143. Vitale GF, Inahara T: Extraperitoneal endarterectomy for iliofemoral occlusive disease. J Vasc Surg 12:409, 1990.
144. Tollefson DFJ, Ernst CB: Natural history of atherosclerotic renal artery stenosis associated with aortic disease. J Vasc Surg 14:327, 1991.
145. Perry MO, Silane MF: Management of renovascular problems during aortic operations. Arch Surg 119:681, 1984.
146. Dean RH, Keyser JE III, Dupont WD, et al: Aortic and renal vascular disease: Factors affecting the value of combined procedures. Ann Surg 200:336, 1984.
147. Tarazi RY, Hertzer NR, Beven EG: Simultaneous aortic reconstruction and renal revascularization: Risk factors and late results in eighty-nine patients. J Vasc Surg 5:707, 1987.
148. Brewster DC, Buth J, Darling RC, et al: Combined aortic and renal artery reconstruction. Am J Surg 131:457, 1976.
149. Stoney RJ, Skioldebrand CG, Qvarfordt PG, et al: Juxtarenal aortic atherosclerosis: Surgical experience and functional result. Ann Surg 200:345, 1984.
150. Stewart MT, Smith RB III, Fulenwider T, et al: Concomitant renal revascularization in patients undergoing aortic surgery. J Vasc Surg 2:400, 1985.
151. Connolly JE, Kwaan JHM: Prophylactic revascularization of the gut. Ann Surg 190:514, 1979.
152. Brewster DC, Darling RC: Splenorenal arterial anastomosis for renovascular hypertension. Ann Surg 189:353, 1979.
153. Moncure AC, Brewster DC, Darling RC, et al: Use of the splenic and hepatic arteries for renal revascularization. J Vasc Surg 3:196, 1986.
154. Brewster DC, Moncure AC: Hepatic and splenic artery for renal revascularization. *In* Bergan JJ, Yao JST (eds): Arterial Surgery: New Diagnostic and Operative Techniques. Orlando, FL, Grune & Stratton, 1988, pp 389–405.
155. Naylor AR, Ah See AK, Engeset J: The morbidity and mortality after aortofemoral grafting for peripheral limb ischemia. J R Coll Surg Edinb 34:215, 1989.
156. Sladen JG, Gilmour JL, Wong RW: Cumulative patency and actual palliation in patients with claudication after aortofemoral bypass. Prospective long-term follow-up of 100 patients. Am J Surg 152:190, 1986.
157. Poulias GE, Polemis L, Skoutas B, et al: Bilateral aorto-femoral bypass in the presence of aorto-iliac occlusive disease and factors determining results: Experience and long term follow up with 500 consecutive cases. J Cardiovasc Surg 26:527, 1985.
158. Perdue GD, Smith RB III, Veazey CR, et al: Revascularization for severe limb ischemia. Arch Surg 115:168, 1980.
159. Brener BJ, Darling RC, Frederick PL, et al: Major venous anomalies complicating abdominal aortic surgery. Arch Surg 108:159, 1974.
160. Effaney PJ, Goldstone J, Chin D, et al: Intraoperative anticoagulation in cardiovascular surgery. Surgery 90:1068, 1981.
161. Brewster DC: Reoperation for aortofemoral graft limb occlusion. *In* Veith F (ed): Current Critical Problems in Vascular Surgery. St. Louis, Quality Medical Publishing, 1989, pp 341–351.
162. Imparato AM: Abdominal aortic surgery: Prevention of lower limb ischemia. Surgery 93:112, 1983.
163. Starr DS, Lawrie GM, Morris GC Jr: Prevention of distal embolism during arterial reconstruction. Am J Surg 138:764, 1979.
164. Comerota AJ, White JV, Grosh JD: Intraoperative intraarterial thrombolytic therapy for salvage of limbs in patients with distal arterial thrombosis. Surg Gynecol Obstet 169:283, 1989.
165. Parent FN III, Bernhard VM, Pabst TS III, et al: Fibrinolytic treatment of residual thrombus after catheter embolectomy for severe lower limb ischemia. J Vasc Surg 9:153, 1989.
166. Diehl JT, Cali RF, Hertzer NR, et al: Complications of abdominal aortic reconstruction: An analysis of perioperative risk factors in 557 patients. Ann Surg 197:50, 1983.
167. Castronuovo JJ, Flanigan DP: Renal failure complicating vascular surgery. *In* Bernhard VM, Towne JB (eds): Complications in Vascular Surgery. Orlando, FL, Grune & Stratton, 1985, pp 258–274.
168. Bush HL, Huse JB, Johnson WC, et al: Prevention of renal insufficiency after abdominal aortic aneurysm resection by optimal volume loading. Arch Surg 116:1517, 1981.
169. Thompson JE, Vollman RW, Austin DJ, et al: Prevention of hypotensive and renal complications of aortic surgery using balanced salt solution: Thirteen year experience with 670 cases. Ann Surg 167:767, 1968.
170. Brewster DC, Franklin DP, Cambria RP, et al: Intestinal ischemia complicating abdominal aortic surgery. Surgery 109:447, 1991.
171. Seeger JM, Doe DA, Kaelin LD, et al: Routine reimplantation of patent inferior mesenteric arteries limits colon infarction after aortic reconstruction. J Vasc Surg 15:635, 1992.
172. Bergman RT, Gloviczki, Welch TJ, et al: The role of intravenous fluorescein in the detection of colon ischemia during aortic reconstruction. Ann Vasc Surg 6:74, 1992.
173. Szilagyi DE, Hageman JH, Smith RF, et al: Spinal cord damage in surgery of the abdominal aorta. Surgery 83:38, 1978.
174. Iliopoulos JI, Howanitz PE, Pierce GE, et al: The critical hypogastric circulation. Am J Surg 154:671, 1987.
175. Elliott JP, Szilagyi DE, Hageman JH, et al: Spinal cord ischemia: Secondary to surgery of the abdominal aorta. *In* Bernhard VM,

Towne JB (eds): Complications in Vascular Surgery. Orlando, FL, Grune & Stratton, 1985, pp 291–310.
176. McCarthy WJ, Flinn WR, Carter MF, et al: Prevention and management of urologic injuries during aortic surgery. *In* Bergan JJ, Yao JST (eds): Aortic Surgery. Philadelphia, WB Saunders, 1989, pp 539–546.
177. Egeblad K, Brochner-Mortensen J, Krarup T, et al: Incidence of ureteral obstruction after aortic grafting: A prospective analysis. Surgery 103:411, 1988.
178. Schubart P, Fortner G, Cummings D, et al: The significance of hydronephrosis after aortofemoral reconstruction. Arch Surg 120:377, 1985.
179. Wright DJ, Ernst CB, Evans JR, et al: Ureteral complications and aortoiliac reconstruction. J Vasc Surg 11:29, 1990.
180. van der Akker PJ, van Schilfgaarde R, Brand R, et al: Long term success of aortoiliac operation for arteriosclerotic obstructive disease. Surg Gynecol Obstet 174:485, 1992.
181. Brewster DC, Meier GH, Darling RC, et al: Reoperation for aortofemoral graft limb occlusion: Optimal methods and long term results. J Vasc Surg 5:363, 1987.
182. Brewster DC: Surgery of late aortic graft occlusion. *In* Bergan JJ, Yao JST (eds): Aortic Surgery. Philadelphia, WB Saunders, 1989, pp 519–538.
183. Nevelsteen A, Suy R: Graft occlusion following aortofemoral Dacron bypass. Ann Vasc Surg 5:32, 1991.
184. Bernhard VM, Ray LI, Towne JB: The reoperation of choice for aortofemoral graft occlusion. Surgery 82:867, 1977.
185. Wray R, DePalma RG, Hunay CH: Late occlusion of aortofemoral bypass grafts: Influence of cigarette smoking. Surgery 70:969, 1971.
186. Greenhalgh RM, Laing SP, Cole PV, et al: Smoking and arterial reconstruction. Br J Surg 68:605, 1981.
187. Robicsek F, Daugherty HK, Mullen DC, et al: The effect of continued cigarette smoking on the patency of synthetic vascular grafts in Leriche syndrome. J Thorac Cardiovasc Surg 70:107, 1975.
188. Provan JL, Sojka SG, Murnaghan JJ, et al: The effect of cigarette smoking on the long term success rates of aortofemoral and femoropopliteal reconstructions. Surg Gynecol Obstet 165:49, 1987.
189. Myers KA, King BB, Scott DF, et al: Effect of smoking on the late patency of arterial reconstructions in the legs. Br J Surg 65:267, 1978.
190. Baird RJ, Ropchan GV, Oates TK, et al: Ascending aorta to bifemoral bypass—A ventral aorta. J Vasc Surg 3:405, 1986.
191. Canepa CS, Schubart PJ, Taylor LM Jr, et al: Supraceliac aortofemoral bypass. Surgery 101:323, 1987.
192. McCarthy WJ, Rubin JR, Flinn WR, et al: Descending thoracic aorta-to-femoral artery bypass. Arch Surg 121:681, 1986.
193. Rosenfeld JC, Savarese RP, DeLaurentis DA: Distal thoracic aorta to femoral artery bypass: A surgical alternative. J Vasc Surg 2:747, 1985.
194. Criado E, Johnson G Jr, Burnham SJ, et al: Descending thoracic aorta-to-iliofemoral artery bypass as an alternative to aortoiliac reconstruction. J Vasc Surg 15:550, 1992.
195. Ernst CB, Daugherty ME: Removal of a thrombotic plug from an occluded limb of an aortofemoral graft. Arch Surg 113:301, 1978.
196. Edwards WH, Jenkins JM, Mulherin JL, et al: Extended profundaplasty to minimize pelvic and distal tissue loss. Ann Surg 211:694, 1990.
197. Sterpetti AV, Feldhaus RJ, Schultz RD: Combined aortofemoral and extended deep femoral artery reconstruction. Arch Surg 123:1269, 1988.
198. Ouriel K, DeWeese JA, Ricotta JJ, et al: Revascularization of the distal profunda femoris artery in the reconstructive treatment of aortoiliac occlusive disease. J Vasc Surg 6:217, 1987.
199. Charlesworth D: The occluded aortic and aortofemoral graft. *In* Bergan JJ, Yao JST (eds): Reoperative Arterial Surgery. Orlando, FL, Grune & Stratton, 1986, pp 271–278.
200. Szilagyi DE, Smith RF, Elliott JP, et al: Anastomotic aneurysms after vascular reconstruction: Problems of incidence, etiology, and treatment. Surgery 78:800, 1975.
201. Satiani B: False aneurysms following arterial reconstruction: Collective review. Surg Gynecol Obstet 152:357, 1981.
202. Edwards JM, Teefey SA, Zierler RE, et al: Intraabdominal paraanastomotic aneurysms after aortic bypass grafting. J Vasc Surg 15:344, 1991.
203. Schellack J, Salam A, Abouzeid MA, et al: Femoral anastomotic aneurysms: A continuing challenge. J Vasc Surg 6:308, 1987.
204. Goldstone J: Anastomotic aneurysms. *In* Bernhard VM, Towne JB (eds): Complications in Vascular Surgery. St. Louis, Quality Medical Publishing, 1991, pp 87–99.
205. Ernst CB, Elliott JP Jr, Ryan CH, et al: Recurrent femoral anastomotic aneurysms: A 30-year experience. Ann Surg 208:401, 1988.
206. Seabrook GR, Schmitt DD, Bandyk DF, et al: Anastomotic femoral pseudoaneurysm: An investigation of occult infection as an etiologic factor. J Vasc Surg 11:629, 1990.
207. Kempczinski RF: Impotence following aortic surgery. *In* Bernhard VM, Towne JB (eds): Complications in Vascular Surgery. St. Louis, Quality Medical Publishing, 1991, pp 160–171.
208. Weinstein MH, Machleder HI: Sexual function after aorto-iliac surgery. Ann Surg 181:787, 1975.
209. DePalma RG, Levine SB, Feldman S: Preservation of erectile function after aortoiliac reconstruction. Arch Surg 113:958, 1978.
210. Cronenwett JL, Gooch JB, Garrett HE: Internal iliac artery revascularization during aortofemoral bypass. Arch Surg 117:838, 1982.
211. Flanigan DP, Sobinsky KR, Schuler JJ, et al: Internal iliac artery revascularization in the treatment of vasculogenic impotence. Arch Surg 120:271, 1985.
212. Moore WS, Cole CW: Infection in prosthetic vascular grafts. *In* Moore WS (ed): Vascular Surgery: A Comprehensive Review. 3rd ed. Philadelphia, WB Saunders, 1991, pp 598–609.
213. Bandyk DF: Aortic graft infection. Semin Vasc Surg 3:122, 1990.
214. O'Hara PJ, Hertzer NR, Beven EG, et al: Surgical management of infected abdominal aortic grafts: Review of a 25-year experience. J Vasc Surg 3:725, 1986.
215. Rubin JR, Malone JM, Goldstone J: The role of the lymphatic system in acute arterial prosthetic graft infections. J Vasc Surg 2:92, 1985.
216. Piotrowski JJ, Bernhard VM: Management of vascular graft infections. *In* Bernhard VM, Towne JB (eds): Complications in Vascular Surgery. St. Louis, Quality Medical Publishing, 1991, pp 235–258.
217. Reilly LM, Altman H, Lusby RJ, et al: Late results following surgical management of vascular graft infection. J Vasc Surg 1:36, 1984.
218. Quiñones-Baldrich WJ, Hernandez JJ, Moore WS: Long-term results following surgical management of aortic graft infection. Arch Surg 126:507, 1991.
219. Yeager RA, Moneta GL, Taylor LM, et al: Improving survival and limb salvage in patients with aortic graft infection. Am J Surg 159:466, 1990.
220. Schmitt DD, Seabrook GR, Bandyk DF, et al: Graft excision and extraanatomic revascularization: The treatment of choice for the septic aortic prosthesis. J Cardiovasc Surg 31:327, 1990.
221. Ricotta JJ, Faggioli GL, Stella A, et al: Total excision and extraanatomic bypass for aortic graft infection. Am J Surg 162:145, 1991.
222. Reilly LM, Stoney RJ, Goldstone J, et al: Improved management of aortic graft infection: The influence of operation sequence and staging. J Vasc Surg 5:421, 1987.
223. Trout HH III, Kozloff L, Giordano JM: Priority of revascularization in patients with graft enteric fistulas, infected arteries, or infected arterial prostheses. Ann Surg 199:669, 1984.
224. Kwann JWM, Connolly JB: Successful management of prosthetic graft infection with continuous povidone-iodine irrigation. Arch Surg 116:716, 1981.
225. Calligaro KD, Veith FJ, Gupta SK, et al: A modified method for management of prosthetic graft infections involving an anastomosis to the common femoral artery. J Vasc Surg 11:485, 1990.
226. Mixter RC, Turnipseed WD, Smith DJ Jr, et al: Rotational muscle flaps: A new technique for covering infected vascular grafts. J Vasc Surg 9:472, 1989.
227. Bernhard VM: Aortoenteric fistula. *In* Bernhard VM, Towne JB (eds): Complications in Vascular Surgery. Orlando, FL, Grune & Stratton, 1985, pp 513–525.
228. Connolly JE, Kwaan JHM, McCart PM, et al: Aortoenteric fistula. Ann Surg 194:402, 1981.
229. Perdue GD Jr, Smith RB III, Ansley JD, et al: Impending aortoenteric hemorrhage: The effect of early recognition on improved outcome. Ann Surg 192:237, 1980.
230. Reilly LM, Ehrenfeld WK, Goldstone J, et al: Gastrointestinal tract involvement by prosthetic graft infection: The significance of gastrointestinal hemorrhage. Ann Surg 202:342, 1985.

231. Seeger JM, Wheeler JR, Gregory RT, et al: Autogenous graft replacement of infected prosthetic graft in the femoral position. Surgery 93:39, 1983.
232. Walker WE, Cooley DA, Duncan JM, et al: The management of aortoduodenal fistula by in situ replacement of the infected abdominal aortic graft. Ann Surg 205:727, 1987.
233. Bandyk DF, Bergamini TM, Kinney EV, et al: In situ replacement of vascular prostheses infected by bacterial biofilms. J Vasc Surg 13:575, 1991.
234. Robinson AJ, Johansen K: Aortic sepsis: Is there a role for in situ graft replacement? J Vasc Surg 13:677, 1991.
235. Jacobs MJHM, Reul G, Gregoric I, et al: In-situ replacement and extraanatomic bypass for the treatment of infected abdominal aortic grafts. Eur J Vasc Surg 5:83, 1991.
236. Kieffer E, Bahnini A, Koskas F, et al: In situ allograft replacement of infected infrarenal aortic prosthetic grafts: Results in 43 patients. J Vasc Surg 17:349, 1993.

53

Infrainguinal Bypass

Anthony D. Whittemore, M.D.

• • •

Arterial reconstruction for infrainguinal peripheral vascular occlusive disease has become increasingly successful with regard to long-term palliation of intermittent claudication and salvage of limbs threatened with critical ischemia. Although primary amputation may represent the most humane solution to irrevocable ischemia when extensive infection or tissue necrosis precludes expeditious limb salvage, an initial attempt at reconstruction is usually indicated in all but the most extenuating circumstances. As numerous improvements in perioperative management and surgical technique have evolved, progressively more distal reconstruction has met the challenge imposed by the more extensive disease characteristic of our aging population. The vast majority of patients with claudication will achieve long-term palliation, as will those with critical ischemia, for whom an 80 to 90 per cent limb salvage rate may be anticipated.

INDICATIONS

The two major indications for intervention during the natural history of peripheral vascular disease consist of claudication and limb-threatening critical ischemia. Claudication is a relative indication because the conditions of the majority of such patients will remain stable throughout their lifetime, with ultimate limb loss limited to 1 per cent per year.[1–4] The conditions of approximately 20 per cent of claudicators will deteriorate to the extent that truly incapacitating symptoms require arterial reconstruction. Whether or not claudication constitutes a significant disability depends on the subjective judgment of both patient and surgeon. Two-block claudication in a younger patient whose livelihood depends on walking tolerance constitutes a more significant disability than the same degree of claudication in an older, retired individual able to attend to his or her daily affairs without significant consequence. Furthermore, the degree of disability cannot be entirely isolated from causative pathologic anatomy. Intervention for relatively moderate symptoms may be justified if excellent results are achieved at low risk. More distal reconstruction associated with less favorable results, higher operative mortality, and increased risk of limb loss may preclude surgery for the same degree of functional impairment. Thus, proximal above-knee reconstruction in a patient with disabling claudication and a patent popliteal artery with excellent runoff may be justified in view of its minimal operative mortality, excellent long-term palliation, and absence of added risk of limb loss beyond that expected from the natural history of the disease process. In contrast, claudicators with diffuse superficial femoropopliteal and tibioperoneal disease are usually not suitable candidates for revascularization because long distal reconstruction will not necessarily provide symptomatic relief and failure of a graft may result in distal arterial thrombosis and a jeopardized limb. Because the majority of claudicants remain stable for years, it is important to allow sufficient time for collaterals to develop, since some patients may improve to such an extent that intervention proves unnecessary. For this reason, a structured exercise program is usually initiated for 6 months following the onset of symptoms prior to reaching a firm decision regarding revascularization.

In contrast, critical ischemia, as evidenced by chronic ischemic rest pain or tissue necrosis, is associated with inevitable amputation for most patients unless surgical correction is undertaken. As is true with claudication, ischemic rest pain must be carefully distinguished from other sources of pain in the elderly population, most commonly arthralgia and neuropathy. Although tissue necrosis and gangrene are usually self-evident when caused by critical ischemia, similar lesions associated with venous stasis, severe anemia, decubitus ulcers, and diabetic neuropathy must be excluded.

Patients with the acute onset of critical ischemia deserve special mention. In the absence of progressive neuromotor or sensory deficit, such patients may be maintained on systemic heparin during preoperative evaluation, which is carried out as it would be for any other patient. The presence of neurologic dysfunction of a progressive nature, however, requires more urgent arteriography and expeditious intervention for limb salvage before irrevocable ischemic nerve damage occurs.

Attempts at revascularization are absolutely contraindicated in the presence of life-threatening sepsis, where adequate drainage may require major amputation.[5] In contrast, extensive foot infection, as commonly seen in the diabetic population, may be amenable to an initial minor drainage procedure and subsequent revascularization following the resolution of sepsis.[6] Well-established flexion contracture and paralysis are additional contraindications, and heroic efforts to salvage a jeopardized limb in a patient with markedly reduced life expectancy are usually not justified.[7, 8] In such individuals, more temporizing procedures such as percutaneous transluminal angioplasty for appropriate localized lesions might be employed.[9] Reconstruction should be delayed in most individuals with significant acute comorbidity, such as a recent myocardial infarction, unless the limb is imminently threatened and higher perioperative morbidity is acceptable.[10]

PREOPERATIVE EVALUATION

Successful infrainguinal reconstruction for ischemic limbs requires the initial recognition and subsequent management of both the underlying systemic atherosclerotic cardiovascular disease and the associated specific manifestation. Significant comorbidity from the various complications of atherosclerosis in vascular surgery patients has been well documented. The Framingham study unequivocally demonstrated that claudicators harbor a significantly higher incidence of coronary artery insufficiency, as well as cerebrovascular and hypertensive disease, than does the nonclaudicating population.[11] Clinically overt cardiac disease is readily apparent in approximately 50 per cent of the vascular surgery population, and an additional 20 per cent have clinically silent but significant coronary artery disease.[12] The use of ambulatory Holter monitoring has confirmed the high prevalence of clinically silent myocardial ischemia in these patients.[13, 14] Because myocardial dysfunction is the overwhelming cause of perioperative morbidity and mortality associated with infrainguinal reconstruction, a thorough understanding of the individual patient's cardiac status is required (see Chapter 22). The approach of the author and his colleagues to preoperative management limits extensive cardiac evaluation to those individuals with clinically overt coronary disease manifested by positive findings on electrocardiography, a history suggestive of coronary insufficiency, or both. Patients with no clinically apparent coronary disease and relatively normal electrocardiographic findings can undergo revascularization without significant cardiac morbidity or mortality.[15] At the other extreme, myocardial revascularization of the patient with unstable angina takes precedence over any attempt at infrainguinal reconstruction. The remaining group of individuals, those with chronic stable angina, sustain the highest incidence of perioperative cardiac morbidity and deserve more exhaustive preoperative evaluation. The author's group routinely employs a combination of ambulatory Holter monitoring and dipyridamole-thallium scanning for risk assessment. Positive Holter monitoring or scanning findings then prompt coronary arteriography, with preliminary coronary revascularization as indicated.[13, 16, 17]

Despite the high prevalence of cigarette smoking in the vascular surgery population, postoperative pulmonary complications are relatively infrequent with routine postoperative pulmonary care. The increased use of regional anesthesia for infrainguinal procedures may contribute to the overall reduction in pulmonary morbidity. It would be ideal for patients to abstain from smoking long before surgery is planned, but until recently this had been an unrealistic goal for most. With the availability of transcutaneous nicotine patches, however, preoperative smoking cessation may become a more reasonable expectation. Routine antihypertensive and cardiac medications are administered as usual until surgery. Patients with chronic renal insufficiency constitute an important group because significant impairment increases operative mortality.[18, 19] Renal function should be optimal before intervention, and patients with end-stage renal disease require dialysis on the day following arteriography and immediately preceding surgery, with reinstitution of dialysis on the 1st postoperative day. Patients with prosthetic valves or atrial dysrhythmia requiring long-term anticoagulation are advised to discontinue oral anticoagulant use 2 or 3 days before angiography. They are maintained perioperatively on intravenous dextran and antiplatelet agents until oral anticoagulation can safely be resumed. Finally, it has been the practice of the author and his colleagues to provide aspirin to their patients during the 2 days immediately preceding surgery to ensure adequate tissue levels of antiplatelet activity at the time of intervention.

Local care of ischemic lesions is primarily directed toward minimizing the impact of associated infection. The use of appropriate drainage procedures and preoperative intravenous antibiotics may be advisable before formal revascularization in an effort to reduce the incidence of postoperative wound and graft infection. Adequate drainage may require minor open amputation with staged revascularization and ultimate revision with primary closure.

Noninvasive evaluation of the lower extremity is often helpful for establishing baseline parameters and for differential diagnosis in the presence of significant comorbidity (see Chapter 5). Segmental Doppler arterial pressure determinations are readily available, as are pulse volume recordings, to interpret spuriously high pressures frequently observed in diabetic patients and in patients in renal failure who have metastatic circumferential calcification. For differentiating patients with significant vascular insufficiency from those with primary arthritic or neurogenic comorbidity, exercise testing may prove helpful in equivocal cases. At present, duplex scanning reliably demonstrates the level of critical lesions but does not provide anatomic resolution to the degree necessary for accurate preoperative planning.[20] Duplex mapping of saphenous or alternative veins, however, may be desirable to establish the presence of adequate vein and to plan incisions more accurately. Information obtained with noninvasive duplex scanning regarding the caliber and quality of vein has not been firmly correlated with actual intraoperative findings or outcome. Thus, this modality appears most useful for establishing the presence or absence of vein, with adequacy best determined intraoperatively.

Comprehensive preoperative arteriography is essential for optimal results. At present, neither duplex scanning nor magnetic resonance imaging techniques provide the degree of resolution required for adequate visualization of the infrainguinal vasculature, especially with regard to the distal tibial vessels and the pedal arch. Reconstruction should not be abandoned, however, in the absence of angiographic visualization of the distal tibioperoneal vasculature because direct exploration may reveal patency sufficient for distal outflow. Patency may be determined either by preliminary intraoperative angiography of the proposed isolated outflow vessel or by cannulation of the vessel with a 25-gauge needle to ascertain the presence of blood flow.[20, 21]

In patients with borderline ischemia in whom the necessity for intervention is in doubt, transcutaneous oxygen determinations may prove helpful.[22] A limb with a transcutaneous partial pressure of oxygen of less than 22 mmHg almost invariably requires revascularization for healing of an ischemic ulcer or a digital amputation site.[23] Reliable measurements, however, require routine use with well-maintained calibrated equipment.

The preoperative administration of intra-arterial thrombolytic therapy remains controversial, and its role is necessarily individualized.[24, 25] Patients with recent onset of acute ischemia and evidence of distal tibioperoneal thrombus may benefit from preoperative lytic therapy to improve outflow from the distal anastomosis. Lysis following thrombosis superimposed on antecedent localized superficial femoral artery stenosis may allow balloon angioplasty in appropriate patients, thereby avoiding the necessity for a surgical procedure. Although this approach will not provide the durability achieved with conventional revascularization, it may prove to be appropriate for selected patients under extraordinary circumstances.

OPERATIVE MANAGEMENT

Exposure

After insertion of appropriate monitoring lines, administration of intravenous antibiotics, and satisfactory induction of anesthesia, the appropriate vessels are exposed, an effort greatly facilitated by a two-team approach when available. The site proposed for the distal anastomosis is initially explored. The above-knee popliteal vessel is easily exposed through a medial thigh incision, with subsequent posterolateral retraction of the sartorius muscle. The underlying deep muscular fascia is incised over the distal adductor canal for exposure of the above-knee popliteal space. The proximal popliteal artery is dissected free of the accompanying structures just posterior to the femur. The artery should be mobilized as far distally as necessary to ensure an optimal anastomotic site determined by external palpation of plaque distribution. The below-knee popliteal artery is usually exposed through a medial calf incision posterior to the medial femoral condyle and extending distally just medial to the tibial crest (Fig. 53–1). The incision should be located directly over the saphenous vein if possible to minimize undermining thin cutaneous flaps. With

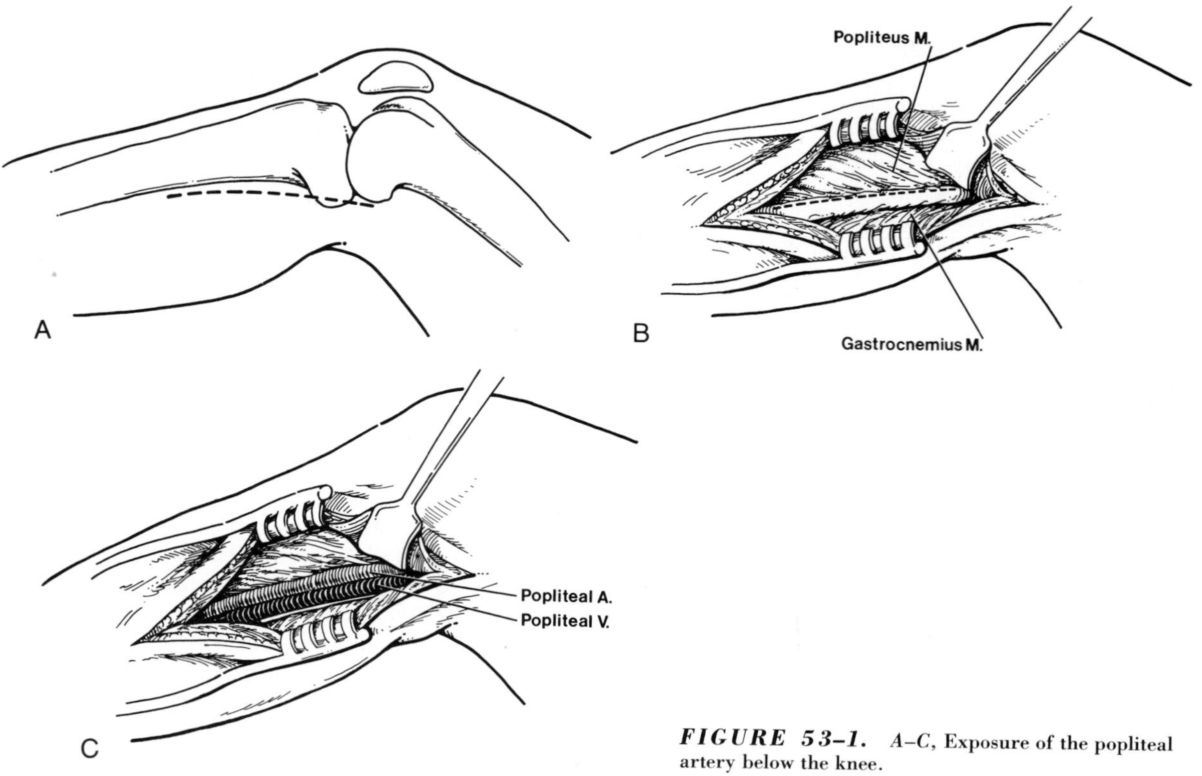

FIGURE 53–1. *A–C,* Exposure of the popliteal artery below the knee.

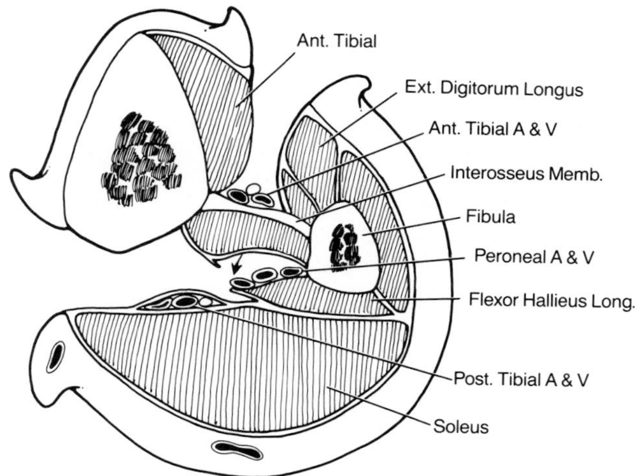

FIGURE 53–2. Anatomic approach to the posterior tibial artery, the anterior tibial artery, and the peroneal artery in the midportion of the leg.

care taken to minimize trauma to the vein during the exposure and division of appropriate tributaries, the deep muscular fascia is incised and the medial head of the gastrocnemius is reflected posterolaterally to expose the popliteal fossa. The distal popliteal artery is mobilized from the posterior tibial nerve posteriorly and the popliteal vein medially. The tibioperoneal trunk can then be exposed if necessary by extending the dissection along the anteromedial surface of the distal popliteal artery and transecting the overlying musculotendinous origin of the soleus muscle. The origin of the anterior tibial artery can also be encircled with a loop for control. The proximal halves of both the posterior tibial and the peroneal vessels are most easily exposed by continued distal dissection beyond the bifurcation of the tibioperoneal trunk (Fig. 53–2). The posterior tibial artery lies more medially on the surface of the reflected soleus muscle or along the posterior tibial muscle. The peroneal artery follows a deeper and more lateral course along the flexor hallucis longus. The peroneal artery at this location is frequently invested with multiple annoying veins that require tedious mobilization for exposure of the desired peroneal segment. The popliteal artery may also be exposed through a lateral incision, a useful approach for patients with prior reconstruction or sepsis.[26] The popliteal space above the knee is entered by incision of the distal fascia lata and posterior retraction of the biceps femoris tendon. The lateral approach to the infragenicular popliteal artery requires division of the biceps femoris tendon and excision of the proximal fibula, with care taken to avoid injury to the peroneal nerve.

More distal exposure of the tibial and peroneal vessels is best obtained through individualized incisions (Fig. 53–3). The distal posterior tibial artery is easily isolated through an incision just posterior to the medial malleolus, and its medial and lateral plantar branches are exposed by extension of the incision onto the medial surface of the foot.[27] The anterior tibial artery is usually approached through a longitudinal incision over the anterior compartment in the distal third of the leg and is exposed by reflecting the anterior tibial muscle anteromedially and the digital extensors and peroneal muscles laterally. The distal third of the peroneal artery is best exposed through a longitudinal incision over the distal fibula (Fig. 53–4). The long peroneal muscle is mobilized from the bone and reflected posteriorly along with the flexor hallucis longus. The periosteum of the fibula is circumferentially scored and elevated, and a 5- to 10-cm length of fibula is resected. The peroneal artery and its accompanying veins lie just deep to the thin layer of fascia directly on the surface of the posterior tibial muscle (see Fig. 53–2). The dorsal pedal artery is easily exposed through an axial incision on the dorsum of the foot just lateral to the extensor hallucis longus tendon (Fig. 53–5). As wide a skin bridge as possible should be provided between the arterial incision and that required for exposure and subsequent mobilization of the distal saphenous vein.[28]

After selection and exposure of the most appropriate site for distal anastomosis, the proximal incision is made most frequently in the groin overlying the medial aspect of the common femoral artery (Fig. 53–6). Care must be taken to direct the inferior aspect of this incision posteriorly to avoid undermining a medial flap prone to subsequent necrosis. The native common femoral artery is exposed from the level of the inguinal ligament at the origin of the epigastric and circumflex iliac branches to its terminal bifurcation. The proximal superficial femoral artery is mobilized sufficiently to allow temporary occlusion, or more distally in the event that it is selected as the site for proximal anastomosis. The profunda femoris is similarly exposed for a distance appropriate for occlusion, or more distally to the level of its first muscular perforating branches in the event that profundaplasty or extensive endarterectomy is required. Although the lateral femoral circumflex branch of the profunda femoris usually originates from the lateral aspect of the proximal profunda, the medial femoral circumflex

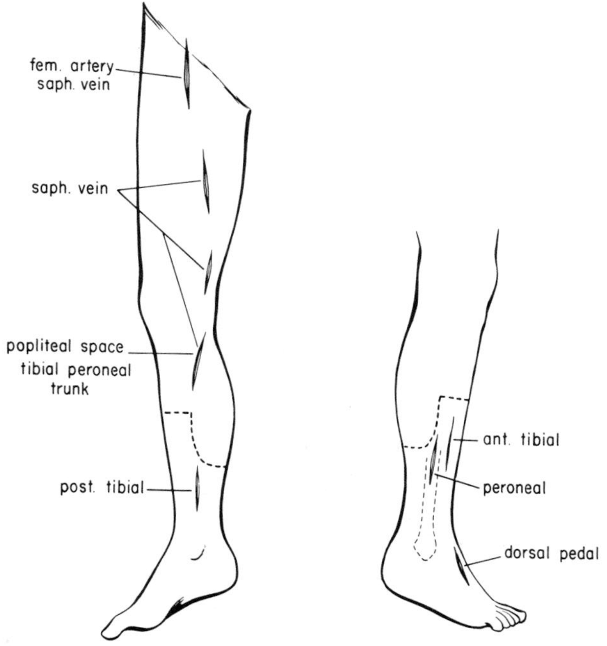

FIGURE 53–3. Placement of incision for femoropopliteal and femorotibial bypass and for saphenous vein harvest. These should avoid the incision lines for a below-knee amputation.

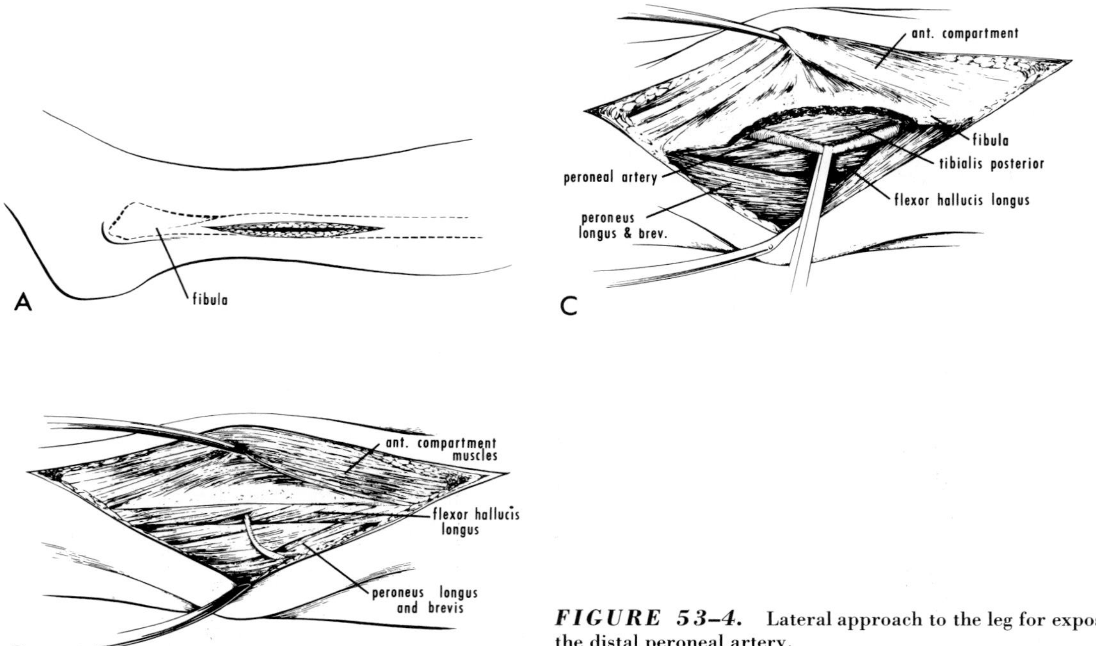

FIGURE 53–4. Lateral approach to the leg for exposure of the distal peroneal artery.

branch often arises posteriorly from the distal common femoral artery as a separate entity necessitating individual control.

Before anticoagulation and construction of the anastomoses, appropriate tunnels are prepared. For reversed or prosthetic conduits, a subsartorial tunnel is usually created between the groin incision and the above-knee popliteal space, either superficial or deep to the deep muscular fascia. Tunnels may be constructed with a variety of instruments, the gentlest of which remain the surgeon's fingers. For below-knee bypass, the tunnel is extended between the heads of the gastrocnemius muscle into the popliteal fossa.

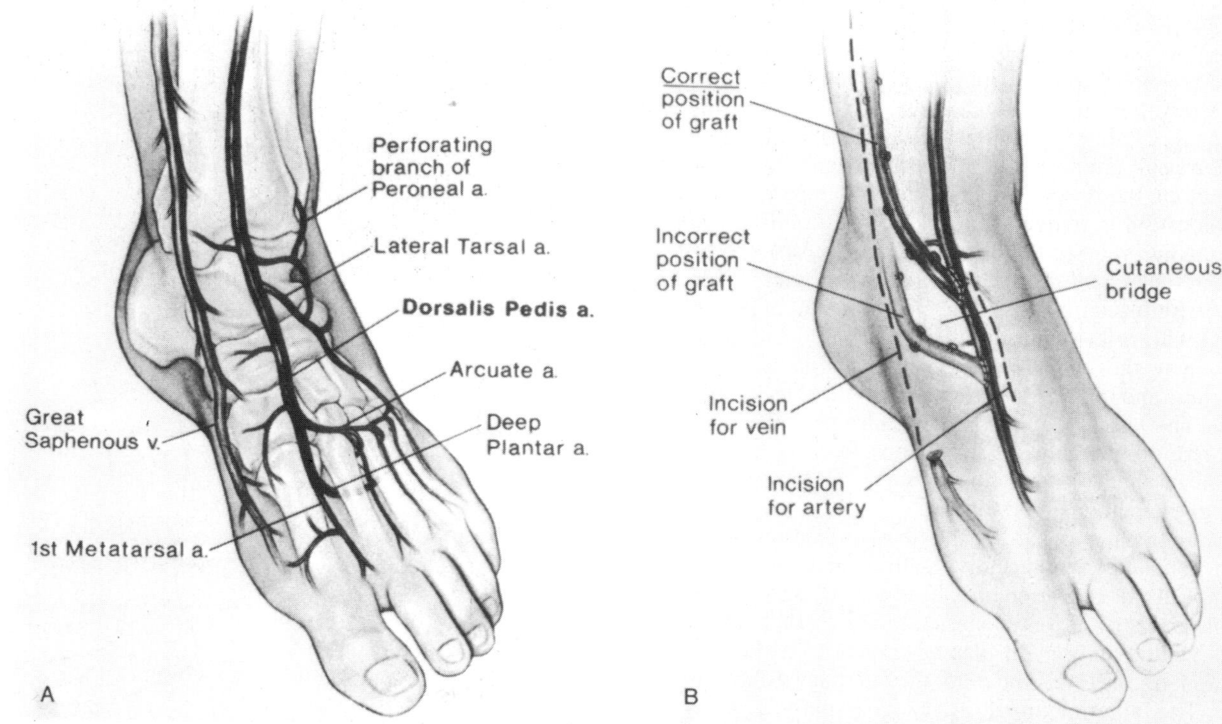

FIGURE 53–5. *A*, The anterior tibial artery continues onto the dorsum of the foot as the dorsal pedal artery, coursing lateral and parallel to the extensor hallucis longus tendon. *B*, Incisions for exposure of both the dorsal pedal artery and the distal greater saphenous vein are illustrated, along with the correct and incorrect tunnels under the skin bridge.

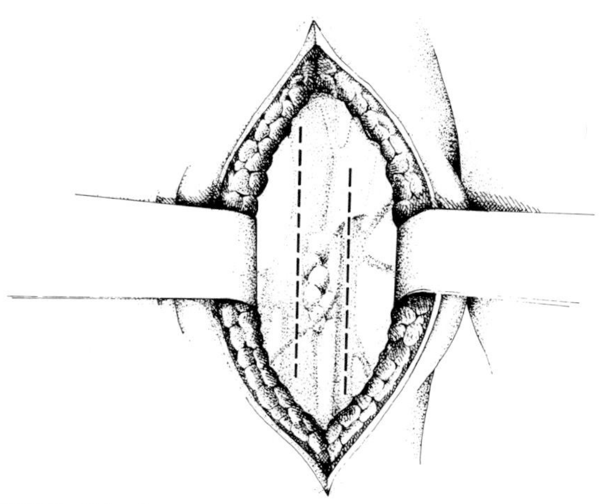

FIGURE 53–6. Separate fascial incisions for exposure of the saphenous vein and common femoral artery in an effort to preserve the lymphatic network.

No further tunneling is necessary for anastomoses to the exposed posterior tibial or proximal peroneal vessels, but the distal peroneal and anterior tibial vessels require a tunnel from the popliteal space through the interosseous membrane into the mid-anterior compartment. Alternatively, subcutaneous tunnels may be constructed from the groin incision, coursing anteriorly over the thigh and the lateral aspect of the knee joint to the anterior compartment. This lateral tunnel is generally reserved for reoperative situations to avoid a scarred popliteal fossa or residual infection near one of the standard medial incisions.

The in situ technique requires no extensive tunneling except when the below-knee popliteal artery is chosen for the site of the distal anastomosis. In this case, the angle of entry of the vein graft into the distal anastomosis may approach 90 degrees if the vein is brought directly from its below-knee subcutaneous position. The vein is best mobilized to the above-knee level and subsequently tunneled distally between the heads of the gastrocnemius muscle to provide a more optimal angle of anastomosis (Fig. 53–7). Special precautions must also be taken when the in situ graft is being tunneled to the dorsal pedal artery to avoid necrosis of the overlying skin bridge (see Fig. 53–5*B*).[28] After the creation of the required tunnels, the patient is customarily anticoagulated with heparin at a dose of 50 to 100 USP units. The sequence of anastomoses varies according to the procedure and the conduit used.

Autogenous Vein Bypass

Reversed Greater Saphenous Vein

Femoropopliteal bypass using autogenous saphenous vein in the reversed position was initially reported by Kunlin in 1949.[29] The vein may be harvested through relatively short longitudinal skin incisions with intervening cutaneous bridges (see Fig. 53–3). Tributaries are divided and ligated, and the vein is harvested and prepared with care to mini-

FIGURE 53–7. A, Intraoperative completion arteriograms illustrating a kinked vein graft at the distal popliteal anastomosis created by a hyperacute angle of entry when the vein graft is anastomosed directly from its subcutaneous position. *B,* This may be avoided by mobilization of the vein and delivery through a popliteal tunnel from the above-knee position.

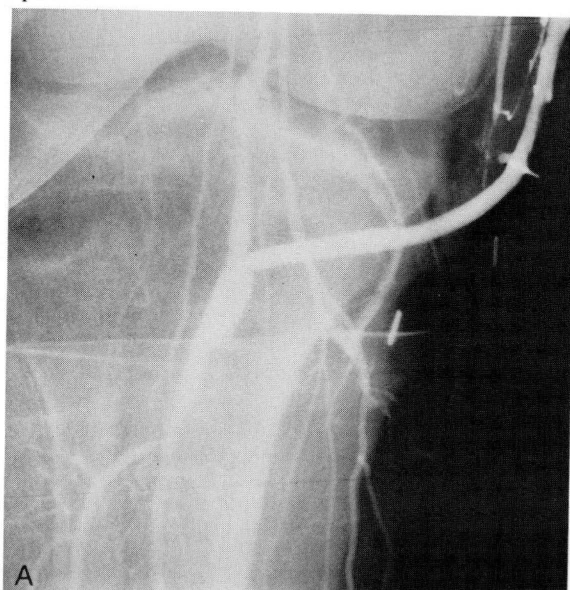

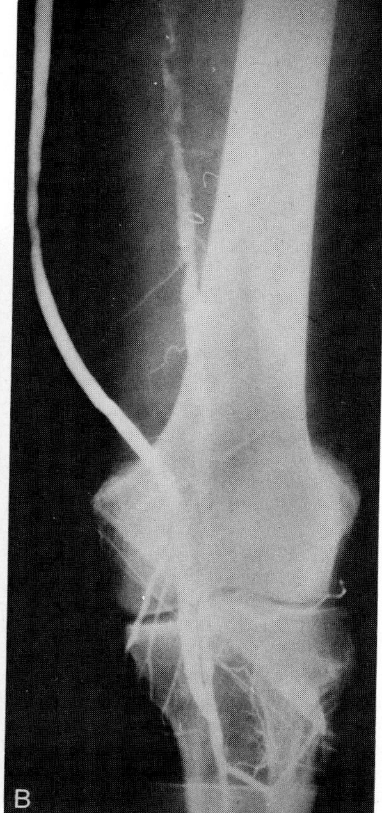

mize mechanical trauma and desiccation. Optimal endothelial preservation may be achieved with external application or perivenous infiltration of a solution containing papaverine.[30] After excision, the reversed vein is gently flushed and subsequently stored in chilled autologous blood, Ringer's lactate, or a combined electrolyte solution (Plasma-Lyte) containing both heparin and papaverine to minimize spasm. The distal anastomosis is usually carried out first using one of several standard techniques (see Chapter 21), and the graft is delivered through the appropriate tunnel to the groin incision. The graft is gently flushed from the proximal end with the vein preservation solution to ensure against mechanical twist or kink and to establish adequate length and appropriate tension with the leg in the extended position. Finally, the proximal anastomosis is constructed, most commonly to the common femoral artery with fine 5–0 or 6–0 monofilament suture, and completed after careful sequential flushing to minimize embolic events.

In Situ Saphenous Vein

The in situ bypass, which was initially advocated by Hall,[31] was further modified and popularized by Leather and associates in 1979.[32, 33] The greater saphenous vein is usually exposed throughout the entire length required. A small-caliber vein may be ligated in the distal aspect of the distal incision and partially transected to allow cannulation and gentle flushing with chilled blood, Ringer's lactate, or a combined electrolyte solution containing both heparin and papaverine. This practice minimizes intraoperative venous spasm and lessens the likelihood of injury during subsequent valvulotomy or angioscopy. Partial transection preserves the rotational alignment and orientation of valve cusps to be subsequently lysed. The exposed vein is covered first with sponges or laparotomy pads soaked in vein preservation solution and then with a barrier to prevent evaporation and desiccation. Alternatively, the skin may be loosely reapproximated over the exposed vein with a stapler during construction of the proximal anastomosis.

Preliminary angioscopy for direct visualization of valve lysis and localization of arteriovenous fistulae has been helpful in some patients by reducing the number of incisions required.[34] Recent experience, however, presents conflicting evidence about whether this practice favorably influences operating time, length of hospital stay, or incidence of wound complications. The primary advantage of routine angioscopy may reside in its ability to demonstrate unsuspected endoluminal pathology such as phlebitic strictures, webs, and fibrotic valve cusps.[35] This technique may prove most useful with arm veins, in which endoluminal pathology is frequently present and is responsible in part for suboptimal results.[36]

In contrast to reversed vein bypass, the in situ method requires the proximal anastomosis to be initially constructed after transection of the saphenofemoral junction and closure of the common femoral venotomy (Fig. 53–8*A*). Ideally, the proximal anastomosis is located in the distal common femoral artery, but the actual site is frequently dictated by the position of the saphenofemoral junction relative to the bifurcation of the common femoral artery (see Fig. 53–8*B*). A portion of the proximal saphenous vein may be mobilized to provide more length and less tension for a distal common femoral anastomosis. To avoid excessive tension, however, the anastomosis must occasionally straddle the common femoral bifurcation. Alternatively, the proximal anastomosis may be located entirely in the proximal superficial femoral artery, which in turn may require preliminary endarterectomy. The cusps of the first venous valve are excised under direct vision in the proximal saphenous vein. After occlusion of the native arteries with atraumatic vascular clamps, an arteriotomy is usually made in the distal common femoral artery and extended either proximally or distally across the origin of the

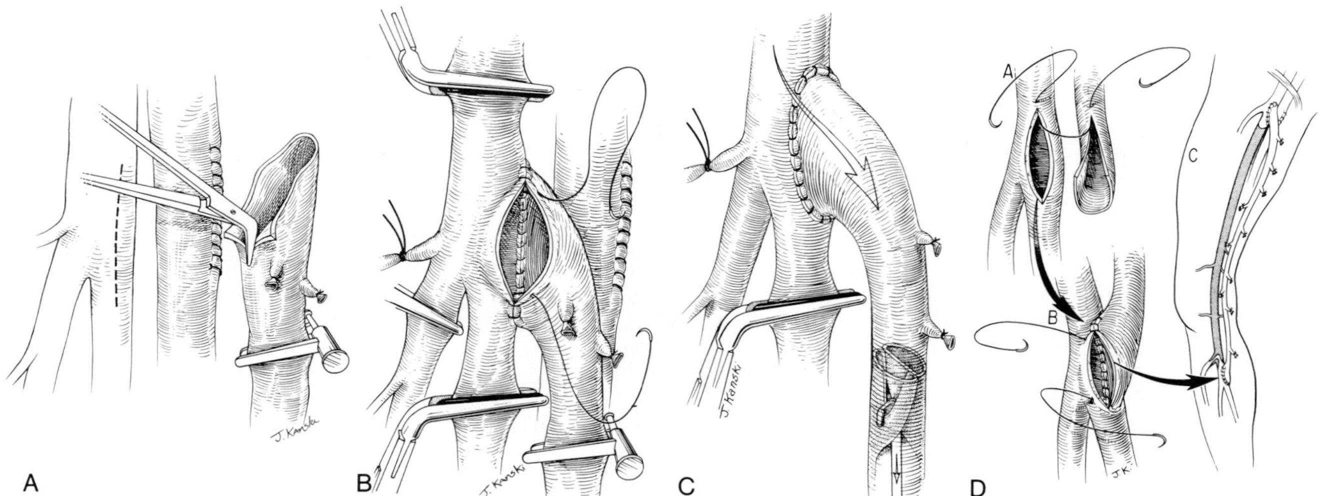

FIGURE 53–8. *A*, In the in situ method of infrainguinal reconstruction, the saphenofemoral junction is transected in the groin, the venotomy in the femoral vein oversewn, and the proximal end of the saphenous vein prepared for anastomosis. *B*, After the first venous valve is excised under direct vision, the graft is anastomosed end-to-side to the femoral artery. *C*, Flow is then restored through the vein graft and the valvulotome inserted through side branches at appropriate intervals to lyse residual valve cusps. *D*, Finally, the distal anastomosis is completed, in this case at the level of the distal tibioperoneal trunk.

superficial femoral artery as indicated by the length of available vein. Preliminary endarterectomy is performed if necessary, and then the proximal anastomosis is constructed with standard techniques. Before completion of the anastomosis, all vessels should be flushed copiously to avoid distal embolization. After all occluding clamps have been removed, arterial flow is established through the vein graft to the level of the first competent valve.

Although various valvulotomes are available for lysis of valve cusps, the preference of the author and his colleagues has been the modified Mills valvulotome used with the entire vein exposed (see Fig. 53–8*C*).[37] Others prefer valvulotomy under direct vision with angioscopic control, but there is little evidence at present to favor one technique over another. Following complete valve lysis and on assurance of satisfactory inflow from the graft, appropriate control of the distal vessel is secured. Methods of control include the application of standard atraumatic external clamps, the use of internal balloon catheters, and the use of a proximal pneumatic tourniquet.[38] An arteriotomy in the distal vessel is initiated, and the distal vein is appropriately trimmed with the leg extended to ensure adequate length without tension. The transected end is spatulated and sutured to the arteriotomy with fine monofilament suture (see Fig. 53–8*D*). Proponents of both the interrupted and the continuous suture technique have yet to provide convincing data that one method is preferable.

Sequential Vein

Prominent among the many reasons for failure of long distal reconstructions is the high peripheral resistance in the distal outflow bed provided by severely diseased runoff. As initially advocated by DeLaurentis and Friedmann in 1972, sequential bypass is designed to enhance flow through the long arterial limb of the graft by providing two or more distal anastomoses, thereby reducing peripheral resistance.[39] That graft flow is significantly augmented has been established in both laboratory and clinical settings, and the technique is believed by some to improve the long-term patency rates of grafts to restricted-outflow tracks.[40, 41] Of the several configurations possible, four are illustrated in Figure 53–9. With an adequate length of autogenous vein available, a side-to-side anastomosis may be interposed between the proximal femoral and distal tibial anastomosis. This interposed anastomosis may be constructed to an isolated segment of the popliteal vessel proximally (see Fig. 53–9*A*) or to a posterior tibial or peroneal vessel distally (see Fig. 53–9*B*). The latter may be constructed with the use of an in situ technique. Similar approaches illustrated in Figures 53–9*C* and *D* are appropriate when shorter segments of vein are available, and the anastomosis may be constructed with either the proximal or distal segment in the in situ configuration. In either case, the interposed sequential anastomosis may be constructed with two separate end-to-side anastomoses or a single side-to-side anastomosis. Alternatively, the distal graft may originate end-to-side from the distal aspect of the proximal graft. These complex reconstructions should clearly be reserved for patients requiring limb salvage and should not be used for palliation of claudication.

Alternative Autogenous Vein

The use of an autogenous conduit may require some creativity in view of the frequency of anatomic variants, endoluminal pathology, and prior use for peripheral or coronary procedures. Whereas a single saphenous vein trunk is present in approximately two thirds of patients, a complete double system is present in some 10 per cent and an incomplete double system is found in an additional 15 per cent.[42] Double systems may be converted to longer lengths after harvesting of the intact saphenofemoral junction, which is subsequently oversewn (Fig. 53–10).[43] One limb of the duplicated system is then reversed, and the other remains nonreversed after lysis of valve cusps with the valvulotome. Similarly, an inadequate length of autogenous vein may ultimately prove to be sufficient if a more distal site for proximal anastomosis is selected.[44, 45] Generally, a minimum caliber of 3.5 mm is required for optimal results with reversed vein, whereas entirely satisfactory results have been obtained with smaller-caliber grafts with the in situ technique.[46]

In the absence of suitable greater saphenous vein, either arm vein or lesser saphenous vein may prove to be adequate (see Chapter 28). If the greater saphenous vein is known to be unavailable preoperatively, the lesser saphenous vein is most easily harvested with the patient initially in the prone position. After closure of the posterior calf incision, the patient is turned, reprepared, and draped. Alternatively, the lesser saphenous vein may be harvested through a medial approach, with the patient in the usual supine position following exposure of arterial anastomotic sites.[47] Both arm and lesser saphenous vein may be used in either the reversed or the nonreversed configuration. The preference of the author and his colleagues is the nonreversed position, which usually provides better size matching at the anastomoses but requires preliminary valve lysis with an appropriate valvulotome. There is no evidence, however, that this practice influences ultimate results.

Prosthetic Bypass

Since the mid-1950s, prosthetic grafts have been used in a variety of locations for arterial reconstruction. The earliest were knitted or woven textile grafts, primarily of Dacron, which provide consistently favorable results in high-flow, large-caliber settings but perform poorly in the more challenging small-caliber, low-flow conditions characteristic of distal infrainguinal reconstruction. As a result, both human umbilical vein and expanded polytetrafluoroethylene (PTFE) were introduced in the 1970s for clinical use as small-caliber arterial substitutes.[48, 49] Because human umbilical vein proved to be cumbersome, PTFE has been more often used as the conduit of choice in the absence of adequate autogenous saphenous vein. Preliminary reports documented impressive early results that were comparable to those obtained with saphenous vein, but these results proved to be overoptimistic as patency data matured.[50–53]

Because results achieved with distal PTFE reconstructions proved to be suboptimal, several modifications of the standard approach to prosthetic infrainguinal bypass have

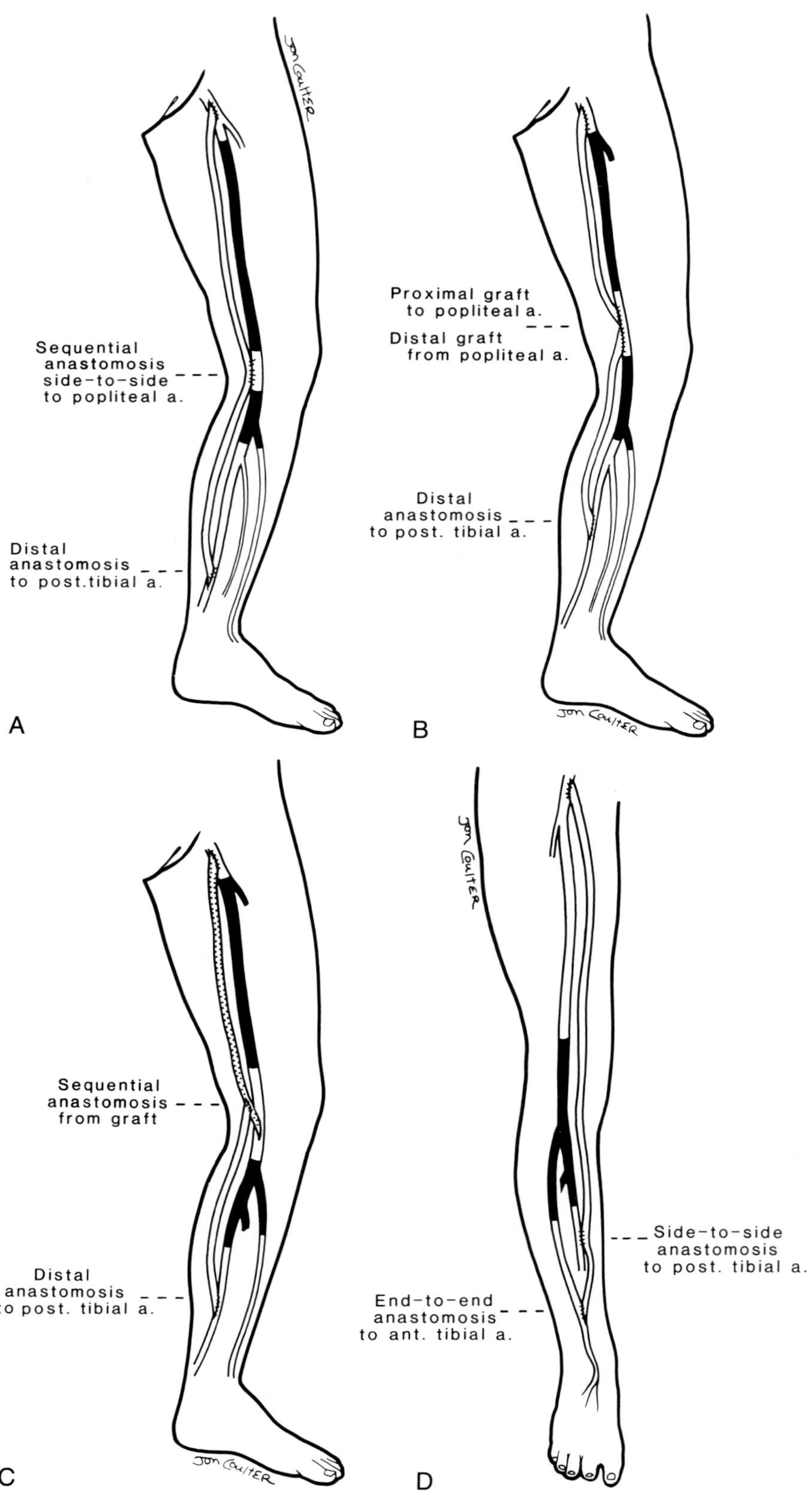

FIGURE 53–9. Four configurations for sequential bypass are possible. In type I *(A)*, a single vein or prosthesis is used and a sequential side-to-side anastomosis is constructed to the popliteal artery. In type II *(B)*, the proximal portion of the graft is anastomosed end-to-side to the popliteal artery and the distal portion (usually autogenous vein) is sewn to the artery just below, and the distal anastomosis sewn end-to-side to a crural vessel. Type III *(C)* is similar, except that the distal portion of the graft takes origin from the prosthesis rather than from the host artery. Type IV *(D)* is usually employed when the popliteal artery is totally occluded. A side-to-side anastomosis is constructed to one crural vessel proximally and an end-to-side to another more distally in the leg.

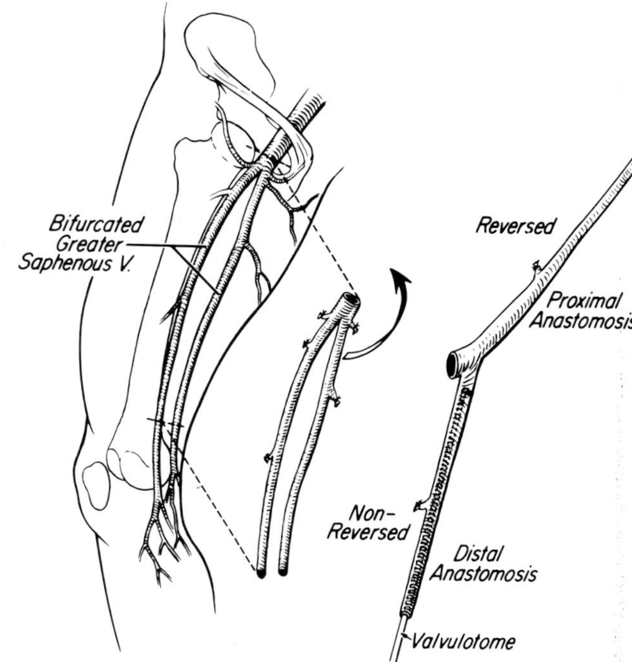

FIGURE 53–10. A short, bifurcated greater superficial saphenous vein may be removed intact and prepared to create a longer vein graft by reversing one limb, lysing the valves in the other nonreversed limb, and oversewing the intervening saphenofemoral junction.

been suggested. Common among several mechanisms of failure associated with PTFE is a particularly vigorous smooth muscle proliferative response at the distal anastomosis, which results in stenosis. A ''collar'' of vein may be interposed between the distal arteriotomy and the distal PTFE graft (Fig. 53–11).[54] It is theorized that when this is done, the kinetic energy stored in the pulse pressure within the noncompliant graft is more effectively dissipated by the relatively elastic properties of autogenous material. As turbulence is reduced, trauma to the arterial endothelium is diminished, thereby minimizing the proliferative response. A similar approach incorporates an autogenous venous ''patch'' across the distal anastomosis (Fig. 53–12).[55] This practice has improved results in the experience of some authors and provides a reasonable alternative for limb salvage in patients who would otherwise have to undergo amputation.[56, 57]

A second modification uses an arteriovenous fistula constructed in conjunction with the distal anastomosis (Fig. 53–13) or at a site more remote from the distal anastomosis (Fig. 53–14) in an effort to augment flow through the prosthetic graft and enhance patency.[58, 59] Preliminary results with this technique are encouraging, but further trials and longer-term data are needed.

The use of a composite prosthetic-vein conduit is a third adjunctive method for enhancing prosthetic performance in patients requiring a long reconstruction with a limited length of vein available (Fig. 53–15). The distal anastomosis of the proximal prosthetic component is constructed end-to-side to a patent popliteal segment, above the knee whenever possible to allow the distal venous component to cross the knee joint through an anatomic tunnel.[60] The proximal vein is anastomosed end-to-side to an elliptical incision excised from the hood of the distal prosthetic anastomosis. The routine use of long-term anticoagulation is another option that is increasingly employed to improve long-term patency in the demanding setting of infrapopliteal prosthetic bypass. Preliminary results in an uncontrolled series suggest that anticoagulation may improve patency rates two- or threefold.[61]

A third prosthetic material with which considerable experience has been gained is human umbilical vein tanned with glutaraldehyde. This prosthesis was introduced in the mid-1970s, at the same time PTFE became popular, and

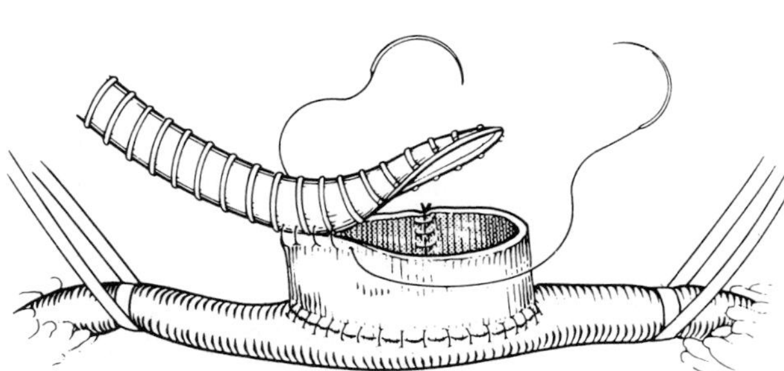

FIGURE 53–11. To minimize the impact of anastomotic intimal hyperplasia, a collar of vein may be interposed between the distal end of the prosthetic graft and the recipient native vessel. (From Miller JH, Foreman RK, Ferguson L, Faris I: Interposition vein cuff for anastomosis of a prosthesis to small artery. Aust NZ J Surg 54:283, 1984.)

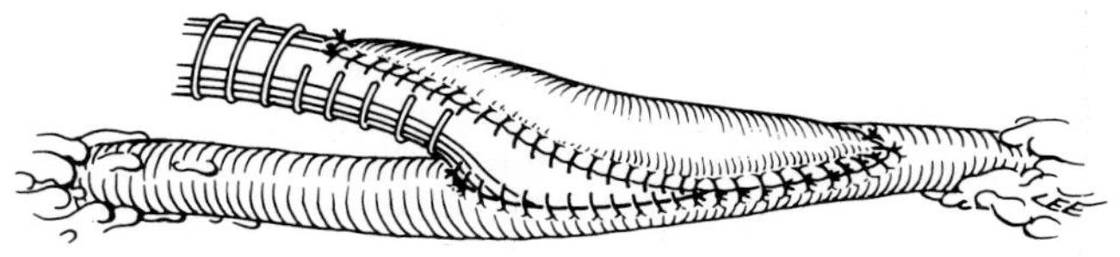

FIGURE 53–12. An alternate method for compensating for inevitable anastomotic intimal hyperplasia consists of a vein patch. (From Taylor RS, McFarland RJ, Cox MI: An investigation into the causes of failure of PTFE grafts. Eur J Vasc Surg 1:335, 1987.)

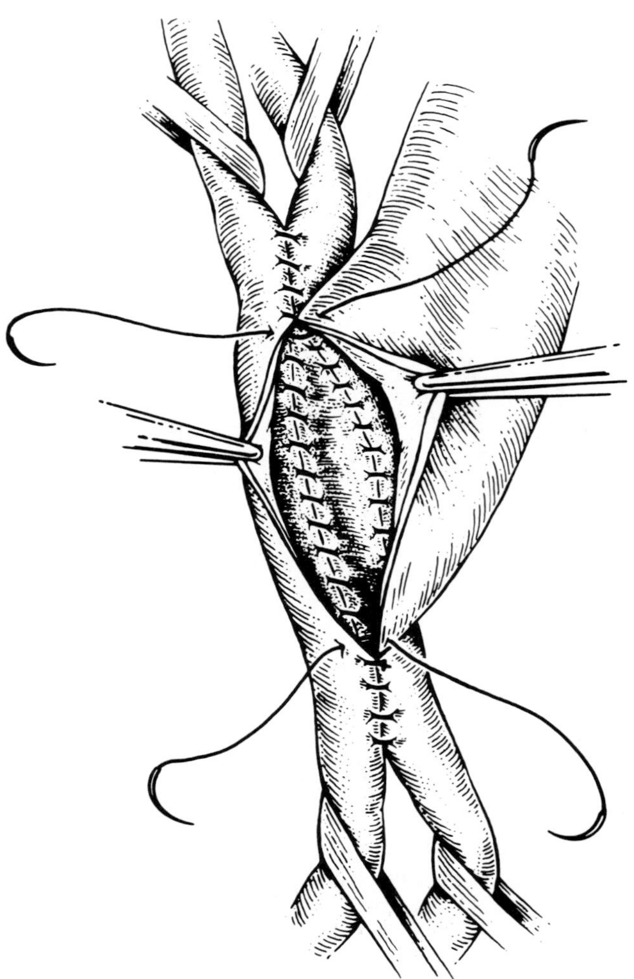

FIGURE 53–13. **In order to increase flow through a prosthetic bypass to limited arterial outflow, an anastomotic arteriovenous fistula may be created to enhance graft flow with diversion into the high-capacitance venous system.**

initially provided similar short-term results.[48] This prosthesis has never gained the popularity associated with PTFE for two major reasons. First, the use of human umbilical vein is technically more demanding because an initial irrigation protocol is necessary to remove residual alcohol and aldehyde and meticulous anastomotic technique is required to incorporate the outer reinforcing mesh (Fig. 53–16).[62] Second, a propensity for dilatation and aneurysm formation has gradually become evident.[63, 64] As longer-term results obtained with PTFE have in most situations proved to be inferior to those achieved with autogenous vein, a resurgence of interest in umbilical vein has developed, particularly with regard to the more favorable location above the knee.[65–67]

Completion Evaluation

After completion of the bypass procedure, an objective assessment of technical adequacy is mandatory (Chapter 24). Completion arteriography is easily performed using a variety of methods (Fig. 53–17). Hand injection of 20 to 25 ml of diluted diatrizoate (Renografin) antegrade into the proximal vein graft with the anastomosis occluded provides excellent visualization. Contrast solution may also be injected retrograde to allow opacification in the presence of normal antegrade blood flow. A single injection is sufficient for an above-knee reconstruction, but two injections are required for assessment of the entire length of longer below-knee or infrapopliteal grafts. Although angiography provides excellent opacification of the distal anastomosis and the outflow vessels, as well as of residual arteriovenous fistulae in the case of in situ grafts, endoluminal pathology may be obscured.[68–71] Completion angioscopy more reliably identifies retained valve cusps and endoluminal pathology. The incidence of retained valve cusps, however, is quite low (4 to 12 per cent), and the most important contribution of angioscopy is the demonstration of unsuspected endoluminal pathology. These short-segment strictures or webs, however, may also be identified with careful duplex evaluation, and transluminal ultrasonography may yet prove to be helpful in the not-too-distant future. Nevertheless, some combination of these techniques is required to ensure a technically satisfactory reconstruction.

If adequate hemostasis is achieved, anticoagulation is not routinely reversed, and the incisions are closed with continuous absorbable subcutaneous suture and skin staples. For excessively thin skin in the distal third of the leg and foot, subcutaneous closure is not necessary and may prove to be detrimental. Closure of the incisions on the

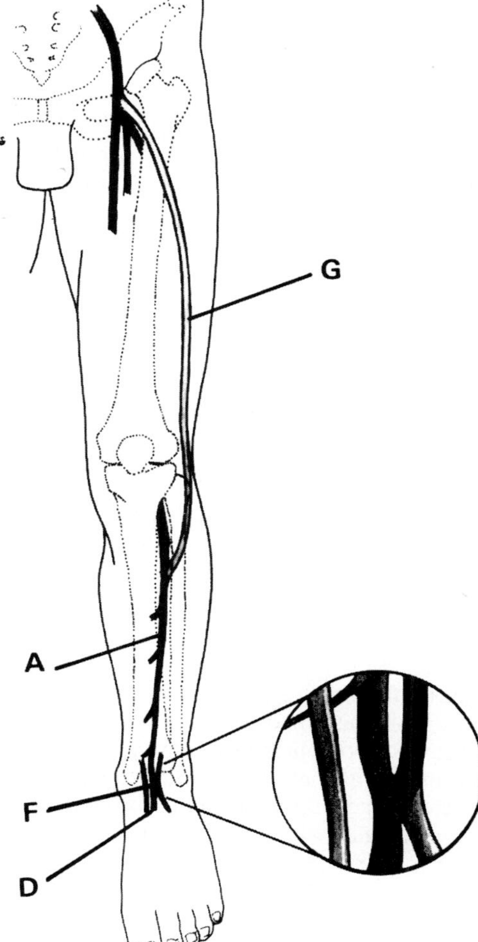

FIGURE 53–14. An alternate approach to enhance flow through a prosthetic graft (G) is the creation of an arteriovenous fistula (F) at a site remote (D) from the distal anastomosis. In theory, flow is also augmented in the intervening arterial segment (A) and its collaterals.

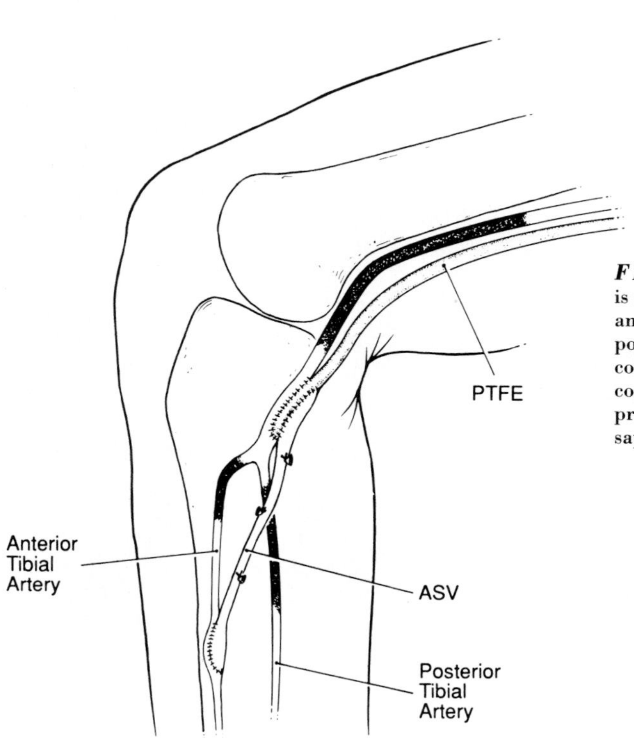

FIGURE 53–15. Composite prosthetic grafting to the popliteal artery is an option in the absence of suitable vein. When possible, the composite anastomosis should be located above the knee, but in some cases a distal popliteal site is required. The distal prosthetic anastomosis is initially constructed end-to-side, and the proximal venous composite anastomosis constructed to an elliptical incision excised from the hood of the distal prosthetic anastomosis. PTFE, polytetrafluoroethylene; ASV, autogenous saphenous vein.

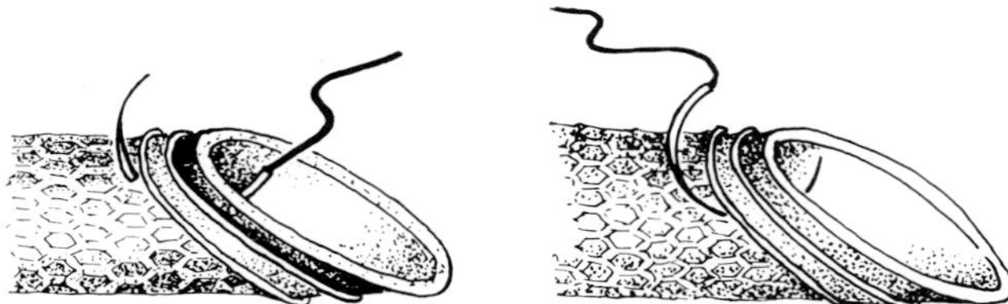

FIGURE 53–16. Proper suture technique for constructing anastomoses with human umbilical vein includes the incorporation of the outer mesh as well as the actual intimal component of the graft in the suture line.

dorsum of the foot required for dorsal pedal in situ bypass is best achieved with continuous absorbable subcuticular suture to minimize excessive countertension.

POSTOPERATIVE MANAGEMENT

Most patients do not require routine admission to an intensive care unit, provided that initial recovery is uneventful. Pulses should be frequently assessed, either by palpation or by monitoring with a Doppler velocity meter during the first 12 hours and several times daily thereafter to ensure sustained patency. In the absence of significant systemic complications, early graft thrombosis should prompt immediate return to the operating room for thrombectomy, angiography, and revision as necessary.

Patients without significant tissue necrosis are routinely ambulated on the 1st postoperative day, and those with healing lesions are ambulated later as indicated. Claudicators who have had uncomplicated procedures are usually discharged by the 5th postoperative day, whereas those with systemic complications or cutaneous distal lesions may require longer hospitalization. Following discharge and the initial postoperative outpatient visit, all grafts require periodic surveillance to identify hemodynamically significant lesions before thrombosis. It has been repeatedly demonstrated that revision of such stenotic lesions results in sustained graft patency, whereas revision of similar lesions following graft thrombosis yields poor results (see Chapter 57).[71–74] At present, there is little clinical evidence available to support the long-term use of oral anticoagulation to maintain graft patency.[75] Preliminary evidence suggests that routine anticoagulation may improve the results with infrapopliteal prosthetic bypass,[61] and a multi-center Veterans Administration study is under way to assess its efficacy in routine autogenous reconstructions. Patients with unexplained graft thrombosis following thrombectomy and those with an identifiable hypercoagulopathy, however, are frequently maintained on oral anticoagulation.

Complications

Perioperative mortality within 30 days of surgery ranges from 2 to 5 per cent and most commonly results from coronary artery disease.[76–82] Overall morbidity rates vary widely depending on inclusion criteria, but major systemic complications, the predominant cause of which is again cardiac, develop in 5 to 10 per cent of patients. Local complications include hemorrhage, graft thrombosis, wound infection, and leg edema. Hemorrhage during the

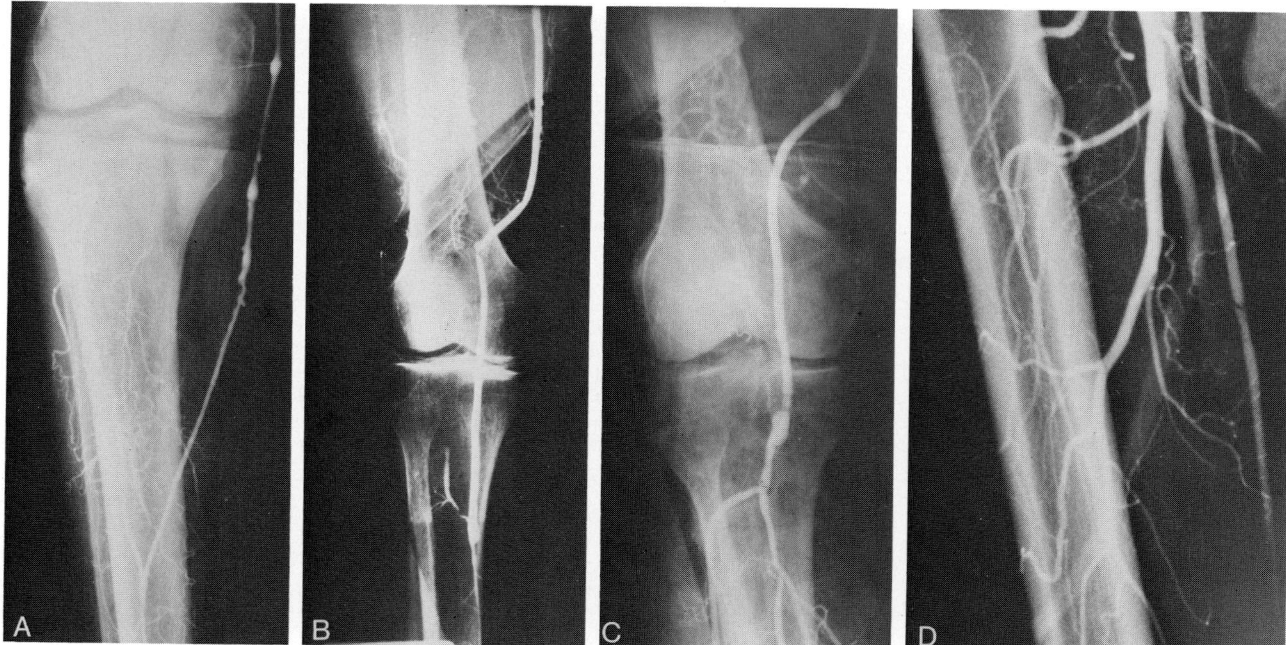

FIGURE 53–17. Intraoperative completion arteriograms demonstrate: an endoluminal lesion in the distal aspect of a femoroperoneal vein graft *(A)*; a kink in a femoroposterior tibial vein graft as the graft enters the popliteal tunnel above the knee *(B)*; a residual platelet plug just proximal to the distal anastomosis in a femoropopliteal vein graft *(C)*; and a retained valve cusp in an in situ femoropopliteal graft with a residual arteriovenous fistula *(D)*.

first 48 hours is an unusual occurrence: the incidence in most series is less than 2 per cent.[77, 78] A significant or an expanding hematoma must be evacuated and a diligent search for its cause undertaken. Of identifiable causes, suture line hemorrhage and insecure ligation of an arterial branch or arterialized venous tributary are frequent culprits. Hemorrhage occurring beyond the immediate postoperative period suggests underlying infection of an anastomotic suture line and usually requires ligation or excision of the graft.

Graft thrombosis within the first 30 days of surgery complicates 2 to 7 per cent of procedures and most often results from technical defects, hypercoagulopathy, inadequate distal runoff, and postoperative hypotension.[83] Technical defects are more common with autogenous reconstructions and are responsible for nearly half of all early failures. Such errors include graft kinks, valvulotome injury, retained leaflets, intimal flaps, significant residual arteriovenous fistulae, and small-caliber vein. Various hypercoagulopathies occur in at least 10 to 14 per cent of the vascular population and are responsible for 20 per cent of early graft thromboses, most commonly resulting from antiphospholipid syndrome and heparin-induced platelet aggregation. Systemic hypotension, which is usually cardiogenic in origin, causes an additional 20 per cent of failures.

Although the majority of wound complications are relatively minor and are limited to superficial skin necrosis along the edges of incisions or an erythematous reaction to sutures or staples, significant wound infection occurs with a reported incidence of 8 to 19 per cent.[78, 81, 84] Infection is usually associated with persistent hematoma, lymphocele, or lymphorrhea and significant superficial necrosis. Lymphocele with or without lymphorrhea from the inguinal incision may result from the transection of unrecognized lymphatics during the initial groin exploration. Although immobility with elevation and local care usually results in spontaneous resolution, copious and persistent lymphorrhea should prompt re-exploration of the groin and ligation of lymph channels to minimize the incidence of secondary infection.[85] An infected incision usually responds to appropriate antibiotics and local drainage with débridement, but if the suture line of an underlying graft becomes involved, especially if complicated with hemorrhage, excision of the graft is required.[86]

Wound healing may be significantly delayed by the inevitable appearance of edema in the leg after successful revascularization. The edema results from increased interstitial fluid accumulation and lymphatic obstruction, and to some degree from venous interruption as well. Of all three potential components, venous interruption seems to be the least important because of the plethora of deep veins available to compensate for ligation during the exposure of distal arteries. In all probability, chronic ischemia attenuates autoregulatory vasomotor responses, which normalize to some extent following reperfusion. Disruption of lymphatic channels, however, is probably the most important factor contributing to lower extremity edema.[87] Patients should be discharged with elastic compression stockings of moderate pressure, with instructions to elevate the legs periodically during early recovery. The edema gradually subsides in most patients over the course of a few weeks, but it may occasionally linger for several months. Delayed wound complications have been reported to occur in as many as 50 per cent of these patients.

RESULTS

General Principles of Interpretation

Comprehensive assessment of the efficacy of infrainguinal reconstruction as reported in the literature is confounded by a frustrating multitude of variables that preclude statistically valid comparisons. Unfortunately, even standardized methods of reporting, as suggested by the ad hoc committee of the International Society for Cardiovascular Surgery/Society for Vascular Surgery (ISCVS/SVS), have not been uniformly adopted.[88] Most authors use life table methods for reporting graft patency, limb salvage, and patient survival, which in turn allows the reader to assess the actuarial probability of the specific end-point after a given interval of time. Graft patency rates are customarily reported as primary or secondary. *Primary patency* usually refers to only those grafts that either require no further intervention after initial bypass or need revision or extension while they are still patent. Some authors consider grafts to be primarily patent even though an acute thrombectomy and revision may have been required for acute thrombosis within 48 hours of the original procedure. Still others consider separately grafts that have required some form of revision while still patent to have ''primary assisted'' or ''primary revised'' patency. *Secondary patency* refers to all grafts that remain primarily patent as well as to thrombosed grafts requiring lysis or thrombectomy with revision. Secondary graft patency rates should not be confused with primary patency rates derived from secondary or reoperative procedures. Successful limb salvage rates customarily include those limbs requiring minor amputation to the transmetatarsal level. Unfortunately, limb salvage rates may be speciously enhanced by inclusion of patients initially operated on for claudication as well as those operated on for critical ischemia. Another common problem in assessing life table analyses are results reported prematurely, with an insufficient number of grafts at risk at longer-term intervals. For instance, the validity of an 80 per cent mean graft patency rate reported for only one or two limbs at risk may be compromised by a large standard error.

Indications for a particular procedure undergoing analysis may demonstrate extraordinary variation. Claudication is a relatively subjective symptom, and although limb viability is clearly threatened by ischemic tissue necrosis, rest pain also remains a subjective complaint that defies quantitation. Patients in the affected age group often have pain from various sources other than ischemia, including arthritis and neuropathy. Broad interpretation of criteria for determining claudication as disabling and rest pain as truly limb threatening contributes to considerable variation in reported results.

The site chosen for the distal anastomosis is also of importance, less so with more tolerant autogenous vein grafts and more so with relatively thrombogenic prosthetic grafts, and it cannot be considered independently from the quality of outflow. Thus, a bypass to a popliteal artery with single-vessel runoff will not fare as well as a similar graft to a popliteal vessel with three unobstructed infrapopliteal vessels for outflow. Although the site of the distal anastomosis is frequently included in analyses of results, the status of the outflow often is not, and it may in fact prove to be the more important variable.[88]

The choice of conduit is a most important determinant of graft patency. In most circumstances, autogenous vein provides a more durable reconstruction than any prosthetic graft, yet several series combine both types of conduit in reporting results.[52] In similar fashion, some reports of all autogenous reconstructions use greater superficial saphenous vein in both reversed and in situ configurations and may include arm, lesser saphenous, and composite vein grafts. Although an appreciable difference between reversed and in situ saphenous vein grafts has not been consistently demonstrated, both usually demonstrate better patency rates than either arm or lesser saphenous vein.[89–94] In addition, the quality and caliber of vein used are important but not easily documented variables.[46, 79] Technical considerations also confound accurate comparison of concurrent reports. Methods of vein preparation, magnification, experience of the surgical team, and intraoperative assessment on completion of the bypass are not necessarily uniform. Although completion arteriography has undoubtedly reduced the number of technical complications resulting in early graft failure, both intraoperative duplex scanning and angioscopy are being used with increasing frequency and may favorably or unfavorably influence the ultimate result.

The extent of significant comorbidity also influences the ultimate outcome. Significant susceptibility to myocardial ischemia increases the risk for perioperative cardiac morbidity and mortality and reduces longer-term survival.[13–17] The presence of diabetes has not significantly altered the results when compared with those observed in nondiabetics; in fact, many series have demonstrated better results in diabetics.[77–79, 95] Patients with mild renal insufficiency and threatened limbs achieve graft patency rates comparable to those of patients with normal renal function, but they sustain higher operative mortality and diminished survival.[96–100] Those with end-stage renal disease, however, especially diabetics, demonstrate lower patency rates. The relatively recent recognition that a significant number of vascular surgery patients harbor a variety of hypercoagulopathies, most commonly antiphospholipid syndrome and heparin-induced platelet aggregation, represents yet another example of significant comorbidity affecting the outcome of bypass results.[101]

Postoperative management of these patients is of critical importance to sustained graft patency. Patients who persist in using tobacco have significantly lower graft patency and limb salvage rates than do patients who abstain from smoking after reconstruction.[81, 95, 102] The role of long-term anticoagulation is currently under investigation with autogenous reconstruction in a cooperative Veterans Administration study, but it has been shown to enhance the primary patency of long prosthetic grafts and is commonly used after secondary intervention for a failed graft.[75] It has been repeatedly shown that repair of vein graft or perianastomotic stenosis before graft thrombosis provides satisfactory sustained patency rates of approximately 80 per cent after 5 years.[71, 103–105] In contrast, similar intervention for recently thrombosed grafts, necessitating initial catheter thrombectomy or thrombolysis, yields much lower patency rates (20 to 30 per cent). This observation has spawned various postoperative graft surveillance protocols, which have demonstrated that neither recurrent ischemic symptoms nor reduced ankle-brachial indices are as reliable in identifying these stenotic lesions, and therefore incipient graft failure, as routine serial duplex evaluation.[73, 106–108] Variations in postoperative surveillance protocols, then, will significantly alter secondary patency results and overall limb salvage rates.

Autogenous Vein Bypass

Four representative series of autogenous infrainguinal bypasses illustrated in Table 53–1 report operative mortality rates of 1 to 3 per cent.[77–79, 109] Primary 5-year patency rates ranged from 63 to 75 per cent, and secondary patency rates ranged from 80 to 83 per cent. Limb salvage rates ranged from 84 to 92 per cent, and overall patient survival rates of 28 to 66 per cent were observed at the end of 5 years. In an attempt to arrive at working figures that enable the practicing clinician to make reasonable decisions and discuss potential outcome with patients, results from several series may be averaged by dividing the sum of the product of the number of limbs and the patency rate (per cent) by the sum of the limbs. This formula represents an effort to correct for variations in the number of patients in each series:

$$\% = \frac{\Sigma(N \times \%)}{\Sigma(N)}$$

Although these four series are relatively comparable, three reports are restricted to experience with in situ greater saphenous vein,[78, 79, 109] and Taylor and coworkers reported experience with reversed autogenous vein including arm and lesser saphenous sources.[77] Claudicators comprised less than 10 per cent of the series reported by Leather and associates[109] and Bergamini and colleagues,[79] and approximately 70 per cent of their bypasses were carried to the tibial level. In contrast, 20 to 30 per cent of procedures reported by Taylor and coworkers[77] and Donaldson and associates[78] were indicated for claudication, and fewer than 50 per cent were infrapopliteal. Table 53–2 illustrates the weighted average of results from these same four series for autogenous reconstructions to above-knee, below-knee, and infrapopliteal levels.

As techniques have improved, allowing the use of smaller-caliber vein, progressively more distal bypasses have been carried out in patients with more extensive disease who would not have been considered appropriate candidates for reconstruction in the early 1980s. This is evidenced by the increasing number of femorotibial bypasses, ranging from 45 to 68 per cent of the series listed in Table 53–1. Bypasses to the peroneal artery, frequently the only suitable alternative in diabetics, have provided results as durable as those of bypasses to the anterior or posterior tibial vessels.[76, 78, 79] Increasing use of the in situ technique

Table 53–1. Infrainguinal Reconstruction With Autogenous Vein

Study	No. of Limbs	Operative Mortality (%)	5-Year Cumulative Rates (%) Graft Patency Primary	Secondary	Limb Salvage	Patient Survival
Taylor et al, 1990[77]	516	1	75	80	90	28
Bergamini et al, 1991[79]	361	3	63	81	86	57
Donaldson et al, 1991[78]	440	2	72	83	84	66
Leather et al, 1992[109]	1688	3	70	81	92	58
Weighted average	3005	2	70	81	90	54

has enabled the use of smaller-caliber veins of 2.5 mm in diameter,[46, 76, 79] and improved methods of exposure and surgical technique allow anastomoses to be constructed as far distally as the plantar branches.[110] Femorotibial bypasses provide primary patency rates ranging from 63 to 69 per cent and secondary patency rates of 72 to 85 per cent after 5 years (see Table 53–2), and acceptable results have also been reported for various subgroups using these distal vessels. For instance, vein grafts beyond the ankle level provide average patency rates of 50 per cent after 4 to 5 years (Table 53–3). In the absence of sufficient length of saphenous vein for conventional femorotibial bypass, a shorter length of residual vein originating from a patent below-knee popliteal artery provides similar 5-year patency rates of 40 to 55 per cent.[111–119] Distal grafts originating from a proximal tibial vessel have also proved satisfactory,[120] as have bypass vein grafts to the plantar vessels, which provide significant salvage of limbs jeopardized by overt distal gangrene.[121, 122]

In the absence of suitable greater saphenous vein, alternative sources include arm and lesser saphenous vein. Primary patency rates associated with arm vein have been reported to range from 40 per cent at 3 years to 50 per cent after 5 years, with secondary patency rates approaching 60 per cent after 5 years and limb salvage rates as high as 82 per cent.[123–125] Arm vein is a less reliable conduit than vein from other sources but provides acceptable results, particularly in the setting of severely compromised outflow, in which prosthetic material has proved unsatisfactory.[126] Evidence suggests that preliminary intraoperative angioscopy may enable correction of unsuspected endoluminal defects more frequently encountered in arm vein than in other venous conduits and thereby improve overall durability.[36] Lesser saphenous vein is yet another autogenous conduit that is associated with primary patency rates of 77 per cent at 2 years and 55 per cent after 3 years. Finally, because of the limited number of patients for whom sequential bypass proves to be appropriate, collective experience has been limited. Reported patency rates, however, have exceeded 80 per cent after 1 year and have ranged from 42 to 64 per cent after 4 years.[127–130]

The deeper femoral and popliteal veins are additional sources of autogenous material and have been used for femoropopliteal reconstruction despite the risk of significant lower extremity edema and the longer operating time required. Harvesting of the shortest possible length of femoral vein with preservation of the deep femoral vein is desirable. In a series of 100 such reconstructions, Shulman and associates reported a 64 per cent 5-year patency rate and a 70 per cent limb salvage rate.[131] These results also reflect adjunctive profundaplasty and secondary interventions. The incidence of early lower extremity edema is significant, but the magnitude of subsequent chronic disability remains unclear at present.

Prosthetic Bypass

Results achieved with infrainguinal bypass using PTFE (Table 53–4) have been less satisfactory than those

Table 53–2. Weighted Average Primary Graft Patency Rates Associated With Infrainguinal Reconstruction Using Autogenous Vein

Site of Distal Anastomosis	Study	Total No. of Limbs	5-Year Cumulative Patency Rates (%) Primary	Secondary
Popliteal				
Above-knee	Donaldson et al, 1991[78] Taylor et al, 1990[77]	155	75	83
Below-knee	Donaldson et al, 1991[78] Taylor et al, 1990[77] Bergamini et al, 1991[79] Leather et al, 1992[109]	952	74	83
Infrapopliteal	Donaldson et al, 1991[78] Taylor et al, 1990[77] Bergamini et al, 1991[79] Leather et al, 1992[109]	1843	67	78

Table 53–3. Paramalleolar Infrapopliteal Reconstruction With Autogenous Vein

Study	No. of Limbs	Primary Patency Rates (%)		4- to 5-Year Limb Salvage Rate (%)
		2- to 3-Year	*4- to 5-Year*	
Andros et al, 1988[114]	224	62	40	71
Klamer et al, 1990[115]	68	81	81	95
Pomposelli et al, 1990[28]	97	80	—	—
Shah et al, 1992[116]	270	74	61	89
Harrington et al, 1992[117]	73	59	50	74
Weighted average	732	70	55	82

Table 53–4. Infrainguinal Reconstruction With Polytetrafluoroethylene

Study	5-Year Primary Patency Rates (%)							
	Femoropopliteal AK and BK		*Femoropopliteal AK*		*Femoropopliteal AK-Claudication*		*Infrapopliteal*	
	No.	Patency	No.	Patency	No.	Patency	No.	Patency
Hobson et al, 1985[132]	80	22					41	12
Charlesworth et al, 1985[133]	134	24	53	39				
Tilanus et al, 1985[134]	24	37						
Sterpetti et al, 1985[135]			90	58	41	76		
Veith et al, 1986[52]	171	38	91	38			98	12
Whittemore et al, 1989[53]	279	37	182	42	64	62	21	12
Patterson et al, 1990[136]			138	54				
Prendiville et al, 1990[81]			114	42	44	57		
Rosenthal et al, 1990[137]					100	65		
Davies et al, 1991[138]			48	63				
Aalders and Van Vroonhoven, 1992[66]			49	39	41	42		
Quiñones-Baldrich et al, 1992[82]	294	59	219	61	110	68	28	22
Pevec et al, 1992[139]	85	27						
Weighted average	1067	40	984	50	400	63	202	14

AK, above-knee; BK, below-knee.

obtained with autogenous vein, with the discrepancy most pronounced in the challenging low-flow conditions of the femorotibial bypass.[52, 53, 66, 81, 82, 132–138] On the basis of these studies, infrapopliteal reconstruction with PTFE provides an average patency rate of 14 per cent, rendering autogenous vein from nearly any source the preferred conduit. In contrast, PTFE in the femoropopliteal position provides 5-year patency rates averaging 40 per cent, less discrepant from those obtained with autogenous vein. As is true with vein, however, better results are achieved with reconstructions indicated for claudication than with those performed in the more challenging setting required for limb salvage. This finding is most pronounced for above-knee reconstructions, for which overall primary patency rates achieved in claudicators ranged from 42 to 68 per cent at the 5-year interval and averaged 63 per cent.

Because surgical technique and graft material are reasonably standardized, and provided that reporting methods are comparable, the significant variation in the results illustrated in Table 53–4 primarily reflects the different patient selection criteria with regard to indication and the quality of the popliteal vessel and its distal runoff. A prosthetic bypass to a compromised popliteal artery with single-vessel runoff cannot be expected to provide the durability of a similar bypass to a relatively disease-free popliteal artery with two- or three-vessel runoff. Most published series represent the summation of some combination of these extremes, but a preponderance of one or the other will shift overall patency rates to the higher or lower end of the range accordingly.

The claim that prosthetic reconstruction with PTFE in the above-knee location is superior to vein with regard to durability has yet to be substantiated by prospectively randomized patients treated by the same group of surgeons using standardized patient selection criteria. Availability of such controlled data is meager and is reviewed in more detail in Chapters 28 and 29.

Initially disappointing results with infrainguinal reconstruction using Dacron prosthetic grafts led to increasing enthusiasm for PTFE shortly after its introduction in the mid-1970s, when preliminary results obtained with PTFE initially appeared comparable to those achieved with saphenous vein. Now that long-term results with PTFE are well documented, it is not clear that it offers any distinct advantage over the textile Dacron material. In a randomized, prospective experience with above-knee infrainguinal reconstruction for claudicators, Rosenthal and coworkers reported a 5-year cumulative primary patency rate of 65 per cent for PTFE grafts and 67 per cent for Dacron, a difference that proved to be statistically insignificant.[137] More dramatic are results reported by Pevec and associates from a nonrandomized but concurrent experience in which the 48 per cent 5-year cumulative patency rate achieved with Dacron proved to be statistically superior to the 27 per cent rate associated with PTFE for femoropopliteal reconstruction, both above and below the knee and for all indications.[139]

Experience with human umbilical vein documents 5-year primary patency rates approximating 60 per cent for femoropopliteal grafts and ranging as high as 81 per cent in the above-knee location.[65, 66, 140–142] In the three randomized series available in the recent literature, umbilical vein demonstrated results that were statistically either comparable or superior to those achieved with PTFE.[65, 66, 138] Because all three series are reporting at 3-year intervals, the overall effect of aneurysmal dilatation of vein grafts cannot be factored into the equation. On the basis of past experience, however, aneurysmal degeneration may be anticipated in as many as 57 per cent of patent grafts after 2 years.[143] Dardik and colleagues reported aneurysmal degeneration in 36 per cent after 5 years and noted dilatation in an additional 21 per cent.[142]

CONCLUSION

Judicious selection of the appropriate method of infrainguinal reconstruction for a given patient requires an appreciation of the results obtained with all available approaches. Although percutaneous transluminal angioplasty may be appropriate for some patients with short-segment lesions and profundaplasty may be an expeditious solution in others, most patients with ischemic limbs require conventional surgical bypass. The majority of claudicators will achieve sustained relief, and 80 to 90 per cent of limbs threatened with critical ischemia are salvaged. Of variables influencing the ultimate outcome, choice of conduit is most important, and every effort must be made to use autogenous vein for optimal results. Additional factors influencing outcome include indications, the site of distal anastomosis and the associated outflow, and the extent of significant comorbidity. Sustained graft patency requires vigilant graft surveillance with secondary intervention before graft thrombosis occurs. A diligent multi-disciplinary approach to the patient with atherosclerosis must coordinate management of individual manifestations of the underlying systemic disease process and reduce predisposing risk factors to further improve results from infrainguinal reconstruction and overall life expectancy.

References

1. Boyd AM: The natural course of arteriosclerosis of lower extremities. Proc R Soc Med 55:591, 1962.
2. Imparato AM, Kim G, Davidson T, et al: Intermittent claudication: Its natural course. Surgery 78:795, 1975.
3. McAllister FF: The fate of patients with intermittent claudication managed non-operatively. Am J Surg 132:593, 1976.
4. Walsh DB, Gilbertson JJ, Zwolak RM, et al: The natural history of superficial femoral artery stenoses. J Vasc Surg 14:299, 1991.
5. McIntyre KE, Bailey SA, Malone JM, Goldstone J: Guillotine amputation in the treatment of nonsalvageable lower extremity infections. Arch Surg 119:450, 1984.
6. Gibbons GW: The diabetic foot; Amputations and drainage of infection. J Vasc Surg 5:791, 1987.
7. Veith FJ, Gupta SK, Samson RH, et al: Progress in limb salvage by reconstructive arterial surgery combined with new or improved adjunctive procedures. Ann Surg 194:386, 1981.
8. Szilagyi DE, Hageman JH, Smith RF, et al: Autogenous vein grafting in femoropopliteal atherosclerosis: The limits of its effectiveness. Surgery 86:836, 1979.
9. Hunink MGM, Donaldson MC, Meyerovitz MF, et al: Risks and benefits of femoral-popliteal percutaneous balloon angioplasty. J Vasc Surg 17:183, 1993.

10. River SP, Scher LA, Gupta SK, Veith FJ: Safety of peripheral vascular surgery after recent acute myocardial infarction. J Vasc Surg 11:70, 1990.
11. Kannel WB, Skinner JJ, Schwartz MJ, et al: Intermittent claudication: Incidence in the Framingham study. Circulation 41:857, 1970.
12. Hertzer NR, Beven EG, Young JR, et al: Coronary artery disease in peripheral vascular patients. A classification of 1000 coronary angiograms and results of surgical management. Ann Surg 199:223, 1984.
13. Raby KE, Goldman L, Creager MA, et al: Correlation between preoperative ischemia and major cardiac events after peripheral vascular surgery. N Engl J Med 321:1296, 1989.
14. Pasternak PF, Grossi EA, Baumann FG, et al: The value of silent myocardial ischemia monitoring in the prediction of perioperative myocardial infarction in patients undergoing peripheral vascular surgery. J Vasc Surg 10:617, 1989.
15. Golden MA, Whittemore AD, Donaldson MC, Mannick JA: Selective evaluation and management of coronary artery disease in patients undergoing repair of abdominal aortic aneurysms: A 16-year experience. Ann Surg 212:415, 1990.
16. Boucher CA, Brewster DC, Darling RC, et al: Determination of cardiac risk by dipyridamole-thallium imaging before peripheral vascular surgery. N Engl J Med 312:389, 1985.
17. Lette J, Waters D, Lassonde J, et al: Multivariate clinical models and quantitative dipyridamole-thallium imaging to predict cardiac morbidity and death after vascular reconstruction. J Vasc Surg 14:160, 1991.
18. Cohen JR, Mannick JA, Couch NP, Whittemore AD: Abdominal aortic aneurysm repair in patients with pre-operative renal failure. J Vasc Surg 3:867, 1986.
19. Whittemore AD, Donaldson MC, Mannick JA: Infrainguinal reconstruction for patients with chronic renal insufficiency. J Vasc Surg 17:32, 1993.
20. Haysukami TS, Primozich JF, Zierler RE, et al: Color Doppler imaging of infrainguinal arterial occlusive disease. J Vasc Surg 16:527, 1992.
21. Flanagan DP, Williams LR, Keifer T, et al: Prebypass operative arteriography. Surgery 92:627, 1982.
22. Ricco JB, Pearce WH, Yao JST, et al: The use of operative prebypass arteriography and Doppler ultrasound recordings to select patients for extended femorodistal bypass. Ann Surg 198:646, 1983.
23. Lalka SA, Anderson G, Bernhard VM, et al: Transcutaneous PO_2 and PCO_2 monitoring to determine severity of limb ischemia and predict surgical outcome. J Vasc Surg 7:507, 1988.
24. Sicard GA, Schier JJ, Totty WG, et al: Thrombolytic therapy for acute arterial occlusion. J Vasc Surg 2:65, 1985.
25. Parent FN, Piotrowski JJ, Bernhard VM, et al: Outcome of intraarterial urokinase for acute vascular occlusion. J Cardiovasc Surg 32:680, 1991.
26. Veith FJ, Ascer E, Gupta SK, et al: Lateral approach to the popliteal artery. J Vasc Surg 6:119, 1987.
27. Ascer E, Veith FJ, Gupta SK: Bypasses to plantar arteries and other tibial branches: An extended approach to limb salvage. J Vasc Surg 8:434, 1988.
28. Pomposelli FB, Jepsen SJ, Gibbons GW, et al: Efficacy of the dorsal pedal bypass for limb salvage in diabetic patients; Short term observations. J Vasc Surg 11:745, 1990.
29. Kunlin J: Le traitment de l'arterite obliterante par la greffe veineuse. Arch Mal Coeur Vaiss 42:371, 1949.
30. LoGerfo FW, Quist WC, Crawshaw HW: An improved technique of preservation of endothelial morphology in vein grafts. Surgery 90:1015, 1981.
31. Hall KV: The great saphenous vein used "in situ" as an arterial shunt after extirpation of vein values. Surgery 51:492, 1962.
32. Leather RP, Powers SR, Karmody AM: A reappraisal of the in situ saphenous vein arterial bypass: Its use in limb salvage. Surgery 86:453, 1979.
33. Leather RP, Shah DM, Chang BB, et al: Resurrection of the in situ saphenous vein bypass: 1000 cases later. Ann Surg 208:435, 1988.
34. Miller A, Stonebridge PA, Tsoukas AI, et al: Angioscopically directed valvulotomy: A new valvulotome and technique. J Vasc Surg 13:813, 1991.
35. Panetta TF, Marin ML, Veith FJ, et al: Unsuspected pre-existing saphenous vein pathology: An unrecognized cause of vein bypass failure. J Vasc Surg 15:102, 1992.
36. Marcaccio EJ, Miller A, Tannenbaum GA, et al: Angioscopically directed interventions improve arm vein bypass grafts. J Vasc Surg 17:994, 1993.
37. Leather RP, Shah DM, Corson JD, Karmody AM: Instrumental evolution of the valve incision method of in situ saphenous vein bypass. J Vasc Surg 1:113, 1984.
38. Bernhard VM, Boren CH, Towne JB: Pneumatic tourniquet as a substitute for vascular clamps in distal bypass surgery. Surgery 87:709, 1980.
39. DeLaurentis DA, Friedmann P: Sequential femoropopliteal bypasses: Another approach to the inadequate saphenous vein problem. Surgery 71:400, 1972.
40. Jarrett F, Berkoff HA, Crummy AB, et al: Femoro-tibial bypass grafts with sequential technique. Arch Surg 116:709, 1981.
41. Jarrett F, Perea A, Begelman K, et al: Hemodynamics of sequential bypass grafts in peripheral arterial occlusion. Surg Gynecol Obstet 150:377, 1980.
42. Shah DM, Chang BB, Leopold PW, et al: The anatomy of the greater saphenous venous system. J Vasc Surg 3:273, 1986.
43. Thompson RW, Mannick JA, Whittemore AD: Arterial reconstruction at diverse sites using nonreversed autogenous vein: An application of venous valvulotomy. Ann Surg 205:747, 1987.
44. Veith FJ, Gupta SK, Samson RH, et al: Superficial femoral and popliteal arteries as inflow sites for distal bypasses. Surgery 90:980, 1981.
45. Ascer E, Veith FJ, Gupta SK, et al: Short vein grafts: A superior option for arterial reconstruction to poor or compromised outflow tracts? J Vasc Surg 7:370, 1988.
46. Wengerter KR, Veith FJ, Gupta SK, et al: Influence of vein size (diameter) on infrapopliteal reversed vein graft patency. J Vasc Surg 11:525, 1990.
47. Chang BB, Paty PSK, Shah DM, Leather RP: The lesser saphenous vein: An under-appreciated source of autogenous vein. J Vasc Surg 15:152, 1992.
48. Dardik H, Ibrahim IM, Dardik I: Evaluation of glutaraldehyde-tanned human umbilical cord vein as a vascular prosthesis for bypass to the popliteal, tibial and peroneal arteries. Surgery 83:577, 1978.
49. Campbell CC, Goldfarb B, Roe R: A small arterial substitute: Expanded microporous polytetrafluoroethylene: Patency versus porosity. Ann Surg 182:138, 1975.
50. Veith FJ, Moss CM, Fell SC, et al: Expanded polytetrafluoroethylene grafts in reconstructive arterial surgery. Preliminary report of the first 100 consecutive cases for limb salvage. JAMA 240:1867, 1978.
51. Bergan JJ, Veith FJ, Bernhard VM, et al: Randomization of autogenous vein and polytetrafluoroethylene grafts in femoral-distal reconstruction. Surgery 92:921, 1982.
52. Veith FJ, Gupta SK, Ascer E, et al: Six-year prospective multicenter randomized comparison of autologous saphenous vein and expanded polytetrafluoroethylene graft in infrainguinal arterial reconstruction. J Vasc Surg 3:104, 1986.
53. Whittemore AD, Kent KC, Donaldson MC, et al: What is the proper role of polytetrafluoroethylene grafts in infrainguinal reconstruction? J Vasc Surg 10:299, 1989.
54. Miller JH, Foreman RK, Ferguson L, Faris I: Interposition vein cuff for anastomosis of prosthesis to small artery. Aust NZ J Surg 54:283, 1984.
55. Taylor RS, McFarland RJ, Cox MI: An investigation into the causes of failure of PTFE grafts. Eur J Vasc Surg 1:335, 1987.
56. Tyrrell MR, Chester JF, Vipond MN, et al: Experimental evidence to support the use of interposition vein collars/patches in distal PTFE anastomoses. Eur J Vasc Surg 4:95, 1990.
57. Tyrrell MR, Grigg MJ, Wolfe JHN: Is arterial reconstruction to the ankle worthwhile in the absence of autologous vein? Eur J Vasc Surg 3:429, 1989.
58. Ibrahim IM, Sussman B, Dardik H, et al: Adjunctive arteriovenous fistula with tibial and peroneal reconstruction for limb salvage. Am J Surg 140:246, 1980.
59. Paty PSK, Shah DM, Saifi J, et al: Remote distal arteriovenous fistula to improve infrapopliteal bypass patency. J Vasc Surg 11:171, 1990.
60. Flinn WR, Ricco JB, Yao JST, et al: Composite sequential grafts in severe ischemia: A comparative study. J Vasc Surg 1:449, 1984.
61. Flinn WR, Rohrer MJ, Yao JST, et al: Improved long-term patency of infragenicular polytetrafluoroethylene grafts. J Vasc Surg 7:685, 1988.

62. Dardik H: The use of glutaraldehyde-stabilized umbilical vein for lower extremity reconstruction. *In* Greenhalgh RM (ed): Vascular Surgical Techniques: An Atlas. London, WB Saunders, 1989.
63. Dardik H, Miller N, Dardik A, et al: A decade of experience with the glutaraldehyde-tanned human umbilical cord vein graft for revascularization of the lower limb. J Vasc Surg 7:336, 1988.
64. Hasson JE, Newton WD, Waltman AC, et al: Mural degeneration in the glutaraldehyde-tanned umbilical vein graft: Incidence and implications J Vasc Surg 4:243, 1986.
65. McCollum C, Kenchington G, Alexander C, et al: PTFE or HUV for femoro-popliteal bypass: A multi-center trial. Eur J Vasc Surg 5:435, 1991.
66. Aalders GJ, van Vroonhoven TJM: PTFE versus HUV in above-knee femoro-popliteal bypass. Six year results of a randomized clinical trial. J Vasc Surg 16:816, 1992.
67. Johnson WC, Lee KK, Bartle E, et al: Comparative evaluation of PTFE, HUV and saphenous vein bypasses in fem-pop AK vascular reconstruction. J Vasc Surg (In press).
68. Baxter BT, Rizzo RJ, Flinn WR, et al: A comparative study of intraoperative angioscopy and completion arteriography following femorodistal bypass. Arch Surg 125:997, 1990.
69. Miller A, Marcaccio E, Tannenbaum GA, et al: Comparison of angioscopy and angiography for monitoring infrainguinal bypass vein grafts: Results of a prospective randomized trial. J Vasc Surg 15:1078, 1992.
70. Gilbertson JJ, Walsh DB, Zwolak RM, et al: A blinded comparison of angiography, angioscopy, and duplex scanning in the intraoperative evaluation of in situ saphenous vein bypass grafts. J Vasc Surg 15:121, 1992.
71. Whittemore AD, Clowes AW, Couch NP, Mannick JA: Secondary femoropopliteal reconstruction. Ann Surg 193:35, 1981.
72. Veith FJ, Weiser RK, Gupta SK, et al: Diagnosis and management of failing lower extremity arterial reconstructions prior to graft occlusion. J Cardiovasc Surg 25:381, 1984.
73. Bandyk DF, Schmitt DD, Seabrook GR, et al: Monitoring functional patency of in situ saphenous vein bypasses: The impact of a surveillance protocol and elective revision. J Vasc Surg 9:286, 1989.
74. Bandyk DF, Bergamini TM, Towne JB: Durability of vein graft revision: The outcome of secondary procedures. J Vasc Surg 113:200, 1991.
75. Kretschmer G, Wenzl E, Piza F, et al: The influence of anticoagulant treatment on the probability of function in femoropopliteal vein bypass surgery: Analysis of a clinical series (1970 to 1985) and interim evaluation of a controlled clinical trial. Surgery 102:453, 1987.
76. Leather RP, Shah DM, Chang BB, Kaufman JL: Resurrection of the in situ saphenous vein bypass. Ann Surg 208:435, 1988.
77. Taylor LM, Edwards JM, Porter JM: Present status of reversed vein bypass grafting: five-year results of a modern series. J Vasc Surg 11:193, 1990.
78. Donaldson MC, Mannick JA, Whittemore AD: Femoral-distal bypass with in situ greater saphenous vein: Long-term results using the Mills valvulotome. Ann Surg 213:457, 1991.
79. Bergamini TM, Towne JB, Bandyk DF, et al: Experience with in situ saphenous vein bypasses during 1981 to 1989: Determinant factors of long-term patency. J Vasc Surg 13:137, 1991.
80. Rafferty TD, Avellone JC, Farrell CJ, et al: A metropolitan experience with infrainguinal revascularization: Operative risk and later results in northeastern Ohio. J Vasc Surg 6:365, 1987.
81. Prendiville EJ, Yeager A, O'Donnell TF, et al: Long-term results with the above-knee popliteal expanded polytetrafluoroethylene graft. J Vasc Surg 11:517, 1990.
82. Quiñones-Baldrich WJ, Prego AA, Ucelay-Gomez R, et al: Long-term results of infrainguinal revascularization with polytetrafluoroethylene: A ten-year experience. J Vasc Surg 16:209, 1992.
83. Donaldson MC, Mannick JA, Whittemore AD: Causes of primary graft failure after in situ saphenous vein bypass grafting. J Vasc Surg 15:113, 1992.
84. Reifsnyder T, Bandyk D, Seabrook G, et al: Wound complications of the in situ saphenous vein bypass technique. J Vasc Surg 15:843, 1992.
85. Schwartz ME, Harrington EB, Schanzer H: Wound complications after in situ bypass. J Vasc Surg 7:802, 1988.
86. Wengrovitz M, Atnip RG, Gifford RRM, et al: Wound complications of autogenous subcutaneous infrainguinal arterial bypass surgery: Predisposing factors and management. J Vasc Surg 11:156, 1990.
87. AbuRahma AF, Woodruff BA, Lucente FC: Edema after femoropopliteal bypass surgery: Lymphatic and venous theories of causation. J Vasc Surg 11:461, 1990.
88. Rutherford RB, Flanigan DP, Gupta SK, et al: Suggested standards for reports dealing with lower extremity ischemia. J Vasc Surg 4:80, 1986.
89. Batson RC, Sottiurai VS: Nonreversed and in situ vein grafts: Clinical and experimental observations. Ann Surg 201:771, 1985.
90. Fogle MA, Whittemore AD, Couch NP, Mannick JA: A comparison of in situ and reversed saphenous vein grafts for infrainguinal reconstruction. J Vasc Surg 5:46, 1987.
91. Veterans Administration Cooperative Study Group 141: Comparative evaluation of prosthetic, reversed, and in situ bypass grafts in distal popliteal and tibial-peroneal revascularization. Arch Surg 123:434, 1988.
92. Harris PL, How TV, Jones DR: Prospectively randomized clinical trial to compare in situ and reversed saphenous vein grafts for femoropopliteal bypass. Br J Surg 74:252, 1987.
93. Wengerter KR, Veith FJ, Gupta SK, et al: Prospective randomized multicenter comparison of in situ and reversed vein infrapopliteal bypasses. J Vasc Surg 13:189, 1991.
94. Moody AP, Edwards PR, Harris PL: In situ versus reversed femoropopliteal vein grafts: Long-term follow-up of a prospective, randomized trial. Br J Surg 79:750, 1992.
95. Rutherford RB, Jones DN, Bergentz SE, et al: Factors affecting the patency of infrainguinal bypass. J Vasc Surg 8:236, 1988.
96. Whittemore AD, Donaldson MC, Mannick JA: Infrainguinal reconstruction for patients with chronic renal insufficiency. J Vasc Surg 17:32, 1993.
97. Edwards JM, Taylor LM, Porter JM: Limb salvage in end-stage renal disease (ESRD): Comparison of modern results in patients with and without ESRD. Arch Surg 123:1164, 1988.
98. Chang BB, Paty PS, Shah DM, et al: Results of infrainguinal bypass for limb salvage in patients with end-stage renal disease. Surgery 108:742, 1990.
99. Harrington EB, Harrington ME, Schanzer H, Haimov M: End-stage renal disease—Is infrainguinal limb revascularization justified? J Vasc Surg 12:691, 1990.
100. Sanchez LA, Goldsmith J, Rivers SP, et al: Limb salvage surgery in end-stage renal disease: Is it worthwhile? J Cardiovasc Surg 33:344, 1992.
101. Donaldson MC, Weinberg DS, Belkin M, et al: Screening for hypercoagulable states in vascular practice: A preliminary study. J Vasc Surg 11:825, 1990.
102. Ameli FM, Stein M, Prosser RJ, et al: Effects of cigarette smoking on outcome of femoral popliteal bypass for limb salvage. J Cardiovasc Surg 30:591, 1989.
103. O'Mara CS, Flinn WR, Johnson ND, et al: Recognition and surgical management of patent but hemodynamically failed arterial grafts. Ann Surg 193:467, 1981.
104. Cohen JR, Mannick JA, Couch NP, Whittemore AD: Recognition and management of impending vein-graft failure. Arch Surg 121:758, 1986.
105. Brewster DC, LaSalle AJ, Robison JG, et al: Femoropopliteal graft failures: Clinical consequences and success of secondary reconstructions. Arch Surg 118:1043, 1983.
106. Wolfe JHN, Thomas ML, Jamieson CW, et al: Early diagnosis of femorodistal graft stenoses. Br J Surg 74:268, 1987.
107. Mills JL, Harris EJ, Taylor LM, et al: The importance of routine surveillance of distal bypass graft with duplex scanning: A study of 379 reversed vein grafts. J Vasc Surg 12:379, 1990.
108. Green RM, McNamara J, Ouriel K, DeWeese JA: Comparison of infrainguinal graft surveillance techniques. J Vasc Surg 11:207, 1990.
109. Leather RP, Fitzgerald K: Personal communication from Vascular Data Registry, Department of Surgery, Albany Medical College, October 19, 1992.
110. Andros G, Harris RW, Salles-Cunha SX, et al: Lateral plantar artery bypass grafting: Defining the limits of foot revascularization. J Vasc Surg 10:511, 1989.
111. Cantelmo NL, Snow JR, Menzoian JO, LoGerfo FW: Successful

vein bypass in patients with an ischemic limb and a palpable popliteal pulse. Arch Surg 121:217, 1986.
112. Rhodes GR, Rollins D, Sidaway A, et al: Popliteal-to-tibial in situ saphenous vein bypass for limb salvage in diabetic patients. Am J Surg 154:245, 1987.
113. Rosenbloom MS, Walsh JJ, Schuler JJ, et al: Long-term results of infragenicular bypasses with autogenous vein originating from the distal superficial femoral and popliteal arteries. J Vasc Surg 7:691, 1988.
114. Andros G, Harris RW, Salles-Cunha SX, et al: Bypass grafts to the ankle and foot. J Vasc Surg 7:785, 1988.
115. Klamer TW, Lambert GE, Richardson JD, et al: Utility of inframalleolar arterial bypass grafting. J Vasc Surg 11:165, 1990.
116. Shah DM, Darling RC, Chang BB, et al: Is long vein bypass from groin to ankle a durable procedure? An analysis of a ten-year experience. J Vasc Surg 15:402, 1992.
117. Harrington EB, Harrington ME, Schanzer H, et al: The dorsalis pedis bypass—Moderate success in difficult situations. J Vasc Surg 15:409, 1992.
118. Marks J, King TA, Baele H, et al: Popliteal-to-distal bypass for limb threatening ischemia. J Vasc Surg 15:755, 1992.
119. Wengerter KR, Yang PM, Veith FJ, et al: A twelve-year experience with the popliteal-to-distal artery bypass: The significance and management of proximal disease. J Vasc Surg 15:143, 1992.
120. Veith FJ, Ascer E, Gupta SK, et al: Tibiotibial vein bypass graft: A new operation for limb salvage. J Vasc Surg 2:552, 1985.
121. Tannenbaum GA, Pomposelli FB, Marcaccio EJ, et al: Safety of vein bypass grafting to the dorsal pedal artery in diabetic patients with foot infections. J Vasc Surg 15:982, 1992.
122. Dalsing MC, White JV, Yao JST, et al: Infrapopliteal bypass for established gangrene of the forefoot or toes. J Vasc Surg 2:669, 1985.
123. Andros G, Harris RW, Salles-Cunha SX, et al: Arm veins for arterial revascularization of the leg: Arteriographic and clinical observations. J Vasc Surg 4:416, 1986.
124. Balshi JD, Cantelmo NL, Menzoian JO, LoGerfo FW: The use of arm veins for infrainguinal bypass in end-stage peripheral vascular disease. Arch Surg 124:1078, 1989.
125. Harward TRS, Coe D, Flynn TC, Seeger JM: The use of arm vein conduits during infrageniculate arterial bypass. J Vasc Surg 16:420, 1992.
126. Sesto ME, Sullivan TM, Hertzer NR, et al: Cephalic vein grafts for lower extremity revascularization. J Vasc Surg 15:543, 1992.
127. Burdick JF, O'Mara C, Ricotta J, et al: The multiple sequential distal bypass graft: Improving nature's alternatives. Surgery 89:536, 1981.
128. Calhoun TR, Wright RM, Wright RM Jr, et al: Sequential bypass grafting for salvage of lower extremities. South Med J 78:41, 1985.
129. Lamberth WC Jr, Karkow WS: Sequential femoropopliteal-tibial bypass grafting: Operative technique and results. Ann Thorac Surg 42:531, 1986.
130. Rosenfeld JC, Savarese RP, Friedman P, et al: Sequential femoropopliteal and femorotibial bypasses: A ten year follow-up study. Arch Surg 116:1538, 1981.
131. Schulman ML, Badhey MR, Yatco R, Pillari G: A saphenous alternative: Preferential use of superficial femoral and popliteal veins as femoropopliteal bypass grafts. Am J Surg 152:231, 1986.
132. Hobson RW II, Lynch TG, Zafar J, et al: Results of revascularization and amputation in severe lower extremity ischemia: A five-year clinical experience. J Vasc Surg 2:174, 1985.
133. Charlesworth PM, Brewster DC, Darling RC, et al: The fate of polytetrafluoroethylene grafts in lower limb bypass surgery: A six-year follow-up. Br J Surg 72:896, 1985.
134. Tilanus HW, Obertop H, Van Urk H: Saphenous vein or PTFE for femoropopliteal bypass. A prospective randomized trial. Ann Surg 202:780, 1985.
135. Sterpetti AV, Schultz RD, Feldhaus RJ, Peetz Jr DJ: Seven-year experience with polytetrafluoroethylene as above-knee femoropopliteal bypass graft. Is it worthwhile to preserve the autologous saphenous vein? J Vasc Surg 2:907, 1985.
136. Patterson RB, Fowl RJ, Kempczinski RF, et al: Preferential use of ePTFE for above-knee femoropopliteal bypass grafts. Ann Vasc Surg 4:338, 1990.
137. Rosenthal D, Evans D, McKinsey J, et al: Prosthetic above-knee femoropopliteal bypass for intermittent claudication. J Cardiovasc Surg 31:462, 1990.
138. Davies MG, Feeley TM, O'Malley MK, et al: Infrainguinal polytetrafluoroethylene grafts: Saved limbs or wasted effort? A report on ten years' experience. Ann Vasc Surg 5:519, 1991.
139. Pevec WC, Darling RC, L'Italien GJ, Abbott WM: Femoropopliteal reconstruction with knitted, nonvelour Dacron versus expanded polytetrafluoroethylene. J Vasc Surg 16:60, 1992.
140. Boontje AH: Aneurysm formation in human umbilical vein grafts used as arterial substitutes. J Vasc Surg 2:524, 1985.
141. Eickoff JH, Broome A, Ericsson BF, et al: Four years' results of a prospective randomized clinical trial comparing polytetrafluoroethylene and modified human umbilical vein for below-knee femoropopliteal bypass. J Vasc Surg 6:506, 1987.
142. Dardik H, Miller N, Dardik A, et al: A decade of experience with the glutaraldehyde-tanned human umbilical cord vein graft for revascularization of the lower limb. J Vasc Surg 7:336, 1988.
143. Hasson JE, Newton WD, Waltman AC, Fallon JT: Mural degeneration in the glutaraldehyde-tanned umbilical vein graft: Incidence and implications. J Vasc Surg 4:243, 1986.

54

Extra-Anatomic Bypass

Robert B. Rutherford, M.D., and Max B. Mitchell, M.D.

• • •

The term *extra-anatomic bypass* has been applied to grafts that pass through a significantly different anatomic pathway than the natural blood vessels they replace. Although correctly criticized by purists as a misnomer, the term has gained practically universal acceptance. Ordinarily, the use of such a bypass implies deliberate avoidance of the natural location of the vascular supply, either because of hostile pathology there or because entering the area adds to the risk of the operation (as in entering the abdomen). The term commonly applies to an axillofemoral or a femorofemoral bypass or to their combination, the so-called axillobifemoral bypass. Other extra-anatomic arterial bypasses, such as carotid-subclavian, axilloaxillary, splenorenal, and crossover femoropopliteal bypass, are dealt with in appropriate chapters elsewhere in this book, as are infrainguinal bypasses, most of which are extra-anatomic to a greater or lesser degree (e.g., the in situ bypass). This chapter focuses on those extra-anatomic routes used to bypass aortoiliac occlusive disease under special circumstances in which the natural inflow has already been or must of necessity be interrupted and in which direct arterial reconstruction, such as aortobifemoral grafting, is precluded by either hostile abdominal pathology or the prohibitive operative risk of this approach as a result of impaired function of one or more vital organs. These operations consist primarily of the femorofemoral, axillounifemoral, and axillobifemoral bypasses, as illustrated in Figure 54–1. In addition, because one of the most common hostile conditions that preclude carrying a proximal bypass down to the usual femoral position is localized infection of a graft previously placed there, obturator foramen bypass, which is primarily used to avoid the infected groin, is also discussed.

HISTORICAL BACKGROUND[6]

In 1952, Freeman and Leeds described the use of a superficial femoral artery to carry blood directly from one femoral artery to another subcutaneously.[18] In 1958, McCaughan sutured a Dacron prosthesis to the left external iliac artery, brought it preperitoneally across to the right groin, and anastomosed it side-to-end to the right profunda femoris artery and end-to-side to the right popliteal artery, bypassing occlusions of the right iliac, common femoral, and superficial femoral arteries. In 1959, Lewis resected an abdominal aortic aneurysm but was unable to anastomose the proximal end of a homograft replacement to the abdominal or even the proximal thoracic aorta because of their involvement with dissecting aneurysm. Therefore, he resected the middle third of the clavicle, sutured a nylon graft end-to-end to the proximal subclavian artery, and brought the graft down the chest wall and into the abdomen at the level of the xiphoid process for anastomosis to the homograft. This somewhat bizarre but ingenious operation demonstrated that arteries in the upper extremity could be used to supply the lower half of the body. Faced with an infected abdominal aortic prosthesis, Blaisdell and associates anastomosed a Dacron graft to the descending thoracic aorta,

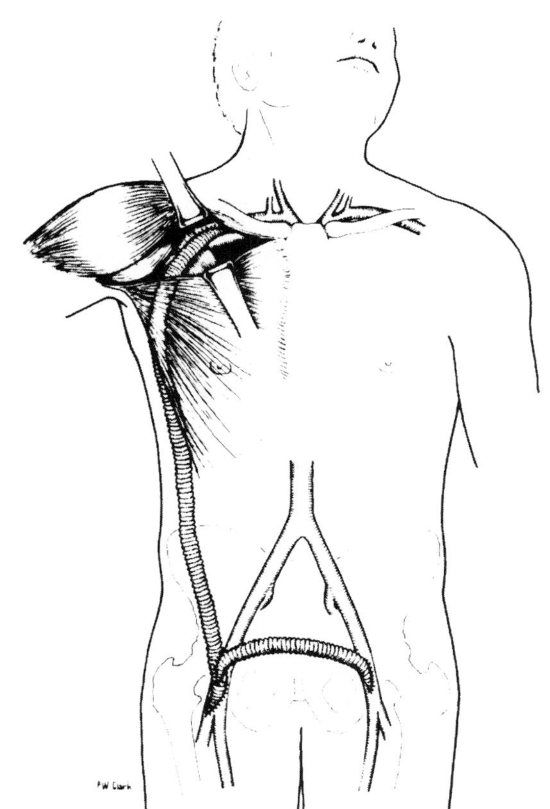

FIGURE 54–1. The axillobifemoral bypass graft represents a combination of axillofemoral and femorofemoral grafts and is employed in preference to bilateral axillofemoral grafts when both lower extremities require revascularization. (From Delaurentis DA, Sala LE, Russell E, McCombs PR: A twelve-year experience with axillofemoral and femorofemoral bypass operations. Surg Gynecol Obstet 147:881–887, 1978. By permission of Surgery, Gynecology & Obstetrics.)

brought it out through the chest below the 12th rib and down the lateral abdominal wall, and sutured it to the left common femoral artery. A ''side-arm'' was then anastomosed to this graft and brought suprapubically across to the right common femoral artery.[4] Warren had earlier reported a bypass between the splenic and iliofemoral arteries.[53] Thus, many surgeons had experimented with ingenious extra-anatomic bypasses before the femorofemoral and axillofemoral grafts were introduced and became the established forms of extra-anatomic bypass in the early 1960s.

In 1962, Vetto reported 10 *transabdominal* subcutaneous femorofemoral graft operations to bypass unilateral iliac occlusive disease in poor-risk patients.[52] The same year, reported almost simultaneously by Blaisdell and Hall and by Louw, Dacron grafts were placed between the axillary and ipsilateral femoral arteries for occlusive disease.[3, 28] Bilateral axillofemoral grafts were placed by Blaisdell and colleagues for revascularization of ischemic extremities after infected aortic prostheses had been removed.[5] Sauvage and Wood are given credit for combining these two procedures into an axillobifemoral graft procedure to avoid the need for bilateral, separate axillofemoral bypasses.[43] The obturator bypass was introduced in 1962 by Shaw and Baue as a means of bypassing graft sepsis localized to the groin.[45]

Originally, the use of extra-anatomic bypass grafts was restricted, for the most part, to cases in which there were complications of aortoiliac reconstruction, although even from the outset, extremely ill patients with impending gangrene were treated with both axillofemoral and femorofemoral grafting. However, within 5 years of the widespread application of these grafts, Alpert and coworkers openly recommended extra-anatomic bypass as the primary reconstructive approach in selected poor-risk patients.[1] By 1970, the same group suggested that the employment of these extra-anatomic bypasses, at least the femorofemoral bypass, had become a matter of ''preference rather than compromise.''[33] In 1972, they suggested that the femorofemoral bypass actually enhanced the continuing patency of the contralateral or ''donor'' iliac artery.[7] By 1977, LoGerfo and associates reported that axillobifemoral grafts had almost twice the flow rate and twice the patency of unilateral axillofemoral grafts.[27] In August of the previous year, this same group had reported that if one allowed for continuing patency achieved with the aid of thrombectomy, the axillobifemoral graft was comparable to the aortofemoral graft in patency but carried only one fourth the mortality rate.[22] However, at the height of this rising enthusiasm for extra-anatomic bypass (in fact, in the same edition of the *Annals of Surgery*), Eugene and coworkers reported a sobering follow-up of the extended experience with extra-anatomic bypass at the San Francisco Veterans Administration Hospital.[16] Subsequent reports of disappointing long-term results with extra-anatomic bypasses, combined with a steadily decreasing risk with direct transabdominal reconstruction (thanks to improved perioperative monitoring and intensive care), resulted in a more conservative, selective application of these procedures. However, more recent reports of improved long-term results have renewed debate about the more liberal application of axillofemoral and axillobifemoral bypasses[55, 56] versus a preference for aortofemoral bypass in all but the highest-risk patients.[57]

The early reported success of axillofemoral bypass ultimately prompted the use of *extended* extra-anatomic bypass procedures for limb-threatening ischemia when use of the femoral arteries was not feasible. Veith and coworkers reported limited success with axillopopliteal bypass in 1978.[58] Connolly and associates subsequently demonstrated modest success with both axillopopliteal and axillotibial bypass for limb salvage.[59] Two larger series with longer follow-up periods have indicated that axillopopliteal bypass can provide limb salvage for a considerable time in a patient population with relatively limited life expectancy.[60, 61]

Axillobifemoral bypass grafting, in conjunction with ligation of the iliac arteries to induce thrombosis of abdominal aortic aneurysms, has been recommended and evaluated as a low-risk alternative to resection in high-risk patients.[72] This is discussed in greater detail in Chapter 75, but it, too, has come under strong criticism based on its poorer patency, difficulty in achieving thrombosis without embolism of patent lumbar arteries, and most alarming, reports of rupture despite successful aneurysm thrombosis.[21, 25, 44] Although there is little argument that extra-anatomic bypass is indispensable when one is dealing with infected grafts, aortoenteric fistulae, and hostile intra-abdominal disease, its elective use as a primary reconstructive procedure, in preference to the direct transabdominal approach, in poor-risk patients with aortoiliac occlusive or aneurysmal disease is still a subject of considerable debate, as is discussed further in the section on indications.

HEMODYNAMIC CONSIDERATIONS

Axillofemoral and femorofemoral bypasses were originally intended only as makeshift or compromise procedures, primarily because it seemed unreasonable to expect one extremity to share its blood supply with another, and particularly when an upper extremity was expected to supply two legs. Furthermore, there was concern that if these grafts did provide more than a modest amount of additional flow to ''recipient'' extremities, this increased demand would produce a significant steal phenomenon in the ''donor'' extremity. However, it was not appreciated initially that the total resistance of parallel circuits, unlike resistances in series, would be less than the sum of its parts. Calculated as the reciprocal sum, the resistance to flow through the donor artery is actually significantly reduced by each extremity that the artery supplies, and its flow is increased accordingly. This has been confirmed by intraoperative electromagnetic flowmeter measurements.[33] Furthermore, in canine models of a femorofemoral bypass graft, flow through the graft to the recipient extremity could be increased 10-fold without producing a steal in the donor extremity.[14, 47] However, all of the foregoing studies were carried out in situations in which there was no outflow obstruction in either extremity.

Although resting ankle pressure in the donor limb is often initially decreased after femorofemoral bypass, it quickly returns to preoperative levels.[48] In fact, in relation to the brachial or systemic pressure, there is no statistically significant decrease: that is, the ankle-brachial *index* remains unchanged. Moreover, even though the ankle pressure in the donor extremity may drop following exercise, if the donor iliac artery is slightly stenosed, this does not constitute a true steal because the contralateral ankle pressure drops an equivalent degree. It is possible to produce a steal in the donor extremity following femorofemoral bypass *if* there is outflow occlusive disease (e.g., superficial femoral artery occlusion) on the *donor* side, but even this is not likely to become clinically manifest unless there is increased flow demand (e.g., with exercise), donor iliac artery stenosis, or poor cardiac function.

Although a steal or, more correctly, a decreased pressure in the donor limb can be demonstrated by noninvasive testing in up to 80 per cent of femorofemoral bypasses, it is rarely clinically significant.[17] However, even though the fear of significant steal in the donor extremity was proved to be unfounded, the same study showed that when either a significant degree of "inflow" stenosis or "outflow" occlusive disease existed, not only were the patency rates of these grafts greatly decreased, but so was their likelihood of relieving claudication or salvaging an extremity, despite continued graft patency. In this study, arteriographically documented inflow and outflow occlusive disease was correlated with the success of femorofemoral bypass. When there was neither inflow nor recipient outflow occlusive disease, the success rate was 90 per cent. When the recipient superficial femoral artery was significantly obstructed, the success rate was more than halved. When the latter was associated with even a moderate degree of obstruction of the donor iliac artery (e.g., 50 per cent), regardless of outflow status, all the grafts either thrombosed or failed to relieve the patient's symptoms. Finally, hemodynamic calculations indicate how little flow augmentation in response to exercise could be expected from a femorofemoral graft in the presence of recipient superficial femoral artery occlusion when there was also some stenosis of the donor iliac artery.[48] These hemodynamic considerations are obviously extremely important in deciding to employ extra-anatomic bypasses.

At one time, before the similarity between the peripheral circulation and electrical circuitry (in terms of the effect on flow of resistances in parallel and in series) was appreciated,[54] it was thought that the reasonably good patency rates of these makeshift grafts were due to their use in limb salvage situations in which there was a *continuous* demand for flow, as opposed to the *intermittent* demand in claudication. Although this argues against using extra-anatomic bypasses for claudication, the matter is not that simple. In fact, most studies have reported better patencies for the claudicator, probably because such patients tend to have better runoff. Furthermore, in 1974, Ernst reported the prophylactic use of an axillofemoral bypass graft before repair of a difficult suprarenal aortic aneurysm.[15] Surprisingly, this bypass remained patent despite the absence of a pressure gradient across the native artery it bypassed and, in fact, had to be closed because of disuse atrophy of that vessel, the ipsilateral iliac artery. Brief and associates have claimed that the crossover femorofemoral bypass is preferable to an ipsilateral iliofemoral bypass because the greater flows it produces in the donor iliac artery protect it against the atheromatous occlusive process that affected the contralateral vessel.[8] Follow-up angiography of femorofemoral bypasses has revealed a tendency toward dilatation of the donor iliac artery, possibly resulting from increased flow.[63] Although other investigators have acknowledged the better than expected long-term patency of the donor iliac artery in large series of femorofemoral bypasses, the senior author has observed its occlusion in 6 per cent of femorofemoral bypasses, which suggests that any protection it affords is certainly not absolute.[34] The final hemodynamic consideration worth comment relates to the observation by LoGerfo and coworkers that both flow and patency rates in axillobifemoral grafts were double those in unilateral axillofemoral grafts.[27] The authors' experience parallels this observation;[40] however, two series have not demonstrated inferior patency rates for unilateral axillofemoral bypass grafts.[56, 64] This is an important consideration because it forms the basis for the practice of making the anastomosis with the crossover femoral graft as low as possible on the axillofemoral graft in order to take maximal advantage of this effect,[16, 36] and for performing an axillobifemoral rather than an axillounifemoral bypass in cases of limb-threatening ischemia on one side only. This is discussed further in the section on technique.

INDICATIONS

Femorofemoral Bypass

The femorofemoral bypass has the best overall patency rate of the extra-anatomic bypasses discussed in this chapter (Table 54–1). It is considered by many to be the operation of choice for unilateral iliac artery occlusion in the elderly. Before one decides in favor of femorofemoral bypass, there are several aspects worth considering: (1) Is the donor iliac artery widely patent? (2) What is the status of the outflow vessels, particularly the superficial femoral artery, and how will this affect patency, likelihood of relief of symptoms, and limb salvage? (3) Is the operation being performed for native iliac artery occlusion or occlusion of one limb of a bifurcation graft? (4) What are the other options, and how do they compare with femorofemoral bypass under the same circumstances? The status of the donor iliac artery may be determined by biplanar arteriography, but physiologic testing may be more accurate. A normal thigh-brachial index, a thigh plethysmographic tracing with a brisk upslope and good excursion, and a triphasic waveform to an analog Doppler tracing recorded over the femoral artery[17] all indicate a wide-open iliofemoral segment. Direct measurement of femoral artery pressure and its response to a papaverine injection (see Chapter 5) is still the most practical and accurate way of detecting occult iliac artery stenosis, and with a little forethought, this should be performed at the time of arteriography.

If the superficial femoral artery is occluded, the patency of a femorofemoral graft is significantly reduced (from 92 to 52 per cent).[40] Further, in the presence of superficial femoral artery occlusion, the likelihood of symptomatic relief or limb salvage is reduced by more than half (from 90 to 41 per cent).[17] In the senior author's experience, the patency rate with femorofemoral bypass performed for native iliac artery occlusive disease was 74 per cent, compared with 39 per cent when bypass was performed for failure of one limb of a bifurcation graft. As seen in Table 54–2, such factors have a major bearing on outcome and

Table 54–1. Variation in Reported Results for Extra-Anatomic Bypass

Procedure	Study	Operative Mortality Rate (%)	5-Year Primary Patency Rate (%)	5-Year Secondary Patency Rate (%)
Femorofemoral	Brief et al, 1975[8]	4	81*	—
	Flanigan et al, 1978[17]	4	74*	—
	Livesay et al, 1979[26]	6	NR	56
	Eugene et al, 1976[16]	15	44	NR
	Rutherford et al, 1987[40]	0	74	82
	Chang, 1986[38]	NR	85	NR
	Hepp et al, 1988[39]	4	80	NR
Axillofemoral	Ray et al, 1979[36]	3	NR	67
	LoGerfo et al, 1977[27]	8	NR	37
	Eugene et al, 1976[16]	8	30	NR
	Rutherford et al, 1987[40]	13	19	37
	Ascer et al, 1985[64]	5	44	71
	Chang, 1986[38]	NR	33	NR
	Hepp et al, 1988[39]	5	NR	46
	El-Massry et al (In press)[56]	5	79	NR
Axillobifemoral	Ray et al, 1979[36]	5	NR	77
	LoGerfo et al, 1977[27]	8	NR	74
	Johnson et al, 1976[22]	2	NR	76
	Eugene et al, 1976[16]	8	33	NR
	Rutherford et al, 1987[40]	11	62	82
	Ascer et al, 1985[64]	5	50	77
	Chang, 1986[38]	NR	75	NR
	Hepp et al, 1988[39]	5	NR	73
	Harris et al, 1990[55]	5	85†	NR
	El-Massry et al (In press)[56]	5	76	NR
Axillopopliteal	Ascer et al, 1989[60]	8	40	59
	Keller et al, 1992[61]	20	43‡	50‡

**Patency not defined.*
†4-year patency.
‡3-year patency.
NR, not reported.

Table 54–2. Overall and Subgroup Patency Rates for Extra-Anatomic Bypasses

Type of Bypass	Occlusive Disease		Superficial Femoral Artery		No.	Patency (%)	
	Yes	*No*	*Patent*	*Occluded*		*Primary*	*Secondary*
Axillounifemoral	+	+	+	+	15	19	37
	+	+	+	−	7	54	54
	+	+	−	+	8	0	0
Axillobifemoral	+	+	+	+	54	62	81
	−	+	+	+	12	91	100
	+	−	+	+	42	47	69
	+	+	+	−	21	95	100
	+	+	−	+	33	46	60
	+	−	+	−	16	92	92
	+	−	−	+	26	41	58
	Native Artery	***Axillobifemoral Graft Limb***					
Femorofemoral	+	+	+	+	60	67	74
	−	+	+	+	13	39	51
	+	−	+	+	47	74	82
	+	+	+	−	22	79	95
	+	+	−	+	38	53	67
	+	−	+	−	19	92	100
	+	−	−	+	28	52	66

From Rutherford RB, Patt A, Pearce WH: Extra-anatomic bypass: A closer view. J Vasc Surg 5:437, 1987.

must be taken into consideration in the risk : benefit analysis that determines the indications for surgery in individual cases.

The options to femorofemoral bypass are iliofemoral bypass (if the ipsilateral common femoral is patent), transluminal angioplasty (if a suitable stenosis is present), unilateral aortofemoral bypass or iliofemoral endarterectomy through a retroperitoneal approach, and aortobifemoral bypass (in a good-risk patient in whom contralateral iliac artery disease is present but not hemodynamically significant). Transluminal angioplasty is preferred for discrete (less than 5 cm) stenoses of the common iliac artery, in which the 5-year patency rate approaches 90 per cent.[41] Multiple stenoses or extensive disease of the iliac segment produces much inferior results, and dilatation of external iliac lesions fares no better than dilatation of femoropopliteal lesions.[23] Iliofemoral bypass is attractive because in trading an oblique retroperitoneal lower quadrant incision for a groin incision, one avoids a higher risk of graft infection and anastomotic aneurysm, leaves the ''normal'' femoral artery untouched, and performs a shorter, more direct bypass graft procedure. Despite these theoretical advantages, in the senior author's experience the iliofemoral bypass has not performed as well as the femorofemoral bypass.[34] This has been predicted by other investigators, who have also pointed out the danger of causing impotence in male patients when the left side is approached.[8] In that same report by one of the authors, aortobifemoral bypass, performed when only one iliac artery was hemodynamically significantly stenosed, did better than femorofemoral bypass in the face of superficial femoral artery occlusion (72 vs. 35 per cent 5-year primary patency, respectively). Patencies were equivalent when runoff was good.[34] In this experience, femorofemoral bypass was performed without mortality, compared with 3 per cent mortality for aortobifemoral bypass. In the presence of unilateral iliac artery occlusion and limited contralateral iliac stenosis, percutaneous transluminal angioplasty of the stenotic iliac artery can provide adequate donor femoral inflow to permit femorofemoral bypass. Patency with this combined approach is comparable to that with femorofemoral bypass in the absence of donor iliac artery stenosis.[34, 40] More recently, however, reports of good results with unilateral aortofemoral bypass[62, 67] and iliac-based proximal reconstructions[69] have added to the number of viable alternatives to femorofemoral bypass.

Suffice it to say, femorofemoral bypass is a safe operation that gives good patency when there is good runoff and can even be performed for disabling claudication in this situation. When superficial femoral artery occlusion is present, this bypass should not be performed for claudication, but it may be performed, with concomitant profundaplasty, for limb salvage in poor-risk patients. Aortofemoral bypass is preferred in good-risk patients whenever the contralateral iliac artery is diseased. When there is forefoot ulceration, gangrene, or infection, concomitant distal bypass is preferable to profundaplasty regardless of the proximal bypass used.[34, 41] Finally, femorofemoral bypass is an acceptable means of handling unilateral bifurcation graft limb occlusion that is not amenable to thrombectomy.[9]

Axillounifemoral Bypass

Because the axillounifemoral bypass has relatively much poorer 5-year patency rates (see Table 54–1), its application should be limited to patients who are clearly in a limb salvage situation, in whom the abdominal approach is strictly prohibited by either severe anesthetic risk or intra-abdominal disease (e.g., sepsis, irradiation, malignant tumor, or stomas) *and* in whom a closer donor artery is not available or cannot be made suitable by percutaneous transluminal angioplasty.[35] Unfortunately, when this procedure is limited to such patients, the results will be poor because of high risk and poor runoff. Thus, in the senior author's experience, the operative mortality rate for this ''low-risk alternative'' was 11 per cent, and no graft placed proximal to a superficial femoral artery occlusion remained patent beyond 30 months.[40] In contrast, when the procedure has been applied with more liberal indications and therefore in a better-risk, better-runoff setting, surprisingly good results have been obtained (e.g., 76 per cent patency[56]). As is seen in Table 54–3, half of the reports in the literature observed a patency difference in favor of axillobifemoral bypass, and the other half found no significant difference. However, in all the latter, the mean difference also favored axillobifemoral bypass. Therefore, it has been the senior author's preference to perform the latter procedure even when there is a *critical* degree of ischemia involving only one limb. Axillounifemoral bypass tends to be applied primarily for graft sepsis, as a temporizing measure, when the septic process prohibits femorofemoral crossover grafting.

Axillobifemoral Bypass

Axillobifemoral bypass has an overall 5-year patency rate ranging from 33 to 85 per cent. In the authors' opinion, it should rarely be performed for claudication, but rather in chronic critical ischemia or other situations in which there are mandatory requirements for femoral inflow and the direct transabdominal reconstructive approach is clearly contraindicated by either prohibitive risk or ''hostile''

Table 54–3. Long-Term Patency Comparison of Axillofemoral Versus Axillobifemoral Bypass

Study	Patency Rate of Axillofemoral Bypass (%)	Patency Rate of Axillobifemoral Bypass (%)
Significant difference observed		
LoGerfo et al, 1977[27]	37	74
Rutherford et al, 1987[40]	19*	62*
Chang, 1986[38]	33*	75*
Hepp et al, 1988[39]	46	73
No significant difference observed		
Ray et al, 1979[36]	67	77
Eugene et al, 1976[16]	30*	33*
Ascer et al, 1985[64]	44*	50*
El-Massry et al (In press)[56]	76*	79*

**Primary patency; others are secondary patency or not defined.*

intra-abdominal pathology. The latter includes an infected aortic graft, aortoenteric fistula, mycotic aneurysm, enteric sources of contamination (diverticulitis, ileocolitis, or stoma), failed high endarterectomy or bypass with juxtarenal occlusion, irradiation, retroperitoneal fibrosis, metastatic malignant disease, multiple abdominal operations with extensive adhesions, complex ventral hernia, massive obesity, and cirrhosis with ascites.

''Prohibitive anesthetic risk'' as an indication for choosing extra-anatomic bypass often requires a subjective decision, but one that should be based as much as possible on objective criteria. Severe cardiac disease (recent myocardial infarction, intractable heart failure, or significant angina pectoris); chronic renal failure (a creatinine clearance rate of less than 40 ml/hr or the need for hemodialysis); severe pulmonary insufficiency (dyspnea at rest, oxygen dependency, or a forced expiratory volume of less than 1 L/sec); morbid obesity (weight greater than 45 kg or at least 100 per cent above ideal body weight); and finally, any uncontrolled malignant or other systemic disease that limits life expectancy to less than 2 years all qualify patients for this indirect form of reconstruction for aortoiliac occlusive disease.

The skilled vascular surgeon, working in an optimal environment with good monitoring and intensive care facilities, should adhere to these more limited indications for axillobifemoral bypass, reserving it for very carefully selected patients, and should continue to treat the majority of patients with aortoiliac occlusive disease with direct transabdominal reconstruction, as detailed in Chapter 52. Extended extra-anatomic bypass (i.e., to the popliteal artery) should be performed only for limb-threatening ischemia. Indications include the previously enumerated factors that favor axillobifemoral bypass in the presence of concomitant occlusive disease of the common femoral or extensive involvement of both the superficial and the deep femoral branches. Subsequent distal revascularization may be required if a prior axillobifemoral bypass remains patent but fails to achieve clinical improvement. Finally, when obturator bypass cannot be performed in patients with either scarring or sepsis of the ipsilateral groin prohibiting a femoral anastomosis, axillopopliteal bypass is indicated.

Obturator Bypass

Although introduced and primarily used as a means of restoring extremity flow when direct vascularization was prohibited by graft sepsis localized to the groin,[37, 45] the ingenious obturator bypass has since been used in the face of crushing injuries to the groin,[29] for bypassing malignancies involving the inguinal nodes, or when irradiation to that area has resulted in occlusive arteritis.[11, 13, 20, 31] More commonly, it has been employed in dealing with infected femoral aneurysms caused by nonsterile technique practiced by drug abusers or physicians performing diagnostic or therapeutic maneuvers through this port of entry (this indication is discussed in detail in Chapter 82.)

It has also been used when the proximal anastomosis of a femorodistal bypass has become infected or would be, if suppurative inguinal nodes from a septic foot were ignored. Thus, almost any hostile groin pathology can force the surgery to bypass through the obturator foramen. The procedure differs from the other extra-anatomic bypasses discussed previously in that one is not using the inflow of another extremity. Because it is rarely applied electively for occlusive disease, the runoff status of the limb below the point of reentry tends to be normal. As a result, better long-term patencies may be achieved than with axillounifemoral bypass.

TECHNIQUES

Extra-anatomic bypasses are normally performed with the patient under light general or balanced endotracheal anesthesia because they involve only relatively superficial dissection and subcutaneous tunneling.[10, 42, 47] Obviously, a femorofemoral bypass can be satisfactorily performed under regional anesthesia (e.g., epidural) or even local anesthesia with sedation. Even axillofemoral grafting has been performed in this manner, with heavy narcotics or brief open-mask anesthesia being used during the tunneling process. Ordinarily this is not necessary, and either light general or balanced anesthesia, supplemented with local lidocaine infiltration for skin incisions, is employed in poor-risk patients.

For an *axillofemoral* or *axillobifemoral* bypass, the patient is placed in the supine position with the donor arm abducted no more than 90 degrees. Alternatively, the arm may be placed at the side but partly flexed at the elbow. This position, which roughly approximates that taken in reaching into one's pants pocket, does not pull the axillary artery into the deeper, more tightly stretched position that occurs with abduction, but it still allows access to the axilla and the upper part of the chest (Fig. 54–2). Ordinarily for an axillobifemoral graft, the axillary artery on the same side as the most severely ischemic lower extremity is selected as the donor. The accuracy of preoperative noninvasive examination of axillary artery inflow is imprecise. Calligaro and associates recommend inflow arteriography because they have found both a higher than expected incidence of inflow disease (25 per cent) and the failure of noninvasive examination to detect disease in 75 per cent of the patients found to have significant stenoses with arteriography.[66] All things being equal, the right subclavian artery is preferred as the donor because it has a much lower risk of eventually developing occlusive disease than the left. If the patient habitually sleeps on a particular side, one might choose to place the graft on the opposite side because a number of these grafts appear to become thrombosed during sleep, presumably when compressed by the patient lying on them. This suspicion has not been confirmed by noninvasive studies; however, the two studies with the highest patency rates for axillofemoral bypass used externally supported graft material, which may protect against thrombosis due to external graft compression.[55, 56] The operative field and the position of the patient for a left axillobifemoral graft are depicted in Figure 54–2.

Axillary exposure is gained through a transverse incision after the fibers of the pectoralis major muscle have been split and the deltipectoral fascia has been opened. The axillary artery, which lies deep and superior to the axillary vein and inferior to the brachial plexus, is identified by

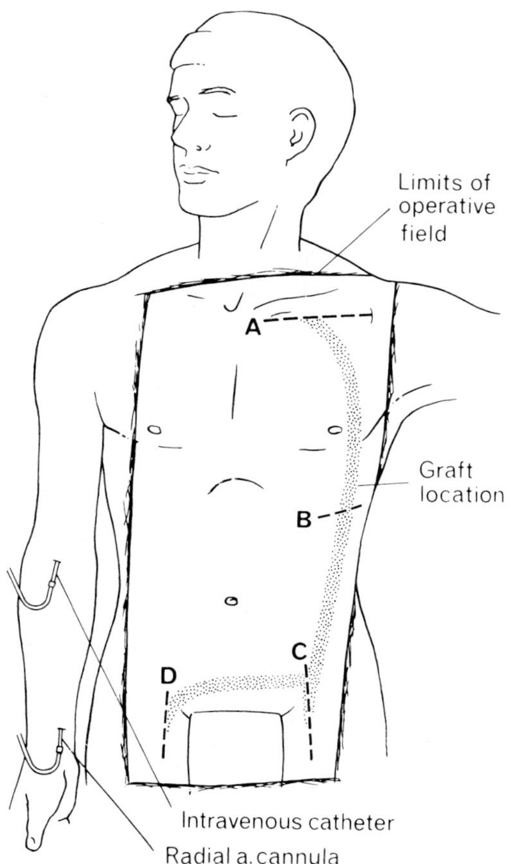

FIGURE 54–2. **The position of patient, extent of operative field, location of incisions (A–D), and subcutaneous course of grafts for axillobifemoral bypass are represented. (From Rutherford RB: Axillary bifemoral bypass graft. *In* Bergan JJ, Yao JST [eds]: Operative Techniques in Vascular Surgery. New York, Grune & Stratton, 1980.)**

dissecting toward the palpable pulse or following a branch of the thoracoacromial trunk. Division of the insertion of the pectoralis minor muscle, which appears in the lateral half of the incision, not only aids exposure but also simplifies tunneling of the graft. Once the axillary artery has been identified, a 5- or 6-cm segment is mobilized. The arteriotomy should be made on the anterior inferior surface of the artery medially near the chest wall so that abduction of the upper extremity does not place tension on the anastomosis. In addition, the angle of entry should not be acute, or at least no less than 75 degrees. Disruption of this anastomosis has been reported when the arm has been abducted too much.[70, 71] Therefore, the previously mentioned precautions are important. For the same reason, the graft should not be pulled down into the subcutaneous tunnel too tightly. This not only threatens the integrity of the anastomosis but can cause the axillary artery to be drawn down into a Y-shaped junction, which can obstruct outflow and contribute to anastomotic stenosis.

Occasionally, a single counterincision placed obliquely over the sixth or seventh intercostal space in the *mid-axillary* line is required between the axillary and femoral incisions. In most patients, particularly those who are average or smaller in stature and whose skin and subcutaneous tissue are relatively loose, a long, hollow metal tunneler can be used to connect the axillary and groin incisions and avoid the need for a counterincision. A more anteriorly placed graft (i.e., in front of the mid-axillary line) not only rides over the costal margin and can give rise to aneurysm formation but also is more likely to kink when the patient bends forward.[30, 32]

The femoral vessels are exposed in standard fashion through vertical incisions. If there is occlusive disease of the superficial femoral artery, the profunda femoris artery is exposed at least down to its first major perforator. An end-to-side anastomosis is then constructed into the appropriate outflow vessel.

The size of the prosthetic graft used should approximate the diameter of the recipient vessel, usually 8 mm. The senior author has used both double-velour knitted Dacron and expanded polytetrafluoroethylene (PTFE) prostheses for this operation, with equally good results. The latter graft has the theoretical advantage that it should be less compressible and thrombectomy should be easier if occlusion occurs. Externally supported grafts have produced apparent improvements in patency when compared with historical controls.[55, 56] However, should thrombosis still occur, the supporting rings make surgical thrombectomy more difficult. The senior author therefore prefers unsupported regular-thickness to externally supported, thin-walled PTFE for these extra-anatomic bypasses.

A *femorofemoral* bypass is performed simply by making two vertical incisions over the femoral vessels and anastomosing the graft in the standard fashion on each side after tunneling it in a gentle upward convex curve through the subcutaneous tissue above the pubis and anterior to the rectus sheath. If there are problems with postirradiation changes or subcutaneous infection or if the patient is morbidly obese, it may be preferable to incise the external oblique aponeurosis and pass the graft in a retrofascial plane. One can even tunnel in the preperitoneal plane behind the rectus muscle, and, by exposing the external iliac artery as "donor" through a somewhat more proximal incision, it is possible to avoid dissecting the groin on that side completely and to obtain a forward-angled end-to-side proximal anastomosis.

The *axillobifemoral* bypass combines the two foregoing operations with the exception that, after completion of the axillofemoral anastomoses, the first anastomosis of the femorofemoral crossover is usually made into the side of the axillofemoral graft distally. Those surgeons who believe that the extra flow associated with the femoral limb of the graft enhances the patency of the axillofemoral limb usually make this anastomosis quite low so that the graft assumes the configuration of an "inverted C."[36] Others construct it in a more natural "lazy S" configuration, with the proximal anastomosis made higher up on the anteromedial surface at the upper edge of the groin incision, which on that side is extended 3 or 4 cm higher than usual. This allows the advantage of an acute-angled antegrade takeoff rather than the retrograde flow characteristic of the inverted C anastomosis. In this regard, the results of the European Axillobifemoral Bypass Trial[68] are interesting. Nineteen vascular centers performed a randomized comparison between an axillobifemoral prosthesis with a right-angled (90 degree) side-arm and a newer prosthesis with an acute-angled, antegrade takeoff ("flow splitter"). At 2 years, the latter prosthesis had better than twice the patency (84 vs. 38 per cent) of the former.

Because both the lazy S and the inverted C configurations have disadvantages, other alternatives have been advocated (Fig. 54–3). To avoid the double "piggyback" anastomoses of the inverted C configuration yet bring the higher flow all the way to the distal end of the axillofemoral limb, Blaisdell and coworkers recommended mobilizing the common femoral and even some of the external iliac proximal to this anastomosis, dividing it and oversewing the upper end, and then using the lower end as the site of the proximal anastomosis of the femorofemoral bypass (see Fig. 54–3, *lower right*).[6] Endarterectomy of this segment may be required to make a suitable donor vessel. If this is not feasible, one can construct the proximal stem as a crossover axillofemoral bypass that swings low across the upper end of the ipsilateral groin incision. This allows a very short, antegrade limb to be anastomosed to the undersurface of the main graft. This anastomosis is easier than the lazy S configuration, the "unprotected" segment is short, and all anastomoses have antegrade flow (see Fig. 54–3, *lower left*).

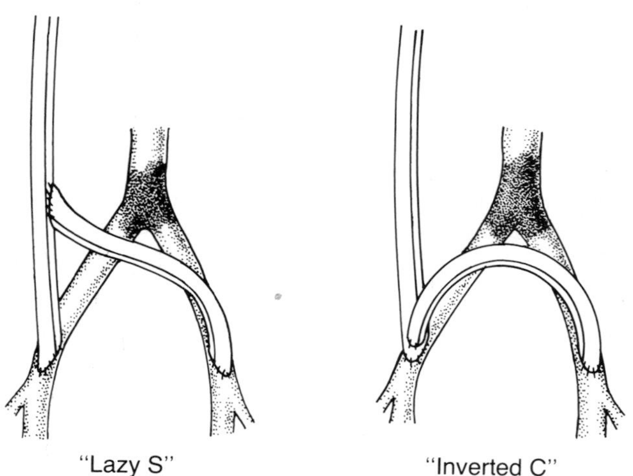

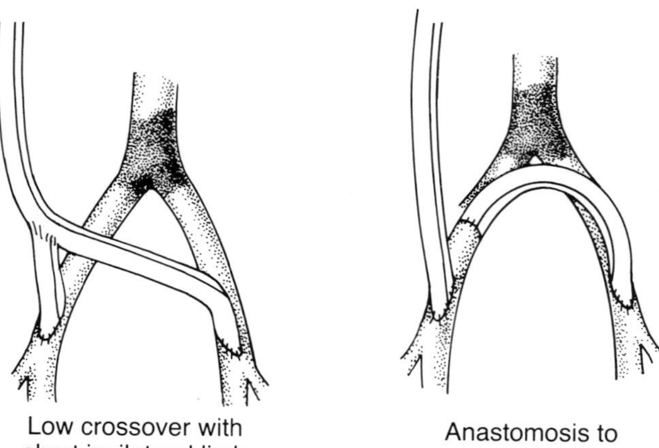

FIGURE 54–3. Some of the more commonly employed configurations for connecting the side limb of an axillobifemoral bypass, as described in the text.

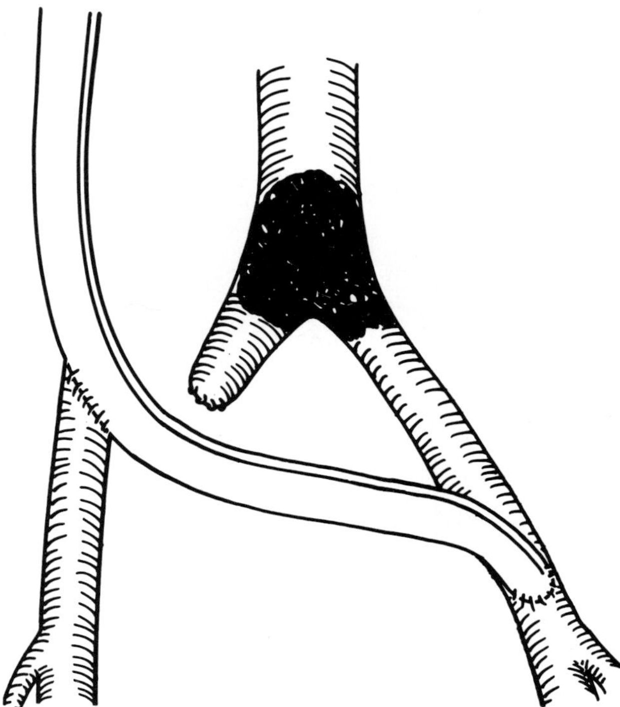

FIGURE 54–4. A modified technique for axillobifemoral bypass in which a single crossover axillofemoral graft is brought down to the contralateral femoral artery and the ipsilateral femoral artery is mobilized, divided, and anastomosed to it. (From Rutherford RB, Rainer WG: A modified technique for axillofemoral bypass [Letter to the Editor]. J Vasc Surg 10:468, 1989.)

The senior author has combined these last two techniques, in suitable cases, into a modification that not only has all antegrade anastomoses *and* brings the higher-flow proximal stem down to the ipsilateral femoral anastomosis but requires only one graft and three, rather than four, anastomoses. This technique, shown in Figure 54–4, involves mobilizing the upper common femoral artery (after severing it from the external iliac artery and closing the latter) and anastomosing it to the underside of an axillary crossover femoral graft as it passes by the upper end of the ipsilateral groin incision.

These extra-anatomic operations are usually well tolerated because there is minimal blood loss or hemodynamic disturbance. Nasogastric intubation is rarely necessary. In fact, patients can usually resume oral intake the day after surgery. Unless contraindicated, sodium warfarin (Coumadin) is administered long term; otherwise, antiplatelet drugs are used. A patency advantage of warfarin in this setting has not been proved at this writing, even though the practice has become popular for this and other long prosthetic grafts (e.g., infrainguinal prosthetic bypasses). The patient is warned against sleeping on the side of the axillofemoral graft. This can be ensured by attaching a loose wrist gauntlet from the donor wrist to the opposite side of the bed at night until the habit is formed. If the patient needs crutches, it is important that the "Canadian" type, with forearm grips, be used rather than the standard variety. The patient should be taught to feel for the pulses in both limbs of the graft every day to detect graft thrombosis and ensure early attention if this complication develops.

Technique of Obturator Bypass

The patient is placed on the operating table in the supine position, with the entire leg prepared and draped so that it can be rotated laterally and abducted and so that the hip can be flexed to relax the thigh musculature.[2, 19] Any groin wound must be carefully covered with an adherent drape and excluded from the operative field of the abdomen and the thigh. Careful preparation of the skin must be carried out because of the likelihood of contamination of the area adjacent to an infection in the groin.

Abdominal exposure may be gained through a right paramedian incision and a transperitoneal approach to the aorta and iliac vessels or the limb of an aortofemoral graft, but a transverse retroperitoneal approach is preferred, if preoperative angiography has confirmed that an iliac artery is suitable as a donor vessel for the graft. This approach allows adequate exposure of the obturator membrane for perforation under direct vision.

If the problem for which the procedure is being carried out is infection in the groin, it is critical at this point to determine whether infection has extended proximal to the inguinal ligament and up the graft. If the graft is still patent, there is a good possibility that infection may not have extended proximally. If the graft is thrombosed, infection will spread to involve the entire thrombosed segment. If the prosthesis shows excellent incorporation by surrounding tissue and overlying peritoneum and if there is no edema, induration, or infected material around it, one can make a reasonable assumption that this portion of the graft is not infected. If time allows, an indium-labeled leukocyte scan or a computed tomographic scan may help with this determination (see Chapter 36). When this has been determined, the patent proximal graft can be used as the proximal inflow for an obturator bypass. If neither the common iliac artery nor the aorta has been previously grafted, either may be selected for the proximal anastomosis. The site selected for anastomosis will, of course, depend on the extent of disease present as determined by palpation and accurate preoperative arteriography. These vessels are then mobilized to obtain proximal and distal control. Care must be taken at this point in the procedure to identify, mobilize, and preserve the ureter in a safe location.

Next, the obturator foramen is located. As shown in Figure 54–5, it lies just posterior to the superior ramus of the pubis. It is exposed by reflecting the peritoneum from its surface, beginning at the external iliac artery and proceeding downward over the pubic ramus. Alternatively, the obturator foramen can be located by identifying the hypogastric artery and determining the origin of the obturator branch, which usually arises from it and courses downward to and through the foramen. Occasionally, the obturator artery arises from the inferior epigastric artery and travels directly posteriorly over the superior ramus of the pubis to the foramen. The obturator artery, vein, and nerve that serve to identify the exact location of the foramen pass through it at the anterolateral border of the obturator fossa in very close apposition to the edge of bone that forms the lateral superior margin of the canal. In addition, by palpation, the obturator fossa can also be felt behind the superior ramus of the pubis. At the upper edge of the obturator fossa, the vas deferens crosses the pubic ramus and runs posteriorly.

An area is now selected for making the tunnel through the foramen. This tunnel should be located some distance from where the obturator artery, vein, and nerve pass through in order to avoid injury to these structures and to traverse the foramen in a relatively avascular location. As shown in Figure 54–5, this point is best located anteriorly and medially, just underneath the superior ramus of the pubis and medial to the vessels. The site for the tunnel should be kept as far anterior as possible to avoid the fleshy, thick muscle of the obturator internus, which is located more inferiorly. From inside the pelvis, blunt dissection and separation of the fibers of the obturator internus are carried out, which will lead to a tough aponeurotic membrane. This is a dense fascial wall lying between the obturator internus and externus, serving as the attachment for these muscles. This membrane is too tough to break through with blunt finger dissection, and it is better incised sharply. An instru-

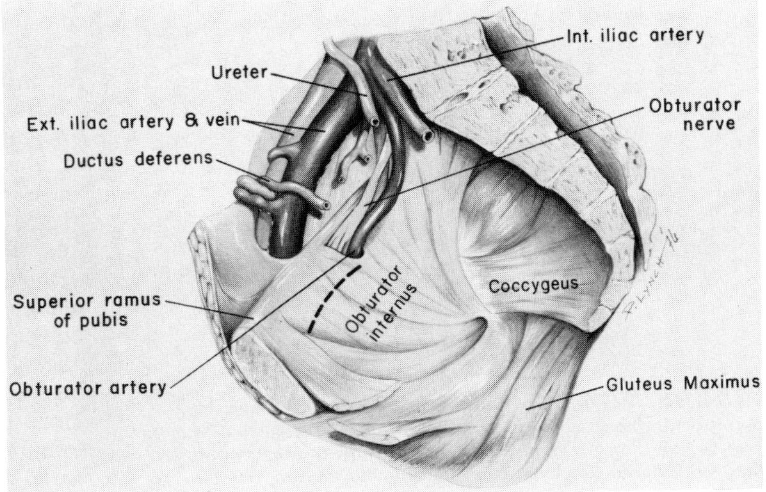

FIGURE 54–5. **Anatomy and exposure of the obturator foramen from within the pelvis. Note particularly the avascular area of the foramen and the superior medial portion where the fibers of the obturator internus muscle are separated and the membranous portion is incised.**

ment can then be passed through the tunnel from the pelvis into the thigh.

Attention is then turned to the thigh. The optimal site for the distal anastomosis depends on the individual patient's disease and other considerations. Use of the popliteal artery above the knee has the advantage that a shorter graft is required, but this segment may be atherosclerotic. The popliteal artery below the knee is more likely to be free of disease, but a longer graft is required. A tunneling instrument may be passed from above downward, to lie along the course of the popliteal artery so that one can begin dissection of the thigh above the knee and medially, well below the infected groin wound. This incision is developed with care to avoid injury to the greater saphenous vein, which may be the best graft to use considering the risk of contamination.

The deep fascia is opened, and the sartorius muscle is retracted to expose the proximal popliteal artery in the groove between the sartorius and the vastus medialis. The tendinous margin of the adductor magnus, which may cover the artery, may be divided to facilitate exposure. The fibrous sheath of the popliteal artery is carefully dissected free of its companion veins. The tunnel is then developed with a conventional tunneling instrument. The pectineus, adductor longus, and adductor brevis arise from the anteromedial rim of the obturator foramen. The anterior surface of these muscles forms the floor and medial boundaries of the femoral triangle. The adductor magnus arises from the posterior rim of the external surface of the foramen, so the tunneler passes through the canal onto the anterior surface of the adductor magnus in the thigh (Fig. 54–6). The tunnel is separated from the superficial femoral artery by the anterior mass of the adductor muscles. With gentle pressure and manipulation, the tunneler passes down easily to the vicinity of the adductor hiatus. The hiatus can then be located by palpation in the area where the superficial femoral artery passes through it, and the tunneler is delivered through the hiatus to lie in the popliteal fossa.

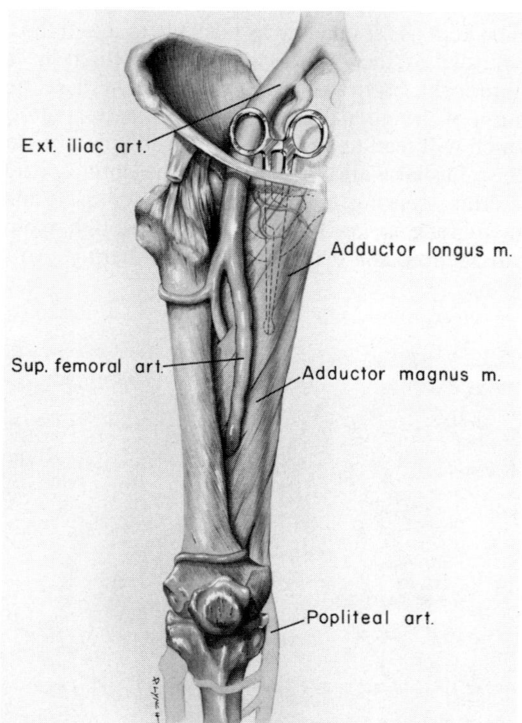

FIGURE 54–6. The tunnel is being created through the obturator foramen, showing the relationships to the pelvis, the major vessels, and the muscles of the thigh. The tunneling instrument lies between the adductor longus and the adductor magnus muscles.

If a previous aortofemoral graft is available to be the donor vessel at the iliac level, the prosthesis is divided and sutured end-to-end to the new graft. The distal end of the old graft is then free to be removed later when the groin is débrided. If the iliac artery is the donor vessel, angled vascular clamps are placed on the artery and then rotated laterally so that the arteriotomy is made with the proper orientation for the graft to pass to the obturator foramen. Finally, the external iliac artery is ligated distal to the takeoff of the graft.

The graft is then carefully passed or drawn through the tunnel using the tunneling device. After application of the popliteal clamps and reapplication of the iliac artery clamp, the distal suture line is made. The popliteal artery is then usually ligated proximal to the graft in order to minimize backbleeding from the superficial femoral artery during the groin dissection.

After restoration of blood flow to the extremity, the peritoneum is closed carefully over the graft. It is best for the new graft to lie along the pelvic wall rather than to run straight across the pelvis. The abdominal and thigh incisions are closed, and dressings are applied. Thereafter, attention is directed to the problem in the groin. If there has been an infected graft, the distal defunctionalized graft limb can now be removed. The divided proximal end is brought down into the field, and the parent artery is closed. Backbleeding from the profunda femoris is controlled by suture ligature, and infected tissue in the groin is débrided thoroughly. A schematic of the completed operation is shown in Figure 54–7. The groin incision is left open for drainage to allow granulation tissue formation and delayed healing. Appropriate antibiotics are continued during this period.

RESULTS AND COMPLICATIONS

These extra-anatomic bypasses can be associated with all the complications encountered following any arterial prosthetic reconstruction: perigraft hemorrhage, thrombosis, infection, and the like. The very nature of these grafts, the extensive subcutaneous tunneling, the need for groin dissections, and the fact that they are often employed *because* of graft sepsis or other inflammatory intra-abdominal conditions all account for a higher than average incidence of each of these complications.[26] On the other hand, the incidence of general or systemic complications (e.g., pneumonia, ileus, pulmonary embolism, myocardial infarction, renal failure), although probably higher than that generally reported for aortobifemoral bypass grafting, is nevertheless lower than if aortobifemoral bypass had been performed on the same group of patients. This also applies to mortality rates, as pointed out later. In addition, there are complications that are more or less specific to these procedures, some primarily involving the upper extremity.[24] The likelihood of a steal has already been discussed. Brachial plexus

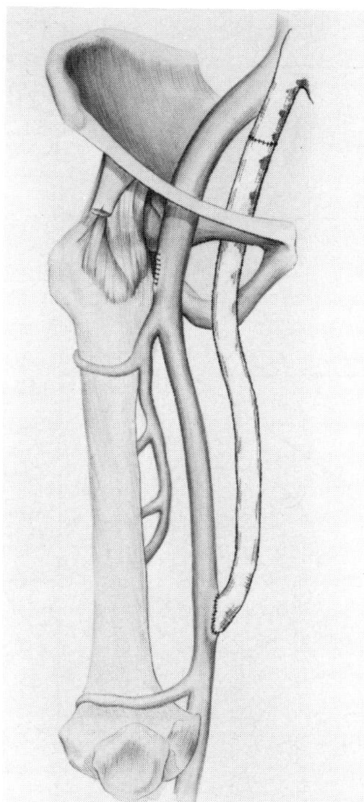

FIGURE 54–7. A graft has been placed from a previous prosthesis and continued down to the proximal popliteal artery. The common femoral artery in the septic area has been closed.

injury, usually because of hyperabduction, has been reported. Occlusion of the subclavian and axillary arteries may result if the graft is inserted under too much tension or becomes tighter as a result of the desmoplastic reaction around it. Occasionally, unrecognized stenoses proximal to the anastomosis result in donor artery thrombosis. The femoral complications are essentially the same as those encountered in aortofemoral bypass grafting.

The results of femorofemoral, axillofemoral, axillobifemoral, and axillopopliteal bypass grafting, as reported in the literature, are summarized in Table 54–1. It demonstrates that roughly fourfold differences in operative mortality and twofold differences in long-term patency are to be found in the literature. Depending on which of these results one accepts, one could take an enthusiastic or a pessimistic position in applying extra-anatomic bypass. Careful reading of the literature indicates that although some of these differences may be due to technical considerations, most can be explained on the basis of case selection (or exclusion) and the criteria for success (or failure).[41] The latter relate mainly to the use of secondary as opposed to primary patency rates, because few grafts present a greater opportunity to test the utility of thrombectomy (i.e., a high thrombosis rate in an accessible [subcutaneous] graft). For example, one reported comparison of axillobifemoral and aortobifemoral procedures showed a 76 per cent secondary patency rate for the former, but this included a 43 per cent rate of thrombectomy or revision.[22] Liberal application of extra-anatomic bypass will result in better mortality and patency rates. At the time of this report, Johnson and associates offered axillobifemoral bypass ''to anyone over the age of 65, regardless of risk.''[22] The majority of axillobifemoral bypasses reported by Ray and colleagues were for claudication.[36] On the other hand, conservative application of axillobifemoral bypass results in a paradoxically higher mortality rate for this ''low-risk option'' than for aortobifemoral bypass (which has benefited by having these high-risk cases removed). By restricting the use of axillofemoral bypass to limb salvage indications, one will also obtain lower patency rates because concomitant superficial femoral artery occlusion will almost uniformly be present. Clearly, ''lumped'' or ''bottom line'' figures can be deceiving. For this reason, one of the authors has published the results for extra-anatomic bypasses broken down according to indications for operation and runoff status and with both primary and secondary patency rates being presented.[40] These are summarized in Table 54–2.

The use of externally supported conduits for axillobifemoral bypass has been associated with markedly improved long-term primary patency rates (76 to 85 per cent). However, these reports are also subject to the influence of patient selection. Thirty-six per cent of the patients reported on by El-Massry and coworkers[56] were claudicators, whereas Harris and associates did not report the incidence of claudication in their series.[55] The only direct comparison of externally supported and nonsupported grafts for extra-anatomic bypass involved the more extended axillopopliteal bypass, in which Keller and coworkers retrospectively reported a nonsignificant trend favoring externally supported grafts.[61] Nevertheless, employing externally supported grafts for axillobifemoral and extended extra-anatomic bypasses is becoming an increasingly popular practice.

Patency rates for obturator bypass range from 66 to 89 per cent.[49] Tilson and Baue[50] and van Det and Brands[51] reported personal series of 10 and 13 cases with 89 per cent and 80 per cent patency rates, respectively. The latter authors collected an additional 66 cases from the literature with an overall patency rate of 68 per cent. Although prosthetic material is often employed, this graft is not subject to acute flexion, and in comparison with femoropopliteal bypasses, it enjoys the advantage of receiving better proximal inflow. Thus, the overall 5-year patency rate of approximately 70 per cent is not surprising. Except for the expected higher risk of graft sepsis, complications have been, for the most part, similar to those experienced with any distal bypass.[46]

Generally, however, extra-anatomic bypasses are usually longer grafts and their extra-anatomic position is more subject to external compression, so lower patency rates here are to be expected. Even in the best series, the patency rates do not approach those reported with direct arterial reconstruction if ''runoff'' and other factors are considered.[22, 36] Mortality will be lower in the same group of high-risk patients, but advances in perioperative monitoring and intensive care have made this a moot consideration in all but the most prohibitive risk patients. Finally, although extra-anatomic bypasses are physiologically much less challenging to the patient, they are usually not technically easier, and they do not significantly reduce operating time. Unlike obturator bypass, which is used when there is little other choice, axillounifemoral, axillobifemoral, and femorofemoral bypasses often compete with other procedures. They rarely compete with each other. The correct choice depends on a number of factors in addition to patient risk and hostile

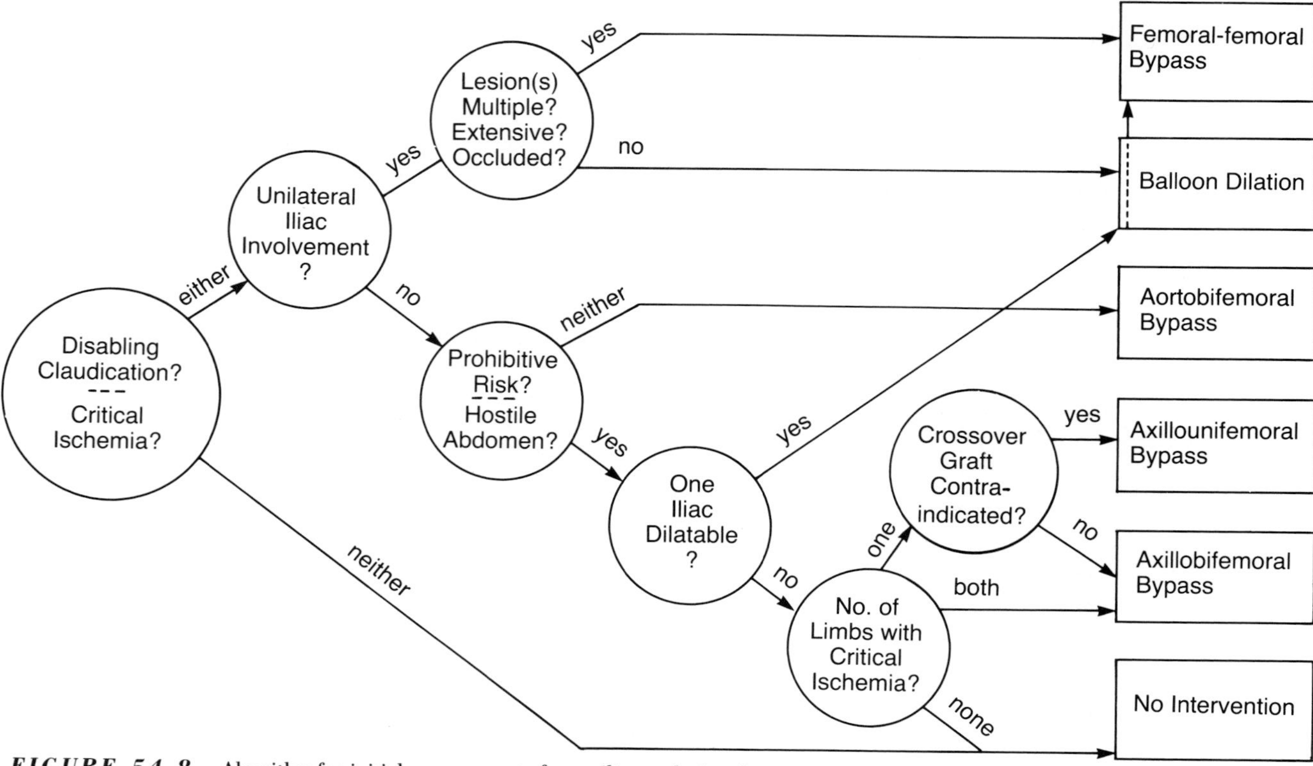

FIGURE 54–8. Algorithm for initial management of aortoiliac occlusive disease.

abdominal pathology. The morphology of the occlusive disease may be important, as in choosing between iliac percutaneous transluminal angioplasty and femorofemoral bypass, and the status of the runoff vessels or the opposite iliac artery may determine the choice between aortobifemoral bypass and femorofemoral bypass (with or without percutaneous transluminal angioplasty). On the basis of the foregoing discussions, these decisions may be approached in a logical way and individualized to the particular patient's benefit. An algorithmic outline of this decision process is offered in Figure 54–8. Although this does not, for simplicity's sake, reflect optional reconstructions to the femorofemoral bypass (aortofemoral bypass, iliofemoral bypass, and endarterectomy, as discussed in the text) and other subtler aspects, it should provide a framework for personal decision making.

References

1. Alpert J, Brief DK, Parsonnet V: Vascular restoration for aortoiliac occlusion and an alternative approach to the poor risk patient. J Newark Beth Israel Hosp 18:4, 1967.
2. Baue AE, Shaw RS: Bypass grafts using the obturator foramen. *In* Haimovici H (ed): Vascular Surgery, Principles and Techniques. New York, McGraw-Hill, 1976.
3. Blaisdell FW, Hall AD: Axillary femoral artery bypass for lower extremity ischemia. Surgery 54:563, 1963.
4. Blaisdell FW, DeMattei GA, Gauder PJ: Extraperitoneal thoracic aorta to femoral bypass graft as replacement for an infected aortic bifurcation prosthesis. Am J Surg 102:583, 1961.
5. Blaisdell FW, Hall AD, Lim RC Jr, et al: Aortoiliac arterial substitution utilizing subcutaneous grafts. Ann Surg 172:775, 1970.
6. Blaisdell FW, Holcroft JW, Ward RE: Axillofemoral and femorofemoral bypass: History and evolution of technique. *In* Greenhalgh RM (ed): Extra-Anatomic and Secondary Arterial Reconstruction. London, Pitman, 1982.
7. Brief DK, Alpert J, Parsonnet V: Crossover femorofemoral grafts: Compromise or preference: A reappraisal. Arch Surg 105:889, 1972.
8. Brief DK, Brener B, Alpert J, et al: Crossover femorofemoral grafts followed up five years or more: An analysis. Arch Surg 110:1294, 1975.
9. Cohn LH, Moore WS, Hall AD: Extra-abdominal management of late aortofemoral graft thrombosis. Surgery 67:775, 1970.
10. Delaurentis DA, Sala LE, Russell E, et al: A twelve-year experience with axillofemoral and femorofemoral bypass operations. Surg Gynecol Obstet 147:881, 1978.
11. DePalma RG, Hubay CA: Arterial bypass via the obturator foramen. Am J Surg 115:323, 1968.
12. Dick LS, Brief DK, Alpert J, et al: A 12 year experience with femorofemoral crossover grafts. Arch Surg 115:1359, 1980.
13. Donahoe PK, Froio RA, Nabseth DC: Obturator bypass graft in radical excision of inguinal neoplasm. Ann Surg 166:147, 1967.
14. Ehrenfeld WK, Harris JD, Wylie EJ: Vascular "steal" phenomenon: An experimental study. Am J Surg 116:192, 1968.
15. Ernst CB: Axillary femoral bypass graft without aortofemoral pressure differential. Ann Surg 181:424, 1974.
16. Eugene J, Goldstone J, Moore WS: Fifteen-year experience with subcutaneous bypass grafts for lower extremity ischemia. Ann Surg 186:177, 1976.
17. Flanigan P, Pratt DG, Goodreau JJ, et al: Hemodynamic and angiographic guidelines in selection of patients for femorofemoral bypass. Arch Surg 113:1257, 1978.
18. Freeman NE, Leeds FH: Operations on large arteries: Application of recent advances. Calif Med 77:229, 1952.
19. Guida PM, Moore SW: Obturator bypass technique. Surg Gynecol Obstet 128:1307, 1969.
20. Hegarty JC, Linton PC, McSweeney ED: Revascularization of the lower extremity through the obturator canal. Arch Surg 98:35, 1969.
21. Inahara T, Geary GL, Mukherjee D, et al: The contrary position to the non-resective treatment of abdominal aortic aneurysm. J Vasc Surg 4:42, 1985.
22. Johnson WC, LoGerfo FW, Vollman RW: Is axillobilateral femoral

graft an effective substitute for aortobilateral iliac femoral graft? Ann Surg 186:123, 1976.
23. Johnston KW, Rae M, Hogg-Johnston SA, et al: 5-year results of a prospective study of percutaneous transluminal angioplasty. Ann Surg 206:403, 1987.
24. Kempczinski RF, Penn I: Upper extremity complications of axillofemoral grafts. Am J Surg 136:209, 1978.
25. Kim L, Kohler T, Johansen K: Non-resective therapy for aortic aneurysm: Results of a survey. J Vasc Surg 4:469, 1986.
26. Livesay JJ, Atkinson JB, Baker JD, et al: Late results of extraanatomic bypass. Arch Surg 114:1402, 1979.
27. LoGerfo FW, Johnson WC, Corson JD, et al: A comparison of the late patency rates of axillobilateral femoral and axillounilateral femoral grafts. Surgery 81:33, 1977.
28. Louw JH: The treatment of combined aortoiliac and femoral popliteal occlusive disease by splenofemoral and axillofemoral bypass grafts. Surgery 55:387, 1963.
29. Mahoney WD, Whelan TJ: Use of the obturator foramen in iliofemoral artery grafting. Ann Surg 163:215, 1966.
30. Mannick JA, Williams LE, Nabseth DC: The late results of axillofemoral grafts. Surgery 68:1038, 1970.
31. Mentha C, Launois B, DeLaere J: Les pontages artériels iliofémoraux par le trou obturator. J Chir (Paris) 90:131, 1965.
32. Orringer MB, Rutherford RB, Skinner DB: An unusual complication of axillary femoral artery bypass. Surgery 72:769, 1972.
33. Parsonnet V, Alpert J, Brief DK: Femorofemoral and axillofemoral grafts: Compromise or preference. Surgery 67:26, 1970.
34. Piotrowski J, Rutherford RB, Jones DN, et al: Aortobifemoral bypass: The operation of choice for unilateral iliac occlusion. J Vasc Surg 8:211, 1988.
35. Porter JM, Eidemiller LR, Dotter CT, et al: Combined arterial dilatation and femorofemoral bypass for limb salvage. Surg Gynecol Obstet 137:409, 1973.
36. Ray LI, O'Connor JB, Davis CC, et al: Axillofemoral bypass: A critical reappraisal of its role in the management of aortoiliac occlusive disease. Am J Surg 138:117, 1979.
37. Rudich M, Gutierrez IZ, Gage AA: Obturator foramen bypass in the management of infected vascular prosthesis. Am J Surg 137:657, 1979.
38. Chang JB: Current state of extraanatomic bypasses. Am J Surg 152:202, 1986.
39. Hepp W, de Jonge K, Pallua N: Late results following extra-anatomic bypass procedures for chronic aortoiliac occlusive disease. J Cardiovasc Surg 29:181, 1988.
40. Rutherford RB, Patt A, Pearce WH: Extra-anatomic bypass: A closer view. J Vasc Surg 5:437, 1987.
41. Rutherford RB, Patt A, Kumpe DA: The current role of percutaneous transluminal angioplasty. *In* Greenhalgh RM, Jamieson CW, Nicolaides AN (eds): Vascular Surgery: Issues in Current Practice. London, Grune & Stratton, 1986.
42. Rutherford RB: Axillary bifemoral bypass graft. *In* Bergan JJ, Yao JST (eds): Operative Techniques in Vascular Surgery. New York, Grune & Stratton, 1980.
43. Sauvage LR, Wood SJ: Unilateral axillary bilateral femoral bifurcation graft: A procedure for the poor risk patient with aortoiliac disease. Surgery 60:573, 1966.
44. Schwartz RA, Nichols WK, Silver D: Is thrombosis of the infrarenal abdominal aortic aneurysm an acceptable alternative? J Vasc Surg 3:448, 1986.
45. Shaw RS, Baue AE: Management of sepsis complicating arterial reconstructive surgery. Surgery 53:75, 1962.
46. Sheiner NM, Sigman H, Stilman A: An unusual complication of obturator foramen arterial bypass. J Cardiovasc Surg 10:324, 1969.
47. Shin CS, Chaudhry AG: The hemodynamics of extra-anatomic bypass grafts. Surg Gynecol Obstet 148:567, 1979.
48. Sumner DS, Strandness DE: The hemodynamics of the femorofemoral shunt. Surg Gynecol Obstet 134:629, 1972.
49. Tilson MD, Sweeney T, Gusberg RJ, et al: Obturator canal bypass grafts for septic lesions of the femoral artery. Arch Surg 114:1031, 1979.
50. Tilson MD, Baue AE: Obturator canal bypass graft for infection of the femoral artery. Surg Rounds 2:14, 1981.
51. van Det RJ, Brands LC: The obturator foramen bypass: An alternative procedure in iliofemoral artery revascularization. Surgery 89:543, 1981.
52. Vetto RM: The treatment of unilateral iliac artery obstruction with a transabdominal subcutaneous femorofemoral graft. Surgery 52:342, 1962.
53. Warren R: Bypass arterial graft between splenic and iliofemoral arteries. Arch Surg 72:57, 1956.
54. Weale FE: The values of series and parallel resistances in steady blood flow. Br J Surg 51:623, 1964.
55. Harris EJ, Taylor LM, McConnell DB, et al: Clinical results of axillobifemoral bypass using externally supported polytetrafluoroethylene. J Vasc Surg 12:416, 1990.
56. El-Massry S, Saad E, Sauvage LR, et al: Axillofemoral bypass using externally-supported, knitted Dacron grafts: A follow-up through twelve years. J Vasc Surg 17:107, 1993.
57. Schneider JR, McDaniel MD, Walsh DB, et al: Axillofemoral bypass: Outcome and hemodynamic results in high-risk patients. J Vasc Surg 15:952, 1992.
58. Veith FJ, Moss CM, Daly V, et al: New approaches to limb salvage by extended extra-anatomic bypasses and prosthetic reconstructions to foot arteries. Surgery 84:764, 1978.
59. Connolly JE, Kwaan JHM, Brownell D, et al: Newer developments of extraanatomic bypass. Surg Gynecol Obstet 158:415, 1984.
60. Ascer E, Veith FJ, Gupta S: Axillopopliteal bypass grafting: Indications, late results, and determinants of long-term patency. J Vasc Surg 10:285, 1989.
61. Keller MP, Hoch JR, Harding AD, et al: Axillopopliteal bypass for limb salvage. J Vasc Surg 15:817, 1992.
62. Cham C, Myers KA, Scott DF, et al: Extraperitoneal unilateral iliac artery bypass for chronic lower limb ischemia. Aust NZ J Surg 58:859, 1988.
63. de Gama AD: The fate of the donor artery in extraanatomic revascularization. J Vasc Surg 8:106, 1988.
64. Ascer E, Veith FJ, Gupta SK, et al: Comparison of axillounifemoral and axillobifemoral bypass operations. Surgery 97:169, 1985.
65. Walker PJ, Harris JP, May J: Combined percutaneous transluminal angioplasty and extraanatomic bypass for symptomatic unilateral iliac artery occlusion with contralateral iliac artery stenosis. Ann Vasc Surg 5:209, 1991.
66. Calligaro KD, Ascer E, Veith FJ, et al: Unsuspected inflow disease in candidates for axillofemoral bypass operations: A prospective study. J Vasc Surg 11:832, 1990.
67. Kram HB, Gupta SK, Veith FJ, Wengerter KR: Unilateral aortofemoral bypass: A safe and effective option for the treatment of unilateral limb-threatening ischemia. Am J Surg 162:155, 1991.
68. Wittens CHA, van Houtte HJKP, van Urk H: European Axillobifemoral (ABF) Bypass Trial: A prospective randomized multicenter study. Presented at the 5th Annual Meeting of the European Society for Vascular Surgery, Warsaw, Poland, September 25–27, 1991.
69. Darling RC, Leather RP, Chang BB, et al: Is the iliac artery a suitable inflow conduit for iliofemoral occlusive disease: An analysis of aortoiliac reconstructions. J Vasc Surg (In press).
70. White GH, Donayre CE, Williams RA, et al: Exertional disruption of axillofemoral graft anastomosis. Arch Surg 125:625, 1990.
71. Sullivan LP, Davidson PG, D'Anna JA, Sithian N: Disruption of the proximal anastomosis of axillobifemoral grafts: Two case reports. J Vasc Surg 10:190, 1989.
72. Karmody AM, Leather RP, Goldman M, et al: The current position of nonresective treatment for abdominal aortic aneurysm. Surgery 94:591, 1983.

55

Profundaplasty

Victor M. Bernhard, M.D.

• • •

The deep femoral artery provides the primary blood supply to the tissues of the thigh and in addition serves as the major collateral channel for bypassing the obstructed superficial femoral artery. Leeds and Gilfillan and Morris and associates were the first to demonstrate that restoration of flow through this vessel alone significantly improves limb perfusion when the superficial femoral is also occluded.[22, 29] Waibel and Wolff established the significance of the profunda femoris as a collateral vessel by measuring the fall in popliteal pressure when it was clamped during femoropopliteal bypass for superficial femoral occlusion.[41] The measurement of blood flow through the profunda femoris after it has achieved its full potential for collateral development around a superficial femoral block further demonstrates the capacity of this vessel to provide sufficient flow to maintain a viable and functional limb.[4, 26] This flow volume was twice that measured through femoropopliteal vein grafts and was frequently equal to flow through the external iliac artery when both superficial and deep femoral vessels were patent (Fig. 55–1).

The anatomy of the profunda femoris artery dictates its role as a major collateral channel and provides the basis for surgical intervention to restore its function (Fig. 55–2). Frequent variations from the usually described picture must be carefully searched for in the preoperative arteriogram and by meticulous dissection at the time of surgery.[3, 21, 27, 42] The main channel is directed posteriorly from its origin at the distal end of the common femoral artery, 2 to 4 cm below the inguinal ligament. It promptly dips behind the very large lateral circumflex femoral vein, which must be divided in order to expose the profunda femoris at this level (Fig. 55–3). The artery runs deep within Hunter's canal under the sartorius and vastus medialis muscles. The distal half of the vessel, at the level of the second perforator, dips posterior to the adductor longus muscle, which must be incised to identify the third perforator branch (Fig. 55–3). Although the lateral and medial circumflex femoral arteries generally arise from the proximal portion of the profunda femoris, these branches occasionally take their origin from the common or superficial femoral vessels. The branches of the lateral circumflex femoral, anastomosing respectively with the inferior gluteal branch of the hypogastric, the first perforator, and the medial circumflex femoral, form the cruciate anastomosis.[42] This constitutes the major collateral complex for bypassing external iliac, common femoral, or proximal profunda obstruction (see Fig. 55–2).[27, 42] The first, second, and third perforator branches pass laterally and posteriorly into the adductor musculature. Interconnecting branches of these vessels form a series of arcades that provide an alternative parallel channel.[21, 42] The terminal branches of the profunda femoris anastomose with this arcade proximally and with the geniculate arteries from the popliteal and recurrent branches of the tibial vessels to complete an extensive collateral network that can bypass the entire femoropopliteal segment (see Fig. 55–2).[42]

The localization of atherosclerosis in the profunda has several characteristic patterns. Most commonly, stenosis is limited to the origin of the artery and is due to extension of plaque on the posterior wall of the common femoral artery into the orifice of the deep femoral. When disease involves the vessel more extensively, it extends to and just beyond a major branch such as the lateral circumflex or the first perforator and less frequently to the second or third perforator. Beyond the point of obstruction, the intima usually reverts to a normal or near-normal appearance. However, in diabetics, there is an increased likelihood for significant

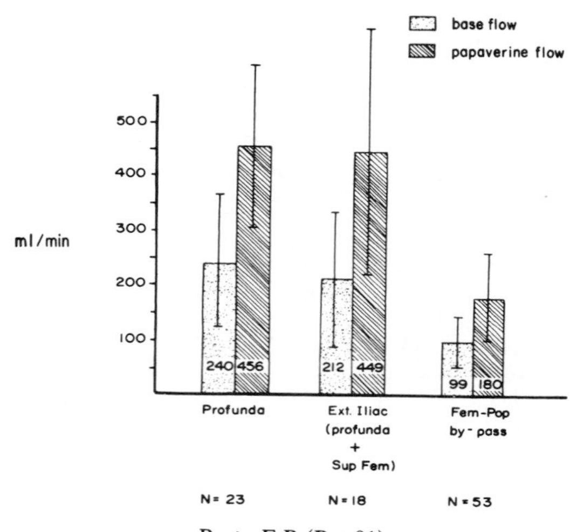

FIGURE 55–1. Blood flow through the unobstructed profunda femoris artery in the presence of chronic superficial femoral occlusion is equal to the flow through the external iliac when both branches of the common femoral are patent. Profunda femoris flow is more than twice that measured through femoropopliteal bypass. These studies demonstrate the capacity for deep femoral collateral development to support perfusion for the entire lower extremity. (From Bernhard VM, Ray LI, Militello JM: The role of angioplasty of the profunda femoris artery in revascularization of the ischemic limb. Surg Gynecol Obstet 142:840, 1976. By permission of Surgery, Gynecology & Obstetrics.)

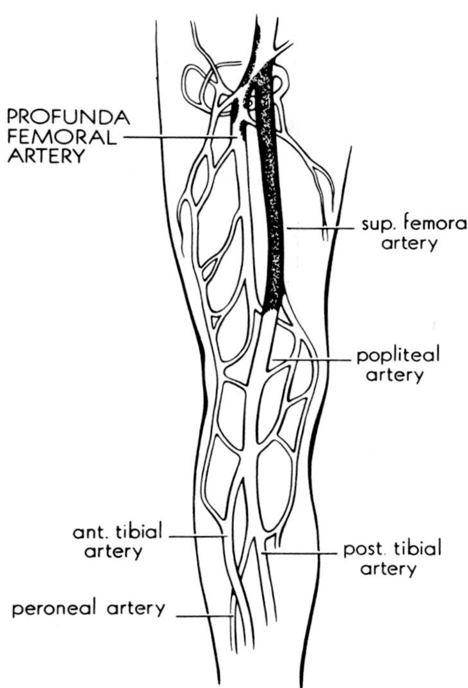

FIGURE 55–2. **The profunda femoris provides the major collateral channel to the leg when the superficial femoral artery is obstructed. Atherosclerosis and thrombosis are usually limited to the origin and proximal third of this vessel. (From Bernhard VM, Militello JM, Geringer AM: Repair of the profunda femoris artery. Am J Surg 127:676, 1974.)**

obstructive disease to involve the distal portion of the profunda femoris and its branches.[19]

Beales and coworkers noted atherosclerotic narrowing of this vessel in 59 per cent of ischemic extremities when arteriograms were performed with the patient in an oblique position.[1] In this projection, the proximal profunda femoris is not obscured by the common and superficial femoral arteries, and the atheromatous plaque that is usually situated posteriorly can be seen in profile.[27] Duplex scanning has been shown to be a reliable technique compared to arteriography for noninvasively demonstrating the presence of significant profunda stenosis.[38] This technique may be useful for identifying patients who may be candidates for profundaplasty, especially when arteriography does not clearly delineate the origin of this artery. Fortuitously, atherosclerotic intimal degeneration is localized to the proximal portion of the profunda in 74 per cent of afflicted limbs, so that surgical intervention to restore circulation through this channel is technically feasible in the majority of limbs in which it may be required.

INDICATIONS FOR PROFUNDAPLASTY

The purpose of profundaplasty is to relieve a significant stenosis or occlusion in the proximal portion of the deep femoral artery in order to restore its function as the major collateral bypass to the popliteal artery or its calf branches when the superficial femoral artery is obstructed. It is most frequently employed as an adjunct to an inflow procedure, such as aortofemoral, femorofemoral, or axillofemoral bypass for the treatment of combined aortoiliac and femoropopliteal occlusive disease.[3, 27, 29, 32, 43] In addition to this primary indication, patients who develop thrombosis of a limb of an aortofemoral graft almost invariably require profunda repair in addition to graft thrombectomy when this multi-level distribution of arterial disease is present.[5, 7, 9, 10, 32]

Profundaplasty is less frequently performed as an isolated procedure to serve as an alternative to femoropopliteal or femorotibial bypass.[4, 8, 21, 27] In some instances when distal bypass is not feasible, deep femoral repair may be the only procedure available to improve perfusion of the end-stage ischemic leg.[4, 8, 21, 34] Although limb salvage may not be achieved in this circumstance, the level of anticipated amputation may be lowered from above to below the knee.[40]

Selection of patients for isolated profundaplasty as an alternative to infrainguinal bypass requires strict adherence to clearly defined criteria. Patients must be critically evaluated both preoperatively and at surgery to determine that sufficient improvement in limb perfusion will be achieved to improve walking tolerance significantly or to heal superficial ulcers, limited areas of pedal necrosis, and minor amputations. Iliac inflow must be hemodynamically unimpaired as determined by the quality of the femoral pulse, the arteriographic appearance of the aortoiliac inflow, and

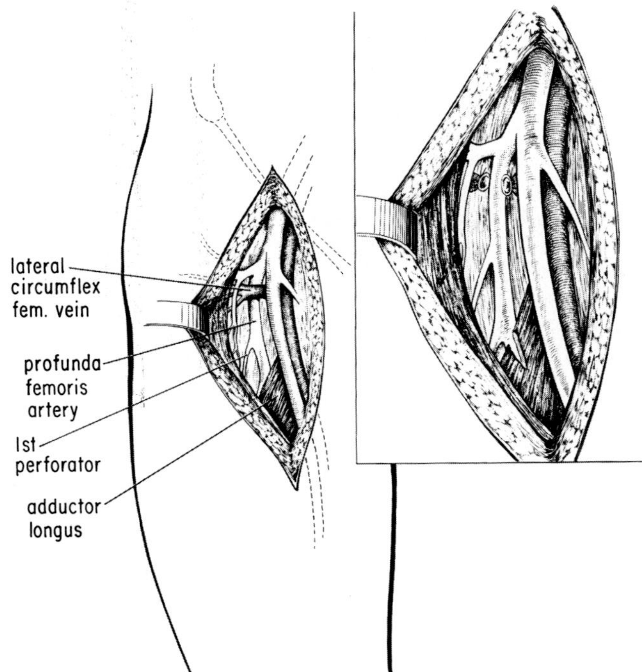

FIGURE 55–3. **Identification of the proximal portion of the profunda femoris artery requires division of the large circumflex femoral vein that lies anterior to it. The distal portion of the profunda at and beyond the level of the second perforator is exposed by incising the adductor longus muscle. (From Bernhard VM: The role of profundaplasty in revascularization of the lower extremities. Surg Clin North Am 59:681, 1979.)**

direct femoral pressure measurement during arteriography or surgery.[4] The development of a systolic pressure gradient of greater than 15 per cent between the brachial and femoral arteries after the femoral injection of 30 mg of papaverine has been determined by Flanigan and colleagues to be a reliable prospective indicator of subcritical iliac stenosis and identifies the need for surgical repair or balloon dilation of the ipsilateral iliac artery in addition to repair of the distal vessels.[2, 14]

Unless stenosis of the deep femoral artery narrows the lumen to less than 50 per cent of its normal diameter, isolated profundaplasty is unlikely to produce a significant improvement in flow to the leg.[2, 28, 35] Arterial repair should extend beyond the area of major stenosis, and every effort should be made to remove atherosclerotic plaques that may be obstructing or narrowing the orifices of profunda femoris branches, especially the lateral circumflex femoral.[2, 8, 21, 32]

Satisfactory collateral connections between the branches of the profunda femoris and the popliteal-tibial runoff vessels are an important prerequisite to success. Although their presence can frequently be visualized by angiography, their hemodynamic value can be more reliably determined by noninvasive measurement of the systolic pressure above (AKSP) and below (BKSP) the knee.[2, 4, 6, 31, 35] A profunda-popliteal collateral index (PPCI) may be calculated from these pressures by using the formula:

$$\mathrm{PPCI} = \frac{\mathrm{AKSP} - \mathrm{BKSP}}{\mathrm{AKSP}}$$

An index of greater than 0.5 due to a high-pressure gradient across the knee suggests poor collateral development and predicts failure of deep femoral repair to salvage a severely ischemic foot, whereas a low index, less than 0.5, indicates a reasonable chance for success.[6, 31, 34]

The angiographic demonstration of a widely patent popliteal-tibial runoff bed usually correlates with significant improvement, whereas extensive occlusive disease in this runoff bed is frequently associated with failure.[2, 4, 35] The presence of diabetes may reduce the chances for success.[2, 21, 35, 40] Gangrene of the toes or forefoot is a poor prognostic sign.[2, 16, 28, 35]

Table 55–1 provides a useful guide for selection of the operation when profunda femoris obstruction is demonstrated in patients with superficial femoral occlusion but unimpaired aortoiliac inflow.

OPERATIVE TECHNIQUE

In the majority of cases, profunda femoris angioplasty is performed as an auxiliary procedure to ensure satisfactory runoff for aortofemoral, axillofemoral, or femorofemoral bypass. However, in approximately 30 per cent of limbs requiring profunda femoris repair, aortoiliac inflow is not obstructed, and profundaplasty is performed as the primary procedure.[40] Occasionally, repair of the deep femoral artery is carried out in conjunction with bypass to the popliteal or tibial arteries when it appears that removal of a modest profunda stenosis by itself will not adequately resolve the ischemic problem.[9, 17, 19, 32]

General anesthesia with full monitoring is mandatory when profundaplasty is carried out in conjunction with aortofemoral bypass. For an isolated procedure performed through a single groin incision, either caudal anesthesia or local lidocaine infiltration with anesthetist standby may be satisfactory and is ideal in the presence of severe cardiopulmonary disease that permits only a limited operation.[3, 21]

A vertical groin incision is made directly over the common femoral artery and is carried 5 cm cephalad of the inguinal crease and 8 cm or more caudally. The distal extension of the incision depends upon the length of the profunda femoris artery that must be exposed. The inguinal ligament is partially or completely divided to facilitate dissection of the distal external iliac artery and its deep epigastric and circumflex iliac branches. The common femoral artery is freed throughout its length and circumference so that anatomic variations can be carefully searched for and all significant branches preserved. The superficial femoral artery is exposed for a variable distance both to facilitate dissection of the profunda and to make the outer wall of this occluded vessel available as an autogenous patch.

The point of origin of the profunda femoris from the posterior aspect of the common femoral is identified. Progressive distal exposure is achieved by incising the enveloping fatty areolar tissue and dividing the large overlying lateral circumflex femoral vein, which lies deep to the superficial femoral and passes over the anterior surface of the

Table 55–1. Choice of Operation (Occluded Superficial Femoral, Normal Aortoiliac Inflow)*

Criteria			
Profunda Femoris Stenosis >50 Per Cent	***Profunda-popliteal Collateral Index <0.5***	***Popliteal Runoff Good (+), Poor (−)***	**Procedure Recommended**
+	+	+	Profundaplasty
+	+	−	Profundaplasty
+	−	+	Femoropopliteal or femorotibial bypass and profundaplasty
+	−	−	Profundaplasty (amputation later?)
−	±	+	Femoropopliteal, femorotibial, or sequential bypass
−	±	−	Amputation

Adapted from Bernhard VM: Limitations of profunda femoris revascularization. In *Veith FJ: Critical Problems in Vascular Surgery. New York, Appleton-Century-Crofts, 1982, p 260.*

profunda 1 to 3 cm distal to its origin (see Fig. 55–3).[3, 8, 21] The length of profunda femoris that must be dissected free depends upon the distal extent of significant atheromatous obstruction. This is readily ascertained by reference to the preoperative arteriogram and direct inspection and palpation of the vessel. The dissection should be carried at least distal to the lateral circumflex femoral and often beyond the first perforating branch. More distal exposure can be facilitated by lateral rotation of the thigh with modest flexion of the knee and hip.[17] Partial or complete division of the adductor longus muscle may be necessary to expose the artery beyond its second perforator branch (see Fig. 55–3).

This direct approach to the profunda may be difficult or impossible to achieve in patients with infection or severe inguinal scar formation due to multiple previous vascular repairs. A simple alternative to this dilemma is to approach the mid-portion of the deep femoral artery through an anterior thigh incision that can be readily located distal to the previous groin incision.[9, 17, 30] The sartorius is retracted laterally to expose the superficial femoral vessels, which are drawn medially. Branches of the femoral nerve in this area should be identified and preserved. The fascia deep to the superficial femoral is incised to expose the deep femoral vessels between the first and second perforator branches. When infection is present, the incision should be placed lateral to the sartorius muscle, which is retracted medially to more effectively separate the operative field from the area of sepsis.[18, 30] The exposed segment of profunda lies distal to the arterial obstruction and can be readily anastomosed to a new or revised inflow graft.[9, 19, 31]

Heparin, 5000 to 7000 units, is given systemically, and thereafter the branches are controlled with microsurgical clips or latex loop slings, and clamps are applied to the common femoral and distal profunda femoris arteries. A vertical incision is made on the anterior aspect of the common femoral artery, and any loose debris and thrombus are removed. Occasionally, the major obstruction is due to a large plaque on the posterior wall of the common femoral artery that obscures the profunda orifice and extends only a few millimeters down the deep femoral lumen. This plaque can be removed entirely through the common femoral incision, and the intima of the distal profunda femoris can be controlled with a few tacking stitches placed from inside the arterial orifice to prevent subsequent dissection (Fig. 55–4*B*). The arteriotomy is then closed with a simple running suture or by end-to-side anastomosis to an inflow graft.

In the majority of cases, however, the obstructing atheroma extends a substantial distance down into the profunda femoris. The common femoral arteriotomy is extended through the profunda orifice and then distally on to the anterior surface of the deep femoral artery. The arteriotomy must be carefully placed to avoid incision into the crotch between the superficial femoral and the deep femoral, and also to skirt the orifices of major branches (Fig. 55–5*A*). The incision should extend a centimeter or more beyond the usually abrupt point of transition between significant atheromatous encroachment and the relatively normal distal intima (Fig. 55–5*A*). This usually occurs just beyond one of the major profunda branches, and at this level the lumen will generally accept a 4- to 5-mm probe.[3, 8, 17, 27] Thromboendarterectomy is carried down to this transition point, which should be at least a few millimeters proximal to the caudal end of the arteriotomy. This will facilitate placement of tacking sutures as needed to prevent further dissection if a clean break from the distal intima cannot be achieved. Extensions of the plaque into branch orifices should be meticulously avulsed so that these branches will remain open and contribute to the collateral function of the profunda femoris.[17]

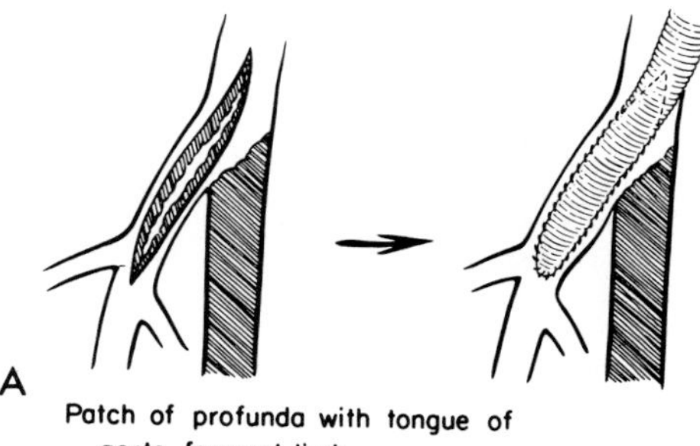

A
Patch of profunda with tongue of aorto femoral limb.

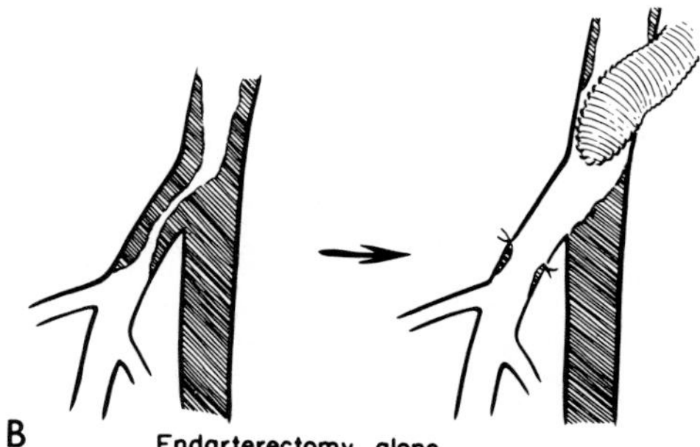

FIGURE 55–4. Operative technique of profundaplasty in association with aortofemoral graft or other procedure for inflow obstruction. *A*, The Dacron limb may be used as an extended tongue to widen a stenotic area in the proximal profunda. *B*, A limited common and deep femoral endarterectomy with suture stabilization of the distal intima can be carried out when the plaque involves only the orifice and not more than 1 cm of the profunda femoris. (*A* and *B*, From Bernhard VM, Militello JM, Geringer AM: Repair of the profunda femoris artery. Am J Surg 127:676, 1974.)

The arteriotomy is then closed with a patch to ensure an adequate lumen without stenosis into the runoff vessel.[3, 8, 17, 21, 27] When profundaplasty is combined with a procedure designed to restore inflow, the Dacron inflow limb can be tailored and sutured over the profunda arteriotomy as an extended tongue for a distance of 2 to 3 cm, as depicted in Figure 55–4*A*. Longer arteriotomies are more reliably closed with a patch of autogenous tissue.[3, 25, 34] A segment of adjacent occluded superficial femoral artery can be filleted and prepared by endarterectomy to make a patch of desired length and width, as diagrammed in Figure 55–5*B* and *C*. Although a major branch of the saphenous also can be used for the patch, the main saphenous trunk should usually be saved in anticipation of its possible future use for distal bypass or coronary revascularization. Regardless of the material employed, the patch should be tailored and sutured in such a way that it produces a gradually tapering lumen, with the caudal end bluntly rounded to produce a funnel into the distal artery (Fig. 55–5*C*). A completion arteriogram should be obtained so that technical defects can be corrected prior to wound closure.

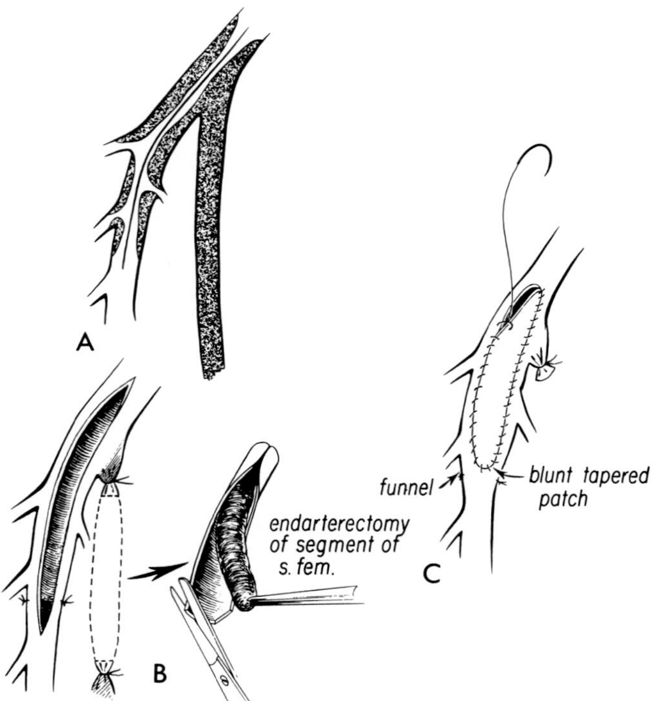

FIGURE 55–5. *A–C*, Technique for long profunda femoris endarterectomy and patch angioplasty utilizing the outer layers of the occluded segment of the superficial femoral artery when a vein is not available for patch.

COMPLICATIONS

Operative complications are similar to those associated with any other vascular reconstructive procedure. Hemorrhage or hematoma formation requires immediate wound exploration to repair a suture line leak and control other bleeding vessels. If early thrombosis occurs, the groin wound should be promptly explored to remove intraluminal clot and correct technical errors.

Lymphorrhea and lymphocele formation are more common following the extended groin incision associated with profundaplasty than with the routine vascular groin incision.[32] The incidence of this complication can be reduced by avoiding the transection of lymph nodes during groin dissection, ligating all observed open lymph ducts, and ensuring meticulous multi-layer closure of the groin wound. Treatment requires bed rest with moderate leg elevation until drainage ceases and groin swelling recedes. Draining fluid should be cultured and appropriate antibiotics given if infection is present. Skin sutures should not be removed until the problem has been resolved, unless the wound is septic. If there is any question of skin edge necrosis, prompt groin exploration should be performed to débride all necrotic tissue and ligate leaking lymphatics.[20]

Superficial wound infections should be drained promptly and treated with local care and antibiotics. Deep infections involving repaired vascular structures or grafts should be managed as described in Chapter 40. To reduce the incidence of wound infection, prophylactic antibiotics are routinely administered, and all wounds are copiously irrigated with antibiotic saline solution before closure.

Late thrombosis of a profunda femoris repair is usually due to progression of the underlying atherosclerotic process in the deep femoral artery or in the aortoiliac inflow vessels.[5] Angiography should be carried out promptly to estimate the feasibility of reoperation on the artery and to determine the need for revision or addition of a procedure for inflow obstruction. If the vessel distal to the occlusive process is still patent, revision and extension of the previous profundaplasty, although tedious, is usually successful.[31] Bypass to the mid-profunda is a reliable alternative when scarring or infection is present.[9, 17, 31] Thrombosis of the associated femoral limb of an aortic bifurcation graft can usually be relieved by Fogarty catheter thrombectomy, and only occasionally is insertion of a new bypass required.[5]

RESULTS

The operative mortality rate for this procedure is low, and deaths occur almost invariably in those patients who are in desperate need of revascularization to prevent major amputation.[40] In the author's experience with 237 profunda

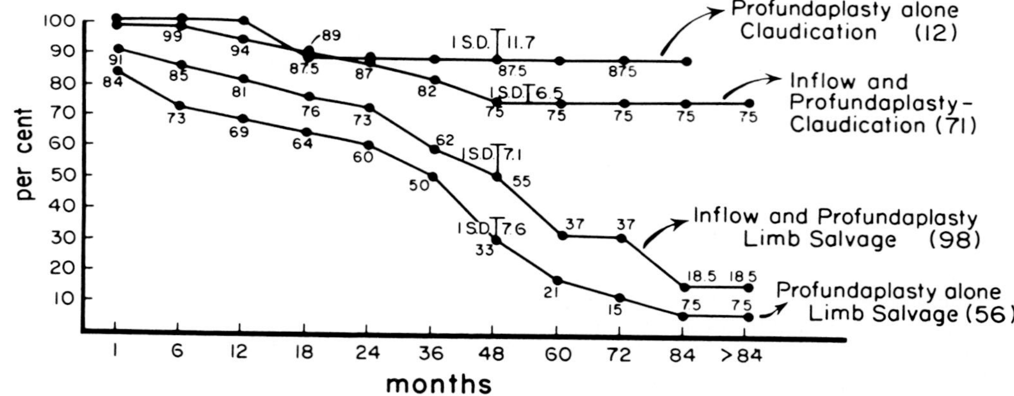

FIGURE 55–6. Cumulative profundaplasty patency of individual groups. (From Towne JB, Bernhard VM, Rollins DL, et al: Profundaplasty in perspective: Limitations in long-term management of limb ischemia. Surgery 90:1037, 1981.)

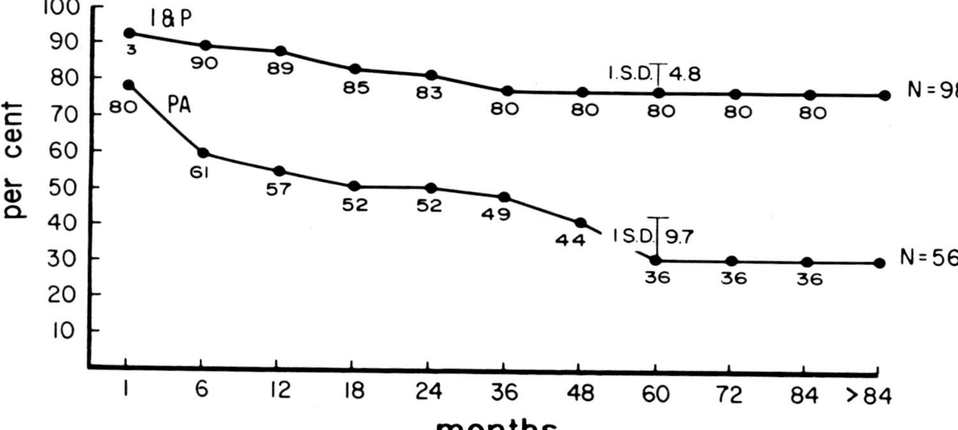

FIGURE 55–7. Cumulative limb salvage of inflow procedure and profundaplasty and profundaplasty alone groups. (From Towne JB, Bernhard VM, Rollins DL et al: Profundaplasty in perspective: Limitations in long-term management of limb ischemia. Surgery 90:1037, 1981.)

repairs in a series of 209 patients, there were no deaths among those operated on for claudication, and five deaths (3 per cent) occurred in the limb salvage group.[40] This difference reflects a more aggressive approach to patients at greater risk in whom the alternative is loss of the limb. Similar results have been reported by others.[8, 10, 21, 27, 31–33, 39, 43]

The improvement in limb perfusion following profundaplasty performed as an adjunct to an inflow procedure is much better than that for profundaplasty alone, because the most important level of obstruction is proximal and the popliteal-tibial runoff is usually relatively good. By comparison, patients with a similar degree of ischemia who have unimpaired aortoiliac inflow and require profunda repair to restore its collateral function generally have more severe disease in the leg and foot.[6, 11, 28, 35, 40]

When the indication for operation in the author's patients was claudication, early patency of the profunda repair was achieved in all patients and was maintained in 77 per cent at 5 years; no significant difference was noted between patients requiring bypass and profundaplasty and those requiring profundaplasty alone (Fig. 55–6).[40] Marked subjective improvement or complete relief of claudication was achieved in 99 per cent of the 82 limbs managed by inflow and profundaplasty or isolated profundaplasty in the author's experience.[40] Similar results have been reported by Martin and coworkers, by Welsh and Repetto, and by others.[7, 12, 13, 26, 27, 29, 31, 33, 37, 43] However, a measurable increase in the ankle-brachial pressure index of more than 0.1 was noted in only 69 per cent of cases in the author's series.[6] Only four of seven patients subjected to isolated profundaplasty had a significant increase in treadmill exercise tolerance in the study reported by Strandness,[37] although Fernandes and associates demonstrated a higher incidence of hemodynamic improvement.[13]

Initial patency in limbs operated upon for salvage was obtained in 88 per cent; however, at 5 years there was progressive attrition in patency of the repair to 37 per cent in patients managed by an inflow procedure and profundaplasty and to 21 per cent in those receiving profundaplasty alone,[40] as noted in Figure 55–6. Nevertheless, limb salvage was achieved initially in 93 per cent and was retained in 80 per cent of the limbs with the combined procedures, but in only 36 per cent of those with profundaplasty alone after 5 years (Fig. 55–7).

There is considerable difference of opinion, on the other hand, regarding the value of isolated profundaplasty for limb salvage; however, criteria for patient selection for this procedure versus a bypass to the popliteal or tibial vessels have not been consistently applied.[2, 11, 16, 21, 28, 35, 40] Relief of rest pain and healing of necrotic lesions or minor amputations are most likely to be achieved in patients who have severe (greater than 50 per cent) stenosis of the profunda, with a patent popliteal segment in continuity with at least one vessel runoff to the pedal arch and a low profunda-popliteal collateral index (PPCI). It is noteworthy that immediate success was achieved[2, 9] in 91 per cent of limbs with a PPCI of less than 0.19. Similar results were achieved by McCoy and associates in patients with a thigh-ankle gradient index (TAGI) of less than .55.[24]

Isolated profundaplasty should be preferred to infrapopliteal bypass as the initial procedure whenever a satisfactory autogenous vein is not available.[24, 40] Furthermore, patients with severe proximal profunda stenosis in whom infrainguinal bypass is not technically feasible should also have profunda revascularization. Although limb salvage is infrequently achieved under these circumstances, amputation at the below-knee level is much more likely to heal if the profunda is patent and well perfused.[40]

Profundaplasty is an important adjunct to aortobifemoral bypass and other inflow procedures when any degree of obstruction in the proximal portion of this artery is identified by arteriography, duplex scanning, or intraoperative assessment. As an isolated procedure, profundaplasty will improve claudication distance, relieve rest pain, and permit healing of minor ischemic lesions in a limited number of patients if the selection criteria outlined in Table 55–1 are routinely employed.

References

1. Beales JSM, Adock FA, Frawley JS, et al: The radiological assessment of disease of the profunda femoris artery. Br J Radiol 44:854, 1971.
2. Bernhard VM: Limitations of profunda femoris revascularization. *In* Veith FJ (ed): Critical Problems in Vascular Surgery. New York, Appleton-Century-Crofts, 1982, pp 251–262.
3. Bernhard VM, Militello JM, Geringer AM: Repair of the profunda femoris artery. Am J Surg 127:676, 1974.
4. Bernhard VM, Ray LI, Militello JM: The role of angioplasty of the

profunda femoris artery in revascularization of the ischemic limb. Surg Gynecol Obstet 142:840, 1976.
5. Bernhard VM, Ray LI, Towne JB: The reoperation of choice for aortofemoral graft occlusion. Surgery 82:867, 1977.
6. Boren CH, Towne JB, Bernhard VM, et al: Profundapopliteal collateral index. A guide to successful profundaplasty. Arch Surg 115:1366, 1980.
7. Brewster DC, Meier GH III, Darling RC, et al: Reoperation for aortofemoral graft limb occlusion: Optimal methods and long-term results. J Vasc Surg 5:363, 1987.
8. David TE, Drezner AD: Extended profundaplasty for limb salvage. Surgery 84:758, 1978.
9. DePalma RG, Malgieri JJ, Rhodes RS, et al: Profunda femoris bypass for secondary revascularization. Surg Gynecol Obstet 151:387, 1980.
10. Goldstone J, Malone JM, Moore WS: Importance of the profunda femoris artery in primary and secondary arterial operations for lower extremity ischemia. Am J Surg 136:215, 1978.
11. Graham AM, Gewertz BL, Zarins CK: Efficacy of isolated profundaplasty. Can J Surg 29:330, 1986.
12. Graziano JL, Olander GA, Lai RB: Significance of the profunda femoris artery in extremities with marked ischemia. Am Surg 35:229, 1969.
13. Fernandes JF, Nicolaides AN, Angelides NA, et al: An objective assessment of common femoral endarterectomy and profundaplasty in patients with superficial femoral occlusion. Surgery 83:313, 1978.
14. Flanigan DP, Ryan TJ, Williams LR, et al: Aortofemoral or femoropopliteal revascularization? A prospective evaluation of the papaverine test. J Vasc Surg 1:215, 1984.
15. Hansen AK, Belle S, Nielson PH, Egeblad K: Profundaplasty as the only reconstructive procedure in patients with severe ischemia of the lower extremity. Surg Gynecol Obstet 171:47, 1990.
16. Harward TR, Bergan JJ, Yao JST, et al: The demise of primary profundaplasty. Am J Surg 156:126, 1988.
17. Hershey FB, Auer AI: Extended surgical approach to the profunda femoris artery. Surg Gynecol Obstet 138:88, 1974.
18. Hurd SP, Jurayj MN, Trippel OH: Innovative applications of extra-anatomic reconstruction. Surg Clin North Am 54:123, 1974.
19. King TA, DePalma RG, Rhodes RS: Diabetes mellitus and atherosclerotic involvement of the profunda femoris artery. Surg Gynecol Obstet 159:553, 1984.
20. Kwaan JHM, Bernstein JM, Connolly JE: Management of lymph fistula in the groin after arterial reconstruction. Arch Surg 114:1416, 1976.
21. Leather RP, Shah DM, Karmody AM: The use of extended profundaplasty in limb salvage. Am J Surg 136:359, 1978.
22. Leeds FH, Gilfillan RS: Revascularization of the ischemic limb. Surgery 82:25, 1961.
23. Lindbom A: Arteriosclerosis and arterial thrombosis in the lower limbs. A roentgenologic study. Acta Radiol Suppl 80, p 1, 1950.
24. McCoy DM, Sawchuk AP, Schuler JJ, et al: The role of isolated profundaplasty for the treatment of rest pain. Arch Surg 124:441, 1989.
25. Malone JM, Goldstone J, Moore WS: Autogenous profundaplasty: The key to long term patency in secondary repair of aortofemoral graft occlusion. Ann Surg 188:818, 1978.
26. Martin P, Jamieson C: The rationale for measurement after profundaplasty. Surg Clin North Am 54:95, 1974.
27. Martin P, Frawley JE, Barabas AP, et al: On the surgery of atherosclerosis of the profunda femoris artery. Surgery 71:182, 1972.
28. Mitchell RA, Bine GE, Bridges R, et al: Patient selection for isolated profundaplasty. Am J Surg 138:912, 1979.
29. Morris GC, Edwards W, Cooley DA, et al: Surgical importance of profunda femoris artery. Arch Surg 82:52, 1961.
30. Nunez AA, Veith JF, Collier P, et al: Direct approaches to the distal portions of the deep femoral artery for limb salvage bypass. J Vasc Surg 8:576, 1988.
31. Ourial K, DeWeese JA, Ricotta JJ, et al: Revascularization of the distal profunda femoris artery in the reconstructive treatment of aortoiliac occlusive disease. J Vasc Surg 6:217, 1987.
32. Pearce WH, Kempczynski RF: Extended autogenous profundaplasty and aortofemoral grafting: An alternative to synchronous distal bypass. J Vasc Surg 1:455, 1984.
33. Prendiville EJ, Burke DE, Colagan MP, et al: The profunda femoris: A durable outflow vessel in aortofemoral surgery. J Vasc Surg 16:23, 1992.
34. Rollins DL, Towne JB, Bernhard VM, et al: Endarterectomized superficial femoral artery as an arterial patch. Arch Surg 120:367, 1985.
35. Sladen JG, Burgess JJ: Profundaplasty: Expectations and ominous signs. Am J Surg 140:242, 1980.
36. Sproul G: Reconstruction of the profunda femoris artery. Surgery 63:871, 1968.
37. Strandness DE Jr: Functional results after revascularization of the profunda femoris artery. Am J Surg 119:240, 1970.
38. Strauss HL, Schaberle W, Rieger H, Roth FJ: Use of duplex scanning in the diagnosis of arteria profunda femoris stenosis. J Vasc Surg 13:698, 1991.
39. Taylor LM Jr, Baur GM, Eidemiller LR, et al: Extended profundaplasty. Indications and techniques with results of 46 procedures. Am J Surg 141:539, 1981.
40. Towne JB, Bernhard VM, Rollins DL, et al: Profundaplasty in perspective. Limitations in long term management of limb ischemia. Surgery 90:1037, 1987.
41. Waibel PP, Wolff G: The collateral circulation in occlusions of the femoral artery: An experimental study. Surgery 60:912, 1966.
42. Warwick R, Williams PE (eds): Gray's Anatomy. 35th British ed. Philadelphia, WB Saunders, 1973, p 677.
43. Welsh P, Repetto R: Revascularization of the profunda femoris artery in aortoiliac occlusive disease. Surgery 78:389, 1975.

56

Femoral and Popliteal Thromboendarterectomy

Toshio Inahara, M.D., and Dipankar Mukherjee, M.D., F.A.C.S.

• • •

Although atherosclerosis is a generalized disease process, arterial circulation is often selectively compromised in a specific organ system or regional watershed area. Because of this selective involvement as well as the segmental distribution of lesions within the diseased vessels, the impaired circulation can usually be corrected surgically utilizing a bypass graft or direct disobliteration by endarterectomy. Endarterectomy is preferentially employed for treatment of the short occlusive lesions encountered in the carotid and renal arteries and, less commonly, in the abdominal aorta and iliac arteries.

HISTORICAL PERSPECTIVE

Thromboendarterectomy was introduced by dos Santos[14] in 1944 and the bypass principle using the autogenous saphenous vein by Kunlin[23] in 1949. Wylie and McGuinness[42] introduced the semi-open technique of endarterectomy of the femoropopliteal arteries in 1953. In 1955, Cannon and Barker[4] advocated the use of arterial loops permitting a semi-closed technique, thus limiting the extent of the arteriotomy. Along similar lines, Sobel and colleagues[33] proposed the technique of gas endarterectomy. In 1950, Edwards[15] described the open technique of endarterectomy with a patch graft of saphenous vein.

The application of endarterectomy for occlusive disease of the femoral and popliteal arteries began in the early 1950s and was widely used in the 1960s. During this period, the operation was performed for occlusions of the entire superficial femoral and popliteal arteries, often in continuity. Such long endarterectomies were accomplished by the semi-open method with multiple arteriotomies or by the open technique with saphenous vein onlay patch graft. The closed method using arterial loops or carbon dioxide gas dissection usually was performed through a proximal and distal arteriotomy.

In the late 1960s and early 1970s, long-term results of endarterectomy were reported.[25, 39, 43] Imparato and coworkers[18] reported 5-year patency rates of 36 per cent by the open technique and 50 per cent by the semi-closed technique. Darling and Linton[10] reported 5-year patency rates of 32 per cent for extended endarterectomy and 72 per cent for the reversed saphenous vein bypass graft. When other reports also confirmed the superiority of the vein bypass,[3, 8, 10, 11, 13, 30] it became the recognized standard of comparison for all other techniques of femoropopliteal reconstruction. Although superficial femoral and popliteal endarterectomy remained a viable option, it was considered only as a last alternative when other techniques for limb salvage were not possible. However, because current prosthetic grafts have failed to achieve results comparable with those of autogenous repair, some authors continued to employ extended femoropopliteal endarterectomy in selected cases.[24, 36, 37]

During this same period, short (less than 15 cm) endarterectomies were successfully performed for occlusive lesions in the common femoral, profunda femoris, superficial femoral, and popliteal arteries.[1, 3, 5, 17, 40] Although the number of patients in whom these techniques were used was relatively small, patency results were more favorable than were those for the extended endarterectomy.[6] Short segmental endarterectomies have been advocated where the saphenous vein is inadequate or the patient is at high risk, since the endarterectomy can be performed more expeditiously than the vein bypass.[17]

Despite the proven success of femoropopliteal endarterectomy for short segmental lesions, it remains infrequently used.[1, 6, 12] Because of the relatively poor results with long segment endarterectomies compared with the reversed saphenous vein grafts, endarterectomy in general was abandoned by many surgeons who failed to distinguish between the results achieved in long occlusions and those seen in short segmental lesions. Because bypass grafts were easily performed with predictably good results, segmental endarterectomies of the superficial femoral artery were not considered. Furthermore, because it was not commonly performed despite appropriate indications and surgical residents were not exposed to this technique, it has not become a part of the armamentarium of many vascular surgeons. Ouriel and associates[28] reported a series of 94 patients in whom superficial femoral endarterectomy was performed over a 25-year period with long-term patency rates of 66 per cent at 3 years and 57 per cent at 7 years with recommendation for endarterectomy of localized adductor canal disease as a viable alternative to the femoropopliteal bypass.

NATURAL HISTORY OF ATHEROSCLEROSIS

Several studies[19, 27, 29, 34, 37, 39] on the natural history of lower extremity atherosclerosis that focused on the progression of symptoms and the incidence of limb loss have demonstrated that (1) symptomatic occlusive disease of the lower extremity is a relatively stable condition, (2) claudication often can be expected to improve with walking and abstinence from smoking, and (3) anticipated limb loss is in the range of 1.1 to 4.4 per cent per year. This has led to a general acceptance of nonoperative treatment for intermittent claudication, and thus few of these patients are referred for diagnostic arteriography. Because arteriography is infrequently performed, the opportunity to identify the early lesion is usually missed. Furthermore, patients rarely seek medical attention when their only symptom is nondisabling claudication, thus contributing further to the difficulty in identifying early segmental lesions.

Two clinical studies provided important objective data on the progression of atherosclerosis in the superficial femoral artery. Strandness and Stahler[34] followed 60 patients with serial measurements of segmental limb pressures. In 58 per cent of these patients, arteriograms were obtained when necessary. Warren and coworkers[39] studied 23 limbs in 17 patients with serial arteriograms performed at intervals over an 8-year period. In this study, short segmental lesions were initially found in 80 per cent of the 23 superficial femoral arteries. In one limb, two segmental lesions were present. Subsequent arteriograms revealed gradual progression of the atherosclerosis in a proximal direction with eventual occlusion of the entire superficial femoral artery.

Both Strandness and Stahler[34] and Warren[39] noted that there was very little correlation between the severity of claudication and its rate of progression, regression, or stability and objective measurements of segmental pressures or anatomic changes documented by arteriography. Objective changes often occurred without symptomatic progression. These studies emphasized two findings: first, that clinical evaluation of atherosclerotic occlusive disease is subjective to a great extent, and often there is not a close relationship to the extent of the disease present; and second, that atherosclerotic disease of the lower extremity is steadily progressive, but the patient's symptoms do not necessarily correlate with the progression. Warren and coworkers'[39] observation represents the most accurate study of anatomic changes reflecting the true natural course of lower extremity atherosclerosis. This study revealed for the first time that within the background of diffuse atherosclerosis, there were segmental sites of accelerated disease that led to eventual short segment occlusions. The distal superficial femoral artery in the adductor canal was not only the earliest site of occlusion but was also the site most frequently involved. From this distal site, there was proximal extension of the disease with eventual total occlusion of the superficial femoral artery. This study is of paramount importance in supporting the concept of segmental endarterectomy.

In 1991, Walsh and colleagues[38] reported their arteriographic observations on the natural history of superficial femoral artery (SFA) stenoses. Twenty-five limbs were studied arteriographically before and after a mean observation period of 25 months. The initial mean stenosis on arteriography was 43 per cent (range, 0 to 100 per cent). After a mean follow-up period of 25 months (range, 7 to 60 months), the mean stenosis had progressed to 56 per cent (range, 0 to 100 per cent). Multi-variate analysis of risk factors for progression of SFA lesions appeared to relate most closely to two factors: the severity of the contralateral SFA disease and the history of significant tobacco usage. This study further corroborates the progressive nature of occlusive disease in the lower extremities.

All vascular surgeons have seen patients with nondisabling claudication as a result of short segmental stenosis or occlusion of the superficial femoral artery who, on subsequent studies, have progressed to complete occlusion. If these segmental lesions are recognized by an early diagnostic approach, it is possible to restore circulation by segmental endarterectomy (Fig. 56–1).

CONCEPT OF SEGMENTAL ENDARTERECTOMY

Segmental endarterectomy is an attempt to maintain patency of the native artery whether it be in the cerebral, visceral, or peripheral circulation. The selection of patients and indications for operation are based mainly upon the symptoms and the potential ischemic threat to the end-organ. Although intermittent claudication may be very inconvenient for the patient, the potential for ischemic limb loss is small; hence, conservative management is commonly recommended. It is at this early stage that arteriographic study is likely to identify a short segmental lesion suitable for endarterectomy. Opportunity for such early appraisal is often lost by patient delay. Similarly, following endarterectomy, periodic longitudinal follow-up is necessary to ascertain changes in symptoms and segmental pressure studies. Early arteriography is the sine qua non for assessing the status and progression of the disease process.

RADIOLOGIC CRITERIA OF OPERABILITY

Selection of a segmental lesion for endarterectomy is based upon the configuration of a relatively compact lesion, either stenosis or an occlusion, isolated between adequate inflow and outflow vessels that preferably are normal in caliber. A diffusely narrow vessel proximal and distal to such a lesion constitutes an unfavorable situation for endarterectomy. Another important consideration for selection is the length of the occlusive lesion. Because of early negative experience with long-segment superficial femoral artery endarterectomy, the authors have arbitrarily selected 15 cm as the maximum length for this procedure, although on occasion longer segments have been disobliterated. In vessels of smaller than normal diameter, it is desirable to decrease the length of the endarterectomy still further. A blind popliteal segment distal to the segmental occlusion may constitute a relative contraindication for endarterec-

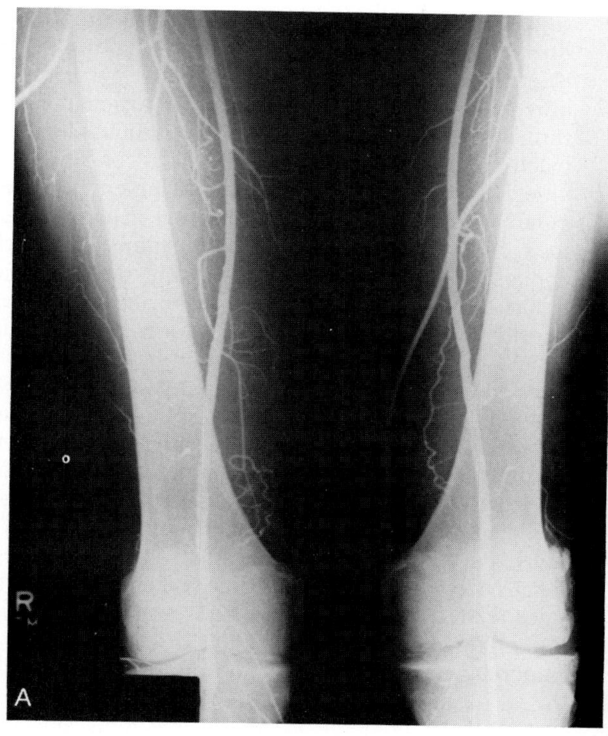

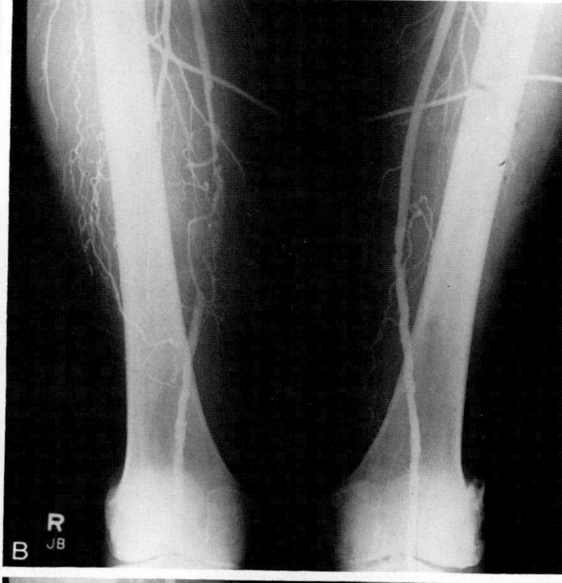

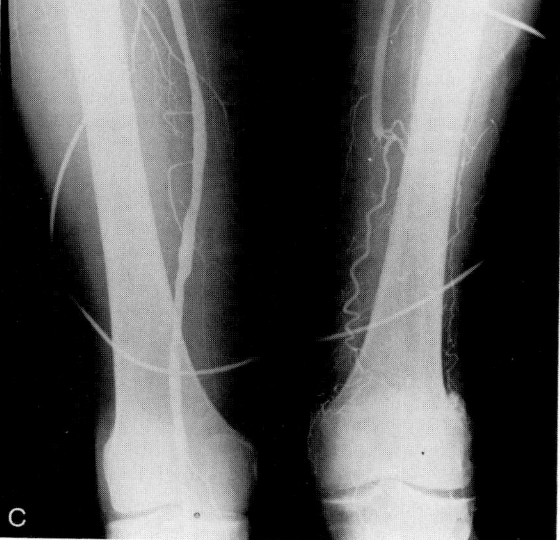

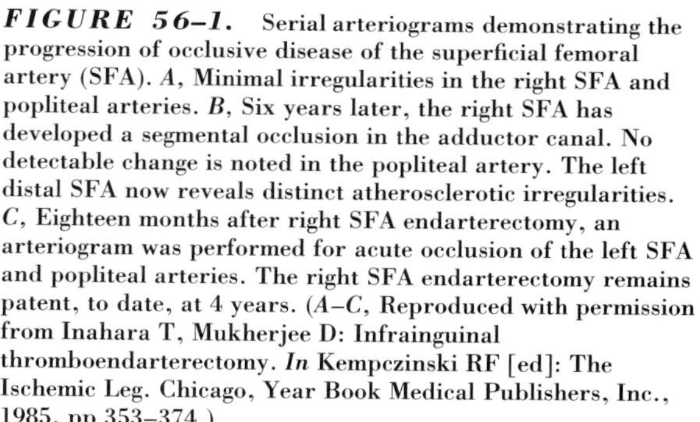

FIGURE 56–1. Serial arteriograms demonstrating the progression of occlusive disease of the superficial femoral artery (SFA). *A*, Minimal irregularities in the right SFA and popliteal arteries. *B*, Six years later, the right SFA has developed a segmental occlusion in the adductor canal. No detectable change is noted in the popliteal artery. The left distal SFA now reveals distinct atherosclerotic irregularities. *C*, Eighteen months after right SFA endarterectomy, an arteriogram was performed for acute occlusion of the left SFA and popliteal arteries. The right SFA endarterectomy remains patent, to date, at 4 years. (*A–C*, Reproduced with permission from Inahara T, Mukherjee D: Infrainguinal thromboendarterectomy. *In* Kempczinski RF [ed]: The Ischemic Leg. Chicago, Year Book Medical Publishers, Inc., 1985, pp 353–374.)

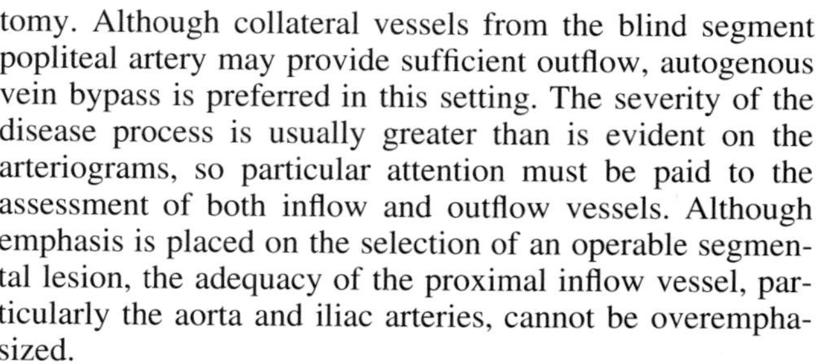

tomy. Although collateral vessels from the blind segment popliteal artery may provide sufficient outflow, autogenous vein bypass is preferred in this setting. The severity of the disease process is usually greater than is evident on the arteriograms, so particular attention must be paid to the assessment of both inflow and outflow vessels. Although emphasis is placed on the selection of an operable segmental lesion, the adequacy of the proximal inflow vessel, particularly the aorta and iliac arteries, cannot be overemphasized.

General measures, such as abstinence from cigarette smoking, control of hypertension, dietary measures, and weight reduction to an ideal body weight, are considered critical in the overall management of these patients. Patients must stop smoking before they are accepted for vascular reconstruction. Patients with hyperlipidemic states are investigated and placed on special dietary modifications (Fig. 56–2).

OPERATIVE TECHNIQUE OF SEGMENTAL ENDARTERECTOMY

Spinal anesthesia was formerly employed for these procedures. However, the authors' preference now is continuous epidural anesthesia[7] with 0.5 per cent bupivacaine hydrochloride (Marcaine). The common femoral artery is exposed through a vertical incision in the groin, whereas the standard medial thigh incision is used for the superficial femoral artery. When one is dealing with the distal superficial femoral artery, the adductor canal is fully released and is not reapproximated. Operative exposure for the popliteal is through a straight posterior incision in the popliteal space with the patient in a prone position. This provides the necessary full exposure of the popliteal artery.

The diseased segment of the artery is exposed using the arteriogram as a guide.[20] The vessel is carefully palpated

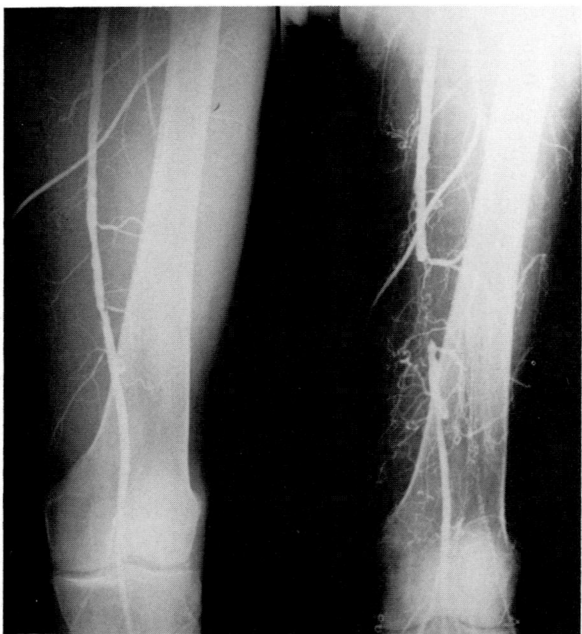

FIGURE 56–2. *Left*, Asymptomatic atherosclerotic lesion of the SFA. *Right*, Segmental occlusion in the same limb 18 months later associated with claudication. Such lesions with adequate inflow and outflow vessels are well suited for endarterectomy. (Reproduced with permission from Inahara T, Mukherjee D: Infrainguinal thromboendarterectomy. *In* Kempczinski RF [ed]: The Ischemic Leg, Chicago, Year Book Medical Publishers, Inc., 1985, pp 353–374.)

to identify the lesion for localization, noting the presence of a thrill or change in the character of the pulse. Noting the pattern of arterial branching is also helpful. Arterial branches are preserved and temporarily occluded with removable metal clips. The patient is anticoagulated for all endarterectomy procedures using 3000 IU intravenous heparin as an initial bolus, followed by hourly supplements of 1000 IU. This low-dose regimen has proved to be adequate and does not require reversal at the completion of the procedure. According to the length of the occlusive segment, endarterectomy is performed through one to three longitudinal arteriotomies. When multiple arteriotomies are employed, the distal one is usually the longest. The distal point of termination is carefully selected at a site showing the least disease, since normal vessel wall is infrequently seen. A smoothly tailored outflow is the most important feature of the reconstruction. Tailoring can be accomplished by transverse or oblique beveling of the end-point. It is helpful to place one's finger behind the vessel as counterpressure for beveling. Use of loupes for magnification is a useful adjunct. Because of its importance, our first preference is to tailor the outflow end-point. The atheromatous disease is next removed proximally through a plane of dissection between the plaque and the media, where it separates readily. The proximal end-point is tailored at this time by a similar beveling technique. After the plaque is removed, the circular fibers of the media are carefully stripped. The smooth muscle layer is quite adherent in the femoral artery, in contrast to that in the iliac vessels, and requires instrument removal to leave a smooth adventitial surface. Careful abrasion with pill sponges removes the remaining filamentous fibers. Finally, interrupted longitudinal mattress sutures (6–0) are placed to secure the beveled edges at both termination points because compression of the residual plaque edge further reduces the profile to improve laminal flow. Venous patch angioplasty is essential in the reconstitution of the vessel. To prevent narrowing of the lumen at the terminal points of the endarterectomy, the vein patch is extended 1 to 2 cm beyond the beveled termination. This technique applies equally to both the distal and the proximal endpoints. It is also important for the reconstructed vessel to be smooth and only slightly fusiform, and the diameter should not be more than 1 to 2 mm larger than the native artery, with the hope that smooth laminar flow will be restored. It is often necessary to split the saphenous vein longitudinally to apply a narrow patch graft. If a tributary of the greater saphenous vein is not available, the ankle segment of the saphenous vein is harvested when there is sufficient collateral venous flow to preserve the main saphenous vein. When a single arteriotomy is employed, its entire length is closed with a vein patch. When multiple arteriotomies are required, the vein patch is applied occasionally to the proximal and always to the distal arteriotomy. It is important to obtain completion arteriograms in all small vessel reconstructions (Fig. 56–3).

Catheter epidural anesthesia injections are continued for an additional 12 to 24 hours. This provides adequate relief of pain, retention of motor function of the extremities, and maximum peripheral vasodilatation. Low-molecular-weight dextran, 250 ml, is given over a 6-hour period immediately postoperatively and again in 12 hours.[41] Aspirin is started with the first oral intake, and is continued for several months.

Lumbar sympathectomy was performed prior to or concomitantly with superficial femoral endarterectomy in 25 patients (19 per cent), with popliteal endarterectomy in 20 patients (19 per cent), and in none of the patients with the common femoral endarterectomy. Lumbar sympathectomy is now infrequently performed.

In patients with adjunctive lumbar sympathectomy, failures of the superficial femoral endarterectomy occurred in seven patients, with one amputation. Failures of the popliteal endarterectomy occurred in five patients, with three amputations. The performance of lumbar sympathectomy did not significantly influence the eventual outcome. Clinical assessment of the long-term effectiveness of sympathectomy is difficult because atherosclerosis is a progressive process.

ANATOMIC SITES

For clinical discussion and analysis of results, the arterial circulation can be divided conveniently into three anatomic areas: the common femoral, the superficial femoral, and the popliteal arteries. Although each anatomic area will be dealt with separately here, it should be noted that occlusive lesions are often contiguous and overlapping. Lesions of the common femoral artery frequently extend into the deep and superficial femoral arteries distally and often are contiguous with the aortoiliac disease proximally. Iso-

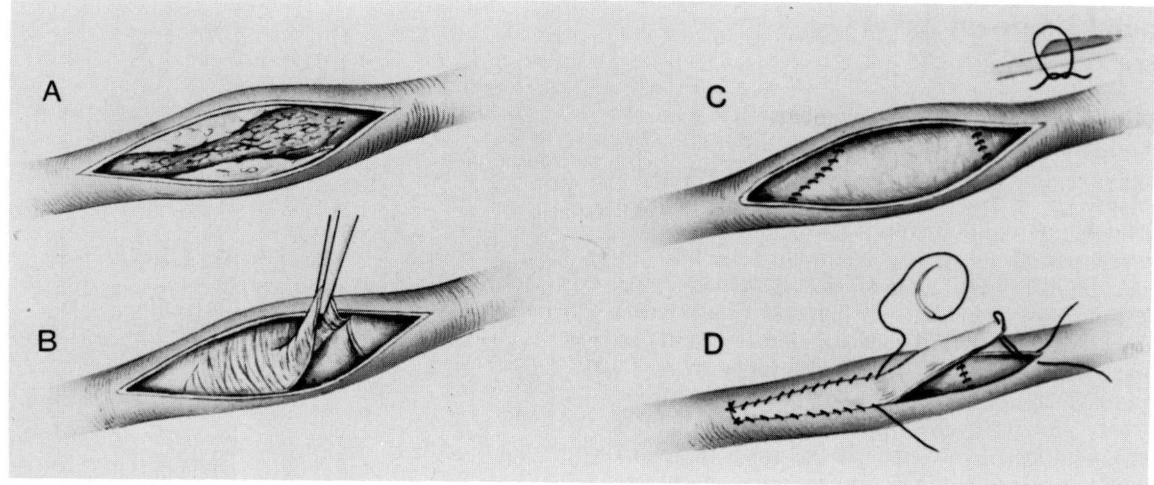

FIGURE 56–3. Technique of segmental endarterectomy. *A*, Arteriotomy is extended beyond the plaque proximally and distally to an area of less disease where the endarterectomy can be terminated. *B*, The adherent circular layer of the media is carefully stripped away, leaving a smooth adventitial surface. *C*, Endarterectomy is terminated by transverse or oblique beveling of the intima. Longitudinal mattress sutures (6–0) are placed at the proximal and distal edges to prevent flap elevation and to reduce profile of endarterectomy to blood flow. *D*, Autogenous vein patch graft is extended proximally and distally, 1 to 2 cm past the end-points of the endarterectomy. (*A–D*, Reproduced with permission from Inahara T, Mukherjee D: Infrainguinal thromboendarterectomy. *In* Kempczinski RF [ed]: The Ischemic Leg. Chicago, Year Book Medical Publishers, Inc., 1985, pp 353–374.)

lated lesions are more frequently seen in the superficial femoral and popliteal arteries.

In the experience of the authors, the approximate incidence of all segmental endarterectomies of the common femoral, superficial femoral, and popliteal arteries (n = 261) relative to the number of patients studied by arteriography (n = 2565) was 10 per cent over a 22-year period. Undoubtedly, there were many other lesions suitable for endarterectomy that were untreated and untabulated. The relative frequency of segmental endarterectomy performed at each of the three anatomic sites being considered was as follows: common femoral artery, 10 per cent; superficial femoral artery, 51 per cent; popliteal artery, 39 per cent.

Common Femoral Endarterectomy

Of the three anatomic sites, surgically treatable localized atherosclerotic disease occurs least frequently in the common femoral artery. Patients often experience claudication of the buttocks and thigh as well as the calf. Not uncommonly, there is accompanying hypoesthesia and paresthesia of the foot and toes because the ischemia is more pronounced in the absence of direct flow into the profunda femoris artery. The femoral pulse is diminished or absent. A strong external iliac pulse just proximal to the inguinal ligament is a clue to the diagnosis. Segmental pressures are evenly diminished throughout the limb, which suggests that the superficial femoral and popliteal vessels are patent.

When the common femoral artery is occluded, arteriography may not visualize adequately the popliteal and its tributaries owing to hemodilution of the contrast media. Percutaneous femoral arteriography distal to the occlusion is necessary to visualize the outflow vessels. Despite the absence of a palpable femoral pulse, a needle can be inserted percutaneously into the superficial or profunda femoris artery for the study (Fig. 56–4).

Results

From 1969 through 1986, 22 patients underwent common femoral endarterectomy (for claudication in 16 and for ischemic ulceration in 6). Ages ranged from 48 to 95 years. Seven patients were women. In 8 patients, endarterectomy was limited to the common femoral artery; in 14, it was carried distally into the deep or superficial femoral artery or both. Nearly all (n = 20) arteriotomies were repaired with vein patch grafts taken from a branch of the saphenous vein or from its distal segment at the ankle.

There were no postoperative complications, and all patients were discharged with patent endarterectomies. There were no amputations among the six patients with ischemic ulcers.

During the follow-up, three patients were lost at 19, 91, and 97 months, respectively, with patent repairs to that time. Six patients with patent endarterectomies died from between 5 and 78 months postoperatively. One patient developed an occlusion of the endarterectomy at 45 months, which required an aortobifemoral graft, of which one limb was to the ipsilateral profunda femoris artery.

The remaining 13 patients are alive at 35 to 206 months with patent endarterectomies at a mean follow-up of 78 months. Cumulative patency rate at 10 years is 94 per cent (Fig. 56–5). No late complications have developed. Subsequent ipsilateral procedures included a popliteal endarterectomy, a femoropopliteal saphenous vein graft, and an aortoiliac endarterectomy. Lumbar sympathectomy was not performed in any of these patients.

Superficial Femoral Artery Endarterectomy

From 1961 through 1985, 147 patients (104 men, 43 women) underwent endarterectomy of the SFA with vein patch angioplasty. The approximate incidence of segmental endarterectomy (n = 147) relative to the number of patients studied by arteriography (n = 2818) was 5.2 per cent for the 24-year period. Presenting symptoms were intermittent claudication in 124 (84 per cent), rest pain in 14 (9 per cent), and ischemic ulceration in 9 patients (7 per cent). There were 13 patients with diabetes mellitus. Twenty-six patients underwent prior (n = 4) or concomitant (n = 22) lumbar sympathectomy. The occlusive disease was most frequently seen in the lower third of the SFA (112 limbs, 76 per cent), with less involvement in the upper two thirds (35 limbs, 24 per cent). When the endarterectomy was performed through a single arteriotomy, a single vein patch was used to repair the vessel (n = 115). However, when multiple arteriotomies were required in longer endarterectomies (n = 25), usually only the distal arteriotomy received the angioplasty (average length 5 cm), although in some instances the proximal arteriotomy was treated similarly. Vein angioplasty was omitted in seven limbs in which the caliber of the reconstructed vessel seemed adequate in size. The average length of the endarterectomy was 9.1 cm (Figs. 56–6 and 56–7).

Atherosclerotic lesions varied in morphology with cavitations, arborized spicules of calcification, focal accumulation of thrombi, ulceration with debris, and intraplaque hemorrhage accentuating the stenosis. Short occlusions were usually the result of thrombosis in a critically stenotic lesion. Two patients presented with the blue toe syndrome, in whom the source of the microembolization was identified from an ulcerated lesion in the SFA.

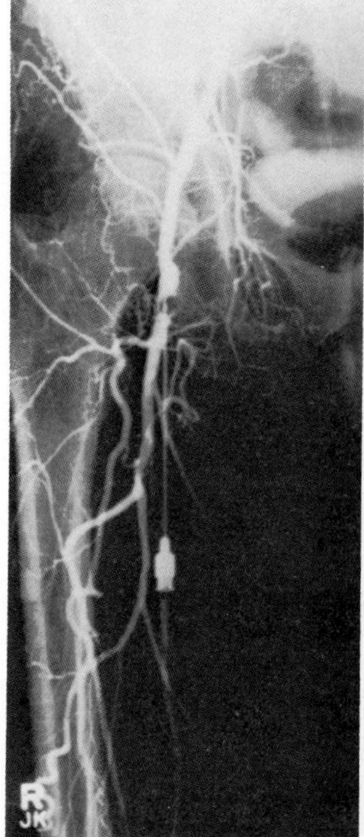

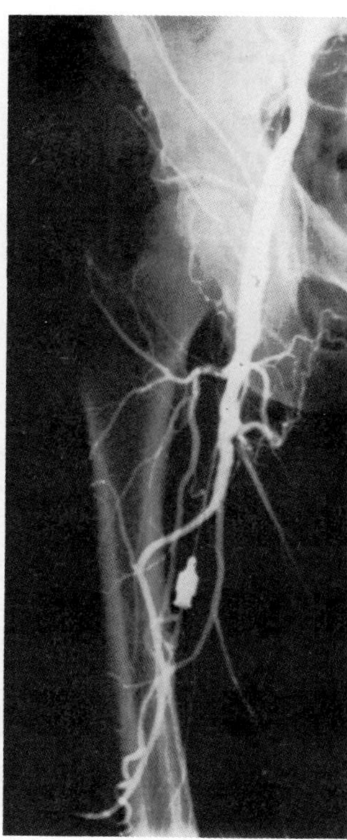

FIGURE 56–4. *Left*, Arteriogram in a 65-year-old man with a segmental occlusion of the right common femoral and entire superficial femoral arteries. *Right*, Repeat arteriogram 2 years after successful endarterectomy with vein patch graft demonstrating continued patency of the reconstructed segment. (Reproduced with permission from Inahara T, Mukherjee D: Infrainguinal thromboendarterectomy. *In* Kempczinski RF [ed]: The Ischemic Leg. Chicago, Year Book Medical Publishers, Inc., 1985, pp 353–374.)

Early and Late Results

All patients were discharged with patent reconstruction. A single postoperative thrombosis, restored immediately by extending the endarterectomy, was the only postoperative complication. There was no early morbidity or mortality.

Reporting the long-term results is based upon the standard life table method of analysis (Fig. 56–8). The cumu-

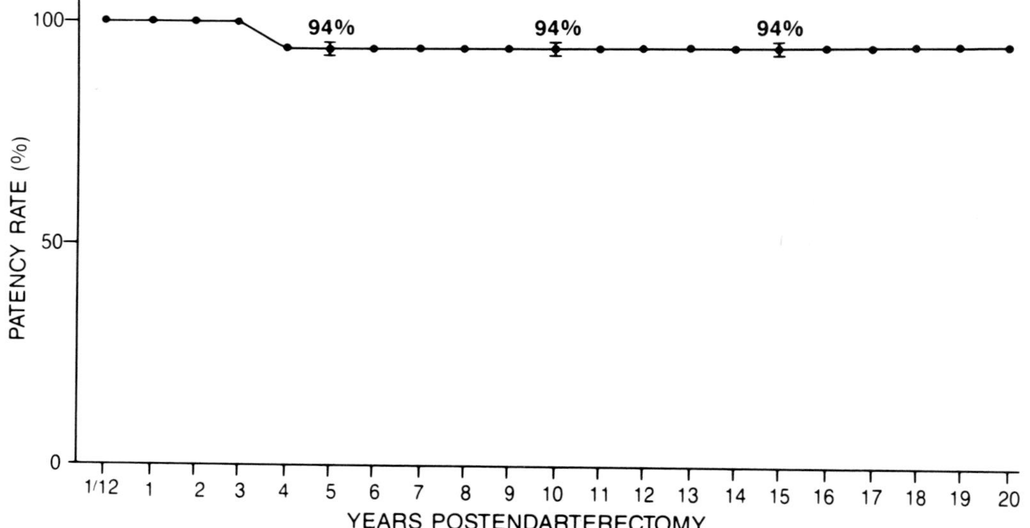

FIGURE 56–5. Life table patency curve for common femoral endarterectomy.

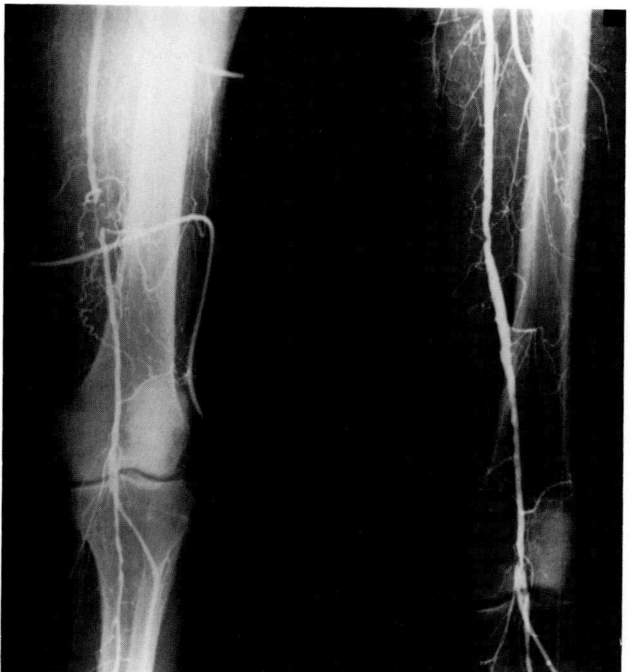

FIGURE 56–6. Arteriogram of an 85-year-old woman with one-block claudication and an ankle : brachial index of 0.6. *Left,* Short segmental occlusion of the SFA in the adductor canal. *Right,* Configuration of the repair by endarterectomy with saphenous vein patch graft at 2½ years with continued patency. (Reproduced with permission from Inahara T, Mukherjee D: Infrainguinal thromboendarterectomy. *In* Kempczinski RF [ed]: The Ischemic Leg. Chicago, Year Book Medical Publishers, Inc., 1985, pp 353–374.)

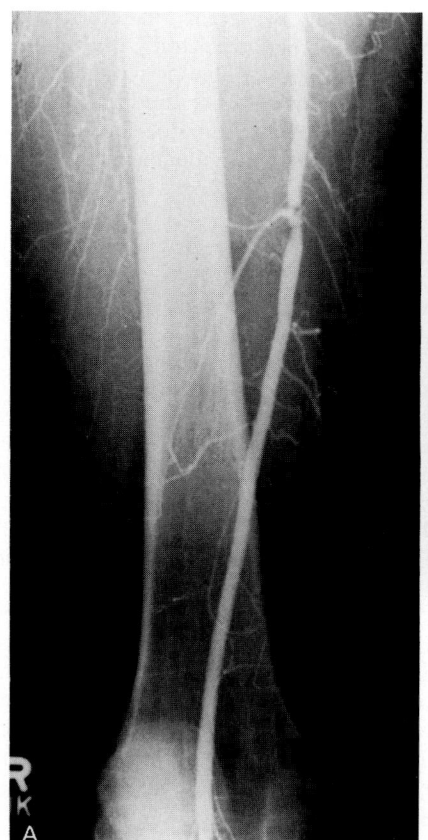

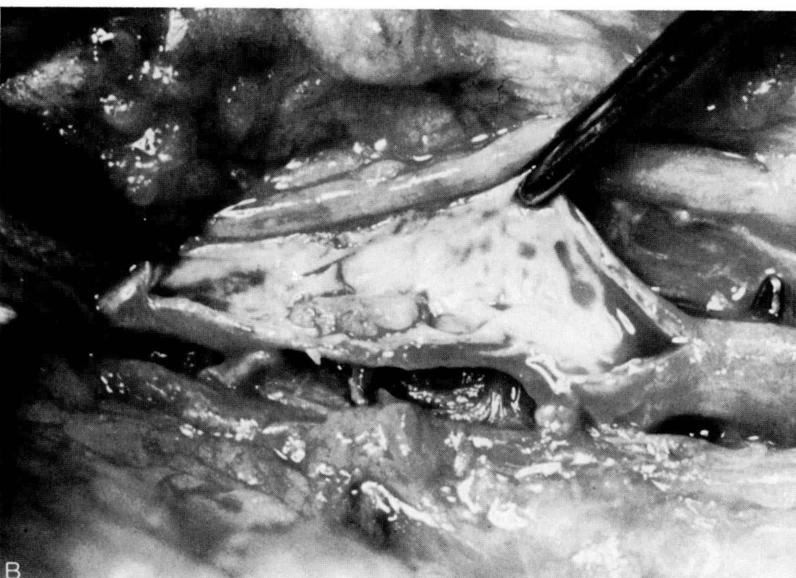

FIGURE 56–7. *A,* Arteriograms of a 55-year-old woman who had a painful blue toe. Localized lesion in the SFA was identified as the probable source of the emboli. *B,* Operative photograph of the lesion prior to endarterectomy. (*A* and *B,* Reproduced with permission from Inahara T, Mukherjee D: Infrainguinal thromboendarterectomy. *In* Kempczinski RF [ed]: The Ischemic Leg. Chicago, Year Book Medical Publishers, Inc., 1985, pp 353–374.)

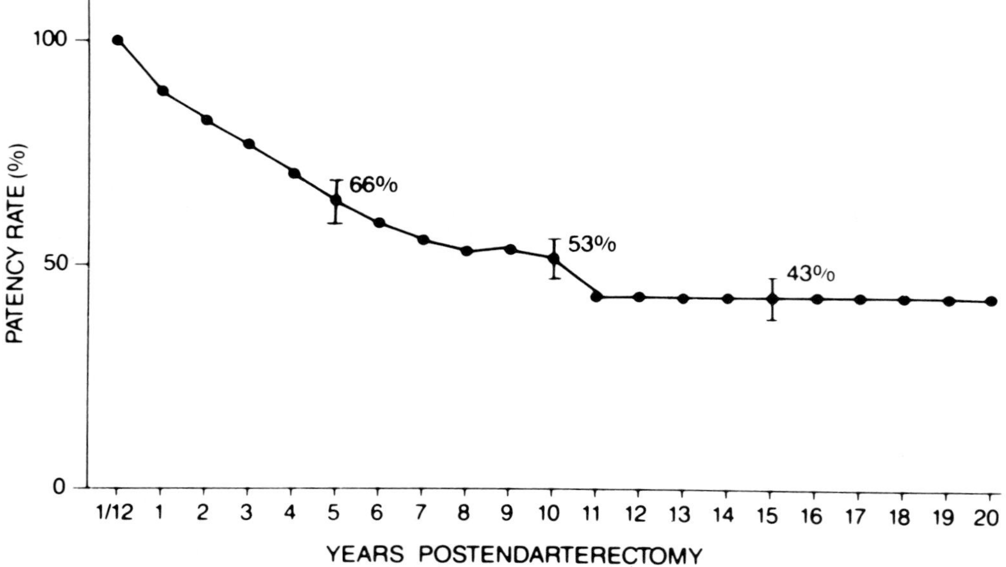

FIGURE 56–8. Life table patency curve for 147 superficial femoral endarterectomies.

lative patency rates were 66 per cent (± 5 per cent) at 5 years, 53 per cent (± 7 per cent) at 10 years, and 43 per cent (± 8 per cent) at 15 years. During the follow-up period, 45 endarterectomies failed. In 19 patients, claudication recurred at the preoperative level and further treatment was deferred to continued follow-up. However, 26 patients underwent additional procedures: femoropopliteal saphenous vein bypass graft (n = 22), femorofemoral bypass graft (n = 2), and aortoiliac reconstruction (n = 3). Of this group, one patient, initially treated for rest pain, underwent above-knee amputation 43 months later with a failed saphenous vein graft from progressive disease.

The group of patients in whom endarterectomies failed were analyzed to determine whether the indications for endarterectomy, location of the lesion, length of the endarterectomy, status of the outflow vessels, serum cholesterol values, and performance of lumbar sympathectomy predisposed the endarterectomy at risk to fail. None of these factors played a significant role in the outcome results except for the location of the lesion. Forty-one (37 per cent) of the endarterectomies in the lower third of the SFA resulted in failure compared with four (11 per cent) in the upper two thirds. This difference is probably significant with a $p < .01$ by chi-square test.

During the late follow-up period, 34 patients required the use of their saphenous vein, which had been preserved by the previous endarterectomy. Femoropopliteal grafts were performed in 26 patients, and coronary grafts were needed in 8 patients. In the 26 patients who received femoropopliteal grafts, the mean duration of the endarterectomy patency was 39 months, during which time these individuals were symptom-free. The secondary procedure with the saphenous vein bypass graft will again provide them with a symptom-free interval.

Endarterectomy with venous patch graft was performed in six patients in whom the saphenous veins were absent. Generally, there are segments of the saphenous vein to be found at the ankle, a saphenous tributary, or the lesser saphenous vein.

Indications for lumbar sympathectomy were based mainly upon the arteriographic demonstration of obliterative disease of the tibioperoneal and distal small vessels as well as the presence of sweating in the foot. All attempts were made to increase the cutaneous blood flow to protect against ischemic ulceration of the skin in these selected patients.

Lumbar sympathectomy was performed prior to or concomitantly with the SFA endarterectomy in 26 patients (19 per cent). In those undergoing lumbar sympathectomy, failure of the SFA endarterectomy occurred in 7 patients, one of whom underwent a late femoropopliteal bypass graft. The performance of lumbar sympathectomy did not influence the results sufficiently to achieve statistical significance.

Other Applications of Superficial Femoral Endarterectomy

In another application, the endarterectomy of the SFA can be treated as the inflow vessel combined with a distal bypass when there is insufficient length of autogenous vein. The technique lends flexibility to the reconstruction because the deficiency of available vein may be compensated for by varying the length of the endarterectomy.

The technique of endarterectomy here may be varied, depending on the vessel diameter and the length to be recanalized. For shorter lengths, endarterectomy can be performed through two or three arteriotomies or by the eversion method. The latter technique requires distal transection and a proximal arteriotomy in the common femoral artery. For longer segments, a semi-closed instrument technique may be suitable. In all instances, the proximal venous anastomosis of the bypass grafts serves as the outflow angioplasty for the endarterectomy.

Over the past 7 years, this procedure was employed in 15 ischemic limbs in 14 patients. Fourteen procedures were performed for advanced ischemia with rest pain or tissue loss and one for incapacitating claudication. The ages of the patients ranged from 45 to 89 years. The lengths of endarterectomy varied from 6 to 30 cm with a mean of 14 cm. The remaining short segments of the greater saphenous vein were utilized in 12 limbs and the lesser saphenous vein in 3. The vein graft originated from the distal end of the endarterectomy of the SFA in 12, from the proximal popliteal in 1, and from the distal popliteal in another.

The distal anastomosis was placed at the upper popliteal in 3, the distal popliteal in 3, the anterior tibial in 1, the posterior tibial in 3, and the peroneal artery in 4. One graft had three crural vessels for runoff; 3 had two-vessel runoff; and 11 had single-vessel runoff, of which 6 were peroneal, 3 posterior tibial, and 2 anterior tibial arteries.

In the review of these reconstructions, there was no correlation between graft patency or lower extremity salvage and the length of the endarterectomy, the length of the vein graft, the location of the distal anastomosis, or the status of the distal outflow. Ten reconstructions remained patent throughout their follow-up. Of these patients, one was lost to follow-up at 18 months and three patients died at 1, 20, and 27 months, respectively. Five endarterectomies became occluded, resulting in three major amputations. However, the two patients with occlusions at 19 and 37 months continued to maintain patency of the distal saphenous vein grafts from collateral vessels. Although these two patients have remained asymptomatic, one underwent a proximal bypass procedure to protect the distal vein graft. With a follow-up period of 1 to 59 months (mean, 22 months), the overall patency rate was 67 per cent, and the limb salvage rate was 80 per cent.

In conclusion, the patency of the combined proximal superficial femoral endarterectomy and distal saphenous vein graft is at least equal to the results of other nonautogenous reconstructions, including polytetrafluoroethylene (PTFE),[35] umbilical vein,[9] and their composite grafts.[15] The combined autogenous reconstruction is less subject to complications that occur with the use of prosthetic materials; hence, the autogenous reconstruction remains our choice.

There are additional uses for the endarterectomized SFA. In restoring flow to the profunda femoral artery, using the eversion technique of endarterectomy, Feldhaus and associates[16] reported 18 SFA bypasses to the distal profunda femoral. Inahara and Mukherjee[21] reported the use of the endarterectomized SFA as a free graft from the common iliac to the profunda femoral artery. Finally, the endarterectomized SFA is frequently used as a patch graft in the repair of the common and profunda femoral arteries.

Extended Femoropopliteal Endarterectomy: Semi-closed Technique

Semi-closed endarterectomy for extensive disease of the superficial femoral or femoropopliteal artery is an alternate technique described by Imparato and colleagues.[18, 37] Patients are selected for this technique based upon the presence of moderate to advanced ischemia, the absence of a suitable saphenous vein, and the presence of anatomically reconstituted popliteal artery with the presence of at least one tibial artery patent to the pedal arch (Fig. 56–9).

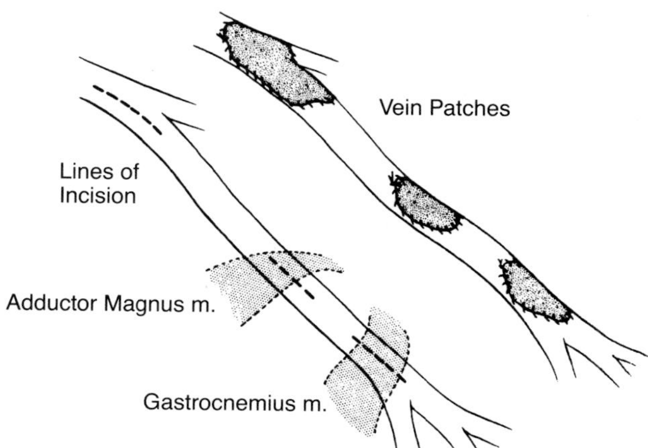

FIGURE 56–9. Technique of semi-closed endarterectomy. (From Imparato AM, Bracco A, Kim GE: Comparison of three technics for femoral-popliteal arterial reconstruction. Ann Surg 177:375, 1973.)

Operative Approach

The operative approach is through an inguinal incision for exposure of the femoral bifurcation and a low medial thigh incision for the upper popliteal artery that can be extended, when indicated, to below the knee.

Following the systemic administration of heparin, endarterectomy is performed through a common or superficial femoral arteriotomy (3 cm) proximally and a popliteal arteriotomy (3 cm) distally. Beginning in the SFA, the plane of dissection is developed between the plaque and the media and, if possible, preferably between the media and the adventitia. A 4-mm ring arterial stripper is passed from the proximal SFA by gentle rotation and infiltration. If the endarterectomy was initiated in the common femoral artery, it is repaired immediately with a venous patch to restore arterial flow to the deep femoral artery. On occasion, the plaque is so densely adherent at the level of the adductor hiatus that a separate arteriotomy is necessary to free the plaque under direct vision. Endarterectomy is terminated at a point of least disease, where the intima is transected and the edge secured with longitudinal mattress sutures to prevent distal dissection. Small cotton sponges are passed through the endarterectomized vessel to facilitate removal of loosened fragments. Clamps are placed at appropriate levels to contain back-bleeding from the reopened branches. After thorough irrigation with heparinized solution, all arteriotomies are closed with venous patch grafts. Completion intraoperative angiography is performed to visualize the disobliterated segment and its runoff vessels. Retained fragments or residual disease must be removed under direct vision with appropriate venous patch graft repair of the arteriotomy.

Results

The results of this technique were reported by Walker and coworkers[37] in 1980. Between 1964 and 1973, 123 semi-closed superficial femoropopliteal endarterectomies were performed on 119 patients. Using the life table method of analysis, the cumulative patency rates for all 123 limbs were 95.7 per cent for immediate patency, 75.9 per cent at 1 year, 46.4 per cent at 5 years, and 26.0 per cent at 10 years. Nine patients died within 30 days of the procedure, with an operative mortality rate of 7.3 per cent. For patients with advanced ischemia, postoperative limb loss occurred more often in 32 diabetic patients (n = 25, 78 per cent) than in the 33 nondiabetic individuals (n = 9, 28.7 per cent). At 5 years, the limb salvage rate (62.9 per cent) was better than the patency rate (46.4 per cent). These results indicate the presence of advanced atherosclerotic disease in these patients.

Similarly, Vericello and associates[36] reported 595 semi-closed endarterectomy procedures performed in 550 patients over a period of 14 years. Indications for operation were claudication in 72.5 per cent and advanced ischemia in 27.5 per cent.

Another technique of semi-closed endarterectomy of the superficial femoral and popliteal arteries employs an oscillating loop (Hall's arterial oscillator).[24] The operative technique differs only with the use of the oscillating instrument. The design of the elliptical loop and the rationale for its oscillating motion were based upon the observation in cadaver arteries that the branches of the femoral and popliteal arteries were occluded only at their orifices. Upon removal of the plaque from the ostia, the distal vessels were patent. The oversized elliptical loop that traverses the plane of dissection displaces the adventitial wall outward to clear the ostia of the branches. This action avoids shearing off the spicules of plaque, which theoretically could occur with a sharp arterial loop stripper. The oscillating motion permits gradual circumferential dilatation and advancement of the loop. To a great extent, the success of the procedure was attributed to the use of antiplatelet and anticoagulant drugs. Using this technique, Lerwick reported on a series of 1091 patients undergoing various combinations of aortoiliac and femoropopliteal endarterectomies, with a cumulative patency rate of 74.4 per cent at 10 years.[24]

Popliteal Endarterectomy

From 1961 through 1986, 101 patients with 106 popliteal occlusive lesions were treated by segmental endarterectomy with vein patch angioplasty.[22] Indications for the operation were claudication in 60 (59 per cent), rest pain in 20 (19 per cent), and ischemic necrosis in 23 (22 per cent). There were 66 men and 35 women. The mean ages were 64 years and 71 years, respectively.

Other criteria for operation included the arteriographic demonstration of a segmental stenosis or an occlusion, as defined earlier, with a relatively disease-free proximal SFA, as well as the visualization of an outflow bed of at least one branch of the popliteal trifurcation. One patient presented with a blue toe syndrome in which the source of the emboli was localized to the popliteal lesion.

A posterior midline incision is routinely employed because this permits access to the entire popliteal artery.

In the majority of patients (n = 76), a single arteriotomy was adequate for the endarterectomy. It averaged 6 cm in length and was repaired with a vein patch graft. In longer endarterectomies (n = 27), in which two or three arteriotomies were used, the average length was 13.3 cm, and usually only the proximal and the distal arteriotomies received the vein patches. In nearly all instances, the lesser saphenous vein was used for the patch graft.

Of the 106 endarterectomies, there were 6 (6 per cent) early failures, of which 5 were restored immediately by secondary procedures that included extension of the endarterectomy to a more suitable outflow site, interposition saphenous vein graft, and a saphenous vein bypass graft. Reoperation was not attempted in the sixth patient, who had juvenile-onset diabetes mellitus with severe outflow vessel disease. This patient later underwent below-knee amputation. One patient died of a myocardial infarction on the fourth postoperative day. Other complications included a subcutaneous hematoma and a superficial wound infection (Figs. 56–10 to 56–12).

There were 45 patients with advanced ischemia, of whom 3 had amputation of the toes (n = 2) and a transmetatarsal amputation (n = 1) for preoperative gangrene, but with limb salvage. Ninety-nine patients (104 limbs) were discharged with patent popliteal reconstructions.

Late Results

The cumulative patency rates were 60 per cent (± 5 per cent) at 5 years and 44 per cent (± 7 per cent) at 10 years. Some patients with patent endarterectomies were followed as long as 25 years. However, beyond 15 years, the numbers were too small (n = 11) to be statistically significant.

There were 39 (38 per cent) late occlusions, the majority (24 limbs) occurring within the first 2 years. This group of patients was analyzed to determine whether the indications for operation, length of the endarterectomy, severity of the outflow disease, or performance of concomitant lumbar sympathectomy predisposed these individuals to endarterectomy failure. None of these factors was found to play a significant role in the outcome. Nineteen patients underwent further repair by femoropopliteal bypass grafts with saphenous vein (n = 16) and PTFE (n = 3). In 7 patients the procedure was required because of subsequent proximal progression of occlusive disease in the SFA. There were 4 late amputations in patients in whom further repair could not be accomplished.

In patients treated for claudication, failures generally resulted in reversion of symptoms to the preoperative level without increased ischemia. For those in the advanced ischemia group (n = 43), there were 18 failures (42 per cent) with 5 amputations (12 per cent), the higher failure rate reflecting the characteristics of terminal vessel disease (Fig. 56–13).

DISCUSSION

Among the many therapeutic approaches to symptomatic occlusive disease of the lower extremities, the results of autogenous saphenous vein bypass grafts remain unexcelled and are the recognized standard for comparison. Several authors have reported their experiences with 5-year cumulative patency rates ranging from 58.3 to 88 per cent and 10-year patency rates ranging from 38 to 52.5 per cent.[11–14]

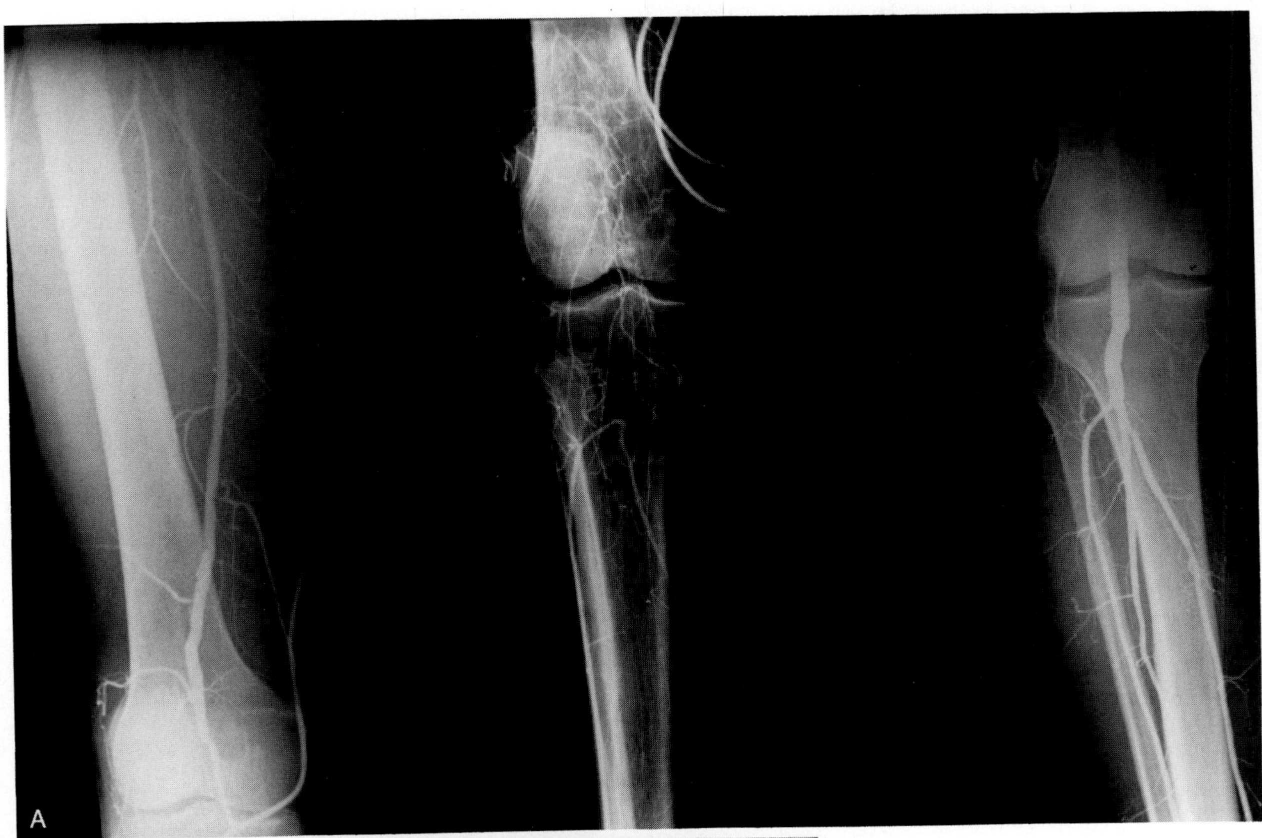

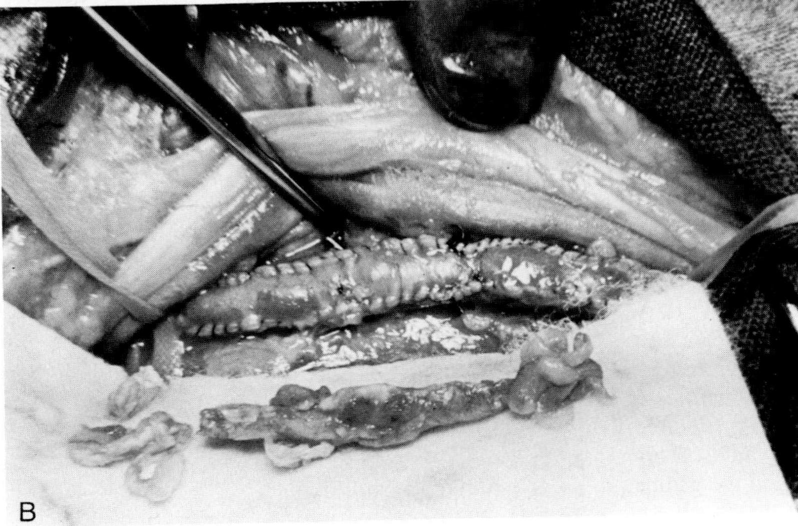

FIGURE 56–10. Arteriograms in a 45-year-old man with ischemic rest pain in the right foot. *A*, Preoperative arteriogram with segmental occlusion in the distal popliteal artery (*left* and *center*); patency was restored by endarterectomy with autogenous vein patch graft (*right*). *B*, Posterior exposure of the popliteal artery demonstrating saphenous vein patch graft and plaque removed by endarterectomy. (*A* and *B*, Reproduced with permission from Inahara T, Mukherjee D: Infrainguinal thromboendarterectomy. *In* Kempczinski RF [ed]: The Ischemic Leg. Chicago, Year Book Medical Publishers, Inc., 1985, pp 353–374.)

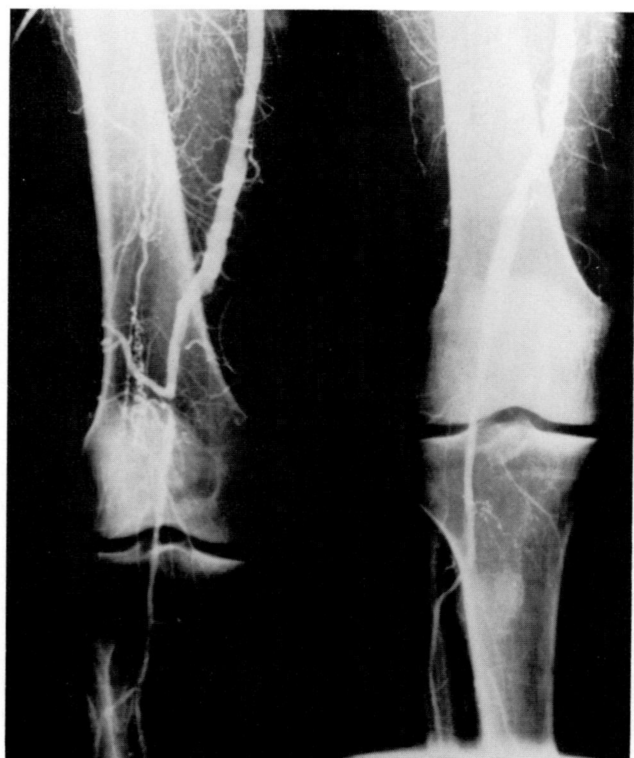

FIGURE 56–11. *Left,* Arteriogram in a 48-year-old man with half-block claudication demonstrating occlusion of the proximal popliteal artery. *Right,* Repeat arteriogram 1 year later shows continued patency of popliteal artery following endarterectomy with saphenous vein patch graft. (Reproduced with permission from Inahara T, Mukherjee D: Infrainguinal thromboendarterectomy. *In* Kempczinski RF [ed]: The Ischemic Leg, Chicago, Year Book Medical Publishers, Inc., 1985, pp 353–374.)

The cumulative patency rate for the common femoral endarterectomy remains at 94 per cent at 10 years. Although a series of 26 patients may not achieve statistical significance, it appears that endarterectomy is ideally suited for disobliteration of occlusive disease of the common femoral artery. This may be due to its larger diameter, relatively short length, and higher-velocity flow with two major outflow vessels. The incidence of disease confined only to the common femoral artery is quite low because it is more frequently involved in continuity with aortoiliac and femoropopliteal disease and is treated in conjunction with them. In either setting, the patency of the common femoral artery is extremely durable following its reconstruction and, in particular, is well suited to segmental endarterectomy.

SFA endarterectomy compares favorably with the saphenous vein graft experience and is particularly notable for its low attendant morbidity and mortality rates. This technique is more successful when it is applied to lesions involving the upper and middle thirds of the artery. When the results of segmental endarterectomy for the upper two thirds and the lower third were evaluated separately, the former (5 years, 92 per cent; 10 years, 92 per cent) showed significantly better patency than the latter (5 years, 65 per cent; 10 years, 43 per cent). Perhaps the natural course of disease that progresses proximally in this vessel influences the results negatively in the lower third. This emphasizes the importance of periodic examination to detect progressive changes, which again may be segmental, in order to institute appropriate procedures toward maintaining patency of the SFA.

The patency rates for popliteal endarterectomy compare favorably with the results of autogenous vein bypass grafts, even though a significantly greater percentage of patients in this group had advanced ischemia (41 per cent) compared with the superficial femoral endarterectomy group (16 per cent) and the common femoral group (27 per cent). Because the popliteal artery is both a vessel of conduction and a vessel of supply, it is less amenable than its proximal counterparts to secondary reconstruction with a bypass or an endarterectomy when thrombosis occurs.

The gradual attrition of patent repairs over time without incidence of failures suggests that the failure of this type of reconstructive operation is a function of progression of the disease process or fibrointimal hyperplasia.

Irregular stenotic lesions are a potential source of microembolization into the terminal vessels of the foot. The blue toe syndrome was associated with SFA and popliteal lesions in which the moth-eaten lesions were detected by arteriography and confirmed by endarterectomy. Localization of such a lesion is an indication for endarterectomy as the procedure of choice. Availability of the greater saphenous vein by its preservation is an immeasurable asset to

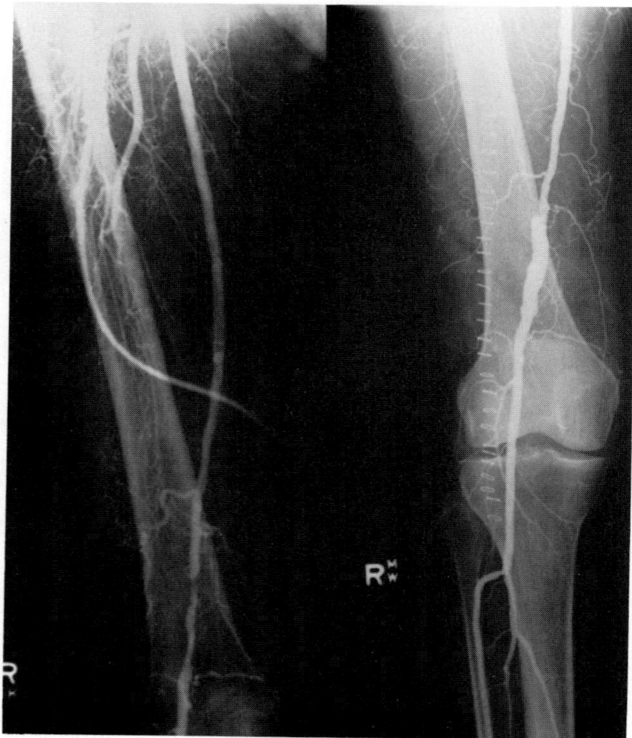

FIGURE 56–12. Arteriogram in an 80-year-old woman with disabling claudication. *Left,* Severe stenosis of proximal popliteal artery. *Right,* Postendarterectomy; angioplasty slightly patulous. (Reproduced with permission from Inahara T, Mukherjee D: Infrainguinal thromboendarterectomy. *In* Kempczinski RF [ed]: The Ischemic Leg, Chicago, Year Book Medical Publishers, Inc., 1985, pp 353–374.)

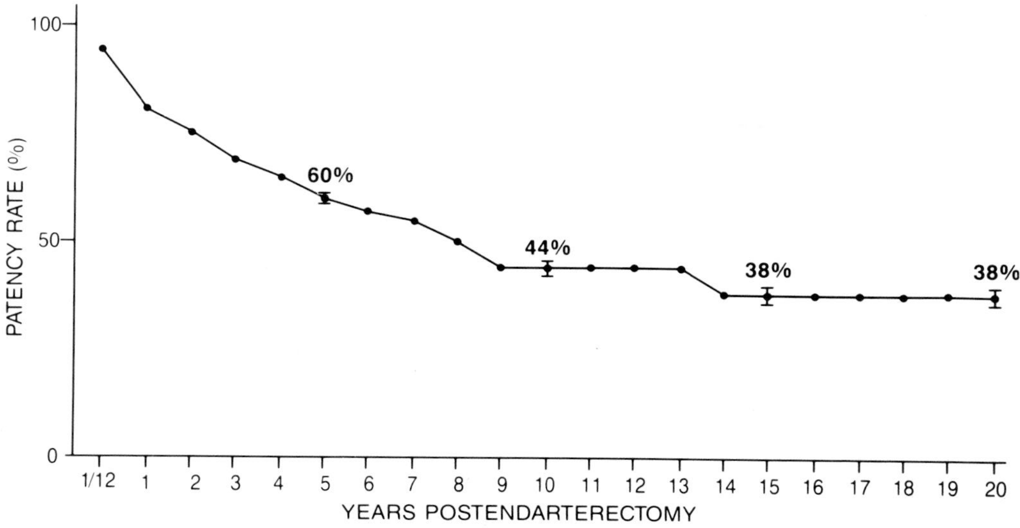

FIGURE 56–13. Life table patency curve for popliteal thromboendarterectomy. (From Inahara T, Mukherjee D. Superficial femoral artery endarterectomy for lower extremity occlusive disease. *In* Ernst CB, Stanley JC [eds]: Current Therapy in Vascular Surgery. Toronto, BC Decker, 1987, p 225.)

the patient. Walker and colleagues[37] emphasized this concept by advocating that the saphenous vein be preserved for myocardial revascularization rather than expended for revascularization of the lower extremity.

The concept of segmental endarterectomy is a conservative approach in the long-term management of arterial disease of the lower extremity. Predictably, this technique allows the circulation to be restored in the native artery and to be maintained for a period of time. The patient is subject to a lesser operative procedure and correspondingly less risk than the bypass operation. Finally, preservation of the greater saphenous vein permits a second opportunity for revascularization. Although infection is infrequent, omission of the bypass graft also avoids a serious prosthetic graft infection.[26]

In the past few years, alternative endovascular procedures have been developed to treat femoral and popliteal arterial lesions. In 1991 a multi-center study[38] (September 1986 to January 1989) of 602 patients undergoing thermal laser-assisted balloon angioplasty of the SFA reported their results. The initial recanalization rate was 89 per cent (538 of 602 patients), as verified by angioscopy or arteriography. Complications occurred in 10 per cent (62 patients), and there was one amputation. Overall life table analysis of the patency rate of 602 patients with SFA thermal laser-assisted balloon angioplasty at a mean follow-up of 11.3 months (range, 1 to 30 months) was 60 per cent. Patients with symptoms only of claudication and short segment noncalcific lesions achieved better results. Long-term results are not known.

In summary, the authors' philosophy concerning the management of the arterial circulation in the lower extremity is based first upon the natural course of atherosclerotic occlusive disease, which in general tends to develop and progress in a segmental fashion with predilection for certain sites. These lesions have proved to be easily accessible for repair. Second, we direct attention toward maintaining the circulation in the native artery, analogous to the practice of maintaining circulation after a bypass reconstruction has taken place. On the other hand, a patient presenting with an occlusion of the entire SFA but with symptoms only of intermittent claudication would most likely be followed conservatively because such occlusions have proved to be symptomatically stable and the conservative treatment has widespread acceptance. For patients with early segmental disease, the authors feel that the risk : reward ratio favors the patient undergoing endarterectomy. In the absence of a suitable saphenous vein, endarterectomy remains a reliable alternative means for reconstruction.

References

1. Baddeley RM, Ashton F, Slaney G: Comparison of autogenous vein bypass grafts with patch angioplasty for short femoropopliteal occlusions. Surg Gynecol Obstet 127:503, 1968.
2. Boyd AM: The natural course of arteriosclerosis of the lower extremities. Proc R Soc Med 55:592, 1962.
3. Brewster DC, LaSalle AJ, Robison JG, et al: Factors affecting patency of femoropopliteal bypass grafts. Surg Gynecol Obstet 157:437, 1983.
4. Cannon JA, Barker WF: Successful management of obstructive femoral arteriosclerosis by endarterectomy. Surgery 38:48, 1955.
5. Catlin R, Movius HJ, Gaspar MR: Femoropopliteal thromboendarterectomy. Am J Surg 112:156, 1966.
6. Conn HJ, Fain WR: Bypass grafts and endarterectomy for femoropopliteal occlusive disease: A 9 year clinical review. Am Surg 32:49, 1966.
7. Cunningham FO, Egan JM, Inahara T: Continuous epidural anesthesia in abdominal vascular surgery: A review of 100 consecutive cases. Am J Surg 139:624, 1980.
8. Cutler BS, Thompson JE, Kleinsasser LJ, et al: Autologous saphenous vein femoropopliteal bypass: Analysis of 298 cases. Surgery 79:325, 1976.
9. Dardik H, Ibrahim IM, Dardik I: Evolution of glutaraldehyde-tanned human umbilical cord vein as a vascular prosthesis for bypass to the popliteal, tibial and peroneal arteries. Surgery 83:577, 1978.
10. Darling CR, Linton RR: Durability of femoropopliteal reconstructions. Am Surg 123:472, 1972.
11. DeWeese JA, Rob CG: Autogenous venous grafts ten years later. Surgery 82:775, 1977.

12. DeWeese JA, Barner HB, Mahoney EB, et al: Autogenous venous bypass grafts and thromboendarterectomies for atherosclerotic lesions of the femoropopliteal arteries. Ann Surg 163:205, 1966.
13. Donaldson MC, Mannick JA: Femoropopliteal bypass grafting for intermittent claudication. Arch Surg 115:724, 1980.
14. dos Santos JC: Sur la desobstruction des thromboses arterielle anciennes. Mem Acad Chir 73:409, 1960.
15. Edwards WS: Composite reconstruction of the femoral artery with saphenous vein after endarterectomy. Surg Gynecol Obstet 111:651, 1960.
16. Feldhaus RJ, Sterpetti AV, Schultz RD, et al: Eversion endarterectomy of the superficial femoral artery and end-to-side anastomosis to the deep femoral artery. Am J Surg 150:748, 1985.
17. Glutelius JR, Kreindler S, Luke JC: Comparative evaluation of autogenous vein bypass graft and endarterectomy in superficial femoral artery reconstruction. Surgery 57:28, 1965.
18. Imparato AM, Bracco A, Kim GE: Comparison of three technics for femoral-popliteal arterial reconstruction. Ann Surg 177:375, 1973.
19. Imparato AM, Kim GE, Davidson T, et al: Intermittent claudication: Its natural course. Surgery 78:795, 1975.
20. Inahara T, Scott CM: Endarterectomy for segmental occlusive disease of the superficial femoral artery. Arch Surg 116:1547, 1981.
21. Inahara T, Mukherjee D: The superficial femoral artery as a conduit: An alternative to prosthetic material. J Vasc Surg 2:739, 1985.
22. Inahara T, Toledo AC: Endarterectomy of the popliteal artery for segmental occlusive disease. Ann Surg 188:43, 1978.
23. Kunlin J: Venous grafts in therapy of endarteritis obliterans [in French]. Arch J Med du Coeur 42:371, 1949.
24. Lerwick ER: Oscillating loop endarterectomy for peripheral vascular reconstruction. Surgery 97:574, 1985.
25. LeVeen HH: Technical features in endarterectomy. Surgery 57:22, 1965.
26. Liekweg WC, Greenfield LJ: Vascular prosthetic-infections: Collected experience and results of treatment. Surgery 81:335, 1977.
27. McAllister FF: The fate of patients with intermittent claudication managed nonoperatively. Am J Surg 132:593, 1976.
28. Ouriel K, Smith CR, DeWeese JA: Endarterectomy for localized lesions of the superficial femoral artery at the adductor canal. J Vasc Surg 3:531, 1986.
29. Peabody CN, Kannel WB, McNamara PM: Intermittent claudication. Arch Surg 109:693, 1974.
30. Reichle FA, Tyson RR: Comparison of long-term results of 364 femoropopliteal or femorotibial bypasses for revascularization of severely ischemic lower extremities. Ann Surg 182:449, 1975.
31. Rosenthal D, Pesa FA, Gottsegen WL, et al: Thermal laser-assisted balloon angioplasty of the superficial femoral artery: A multicenter review of 602 cases. J Vasc Surg 14:152, 1991.
32. Sapirstein W, Bottomley MG, Baker CB: Thromboendarterectomy in the treatment of femoropopliteal occlusions. Can J Surg 9:231, 1966.
33. Sobel S, Kaplitt MJ, Reingold M, et al: Gas endarterectomy. Surgery 59:519, 1966.
34. Strandness DE, Stahler C: Arteriosclerosis obliterans: Manner and rate of progression. JAMA 196:121, 1966.
35. Veith FJ, Moss CM, Fell SC, et al: Comparison of expanded polytetrafluoroethylene and autologous saphenous vein grafts in high risk arterial reconstruction for limb salvage. Surg Gynecol Obstet 147:749, 1978.
36. Vericello G, Castelli P, Colleti M, et al: Semiclosed thromboendarterectomy on femoropopliteal tract revisited after fourteen years experience on 595 cases. Int Surg 71:59, 1986.
37. Walker PM, Imparato AM, Riles TS, et al: Long-term results in superficial femoral artery endarterectomy. Surgery 89:231, 1981.
38. Walsh DB, Gilbertson JJ, Zwolak RM, et al: The natural history of superficial femoral artery stenoses. J Vasc Surg 14:299, 1991.
39. Warren R, Gomez RL, Marston JAP, et al: Femoropopliteal arteriosclerosis obliterans: Arteriographic patterns and rates of progression. Surgery 55:135, 1964.
40. Warren R: Evaluation of thromboendarterectomy for arteriosclerosis obliterans of the femoral artery. Surg Gynecol Obstet 104:503, 1957.
41. Winfrey EW, Foster JH: Low molecular weight dextran in small artery surgery. Arch Surg 88:100, 1964.
42. Wylie EJ, McGuinness JS: The recognition and treatment of arteriosclerotic stenosis of major arteries. Surg Gynecol Obstet 97:425, 1953.
43. Wylie EJ, Binkley FM, Albo RJ: Femoropopliteal endarterectomy. Am Surg 108:215, 1964.

57

Secondary Arterial Reconstructions in the Lower Extremity

Frank J. Veith, M.D., Enrico Ascer, M.D., Sushil K. Gupta, M.D., Kurt R. Wengerter, M.D., and Thomas F. Panetta, M.D.

• • •

Arterial reconstructions for lower extremity ischemia include aortoiliac, aortofemoral, axillofemoral, and femorofemoral procedures and bypasses to the popliteal and infrapopliteal arteries. As indicated by the life table patency rates shown in other chapters of this volume, all these operations have an intrinsic tendency to fail or become ineffective as time elapses. The proportion of such operations undergoing this fate increases with time and is greater at all times for reconstructions terminating more distally in the arterial tree. Because a sizable minority of patients undergoing these operations have circulatory deterioration in their lifetimes and because this deterioration often is associated with disabling or limb-threatening manifestations, appropriate management of this condition has become an extremely important aspect of vascular surgery and one to which the competent vascular surgeon must be committed in order to serve the patients' interests well. The purpose of this chapter is to discuss the general principles and strategies of this management with a specific focus on the aspects of reoperative vascular surgery that differ from a primary approach to lower extremity ischemia.

INDICATIONS

In general, we believe that arterial reconstructions should rarely be performed for intermittent claudication.[1] Our reason for this attitude is the relatively high inevitable failure rate of these operations and the fact that failure may be associated with ischemia worse than that prompting the original operation. These factors and the increased difficulty and complication rate associated with most secondary operations, particularly if the involved arteries have been dissected, seem to justify our conservative attitude toward *primary* operations for intermittent claudication. This attitude, however, is by no means universal, and present practice accepts ''truly disabling'' claudication as an indication for primary arterial reconstruction to at least the popliteal level. In contrast, almost all present-day vascular surgeons tend to avoid secondary arterial operations for intermittent claudication. Thus gangrene, a nonhealing ischemic ulcer, or severe ischemic rest pain should be the indication for most *secondary* arterial reconstructions, especially those below the inguinal ligament. Interestingly, occasional patients with these classic limb-threatening manifestations and poor noninvasive indices can be effectively managed by conservative measures for protracted periods[2] and such treatment, if possible, is particularly appropriate in patients who are faced with the need for a difficult distal reoperation. Thus, except for the special circumstances occurring with a ''failing graft'' (see later discussion), most patients undergoing secondary arterial reconstruction should have as their indication for operation unquestionable immediate limb salvage.

ETIOLOGY OF PROCEDURE FAILURE

Early Reoperations (Within 30 Days). The need to reintervene soon after a primary arterial reconstruction may be generated by several situations.[3] First, the original repair may thrombose or fail in the early postoperative period (i.e., within 30 days). Generally this is due to a technical flaw in the operation or to a poor choice of inflow or outflow sites. In addition, thrombosis may occur for no apparent reason, presumably owing to the inherent thrombogenicity of the graft in a low-flow setting. Usually this occurs only with polytetrafluoroethylene (PTFE) and other prosthetic grafts, but rarely it can occur with a vein graft also. A transient fall in cardiac output or hypotension can contribute to such unexplained thrombosis. Second, the original operation, although technically satisfactory and associated with a patent bypass graft, may fail to provide hemodynamic improvement sufficient to relieve the patient's symptoms. This in turn may be due to the choice of the wrong operation (e.g., the performance of an aortofemoral bypass in a patient whose femoral artery pressure was normal and who actually needed a femoropopliteal bypass). Alternatively, such hemodynamic failure may also occur in the presence of multisegment disease and extensive foot gangrene or infection. In this setting, uninterrupted arterial circulation to the foot may be required and a primary or secondary sequential bypass may be indicated.[1, 4, 5]

Late Reoperations (After 30 Days). Failure with graft thrombosis can occur at any time after the first postoperative month. This may be due to some of the factors already mentioned. However, it is usually due to the development of some flow-reducing lesion within the bypass graft or its inflow or outflow tract. Intimal hyperplasia is a prominent cause of failure and graft thrombosis. This may occur with all kinds of grafts in all positions. The etiology of this process is poorly understood, and fortunately it does not affect most arterial reconstructions. When intimal hyperplasia does occur, it usually produces infrainguinal graft failure between 2 and 18 months after operation.[3, 6, 7] It can involve any portion of a vein graft in a focal or diffuse manner and either anastomosis of vein or prosthetic grafts. Because the lumen of the distal artery is smaller, this site is most vulnerable to flow reduction by this process. After 18 months, progression of the atherosclerotic disease process involving the inflow or outflow tract of the arterial reconstruction becomes the predominant cause of failure and graft thrombosis. After 3 to 4 years, a variety of other degenerative lesions may also afflict autogenous vein grafts and umbilical vein grafts.[6, 8, 9] These processes, which are rare in autogenous vein grafts but extremely common in umbilical vein grafts, may lead to wall changes and aneurysm formation with thrombosis or embolization.

FAILING GRAFT CONCEPT

Intimal hyperplasia, progression of proximal or distal disease, or lesions within the graft itself can produce signs and symptoms of hemodynamic deterioration in patients with a prior arterial reconstruction without producing concomitant thrombosis of the bypass graft.[10–13] The authors refer to this condition as a ''failing graft'' because, if the lesion is not corrected, graft thrombosis will almost certainly occur.[10] The importance of this failing graft concept lies in the fact that many difficult lower extremity revascularizations can be salvaged for protracted periods by relatively simple interventions if the lesion responsible for the circulatory deterioration and diminished graft blood flow can be detected before graft thrombosis occurs.

The authors have now been able to detect more than 220 failing grafts and to correct these lesions before graft thrombosis occurred.[10, 14, 15] The majority of these grafts were vein grafts, but approximately one third were PTFE or Dacron grafts (Figs. 57–1 and 57–2). Invariably, the corrective procedure was simpler than the secondary operation that would be required if the bypass went on to thrombose. Many lesions responsible for the failing state were remedied by percutaneous transluminal angioplasty (PTA), although some required a vein patch angioplasty, a short bypass of a graft lesion, or a proximal or distal graft extension.[10, 14, 15] Some of the angioplasties of these lesions have

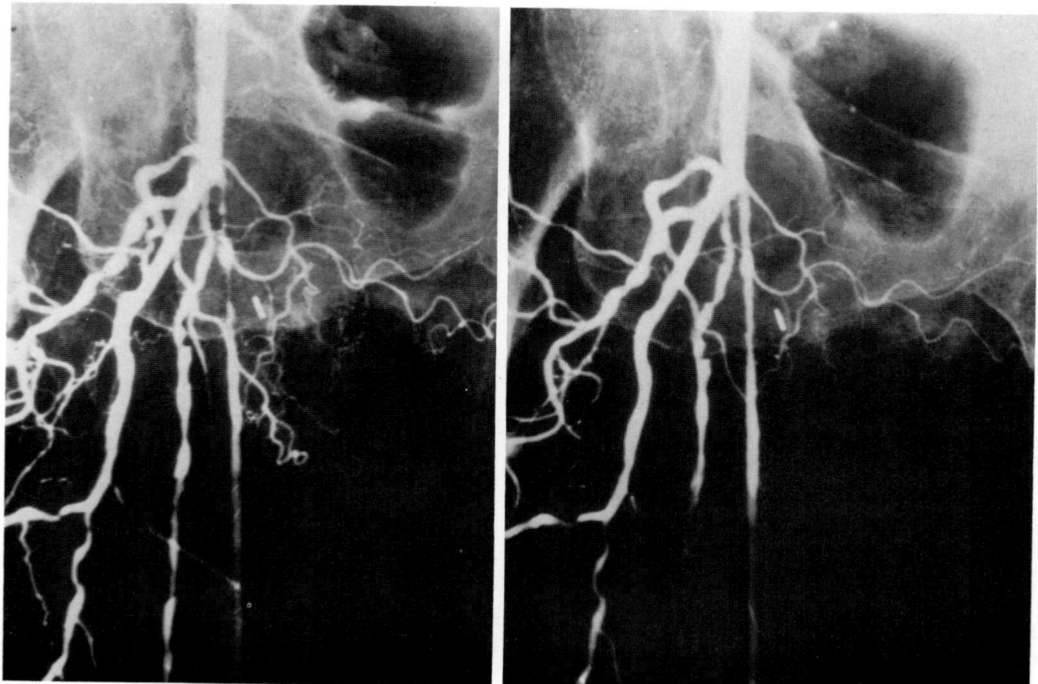

FIGURE 57–1. *Left*, Arteriogram 18 months after a common femoral–to–anterior tibial bypass. A proximal stenosis produced the "failing state." *Right*, An arteriogram 2 years after the stenosis was corrected by percutaneous transluminal angioplasty. The graft remained patent 5 years later.

failed and required a second reintervention; others have remained effective in correcting the responsible lesion as documented by arteriography more than 2 to 5 years later (Fig. 57–1). However, the role of PTA for vein graft lesions remains controversial. Although the authors and Berkowitz and colleagues[13] have had many excellent results with PTA of vein graft stenoses, other groups have not. Moreover, the authors have had some recent failures with limb loss. The authors, therefore, currently restrict the use of PTA to lesions of less than 1.5 cm in length when they are located in an inaccessible part of the vein. PTA has also been useful in the treatment of some inflow and outflow lesions.[15] Most important, the results of reinterventions for failing grafts, in terms of both continued cumulative patency and limb salvage rates, have been far superior to the results of reinterventions for grafts that have thrombosed and failed (Fig. 57–3).[7, 10, 12, 14, 15]

This difference in results, together with the ease of reintervention for failing grafts, mandates that surgeons performing infrainguinal bypass operations follow their patients closely in the postoperative period and indefinitely thereafter. In the authors' practice, the surgeon examines the peripheral pulses of patients at 6- to 8-week intervals for the first 6 months and every 2 to 4 months thereafter. Ideally, noninvasive laboratory tests, including duplex scans of vein grafts, should be performed with similar frequency, but the authors have found them to be expensive and sometimes impractical to perform in all patients.

If the patient has any recurrence of symptoms or the surgeon detects *any* change in peripheral pulse examination or other manifestations of ischemia, the circulatory deterioration is confirmed by noninvasive parameters, and the patient is admitted for urgent anticoagulation and arteriography. If a lesion is detected as a cause of the failing state, it is corrected urgently by PTA or operation. Our aggressive prophylactic intervention for these lesions, even if they are asymptomatic, is based on their dire prognosis if left untreated and the greater difficulty and worse outcome that result if the lesion is untreated and the graft goes on to thrombose, as it almost certainly will.[10, 14] Moreover, if the failing graft is a vein bypass, detection of the failing state permits accurate localization and definition of the responsible lesion by arteriography and salvage of any undiseased vein. In contrast, if the graft is permitted to thrombose, the responsible lesion may be difficult to identify; it may be difficult or impossible to clear the vein with thrombectomy; the results of lytic therapy are poor; and the patient's best graft, the ipsilateral greater saphenous vein, may have to be sacrificed, rendering the secondary operation even more difficult and more likely to fail with associated limb loss.

MANAGEMENT STRATEGIES FOR PRESUMED INFRAINGUINAL GRAFT FAILURE

Patients with circulatory deterioration after an infrainguinal arterial reconstruction present with recurrent symptoms, a decrease in pulses in the involved limb, other changes on physical examination, or a decrease in noninvasive vascular laboratory values. These manifestations may occur at any time after operation and are presumptive evidence that the arterial reconstruction has thrombosed, although they may also occur in the absence of graft throm-

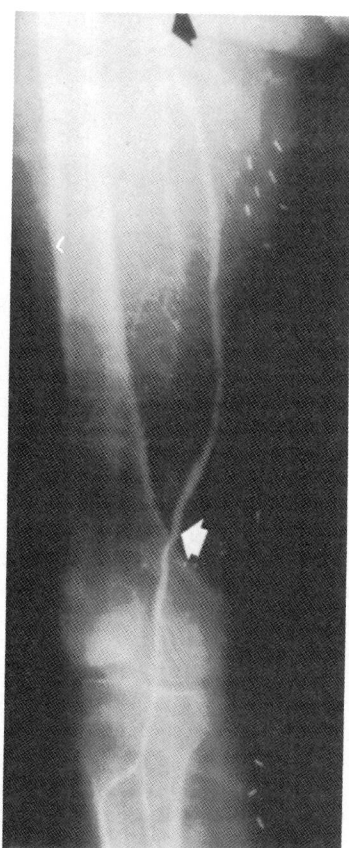

FIGURE 57–2. Arteriogram of a patient with a failing polytetrafluoroethylene (PTFE) femoropopliteal graft 2 years after the initial operation. The arteriogram was performed because of a return of rest pain and the loss of distal pulses. The graft (*between arrows*) was patent despite a proximal occlusion of the common femoral artery and an inflow pressure of only 40 mmHg. A bypass from the external iliac artery to the original graft was performed, and the original graft remained patent until the patient's death 6 years later.

bosis if some lesion is present in, proximal to, or distal to the bypass graft (i.e., with a failing graft).

Presumed Early Graft Failure (Within 30 Days of Operation)

If the primary operation was originally justified, a secondary procedure is also mandated. If the primary operation was performed for limb salvage, early graft failure or thrombosis is always associated with a renewed threat or even a worse threat to the limb. If the original preoperative arteriogram was satisfactory, repeat arteriography is not necessary. The patient is given intravenous heparin and returned to the operating room as expeditiously as possible. Because vein grafts can be injured by the ischemia associated with intraluminal clot and because it may be more difficult to remove solid thrombotic material from vein grafts, there is greater urgency to reoperate on a patient with a failed autogenous vein graft than one with a PTFE graft. In any event, reoperation should be undertaken within less than 12 hours of the detection of failure. Even greater urgency is required if calf muscle tenderness or neurologic changes are associated with graft failure.

Vein Grafts. The distal incision over the arterial reconstruction is reopened. The graft thrombosis is confirmed by palpation. Control of the artery proximal and distal to the distal anastomosis is obtained, and a full anticoagulating dose of intravenous heparin (7500 IU) is given. A linear incision is made in the hood of the graft (Fig. 57–4) to visualize the interior of the distal anastomosis.[3] Balloon catheters are gently passed retrograde in the graft to remove clot (Fig. 57–5). If necessary, any clot is similarly removed from the proximal and distal adjacent host artery, and any visualized anastomotic defect is repaired. Valves in the vein graft may prevent retrograde passage of the catheter, or it may be impossible to restore adequate, normal prograde arterial flow through the graft. In either event, the proximal incision is opened, and the same procedures are performed at the proximal anastomosis. With flow restored and all openings in the graft closed with fine running monofilament sutures, an intraoperative arteriogram is performed to visualize the graft and the outflow tract. If no defect is seen, adequacy of the reconstruction and the inflow tract is demonstrated by direct arterial pressure measurements, which should reveal no gradient in excess of 15 to 20 mmHg between the distal end of the graft and the brachial or radial artery. Any gradient in excess of 30 mmHg should be localized to the inflow tract or the graft by appropriate needle placement. If there is a gradient in the vein graft, it should be eliminated by revision. If this is impossible, the graft should be replaced by a prosthetic (PTFE) graft. Often such unexplained gradients are due to recanalized, throm-

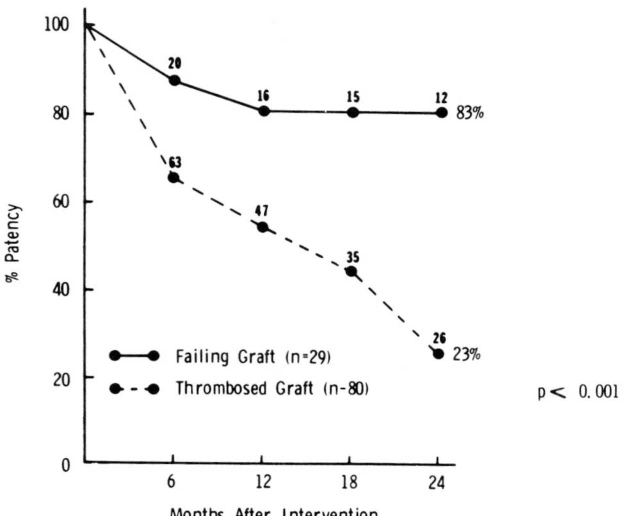

FIGURE 57–3. Comparison of patency rates after reintervention or reoperation for failing and failed (thrombosed) below-knee femoropopliteal and femorodistal PTFE grafts. Numbers of grafts at risk are shown at 6-month intervals. Standard error for all points is less than 10 per cent. (From Ascer E, Collier PE, Gupta SK, Veith FJ: Reoperation for PTFE bypass failure: The importance of distal outflow site and operative technique in determining outcome. J Vasc Surg 5:298, 1987.)

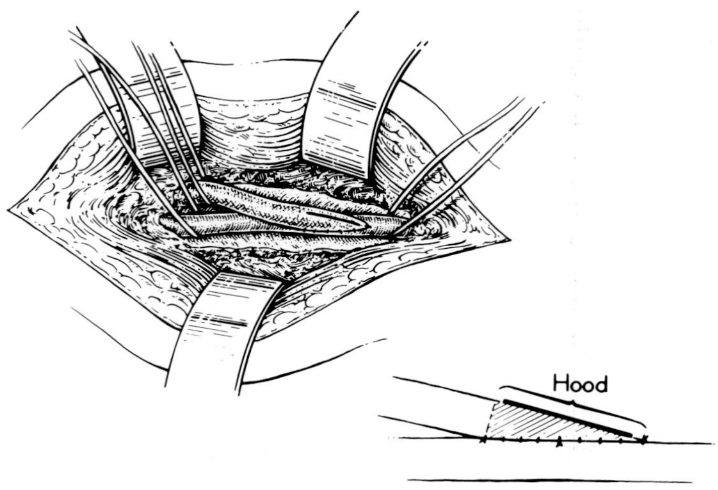

FIGURE 57–4. Operative exposure of the distal anastomosis. The incision in the hood of the graft is made to within 1 mm of the distal end of the graft. This provides optimal exposure of the distal anastomosis and facilitates thrombectomy. (From Ascer E, Collier PE, Gupta SK, Veith FJ: Reoperation for PTFE bypass failure: The importance of distal outflow site and operative technique in determining outcome. J Vasc Surg 5:298, 1987.)

bophlebitic segments of vein.[16] Unless removed, such segments will cause recurrent failure. If an inflow gradient is present, it should be eliminated by a suitable inflow bypass (aortofemoral, femorofemoral, or axillofemoral) or occasionally by an intraoperative or postoperative balloon angioplasty.

If disease in the outflow tract is detected and is the presumed cause of graft failure, it generally is best treated by an extension to a more distal, less-diseased segment of the same or another outflow artery (Fig. 57–6).

If no defect is detected by arteriography or pressure measurements, the procedure is terminated. Despite older evidence to the contrary,[17] an occasional vein graft undergoes early failure for no apparent reason and remains patent indefinitely after simple thrombectomy. Perhaps the unexplained thrombosis is due to undetected decreased cardiac output with hypotension and decreased arterial flow.

With our increasing ability to perform distal bypasses to disadvantaged outflow tracts,[1, 18, 19] the authors have encountered some patients whose distal grafts failed early for no apparent reason other than high-outflow resistance. In some of these instances, thrombectomy and extension of the graft to another outflow vessel as a sequential graft have resulted in long-term graft patency and limb salvage.[20]

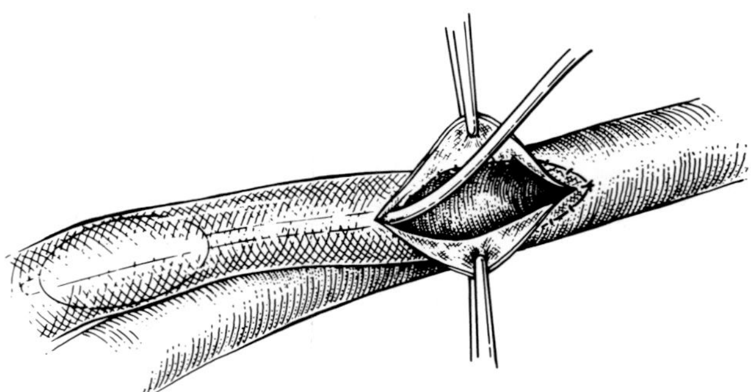

FIGURE 57–5. Thrombectomy alone is performed through the distal graft incision when no cause for graft failure is identified. Clot is removed from the graft and, if needed, from the artery both proximally and distally. (From Ascer E, Collier PE, Gupta SK, Veith FJ: Reoperation for PTFE bypass failure: The importance of distal outflow site and operative technique in determining outcome. J Vasc Surg 5:298, 1987.)

PTFE and Other Prosthetic Grafts. Early thrombosis of PTFE grafts is managed in essentially the same fashion as that already described for early failure of vein grafts.[3, 14] Differences include the almost complete freedom from graft defects as a cause of failure, although occasionally a PTFE graft will be compressed, kinked, or twisted because of poor tunneling technique and malposition around or through some of the tendinous structures in the region of the knee. In addition, graft thrombosis for no apparent reason is more common with PTFE grafts than vein grafts and occurred in 56 per cent of the authors' 61 early failures in a series of 822 PTFE infrainguinal grafts (Table 57–1).[21] Simple thrombectomy of the graft by the techniques already described results in patency rates in excess of 50 per cent after 3 years, if no other defect is found and if the distal end of the graft is above the knee joint.[3, 14] The secondary operative treatment in all of these 61 cases was based on the cause of early failure, as shown in Table 57–1. Management techniques were similar to those described for vein grafts except that in one case disease just beyond the distal anastomosis was treated by a patch graft angioplasty (Fig. 57–7) rather than by a distal graft extension.

Presumed Late Graft Failure (1 Month or More After Operation)

All patients with presumed late graft failure should undergo a standard transfemoral or translumbar arteriogram with visualization of all arteries from the renals to the forefoot.[1] If a failing graft is found, it is urgently treated by a reintervention, as already discussed. If a failed or thrombosed graft is present, the patient is not subjected to reinterventional treatment unless the limb is unequivocally rethreatened. Surprisingly, even if the original operation was performed for limb salvage with critical ischemia,[22] the limb may not be rethreatened when the original arterial reconstruction occludes.[3] Ten to 25 per cent of patients are able to tolerate occlusion of a limb salvage bypass and

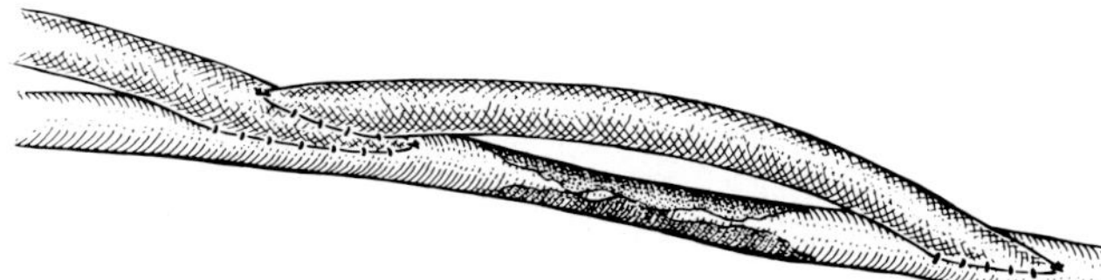

FIGURE 57–6. If disease in the outflow tract is detected, particularly a distal arteriosclerotic lesion, a graft extension is performed. (From Ascer E, Collier PE, Gupta SK, Veith FJ: Reoperation for PTFE bypass failure: The importance of distal outflow site and operative technique in determining outcome. J Vasc Surg 5:298, 1987.)

function effectively indefinitely. This proportion seems to increase as the interval between the primary operation and its failure increases. Presumably, this phenomenon occurs because the original limb-threatening lesion has healed by virtue of the bypass and does not recur with the renewed ischemia. Alternatively, improved collaterals maintain the limb better after some graft failures than before the operation for reasons that remain obscure.

When graft thrombosis *is* associated with renewed critical ischemia and an imminently endangered lower extremity, aggressive reintervention is indicated and is very important in achieving optimal limb salvage results.[1, 23] Management strategies differ, depending on the type of graft and its location. In all instances, complete arteriography should precede any reintervention.

Axillofemoral and Femorofemoral Grafts. When failure of one of these grafts occurs, the inflow tract of the graft should be examined angiographically. With axillofemoral grafts, it is possible to perform an arch arteriogram by the transfemoral or translumbar route.[24] Similar examination should be used to evaluate the inflow or donor iliac system with failed femorofemoral grafts. If significant inflow disease is found, it can be corrected by PTA, or a new bypass from an alternate site must be performed. If, for example, inflow iliac disease has caused failure of a femorofemoral graft, it can be corrected by PTA or an aortobifemoral bypass, or an aortic limb can be brought to the thrombectomized femorofemoral graft.

The same arteriogram should also be used to seek evidence of progression of outflow disease and should define patent distal segments that can be used to bypass such outflow disease if necessary. An example of this is progression of deep femoral artery disease in a patient for whom that vessel is providing outflow for an axillofemoral or femorofemoral bypass. In this circumstance, the popliteal artery should be evaluated angiographically, and thrombectomy of the graft should be followed by a profundaplasty or graft extension to the undiseased deep femoral or popliteal artery.

Table 57–1. Early (<1 Month) PTFE Bypass Graft Occlusion in 61 Failed Grafts

Cause	Treatment	Number	Incidence (Per Cent)
None found	Thrombectomy alone	34	56
Hypotension	Thrombectomy alone	2	3
Embolus	Thrombectomy alone	2	3
Technical*	Patch graft	1	2
Inflow stenosis	Proximal extension	3	5
Distal disease	Distal extension	19	31

**Unrecognized stenotic lesion just beyond distal anastomosis.*

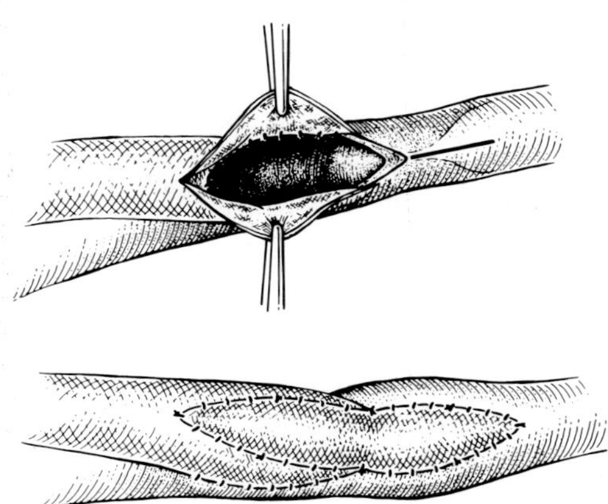

FIGURE 57–7. Stenosis just distal to the anastomosis can be caused by an unrecognized atherosclerotic lesion. This can be corrected by extending the graft incision distally across its apex and down the recipient artery until its lumen is no longer narrowed. A patch of PTFE or vein is then inserted across the stenosis to widen the lumen. Similar treatment is appropriate for intimal hyperplasia that causes late graft occlusion. (From Ascer E, Collier PE, Gupta SK, Veith FJ: Reoperation for PTFE bypass failure: The importance of distal outflow site and operative technique in determining outcome. J Vasc Surg 5:298, 1987.)

After suitable arteriographic examination, the patient is subjected to a secondary operation. The graft is opened over the hood or hoods of the distal anastomoses so that the interior of the distal anastomosis can be inspected (Fig. 57–8). With axillofemoral grafts, this is facilitated if the original femorofemoral limb is placed over the distal end of the axillary limb (Fig. 57–9). In this way, a single opening in the graft permits thrombectomy of all prosthetic grafts, thrombectomy of arteries in one groin, and diagnosis and correction of anastomotic problems at one distal anastomosis (Fig. 57–8). Although blind balloon catheter thrombectomy of any distal anastomosis via an opening in the graft remote from the anastomosis is occasionally successful, the authors object strongly to the practice. The chance of damage to the anastomosis, intimal injury, or plaque disruption in the adjacent artery is too great. Although it is true that the anastomosis and adjacent arteries must be dissected free and controlled and that this procedure may be difficult because of scarring, it is clearly worth the effort. If distal anastomotic intimal hyperplasia is detected as the cause of graft failure, it is treated by a graft extension or by incising across the hyperplastic lesion and inserting a patch graft (see Fig. 57–7). In the latter circumstance, the incision and patch are usually placed across the origin of the deep femoral artery.

If no cause of failure is found on preoperative arteriography or intraoperative inspection, an intraoperative arteriogram is performed. If no defects or partially obstructing lesions are found, as is often the case with failed

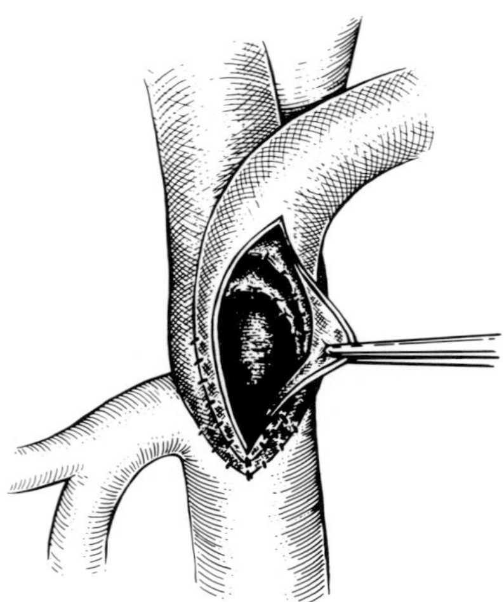

FIGURE 57–8. Approach to a failed axillobifemoral bypass. The distal anastomosis and adjacent vessels are dissected free and controlled. An opening is made in the hood of the graft to permit proximal thrombectomy and visualization of the interior of this anastomosis.

axillofemoral grafts, the reoperative procedure is terminated, and good results can be expected.

The value of these reoperations for failed extra-anatomic bypasses is substantially increased late patency rates[25] with a 3-year *additional* patency rate, calculated from the time of reoperation, of 75 per cent.[14]

Reoperations or Secondary Operations After Failed Femoropopliteal or Infrapopliteal Bypasses

General Observations

In these circumstances, if the graft is confirmed by arteriography to be thrombosed, reintervention is undertaken only if the limb is in immediate jeopardy. If this is the case, complete contrast arteriography must precede any secondary operation to provide some information, albeit perhaps incomplete, as to why the graft failed and to define possible therapeutic options by demonstrating remaining patent distal arterial segments and the quality of undissected proximal arteries that may be used for bypass origin, such as the mid- or distal portions of the deep femoral artery.[26, 27]

Bilateral contrast venography should also precede reoperation to define the length and quality of the remaining superficial veins.[28] This can be helpful in patients with failed vein grafts by revealing unused accessory greater saphenous veins, unused short saphenous veins, and occasionally a main saphenous trunk. The authors have also found that duplex ultrasonography can be useful in predicting the length and diameter of residual venous segments. However, neither technique of preoperative evaluation is totally accurate, and surgical exploration may be the only way to assess vein suitability with certainty. Venography or duplex ultrasonography is also indicated preoperatively in patients who have previously had a prosthetic bypass. The authors have been surprised by how often the greater saphenous vein in such cases has been damaged at the first operation or by scarring.

The usual standard surgical approaches to arteries in patients who have failed bypasses are often rendered more difficult or even impossible to use because of surgical scarring or infection. For that reason, the authors have developed a variety of new or unusual approaches to all the infrainguinal arteries, which allow these vessels to be reached through virginal tissue planes.[26] These approaches can be helpful in avoiding the scarred standard access routes and can be essential if a previous operation was complicated by infection. These unusual routes include direct approaches to the distal part or second and third portions of the deep femoral artery medial or lateral to the sartorius muscle.[26, 27] These approaches obviate the need to use a scarred or infected groin to trace the deep femoral artery down from its origin. They also permit the distal portions of the artery to be used to provide inflow for a distal shorter vein graft. The authors have now used these direct distal routes to the deep femoral artery in more than 80 secondary cases. Another set of unusual approaches comprises approaches to the above-knee or below-knee popliteal artery.[29] These approaches are particularly useful in the presence of medial incision sepsis and permit use of the popliteal artery for bypass inflow or outflow even in the presence of groin and medial thigh infection.[29] In addition, all three leg arteries can be reached medially or laterally, and adequate exposure can be obtained to perform an anastomosis. The lateral approach involves fibula resection through which all parts of the tibial and peroneal arteries can be reached.[26, 30–32] The authors have devised a method for exposing the lower third of the peroneal artery from a medial approach. This technique involves division of the long flexor muscles and tendons to the toes and foot and is particularly suited if an in situ bypass to the distal third of the peroneal artery is to be performed. Finally, the authors have developed surgical approaches to the terminal branches of the posterior tibial artery and the dorsalis pedis artery.[26, 32] Any of these branches, which include the medial

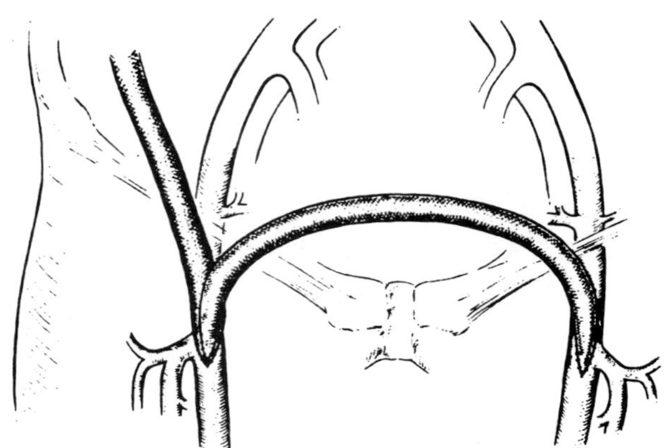

FIGURE 57–9. Crossover portion of axillobifemoral procedure is placed directly over the first femoral anastomosis. (From Ascer E, Collier PE, Gupta SK, Veith FJ: Reoperation for PTFE bypass failure: The importance of distal outflow site and operative technique in determining outcome. J Vasc Surg 5:298, 1987.)

and lateral plantar branches of the posterior tibial artery and the lateral tarsal and deep metatarsal arch branches of the dorsalis pedis artery, can be used for secondary bypass operations.[18] The deep metatarsal arch is accessed via a dorsal incision with removal of portions of the shaft of the second and perhaps third metatarsal bones.

Another principle that is particularly useful to the vascular surgeon planning a secondary procedure is the short vein graft or distal origin bypass concept. Every bypass to the popliteal or infrapopliteal vessels need not originate from the common femoral artery.[33] Grafts to these distal arteries may originate from the superficial femoral, popliteal, or even tibial arteries without compromising late patency results (Fig. 57–10).[18, 33] Such short vein grafts are particularly useful in secondary bypass operations because they allow the surgeon to avoid previously scarred or infected areas and facilitate the use of the limited remaining superficial veins as bypass conduits.[18, 33] Certainly, they are better than prosthetic grafts.[34] Moreover, the authors have shown that short vein grafts probably have better patency rates than long vein grafts, particularly when they are used as bypasses to disadvantaged outflow tracts.[18, 19]

Two types of secondary arterial reconstruction are available to the vascular surgeon who is planning a reintervention for a failed infrainguinal bypass. The first, termed by the authors a ''reoperation,'' employs some form of graft thrombectomy and revision or extension in an effort to save all or as much of the original graft as possible. The other type of secondary operation involves placement of a totally new secondary bypass graft preferably but not necessarily using previously undissected patent arteries for the origin and insertion of the bypass. The choice of which type of secondary bypass to employ is dependent on a number of variables, including the type of primary bypass (PTFE or autogenous vein), the nature and location of the lesion responsible for the failure of the primary operation, the surgeon's training and experience, the residual arterial and superficial venous anatomy, and, most important, the location of the primary bypass. Because of the importance of the last factor, the management of different kinds of failed primary operations that require reintervention is considered separately.

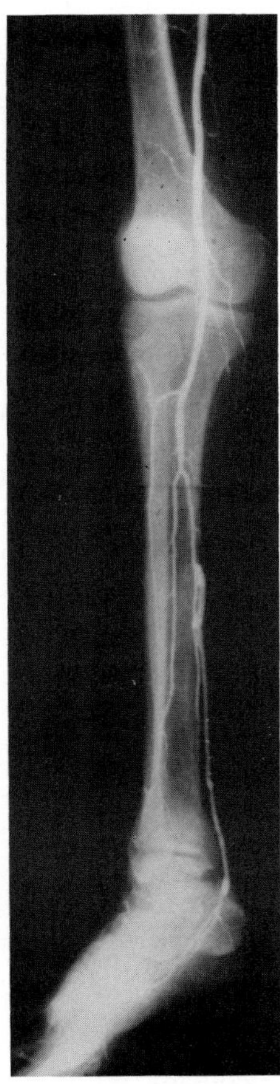

FIGURE 57–10. Arteriogram showing a posterior tibial to posterior tibial bypass, which has now remained patent for more than 6 years. (From Veith FJ, Ascer E, Gupta SK, et al: Tibiotibial vein bypass grafts: A new operation for limb salvage. J Vasc Surg 2:552, 1985.)

Failed Femoropopliteal or Infrapopliteal Autogenous Vein Grafts. In this setting, thrombectomy of the occluded vein graft is not attempted. If a patent albeit isolated popliteal segment is present, a bypass to that segment is attempted. An effort to perform this with a vein graft from the ipsilateral extremity is made using a remnant of the greater saphenous or the lesser saphenous vein. This is facilitated by using the distal deep femoral or superficial femoral artery for inflow, if possible, and by keeping the vein graft short. If no ipsilateral lower extremity vein of adequate length is available, a PTFE graft has good prospects of remaining patent and providing long-term limb salvage, particularly if it is inserted above the knee,[34] and the authors use it in preference to vein from the opposite leg or upper extremities. If foot necrosis or infection is extensive in this setting, a sequential femoral-to-popliteal-to-tibial bypass should be performed using a short distal vein graft obtained from any extremity of the patient. If no patent popliteal segment is present, as short a vein graft as possible is performed, extending from the distal-most artery with unobstructed proximal flow (i.e., deep or superficial femoral, popliteal, or tibial artery) to the most proximal patent infrapopliteal artery that courses without significant obstruction to its terminal end. For such procedures, autogenous vein from any extremity is used even if it is only 2.5 to 3 mm in diameter when distended.[18, 35] PTFE grafts should only be used for bypasses to infrapopliteal arteries if absolutely no autogenous vein is available. However, a secondary arterial reconstruction with such a prosthetic graft has a chance of remaining patent for several years and has a moderate chance of saving the involved limb.[34] Accordingly, use of such a graft, though not ideal, is a better option than an amputation.

Failed Femoral-to-Above-Knee Popliteal PTFE Bypass. When failure of such a bypass results in a threatened limb and a secondary intervention is required, it is the authors' present belief that a reoperation with an attempt at graft salvage is justified and indicated (Table 57–2).[3, 14] If the preoperative arteriogram indicates an inflow problem, this is treated appropriately by PTA or a proximal extension. The distal end of the graft is redissected along with its adjacent arteries (see Fig. 57–4), and, after administration of 7500 IU of heparin, a vertical incision is made in

Table 57–2. Cause, Incidence, and Management of Late PTFE Bypass Graft Occlusions (n = 104)

Cause of Failure	Number of Cases	Per Cent of Total	Treatment
Progression of distal disease	39	37	Thrombectomy and distal graft extension (30) or new bypass to more distal artery (9)
None found	29	28	Thrombectomy alone
Intimal hyperplasia	22	21	Thrombectomy and patch angioplasty
Progression of proximal disease	12	12	Thrombectomy and proximal graft extension
Hypotension/technical	2	2	Thrombectomy alone

the distal hood of the graft to permit balloon catheter thrombectomy of the graft and the popliteal artery proximally and distally (see Figs. 57–4 and 57–5). Great care is exercised and minimal balloon inflation is used when passing the catheter in arteries to avoid intimal injury. Only if necessary is a proximal incision made. If the presence of a distal lesion is detected on inspection of the anastomosis or by preoperative arteriography, it is treated. The authors still believe that an incision across the lesion and patch angioplasty are best for intimal hyperplasia (see Fig. 57–7), and a graft extension to a distal patent artery with a PTFE or vein graft (see Fig. 57–6) is best for distal disease progression. Although this approach requires a difficult redissection of the distal anastomosis (which may be more technically demanding than performance of a totally new bypass), the authors believe it is justified and indicated in view of the acceptable 3-year patency results (Fig. 57–11) and the fact that it preserves the maximal amount of undissected patent distal arterial tree should further problems develop.

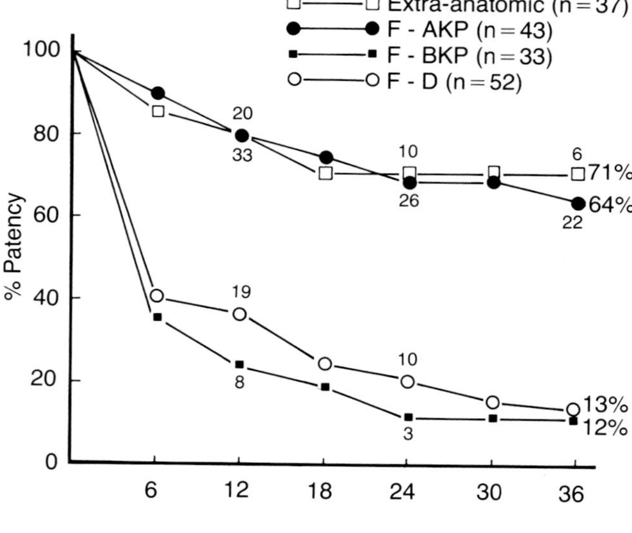

FIGURE 57–11. Cumulative life table patency rates for various types of PTFE bypasses subjected to one or more reoperations with salvage of the original graft. Numbers of grafts at risk are shown at yearly intervals. Extra-anatomic procedures include axillofemoral and femorofemoral grafts. F-AKP, femoral to above-knee popliteal grafts; F-BKP, femoral to below-knee popliteal grafts; F-D, femoral to infrapopliteal artery grafts. (From Ascer E, Collier PE, Gupta SK, Veith FJ: Reoperation for PTFE bypass failure: The importance of distal outflow site and operative technique in determining outcome. J Vasc Surg 5:298, 1987.)

Failed Femoral-to-Below-Knee Popliteal or Infrapopliteal PTFE Bypass. When failure of such a procedure results in the need for a secondary arterial reconstruction, at present the authors perform an entirely new secondary bypass, preferably employing an autogenous vein graft using some of the strategies already discussed that minimize graft length and permit use of previously unused segments of arteries or segments approached through virginal tissue planes.[26, 27, 29] The authors' primary reason for departing from the previous strategy[3] of performing a reoperation with an attempt at graft salvage is the poorer additional patency that is obtained with reoperations on these below-knee grafts (Fig. 57–11), compared with better results (over 40 per cent 2-year patency) when a totally new secondary bypass is employed.[14] A second reason for not using the reoperation strategy is the high infection rate of 6 per cent with such procedures, whereas the infection rate with a new secondary bypass is less than 1 per cent.[14]

Failure of Secondary Arterial Reconstructions. Although some vascular surgeons are reluctant to undertake multiple attempts at arterial reconstruction to salvage a threatened limb in the belief that the risks of infection and knee loss outweigh the potential benefits, the authors and others disagree.[1, 3, 7, 14, 23, 36] The results show that many patients can benefit from multiple limb salvage operations and that the benefits outweigh the risks and disadvantages, if the principles and strategies already advocated are employed.[1, 3, 7, 14, 23, 36]

Use of Fibrinolytic Agents

In the last several years, there has been renewed interest in the use of streptokinase and particularly urokinase to lyse intravascular clots (see Chapters 19, 35, 43, and 134), and the administration of low-dose streptokinase or high-dose urokinase by intra-arterial injection directly into thrombosed vein and PTFE bypass grafts has been found to be effective in restoring patency.[37–39] With restored bypass patency, any flow-reducing lesion contributing to the thrombosis can be identified and corrected by an appropriate PTA or a relatively minor operation. The authors' experience with this approach for thrombosed vein grafts was at first encouraging. However, our group and many others have found that patency of thrombosed vein grafts treated by lysis and revision has been poor.[40] Moreover, use of lytic agents is time consuming and complex and should not be used if the patient has severe ischemia with muscle tenderness and loss of foot motion or sensation. However, the authors and several other groups continue to use urokinase for thrombosed PTFE grafts with promising results, and this agent plus the newer human tissue plasminogen activator should continue to be regarded with interest. Nevertheless, more experience is needed before a final conclusion can be reached about the general usefulness of these agents in the management of failed infrainguinal arterial reconstructions.

CONCLUSIONS

Secondary arterial reconstructions play an important role in achieving the ultimate goal of limb salvage after primary infrainguinal interventions fail. By employing the strategies and principles outlined in this chapter, the surgeon can obtain good results in terms of patency of the reoperated primary reconstruction or the secondary reconstruction with significantly augmented limb salvage at a low cost in operative morbidity and mortality.[23] These results mandate that vascular surgeons maintain an aggressive attitude toward the use of these secondary operations when a primary procedure fails to achieve or maintain its intended goal and when a patient is faced with the imminent loss of a lower limb because of distal ischemia.

References

1. Veith FJ, Gupta SK, Samson RH, et al: Progress in limb salvage by reconstructive arterial surgery combined with new or improved adjunctive procedures. Ann Surg 194:386, 1981.
2. Rivers SP, Veith FJ, Ascer E, et al: Successful conservative therapy of severe limb-threatening ischemia: The value of nonsympathectomy. Surgery 99:759, 1986.
3. Veith FJ, Gupta SK, Daly V: Management of early and late thrombosis of expanded polytetrafluoroethylene (PTFE) femoropopliteal bypass grafts: Favorable prognosis with appropriate reoperation. Surgery 87:581, 1980.
4. Veith FJ, Gupta SK, Daly V: Femoropopliteal bypass to the isolated popliteal segment: Is polytetrafluoroethylene graft acceptable? Surgery 89:296, 1981.
5. Flinn WR, Flanigan DP, Verta MJ, et al: Sequential femoral-tibial bypass for severe limb ischemia. Surgery 88:357, 1980.
6. Szilagyi DE, Smith RF, Elliott JP, et al: The biologic fate of autogenous vein implants as arterial substitutes: Clinical, angiographic and histopathologic observations in femoropopliteal operations for atherosclerosis. Ann Surg 178:232, 1973.
7. Whittemore AD, Clowes AW, Couch NP, et al: Secondary femoropopliteal reconstruction. Ann Surg 193:35, 1981.
8. Karkow WS, Cranley JJ, Cranley RD, et al: Extended study of aneurysm formation in umbilical grafts. J Vasc Surg 4:486, 1986.
9. Hasson JE, Newton WD, Waltman AC, et al: Mural degeneration in the glutaraldehyde tanned umbilical vein graft: Incidence and implications. J Vasc Surg 4:243, 1986.
10. Veith FJ, Weiser RK, Gupta SK, et al: Diagnosis and management of failing lower extremity arterial reconstructions. J Cardiovasc Surg 23:381, 1984.
11. O'Mara CS, Flinn WR, Johnson ND, et al: Recognition and surgical management of patent but hemodynamically failed arterial grafts. Ann Surg 193:467, 1981.
12. Smith CR, Green RM, DeWeese JA: Pseudoocclusion of femoropopliteal bypass grafts. Circulation 68 (Suppl II):88, 1983.
13. Berkowitz HD, Hobbs CL, Roberts B, et al: Value of routine vascular laboratory studies to identify vein graft stenosis. Surgery 90:971, 1981.
14. Ascer E, Collier P, Gupta SK, Veith FJ: Reoperation for PTFE bypass failure: The importance of distal outflow site and operative technique in determining outcome. J Vasc Surg 5:298, 1987.
15. Sanchez L, Gupta SK, Veith FJ, et al: A ten-year experience with one hundred fifty failing or threatened vein and polytetrafluoroethylene arterial bypass grafts. J Vasc Surg 14:729, 1991.
16. Panetta TF, Marin ML, Veith FJ, et al: Unsuspected pre-existing saphenous vein disease: An unrecognized cause of vein bypass failure. J Vasc Surg 15:102, 1991.
17. Craver JM, Ottinger LW, Darling C, et al: Hemorrhage and thrombosis as early complications of femoropopliteal bypass grafts: Causes, treatment, and prognostic implications. Surgery 74:839, 1973.
18. Veith FJ, Ascer E, Gupta SK, et al: Tibiotibial vein bypass grafts: A new operation for limb salvage. J Vasc Surg 2:552, 1985.
19. Ascer E, Veith FJ, Gupta SK, et al: Short vein grafts: A superior option for arterial reconstructions to poor or compromised outflow tracts? J Vasc Surg 7:370, 1988.
20. Ascer E, Veith FJ, Morin L, et al: Components of outflow resistance and their correlation with graft patency in lower extremity arterial reconstructions. J Vasc Surg 1:817, 1984.
21. Collier P, Ascer E, Veith FJ, et al: Acute thrombosis of arterial grafts. *In* Bergan JJ, Yao JST (eds): Vascular Surgical Emergencies. New York, Grune and Stratton, 1987, pp 517–528.
22. Working Party of the International Vascular Symposium: The definition of critical ischaemia of a limb. Br J Surg 69(Suppl):S2, 1982.
23. Veith FJ, Gupta SK, Wengerter KR, et al: Changing arteriosclerotic disease patterns and management strategies in lower limb-threatening ischemia. Ann Surg 212:402, 1990.
24. Calligaro KD, Ascer E, Veith FJ, et al: Unsuspected inflow disease in candidates for axillofemoral bypass operations: A prospective study. J Vasc Surg 11:832, 1990.
25. Ascer E, Veith FJ, Gupta SK, et al: Comparison of axillounifemoral and axillobifemoral bypass operations. Surgery 97:169, 1985.
26. Veith FJ, Ascer E, Nunez A, et al: Unusual approaches to infrainguinal arteries. J Cardiovasc Surg 28:58, 1987.
27. Nunez A, Veith FJ, Collier P, et al: Direct approaches to the distal portions of the deep femoral artery for limb salvage bypasses. J Vasc Surg 8:576, 1988.
28. Veith FJ, Moss CM, Sprayregen S, et al: Preoperative saphenous venography in arterial reconstructive surgery of the lower extremity. Surgery 85:253, 1979.
29. Veith FJ, Ascer E, Gupta SK, et al: Lateral approach to the popliteal artery. J Vasc Surg 6:119, 1987.
30. Veith FJ, Gupta SK: Femoral-distal artery bypasses. *In* Bergan JJ, Yao JST (eds): Operative Techniques in Vascular Surgery. New York, Grune and Stratton, 1980, pp 141–150.
31. Dardik H, Dardik I, Veith FJ: Exposure of the tibial-peroneal arteries by a single lateral approach. Surgery 75:337, 1974.
32. Ascer E, Veith FJ, Gupta SK: Bypasses to plantar arteries and other tibial branches: An extended approach to limb salvage. J Vasc Surg 8:434, 1988.
33. Veith FJ, Gupta SK, Samson RH, et al: Superficial femoral and popliteal arteries as inflow sites for distal bypasses. Surgery 90:980, 1981.
34. Veith FJ, Gupta SK, Ascer E, et al: Six-year prospective multicenter randomized comparison of autologous saphenous vein and expanded polytetrafluoroethylene grafts in infrainguinal arterial reconstructions. J Vasc Surg 3:104, 1986.
35. Wengerter KR, Veith FJ, Gupta SK: Influence of vein size (diameter) on infrapopliteal reversed vein graft patency. J Vasc Surg 11:525, 1990.
36. Bartlett ST, Olinde AJ, Flinn WR, et al: The reoperative potential of infrainguinal bypass: Long-term limb and patient survival. J Vasc Surg 5:170, 1987.
37. Hargrove WC III, Barker CF, Berkowitz HD, et al: Treatment of acute peripheral arterial and graft thromboses with low dose streptokinase. Surgery 92:981, 1982.
38. van Breda A, Robison JC, Feldman L, et al: Local thrombolysis in the treatment of arterial graft occlusions. J Vasc Surg 1:103, 1984.
39. McNamara TO, Fisher JR: Thrombolysis of peripheral arterial and graft occlusions: Improved results using high-dose urokinase. Am J Roentgenol 144:769, 1985.
40. Veith FJ, Gupta SK, Ascer E, et al: Reoperations and other reinterventions for thrombosed and failing polytetrafluoroethylene grafts. *In* Yao JST, Bergan JJ (eds): Reoperative Arterial Surgery. New York, Grune and Stratton, 1986, pp 337–392.

58

Endovascular Interventions for Lower Extremity Ischemia

Robert B. Rutherford, M.D., Janette D. Durham, M.D., and David A. Kumpe, M.D.

• • •

Balloon catheters for percutaneous transluminal angioplasty (PTA) became widely available in the late 1970s, and the North American experience with PTA largely began at that time. After more than 15 years of experience, the current role of PTA in the treatment of the patient with peripheral vascular disease has become fairly well defined. In 1985 Ginsburg and colleagues first introduced the laser in an attempt to disobliterate peripheral arteries. Problems with surface charring by coagulated blood, thermal injury, and perforation of the vessel wall combined to make bare fiber use unfeasible.[37] By 1987 laser-assisted balloon angioplasty (LABA) was introduced clinically, using a laser-heated, hot-tipped probe to provide a channel for the introduction of a dilating balloon. In the ensuing years a startling array of laser and atherectomy devices has appeared whose application is encompassed by the term endovascular surgery, although many interventional radiologists and cardiologists prefer to use the term PTA in the broader sense. For simplicity, PTA is used in this chapter as the generic term, and standard percutaneous transluminal balloon dilatation is identified as PTBA. Chapter 20 reviews many of the fundamental considerations associated with PTA, including the mechanisms and techniques of PTBA, LABA, and other laser modalities plus current atherectomy devices as well as the adjunctive use of intravascular stents, current catheter usage, complications, and future directions for intraluminal therapy. This chapter analyzes the current role of all these forms of endovascular intervention in the treatment of lower extremity ischemia as the sole or initial treatment of arteriosclerosis obliterans, as an adjunct to arterial reconstruction, in preserving graft patency, and in combination with thrombolytic therapy. This last topic is dealt with in more detail in Chapter 19.

Finally, because PTBA now has an established role in the management of peripheral arterial occlusive disease (PAOD) and is for the most part complementary to rather than competitive with bypass and other arterial reconstructive techniques, the major part of this chapter is devoted to defining that role. The other devices that have been touted (and justified to the Food and Drug Administration [FDA]) as improving on the "disappointing" results of PTBA, allowing PTA to be extended to longer and more complex lesions, are discussed last. This order is particularly appropriate because PTBA, not bypass, should serve as the gold standard for these new techniques.

PATIENT EVALUATION AND SELECTION

The initial decision as to whether a patient with lower extremity ischemia should undergo any interventional procedure—surgery or PTA—is primarily based on the history, physical examination, and noninvasive vascular testing, supplemented as needed with evaluation of the severity of other vascular or organ-system disease. This initial clinical evaluation usually establishes the degree of disability, the threat to limb viability, the general location and severity of the occlusive lesions, the anesthetic risk, and the patient's prospects for long-term survival. Almost any patient who is deemed to be a candidate for interventional treatment should then also be considered a *potential* candidate for PTA. However, as the results of PTA in general and PTBA in particular, have become more apparent, it has become clear that the reverse is not the case because there are some patients who are candidates for PTA who would *not* be considered candidates for bypass surgery. Obtaining arteriograms in all patients with PAOD in the hope that they might have a lesion favorable to PTA is not cost-effective, but this dilemma has been nicely solved for femoral popliteal lesions, at least, by using color flow duplex scanning as a preliminary screening device. Arteriography may well be justified for those in whom noninvasive testing indicates an iliac stenosis. However, patients who are not candidates for bypass, typically claudicators with discrete, localized iliac or superficial femoral artery (SFA) stenoses and short SFA occlusions, may well be candidates for an exercise program, and the choice between this option and PTA, which is discussed later in this chapter, needs to be made before proceeding with arteriography. If, on the other hand, the choice is between PTA and bypass, it is usually based on morphologic criteria. Arteriography must then be performed in a manner that facilitates performing PTA during the same procedure should this option be considered most appropriate. From the morphologic characteristics and location of the lesion(s), one can generally predict the outcome of PTA and compare this with the anticipated results of arterial reconstruction for the same lesion. When the greater cost and risk of surgery are balanced against the lower durability and more limited applicability of PTA, the choice is almost always clear. To provide a background for this decision, the next sections will review the results of

PTBA in regard to relevant outcome variables. Later in this chapter the early experiences with other forms of PTA will be reviewed against this background.

FACTORS AFFECTING THE REPORTED OUTCOME OF BALLOON ANGIOPLASTY

Patient Selection. Initial and long-term results are affected by the morphologic selection criteria for PTBA that are followed by the angiographer and the vascular surgeon. The best results are obtained if only the most favorable lesions (i.e., short focal stenoses) are dilated. At the other extreme, if the angiographer and surgeon insist that PTBA be used only in cases in which surgery would be performed if PTBA failed, the high proportion of cases with multi-segmental or diffuse disease with poor runoff will result in poorer overall PTBA results. These two "conservative" attitudes thus cause contrastingly different results and striking differences in the proportion of patients subjected to PTBA. Martin, in considering the strategy of limiting PTBA to the shorter (< 5 cm) favorable lesions, observed from the study of a large number of arteriograms obtained during a multi-center trial, that whereas 94 per cent of iliac and 79 per cent of femoropopliteal stenoses fit under this limit, only 30 per cent of iliac and 9 per cent of femoropopliteal occlusions qualified.[38] Thus, although femoropopliteal lesions outnumber iliac occlusive lesions by 2 to 4 times in patients presenting for treatment, in most PTBA series iliac lesions far outnumber femoropopliteal lesions.[16] On the other hand, if one is relatively "liberal" in the application of PTBA, one will perform PTBA both on "favorable" isolated lesions producing lesser symptoms, for which surgery and its greater attendant risk cannot be justified, and, at the other extreme of the spectrum of disease, on "unfavorable," more extensive lesions in an attempt to avoid surgery in high-risk patients with limb-threatening ischemia. This liberal application assumes that, in skilled hands, PTBA is a safe procedure that rarely makes matters worse.[15] It allows a wider spectrum of patients to be treated by using combinations of PTBA and surgery and, by treating patients at both extremes, produces intermediate overall results.

Location of Lesion. The long-term patency following PTBA is more dependent on the dilatation site than on any other single factor. Proximal, larger-caliber arteries offer the best initial and long-term results, so it has become a convention to separate the results of iliac and femoropopliteal PTBA.

Rutherford and Durham[39] recently reviewed the literature to define the long-term patency rate of PTBA and, for the reasons just cited, presented the results for iliac and femoropopliteal lesions separately. Figure 58–1 summarizes that analysis. It will be noted that femoropopliteal PTBA has twice the initial failure rate of iliac PTBA (16 per cent vs. 8 per cent) and twice the early failure rate (20 per cent/year vs. 10 per cent/year), but after the first year they both enjoyed the same modest rate of failure (3 per cent/year), ending with 5-year patencies (including initial failures) of 52 per cent and 70 per cent, respectively. As will be apparent from the following discussion, the degree of occlusion, length of lesion, extent of disease, and runoff status all influence these overall results.

Stenoses Versus Occlusion and Extent of Atheromatous Disease. In the iliac arteries, usually only discrete stenotic lesions and very short occlusions are treated by PTBA *alone* (i.e., without stents). In femoropopliteal angioplasties, one series has shown a 20 per cent difference in late outcome favoring femoropopliteal stenoses versus occlusions,[21] although in this series the length of the lesion was not considered. Others[20, 21, 26] found no difference. In fact, in the series reported by Murray and colleagues,[26] the long-term patency rate for femoropopliteal occlusion was higher than for stenosis. The extent of the atheromatous disease—i.e., length of lesion and whether there is focal or diffuse involvement of the artery—is a more important determinant of long-term patency than whether the arterial segment is stenotic or occluded. Results worsen when longer and/or multiple segments are dilated, as documented in the section on long-term results.

Runoff Status. Although initial experience with angioplasty suggested that long-term patency of the dilated segment was not affected by the presence of distal occlusive disease, subsequent reports have suggested that poor runoff

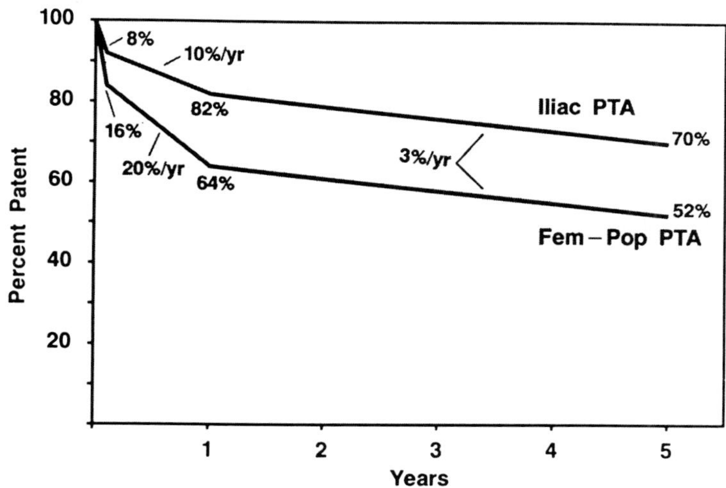

FIGURE 58–1. Composite patency curve for iliac and femoropopliteal PTA. Note that the initial and early failure rates for the femoropopliteal group are twice those of the iliac group; however, after the first year, the failure rates for both groups are similar. (From Rutherford RB, Durham J: Percutaneous balloon angioplasty for arteriosclerosis obliterans: Long-term results. *In* Yao JST, Pearce WH [eds]: Technologies in Vascular Surgery. Philadelphia, WB Saunders, 1992, pp 329–345.)

does negatively affect patency. In our initial series, the difference between iliac dilatations performed with open runoff versus those with superficial femoral occlusion was not statistically significant (92 vs. 83 per cent, respectively). Johnston and associates[16] reported 5-year patencies of 63 per cent for iliac stenoses with good runoff and 51 per cent for iliac stenoses with poor runoff. Their reported patency rate is lower than others because their patency criteria rely on the ankle-brachial index (ABI) and thus include the effect of distal occlusive disease (see later discussion). This difference is accentuated in diabetic patients, who often have severe infrapopliteal occlusive disease. Stokes and colleagues, in a study of PTBA in diabetic patients, observed a 19 per cent difference between good and poor runoff groups at 1 year (95 vs. 76 per cent), but at 5 years there was an almost fourfold difference in patency (77 vs. 20 per cent).[40]

For femoropopliteal dilatations, one series found that runoff status had no influence, whereas several others did.[8, 10, 20] Krepel and coworkers reported 5-year success rates of 77 versus 59 per cent for good versus poor runoff cases, respectively.[20] Gallino and colleagues,[8] who included initial failures in their patency results, reported better early (2-day) and late (2-year) success among patients with two or three patent crural arteries (86 and 71 per cent, respectively) compared with patients with one or no crural artery patent (43 and 36 per cent). In Johnston's series, which also included initial failures, 5-year primary patency was 50 per cent for stenoses with good runoff, 38 per cent for stenoses with poor runoff, 34 per cent for occlusions with good runoff, and 20 per cent for occlusions with poor runoff. Again, the length of lesion treated was not taken into account.[16] In this regard, Jeans and associates[41] have provided a more detailed breakdown, with steadily decreasing 5-year success rates for longer occlusions (37 per cent for occlusions of 0 to 4 cm, 43 per cent for those of 4 to 9 cm, 29 per cent for those of 9 to 14 cm, and 17 per cent for those greater than 14 cm). These figures include initial failures.

Initial Hemodynamic Response. There is evidence[11, 29] that the initial hemodynamic improvement after angioplasty does not equal that following surgical bypass of a similar lesion, but such differences are relative, not absolute, and should not influence pretreatment decision making, since both PTBA and surgical bypass usually produce sufficient hemodynamic improvement to achieve initial success. After angioplasty, the degree of improvement in the ABI serves not only as a gauge of the immediate clinical improvement to be expected and as a baseline for follow-up studies, but also, in the case of iliac PTBA, as a prognostic indicator. Improvement in the ABI after iliac PTBA had a strongly favorable prognostic significance for sustained patency in the authors' initial series,[21] whereas improvement in the thigh-brachial index (TBI) alone, by greater than 0.2, was also a positive prognostic sign, though not as strong as the ABI (Table 58–1). The authors did not find a similar prognostic value for the change in the ABI following femoropopliteal PTBA.

It is important to recognize that the initial hemodynamic response following PTBA may not be fully appreciated for several days. Hemodynamic deterioration rarely occurs in the first several days after a good initial hemodynamic result, but, in cases in which the initial hemodynamic improvement is only modest, it is not unusual to see further improvement within several days. It is important, therefore, to wait several days before judging the end-result of an angioplasty, particularly if the placement of a femoropopliteal or femorofemoral graft distal to an iliac angioplasty is contemplated.

Table 58–1. Predictive Value of Change in TBI and ABI Following Iliac Angioplasty in 68 Patients[26]

	n	Late Deterioration
$\Delta TBI < 0.2$	15	5 (33 per cent)
$\Delta TBI > 0.2$	53	4 (7.6 per cent) $p = .02$
$\Delta ABI < 0.1$	27	8 (29.6 per cent)
$\Delta ABI > 0.1$	41	1 (2.4 per cent) $p = .002$

Diabetes. In some series, the presence of diabetes correlates with poorer results,[8, 16, 30, 35] although if a negative effect exists, it is probably due to the characteristically different distribution of occlusive lesions in diabetic patients—they have proportionally fewer favorable proximal iliac lesions and a high frequency of infrapopliteal occlusive lesions, that is, poor runoff. *For the same combination of occlusive lesions,* there is no difference between diabetic and nondiabetic patients in outcome following angioplasty, just as has been observed following reconstructive surgery.

Redilatation. Comparatively few reports on the long-term results of redilatation following failed angioplasties are available.[8, 25, 31, 35] Gallino and associates[8] and Johnston and colleagues[16] found similar initial and long-term success rates following first and second dilatations. Schmidtke and Roth[31] found that redilatation results were best for iliac lesions with restenosis (82 per cent success), intermediate for femoropopliteal lesions associated with claudication (63 per cent success), and worst for patients with gangrene and recurrent femoropopliteal disease (47 per cent improvement after one repeat dilatation, 20 per cent after second redilatation).

Thus, restenosis following PTBA is *not* automatic grounds for proceeding with arterial reconstruction. As discussed later, it may be an indication for redilatation with the adjunctive use of an intraluminal stent. Recurrent stenosis at a PTBA site or a new stenosis in the same segment should be redilated if the occlusive process is not extensive or the location is favorable (see Figs. 58–4*C* and *D* and 58–7*C–E*). This is particularly true if the reasons for choosing dilatation over surgery in the first place still pertain. Some authors have even included redilatation in reporting long-term results and are therefore reporting secondary patency rates.[2, 26, 27, 34]

Other Morphologic Features. Calcification of the stenotic lesion does not appear to affect long-term patency, although initial success rates may be lower for complete femoropopliteal occlusions that are heavily calcified. Eccentricity versus concentricity of the lesion is probably not important provided that a good hemodynamic correction has been achieved.[20]

INDICATIONS FOR TRANSLUMINAL BALLOON ANGIOPLASTY

Assuming that there are symptoms that justify intervention, transluminal angioplasty is the initial choice of interventional therapy for *discrete* (less than 5 cm) stenoses in either the iliac or the femoropopliteal segment and for occlusions of less than 10 cm in otherwise normal femoropopliteal arteries. This also assumes that attention has been given to control of risk factors (e.g., smoking, hyperlipidemia, hypertension) and that *serious* consideration has been given to exercise training as an option (see later discussion of angioplasty vs. nonoperative management).

The remaining majority of occlusive lesions—long stenoses or occlusions, or multiple short stenoses in the same segment, or a single critical stenosis in a diffusely involved irregular segment—are all best treated by arterial reconstruction, presuming the balance between operative risk and the threat of limb loss or restriction in essential activities justifies such intervention. When the balance does not clearly favor surgery, adjunctive use of stents with PTBA may be justified, as discussed later.

If a discrete iliac stenosis exists on the side opposite an extensively diseased or totally occluded contralateral iliac artery or proximal to an ipsilateral superficial femoral artery lesion, the iliac stenosis should be dilated several days prior to a femorofemoral or femoropopliteal bypass, respectively.[42] Only very limited experience with concomitant intraoperative dilatation of stenoses, proximal or distal to a reconstruction, has been reported at this time. However, the authors do not recommend dilating iliac lesions *intraoperatively* before proceeding with femoropopliteal or femorofemoral bypass, not only because the maximum hemodynamic improvement following angioplasty may not become apparent for several days but also because delayed occlusion, though rare, would also condemn the bypass to failure.

Stenoses developing adjacent to or in a bypass graft, and recurrent stenoses in previously dilated arterial segments, can be detected early by serial noninvasive testing. Balloon dilatation of such lesions can add significantly to the cumulative patency rate of grafts and arteries. Some of these lesions may not have as durable a response to angioplasty as the original atherosclerotic lesions,[43, 44] but this is easily recognized with continued follow-up, allowing surgical revision to be performed electively.

Finally, in categorically poor-risk patients who have limb-threatening ischemia, transluminal angioplasty can be performed on extensive lesions, with or without the aid of intra-arterial infusions of thrombolytic drugs (and, more recently, stents), in an attempt to avoid a high-risk operation or an otherwise inevitable amputation.[1, 12, 36]

CRITERIA FOR REPORTING RESULTS

Reported results will obviously vary, depending on the criteria used to consider a procedure successful, as discussed in Chapter 25. Except as noted, the results discussed in the following section are from series that have demanded an increase in the arterial luminal diameter after dilatation, categorical improvement in clinical status, and improvement in the appropriate segmental limb pressure index for the procedure to be counted successful initially and during follow-up. Patency is estimated using life table analysis or the Kaplan-Meier product-limit method. In assessing results of iliac angioplasty, it is important to note whether the TBI or ABI is used to gauge outcome. The former is appropriate for determining patency; the latter correlates with overall clinical improvement. For example, in our initial report,[21] 3 years following iliac dilatation, there was sustained improvement in the TBI in 82 per cent of patients, whereas the ABI remained improved in only 55 per cent owing to progression of distal occlusive disease. If the ABI is used to assess outcome following iliac dilatation, as in the Toronto series,[15, 16, 25] a lower success rate will be reported (e.g., 59 per cent for common iliac stenoses at 5 years) than in studies in which patency is the main criterion.

Because the initial failure rate of angioplasty can be substantial, up to 10 per cent for iliac lesions and 25 per cent for femoropopliteal lesions, a nearly universal convention among angiographers has been to report long-term durability of only the successful dilatations. Fortunately, interventional radiologists are now accepting the need to observe the same reporting standards used for bypass surgery.[45] The Journal of Vascular Interventional Radiology now requires compliance with these standards.[46] Unfortunately, these standards are not reflected in all reports cited in the following section.

RESULTS OF BALLOON ANGIOPLASTY

Iliac Stenoses. Unquestionably, iliac arteries give the best initial and long-term results with balloon angioplasty. Optimal iliac lesions for dilatation are short (less than 2 cm), hemodynamically significant stenoses in otherwise relatively normal arteries. In these, an *initial* success rate of around 95 per cent can be anticipated. Slightly longer stenoses (2 to 5 cm) also respond well to dilatation (Fig. 58–2) but will have a lower long-term primary patency rate. *Initial* success in most series ranges between 90 and 95 per cent for iliac dilations (Table 58–2).

Table 58–2 contains the long-term results following iliac angioplasty from six different series in which long-term patencies have been reported using life table analysis or the Kaplan-Meier product-limit method. Figure 58–3 attempts to simplify these data and present a composite patency curve derived from it. The initial technical success of aortoiliac angioplasty in these six studies ranged from 94 to 96 per cent. The easy access to the lesion from a retrograde femoral approach, the large vessel diameter, the rapid blood flow through the iliac artery, and the low thrombosis rate following dilatation all contributed to this high success rate. Initial clinical success, based on improvement in leg hemodynamics after a technically successful angioplasty, ranged from 89 to 97 per cent, resulting in a mean overall success rate (30 days) for all six studies of 92 per cent. One-, 3-, and 5-year cumulative patency rates, *including*

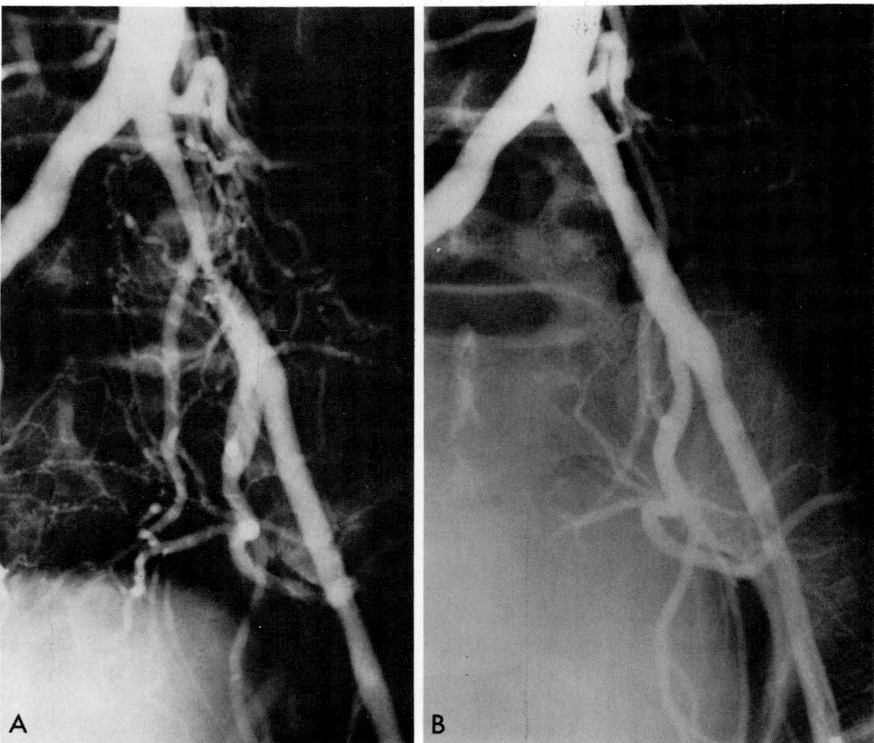

FIGURE 58–2. *A*, Isolated 4.5-cm stenosis of common iliac artery in a 40-year-old man with claudication. *B*, Normal hemodynamics were restored by successful dilatation.

initial failures, ranged from 74 to 96 per cent (mean, 84 per cent), 61 to 89 per cent (mean, 76 per cent), and 59 to 83 per cent (mean, 74 per cent), respectively. Differences in primary patency, reporting methods, and patient selection explain these wide ranges in long-term data. To generalize, one can expect a 4 per cent technical failure rate, compounded by an additional hemodynamic failure rate of 4 per cent, for an overall initial success rate of 92 per cent. During the first year, there is a further 10 per cent failure rate, and approximately 3 per cent failure per year in subsequent years can be expected.

Longer stenoses and multiple stenoses carry lower long-term primary patency rates. Spence and colleagues[34] reported a 10 per cent lower patency rate at 2 years for lesions 2 to 5 cm long than for lesions 1 cm long (74.6 vs. 85.8 per cent, respectively). In the authors' initial experience, single discrete iliac stenoses had a 3-year patency rate of 91 per cent compared with 56 per cent when two or more ipsilateral iliac lesions required dilatation.[29] Similar findings were reported by Johnston and coworkers,[15, 16] who also found a lower long-term primary patency rate for external iliac lesions than for common iliac lesions.

Table 58–2. Patency Following Iliac Angioplasty

Study Number	Author (Year)	Number of Patients	Initial Success (Technical/Clinical)	Cumulative Patency Reported (Corrected) in Years			
				1	*2*	*3*	*5*
1.	Kumpe[21] (1982)*	71 A	.96/.93	.88(.82)	.82(.76)	.82(.76)	
		B	.96/.85	.73(.62)	.55(.47)		
2.	Van Andel[35] (1985)	154	.96/NR	.98(.94)	.93(.89)	.91(.87)	.86(.83)
3.	Johnston[16] (1987)†	684	NR/.91 A	.80	.80	.70	
			CI	.79	.69	.65	.59
			EI	.74	.62	.51	.48
4.	Wilson[47] (1989)	81	.89	.74	.71	.61	
5.	In der Maur[48] (1990)	157	NR/.97	.99(.96)	.96(.93)	.92(.89)	.84(.81)
6.	Stokes[40] (1990)	70	.94/.89	.85(.79)	.74(.69)	.67(.63)	.34(.32)

From Rutherford RB, Durham J: Percutaneous balloon angioplasty for arteriosclerosis obliterans: Long-term results. In *Yao JST, Pearce WH (eds): Technologies in Vascular Surgery. Philadelphia, WB Saunders, 1992, pp 329–345.*

**Reported same patients by thigh-brachial index (A) and ankle-brachial index (B) criteria.*

†Reported separately aortic (A), common iliac (CI), and external iliac (EI) lesions.

NR, Not reported. The last study applies to diabetics only.

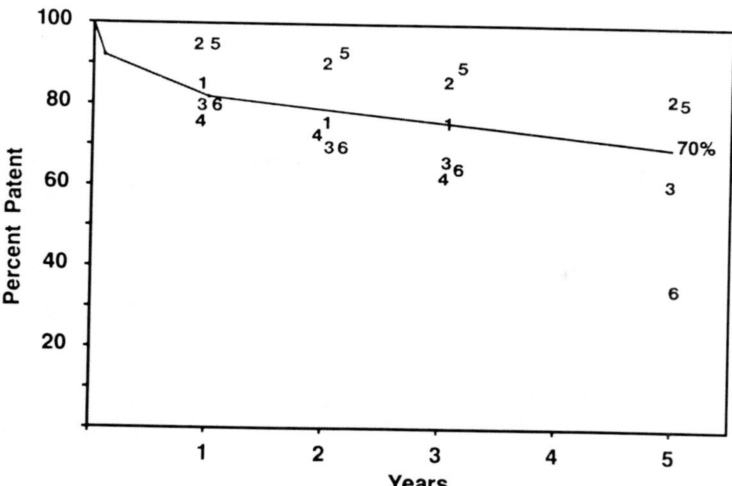

FIGURE 58–3. Composite patency curve for iliac percutaneous transluminal angioplasty (PTA), based on the six best references from the literature, as detailed in Table 58–2. (From Rutherford RB, Durham J: Percutaneous balloon angioplasty for arteriosclerosis obliterans: Long-term results. *In* Yao JST, Pearce WH [eds]: Technologies in Vascular Surgery. Philadelphia, WB Saunders, 1992, pp 329–345.)

Chronic Iliac Occlusion. The role of angioplasty in the treatment of chronic iliac occlusions is not yet established. One large series deserves attention. Colapinto and coworkers reported a very favorable experience in recanalization of 64 chronic iliac obstructions of 1 to 19 cm in 59 patients.[4] Initial success was obtained in 78 per cent overall, with a cumulative 4-year patency rate of 78 per cent in these. Initial success was achieved in 90 per cent of patients whose occlusions were 5 cm or less, and in 70 per cent of those whose obstructions were more than 5 cm long. Four-year patencies were 72 and 86 per cent, respectively, for the shorter and longer occlusions. Only 3.1 per cent of their patients had distal embolization that required surgery. These authors concluded that PTBA was more likely to be successful in shorter occlusions (< 5 cm) affecting only one iliac arterial segment, either the common or external iliac artery, but that long-term patency was not affected by the length of the lesion. Other investigators, in considerably smaller series, have found the rate of major embolization requiring surgery to be 20 to 50 per cent and do not routinely dilate longer iliac occlusions.[21, 28] Short iliac occlusions (Fig. 58–4*A* and *B*) are well treated with a lesser chance of embolization.

There are preliminary experiences[1, 12, 36] suggesting that chronic iliac occlusions can be treated by initial thrombolysis, using transcatheter administration of a fibrinolytic agent (preferably urokinase), followed by angioplasty of the underlying stenosis, with a 60 to 75 per cent success rate. More recently, this approach has been reinforced with the adjunctive use of stents, but results are too preliminary to warrant wholesale endorsement, although some early reports have been encouraging.[39] Unless there is a prohibitive risk, bypass surgery is still the choice here.

To summarize with a simpler view of iliac PTBA results, overall results have shown a 70 per cent 5-year patency rate, but consideration of certain characteristics that affect outcome helps in decision making.[39] Thus, there is a best case–worst case scenario for which long-term patency rates range between 85 per cent and 45 per cent with increments of roughly 10 per cent being accounted for by *location* (common vs. external iliac), *runoff status* (superficial femoral patency or occlusion), *discreteness of lesion* (short vs. multiple or long lesions), and *clinical stage* (claudication vs. limb salvage). These factors are similar to those detailed in Johnston's report,[16] but there is a higher range of success because for iliac PTBA the ABI is not reliable as the major criterion for success.

Femoropopliteal Lesions. Neither the initial success rate nor the long-term patency is as high for femoropopliteal angioplasty as it is for iliac lesions. Optimal lesions for femoropopliteal angioplasty are short stenoses and occlusions (< 3 cm). The initial success rate is somewhat lower for occlusions than for stenoses. Longer stenoses and occlusions can be treated by angioplasty (Fig. 58–5), but these have a lower initial success and long-term primary patency.

There are more than 40 articles in the literature that present the results of femoropopliteal (FP) PTBA, and although some contribute worthwhile information on specific aspects, less than a third yield meaningful data on long-term patency. Some of these results, primarily those with serial data compiled over time, are summarized in Table 58–3. In studying PTBA results, two North American series are particularly noteworthy because of their large number of patients and their careful, in-depth analysis using objective criteria: the University of Toronto series reported by Johnston and colleagues[16] and the University of Pennsylvania experience summarized by Berkowitz and his associates.[43, 44] In addition, Adar and associates[51] have made a meaningful contribution to our understanding of FP-PTBA results by subjecting what they considered the most complete and informative results to confidence profile analysis, producing a composite estimate of the durability of FP-PTBA success over time, including a separate breakdown for patients treated for claudication and those treated for limb salvage (Table 58–4). Estimates from these combined data projected an early (30-day) overall success rate of 86 ± 3 per cent with continuing "patency at 6 months of 73 ± 4 per cent, at 1 year of 66 ± 5 per cent, at 2 years of 61 ± 4 per cent, at 3 years of 58 ± 6 per cent, and at 5 years of 60 ± 5 per cent." In general, reports from European centers present a more favorable impression of PTBA durability than those from North America, and this is reflected in Adar's projections. The suggested explanations

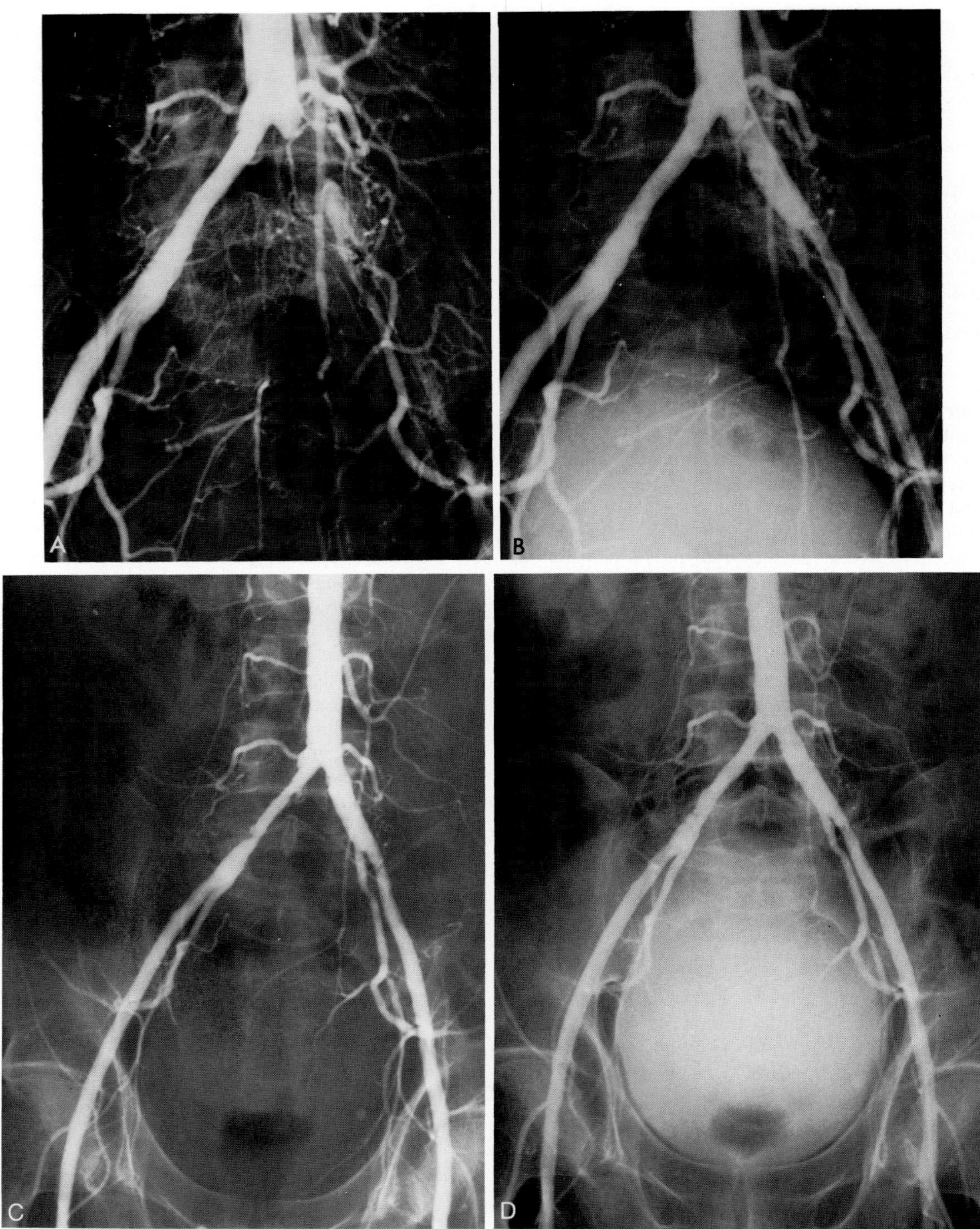

FIGURE 58–4. *A*, A 2.5-cm common iliac artery occlusion in a 55-year-old man with claudication. *B*, Successful recanalization produced normal hemodynamics. Leg hemodynamics and the arteriographic appearance of the treated segment were normal 25 months after dilatation. *C*, Appearance 31 months later. Continued patency of the dilated left common iliac segment is seen despite interval development of new stenoses in the right common iliac and left proximal external iliac segments. *D*, After dilatation of the new stenoses.

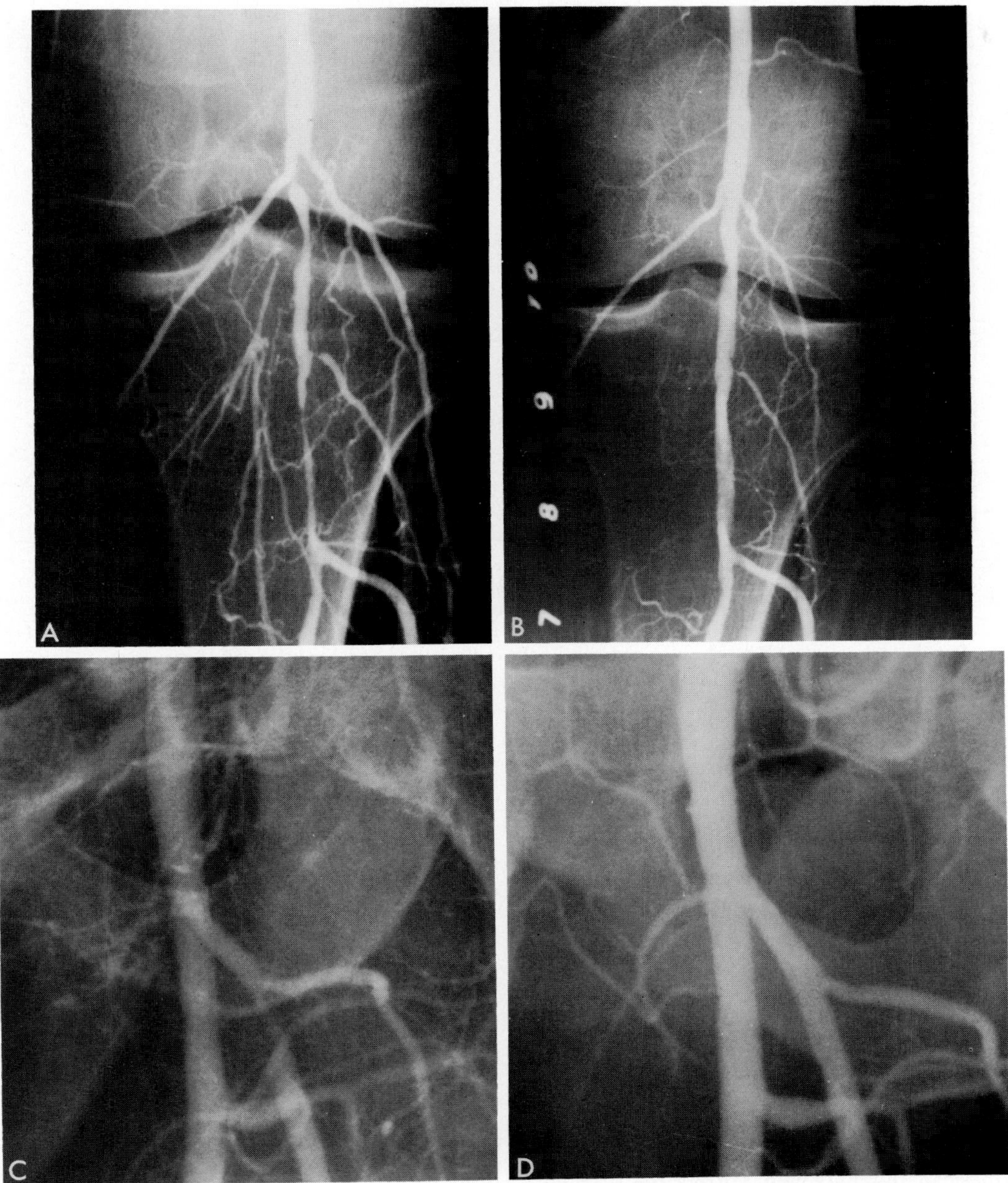

FIGURE 58–5. *A*, An 8-cm popliteal stenosis in an active 42-year-old-man, a smoker with juvenile diabetes and three prior myocardial infarctions. *B*, Following successful dilatation. *C*, Associated profunda femoris stenosis in the same patient. *D*, Following successful dilatation. Patient has normal hemodynamics 20 months after treatment.

Illustration continued on following page

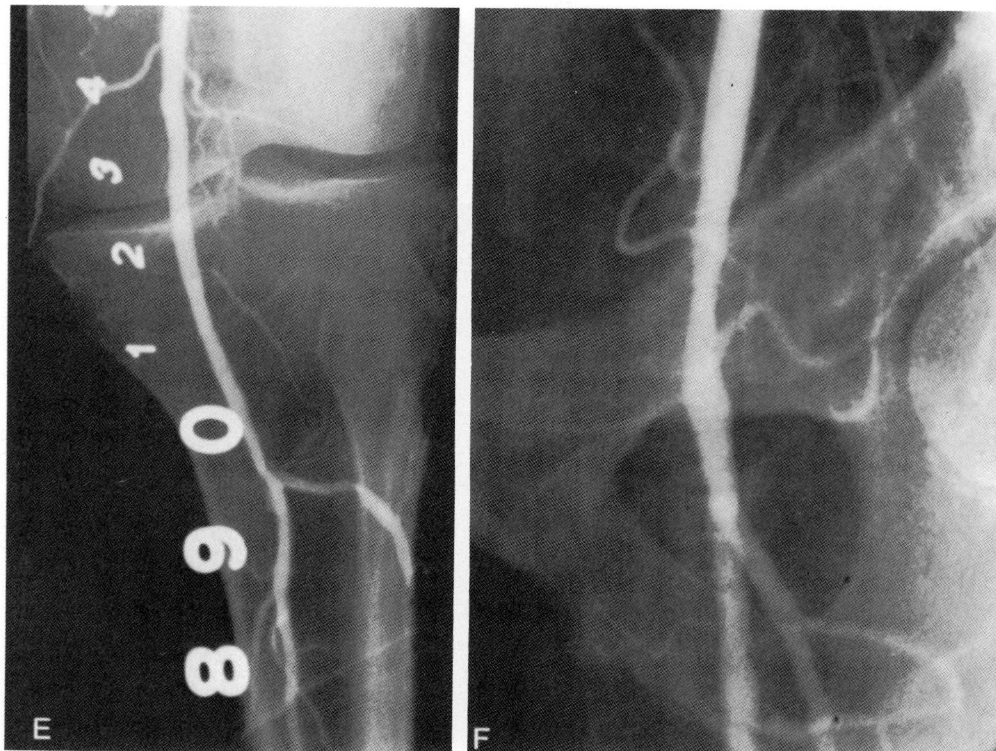

FIGURE 58–5. *Continued* *E* and *F*, Arteriogram of the left leg performed 6¾ years later. There is continued patency of the previously dilated segments of the profunda femoris and popliteal arteries. Multiple distal tibial artery occlusions had developed in the interval. A transmetatarsal amputation was necessary even though technically successful iliac and proximal anterior tibial angioplasties were performed after this arteriogram. Below-knee amputation of the contralateral leg was performed at same time.

for these differences—greater skill or selectivity versus more demanding criteria of success or treating more difficult lesions—cannot be easily reconciled. What is apparent from the figures of Adar and associates, however, is that there is still a much greater technical failure rate compared to that for dilating iliac stenoses and that after a high restenosis rate during the first year, averaging 13 per cent at 6 months and 20 per cent by 12 months, the patency curve flattens out to the range of 60 per cent by 2 years with minimal additional fall thereafter. In most North American experiences, this late plateau is closer to 40 per cent. Figure 58–6 shows a composite patency curve for femoropopliteal PTBAs using data and taking the differences previously described (between North American and European results) into consideration. The 52 per cent 5-year patency rate represents a compromise between data from the European and North American literature and reflects the gradually improving results from more discriminating patient selection and improving technique.

Although angioplasty of more extensively diseased femoropopliteal segments, either occluded or diffusely stenotic, is much less durable, it may be reasonable to dilate such lesions for limb salvage indications in patients who are *prohibitive* surgical risks, especially if the rest pain is recent or the ischemic ulcer superficial.[23] In these circumstances, although the improved arterial circulation is often short lived (several months), it may save the extremity without surgical intervention. Rush and associates[30] have reported a large experience with such cases. They treated 97 limbs in 86 patients with end-stage arterial occlusive disease in whom vascular reconstruction was not considered either appropriate or possible. Limb salvage was 76 per cent at intervals ranging from 1 to 45 months. The 1-year restenosis rate was 57 per cent, and repeat PTBA successfully maintained patency in only 10 limbs.

Although not yet documented, it is our impression that longer (10 to 25 cm) segmental occlusions in otherwise "clean" femoropopliteal segments in which the underlying stenosis is actually quite short may represent a subgroup that has a potentially better long-term patency following angioplasty, with or without the aid of local thrombolysis (Fig. 58–7*A* and *B*). In such patients, serial dilatation may be required (Fig. 58–7*C–E*).

To summarize, femoropopliteal PTBA carries an overall 5-year success rate in the range of 50 per cent, but for decision-making purposes, one should consider those characteristics that affect outcome and adjust the prognosis accordingly. As suggested for iliac PTBA but with a lower and wider range, one can consider best- and worst-case scenarios ranging from 70 per cent to 20 per cent, with increments accounted for by *clinical stage* (20 per cent, claudication vs. limb salvage), *degree of occlusion* (10 per cent, occlusion vs. stenosis), *runoff* (20 per cent, 2 to 3 vs. 0 to 1 vessels patent), and *length of lesion* (20 per cent, less than or greater than 10 cm). Obviously, there is some overlap here, so that one should subtract for no more than three

Table 58–3. Long-Term Patency of Femoropopliteal PTA

Study Number	Author	Years 1	2	3	4	5
Initial failures excluded						
	Krepel[20]		.77			
	Gallino[8]		.71	.70		
	Schneider[88]	(.74)*	.70			.70
	Waltman[87]	.86	.84		.70	(.67)*
	Greenfield[55]	.89	.84	.73	.69	.68
Initial failures included						
1.	†Gallino[8]	.63	.62			
2.	Berkowitz[43]		.67	.61		
3.	†Waltman[87]	.73	.70	.63		
4.	†Greenfield[55]	.72	.68	.62		.58
5.	‡Adar[51]	.66	.61	.58		.59
6.	¶Johnston[16]	.63	.53	.50	.44	.40

Modified from Stokes KR, Strunk HM, Campbell DR, et al: Five-year results of iliac and femoropopliteal angioplasty in diabetic patients. Radiology 174:977–982, 1990.

**From other article by same author(s).*

†Adjusted for initial failure rate by Adar R, Critchfield GC, Eddy DM: A confidence profile analysis of the results of femoropopliteal percutaneous transluminal angioplasty in the treatment of lower-extremity ischemia. J Vasc Surg 10:57, 1989.

‡Estimated from the literature (including most of the above studies) using confidence profile analysis.

¶Also required improvement in clinical grade.

negative factors in estimating long-term success rates. These rough guidelines suffice for most clinical decision making, but for more accurate estimates (of femoropopliteal PTBA) the reader is referred to the report of Johnston and colleagues,[16] who originally suggested this approach.

PTBA for Infrapopliteal Arterial Occlusive Disease. Now that the soft, low-profile catheters developed for coronary dilatation have been modified for tibial use, PTBA of infrapopliteal arteries is becoming increasingly common, but to date only about a half dozen series have been reported, and even those have only 1 to 3 years follow-up. Horvath and associates, from Linz, Austria,[52] reported on dilatation of 103 tibial lesions, noting a 96 per cent technical success rate and a cumulative patency rate of 80 per

Table 58–4. Comparison of Success/Patency Rates for Femoropopliteal PTA: Claudication Versus Limb Threat

Length of Follow-up	Claudication (%)	Limb Threat (%)
30 days	89.1 ± 2.5	76.8 ± 4.0
6 mo	81.1 ± 2.7	60.7 ± 4.4
1 yr	69.8 ± 4.2	50.3 ± 6.4
2 yr	63.7 ± 8.1	46.6 ± 6.5
3 yr	62.4 ± 9.1	43.1 ± 7.2

Adapted with permission from Adar R, Critchfield GC, Eddy DM: A confidence profile analysis of the results of femoropopliteal percutaneous transluminal angioplasty in the treatment of lower-extremity ischemia. J Vasc Surg 10:57, 1989.

cent at 1 year, 75 per cent at 2 years, and 65 per cent at 3 years. Schwarten[53] reported a 97 per cent technical success rate and an 83 per cent 2-year limb salvage rate in a group of patients who were essentially all smokers with threatened limbs, two thirds of whom were diabetics. Brown and coworkers[54] and Greenfield[55] reported 75 per cent and 81 per cent 1-year limb salvage rates, respectively, but Sprayregen and colleagues[56] and Tamura and associates[57] reported only 40 and 33 per cent success rates at 1.5 and 2 years, respectively. The reason for these marked differences is not clear, but it is suspected that the latter reports focused on evidence of patency (i.e., continued improvement) and not on mere avoidance of amputation. Unfortunately, many tibial PTBA procedures are done as one or more of several dilatations performed for multi-level disease.[58] This, and the difficulty of assessing the individual patency of one of three peroneal-tibial vessels, precludes accurate appraisal of the patency of tibial PTBA from the current literature.

COMPARISON OF BALLOON ANGIOPLASTY WITH SURGERY AND NONOPERATIVE TREATMENT

Comparison of balloon angioplasty with bypass on the one hand and nonoperative management on the other must

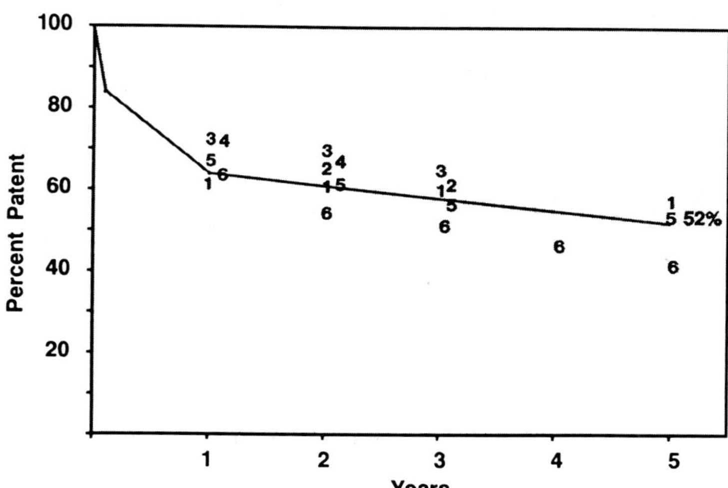

FIGURE 58–6. Composite patency curve for femoropopliteal PTA, based on the six best studies from the literature as detailed in Table 58–3. (From Rutherford RB, Durham J: Percutaneous balloon angioplasty for arteriosclerosis obliterans: Long-term results. *In* Yao JST, Pearce WH [eds]: Technologies in Vascular Surgery. Philadelphia, WB Saunders, 1992, pp 326–345.

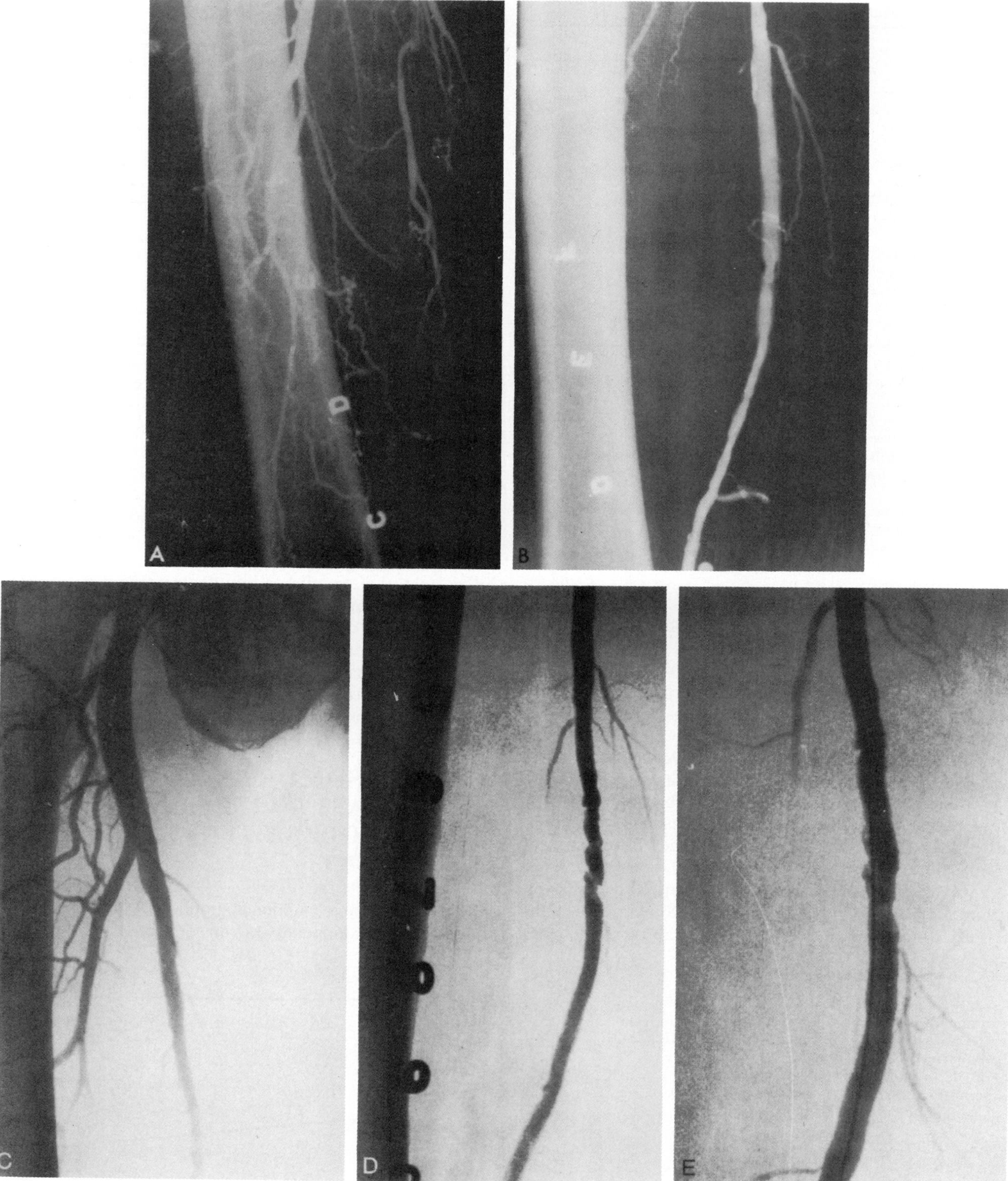

FIGURE 58–7. *A*, An 18-cm occlusion in a 43-year-old man with bilateral calf claudications and symmetric superficial femoral occlusions. He had had previous coronary artery bypass surgery. *B*, Following successful bilateral dilatation. *C*, Arteriogram performed 55 months later, when the patient developed recurrent claudication. The previously occluded segment remains patent, and there is recurrent stenosis at its distal end (*D*). This stenosis was redilated (*E*), restoring a normal ABI. A similar recurrent stenosis was treated on the contralateral side at the same time.

With femoropopliteal lesions, repeat dilatations are required in 30 to 50 per cent of cases, depending on the length of the initially treated segment, and should be regarded as part of the treatment.

take many factors into account—initial and long-term success rates, risk (mortality and morbidity), cost-effectiveness, and the consequences of failure. As a generalization, PTBA stands between surgery and nonoperative management based on these factors. For the claudicator, PTBA is less expensive per procedure than bypass, with hospital stay being mainly responsible for the difference.[7, 14, 19] On the other hand, it is obviously more expensive than nonoperative management. Considering overall health care costs, to the extent that PTBA removes patients from surgery (assuming careful patient selection to minimize failure and the likelihood of either redilatation or eventual bypass), PTBA decreases health care costs; to the extent that it removes nonsurgical candidates from the ranks of those traditionally treated nonoperatively, it increases *overall* health care costs.

This additional cost of PTBA compared with exercise training could be justified if functional improvement following PTBA were significantly greater and if it were reasonably durable. This is clearly the case for iliac PTBA if favorable lesions are selected but is not indisputable for femoropopliteal PTBA, judging from comparative randomized trials. For example, in the Oxford study reported by Creasy and colleagues,[59] in which claudicants with discrete femoropopliteal disease were prospectively randomized into two well-matched groups (by ABI and walking distance) to receive exercise training or PTBA, the initial (3-month) advantage of PTBA was lost by 12 months, at which time not only was the ABI of the PTBA group no longer better by statistical significance, but the exercise-trained group was walking significantly further before claudication occurred, almost three times their pretreatment distance.

On the other hand, there are many patients with truly disabling claudication who by temperament will not participate in or persist with an exercise program. Others may need to more than double the distance to claudication to resume normal activities or return to work. Here, the choice rests between PTBA and bypass and depends primarily on the location and morphology of the responsible lesions and the patient's operative risk and longevity outlook.

The advantages of arterial reconstruction are primarily its greater durability and better hemodynamic response and also the fact that it can be applied to a much wider spectrum of patients, regardless of the degree and extent of occlusive disease.

However, durability is not the only standard by which to judge a vascular reconstructive procedure. Patients with peripheral vascular disease have a high mortality rate in follow-up, ranging from 25 to 50 per cent at 5 years and from 60 to 90 per cent at 10 years.[3, 5] In view of such high late death rates, the initial advantages of PTBA become more significant and may well counterbalance its lesser degree and duration of benefit.

Furthermore, there appears to be a difference in the pattern of failure of surgery and angioplasty. Thrombosis of some bypass grafts is associated with propagation of thrombus or progression of disease into the adjacent native artery, leaving the patient with a worse clinical status than before the bypass. The management of a failed graft with some combination of fibrinolysis, balloon angioplasty, surgical thrombectomy, and surgical revision or secondary reconstruction is usually more complex and expensive than the original operation and requires an extended hospitalization and convalescence. In thrombosed femoropopliteal and femorotibial grafts, a precious nonrenewable resource, the saphenous vein, may be lost.[2] This is not the case with angioplasty, in which redilatation of recurrent stenosis or a new stenosis in the same arterial segment is usually possible.

Kalman and Johnston[18] have documented that the implications of a failed angioplasty are less ominous than those of a failed graft, and that recurrent stenosis at the dilatation site or new stenosis in the same arterial segment usually returns the patient to the predilatation clinical level. They studied 223 eventual failures among 631 angioplasties. Eighty-five per cent of these patients with failure returned to their original level of symptoms, 5.5 per cent remained better off than they were originally, and only 9.5 per cent were clinically worse than before PTBA. The 12 amputations in this series were due to advanced atheromatous disease and in no instance were attributed to failure of the PTBA. Among those patients undergoing subsequent reconstructive surgery, a failed PTBA had little effect on the type and outcome of the operation, although vascular reconstruction was often technically more demanding because of fibrosis at the puncture site and/or perivascular inflammation at the dilatation site.

In patients with chronic critical ischemia, nonoperative therapy is not usually a competitive option, although the authors have learned from control groups in clinical trials of prostanoids that up to 40 per cent of those with rest pain or shallow ischemic ulcers can be relieved or healed, respectively, without intervention (see Chapter 51). However, in this setting, bypass is clearly much more effective than PTBA because the occlusive disease is characteristically much more extensive and the degree of hemodynamic improvement required is also greater. Nevertheless, even here there may be key lesions that are amenable to PTBA performed either as an adjunctive procedure or, in high-risk patients, as the sole therapy. In high-risk patients in whom there is adequate circulation to keep intact tissues viable but not enough to meet the increased demands of wound healing, PTBA is a reasonable option even when longer lesions are involved and predicted durability is more limited. In these cases even a few months of improved flow are often enough to achieve limb salvage.

Thus, although well-designed overall comparisons among these three modalities for claudicators and for those with chronic critical ischemia are valuable, they are unlikely to produce absolute answers or establish exclusive superiority of one treatment over another. However, knowledge of their relative merits in these settings allows appropriate choices to be made in individual patients.

It is a mistake to dwell too heavily on the competitive aspect of these three modes of therapy, particularly if it fosters a tendency among vascular surgeons to defend, promote, and invariably recommend bypass, and among interventional radiologists and vascular internists to apply PTBA and exercise training, respectively, in a biased fashion. These three forms of therapy each contain obvious strengths and weaknesses, and the authors continue to be impressed by how often the choice in *individual* patients is obvious when all factors are considered.

THE ROLE OF LASER THERAPY, ATHERECTOMY DEVICES, AND STENTS

Five years ago, when this chapter was written for the previous edition, nothing much was said about these other endovascular techniques, and by the time that edition was in print, there was concern that it might be quickly outdated, such was the speed and enthusiasm with which these new techniques were being developed and applied. Now, although PTBA has settled nicely into a valuable role, the other techniques of endovascular surgery are going through a ''boom or bust'' crisis. On the one hand, laser therapy appears to be a ''bust'' in terms of its application to the management of peripheral arterial occlusive disease. Its apparent demise would not have produced so few mourners (and so many celebrants) had it not been for the shameful commercialism with which it was promoted. Atherectomy devices, with pointed exceptions to be discussed, also have been disappointing although each new device is greeted with enthusiasm by those whose previous interventional device has run its course. The laser and the various atherectomy devices were introduced ostensibly to extend the scope of endovascular intervention to the treatment of more extensive occlusive lesions than those favorable for PTBA. Some, in fact most, simply provide a channel that allows introduction of the balloon catheter for transluminal dilatation. Others have effectively removed plaque, and, to the extent that the residual luminal narrowing has been significantly reduced (e.g., to less than 30 per cent in diameter), they have achieved a degree of lasting success. But all are more or less traumatic, and we have learned from their clinical results that the universal response to endovascular trauma is neointimal hyperplasia. This response has been largely responsible for restenosis rates in the range of 30 to 50 per cent within 6 to 12 months for most devices. With better angiographic techniques (steerable guidewires, ''roadmapping,'' and so on) and better guidance and monitoring systems (intraluminal ultrasound and angioscopy), the *potential* role for these devices has been enhanced and now depends primarily on control of neointimal hyperplasia, where some progress is being made (see Chapter 15). In the meantime, there is much work to be done resolving unpleasant ''political issues'' (e.g., credentialling and training, turf battles, self-serving reporting practices, premature release of these devices for open clinical application, and uncontrolled commercial promotion by corporations, hospital boards, and individual interventionalists.[85, 86] At the moment, intravascular stents are enjoying a boom and show promise of extending the role of PTBA in patients with iliac disease and possibly atherectomy. However, it is predictable, given the increasing public recognition of the limited resources that can be applied to health care, that the costs of these latest approaches (e.g., thrombolysis and stenting) may soon be considered prohibitive, especially when they are compared with such inexpensive treatments as exercise training and abstinence from tobacco.

Laser Therapy. Ginsburg and colleagues[37] first introduced the laser to treat PAOD in 1987. There were three perforations with this method, and only 8 of 16 cases were successfully ''recanalized.'' It soon became apparent that unguided, bare-fiber laser application carried too high a risk of thermal injury and perforation. Subsequently, laser energy was used to produce hot-tip probes that penetrated occluded segments and produced a channel adequate for the introduction of balloon dilators. This mode of balloon angioplasty (LABA) was claimed by Sanborn and associates[60] to produce better results than PTBA alone. An overall 82 per cent 1-year patency rate was claimed, but initial failures were excluded; otherwise, only a 63 per cent patency rate was achieved. Although this figure is essentially identical to the PTBA results achieved at 1 year in the analyses by Adar and colleagues[51] and the authors (see Fig. 58–1), similar combined 1-year data (77 per cent success with and 59 per cent without initial failures excluded) gained FDA release for LABA.[61] It was also claimed that such results were obtained in patients in whom a guidewire could not be passed, but these ordinarily include only 10 to 15 per cent of cases (and possibly less with the addition of the Terumo guidewire), and yet a significant number of short lesions were included, and the *1-year* overall success rate of lesions longer than 7 cm was under 50 per cent! In less than 2 years, 20,000 LABAs were performed, reaching a rate of over 1500 a month, and more than 300 self-proclaimed ''laser centers'' appeared in the United States alone. Quickly, the pendulum swung back as negative reports emerged documenting high technical failure rates (16 to 33 per cent), high initial hemodynamic failure rates (13 to 36 per cent), low overall patency rates (22 to 50 per cent at 6 to 12 months), and a higher complication rate than achieved with PTBA alone (e.g., 4 to 9 per cent perforation, 5 to 11 per cent hemorrhage, 5 to 17 per cent dissection, and 1.5 to 8.7 per cent amputation).[62–66] In AbuRahma and associates' experience, *initial* success rates of 86 per cent, 60 per cent, and 27 per cent, respectively, were reported for lesions of less than 5 cm, 5 to 10 cm, and over 10 cm long, respectively.[66] However, the 1-year patency rate in the *favorable* (less than 5 cm group) was 59 per cent, but for lesions more than 10 cm long, it was only 9 per cent!

Larger hot-tip probes were tried as sole therapy and underwent a multi-center trial with overall success rates for femoral artery lesions at 1 year of 50 per cent with a range of 31 to 70 per cent depending on length of the lesion and degree of occlusion.[67] Subsequently, there have been trials with the Eximer (cool) laser[68, 69] and the computer-guided ''Smart'' laser,[70, 71] both of which proved disappointing despite their theoretical advantages. At the moment, none of the laser devices appear to have improved on the results of PTBA alone, and the laser is not necessary to produce hot-tip probes, which can be made safer and less expensive by using radiofrequency heating. Lasers carry a significantly higher cost in terms of equipment and actual procedural costs in addition to their complication rate. It is hoped that this cost will be partially repaid by important lessons learned.

Atherectomy Devices. A number of clever devices have been designed, developed, and tested for their ability to remove rather than displace plaque; they have the potential advantages over PTBA of reducing the likelihood of restenosis, managing greater degrees and lengths of occlusion, and avoiding initial subintimal dissection with resultant thrombosis. To date, four have been approved by the FDA for clinical use.

The *Kensey Atherectomy* (now the TracWright System) has a flexible catheter with a central drive shaft that rotates a sharp distal cam tip at 100,000 rpm and pulverizes the atheromatous plaque. It has no coaxial guidewire, and the procedure is carried out under fluoroscopy through a femoral arteriotomy. Snyder and colleagues[72] reported initial success with 14 of 23 SFA occlusions, but PTBA was also used in 11. Of the 9 initial failures, 8 were caused by perforation, 1 by early occlusion, and all required arterial reconstruction. Long-term follow-up was not available, but in a subsequent multi-center trial organized by Snyder[73] the *overall* 1-year success rate was just under 40 per cent. Desbrosses and associates[74] reported an encouraging experience with 46 long (up to 24 cm) total SFA occlusions with an 87 per cent initial success rate (also using concomitant PTBA). There were 5 early occlusions and 3 perforations, but 14 of 20 arteries beyond that point (70 per cent) were still patent at 1 year (less than one third of the total). Currently, this device is not being used much for its original intended purpose but is being considered as a means of removing thrombus material in patients with early and subacute arterial thromboses.

The *Auth Rotablator* atherectomy device comes with variably sized, olive-shaped tips (1.25 to 5.0 mm in diameter), on the surface of which are embedded multiple diamond chips ranging from 22 to 45 μ in size. Introduced over a central guidewire, the tip is rotated at 100,000 to 200,000 rpm as it traverses the lesion. It preferentially pulverizes calcified plaque while deflecting the softer and more elastic underlying arterial wall. Surprisingly, it appears to treat tibial occlusive lesions much better (2 times) than popliteal or SFA lesions. Its use has been marked by transient hemoglobinuria, perforations, equipment breakage, and thrombosis. Early (6-month) follow-up of the Stanford experience[75] comprising 42 procedures showed a 24 per cent incidence of *major* complications (with a 5 per cent amputation rate), 24 per cent hemodynamic failures, and 5 per cent technical failures. Eighteen procedures (47 per cent) were deemed initial successes, but only 11 of 18 (29 per cent) were patent at 6 months, and 3 of 7 patients were worse than before the procedure. In the most recent UCLA experience reported by Ahn and coworkers,[76] which primarily covered intraoperative use of the Auth device (60 per cent use as an adjunctive measure), the results showed 93 per cent initial technical success, 72 per cent in-hospital success, and 32 per cent improved at last follow-up (20 per cent at 2 years). Initial complications included hemoglobinuria (16 per cent), embolism (16 per cent), thormbosis (20 per cent), and amputation (6 per cent).

The *Simpson Atherocath* has a circular cutter spinning at 2000 rpm inside a metal capsule with a longitudinal slit or window on one side that can be pressed against the plaque by inflating a balloon located on its opposite side, thereby slicing off strips of plaque and depositing them inside the chamber of the capsule. Because of the size of the device and the need to evacuate it periodically, the process is so time-consuming and labor-intensive that it can only be used in practice for short (and ideally eccentric) occlusive lesions. Nevertheless, complication rates are lower and patency rates higher than those reported with other devices (possibly because its use is limited to more discrete favorable lesions).

In Simpson and associates' initial experience,[77] there was an 87 per cent initial success rate, but only 69 per cent of these patients had continued relief of claudication by 6 months. Those with follow-up angiograms showed a 36 per cent restenosis rate. Polnitz and colleagues[78] reported an 82 per cent initial success rate and a 72 per cent 1-year patency rate (about 60 per cent overall patency). Graor and Whitlow[79] reported 93 per cent and 76 per cent 1-year (overall) patency rates in under 5-cm and over 5-cm lesions, respectively, with a 7 per cent major complication rate and one fatal myocardial infarction. However, Dorros and coworkers[50] reported an angiographic and clinical follow-up of 126 patients in whom restenosis or occlusion occurred in more than 50 per cent of those followed for more than 5 months.[50]

The *Transluminal Extraction Catheter* (TEC) system utilizes hollow 5-Fr to 9-Fr catheters introduced through a sheath and over a guidewire. The conical tip contains cutting blades that rotate at 700 rpm. Suction carries the plaque cuttings through the housing while a heparin solution is introduced as irrigation. Because of its size relative to the arterial lumen, it often requires ''adjunctive'' PTBA. In a multi-center trial, Wholey and Jarmolowski reported a 92 per cent success rate in treating 126 lesions in 95 patients.[80] Almost half (47 per cent) required PTBA. Only 16 patients had follow-up angiography at 6 months with a 25 per cent rate of reocclusion. Problems with excessive blood loss (suction) or embolization (when the suction bottles became filled) are unique to this device, whereas other complications such as perforation have been less. It may be the best of the four atherectomy devices for *long* SFA occlusions.

In summary, at this point in time, the laser and various atherectomy devices have not succeeded in extending the application of PTA to longer or more complex lesions than can be managed by PTBA alone because of unacceptable restenosis rates or greater morbidity. Whether other, newer devices can succeed where these have failed remains doubtful in view of the almost universal myointimal proliferative response to endovascular trauma. Only a means of preventing or minimizing neointimal hyperplasia can be expected to change this picture.

Vascular Stents. Although intraluminal vascular stents were developed and tested more than 5 years ago and there are at least five stents being actively used and evaluated for various applications around the world, clinical data on these experiences are still very preliminary. The Palmaz stent is the only one currently approved for clinical use in the United States (as an adjunct to iliac PTBA); the Strecker, Sigwort, and Wallstents are used primarily in Europe, although the latter has had special-purpose applications in the United States and is under trial here.

Stents vary in size, length, material (rigidity), and method of expansion. For example, the Palmaz-Schatz stent is rigid and balloon-expandable, the Strecker stent is flexible and balloon-expandable, and the Wallstent is flexible and self-expandable. Because of the availability of clinical data, only placement of the Palmaz stent in the iliac arteries will be discussed at length here. More distal stent placement in peripheral arteries has been plagued by high thrombosis and restenosis rates.

Palmaz and coworkers coordinated a multi-center trial with the Palmaz stent several years ago.[81] There was an initial 97 per cent successful iliac stent placement in 165 limbs in 146 patients, with "excellent" patency for up to 6 months. This ongoing prospective clinical trial, updated at 171 patients,[82] at last report had over 200 patients enrolled. In the initial report there was no significant difference between stented and nonstented PTBA results, but now, 24-month data show a more than 10 per cent advantage for primary stenting, which is said to be statistically significant. Recently, Richter[83] reported on the progress of the German multi-center trial with this stent (185 prospectively randomized patients). Stenting produced a significantly better hemodynamic result as judged by pressure gradients. Luminal narrowing stabilized between 12 and 24 months at 14 to 15 per cent in the stented group, whereas those with PTBA alone continued to show narrowing (average, 27 per cent at 24 months). Twenty-eight per cent of those with iliac PTBA alone required further intervention by 36 months compared with only 2 per cent of the stented group. Dalsing and colleagues reported a longer term follow-up of the original Indiana University experience.[84] The 2-year life table patency was 87.4 per cent, which is quite good considering that it was applied to more difficult iliac lesions. There was a 6 per cent mortality and a 19 per cent complication rate (11 per cent requiring surgery).

At this point the use of iliac stents with PTBA is clearly justified, when there has been an acute dissection or when there is immediate elastic recoil, to reduce the technical and hemodynamic failure rates, respectively. Although there is still no proof, the use of stents in redilatations to prevent restenosis has also been generally accepted again. Justification for using stents *primarily* to reduce stenosis following PTBA will depend on the results of the trials mentioned previously and on their cost-effectiveness. The use of stents to extend the application of PTBA to lesions currently considered unfavorable for PTBA alone (e.g., long or multiple stenoses or complete occlusions [with or without thrombolytic therapy]), is a matter that will be settled in future trials. In this regard, it must be remembered that stents (and urokinase) are very expensive ($800 to $1000 per stent with multiple [2 to 4] stents commonly being used). Unless significant short- and long-term advantages over simple unilateral bypass (femorofemoral or iliofemoral) can be shown, iliac stenting for these more complex lesions will likely be justified only for patients who are *prohibitive* surgical risks.

SUMMARY

Although PTBA has established its place in the management of patients with lower extremity ischemia and clearly plays useful primary and adjunctive roles in specific settings, percutaneous attempts to extend the role of PTA by laser and atherectomy devices, thrombolytic therapy, and stents, to longer and more extensive lesions have been generally disappointing. The use of open techniques that allow intraluminal ultrasound and angioscopy and the larger atherectomy devices employed *may* produce a more complete debulking and lower restenosis rate, but this is of doubtful value because it also requires general or regional anesthesia, dissection and control of vessels, and frequent need for patch angioplasty. Thus, these improvements would have no practical advantage over arterial reconstruction, although the same techniques could be justified as adjunctive measures to arterial reconstruction, assuming that anesthesia and a surgical procedure were already indicated.

References

1. Auster M, Kadir S, Mitchell SE, et al: Iliac artery occlusion: Management with intrathrombus streptokinase infusion and angioplasty. Radiology 153:385, 1984.
2. Berkowitz HO, Spence RK, Freiman DB, et al: Long-term results of transluminal angioplasty of the femoral arteries. *In* Dotter CT, Gruntzig AR, Schoop W, et al (eds): Percutaneous Transluminal Angioplasty. Technique, Early and Late Results. Berlin, Springer-Verlag, 1983, pp 207–214.
3. Boyd AM: The natural course of arteriosclerosis of the lower extremities. Angiology 11:10, 1960.
4. Colapinto RF, Stronell RD, Johnston KW: Transluminal angioplasty of complete iliac obstructions. AJR 146:859, 1986.
5. DeWeese JA, Rob CG: Autogenous venous grafts ten years later. Surgery 82:775, 1977.
6. Doubilet P, Abrams HL: The cost of underutilization. Percutaneous transluminal angioplasty for peripheral vascular disease. N Engl J Med 310:95, 1984.
7. Freiman DB, Freiman MP, Spence RK, et al: Economic impact of transluminal angioplasty. Angiology 36:772, 1985.
8. Gallino A, Mahler F, Probst P, et al: Percutaneous transluminal angioplasty of the arteries of the lower limbs: A 5 year follow-up. Circulation 70:619, 1984.
9. Gardiner GA Jr, Meyerovitz MF, Stokes KR, et al: Complications of transluminal angioplasty. Radiology 159:201, 1986.
10. Graor RA, Young JR, McCandless M, et al: Percutaneous transluminal angioplasty: Review of iliac and femoral dilatations at Cleveland Clinic. Cleve Clin Q 51:149, 1984.
11. Grüntzig A: Die perkutane transluminale Rekanalisation chronischer Arterienverschlüsse mit einer neuen Dilatations-technik. Baden-Baden, Verlag Gerhard Witzstock, 1977, p 43.
12. Griffin DJ, Kumpe DA, Seibert CE, et al: Iliac recanalization: A new approach. Presented at the 72nd Annual Meeting, Radiological Society of North America, Chicago, December 1, 1986.
13. Hewes RC, White RI, Murray RR, et al: Long-term results of superficial femoral artery angioplasty. AJR 146:1025, 1986.
14. Jeans WD, Danton RM, Baird RN, et al: A comparison of the costs of vascular surgery and balloon dilatation in lower limb ischaemic disease. Br J Radiol 59:453, 1986.
15. Johnston KW, Kalman PG: Percutaneous transluminal angioplasty. *In* Kempczinski RF: The Ischemic Leg. Chicago, Year Book Medical Publishers, 1985, pp 269–278.
16. Johnston KW, Rae M, Hogg-Johnston SA, et al: Five year results of a prospective study of percutaneous transluminal angioplasty. Ann Surg 206:403, 1987.
17. Jones BA, Maggisano R, Robb C et al: Transluminal angioplasty results in high risk patients with advanced peripheral vascular disease. Can J Surg 28:150, 1985.
18. Kalman PG, Johnston KW: Outcome of a failed percutaneous transluminal dilation. Surg Gynecol Obstet 161:43, 1985.
19. Kinnison ML, White RI, Bowers WP, et al: Cost incentives for peripheral angioplasty. AJR 145:1241, 1985.
20. Krepel VM, van Andel GJ, van Erp WFM, et al: Percutaneous transluminal angioplasty of the femoropopliteal artery: Initial and long-term results. Radiology 156:325, 1985.
21. Kumpe DA, Jones DN: Percutaneous transluminal angioplasty: Radiological viewpoint. Vasc Diagn Ther 3:19, 1982.
22. Lally ME, Johnston KW: Percutaneous transluminal dilatation of peripheral arteries: An analysis of factors predicting early success. J Vasc Surg 1:704, 1984.

23. Lu CT, Zarins CF, Yang CF, et al: Percutaneous transluminal angioplasty for limb salvage. Radiology 142:337, 1982.
24. Martin EC, Frankuchen EI, Karlson KB, et al: Angioplasty for femoral artery occlusion: Comparison with surgery. AJR 137:915, 1981.
25. Morin JF, Johnston KW, Wasserman L, et al: Factors that determine the long-term results of percutaneous transluminal dilatation for peripheral arterial occlusive disease. J Vasc Surg 4:68, 1986.
26. Murray RR, Hewes RC, White RI, et al: Long-segment femoropopliteal stenoses: Is angioplasty a boon or a bust? Radiology 162:473, 1987.
27. Neiman HL, Bergan JJ, Yao JST, et al: Hemodynamic assessment of transluminal angioplasty for lower extremity ischemia. Radiology 143:639, 1982.
28. Ring EJ, Freiman DB, McLean GK, et al: Percutaneous recanalization of common iliac artery occlusions: An unacceptable complication rate? AJR 139:587, 1982.
29. Rutherford RB, Patt A, Kumpe DA: The current role of percutaneous transluminal angioplasty. *In* Greenlagh KM (ed): Vascular Surgery: Issues in Current Practice. New York, Grune & Stratton, 1986, pp 229–244.
30. Rush DS, Grewertz BL, Lu CT, et al: Limb salvage in poor-risk patients using transluminal angioplasty. Arch Surg 118:1209, 1983.
31. Schmidtke I, Roth F-J: Relapse treatment by percutaneous transluminal dilatation. *In* Dotter CT, Grüntzig AR, Schoop W, et al (eds): Percutaneous Transluminal Angioplasty. Technique, Early and Late Results. Berlin, Springer-Verlag, 1983, pp 131–139.
32. Schneider E, Grüntzig A, Bollinger A: Long-term patency rates after percutaneous transluminal angioplasty for iliac and femoropopliteal obstructions. *In* Dotter CT, Grüntzig AR, Schoop W, et al (eds): Percutaneous Transluminal Angioplasty. Technique, Early and Late Results. Berlin, Springer-Verlag, 1983, pp 175–180.
33. Schneider E, Grüntzig A, Bollinger A: Langzeitergebnisse nach perkutaner transluminale Angioplastie (PTA) bei 882 consekutiven Patienten mit iliaken und femoro-poplitealen Obstrucktionen. Vasa 11:322, 1982.
34. Spence RK, Freeman DB, Gatenby R, et al: Long term results of transluminal angioplasty of the iliac and femoral arteries. Arch Surg 116:1377, 1981.
35. van Andel GJ, van Erp WFM, Krepel VM, et al: Percutaneous transluminal dilatation of the iliac artery: Long-term results. Radiology 156:321, 1985.
36. van Breda A, Katzen BT, Picus D, et al: Intraarterial urokinase infusion for treatment of acute and chronic arterial occlusions. Presented at the 72nd Annual Meeting, Radiological Society of North America, Chicago, December 1, 1986.
37. Ginsburg R, Wexler L, Mitchell RS, et al: Percutaneous transluminal laser angioplasty for treatment of peripheral vascular disease. Radiology 156:619, 1985.
38. Martin EC: Introduction. Circulation 83(2)(Suppl I):1, 1991.
39. Rutherford RB, Durham J: Percutaneous balloon angioplasty for arteriosclerosis obliterans: Long-term results. *In* Yao JST, Pearce WH (eds): Technologies in Vascular Surgery. Philadelphia, WB Saunders, 1992, pp 329–345.
40. Stokes KR, Strunk HM, Campbell DR, et al: Five-year results of iliac and femoropopliteal angioplasty in diabetic patients. Radiology 174:977, 1990.
41. Jeans WD, Armstrong S, Cole SE, et al: Fate of patients undergoing transluminal angioplasty for lower limb ischemia. Radiology 177(2):559, 1990.
42. Brewster DC, Cambria RP, Darling RC, et al: Long-term results of combined iliac balloon angioplasty and distal surgical revascularization. Ann Surg 210:324, 1989.
43. Berkowitz HD, Spence RK, Frieman DB, et al: Long-term results of transluminal angioplasty of the femoral arteries. *In* Dotter CT, Grüntzig A, Schoop W, Zietler E (eds): Percutaneous Transluminal Angioplasty. Berlin, Springer-Verlag, 1983, pp 207–214.
44. Berkowitz HD: Percutaneous arterial dilation for atherosclerotic lower extremity occlusive disease. *In* Ernst CB, Stanley JC (eds): Current Therapy in Vascular Surgery. 2nd ed. Philadelphia, BC Decker, 1991, pp 473–475.
45. Rutherford RB, Flanigan DP, Gupta SK, et al: Suggested standards for reports dealing with lower extremity ischemia. J Vasc Surg 4:80, 1986.
46. Rutherford RB, Becker GJ: Standards for evaluating and reporting the results of surgical and percutaneous therapy for peripheral arterial disease. J Vasc Interv Radiol 2:169, 1991.
47. Wilson SE, Wolf GL, Cross AP: Percutaneous transluminal angioplasty versus operation for peripheral arteriosclerosis. Report of a prospective randomized trial in a selected group of patients. J Vasc Surg 9:1, 1989.
48. In der Maur GTD, Boeve J, Kerdel MC, et al: Angioplasty of the iliac and femoral arteries. Initial and long-term results in short stenotic lesions. Eur J Radiol 11:163, 1990.
49. Benenati JF, Becker GJ, Katzen BT, Zemel G: Chronic iliac artery occlusions: Treatment with percutaneous endoluminal stents. Presented at the Radiological Society of North America meeting in Chicago, 1991.
50. Dorros G, Iyer S, Lewin R, et al: Angiographic follow-up and clinical outcome of 126 patients after percutaneous directional atherectomy (Simpson AtheroCath) for occlusive peripheral vascular disease. Cathet Cardiovasc Diagn 22:79, 1991.
51. Adar R, Critchfield GC, Eddy DM: A confidence profile analysis of the results of femoropopliteal percutaneous transluminal angioplasty in the treatment of lower extremity ischemia. J Vasc Surg 10:57, 1989.
52. Horvath W, Oertl M, Haidinger D: Percutaneous transluminal angioplasty of crural arteries. Radiology 177(2):565, 1990.
53. Schwarten DE: Clinical and anatomical considerations for nonoperative therapy in tibial disease and the results of angioplasty. Circulation 83 (Suppl I):86, 1991.
54. Brown KT, Schoenbert NY, Moore ED, et al: Percutaneous transluminal angioplasty of infrapopliteal vessels: Preliminary results and technical considerations. Radiology 169:75, 1988.
55. Greenfield AJ: Femoral, popliteal, and tibial arteries: Percutaneous transluminal angioplasty. AJR 135:927, 1980.
56. Sprayregen S, Sniderman KW, Sos TA, et al: Popliteal artery branches: Percutaneous transluminal angioplasty. AJR 135:945, 1980.
57. Tamura S, Sniderman KW, Beinart C, et al: Percutaneous transluminal angioplasty of the popliteal artery and its branches. Radiology 143:645, 1982.
58. Dake MD, Katzen BT: The current state of percutaneous transluminal angioplasty in peripheral vascular disease. *In* Veith FJ (ed): Current Critical Problems in Vascular Surgery. St. Louis, Quality Medical Publishing, 1990, vol. 2, pp 145–154.
59. Creasy TS, McMillan PJ, Fletcher EWL, et al: Is percutaneous transluminal angioplasty better than exercise for claudication? Preliminary results from a prospective randomized trial. Eur J Vasc Surg 4:135, 1990.
60. Sanborn TA, Cumberland DC, Greenfield AJ, et al: Percutaneous laser thermal angioplasty: Initial results and 1-year follow-up in 129 femoropopliteal lesions. Radiology 168:121, 1988.
61. Sanborn TA, Cumberland DC, Greenfield AJ, et al: Peripheral laser-assisted balloon angioplasty: Initial multicenter experience in 219 peripheral arteries. Arch Surg 124:1099, 1989.
62. Blebea J, Ouriel K, Green RM, et al: Laser angioplasty in peripheral vascular disease: Symptomatic versus hemodynamic results. J Vasc Surg 13:222, 1991.
63. Harrington ME, Schwartz ME, Sanborn TA, et al: Expanded indications for laser-assisted balloon angioplasty in peripheral arterial disease. J Vasc Surg 11:146, 1990.
64. Perler BA, Osterman FA, White RI, et al: Percutaneous laser probe femoropopliteal angioplasty: A preliminary experience. J Vasc Surg 10:351, 1989.
65. Wright JG, Belkin M, Greenfield AJ, et al: Laser angioplasty for limb salvage: Observations on early results. J Vasc Surg 10:29, 1989.
66. AbuRahma AF, Robinson PA, Kennard W, Boland JP: Intra-operative peripheral Nd:YAG laser-assisted thermal balloon angioplasty: Short-term and intermediate-term follow-up. J Vasc Surg 12:566, 1990.
67. Rosenthal D, Wheeler WG, Seagraves A, et al: Nd:YAG iliac and femoropopliteal laser angioplasty: Results with large probes as "sole therapy." J Cardiovasc Surg 32:186, 1991.
68. Grundfest WS, Litvak IF, Goldenberg T, et al: Pulsed ultraviolet lasers and the potential for safe laser angioplasty. Am J Surg 150:220, 1985.
69. McCarthy WJ, Vogelzang RL, Pearce WH, et al: Excimer laser treatment of femoral artery atherosclerosis. *In* Yao JST, Pearce WH (eds): Technologies in Vascular Surgery. Philadelphia, WB Saunders, 1992, pp 346–356.
70. Geschwind HJ, Dubois-Rande J, Shafton E, et al: Percutaneous pulsed laser-assisted balloon angioplasty guided by spectroscopy. Am Heart J 117:1147, 1989.
71. Leon MB, Almagor Y, Bartorelli AL, et al: Fluorescence-guided laser-

assisted balloon angioplasty in patients with femoropopliteal occlusions. Circulation 81:143, 1990.
72. Snyder SO, Wheeler JR, Gregory RT, et al: Kensey catheter: Early results with a transluminal endarterectomy tool. J Vasc Surg 8:541, 1988.
73. Snyder SO: Results of a multi-center study of TracWright Systems. Unpublished data.
74. Desbrosses D, Petit H, Torres E, et al: Percutaneous atherectomy with the Kensey catheter: Early and midterm results in femoropopliteal occlusions unsuitable for conventional angioplasty. Ann Vasc Surg 4(6):550, 1990.
75. Jennings LJ, Mehigan JT, Ginsberg R, et al: Rotablator atherectomy: Early experience and six-month follow-up. Presented at the Western Vascular Society, Rancho Mirage, CA, January 1991.
76. Ahn SS, Yeatman LR, Deutsch LS, et al: Intraoperative peripheral atherectomy: Preliminary clinical results. Presented at the Western Vascular Society, Rancho Mirage, CA, January 1991.
77. Simpson JB, Selman MR, Roberson GC, et al: Transluminal atherectomy for occlusive peripheral vascular disease. J Am Coll Cardiol 61:96, 1988.
78. Polnitz A, Nerlich A, Berger H, et al: Percutaneous peripheral atherectomy. J Am Coll Cardiol 15:682, 1990.
79. Graor R, Whitlow P: Transluminal atherectomy for occlusive peripheral vascular disease. J Am Coll Cardiol 15(7):1551, 1990.
80. Wholey MH, Jarmolowski CR: New reperfusion devices: The Kensey catheter, the atherolytic reperfusion wire device, and the transluminal extraction catheter. Radiology 172:947, 1989.
81. Palmaz JC, Richter GM, Noeldge G, et al: Intraluminal stents in atherosclerotic iliac artery stenosis: Preliminary report of a multicenter study. Radiology 168:727, 1988.
82. Palmaz JC, Garcia OJ, Schatz RA, et al: Placement of balloon-expandable intraluminal stents in iliac arteries: First 171 procedures. Radiology 174:969, 1990.
83. Richter G: Balloon-expandable Palmaz Stent placement versus PTA in iliac artery stenoses and occlusions: Long term results of a randomized trial. Presented at the Society of Cardiovascular and Interventional Radiologists' annual meeting in Washington, DC, 1992.
84. Dalsing MC, Ehrman KO, Cikrit DF, et al: Iliac artery angioplasty and stents: A current experience. *In* Yao JST, Pearce WH (eds): Technology in Vascular Surgery. Philadelphia, WB Saunders, 1992, pp 373–386.
85. Rutherford RB: Political issues in endovascular surgery. Surg Clin North Am 72(4):757, 1992.
86. Rutherford RB: Endovascular surgery: A critical overview and standards to live up to. *In* Ahn SS, Moore WS (eds): Endovascular Surgery. 2nd ed. Philadelphia, WB Saunders, 1992, pp 5–11.
87. Waltman AC, Greenfield AJ, Novelline RA, et al: Transluminal angioplasty of the iliac and femoropopliteal arteries. Arch Surg 117:1218, 1982.
88. Schneider E, Grüntzig A, Bollinger A: Long-term patency rates after percutaneous transluminal angioplasty for iliac and femoropopliteal obstructions. *In* Dotter CT, Grüntzig A, Schoop W, Zeitler E (eds): Percutaneous Transluminal Angioplasty. Berlin, Springer-Verlag, 1983, pp 175–180.

59

Lumbar Sympathectomy: Indications and Technique

Robert B. Rutherford, M.D., and Francis L. Shannon, M.D.

• • •

HISTORICAL BACKGROUND

The concept of sympathetic denervation as a mode of therapy for arterial occlusive disease was first elaborated and tested by Leriche and Jaboulay in 1913.[18] Their experience with periarterial sympathectomy was disappointing because reinnervation and vasospasm recurred within weeks of operation. Adopting the lumbar sympathetic ganglionectomy technique of Royle and Hunter, Adson and Brown in the United States and Diez in South America secured more lasting relief among patients with symptomatic vasospasm in the 1920s.[1, 16] These reports marked the beginning of an era in which sympathetic denervation was widely used for occlusive arterial disease, often as the only surgical alternative to amputation. During the next 30 years, variable results were reported, but the use of the procedure was not seriously questioned because alternative methods of improving limb perfusion were unavailable. With the development of arterial reconstructive techniques, direct vascularization had supplanted sympathectomy as optimal surgical therapy by the 1960s. This transition was aided by experimental studies of the effects of sympathetic denervation that confirmed the growing clinical impression that significant hemodynamic improvement could *not* be achieved with this approach alone. With further improvement in reconstructive techniques, vascular indications for lumbar sympathectomy have become very limited. During this transition, many surgeons persisted in using sympathectomy, admitting its lesser degree of benefit but preferring its lower risk. Currently, noninvasive vascular testing, performed before and after sympathetic blockade, is being increasingly utilized preoperatively to provide objective evidence for a potential benefit of sympathectomy rather than being applied empirically in the hope that it might help. In this chapter, the physiologic consequences and the results of lumbar sympathectomy in different clinical settings are presented as the basis for our recommended indications and techniques.

PHYSIOLOGIC CONSEQUENCES

Critical understanding of the effects of lumbar sympathectomy requires synthesis of both clinical and experimental data. Although sympathetic denervation clearly increases blood flow to a normal limb, its impact on an extremity afflicted with arterial occlusive disease is less clear. Elucidation of its role in improving microcirculatory hemodynamics and relieving ischemic symptoms can be considered in regard to several aspects: (1) the magnitude, distribution, and duration of the blood flow increase; (2) its effect on collateral perfusion in acute and chronic ischemia; (3) the nutritive value of the observed flow increases; and (4) the alteration of pain impulse transmission. The effect of sympathectomy on each of these factors will be examined within the context of more recent studies that attempt to define better the potential benefit of sympathectomy in limb ischemia.

Increase in Blood Flow. Lumbar sympathectomy increases total blood flow to an extremity by abolishing both basal and reflex constriction of arterioles and precapillary sphincters. Flow increases ranging from 10 to 200 per cent have been observed and vary with the degree of arterial occlusive disease involving the limb.[2, 10, 36, 61] Indeed, patients with severe, multi-level occlusions may receive no benefit from sympathectomy because their muscular and cutaneous arteries are already maximally dilated at rest. In both normal and diseased limbs, the majority of the observed flow increase is shunted through cutaneous arteriovenous anastomoses (AVA) without significantly increased tissue perfusion.[12] This alteration in blood flow distribution is due to elimination of the primary sympathetic function of modulating the musculocutaneous distribution in response to thermal regulatory requirements. Following sympathectomy, the positive distributional effects are maximal for the distal cutaneous circulation and characteristically produce the warm, pink foot or hand that was long felt to reflect the net improvement in limb perfusion.

This phenomenon of extremity blood flow redistribution is important because improved muscular perfusion was once presumed to parallel increased cutaneous blood flow and justify the application of sympathectomy for claudication. Radioactively labeled microsphere studies by Rutherford and Valenta in a canine arterial occlusion model showed that both resting and exertional muscle perfusion is *not* improved by sympathectomy.[50] Using a similar technique in a canine hindlimb study, Cronenwett and Lindenauer[11] corroborated this finding in subjects with both patent and acutely obstructed femoral arteries. This phenomenon is explained by the relative sensitivities of precapillary sphincters in muscle and skin to adrenergic tone; cutaneous sphincters have low resting myogenic tone and are exclusively controlled by sympathetic impulses. Precapillary sphincters in muscle, however, have high resting myogenic tone and respond almost exclusively to local, primarily metabolic, humoral factors.[61] In patients in whom proximal occlusive disease places relatively fixed limitations on arterial inflow, sympathectomy can actually adversely affect the natural redistribution of blood flow to exercising muscle by lowering cutaneous vascular resistance.[50, 56]

Regardless of the patency of the arterial tree, maximum vasodilation is noted immediately following sympathectomy and begins to taper off within 5 to 7 days of denervation. This ''fifth day phenomenon'' is more noticeable following dorsal sympathectomy, but it occurs in the lower extremities as well. Although at a much lesser level than initially observed, peripheral cutaneous vasodilation and blood flow remain elevated over basal levels for months, persisting in the face of stimuli that provoke vasoconstriction through centrally mediated reflexes (e.g., vasoconstrictor cold response test).[64] Resting vasomotor tone usually returns to normal levels from 2 weeks to 6 months after sympathectomy. Previous explanations for this return of sympathetic vasomotor tone have included anatomically incomplete denervation, crossover reinnervation, and vascular hyperreactivity to circulating catecholamines. Isolated rabbit ear sympathectomy studies have shown that arteriolar smooth muscle cells are 1.5 times more sensitive to exogenous norepinephrine but are unable to constrict maximally owing to viscoelastic changes in the vessel wall.[3] In addition, study of canine adrenergic receptors demonstrates no change in the concentration of extrasynaptic, alpha$_2$-receptors that initiate vasoconstriction in response to blood-borne catecholamines.[6] Although attenuated, the capacity for vasoconstriction and its mediators is *not* obliterated by sympathectomy. The degree of recovery of vasomotor tone following sympathectomy depends on circulating norepinephrine levels and the degree of vascular adaptation to loss of physiologic constriction.

Effect on Collateral Perfusion. The effect of lumbar sympathectomy on resting collateral blood flow in response to both acute and chronic arterial occlusion has been studied in human as well as canine models. Using a canine model of acute popliteal arterial occlusion, Dalessandri and associates[14] have shown that lumbar sympathectomy produces a temporary but significant increase in paw blood flow as measured by plethysmographic tracings. This effect was noted after sufficient time had elapsed to allow maximal vasodilation of collaterals around the knee. Among patients with chronic foot ischemia as a result of multi-level arterial occlusions, Ludbrook observed submaximal collateral blood flow at rest in 30 per cent. Sympathectomy produced an average 11 per cent increase in distal perfusion among these patients with inappropriate resting vasoconstriction.[35] Van der Stricht reported a similar phenomenon and postulates that sympathectomy increases collateral flow by increasing the pressure gradient across fixed obstructions at the femoral and popliteal levels.[61] Although this improvement is relatively small and transient, sympathectomy does seem to increase distal perfusion around proximal obstructions in patients with inappropriate resting vasoconstriction. However, in the *majority* of patients with ischemia at rest, locally released humoral factors maximize flow through existing and newly formed collateral channels.

Nutritive Value of Blood Flow Increase. Central to the debate concerning the utility of sympathectomy is determination of the nutritive value of whatever blood flow increase is observed following denervation. Presuming that cutaneous AVA flow is non-nutritive because capillary perfusion is bypassed, Cronenwett and colleagues[12] maintain that sympathectomy does not increase blood flow to ischemic skin and therefore should have no effect on rest pain or ischemic ulcers. This contention is supported by Welch and Leiberman's studies of cutaneous capillary perfusion using iodine-125–iodoantipyrine clearance in patients with peripheral vascular disease following lumbar sympathectomy or arterial reconstruction; no improved clearance was found in denervated limbs in contrast to accelerated clearance seen following arterial reconstruction.[66]

Perry and Horton, likewise, found no difference in spectrophotometric measurements of transcutaneous oxygen tensions in patients before and after lumbar sympathectomy.[41] Using intradermal xenon-133 clearance, however, Moore and Hall showed improved skin capillary perfusion and observed ischemic ulcer healing after lumbar sympathectomy in patients with severe vascular disease.[38] Uncontrolled clinical series further corroborate Moore and Hall's study in noting ischemic ulcer healing in 40 to 67 per cent of patients following sympathectomy.[5, 9, 29, 42] In the face of these conflicting data, it seems fair to concede that in some patients sympathectomy may produce a small but sufficient increase in nutritive perfusion to facilitate healing of small ulcers or relieve ischemic rest pain.

Alteration of Pain Impulse Transmission. An alternative mechanism for relief of ischemic rest pain is both central and peripheral attenuation of painful stimulus transmission by sensory nerves. Although objective assessment of pain threshold changes is difficult, aversive stimuli studies in cats have shown that lumbar sympathectomy enhances tolerance of hindlimb noxious stimuli.[43] Theories concerning a relationship between sympathetic innervation and pain threshold suggest that sympathectomy decreases noxious stimulus perception by both decreasing tissue norepinephrine levels and reducing spinal augmentation of painful stimulus transmission to cerebral centers.[34] This may also explain clinical series reporting a significant portion of patients afflicted with either disabling claudication or rest pain who were subjectively relieved without hemodynamic evidence of improved perfusion.[13] Among the subset with rest pain, Owens suggests that clear differentiation of neuropathic from ischemic pain in patients with absent ankle pulses is not made.[39] Including patients with causalgic-type pain in the clinical group with ischemic rest pain would spuriously increase the sympathectomy response rate. Despite this possible flaw in inclusion criteria, both clinical and experimental evidence suggests that lumbar sympathectomy can be efficacious in attenuating pain perception in patients with ischemic rest pain.

Summary of Physiologic Effect. In summary, sympathectomy increases peripheral blood flow by the vasodilation of arterioles primarily in cutaneous vascular beds. Much of this increased flow passes through naturally occurring AVAs. Thus, although overall extremity blood flow may be increased, for all intents and purposes, significant increases in nutritive flow occur only in distal cutaneous beds. Limitations in arterial inflow imposed by proximal occlusive lesions may mitigate this increase, and the return of vasomotor tone toward normal with time may further diminish it. Nevertheless, some patients *may* receive sufficient increases to help heal superficial ischemic ulcers and relieve ischemic rest pain. In addition, although increases in blood perfusion are relatively small in the long run in patients with organic occlusive disease, protection against an exaggerated vasoconstrictor response to cold, amelioration of sympathetic pain, and suppression of sweating are long lasting. These observations determine the appropriate indications for sympathectomy.

INDICATIONS AND RESULTS

It can be said that indications determine results and results determine indications. Nowhere is this more true than in an operation like sympathectomy, which has been performed for a variety of diverse indications with such markedly differing success rates that quoting overall results has little meaning. It is its results in the individual situations in which it has been tried that have gradually defined its indications. With the passage of time, its application for some indications has gradually become more limited and selective with the increasing use of trial blocks, noninvasive testing, and improvement in competitive forms of therapy. For example, better pharmacologic management of the initial stage causalgia and pure vasospastic disorders has significantly reduced the number of patients now being referred for sympathectomy.[22, 45] Furthermore, increasing success with infrapopliteal bypass has further reduced the number of patients in which sympathectomy is considered because direct revascularization is not feasible. Even in these cases, selection criteria have been tightened by noninvasive testing before and after trial blocks. Attempts at sympathetic denervation for previously inoperable occlusive disease by injections of phenol or alcohol have become increasingly popular, especially in Europe.[47] More recently, radiofrequency ablation has been tried with some success.[70] However, at the present time, the incidence of incomplete or transient sympathetic denervation is still significant using these methods. Furthermore, the injection of phenol and alcohol can result in painful complications, and all such attempts, even multiple blocks using local anesthetic agents, ultimately can create enough inflammation and scarring to make subsequent surgical sympathectomy difficult, if not dangerous. Although further progress may change this perspective, it must be kept in mind that surgical sympathectomy today can be carried out with minimal risk. This current perspective makes it appropriate to recommend the performance of *no* percutaneous technique that cannot achieve a complete and durable sympathectomy in almost all patients who might otherwise be considered potential candidates for surgical sympathectomy.

Intermittent Claudication

As previously discussed, there is no objective evidence that sympathectomy improves muscular blood flow in patients with ischemic muscle pain induced by exercise.[57] Muscular perfusion is primarily increased by vasodilation mediated by the acidic products of anaerobic metabolism. Despite this dictum, clinical reviews from Europe continue to report improvement in walking time among claudicants who show neither hemodynamic improvement following sympathectomy nor enhanced muscular perfusion.[44] These results from nonrandomized studies may simply reflect the natural history of claudication or the known pain-modulating effects of sympathectomy. However, there is *no* physiologic or clinical rationale for performing lumbar sympathectomy for claudication.

Causalgia

The central role of the sympathetic nervous system in perpetuating causalgic pain makes sympathetic denervation particularly suitable for this entity. Uniform success is obtained when the diagnosis and therapeutic potential of sympathectomy are confirmed by trial block. In the authors' more recent experience, early postoperative pain relief was obtained in 96 per cent of patients by trial block with 84 per cent remaining asymptomatic after a median follow-up interval of 28 months.[37] Similar results have been obtained by other investigators and are superior to those of repeated transcutaneous sympathetic blocks alone.[28] In an unpublished report by AbuRahma and colleagues,[71] initial and late satisfactory results of 100 and 95 per cent, respectively, were achieved in patients who showed an excellent response to a trial sympathetic block. This indication is discussed in detail in Chapter 49.

Peripheral Vasospasm

Most patients with Raynaud's phenomenon secondary to vasospasm complain more of upper extremity than of lower extremity discomfort; therefore, this indication is discussed in greater detail in Chapters 68 and 72. Occasionally, however, the reverse is true, particularly for patients in colder climates, possibly because it is easier to warm the hands periodically than the feet. Thus, although the procedure is uncommonly needed, lower extremity vasospasm and cold intolerance respond remarkably well to lumbar sympathectomy, apparently more so than with upper extremity involvement. Janoff and colleagues reported their experience with 10 patients suffering from episodic distal vasospasm that was refractory to maximal medical management.[27] Pernio was noted in each patient and did not recur following lumbar sympathectomy. Hypothermic toe plethysmographic testing normalized, and all patients remained asymptomatic after 4 years mean follow-up. Both Felder and Gifford and their associates reported similarly good and lasting symptom relief among a larger group of patients.[20, 23] Despite loss of resting cutaneous vasodilation, reflex digital vasoconstriction in response to regional or remote cold stimuli did not recur in any of the more recently studied patients.

Ischemic Rest Pain

Critical assessment of clinical reports on the efficacy of lumbar sympathectomy for ischemic rest pain is limited by variations in the severity and anatomic distribution of occlusive disease, failure to differentiate this from other forms of lower extremity pain, and differing criteria for determining "inoperability" for distal bypass. With this in mind, the more recent reports cited, it is hoped, better reflect progress in infrapopliteal revascularization, pharmacologic manipulation, and noninvasive testing. Nevertheless, most share the same flaw, that is, they were not prospectively randomized against conservatively treated controls.

Of the two manifestations of critical lower limb ischemia that may be considered categorical indications for lumbar sympathectomy, rest pain has a higher response rate than ischemic ulceration for two reasons: (1) the blood flow increase needed to satisfy oxygen demands at rest is less than the inflammatory response required for tissue healing, and (2) pain impulse attenuation may enhance tolerance of ischemic pain even if perfusion is not very significantly increased. It has been suggested that selection of patients for lumbar sympathectomy for both of these indications be based on three simple assessment criteria, which were derived from retrospective, multi-factorial analysis designed to differentiate responders from nonresponders. These criteria are (1) an ankle-brachial index (ABI) of greater than 0.3, (2) absent neuropathy on physical examination, and (3) limited forefoot tissue loss.[42, 63] To this may be added relief of pain associated with plethysmographic or other objective evidence of improved flow in response to sympathetic blockade.[58]

Critical to the success of lumbar sympathectomy is adequate arterial inflow as indirectly measured by Doppler segmental limb pressures. Designation of a threshold ABI of 0.3 is based on Yao and Bergan's original observation that arterial inflow below this level was insufficient to allow perfusion augmentation or symptom relief with sympathectomy in 90 per cent of patients.[68] Subsequent studies have defined a range of ABIs centered around 0.3 when patients with spuriously high ankle pressures as a result of incompressible vessels are excluded. In the minds of some investigators, this ABI threshold cast doubt on the efficacy of sympathectomy because the natural history of rest pain alone in a patient with an ABI greater than 0.3 might not be significantly different from the response to sympathectomy. This question was addressed and partially answered in a prospective, randomized clinical trial conducted by Cross and Cotton in which transcutaneous phenol lumbar sympatholysis was compared with saline sham lumbar injections.[13] Forty-one limbs in 37 patients were objectively and subjectively analyzed at regular intervals up to 6 months following treatment. Among the control group, only 24 per cent of patients reported symptomatic relief, as shown by a decrease in narcotic requirements, in comparison with 84 per cent in the treatment group. This highly significant subjective difference was *not* associated with objective signs of improved perfusion as measured by segmental limb pressures or blood flow and galvanic skin response monitored on the dorsum of the foot. This study reflects both the natural history of ischemic rest pain in "inoperable" patients (one quarter of whom were spontaneously improved) and the pain impulse modulation effect of sympathetic denervation. Other clinical series report similar symptomatic response rates ranging from 47 to 78 per cent, with early "limb salvage" rates of 60 to 94 per cent.[5, 9, 29] Persson and colleagues[42] report the best results for sympathectomy for this indication. In patients followed up to 82 months following lumbar sympathectomy, 30 of 35 limbs with an ABI greater than 0.3 (86 per cent) experienced early and sustained elimination or improvement of rest pain, compared with 5 patients who received no relief and required early amputation. Again, no significant overall improvement in limb perfusion was noted and, reflective of the severity of their systemic atherosclerosis, nearly 50 per cent of the patients suffered myocardial infarction from 6 months to 4 years after operation. These results support a limited role for sympathectomy as a pain control procedure for patients with ischemic rest pain whose occlusive arterial disease is truly not amenable to direct revascularization or transluminal angioplasty and is refractory to maximal medical management (see Chapter 51).

An unfortunate subgroup of patients are diabetics who have not only end-stage extremity arterial disease but also an "autosympathectomy" that is due to progressive diabetic neuropathy. Rest pain in this group is rarely, if ever, responsive to sympathectomy. Not only can increased distal perfusion not be expected, but also the prospects of enhanced pain tolerance is negligible. Imparato first noted the relationship between diabetic neuropathy and lack of responsiveness to surgical sympathectomy. He demonstrated the histologic equivalence of diabetic autosympathectomy and surgical lumbar sympathetic ganglionectomy by finding no difference in the number of periarterial sympathetic fibers in lower extremity amputation specimens from both groups.[24] Other clinical series have confirmed that the high frequency of a sensory and sympathetic neuropathy in diabetic patients with limb-threatening ischemia is associated with autosympathectomy and an unresponsiveness to lumbar sympathetic ganglionectomy in the majority of patients.[15]

Finally, the results of sympathectomy in patients with Buerger's disease, and patient selection, are discussed in Chapter 11.

Ischemic Ulceration or Tissue Loss

Assessment of the results of lumbar sympathectomy for distal ischemic ulceration or focal gangrene is subject to the same limitations as were described for rest pain. The additional flow above basal requirements, needed to heal wounds and combat infection, creates even greater demands of sympathectomy than combating ischemic rest pain. Radionuclide perfusion studies show that close to a twofold increase in blood flow around the ulcer (hyperemic response) is necessary for healing.[55] Infected or deeper ulcers require even greater increases in regional perfusion. As expected, both clinical and experimental studies indicate that sympathectomy rarely provides sufficiently increased nutritive perfusion to allow healing of deep ulcers or large areas of skin necrosis, even when secondary infection is not prominent.

Clinical reports, noting partial or complete healing in 35 to 62 per cent of patients with forefoot tissue loss, corroborate the intrinsic limitations of sympathectomy.[5, 9, 29] Again, the best results are reported by Persson and coworkers, who performed sympathectomy on 22 limbs with adequate inflow but, importantly, with no evidence of neuropathy or subcutaneous infection; 77 per cent demonstrated complete ulcer healing, whereas only 22 per cent required amputation.[42] Lee and colleagues reported somewhat lower healing rates for patients with superficial toe gangrene, with 56 per cent of the involved digits "salvaged" by sympathectomy and a 40 per cent toe salvage rate among those with three or more digits involved.[31] Among "nonresponders" in such reports, the immediate amputation rate ranged from 27 to 38 per cent, suggesting that not all these cases were doomed without therapeutic intervention and that the level of amputation required was not improved by sympathectomy.

Precise characterization of the ischemic forefoot lesion that is most likely to respond to sympathectomy is difficult to glean from this literature. From a conceptual and practical point of view, however, use of sympathectomy should be confined to small, shallow, uninfected forefoot ulcers or single-digit superficial gangrene in patients with an ABI greater than 0.3 and absent neuropathy. One might expect successful healing in at least 35 per cent of such patients, but no change in amputation level can be anticipated should amputation ultimately be required.

Sympathectomy as an Adjunct to Arterial Reconstruction

There is experimental evidence that sympathectomy improves patency of small vessel anastomoses and the repair of traumatized arteries.[7, 52] Some authors have even reported better patency rates for both proximal and distal arterial reconstructions when concomitant sympathectomy is performed.[19, 51] It is difficult, however, to predict which reconstructions would be protected by sympathectomy. Its application in proximal reconstructions that have been performed in the face of distal thromboembolism, poor runoff, or small "hypoplastic" vessels is less problematic because the sympathetic chain can often be exposed through the same incision. With distal reconstruction, however, sympathectomy would constitute an entirely separate surgical procedure and therefore is harder to justify. Preferably, intraoperative electromagnetic flowmeter studies, documenting low graft blood flow that significantly increases in response to intra-arterial papaverine or tolazoline (Priscoline), should be used to justify the addition of lumbar sympathectomy. However, a multi-center trial has shown that dextran 40 infusions can produce a threefold decrease in early postoperative thrombosis of difficult distal bypass operations.[49] This results from both an increase in flow and a decrease in coagulability and would seem to provide a better alternative to sympathectomy. Prostanoids and hemorrheologic agents may offer future promise in this situation, and it is anticipated that the appreciation of sympathectomy for this indication will be negligible.

Sympathectomy to Speed Up Development of Collateral Circulation

This is a commonly mentioned indication for which there is little scientific proof. Ludbrook has shown that collateral arteries contributed 23 per cent of the resistance at rest and 73 per cent at peak flows in patients with claudication, and 52 per cent of the resistance at rest and 89 per cent at peak flows in patients with rest pain.[35] Decreasing the resistance of the peripheral vascular bed distal to the obstruction by sympathectomy would not greatly decrease overall resistance or increase flow, particularly if the occlusive process was a severe one. In the same situation, however, an equal decrease in the collateral artery resistance would have a very significant effect on overall blood flow. Therefore, the critical question is, to what extent are the collateral arteries under sympathetic control? Shepherd, using indirect methods of evaluating the collateral circulation, concluded that collateral vessels are indeed under the control of the sympathetic nervous system.[53] However, Dornhorst and Sharpey-Shafer studied the effect of lumbar sympathectomy in 10 patients and found that although the collateral resistance fell in 7 cases, the decreases were quite transient.[17] Similar findings were reported by Barcroft and Swan.[2] Thus, there probably is some improvement in the speed but not in the magnitude of development of collateral circulation following sympathectomy, *if* it is performed early enough (i.e., the first few weeks after occlusion). This benefit may result from either vasodilation of the collateral channels themselves or the increased pressure gradient produced across the block by the decrease in distal resistance that results from sympathectomy.

Summary of Recommended Indications

Within the context of its physiologic consequences and the clinical results just presented, lumbar sympathectomy should obviously be applied rarely and very selectively to patients with lower extremity pain or ischemic syndromes and only to those who are refractory to medical management and are not candidates for more effective revascularization techniques. Regardless of the indication, both subjective and objective preoperative assessment of response to sympathetic blockade greatly enhances the probability of therapeutic success. With these considerations in mind, lumbar sympathectomy may be indicated for the following conditions, using the recommended selection criteria: (1) causalgia; (2) inoperable arterial occlusive disease with limb-threatening ischemia causing rest pain, limited ulceration, or superficial digital gangrene; and (3) symptomatic vasospastic disorders.

Causalgia. When diagnosed and treated early, in stage I, post-traumatic pain syndromes respond to intensive medical therapy in 40 to 60 per cent of cases.[60] Such nonoperative treatment consists of mild analgesics, physiotherapy, tricyclic antidepressants, anticonvulsants, and alpha$_2$-adrenergic blockers administered in a stepwise manner according to symptom responsiveness.[22] Consideration of surgical sympathectomy usually is withheld until conscientious participation in medical therapy has continued for 3 months. Multiple translumbar sympathetic blocks with local anesthetics are used to obtain and observe symptom relief, particularly its degree and duration.[54] Among patients with chronic pain or atypical pain and a "learned helplessness" personality profile, saline placebo injections may help confirm or rule out a true cause-effect relationship for the reported symptomatic relief.[8] If reproducible pain relief is achieved, lumbar sympathectomy yields a uniformly gratifying and sustained response rate.[37] It should be applied as soon as the patient's relief from sympathetic blockade, which lasts only as long as the effect of the local anesthetic used. This corresponds to stage II. Patients allowed to progress to stage III do not respond to sympathectomy (see Chapter 49 for a more detailed discussion of this indication).

Inoperable Arterial Occlusive Disease. Prior to the discussion of specific selection criteria, the term inoperable requires definition. In general, the application of direct revascularization techniques for ischemic limbs with severe infrapopliteal occlusive disease is limited by the level and characteristics of the recipient artery, the adequacy of distal runoff, the conduit available for arterial bypass, and the technical expertise of the surgeon. Inadequate runoff (i.e., no distal arteries to bypass) is becoming an infrequent indication thanks to intra-arterial digital subtraction, color Doppler scanning, and, more recently, magnetic resonance arteriography. Improved application of in situ, translocated, or reversed saphenous vein grafting techniques permits bypass to suitable arteries in the lower calf, ankle, and foot with very acceptable limb salvage rates.[30] With available autogenous vein and patent distal arteries, "inoperability" is determined by the technical proficiency of the surgeon (see Chapter 53).

Rest Pain. Assuming that a critical degree of forefoot ischemia has been demonstrated by objective criteria to confirm the clinical diagnosis of ischemic rest pain, lumbar sympathectomy is preferable to amputation if the following criteria are met: (1) ankle-brachial index (ABI) greater than 0.3, (2) absent neuropathy, and (3) symptomatic relief obtained by trial block. Relief of rest pain from lumbar sympathectomy can be expected in 50 to 85 per cent of patients meeting these criteria.

Limited Tissue Loss. Initial evaluation includes definition of the extent and depth of tissue loss, treatment of secondary infection with limited débridement, topical care, and culture-specific antibiotic therapy. In addition to noninvasive testing, perfusion scans with injections of intravenous thallium or intra-arterial technetium-99m–labeled albumen microspheres permit determination of the hyperemic ratio surrounding the lesion and prediction of healing potential (see Chapter 5).[55] Such studies or the absence of signs of healing after 6 weeks of intensive wound management warrant obtaining arteriograms using special timing or digital subtraction methods to demonstrate "operability." Other selection criteria for sympathectomy are similar to those used for determining rest pain and include (1) ABI greater than 0.3, (2) absent neuropathy, (3) limited ulceration or superficial single-digit gangrene, and (4) absence of major deep infection. Strict adherence to these criteria can be expected to result in healing in 35 to 65 per cent of patients following lumbar sympathectomy.[42, 63]

Lower Extremity Vasospasm. Symptomatic vasospasm of the lower extremity primarily affects patients with

Raynaud's phenomenon or victims of frostbite. Discomfort and typical color changes in response to mild environmental cold with painful rewarming hyperemia or even a mild superficial dermatitis (pernio) are noted. Severe vasospasm may produce digital ulcerations in the presence of readily palpable pedal pulses. Digital photoplethysmography discloses either artifactually peaked pulse volume recordings or sustained loss of pulsatile flow in response to a local or distant hypothermic challenge.[27] A good response to sympathectomy can be predicted by demonstrating at least a 50 per cent increase in amplitude of the digital pulse volume recording with cold exposure following chemical sympathetic blockade.[58] Prior to consideration of lumbar sympathectomy, maximal medical therapy with calcium-channel blockers, cold avoidance, and cessation of smoking must be earnestly pursued. Vasospasm refractory to these measures warrants lumbar sympathectomy; immediate and lasting symptom resolution has been noted in nearly 90 per cent of patients managed in this stepwise fashion.[20, 23, 27]

PERFORMANCE OF LUMBAR SYMPATHECTOMY

Anatomic Considerations

Proper performance of lumbar sympathectomy requires appreciation of the anatomic characteristics of the lumbar sympathetic chain. Preganglionic neurons are located in the anteromedial aspect of the thoracolumbar spinal cord. At segmental levels, efferent fibers from preganglionic neurons synapse with postganglionic neurons in paravertebral ganglia via white rami communicantes. A small percentage of preganglionic efferent fibers either bypass the paravertebral ganglia to synapse in more peripherally located intermediate ganglia or cross over to innervate contralateral regions via conventional pathways. Characteristically, preganglionic fibers that supply a specific somatic region either synapse with multiple postganglionic fibers in paravertebral ganglia or proceed more peripherally to synapse in intermediate ganglia that are at a distance from their segmental source. Therefore, complete sympathetic denervation of an extremity requires division of preganglionic fibers along their segmental origin as well as resection of their corresponding relay ganglia and intercommunicating fibers.

Sympathetic outflow to the lower extremities originates in spinal cord segments from T10 to L3. Preganglionic fibers from these segments form extensive synaptic connections in paravertebral ganglia from L1 to S3 for innervation of the entire lower extremity and pelvic region. Sympathetic innervation of the foot and lower leg is primarily conveyed through the L2 and L3 ganglia; the proximal leg region is primarily innervated from the L1 to the L4 ganglia. Variations in the number and location of sympathetic ganglia are most common in the lumbar region, with the majority occurring at the L1, L4, and L5 levels. Overall, three lumbar ganglia are most commonly found, with the fusion of the L1 and L2 ganglia most commonly accounting for the reduced number.[69] Crossover fibers occur in 15 per cent of patients, with most leaving via the fourth and fifth lumbar ganglia.[65] For most clinical indications, L2 and L3 ganglionectomy is sufficient, but also removing L4 is advised to reduce the possibility of collateral reinnervation. Imparato advocates removal of all encountered lumbar ganglia to ensure that complete lower extremity sympathectomy is accomplished.[26] However, such extensive ganglionectomy is not usually warranted and may result in ejaculatory disturbances in preclimacteric males when bilateral high ganglionectomies (i.e., including L1) are performed. Impotence is also claimed to occur under these circumstances but has no known physiologic basis at this level. It is more likely to be produced by extensive dissection of the distal aorta, particularly around the origin of the left common iliac artery.

Technique

Lumbar sympathectomy begins with proper positioning of the patient so that the interval between the costal margin and iliac crest is "opened." This objective is accomplished by raising the flank region approximately 30 degrees by placing padded rolls beneath the hip and thorax. With the mid-flank region centered over the kidney rest, the table is flexed approximately 10 to 15 degrees to widen the distance between the costal margin and the iliac crest. Tension on the ipsilateral psoas muscle is relieved by flexing the upper (ipsilateral) thigh with appropriate padding beneath and between each leg.

An oblique incision is begun at the lateral edge of the rectus muscle, extended toward the middle of the space between the ribs and iliac crest and ending at the anterior axillary line. The musculofascial layers of the internal and external oblique as well as the transversalis are split in the direction of their fibers or divided in line with the incision. The transversalis fascia should be divided laterally where the peritoneum is stronger, less adherent, and more easily separated from the fascial undersurface. The lateral plane between the transversalis fascia and the peritoneum is easily developed by blunt finger dissection directed toward the vertebral column. Continued separation of the peritoneum is gently performed in medial, caudal, and cephalad directions to maximize retroperitoneal exposure through the relatively small anterior flank incision.

With continued dissection toward the posterior midline, care should be taken to remain close to the peritoneum and anterior to the psoas muscle rather than dropping back into the retroperitoneal fat or posterolateral flank muscles, where bleeding may be encountered. The ureter and gonadal vessels are left attached to overlying peritoneum and are lifted off the psoas muscle as the dissection proceeds medially. The ureter should always be clearly visualized to avoid inadvertent injury.

The lumbar sympathetic chain is located medial to the psoas muscle and lies over the transverse processes of the lumbar spine. The lumbar chain should not be confused with the genitofemoral nerve, which lies more laterally over the medial third of the psoas muscle itself. On the left, the lumbar ganglia lie adjacent and lateral to the abdominal aorta; on the right, the chain lies just beneath the edge of the inferior vena cava.

Tactile identification of the lumbar chain by plucking

discloses a characteristic ''snap'' as a result of tethering of the nodular chain by rami communicantes. Other vertical, band-like structures in this region (genitofemoral nerve, paravertebral lymph nodes, or ureter) do not recoil as briskly. Once identified, the mid-portion of the sympathetic chain is dissected free of surrounding tissues and retracted with a right angle clamp or a nerve hook to draw it up under tension from the surrounding tissue. The ganglia are mobilized by division of tethering rami with prior metal clip application. Orientation and ganglion numbering is facilitated by identifying the sacral promontory and an adjacent lumbar vein that usually crosses the sympathetic chain in front of or behind the third lumbar ganglion. A large space between the first and second lumbar ganglia is often found with the first ganglion partially obscured by the lumbocostal arch. Metal clip application to all elements of the sympathetic chain prior to division prevents unexpected bleeding from vessels mistaken for rami or injury to nonneural structures during attempts to control the latter. Once the chain, with at least two lumbar ganglia, is removed, hemostasis is secured, and the incision is closed in layers after the table is flexed.

This anterolateral approach of Flowthow is most popular because the incision is well tolerated, dissection remains retroperitoneal, and exposure is adequate.[21] The posterior approach of Royle is not favored because of significant postoperative paraspinal muscle spasms.[48] The anterior approach of Adson is applicable only for sympathectomy combined with an abdominal aortic or other intraperitoneal procedure.[1] Using this anterior, transperitoneal approach, the right lumbar chain is identified by dissecting along the right lateral aspect of the inferior vena cava. Exposure of the left lumbar chain is best accomplished by mobilization and medial reflection of the left colon along the white line of Toldt. This approach avoids dissection through lymphatic and vascular tissue immediately lateral to the aorta.

Complications

Major complications result from failure to appreciate normal anatomic relationships with resultant injury to the genitofemoral nerve, ureter, lumbar veins, aorta, and inferior vena cava. Although reported, such injuries are avoidable by attention to anatomic detail and prevention of hemorrhage from vessels lying outside the proper plane of dissection.

The most common complication following lumbar sympathectomy is postsympathectomy neuralgia. This appears in up to 50 per cent of patients from 5 to 20 days following sympathectomy.[33, 37] The pain is characterized as an annoying ''ache'' in the anterolateral thigh region that is worse at night and is unaffected by activity or level of cutaneous stimulation. The discomfort responds to moderate analgesics and spontaneously remits within 8 to 12 weeks after onset. Counseling preoperative patients about this complication is essential and often attenuates overreaction to this annoying sequela. The cause of this neuralgia is still speculative, and various technical maneuvers have not reduced its overall incidence.

Sexual derangement in the male consists of retrograde ejaculation occurring in 25 to 50 per cent of patients undergoing bilateral L1 sympathetic ganglionectomy.[46, 67] This complication rarely occurs following unilateral ganglionectomy, especially when care is used to preserve the first lumbar ganglion. Although potency should not be affected, many older surgeons insist that such derangements in sexual function in the male do occur. Careful preoperative questioning about sexual function is important to evaluate any changes reported after lumbar sympathectomy.

Systemic arterial steal syndromes resulting from lumbar sympathectomy have been reported but are largely unsubstantiated by careful analysis. Nonetheless, paradoxical gangrene of the contralateral extremity has been reported but was shown to be due to intrinsic arterial occlusion of the affected leg rather than to selective hypoperfusion at the aortoiliac level.[4] Similarly, mesenteric arterial insufficiency with bowel infarction has likewise been attributed to intrinsic mesenteric occlusive disease rather than to aortoiliac steal.

Apart from postsympathectomy neuralgia, the second most common ''complication'' is failure to achieve the desired objectives of pain relief or tissue healing. Additionally, attenuation of initially favorable results have been previously considered to be secondary to technical errors or inadequate sympathectomy. Better elucidation of the consequences of lumbar sympathectomy as well as its intrinsic limitations has shown that these sequelae are unavoidable. However, within the context of the criteria and indications outlined in this chapter, ''complications'' of this nature should be infrequent.

Proper patient selection for operation, and evaluation, in terms of standard anesthetic risk factors, as well as improvement in perioperative management protocols has markedly reduced the mortality of this procedure. Although Haimovici and associates,[25] Palumbro and Lulu,[40] and Taylor[59] have reported mortality rates ranging from 2.9 to 6.0 per cent in older series, the authors and others have had no operative deaths among a large series of high-risk patients.[9, 29, 37, 42] Modern surgical care, therefore, permits performance of lumbar sympathectomy with an almost negligible risk of perioperative death.

CONCLUSION

The role of lumbar sympathectomy in the modern management of lower extremity vascular disease is quite minor. However, in carefully selected patients with no other surgical options, sympathetic denervation may sufficiently increase distal perfusion and cutaneous capillary nutritive flow to allow healing in situations of lumbar tissue loss, as well as decrease ischemic pain perception. Causalgic pain remains its best indication, and though the procedure is also effective in cold-induced vasospasm, the level of disability caused is so low and the success of nonoperative management is so high that it is rarely warranted here. Although very effective in controlling hyperhidrosis, this is uncommonly a consideration in the lower extremities (in contrast to the upper extremities), where desiccating foot powders are quite effective. Further elucidation of the influence of lumbar sympathectomy on microcirculatory hemodynamics in patients with end-stage arterial occlusive disease may refine criteria and indications for future usage, but it is more likely that pharmacologic agents (e.g., prostacyclin analogues) will fill this void rather than an increased application of sympathectomy.

References

1. Adson AW, Brown CE: Treatment of Raynaud's disease by lumbar ramisection and ganglionectomy and perivascular sympathectomy neurectomy of the common iliacs. JAMA 84:1908, 1925.
2. Barcroft H, Swan HJC: Sympathetic Control of Human Blood Vessels. London, Arnold and Co, 1953.
3. Beran RD, Tsuru H: Functional and structural changes in the rabbit ear artery after sympathetic denervation. Circ Res 49:478, 1981.
4. Bergan JJ, Trippell OH: Arteriograms in ischemic limbs worsened after lumbar sympathectomy. Arch Surg 85:135, 1962.
5. Blumenberg RM, Gelfand L: Lumbar sympathectomy for limb salvage: A goal-line stand. Am J Surg 138:241, 1979.
6. Bobik A, Anderson WP: Influence of sympathectomy on alpha-2 adrenoreceptor binding sites in canine blood vessels. Life Sci 33:331, 1983.
7. Casten DF, Sadler AH, Furman D: An experimental study of the effect of sympathectomy on patency of small blood vessel anastomoses. Surg Gynecol Obstet 115:462, 1962.
8. Chapman SL, Brena SF: Learned helplessness and responses to nerve blocks in chronic low back pain patients. Pain 14:355, 1982.
9. Collins GI, Rich NM, Claggett GP, et al: Clinical results of lumbar sympathectomy. Am Surg 47:31, 1981.
10. Cronenwett JL, Lindenauer SM: Direct measurement of arteriovenous anastomotic blood flow after lumbar sympathectomy. Surgery 82:82, 1977.
11. Cronenwett JL, Lindenauer SM: Hemodynamic effects of sympathectomy in ischemic canine hind limbs. Surgery 87:417, 1980.
12. Cronenwett JL, Zelenock GB, Whitehouse W Jr, et al: The effect of sympathetic innervation of canine muscle and skin blood flow. Arch Surg 118:420, 1983.
13. Cross FW, Cotton LT: Chemical lumbar sympathectomy for ischemic rest pain. A randomized, prospective controlled clinical trial. Am J Surg 150:341, 1985.
14. Dalessandri KM, Carson SM, Tillman P, et al: Effect of lumbar sympathectomy in distal arterial obstruction. Arch Surg 118:1157, 1983.
15. DaValle MJ, Bauman FG, Mintzer R, et al: Limited success of lumbar sympathectomy in the prevention of ischemic limb loss in diabetic patients. Surg Gynecol Obstet 152:784, 1981.
16. Diez J: Un nuevo metodo de simpatectomia periferica para el tratamiento de affecionas trofilas y gangrenosas de los miembros. Bol Soc Cir Buenos Aires 8:10, 1924.
17. Dornhorst AC, Sharpey-Schafer EP: Collateral resistance in limbs with arterial obstruction: Spontaneous changes and effects of sympathectomy. Clin Sci 10:371, 1951.
18. Ewing M: The history of lumbar sympathectomy. Surgery 70:791, 1971.
19. Faenza A, Splare R, Lapilli A, et al: Clinical results of lumbar sympathectomy alone or as a complement to direct arterial surgery. Acta Chir Belg 76:101, 1977.
20. Felder DA, Simeone FA, Linton RR, et al: Evaluation of sympathetic neurectomy in Raynaud's disease. Surgery 26:1014, 1949.
21. Flowthow PG: Anterior extraperitoneal approach to the lumbar sympathetic nerves. Am J Surg 127:953, 1948.
22. Ghostine SY, Gomair YG, Turner DM, et al: Phenoxybenzamine in the treatment of causalgia: Report of 40 cases. J Neurosurg 60:1263, 1984.
23. Gifford RS Jr, Hines EA Jr, Craig WM: Sympathectomy for Raynaud's phenomenon: Follow-up study of 70 women with Raynaud's disease and 54 women with secondary Raynaud's phenomenon. Circulation 17:5, 1958.
24. Groch JM, Bauman FG, Riles TS, et al: Effect of surgical lumbar sympathectomy on innervation of arterioles in the lower limb of patients with diabetes. Surg Gynecol Obstet 153:39, 1981.
25. Haimovici H, Steenman C, Karson IH: Evaluation of lumbar sympathectomy. Arch Surg 89:1089, 1964.
26. Imparato AM: Lumbar sympathectomy. Role in the treatment of occlusive arterial disease in the lower extremities. Surg Clin North Am 59:719, 1979.
27. Janoff KA, Phinney ES, Porter JM: Lumbar sympathectomy for lower extremity vasospasm. Am J Surg 150:147, 1985.
28. Je'bara VA, Saade B: Causalgia: A wartime experience—report of twenty treated cases. J Trauma 27:519, 1987.
29. Kim GE, Ibrahim IM, Imparato AM: Lumbar sympathectomy in end-stage arterial occlusive disease. Am Surg 183:157, 1976.
30. Leather RP, Karmody AM: In-situ saphenous vein arterial bypass for the treatment of limb ischemia. Adv Surg 19:175, 1986.
31. Lee BY, Madden JL, Tuoden WR, et al: Lumbar sympathectomy for toe gangrene. Long-term follow-up. Am J Surg 145:398, 1983.
32. Lindenauer SM, Cronenwett JL: What is the place of lumbar sympathectomy? Br J Surg Suppl 69, p 532, 1982.
33. Litwin MS: Post-sympathectomy neuralgia. Arch Surg 84:591, 1962.
34. Loh L, Nathan PW: Painful peripheral states and sympathetic blocks. J Neurol Neurosurg Psychiatry 41:664, 1978.
35. Ludbrook J: Collateral arterial resistance in human lower limbs. J Surg Res 6:423, 1966.
36. May AG, DeWeese JA, Rob CG: Effect of sympathectomy on blood flow in arterial stenosis. Ann Surg 158:182, 1968.
37. Mockus MB, Rutherford RB, Rosales C, et al: Sympathectomy for causalgia. Arch Surg 122:668, 1987.
38. Moore WS, Hall AD: Effects of lumbar sympathectomy on skin capillary blood flow in arterial occlusive disease. J Surg Res 14:151, 1973.
39. Owens JC: Causalgia. Am Surg 23:636, 1957.
40. Palumbro LT, Lulu DJ: Lumbar sympathectomy in peripheral vascular disease. Arch Surg 86:182, 1963.
41. Perry MO, Horton J: Muscle and subcutaneous oxygen tension. Measurements by mass spectrometry after sympathectomy. Arch Surg 113:176, 1973.
42. Persson AV, Anderson LA, Padberg FT Jr: Selection of patients for lumbar sympathectomy. Surg Clin North Am 65:393, 1985.
43. Petten CV, Roberts WJ, Rhodes DL: Behavioral test of tolerance for aversive mechanical stimuli in sympathectomized cats. Pain 15:177, 1983.
44. Pistolese GR, Speziale F, Taurino M, et al: Criteria for prognostic evaluation of the results of lumbar sympathectomy: Clinical, hemodynamic and angiographic findings. J Cardiovasc Surg 23:411, 1982.
45. Porter JM, Rivers SP: Management of Raynaud's syndrome. *In* Bergan JJ, Yao JST (eds): Evaluation and Treatment of Upper and Lower Extremity Circulatory Disorders. New York, Grune and Stratton, 1983, pp 181–202.
46. Quale JB: Sexual function after bilateral lumbar sympathectomy and aortoiliac bypass surgery. J Cardiovasc Surg 21:215, 1980.
47. Ramos M, Almazán A, Lozano F, et al: Phenol lumbar sympathectomy in severe arterial disease of the lower limb: A hemodynamic study. Int Surg 68:127, 1983.
48. Royle ND: A new operative procedure in the treatment of spastic paralysis and its experimental basis. Med J Aust 1:77, 1924.
49. Rutherford RB, Jones DH, Bergentz SE, et al: The efficacy of dextran-40 in preventing early postoperative thrombosis following difficult lower extremity bypass. J Vasc Surg 1:776, 1984.
50. Rutherford RB, Valenta J: Extremity blood flow and distribution: The effects of arterial occlusion, sympathectomy and exercise. Surgery 69:332, 1971.
51. Satiani B, Liapsis CD, Hayes JP, et al: Prospective randomized study of concomitant lumbar sympathectomy with aortoiliac reconstruction. Am J Surg 143:755, 1982.
52. Sandmann W, Kremer K, Wust H, et al: Postoperative control of blood flow in arterial surgery and results of electromagnetic blood flow measurement. Thoraxchir 25:427, 1977.
53. Shepherd JT: The effects of acute occlusion of the femoral artery on the blood supply to the calf of the leg before and after release of sympathetic vasomotor tone. Chir Sci 9:355, 1950.
54. Shumacker HB Jr: A personal overview of causalgia and other reflex dystrophies. Ann Surg 201:278, 1985.
55. Siegel ME, William GM, Giargiano FA Jr, et al: A useful objective criterion for determining the healing potential of an ischemic ulcer. J Nucl Med 21:993, 1975.
56. Smith RB, Dratz AF, Coberly JC, et al: Effect of lumbar sympathectomy on muscle blood flow in advanced occlusive vascular disease. Ann Surg 37:247, 1971.

57. Strandness DE, Bell JW: Critical evaluation of the results of lumbar sympathectomy. Ann Surg 160:1021, 1964.
58. Sumner DS, Strandness DE Jr: An abnormal finger pulse associated with cold sensitivity. Ann Surg 175:294, 1972.
59. Taylor I: Lumbar sympathectomy for intermittent claudication. Br J Clin Pract 27:39, 1973.
60. Thompson JE: The diagnosis and management of post-traumatic pain syndromes (causalgia). Aust NZ J Surg 49:299, 1979.
61. van der Stricht J: Lumbar sympathectomy in occlusive diseases. Int Angiol 4:345, 1985.
62. Vautinnen E, Luberg MV, Sotaranta M: The immediate effect of lumbar sympathectomy on arterial blood flow measured by electromagnetic flowmetry. Scand J Thorac Cardiovasc Surg 12:101, 1978.
63. Walker PM, Johnston KW: Predicting the success of a sympathectomy: A retrospective study using discriminant function and multiple regression analysis. Surgery 87:216, 1980.
64. Walsh JA, Glynn CJ, Cousins MJ, et al: Blood flow, sympathetic activity and pain relief following lumbar sympathetic blockade or surgical sympathectomy. Anaesth Intensive Care 13:18, 1985.
65. Webber RH: An analysis of the cross communications between the sympathetic trunks in the lumbar region in man. Ann Surg 145:365, 1957.
66. Welch GH, Leiberman DP: Cutaneous blood flow in the foot following lumbar sympathectomy. Scand J Clin Lab Invest 45:621, 1985.
67. Whitelaw GP, Smithwick RH: Some secondary effects of sympathectomy, with particular reference to disturbance of sexual dysfunction. N Engl J Med 245:121, 1951.
68. Yao JST, Bergan JJ: Predictability of vascular reactivity relative to sympathetic ablation. Arch Surg 107:676, 1973.
69. Yeager GH, Cowley RA: Anatomical observations on the lumbar sympathetics with evaluation of sympathectomies in organic peripheral vascular disease. Ann Surg 127:953, 1948.
70. Noe CE, Haynsworth RF Jr.: Lumbar radiofrequency sympatholysis. J Vasc Surg 17:801, 1993.

60

Adventitial Cystic Disease of the Popliteal Artery

John J. Bergan, M.D.

• • •

Occlusion of the popliteal artery caused by adventitial cystic disease is a rare and obscure entity. Little more is known about it today than when the condition was first encountered more than 35 years ago.

HISTORICAL BACKGROUND

It is unlikely that adventitial cystic degeneration of arteries was unrecognized prior to 1946; however, the report of Atkins and Key appearing in that year is truly the first.[3] Their patient, a 40-year-old man, was admitted to Guy's Hospital with intermittent claudication involving the quadriceps and calf muscles, which had become progressively worse over a 4-month period. A painless lump eventually appeared above the inguinal ligament in the line of the external iliac artery. At operation, a grayish-red growth that had the characteristics of a typical ganglion containing myxomatous tissue was found arising from the posterior aspect and investing the middle third of the external iliac artery.

Eight years after this first observation, Ejrup and Hiertonn encountered a similar condition in what was subsequently found to be its most common location, the popliteal artery.[26] By 1957, Hiertonn and associates were able to collect a total of only four cases of cystic degeneration of this artery.[40] Characteristically, the patients were young men complaining of intermittent claudication that was found to be due to a popliteal artery cyst containing a peculiar jelly-like material. Microscopic examination revealed that the main lesion was a cyst resembling a ganglion lying within the adventitial layer of the artery (Fig. 60–1). The intramural mucinous degeneration was clearly differentiated from Erdheim's cystic medial necrosis. Hiertonn and Lindberg likened the external appearance of the lesion to that of a hot dog.[39] Hiertonn and Hemmingsson reported the follow-up examination of these patients in 1984, some 27 to 30 years after insertion of the grafts. The veins were patent, though widened and irregular.[38]

Ishikawa and colleagues contributed an important diagnostic sign when they noted that normal distal pulsations are obliterated when the knee is sharply flexed in patients whose cystic disease produces stenosis without total occlusion.[43] Jacquet and Meyer-Burgdorff pointed out that the cyst might be manifested as a localized stenosis allowing passage of blood only at the very peak of systolic pressure.[44] Subsequently, Eastcott suggested that an arterial murmur over the popliteal fossa was an important sign for establishing the diagnosis in a young nonsmoker with intermittent claudication.[23]

By 1963, cases had been reported from California, Le Havre, Auckland, Belgium, Paris, and Heidelberg; however, the true cause of the cystic degeneration had not been identified.[42, 59, 63, 70, 77, 79] In 1961, Parkes of Glasgow and

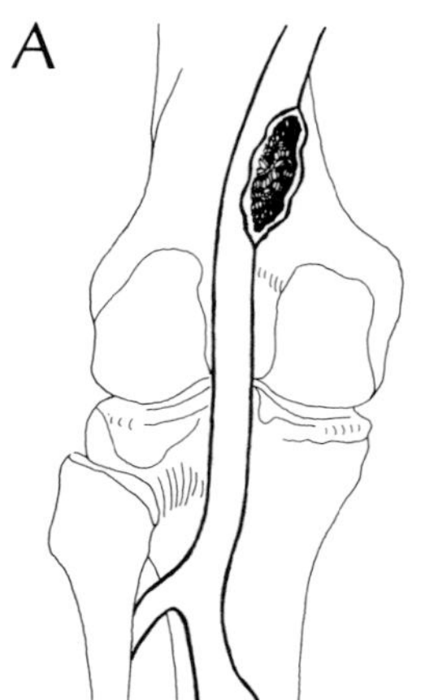

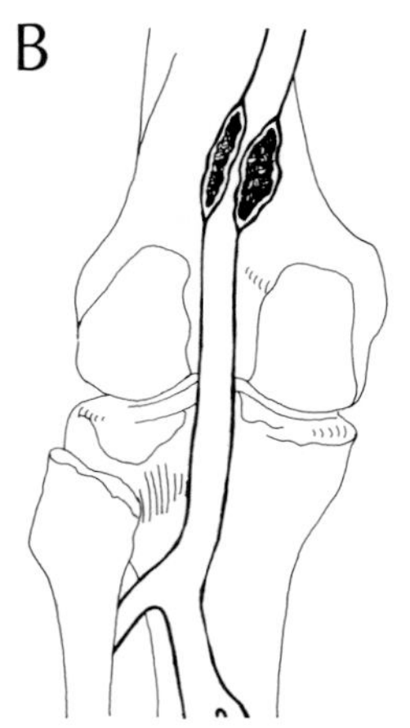

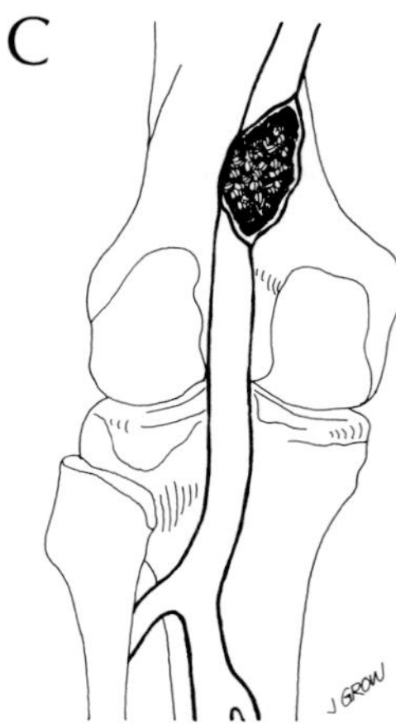

FIGURE 60–1. Adventitial cysts will present in variable locations on the popliteal artery. The expanding cyst may indent the artery (*A*), the scimitar sign; encircle the artery (*B*), the hourglass sign; or completely occlude the vessel (*C*).

Clark of Stoke-on-Trent, England, described cysts containing mucoid material involving the lateral popliteal nerve.[45, 57] Parkes suggested that the ganglion initially arose from the fibular joint and traced along the sheath of the small recurrent articular branch, coming to lie within the sheath of the main nerve itself. He related these findings to the demonstration in two cases of a dissecting ganglion within the adventitia of a radial and an ulnar artery, in each instance connected by a pedicle to a joint space in the wrist. In an annotation in the American Heart Journal in 1964, Bliss indicated that the cause of the lesion was still unknown but that the clinical picture, pathologic features, and treatment were well defined.[9] That the cyst is indeed of joint origin is strongly suggested by reports of connection of the cavity to the joint space by fibrous strands or tubes. This suggests that disconnection of the cyst from the adjacent joint is an important part of surgical therapy.[12]

By 1970, after 40 cases had been reported, Bergan surveyed the authors of these reports to obtain long-term follow-up, and 4 new cases were added.[30] The incidence of popliteal cystic disease was found to be approximately 1 in 1200 cases of claudication, or 1 in 1000 femoral arteriograms.[48] It was suggested that the most likely theory of origin of the condition was developmental inclusion of mucin-secreting cells within the adventitia of the artery: that is, that these cells arising from adjacent joint or tendon structures were enclosed within the adventitia during embryologic formation. As the cells secreted mucin, cysts developed that by pressure could occlude the arterial lumen. The observation that cystic degeneration of the popliteal nerve had been encountered in the same area supported this hypothesis. However, direct communications with adjacent joints have now been reported, thus suggesting a more direct contact as a cause of the cyst.

In the follow-up evaluation, all but six cases were traced, and 27 patients were observed for more than 2 years. The longest follow-up time was 30 years. No serious disability was found, no amputations resulted, and in no instance had there been development of the condition in the contralateral popliteal artery. Cystic adventitial disease of another artery had not occurred, none of these 27 patients had a generalized connective tissue disorder, and no joint disease was found.

By 1987, Ishikawa had collected a total of 195 cases from the world literature, and his review reaffirmed the findings described previously.[43a] Adventitial cystic disease has been reported in other arteries and veins in 39 cases. Twenty-eight of these have involved the external iliac artery or vein or the femoral artery or vein. These lesions have been in close proximity to the hip joint and its capsule.[2]

PATHOPHYSIOLOGY

The condition of cystic adventitial disease of the popliteal artery chiefly affects males in the ratio of approximately 15 : 1, and it appears in the 4th and 5th decades. The youngest patient was 10 years old, and the oldest a man of 77. In women, the condition appears in the 6th decade.[30]

The onset of symptoms is usually sudden, but it is probable that the cyst arises over a long period, producing stenosis of the artery with preservation of patency. Once the intracystic pressure exceeds that of the adjacent artery, occlusion of the affected vessel occurs, although thrombosis may not be superimposed. Evidence for this is the fact that simple cyst evacuation may result in full arterial patency, even in cases of arteriographically proven arterial occlusion. The pathophysiologic appearance subsequent to this single arterial occlusion is no different from that produced by other causes of arterial constriction. Claudication without severe ischemia is a regular finding in these cases.

ETIOLOGY

Although the exact cause of cystic degeneration of the adventitia of the popliteal artery is unknown, there are three theories of causation. The theory first proposed was that repetitive trauma caused arterial wall destruction and cystic degeneration of the adventitia.[53] However, the theory of trauma as a possible cause seems unlikely. Similarly, the name myxomatous cystic degeneration seems to be a misnomer.[48]

The second theory of origin is that the adventitial degenerative process is a mucinous or myxomatous condition associated with a generalized body disorder.[49] Long-term follow-up has shown that the condition has not developed contralaterally, nor has generalized connective tissue disorder appeared in any of the patients.[35, 48] This theory seems untenable because it is unlikely that a generalized disorder should be so frequently isolated to the popliteal artery.

The third theory of causation, which is attractive but unproved, assumes the developmental inclusion of mucin-secreting cells within the adventitia of the artery, allowing cysts to develop within the adventitia.[35] This mechanism does not explain all cases; cysts are often well encapsulated and, on being removed, leave a fairly intact artery behind. Demonstration that cyst fluid is often crystal clear and similar in chemical content to ganglia suggests a common origin and an attractive alternative to support the inclusion theory. It was suggested by Richards that more definitive evidence for a similar origin of cysts and ganglia would demonstrate a communication between the cysts and neighboring joint structures.[62] Such a demonstration was reported in 1973 by Shute and Rothnie, who described two cases in which communication could be proved surgically.[69] Within a few years, other cases were reported in which the cyst communicated with the joint capsule.[21, 33] Parkes previously had noted connections between cysts of the radial and ulnar arteries and carpal joints.[57] Other investigators had noted a tight adherence of the popliteal cyst to the knee joint.[34]

Invoking a pathogenesis similar to that of a simple ganglion and postulating two mechanisms for inclusion in an arterial wall provide a concept of development consistent with surgical experience. Either capsular synovial cysts enlarge and track along a genicular artery to involve the adventitia of the popliteal artery; or synovial rests are sequestered into the arterial wall during development, there to secrete and enlarge over many years. When the cyst is entirely adventitial, it is readily removed, leaving the intact artery. Otherwise, when sequestered cells are the cause of cystic formation, enucleation is impossible, and resection of the affected arterial segment is necessary. Further support for the theory of ganglion involvement of adjacent structures is provided by case reports in which such cystic lesions have involved adjacent vascular structures. These cases include adventitial cystic disease involving the lesser saphenous vein,[81] lesions connected to Baker's cyst,[82] and further reports of adventitial cystic disease involving the radial artery.[83]

CYST CONTENT

Chemical analysis of cyst fluid by Hiertonn and Lindberg showed that the viscous mucinous substance, when incubated with hyaluronidase, turned into a thin, cloudy fluid.[39] Paper chromatography revealed amino acids but no carbohydrates. Cholesterin and calcium could not be detected. Other authors reported that mucoproteins or mucopolysaccharides were the most common finding.[26, 37, 48, 77] Hyaluronic acid and hydroxyproline were also found, and these, of course, indicated a connective tissue origin for the fluid.[18, 37] Table 60–1 indicates the result of chemical studies reported by Leaf from case 2 of Lewis and coworkers.[47, 48] Although it has been suggested that the material originates from collagen tissue because of the significant amounts of hydroxyproline present, this hypothesis was not confirmed.

Table 60–1. Amino Acid Composition of Protein From Popliteal Cyst Compared With Collagen and Elastin*

	Cyst Protein	Collagen	Elastin
Aspartic acid	38.4	50.5	15.6
Threonine	24.4	19.3	13.4
Serine	23.2	38.5	10.5
Glutamic acid	52.9	75.5	23.1
Proline	23.6	127.2	117.3
Hydroxyproline	0	96.2	11.4
Glycine	87.0	338.0	318.7
Alanine	41.0	115.6	223.6
Cystine	19.0	0	0
Valine	29.0	26.5	136.7
Methionine	4.3	6.0	2.0
Isoleucine	6.4	9.5	30.5
Leucine	32.3	27.2	67.2
Tyrosine	11.2	3.8	12.7
Phenylalanine	18.8	14.8	36.4
Lysine	42.3	22.5	8.2
Histidine	9.5	5.6	1.9
Arginine	19.9	51.2	9.8
Glucosamine	29.2	—	—
Hydroxylysine	0	9.3	—

From Leaf G.: Amino acid analysis of protein present in a popliteal artery cyst. Br Med J 3:415, 1967.

**Values are expressed as μ moles amino acid per 10^5 gm dry matter for the unknown protein, and μ moles per 10^5 gm protein for collagen (human tendon) and elastin (bovine aorta).*

The chemical and histologic analyses indicate that ganglia and adventitial cysts are quite similar.[47, 48] After sophisticated investigation, Endo and coworkers indicated the degree of confusion regarding the origin of the cyst and its contents:

> The results of the chemical, enzymatic, and electrophoretic studies together with infrared spectrum indicated that the major component (0.5 M Fr) in the cyst of mucoid degeneration was proteohyaluronic acid. Although the substance separated from the cyst of cystic mucoid degeneration is shown to be identical to the proteohyaluronic acid obtained from normal human umbilical cord, the mechanism of the accumulation of proteohyaluronic acid in the cyst of this disease remains to be solved.[27]

CLINICAL FINDINGS

The typical patient with symptoms from cystic adventitial disease of the popliteal artery is a man in his mid-forties seeking medical consultation because of sudden onset of claudication, with or without ischemic neuropathy. Usually, there is a short history of symptoms, measured in days to weeks rather than in months to years. The claudication is usually severe, limiting walking distance to 50 meters or less. Occasionally, ischemic neuropathy may cause paresthesias, burning pain, or coldness.

Absence of popliteal and foot pulses is characteristic; however, if the lesion is producing only stenosis, a bruit is heard in the popliteal fossa and evidence of total occlusion appears only during acute knee flexion, when distal pulses disappear. Stenosis rather than occlusion is present in approximately two thirds of cases. Lewis has reported that a bruit could be heard over the popliteal artery of one of his patients in whom the symptoms had recurred after the cyst had been incompletely excised.[48]

The phenomenon of disappearing distal arterial pulses was noted by Barnett and associates in their 61-year-old patient who had normal limb pulses and oscillometric readings.[6] Ankle pulses disappeared on exercise, and a loud murmur appeared over the popliteal artery at that time. Other investigators have reported hemodynamic alterations produced by exercise.[72]

Imaging of the cyst and its relationship to the parent artery is easily achieved by ultrasonography. B-mode scans allow determination of the shape, dimensions, and number of cysts that are present. The boundary between the cyst contents and vessel lumen is seen as a fine bright line that pulsates in real-time. The absence of atherosclerotic plaques and absence of flow signals within the cyst in the presence of a distinctive sign of aneurysmal enlargement of the artery can be considered signs that are pathognomonic for adventitial cystic disease.[84] Computed tomography (CT) can show circumferential involvement of the artery and even cyst recurrence after supposedly successful primary resection.[85] CT guidance lends itself to percutaneous cyst aspiration.[28] However, this approach should be viewed cautiously because complete decompression may be difficult to achieve, and ultimate recurrence is possible.[86]

ARTERIOGRAPHIC FINDINGS

Early in the course of the condition, arteriography will show stenosis of the artery.[1] The lesion is usually in the mid-portion of the vessel, extending from 1 to 8 cm in length. The vessel above and below the lesion is surprisingly free of atheromatous degeneration. There are a few marginal irregularities.[25] When the smooth tapering is concentric, the lesion is described as having an ''hourglass'' appearance (Fig. 60–2). If the cyst is eccentrically located, the artery tapers smoothly above and below the cyst. This shape has also been described as a ''scimitar sign.'' The artery may be displaced medially or, more commonly, laterally.

The stenosis may be missed on conventional anteroposterior films, and it may appear only on lateral exposures.[6] The arteriographic findings are sufficiently characteristic to be diagnostic. The condition is easily differentiated from atherosclerosis and from the several popliteal artery entrapment syndromes. It should not be confused with hematoma or occlusion of the artery from true joint cyst.[66, 67]

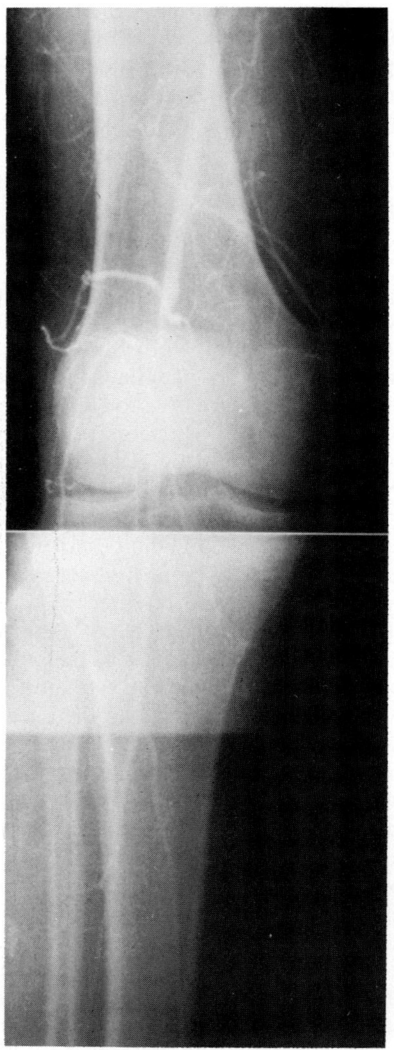

FIGURE 60–2. Composite angiogram showing the curvilinear appearance of the popliteal cyst occluding the main artery, the profuse collateral network, and the normal arterial tree above and below the lesion.

TREATMENT

Optimal treatment of this condition is surgical, but it is surprising how often conservative surgical approaches such as aspiration have been successful in eradicating the arterial occlusion. However, percutaneous transluminal angioplasty (PTA) has proved manifestly unsatisfactory simply because, unlike atherosclerosis, in cystic disease the intima is normal, and it is the arterial wall that is compliant.[31] The operative findings are relatively uniform. On exposure, the artery is found to be enlarged and sausage-shaped. Adhesions may be present, binding the cystic adventitial structure to adjacent vein or to the posterior aspect of the joint capsule. The cyst itself is usually unilocular but may be multi-ocular with septa. The fluid is usually crystal clear but may be faintly yellow or even the color of currant jelly, depending on the amount of recent or old hemorrhage.

Incision into the cyst and evacuation of its contents usually restore arterial patency. Because the condition is rare and preoperative diagnosis was rarely made in the past, a number of cases have been treated by excision of the cyst with its adjacent artery and interpolations of various grafts, with good results. Cyst evacuation, however, is the preferred treatment if the artery has not become occluded. Now that the condition is becoming better known, this method is being used with increasing frequency. However, if the process has proceeded to total arterial occlusion, graft replacement or bypass is preferred, using adjacent long or short saphenous vein as the arterial substitute.

Lytic therapy may be employed, and because such therapy is used to clear an arterial segment to perform minimally invasive correction of the underlying arterial occlusion, it is predictable that cystic adventitial disease will be diagnosed.[87] In such a situation, it might be tempting to aspirate the cyst under ultrasound or CT guidance. However, after total occlusion of the artery, operative intervention has proved to be the most successful method of restoring arterial flow permanently. Continuing reports suggest that both short-term and long-term outcomes are better after complete cyst removal. Although some have treated this condition without arterial reconstruction, majority opinion holds that autogenous arterial repair remains the treatment of choice.[88]

A review of 115 case reports has been completed to allow an evaluation of treatment procedures.[30] Simple cyst evacuation has restored arterial blood flow in 56 instances. Prosthetic grafts, homografts, and autogenous vein grafts were used to restore flow in 42 patients. Patches were used to perform angioplasty in some cases, and in a patient who refused other surgery, rest pain was relieved with a sympathectomy. Curiously, the popliteal fossa in this instance was punctured, and a quantity of jelly was aspirated from the cyst.[55] Cyst aspiration under CT guidance has been accomplished.[20] Disappointing results and rapid reaccumulation of cyst fluid have been experienced repeatedly.

Recurrent occlusions due to the cysts have been treated by needle aspiration, with recovery of varying amounts of gelatinous material and subsequent restoration of arterial flow.[48] Because simple cyst evacuation is effective treatment, it should be employed in situations in which the afflicted artery has not become occluded.[30] If simple cyst evacuation cannot be done, local angioplasties should be avoided. None of the various procedures tried has been as effective as replacement of the vessel by grafting. When total occlusion of the popliteal artery by the cyst is encountered, replacement of the artery or bypass should be performed using the best surgical techniques available.

DISCUSSION

Cystic adventitial disease of arteries remains a rare and interesting cause of stenosis and occlusion. Naturally, one wonders at the cause of such an anomaly. It is an unforgettable experience to apply atraumatic clamps to a pulsating vessel, incise its adventitia, and be treated to the vision of crystal-clear fluid instead of blood pouring under pressure from the arteriotomy. In such a circumstance, the relation to simple ganglia seems irrefutable. Whereas ganglia of nonpopliteal location are common, cystic arterial disease itself is rare and, in volar or dorsal carpal locations rare indeed (five cases). The location of cystic arterial disease in the popliteal fossa and along the external iliac artery is remote from the usual locations of ganglia. Logical as these facts are, however, the fluid remains crystal clear, tantalizing in its similarity to the familiar content of a simple ganglion. The cause, therefore, remains obscure, even though dissections performed meticulously in recent years have shown connection of cyst wall to the knee joint.[68]

Treatment of this condition is as illogical as the lesion is curious. What could be less likely to cure an arterial occlusion than evacuation of the cyst? To a vascular surgeon trained in performing bypass or vein grafts to restore arterial patency, simple cystotomy seems too easy. Yet there is no doubt now that this, rather than resection, is the treatment of choice if the artery is not occluded.[16] If total evacuation can be accomplished without violating the integrity of the arterial intima, cystotomy will suffice. Otherwise, if the artery is completely blocked, arterial bypass must be performed. Although spontaneous resolution of cystic adventitial disease has been reported, such an outcome is not to be expected regularly.[89]

References

1. Andersson T, Gothman B, Lindberg K. Mucinous cystic dissecting intramural degeneration of the popliteal artery. Acta Radiol 52:455, 1959.
2. Annetts DL, Graham AR: Cystic degeneration of the femoral vein. Br J Surg 67:287, 1980.
3. Atkins HJB, Key JA: A case of myxomatous tumor arising in the adventitia of the left external iliac artery. Br J Surg 34:426, 1947.
4. Backstrom CG, Linell F, Ostberg G: Cystic myxomatous adventitial degeneration of the radial artery with development in the connective tissue. Acta Chir Scand 129:447, 1965.
5. Barnett AJ, Morris KN: Cystic myxomatous degeneration of the popliteal artery. Med J Aust 2:793, 1964.
6. Barnett AJ, Dugdale L, Ferguson I: Disappearing pulse syndrome due to myxomatous degeneration of the popliteal artery. Med J Aust 2:355, 1966.
7. Bartos J, Kalus M, Possner J: Cystische adventitielle Degeneration der Arteria poplitea. Langenbecks Arch Klin Chir 314:177, 1966.
8. Baumann G, Schmidt FC, Becker HM, et al: Cystische Wanddegeneration der Arteria iliaca externa und Arteria femoralis communis. Chirurg 38:520, 1967.
9. Bliss BP: Cystic myxomatous degeneration of the popliteal artery. Am Heart J 68:838, 1964.
10. Bliss BP, Rhodes J, Harding Rains AJ: Cystic myxomatous degeneration of the popliteal artery. Br Med J 2:847, 1963.
11. Campbell RT, McCluskey BC, Andrews MIJ: A case of polycystic adventitial disease of the left external iliac and femoral artery. Br J Surg 57:865, 1970.
12. Campbell WB, Millar AW: Cystic adventitial disease of the common femoral artery communicating with the hip joint. Br J Surg 72:537, 1985.
13. Chandler JJ: Popliteal artery occlusion by subadventitial pseudocyst. Surgery 69:474, 1971.
14. Chevrier JL: Un cas de dégénérescence colloide de l'adventice de l'artère poplitée. Mem Acad Chir 88:261, 1962.
15. Clark K: Ganglion of the lateral popliteal nerve. J Bone Joint Surg 43:778, 1961.
16. Cystic degeneration of the popliteal artery [Leading Article]. Br Med J 4:699, 1970.
17. Delannoy E, Martinot M: Dégénérescence colloide de l'adventice de l'artère poplitée. Mem Acad Chir 86:824, 1962.
18. DeLaurentis DA, Wolferth CC Jr, Wolf FM, et al: Mucinous adventitial cysts of the popliteal artery in an 11 year old girl. Surgery 74:456, 1973.
19. Descotes J, Grobert J, Chavent J, et al: Dégénérescence colloide de l'adventice de l'artère poplitée. Lyon Chir 62:898, 1966.
20. Deutsch AL, Hyde J, Miller SM, et al: Cystic adventitial degeneration of the popliteal artery: CT demonstration and directed percutaneous therapy. Am J Roentgenol 145:117, 1985.
21. Devereux D, Forrest H, McLeod T, et al: The non-arterial origin of cystic adventitial disease of the popliteal artery in two patients. Surgery 88:723, 1980.
22. Dunant JH, Eugenidis N: Cystic degeneration of the popliteal artery. Vasa 2:156, 1973.
23. Eastcott HHG: Cystic myxomatous degeneration of popliteal artery. Br Med J 2:1270, 1963.

24. Eastcott HHG: Cystic degeneration of the popliteal artery. Br Med J 1:111, 1971.
25. Ehringer VH, Denck H: Zystische Adventitiadegeneration. Wien Med Wochenschr 120:49, 1970.
26. Ejrup B, Hiertonn T: Intermittent claudication. Three cases treated by free vein graft. Acta Chir Scand 108:217, 1954.
27. Endo M, Tamura S, Minakuchi S, et al: Isolation and identification of proteohyaluronic acid from a cyst of cystic mucoid degeneration. Clin Chim Acta 47:417, 1973.
28. Fitzjohn TP, White FE, Loose HW, et al: Computed tomography and sonography of cystic adventitial disease. Br J Radiol 59:933, 1986.
29. Flanc C: Cystic degeneration of the popliteal artery. Aust NZ J Surg 36:243, 1967.
30. Flanigan DP, Burnham SJ, Goodreau JJ, et al: Summary of cases of adventitial cystic disease of the popliteal artery. Ann Surg 189:165, 1979.
31. Fox RL, Kahn M, Alder J: Adventitial cystic disease of the popliteal artery: Failure of percutaneous transluminal angioplasty. J Vasc Surg 2:464, 1985.
32. Fyfe NCM, Silcocks PB, Browse NC: Cystic mucoid degeneration in the wall of the femoral vein. J Cardiovasc Surg 21:703, 1980.
33. Gertsch P, Stamm B, Burri B, et al: Die arterielle Adventitiazyste der Arteria poplitea. Angio 3:191, 1980.
34. Gripe K: Intramural cystisk arterial mukoiddegeneration. Nord Med 70:1381, 1963.
35. Haid SP, Conn J Jr, Bergan JJ: Cystic adventitial disease of the popliteal artery. Arch Surg 101:765, 1970.
36. Hansen JPH: Cystic mucoid degeneration of the popliteal artery. Acta Chir Scand 131:171, 1966.
37. Harris JD, Jepson RP: Cystic degeneration of the popliteal artery. Aust NZ J Surg 34:265, 1965.
38. Hiertonn T, Hemmingsson A: The autogenous vein graft as a popliteal artery substitute. Acta Chir Scand 150:377, 1984.
39. Hiertonn T, Lindberg K: Cystic adventitial degeneration of the popliteal artery. Acta Chir Scand 113:72, 1957.
40. Hiertonn T, Lindberg K, Rob C: Cystic degeneration of the popliteal artery. Br J Surg 44:348, 1957.
41. Hofmann KT, Consiglio L, Hofmeier G, et al: Die zystische Gefassdegeneration. Brun's Beitr Klin Chir 217:284, 1969.
42. Holmes JG: Cystic adventitial degeneration of the popliteal artery. JAMA 173:654, 1960.
43. Ishikawa K, Mishima Y, Kobayashi S: Cystic adventitial disease of the popliteal artery. Angiology 12:357, 1961.
43a. Ishikawa K: Cystic adventitial disease of the popliteal artery and of other stem vessels in the extremities. Jpn Surg 17:221, 1987.
44. Jacquet GH, Meyer-Burgdorff G: Arterielle Durchblutungsstörung infolge cysticher Degeneration der Adventitia. Chirurg 31:481, 1960.
45. Kuijpers PJ, Mol PCM, Hoefsloot FAM: Idiopathic cystic degeneration of the left common femoral artery. Arch Chir Neerl 21:77, 1969.
46. Lambley DG: Intermittent claudication due to cystic degeneration of popliteal artery. Br Med J 2:849, 1963.
47. Leaf G: Amino-acid analysis of protein present in a popliteal artery cyst. Br Med J 3:415, 1967.
48. Lewis GJT, Douglas DM, Reid W, et al: Cystic adventitial disease of the popliteal artery. Br Med J 3:411, 1967.
49. Linquette M, Mesmacque R, Beghin B, et al: Dégénérescence kystique de l'adventice de l'artère poplitée. Semaine Hôp (Paris) 43:3005, 1967.
50. Little JM, Goodman AH: Cystic adventitial disease of the popliteal artery. Br J Surg 57:708, 1970.
51. Lord JW: *In* Haid SP, Conn J Jr, Bergan JJ: Cystic adventitial disease of the popliteal artery. Arch Surg 101:765, 1970.
52. Lowe DK, Winegarner FG, Jesseph JE: Cystic adventitial degeneration of the common femoral artery. Surgery 76:511, 1974.
53. Marzoli GP, Meyer-Burgdorff G, Jacquet GH: Sulle pseudocisti dell parete arteriosa. Chirurgia Italiana 14:291, 1962.
54. Mentha C: La dégénérescence mucoide des veines. Presse Med 71:2205, 1963.
55. Mentha C: Dégénérscence kystique adventitielle ou bursite de l'artère poplitée. J Chir 89:173, 1965.
56. Milliken JC: Cystic degeneration of the popliteal artery in a female. Br Med J 2:769, 1971.
57. Parkes A: Intraneural ganglion of the lateral popliteal nerve. J Bone Joint Surg 43B:784, 1961.
58. Patel J, Cormier JM: La dégénérescence kystique ou colloide de l'adventice artériel. Presse Med 71:244, 1963.
59. Patel J, Facquet J, Piwnica A: Dégénérescence kystique ou colloide de l'adventice. Presse Med 66:1164, 1958.
60. Pierangeli A, De Rubertis C: Degenerazione cistica avientiziale dell'arteria poplitea. Arch Ital Chir 92:108, 1966.
61. Powis SJA, Morrissey DM, Jones EL: Cystic degeneration of the popliteal artery. Surgery 67:891, 1970.
62. Richards RL: Cystic degeneration. Br Med J 3:997, 1963.
63. Robb D: Obstruction of popliteal artery by synovial cyst. Br J Surg 48:221, 1960.
64. Savage PEA: Cystic disease of the popliteal artery. Br J Surg 56:77, 1969.
65. Savage PEA: Arterial cystic degeneration. Postgrad Med J 48:603, 1972.
66. Schlenker JD, Johnston K, Wolkoff JS: Occlusion of popliteal artery caused by popliteal cysts. Surgery 76:833, 1974.
67. Schramek A, Hashmonai M: Subadventitial haematoma of the popliteal artery. J Cardiovasc Surg 14:447, 1973.
68. Shannon R: Cystic degeneration of the popliteal artery. Aust NZ J Surg 40:290, 1971.
69. Shute K, Rothnie NG: The aetiology of cystic arterial disease. Br J Surg 60:397, 1973.
70. Simon R: Dégénérescence colloide de l'adventice de l'artère poplitée traitée par prosthèse en dacron. Mem Acad Chir 89:849, 1963.
71. Sperling M, Schott H, Rüppell V: Die cystische Adventitiadegeneration der Blutgefässe. Chirurg 43:37, 1972.
72. Stallworth JM, Brown AG, Burges GE, et al: Cystic adventitial disease of the popliteal artery. Am Surg 51:455, 1985.
73. Stirling GR, Aarons BJ: Cystic myxomatous degeneration of the popliteal artery. Alfred Hosp Clin Rep 14:91, 1967.
74. Suy R, Van Osselaer G, Pakdaman A, et al: The pseudocyst of the adventitia of the popliteal artery. J Cardiovasc Surg 11:103, 1970.
75. Taylor H, Taylor RS, Ramsay CA: Cyst of popliteal artery. Br Med J 4:109, 1967.
76. Tracy GD, Ludbrook J, Rundle FF: Cystic adventitial disease of the popliteal artery. Vasc Surg 3:10, 1969.
77. Tytgat H, Derom F, Galinsky A: Dégénérescence kystique de l'artère poplitée traitée par greffe en nylon. Acta Chir Belg 57:188, 1958.
78. Velasques G, Zollikofer C, Nath HP, et al: Cystic adventitial arterial degeneration. Radiology 134:19, 1980.
79. Vollmar J: Die zystische Adventitiadegeneration der Schlagadern. Z Kreislaufforsch 52:1028, 1963.
80. Zinicola N, Ferrero S, Odero A: Adventitial cyst of the popliteal artery. Case report. Minerva Cardioangiol 21:474, 1973.
81. Lie JT, Jensen PL, Smith RW: Adventitial cystic disease of the lesser saphenous vein. Arch Pathol Lab Med 115(9):946, 1991.
82. Schroe H, Van Opstal C, De Leersnijder J, et al: Baker's cyst connected to popliteal artery cyst. Ann Vasc Surg 4:385, 1988.
83. Durham JR, McIntyre KE Jr: Adventitial cystic disease of the radial artery. J Cardiovasc Surg 30:517, 1989.
84. Stapff M, Zoller WG, Spengel FA: Image-directed Doppler ultrasound findings in adventitial cystic disease of the popliteal artery. J Clin Ultrasound 17:689, 1989.
85. Rizzo RJ, Flinn WR, Yao JST, et al: Computed tomography for evaluation of arterial disease in the popliteal fossa. J Vasc Surg 11:112, 1990.
86. Sieunarine K, Lawrence-Brown M, Kelsey P: Adventitial cystic disease of the popliteal artery: Early recurrence after CT-guided percutaneous aspiration. J Cardiovasc Surg 32:702, 1991.
87. Samson RH, Willis PD: Popliteal artery occlusion caused by cystic adventitial disease: Successful treatment by urokinase followed by nonresectional cystotomy. J Vasc Surg 12:591, 1990.
88. Melliere D, Ecollan P, Kassab M, Becqemin JP: Adventitial cystic disease of the popliteal artery: Treatment by cyst removal. J Vasc Surg 8:638, 1988.
89. Owen ERTC, Speechly-Dick EM, Kour NE, et al: Cystic adventitial disease of the popliteal artery—A case of spontaneous resolution. Eur J Vasc Surg 4:319, 1990.

61

Popliteal Artery Entrapment

Richard J. Fowl, M.D., Richard F. Kempczinski, M.D., and Thomas J. Whelan, Jr., M.D.

In 1879, T. P. Anderson Stuart,[1] a medical student at the University of Edinburgh, in writing a "Note on a Variation of the Popliteal Artery," concisely described the anomaly that may result in popliteal entrapment by stating, "The popliteal artery, after passing through the opening in the adductor magnus, instead of, as it usually does, coursing downwards and outward towards the middle of the popliteal space, so as to lie between the two heads of the gastrocnemius muscle, passes almost vertically downwards internally to the inner head of the gastrocnemius. It reaches the bottom of the space by turning round the inner border of that head, and then passes downwards beneath it—between it and the lower end of the shaft of the femur." It was not until almost a century later, in 1959, that the clinical significance of this anomaly was recognized and its management was described by Hamming of the Netherlands. Additional cases were later reported by Servello in Italy in 1962, Carter and Eban in England in 1964, and Love and Whelan in the United States in 1965. A recent review of the English literature on popliteal entrapment disclosed 249 reported cases of this anomaly.[2]

ANATOMIC FEATURES AND CLASSIFICATION

This entity results from a developmental defect in which the popliteal artery passes medial to and beneath the medial head of the gastrocnemius muscle or a slip of that muscle, with consequent compression of the artery. Rarely, an anomolus fibrous band or the popliteus muscle deep to the medial head of the gastrocnemius is the compressing structure.[3] Concomitant entrapment of the popliteal vein with the artery has been reported in only 7.6 per cent of cases.[2]

The most widely accepted classification recognizes five types of popliteal entrapment.[4]

Type I. The medial head of the gastrocnemius arises normally, and the artery is displaced in an exaggerated loop that passes medially around and beneath the muscle origin (Fig. 61–1).

Type II. The medial head of the gastrocnemius arises from a point more lateral than its normal origin. The popliteal artery descends in a relatively straight course but still passes medial and beneath the muscular origin (Fig. 61–2).

Type III. The popliteal artery is compressed by an accessory slip of muscle from the medial head of the gastrocnemius, which arises more laterally than the medial head. The artery descends in a relatively straight course, as in type II (Fig. 61–3).

Type IV. The popliteal artery is entrapped by the deeper popliteus muscle or by a fibrous band in the same location.[5] The artery in this type may or may not pass medially around the medial head of the gastrocnemius (Fig. 61–4).

Type V. This includes any of the above variants in which the popliteal vein is entrapped along with the popliteal artery.

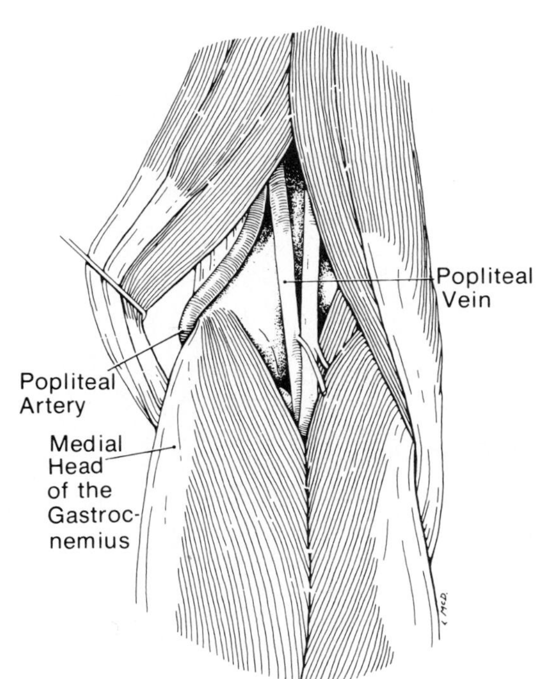

FIGURE 61–1. Type I anomaly: Exaggerated medial looping of the popliteal artery around and under the normally arising head of the gastrocnemius. Medial hamstring muscles have been retracted. (From Haimovici H: Vascular Surgery: Principles and Techniques. 2nd ed. New York, McGraw-Hill, 1984.)

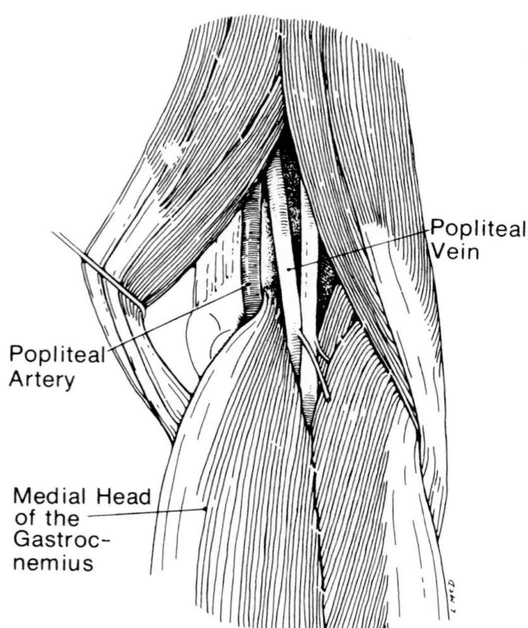

FIGURE 61–2. Type II anomaly: Course of popliteal artery is straighter but still medial and beneath the medial head of the gastrocnemius, which arises more laterally than normal. (From Haimovici H: Vascular Surgery: Principles and Techniques. 2nd ed. New York, McGraw-Hill, 1984.)

Other variations are rare and consist of hypertrophied gastrocnemius, plantaris, or semimembranosus muscles in highly trained and athletic individuals.[6, 7] Soleus and plantaris muscle entrapment of the popliteal artery in well-conditioned athletes has also been reported.[8]

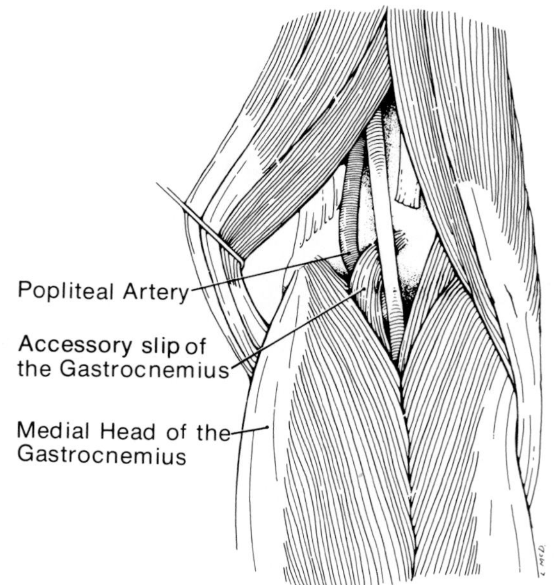

FIGURE 61–3. Type III anomaly: The structure compressing the popliteal artery is an accessory muscle or fascial slip arising more laterally than the medial head of the gastrocnemius. (From Haimovici H: Vascular Surgery: Principles and Techniques. 2nd ed. New York, McGraw-Hill, 1984.)

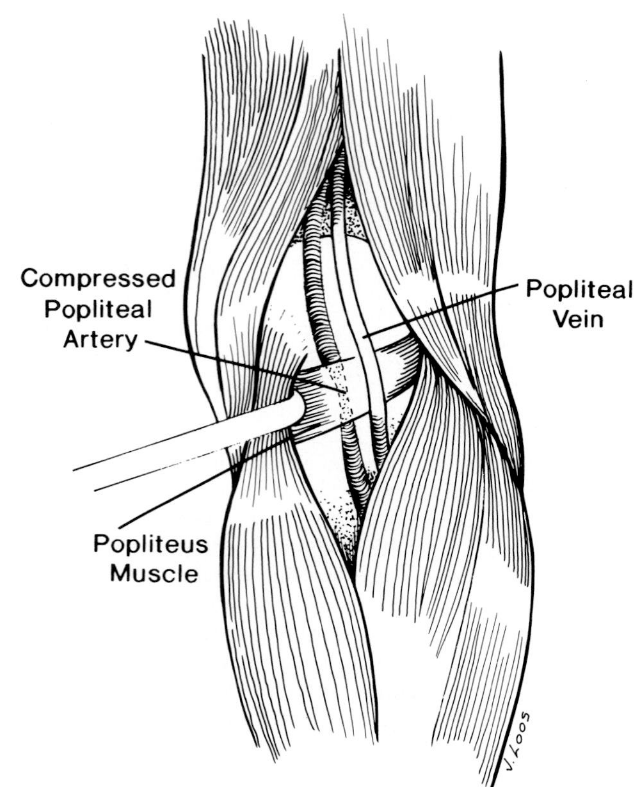

FIGURE 61–4. Type IV anomaly: The popliteal artery is entrapped by the popliteus muscle or a fibrous band in this location. The artery may or may not pass medially around the medial head of the gastrocnemius.

INCIDENCE

Hamming and Vink, who reported the first surgical case, reported four additional cases and claimed that the incidence of popliteal artery entrapment was 40 per cent in patients less than 30 years of age with calf and foot claudication.[9] In their overall population of 1200 patients with claudication, 12 were less than 30 years of age, and of these, 5 had popliteal artery entrapment. The condition, although described infrequently in the literature, is more common than originally thought.[6, 10, 11] Gibson and colleagues, in a study of 86 autopsy specimens, demonstrated the anomaly in 4 cases (3.5 per cent),[10] and Bouhoutsos and Daskalakis found 45 instances of the anomaly in 33 patients in a review of 20,000 Greek soldiers (0.17 per cent).[6]

CLINICAL FINDINGS

Claudication in the calf and foot of a young man should suggest popliteal artery entrapment syndrome. Table 61–1 summarizes the pertinent clinical data from a review of the literature comprising 249 cases. It occurs nine times more frequently in males. The onset of symptoms is often sudden, occurring during an episode of intense lower extremity activity (e.g., during the running of an obstacle course).[12–14] Although claudication is the only symptom in 69 per cent of patients, paresthesias occur in 14 per cent

Table 61–1. Characteristics of Popliteal Artery Entrapment

	No. Patients*	Sex	Age	Age Range	Distribution
Demographics	189	M = 90% F = 10%	> 30 yr = 67% < 30 yr = 33%	M 12–63 yr F 14–53 yr	Unilateral = 66%; R = 50%; L = 50% Bilateral = 34%
Symptoms	159	Claudication 69%	Paresthesias 14%	Rest pain/ulcer 11%	Other 6%
Pedal Pulse Findings	88	Absent 63%	Decreased 10%	Palpable 16%	Absent with plantar flexion 11%
Popliteal Artery Angiogram	199	Occlusion 53%	Stenosis 34%	Normal 13%	Occl/Sten with plantar flexion 24%
Operative Approach	122	Posterior 79%	Medial 21%		
Operative Procedure	196	Myectomy only 32%	Myectomy and arterial repair 37%	Vein graft arterial repair only 20%	TEA ± Patch 5% Other 6%

Data from Persky JM, Kempczinski RF, Fowl RJ: Entrapment of the popliteal artery. Surg Gynecol Obstet 173:84, 1991.
**Number of patients for whom data were provided because information on each characteristic was not available for all patients.*
M, Male; F, female; Occ, occlusion; Sten, stenosis; TEA, thromboendarterectomy.

and rest pain or ulcer is present in 11 per cent.[2] The latter symptoms usually are correlated with the development of segmental occlusion of the mid-popliteal artery, which was seen in 53 per cent of reported cases.[2] In the remainder, the patients had symptoms even though their arteries were patent, albeit compressed or stenotic (see Table 61–1).

The symptoms described by these patients include cramping in the calf and foot and coldness, blanching, paresthesias, and numbness in the foot associated with walking and relieved by rest. Symptoms are generally unilateral despite the common occurrence of bilateral involvement.[5] In a few patients with arterial compression but without occluding thrombus, claudication has had some unusual characteristics, for example, calf pain with walking but not with running, or pain beginning immediately with the first step rather than after walking a finite distance.[13, 15] Some patients present with frank popliteal artery aneurysms distal to the site of arterial compression.[13]

In most cases the anomaly is suspected from the patient's history, but certain physical findings may reinforce the suspicion. Pedal pulses are absent in 63 per cent, diminished in 10 per cent, and palpable in 16 per cent, but in 11 per cent pulses palpable at rest disappear with passive dorsiflexion or active plantar flexion (see Table 61–1). In addition, there may be evidence of increased collateral circulation around the knee. Geniculate arteries are palpable over the anteromedial and anterolateral aspects of the knee, which may be warm.

In patients who have characteristic symptoms but palpable popliteal and pedal pulses, the pathophysiologic finding is a compressed but nonoccluded popliteal artery. In this situation, two maneuvers must be added during palpation of the pedal pulses: passive dorsiflexion of the foot and active plantar flexion against resistance. With these maneuvers, the gastrocnemius compresses the popliteal artery, thus causing obliteration of the pedal pulses. This portion of the physical examination may be quantitated using an ankle pulse volume recording (PVR), which can document a decrease in PVR amplitude as evidence of arterial compression with the stress maneuvers (Fig. 61–5). Auscultation of the popliteal artery may reveal a systolic bruit if the artery is sufficiently compressed. The maneuvers just described should also be performed on the opposite asymptomatic limb because the predisposing anatomic abnormality may be bilateral.

Palpation of a popliteal artery aneurysm in a young male should suggest the presence of the anomaly. Evaluation of the venous system for evidence of obstruction at the popliteal level, namely, distended superficial veins, edema, and dependent cyanosis, completes the evaluation of the lower extremities.

The remainder of the evaluation consists of efforts to exclude diffuse arterial disease (i.e., arteriosclerosis, arteritis, collagen vascular disease, or a proximal source of arterial embolus). If the more usual causes of popliteal artery occlusion have been eliminated by careful examination, a localized anomaly in the popliteal artery is likely.

DIAGNOSTIC EVALUATION

The critical examination is bilateral femoral arteriography. The diagnosis of popliteal artery entrapment is unequivocally established when two or more of the following findings are noted on neutral, nonstressed views: (1) medial deviation of the proximal popliteal artery, (2) segmental occlusion of the mid-popliteal artery, and (3) post-stenotic dilatation. In addition, "stress arteriograms" should be performed with the leg actively plantar flexed against resistance or passively dorsiflexed to show compression that may not be seen in the neutral position (see Fig. 61–5).[16]

The most characteristic radiologic feature of the anomaly is the medial deviation. Segmental occlusion of the mid-popliteal artery is usually confused with only one other entity, cystic adventitial degeneration (popliteal artery cyst) with *thrombosis* (see Chapter 60). This same segment of the artery is involved in both entities, whereas degenerative disease or inflammatory diseases of arteries are almost never so focal or located in the mid-popliteal artery. Prior to thrombosis, a popliteal artery cyst presents the arteriographic picture of a smooth curvilinear filling defect encroaching upon the arterial lumen. Another important find-

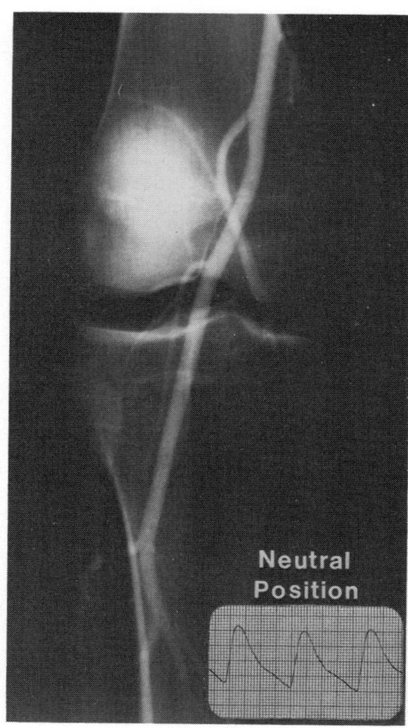

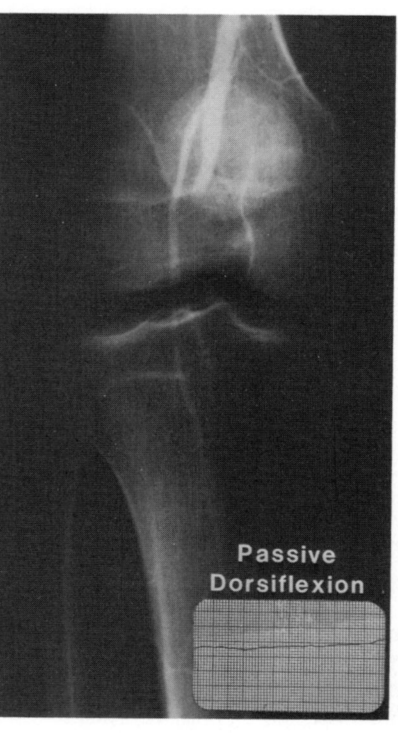

FIGURE 61–5. *Left*, Angiogram reveals a normal course of the popliteal artery with a normal ankle pulse volume recording (PVR) (*inset*) when the foot is in the neutral position. *Right*, With passive dorsiflexion of the foot, the popliteal artery becomes occluded and the ankle PVR becomes flat (*inset*).

ing is post-stenotic dilatation, which is present in 12 per cent of patients with this anomaly.[2]

Duplex scanning of the popliteal artery may be used to identify popliteal compression. A baseline scan is first obtained of the popliteal artery. If popliteal artery flow decreases or disappears with active plantar flexion, this suggests popliteal entrapment.[17]

Computed tomography (CT) has been utilized to determine relationships in the popliteal fossa when the artery is thrombosed because the arterial anatomy in the crucial area cannot be delineated by arteriograms in this instance. Popliteal artery cysts as well as anomalous insertion of muscle can be delineated by CT scan.[18] Magnetic resonance imaging (MRI) has also been able to define the anatomy preoperatively.[19]

If the remaining patent distal arteries and proximal femoral arteries are normal, the characteristic radiologic findings are present, and the physical findings are not suggestive of generalized arterial disease, preparation can be made for operative correction of the occluded artery, if present, and resection of the anomalous anatomy.

If there is any question about the presence of more generalized arterial disease, additional arteriography and appropriate tests to rule out metabolic or hematologic aberrations may be required. However, these procedures are seldom necessary in patients with popliteal artery entrapment syndrome. The localized symptoms of calf and foot claudication on one side usually occur in a young individual who is otherwise perfectly well.

OPERATIVE INTERVENTION

All cases of popliteal artery entrapment should be surgically corrected whether the artery is occluded or not. This philosophy applies not only to symptomatic limbs but also to asymptomatic limbs in which the anomaly is incidentally identified by routine bilateral arteriography. To risk progression to popliteal occlusion and potential lower extremity ischemic injury in such young, healthy individuals is unacceptable. The various procedures that have been performed in 196 patients are listed in Table 61–1.

The posterior approach to the popliteal artery has been most commonly used because it most clearly delineates all variations of this anomaly. Although the medial calf approach (Szilagyi incision) has been utilized and is satisfactory for type I lesions, it may be cumbersome and may pose problems in the management of type II, III, and IV lesions. When the occlusion extends to the popliteal bifurcation, medial incision may be more appropriate. Table 61–2 emphasizes the advantages and disadvantages of each approach.

Either subarachnoid block, epidural block, or endotracheal general anesthesia is applicable. The patient lies prone on the operating table with the leg slightly flexed to 10 to 15 degrees. The incision is S-shaped, with the cephalad vertical portion of the S placed over the posteromedial thigh, the caudad vertical portion on the posterolateral aspect of the calf, and the horizontal limb in the popliteal crease (Fig. 61–6*A*).

Wide flaps are raised in the subcutaneous tissue, exposing the deep fascia; the deep fascia is then incised longitudinally, avoiding injury to the median cutaneous sural nerve, which lies immediately subfascial at this level. The accompanying lesser saphenous vein may be sacrificed to obtain better exposure.

The first of the deep structures to be identified is the tibial nerve, which is mobilized as the vessels are approached (Fig. 61–6*B*). The vein, unless it participates in the anomaly, is found in the deep popliteal fossa passing

Table 61–2. Operative Approaches to the Popliteal Artery

Posterior Approach	Medial Approach
Better identification of the anomaly; surgeon does not miss it	May miss the anomaly; recurrences more likely
Adequate exposure for most cases	Better exposure for infrapopliteal vessel involvement
Limited access to saphenous vein	Better access to saphenous vein

between the heads of the gastrocnemius. The artery is not present in the normal location but is identified high in the popliteal space as it exits from the adductor canal. By distal dissection along the arterial adventitia, the anomalous course medial to the medial head of the gastrocnemius is verified. Transection of the compressing muscle or fascial band is begun at the point where the artery passes deep to it. The tight compression of the artery between the muscle and the posterior femur and knee joint capsule is remarkable. The transection must be complete and the entire artery must be mobilized. If the artery is compressed but not occluded, and secondary fibrotic changes have not taken place in the arterial wall, nothing further is necessary. The medial head of the gastrocnemius may be resected without disturbing function, or, if desired, the transected head may be attached to the femur medial to the corrected course of the artery.[13] Turnipseed and Pozniak described an unusual variant of popliteal entrapment in which the popliteal artery was compressed by hypertrophied soleus and plantaris muscles in well-conditioned athletes. Symptoms were relieved by surgical release of the soleus muscle from the tibia and resection of the plantaris muscle.[8]

Thrombectomy is required when the popliteal artery is occluded by fresh thrombus. Heparin (5000 to 7500 units) is given systemically prior to occluding the artery with vascular clamps. Through a longitudinal or transverse arteriotomy, thrombus is extracted, and a Fogarty catheter is passed to the ankle to remove distal clots or emboli. The arteriotomy is closed with a continuous 6–0 polypropylene suture. If pedal pulses are present, no further evaluation is necessary. If not, intraoperative arteriograms are indicated to demonstrate the point of obstruction, and either Fogarty catheterization of the distal artery is repeated or the arteriotomy closure is revised.

Intra-arterial thrombolytic agents have been utilized to disobliterate a recently clotted artery.[16] However, arterial bypass or replacement is still necessary for a patent artery in which thrombus has been successfully lysed because of the arterial wall injury and subsequent fibrosis and thickening due to the longstanding entrapment. If organized thrombus with a poor line of cleavage between thrombus and vessel wall is present, or if the vessel is narrowed owing to fibrosis, resection and vein graft interposition are indicated.[11] The graft can be obtained from the greater saphenous vein in the medial flap in the lower thigh. Alternatively, a short bypass vein graft can be utilized without resection of the thrombosed segment.

If a popliteal aneurysm has developed as an extension of the process of post-stenotic dilatation, resection and replacement vein graft with ligation of the aneurysmal segment should be performed.[15] It should be emphasized that in all operations on the artery, it is necessary to relieve the entrapment first by transection of the offending muscle. The wound is closed without drainage, using interrupted silk sutures in the deep fascia, subcutaneous tissues, and skin. Quadriceps setting exercises should be performed hourly until the 2nd to 3rd postoperative day, when the patient is allowed to ambulate.

RESULTS

Table 61–1 summarizes the frequency with which various operative procedures have been used. For patients requiring arterial reconstructions, the most successful procedure is vein graft bypass. Of 40 such procedures reported, only 2 (5 per cent) became occluded in the immediate postoperative period. Thromboendarterectomy, with or without a patch, has had the poorest results, with five of nine patients (55 per cent) developing acute postoperative thrombosis. Of 119 patients in whom results of surgical treatment were available, 103 (87 per cent) had results

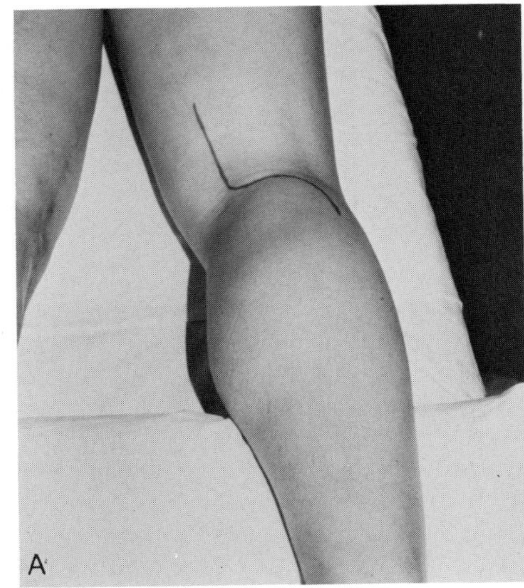

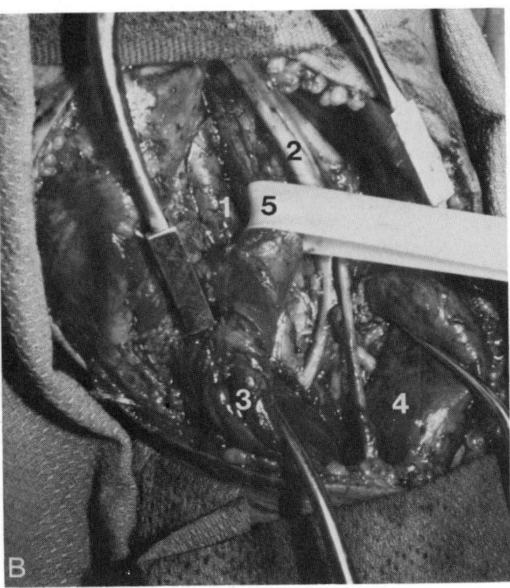

FIGURE 61–6. *A*, The S-shaped incision in the popliteal fossa is used for the posterior approach. *B*, Anatomic structures identified through the posterior incision are: (1) popliteal artery, (2) tibial nerve, (3) medial head of gastrocnemius muscle, (4) lateral head of gastrocnemius muscle, (5) Penrose drain wrapped around accessory slip of gastrocnemius muscle causing arterial compression.

described as "good." Eight required early reoperation, and in another 8 problems developed more than 1 month postoperatively.[2]

Complications that may follow operation for popliteal artery entrapment are thrombosis of the graft, bleeding, infection, and deep venous thrombosis. Graft thrombosis is indicated by loss of pedal pulses and is confirmed by arteriography. Reoperation should be carried out promptly to rectify the technical error and restore circulation. Although bleeding is seldom a problem, hematoma developing shortly after operation should be evacuated in the operating room under sterile conditions, with control of all bleeding points and thorough irrigation of the wound with saline or antibiotic (kanamycin) solution.

Deep venous thrombosis is the only indication for anticoagulation in the immediate postoperative period. Because adequate heparinization in the early postoperative period predisposes the patient to bleeding and hematoma formation, anticoagulation should be instituted only when venous thrombosis is confirmed. As in most vascular surgical procedures, prophylactic antibiotics should be used appropriately.

SUMMARY

Although popliteal entrapment is uncommon, it is an important cause of arterial insufficiency in younger patients. Accurate diagnosis depends on a high index of suspicion combined with dynamic noninvasive testing and "stress angiography." Although angiographic demonstration of medial deviation of the artery is diagnostic, absence of this finding does not exclude the diagnosis. Positional angiography may be necessary in such cases. Surgical exploration should be performed through a posterior approach because this facilitates identification of the precise anatomic variant while allowing easy arterial repair if necessary. The condition of the popliteal artery must dictate the extent of the surgical procedure. If the artery is normal, relief of the constricting lesion alone will suffice. If the artery appears diseased or is thrombosed, myotomy and arterial reconstruction must be undertaken. This is best accomplished by bypass grafting using autogenous vein or artery. If thromboendarterectomy is employed, the surgeon can expect a higher percentage of acute postoperative thromboses.

References

1. Stuart TPA: Note on a variation in the course of the popliteal artery. J Anat Physiol 13:162, 1879.
2. Persky JM, Kempczinski RF, Fowl RJ: Entrapment of the popliteal artery. Surg Gynecol Obstet 173:84, 1991.
3. Haimovici H, Sprayregen S, Johnson F: Popliteal artery entrapment by fibrous band. Surgery 72:789, 1972.
4. Rich NM, Collins GJ Jr, McDonald PT, et al: Popliteal vascular entrapment. Arch Surg 114:1377, 1979.
5. Ezzet F, Yettra M: Bilateral popliteal artery entrapment: Case report and observations. J Cardiovasc Surg 12:71, 1971.
6. Bouhoutsos J, Daskalakis E: Muscular abnormalities affecting the popliteal vessels. Br J Surg 68:501, 1981.
7. Rignault DP, Pailler JL, Lunely F: The "functional" popliteal artery syndrome. Int Angiol 4:341, 1985.
8. Turnipseed WD, Pozniak M: Popliteal entrapment as a result of neurovascular compression by the soleus and plantaris muscles. J Vasc Surg 15:285, 1992.
9. Hamming JJ, Vink M: Obstruction of the popliteal artery at early age. J Cardiovasc Surg 6:516, 1965.
10. Gibson MHL, Mills JG, Johnson GE, et al: Popliteal entrapment syndrome. Ann Surg 185:341, 1977.
11. Insua JA, Young JR, Humphries AW: Popliteal artery entrapment syndrome. Arch Surg 101:771, 1970.
12. Brightmore TGJ, Smellie WAB: Popliteal artery entrapment. Br J Surg 58:481, 1971.
13. Darling RC, Buckley CJ, Abbott WM, et al: Intermittent claudication in young athletes: Popliteal artery entrapment syndrome. J Trauma 14:543, 1974.
14. Love JW, Whelan TJ: Popliteal artery entrapment syndrome. Am J Surg 109:620, 1965.
15. Carter AE, Eban R: A case of bilateral developmental abnormality of the popliteal arteries and gastrocnemius muscles. Br J Surg 51:518, 1964.
16. Greenwood LH, Yiezarry JM, Hallett JW: Popliteal artery entrapment: Importance of the stress run-off for diagnosis. Cardiovasc Intervent Radiol 9:93, 1986.
17. di Marzo L, Cavallaro A, Sciacca V, et al: Diagnosis of popliteal artery entrapment syndrome: The role of duplex scanning. J Vasc Surg 13:434, 1991.
18. Williams LR, Flinn WR, McCarthy WJ, et al: Popliteal artery entrapment: Diagnosis by computed tomography. J Vasc Surg 3:360, 1986.
19. Fujiwara H, Sugano T, Fujii N: Popliteal artery syndrome: Accurate morphological diagnosis utilizing MRI. J Cardiovasc Surg 33:160, 1992.

62

Management of Foot Lesions in the Diabetic Patient

Jonathan B. Towne, M.D.

• • •

BACKGROUND

Because of the unique consequences of their disease, patients with diabetes mellitus are vulnerable to foot complications. In addition to being at risk for rampant and often widespread arteriosclerosis of the popliteal and tibial vessels, the diabetic also is subject to peripheral neuropathy with its resultant anesthesia, sympathetic denervation, autonomic neuropathy, and motor paralysis of the intrinsic muscles of the foot. This combination of occlusive disease and neuropathy makes these patients susceptible to foot ulcerations, infection, and gangrene. The magnitude of this problem is illustrated by the observation that gangrene occurred 53 times as frequently in diabetic men and 71 times as frequently in diabetic women as in their nondiabetic counterparts.[5] A similar increased incidence of atherosclerotic gangrene was also seen in diabetic women, and the usual male predominance seen in atherosclerotic patients was absent in diabetic patients. A knowledge of the pathophysiologic changes caused by diabetes mellitus is essential for the proper understanding and treatment of foot problems in these patients.

ARTERIAL OCCLUSIVE DISEASE

Diabetic arterial occlusive disease can be divided into four categories: (1) that of the aortoiliac system; (2) that of the femoral, popliteal, and tibial vessels; (3) that of the large vessels of the foot, namely the dorsal pedal, pedal arch, and metatarsal arteries; and (4) that of the small arteries, arterioles, and capillaries. The aortoiliac system is usually relatively uninvolved in the diabetic, and occlusive disease is usually most severe at the distal superficial femoral, popliteal, and tibial levels. Grossly and microscopically, the disease process is not dissimilar to that seen in nondiabetic patients with advanced atherosclerosis. In the diabetic, however, it is generally more widespread and rapidly progressive.[20, 25, 47] In a study of limbs amputated for ischemia in both diabetics and nondiabetics, no difference was found in the incidence of occlusive disease of the popliteal, tibial, or large vessels of the pedal arch.[12] Increased calcification was deposited adjacent to the internal elastic lamina in the smaller vessels of the foot, including the pedal arch and the metatarsal vessels, and a higher incidence of occlusive disease in the metatarsal vessels of the diabetic. Sixty per cent of the metatarsal arteries from diabetic patients had significant occlusive disease, compared with only 21 per cent of vessels from those without diabetes. There was also more involvement in the digital vessels of diabetics, in whom 19 per cent of digital arteries were obstructed compared with 10 per cent in nondiabetics. Calcification of digital vessels in this series was seen only in diabetics and was primarily limited to the proximal digital vessel, and atherosclerotic involvement of the distal digital vessels was rare.

Diabetics also have a microangiopathy that histologically appears as intimal thickening. On electron microscopic examination, this consists primarily of thickening of the basement membrane. Banson and Lacy found it in 88 per cent of diabetics compared with only 23 per cent of nondiabetics.[3] Its distribution was patchy, with normal capillaries often interspersed with diseased ones. Basement membrane width increased as one proceeded distally in the leg, suggesting an effect of venous hydrostatic pressure in its formation.[27] Siperstein and his colleagues, in a study of muscle capillary basement membranes by electron microscopy in human subjects, noted that the average width in diabetic patients was twice that in nondiabetics.[51] Increase in basement membrane thickness was common in diabetic patients, with 98 per cent demonstrating this lesion. Of interest was the fact that this thickening was seen in 50 per cent of patients who are genetically prediabetic but do not yet have any manifest problems with carbohydrate metabolism. This work suggests that basement membrane thickening is an early lesion of diabetic microangiopathy and is not a result of disturbance of carbohydrate metabolism.[51] This thickening usually did not occlude the lumen, however, and its role in selective capillary permeability and its effect on endothelial metabolism remain hypothetical. Some investigators have suggested that basement membrane thickening impedes the diffusion of nutrients through the capillary wall and limits the movement of leukocytes into areas of infection.[3] Goldenberg and associates reported endothelial proliferation of such magnitude that it occluded the lumen in digital and smaller vessels.[15] Other investigators, however, have failed to confirm this observation, and the importance of this thickening remains questionable.[3, 12, 20, 47] The thickening of the basement membrane tends to increase with duration of diabetes mellitus, suggesting that it may be related to carbohydrate intolerance.[56] However, the thickness of the basement membrane does not correlate with the severity or the regulation of the diabetes, and it is seen in patients with medically controlled as well as insulin-dependent diabetes.

Peripheral Neuropathy

Neuropathy is a unique complication of diabetes mellitus that predisposes these patients to foot injury and infection. The nerve lesion is a segmental demyelination that some investigators believe is due to a defect in the metabolism of the Schwann cell resulting in delayed nerve conduction velocity.[7] As noted in the capillary, there is a thickening of the basement membrane surrounding the Schwann cell, and in advanced stages there is a breakdown in the medullary sheath into separate concentric conglomerates. Nerves of the distal part of the leg were more commonly affected, with involvement of both medullated and nonmedullated fibers. There is diminution of anterior horn cells in the spinal cords of some diabetic patients.[10, 17] Degeneration of the dorsal columns is also commonly found and is most marked in the lower segments, resulting in scattered destruction and gliosis.[36]

When peripheral nerves are examined, the more distal portion of the nerve shows greater demyelinations than the proximal portion.[10] Neuropathy generally develops slowly, initially consisting of night cramps and paresthesias, progressing to a loss of vibration sense and perception of light touch and pain, and finally to a loss of deep tendon reflexes. Because motor nerves are also involved, diabetics often develop a weakness in the intrinsic muscles of the feet that results in pes cavus deformity, hammer toe with extensor subluxation of toes, and concomitant plantar prominence of the metatarsal heads and proximal migration of the metatarsal fat pads. The denervation of the intrinsic muscles of the foot disrupts the normal fine balance between the toe flexors and extensors, which is necessary for proper weight distribution while walking.[46] The protrusion of the metatarsal heads causes an overload on the protruding bone prominences during ambulation. There is also a decrease in the proportion of weight borne by the toes, this weight being shifted proximally to the metatarsal area.[27] Instead of the weight being distributed over a wide area, the protruding metatarsal heads, primarily the first metatarsal, carry the brunt of it during walking. There is a correlation between the site of an ulcer and the point at which maximum force is exerted while walking.[8] The increase in vertical force seen with abnormal sensation makes the diabetic patient more prone to develop ulceration in this area.

Another effect of the shift in weight bearing is to render these areas more susceptible to bacterial infection. Experimentally, it has been shown that bacteria localize in areas of compression, where their multiplication rate is markedly increased.[18, 41] Ischemia results in a decreased supply of phagocytes to an infected area.[34] In the animal model, denervation of a limb also results in increased bacterial growth in soft tissue following inoculation compared with growth in the normally innervated extremity.[40] It is unclear whether this effect is secondary to the presence of edema in the paralyzed extremity or to some other factor. The combination of metatarsal protrusion with the resulting increased load bearing and neuropathy with its loss of sensation makes the diabetic patient more prone to develop ulceration and subsequent infection. The pressure points encourage bacterial proliferation, and the decreased sensation allows the infection to progress without normal pain.

The etiology of the autosympathectomy often seen in diabetics is related to a decrease in the number of vasomotor nerves in lower limb arterioles. Electron microscopic evaluation of arterioles of diabetics demonstrates fewer axons in arteriolar smooth muscle than in similarly ischemic legs of patients without diabetes.[19] The mechanism of the obliteration of neural fibers is unknown, but the concept provides a theoretical basis for the lack of efficacy of lumbar sympathectomy in the treatment of ischemic lesions in the diabetic.

Infection

Although it is a common belief that infections are more common in diabetic patients, data supporting this contention remain controversial. Only bacteriuria can be documented to occur with increased frequency in diabetic patients.[54] When infections do occur, they tend to be more rapidly progressive and involve greater limb loss and a higher mortality rate.

Because of the immunosuppressive effects of diabetes mellitus, which lead to defective granulocyte and cell-mediated immunity, infections in diabetic patients are often due to different principal bacterial species than those seen in nondiabetic patients. Lye and colleagues demonstrated that urinary tract infections in diabetics were more likely to be caused by *Klebsiella,* and the contribution of *Escherichia coli* was much less than that seen in nondiabetic patients.[31] This was true for both community-acquired and nosocomial infections. The bacteria were also more likely to be resistant to commonly used antibiotics.

EVALUATION

The most important aspect of evaluation of the diabetic foot is the clinical examination. A careful neurologic examination should be performed with assessment of vibratory sense, proprioception, and light touch. The proximal extent of the neuropathy should be documented because it is common for only the forefoot to have significant neuropathy while the hindfoot and lower leg have relatively normal sensation.

The diabetic patient poses unique problems in the application of noninvasive techniques to quantitate lower extremity arterial flow. Because of increased vessel wall calcification in the medium-sized and small arteries, there is difficulty in compressing the vessels when arterial segmental limb pressures are measured. This is most marked in long-standing insulin-dependent diabetics and results in erroneously high pressure readings. As noted previously, there is much less calcification of the digital vessels than in proximal metatarsal, plantar, and tibial vessels; thus, toe pressures can be measured accurately.[12] The author and his associates use a photoplethysmograph attached to the toe distal to a small digital pneumatic pressure cuff. Accurate, reproducible pressures can be obtained, which correlate well with ankle pressures in patients with compressible vessels. These noninvasive tests are of greatest value in assessing the vascular supply of the foot and in evaluating the healing potential of local amputations or ulcerations.[6, 14] Holstein and Lassen reported successful healing of local amputations when the toe pressures were greater than 30 mmHg.[21] Only 9 per cent of toe amputations healed when digital pressure was 20 mmHg or less, whereas all 33 patients with pressures greater than 30 mmHg healed. Barnes reported successful healing in those patients with digital pressure greater than 25 mmHg.[4] Karanfilian and his colleagues reported improved ability to predict healing in patients with ischemic ulceration of the forefoot or digital gangrene by using laser Doppler velocimetry and by measuring transcutaneous oxygen tension. A transcutaneous Po_2 of greater than 10 mmHg was associated with healing in 95 per cent of patients. Laser Doppler velocimetry to measure skin blood flow velocity and pulse wave amplitude was also a reliable predictor of healing. A skin blood flow velocity of greater than 40 mV and pulse wave amplitude greater than 4 mV predicted healing in 87 per cent of patients.[22]

All other factors being equal, the pressure necessary for healing in diabetics is higher than that needed in nondiabetics. This is due in part to the aggregate effect of occlusive disease of both large and small vessels, which results in greater resistance and lower arterial flow at any given pressure.[53] Toe pressures have also been helpful in evaluating patients who have combined popliteal and tibial occlusive disease as well as occlusive disease of the small vessels of the foot. By quantitating the digital blood pressure, we can select those patients who will require bypass surgery sooner and avoid unsuccessful attempts at more conservative therapy, thereby shortening the patient's hospital stay. Toe pressures also give an objective measurement of the amount of occlusive disease between the ankle and the toe. However, ankle pressures that are falsely elevated because of calcified, incompressible vessels can skew these results. The author's normal toe-brachial index is 0.75, and an index of less than 0.25 represents severe occlusive disease. By calculating the toe-brachial index and measuring segmental pressures, the surgeon can evaluate the various segments of the vascular tree from the femoral artery to the digital artery and can quantitate the relative contributions of arterial obstruction at each level.

FOOT ULCERS

Ulcers in the diabetic patient can be divided into three groups: ulcers secondary to arterial insufficiency, ulcers in feet with normal vascularity but with severe diabetic neuropathy, and those in feet with both neuropathy and arterial insufficiency. Ischemic foot and leg ulcers in diabetics should be treated in the same way as ulcers in nondiabetic patients. These ulcers are typically the result of trauma: for example, striking the lateral malleolus, cutting the soft tissue while trimming toenails, or blistering caused by malfitting shoes. There is usually evidence of proximal occlusive disease, most commonly in the distal superficial femoral, popliteal, and tibial vessels and only occasionally in the aortoiliac segments. Noninvasive evaluation is diagnostic, with toe pressures usually measuring less than 20 mmHg; not uncommonly they are undetectable. Classic physical findings such as delayed capillary filling time, ischemic rubor, and collapsed veins are also found. The treatment of these ischemic ulcers begins with angiography. Distal grafting is performed if a suitable vessel is found. If no reconstructible distal vessel is detected on angiography, a below-knee amputation is necessary.

Patients with ulcers secondary to peripheral neuropathy present a different problem. They often have palpable dorsal pedal or posterior tibial pulses, and the tissues surrounding the ulcer are usually warm and well perfused. The neurologic examination will reveal a decrease in perception of light touch and an absence of proprioception in a dry, warm foot, suggesting autosympathectomy. Denervation of the intrinsic muscles is common, with protrusion of the metatarsal heads that causes a pes cavus deformity of the foot. The ulcerations are generally over the metatarsal heads, most commonly the first. Treatment begins by assessing the depth of the ulceration to determine whether tendon, bone, or joints are involved. Roentgenograms of the foot, especially magnification views, are helpful in determining whether osteomyelitis is present. It is important to note that both radiography and bone scans are often inaccurate for detecting bone involvement. Shults and colleagues found positive bone cultures and negative radiographs in 48 per cent of diabetic patients with foot ulcers.[50] Bone scans were negative in 33 per cent of patients with positive bone cultures. Excellent results with CT scan for detecting bone involvement have been reported by Williamson and colleagues, and CT scans or MRI should be considered if the status of bone involvement is in doubt.[55]

Sinograms are also useful to detect subfascial plantar extension and involvement of the joint space.[39] If the ulcer is limited to the skin and subcutaneous tissue, avoidance of weight bearing and local care are recommended. Because patient compliance may be poor, this treatment is often best done in the hospital. If the sinogram demonstrates a sinus tract, it must be unroofed, and all necrotic debris must be excised. Any infected bone adjacent to an ulcer should be removed as well. The success of conservative treatment is inversely proportional to the extent of peripheral neuropathy. If neuropathy is minimal, the ulcers heal like those in nondiabetic patients. If there is no osteomyelitis and no cellulitis in the surrounding tissues, the author does not prescribe antibiotics for these patients because studies have demonstrated the failure of parenteral antibiotics to influence the bacterial flora in granulation tissue.[42] Following successful healing of these ulcers, it is important for patients with severe neuropathy and orthopedic deformation of the feet to have special shoes constructed to distribute the weight as evenly as possible on the plantar surface and to avoid overloading the protruding metatarsal heads. The application of a total contact cast is an effective therapeutic option for treating diabetic foot ulcers. This technique has been championed by Brand and his colleagues at the Gillis

W. Long Hansen's Disease Center and often can result in healing of chronic ulcers.[11] Contraindications for cast treatment include acute infection, ischemia, deep ulcers, and draining wounds. When patients have multiple plantar ulcers or when peripheral neuropathy is limited to the forefoot, consideration should be given to transmetatarsal amputation. This accomplishes two objectives: it removes the area of ulceration and it places the insensate skin on the non–weight-bearing surface of the foot, as stressed by McKittrick and associates.[33] When there is adequate blood supply, these amputations usually heal without difficulty. Prior to any operative procedure, precise bacteriologic identification should be obtained so that preoperative antibiotics specific for the infecting organisms can be prescribed.

Conservative treatment of diabetic ulcers is frustrating because the absence of pain in the ulcer makes patient compliance less likely. These patients also frequently practice poor hygiene, in part because of poor vision secondary to retinopathy. Congestive heart failure with its resultant leg edema also complicates ulcer healing. Careful follow-up is necessary to detect the development of a plantar space infection and occasionally extension of infection above the ankle with septicemia and hyperglycemia.

Treatment of patients with combined neuropathy and popliteotibial occlusive disease is most difficult. The author relies on the clinical examination to evaluate foot perfusion: for example, capillary filling time, the warmth of the surrounding tissue, and digital pressures. Conservative therapy is not recommended in patients with a digital pressure of less than 30 mmHg. Arteriography and vascular reconstruction, if technically feasible, are performed.

SEPTIC FOOT

The most dreaded complication in the diabetic is the development of a septic foot. Often the patient gives a long history of an inadequately treated plantar ulcer culminating in extension of the infection into the subplantar space. A second predisposing factor is a superficial abrasion that becomes secondarily infected. The third and most common presentation is the secondary bacterial invasion of gangrenous tissue, most commonly the toe. The combination of vascular insufficiency with peripheral neuropathy allows the infection to progress without causing any significant local symptoms. These patients often present to the emergency room in a septic state, with their diabetes out of control and with coexistent congestive heart failure. Treatment must be prompt and aggressive if there is any hope of salvaging the patient's limb—and avoiding death from septic complications.

Bacteriology

Unlike infected gangrene in the nondiabetic, foot sepsis in the diabetic patient is usually due to infection with multiple organisms, both gram-negative and gram-positive, aerobic as well as anaerobic.[37] Louie and coworkers identified an average of 5.8 bacterial species per specimen from a diabetic patient's infected foot—among them, on average, 2.3 aerobic organisms and 2.6 anaerobic organisms.[30] When the subgroup with cellulitis was studied, these investigators found an average of 7.3 isolated organisms per specimen compared with 4.9 for patients with chronic ulcers. The incidence and distribution of the various bacterial species in this series are listed in Table 62–1. The prevalence of anaerobic bacteria in diabetic gangrene was disputed by Sharp and Bessman, who found only a 7.5 per cent incidence in deep wound cultures obtained at amputation.[48] Sapico and associates, in a study of 13 patients with diabetic foot infections, noted an average of 4.7 strains of bacteria isolated. Only 2 of 13 patients did not have anaerobic bacteria isolated from deep tissue.[43] In a more recent series of 26 patients with diabetic foot infections, the author identified 172 bacterial isolates including 95 aerobes and 77 anaerobes (mean, 6.6 isolates per patient).[45]

The organisms cultured from deep within the wound often differ from those obtained superficially. In the study of 58 diabetic foot infections that came to surgery, for which superficial cultures were obtained prior to surgery and compared with cultures obtained deep within the wound at surgery, Sharp and coworkers demonstrated that superficial cultures alone gave imprecise identification of causative bacteria (Table 62–2).[49] The averages for this study were 2.3 organisms for each superficial site and 2.2 organisms from each deep site. *Proteus* species and enterococci were the most common organisms cultured from both sites. When only the deep cultures were evaluated, there were only 13 that were pure (27 per cent of the total studied); four of these were *Staphylococcus aureus,* four were *Proteus* species, two were *Pseudomonas aeruginosa,* and there were one each of *Escherichia coli, Klebsiella,* and *Streptococcus.* Seventy-eight per cent of the patients had two or more organisms isolated from the deep wound. In another study, Sapico also demonstrated poor concordance of culture results between deep and superficial culture. Of all the techniques for obtaining superficial cultures, curettage of the ulcer and needle aspiration after normal saline injection into a site with demonstrable fluctuance or bogginess correlated best with deep cultures.[44] There is also poor

Table 62–1. Organisms Most Commonly Found in Foot Ulcers in Diabetic Patients

Organism	Per Cent
Gram-negative, aerobic	
Proteus species	55
Escherichia coli	30
Klebsiella species	20
Pseudomonas aeruginosa	15
Gram-positive, aerobic	
Streptococcus faecalis	45
Staphylococcus aureus	35
Streptococci (nongroup A or D)	35
Staphylococcus epidermidis	30
Gram-negative, anaerobic	
Bacteroides fragilis	45
Bacteroides melaninogenicus	35
Gram-positive, anaerobic	
Peptococcus species	80
Clostridium species	35
Propionibacterium species	25

Data from Louie TJ, Bartlett JG, Tally FP, Gorbach SL: Aerobic and anaerobic bacteria in diabetic foot ulcers. Ann Intern Med 85:461, 1976.

Table 62–2. Culture Results at Deep and Superficial Sites in Foot Sepsis in Diabetes

	Per Cent
Same organism cultured from both deep and superficial sites	17
No common organism	22
All organisms isolated in superficial sites found in deep sites plus additional organisms in deep sites	16
All organisms isolated in deep sites found in superficial sites plus additional organisms in superficial sites	14
Common organisms as well as species limited to deep sites alone and superficial sites alone	31
	100

Data from Sharp CS, Bessman AN, Wagner FW Jr, et al: Microbiology of superficial and deep tissues in infected diabetic gangrene. Surg Gynecol Obstet 149:217, 1979.

concordance between sinus tract cultures and the organisms cultured from operative specimens in patients with chronic osteomyelitis and draining sinus tracts. Mackowiak and his associates were able to isolate the pathogen by surgery in only 44 per cent of the sinus tract cultures.[32] The presence of multiple organisms, including both gram-positive and gram-negative as well as anaerobic bacteria, emphasizes the importance of broad-spectrum antibiotics in treating the diabetic patient with an infected foot. Traditional antibiotic therapy includes an aminoglycoside for aerobic bacteria, adding ampicillin to cover enterococci and using clindamycin or metronidazole for anaerobic bacteria. The renal toxicity of the aminoglycosides has been a major concern, especially in diabetics with deteriorating renal function. The author has determined that combining a semi-synthetic penicillin with a beta-lactamase inhibitor provides adequate coverage. Combinations of ticarcillin with clavulanate or ampicillin with sulbactam effectively provide broad-spectrum coverage without the renal toxicity related to aminoglycosides. Approximately half of the anaerobic cultures in the author's study grew *Peptostreptococcus magnus.* This organism has recently been shown to be a virulent pathogen in soft tissue infections, producing a collagenase enzyme that contributes to the rapid and extensive tissue destruction that is a clinical hallmark of diabetes-related foot infections.[24]

Treatment

The diabetic patient with a septic foot represents a surgical emergency. These patients are admitted immediately to the hospital, and administration of intravenous broad-spectrum antibiotics is begun. Their diabetes is often out of control, and occasionally they present in septic shock. If there is any evidence of septicemia or cardiac instability, a Swan-Ganz catheter is inserted for monitoring fluid resuscitation. Generally, 8 to 12 hours are required to prepare the patient for surgery. During this interval, hyperglycemia is controlled, any cardiovascular instability is corrected, and adequate blood levels of antibiotics are achieved.

An assessment of the vascular supply of the foot is made. If the patient has diffuse popliteotibial occlusive disease and an ischemic hindfoot, a guillotine amputation at the supramalleolar level is performed. In patients with a good blood supply (e.g., pedal or posterior tibial pulses) or in whom the hindfoot is warm and capillary filling is prompt, consideration is given to a foot salvage procedure. The initial procedure consists of extensive débridement of all infected and necrotic tissues, which must be excised without regard for subsequent reconstruction of the foot. This often includes several digits and metatarsals and occasionally extends to the level of the tarsal bones. All pockets of purulent material must be opened widely. The amount of devitalized infected tissue is generally much greater than the amount initially appearing on examination of the wound. The best indication for extension above the malleolar level is pain in the calf, which is accompanied by crepitation in late cases. At the conclusion of the débridement, all necrotic and devitalized tissue should be removed, and all the wound surfaces should be bleeding. In general, the author prefers to leave the cartilage intact over exposed bones to prevent spread of infection into the marrow cavity. The wounds are then reexamined in 24 hours. If there has been any progressive necrosis with new areas of gangrene of the skin edge and particularly the exposed muscle, the author proceeds with a below-knee amputation. Primary closure of the below-knee amputation is usually possible if there has been no evidence of any spread of the cellulitis to the supramalleolar level. Most wounds in which salvage of the foot is going to be successful develop a granulating base rather promptly, and by the third postoperative day, whirlpool treatment is begun to facilitate wound care. When the wounds are granulating well, consideration should be given to secondary closure. Although the wounds generally fill in quite well, there is usually a need for additional skin coverage to shorten the period of recovery, which is most often accomplished by the application of split-thickness skin grafts (Fig. 62–1). Prior to the application of skin grafts, the author obtains quantitative cultures to ensure that the bacterial count is 10^5/gm tissue or less. If the bacterial count is greater than that, he applies an amnion dressing or mafenide (Sulfamylon) cream to decrease the surface bacteria count. In resistant cases, however, he occasionally excises the granulation tissue. He does not recommend formal transmetatarsal amputation unless the medial three toes have already been removed.

One technique of obtaining skin coverage is to use one of the remaining toes as a pedicle graft (Fig. 62–2). The toe is incised on its medial or lateral side, taking care to protect the neurovascular bundle on its contralateral side. The proximal and distal phalanges are removed, and the remaining tissue is used as a full-thickness pedicle graft to cover the defect. It is important that the wound have a good granulating bed and that appropriate antibiotic coverage be selected. This technique provides a sensate full-thickness flap that helps to close rather large defects (Fig. 62–3).

In an attempt to salvage the foot, the surgeon must be vigilant not to overlook pockets of undrained purulent material. Postoperatively, any purulent material on the dressings generally indicates an incompletely drained abscess pocket, which must be incised and widely opened in the operating room. Often pain in the heel or above the ankle is the only symptom of extension of the infectious process. In an occasional patient, the infection clears with this treat-

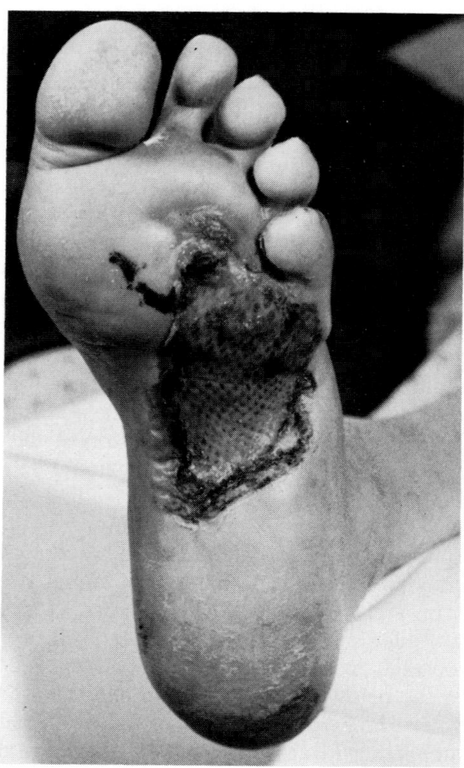

FIGURE 62–1. Split-thickness skin graft successfully applied to the plantar surface of the foot 3 weeks after excision and débridement of septic foot in a diabetic patient.

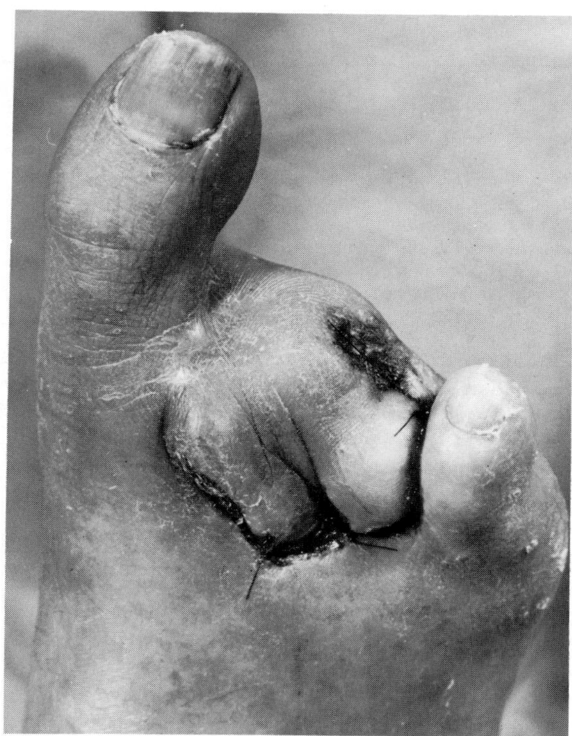

FIGURE 62–3. The patient's second toe was used as a full-thickness flap to close the large defect on the foot following débridement for sepsis.

ment, but there is not sufficient blood supply to heal the resulting wounds. In such patients, angiography is obtained, and the appropriate vascular reconstruction is done. The author is reluctant to perform bypass grafting even with autogenous vein in patients with active lower extremity sepsis in the belief that a primary amputation is preferable to exposing the patient to the risk of an infected vascular prosthesis. Because of the possibility that a toe may be used as a subsequent flap for closure, the author does not amputate a viable digit at the initial procedure even if its metatarsal is excised. On occasion, he performs a transmetatarsal amputation, usually as a secondary procedure to facilitate wound closure following control of the initial infection. These are often variants of the classic procedure because it is not unusual for several metatarsals to have been com-

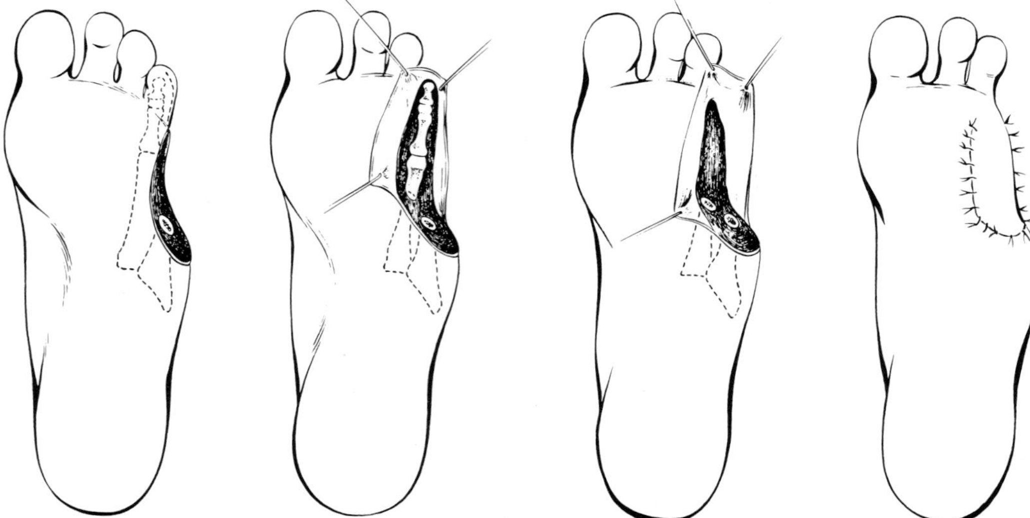

FIGURE 62–2. Technique for obtaining skin coverage following débridement of septic foot in a diabetic patient. An incision is made along the lateral aspect of the digit. The phalanges and distal metatarsal are dissected free and excised. The full-thickness flap is then sutured to close the defect.

pletely resected on the medial or lateral aspect of the foot. The author has found that this causes these patients no problem with subsequent ambulation. Generally, a minimum of two and often three procedures is required to achieve complete coverage of the foot.

ISCHEMIC GANGRENE

The diabetic patient who presents with uninfected gangrene of the toe or distal portion of the foot requires careful assessment to determine the best treatment. Depending on the blood supply, one of several types of procedures is performed. The first group of patients includes those who require additional inflow into the foot for healing. If there is no suitable vessel, a major amputation, usually below the knee, is performed. The second group comprises those in whom a transmetatarsal or toe amputation will heal. Those who present with pedal pulses obviously do well with digital amputations, but they are generally a minority of patients. Other criteria used to determine the level of amputation include the temperature of the forefoot adjacent to the gangrenous area, the presence of a relatively normal capillary filling time in the forefoot, and the results of noninvasive testing, as mentioned earlier in this chapter.

Toe pressure of 30 mmHg or more in the adjacent toes generally augers well for a successful toe amputation. If several toes are gangrenous and the distal foot is neurotrophic, transmetatarsal amputation is often preferable. The clinical indications for a transmetatarsal amputation remain similar to those listed by McKittrick and associates in 1949.[33] These include gangrene of all or part of one or more toes provided that the accompanying infection is stabilized and the gangrene does not involve the plantar or dorsal aspect of the foot, and an open wound involving the distal portion of the foot that can be totally excised. In general, lumbar sympathectomy is seldom of value in these patients. In questionable cases, this author looks for evidence of sympathetic activity by examining patients for sweat gland activity on the foot. This is accomplished by placing an occlusive plastic bag around the foot and lower leg for approximately 1 hour. If sweating is present, a sympathetic block is performed. In those few patients in whom a favorable response is obtained, a lumbar sympathectomy is subsequently performed. As noted by DaValle and associates, this procedure has limited success in the diabetic patient.[9] After 5 years, diabetic patients had a cumulative success rate of 19.1 per cent compared with 51 per cent for a general atherosclerotic population following lumbar sympathectomy for similar indications.

No patient should be denied a conservative amputation solely on the basis of noninvasive evaluation. The decision for amputation must consider a multitude of factors, including the noninvasive laboratory assessment, clinical examination of the extremity, and overall status of the patient. Gibbons and colleagues reported healing of amputations in 38 per cent of the patients in whom failure was predicted by ankle systolic pressure.[13] This group did not use toe pressures, however, which would probably have increased their diagnostic accuracy. There is no noninvasive evaluation that guarantees successful amputation because patients who have amputations may develop secondary progressive infection that further compromises their blood supply, resulting in advancing gangrene. The ankle pressure that is generally thought to be adequate for healing of digital or transmetatarsal amputation is 70 mmHg or greater.

There are obviously many factors that affect the development of digital or forefoot gangrene in the diabetic patient. Of special interest is the deleterious effect of edema secondary to congestive heart failure or venous insufficiency. Lithner and Törnbloom noted a close temporal relationship between the development of edema and the development of gangrene in 66 per cent of 247 patients who developed gangrene.[28] They also noted multiple lesions more often in patients with edema secondary to cardiac decompensation.[29] Edema causes increased tissue pressure, which makes it more difficult for the collateral flow to reach the tissues. Also, edema secondary to congestive heart failure often is associated with a decrease in cardiac output, which will affect the involved extremity more adversely than it does other parts of the body.

Bailey and coworkers noted a correlation between high hemoglobin levels, even within the normal range, and increased failure rate of digital metatarsal or transmetatarsal amputations.[1] Patients with successful amputations had a hemoglobin level of 11.3 ± 0.8 gm/100 ml, whereas those whose operations failed had a hemoglobin level of 14.0 ± 0.9 gm/100 ml. All 18 amputations in their series of patients with hemoglobin levels of less than 12 gm/100 ml were successful, whereas all 30 amputations in the group with preoperative hemoglobin levels greater than 13 gm/100 ml failed. This was probably related to a change in the viscosity of blood with increasing hemoglobin levels because an increase in hemoglobin of 2.7 gm/100 ml is accompanied by an increase in blood viscosity of approximately 25 per cent at high shear rates. Although this work has yet to be confirmed, hemodilution of some patients may be a useful adjunct prior to a localized amputation.

An innovative technique used to select the proper level of amputation is xenon-133 clearance. Blood flow of 2.6 ml/100 gm is sufficient for healing.[35] Although this technique is relatively new, its early success warrants further study.

The diabetic patient who requires vascular reconstruction generally has results comparable with those of nondiabetic patients. Reichle and associates reported a 5-year limb salvage rate for femoral distal popliteal autogenous vein bypass of 44.1 per cent in diabetics compared with 51.4 per cent in nondiabetics.[38] Throughout the follow-up period of their study, up to 10 years, the diabetic patients did slightly less well than the nondiabetic patients. In a series of in situ bypasses performed primarily for limb salvage, there was no significant difference in patency in nondiabetic versus diabetic patients.[26] These excellent short-term results have held up in long-term follow-up, indicating the durability of the in situ saphenous vein bypass.[2] In a more current series, Tannenbaum and associates reported a 92 per cent graft patency at 36 months in diabetic patients with foot infections.[52] These studies demonstrate that the revascularization procedures in the diabetic are durable and should be performed if technically feasible.

The importance of attempting to salvage a viable extremity in the diabetic patient is emphasized by the presence of contralateral disease that soon jeopardizes the other extremity. Goldner reported that 50 per cent of his patients who had a unilateral amputation developed an ischemic lesion in the contralateral leg within 2 years of the amputation, stressing the need for a conservative approach in dealing with these patients.[16]

In order to understand the relative contribution of infection and ischemia, the two major components of diabetic foot infections, the author's group stratified their patients into three groups classified according to the severity of infection and degree of ischemia. Group I patients required urgent operation within 24 hours of admission for débridement of infected gangrene, drainage of abscesses, and control of systemic sepsis. Group II patients presented with cellulitis only, did not require urgent operation, and usually were treated initially with systemic antibiotics. Group III patients presented with chronic nonhealing ulceration or dry gangrene, indicating that ischemia was the principal problem.

Forty-six per cent of the patients developed a lesion on the contralateral extremity in the follow-up period, occurring at a mean of 27 months following presentation of the original lesion. Of this group, 18 per cent required a major amputation of the original extremity, 10 per cent of the contralateral extremity, and 20 per cent of both extremities.

The incidence of early major amputation was greatest in group I (16 per cent), compared with 0 per cent and 1.2 per cent in groups II and III, respectively, indicating that foot sepsis is the major factor in early limb loss. Long-term limb loss varied from 20 per cent in group I to 18 per cent in group II and 39 per cent in group III, resulting in overall limb loss of 36 per cent in group I, 18 per cent in group II, and 40.5 per cent in group III. In the long term, both sepsis and ischemia affect limb salvage equally, with ischemia primarily causing problems in the follow-up period. The operative mortality rate was 3 per cent for major amputations and 2 per cent for revascularization procedures, demonstrating that these procedures can be performed safely.

These data emphasize the need for long-term follow-up of such patients. The role of education of the patient and the primary physician is necessary to detect problems early. Aggressive surgical care provides the best chance of avoiding major amputation.[23]

References

1. Bailey MJ, Johnston CLW, Yates CJP, et al: Preoperative haemoglobin as predictor of outcome of diabetic amputations. Lancet 2:168, 1979.
2. Bandyk DF, Kaebnick HW, Stewart GW, et al: Durability of the in situ saphenous vein bypass: A comparison of primary and secondary patency. J Vasc Surg 5:256, 1987.
3. Banson BB, Lacy PE: Diabetic microangiopathy in human toes. Am J Pathol 45:41, 1964.
4. Barnes RW: Discussion of Gibbons GW, Wheelock FC Jr, Siembieda C, et al: Noninvasive prediction of amputation levels in diabetics. Arch Surg 114:1253, 1979.
5. Bell ET: Atherosclerotic gangrene of the lower extremities in diabetic and nondiabetic persons. Am J Clin Pathol 28:27, 1957.
6. Bone GE, Pomajzl MJ: Toe blood pressure by photoplethysmography: An index of healing in forefoot amputation. Surgery 89:569, 1981.
7. Chopra JS, Hurwith LJ, Montgomery DAD: The pathogenesis of sural nerve changes in diabetes mellitus. Brain 92:381, 1969.
8. Ctercteko GC, Dhanondran M, Hutton WC, et al: Vertical forces acting on the feet of diabetic patients with neuropathic ulceration. Br J Surg 68:608, 1981.
9. DaValle MJ, Baumann FG, Mintzer R, et al: Limited success of lumbar sympathectomy in the prevention of ischemic limb loss in diabetic patients. Surg Gynecol Obstet 152:784, 1981.
10. Dolman CL: The morbid anatomy of diabetic neuropathy. Neurology (Minneap) 13:135, 1963.
11. Duffy JC, Patout CA Jr: Management of the insensitive foot in diabetes: Lessons learned from Hansen's disease. Mil Med 155:575, 1990.
12. Ferrier TM: Comparative study of arterial disease in amputated lower limbs from diabetics and nondiabetics. Med J Aust 1:5, 1967.
13. Gibbons GW, Wheelock FC Jr, Hoar CS, et al: Predicting success of forefoot amputations in diabetics by noninvasive testing. Arch Surg 114:1034, 1979.
14. Gibbons GW, Wheelock FC Jr, Siembieda C, et al: Noninvasive prediction of amputation levels in diabetics. Arch Surg 114:1253, 1979.
15. Goldenberg S, Alex M, Ram AJ, et al: Nonatheromatous peripheral vascular disease of the lower extremity in diabetes mellitus. Diabetes 8:261, 1959.
16. Goldner MG: The fate of the second leg in the diabetic amputee. Diabetes 9:100, 1960.
17. Greenbaum D, Richardson PC, Salmon MJ, et al: Pathological observation on six cases of diabetic neuropathy. Brain 87:201, 1964.
18. Groth KE: Clinical observations and experimental studies of the pathogens of decubitus ulcers. Acta Chir Scand (Suppl) 87(76):207, 1942.
19. Grover-Johnson N, Baumann FG, Riles TS, et al: Effects of surgical sympathectomy on innervation of arterioles in the lower limb of patients with diabetes. Surg Gynecol Obstet 153:39, 1981.
20. Guggenheim W, Koch G, Adams AP, et al: Femoral and popliteal occlusive vascular disease. Diabetes 18:428, 1969.
21. Holstein P, Lassen NA: Healing of ulcers on the feet correlated with distal blood pressure measurements in occlusive arterial disease. Acta Orthop Scand 51:995, 1980.
22. Karanfilian RG, Lynch TG, Ziral VT, et al: The value of laser Doppler velocimetry and transcutaneous oxygen tension determination in predicting healing of ischemic forefoot ulcerations and amputations in diabetic and nondiabetic patients. J Vasc Surg 4:511, 1986.
23. Klamer TW, Towne JB, Bandyk DF, et al: The influence of sepsis and ischemia on the natural history of the diabetic foot. Am Surg 53:490, 1987.
24. Krepel CJ, Gohr CM, Edmiston CE: Anaerobic pathogenesis: Collagenase production by *Peptostreptococcus magnus* and its relationship to site of infection. J Infec Dis 163:1148, 1991.
25. Levin ME, O'Neal LW (eds): The Diabetic Foot. St. Louis, CV Mosby, 1973.
26. Levine AW, Bandyk DF, Bonier PH, et al: Lessons learned in adopting the in situ saphenous vein bypass. J Vasc Surg 2:145, 1985.
27. Lippman HI: Prevention of amputation in diabetics. Angiology 30:649, 1979.
28. Lithner F, Tornbloom N: Gangrene localized to the lower limbs in diabetics. Acta Med Scand 208:315, 1980.
29. Lithner F, Tornbloom N: Gangrene localized to the feet in diabetics. Acta Med Scand 215:754, 1985.
30. Louie TJ, Bartlett JG, Tally FP, et al: Aerobic and anaerobic bacteria in diabetic foot ulcers. Ann Intern Med 85:461, 1976.
31. Lye WC, Chan RKT, Lee EJC, Kumarasinghe G: Urinary tract infections in patients with diabetes mellitus. J Infect 24:169, 1992.
32. Mackowiak PA, Jones SR, Smith JW: Diagnostic value of sinus tract cultures in chronic osteomyelitis. JAMA 239:2772, 1972.
33. McKittrick LS, McKittrick JB, Risley TS: Transmetatarsal amputation for infection or gangrene in patients with diabetes mellitus. Ann Surg 130:826, 1948.
34. Miles AA: Nonspecific defense reactions in bacterial infections. Ann NY Acad Sci 66:356, 1956.
35. Moore WS, Henry RE, Malone JM, et al: Prospective use of xenon Xe-133 clearance for amputation level selection. Arch Surg 116:86, 1981.
36. Olsson Y, Save-Soderbergh J, Sourander P, et al: A pathoanatomical study of the central and peripheral nervous system in diabetics of early onset and long duration. Pathol Eur 3:62, 1968.

37. Pratt TC: Gangrene and infection in the diabetic. Med Clin North Am 49:987, 1965.
38. Reichle FA, Rankin KP, Tyson RR, et al: Long-term results of femoro-infrapopliteal bypass in diabetic patients with severe ischemia of the lower extremity. Am J Surg 137:653, 1979.
39. Robertson C: Diabetic neuropathic foot sinuses. Proc R Soc Med 62:271, 1969.
40. Robson MC: Difficult wounds: Pressure ulcerations and leg ulcers. Clin Plast Surg 6:537, 1979.
41. Robson MC, Krizek TJ: The role of infection in chronic pressure ulcerations. *In* Fredericks S, Brody GS: Symposium on the Neurologic Aspects of Plastic Surgery. St. Louis, CV Mosby, 1978.
42. Robson MC, Edstrom LE, Krizek TJ, et al: The efficacy of systemic antibiotics in the treatment of granulating wounds. J Surg Res 16:299, 1974.
43. Sapico FL, Conewati HN, Witte JL, et al: Qualitative aerobic and anaerobic bacteriology of the infected diabetic foot. J Clin Microbiol 12:413, 1980.
44. Sapico FL, Witte JL, Conewati HN, et al: The infected foot of the diabetic patient: Quantitative microbiology and analysis of clinical features. Rev Infect Dis Suppl 7, p 5171, 1984.
45. Seabrook GR, Edmiston CE, Schmitt DD, et al: Comparison of serum and tissue antibiotic levels in diabetes-related foot infections. Surgery 110:671, 1991.
46. Sella EJ: Diabetic neuro-osteoarthropathy of the tarsus. Conn Med 43:70, 1979.
47. Semple R: Diabetes and peripheral arterial disease. Lancet 1:1064, 1953.
48. Sharp C, Bessman AN: Microbiology of deep wound cultures in diabetic gangrene. Diabetes Suppl 25, p 385, 1976.
49. Sharp CS, Bessman AN, Wagner FW Jr, et al: Microbiology of superficial and deep tissues in infected diabetic gangrene. Surg Gynecol Obstet 149:217, 1979.
50. Shults DW, Hunter GC, McIntyre KE, et al: Value of radiographs and bone scans in determining the need for therapy in diabetic patients with foot ulcers. Am J Surg 158:525, 1989.
51. Siperstein MD, Unger RH, Madison LL: Studies of muscle capillary basement membranes in normal subjects, diabetics and prediabetic patients. J Clin Invest 47:1973, 1968.
52. Tannenbaum GA, Pomposelli FB Jr, Marcaccio EJ, et al: Safety of vein bypass grafting to the dorsal pedal artery in diabetic patients with foot infections. J Vasc Surg 15:982, 1992.
53. Tenembaum MM, Rayfield E, Junior J, et al: Altered pressure flow relationship in the diabetic foot. J Surg Res 31:307, 1981.
54. Wheat LJ: Infection and diabetes mellitus. Diabetes Care 3:187, 1980.
55. Williamson BRJ, Teates CD, Phillips CD, Croft BY: Computed tomography as a diagnostic aid in diabetic and other problem feet. Clin Imag 13:159, 1989.
56. Williamson JR, Vogler NJ, Kilo C: Regional variations in the width of the basement membrane of muscle capillaries in man and giraffe. Am J Pathol 63:359, 1971.

63

Vasculogenic Impotence

Richard F. Kempczinski, M.D.

• • •

Leriche and Morel first described the association between impotence and distal aortic occlusion,[25] but Harris and Jepson were the first to report erectile dysfunction as a complication of aortic surgery.[20] These pioneering studies called attention to the entity of vasculogenic erectile dysfunction, but a true appreciation of the magnitude of this problem awaited more refined diagnostic techniques and a better understanding of the mechanism of erection.

Impotence, the inability to achieve or maintain an erection adequate for satisfactory coitus, must be distinguished from retrograde ejaculation, which is primarily a neurogenic disorder in which bladder neck closure does not occur and semen is deposited into the bladder. In such cases, the patient is still able to complete coitus and achieve an orgasm. Although impotence, by the preceding definition, appears to be a disorder limited to men, women with an aortoiliac arterial obstructive disease may complain of insufficient vaginal lubrication and loss of orgasm.[11] However, this is a much less common problem because female genital sensation depends, in great part, upon the integrity of the somatic pudendal nerves and their efferent sensory fibers. These are situated deep within the pelvis and are protected by the thick layer of endopelvic fascia. Secondly, collateral arterial blood supply to the female sexual organs is quite extensive. As a result, female organic "impotence" is extremely uncommon.[35]

This chapter provides a detailed description of the physiology of erection, as it is currently understood, and explains how the normal, delicate interplay of neural and vascular elements of this process can be disturbed by the patient's own arterial occlusive disease or by surgical attempts to correct it. Because vascular surgeons are often consulted by patients with erectile dysfunction, this chapter emphasizes the various diagnostic techniques that are useful in these patients. Finally, those technical modifications that should be employed during aortic surgery to prevent iatrogenic impotence, as well as the most effective treatment for established impotence, are discussed.

PHYSIOLOGY OF ERECTION

Since 1948, when Leriche and Morel first described the association between aortoiliac arterial occlusive disease and impotence, medical research has broadened physicians' understanding of the complex interplay among psychological, hormonal, neurologic, and vascular elements that is required to achieve an adequate erection.

Satisfactory male sexual function requires the presence of anatomically normal male genitalia, an appropriate hormonal milieu, intact nerve and blood supply to the genitalia, and appropriate physical or psychic stimulation, or both. Elimination of any single one of these elements or moderate dysfunction in several of them may result in impotence.

Neurophysiology

The precise neurophysiologic basis for erection remains unknown. The afferent and efferent neural pathways that appear to be involved in erection are depicted in Figure 63–1. Thoracolumbar sympathetic nerves (T12–L4) are believed to be important in mediating the psychogenic erections that can occur even in patients with complete sacral cord destruction.[39] However, younger individuals undergoing bilateral radical retroperitoneal node dissection in which both sympathetic nerve chains are usually removed rarely become impotent.[22] Therefore, sacral efferent outflow (parasympathetic) appears to be capable of mediating both psychogenic and reflex erections. Clearly, bilateral resection of the T12–L1 sympathetic ganglia can result in retrograde ejaculation. However, this should not be confused with erectile dysfunction.

Based on current neurophysiologic research, erection appears to develop as a result of neural transmissions that reach the genitalia via the pelvic parasympathetic nerves. Destruction of the parasympathetic outflow from the sacral cord will cause impotence. Clinically, pelvic operations, such as radical prostatectomy or abdominal perineal resection of the rectum in which parasympathetic nerve damage often occurs, have been associated with postoperative impotence in 70 to 100 per cent of cases.[24] The final common pathway for this hemodynamic control appears to be short adrenergic nerves within the penis. In the flaccid state, baseline adrenergic neurotransmission via these nerves results in contraction of the corporal lacunar and helicine arteriolar smooth muscle. Interruption of this adrenergic tone (e.g., with alpha-blocking vasodilators) results in shunting of arterial blood into the corpora and triggers erection. Pelvic nerve stimulation results in the release of acetylcholine and possibly vasoactive intestinal peptide (VIP) at the site of the corporal lacunae and helicine arterioles. Approximately 30 to 70 per cent of the neurotransmitter response is cholinergic, with the remainder possibly being VIPergic. Thus, erection can no longer be considered a purely cholinergic event, and acetylcholine is not the final neural transmitter.

The central nervous system loci that initiate erection in men have not been precisely identified. However, because these signals must reach the genitalia via the spinal cord, injury or transection of the cord may result in impotence. Reflex erections are possible in a high percentage of patients with lesions of the upper spinal cord, but the level of injury largely determines the preservation of erectile

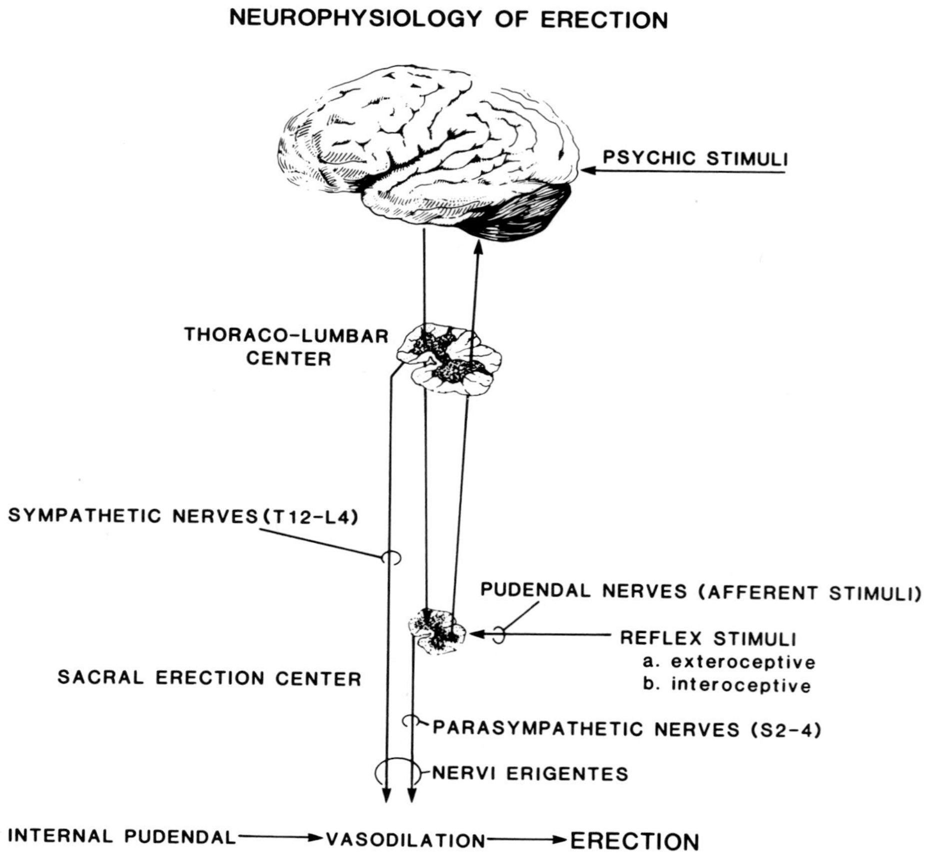

FIGURE 63–1. Diagrammatic representation of the neural pathways involved in penile erection.

potency. These reflex erections appear to require the integrity of the afferent pudendal nerves because pudendal neurectomies in such patients result in impotence.

Most drugs that produce impotence do so by their actions on these neurophysiologic pathways. However, it is difficult to determine whether their actions are peripheral or central. Ganglion-blocking agents, such as hexamethonium, are a well-known cause of impotence and ejaculation disturbances. Propranolol frequently causes impotence when administered in doses greater than 200 mg/day. Drugs such as reserpine, methyldopa, and tricyclic antidepressants probably produce impotence by their action on the central nervous system.

In summary, normal erectile function appears to involve both pelvic parasympathetic nerves and penile corporeal short adrenergic receptors. Although both alpha- and beta-receptors are present within the penis, alpha-receptors are believed to predominate in a 10:1 ratio. In addition, studies have suggested that VIP, either alone[40] or in synergy with alpha-adrenergic blockade[2] or acetylcholine,[3,4] may be responsible for erection. Thus, many questions remain regarding the neurophysiology of erection.

Penile Blood Supply

When neural pathways are intact, the ability to achieve an erection is largely determined by the adequacy of arterial inflow. The blood supply of the penis arises from the internal pudendal artery, which in turn is one of the terminal branches of the internal iliac artery. The paired internal pudendal arteries enter the male perineum through the lesser sciatic foramina. Each of the internal pudendal arteries, in turn, gives rise to a dorsal penile artery, a more laterally placed deep artery of the penis that supplies the corpus cavernosum, and a bulbourethral artery that supplies the corpus spongiosum (Fig. 63–2). Terminal branches of the penile arteries and the penile vessels themselves appear to communicate with the cavernous spaces via structures previously called polsters, Ebner's pads, or coussinets.[9]

Investigations in animal models and human volunteers have settled some of the long-standing controversy regarding the precise sequence of events in erection.[27] In the flaccid state, the arterioles are constricted and the venous sinusoids are contracted. Together, they exert maximal resistance against arterial flow, thus allowing only a small amount of nutrient blood to enter the corpora. The venules in the periphery of the corpora run between the adjacent sinusoidal wall, whereas the larger intermediary venules traverse the sinusoidal wall and tunica albuginea for some distance before exiting as the emissary veins. While the sinusoids are contracted, these venules drain freely to extrapenile veins.

During erection, the smooth muscles of the sinusoids and arterioles relax, which in turn increases sinusoidal compliance and causes a maximal decrease in the peripheral resistance. This results in an immediate increase in arterial flow and filling of the sinusoids. The resulting dilation of the arterial tree not only allows blood to enter rapidly but also permits transmission of the approximately 80 per cent of the arterial systolic pressure to the sinusoidal spaces (vascular or full erection phase). Subsequent contraction of the bulbocavernosus and ischiocavernosus muscles either spontaneously or reflexly compresses the proximal corpora and culminates in cavernosal rigidity with further engorgement of the glans penis as seen during intercourse (skeletal muscle or rigid erection phase). In the full erection phase, mean pressure in the corpora cavernosa is approximately 90 to 100 mmHg. In the rigid erection phase, compression of the blood-distended corpora can increase the intracavernous pressure well above arterial systolic pressure.

This proposed sequence of events is further supported by the work of Newman and colleagues, who infused the pudendal arteries of human cadavers at a pressure of 200

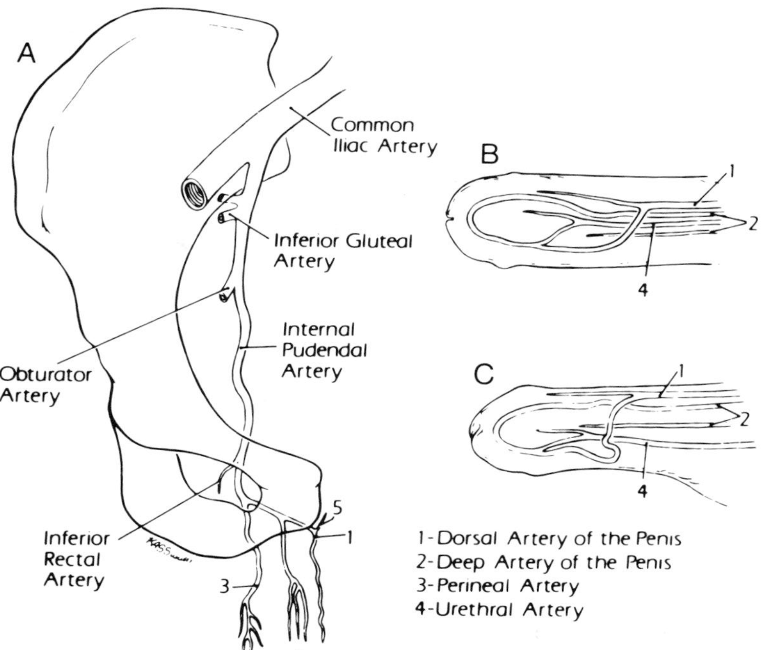

FIGURE 63–2. Major blood supply to the penis is from the deep and dorsal penile arteries and the urethral artery. These are branches of the internal pudendal artery, which in turn is a branch of the internal iliac artery. (From Queral LA, Flinn WR, Bergan JJ, et al: *In* Bergan JJ, Yao JST [eds]: Surgery of the Aorta and Its Body Branches. New York, Grune & Stratton, 1979.)

mmHg but were unable to produce a normal erection.[34] Subsequently, direct infusion of the corpora cavernosa at rates ranging from 20 to 50 ml/min resulted in a normal erection. Once an erection was obtained, it was possible to maintain turgidity with decreased infusion rates. These results are similar to studies by Michal, who demonstrated that a mean infusion rate of 90 ml/min directly into the corpora was initially necessary to produce erections in normal human subjects, but once an erection was achieved, maintenance flow rates of 62 ml/min were satisfactory to maintain erection.[30]

By injecting microspheres into the internal pudendal arteries in cadavers, investigators have confirmed the presence of arteriovenous shunts measuring 100 millimicra in diameter.[34] They also noted that occlusion of the dorsal vein of the penis failed to result in an erection. Thus, erection appears to occur as the result of preferential redirection of increased arterial flow into the corporeal spaces and active venoconstriction is apparently unnecessary.

Psychic Influences

Although more recent work has emphasized the frequent organic nature of postoperative impotence, the contribution of psychogenic factors should not be lightly dismissed. Following major surgical procedures, the patient and his sexual partner may be concerned that resumption of normal sexual activity could be potentially harmful, thus resulting in decreased libido and functional impotence. Even if such subconscious fears alone may be inadequate to cause erectile dysfunction, in the presence of marginal penile perfusion, they may be contributory. When initial attempts at resumption of normal sexual activity in the postoperative period meet with failure, a reactive depression may result, which can prolong the problem. If appropriate neurologic and vascular causes of impotence have been excluded in the postoperative patient, complete evaluation of the patient and, if possible, his sexual partner, by an interested and knowledgeable psychiatrist may be helpful.

DIAGNOSIS

Because so many factors can result in erectile dysfunction, a multi-modal diagnostic approach to the problem is essential (Fig. 63–3). Even in cases in which the underlying defect cannot be directly corrected, confirmation of the organic nature of the patient's impotence is vital in preventing the emotional havoc that this problem can wreak on his personal life. Furthermore, once the diagnosis of organic impotence is established, the patient can be referred for a penile implant, if appropriate correction of the specific problem is impossible.

History

Although many of the barriers that previously precluded frank discussion of erectile dysfunction have been dismantled, some patients are still reluctant to broach this problem with their physician. Because in some series 70 to 80 per cent of patients with aortoiliac arterial occlusive disease have been impotent[28, 33] and as many as 50 per cent of diabetics under the age of 40 may be similarly disabled,[14] vascular surgeons must be prepared to initiate such discussions with their patients. This is especially vital in preoper-

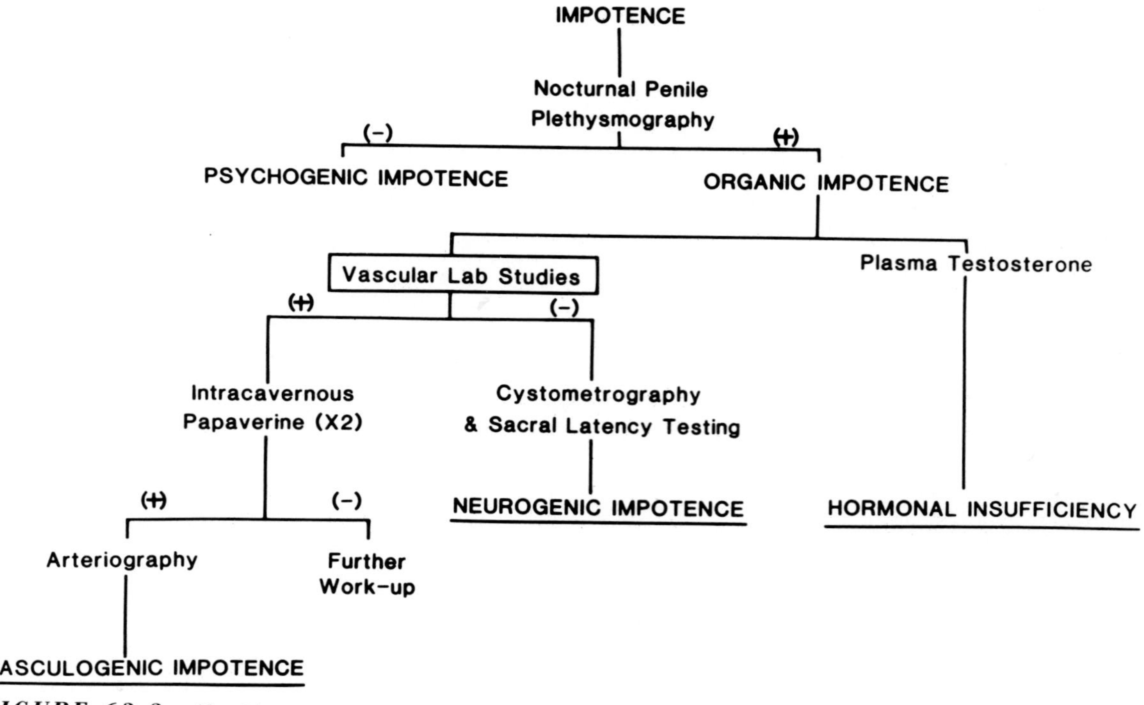

FIGURE 63–3. Algorithm suggesting a diagnostic approach to the impotent patient (see text for details).

ative patients, not only to permit modification of the operation to relieve their impotence, when possible, but also to document that it antedated the surgical procedure.

A careful and detailed history of the patient's sexual dysfunction may suggest its cause. *Organic* impotence is typically of gradual onset and results in complete inability to achieve erection. It is not partner specific, and masturbatory and morning erections are absent. The onset of the patient's symptoms cannot be related to any identifiable emotional stress, and libido is typically retained. By contrast, *psychogenic* impotence may be rapid in onset, frequently less than 1 month, and may be intermittent in pattern. Partner specificity may be present, and erection can be achieved during masturbation. Morning erections occur, and the onset of the patient's symptoms frequently can be related to an identifiable emotional stress. The presence of normal sexual drive may be quite variable.

In patients with known organic impotence, certain historical features help to differentiate those with a neurogenic from those with a vasculogenic impotence. Patients suffering from *neurogenic* impotence are usually unable to achieve erections at all and may have decreased testicular sensation upon palpation. Ejaculation with masturbation in such patients is generally absent. On the other hand, patients with *vasculogenic* impotence may be able to achieve an erection temporarily, but it is short lived. Testicular pain on palpation is normal, and masturbatory ejaculations are present. In patients with external iliac artery occlusion, the ipsilateral internal iliac artery may be the major collateral blood supply to the lower extremity. Some of these patients may complain that although they are able to achieve a satisfactory erection during foreplay, when thrusting is initiated, the penis becomes flaccid and coitus becomes impossible. Presumably, the increased demand for blood by the buttock and thigh muscles during active coitus shunts blood away from the genitalia, causing loss of erection.[33]

Nocturnal Penile Tumescence

A study, based upon the observation that sexually potent males have regular erections during the rapid eye movement (REM) phase of sleep,[6] found that the complete absence of tumescence during an adequate sleep study is strong evidence of organic impotence. Unfortunately, the failure of erection is often qualitative rather than complete, and it has been difficult to standardize the *quality* of erections. Such studies are difficult to perform properly and are best carried out on an inpatient basis in specially equipped sleep laboratories.[21] Changes in penile circumference are monitored by means of mercury-filled strain gauges or video camera characterizations of the quality of the erection. The documentation of normal erections during REM sleep clearly establishes the psychogenic basis of the patient's erectile dysfunction and allows appropriate therapy.

Noninvasive Vascular Testing

Canning and colleagues first emphasized that vascular insufficiency of the pelvic vessels, even in the presence of normal femoral pulses, could result in impotence.[8] They attempted to identify such patients by palpating penile pulses and performing impedance plethysmography. Subsequently, other investigators assessed penile blood flow using mercury strain gauge plethysmography, spectrographic or ultrasonic measurement of penile systolic pressure, and pulse volume recordings.[1, 7, 18, 23] When such studies are abnormal and the possibility of vasculogenic impotence is likely, more traditional noninvasive tests to exclude aortoiliac arterial occlusive disease should be performed (see Chapter 5).

Kempczinski studied 134 patients using the Doppler velocity meter to measure penile systolic pressure.[23] This, in turn, was divided by brachial systolic pressure to obtain a penile-brachial index (PBI). Pulse volume waveforms (PVW) of penile volume change with each systolic ejection were also recorded. The influence of both sexual function and patient age on each of these parameters was then determined.

Age exerted a deleterious influence on all variables of penile blood flow independent of the status of sexual potency. Patients under the age of 40 had a mean PBI of 0.99 compared with a PBI of 0.74 for equally potent males over the age of 40. This difference was statistically significant. By contrast, impotent males over the age of 40 had a mean PBI of 0.58, which was also a statistically significant difference (Fig. 63–4).

The PVW of patients under the age of 40 was of good to fair quality, and no poor quality waveforms were observed. With increasing age and sexual dysfunction, a greater percentage of patients had poor quality waveforms, but this difference was not statistically significant. The validity of these findings has been confirmed by numerous other investigators, who have emphasized the importance

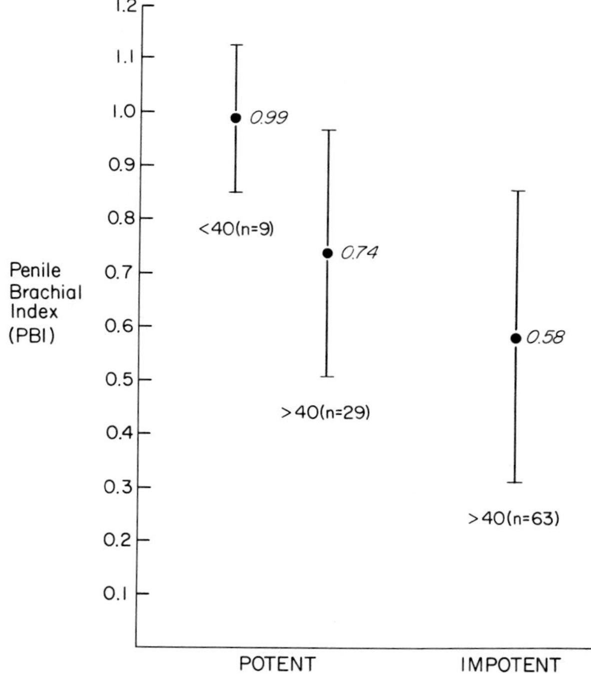

FIGURE 63–4. Distribution of penile : brachial index (mean ± SD) in patients by age and sexual potency. (Based on data from Kempczinski RF: Role of the vascular diagnostic laboratory in the evaluation of male impotence. Am J Surg 138:278, 1979.)

of this type of testing in the evaluation of patients with erectile dysfunction.[29, 36] However, the diagnosis of vasculogenic impotence cannot be established solely on the basis of such noninvasive measurements. Although mean PBIs differed significantly among the three groups, there was a great deal of overlap, and several male patients were fully potent despite PBIs of less than 0.6. Other investigators have similarly confirmed a lack of correlation between the PBI and the degree of erectile dysfunction.[33] Although a low PBI is not sufficient to establish the diagnosis of vasculogenic impotence, the finding of a PBI of greater than 0.8 confirms the adequacy of penile blood flow and suggests that vasculogenic impotence is extremely unlikely.

DePalma and associates placed greater emphasis on the diagnostic importance of the penile PVW.[10] Using a pneumoplethysmographic cuff containing a pressure transducer, they inflated the cuff to mean arterial pressure and recorded waveforms on a polygraph. A waveform amplitude of more than 6 mm and a systolic upstroke rate of 4 to 6 mm at a chart speed of 25 mm/sec were considered normal. Marked flattening of the waveforms with delayed upstroke greater than 6 mm and rounded waveforms were considered abnormal. Although they noted certain borderline categories in which diagnosis was equivocal, the technique was particularly helpful in cases in which the PBI was between 0.6 and 0.7.

Lue and colleagues reported the use of ultrasonography and pulsed Doppler spectrum analysis in the evaluation of vasculogenic impotence.[26] Using a high-resolution 10-MHz ultrasound probe, they were able to visualize the cavernous arteries, dorsal veins, tunica albuginea, corpora cavernosa, and corpus spongiosum clearly. The diameter of the arterial lumina, the thickness of the arterial walls, and the quality of their pulsations were assessed before and after papaverine injection. The pulsed Doppler was then used to study the blood flow through each of the penile arteries. Because this test can only be performed on the vessels distal to the pubis, further visualization with internal pudendal arteriography was required when ultrasonography suggested arterial disease.

In a more recent study, Kornick and colleagues used the color flow Doppler to study a group of 70 male patients with erectile dysfunction.[41] By analyzing flow velocities and volumes within the penile arteries before and after an intracorporeal injection of papaverine, they were easily able to identify such anatomic abnormalities as venous leaks (19 per cent), arteriovenous malformations (1.4 per cent), and arterial occlusive disease (53 per cent) as the cause of the impotence in their patients. The remaining 27 per cent of patients were impotent owing to nonvascular causes.

Neurologic Testing

Because there are no direct measures of the neural pathways involved in erection, indirect measures must be employed. Fortunately, the autonomic pathways involved in micturition and erection are similar, and *cystometrography* with measurement of bladder capacity and residual urine can be used as an indirect measure of penile innervation, assuming that involvement of the appropriate pelvic nerves would be reflected by abnormalities in both areas. Using this technique, Ellenberg was able to confirm neuropathy in 82 per cent of impotent diabetic subjects.[14]

The bulbocavernosus reflex may be quantified by indirect measurement of pudendal nerve velocity (*sacral latency testing*). Because this examination requires electrical stimulation of the penile skin with simultaneous electromyographic recording of the response in the bulbocavernosus muscle, it must usually be performed under general anesthesia. The technique has been modified by using surface-mounted perineal electrodes, thus making measurement of somatosensory-evoked potentials (SEP) from the dorsal penile and posterior tibial nerves more comfortable. Values of three standard deviations above the mean are considered abnormal.[10]

Intracavernous Papaverine

This technique is useful in differentiating vasculogenic from psychogenic impotence.[27] However, it cannot distinguish psychogenic erectile dysfunction from neurogenic or hormonal impotence. It should be used only to supplement a careful history and physical examination, not to supplant them.

In patients with a penis of average size, 60 mg of papaverine diluted with 2 to 5 ml of normal saline are injected into the corpus cavernosum. A rubber band is wrapped tightly around the base of the penis before the injection to ensure that most of the drug remains in the corpus, and it is left in place for 2 minutes after injection. The dose of papaverine may need to be adjusted in patients with an unusually large or small penis. In patients suspected of having neurogenic impotence, an initial test dose of 15 mg of papaverine should be used because these individuals are prone to suffer priapism.

After the rubber band is removed, the patient is asked to stand to increase the venous pressure in the pelvis and to further reduce the entry of papaverine into the systemic circulation. If the patient develops a full erection within 10 minutes and if it lasts for more than 30 minutes, the arterial, venous, and sinusoidal mechanisms can be assumed to be normal, and vasculogenic impotence can be excluded. However, because a nervous or anxious patient may not develop a full erection under the conditions of testing, a poor response does not infallibly confirm vasculogenic impotence.[27] When two or more injections fail to produce an adequate erection, an angiogram should be considered.

Angiography

The pelvic vasculature can be visualized using standard angiographic techniques with appropriate oblique projections. This should be the first procedure performed when large vessel arterial occlusive disease or aortic aneurysm is suspected. Patency of the internal iliac artery on each side should be determined, and the presence of significant lesions should be noted. Unfortunately, arteriographic findings correlate poorly with the patient's erectile function. In one study in which these were compared, 23 per cent of potent males undergoing aortic operation were noted to

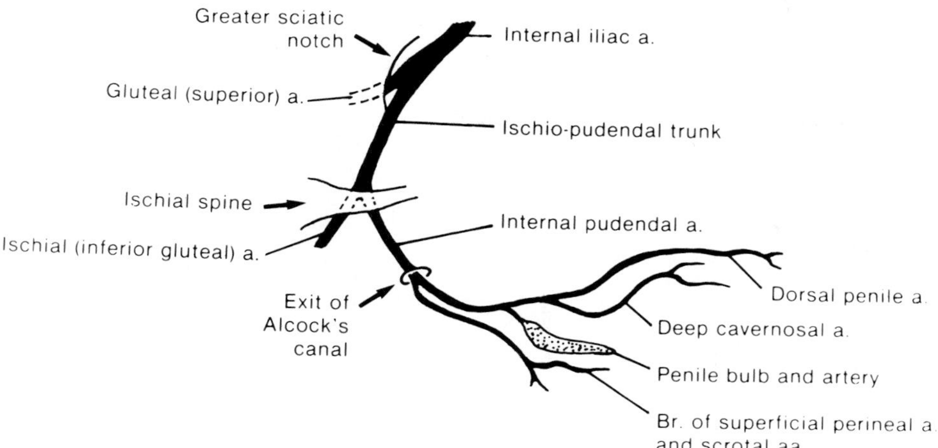

FIGURE 63–5. Idealized normal subselective angiogram. Note filling of dorsal and deep penile arteries. The arteries of the corpus spongiosum do not visualize. (Reproduced with permission from DePalma RG, Emsellem HA, Edwards CM, et al: A screening sequence for vasculogenic impotence. J Vasc Surg 5:228, 1987.)

have bilateral iliac artery occlusions, and an additional 36 per cent had unilateral occlusion.[16] This should not be surprising because routine angiograms rarely provide complete definition of the distal penile vasculature and cannot assess the adequacy of collateral blood flow around arterial occlusive lesions.

When no flow-reducing lesions are identified in the hypogastric arteries or their major branches, selective cannulation of the internal pudendal artery with the patient positioned in the appropriate degree of obliquity may be necessary. Because selective cannulation of this vessel may be difficult and the subsequent injection of dye may be painful, such studies are usually performed under epidural anesthesia.[19] Intra-arterial vasodilators, prior to the injection of contrast, are important for improving visualization of the penile arteries (Fig. 63–5).

Corpus cavernosography, which can usually be performed under local anesthesia, may be used in the assessment of patients with erectile dysfunction that is thought to be secondary to venous outflow problems. However, pulsed Doppler sonography should routinely be performed in such patients because only those with a normal sinusoidal system and arterial tree will have a good arterial response to papaverine.[27] If they do not achieve a full erection, their problem can be attributed to abnormal venous channels rather than to sinusoidal fibrosis. In addition, patients with congenital or acquired chordee may require cavernosography.[15]

PREVENTION

In order to ensure preservation of erectile function, surgical correction of aortoiliac occlusive disease must accomplish the following objectives: minimal disturbance of genital autonomic function, maintenance of adequate pelvic blood flow, and successful revascularization of the ischemic extremity. DePalma and colleagues[12] popularized a nerve-sparing procedure for the infrarenal aorta that emphasizes approaching the abdominal aorta along its right lateral aspect, minimal division of longitudinal periaortic tissues to the left of the infrarenal aorta, avoidance of dissection at the base of the inferior mesenteric artery, and sparing of the nerve plexuses that cross the left common iliac artery (Fig. 63–6). Using such a nerve-sparing approach, several authors have achieved a notable reduction in postoperative impotence.[13, 16, 32, 38]

Although the findings on preoperative angiograms correlate poorly with erectile function, preservation of adequate perfusion into at least one hypogastric artery appears to be a vital component of all operations that are successful in minimizing iatrogenic erectile dysfunction. When possible, direct antegrade perfusion of the internal iliac artery should be ensured. This may require thromboendarterectomy of the hypogastric artery orifice, when appropriate. If both external iliac arteries are occluded or stenotic, and bypass into the common femoral arteries is anticipated, proximal aortic anastomoses should be performed in an end-to-side fashion because retrograde perfusion of the internal iliac artery would be impossible in such circumstances and significant reduction of pelvic blood flow would be likely. When proximal disease is so extensive that thromboendarterectomy is impractical and preoperative noninvasive testing has confirmed decreased penile perfusion, simple aortofemoral grafting may not always restore a pelvic collateral blood flow that is adequate to relieve vasculogenic impotence. Although preoperative recognition of such cases is not easy, when the probability seems likely, the surgeon should consider reimplanting the hypogastric artery into one limb of the aortofemoral graft or adding a jump graft into the distal hypogastric artery.[5]

In patients with unilateral iliac artery occlusive disease, the objectives of nerve sparing, extremity revascularization, and increased hypogastric artery perfusion may all be accomplished using femorofemoral bypass. Several investigators have confirmed the success of this procedure in improving penile blood flow and restoring erection.[29, 37] Femorofemoral bypass is especially appropriate for young, sexually active males with unilateral disease because it avoids the necessity for *any* periaortic dissection.

When direct aortic reconstruction is necessary, it is important to avoid flushing atheromatous debris down the hypogastric artery.[16] Operative technique should be modified to backbleed the hypogastric arteries adequately prior to completion of anastomoses. Unfortunately, emergent aortic surgery, such as the resection of a ruptured abdominal

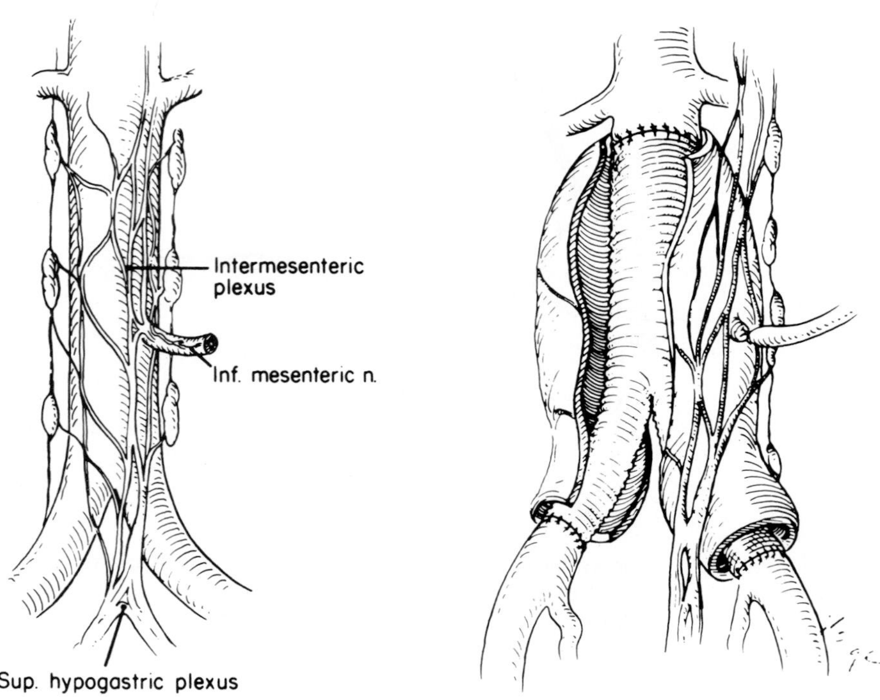

FIGURE 63–6. Diagrammatic representation of the autonomic nerve supply to the penis (*left*) and suggested modification of the surgical approach to the aorta during resection of abdominal aortic aneurysms (*right*) to minimize damage to these structures. (From Weinstein MH, Machleder HI: Sexual function after aortoiliac surgery. Ann Surg 181:787, 1975.)

aortic aneurysm, rarely allows time for the careful anatomic dissection necessary to avoid nerve damage, and the incidence of iatrogenic impotence is, accordingly, higher.[17] Although rarely under the control of the vascular surgeon, emergent operations should be avoided whenever possible.

TREATMENT

Once organic impotence is confirmed, a precise etiologic diagnosis is essential prior to initiating appropriate therapy. If arteriograms confirm occlusion of the proximal pelvic arteries and the measured PBI is less than 0.6, bypass into a distal patent branch of the hypogastric artery on at least one side should be considered. If the PBI is less than 0.6 but no large vessel occlusive lesions are identified, selective angiograms of the internal pudendal artery may document more distal occlusive lesions. If patent deep penile or dorsal penile arteries can be confirmed, consideration should be given to direct revascularization of the penis using the inferior epigastric artery and microvascular anastomosis into one of these vessels. Although the long-term durability of such procedures has not been documented, initial success has been reported in approximately 70 per cent of such procedures.[31]

When neurogenic impotence is documented, patients may be managed by teaching them to perform self-injection of intracorporeal papaverine or by implantation of a suitable penile prosthesis. In hypertensive patients who require ganglion-blocking drugs to control their disease and who develop impotence secondary to such medications, alternate forms of treatment should be found. If hypertension is secondary to renal artery stenosis, renal revascularization should be considered.

RESULTS

In a collected series of 138 patients undergoing aortic reconstruction using standard vascular surgical techniques, Flanigan and associates documented a 25 per cent incidence of iatrogenic impotence.[16] By minimizing periaortic dissection and emphasizing a nerve-sparing technique as well as attempting to ensure perfusion of at least one hypogastric artery during the arterial reconstruction, they were able to eliminate this complication. Furthermore, retrograde ejaculation was reduced from 43 per cent in the collected series to only 3 per cent in the control group.

Because 80 per cent of patients who present with aortoiliac arterial occlusive disease have significant erectile dysfunction, careful planning of the operative reconstruction to ensure hypogastric artery perfusion is essential if this symptom is to be relieved. Excluding patients with diabetes mellitus in whom neurogenic impotence is most likely, relief of preoperative erectile dysfunction can be anticipated in 30 per cent of patients so afflicted.[16, 28] Half of the patients who regained potency following revascularization were noted to have bilateral iliac artery occlusion on their preoperative arteriograms.[16]

CONCLUSIONS

A multi-modal diagnostic approach to the impotent patient is essential to ensure precise etiologic diagnosis and appropriate therapy. Furthermore, an understanding of the multiple factors involved in achieving a normal erection is essential if potency is to be preserved during the course of aortic surgery. Because nearly 25 per cent of patients undergoing direct aortic reconstruction will suffer iatrogenic erectile dysfunction if appropriate technical modifications are not employed, the problem of iatrogenic impotence is not inconsequential. By appropriate nerve-sparing dissection of the infrarenal aorta and preservation of hypogastric-perfusion, the postoperative development of erectile dysfunction can be virtually eliminated, and improvement in preoperative impotence can be maximized. When postoperative impotence occurs despite every precaution, an attentive and objective approach can offer much comfort to the patient and his sexual partners. In only a small percentage of such cases will additional revascularization be necessary.

References

1. Abelson D: Diagnostic value of the penile pulse and blood pressure: A Doppler study of impotence in diabetics. J Urol 113:636, 1975.
2. Adaikan PG, Kottegoda SR, Ratnam SS: Is vasoactive intestinal polypeptide the principal transmitter involved in human penile erection? J Urol 135:638, 1986.
3. Benson GS: Penile erection: In search of a neurotransmitter. World J Urol 1:209, 1983.
4. Benson GS, McConnell J, Lipshultz LI: Neuromorphology and neuropharmacology of the human penis. J Clin Invest 65:506, 1980.
5. Billet A, Dagher FJ, Queral LA: Surgical correction of vasculogenic impotence in a patient after bilateral renal transplantation. Surgery 91:108, 1982.
6. Bohlen JG: Sleep erection monitoring in the evaluation of male erectile failure. Urol Clin 8:119, 1981.
7. Britt DB, Kemmerer WT, Robison JR: Penile blood flow determination by mercury strain gauge plethysmography. Invest Urol 8:673, 1971.
8. Canning JR, Bowers LM, Lloyd FA, et al: Genital vascular insufficiency and impotence. Surg Forum 14:298, 1963.
9. Conti G: L'erection du penis humain et ses bases morphologico vascularies. Acta Anat 14:17, 1952.
10. DePalma RG, Emsellem HA, Edwards CM, et al: A screening sequence for vasculogenic impotence. J Vasc Surg 5:228, 1987.
11. DePalma RG, Kedia K, Persky L: Vascular operations for preservation of sexual function. *In* Bergan JJ, Yao JST (eds): Surgery of the Aorta and Its Body Branches, New York, Grune & Stratton, 1979.
12. DePalma RG: Impotence in vascular disease: Relationship to vascular surgery. Br J Surg 69:514, 1982.
13. DePalma RG, Levine SB, Feldman S: Preservation of erectile function after aortoiliac reconstruction. Arch Surg 113:958, 1978.
14. Ellenberg M: Impotence in diabetes: The neurologic factor. Ann Intern Med 75:213, 1971.
15. Fitzpatrick T: The corpus cavernosum intercommunicating venous drainage system. J Urol 113:494, 1975.
16. Flanigan DP, Schuler JJ, Keifer T, et al: Elimination of iatrogenic impotence and improvement of sexual function after aortoiliac revascularization. Arch Surg 117:544, 1982.
17. Flanigan DP, Pratt DG, Goodreau JJ, et al: Hemodynamic and angiographic guidelines in selection of patients for femorofemoral bypass. Arch Surg 113:1257, 1978.
18. Gaskell P: The importance of penile blood pressure in cases of impotence. Can Med Assoc J 105:1047, 1971.
19. Ginestie JF, Romieu A: Radiologic Exploration of Impotence. The Hague, Martinus Nijhoff, 1978.
20. Harris JD, Jepson RP: Aorto-iliac stenosis: A comparison of two procedures. Aust NZ J Surg 34:211, 1965.
21. Karacan I, Salis PJ, Ware JC, et al: Nocturnal penile tumescence and diagnosis in diabetic impotence. Am J Psychiatry 135:191, 1978.
22. Kedia KR, Markland C, Fraley EE: Sexual function following high retroperitoneal lymphadenectomy. J Urol 114:237, 1975.
23. Kempczinski RF: Role of the vascular diagnostic laboratory in the evaluation of male impotence. Am J Surg 138:278, 1979.
24. Krane RJ, Siroky MB: Neurophysiology of erection. Urol Clin 8:91, 1981.
25. Leriche R, Morel A: The syndrome of thrombotic obliteration of the aortic bifurcation. Ann Surg 127:193, 1948.
26. Lue TF, Hricak H, Marick KW, et al: Vasculogenic impotence evaluated by high-resolution ultrasonography and pulsed Doppler spectrum analysis. Radiology 155:777, 1985.
27. Lue TF, Tanagho EA: Physiology of erection and pharmacological management of impotence. J Urol 137:829, 1987.
28. May AG, DeWeese JA, Rob CG: Changes in sexual function following operation on the abdominal aorta. Surgery 65:41, 1969.
29. Merchant RF Jr, DePalma RG: Effects of femorofemoral grafts on postoperative sexual function: Correlation with penile pulse volume recordings. Surgery 90:962, 1981.
30. Michal V, Pospichal J: Phalloarteriography in the diagnosis of erectile impotence. World J Surg 2:239, 1978.
31. Michal V, Kramar R, Hejhal L: Revascularization procedure of the cavernous bodies. *In* Zorgomotti AW, Rossi G (eds): Vasculogenic Impotence: Proceedings of the First International Conference on Corpus Cavernosum Revascularization. Springfield, IL, Charles C Thomas, 1980.
32. Miles JR, Miles DG, Johnson G: Aortoiliac operations and sexual dysfunction. Arch Surg 117:1177, 1982.
33. Nath RL, Menzoian JO, Kaplan KH, et al: The multidisciplinary approach to vasculogenic impotence. Surgery 89:124, 1981.
34. Newman HF, Northrup JD, Devlin J: Mechanism of human penile erection. Invest Urol 1:350, 1964.
35. Queral LA, Flinn WR, Bergan JJ, et al: Sexual function and aortic surgery. *In* Bergan JJ, Yao JST (eds): Surgery of the Aorta and Its Body Branches. New York, Grune & Stratton, 1979.
36. Queral LA, Whitehouse WM, Flinn WR, et al: Pelvic hemodynamics after aortoiliac reconstruction. Surgery 86:799, 1979.
37. Schuler JJ, Gray B, Flanigan DP, et al: Increased penile perfusion and reversal of vasculogenic impotence following femorofemoral bypass. Br J Surg 69:S7, 1982.
38. Weinsten MH, Machleder HI: Sexual function after aorto-iliac surgery. Ann Surg 181:787, 1975.
39. Weiss HD: The physiology of human penile erection. Ann Intern Med 76:793, 1972.
40. Willis EM, Ottesen B, Wagner G, et al: Vasoactive intestinal polypeptide (VIP) as a possible neurotransmitter involved in penile erection. Acta Physiol Scand 113:545, 1981.
41. Kornick AL, Villemarette PY, Baum N, Hower JF: Vasculogenic impotence: Diagnostic applications of color flow Doppler. J Vasc Tech 14:173, 1990.

SECTION IX

Neurovascular Conditions Involving the Upper Extremity

Edited by K. Wayne Johnston, M.D., F.R.C.S.(C.)

64

Overview

K. Wayne Johnston, M.D., F.R.C.S.(C.)

• • •

In comparison to those involving the lower extremity, symptomatic vascular diseases involving the upper extremity are quite rare; however, when present, they may be very disabling because they affect the function of the hand and may have a poor prognosis because they may be a manifestation of a systemic disorder. Intermittent claudication is the most common symptom associated with lower extremity arterial occlusive disease; however, in the upper extremity, coldness and color changes of the digits are more common than complaints of tiredness, claudication, or ulceration and gangrene. These differences in the upper extremity symptoms are related to the more frequent distal distribution of the arterial disease and the excellent collateral supply around the shoulder and elbow.

Diagnosis of the anatomic location of the upper extremity arterial occlusive disease is often straightforward and is based on (1) careful vascular examination, including blood pressure measurements, pulse palpation, Allen's test, and thoracic outlet maneuvers; (2) noninvasive tests to detect obstruction of large arteries (segmental blood pressure measurements, Doppler recordings, or duplex Doppler studies) and small arteries (digital blood pressure measurements, Doppler recordings, or plethysmographic recordings); and (3) angiography. However, establishing the etiologic diagnosis is often difficult unless there are digital or general manifestations of a systemic disease. Acute ischemia due to obstruction of the subclavian, axillary, brachial, or forearm arteries is usually caused by trauma (blunt, penetrating, or iatrogenic) or emboli from the heart (atrial fibrillation, valvular disease, myocardial infarction, ventricular aneurysm, cardiomyopathy, or subacute bacterial endocarditis) or from the large proximal arteries (atherosclerosis, aneurysm, or thoracic outlet compression). Acute digital arterial occlusion may be the result of microemboli or acute manifestations of collagen vascular diseases. The etiologic diagnosis of chronic ischemia can often be strongly suspected on the basis of (1) the anatomic localization of the arterial occlusive disease, (2) whether ischemia is constantly present or is intermittent, and (3) evidence of systemic findings. Table 64–1 summarizes the common causes of chronic upper extremity ischemia based on the anatomic localization of the pathology. Note the important distinction between vasospasm and fixed arterial obstruction of the digital arteries.

The following topics relevant to upper extremity vascular disease are covered elsewhere in this text: Takayasu's disease (see Chapter 12), Buerger's disease (see Chapter 11), vasculitis (see Chapter 16), causalgia (see Chapter 49), cold injury, and proximal arterial injuries (see Chapter 46).

The chapters in this section describe the neurovascular diseases of the upper extremity. The following sections summarize the most important aspects of the pathogenesis, diagnosis, and management of these diseases.

EVALUATION OF UPPER EXTREMITY ISCHEMIA

(see Chapter 65)

The assessment of the ischemic upper extremity by clinical evaluation, noninvasive assessment, and arteriography aims to determine (1) the anatomic site of the arterial disease, (2) the severity of the ischemia, and (3) the etiology. The diagnostic approach depends on the results of a comprehensive history taking and a careful physical examination because it will usually determine the site of obstruction and may suggest the possible etiology.

Further evaluation of arterial disease involving the arch vessels and the subclavian arteries includes segmental

Table 64–1. Etiologic Causes of Chronic Upper Extremity Ischemia Classified According to the Anatomic Site of the Pathology

Anatomic Site	Etiology
Arch arteries	Atherosclerosis Takayasu's disease Giant cell arteritis (temporal arteritis) Aneurysmal disease with emboli
Subclavian and axillary arteries	Thoracic outlet arterial damage Crutch trauma Atherosclerosis
Brachial, radial, ulnar, and palmar arteries	Buerger's disease Collagen vascular diseases (see below) Atherosclerosis
Digital arteries	Vasospasm Fixed arterial obstruction Collagen vascular diseases (scleroderma, CREST variant, systemic lupus erythematosus, mixed connective tissue disorder, rheumatoid arthritis, Sjögren's syndrome, dermatomyositis, polyarteritis nodosa) Microemboli (e.g., from thoracic outlet compression) Vibration-induced injury Occupational trauma (e.g., hypothenar hammer syndrome) Cold injury (frostbite, immersion foot) Drug-induced (e.g., ergot) Hematologic (thrombocytosis, polycythemia, dysproteinemia, cryoglobulinemia, cold agglutinins, hypercoagulable state [e.g., antithrombin III deficiency, malignancy, or ulcerative colitis])

blood pressure measurements; Doppler recordings, duplex scanning, or both; and arteriography. Significant thoracic outlet arterial compression can be detected by palpation of the radial pulse and auscultation for bruits in the infraclavicular area during the various thoracic outlet maneuvers or by noninvasively recording changes in radial artery flow with a Doppler flowmeter or changes in digital flow with a photoplethysmograph.

Acute or chronic obstruction of the axillary, brachial, or forearm arteries can usually be evaluated by clinical examination, segmental blood pressure measurement, Doppler recordings, and occasionally arteriography.

Digital artery involvement may be due to primary vasospasm and present as episodic vasospasm on exposure to cold or emotional stimuli, or it may be due to fixed arterial obstruction (see Table 64–1) and present as similar cold intolerance or more advanced ischemic sequelae. A cold tolerance test will verify the symptoms but does little to establish the anatomic or etiologic diagnosis. Noninvasive tests distinguish between primary vasospasm and fixed arterial obstruction. The most useful are digital pressure measurements, Doppler recordings, and digital plethysmographic waveform recordings. Arteriography is necessary if the results of the clinical and noninvasive tests are equivocal.

ATHEROSCLEROTIC DISEASES OF THE ARCH BRANCHES

(see Chapter 66)

Arterial occlusive disease of the brachiocephalic and aortic arch vessels may be due to atherosclerosis, inflammatory arteritis, or trauma. Chapter 66 describes atherosclerotic occlusive disease, Chapter 12 Takayasu's disease, Chapter 16 arteritis, and Chapter 46 trauma.

Because of the abundant collateral blood supply around the shoulder, most frequently lesions of the brachiocephalic vessels are asymptomatic, but some patients will present with arm claudication or cerebral symptoms resulting from changes in perfusion. Less commonly, if the lesions ulcerate, they may become symptomatic because of platelet or atheromatous embolization to the upper extremities or the brain.

In general, patients complaining of arm claudication or symptoms of cerebral hypoperfusion can be treated conservatively unless their quality of life is adversely affected. In contrast, if the symptoms are the result of emboli to either the arm or the brain, surgical repair is required. Selected extrathoracic operations provide satisfactory long-term results and have a low operative mortality; however, Chapter 70 indicates that direct repair can be accomplished with a low risk. Many surgeons prefer extrathoracic procedures to intrathoracic endarterectomy or bypass procedures, except for the management of complex occlusive disease of two or more major vessels.

The options for repairing an innominate lesion include endarterectomy, aortoinnominate (or carotid or subclavian) bypass through a median sternotomy, and axilloaxillary bypass. A left subclavian lesion can be repaired by carotid-subclavian bypass or subclavian-carotid reimplantation. On the right side, subclavian endarterectomy and carotid-subclavian bypass are possible alternatives. Common carotid occlusion can be repaired by endarterectomy on the right side, but subclavian-carotid bypass is usually a simpler operation. Multiple lesions of the arch vessels are bypassed from the aortic arch.

UPPER EXTREMITY REVASCULARIZATION

(see Chapter 67)

In Chapter 67, the surgical treatment of occlusive disease affecting the axillary, brachial, radial, and ulnar arteries is discussed. The most common problems involving these vessels include emboli, trauma, and iatrogenic injury.

In general, except for occlusion of one of the two forearm arteries, acute arterial occlusions should be repaired in order to minimize the risk of late symptoms. The decision to repair a chronic arterial occlusion is based on the presence of disabling forearm and hand claudication with minimal exercise or the presence of severe ischemic sequelae.

Brachial artery thrombosis following cardiac catheterization is often associated with few symptoms during the acute stage because of the extensive collateral circulation around the elbow; however, late symptoms are present in up to 45 per cent of patients. Furthermore, because repair is usually straightforward and requires thrombectomy or local resection and anastomosis, early repair is advised.

Thrombosis following transaxillary angiography should be repaired promptly, and the hematoma in the axillary sheath should be decompressed before neurologic sequelae develop.

The ischemic consequences of radial artery thrombosis following cannulation for blood pressure monitoring can be minimized by ensuring that the palmar arch is patent, using the Allen test. In rare cases of acute ischemia, thrombectomy of the radial artery and the palmar arch may be successful.

Embolic occlusion of the axillary or the brachial artery can usually be treated by embolectomy through the brachial artery at the supracondylar level.

Penetrating traumatic injuries are approached directly. Injuries to the proximal axillary artery can usually be approached through an incision in the deltopectoral groove; however, it may be necessary to control the subclavian artery through a supraclavicular incision or by removal of the middle third of the clavicle to optimize exposure.

Chronic upper extremity arterial occlusions are repaired by saphenous vein bypass grafting if the patient's symptoms are disabling.

RAYNAUD'S SYNDROME

(see Chapter 68)

The clinical manifestations of diseases of the distal small arteries of the upper extremity span the spectrum from episodic vasospasm on exposure to cold or emotional stimuli to digital ulceration and gangrene. Episodic spasm of the small arteries and arterioles may affect 20 to 30 per cent of certain patient populations. It results from increased force of vasoconstriction owing to altered sensitivity of the adrenergic receptors in smooth muscle cells, and it may be an early manifestation of diseases that cause fixed arterial obstruction. Ulceration or gangrene is invariably the consequence of fixed organic arterial occlusions, most commonly arteritis associated with autoimmune diseases (scleroderma or a CREST variant, mixed connective tissue disease, rheumatoid arthritis, systemic lupus erythematosus, Sjögren's syndrome, or unclassified connective tissue disease) or arteriosclerosis. Early in the course of connective tissue diseases, the patient's arteries may exhibit excessive vasospasm, but later, diffuse small artery obstruction is present as the consequence of vasculitis and subsequent inflammatory thrombosis.

The clinical picture of cold- or emotion-induced episodic digital ischemia is best referred to as Raynaud's syndrome because the original classification into Raynaud's disease and Raynaud's phenomenon is difficult and has not proved to be of prognostic significance.

Raynaud's syndrome is diagnosed by a clinical history of episodic digital ischemia, usually associated with color changes (pallor, cyanosis, and the rubor of hyperemia). The proximal arteries are evaluated by measuring systolic blood pressures at three levels and recording Doppler waveforms from the brachial, radial, ulnar, and digital arteries. Obstructive diseases of the small arteries may be diagnosed clinically and are invariably present if there is ulceration, but they are most accurately assessed by digital plethysmography with waveform analysis, digital blood pressure measurements, the occlusive digital hypothermic challenge test, magnification arteriography, or a combination. Associated diseases causing fixed arterial obstruction are diagnosed on the basis of history, physical examination, and baseline laboratory investigations, including complete blood count, erythrocyte sedimentation rate, chemistry profile, urinalysis, rheumatoid factor, and antinuclear antibody. In selected patients, more detailed investigations may be necessary to detect autoimmune diseases. Because the symptoms associated with Raynaud's syndrome may precede the detection of associated diseases by many months or years, careful follow-up with repeated investigation is justified.

In addition to avoidance of cigarette smoking and cold exposure, the vasospastic symptoms of patients with Raynaud's syndrome are most often treated with calcium channel blocking agents (nifedipine). Other methods of treatment, including intra-arterial reserpine, infusion of prostaglandins, plasmaphoresis, and cervical sympathectomy, are not recommended because symptomatic recurrence almost invariably follows the initial period of improvement. Digital ulcers usually respond to conservative therapy, including soaks, débridement, antibiotics, and length-conserving digital amputation. Specific treatment of the collagen vascular disease may be possible.

NEUROGENIC THORACIC OUTLET SYNDROME

(see Chapter 69)

Thoracic outlet syndromes are due to compression of the brachial plexus, the subclavian artery, or the subclavian vein as these structures pass through the thoracic outlet. The anatomic abnormalities are generally congenital in origin and include skeletal abnormalities that can be seen on x-ray studies (e.g., a cervical rib, an elongated transverse process of C7, callus formation from a fractured first rib or clavicle, or hypoplastic first rib) and, more often, soft tissue abnormalities (e.g., fibromuscular bands or scalene muscle anomalies). Patients with an anatomic defect may develop thoracic outlet syndrome as the result of postural abnormalities, musculoskeletal injury, or a spasm secondary to injury.

In Chapter 69, neurologic thoracic outlet syndrome is described. Controversy surrounds the etiology and treatment of the symptoms of brachial plexus irritation due to mechanical abnormalities of the thoracic outlet. Presenting complaints may include pain, paresthesias, and weakness, which are usually aggravated by the overhead posture. Autonomic disturbances are rare. The differential diagnosis includes musculoskeletal disorders of the neck and shoulder and nerve root compression (cervical root, ulnar nerve, or carpal tunnel). Diagnosis is made on the basis of a careful clinical examination and the use of ancillary tests, which are used primarily to exclude other causes of the complaints.

Conservative measures are usually tried first, and surgical decompression is reserved for patients with disabling complaints. Of the possible alternative operative approaches (supraclavicular, transaxillary, infraclavicular, and parascapular), the approach used depends on which anatomic structure is considered to be the most important cause of compression (congenital or acquired abnormalities of the scalene muscle, cervical rib, an abnormal transverse process of a cervical vertebra, the first rib, congenital or acquired fibromuscular bands, and others). Chapter 69 discusses the controversy that surrounds surgical treatment. Although osseous abnormalities are not a common cause of compression, it is agreed that any such abnormality should be removed. First rib resection plus transaxillary decompression of the thoracic outlet is a common approach; however, the authors recommend a supraclavicular approach to total removal of the scalene muscles, brachial plexus neurolysis, and excision of congenital and acquired fibromuscular bands.

ARTERIAL COMPLICATIONS OF THORACIC OUTLET COMPRESSION (see Chapter 70)

Although less common than neurologic complications, arterial complications of thoracic outlet syndrome may have serious sequelae. Most often, the compression is due to a congenital bony abnormality (a complete cervical rib or an incomplete rib associated with a fibrous band, an elongated transverse process of C7, a congenital anomaly of the first thoracic rib, or malunion or hypertrophic callus following fracture of the clavicle or first rib); the compression is rarely associated with a fibrous band. The compression produces subclavian artery stenosis, which is followed in time by post-stenotic dilatation, aneurysm formation, or the development of an intimal lesion. Complications include subclavian artery thrombosis, embolization of mural thrombi, and embolization of platelet aggregates.

Most often, patients complain of symptoms of Raynaud's syndrome that are the result of microembolization to digital arteries or of reduced forearm blood flow due to progressive occlusion of large arteries. A large embolus may produce acute ischemic symptoms and must be distinguished from emboli of cardiac origin.

Although clinical findings of a cervical rib, subclavian aneurysm, or supraclavicular bruit or a history of a fractured clavicle or first rib may lead to the correct diagnosis, most often the diagnosis is established by a combination of cervical and upper thoracic spine x-ray studies, noninvasive tests, and arteriography, which demonstrates abnormalities of the subclavian artery (displacement, stenosis, post-stenotic dilatation, aneurysm, an irregular wall, or filling defects).

Because the thoracic outlet must be decompressed and the artery repaired, the optimal surgical exposure is usually the supraclavicular approach. Surgical repair is considered in three steps.

1. The thoracic outlet decompression usually involves complete removal of a cervical rib and its accompanying muscular or fibrous tissue or clavicular resection if malunion, hypertrophic callus, or both are present after a fracture. Simultaneous first rib removal is recommended by some surgeons.
2. Arterial reconstruction is necessary if mural thrombus or an aneurysm is present. The treatment of mild post-stenotic dilatation is controversial; some surgeons believe that this lesion will regress after removal of the compression, whereas others believe that arterial repair is necessary.
3. Distal embolic occlusions are difficult to manage, but the ischemic sequelae may decrease in severity after cervical sympathectomy. Proximal embolic occlusions can be managed conservatively if the collateral blood supply is adequate; however, if significant ischemic symptoms are present, sympathectomy, embolectomy, or bypass grafting should be considered. The prognosis depends on the extent of distal embolization.

AXILLARY-SUBCLAVIAN VEIN THROMBOSIS (see Chapter 71)

Primary (effort) thrombosis may result from reduced flow through the subclavian vein due to intrinsic venous abnormalities (a congenital web or a valve in the subclavian vein at the border of the first rib that may become thickened by repetitive compression); from venous damage due to extrinsic compression (by the subclavius muscle and tendon, the costoclavicular ligament, or the anterior scalene muscle; by callus from a fractured clavicle or first rib; or by congenital fibromuscular bands) that is aggravated by performing repetitive tasks or heavy work with the arm in the elevated position; or less likely, from coagulation abnormalities. Thus, these patients frequently have a history of recent physical exertion or trauma, and they often have an abrupt onset of swelling and venous engorgement and visible shoulder collaterals. Venography is diagnostic.

If the diagnosis is delayed, a conservative approach (heparin, elevation, and long-term oral anticoagulants) is justified to reduce the risk of pulmonary embolism and the late incidence of symptoms. However, because many patients will have persistent symptoms, especially with vigorous upper extremity activity, an aggressive approach to the management of early disease, which consists of clot removal followed by correction of the predisposing factors, is considered. Although there is no universal agreement on the optimum method of treatment, systemic or, preferably, catheter-directed local fibrinolytic therapy is recommended, followed by the administration of heparin and warfarin.

Subsequent balloon angioplasty of residual vein stenosis and thoracic outlet decompression (division of a prominent subclavius muscle, the costoclavicular ligament, congenital fibromuscular bands, or the anterior scalene muscle) are considered.

Axillary-subclavian vein thrombosis may be due to local trauma from a central venous catheter, a pacemaker lead, a diagnostic catheter, or a dialysis catheter. These patients often have localized thrombosis with good collateralization and few symptoms. If the patient is asymptomatic and the thrombus is discovered coincidentally, no specific treatment is necessary. On the other hand, if edema or enlarging collaterals suggest propagation of the thrombus, anticoagulation, infusion of fibrinolytic agents directly into the thrombus through the partially withdrawn indwelling catheter, or both may be of benefit.

UPPER EXTREMITY SYMPATHECTOMY (see Chapter 72)

Although performed less frequently than in the past, upper extremity sympathectomy is still indicated in the treatment of selected patients with hyperhidrosis, ischemia, and post-traumatic pain syndromes.

If excessive debilitating sweating of the hands and axillae is not secondary to a systemic disorder such as hyperthyroidism and does not respond to atropine-like drugs or topical antiperspirant medication, sympathectomy is indicated. It usually results in complete relief of symptoms.

The role of sympathectomy in upper extremity ischemic syndromes is controversial. Patients with Raynaud's syndrome not associated with digital artery occlusion usually have a transient benefit, perhaps because many will later prove to have a collagen vascular disease. Although Porter and Edwards (see Chapter 68) describe their experience, which indicates that most patients with severe digital ischemia can be treated conservatively, the observations by Harris and colleagues in Chapter 72 suggest that sympathectomy will relieve pain, improve digital perfusion, and decrease the need for amputation.

Although most patients with a post-traumatic pain syndrome (sympathectomy dystrophy) will respond to conservative therapy, those without evidence of atrophic changes may show improvement after sympathectomy.

The upper extremity can be denervated by cutting the sympathetic trunk below the third thoracic ganglion and severing the rami communicantes of the second and third thoracic ganglia. It is unnecessary to excise any portion of the stellate ganglion or to divide the rami to the first thoracic ganglion. To denervate the axilla, it is necessary to divide the sympathetic chain below the fourth thoracic ganglion and its associated rami.

Of the alternative surgical approaches, the supraclavicular and axillary transthoracic approaches are the most popular. Complications following supraclavicular sympathectomy may include Horner's syndrome, lymphatic interruption, and incisional pain. Respiratory complications are the most frequent when a transthoracic approach is used, but a winged scapula can occur from injury to the long thoracic nerve to the serratus anterior. After either procedure, postsympathectomy neuralgia and compensatory hyperhidrosis may occur. The choice between the two operations is made by balancing these relative risks in the hands of the individual surgeon.

After more experience has been obtained with transthoracic endoscopic sympathectomy, this less invasive procedure may gain widespread acceptance.

OCCUPATIONAL VASCULAR PROBLEMS (see Chapter 73)

Arterial and venous injuries occur in the work environment as a result of excessive physical force to the shoulder or hand. Vibration-induced white finger syndrome is due to vasospasm and segmental occlusion of digital arteries caused by the prolonged use of vibrating tools such as pneumatic drills and chain saws. In the early stages, the worker presents with numbness and tingling, but later attacks of cold-induced Raynaud's syndrome predominate. Prevention is important; treatment of established cases by a change of job or the use of a calcium channel blocker may be effective.

The hypothenar hammer syndrome is caused by injury to the ulnar artery in its vulnerable subcutaneous position in the area of the hypothenar eminence owing to repetitive injury to the palm of the hand. The symptoms of Raynaud's syndrome are due to ulnar and digital arterial spasm, ulnar artery thrombosis, or digital artery occlusion secondary to emboli from an ulnar artery aneurysm. Treatment is often supportive, but it may be possible to resect an ulnar artery aneurysm.

Workers exposed to polyvinylchloride may develop occupational acro-osteolysis and present with symptoms of Raynaud's syndrome, owing to multiple digital arterial occlusions; tapering of the tips of the fingers similar to that observed in scleroderma, resulting from resorption of the distal phalangeal tufts; or clubbing secondary to hypervascularity adjacent to the areas of bony resorption.

High-voltage (more than 1000 volts) electrical injuries are associated with widespread tissue damage, but arterial necrosis, thrombosis, stenosis, and aneurysm formation may be observed at any site between the point of entrance and the point of exit during early or late follow-up.

Athletes may suffer from hand ischemia due to the arterial damage that results from repeated local trauma associated with such sports as handball, baseball, and karate, or from thoracic outlet syndrome if shoulder movement is overextended, as in baseball pitchers and butterfly swimmers.

65

Evaluation of Acute and Chronic Ischemia of the Upper Extremity

David S. Sumner, M.D.

• • •

The evaluation of ischemic disorders of the upper extremity often challenges the diagnostic ability of even the most experienced clinician.[22, 53, 68] Not only are there multiple causes, but many of the disease processes are poorly understood. Ischemia may be constant or intermittent; may be a manifestation of a fixed arterial obstruction, vasospasm, or both; and may reflect involvement of large proximal arteries, small distal arteries, or the microvasculature. Although much can be learned from the history and physical examination, simple noninvasive tests contribute important diagnostic information that can prove useful in selecting further investigative modalities, such as arteriography, blood tests, or nerve blocks.[81] They provide an accurate assessment of the severity of the circulatory impairment, locate the site or sites of obstruction, differentiate between obstruction and vasospasm, and may also suggest a cause. Finally, noninvasive tests help define the natural history of the disease process and lend objectivity to the evaluation of the results of medical and surgical treatment.

PATHOPHYSIOLOGY

Some knowledge of the pathophysiology of upper extremity ischemic syndromes is necessary in order to understand the results of noninvasive testing. Analogous to the situation in the lower extremity, the system responsible for delivering blood to the tissues of the arm and hand consists of inflow arteries (innominate and subclavian); intrinsic arteries (axillary, brachial, antecubital, radial, ulnar, palmar, and digital); and arterioles, which terminate in sphincters that control flow into the capillaries. The collateral circulation around the shoulder, axilla, and elbow is particularly well developed; also, within the forearm, hand, and fingers, the radial and ulnar arteries, the deep and superficial palmar arches, and the paired proper digital arteries provide parallel systems in which either one of the pair can usually sustain circulation independent of the other. Arteriovenous anastomoses, which are situated proximal to the capillary bed and which divert blood away from the capillaries, are more frequent than in the lower extremity and are especially numerous in the tips of the fingers. They are also found in the volar surface of the finger and hand but are essentially absent in the forearm.

Fixed Arterial Obstruction

The term fixed is used to designate obstructions that are due to well-defined anatomic changes involving the wall or lumen of the artery. A host of disparate entities can produce fixed obstruction of the upper extremity arteries, including atherosclerosis; thrombosis; emboli; dissection; toxins; autoimmune disorders (connective tissue diseases); Buerger's disease (thromboangiitis obliterans); and vibratory, blunt, and penetrating trauma. As discussed in Chapter 3, lesions seldom produce recognizable hemodynamic changes unless the cross-sectional area of the arterial lumen is diminished by more than 75 per cent. Disturbances of pressure and flow are less severe when the process is localized and when collaterals are well developed. Impairment is more severe when the disease is extensive or multisegmental, when the entrance or exit of collaterals is blocked, or when terminal arteries or those without efficient collateral beds are involved. Lesions that are asymptomatic under normal resting conditions may become symptomatic during exercise or when stimuli that produce vasospasm are superimposed.

Chronic stenoses or occlusions isolated to the subclavian, axillary, or brachial arteries are usually well tolerated because of the abundant collateral circulation. Although peripheral blood pressures are reduced, blood flow at rest remains normal. Exercise, however, may produce claudication. In the forearm, hand, and fingers, chronic and even some acute occlusions limited to either one of the paired arteries may cause little or no hemodynamic change. Lesions in these areas are often completely asymptomatic. Multiple occlusions, on the other hand, may be so extensive or so critically located that they overwhelm the compensatory mechanisms, resulting in ischemia. Chronic obstruction of an end-artery, such as the common digital, or of both proper digital arteries frequently causes ischemia of the involved finger.

As a rule, acute occlusions, especially those involving unpaired or terminal arteries, prove to be more devastating. Owing to the instantaneous nature of the obstruction, blood flow distal to the site of trauma or an embolic occlusion must be maintained by preexisting collaterals, which may not be adequate to sustain tissue viability. Moreover, emboli tend to lodge at bifurcations, where they obstruct both the main arterial channel and the collateral input. Consequently, peripheral arterial pressure is usually severely reduced and may not be measurable.

Intermittent Obstruction

The two major causes of intermittent episodes of arm or hand ischemia are (1) extrinsic compression of the large inflow arteries and (2) vasospasm of the digital arteries. Although the two sometimes occur together, their clinical manifestations and pathophysiology are radically different. Both may also occur in conjunction with fixed arterial obstruction.

Extrinsic Compression

The structures responsible for extrinsic arterial compression include bones, muscles, tendons, and ligaments. In the upper extremity, compression is most likely to occur at the thoracic outlet, where the subclavian artery must traverse a narrow triangular opening bounded by the first rib, the scalenus anticus and medius muscles, and their associated ligaments. It may also occur around the pectoralis minor muscle. In these areas, obstruction is related to the position of the arm. Unless emboli arising from a poststenotic dilatation of the subclavian artery have lodged in the more peripheral arteries of the arm, hemodynamic changes are evident only while the artery is actually being compressed.

Vasospasm

The peripheral arterioles of the upper extremity, especially those located in the fingertips, are normally quite sensitive to sympathetic or alpha-adrenergic stimuli. Emotional factors, pain, respiratory reflexes, local cold exposure, and total body cooling all cause arteriolar constriction. Release of arteriolar constriction by local or total body heating, administration of sympatholytic agents or vasodilating drugs, or surgical or pharmacologic sympathectomy ordinarily causes a great increase in blood flow. Much of this increase is due to the opening of arteriovenous shunts, which, as mentioned previously, are abundant in the fingertips. Flow through the capillaries is less affected. Fingertip blood flow is therefore quite variable, ranging from 1.0 ml/100 ml/min to as much as 150 ml/100 ml/min in normal individuals.[54]

Ischemia caused by vasospasm is much more common in the upper extremities than it is in the lower extremities. The episodic color changes that occur in the fingers and toes of patients with cold sensitivity are known as Raynaud's phenomenon, after the French physician who initially described the condition in 1862. Classically, in response to cold exposure, the fingers initially become pallid, then cyanotic, and finally red as the vasospasm subsides. Variations are common, and many patients never experience the typical triphasic color change. The etiology of Raynaud's phenomenon is multi-factorial and, despite intensive investigation, remains incompletely understood. Although many classifications have been proposed, none is entirely satisfactory. For the purpose of discussing the hemodynamics of vasospastic disease, this chapter employs the term secondary Raynaud's phenomenon to designate conditions in which a fixed anatomic obstruction has been identified (or is strongly suspected) and the term primary Raynaud's disease to identify conditions in which the cause remains obscure.[3, 5, 37, 78]

Secondary Raynaud's Phenomenon. Arteriolar constriction is usually well tolerated, but when it is superimposed on a substrate of fixed arterial obstruction, the previously adequately perfused fingers may become ischemic (Fig. 65–1).[30, 55, 78] This is the mechanism primarily respon-

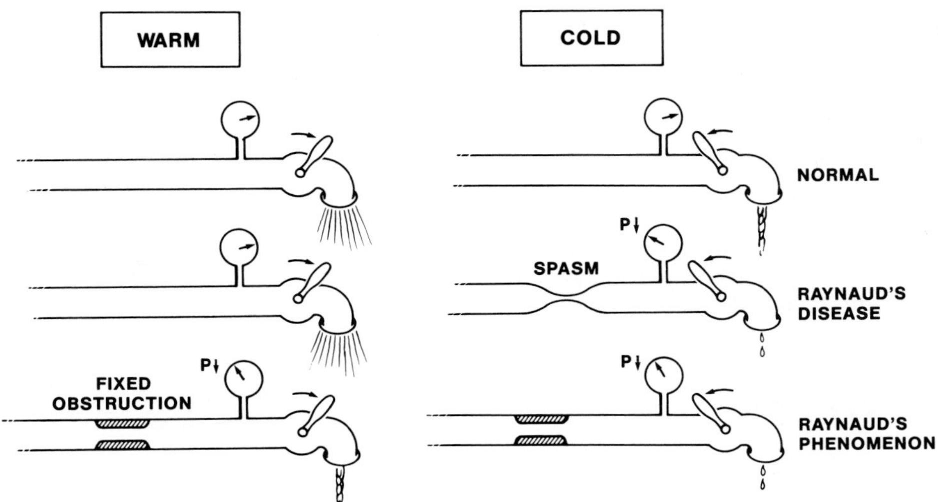

FIGURE 65–1. Effect of cold exposure on normal fingers, fingers with primary Raynaud's disease, and fingers with Raynaud's phenomenon secondary to fixed arterial obstruction. Faucets represent arteriolar sphincters. When the handle is turned to the right, the arterioles are dilated; when it is turned to the left, the arterioles are constricted. Gauges represent digital arterial pressure, with increasing pressure being indicated by clockwise rotation of the hand. Digital blood flow is represented by the output of the faucets.

sible for the appearance of Raynaud's phenomenon in patients with autoimmune diseases (e.g., scleroderma), Buerger's disease, and traumatic arteritis. Although these fingers typically display hemodynamic alterations even when they are warm, the changes become more marked with cold exposure.

Primary Raynaud's Disease. Although the digital arteries in patients suffering from this form of episodic ischemia may be histologically normal, they are hypersensitive to cold and to alpha-adrenergic stimuli.[11, 19, 24, 38, 46, 47] Unlike the digital arteries of normal individuals, which are relatively nonresponsive to cold, those of patients with primary Raynaud's disease display a remarkable ability to constrict. This, together with cold-induced arteriolar constriction, produces profound but temporary digital ischemia (see Fig. 65–1).[43, 64, 75] Even when the hands are warm, there is evidence of enhanced sympathetic activity. Although the digital arterial pressure is normal, blood flow in the fingers is moderately reduced.[64, 71] Whereas the arterioles are sensitive both to local and to remote cold exposure, the digital arteries respond almost exclusively to local cold.[64]

Comment. Admittedly, this classification into secondary Raynaud's phenomenon and primary Raynaud's disease is arbitrary. Not infrequently, patients in one category show responses consistent with the other. For example, digital artery vasospasm may occur in patients with histologic features of autoimmune disease; in addition, autoimmune phenomena have been proposed as the mechanism underlying the hypersensitivity of the anatomically normal digital arteries in patients with primary Raynaud's disease.[68] There may well be a continuum of pathophysiologic features extending from one classification to the other. This is supported by the observation that patients who initially appear to have the more benign primary Raynaud's disease are eventually diagnosed as having scleroderma or some other autoimmune problem. Nonetheless, for the purposes of the initial hemodynamic evaluation, the author has found the classification to be quite useful.

On the other hand, the dichotomous classification proposed by Edwards and Porter has considerable merit because it makes no assumptions about the presence or absence of a currently diagnosable associated disease in patients with no demonstrable organic obstruction of the digital or palmar arteries.[21] Patients who have normal digital blood pressures between attacks are said to have vasospastic Raynaud's syndrome. Patients in whom the resting digital blood pressure is reduced and who by definition have an associated disease are said to have obstructive Raynaud's syndrome.

NONINVASIVE STUDIES

Noninvasive studies are designed to answer the following questions: (1) Is there fixed arterial obstruction? If so, what is its location and how severe is the hemodynamic impairment? (2) Is there intermittent obstruction related to arm position? (3) Is there cold-induced vasospasm? (4) Do the arterioles retain the ability to dilate? (5) Is sympathetic activity present? Answers to the first three questions help determine the cause of the patient's complaints, and answers to the last two aid in selecting therapy.

Segmental Pressure Measurements

The examination of any patient with complaints suggesting upper extremity ischemia should begin with the measurement of segmental arterial pressures. Techniques for noninvasive pressure measurements are described in Chapter 4. Pneumatic cuffs are placed around the brachial area, the upper forearm, and the wrist; each cuff in turn is inflated above the systolic pressure and then slowly deflated while the return of flow signifying the pressure at each level is detected by a Doppler probe placed over the radial or ulnar arteries or the palmar arch. In the absence of an arterial signal, the return of flow can be monitored plethysmographically.

At each of the three anatomic levels, the pressure in one arm is compared with that in the other.[82] Normally, the difference in pressure between the two arms at any given site seldom exceeds 15 to 20 mmHg and is usually considerably less, averaging about 5 to 8 mmHg (Table 65–1). Indices obtained by dividing the lower of the two pressures by the higher average about 0.95 and are rarely less than 0.85 (see Table 65–1). Pressure gradients between adjacent levels of the same arm are usually less than 15 mmHg, with a mean in the range of 5 to 7 mmHg (Table 65–2). Because the relationship between cuff width and arm diameter varies between levels and perhaps because peripheral augmentation of systolic pressure may occur, the gradients may occasionally be reversed, with pressures at the more distal sites exceeding those measured further up the arm (see Chapters 3 and 4). Indices obtained by dividing the pressure at the forearm or wrist by the ipsilateral brachial pressure fluctuate around 1.0 and almost always exceed 0.85 (see Table 65–2).

Table 65–1. Pressure Data: Normal Arms*

	Difference (mmHg) *Higher Pressure Minus Lower Pressure*	
	MEAN ± SD	RANGE
Brachial	5.4 ± 4.6	0–16
Forearm	7.6 ± 4.6	2–16
Wrist	7.2 ± 6.1	0–22
	Index *Lower Pressure Divided by Higher Pressure*	
	MEAN ± SD	RANGE
Brachial	0.96 ± 0.03	0.88–1.00
Forearm	0.93 ± 0.04	0.85–0.98
Wrist	0.94 ± 0.05	0.83–1.00

Data from Sumner DS, Lambeth A, Russell JB: Diagnosis of upper extremity obstructive and vasospastic syndromes by Doppler ultrasound, plethysmography, and temperature profiles. In *Puel P, Boccalon H, Enjalbert A (eds): Hemodynamics of the Limbs 1. Toulouse, France, GEPESC, 1979, pp 365–373.*

**Pressures in one arm compared with those in the other arm at the same level.*

Table 65–2. Pressure Data: Normal Arms*

	Gradient (mmHg)	
Brachial-forearm	5.0 ± 4.8	−6 to + 15
Forearm-wrist	6.6 ± 4.6	−19 to + 14
	Index	
Forearm-brachial	0.97 ± 0.06	0.87 to 1.06
Wrist-brachial	0.99 ± 0.06	0.89 to 1.15

Data from Sumner DS, Lambeth A, Russell JB: Diagnosis of upper extremity obstructive and vasospastic syndromes by Doppler ultrasound, plethysmography, and temperature profiles. In *Puel P, Boccalon H, Enjalbert A (eds): Hemodynamics of the Limbs 1. Toulouse, France, GEPESC, 1979, pp 365–373.*

**Pressures at different levels compared in the same arm.*

A reduction in the brachial pressure indicates occlusive disease of the ipsilateral innominate, subclavian, axillary, or upper brachial artery.[26, 88] In a series of patients with lesions in one or more of these arteries, the author's group observed that the brachial pressures in the involved arms were 20 to 124 mmHg less than those in the control arms, with a mean difference of 50 ± 33 mmHg.[82] The average ipsilateral-contralateral pressure index was 0.65 ± 0.15, with a range of 0.38 to 0.81. Because bilateral subclavian artery obstruction is not uncommon, both brachial pressures may be reduced. Bilateral disease is suggested by the presence of bruits over both subclavian arteries and may be confirmed by the detection of abnormal Doppler signals from the subclavian arteries. In such cases, the ankle pressure can be used as a reference value, provided there is no evidence of arterial obstruction in the lower limbs.

An abnormally large pressure gradient between any two adjacent levels in the arm implies significant obstructive disease of the arteries in the intervening segment.[6] As is the case with similar studies in the leg, segmental pressure measurements lack sensitivity and specificity (see Chapter 5). Gradients, for example, may be reduced when the ipsilateral brachial pressure is also low. The author's group measured gradients of 42 ± 30 mmHg in a series of arms with occlusions of the distal brachial, antecubital, radial, and ulnar arteries.[82] The range, however, was large (12 to 114 mmHg). Forearm-brachial and wrist-brachial indices in these patients ranged from 0.37 to 0.86, with a mean of 0.68 ± 0.16. A marked difference between the pressure measured at the wrist with the Doppler probe over the radial artery and that obtained with the probe over the ulnar artery indicates which of these two vessels is the more severely diseased.

Finger Pressure Measurements

The technique for measuring systolic blood pressures in the fingers is analogous to that employed in the arms (see Chapter 4).[18, 27, 29, 61] To avoid vasoconstriction, all measurements should be performed in a warm (about 25° C), draft-free room. The patient should be relaxed, and efforts should be made to allay apprehension. A pneumatic cuff with a width of at least 1.2 times the diameter of the finger is wrapped around the proximal phalanx. A Doppler probe applied to a volar digital artery at the distal interphalangeal joint may be used to detect the return of blood flow as the cuff is deflated. Alternatively, a mercury strain-gauge or a photoplethysmograph placed over the distal phalanx can be used (see Fig. 4–15). The values obtained with the cuff at the proximal phalangeal level reflect pressures in the common and proximal proper digital arteries. When it is necessary to record pressures at the middle phalangeal level, the cuff may be moved to this position. By wrapping the cuff around both the distal phalanx and a photoplethysmographic sensor, one can even obtain reasonably accurate pressure measurements at the fingertip. Hirai and colleagues have devised a bladder-free cuff specifically for this purpose.[32]

Nielsen and colleagues, using a 2.4-cm cuff, found that finger pressures exceeded brachial pressures by 9 ± 7 mmHg in subjects 17 to 31 years of age.[61] The range was from 3 mmHg lower to 21 mmHg higher. In normal older subjects (43 to 57 years of age), the average pressure difference was approximately 0, with a standard deviation of ± 7 mmHg. Using a somewhat larger cuff (3.8 cm), Downs and associates observed that simultaneously measured pressures in corresponding fingers of both hands differed by only 3.5 ± 3.2 mmHg.[18] Only 3 per cent had a difference greater than 9 mmHg. In their study, finger pressures averaged 9.5 ± 6.8 mmHg less than wrist pressures, which in turn were 9.6 ± 7.0 mmHg lower than those at the brachial level. They considered a pressure difference exceeding 15 mmHg between corresponding fingers, a wrist-digital gradient of greater than 30 mmHg, and an absolute finger pressure of less than 70 mmHg to be abnormal. Hirai, whose results were similar to those of Nielsen and colleagues, considers any arm-finger pressure gradient to be abnormal if it exceeds 19 mmHg in subjects under the age of 50, or 25 mmHg in older subjects.[29]

In a series of normal subjects, the author's group found the mean finger–ipsilateral brachial index to be 0.97 ± 0.09. Values ranged from 0.78 to 1.27 (Fig. 65–2).[82] Finger–ipsilateral brachial indices in patients thought to have primary Raynaud's disease on the basis of clinical criteria and laboratory test findings were similar to those of normal individuals (mean, 0.96 ± 0.11; range, 0.60 to 1.23). When, however, there was evidence of proximal digital or palmar arterial obstruction in limbs with no inflow disease, the finger–ipsilateral brachial indices were markedly decreased, averaging 0.56 ± 0.27 with a range extending from 0 to 0.95 (see Fig. 65–2). Low pressures were found in the fingers of both hands in 57 per cent of the patients. Only one finger was affected in 17 per cent of the hands, two fingers were affected in 11 per cent, three or four were affected in 39 per cent, and all five were affected in 33 per cent. As shown in Figure 65–3, finger pressures accurately predict arteriographic findings.

Interpretation

Pressures in all fingers will be reduced in proportion to any reduction in the ipsilateral brachial, forearm, or wrist pressure. When the disease is confined to the arm arteries and the palmar or digital arteries are spared, pressures in all fingers will be approximately equal and the wrist-finger gradient will be within normal limits. If, however, the pressure in one or more fingers is distinctly lower than that in

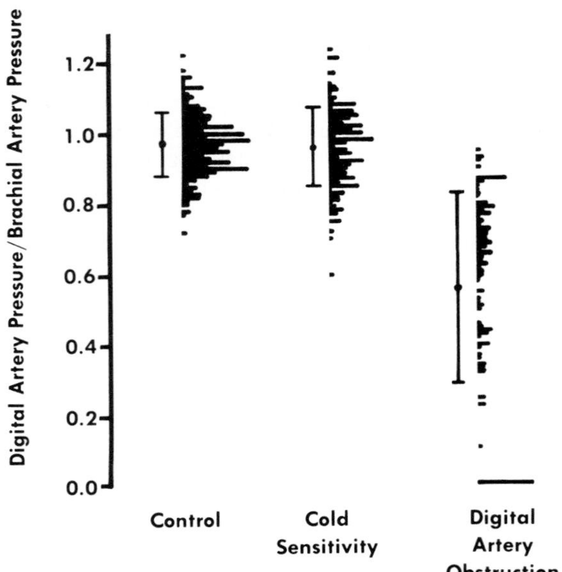

FIGURE 65–2. Finger pressure indices (mean ± 1 SD). Data for cold sensitivity are derived from patients with primary Raynaud's disease. Those in the digital artery obstruction category are from patients who may or may not have secondary Raynaud's phenomenon. (From Sumner DS, Lambeth A, Russell JB: Diagnosis of upper extremity obstructive and vasospastic syndromes by Doppler ultrasound, plethysmography, and temperature profiles. *In* Puel P, Boccalon H, Enjalbert A [eds]: Hemodynamics of the Limbs 1. Toulouse, France, GEPESC, 1979, pp 365–373.)

the others, obstruction of the palmar or digital arteries must also be present.

When arm pressures are normal at all levels, a reduction in finger pressure indicates the presence of disease in the palmar or digital arteries. If pressures in all fingers are equally decreased, the lesion must involve the palmar arch or the terminal portions of both the radial and the ulnar arteries. A reduction in pressure limited to the fingers on one side of the hand suggests that the palmar arch is incomplete or occluded at some point. Isolated obstruction of a common digital artery is implied when the pressure reduction is confined to a single finger and pressures in adjacent fingers remain normal.

Occlusion of only one of the paired proper digital arteries may have no perceptible effect on finger pressure.[18, 29] Not infrequently, the disease process is confined to arteries in the middle or distal phalanx, in which case the pressure measured at the base of the finger is likely to be normal.[18] In such cases, pressures representing the true perfusion potential can be obtained by moving the cuff to the middle or the terminal phalanx.[29, 32, 49]

Doppler Flow Studies

The contour of the blood flow pulse in the upper extremity is similar to that in the lower (see Chapters 3 to 5). Normally, the velocity rises rapidly to a peak in early systole. It then falls abruptly to the baseline, frequently reversing in early diastole (Fig. 65–4). In late diastole, a final, low-level forward flow phase may be present. This gives rise to the typical bi- or triphasic audible signal that is easily recognized by the experienced observer. Below an obstruction or a high-grade stenosis, the signals become attenuated and have a slower upslope, a more rounded peak, and a downslope that continues throughout diastole. Flow reversal no longer occurs (see Fig. 65–4). Audible signals have a low frequency and are monophasic. When the probe is placed over or just distal to a stenosis, noisy, high-frequency signals are obtained, reflecting the presence of disturbed high-velocity flow. No signals are obtained over a totally occluded artery.

An examination of the subclavian, axillary, brachial, radial, and proper digital arteries will often identify the exact location of the obstruction.[4, 88] In most cases, the audible signal suffices; recordings are seldom required. Occasionally, however, it is helpful to use a duplex scanner to interrogate the more proximal vessels.

Because of the extensive collateral network in the forearm and hand, signals obtained from the radial and ulnar arteries at the wrist may sound normal even though one of the pair may be occluded proximally. Clues to the true condition of either one of the two arteries can be obtained by observing the direction of flow and the effect of compression of the other major artery. For example, if flow in the radial artery at the wrist is reversed or if compression of the ulnar artery obliterates the signal, it is evident that an obstruction of the proximal radial artery is present. Patency of the distal radial and ulnar arteries and the palmar

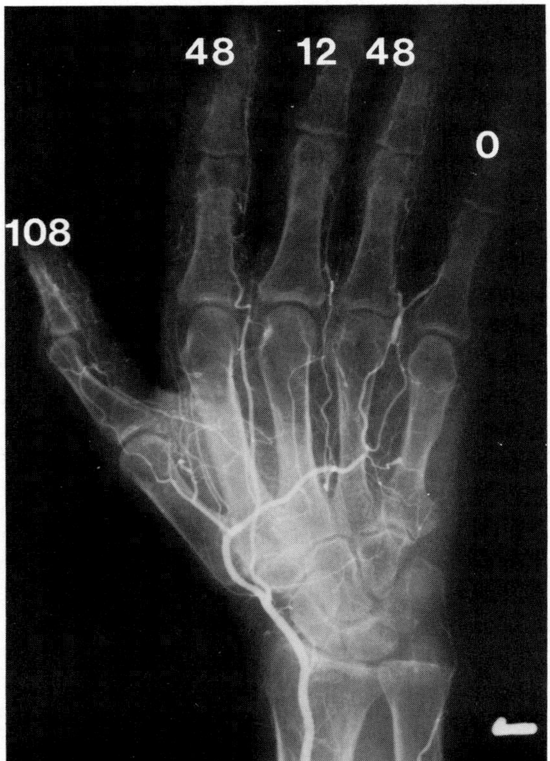

FIGURE 65–3. Digital artery pressures from the proximal phalanges of a 49-year-old man with an ischemic ulcer on the tip of the middle finger. The ipsilateral brachial pressure was 108 mmHg. The arteriogram shows major obstruction of the proper digital arteries to all fingers except the thumb, which has a normal pressure. Pressures in all the other fingers are markedly reduced.

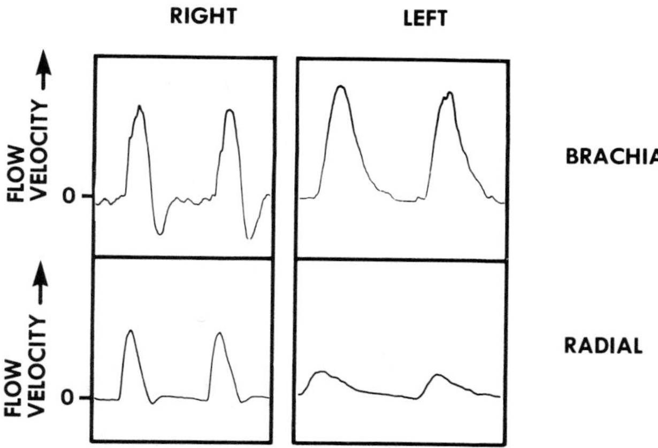

FIGURE 65–4. Analog recordings of Doppler flow signals from the right and left brachial and radial arteries of an 89-year-old woman with occlusion of the left subclavian artery. Brachial pressure: right, 164 mmHg; left, 101 mmHg. Wrist pressure: right, 154 mmHg; left, 77 mmHg. (From Sumner DS: Vascular laboratory diagnosis and assessment of upper extremity vascular disorders. *In* Machleder HI [ed]: Vascular Disorders of the Upper Extremity. 2nd ed. Mount Kisco, NY, Futura Publishing Company, 1989, pp 9–57. Reprinted by permission.)

arch can be ascertained by noting the effect of sequential compression of the radial and ulnar arteries on the mid-palmar signal.[59] Normally, there should be no interruption of flow when either one of the arteries is compressed. When both arteries are compressed simultaneously, flow in the palm should disappear or be markedly decreased, unless a well-developed interosseous arterial communication exists. Flow should resume with release of the compression, provided that the artery being compressed was patent and communicated with the palmar arch. This test is easy to interpret, can be performed rapidly, and is more objective and more informative than the classic Allen test. With the probe placed over a digital artery, similar compression maneuvers can be used to determine the primary source of the blood supply to any one of the fingers.

The hands must be warm when the digital arteries are being studied in order to avoid vasoconstriction, which could lead to a false-positive interpretation.[4] A complete examination requires interrogation of the volar proper digital arteries on both sides of each finger at the proximal and distal interphalangeal joints. Signals from each finger should be compared with those obtained from other fingers on both hands. It is not unusual to detect a signal at the distal interphalangeal joint in the absence of a signal at the proximal interphalangeal joint or at the base of the finger.[4, 82] In this event, compression of the proximal digital artery on the other side of the finger will often obliterate the signal, thus confirming the existence of a crossover collateral derived from the contralateral artery (Fig. 65–5). Examination of the signal over the volar surface of the fingertip is also often informative. A loud signal in this area signifies good perfusion and is typical of the hyperemic phase of primary Raynaud's disease. Poor or absent signals imply vasospasm or fixed arterial obstruction.

A complete Doppler survey of the upper extremities is time consuming and need not be performed in most cases. The history and physical examination findings, coupled with pressure data, will usually permit the examiner to focus on a particular artery. For example, extensive digital artery surveys are required only when digital pressure study results are normal and do not coincide with the clinical assessment.

Duplex and Color Flow Scanning

As it has in all other areas of the peripheral circulation, duplex scanning has had a significant impact on the evaluation of upper extremity arterial disease. The addition of color facilitates scanning by making vessels easier to locate and to follow longitudinally. Small arteries of the forearm, wrist, and hand are readily identified, and even those in the digits can usually be studied. Absence of color in an artery clearly visualized by B-mode scanning is diagnostic of total obstruction, and a color shift from red to white identifies stenotic sites, where flow velocities are increased. This feature reduces the need for serial Doppler interrogation of flow patterns. Because these instruments not only locate lesions precisely but also determine their longitudinal extent, arteriography is less often required. Aneurysms of the radial and ulnar arteries and elsewhere in the upper extremity are easily recognized and differentiated from other masses.[1] Lastly, duplex and color flow scanning are excellent methods for evaluating trauma due to intra-arterial cannulation and for determining the patency of arterial reconstructions in the arm or hand.[40, 60] Indeed, these versatile

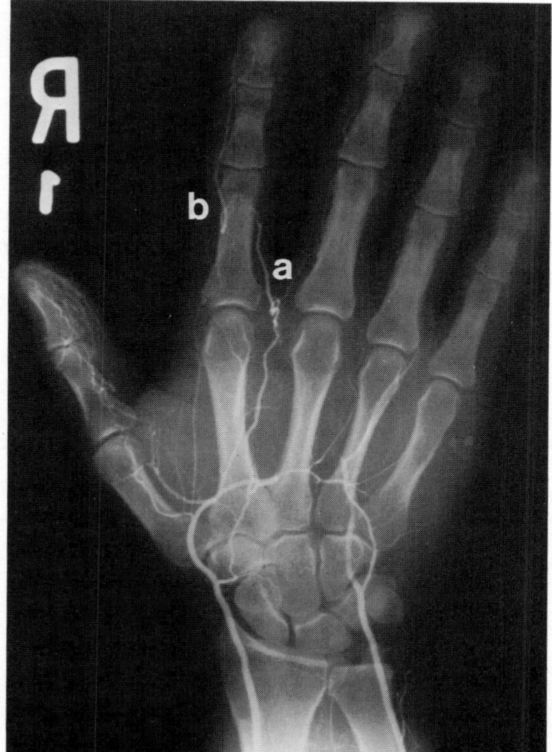

FIGURE 65–5. Arteriogram showing a crossover collateral from the proximal ulnar proper digital artery (a) to the distal radial proper digital artery (b) at the level of the proximal phalanx of the index finger. Compression of the ulnar digital artery at the base of the finger obliterated the Doppler signal heard on the radial side at the level of the middle phalanx.

modalities are fast replacing many of the more cumbersome and less specific noninvasive tests—especially when the information required is largely anatomic.

Plethysmographic Studies

As described in Chapter 4, volume pulses can be recorded from the tips of the fingers with a variety of plethysmographs. For most clinical studies, the photoplethysmograph is entirely satisfactory and is somewhat easier to use than the mercury strain-gauge. Quantification, however, requires the use of a strain-gauge.[80] Although venous occlusion plethysmography can be used to measure digit volume flow (see Chapter 4), these measurements are cumbersome and are reserved for research purposes.[17, 24, 64, 72] For diagnostic evaluations, recording the pulse volume and contour is sufficient.

Pulse Contour

Like the toe pulse, the normal fingertip pulse has a rapid upslope, a sharp systolic peak, and a downslope that bows toward the baseline. A dicrotic notch or wave is usually present on the downslope (Fig. 65–6*A*). The pulse recorded distal to a hemodynamically significant stenosis or occlusion has a delayed upslope, a rounded peak, and a downslope that bows away from the baseline (Fig. 65–6*C*). No dicrotic wave is present on the downslope. An intermediate form, characterized by a rapid ascending limb, an anacrotic notch or an abrupt bend terminating in a systolic peak, and a dicrotic notch high on the downslope, has been called a peaked pulse (Fig. 65–6*B*).[83] Another variant resembles the normal pulse but has a dicrotic notch high on the downslope just after the systolic peak.[65, 84]

Initial studies should be conducted with the fingers warm to obviate the effects of vasoconstriction. Not only must the room temperature be warm, but it may also be necessary to warm the hands by immersing them in warm water. Although mild vasoconstriction merely decreases the pulse amplitude, more severe vasoconstriction may alter the contour of the pulse or result in its disappearance.[28]

Absence of a fingertip pulse or an obstructed pulse recorded under conditions conducive to vasodilatation implies the presence of fixed arterial obstruction somewhere in the vascular pathway supplying the terminal phalanx.[67]

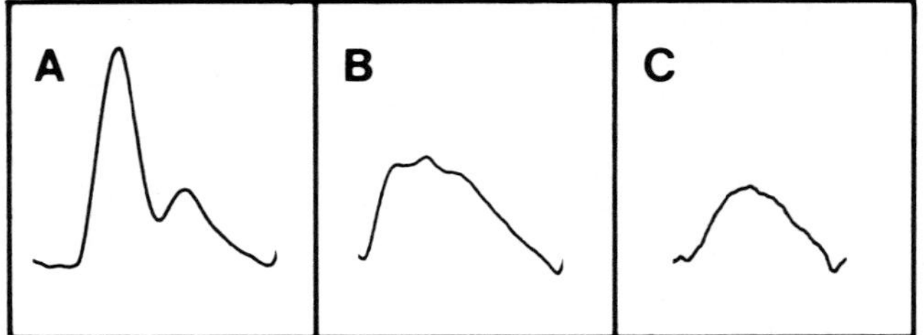

FIGURE 65–6. Plethysmographic pulse contours. *A*, Normal. *B*, Peaked. *C*, Obstructed. (*A–C*, From Sumner DS: Noninvasive assessment of upper extremity ischemia. *In* Bergan JJ, Yao JST [eds]: Evaluation and Treatment of Upper and Lower Extremity Circulatory Disorders. Orlando, FL, Grune & Stratton, 1984, pp 75–95.)

The obstruction may be confined to the digital arteries or the palmar arch, or it may involve the forearm, brachial, axillary, or subclavian arteries. Multi-level disease may be present. Obstructions limited to one of the paired digital arteries or one of the forearm arteries may not produce an obstructed pulse, provided that collateral channels are well developed. This, of course, is not unexpected: to affect the contour of the plethysmographic pulse adversely, a stenosis must be hemodynamically significant and all vessels feeding the fingertip must be involved. As a rule, plethysmographic pulses tend to be less sensitive than pressure measurements to the presence of disease. Normal pulses, on the other hand, are highly specific for the absence of fixed arterial disease.

Owing to the lack of sensitivity, some patients with secondary Raynaud's phenomenon may have relatively normal pulse contours in one or more fingers and occasionally in all.[89] Thus, the negative predictive value of a normal pulse may not be high, particularly if the population has a high prevalence of obstructive disease. Nonetheless, in the author's experience, finding a normal pulse in all fingers of both hands in a patient complaining of cold sensitivity is highly suggestive of primary Raynaud's disease.

Although the significance of peaked pulses remains uncertain, they have been observed frequently in patients with autoimmune (collagen) disorders who do not have major arterial obstruction proximal to the terminal phalanges.[2, 36, 78, 83] They may also be present in a significant number of patients thought on the basis of other criteria to have primary Raynaud's disease. Ohgi and associates showed that normal pulses can be converted to peaked pulses by both direct and indirect cold exposure, even in subjects with no history of cold sensitivity.[65] Peaked pulses, therefore, appear—at least in some cases—to be associated with vasospasm of the digital arteries and arterioles.[2]

Additional diagnostic information can be obtained by observing the effect of cold exposure and spontaneous rewarming on the amplitude of the finger pulse.[34] Cooling of normal fingers to 20° C or below markedly reduces the pulse amplitude, which, on rewarming, rapidly and steadily returns to pre-exposure levels. Similarly, in patients with secondary Raynaud's phenomenon, exposure to cold causes the pulse to either disappear or become barely detectable; recovery to pre-exposure levels is gradual, requiring a longer time than it does in normal subjects. Reflecting the critical closure phenomenon that characterizes the vasospastic response in patients with primary Raynaud's disease, plethysmographic pulses in patients with this condition disappear entirely on cold exposure and remain undetectable until the finger temperature rises above 24 to 26° C; a normal waveform then suddenly reappears. Other investigators have found this test to be of more value in the foot than in the hand for assessing vasospasm.[20, 39]

Responses to Sympathetic Stimuli

In normal limbs, both the amplitude of the digital pulse and the volume of the fingertip vary with respiration (see Fig. 4–2). Respiratory waves are superimposed on larger, but less frequent, alpha-, beta-, and gamma-waves.[10, 35, 78] For these responses to occur, the sympathetic innervation must be intact. Absence of these waves is therefore

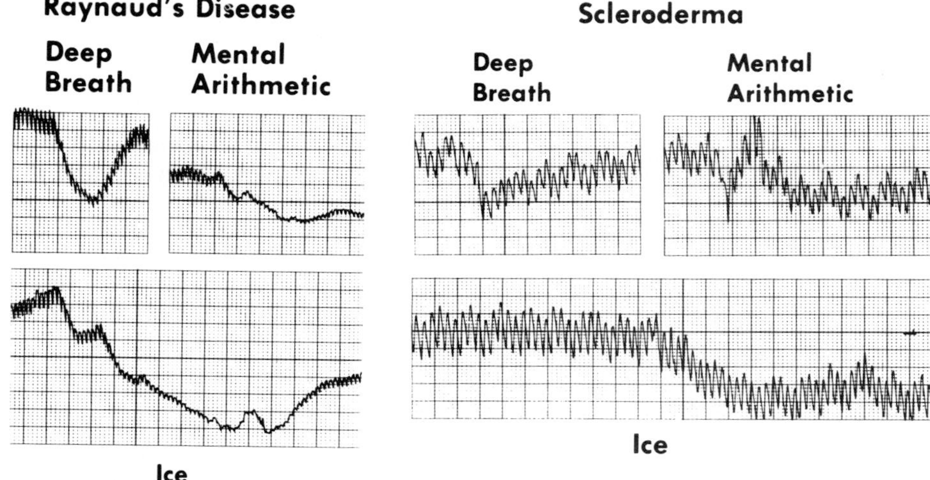

FIGURE 65–7. Effect of sympathetic stimuli on digit volume and digital pulse amplitude in a patient with primary Raynaud's disease and in a patient with scleroderma. Recordings in the right-hand panels were made at a higher sensitivity than those in the left. The patient with scleroderma shows little or no response. (From Sumner DS, Lambeth A, Russell JB: Diagnosis of upper extremity obstructive and vasospastic syndromes by Doppler ultrasound, plethysmography, and temperature profiles. *In* Puel P, Boccalon H, Enjalbert A [eds]: Hemodynamics of the Limbs 1. Toulouse, France, GEPESC, 1979, pp 365–373.)

abnormal, implying lack of sympathetic activity. Sympathetic activity can also be monitored by recording the response of the pulse amplitude and fingertip volume to a deep breath, mental arithmetic, or ice placed on the chest or forehead (Fig. 65–7, *left*).[9, 16, 38, 82] Normally, these maneuvers cause significant vasoconstriction. Reduction of the pulse amplitude reflects a comparable decrease in digital blood flow, and a reduction in fingertip volume reflects both a decrease in arterial inflow and constriction of the terminal arteries and veins. A diminished or an absent response (commonly seen in patients with collagen diseases) is indicative of impaired sympathetic activity (see Fig. 65–7, *right*). Sympathectomy is unlikely to be effective in limbs that display little evidence of sympathetic activity.

To record the larger, slower changes in fingertip volume, it is necessary to employ DC coupling; the more rapid changes in digital pulse amplitude are more conveniently recorded with an AC-coupled plethysmograph (see Chapter 4).[80]

Reactive Hyperemia

The capacity of the digital arterioles to dilate can be determined by monitoring the response of the pulse amplitude to a short period of ischemia (reactive hyperemia test).[80] A pneumatic cuff is placed around the arm, inflated for 5 minutes to a suprasystolic pressure, and then rapidly deflated. In normal limbs and in limbs with purely vasospastic disease, the finger pulse returns promptly and its amplitude increases rapidly (within 30 seconds) to double that of the control pulse (Fig. 65–8).[82] On the other hand, when the peripheral arterioles have dilated maximally to compensate for an increased proximal resistance imposed by a fixed arterial lesion, little or no increase in pulse amplitude will be observed. A similarly poor response is also frequently observed in the limbs of patients whose microvasculature has been stiffened by autoimmune disease.[82] Although sympathectomized limbs may continue to display reactive hyperemia, lack of vasodilatation following a period of ischemia is usually associated with a similarly poor response to a surgical sympathectomy or to the administration of vasodilator drugs.

Vasodilatation can also be induced by warming the patient with an electric blanket, by the oral administration of alcohol, or by immersing the hands in warm water.

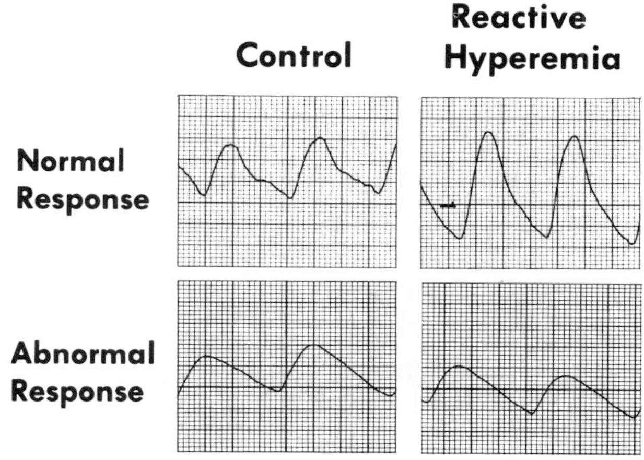

FIGURE 65–8. Normal and abnormal reactive hyperemia responses in a patient with primary Raynaud's disease *(upper panels)* and a patient with scleroderma *(lower panels)*. Both patients had normal digital pressures at the level of the proximal phalanges. (From Sumner DS, Lambeth A, Russell JB: Diagnosis of upper extremity obstructive and vasospastic syndromes by Doppler ultrasound, plethysmography, and temperature profiles. *In* Puel P, Boccalon H, Enjalbert A [eds]: Hemodynamics of the Limbs 1. Toulouse, France, GEPESC, 1979, pp 365–373.)

Laser Doppler Examination

Although laser Doppler recordings do not permit quantitative measurement of blood flow, the output is related to changes in microcirculatory blood flux (see Chapter 4). Results are expressed in millivolts or in arbitrary units. Direct and indirect cooling cause a more profound reduction in fingertip laser Doppler flux in patients with Raynaud's syndrome than they do in subjects without cold sensitivity.[44] Recovery to baseline levels is also delayed. Results, therefore, are similar to those obtained with photoplethysmography. Recordings of laser Doppler flux have proved useful as an adjunct to physiologic studies of Raynaud's disease and as an objective method of documenting the efficacy of drug therapy.[25, 72]

Cold Tolerance Tests

Although the testimony of a reliable patient may be sufficient to establish the diagnosis of cold sensitivity, there are cases—especially those involving industrial injury or compensation—when a more objective method is desirable. Moreover, an accurate assessment of the results of therapy requires objective documentation. All investigators who have attempted to reproduce the typical triphasic changes in the laboratory are aware of how frustrating such efforts may be.

The simple cold tolerance test described by Porter and associates has, in the author's experience, proved to be reasonably reliable.[69] Thermistors are taped to the fingertips, and pre-exposure temperatures are noted. The hands are immersed in ice water for 20 seconds and then removed and dried; post-exposure temperatures are monitored for 20 minutes or until temperatures return to pre-exposure levels. Because the relationship between skin temperature and digit blood flow is so markedly curvilinear, temperature measurements do not accurately reflect blood flow (see Fig. 4–13).[64] Recovery times after cold exposure are, however, roughly comparable, signifying the end of vasoconstriction.

Under the same environmental conditions, fingertip temperatures in normal subjects tend to be several degrees higher than those in patients with cold sensitivity (Fig. 65–9). Immersion in ice water cools the fingertips of both groups to similar levels; however, within 10 minutes after exposure, most normal fingers recover to pre-exposure temperatures, whereas relatively few cold-sensitive fingers do.[82] Recovery in cold-sensitive fingers is often delayed for 20 minutes or more.

In the author's laboratory, this test was 87 per cent sensitive and 79 per cent specific for detecting or ruling out cold-induced vasospasm (when, after a 20-second cold exposure, a 10-minute recovery time was used to divide normal from abnormal responses).[82] Using a modification of their original protocol (in which cold exposure was limited to 5 to 10 seconds and a 5-minute recovery time was taken as the upper limit of normal), Edwards and Porter reported a specificity of 95 per cent but a disappointingly low sensitivity of 50 to 60 per cent.[20]

Nielsen and Lassen have devised a more elegant test that measures the decrease in digital blood pressure as the finger is cooled.[33, 43, 62] A cuff with a double inlet, placed around the middle phalanx, is used first to cool the finger and the underlying arteries to the desired temperature and then to measure blood pressure at that level. To ensure rapid and complete cooling, the finger is made ischemic by inflating a cuff placed around the proximal phalanx to suprasystolic pressure while a cooling solution is circulated through the more distal cuff. When the desired temperature has been attained, the distal cuff is inflated, the proximal

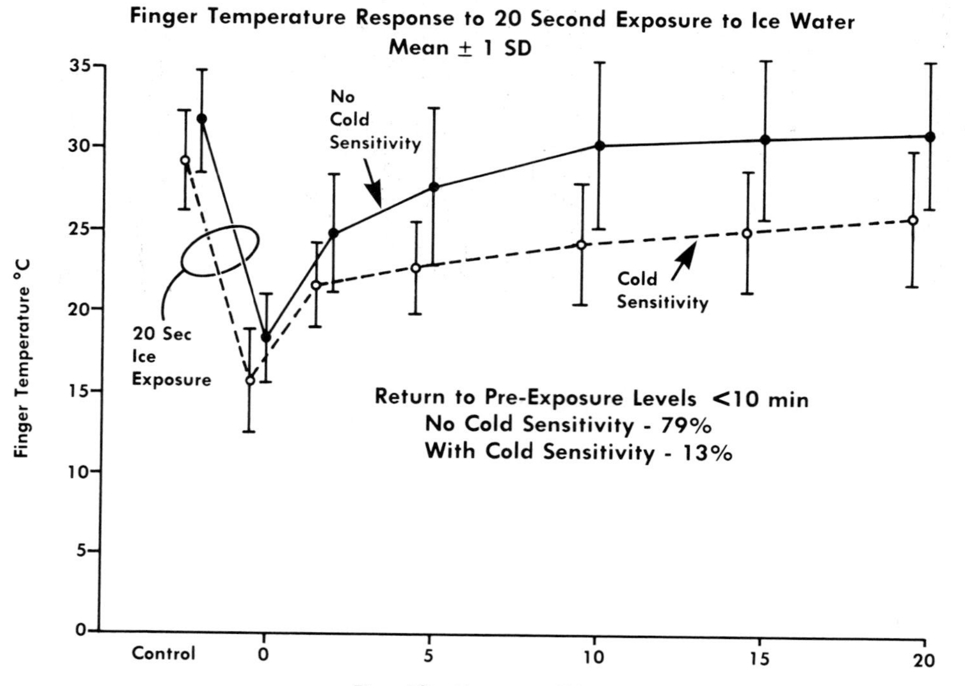

FIGURE 65–9. Fingertip temperatures before, during, and after 20-second immersion of the hands in ice water. (From Sumner DS, Lambeth A, Russell JB: Diagnosis of upper extremity obstructive and vasospastic syndromes by Doppler ultrasound, plethysmography, and temperature profiles. *In* Puel P, Boccalon H, Enjalbert A [eds]: Hemodynamics of the Limbs 1. Toulouse, France, GEPESC, 1979, pp 365–373.)

occluding cuff is deflated, and finger pressure is measured by noting the return of blood flow with a mercury strain-gauge or photoplethysmograph placed around the fingertip as the distal cuff is gradually deflated. The process is repeated at progressively lower temperatures until 10° C is reached. (Newer instruments use the same cuff for producing ischemia, cooling the finger, and measuring pressure. Two fingers may be examined simultaneously; one, which is not cooled, serves as the reference finger.)

Whereas the digital artery pressure in normal subjects decreases only 16 ± 3 per cent at a skin temperature of 10° C, the pressure in patients with primary Raynaud's disease falls rapidly with decreasing temperature and then precipitously to undetectable levels as a "trigger point" is reached. The trigger point at which zero pressures are reached varies from 10 to 20° C, depending on the individual patient, but is reproducible in the same patient. This test, according to Alexander and colleagues, has a sensitivity of 100 per cent, a specificity of 79 per cent, a positive predictive value of 95 per cent, and a negative predictive value of 100 per cent for identifying the presence or absence of digital artery vasospasm in patients with primary Raynaud's disease and secondary Raynaud's phenomenon.[2] According to Carter and associates, this test is most sensitive during total body cooling and is more accurate in patients with secondary Raynaud's phenomenon than it is in patients with primary disease.[11] Corbin and coworkers also noted a low sensitivity in patients with primary Raynaud's disease.[12] Unfortunately, the test is time consuming, requires special equipment not available in most vascular laboratories, and is somewhat artificial in that ischemia is a necessary adjuvant to ensure local cooling.[11] In fact, the lowered pressure measured in the cooled finger may be due in part to prolonged digital artery contraction or delayed relaxation caused by the combined effects of suprasystolic cuff pressure and increased stiffness of the cooled digital artery. For this reason, the measurements are more appropriately termed apparent systolic pressures.[11]

Another, and perhaps more physiologic, method of studying the effect of cold on finger pressures is to make the measurements while the entire hand is immersed in a water bath at progressively lower temperatures (Fig. 65–10).[64] Arterial occlusion is not used. In normal fingers, there is little change in pressure at 10° C, but in cold-sensitive fingers, blood pressure drops precipitously, reaching 0 in about half of the subjects. In the study by DiGiacomo and associates, finger pressures in patients with primary Raynaud's disease averaged 105 ± 24 mmHg in 40° C water and 13 ± 38 mmHg in 10° C water.[17]

Lafferty and associates have devised a test for digital vasospasm based on the principle of *thermal entrainment*.[45] This test attempts to synchronize thermal stimuli with the natural oscillatory frequency of digital blood flow. Recordings of pulse amplitude are made with a photoplethysmograph applied to a finger on one hand while the other hand is alternately placed in a hot (40° C) and a cold (15° C) water bath over a period of 10 minutes. The optimum duration of exposure to each temperature was found to be 40 seconds. A computer is used to analyze the ratio of blood flow response to the temperature stimulus, and the result is referred to as the gain. Gains in patients with Raynaud's phenomenon are significantly higher than those

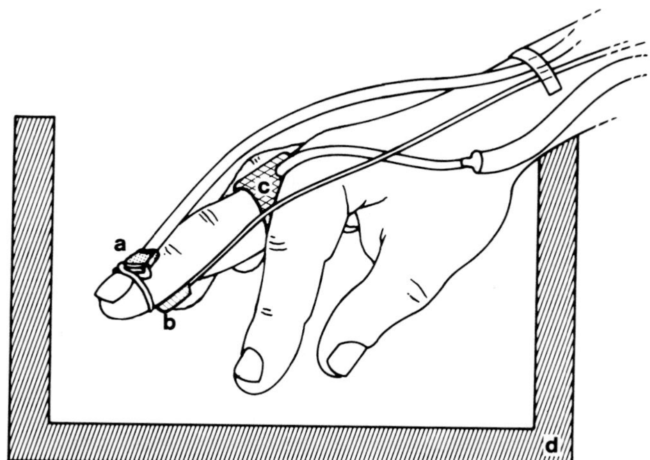

FIGURE 65–10. Apparatus for measuring skin temperature, finger blood flow, and finger pressure during local cold exposure. The apparatus consists of a mercury-in-Silastic strain-gauge (a), an insulated thermistor probe (b), a digital blood pressure cuff (c), and an insulated water bath (d). (From Ohgi S, Moore DJ, Miles RD, et al: The effect of cold on circulation in normal and cold-sensitive fingers. Bruit 9:9, 1985.)

recorded from control subjects. Although this test is objective and appears to be as sensitive as the cold-occlusion pressure test described previously, it is considerably more cumbersome and has not been widely used.[20]

Capillary Microscopy

Capillary loops can be observed in the nailfold with a microscope adjusted to magnify 20 to 40 times. If photographs are not required, a standard ophthalmoscope set at the highest magnification (+40) may suffice. To facilitate visualization, a drop of immersion oil is placed on the skin. Normally, the loops are uniformly distributed and are similar in size and morphology. Findings associated with connective tissue diseases include enlarged, dilated, distorted loops with dropout of adjacent capillaries and areas of avascularity. About 90 per cent of patients with scleroderma have abnormal nailfold capillary patterns.[50] Priollet and associates noted abnormal nailfold capillary patterns in 13 of 14 patients originally classified as having primary Raynaud's disease who on follow-up were later diagnosed as having scleroderma or other connective tissue diseases.[70] Similarly, in a prospective study of patients who had Raynaud's phenomenon without an associated illness, Fitzgerald and associates found abnormal results on capillary microscopy to be the variable most strongly associated with the subsequent development of a connective tissue disease.[23] The odds ratio was 27:1. Thus, capillary microscopy provides important prognostic information.

APPLICATION OF NONINVASIVE TESTS

A careful history and physical examination will often suggest a diagnosis or at least eliminate a number of disease categories. This information will enable the examiner to select those noninvasive tests that are apt to be most productive. In most cases, only a few tests are required. The diagnostic approach should be modified according to the suspected site of obstruction, the duration of symptoms, the presence or absence of cold sensitivity or vasospasm, and the constant or intermittent character of the complaints. Simple algorithms, such as those in Figure 65–11, serve as rough guidelines for the efficient use of noninvasive diagnostic tests.[81]

Obstruction of Arm and Forearm Arteries

When symptoms suggest ischemia of the arm or forearm, the diagnosis of obstruction involving the subclavian, axillary, brachial, radial, or ulnar arteries is usually easily established by measuring and comparing the segmental pressures in both arms. Pressure levels also serve to define the severity of the circulatory impairment. A rapid survey with a Doppler flow detector will often localize the obstruction to one or more of these arteries and may indicate the approximate site of obstruction. More precise definition of the problem can be obtained with a duplex scanner or with a real-time, color-coded Doppler flow-mapping device. Unless intermittent obstruction or hand involvement is suspected, additional noninvasive tests are not required (see Fig. 65–11).

Acute Obstruction

Acute ischemia of the arm may be caused by emboli originating from the heart or ipsilateral subclavian artery or by penetrating, blunt, or iatrogenic trauma. When symptoms are compatible with an embolus, especially in patients with atrial fibrillation or a recent myocardial infarction, noninvasive tests will confirm the diagnosis and help the surgeon chose the appropriate incision. Preoperative arteriography is seldom necessary, but intraoperative arteriography should be employed to confirm the patency of the distal vessels after the embolus has been extracted.

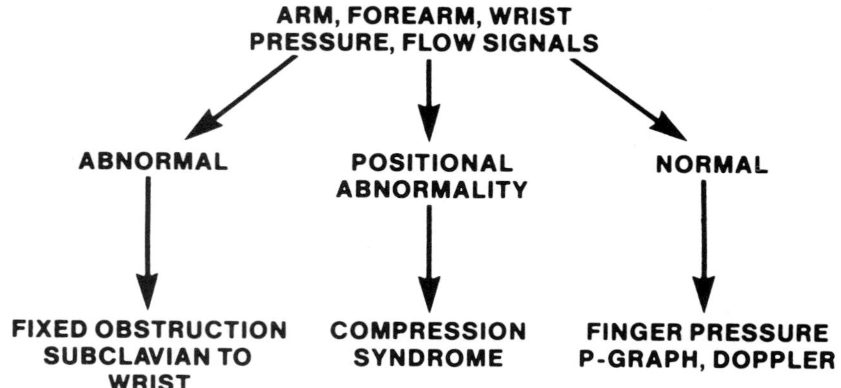

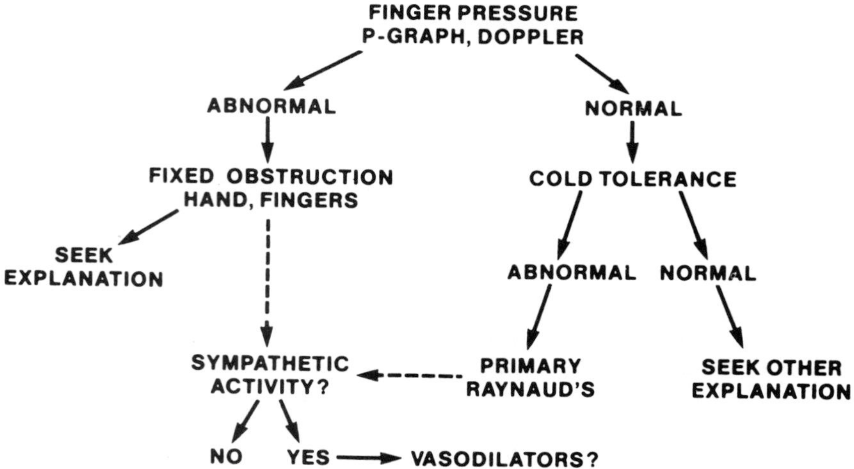

FIGURE 65–11. Approach to noninvasive diagnosis of upper extremity ischemia. (From Sumner DS: Noninvasive assessment of upper extremity and hand ischemia. P-graph, plethysmograph. J Vasc Surg 3:560, 1986.)

Although a decreased pressure or an abnormal Doppler signal distal to the site of penetrating trauma establishes the diagnosis of arterial injury, a normal distal pressure does not necessarily rule out the diagnosis. In all cases in which there is overt bleeding or extensive hematoma formation, arteriography or surgical exploration should be performed even when noninvasive test results are normal. Arterial obstruction caused by blunt trauma, fractured bones, joint dislocations (especially at the elbow), or prolonged extrinsic pressure (e.g., crutch injuries) can be recognized by a reduction in arterial pressure distal to the site of the injury. It must be emphasized that the presence of an audible Doppler signal or even a palpable pulse does not exclude an injury because collateral development may continue to supply some blood flow to the peripheral tissues. Careful pressure measurements are necessary to avoid overlooking a potentially disastrous injury. Depending on the clinical presentation, the nature of the trauma, and the certainty of the noninvasive diagnosis, arteriography may or may not be required.

Cardiac catheterization, diagnostic venous or arterial puncture, and radial artery pressure monitoring are frequent causes of iatrogenic injuries.[6, 40, 48] Many of these mishaps may initially be attributed to spasm. True vasospasm, however, usually causes relatively little reduction in distal arterial pressure despite the fact that the radial or ulnar pulses may be difficult to palpate. A distinct reduction in pressure implies mechanical obstruction. If the pressure is only moderately reduced, it is safe to delay further investigation for a few hours. In the event that vasospasm was indeed the culprit, the pressure will return to normal levels. Some transient obstructions attributed to vasospasm are in reality due to thrombi that undergo lysis or fragmentation, with the fragments having been dispersed to ''silent'' areas of the forearm or hand.

Although prompt operative intervention is the recommended approach in most cases of acute obstruction of the arteries of the upper extremity, it is possible to temporize when the patient's condition makes immediate surgery hazardous or otherwise inadvisable and the noninvasive findings are compatible with continued viability of the arm and hand. As long as distal pressures exceed 40 mmHg, digital plethysmographic pulses are present, and Doppler signals can be detected in the hand and fingers, the potential for tissue survival is good. Because the condition can deteriorate at any time, these parameters must be monitored frequently until it is certain that the limb is out of danger.

Chronic Obstruction

Although atherosclerosis is infrequently responsible for obstruction of the axillary, brachial, or forearm arteries, it is a common cause of proximal subclavian artery obstruction. Beyond the origin of the subclavian artery, retained emboli and neglected trauma are other etiologic factors to be considered. Rarely, giant cell arteritis or Takayasu's disease may affect the subclavian or brachial arteries. Thromboangiitis obliterans (Buerger's disease), another rare condition, tends to involve the distal arteries of the forearm, sparing those in the more proximal parts of the extremity. Segmental pressure measurements will establish the diagnosis, determine the severity of the circulatory deprivation, and usually provide some insight into the site of obstruction. More information regarding the location of the obstructive process can be obtained with the Doppler flow detector or with duplex scanning. Digital plethysmography and finger pressure measurements are necessary only when involvement of the hand arteries is also suspected. Arteriography is required only when operative intervention is being considered. As with similar diseases of the lower extremity, the decision to intervene surgically should be based primarily on symptoms and the degree to which the patient is incapacitated; however, regardless of the symptoms, finding a distal pressure within the ischemic range (less than 40 mmHg) provides a strong impetus.

Intermittent Claudication. An occasional patient with symptoms compatible with arm claudication may have essentially normal segmental pressures at rest. In such cases, a distinct fall in arm pressure after exercise of sufficient intensity to duplicate the symptoms provides confirmation of the diagnosis.[26, 88] Comparing the effect of reactive hyperemia on the blood pressure in both arms is another technique for demonstrating subtle degrees of arterial obstruction. If the pressure drop in the symptomatic arm is significantly greater (20 mmHg or more) than that in the asymptomatic arm, arterial obstruction is the likely explanation for the patient's complaints. Most patients, however, tolerate chronic upper extremity arterial obstruction quite well, especially when the lesion is confined to the proximal subclavian artery. In fact, pressure differentials between the arms that exceed 20 mmHg are frequently observed in completely asymptomatic patients.

Subclavian Steal. Although a normal brachial artery pressure essentially eliminates the diagnosis of subclavian steal, a decreased pressure does not establish the diagnosis because the obstruction responsible for the pressure drop may be distal to the origin of the vertebral artery. If a normal Doppler signal is obtained from the infraclavicular axillary artery, the obstruction responsible for the pressure drop must lie further distally in the arm, thus ruling out the diagnosis of subclavian steal. Finding an abnormal Doppler signal in the supraclavicular subclavian artery increases the likelihood that a subclavian steal is present. To confirm the diagnosis, reversed flow must be demonstrated in the vertebral artery. This is best accomplished with duplex scanning or with arteriography.[8, 13, 58]

Intermittent Obstruction

The first rib, the scalene muscles, the pectoralis minor muscle, and associated ligaments may cause intermittent compression of the subclavian and axillary arteries. When the arm is subjected to the various thoracic outlet maneuvers, a reduction in the arterial cross section of 75 per cent or more can be detected noninvasively by monitoring changes in the radial artery flow pattern, the brachial blood pressure, and the digital plethysmographic pulse (Fig. 65–12).[76, 88] Because compression of a lesser degree will go undetected and because pressure on the brachial plexus is responsible for most of the arm symptoms, negative test findings do not exclude the diagnosis of a thoracic outlet syndrome. On the other hand, positive test results do not

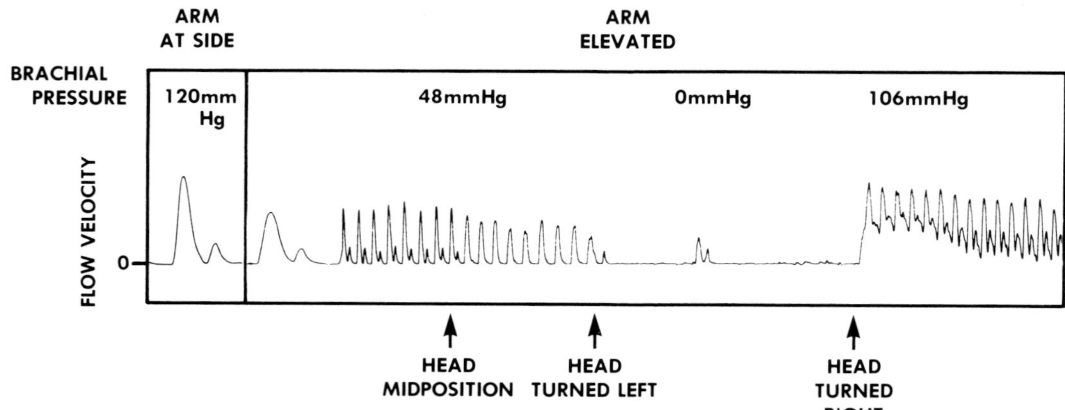

FIGURE 65–12. Doppler flow signals from the right radial artery of a 34-year-old man with thoracic outlet syndrome. Signals decrease with arm elevation and disappear when the head is turned to the left. Hyperemia appears when the head is turned to the right. The brachial blood pressure shows similar changes. (From Sumner DS: Vascular laboratory diagnosis and assessment of upper extremity vascular disorders. *In* Machleder HI [ed]: Vascular Disorders of the Upper Extremity, 2nd ed. Mount Kisco, NY, Futura Publishing Company, 1989, pp 9–57. Reprinted by permission.)

confirm the diagnosis because some degree of arterial compression is often present during these maneuvers, even in normal subjects. In the author's opinion, noninvasive tests add little to a carefully performed physical examination during which the radial pulses are palpated and the infraclavicular area is auscultated for bruits as the arm is manipulated. Objective tests are valuable, however, for detecting emboli originating from post-stenotic subclavian dilatation that obstruct arteries further distally in the arm or hand.

Repeated trauma to the vessels of the shoulder girdle resulting from strenuous athletic activities, such as pitching a baseball or passing a football, may also cause local thrombosis and emboli to the distal arm arteries. Because these highly motivated individuals tend to minimize their symptoms or attribute them to muscle strain, the diagnosis may be overlooked. Noninvasive tests provide an easy way of making the diagnosis and avoiding a result that may prove disastrous to their careers.[52]

Obstruction of Hand and Finger Arteries

Conditions responsible for obstruction of the arteries of the hand and fingers include emboli, vibratory trauma (in chain saw or jackhammer operators), repetitive percussive trauma (hypothenar hammer syndrome, baseball catchers), frostbite, autoimmune diseases (scleroderma or rheumatoid arthritis), Buerger's disease, intra-arterial drug administration, and exposure to various toxins. Patients with end-stage renal disease may have heavily calcified obstructed digital arteries. Atherosclerotic involvement does occur but is relatively rare. In many cases, the cause remains unclear despite extensive investigation. Fixed obstruction of the arteries of the hand or fingers may be entirely asymptomatic; may be symptomatic only during cold exposure (secondary Raynaud's phenomenon); or may cause continued pain, fingertip ulcers, or gangrene.

Noninvasive detection of arterial obstruction is usually not difficult.[7] Even when symptoms are confined to the hand or fingers, the first step is to ascertain whether disease is present in the more proximal arteries (see Fig. 65–11). If lesions are demonstrated in the subclavian, brachial, or forearm arteries, it is likely that any additional obstructions in the hand are part of the same pathologic process. When the proximal examination is normal, the next step is to determine whether the hand symptoms are indeed due to arterial obstruction or whether they represent an exclusively vasospastic process (see Fig. 65–11). This differentiation is important because vasospasm generally has a benign prognosis, whereas that of arterial obstruction is more ominous.

The patency of the palmar arch should be investigated in all cases, and the relative contributions of the radial, ulnar, and interosseous arteries should be determined. Blood pressure at the proximal phalangeal level should be measured in all 10 fingers, especially when symptoms are bilateral.[29, 82] If measurements are restricted to the symptomatic finger or fingers, the presence of more generalized involvement may be overlooked. Similarly, digital pulse waveforms should be recorded from the tips of all fingers. When proximal finger pressures are normal, this step is particularly important in order to avoid missing disease of the intervening arteries. Measurement of pressure at the middle or distal phalangeal level may be revealing in fingers with normal proximal digital pressures and abnormal plethysmographic pulses. Because extensive Doppler surveys of the digital arteries are time consuming and may not be rewarding, this test ordinarily need not be performed on all fingers; however, selective studies of individual fingers may be quite informative. As emphasized previously, to prevent vasospasm and arteriolar constriction, studies designed to detect fixed arterial obstruction should be undertaken only when the hands are warm.

The distribution of the lesions identified by noninvasive testing may suggest a cause. An incomplete palmar arch may represent a common congenital variant, in which case the digital pressures and plethysmographic waveforms in all fingers will be normal, or it may be due to a host of pathologic entities, including trauma, atherosclerosis, emboli, or collagen diseases. If pressures are decreased and pulses are abnormal in the fourth and fifth fingers and the patient gives a history of repetitive percussive trauma to the palm of the hand, the hypothenar hammer syndrome is a strong possibility.[1, 7, 42, 53] In this event, compression of the radial artery at the wrist will obliterate Doppler signals and reduce pressures in the involved fingers, whereas compression of the ulnar artery will have no effect.[31]

Patients often present with symptoms and signs confined to one finger. Noninvasive tests, however, may disclose widespread subclinical lesions in both hands, confirming the presence of a generalized process such as scleroderma or another autoimmune disease. Given sufficient time, more fingers will inevitably become symptomatic.[89] If the obstructions are diffuse but are confined to one hand, a traumatic or embolic cause should be considered. Possible causes include the use of a jackhammer or chain saw or an unrecognized proximal lesion that serves as a source of emboli. When, after all fingers have been carefully studied, the obstruction appears to be localized to a single finger, it is reasonable to postulate that isolated trauma or a single small embolus might be responsible. Nonetheless, the clinician should never discount the possibility that the disease process is generalized and that other lesions may eventually appear.

Abnormalities of the plethysmographic pulses may be the only objective evidence of arterial disease. When all other study results are negative, obstructive or peaked pulses imply disease localized to the terminal vasculature. Autoimmune diseases can present in this fashion.[15, 83]

Arteriography is necessary only in those patients in whom an occult embolic focus is suspected and in those relatively rare situations in which microsurgical arterial reconstruction is contemplated. Revascularization may be feasible when noninvasive tests reveal patent digital arteries lying distal to an occluded palmar arch (as in the hypothenar hammer syndrome). Doppler surveys are especially useful for mapping out the extent of arterial involvement. When hand ischemia is due to diffuse arterial involvement, extensive blood tests are required to identify the cause (see Chapter 68).

Although unrelenting pain, digital ulceration, and gangrene are indicative of severe ischemia, in other, less obvious situations, objective methods may be necessary to define the degree of circulatory impairment. During the acute phase of the disease, digital pressures may lie in the ischemic range and plethysmographic pulses may be absent. Over a period of a few days or weeks, digital pressures often rise and plethysmographic pulses become more nearly normal. Not infrequently, improvement in the circulation of one finger parallels deterioration in the circulation of another. Once the dynamic phase of the disease runs its course, noninvasive findings may remain remarkably stable for prolonged periods. For this reason, the surgeon should avoid precipitous action and adopt a wait-and-see attitude. Because the natural history of digital arterial disease is ordinarily one of fluctuating degrees of ischemia, the clinician must be cautious in attributing improvement to vasodilating drugs, surgical sympathectomy, or other therapeutic measures.[56]

Vasospasm: Intermittent Digital Ischemia

Episodic ischemia of the fingers occurring in response to cold exposure or emotional stimuli (Raynaud's phenomenon) is a frequent complaint of patients referred for vascular evaluation. Estimates of the prevalence of this condition in the general population vary widely, from less than 1.0 per cent to as much as 20 per cent. Ten per cent of 1752 randomly selected subjects from South Carolina complained of cold sensitivity.[51] About 5 per cent reported color changes and 3 per cent sought medical attention. Although the apparent prevalence may be considerably higher in other regions of the world where the climate is colder and damper, this may reflect more frequent exposure to the triggering stimulus rather than a difference in the prevalence of the underlying disorder.

An attempt to classify the patient's disease process is made in order to formulate a treatment plan and to offer a short-term prognosis. If, in addition to cold sensitivity, the patient has symptoms or signs of fixed arterial obstruction (e.g., trophic skin changes, ulcers, or severe pain) or if results of noninvasive tests are positive for arterial obstruction, the process is classified as secondary Raynaud's phenomenon (see Fig. 65–11).[30, 82] In most of these patients, cold sensitivity is overshadowed by other complaints. One or both hands may be symptomatic, but digital involvement is seldom symmetric.

If digital pressures, pulses, and Doppler study results are normal when the hands are warm, a diagnosis of primary Raynaud's disease or vasospastic Raynaud's syndrome can be made, provided that the existence of cold sensitivity can be documented by history, direct observation, or cold tolerance tests (see Fig. 65–11).[30, 83, 85] Patients with primary Raynaud's disease are usually young, and the majority are female. Although these patients may complain of discomfort during the attacks, severe pain is rare. Symptoms are bilateral and symmetric, and there are no skin changes. Responses to sympathetic stimuli are active, and reactive hyperemia studies demonstrate a normal capacity for vasodilatation.[82] In the author's experience, blood test results in all patients with this constellation of symptoms, signs, and normal noninvasive findings have consistently been normal.

Between these two extremes is a group of patients in whom the history and physical examination are consistent with primary Raynaud's disease but whose noninvasive test results suggest an underlying disorder.[5, 15, 83, 89] In some or all of the fingers, digital artery pressures may be moderately decreased and plethysmographic pulses may be peaked or have a high dicrotic notch. The Doppler survey may reveal isolated abnormalities. Laboratory tests may disclose abnormalities in the sedimentation rate, antinuclear antibody (ANA) titers, or serum immunoelectrophoretic patterns; however, in the majority of these patients, the results are normal. Although it is likely that some of these patients will ultimately prove to have scleroderma or another connective tissue disease, the data currently available are insufficient to substantiate this prediction.

Among the criteria proposed in the early 1930s by

Allen and Brown for primary Raynaud's disease was the stipulation that episodic cold sensitivity must be present for 2 years without the appearance of any associated disease.[3] Subsequently, many investigations have shown that this period is too short and that Raynaud's syndrome may be present for as long as 30 years before an associated disease becomes apparent. Indeed, there seems to be no clearly defined upper limit. Although it is impossible to predict which patients will ultimately develop a connective tissue disease, the likelihood that such diseases will become manifest during follow-up appears to be related to the initial clinical and laboratory findings. If the cumulative results of those articles published after 1980 are extracted from Edwards and Porter's literature review, only 12 of 408 patients (2.9 per cent) classified on the basis of serologic and clinical evaluations as having primary Raynaud's disease developed a connective tissue disease over a follow-up period averaging 3.7 years.[21] In contrast, 60 of 184 patients (32.6 per cent) with one or more clinical or serologic abnormalities but without all the necessary criteria for a definitive diagnosis of connective tissue disease as promulgated by the American Rheumatism Association[79] developed a connective tissue disease over an average follow-up period of 4.0 years. The term *suspected secondary Raynaud's phenomenon* has been proposed to differentiate this high-risk group from the group without evident abnormalities.[41, 70]

Among the clinical features that suggest the diagnosis of connective tissue disease in patients with Raynaud's syndrome are sclerodactyly, digital pitting scars, puffy fingers, telangiectasias, pulmonary fibrosis, and esophageal dysmobility. Although elevated ANA titers often correlate with the subsequent appearance of an associated disease, positive antinuclear antibody findings have been reported in 12 per cent of otherwise normal women in whom no connective tissue disease developed over a period of 5 years.[21, 87] Perhaps the test with the greatest prognostic value is capillary microscopy.[23, 37, 70] It seems reasonable to speculate that many, if not most, patients classified as having suspected secondary Raynaud's phenomenon will also demonstrate some changes in digital pulse waveforms, Doppler signals, or digital pressures.

THERAPY

When lesions involve the subclavian, axillary, brachial, radial, or ulnar arteries, vascular reconstruction is usually possible. With microvascular techniques, reconstruction of the small arteries of the hand is often feasible.[1, 60, 77] Emboli and thrombi can be treated surgically or with thrombolytic therapy. As discussed previously, noninvasive tests are helpful in identifying those lesions that compromise the circulation sufficiently to require direct therapy. After treatment, these tests are valuable not only for assessing the degree of immediate physiologic improvement but also for following the results longitudinally (Table 65–3).[52, 60] Restoration of flow to completely or partially severed arms, hands, and fingers is now being performed routinely in many centers. Although continued viability of the severed part confirms the patency of the vascular anastomoses, noninvasive measurement of digital pulses, blood flow, and digital pressures provides objective data concerning the adequacy of the blood supply. The author's group showed that perfusion of tissues surviving reimplantation is usually within normal limits but is often lower than that in normal tissues of the same individual (Fig. 65–13).[49]

Many patients, however, have lesions that are situated too far distally or are too extensive to be amenable to vascular reconstruction. Included in this group are patients with autoimmune and connective tissue diseases, vibratory trauma, frostbite, Buerger's disease, and a host of other problems. To increase blood flow, the physician may turn to vasodilating drugs, calcium channel blockers, prostaglandins, hemorrheologic agents, fish oil supplements, or surgical sympathectomy.[17, 56, 66, 72–74, 86] All of these methods have been reported to be successful by some investigators and unsuccessful by others, but few controlled studies have been performed. As mentioned previously, given sufficient time, the circulation of most ischemic fingers will improve spontaneously, although the improvement may be temporary and may occur concurrently with decreasing circulation to another finger.[56] Noninvasive tests, therefore, provide an objective method of assessing the effect of a specific therapy and of documenting the natural history of the disease.[17, 25, 56, 57, 63, 66, 73] Although alleviation of symptoms is the primary goal, subjective evaluations are notoriously unreliable.

Vasodilating drugs and sympathectomy are likely to be beneficial only when the terminal vasculature is capable of vasodilatation. Noninvasive tests designed to evaluate sympathetic activity should be performed when these forms of therapy are contemplated (see Fig. 65–11). If, in response to a reactive hyperemia test, the digital pulse volume does not increase appreciably, it is doubtful that these measures will be successful (see Fig. 65–8). Even when reactive hyperemia develops, sympathectomy or the use of sympatholytic drugs would not be expected to increase blood flow in the absence of a positive response to a deep breath test (see Fig. 65–7). Before the patient is subjected to a sympathectomy, plethysmographic pulses should be monitored both before and after a sympathetic block to confirm that vasodilatation is possible.

Patients with primary Raynaud's disease almost invariably demonstrate reactive hyperemia and an active re-

Table 65–3. Pressure Data (mmHg) Before and After Revascularization in Patients With Obstructions of the Brachial, Radial, and Ulnar Arteries

	Site of Obstruction					
	Brachial		*Radial (Forearm)*		*Ulnar, Palmar Arch*	
	BEFORE	AFTER*	BEFORE	AFTER†	BEFORE	AFTER‡
Brachial	100	110	90	100	132	130
Forearm	88	102	70	104	—	—
Wrist	86	94	—	—	—	—
Finger (1)	0	106	22	98	126	128
(2)	46	100	25	82	130	136
(3)	30	102	—	—	130	128
(4)	55	87	—	--	100	124
(5)	25	103	—	—	60	118

*Proximal brachial–antecubital bypass graft.
†Distal brachial–distal radial bypass graft.
‡Distal ulnar–common digital bypass graft.

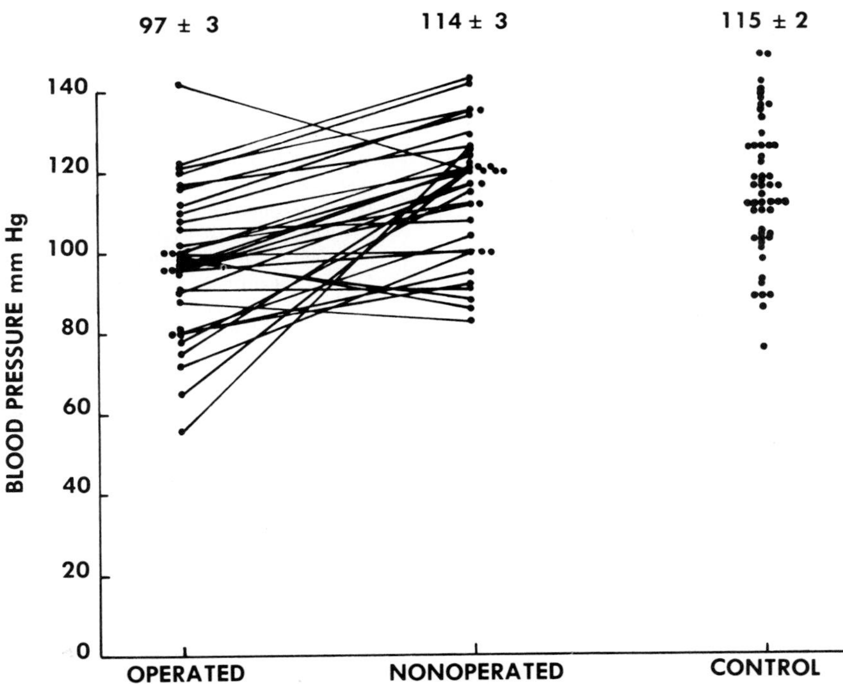

FIGURE 65–13. Blood pressures in the distal phalanges of 32 replanted fingers (operated) compared with those of the comparable fingers of the other hand (nonoperated). Control pressures are from 52 normal fingers. (From Manke DA, Sumner DS, Van Beek AL, et al: Hemodynamic studies of digital and extremity replants or revascularizations. Surgery 88:445, 1980.)

sponse to a deep breath (see Figs. 65–7 and 65–8). Although sympathectomy usually increases blood flow (at least temporarily), it is seldom if ever indicated in these patients because symptoms are rarely severe and the disease does not jeopardize tissue survival. Vasodilators may, however, be helpful. Unfortunately, sympathectomy and sympatholytic drugs are least efficacious in those cases in which an increased level of perfusion is most needed because the arterioles are often maximally dilated to compensate for a proximal obstruction and the compliance of the terminal vessels is impaired by the disease process responsible for the ischemia.[56] A few drugs—particularly calcium channel blockers—do seem to afford some relief, but noninvasive tests show little objective evidence of increased perfusion.[14, 56, 57, 66, 72–74]

CONCLUSIONS

The evaluation of acute and chronic ischemia of the upper extremity is facilitated by the selective use of simple noninvasive methods available in most vascular laboratories. They detect the presence of arterial obstruction, help locate the site or sites of obstruction, assess the severity of the circulatory impairment, and distinguish between primarily obstructive and vasospastic disease. Although noninvasive tests do not establish a cause, they clarify the need for further laboratory tests or arteriography. Finally, they provide an objective method of evaluating the results of therapeutic intervention and of defining the natural history of the disease process.

References

1. Abshire J, Fruscha JD, Jones TR, Schellack JV: Demonstration of hypothenar hammer syndrome by duplex ultrasound. J Vasc Technol 16:39, 1992.
2. Alexander S, Cummings C, Figg-Hoblyn L, et al: Usefulness of digital peaked pulse for diagnosis of Raynaud's syndrome. J Vasc Technol 12:71, 1988.
3. Allen E, Brown G: Raynaud's disease: A critical review of minimal requisites for diagnosis. Am J Med Sci 183:187, 1932.
4. Balas P, Katsogiannis A, Katsiotis P, et al: Comparative study of evaluation of digital arterial circulation by Doppler ultrasonic tracing and hand arteriography. J Cardiovasc Surg 21:455, 1980.
5. Balas P, Tripolitis AJ, Kaklamanis P, et al: Raynaud's phenomenon. Primary and secondary causes. Arch Surg 114:1174, 1979.
6. Barnes RW, Peterson JL, Krugmire RB, et al: Complications of brachial artery catheterization: Prospective evaluation with the Doppler velocity detector. Chest 66:363, 1974.
7. Bartel P, Blackburn D, Peterson L, et al: The value of non-invasive tests in occupational trauma of the hands and fingers. Bruit 8:15, 1984.
8. Berguer R, Higgins R, Nelson R: Noninvasive diagnosis of reversal of vertebral-artery blood flow. N Engl J Med 302:1349, 1980.
9. Browse NL, Hardwick PJ: The deep breath–venoconstriction reflex. Clin Sci 37:125, 1969.
10. Burch GE: Digital Plethysmography. New York, Grune & Stratton, 1954.
11. Carter SA, Dean E, Kroeger EA: Apparent finger systolic pressures

during cooling in patients with Raynaud's syndrome. Circulation 77:988, 1988.
12. Corbin DOC, Wood DA, Housley E: An evaluation of finger systolic-pressure response to local cooling in the diagnosis of primary Raynaud's phenomenon. Clin Physiol 5:383, 1985.
13. Corson JD, Menzoian JO, LoGerfo FW: Reversal of vertebral artery blood flow demonstrated by Doppler ultrasound. Arch Surg 112:715, 1977.
14. Creager MA, Pariser KM, Winston EM, et al: Nifedipine-induced fingertip vasodilation in patients with Raynaud's phenomenon. Am Heart J 108:370, 1984.
15. Dabich L, Bookstein JJ, Zweifler A, et al: Digital arteries in patients with scleroderma. Arteriographic and plethysmographic study. Arch Intern Med 130:708, 1972.
16. Delius W, Kellerova E: Reactions of arterial and venous vessels in the human forearm and hand to deep breath or mental strain. Clin Sci 40:271, 1971.
17. DiGiacomo RA, Kremer JM, Shah DM: Fish-oil dietary supplementation in patients with Raynaud's phenomenon: A double-blind, controlled, prospective study. Am J Med 86:158, 1989.
18. Downs AR, Gaskell P, Morrow I, et al: Assessment of arterial obstruction in vessels supplying the fingers by measurement of local blood pressures and the skin temperature response test: Correlation with angiographic evidence. Surgery 77:530, 1975.
19. Edwards JM, Phinney ES, Taylor LM, et al: α2-adrenergic receptor levels in obstructive and spastic Raynaud's syndrome. J Vasc Surg 5:38, 1987.
20. Edwards JM, Porter JM: Diagnosis of upper extremity vasospastic disease. *In* Ernst CB, Stanley JC (eds): Current Therapy in Vascular Surgery. 2nd ed. Philadelphia, BC Decker, 1991, pp 186–190.
21. Edwards JM, Porter JM: Long-term outcome of Raynaud's syndrome. *In* Yao JST, Pearce WH (eds): Long-Term Results in Vascular Surgery. Norwalk, CT, Appleton & Lange, 1993, pp 345–352.
22. Erlandson EE, Forrest ME, Shields JJ, et al: Discriminant arteriographic criteria in the management of forearm and hand ischemia. Surgery 90:1025, 1981.
23. Fitzgerald O, O'Connor GT, Spencer-Green G: Prospective study of the evolution of Raynaud's phenomenon. Am J Med 84:718, 1988.
24. Freedman RR, Mayes MD, Sabharwal SC: Induction of vasospastic attacks despite digital nerve blood in Raynaud's disease and phenomenon. Circulation 80:859, 1989.
25. Graafsma SJ, Wollersheim H, Droste HT, et al: Adrenoceptors on blood cells from patients with primary Raynaud's phenomenon. Clin Sci 80:325, 1991.
26. Gross WS, Flanigan P, Kraft RO, et al: Chronic upper extremity arterial insufficiency. Arch Surg 113:419, 1978.
27. Gundersen J: Segmental measurements of systolic blood pressure in the extremities including the thumb and the great toe. Acta Chir Scand 426(Suppl):1, 1972.
28. Hertzman AB, Roth LW: The reactions of the digital artery and minute pad arteries to local cold. Am J Physiol 136:680, 1942.
29. Hirai M: Arterial insufficiency of the hand evaluated by digital blood pressure and arteriographic findings. Circulation 58:902, 1978.
30. Hirai M: Cold sensitivity of the hand in arterial occlusive disease. Surgery 85:140, 1979.
31. Hirai M: Digital blood pressure and arteriographic findings under selective compression of the radial and ulnar arteries. Angiology 31:21, 1980.
32. Hirai M, Ohta T, Shionoya S: Development of a bladder-free cuff for measuring the blood pressure of the fingers and toes. Circulation 61:704, 1980.
33. Hoare M, Miles C, Girvan R, et al: The effect of local cooling on digital systolic pressure in patients with Raynaud's syndrome. Br J Surg 69(Suppl):527, 1982.
34. Holmgren K, Bauer GM, Porter JM: Vascular laboratory evaluation of Raynaud's syndrome. Bruit 5:19, 1981.
35. Honda N: The periodicity in volume fluctuations and blood flow in the human finger. Angiology 21:442, 1970.
36. Huff SE: Observations on peripheral circulation in various dermatoses. Arch Dermatol 71:575, 1955.
37. Jacobs MJHM, Breslau PJ, Slaaf DW, et al: Nomenclature of Raynaud's phenomenon: A capillary microscopic and hemorrheologic study. Surgery 101:136, 1987.
38. Jamieson GG, Ludbrook J, Wilson A: Cold hypersensitivity in Raynaud's phenomenon. Circulation 44:254, 1971.
39. Janoff KA, Phinney ES, Porter JM: Lumbar sympathectomy for lower extremity vasospasm. Am J Surg 150:147, 1985.
40. Jones CE, Anderson FA Jr, Cardullo PA: Duplex ultrasound evaluation of radial artery diameter and hemodynamics before and after placement of a radial artery cannula. J Vasc Technol 15:181, 1991.
41. Kallenberg CGM, Pastoor GW, Wouda AA, et al: Antinuclear antibodies in patients with Raynaud's phenomenon: Clinical significance of anticentromere antibodies. Ann Rheum Dis 41:382, 1982.
42. Koman LA, Urbaniak JR: Ulnar artery insufficiency: A guide to treatment. J Hand Surg 6:16, 1981.
43. Krähenbühl B, Nielsen SL, Lassen NA: Closure of digital arteries in high vascular tone states as demonstrated by measurement of systolic blood pressure in the fingers. Scand J Clin Lab Invest 37:71, 1977.
44. Kristensen JK, Engelhart M, Nielsen T: Laser-Doppler measurement of digital blood flow regulation in normals and in patients with Raynaud's phenomenon. Acta Derm Venereol (Stockh) 63:43, 1983.
45. Lafferty K, de Trafford JC, Roberts VC, Cotton LT: Raynaud's phenomenon and thermal entrainment: An objective test. Br Med J 286:90, 1983.
46. Lewis T: Experiments relating to the peripheral mechanism involved in spasmodic arrest of circulation in fingers, a variety of Raynaud's disease. Heart 15:7, 1929.
47. Lynn RB, Steiner RE, Van Wyk FAK: Arteriographic appearances of the digital arteries of the hands in Raynaud's disease. Lancet 1:471, 1955.
48. Machleder HI, Sweeney JP, Barker WF: Pulseless arm after brachial artery catheterization. Lancet 1:407, 1972.
49. Manke DA, Sumner DS, Van Beek AL, et al: Hemodynamic studies of digital and extremity replants or revascularizations. Surgery 88:445, 1980.
50. Maricq HR, Spencer-Green G, LeRoy EC: Skin capillary abnormalities as indicators of organ involvement in scleroderma (systemic sclerosis), Raynaud's syndrome and dermatomyositis. Am J Med 61:862, 1976.
51. Maricq HR, Weinrich MC, Keil JE, et al: Prevalence of Raynaud phenomenon in the general population. A preliminary study by questionnaire. J Chron Dis 39:423, 1986.
52. McCarthy WJ, Yao JST, Schafer MF, et al: Upper extremity arterial injury in athletes. J Vasc Surg 9:317, 1989.
53. McNamara MF, Takaki HS, Yao JST, et al: A systematic approach to severe hand ischemia. Surgery 83:1, 1978.
54. Mead J, Schoenfeld RC: Character of blood flow in the vasodilated fingers. J Appl Physiol 2:680, 1950.
55. Mendlowitz M, Naftchi N: The digital circulation in Raynaud's disease. Am J Cardiol 4:580, 1959.
56. Mills JL, Friedman EI, Taylor LM Jr, et al: Upper extremity ischemia caused by small artery disease. Ann Surg 206:521, 1987.
57. Mohrland JS, Porter JM, Kahaleh MB, et al: A multiclinic, placebo-controlled, double-blind study of prostaglandin E1 in Raynaud's syndrome. Ann Rheum Dis 44:754, 1985.
58. Mozersky DJ, Barnes RW, Sumner DS, et al: Hemodynamics of innominate artery occlusion. Ann Surg 178:123, 1973.
59. Mozersky DJ, Buckley CJ, Hagood CO Jr, et al: Ultrasonic evaluation of the palmar circulation. A useful adjunct to radial artery cannulation. Am J Surg 126:810, 1973.
60. Nehler MR, Dalman RL, Harris EJ, et al: Upper extremity arterial bypass distal to the wrist. J Vasc Surg 16:633, 1992.
61. Nielsen PE, Bell G, Lassen NA: The measurement of digital systolic blood pressure by strain gauge technique. Scand J Clin Lab Invest 29:371, 1972.
62. Nielsen SL, Lassen NA: Measurement of digital blood pressure after local cooling. J Appl Physiol 43:907, 1977.
63. Nobin BA, Nielsen SL, Eklov B, et al: Reserpine treatment of Raynaud's disease. Ann Surg 87:12, 1978.
64. Ohgi S, Moore DJ, Miles RD, et al: The effect of cold on circulation in normal and cold sensitive fingers. Bruit 9:9, 1985.
65. Ohgi S, Moore DJ, Miles RD, et al: Physiology of the peaked finger pulse in normal and cold-sensitive subjects. J Vasc Surg 3:516, 1986.
66. Pardy BJ, Hoare MC, Eastcott HHG, et al: Prostaglandin E1 in severe Raynaud's phenomenon. Surgery 92:953, 1982.
67. Peller JS, Gabor GT, Porter JM, et al: Angiographic findings in mixed connective tissue disease. Correlation with fingernail capillary photomicroscopy and digital photoplethysmography findings. Arthritis Rheum 28:768, 1985.
68. Porter JM, Rivers SP, Anderson CJ, et al: Evaluation and management of patients with Raynaud's syndrome. Am J Surg 142:183, 1981.

69. Porter JM, Snider RL, Bardana EJ, et al: The diagnosis and treatment of Raynaud's phenomenon. Surgery 77:11, 1975.
70. Priollet P, Vayssairat M, Housset E: How to classify Raynaud's phenomenon. Long-term follow-up study of 73 cases. Am J Med 83:494, 1987.
71. Pyykkö I, Kolari P, Fäkkilä M, et al: Finger peripheral resistance during local cold provocation in vasospastic disease. Scand J Work Environ Health 12:395, 1986.
72. Rademaker M, Cooke ED, Almond NE, et al: Comparison of intravenous infusions of iloprost and oral nifedipine in treatment of Raynaud's phenomenon in patients with systemic sclerosis: A double blind randomized study. Br Med J 298:561, 1989.
73. Roald OK, Seem E: Treatment of Raynaud's phenomenon with ketanserin in patients with connective tissue disorders. Br Med J 289:577, 1984.
74. Rodeheffer RJ, Rommer JA, Wigley F, et al: Controlled double-blind trial of nifedipine in the treatment of Raynaud's phenomenon. N Engl J Med 308:880, 1983.
75. Rösch J, Porter JM, Gralino BJ: Cryodynamic hand angiography in the diagnosis and management of Raynaud's syndrome. Circulation 55:807, 1977.
76. Sanders RJ, Monsour JW, Baer SB: Transaxillary first rib resection for the thoracic outlet syndrome. Arch Surg 97:1014, 1968.
77. Silcott GR, Polich VL: Palmar arch arterial reconstruction for the salvage of ischemic fingers. Am J Surg 142:219, 1981.
78. Strandness DE Jr, Sumner DS: Raynaud's disease and Raynaud's phenomenon. *In* Hemodynamics for Surgeons. New York, Grune & Stratton, 1975, pp 543–581.
79. Subcommittee for scleroderma criteria of the American Rheumatism Association Diagnostic and Therapeutic Criteria Committee: Preliminary criteria for the classification of systemic sclerosis (scleroderma). Arthritis Rheum 23:581, 1980.
80. Sumner DS: Mercury strain-gauge plethysmography. *In* Bernstein EF (ed): Noninvasive Diagnostic Techniques in Vascular Disease. 3rd ed. St. Louis, CV Mosby, 1985, pp 133–150.
81. Sumner DS: Noninvasive assessment of upper extremity and hand ischemia. J Vasc Surg 3:560, 1986.
82. Sumner DS, Lambeth A, Russell JB: Diagnosis of upper extremity obstructive and vasospastic syndromes by Doppler ultrasound, plethysmography, and temperature profiles. *In* Puel P, Boccalon H, Enjalbert A (eds): Hemodynamics of the Limbs 1. Toulouse, France, GEPESC, 1979, pp 365–373.
83. Sumner DS, Strandness DE Jr: An abnormal finger pulse associated with cold sensitivity. Ann Surg 175:294, 1972.
84. Thulesius O: Methods for the evaluation of peripheral vascular function in the upper extremities. Acta Chir Scand 465(Suppl):53, 1975.
85. Tordoir JHM, Haeck LB, Winterkamp H, et al: Multifinger photoplethysmography and digital blood pressure measurement in patients with Raynaud's phenomenon of the hand. J Vasc Surg 3:456, 1986.
86. Welling RE, Cranley JJ, Krause RJ, et al: Obliterative arterial disease of the upper extremity. Arch Surg 116:1593, 1981.
87. Yadin O, Sarov B, Naggan L, et al: Natural autoantibodies in the serum of healthy women—A five-year follow-up. Clin Exp Immunol 75:402, 1989.
88. Yao JST, Gourmos C, Pathanasiou K, et al: A method for assessing ischemia of the hands and fingers. Surg Gynecol Obstet 135:373, 1972.
89. Zweifler AJ, Trinkaus P: Occlusive digital artery disease in patients with Raynaud's phenomenon. Am J Med 77:995, 1984.

66

Arteriosclerotic Occlusive Disease of Brachiocephalic Arteries

Kenneth J. Cherry, Jr., M.D.

• • •

Occlusive lesions of the innominate, common carotid, and subclavian arteries requiring reconstruction occur much less frequently than those encountered at the carotid bifurcations. The Joint Study of Arterial Occlusion reported that only 17 per cent of lesions demonstrated on arteriography involved the innominate artery and the proximal subclavian arteries.[1] Wylie and Effeney reported that of the 1961 operations performed at the University of California–San Francisco for carotid bifurcation, vertebral artery, or great vessel disease, only 7.5 per cent were performed for innominate, common carotid, or subclavian artery lesions.[2] The relative rarity of these lesions has meant that their natural history is unknown and that data concerning operations to correct brachiocephalic stenoses and occlusions, especially of the innominate and common carotid arteries, have come from retrospective studies at large referral centers.[3–10]

Innominate artery and other brachiocephalic occlusive lesions occur in an age group relatively younger than that seen for other sites of vascular disease, with mean or median ages ranging from 50 through 57 years.[3–10] Men predominate slightly. However, in women such lesions are relatively more common than atherosclerotic lesions of the lower extremities. In most reports from the United States, women comprise 45 to 49 per cent of the patients,[3–5, 7, 10] and in three series, they represent a majority.[6, 8, 9] Atherosclerosis is the predominant etiology in North America, with Takayasu's arteritis a distant second. These latter patients are more often female and younger. Radiation-induced atherosclerosis obliterans accounts for a minor fraction of the cases seen.[11, 12] Patients with atherosclerosis may present with either occlusive or atheroembolic symptoms, whereas the symptoms in patients with arteritis are occlusive.

Smoking has been identified as a risk factor in 78 to

100 per cent of patients with brachiocephalic arterial occlusive disease.[4, 7–10] Concomitant coronary artery disease is an association in 27 to 65 per cent of these patients.[4, 7–10] Three of the larger series of aortic arch reconstructions reported coronary disease in approximately 45 per cent of patients.[4, 7, 8]

A HISTORY

The first patient described with signs and symptoms referable to multiple occlusive lesions of the brachiocephalic vessels was a woman reported by Savory in 1856.[13] In 1875, Broadbent reported chronic occlusive lesions of the innominate and left subclavian arteries, which he termed nonpulsating radial arteries, in a man. The localized nature of such lesions was described and confirmed by postmortem examination.[14] In 1908, Takayasu described the ophthalmologic findings in a patient with the disease that now bears his name.[15] In 1926, Harbitz and Raeder reported a case of arteritis in a non-Asian woman.[16] In 1944, Martorell and Fabre described what was for a time called the Martorell syndrome in a patient with occlusive disease of all great vessels.[17] In 1951, Shimizu and Sano's article "Pulseless disease" was published and excited new interest.[18] Caccamise and Whitman, 1 year later, described the first patient with arteritis in the United States and again used the term pulseless disease.[19] Ross and McKusick analyzed 100 cases of aortic arch syndrome from the literature in 1953.[20] In 1957, Kalmansohn and Kalmansohn reviewed 90 cases from the literature.[21] In 1960, Contorni described a radiologic subclavian steal for the first time.[22]

Sporadic attempts at sympathectomy and thrombectomy for the treatment of symptoms of occlusive disease of the great vessels were made in these early years, with predictably poor results. In 1950, Murray of Toronto performed a retrograde endarterectomy of the common carotid arteries, presumably through supraclavicular or cervical incisions, in a patient with syphilitic aortitis presenting with occlusion of all great vessels.[20] The symptoms recurred after 4½ months, and in 1953, Bahnson, in Baltimore, performed an ascending aorta–innominate artery bypass on this same patient, using a pediatric aortic homograft. The patient was known to have done well for 5 years.[20, 23] Davis and colleagues reported the first thromboendarterectomy of the innominate artery, performed through a right anterior thoracotomy, in 1954.[24] The operation successfully restored flow to the right carotid artery but not to the right upper extremity. The patient was known to have relief of his neurologic symptoms for at least 1 year. In 1956, Lyons and Galbraith of Alabama reported four subclavian-carotid artery bypass procedures performed for disease of the carotid bifurcation.[25] DeBakey and colleagues reported the first prosthetic aortic-origin grafting in 1958.[26] A bifurcated nylon graft originating from the ascending aorta was successfully placed end-to-side to the right subclavian artery and end-to-end to the right common carotid artery in 1957. This same article reported the first left subclavian artery endarterectomy, performed through combined thoracotomy and supraclavicular incisions. Wylie performed the first of his remarkable series of innominate artery endarterectomies in 1960.[3] By 1961, the Houston group had also reported subclavian-carotid artery bypass grafting.[27] In 1964, Parrott of Minneapolis described subclavian artery transposition for disease of the right subclavian artery in two patients.[28] In 1965, Javid and associates reported a series of 44 patients undergoing a combination of innominate endarterectomy and aortic-origin grafting to the carotid, subclavian, and innominate arteries.[29] In 1967, Diethrich and coworkers analyzed the Houston group's experience with 125 cases of carotid-subclavian artery bypass grafting,[30] thereby popularizing that operation. In their report of 1961, De Bakey and colleagues mentioned but did not detail 49 subclavian, 23 innominate, and 22 common carotid artery operations.[27] That experience was detailed in 1969 by Crawford and colleagues.[31]

Axilloaxillary artery grafting was first reported for treatment of innominate or subclavian artery lesions in 1971 by Myers and coworkers from the Marshfield Clinic.[32] That same year, femoroaxillary artery bypass grafting was also reported as a method of avoiding direct reconstruction of the great vessels.[33]

Interest in direct reconstruction of the brachiocephalic vessels waned in all but a few centers during the 1970s, in large part because of the mortality and morbidity associated with the early reconstructions.[31, 34] Direct brachiocephalic reconstructions either were omitted or were discussed only in passing in textbooks from that era. However, the more recent cumulative experience of several centers,[3–10] which has detailed very acceptable morbidity and mortality rates for direct reconstruction, coupled with the suspect patency and unappealing placement of extra-anatomic grafts crossing the neck or anterior chest, has revived interest in direct repair of these lesions.

INNOMINATE ARTERY

Innominate artery lesions are uncommon. Wylie and Effeney found that procedures for these lesions represented only 1.7 per cent of the 1961 operations performed at the University of California–San Francisco for occlusive lesions of the brachiocephalic vessels, vertebral arteries, and carotid bifurcations over a 20-year period.[2]

Presentation

Innominate artery lesions may be asymptomatic, although this is an uncommon indication in operative series.[3–6, 8–10] Patients may present with (1) ischemia of the right upper extremity, (2) symptoms referable to the anterior (carotid artery) or the posterior (vertebral artery) circulation, or (3) combined upper extremity and neurologic symptoms. In the Mayo Clinic series, 76.9 per cent of patients had neurologic symptoms.[9] Fifty per cent of these symptoms were referable to the anterior cerebral circulation alone, 40 per cent were referable to the vertebrobasilar distribution, and 10 per cent were referable to both. Of the 10 patients with anterior cerebral circulation symptoms, 6 had right amaurosis fugax and 4 had right-hemispheric transient ischemic attacks. None presented with stroke.

In the large 1991 Texas Heart Institute series, 77.8 per cent of patients had neurologic symptoms.[10] Three of the 54 patients in this series presented with stroke or a history of stroke. The percentage of patients presenting with neurologic symptoms ranges from 5 to 90 per cent.[3–10] Upper extremity symptoms have been reported in 5.9 to 63.8 per cent of patients.[3, 6, 7, 9, 10] In the Mayo Clinic series, 63.8 per cent of patients had symptoms of the right upper extremity, with 5 of the 14 having microembolization and 9 having claudication.[9] By and large, patients with claudication had tightly stenotic lesions, as opposed to the less stenotic but ulcerative lesions seen with microembolization. In contrast, only 14.8 per cent of the patients in the Houston series had arm ischemia.[10] Combined upper extremity and neurologic symptoms occurred in 38.5 per cent of the Mayo Clinic patients[9] and in 32 per cent of the Texas Heart Institute patients.[10] All series report few operations for asymptomatic lesions. Generally, these procedures are performed concomitantly in patients requiring coronary artery bypass or prophylactically in patients needing renal artery or infrarenal aortic reconstructions. A few patients with multiple, albeit asymptomatic, extracranial lesions have also undergone innominate artery reconstruction in this setting.

Diagnosis

Diagnosis may be aided by duplex scanning of the carotid and subclavian arteries and by waveform analysis of the upper extremity circulation. The bases of diagnosis, however, remain physical examination and aortic arch arteriography. Physical examination should include palpation and auscultation of the proximal and mid-cervical carotid artery pulses, as well as the superficial temporal, subclavian, brachial, radial, and ulnar artery pulses. Proximal carotid and subclavian artery bruits or thrills should arouse suspicion of innominate artery or other great vessel stenotic lesions. Absent proximal cervical or subclavian pulses are evidence of occlusive lesions. Allen's test or its variations may reveal digital artery occlusions. Blood pressure comparison in both upper extremities is mandatory. If evidence of bilateral upper extremity occlusive disease is present, pressure in the upper extremities should be compared with that in the lower extremities. The presence of bluish, painful discolorations in the fingertips, subungual splinter hemorrhages, or livedo reticularis may be indicative of innominate artery or subclavian artery atheroembolic lesions. Unilaterality of symptoms may help differentiate atherosclerosis of the innominate or the subclavian artery from systemic causes of upper extremity ischemia.

Arch aortography with runoff views of the carotid, subclavian, and vertebral artery circulations is the sine qua non of diagnosis. Aortography is necessary to confirm the diagnosis, to localize the lesions, to determine etiology, and to plan surgery. In the Mayo Clinic series of 26 patients with innominate artery lesions, 73 per cent had multiple arch lesions and another 11.5 per cent had concomitant vertebral artery or carotid bifurcation lesions.[9] Of the patients treated at the Texas Heart Institute, 61 per cent had concomitant arch or bifurcation lesions.[10] If direct reconstruction is anticipated, the aortogram provides essential information about the feasibility of endarterectomy or bypass grafting and allows planning for the reconstruction of multiple arch vessels and concomitant carotid endarterectomy.

Operative Approaches

Stenotic lesions of the innominate artery requiring reconstruction may be approached directly via arch reconstruction or indirectly via extra-anatomic methods, such as subclavian-subclavian artery bypass, axilloaxillary artery bypass, or contralateral carotid-carotid or carotid-subclavian artery bypass.

Extra-Anatomic Methods

Extra-anatomic methods came into vogue as a means of reducing the high morbidity and mortality encountered in the early experience with direct reconstruction.[31] It should be noted, however, that the extra-anatomic operations espoused by Crawford and colleagues in that report (i.e., carotid-subclavian artery and subclavian-carotid artery bypass grafting) have endured and that they were proposed for a subset of great vessel lesions, not for all great vessel lesions. Nonetheless, median sternotomy has proved over the course of the past 2 decades to be a safe procedure with low inherent morbidity and mortality.

Brewster and associates reported a 50 per cent failure rate for axilloaxillary artery grafts.[7] Criado, in a review of the English language literature on extrathoracic operations, found axilloaxillary artery grafts to have the worst patency and recommended against their use.[35] Nonetheless, selected series have reported excellent results with axilloaxillary artery bypass grafts.[36–39] All of the 112 patients in these four reports were treated for subclavian artery disease; none were operated for occlusive disease of the innominate artery. One group has reported less morbidity and better patency with axilloaxillary artery grafts than with carotid-subclavian artery grafts for symptomatic subclavian artery disease.[40]

The routes of extra-anatomic bypasses performed for innominate artery disease crossing the trachea or sternum make these prone to skin erosion and infection. Further, they complicate tracheostomy, coronary artery bypass grafting, or subsequent arch reconstructions if any of these become necessary (Fig. 66–1). If the patient is dependent on the graft for cerebral flow, the presence of a graft crossing the sternum complicates and alters repair. Because approximately 45 per cent of patients with brachiocephalic occlusive disease may be expected to have associated coronary artery disease[4, 7, 8] and because these patients are relatively young, this is a practical and valid concern. Furthermore, 5.2 per cent of patients undergoing brachiocephalic revascularization in the best of hands may be expected to need repeated arch reconstruction.[41]

Three other arguments or situations mitigate against extra-anatomic reconstructions. The retrograde origins of extra-anatomic bypass grafts are, at least theoretically, less appealing than prograde reconstructions. Atheroembolic lesions require direct repair rather than extra-anatomic reconstruction if the atheroembolic source is to be removed from the circulation. Finally, multiple great vessel occlusive lesions are better treated by direct arch reconstruction because the aorta offers an excellent source of inflow and diseased arch vessels do not.

Poor patency may be expected from even more com-

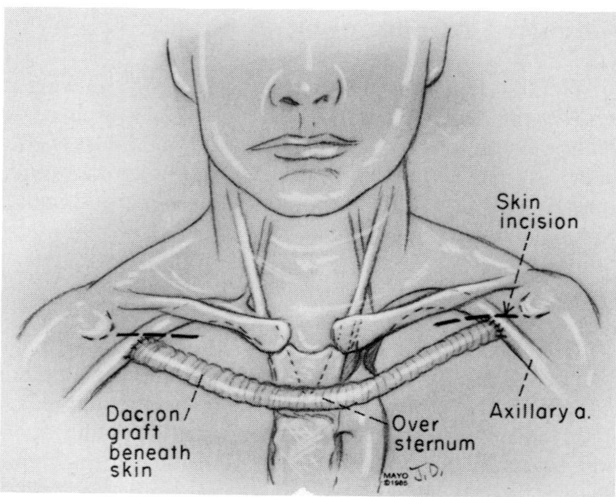

FIGURE 66–1. Drawing of an axilloaxillary graft demonstrates its position overlying the sternum. (By permission of Mayo Foundation.)

plicated and involved attempts to avoid direct repair, such as femoroaxillary artery bypass grafts.[33]

Direct Reconstruction

Direct reconstruction may be accomplished by aortic-origin grafting or by innominate artery endarterectomy (Fig. 66–2). Each has its proponents and gives excellent results in properly selected patients. The Mayo Clinic group found no difference in early reconstructive failures for bypass and endarterectomy with no early failures in either group.[9] Similarly, no significant differences were reported in the patients from the Massachusetts General Hospital and the Texas Heart Institute.[7, 10] The Texas Heart Institute group reported four late failures, all of which were graft related except for one carotid bifurcation endarterectomy.[10] The Mayo Clinic group found no difference in late symptomatic recurrences for patients undergoing direct repair by either grafting or endarterectomy with 2 of 14 patients undergoing bypass having recurrence (14.3 per cent) and 1 of 9 patients with endarterectomy experiencing recurrence (11.1 per cent).[9] It appears from the literature that most centers favor direct bypass grafting as a technically less demanding operation that is suitable for all good-risk patients,[5, 7] whereas innominate artery endarterectomy is somewhat limited in its applicability, being suitable only for patients with atherosclerotic lesions whose anatomy and extent of disease permit it.

Direct bypass grafting is preferred for patients with Takayasu's arteritis (Fig. 66–3), radiation injury, or recurrent innominate disease. The inflammatory arteritides, by nature of their panmural involvement, are generally not suitable for endarterectomy. Multiple arch lesions are probably more easily handled by bypass than endarterectomy. The extent of the atherosclerotic process and the patient's anatomy may mitigate against endarterectomy of the innominate artery. Atherosclerosis involving the aortic arch at the base of the innominate artery was identified by Carlson and associates as a contraindication to innominate artery endarterectomy.[3] Atherosclerosis or calcification in this location precludes safe, hemostatic clamping of the base of the innominate artery without undue risk of intimal disruption, dissection, or embolization. Aortic dissection with innominate artery reconstruction has been reported, albeit with bypass rather than endarterectomy.[8] The San Francisco group also identified the close proximity of the origin of the left common carotid artery to that of the innominate artery as a relative contraindication to endarterectomy because clamping of the latter would not be possible without impinging on the blood flow to the left hemisphere.[3] A common brachiocephalic trunk would, therefore, require grafting. One other relative contraindication has emerged from the literature. Crawford and associates advocated endarterectomy for patients with lesions of the distal innominate artery, whereas proximal innominate artery lesions were thought to be better treated by direct bypass grafting.[5] Not all authors, however, agree with this view.[3, 9]

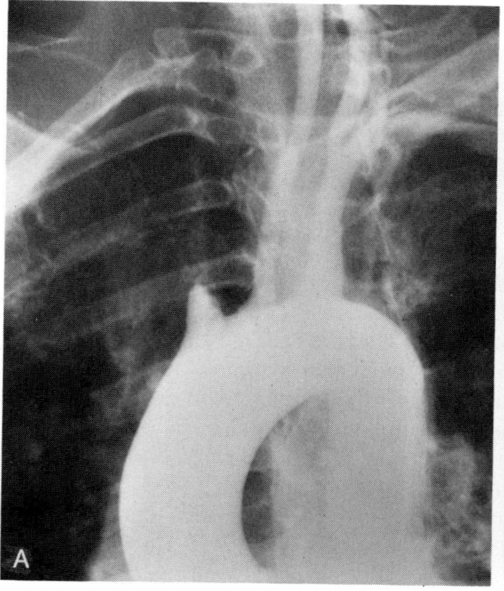

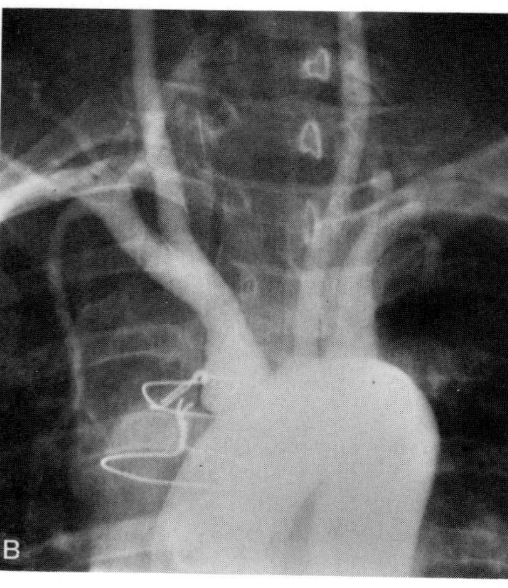

FIGURE 66–2. *A*, Preoperative arteriogram of a 47-year-old white woman with innominate artery occlusion and global ischemia. *B*, Postoperative arteriogram of the same patient after innominate artery endarterectomy.

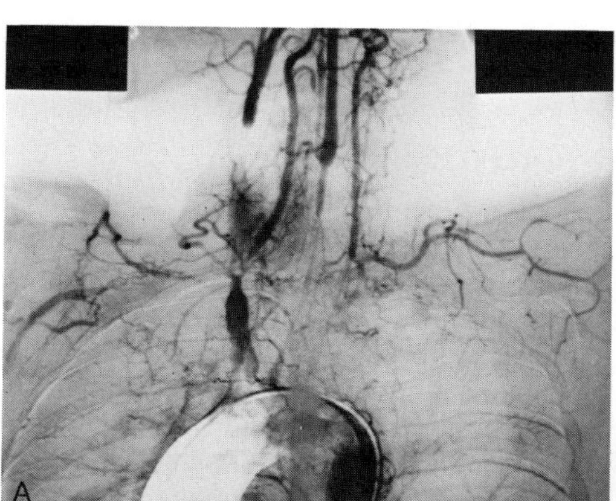

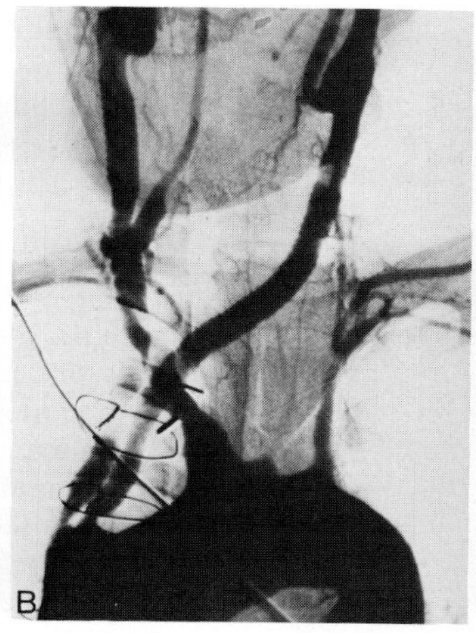

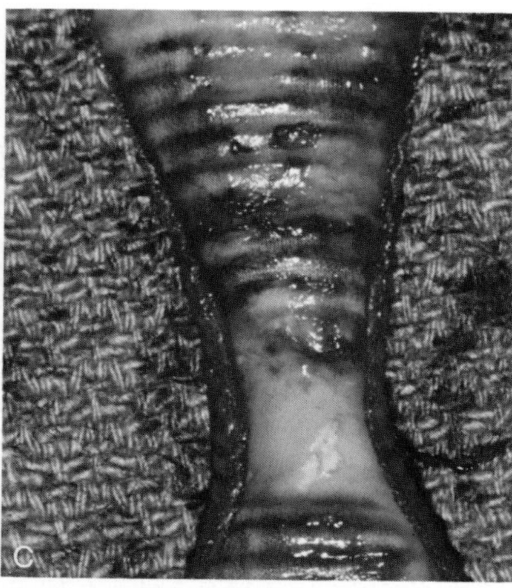

FIGURE 66–3. *A*, Arteriogram of a 19-year-old white woman with Takayasu's arteritis who presented with global cerebral ischemia and bilateral upper extremity claudication. *B*, Arteriogram obtained 16 months postoperatively demonstrates stenoses at the origins of the limbs of the bifurcated graft. Her claudication was relieved despite the fact that the subclavian arteries were not directly reconstructed. *C*, Photograph of the resected graft limb demonstrates fibrous stenosis. (*B*, From Cherry KJ Jr, McCullough JL, Hallet J Jr, et al: Technical principles of direct innominate artery revascularization: A comparison of endarterectomy and bypass grafts. J Vasc Surg 9[5]:718, 1989.)

Aortic-origin grafting to the innominate, subclavian, or common carotid arteries presents the vascular surgeon with several choices. Simple grafting to the distal innominate artery may be accomplished using an 8- or 10-mm Dacron graft. Woven grafts are usually used in this location, although collagen-coated knitted grafts may prove to be preferable in the coming years. If multiple arteries are to be bypassed, two methods of reconstruction are advocated. Compression of the graft by mediastinal contents and the reapproximated sternum has long been recognized as a mechanism of graft failure, of venous compression, and even of death by tracheal compression.[5] Crawford and colleagues proposed the use of single-limb grafts with necessary side arms added as an efficient method of reducing bulk in the mediastinum while reconstructing multiple great vessels (Fig. 66–4).[34] The author's group supports this view, having had at least one failure secondary to the use of a bifurcated graft[9] (Fig. 66–3). Surgeons from the Texas Heart Institute, however, use bifurcated grafts with excellent results.[10] One noticeable difference that may account for this success is their use of a long segment of graft trunk, as opposed to the use of a short segment (Fig. 66–5). The use of a short trunk is common practice in infrarenal aortic operations but may not be preferred in this setting. The longer trunk probably reduces turbulence at the divergence of the limbs. The two methods, the use of bifurcated grafts and the use of single-limb grafts with added side arms, are in all probability equivalent in terms of hemodynamics. The use of the longer trunk places the second limb in approximately the position that an added side arm would take. The use of single graft limbs with added side arms probably does reduce mediastinal bulk more readily than does the use of bifurcated grafts. Other measures that may be taken to reduce the volume of the mediastinal contents include resection of the diseased innominate artery following bypass, and division and ligation of the left brachiocephalic vein. The latter maneuver has been safe in the author's experience, with only transient left upper extremity swelling. Kieffer uses it and has had no significant problems with it,[42] although permanent left upper extremity swelling has been noted by others.[43] Alternatively, the vein is mobilized by division and ligation of its tributaries and the graft is placed behind it. In either circumstance, monitoring lines should not be placed from the left side of the neck or the left upper extremity as the vein is either divided or mobilized extensively.

Another decision to be made at the time of grafting is the extent of reconstruction in patients with multiple lesions. There are two schools of thought. The first, best expressed by the surgeons from the Texas Heart Institute, is to bypass all diseased vessels.[10] This approach results in placement of multiple grafts (see Fig. 66–5) and has provided excellent results in their hands. The philosophy of the author's group has been to reconstruct symptomatic lesions and those lesions needing repair by virtue of their anatomy, such as a left common carotid artery arising from a common brachiocephalic trunk. Adherents of either philosophy would repair concomitant asymptomatic stenotic lesions of the left common carotid artery arising in the usual location from the aorta. Synchronous highly stenotic carotid bifurcation lesions would also probably undergo concomitant repair by all surgeons performing direct reconstruction. It is the concomitant subclavian artery lesion, especially of the left subclavian artery, that is the point of difference. The experience of the author's group has been that restoration of flow to the carotid arteries has resulted in relief of upper extremity claudication even in the most severe cases (see Fig. 66–3). Subsequent left carotid-subclavian artery bypass may be an easier operation than ascending aorta–left subclavian artery grafting because the left subclavian artery lies far posterior in the mediastinum. Both approaches work, however, and the choice remains the prerogative of the surgeon.

Results of innominate artery reconstructions are excellent, with early relief of symptoms in 95 per cent of patients[3–10] and long-term relief in 87 to 90 per cent of patients

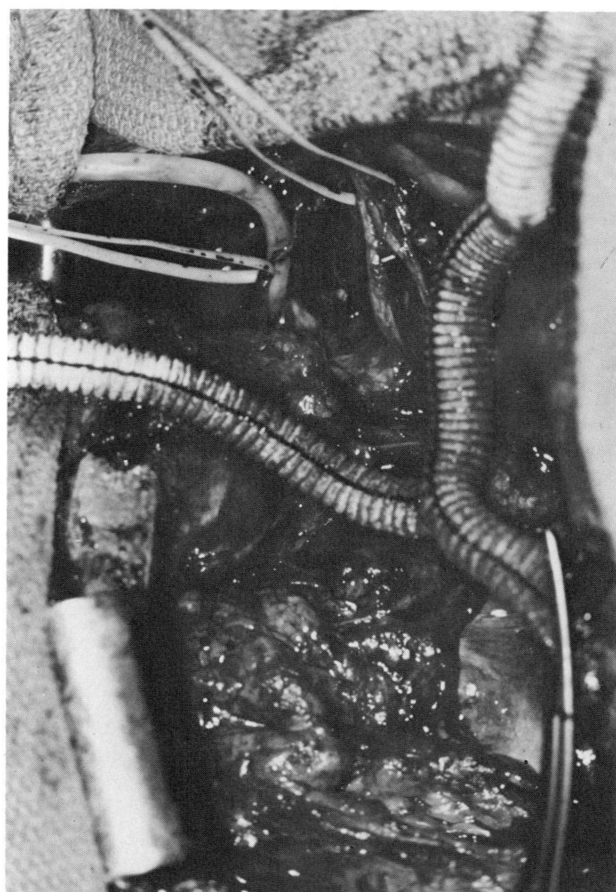

FIGURE 66–4. Anastomosis of an added graft limb to a single-limb graft originating from the ascending aorta with a clamp placed proximally.

(Table 66–1).[3–10] Perioperative stroke rates range from 0 to 7.6 per cent; mortality rates range from 0 to 14.7 per cent.[3–10] The Cleveland Clinic group reported a 14.7 per cent mortality rate.[4] These patients had a high percentage of coronary artery and valvular disease. The only deaths in the University of California and the Mayo Clinic series were cardiac related.[3, 9] These deaths underscore the necessity for evaluating the status of the coronary circulation and cardiac function in these patients. Concomitant coronary artery bypass grafting has been performed successfully,[5, 8, 44] and it is probably preferable to staged operations with the necessity of repeated sternotomy. The absolute number of reconstructive failures is unknown because generally only symptomatic patients undergo repeated aortography and operation.

Operative Technique

General anesthesia is employed for all the operations described in this chapter. Assessment of the need to shunt blood to the distal carotid artery circulation may be made by the same criteria the surgeon usually employs for carotid artery endarterectomy. Fortunately, these more proximal brachiocephalic lesions seldom require shunting. Determining the site of placement of arterial lines for blood pressure monitoring in patients with multiple arch lesions requires close communication between the surgeon and the anesthesiologist.

Innominate Artery Endarterectomy

The patient is placed supine on the operating table, with the arms at the side. The patient's back is elevated on rolls placed vertically between the scapulae, and the head is supported in an extended position and turned to the left. The neck, chest, and upper abdomen are prepared and draped into the operative field. A mid-line incision is made, dividing the entire sternum and extending a short distance into the right side of the neck along the anterior border of the sternocleidomastoid muscle (Fig. 66–6*A*). The sternal attachments of this muscle are divided, if necessary. The thymus and pericardial fat are mobilized, exposing the left innominate or brachiocephalic vein, which is then either mobilized by division and ligation of its tributaries or divided primarily (see Fig. 66–6*B*). The ascending aortic arch proximal to the innominate artery and the origins of the innominate and left common carotid arteries are dissected free. The aorta at the base of the innominate artery is inspected, and the distance between the innominate artery and the left common carotid artery is ascertained. If the aorta is normal at the base of the innominate artery and the origin of the left common carotid artery is sufficiently distant from the innominate artery (1.5 to 2 cm), endarterectomy is feasible.

The innominate artery is mobilized past the origins of the right common carotid and subclavian arteries. If the disease continues distal to the innominate artery, the atherosclerotic plaque will usually extend into the subclavian rather than the common carotid artery. The vagus and recurrent laryngeal nerves are identified and preserved. If more distal dissection of the subclavian artery is necessary, the phrenic nerve must be identified and preserved also.

The patient is systemically heparinized. Control is obtained of the subclavian and common carotid arteries first to prevent distal atheroembolization. The origin of the in-

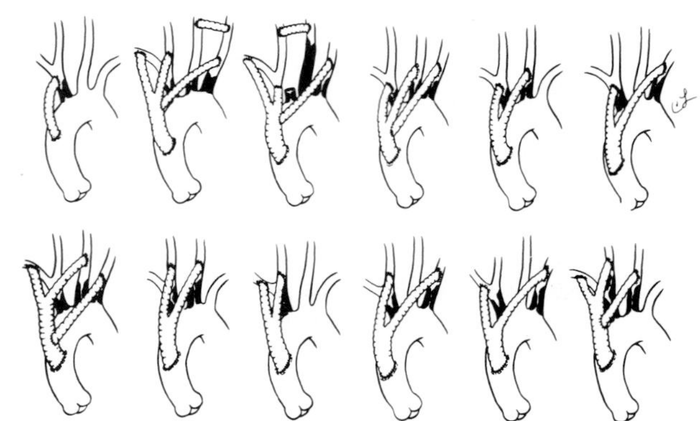

FIGURE 66–5. Texas Heart Institute's method of innominate artery and multiple brachiocephalic artery reconstructions. Note the length of the graft trunk and the reconstruction of all diseased vessels. (From Reul GJ, Jacobs MJ, Gregoric ID, et al: Innominate artery occlusive disease: Surgical approach and long-term results. J Vasc Surg 14:405, 1991.)

Table 66–1. Results of Innominate Artery Reconstructions

Institution	No. of Patients	Perioperative Transient Ischemic Attack or Stroke (%)	Mortality (%)	Relief of Symptoms (%)
University of California, San Francisco, 1977	37	2.9	6.0	94
Cleveland Clinic, 1982	34	0	14.7	82
Baylor, 1983	43	5.5	4.7	94
University of Michigan, 1985	17	5.9	0	100
Massachusetts General Hospital, 1985*	29	6.9	3.4	88
Ohio State University, St. Anthony, 1988	26	7.6	7.6	96
Mayo Clinic, 1989	26	0.0	3.8	96
Texas Heart Institute, 1991	38	2.7	0	92

Data from Cherry KJ Jr, McCullough JL, Hallett JW Jr, Pairolero P: Technical principles of direct innominate artery revascularization: A comparison of endarterectomy and bypass grafts. J Vasc Surg 9:718, 1989.

**Intrathoracic approach.*

nominate artery is then clamped with a narrow, deep partial-occlusion clamp, such as the Wylie J-clamp (Pilling). Satisfactory flow into the left common carotid artery should be ascertained by pulse examination. A vertical innominate arteriotomy is made. If necessary, the arteriotomy is extended into the right subclavian artery or, more rarely, into the right common carotid artery. Proximally, the incision is carried down into the aorta (Fig. 66–7). If the proximal innominate artery is free of disease, the endarterectomy plane is started just distal to the origin of the innominate artery. It is developed circumferentially at this point, and the specimen is divided. Using an arterial elevator, the surgeon dissects the diseased intima and the inner media free. The plaque usually has a nice tapered end-point. Tacking sutures of fine polypropylene may be used distally if necessary. If disease is present at the origin of the innominate artery, it is removed by judicious use of the arterial elevator and fine, sharply pointed scissors. Tacking sutures may be necessary or preferred on the aortic intima at the medial side (carotid artery side) of the endarterectomy. The operative site is inspected for any remnants of atherosclerotic debris and is thoroughly rinsed. If the artery is small, it may be patched with a woven Dacron graft using running 5–0 or 6–0 polypropylene sutures. In the author's experience, most arteries may be closed primarily with these same fine polypropylene sutures. The innominate artery, like the subclavian artery, is fragile, and braided sutures should not be used. Just before the closure is completed, the proximal

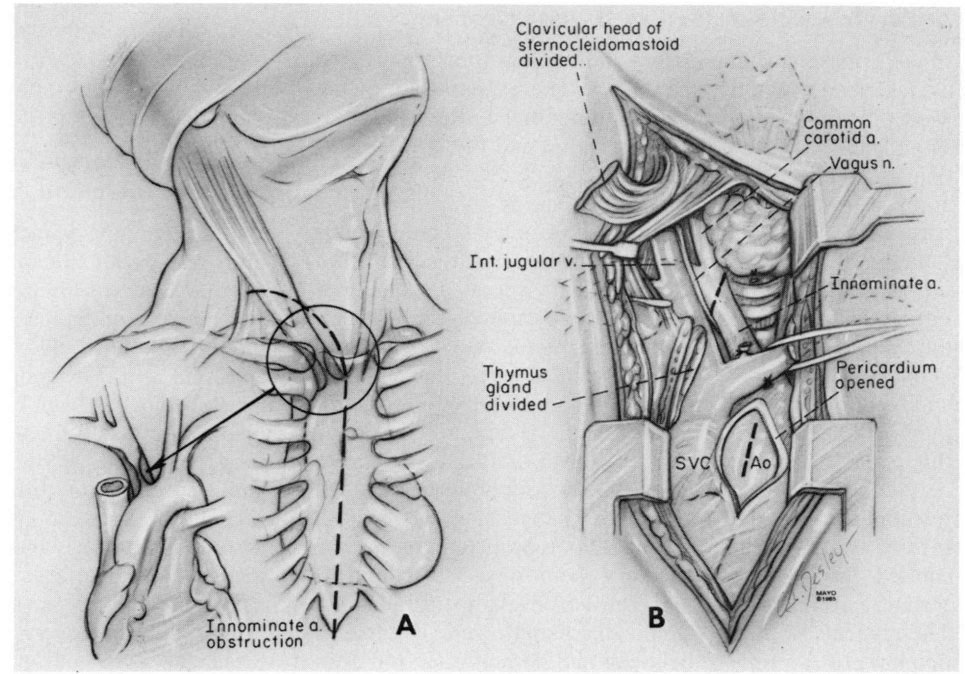

FIGURE 66–6. *A*, Full median sternotomy with extension into the right side of the neck. *B*, Sites of anastomosis for aorta–innominate artery grafting *(heavy dashed lines)*. The vein may be mobilized or divided. The intrapericardial ascending aorta is usually free of atherosclerotic disease. Ao, aorta; SVC, superior vena cava. (*A* and *B*, By permission of Mayo Foundation.)

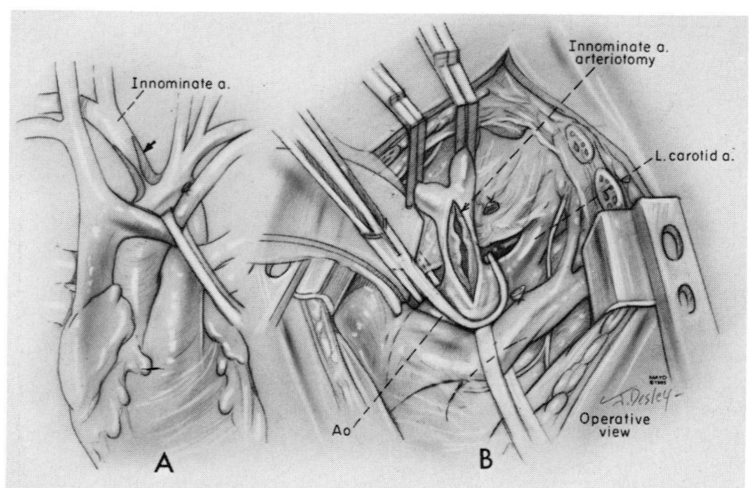

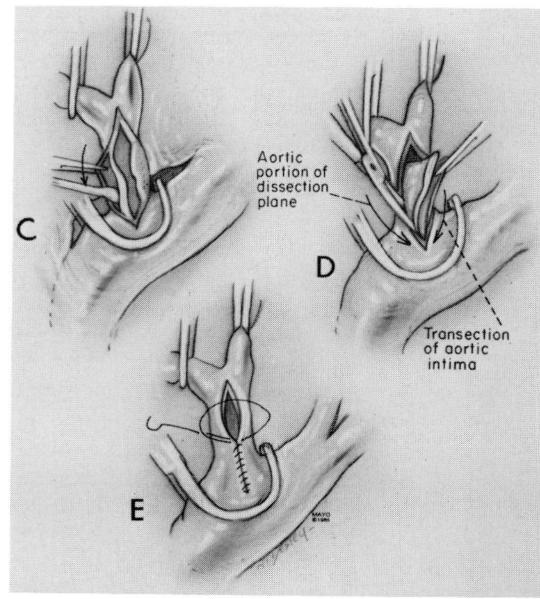

FIGURE 66–7. Innominate artery endarterectomy. *A*, Endarterectomy is suitable for patients with a soft aorta at the base of the innominate artery and flow through the left common carotid artery unimpaired by clamping. *Arrow* indicates innominate artery occlusive lesion. *B*, Application of clamps and extension of the incision onto the aortic arch. *C*, Initiation of the endarterectomy. *D*, Precise division of the innominate plaque. *E*, Closure with polypropylene sutures. (*A–E*, By permission of Mayo Foundation.)

clamp is partially opened and reapproximated. Back-bleeding is allowed from the subclavian artery and, finally, from the common carotid artery. After closure of the arteriotomy, the subclavian artery clamp is removed, and hemostasis is evaluated. If the closure is hemostatic, flow is restored first to the right subclavian artery and then to the right common carotid artery. Protamine sulfate may be given at this point. Mediastinal and chest tubes are placed, and the wound is closed in the standard manner with wire reapproximation of the sternum.

Aorta–Innominate Artery Bypass Grafting

Positioning of the patient and the incision are the same as described previously. A more extensive exposure of the ascending aorta proximal to the innominate artery is necessary. The pericardium may be entered and the intrapericardial ascending aorta dissected free (see Fig. 66–6*B*). The aorta is usually free of atherosclerosis in this location. A partial-occlusion clamp, such as the Cooley Curved Multi-Purpose clamp (V. Mueller), is placed as far laterally on the ascending aorta as possible. This lateral placement is important to minimize direct compression of the graft by the reapproximated sternum. The administration of heparin is not necessary at this point. A vertical aortotomy is made, and the aortic wall is separated with guy sutures of polypropylene. Woven Dacron grafts of 8 or 10 mm are chosen for this bypass; however, collagen-coated grafts may prove to be equally satisfactory. The graft is widely spatulated and fashioned to fit the aortotomy. The anastomosis is performed using running 3–0 or 4–0 polypropylene or Dacron sutures. Following satisfactory hemostasis, a clamp is placed across the graft and the aortic clamp is removed. The patient is now systemically heparinized. Control is obtained of the right subclavian and common carotid arteries and lastly of the innominate artery to prevent distal embolization. The innominate artery is divided distally. If necessary, the distal artery is spatulated for anastomosis. If the disease process extends into the subclavian artery, this must be dealt with appropriately. The distal anastomosis is performed in an end-to-end manner with running 4–0 or 5–0 polypropylene sutures. Appropriate antegrade bleeding and retrograde bleeding are allowed, and the anastomosis is completed. Flow is restored first to the subclavian and then to the common carotid artery (Fig. 66–8).

As much of the innominate artery is excised as feasible to help decompress the mediastinum. The stump is oversewn with horizontal and over-and-over polypropylene sutures. The conduct of the remainder of the operation is identical to that of innominate artery endarterectomy.

Ascending Aorta–Carotid Artery and Aorta–Subclavian Artery Bypass

As previously mentioned, bifurcated grafts or single-limb grafts with side arms attached may be used. If the left common carotid artery is to be reconstructed at the same time as the innominate artery, a Dacron graft may be sutured to the left lateral wall of the innominate artery graft as a side arm. This side arm is attached after the proximal anastomosis has been completed. It should lie in the upper mediastinum, and the anastomosis is performed with a running permanent suture. To determine the most advantageous location for this graft, the sternal retractor may be relaxed to allow the grafts and the mediastinal contents to assume more nearly their permanent positions. Side arms to the subclavian artery, most often to the right subclavian artery, are attached in the same manner.

If it is necessary to expose the carotid bifurcations, these exposures are performed through standard vertical

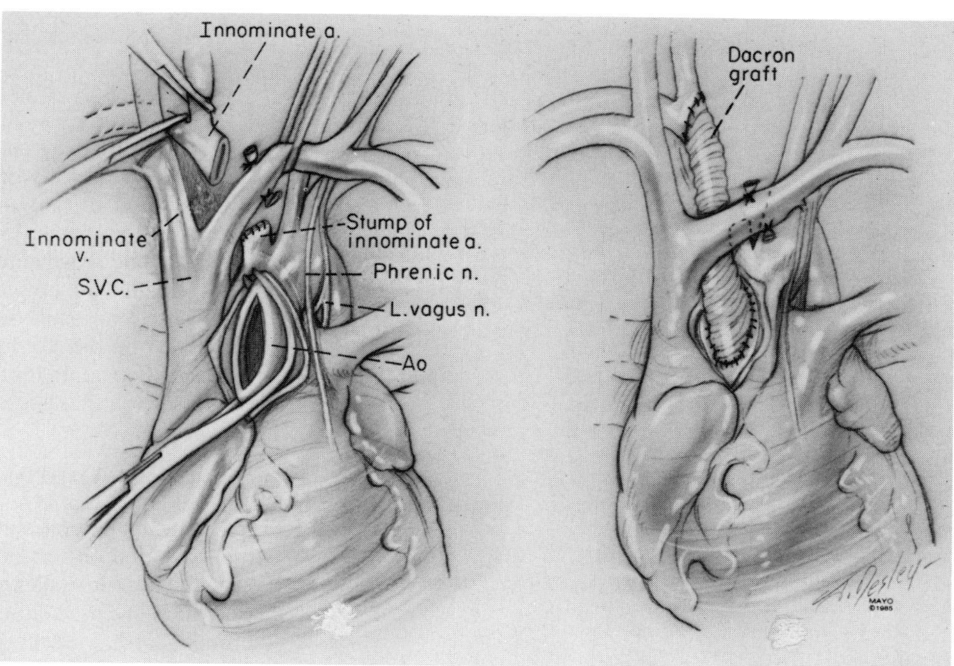

FIGURE 66–8. Aortotomy and division of the innominate artery. If the left brachiocephalic vein is mobilized, the graft is placed behind it. The innominate artery is resected after bypass. (By permission of Mayo Foundation.)

incisions. On the right side, the sternal incision may simply be extended. On the left side, a separate cervical incision is usually made.

If the distal anastomosis is to the carotid bifurcation, it is generally performed in an end-to-side manner as an angioplasty. Proximal ties on the common carotid artery or end-to-end anastomosis may be necessary in some cases, especially those involving distal embolization. If endarterectomy of the carotid bifurcation is necessary, it is performed in the standard manner.

The closure of the mediastinal wound is identical to that of innominate artery endarterectomy. The cervical wounds are closed in the standard manner.

COMMON CAROTID ARTERY

Occlusive lesions of the common carotid arteries necessitating repair are encountered less frequently than those of the carotid bifurcations. Toole reported that only 1 per cent of patients with carotid artery syndrome had common carotid artery occlusions and that the right side was involved much less frequently than the left.[45] Riles and colleagues stated that 2 per cent of patients with symptomatic carotid artery disease would be found to have occlusions of the common carotid artery.[46] Wylie and Effeney, in their review of surgery of the aortic arch branches, found only 32 of 1961 patients (1.6 per cent) with great vessel, carotid bifurcation, or vertebral artery disease to have common carotid artery lesions.[2] Lesions of the right common carotid artery are seen only rarely in the absence of innominate artery lesions and far less frequently than those of the left common carotid artery. Atherosclerosis, Takayasu's arteritis, and very infrequently, radiation-induced atherosclerosis are the etiologies.

Most of the reports dealing with common carotid artery disease focus on occlusions rather than stenoses,[46–48] although stenoses as well as occlusions may give rise to symptoms. A more thorough understanding of the natural history of common carotid artery lesions and the best methods of repair has been hindered by the relative rarity of these lesions, especially those requiring surgery, and a lack of long-term evaluation. Further hampering the acquisition of precise knowledge about these lesions and their treatment has been the grouping of these patients with patients undergoing either reconstruction for subclavian artery lesions or arch reconstruction for multiple lesions.

Diagnosis

Physical examination may reveal reduced carotid artery pulses or the presence of a proximal bruit distinct from a bifurcation bruit. No pulse would be palpable with common carotid artery occlusion. Duplex scanning may be expected to demonstrate proximal flow disturbances and dampened waveforms, even if the lesion cannot be visualized. Oculoplethysmography may demonstrate hemodynamically significant lesions. Patients suspected of having strokes should undergo computed tomography of the head, and the timing of the operation should be based on the presence or absence of infarction. Arch aortography with four-vessel runoff should be performed in all patients to localize disease, determine etiology, facilitate the planning of surgery, and determine the presence of synchronous extracranial vessel lesions.

Common carotid artery lesions may give rise to symptoms because of a reduction in flow or because of embolization. The indications for operation are the same as those with bifurcation disease: amaurosis fugax, transient ischemic attack, and stroke. High-grade asymptomatic stenotic lesions in good-risk patients have also undergone reconstruction. If tandem lesions of both the common carotid artery and the carotid bifurcation exist, it is difficult, if not

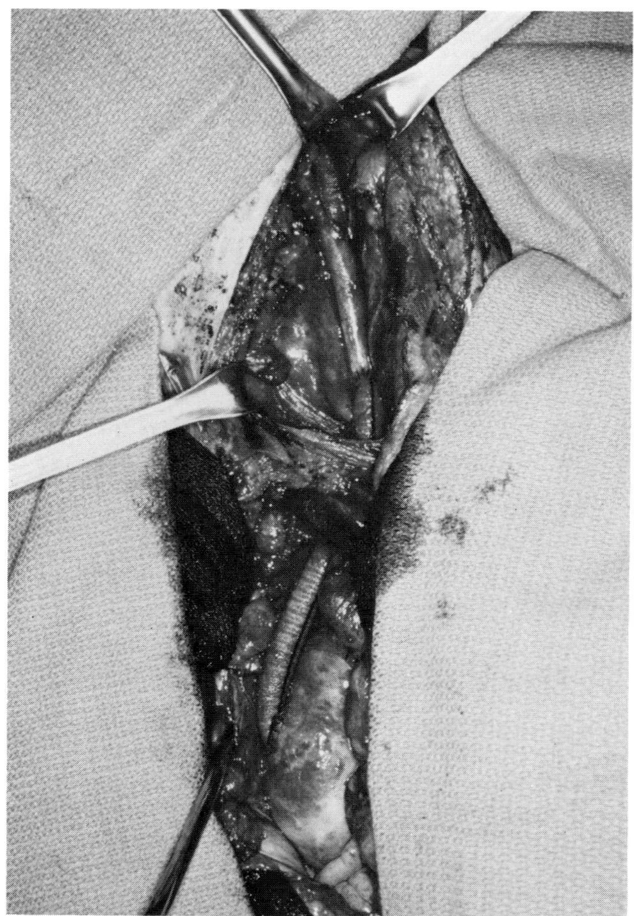

FIGURE 66–9. Intraoperative photograph of aorta–left common carotid artery grafting and left carotid bifurcation endarterectomy in a 68-year-old white man 6 weeks after left hemispheric stroke. Both the origin of the left common carotid artery and the left carotid bifurcation had 90 per cent stenosis, and the left subclavian artery was occluded.

impossible, to determine which stenosis is the source of the presenting problem. As a consequence, both lesions require repair to ensure high flow rates and removal of both potential sources of symptoms (Fig. 66–9). Isolated asymptomatic, highly stenotic lesions of the common carotid artery have been repaired, the assumption being that they have the same propensity for giving rise to symptoms as asymptomatic bifurcation lesions. The data for this assumption are admittedly lacking.

Occlusions of the common carotid artery may originate at either end of the artery: ostial stenosis may progress to occlusion with prograde thrombosis, or bifurcation disease may advance to occlusion with retrograde thrombosis. Patients with recurrent or persistent symptoms and common carotid artery occlusions merit careful evaluation because conventional arteriography may fail to demonstrate patent external or internal carotid arteries. Either of these arteries is a suitable recipient vessel. Riles and colleagues used rapid-sequence computed tomography with good results.[46] Podore and associates reported their early experience with directional Doppler investigations to determine internal carotid artery patency.[47] Keller and associates combined Doppler examinations and sequential computed tomography to evaluate external carotid artery and internal carotid artery patency.[48] Magnetic resonance angiography is proving useful in this setting. Asymptomatic patients with common carotid artery occlusions, in comparison to stenoses, are usually observed. If symptoms persist or recur and if arteriography fails to demonstrate patent internal or external carotid arteries, computed tomography, Doppler examination, magnetic resonance angiography, or some other method should be employed to ascertain the patency of these bifurcation vessels. Exploration with reconstruction, if possible, of the common, internal, or external carotid arteries, or formal ligation of the internal carotid artery may be necessary in these situations.

Operative Approaches

If the ipsilateral subclavian artery is patent, a reconstruction based on this artery is the easiest, safest, and best method. These lesions are treated by subclavian-carotid artery bypass or, less commonly, by transposition of the distal common carotid artery onto the subclavian artery. Such repairs are feasible, of course, only if the ipsilateral subclavian artery is a normal vessel.

If the common carotid artery distal to a stenosis is healthy and the ipsilateral subclavian artery is widely patent, transposition of the distal common carotid artery onto the subclavian artery is an easily performed and attractive procedure. Its only drawback is the necessity of more proximal dissection of the common carotid artery than would be required if bypass was performed. Wylie and Effeney[2] and Ehrenfeld and coworkers[49] described a small number of patients who had transposition of the carotid artery onto the subclavian artery with good results. The author's group has had similar results in the few patients in whom this procedure has been performed (Fig. 66–10). Stenotic disease

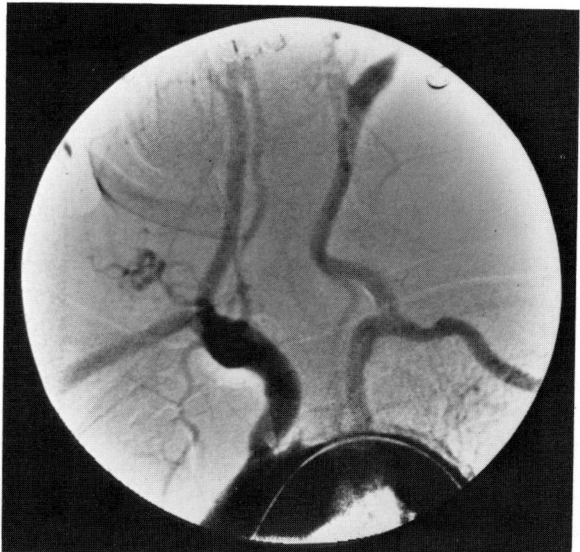

FIGURE 66–10. Postoperative digital subtraction angiogram of a 66-year-old white woman demonstrates a patent left common carotid artery transposed 57 months earlier for a stenosis of the proximal artery and a reversible ischemic neurologic deficit. The left vertebral artery arises from the aortic arch.

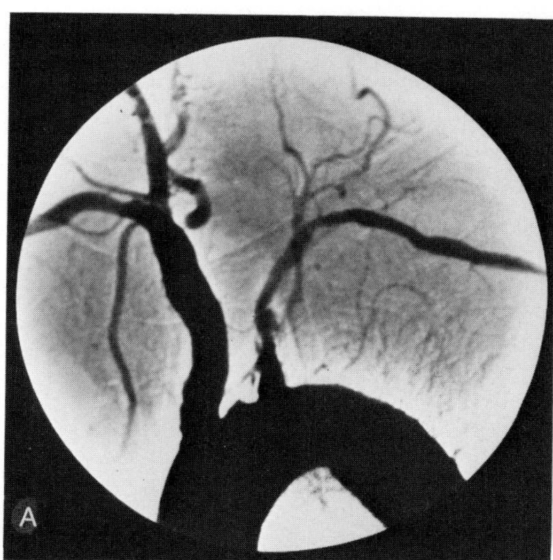

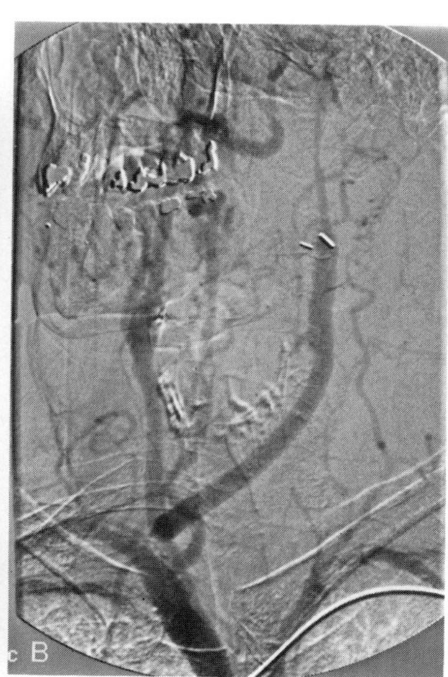

FIGURE 66–11. *A*, Arteriogram of a 67-year-old white woman with left amaurosis fugax. Note the occluded left common carotid artery and the markedly diseased left subclavian artery. *B*, Postoperative digital subtraction arteriogram obtained after carotid-carotid artery bypass grafting and left carotid endarterectomy. Arterial outflow is through the internal carotid artery. The patient's symptoms were relieved.

extending the length of the common carotid artery or occlusions with thrombosis mitigate against transposition.

Subclavian-carotid artery bypass grafting is the most commonly performed reconstructive operation for common carotid artery disease. Fry and associates reported 20 patients, treated over a 12-year period.[50] These authors analyzed their patients separately and did not group them with patients who had carotid-subclavian artery grafts or repair of multiple arch lesions. Their results were excellent, with no strokes and one death. Four patients underwent concomitant ipsilateral bifurcation endarterectomy. Saphenous vein grafts were used in 15 patients, and prosthetic grafts in the other 5. In follow-up ranging to 55 months, all grafts were patent. Only 1 patient had cerebrovascular symptoms, and these symptoms were of the posterior circulation. Unlike the experience with carotid-subclavian artery grafts,[51] the use of saphenous vein in this series of subclavian-carotid artery bypass grafts provided the same long-term patency as that of prosthetic grafts. Of interest, the majority of patients in this series had right common carotid artery lesions. All the grafts in this series were to the level of the carotid bifurcation or beyond. Five of the 20 had external carotid artery outflow only. None were placed horizontal to the common carotid artery at the same level as the subclavian artery. The vertical orientation[50] and the decreased resistance of the cerebral vasculature[52] were proposed as possible reasons for the better results with vein grafts in this setting than in carotid-subclavian artery bypass grafting. Subclavian-carotid artery bypasses with a horizontal orientation (e.g., for a symptomatic common carotid origin stenosis) may have rates of patency similar to those of carotid-subclavian artery grafts. The data to determine this are not available.

If the ipsilateral subclavian artery is also involved in the atherosclerotic process, aortic-origin grafting (see Fig. 66–9) or contralateral carotid-carotid artery grafting (Fig. 66–11) is necessary. Disease of the innominate artery in this setting would mandate sternotomy and aortic-origin repair. Common carotid artery lesions in association with multiple other arch lesions are best treated by direct arch reconstruction in good-risk patients.[5, 6, 8–10]

Concomitant ipsilateral bifurcation lesions are repaired at the same time for the reasons given earlier. It is a matter of personal choice whether the anastomosis is distal to the carotid bifurcation endarterectomy site (as an angioplasty) or proximal to it. The latter may be more appealing in appearance and in the relative shortness of the graft needed. It does, however, require another anastomosis and the need to interrupt blood flow to the carotid circulation twice instead of once. A horizontal orientation, as discussed previously, may be less advantageous in this instance than a vertical one.

Operative Technique

Subclavian-Carotid Artery Bypass Grafting

The patient is placed supine on the operating table, with a roll placed vertically between the scapulae to elevate the shoulders. The neck is extended as much as feasible, and the head is turned away from the side of the lesion. A supraclavicular incision 2 to 3 cm above and parallel to the clavicle is made, with its medial extent overlying the clavicular head of the sternocleidomastoid muscle. After the platysma is incised, the clavicular head of the sternocleidomastoid muscle may be transected if necessary. The scalene fat pad is mobilized by clamping, division, and ligation and is reflected superiorly. The thoracic duct or the right lymphatic duct may be sought at this time and formally ligated if necessary. Because the subclavian veins lie more inferiorly than the arteries, the surgeon may elect not to ligate but simply to avoid avulsion injuries by careful dissection. The anterior scalene muscle is identified, the phrenic nerve coursing medially along its anterior surface is identified and protected, and the muscle is transected. Some surgeons elect not to transect this muscle but to retract it. The subclavian artery is identified just posterior to the muscle (Fig.

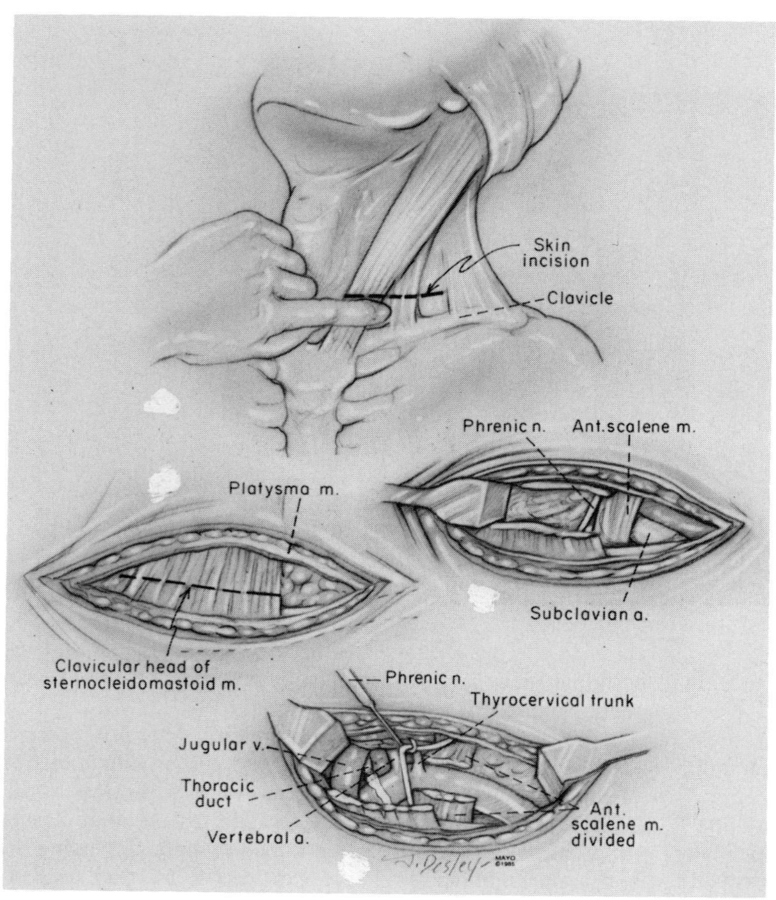

FIGURE 66–12. Left supraclavicular incision and exposure of the subclavian artery. (By permission of Mayo Foundation.)

66–12). Adequate length is mobilized to allow proximal and distal control. Its branches may be divided and ligated to facilitate mobilization. The vertebral artery must be preserved, and the internal mammary artery should be preserved, if at all possible, for possible subsequent coronary artery revascularization.

If the anastomosis is to be made to the common carotid artery at the same level, this artery may be exposed through the same incision. Medial retraction allows dissection. The jugular vein and the vagus nerve are identified and protected. In most instances, a tunnel is made posterior to the jugular vein. The positions of the vagus and phrenic nerves may vary, depending on the patient's anatomy, and any variations should be noted in the operative report.

If the distal anastomosis is to be made to the carotid bifurcation, that area is exposed through a vertical incision and the bifurcation is dissected free in the standard manner. The tunnel is made posterior to the jugular vein and the sternocleidomastoid muscle.

The patient is systemically heparinized. Control is obtained of the subclavian artery, and a vertical arteriotomy is made at the dome of the artery. Usually a 7- or 8-mm preclotted knitted Dacron graft is employed. Expanded polytetrafluoroethylene (ePTFE) or venous autografts may also be used. The anastomosis is performed end-to-side to the artery using running 4–0 or 5–0 Prolene sutures. The subclavian artery is fragile, and braided permanent sutures are not as desirable as monofilament sutures. After appropriate flushing, the anastomosis is completed and a clamp is placed across the origin of the graft. Flow is restored to the extremity. The graft is brought through the tunnel, and control is obtained of the carotid artery. If the anastomosis is to the common carotid artery at the same level, the arteriotomy is made in the lateral wall. The arteriotomy should not be too long because the graft will be joining the carotid artery at a right angle. A long arteriotomy will cause the anastomosis to be elongated and flattened. If the distal anastomosis is to the carotid bifurcation or either of its two branches, the incision is made in the usual location. This distal anastomosis may be combined with carotid endarterectomy if indicated (Fig. 66–13). The wound or wounds are closed in the standard manner. The platysma is reapproximated with Vicryl sutures, and the skin with subcuticular sutures or horizontal mattress nylon sutures.

Transposition of the Common Carotid Artery

Positioning of the patient, the incision, and the exposure are as described previously. The common carotid artery is dissected free into the mediastinum until adequate length is obtained. After systemic heparinization, the *distal* clamp is placed first on the carotid artery to prevent clamp injury to the proximal lesion and embolization. The *proximal* clamp is then applied, and the artery is divided. The proximal stump is oversewn with horizontal and over-and-

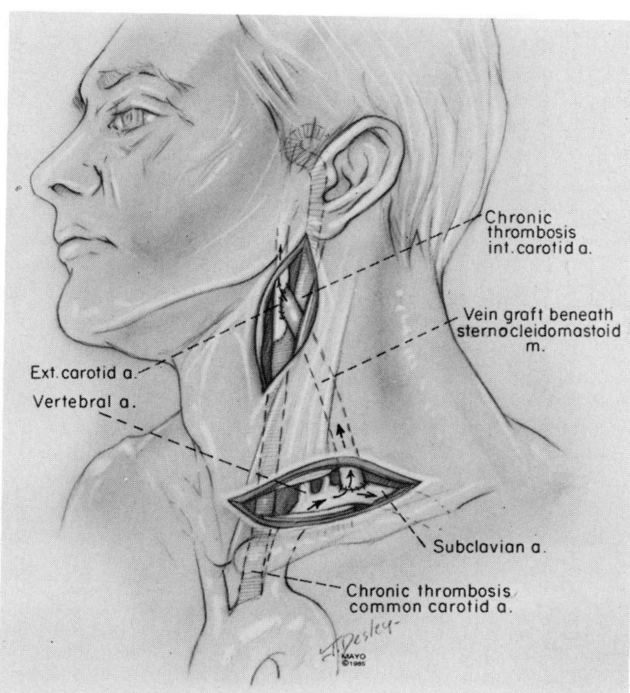

FIGURE 66–13. Left subclavian-carotid artery bypass. In this instance, outflow is through the external carotid artery. (By permission of Mayo Foundation.)

over Prolene sutures. Control is obtained at the subclavian artery, and a vertical arteriotomy is made at its apex. The carotid artery is cut to length and sutured end-to-side to the subclavian artery with running 4–0 or 5–0 Prolene sutures. Again, care should be taken that the arteriotomy not be too long, to avoid narrowing of this anastomosis. The wound is closed as described earlier (Fig. 66–14*A*).

SUBCLAVIAN ARTERY

Lesions of the subclavian artery requiring arterial reconstruction are relatively uncommon, but they are encountered more frequently than lesions of the innominate artery or common carotid artery. Wylie and Effeney found these lesions to account for 4.3 per cent of the 1961 operative cases they reviewed of carotid bifurcation, vertebral artery, and great vessel reconstructions.[2] Crawford and associates reported 80 subclavian artery repairs in their review of 142 great vessel reconstructions.[5] The left subclavian artery is more often atherosclerotic than the right, being involved in approximately 70 per cent of symptomatic cases.

Isolated occlusive lesions of the subclavian artery are usually asymptomatic because of the rich arterial collateral supply of the head, neck, and shoulder. These lesions may give rise to ischemia of either the upper extremity or the posterior cerebral circulation. The mechanism for symptomatology may be hemodynamic or atheroembolic. The latter is especially notable with upper extremity ischemia.

In 1960, Contorni described a radiographically observed subclavian steal (i.e., reversal of flow in the ipsilateral vertebral artery distal to a proximal lesion) in an asymptomatic patient.[22] The term subclavian steal was coined the following year.[53] The so-called subclavian steal syndrome has been stated to occur when use of the upper extremity increases its demand for blood and the extremity ''steals'' it from the cerebral circulation through the ipsilat-

FIGURE 66–14. *A*, Transposition of the left common carotid artery. (The interposition Dacron graft pictured here is seldom necessary if the proximal common carotid artery is mobilized sufficiently.) *B*, Left subclavian artery transposition. (*A* and *B*, By permission of Mayo Foundation.)

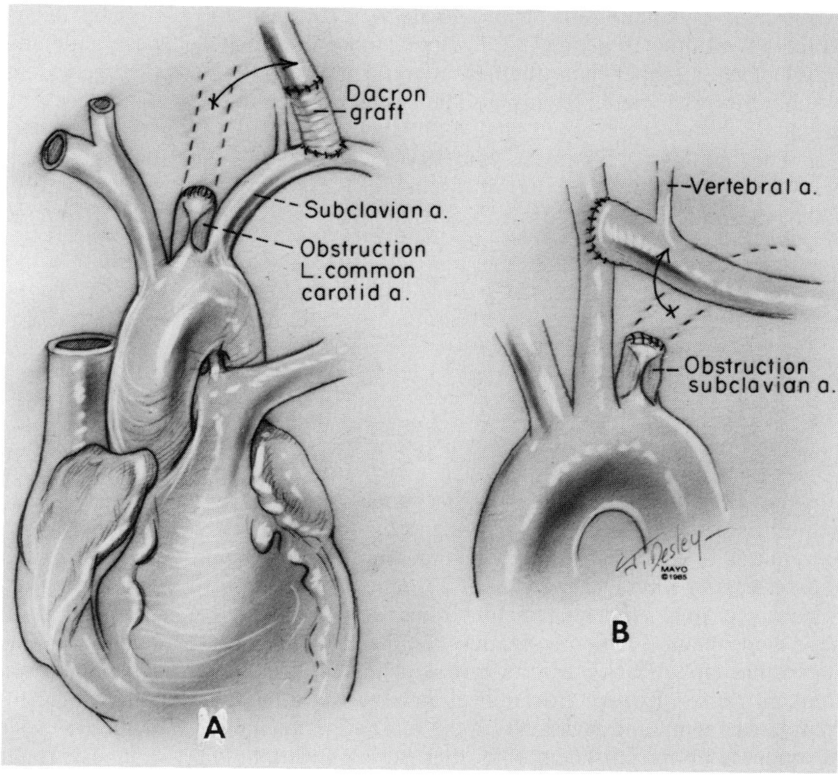

eral vertebral artery distal to the proximal subclavian (or rarely the innominate) artery lesion. Despite its simplistic anatomic appeal, however, the existence of such a clinical syndrome, in distinction to radiographic or duplex scanning findings, has been seriously questioned by vascular surgeons,[5, 49] especially in the absence of concomitant extracranial arterial occlusive lesions. Reversal of vertebral artery flow, documented by arteriography or duplex scanning, usually represents a normal pattern of collateral response to a proximal subclavian artery lesion and is not by itself an indication for surgery.

Symptomatic subclavian artery lesions are associated with concomitant lesions of the contralateral vertebral artery or of one or both carotid arteries in 35 to 85 per cent of patients.[1, 5, 54, 55] The Joint Study of Extracranial Arterial Occlusion found 80 per cent of patients with cerebral steal to have concomitant lesions.[1] Walker and coworkers found 72 per cent of 157 patients to have such concomitant lesions.[55] Further, they were unable to correlate symptoms with the presence or absence of reversed flow in the ipsilateral vertebral artery. It is most probable that subclavian artery lesions cause vertebrobasilar insufficiency by virtue of flow reduction, thrombosis, or embolization rather than steal and that a majority are associated with synchronous lesions of the great vessels, vertebral arteries, or carotid bifurcations.

Vertebrobasilar insufficiency may present as multiple and diverse symptoms that are often obscure. They include visual disturbances (often bilateral), vertigo, ataxia, syncope, dysphasia, dysarthria, sensory deficits of the face, and motor and sensory deficits of the extremities.

Symptomatic occlusive disease of the upper extremities, which may include muscle fatigue or ''claudication,'' ischemic rest pain, ulcers, digital necrosis, and atheroembolization, is much less common than that of the lower extremities, accounting for approximately 5 per cent of patients with limb ischemia.[56–58] The prevalence of subclavian lesions is higher than this figure would indicate, with the majority of patients having no symptoms or very mild ones.

The etiology of upper extremity ischemia is diverse; in contrast, lower extremity ischemia is most often atherosclerotic in origin. In addition to atherosclerosis, vasospastic disorders, thoracic outlet syndrome with arterial involvement, arteritis, autoimmune diseases, trauma, and cardiac-source embolization may all produce ischemia of the upper extremity. These causes and their management are discussed elsewhere.

In addition to the presence of synchronous lesions of the arch vessels, vertebral arteries, or carotid bifurcations as a contributing cause of more severe ischemia, atheroembolization from proximal subclavian artery ulcerative lesions is noteworthy (Fig. 66–15). Ischemia of the upper extremities is much more likely than that of the lower extremities to manifest itself by microembolization. Rapp and colleagues found 47 per cent of 17 patients with symptomatic proximal subclavian or innominate artery disease to have evidence of microembolization.[59] Although it has been stated that embolization from a cardiac source is the most frequent cause of upper extremity ischemia, proximal atherosclerosis with embolization was the most common cause of upper extremity ischemia in that series.[59] Similarly,

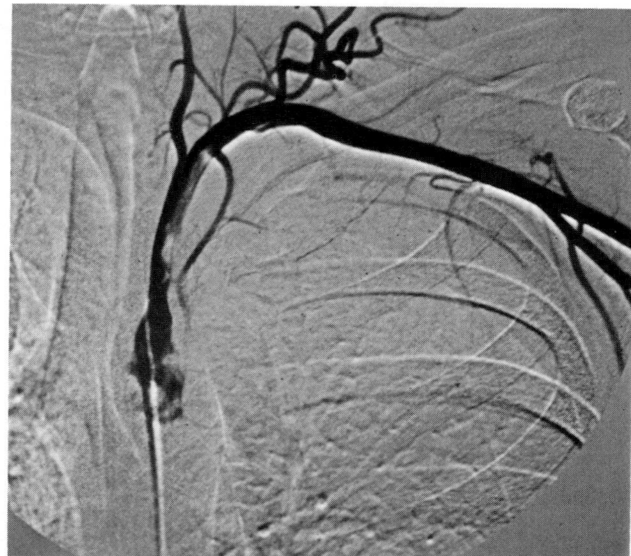

FIGURE 66–15. Arteriogram of a 50-year-old white woman who has atheroembolization to the left upper extremity and rest pain demonstrates a proximal left subclavian artery lesion and tailing thrombus. Embolic lesions were demonstrated distally.

Kadwa and Robbs found 13 patients with atheroembolization and 2 with cardiac-source embolization in their review of 35 patients with gangrenous fingers presenting over 7 years.[58] Atheroemboli may rise from highly stenotic lesions or from those that are ulcerated but not hemodynamically significant. In the latter situation, radial and ulnar pulses may be readily palpable, and blood pressures in the upper extremities may be equal. Palpable pulses may mislead physicians and prompt a search for systemic disorders, thereby delaying diagnosis. In more advanced cases that have gone undiagnosed or untreated, radial and ulnar pulses may be absent because the digital and palmar arteries have occluded with atheroembolic debris. This low-flow state results in occlusion of the radial and ulnar arteries. That this is a potentially limb-threatening problem is borne out by the study from San Francisco, in which four major limb amputations were reported following atheroembolization to the upper extremity.[59]

Diagnosis

The salient features of the history and physical examination are the same as those described in the section on the innominate artery. Computed tomography of the head should be performed for patients thought to have had a stroke. The localization of infarction may help to determine the source of injury (i.e., carotid or vertebrobasilar artery origin). Aortic arch aortography with four-vessel views is necessary in all patients. Runoff views of the arteries of the involved extremity may be necessary to localize embolic occlusions. Selective catheters should not be placed in the subclavian artery before a film of the artery's origin has been obtained, because hemodynamically insignificant but ulcerative lesions may be missed.

The diagnosis of a subclavian artery occlusive lesion

as the source of symptoms of upper extremity ischemia is usually evident after arteriography. The etiologic association between a subclavian artery lesion and vertebrobasilar symptoms may be less clear, especially in the presence of synchronous carotid lesions, vertebral artery lesions, or both. Patients presenting with vertebrobasilar symptoms in the presence of both significant subclavian artery and carotid bifucation disease are usually offered carotid artery endarterectomy as a first operation or in combination with ipsilateral carotid-subclavian artery bypass. Synchronous lesions may adversely affect the results of surgery. The author's group found that the rate of morbidity for carotid-subclavian artery bypass (i.e., the stroke rate) increased when this procedure was performed in the presence of significant concomitant bifurcation disease.[54] Crawford and associates found that the stroke rate increased in the presence of multiple lesions.[5]

Operative Approaches

The operative management of subclavian artery lesions causing both vertebrobasilar symptoms and upper extremity ischemia is technically the same. Adjunctive measures, such as shunting of the carotid artery, Fogarty embolectomy, or cervical sympathectomy, are dependent on the particular situation. In some cases, especially those involving the right subclavian artery, localized endarterectomy of the subclavian artery may be an appropriate option. The left subclavian artery is involved far more often than the right, and in most instances subclavian artery endarterectomy will not suffice. If the ipsilateral common carotid artery is healthy, a reconstruction based on this vessel is the preferred method of revascularization. Carotid-subclavian artery bypass using prosthetic material is the most commonly performed operation. The report of Diethrich and colleagues on 125 patients in 1967 brought this extra-anatomic reconstruction into the forefront.[30] Synthetic grafts, usually of Dacron, have been found to have better patency rates than saphenous vein grafts when used in carotid-subclavian artery bypass.[51, 60] It is thought that the size mismatch of the vein and the arteries and the axial forces generated by movement in the neck and shoulder regions contribute to the decreased patency rates of venous grafts in this location. Carotid-subclavian artery bypass grafting yields good results, with acceptable morbidity and mortality rates. Crawford and associates reported no deaths and a 1.3 per cent stroke rate for 80 patients who had subclavian artery reconstruction.[5] Perler and Williams reported no operative mortality in 31 patients (3 of whom had transposition). There were no early graft thromboses, although three grafts occluded during follow-up. Long-term patency rates (including the transposition patients) were 92 per cent at 5 years and 83 per cent at 8 years. One stroke occurred in this series.[61] Kretschmer and colleagues reported no deaths and one stroke for 19 patients undergoing carotid-subclavian artery bypass grafting.[62] At the author's institution, there were no deaths in 40 patients, but there were two strokes.[54] A peculiar mechanism of stroke in these patients is thrombosis of the synthetic graft in the early postoperative period, with protrusion of the thrombus into the common carotid artery and distal embolization into the cerebral circulation. The Houston group reported such a case,[5] and one was found at the Mayo Clinic.[54] For this reason, the author's group believes that thrombosis of carotid-subclavian artery grafts should be aggressively managed with full anticoagulation while the patient is being readied for reoperation, or as definitive treatment if reoperation is not planned.

Parrott first reported transposition of the subclavian artery onto the common carotid artery in 1964.[28] Interest in this operation was excited by the series from Germany by Sandmann and coworkers.[63] Subclavian artery transposition avoids the use of prosthetics in these relatively young patients. It does require more proximal dissection of the subclavian artery, but this requirement appears to be its only drawback. It is necessary to dissect the artery proximal to the vertebral and internal mammary arteries so that prograde flow into these two important branches may be maintained (Fig. 66–16). Origination of the vertebral artery from the proximal subclavian artery instead of its usual location may mitigate against transposition. The operation may be superior to bypass. Several retrospective reviews indicate that this procedure results in less morbidity and improved patency.[62–65] Sandmann and coworkers reported a 1.4 per cent mortality rate and a 95 per cent late patency rate for 72 patients undergoing transposition.[63] Sterpetti and associates compared carotid-subclavian artery bypass and subclavian artery transposition in 46 patients, with a mean follow-

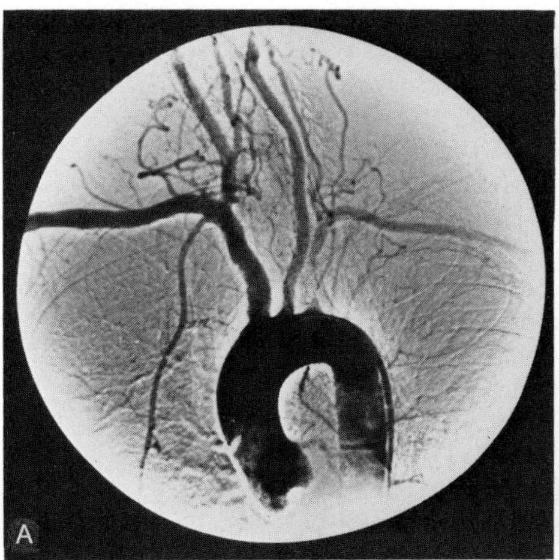

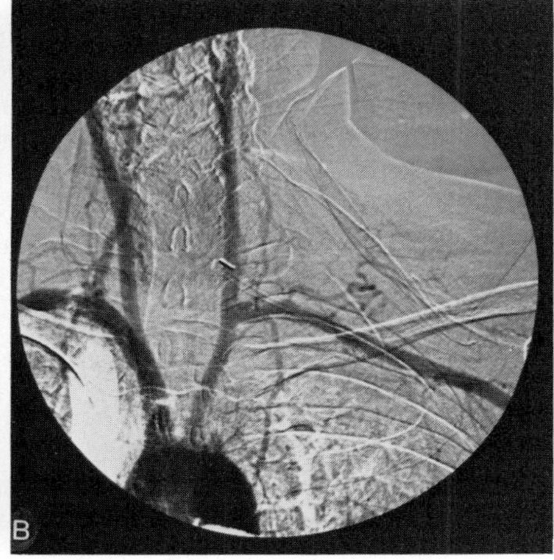

FIGURE 66–16. *A*, Arteriogram of a 59-year-old white woman who has incapacitating left upper extremity claudication demonstrates left subclavian artery occlusion and reconstitution via retrograde flow through the vertebral artery. *B*, Postoperative digital subtraction angiogram demonstrates a patent transposed subclavian artery, with prograde flow through the vertebral artery and the internal mammary artery.

up of 46.9 months.[64] The 7-year actuarial patency rate was 100 per cent for transpositions and 85 per cent for bypasses. Dacron, ePTFE, and vein grafts were all used. Dacron grafts had better patency rates than either ePTFE or vein grafts. Kretschmer and colleagues from Vienna, analyzing 52 patients, found the 33 transpositions to have 100 per cent patency, whereas there were five occlusions in the 19 patients who underwent bypass.[62] Ziomek and colleagues from the University of California–Los Angeles found transpositions to have better actuarial patency (100 per cent) than prosthetic grafts (94.1 per cent) or vein grafts (58.3 per cent), although only five transpositions were included in this group of 36 patients.[51] Weimann and associates reported no occlusions in 38 transpositions.[65]

The risk of perioperative stroke may be less with transpositions. Perler and Williams reported a 3.6 per cent stroke rate for 28 patients undergoing bypass.[61] Kretschmer and colleagues had a 5.3 per cent stroke rate for 19 bypass patients and a rate of 0 per cent for 32 transposition patients.[62] Sandmann and coworkers had no strokes in 72 patients undergoing transposition.[63] Sterpetti and associates reported more neurologic complications with bypass patients than with those undergoing transposition, but all of the patients who had neurologic problems had concomitant carotid endarterectomy.[64] The mechanism of synthetic graft thrombosis and distal embolization may account for the difference in the stroke rates for the two operations.

Operative Technique

Carotid-Subclavian Artery Bypass Grafting

The patient is placed supine on the operating room table, with a vertical roll between the scapulae to elevate the shoulders. The neck is extended, and the head is turned away from the side of the lesion. A supraclavicular incision is made parallel to the clavicle and 2 to 3 cm above it, with its medial extent overlying the clavicular head of the sternocleidomastoid muscle. The clavicular head is completely or partially incised. The scalene fat pad is mobilized by division and ligation and is reflected superiorly. The thoracic duct may be formally ligated or carefully avoided. The phrenic nerve is identified anterior to the scalene muscle and protected. The anterior scalene muscle is transected, and the subclavian artery, located posteriorly, is identified (see Fig. 66–12). It is dissected free. Its branches may be divided and ligated to facilitate mobilization. The vertebral and internal mammary arteries should be preserved. Through the same incision, the common carotid artery is dissected free. The vagus nerve is identified and protected. A tunnel is made, usually posterior to the jugular vein. The positions of the vagus and phrenic nerves relative to the tunnel may vary, depending on the patient's anatomy, and these positions should be documented in the operative note. A 7- or 8-mm prosthetic graft, either of knitted Dacron or ePTFE, is chosen. There is some evidence that Dacron may provide better patency than ePTFE.[64] The patient is systemically heparinized. Control is obtained of the common carotid artery, and a lateral arteriotomy is made. The graft will arise at a right angle, and care must be taken not to make the arteriotomy too long, lest the anastomosis be elongated and narrowed. The anastomosis is performed using running 4–0 or 5–0 polypropylene or Dacron sutures. After appropriate forward and backward bleeding is allowed, a clamp is placed across the proximal graft and flow is restored to the carotid circulation. Shunting is rarely necessary. The graft is brought through the tunnel, and control is obtained of the subclavian artery. A vertical arteriotomy is made at the dome of the artery. The graft is fashioned to fit and is sutured end-to-side with running 4–0 or 5–0 polypropylene sutures. Braided suture should probably not be used on the subclavian artery. Appropriate flushing is allowed, and flow is instituted to the subclavian artery circulation (Fig. 66–17). If necessary, a tie should be placed about the subclavian artery proximal to the vertebral artery. This is especially vital if the presenting problem is one of atheroembolization and if the lesion is not hemodynamically significant. The platysma is closed with Vicryl sutures and the skin with subcuticular Vicryl sutures.

Transposition of the Subclavian Artery

Positioning of the patient, the incision, and the exposure are essentially the same as in the preceding operation. The subclavian artery must be dissected and mobilized more extensively into the mediastinum and proximal to the origins of the vertebral and internal mammary arteries. Branches other than these may be divided and ligated as necessary to facilitate exposure and mobilization. The patient is systemically heparinized. Control is obtained first of the distal subclavian, vertebral, and internal mammary arteries and then of the proximal subclavian artery, to avoid embolization from the lesion into the distal circulation. The subclavian artery is divided, and the proximal stump is oversewn with horizontal and over-and-over polypropylene

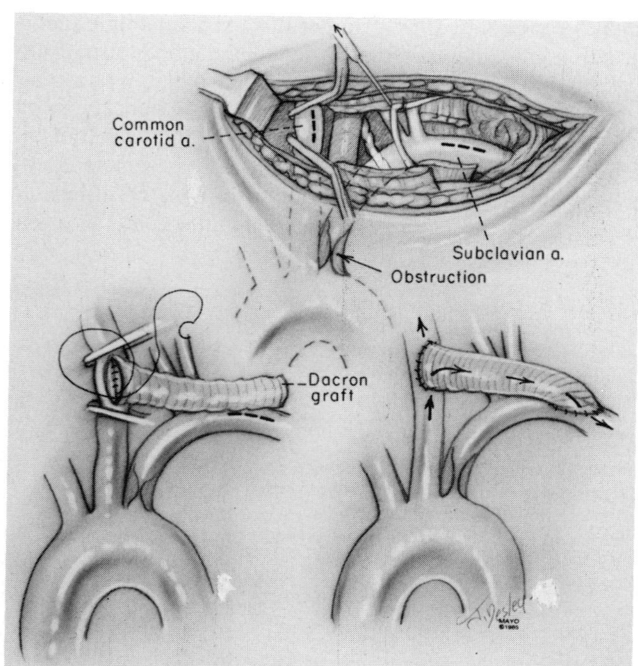

FIGURE 66–17. Left carotid-subclavian artery bypass grafting. (By permission of Mayo Foundation.)

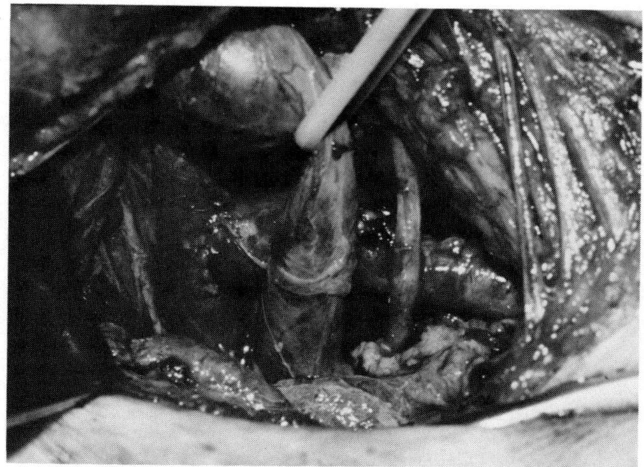

FIGURE 66–18. Intraoperative photograph of left subclavian artery transposition. The subclavian artery is posterior to the jugular vein and the phrenic nerve and anterior to the vagus nerve in this patient. The vertebral artery and the internal mammary artery are obscured by the jugular vein.

sutures. The artery is then brought into approximation with the carotid artery, usually posterior to the jugular vein (Fig. 66–18; see also Fig. 66–14*B*). The phrenic nerve will lie anterior to the artery in this operation. Control is obtained of the carotid artery, and a lateral arteriotomy is made. Because the subclavian artery will arise at a right angle to the carotid artery, the arteriotomy must not be too long so that narrowing of the anastomosis is avoided. After the anastomosis is performed using running 4–0 or 5–0 polypropylene sutures and after appropriate flushing, flow is restored or instituted to the subclavian, internal mammary, vertebral, and carotid arteries. The conduct of the remaining portion of the procedure is the same as that for carotid-subclavian artery bypass.

PERCUTANEOUS TRANSLUMINAL BALLOON ANGIOPLASTY

Percutaneous transluminal balloon angioplasty (PTA) of the great vessels, especially of the subclavian artery, is being performed with increasing frequency. Most reports emanate from Europe,[66–71] but some centers in the United States perform these procedures.[72] Patients with Takayasu's arteritis have undergone PTA,[72, 73] as have patients with atherosclerotic lesions. These reports chronicle high early success rates and moderate long-term success. However, close scrutiny of many of these reports raises questions about the understanding of the mechanisms of disease involved and the objectivity of reporting.

Common carotid and innominate artery PTA have been performed infrequently. Kachel and colleagues of Erfurt, Germany, reported on 105 patients undergoing balloon angioplasty of the internal carotid, external carotid, common carotid, vertebral, subclavian, and innominate arteries.[68] Fifty-one occlusions or stenoses of the subclavian artery were dilated. In contrast, there were 3 stenoses of the innominate artery and 2 of the common carotid artery in this series. The authors reported ''no major complications''; however, a postprocedure transient ischemic attack and a carotid thrombosis necessitating operation occurred, both of which were termed ''minor.'' In their summation of the literature, these authors classified puncture site hematomas, thrombosis of the subclavian artery, thromboembolism to the fingers, and transient ischemic attacks as minor complications. These same authors found that only 1 of 7 occluded subclavian vessels was successfully opened.[68] Forty-four stenotic subclavian vessels were dilated ''successfully,'' with 2 late restenoses. These authors recommended dilatation of the arch aortic vessels when there was ''smooth delineation of the stenoses with no indication of ulceration, heavy calcification or thrombotic deposits.'' Further, they believed that ulcerated stenoses of the carotid arteries were contraindications to PTA, as were occlusions of all brachiocephalic vessels. Other authors have not agreed with these contraindications. Romanowski and associates, in their report on subclavian and axillary artery PTA, stated that they had no problems performing dilatation in patients with evidence of microembolization.[71] Despite this statement, they reported multiple occlusive episodes distal to the angioplasty site resulting in limb amputation in one patient and the loss of a previously present radial pulse in another patient. They reported an 84.2 per cent early success rate and a 68 per cent long-term success rate.

Düber and colleagues from Mainz, Germany, reported a long-term patency rate after subclavian artery PTA of less than 50 per cent.[70] Farina and colleagues retrospectively compared patients who underwent PTA in Rome with patients who had subclavian artery reconstructions in Omaha.[67] The groups were dissimilar in other respects, and 18 subclavian reconstructions were excluded from analysis. The actuarial patency rate was 87 per cent for reconstruction and 54 per cent for subclavian artery PTA.

Much of the literature from interventionalists may be criticized for its failure to differentiate between radiologic and clinical subclavian steals, to detail presenting symptoms, and to place the presence of the arch vessel occlusion or stenosis in context. Patients have been described as undergoing PTA for subclavian steal, without further clarification.[66] The presence of concomitant aortic arch and carotid bifurcation lesions and the presence of associated coronary disease would be expected to influence patient outcome with brachiocephalic vessel PTA, just as they do with operative reconstructions.[3–5, 9, 54] These associated arterial lesions are seldom detailed in the PTA literature. Some series have listed limb ischemia as an indication without stratification (i.e., claudication, ischemic rest pain, or gangrene).[67] The early and long-term results of PTA for each of the various arch lesions should be carefully assessed in terms of the patient's general health, specific risk factors, and concomitant associated aortic arch and bifurcation lesions. To allow meaningful comparison with reports from the surgical literature, the symptoms prompting PTA must be clearly set forth. Complications such as transient ischemic attacks, occluded arteries, and digital embolization must be considered major. Occlusive lesions should be differentiated from atheroembolic ones. The fact that atheroembolic lesions may result in limb loss[59] should mitigate against balloon disruption of these fragile and treacherous lesions. No doubt stenting of these vessels in addition to balloon dilatation will be performed with increasing frequency in the coming years. Careful patient selection, with categorization of risk factors and associated atherosclerotic lesions, precise identification of presenting symptoms, close follow-up, and careful analysis will be necessary to determine the proper place of these procedures in the treatment of patients with atherosclerotic lesions of the brachiocephalic vessels.

References

1. Fields WS, Lemak NA: Joint Study of Extracranial Arterial Occlusion. VII. Subclavian steal—A review of 168 cases. JAMA 222:1139, 1972.
2. Wylie EJ, Effeney DJ: Surgery of the aortic arch branches and vertebral arteries. Surg Clin North Am 59:669, 1979.
3. Carlson RE, Ehrenfeld WK, Stoney RJ, Wylie EJ: Innominate artery endarterectomy: A 16-year history. Arch Surg 112:1389, 1977.
4. Vogt DP, Hertzer NR, O'Hara PJ, Beven EG: Brachiocephalic arterial reconstruction. Ann Surg 196:541, 1982.
5. Crawford ES, Stowe CL, Powers RW Jr: Occlusion of the innominate, common carotid, and subclavian arteries: Long-term results of surgical treatment. Surgery 94:781, 1983.
6. Zelenock GB, Cronenwett JL, Graham LM, et al: Brachiocephalic arterial occlusions and stenoses: Manifestations and management of complex lesions. Arch Surg 120:370, 1985.
7. Brewster DC, Moncure AC, Darling RC, et al: Innominate artery lesions: Problems encountered and lessons learned. J Vasc Surg 2:99, 1985.
8. Evans WE, Williams TE, Hayes JP: Aortobrachiocephalic reconstruction. Am J Surg 156:100, 1988.
9. Cherry KJ Jr, McCullough JL, Hallett JW Jr, Pairolero P: Technical principles of direct innominate artery revascularization: A comparison of endarterectomy and bypass grafts. J Vasc Surg 9:718, 1989.
10. Reul GJ, Jacobs MJHM, Gregoric ID, et al: Innominate artery occlusive disease: Surgical approach and long-term results. J Vasc Surg 14:405, 1991.
11. McCready RA, Hyde GL, Bivins BA, et al: Radiation-induced arterial injuries. Surgery 93:306, 1983.
12. Levinson SA, Close MB, Ehrenfeld WK, Stoney RJ: Carotid artery occlusive disease following external cervical irradiation. Arch Surg 107:395, 1973.
13. Savory WS: Case of a young woman in whom the main arteries of both upper extremities, and of the left side of the neck were throughout completely obliterated. Med Chir Trans 39:205, 1856.
14. Broadbent WH: Absence of pulsation in both radial arteries, the vessels being full of blood. Trans Clin Soc Lond 8:165, 1875.
15. Takayasu M: Case of queer changes in central blood vessels of retina. Acta Soc Ophthalmol Jpn 12:554, 1908.
16. Harbitz F, Raeder JG: Ansigts- og orienatrofi foraarsaget av symmetrisk karotisaffektion. Norsk Mag Laegevidensk 87:529, 1926.
17. Martorell F, Fabre J: El sindrome de obliteration de los trancos supraaorticos. Med Clin (Barc) 2:26, 1944.
18. Shimizu K, Sano K: Pulseless disease. J Neuropathol Clin Neurol 145:1095, 1951.
19. Caccamise WC, Whitman JF: Pulseless disease. Am Heart J 44:629, 1952.
20. Ross RS, McKusick VA: Progress in internal medicine: Aortic arch syndromes—Diminished or absent pulses in arteries arising from arch of aorta. AMA Arch Intern Med 92:701, 1953.
21. Kalmansohn RB, Kalmansohn RW: Thrombotic obliteration of branches of aortic arch. Circulation 15:237, 1957.
22. Contorni L: Il circolo collaterale vertebro-vertebrale nella obliterazione dell'arteria succlavia alla sua origine. Minerva Chir 15:268, 1960.
23. Bahnson HT, Spencer FC, Quattlebaum JK Jr: Surgical treatment of occlusive disease of the carotid artery. Ann Surg 149:711, 1959.
24. Davis JB, Grove WJ, Julian OC: Thrombic occlusion of the branches of the aortic arch, Martorell's syndrome: Report of a case treated surgically. Ann Surg 144:124, 1956.
25. Lyons C, Galbraith G: Surgical treatment of atherosclerotic occlusion of the internal carotid artery. Ann Surg 146:487, 1957.
26. De Bakey ME, Morris GC Jr, Jordan GL Jr, Cooley DA: Segmental thrombo-obliterative disease of branches of aortic arch. JAMA 166:998, 1958.
27. De Bakey ME, Crawford ES, Morris GC, Cooley DA: Surgical considerations of occlusive disease of the innominate, carotid, subclavian, and vertebral arteries. Ann Surg 154:698, 1961.
28. Parrott JC: The subclavian steal syndrome. Arch Surg 88:661, 1964.
29. Javid H, Julian O, Dye WS, Hunter JA: Management of cerebral arterial insufficiency caused by reversal of flow. Arch Surg 90:634, 1965.
30. Diethrich EB, Garrett HE, Ameriso J, et al: Occlusive disease of the common carotid and subclavian arteries treated by carotid-subclavian bypass: Analysis of 125 cases. Am J Surg 114:800, 1967.
31. Crawford ES, De Bakey ME, Morris GC, Howell JF: Surgical treatment of occlusion of the innominate, common carotid, and subclavian arteries: A 10-year experience. Surgery 65:17, 1969.
32. Myers WO, Lawton BR, Sautter RD: Axillo-axillary bypass graft. JAMA 217:826, 1971.
33. Sproul G: Femoral-axillary bypass for cerebral vascular insufficiency. Arch Surg 103:746, 1971.
34. Crawford ES, De Bakey ME, Morris GC Jr, Cooley DA: Thrombo-obliterative disease of the great vessels arising from the aortic arch. J Thorac Cardiovasc Surg 43:38, 1962.
35. Criado FJ: Extrathoracic management of aortic arch syndrome. Br J Surg 69(Suppl):45, 1982.
36. Posner MP, Riles TS, Ramirez AA, et al: Axilloaxillary bypass for symptomatic stenosis of the subclavian artery. Am J Surg 145:644, 1983.
37. Schanzer H, Chung-Loy H, Kotok M, et al: Evaluation of axillo-axillary artery bypass for the treatment of subclavian or innominate artery occlusive disease. J Card Surg 28:258, 1987.
38. Rosenthal D, Ellison RG Jr, Clark MD, et al: Axilloaxillary bypass: Is it worthwhile? J Card Surg 29:191, 1988.
39. Weiner RI, Deterling RA Jr, Sentissi J, O'Donnell TF Jr: Subclavian artery insufficiency: Treatment with axilloaxillary bypass. Arch Surg 122:876, 1987.
40. Mingoli A, Feldhaus RJ, Farina C, et al: Comparative results of carotid-subclavian bypass and axillo-axillary bypass in patients with symptomatic subclavian disease. Eur J Vasc Surg 6:26, 1992.
41. Kieffer E, Petitjean C, Bahnini A: Surgery of failed brachiocephalic reconstructions. *In* Bergan JJ, Yao JST (eds): Reoperative Arterial Surgery. Orlando, FL, Grune & Stratton, 1986, pp 581–607.
42. Kieffer E: Personal communication.
43. Berguer R: Personal communication.
44. Selle JG, Cook JW, Elliott CM, et al: Simultaneous revascularization for complex brachiocephalic and coronary artery disease. Surgery 90:91, 1981.
45. Toole JF: Syndromes of the carotid artery and its branches. *In* Toole JF (ed): Cerebrovascular Disorders. 3rd ed. New York, Raven Press, 1984, pp 60–61.
46. Riles TS, Imparato AM, Posner MP, Eikelboom BC: Common carotid occlusion: Assessment of the distal vessels. Ann Surg 199:363, 1984.
47. Podore PC, Rob CG, DeWeese JA, Green RM: Chronic common carotid occlusion. Stroke 12:98, 1981.
48. Keller HM, Valavanis A, Imhof HG, Turina M: Patency of external and internal carotid artery in the presence of an occluded common carotid artery: Noninvasive evaluation with combined cerebrovascular Doppler examination and sequential computertomography. Stroke 15:149, 1984.
49. Ehrenfeld WK, Chapman RD, Wylie EJ: Management of occlusive lesions of the branches of the aortic arch. Am J Surg 118:236, 1969.
50. Fry WR, Martin JD, Clagett P, Fry WJ: Extrathoracic carotid reconstruction: The subclavian-carotid artery bypass. J Vasc Surg 15:83, 1992.
51. Ziomek S, Quiñones-Baldrich WJ, Busuttil RW, et al: The superiority of synthetic arterial grafts over autologous veins in carotid-subclavian bypass. J Vasc Surg 3:140, 1986.
52. Fry WR, Martin JD, Clagett P, Fry WJ: Extrathoracic carotid reconstruction: The subclavian-carotid artery bypass. J Vasc Surg 15:83; discussion 89, 1992.
53. Fisher CM: A new vascular syndrome—''The subclavian steal.'' N Engl J Med 265:912, 1961.

54. Hallett JW, Knight CD Jr, Hollier LH, et al: Early and late results of carotid-subclavian grafts: A 26-year review. Unpublished report.
55. Walker PM, Paley D, Harris KA, et al: What determines the symptoms associated with subclavian artery occlusive disease? J Vasc Surg 2:154, 1985.
56. Whitehouse WM, Zelenock GB, Wakefield TW, et al: Arterial bypass grafts for upper extremity ischemia. *In* Symposium: Surgical Treatment of Upper Extremity Ischemia. J Vasc Surg 3:569, 1986.
57. McCarthy WJ, Flinn WR, Yao JST, et al: Result of bypass grafting for upper limb ischemia. J Vasc Surg 3:741, 1986.
58. Kadwa AM, Robbs JV: Gangrenous fingers: The tip of the iceberg. J R Coll Surg Edinb 35:71, 1990.
59. Rapp JH, Reilly LM, Goldstone J, et al: Ischemia of the upper extremity: Significance of proximal arterial disease. Am J Surg 152:122, 1986.
60. Wylie EJ: Personal communication.
61. Perler BA, Williams GM: Carotid-subclavian bypass—A decade of experience. J Vasc Surg 12:716, 1990.
62. Kretschmer G, Teleky B, Marosi L, et al: Obliterations of the proximal subclavian artery: To bypass or to anastomose? J Card Surg 32:334, 1991.
63. Sandmann W, Kniemeyer HW, Jaeschock R, et al: The role of subclavian-carotid transposition in surgery for supra-aortic occlusive disease. J Vasc Surg 5:53, 1987.
64. Sterpetti AV, Schultz RD, Farina C, Feldhaus RJ: Subclavian artery revascularization: A comparison between carotid-subclavian artery bypass and subclavian-carotid transposition. Surgery 106:624, 1989.
65. Weimann S, Willeit H, Flora G: Direct subclavian-carotid anastomosis for the subclavian steal syndrome. Eur J Vasc Surg 1:305, 1987.
66. Jaschke W, Menges HW, Ockert D, et al: PTA of the subclavian and innominate artery: Short- and long-term results. Ann Radiol (Paris) 32:29, 1989.
67. Farina C, Mingoli A, Schultz RD, et al: Percutaneous transluminal angioplasty versus surgery for subclavian artery occlusive disease. Am J Surg 158:511, 1989.
68. Kachel R, Basche ST, Heerklotz I, et al: Percutaneous transluminal angioplasty (PTA) of supra-aortic arteries, especially the internal carotid artery. AJNR 33:191, 1991.
69. Nicholson AA, Kennan NM, Sheridan WG, Ruttley MS: Percutaneous transluminal angioplasty of the subclavian artery. Ann R Coll Surg 73:46, 1991.
70. Düber C, Klose KJ, Kopp H, Schmiedt W: Percutaneous transluminal angioplasty for occlusion of the subclavian artery: Short- and long-term results. Cardiovasc Intervent Radiol 15:205, 1992.
71. Romanowski CAJ, Fairlie NC, Procter AE, Cumberland DC: Percutaneous transluminal angioplasty of the subclavian and axillary arteries: Initial results and long term follow-up. Clin Radiol 46:104, 1992.
72. Staller BJ, Maleki M: Percutaneous transluminal angioplasty for innominate artery stenosis and total occlusion of subclavian artery in Takayasu's type arteritis. Cathet Cardiovasc Diagn 16:91, 1989.
73. Kumar S, Mandalam KR, Rao VRK, et al: Percutaneous transluminal angioplasty in nonspecific aortoarteritis (Takayasu's disease): Experience of 16 cases. Cardiovasc Intervent Radiol 12:321, 1990.

67

Upper Extremity Revascularization

Walter M. Whitehouse, Jr., M.D., and Errol E. Erlandson, M.D.

• • •

Occlusive arterial disease resulting in symptomatic upper extremity ischemia occurs much less frequently than that affecting the lower extremities. Arterial reconstructions involving the upper extremity represent only 4 per cent of peripheral arterial procedures performed in contemporary practice. Diseases causing upper extremity ischemia are similar to those affecting the lower limbs; however, significant differences exist in the incidence, symptomatology, complications, and severity of associated disability. Some of these differences relate to the anatomic and functional differences between the upper and the lower extremities. The collateral circulation of the upper extremity is superior to that of the lower extremity. The upper extremity muscle mass is less and is ordinarily subjected to less work. Additionally, the functional importance of the hand in activities of daily living and employment is of major concern to affected patients.

Direct surgical treatment of upper extremity arterial insufficiency was first reported in 1956.[20] Improvement in arteriography and refinement of vascular surgical techniques since that time have contributed to the evolution of surgical treatment of the ischemic upper extremity. In this chapter, discussion is limited to diseases affecting the axillary, brachial, radial, and ulnar arteries that may be treated successfully by direct revascularization. Brachiocephalic occlusive disease is described in Chapter 66; diseases affecting the more distal vasculature are discussed in Chapter 68.

ANATOMY

The major blood supply for the upper extremity comes from the subclavian artery.[46, 71] As this vessel passes over the first rib, it becomes the axillary artery, which extends to the lower border of the teres major muscle. Throughout its 15-cm course, the axillary artery gives off six branches of major significance, including the highest thoracic, thoracoacromial, lateral thoracic, subscapular, and anterior and posterior circumflex humeral arteries. All but the first may serve as major collateral vessels around the shoulder girdle. The brachial artery extends from the lower border of the teres major muscle to its bifurcation, which is adjacent to the head of the radius. It is single in approximately 80 per cent of cases. An additional superficial brachial artery occurs in the remaining 20 per cent of cases. It begins at the upper brachial level and descends through the arm superficial to the median nerve. The superficial brachial artery constitutes a high radial or ulnar artery in 10 to 15 per cent and 2 to 3 per cent of cases, respectively. The deep brachial artery, which is the largest branch of the brachial artery, usually originates just below the level of the teres major muscle. Other important branches include the superior and inferior ulnar collateral arteries. The radial and ulnar arteries are the terminal branches of the brachial artery, with the interosseous artery originating from the ulnar artery. The ulnar recurrent, radial recurrent, and interosseous recurrent arteries anastomose with the collateral arteries of the brachial artery to form a rich collateral bed around the elbow. The superficial palmar arch, the major source of blood flow to the digits, is primarily derived from the ulnar artery. The radial artery supplies the smaller deep palmar arch and dorsal arches of the hand. Superficial and deep palmar arch anatomy is quite variable and has been well described on the basis of both anatomic dissection and analysis of hand arteriograms.[17, 34] An incomplete palmar arch without significant retrograde collateral circulation, such that the hand is perfused primarily by the radial artery, has been reported in 1.6 per cent of patients.[4] Other studies have demonstrated a higher incidence of radial artery dominance.[43]

The abundance of collateral supply at both the shoulder and the elbow levels is responsible for the low incidence of symptomatic ischemia associated with segmental arterial occlusion at these levels. Except for occlusion of a digital vessel, chronic single-artery occlusion rarely results in severe distal ischemia with tissue loss. Gangrene results from ligation of the axillary artery in approximately 10 to 15 per cent of cases and after brachial artery ligation distal to the deep brachial origin in 3 to 4 per cent of cases.[39]

CLINICAL MANIFESTATIONS

Patients with acute arterial insufficiency of the upper extremity present with the same dramatic signs and symptoms seen with acute arterial insufficiency of the lower extremity, including pulselessness, pallor, pain, paresthesia, and paralysis. Chronic arterial insufficiency of the upper extremity is more subtle. Disabling exertional forearm and hand discomfort is a common manifestation of chronic ischemia and is reported to be the most common indication for surgical treatment in one series.[26] Such discomfort may occur with minimal exercise, such as shaving or combing hair, whereas that associated with less severe ischemia occurs only with prolonged repetitive activity. The degree of disability is directly related to the severity of ischemia and to whether the dominant hand is involved. Rest pain and gangrene may be less common manifestations, although one review reported these to be the most frequent indications for surgical treatment.[44] Tissue loss implies the presence of severe distal arterial obstruction, usually involving the palmar arch or digital vessels, but it may also occur with multi-segment disease.

ETIOLOGY, DIAGNOSIS, AND TREATMENT

Acute and chronic upper extremity ischemia amenable to direct revascularization result from a multitude of causes. As discussed in the following sections, these include iatrogenic injury (cannulation of the axillary, brachial, and radial arteries for a cardiac or peripheral arteriographic study or blood pressure monitoring), emboli, and noniatrogenic trauma. Atherosclerosis, a major cause of occlusive disease of the innominate and subclavian arteries, rarely involves the more distal vasculature to such a degree that clinically significant ischemia results. Other disease entities, such as thromboangiitis obliterans and collagen vascular diseases, are important causes of hand ischemia but are seldom successfully treated by direct revascularization. Severe forearm and hand occlusive disease seen in patients with end-stage renal failure has been treated with arterial bypass distal to the wrist.[19] Giant cell arteritis may involve the axillobrachial arterial segment but ordinarily responds to medical therapy.[59] Radiation arteritis may rarely require bypass.[12, 42]

Iatrogenic Injury

Cardiac Catheterization via the Brachial Artery

Brachial arteriotomy for cardiac catheterization is the most common iatrogenic cause of upper extremity ischemia (Fig. 67–1).[1, 8, 11, 13, 21, 36, 40, 41, 49, 50, 52, 54, 56, 58, 62, 68] The incidence of thrombotic complications from this procedure is quite variable, ranging from 0.3 per cent[60] to 28 per cent.[11] The incidence reported in most large contemporary experiences ranges from 0.9 to 4 per cent.[40, 41, 45, 49, 52] This is significantly higher than the 0.4 per cent incidence of thrombotic complications reported with the transfemoral Judkins technique.[21] The transfemoral approach is currently the preferred method of arterial access for cardiac catheterization and coronary angioplasty in most institutions. As a result, the frequency of this form of brachial artery injury has declined. Because of the extensive collateral circulation surrounding the site of brachial arteriotomy, patients may remain asymptomatic despite brachial artery occlusion. Thus, the true incidence of this complication may exceed that reported.

Brachial artery injuries may account for both acute and chronic symptoms. Thrombosis of a long segment of the artery may jeopardize collateral flow and result in acute symptomatology requiring immediate surgical intervention. On the other hand, occlusion of a short segment may not produce significant acute ischemia, and symptoms of chronic ischemia may become apparent only after discharge, when upper extremity exercise becomes more vigorous. Because the right brachial artery is ordinarily used for these studies, most patients with significant ischemia are rendered symptomatic in their dominant hand.

Certain factors that predispose to brachial artery thrombosis after cardiac catheterization have been recognized. The method of arteriotomy closure is of importance: pursestring or longitudinal closure may be associated with a higher incidence of complications than a more precise

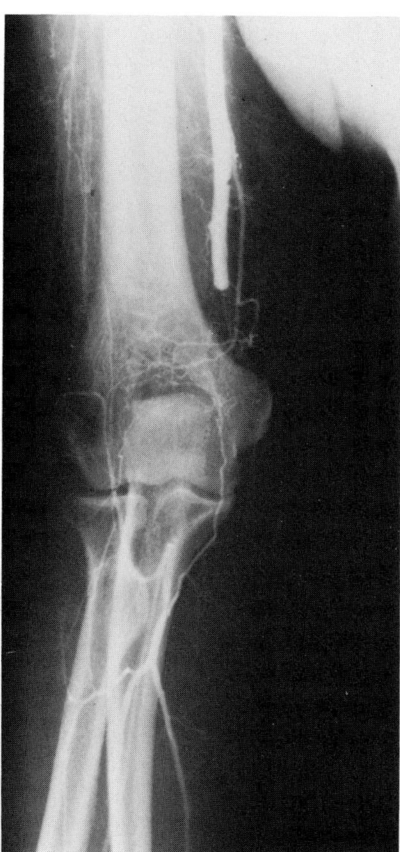

FIGURE 67–1. Acute brachial artery thrombosis following cardiac catheterization. (From Whitehouse WM Jr: Direct revascularization for forearm and hand ischemia. *In* Bergan JJ, Yao JST [eds]: Evaluation and Treatment of Upper and Lower Extremity Circulatory Disorders. Orlando, FL, Grune & Stratton, 1984, pp 231–248.)

transverse closure. Other factors include multiple catheter changes, duration of catheterization, the presence of brachial artery atherosclerosis, female gender, experience of the cardiologist, and lack of anticoagulation during the procedure.

The diagnosis of brachial artery thrombosis is ordinarily apparent with reduction in or complete absence of the radial pulse on physical examination. This finding may be accompanied by symptoms of hand ischemia. Assessment of the axillary and proximal brachial artery pulses and measurement of the perfusion pressure of the arm and forearm will aid in the localization of the obstructing lesion.[6] Most lesions are limited to the arteriotomy site; however, proximal axillary or subclavian dissections may result from difficult catheterizations (Fig. 67–2). Although this rarely occurs, failure to recognize this lesion promptly may result in recurrent thrombosis after a local brachial procedure has been performed. If a proximal dissection is suspected because of a reduction in arm perfusion pressure or abnormal Doppler waveforms, preoperative arteriography is essential. Radiographic examination should include an arch aortogram followed by a selective subclavian injection. The importance of a complete arteriographic study cannot be overemphasized.[23] Major surgical misadventures leading to amputation may be avoided with early diagnosis and treatment of such proximal lesions.

Management of Acute Ischemia. Operative repair is indicated in the presence of acute symptoms of forearm and hand ischemia. Management of the asymptomatic patient has been controversial in the past. Some authors have suggested conservative treatment in patients with forearm pressures exceeding 60 mmHg. However, as many as 45 per cent of patients who are initially asymptomatic despite brachial artery occlusion will develop late symptomatology.[49] One half of these patients will require late arterial reconstruction. Early surgical therapy usually requires only thrombectomy or local resection, whereas procedures performed later require more complex bypass procedures. Further, the brachial and radial arteries may be required for repeated cardiac catheterization or blood pressure monitoring at a later date. Thus, an aggressive approach of re-exploration for all occlusions in the absence of significant contraindications to operation is recommended.

Brachial artery exploration may be performed under local anesthesia either in the cardiac study unit or in the operating room. The latter is usually preferable because of better instrumentation, lighting, and assistance. Preoperative heparinization (150 U/kg) is advisable to limit thrombus propagation. The previously made transverse antecubital incision is extended medially and laterally because the initial exposure is almost always inadequate for proper repair. If further exposure is required, the incision may be extended proximally along the bicipital groove and distally at the lateral extent of the transverse incision. Sufficient mobilization of the brachial artery is gained proximal and distal to the arteriotomy. Care is taken to protect the median nerve during this dissection. After the suture line is opened, proximal and distal thrombectomy is performed using a 3 Fr balloon catheter. If adequate inflow cannot be established, a proximal intimal flap must be suspected. In this case, transfemoral aortography will be required to define the proximal pathology. Following thrombectomy, the vessel is débrided and then closed transversely with 6–0 monofilament suture. Interrupted suture technique facilitates a precise closure. Alternatively, if the vessel is significantly damaged, segmental resection with primary spatulated end-to-end anastomosis may be required. The technique should include anterior spatulation of the distal artery to ensure direct visualization of the intima at the time of suture placement. If a long segment is damaged, reversed saphenous vein interposition grafting may be necessary.

If preoperative arteriography has demonstrated a proximal intimal dissection, a more complex reconstruction is necessary, using a reversed saphenous vein or prosthetic conduit to bypass the diseased segment. Depending on the location of the arterial injury, this may require a carotid-axillary, carotid-brachial, or axillary-brachial bypass. Although prosthetic conduits function well for short, proximal bypasses, saphenous vein appears to be preferable for longer, more distal reconstructions. Such procedures are best performed before brachial artery repair.

Surgical results appear to justify an aggressive approach to postcatheterization brachial artery thrombosis. Thrombectomy alone may be feasible in 34 to 90 per cent

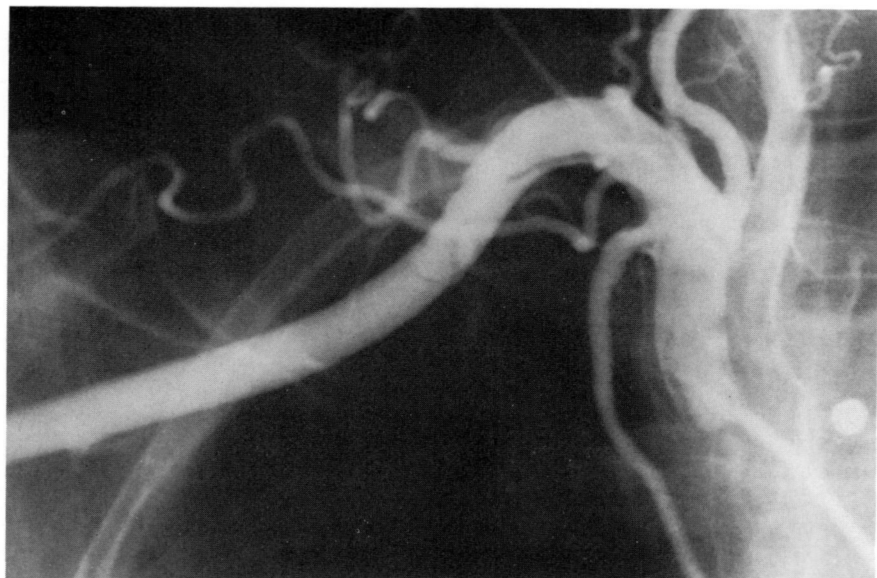

FIGURE 67–2. Intimal dissection of the subclavian artery following cardiac catheterization. This lesion would have gone undetected with a more distal selective injection of contrast. (From Whitehouse WM Jr: Direct revascularization for forearm and hand ischemia. *In* Bergan JJ, Yao JST [eds]: Evaluation and Treatment of Upper and Lower Extremity Circulatory Disorders. Orlando, FL, Grune & Stratton, 1984, pp 231–248.)

of cases, with resection and reanastomosis or vein interposition grafting required in the other 10 to 66 per cent.[36, 40, 41, 45] Early occlusion occurs in approximately 5 per cent of cases; however, even if re-exploration is required, as many as 99 per cent of patients have been reported to leave the hospital with patent reconstructions.[40, 41, 45] The use of short-term postoperative heparinization has been reported to reduce the incidence of early occlusion.[41]

Management of Chronic Ischemia. Symptomatic chronic arterial insufficiency may develop if acute occlusions following cardiac catheterization are not repaired. As many as 45 per cent of such patients may become symptomatic, and half of these patients may develop symptoms severe enough to require vascular reconstruction.[49] Generally, symptomatology is limited to exercise intolerance, although rest pain may occur. When exercise intolerance significantly limits the patient's lifestyle, consideration should be given to surgical intervention. Rest pain and tissue loss are absolute indications for surgical treatment.

Evaluation of the chronically ischemic upper extremity must include noninvasive laboratory assessment and arteriography if surgical treatment is planned.[6] Exercise studies may occasionally assist the clinician in determining the severity of ischemia. In addition to delimiting the obstructed segment, arteriography demonstrates distal runoff, which is important in planning an optimal procedure. Complete arteriographic studies should include arch aortography in addition to selective views of the entire extremity, including the hand.[23]

Surgical treatment of chronic lesions requires bypassing of the occluded arterial segment. Autogenous saphenous vein is the conduit of choice.[25, 26, 44, 72] Upper extremity veins may be used as alternatives in the absence of an adequate saphenous vein. The use of an in situ cephalic vein graft has recently been reported.[16] There are no large clinical series reporting the late results of the use of prosthetic conduits in this position. Prosthetic material should be used only in rare instances when an adequate autogenous vein is not available. The proximal end-to-side anastomosis is created just proximal to the site of occlusion, and the distal end-to-side anastomosis is created distal to the occlusion, usually just proximal to the bifurcation of the brachial artery. This may include an angioplasty of the bifurcation with the hood of the graft. Direct anastomosis to either the radial or the ulnar artery will occasionally be required (Fig. 67–3). Rarely, the interosseous artery may be the only forearm vessel that is patent; anastomosis to this vessel or its anterior or posterior branch is required. The importance of the interosseous artery in this setting has recently been emphasized.[44] Completion arteriography is recommended for distal reconstructions. These upper extremity arterial bypass procedures are associated with success rates of greater than 90 per cent, with few early failures.[26, 32, 44, 64, 69, 70] Early failure is usually associated with limited outflow. Late failures are more common when the distal anastomosis is below the brachial bifurcation.[44]

Transaxillary Arteriography

Percutaneous transaxillary arteriographic studies account for additional cases of upper extremity ischemia. Axillary artery thrombosis is reported to occur in 0.8 per cent of patients studied.[30] This is five times the rate associated with transfemoral studies but less than that associated with brachial cutdown techniques used for cardiac catheterization. Such axillary artery occlusions are likely to render the patient acutely symptomatic, and as a result, the diagnosis is usually obvious. Noninvasive arterial studies are used for confirmation, and arteriography is seldom required.

Surgical treatment is generally indicated when the diagnosis is made. Immediate heparinization is recommended. A longitudinal incision is made over the upper bicipital groove and extended proximally. Arterial control is obtained proximal and distal to the injury. A transverse arteriotomy is made at the puncture site, and proximal and distal thrombectomy is performed with a 3 Fr balloon catheter. This usually suffices, and the arteriotomy is closed

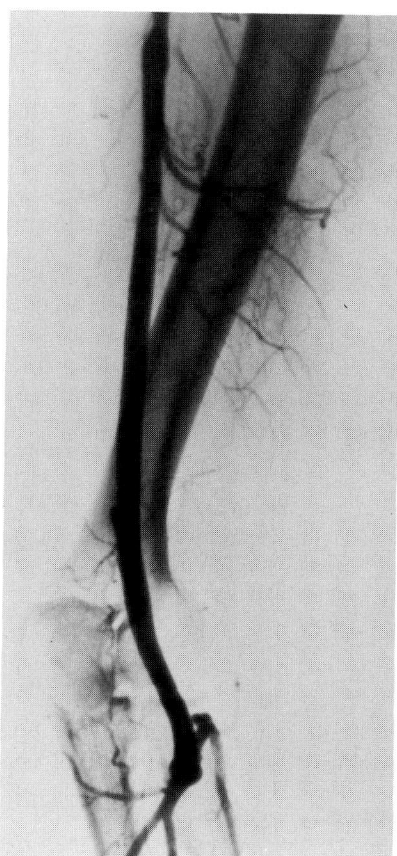

FIGURE 67–3. Reversed saphenous vein brachioulnar bypass in a patient with chronic hand ischemia secondary to cardiac catheterization (postoperative arteriogram).

transversely. Occasionally, resection with primary anastomosis or vein interposition grafting is necessary.

Morbidity is more often the consequence of neurologic complications from an axillary sheath hematoma than the result of the vascular injury itself. Many radiologists now prefer to perform percutaneous cannulation of the mid–brachial artery distal to the deep brachial origin rather than cannulation of the axillary artery in order to lessen the potential ischemic and neurologic sequelae of such injuries.

Radial Artery Cannulation

Cannulation of the radial artery is a rare iatrogenic cause of upper extremity ischemia.[4, 7, 24, 38] This technique is frequently used for continuous blood pressure monitoring and arterial blood sampling, both intraoperatively and in critical care units. Demonstration of a patent palmar arch using the Allen test[2] is a prerequisite for radial artery cannulation. More precise assessment may be performed using a Doppler probe to map out the palmar arch and digital arteries, with and without ulnar and radial artery compression.[31, 35, 51]

Radial artery thrombosis has been shown to occur in as many as 40 per cent of cases of radial artery cannulation.[7] Factors recognized to predispose to thrombosis include a prolonged period of cannulation, spasm secondary to repeated arterial puncture, diminished systemic perfusion pressure, large catheter size, underlying arterial disease, and sustained local pressure to arrest hemorrhage from the catheter site at the time of removal.[4] Authors have estimated the incidence of severe ischemic complications as a result of radial artery cannulation to be only 0.3 to 0.5 per cent in patients at risk.[51] This complication rate may be significantly higher if underlying palmar arch disease is unrecognized. After the appearance of severe ischemia, tissue loss may occur in as many as 80 per cent of patients.

Severe hand ischemia secondary to radial artery cannulation is significantly more difficult to treat by revascularization than are the more proximal axillary or brachial artery lesions. Propagation of thrombus into the palmar arch may complicate attempted revascularization. Nonetheless, in view of the high incidence of tissue loss, an aggressive surgical approach is justified when significant ischemic changes are apparent. Arteriography may be of assistance in some specific instances but is generally not beneficial. Exposure of the vessel is obtained through a longitudinal incision at the level of cannulation. Proximal and distal thrombectomy is performed carefully using 2 Fr and 3 Fr balloon thrombectomy catheters. Use of 2 Fr catheters may enable the surgeon to maximize distal thrombectomy within the palmar arch. If significant arterial damage is noted at the site of cannulation, segmental resection and primary spatulated end-to-end anastomosis may be required. Optical magnification and the use of interrupted 7–0 monofilament sutures facilitate the creation of a precise anastomosis. Results of this rare procedure are not well documented in the literature. A successful outcome is unlikely if thrombosis of arch and digital arteries is present. The administration of intra-arterial thrombolytic agents for the treatment of palmar arch and digital thrombus has been used in the past.[37] The combination of catheter thrombectomy and intraoperative intra-arterial lytic therapy has been reported, particularly in the lower extremity.[18, 53, 55, 57] Both streptokinase and urokinase have been used for this purpose. Urokinase is probably the agent of choice, although reported series are too limited in numbers to draw meaningful conclusions about the comparative efficacy or the best method of administration. Slow intra-arterial bolus infusion with up to 150,000 units of urokinase has been successful in lysing residual thrombus inaccessible to balloon catheters. The application of this technique in the upper extremity has been extremely limited. In combination with the use of vasodilators, intra-arterial thrombolytic therapy has been used in the treatment of acute thrombosis of the distal arteries following inadvertent arterial injections by drug abusers (see Chapter 45).

Placement of Chemotherapeutic Infusion Catheters

Percutaneous transbrachial or axillary placement of long-term chemotherapy infusion catheters is an additional although infrequent cause of upper extremity ischemia. The exact incidence of such complications is not well defined, but they may occur in as many as 24 per cent of patients undergoing such treatment.[15] The use of implantable infusion pumps and a trend away from hepatic chemotherapy infusion altogether will reduce the number of these complications. Nonetheless, when upper extremity ischemia is recognized, the catheter should be removed and the patient heparinized. Unless significant resolution of ischemia is noted, local exploration with thrombectomy, with or without segmental resection and primary reanastomosis, is appropriate. Results are variable and poorly documented. Duration of catheterization is an important factor influencing outcome.

Emboli

Embolic arterial occlusion is an additional cause of upper extremity ischemia.[3, 5, 27, 33, 63] Emboli involving the upper extremity arterial tree are uncommon and represent 15 to 32 per cent of all peripheral emboli.[27] Cardiac origin is reported in approximately 90 per cent of cases. Rheumatic heart disease, less common today than in the past, has been replaced by arteriosclerotic heart disease and myocardial infarction as the most common underlying cardiac disease responsible for the embolic event. Atrial fibrillation is present in approximately 80 per cent of these patients.

The brachial artery is the most frequently involved upper extremity vessel: it is the site of the embolus in approximately 60 per cent of patients. The three characteristic locations of lodgment include the upper third of the arm just proximal to the origin of the deep brachial artery, the mid-arm at the origin of the superior ulnar collateral artery, and the brachial bifurcation. The axillary (23 per cent) and subclavian arteries (12 per cent) are less frequently involved.[27] The radial and ulnar arteries are rarely the sites of cardiac embolic occlusion but are more frequently involved with emboli of arterial origin. Such embolic sources include proximal atherosclerotic plaques, aneurysms of the subclavian or axillary artery, and complications of thoracic outlet syndrome.

Although the onset of ischemic symptoms secondary to embolic arterial occlusion may be quite dramatic, symptoms may also develop slowly over a matter of hours. The level of occlusion is ordinarily detectable by physical examination. The site of disappearance of the axillary or brachial pulse is usually easily assessed by palpation. Doppler studies may also be of assistance in localizing the level of occlusion and assessing the degree of peripheral ischemia. Preoperative arteriography is particularly useful in ruling out a proximal arterial embolic source and is indicated if a cardiac source is not evident.

Embolectomy is indicated in all but the moribund patient. Without treatment, morbidity and mortality may be significant.[27] Prompt systemic heparinization is important not only to limit the propagation of thrombus but also to prevent recurrent embolism. Standard techniques using balloon embolectomy catheters are employed. Exposure for axillary embolectomy may be obtained through a longitudinal incision in the upper third of the arm over the bicipital groove. This approach may be of particular value with embolic involvement at the level of the deep brachial artery. An alternative approach involves exposure of the brachial artery in the antecubital fossa, with antegrade embolectomy being performed from that location. This is the procedure of choice for mid- and distal brachial lesions. The embolectomy technique should include transverse arteriotomy with interrupted closure. Occasionally, exposure of the brachial artery to its bifurcation will be necessary in order to pass catheters selectively down the radial and ulnar arteries. In certain cases with distal thrombus propagation, palmar arch thrombectomy using 2 Fr thrombectomy catheters may be required through incisions in the radial and ulnar arteries at the wrist. A transverse arteriotomy is used. Following the thrombectomy, closure is accomplished using interrupted 7–0 monofilament sutures. Optical magnification facilitates this closure. After embolectomy, fasciotomy is rarely necessary. Intraoperative arteriography should be used if there is any question about the adequacy of distal thrombectomy. The intraoperative use of thrombolytic agents may be efficacious in this setting, as previously described.

Operative mortality rates range from 0 to 19 per cent in this group of patients. Generally, mortality results from associated cardiac disease. Limb salvage rates range from 81 to 100 per cent.[3, 5, 27, 33, 48] Gangrene may occur in up to 37 per cent of patients treated conservatively without embolectomy.[27] In certain carefully selected cases, thrombolytic therapy may play an important role in the nonoperative management of upper extremity embolism.

Trauma

Noniatrogenic injury of the axillary, brachial, radial, and ulnar arteries is an important cause of upper extremity ischemia.[10, 14, 48, 56, 62, 65–67] These injuries are not infrequently encountered by a vascular surgeon associated with a busy trauma service. In civilian experience, the incidence of axillary artery injury is reported to range from 5 to 9 per cent,[22, 56] the incidence of brachial artery injury is approximately 30 per cent,[22, 56] and injuries of the radial and ulnar arteries make up 7 to 20 per cent[9, 22, 29, 56, 65] of all arterial injuries. Some series suggest that injuries of the radial and ulnar arteries are more common, but they are rarely of clinical significance if only one vessel is involved. When both vessels are injured, hand viability may be threatened.

Axillary artery injuries range from intimal damage resulting from blunt shoulder girdle trauma and shoulder dislocation to complete transection from a high-velocity missile. Findings associated with axillary artery injury range from an ischemic upper extremity without other significant clinical findings to a rapidly expanding axillary hematoma or hemorrhage from a penetrating axillary wound. Because of the proximity of the brachial plexus and the axillary artery and veins, there is a high incidence of concomitant neurologic and venous injuries; brachial plexus injury in the presence of normal vascular examination findings should raise the possibility of a subclinical arterial injury.

Diagnosis is obvious in the presence of frank distal ischemia or hemorrhage; however, palpable distal pulses do not preclude proximal arterial injury and are present in up to 30 per cent of patients.[9, 61, 65, 67] Arteriography is the most precise diagnostic modality, but in the face of frank ischemia and an obvious site of injury, arteriography may only postpone necessary expeditious surgery. Its use is of particular importance in ruling out subclinical vascular injury in the face of brachial plexus injury without obvious arterial damage. In addition, if there is a possibility of intrathoracic arterial injury, arteriography is mandatory.

Surgical treatment is indicated whenever axillary arterial injury is identified. The choice of incision depends on the location of the injury. Proximal lesions are best approached through an incision over the deltopectoral groove, whereas distal lesions are approached through a more lateral incision. Occasionally, proximal subclavian artery control through a supraclavicular incision may be necessary before distal exposure. Resection of the middle third of the clavicle may optimize exposure in selected cases. The pectoralis minor and major tendons may be transected if necessary for adequate exposure of more distal lesions. Although expeditious control of hemorrhage is necessary, hasty arterial clamping should be avoided because of the proximity of the brachial plexus. Digital pressure on the vessel as it exits under the clavicle will usually provide hemostasis until the vessel can be carefully dissected free of surrounding soft tissue. Only then, under direct vision, should clamps be carefully applied. The ends of the vessel are débrided, and contused vessel segments are resected. Following thrombectomy with a balloon catheter, a primary end-to-end spatulated anastomosis is usually sufficient. A reversed vein interposition graft may be required to replace excised segments. Forearm fasciotomy may be required when prolonged ischemia has occurred.

The results of surgical repair of axillary artery injuries should be excellent. The vessel is of satisfactory caliber and sufficiently mobile. Surgical failures are ordinarily due to preventable errors such as inadequate vessel débridement or incomplete distal thrombectomy. Amputation rates range from 0 to 10 per cent.[9, 22, 56] Although gangrene does not occur frequently following ligation, this is not the preferred approach. In fact, in cases in which this approach would be most applicable, namely those with significant adjacent soft tissue destruction, a higher incidence of gangrene is likely because of collateral vessel destruction. Associated residual neurologic damage is of major importance because it is a greater factor in long-term disability than the consequences of arterial insufficiency.[28, 47, 65]

Most brachial artery injuries are caused by low-velocity missiles or lacerations from glass or knives,[2, 48] but fractures, particularly a supracondylar fracture of the humerus, or dislocations of the humerus and elbow are also causes (Fig. 67–4). Blunt injury of the brachial artery is unusual. Associated injuries include median nerve damage, bone fracture, and venous injury.

Brachial artery injuries are usually obvious, and the diagnosis can be made on the basis of physical examination. Doppler studies are used to document the degree of distal ischemia. Arteriography may be appropriate when the diagnosis is unclear and may be of particular assistance in dealing with blunt trauma.

Surgery is generally indicated for all brachial artery injuries. Sufficient surgical exposure is afforded with an incision along the bicipital groove. If necessary, this can be extended transversely across the antecubital fossa and then farther distally. Care must be taken to avoid injury to the median nerve during exposure. Lateral repair is seldom appropriate. Because this vessel lacks many major branches, adequate length of the vessel can usually be mobilized, and primary spatulated end-to-end anastomoses can be performed. If interposition grafting is necessary, autogenous saphenous vein is the conduit of choice. Amputation rates range from 0 to 2.5 per cent.[9, 10, 22, 56, 65]

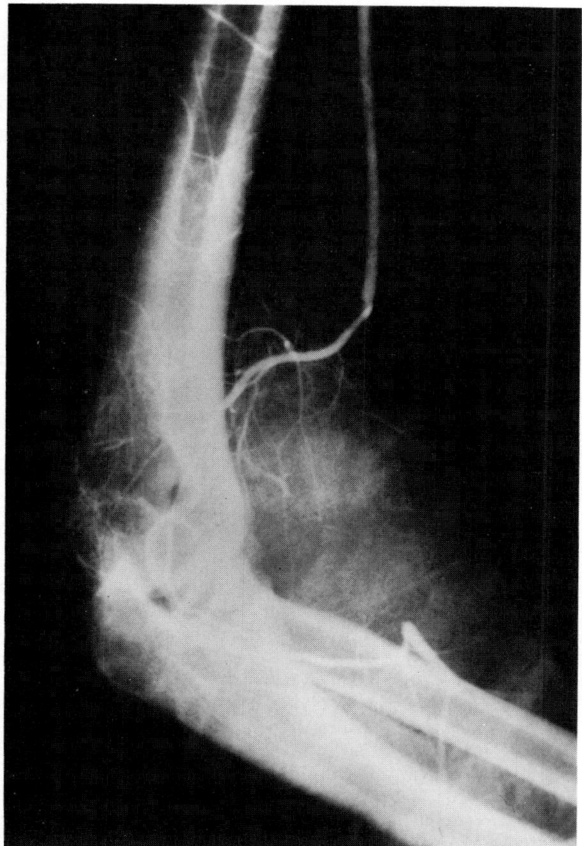

FIGURE 67–4. Brachial artery thrombosis secondary to a fracture-dislocation of the elbow. (From Whitehouse WM Jr: Direct revascularization for forearm and hand ischemia. *In* Bergan JJ, Yao JST [eds]: Evaluation and Treatment of Upper and Lower Extremity Circulatory Disorders. Orlando, FL, Grune & Stratton, 1984, pp 231–248.)

Radial and ulnar artery injuries are frequently deemphasized in reports dealing with vascular trauma. This is due in part to the fact that ligation of one of these vessels is ordinarily of no clinical significance. When the vessels are considered in clinical reports, such injuries represent up to 20 per cent of vascular injuries and up to 67 per cent of upper extremity arterial injuries.[65] Lacerations and transections from sharp objects are most frequently reported. Contusion with resulting intimal flaps and thrombosis from blunt trauma may also occur. Diagnosis can usually be established on the basis of physical examination and Doppler studies. Arteriography may be useful in certain select clinical settings but is seldom used.

Surgery is indicated in the presence of significant hand ischemia. Hemorrhage, if present, can ordinarily be controlled with pressure over the vessel proximal to or at the site of injury. Exposure of the proximal radial and ulnar arteries can be accomplished through the same Z-shaped incision in the antecubital fossa used for exposure of the distal brachial artery. Distal exposure is best afforded by longitudinal incisions overlying the vessels. When only one vessel is injured and collateral flow is satisfactory, ligation is appropriate. When both vessels are injured, however, repair of at least one artery is required. Generally, the ulnar is largest and should be repaired if possible. Small defects may be repaired with resection and primary end-to-end anastomoses using interrupted 6–0 or 7–0 monofilament sutures. If interposition grafting is required, the distal saphenous vein or cephalic vein serves as a satisfactory conduit. Thrombectomy using 2 Fr and 3 Fr catheters should be performed before repair to remove any residual thrombus. Optical magnification facilitates such repairs.

Chronic ischemia of the hand and forearm may occur as a late sequela of traumatic injuries of the axillary, brachial, radial, and ulnar arteries. Surgery is indicated when ischemia causes severe exercise intolerance, tissue loss, or rest pain. The standard surgical approach to these problems includes preoperative arteriography and bypass procedures using saphenous vein, as previously described. In the absence of distal arterial disease, results from such reconstructions are satisfactory.[26, 44] Early failures are associated with limited outflow; late failures are uncommon.

References

1. Armstrong PW, Parker JO: The complications of brachial arteriotomy. J Thorac Cardiovasc Surg 61:424, 1973.
2. Ashbell TS, Keinert HE, Kutz JE: Vascular injuries about the elbow. Clin Orthop 50:107, 1967.
3. Baird RJ, Lajos TZ: Emboli to the arm. Ann Surg 160:905, 1964.
4. Baker RJ, Chunprapaph B, Nyhus IM: Severe ischemia of the hand following radial artery catheterization. Surgery 80:449, 1976.
5. Banis JC, Rich N, Whelan TJ: Ischemia of the upper extremity due to noncardiac emboli. Am J Surg 134:131, 1977.
6. Baxter BT, Blackburn D, Payne K, et al: Noninvasive evaluation of the upper extremity. Surg Clin North Am 70:87, 1990.
7. Bedford RF, Wollman H: Complications of percutaneous radial-artery cannulation. Anesthesiology 38:228, 1973.
8. Bergqvist D, Ericsson BF, Konrad P, Bergentz SE: Arterial surgery of the upper extremity. World J Surg 7:786, 1983.
9. Bole PV, Purdy RT, Munda RT, et al: Civilian arterial injuries. Ann Surg 183:13, 1976.
10. Borman KR, Snyder WH, Weigelt JA: Civilian arterial trauma of the upper extremity: An 11 year experience in 267 patients. Am J Surg 148:796, 1984.
11. Brener BJ, Couch NP: Peripheral arterial complications of left heart catheterization and their management. Am J Surg 125:521, 1973.
12. Butler MJ, Lane RHS, Webster JHH: Irradiation injury to large arteries. Br J Surg 67:341, 1980.
13. Campion BC, Frye RL, Pluth JR, et al: Arterial complications of retrograde brachial arterial catheterization. Mayo Clin Proc 46:589, 1971.
14. Cheek RC, Pope JC, Smith HF, et al: Diagnosis and management of major vascular injuries: A review of 200 operative cases. Am Surg 41:755, 1975.
15. Clouse ME, Ahmed R, Ryan RB, et al: Complications of long term transbrachial hepatic arterial infusion chemotherapy. Am J Roentgenol 129:797, 1977.
16. Cohen ES, Holtzman RB, Johnson GW: Axillobrachial artery bypass grafting with in situ cephalic vein for axillary artery occlusion: A case report. J Vasc Surg 10:683, 1989.
17. Coleman SS, Ansun BJ: Arterial patterns of the hand based upon a study of 650 specimens. Surg Gynecol Obstet 113:409, 1961.
18. Comerota AJ, White JV, Grosh JD: Intraoperative intra-arterial thrombolytic therapy for salvage of limbs in patients with distal arterial thrombosis. Surg Gynecol Obstet 169:283, 1989.
19. Dalman RL, Nehler MR, Harris EJ, et al: Upper extremity arterial bypass distal to the wrist. J Vasc Surg 16:633, 1992.
20. Davis JB, Grove WJ, Julian OC: Thrombotic occlusion of the aortic arch, Martorell's syndrome: Report of a case treated surgically. Ann Surg 144:124, 1956.
21. Davis K, Kennedy JW, Kemp HG Jr: Complications of coronary arteriography from the collaborative study of coronary artery surgery. Circulation 59:1105, 1979.
22. Drapanas T, Hewitt RL, Weichert RF, et al: Civilian vascular injuries: A critical appraisal of three decades of management. Ann Surg 172:351, 1970.
23. Erlandson EE, Forrest ME, Shields JJ, et al: Discriminant arteriographic criteria in the management of forearm and hand ischemia. Surgery 90:1025, 1981.
24. Evans PJD, Kerr JH: Arterial occlusion after cannulation. Br Med J 3:197, 1975.
25. Garret HE, Morris GC, Howell JE, et al: Revascularization of upper extremity with autogenous vein bypass graft. Arch Surg 91:751, 1965.
26. Gross WS, Flanigan DP, Kraft RO, et al: Chronic upper extremity arterial insufficiency. Arch Surg 113:419, 1978.
27. Haimoviei H: Cardiogenic embolism of the upper extremity. J Cardiovasc Surg 23:209, 1982.
28. Hardin WD, O'Connell RC, Adinolfi MF, et al: Traumatic arterial injuries of the upper extremity: Determinants of disability. Am J Surg 150:266, 1985.
29. Hardy JD, Raju S, Neely WA, et al: Aortic and other arterial injuries. Ann Surg 181:640, 1975.
30. Hessel SJ, Adams DF, Abrams HL: Complications of angiography. Radiology 138:273, 1981.
31. Hirai M: Arterial insufficiency of the hand evaluated by digital blood pressure and arteriographic findings. Circulation 58:902, 1978.
32. Holleman JH, Hardy JD, Williamson JW, et al: Arterial surgery for arm ischemia: A survey of 136 patients. Ann Surg 191:727, 1980.
33. James EC, Khuri NT, Fedde CW, et al: Upper limb ischemia resulting from arterial thromboembolism. Am J Surg 137:739, 1979.
34. Javenski BK: Angiography of the Upper Extremity. The Hague, Martinus Nijhoff Publishers, 1982.
35. Kamienski RW, Barnes RW: Critique of the Allen test for continuity of the palmar arch assessed by Doppler ultrasound. Surg Gynecol Obstet 142:861, 1976.
36. Karmody AM, Zaman SN, Mirza RA, et al: The surgical management of catheter injuries of the brachial artery. J Thorac Cardiovasc Surg 73:149, 1977.
37. Kartchner MM, Wilcox WC: Thrombolysis of palmar and digital arterial thrombosis by intraarterial thrombolysin. J Hand Surg 1:67, 1976.
38. Katz AM, Birnbaum M, Moylan J, et al: Gangrene of the hand and forearm: A complication of radial artery cannulation. Crit Care Med 2:270, 1974.
39. Key E: Embolectomy of the vessels of the extremities. Br J Surg 24:350, 1936.
40. Kitzmiller JW, Hertzer NR, Beven EG: Routine surgical management of brachial artery occlusion after cardiac catheterization. Arch Surg 117:1066, 1982.
41. Kline RM, Hertzer NR, Beven EG, et al: Surgical treatment of brachial artery injuries after cardiac catheterization. J Vasc Surg 12:20, 1990.
42. Kretschmer G, Niederle B, Polterauer P, et al: Irradiation-induced changes in the subclavian and axillary arteries after radiotherapy for carcinoma of the breast. Surgery 99:658, 1986.
43. Little JM, Zylstra PL, West J, et al: Circulatory patterns in the normal hand. Br J Surg 60:652, 1973.
44. McCarthy WJ, Flinn WR, Yao JST, et al: Result of bypass grafting for upper limb ischemia. J Vasc Surg 3:741, 1986.
45. McCollum CH, Mavor E: Brachial artery injury after cardiac catheterization. J Vasc Surg 4:355, 1986.
46. McCormack LJ, Cauldwell EW, Anson BJ: Brachial and antebrachial arterial patterns: A study of 750 extremities. Surg Gynecol Obstet 96:44, 1953.
47. McCready RA, Procter CD, Hyde GL: Subclavian-axillary vascular trauma. J Vasc Surg 3:24, 1986.
48. McCroskey BL, Moore EE, Pearce WH, et al: Traumatic injuries of the brachial artery. Am J Surg 156:553, 1988.
49. Menzoian JO, Corson JD, Bush HL, et al: Management of the upper extremity with absent pulses after cardiac catheterization. Am J Surg 135:484, 1978.
50. Menzoian JO, Doyle JE, Cantelmo NL, et al: A comprehensive approach to extremity vascular trauma. Arch Surg 120:801, 1985.
51. Mozersky DJ, Buckley CJ, Hagood CO, et al: Ultrasonic evaluation of the palmar circulation. Am J Surg 126:812, 1973.
52. Nicholas GG, DeMuth WE Jr: Long-term results of brachial thrombectomy following cardiac catheterization. Ann Surg 183:436, 1976.
53. Norem RF, Short DH, Kerstein MD: Role of intraoperative fibrino-

lytic therapy in acute arterial occlusion. Surg Gynecol Obstet 167:87, 1988.
54. Page CP, Hagood CO, Kemmerer WT: Management of post-catheterization brachial artery thrombosis. Surgery 72:619, 1972.
55. Parent FN, Bernhard VM, Pabst TS, et al: Fibrinolytic treatment of residual thrombus after catheter embolectomy for severe lower limb ischemia. J Vasc Surg 9:153, 1989.
56. Perry MO, Thal ER, Shires GT: Management of arterial injuries. Ann Surg 173:403, 1971.
57. Quiñones-Baldrich WJ, Zierler RE, Hiatt JC: Intraoperative fibrinolytic therapy: An adjunct to catheter thromboembolectomy. J Vasc Surg 2:319, 1985.
58. Rich NM, Hobson RW, Fedde CW: Vascular trauma secondary to diagnostic and therapeutic procedures. Am J Surg 128:715, 1974.
59. Rivers SP, Baur GM, Inahara T, et al: Arm ischemia secondary to giant cell arteritis. Am J Surg 143:554, 1982.
60. Ross RS: Arterial complications. Circulation 37 (Suppl III):39, 1968.
61. Rutherford RB: Diagnostic evaluation of extremity vascular injuries. Surg Clin North Am 68:683, 1988.
62. Sachatello GR, Ernst CB, Griffen WO Jr: The acutely ischemic upper extremity: Selective management. Surgery 76:1002, 1974.
63. Savelyev VS, Zatevakhin JJ, Stepano NV: Artery embolism of the upper limbs. Surgery 81:367, 1977.
64. Schmidt FE, Hewitt RL: Severe upper limb ischemia. Arch Surg 115:1188, 1980.
65. Sitzman JV, Ernst CB: Management of arm arterial injuries. Surgery 96:895, 1984.
66. Smith RF, Szilagyi DE, Elliott JP Jr: Fracture of long bones with arterial injury due to blunt trauma. Arch Surg 99:315, 1969.
67. Smith RF, Elliott JP, Hageman JH, et al: Acute penetrating arterial injuries of the neck and limbs. Arch Surg 109:198, 1974.
68. Tuzzeo S, Saad SA, Hastings OM, et al: Management of brachial artery injuries. Surg Gynecol Obstet 146:21, 1978.
69. Welling RE, Cranley JJ, Krause RJ, et al: Obliterative arterial disease of the upper extremity. Arch Surg 116:1593, 1981.
70. Wood PB: Vein graft bypass in axillary and brachial artery occlusions causing claudication. Br J Surg 60:29, 1973.
71. Woodburne RT: Essentials of Human Anatomy. New York, Oxford University Press, 1983, pp 91–92.
72. Yao JST, Pearce WH: Reconstructive surgery for chronic upper extremity ischemia. Semin Vasc Surg 3:258, 1990.

68

Occlusive and Vasospastic Diseases Involving Distal Upper Extremity Arteries —Raynaud's Syndrome

John M. Porter, M.D., and James M. Edwards, M.D.

• • •

Many disparate disease processes may affect the distal small arteries of the upper extremities. The clinical manifestations of these disease processes range from episodic digital vasospasm to severe hand ischemia with rest pain and gangrene. Although fixed arterial occlusions are uniformly present in the distal extremity arteries of patients with digital ulceration and gangrene, patients with episodic digital vasospasm frequently have no identifiable morphologic arterial abnormality. These patients experience excessive digital artery vasospasm on cold provocation or emotional stimulation and are completely normal between attacks. Digital vasospasm and digital arterial occlusion are clearly not mutually exclusive. Many patients with digital ischemia have elements of both arterial obstruction and vasospasm. Additionally, during long-term follow-up, a number of patients with episodic digital vasospasm subsequently develop diffuse palmar and digital arterial occlusions in conjunction with one or more of various associated diseases. Thus, it appears clear that episodic digital vasospasm and ischemic digital ulceration exist as components of a continuous clinical spectrum of disease entities that may affect the distal small arteries of the upper extremity.

This chapter reviews the clinical presentation, pathophysiology, diagnosis, and treatment of spastic and obstructive upper extremity small artery diseases. The Division of Vascular Surgery at the Oregon Health Sciences University is conducting an ongoing prospective clinical study of upper extremity small artery diseases. To date, more than 900 patients have been enrolled, two thirds of whom have been fully analyzed. The contents of this chapter are, in large part, derived from the authors' experience with this patient population.

RAYNAUD'S SYNDROME

Raynaud's syndrome (RS) is a clinical condition characterized by episodic attacks of vasospasm caused by closure of the small arteries and arterioles of the most distal parts of the extremities in response to cold or emotional stress. The fingers and hands are most frequently affected, although in certain patients, the toes and feet may be involved. Classically, the episodes of vasospasm consist of an intense pallor of the distal extremities followed in sequence by cyanosis and rubor on rewarming. Generally, the attacks are completed within 30 to 60 minutes, although many patients describe attacks induced by cold exposure that persist until they enter a warm area. It is important to note that most patients do not experience the complete triple-color response but note only pallor or cyanosis during attacks. The authors have encountered a number of patients who complain of cold hands without color changes and demonstrate abnormal digital arteriographic and blood flow changes that are indistinguishable from those in patients with classic triple-color Raynaud's attacks. Thus, it is questionable whether any color change should be required for diagnosis.

Historical Background

The first description of a group of patients with finger ischemia presumably caused by digital artery vasospasm was presented by Maurice Raynaud in 1862.[106] He reported on 25 patients with varying degrees of episodic digital pallor and cyanosis frequently associated with localized finger gangrene. Raynaud proposed that the observed changes were caused by vasospasm produced by sympathetic overactivity because in most of his patients, the wrist pulses were palpable, and in some of them, large artery patency was documented at autopsy. It is now known that vasospasm alone is insufficient to produce gangrene, and it appears likely that most if not all of Raynaud's original patients had far advanced, unrecognized fixed small artery occlusive disease in addition to episodic vasospasm.

Raynaud's vasospastic hypothesis was challenged by Hutchinson at the turn of the century.[56] He recognized that digital gangrene, as well as episodic digital ischemia, may be associated with many conditions, such as arteriosclerosis, scleroderma, and heart failure. Hutchinson suggested that the term Raynaud's phenomenon be applied to episodic digital vasoconstriction and that this was a clinical sign common to diseases with diverse etiologies.

The clinical approach to RS was substantially influenced by the publication of Allen and Brown in 1932.[6] They clearly recognized that the Raynaud's event, namely episodic digital artery vasoconstriction, may occur with a variety of associated disorders, particularly digital artery occlusive diseases. They proposed division of the syndrome into Raynaud's disease, which was benign, idiopathic, and unassociated with systemic diseases, and Raynaud's phenomenon, which had a similar symptom complex but occurred in association with various systemic diseases. They presented rigid diagnostic criteria, supposedly allowing the categorization of an individual patient as having either Raynaud's phenomenon or idiopathic Raynaud's disease.

From 1932 to the present, the attempted separation of Raynaud's disease from Raynaud's phenomenon has dominated the medical literature concerning this topic. This approach has done little to further understanding of this syndrome because many authors have varied the diagnostic criteria without changing the terminology. Additionally, this conceptual framework retarded the recognition of changing clinical patterns in an individual patient.

Since Allen and Brown's article appeared, many investigators have examined the natural history and clinical significance of RS. Lewis and Pickering reported that most of their patients had a benign clinical course.[71] This position was challenged in 1957 by Gifford and Hines, who first described the occurrence of associated disorders in certain patients long after the onset of typical RS.[37] Several years later, deTakats and Fowler accurately noted that a long period of clinical observation is often required before an associated disease can be recognized and that methods available to earlier investigators for identification of these diseases were unsophisticated by present standards.[24] These deficiencies undoubtedly led to the erroneous conclusion in the older literature that RS without any associated disease occurred more frequently than was actually the case. The striking frequency of associated disease has been confirmed in reports from the authors' service, which, as noted, is conducting an ongoing prospective clinical investigation of small artery and vasospastic diseases.[11, 96–99, 107–109, 134]

The information obtained from their investigations has led the authors to abandon the older terminology of Raynaud's disease and phenomenon, which often implied more than was actually understood about the patient's condition. The authors prefer to use the term *Raynaud's syndrome* to define cold-induced or emotionally induced episodic digital ischemia. Available evidence clearly shows that patients with RS are not easily separated into a benign "disease" group and a virulent "phenomenon" group, as suggested by Allen and Brown. The increasing sophistication of clinical, radiologic, and immunologic diagnostic techniques is allowing the unequivocal diagnosis of autoimmune and other associated diseases in many patients with mild symptoms who would have undoubtedly been categorized as having Raynaud's disease by the Allen and Brown criteria.[96–98]

Epidemiology

Surprisingly little information is available on the incidence of RS in the general population. Lewis and Pickering questioned 122 individuals selected at random and found that 25 per cent of the males and 30 per cent of the females had a history of Raynaud's attacks.[71] Taylor and Pelmear, as part of a study on vibration-induced RS, questioned 254 working men without vibration exposure and found a 5.3 per cent incidence of RS.[129] Olsen and Nielsen questioned a group of apparently healthy women between the ages of 21 and 50 years in Copenhagen and found that 22 per cent reported symptoms of RS.[90] Heslop and associates found a 17.6 per cent incidence of RS in females and an 8.3 per cent incidence in males who were seen in a stratified random sample of patients selected from a general practice in Hampshire, England. Only about half had sought medical attention for digital ischemia.[49] Maricq and colleagues conducted a population-based survey in South Carolina to attempt to determine the incidence of RS in the general population.[74] They found an incidence of RS of 5.1 per cent in females and 3.5 per cent in males. Leppert and coworkers sent questionnaires to a random sample of 3000 women in Sweden.[69] They found an incidence of RS of 15.6 per cent in the 2705 patients who responded. Silman and associates found an incidence of RS of 19 per cent in females and 11 per cent in males who responded to their questionnaire.[118]

The authors questioned 150 individuals selected at random in their institution and found that 30 per cent described symptoms suggestive of RS.[96–98] Combining all these studies yields an incidence of RS of 11.8 per cent (13.5 per cent in females [n = 4320] and 6.7 per cent in males [n = 1443]). It appears that a large number of patients in cool, damp climates such as Denmark, England, and Oregon have mild but definite cold sensitivity, whereas only a small percentage of this group seeks treatment for the condition. Holling stated that cool climates should result in an increase both in the frequency and in the severity of RS in the population.[54] This intuitive reasoning, however, remains unsupported by firm data.

Between 70 and 90 per cent of all reported patients with RS are women. The reason for this gender predominance is unknown. As noted previously, random population surveys have revealed that RS affects 20 to 30 per cent of the population in certain geographic areas. It must be remembered that the literature concerning RS has exclusively reported patients with vasospastic symptoms of sufficient severity and persistence that they have sought medical treatment. It is unclear whether conclusions derived from these more severely symptomatic patients can be applied accurately to less symptomatic patients who do not seek treatment. This seems especially unlikely in the important epidemiologic areas of frequency and type of associated diseases.

Of considerable interest are several population groups in whom RS appears to occur as a complication of employment.[89, 128] The best-studied groups of such patients are those whose work requires the frequent use of vibratory equipment, such as chain saw and pneumatic drill operators. A number of studies have shown that more than 50 per cent of persons routinely employed in such activities will ultimately experience RS.[14, 129] The exact mechanism of the production of RS in these patients is not understood. Laboratory studies have shown that a vibration frequency of about 125 Hz causes severe shear stresses on the arteries of the hands and fingers.[114] Limited pathologic studies have shown increasing subintimal fibrosis after prolonged exposure to vibrating instruments. One study described the angiographic pattern of vibration white finger as one of widespread palmar and digital arterial obstruction.[58] Available data suggest that the incidence of RS in chain saw operators has decreased significantly since the introduction of the antivibration chain saw in the early 1980s.

The relationship of chronic industrial cold exposure to the production of RS is of great potential importance. One report indicated that 50 per cent of workers in a food-processing industry who were exposed to alternate hot and cold temperatures noted some degree of RS.[73] Control workers for both the vibration and the cold food-processing study groups showed an approximate 5 per cent incidence of RS.[3, 12] Future clarification of the precise relationship between RS and specific employment is required and will have great potential medicolegal significance.

Pathophysiology

The events of a classic triphasic Raynaud's attack begin with profound blanching of the digits and occasionally the proximal part of the hand on cold exposure or emotional stress. This is produced by complete closure of the palmar and digital arteries and possibly of the arterioles, which results in the cessation of capillary perfusion. The blanching may be accompanied by a feeling of relative numbness or paresthesias, and both generally persist as long as the exposure continues. Attacks may terminate spontaneously or when the patient enters a warm environment. The capillaries and probably the venules reflexively dilate secondary to regional hypoxia, possibly influenced by an accumulation of the local by-products of anaerobic metabolism. Eventually, a slight relaxation of arterial spasm occurs, which permits the entry of a trickle of blood into the dilated capillary bed, where it rapidly desaturates, producing cyanosis. Subsequently, the digits may become ruborous, reflecting reactive hyperemia following transient digital ischemia[95] as increasing amounts of blood enter the dilated capillaries. The attack terminates with the relaxation of the arterial spasm and the return of baseline arterial inflow and capillary perfusion.

The search for the mechanism responsible for the vasoconstriction occurring during a Raynaud's attack has occupied investigators for more than a century. The suggestion of Raynaud that abnormal nervous system function caused the attacks was substantially disproved by the methodical evaluations of Lewis in the 1920s and 1930s.[70, 71] He repeatedly observed that autonomic and somatic nerve blocks with local anesthesia did not prevent the Raynaud's attacks. He therefore proposed that a "local vascular fault" was responsible for the observed vascular wall hyperresponsiveness to cold exclusive of sympathetic innervation.

Blood flow in an artery ceases when the constrictive force in the arterial wall exceeds the intraluminal distending pressure, the so-called critical closing pressure. Lewis showed that complete digital artery closure occurs during a Raynaud's attack,[70] and the measured digital artery pressure is actually in the range of 5 mmHg.[52] Abundant clinical observations suggest that the critical arterial closing pressure required to produce a Raynaud's attack may be achieved by two distinct pathophysiologic mechanisms, which the authors have termed obstructive and vasospastic,[21, 98, 142] although a number of patients appear to manifest elements of both mechanisms. This further reinforces the tenet that vasospastic and obstructive RS represent a continuum of disease rather than two separate entities.

Obstructive RS occurs in the presence of fixed organic obstruction of the palmar or digital arteries, with a resultant decrease in the intraluminal distending pressure. In the face of a normal vasoconstrictive response to cold or emotional stimuli, complete digital artery closure occurs and blood flow ceases, thus producing an attack. These small artery obstructions may be caused by a variety of disorders; two of the most common are arteriosclerosis and chronic arteritis associated with autoimmune connective tissue disease.[22] A systolic brachial-finger pressure gradient of up to 10 to 15 mmHg is present in normal persons. A brachial-finger gradient of more than 15 mmHg, an absolute finger blood pressure of less than 70 mmHg, or a difference of more than 15 mmHg between any two fingers indicates the presence of significant palmar or digital artery obstruction.[26] The relationship between arterial occlusive disease and cold sensitivity is a quantitative one. Hirai studied a group of patients who had palmar and digital artery obstruction with plethysmography and digital blood pressure measurements.[52] He found that mild degrees of digital artery obstruction were not associated with RS. The production of an obstructive Raynaud's attack required arterial occlusive disease of sufficient severity to produce a significant reduction in resting digital artery pressure—a condition that occurred only with obstruction of both arteries in a single digit. When this degree of occlusive disease was present, a Raynaud's attack was always observed during cooling. A corollary of this observation is the prediction that anyone with palmar or digital artery obstruction capable of causing a significant decrease in digital artery pressure should experience RS. Analysis of the more than 900 patients undergoing investigation at the authors' center confirms this hypothesis.

In contrast to the relatively straightforward and quantitative relationship between digital artery occlusive disease and RS, the pathophysiology of *vasospastic RS* remains incompletely understood. Patients with vasospastic RS do not have significant palmar or digital artery obstruction and have normal digital artery pressure at room temperature. Plethysmographic and angiographic studies in affected patients demonstrate complete digital artery closure after cold provocation despite the previously normal finger systolic blood pressure and the absence of significant arterial obstruction.[67, 90, 111] Krahenbuhl and associates examined a group of patients with vasospastic RS by measuring digital artery blood pressure changes induced by external finger cooling.[67] These patients showed a moderate decline in digital artery pressure until a critical temperature of approximately 28° C was reached, at which point total digital artery closure suddenly occurred, with an abrupt decline in the finger blood pressure to unmeasurable levels (Fig. 68–1).

The cause of this increased force of arterial vasoconstriction, the "local vascular fault" of Lewis, is unknown. Evidence of enhanced adrenergic neuroeffector activity has been suggested by the successful clinical use of sympathetic blocking agents and experimentally by radioisotope clearance studies. Coffman and Cohen performed detailed studies of finger blood flow before and after cooling in a group of controls and patients with RS.[19, 21] Normal fingers subjected to hypothermia showed a decrease in arteriovenous shunt flow without alterations in nutrient capillary flow. In patients with RS, however, both shunt flow and capillary nutritive flow were reduced at room temperature and after cooling. Pretreatment with the sympathetic blocking agent reserpine significantly increased the capillary flow in patients with RS both at room temperature and after cooling. These findings suggest that enhanced adrenergic neuroeffector activity may be a major factor in the pathophysiology of RS.

The existence of a local fault resulting in intermittent vasospasm is suggested by several observations. The persistence or recurrence of vasospastic symptoms often seen following the performance of a sympathectomy may be explained by an unaltered defect in the vessel wall responding to circulating catecholamines, possibly in association with receptor denervation hypersensitivity. Additionally, vasospastic events are known to occur in isolated and seemingly unrelated vessels, producing such disparate clinical entities as variant angina, classic migraine, abdominal migraine, and RS. Indeed, RS has been observed five times more frequently in patients with variant angina than in a control group.[79]

Alteration of the alpha-adrenergic receptors in vascular smooth muscle, possibly related to repeated exposure to cool temperatures, has also been implicated in the pathophysiology of vasospastic RS.[59] Experimental studies have provided evidence in support of this theory. Keenan and Porter found significantly higher levels of alpha$_2$-adrenergic receptors in circulating platelets of patients with vasospastic RS than in either patients with obstructive RS or normal controls.[64] This observation was subsequently confirmed, and a subset of patients with subnormal alpha$_2$-adrenergic receptor levels was identified.[28] When serum from patients with vasospastic RS was incubated with platelets from controls, an absolute decrease occurred in the measured alpha$_2$-adrenoreceptor levels of the control platelets that was not observed following a control incubation. This observation suggested receptor modulation as a mechanism of increased cellular receptor synthesis. Although the relationship between receptor levels in platelet membranes, which contain a pure population of alpha$_2$-adrenergic receptors, and vascular smooth muscle remains to be quantitated in humans, extrapolation from other experimental and clinical models supports a direct correlation. The existence of an altered receptor population may prove to be the fundamental abnormality through which any one of a number of factors, such as neurogenic activity, immunologic mediators, or elevated serotonin levels, may act to result in vasospasm. This may also help explain the observation that sympathetic nerve transection with resultant adrenoreceptor hypersensi-

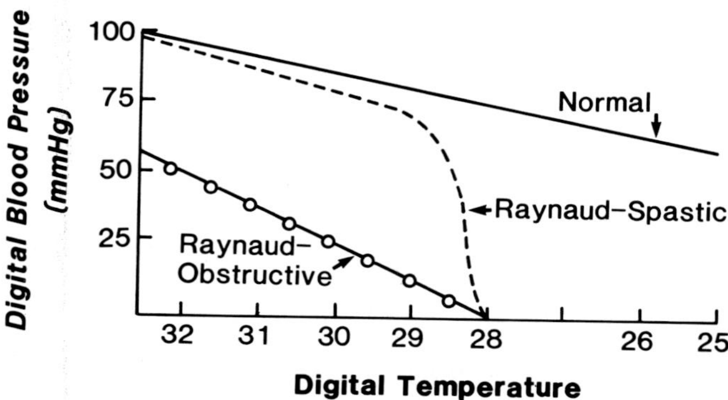

FIGURE 68–1. Alterations in digital artery blood pressure with a decrease in temperature. (From Edwards JM, Porter JM: Raynaud's syndrome. *In* Sabiston DC Jr [ed]: Textbook of Surgery. 14th ed. Philadelphia, WB Saunders, 1991, p 1645.)

tivity is not as effective as adrenergic receptor blockade in the relief of vasospastic symptoms.

Many other factors have been considered in the pathophysiology of vasospastic RS. Alterations in blood viscosity,[41, 131] abnormal serum proteins,[40, 131] elevated serotonin levels,[45] and altered shear stress[85, 114] have all been demonstrated in certain patients with RS. More recently, abnormalities in vasoactive peptides such as calcitonin gene–related peptide and endothelin have been described in patients with RS.[13, 32, 115, 141] Although certain of these factors may occasionally play a significant role in the pathogenesis of symptomatic cold-induced vasospasm in patients, their presence is uncommon, inconsistently observed, and unlikely to be a major factor in a majority of patients.[11, 44, 64, 98]

Clinical Presentation

RS consists of episodic digital coldness associated with pallor or cyanosis brought on by cold exposure or emotional stimuli. Mild pain, paresthesias, and numbness are frequent complaints, but severe pain is rare. RS may coexist with persistent or chronic digital ischemia. Persistent digital cyanosis or painful digital ischemic ulceration may infrequently dominate the clinical picture and be the presenting complaint in patients with previous long-standing, stable RS.[98] Conversely, previously asymptomatic patients may present with the abrupt onset of digital ischemia and then manifest chronic RS following resolution of the initial ischemic symptoms.[9, 80, 125] It is important to note that digital ulceration is never caused by vasospasm alone. Ischemic digital ulceration always implies widespread palmar and digital artery obstruction.

Clinical and Laboratory Evaluation

The only absolute requirement for the diagnosis of RS is the history of cold-induced or emotionally induced episodic digital ischemia, usually manifested by color changes. Diagnostic studies should therefore be directed toward precise quantification of the degree of ischemia and identification of associated disorders. The history taking is the most important initial diagnostic modality and will substantially direct the course and extent of subsequent investigations. A history of arthralgia, dysphagia, xerostomia, or xerophthalmia suggests a connective tissue disorder. Symptoms relative to large vessel arterial occlusive disease, exposure to trauma, or a history of malignancy should be sought because all these disorders may be associated with digital ischemia. A complete medication profile is essential. The physical examination findings are frequently unremarkable; however, specific attention should be directed to the quality of the peripheral pulses, the presence of digital ulcerations, evidence of prior tissue loss, and joint changes. The skin should be evaluated for the presence of telangiectasias or rashes, or thinning and tightening suggestive of scleroderma; the latter is most easily seen in the face and hands.

The extent of laboratory testing will vary depending on initial clinical suspicions. Minimal evaluation performed on all patients with suspected RS includes a complete blood count, determination of the erythrocyte sedimentation rate, a chemistry profile, and urinalysis. A serum rheumatoid factor assay and a screening antinuclear antibody titer are of sufficient value to warrant inclusion in a baseline evaluation. The antinuclear antibody test is most sensitive when performed on two different substrates.[7] These tests are most helpful in the diagnosis of rheumatoid arthritis, systemic lupus erythematosus, mixed connective tissue disease, and scleroderma. Additional laboratory testing should be pursued in selected patients as indicated by the results of the screening tests (Table 68–1).

Table 68–1. Laboratory Evaluation of Raynaud's Syndrome

Baseline Tests (routine)	Adjunctive Tests (in selected patients)
Complete blood count	Serum protein electrophoresis
Erythrocyte sedimentation rate	Extractable nuclear antibody
Chemistry profile	Anti–native DNA antibody
Urinalysis	HEP-2 antinuclear antibody
Rheumatoid factor	Cryoglobulins
Antinuclear antibody	Complement levels
	Hepatitis B screen
	Anticentromere antibody

Vascular Laboratory and Arteriographic Evaluation

The objective vascular laboratory documentation of RS, although not essential for diagnosis in most patients, is of great value in certain situations. It is especially useful in the evaluation of symptomatic patients who do not manifest typical color changes, in certain patients with medicolegal claims, and in an attempt to quantitate objectively the results of treatment.

The simplest vascular laboratory test for detection of RS is the hand *ice water immersion test* with determination of fingertip temperatures with a thermistor probe. The patient's hand is immersed in a container of ice water for 30 seconds. The hand is then dried, and fingertip pulp temperatures are measured every 5 minutes for 45 minutes, or until the temperature returns to preimmersion levels. The test requires body warming so that the preimmersion digital temperature is above 30° C. The digital temperature of normal persons returns to normal in 10 minutes or less, whereas patients with RS have a much longer temperature recovery. This test appears quite specific for RS but, unfortunately, appears to have low sensitivity.[99] A representative temperature recovery curve appears in Figure 68–2.

Sumner and Strandness described a distinctive peaked appearance of the *digital photoplethysmographic waveform* in 78 per cent of patients with cold sensitivity and RS.[122] This peaked waveform was found in only 3 per cent of asymptomatic individuals. A detailed assessment of the use of the plethysmographic peaked digital pulse waveform in the diagnosis of RS indicated that presence of the peaked pulse was 66 per cent sensitive and 100 per cent specific and had an overall accuracy rate of 70 per cent in the objective diagnosis of RS.[4]

The *occlusive digital hypothermic challenge test* described by Nielsen and Lassen is the most sensitive and

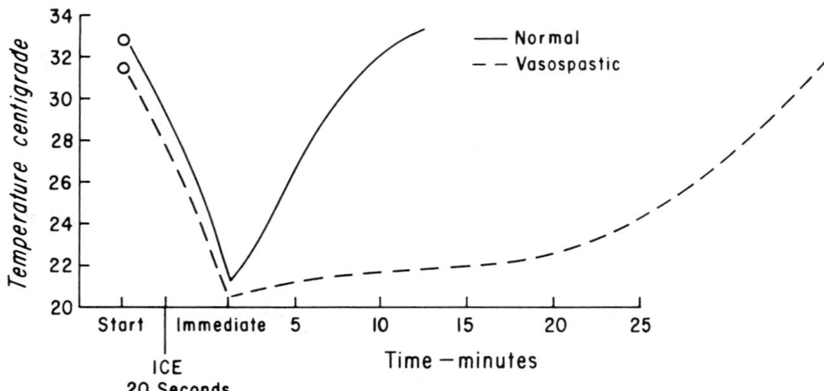

FIGURE 68–2. Digital temperature recovery after ice water exposure. The different curves for the normal and the vasospastic digit are indicated. (From Porter JM, Snider RL, Bardana EJ, et al: The diagnosis and treatment of Raynaud's phenomenon. Surgery 77:11, 1975.)

specific test currently available for the diagnosis of RS.[86] Patients are examined at a room temperature of 21° C. A double-inlet cuff for local cooling is placed over the proximal phalanx of the test finger (most commonly the right second digit). Baseline digital artery pressures are obtained in the reference and test fingers using a mercury-in-rubber strain-gauge distal to the occlusive finger cuff; this is followed by 5 minutes of ischemic hypothermic perfusion of the test finger. After tourniquet release following cooling, the digital blood pressure recovery is recorded. Results are expressed as the percentage of decrease in the cool finger systolic pressure on reperfusion compared with the reference finger. A decrease in digital blood pressure of 20 per cent or greater is considered positive for RS. In the authors' vascular laboratory, this test is 100 per cent sensitive and 80 per cent specific, with an accuracy of 97 per cent in the diagnosis of RS.[4, 33]

Several *other diagnostic tests* have been used for the detection of RS, although none appear equal to the digital hypothermic challenge test. These have included thermal entrainment,[68] digital thermography,[15] venous occlusion plethysmography, digital artery caliber measurement,[119] and other methods of digital blood flow measurement.[21, 140]

Digital plethysmography with waveform analysis and *digital blood pressure determination* provide an accurate assessment of the status of the digital arterial circulation.[39, 55] The information obtained with these noninvasive examinations is essential in differentiating between vasospastic and obstructive RS in the individual patient and is frequently important in establishing the diagnosis of an associated disease. Examples of a normal and an abnormal digital photoplethysmographic tracing are seen in Figure 68–3.

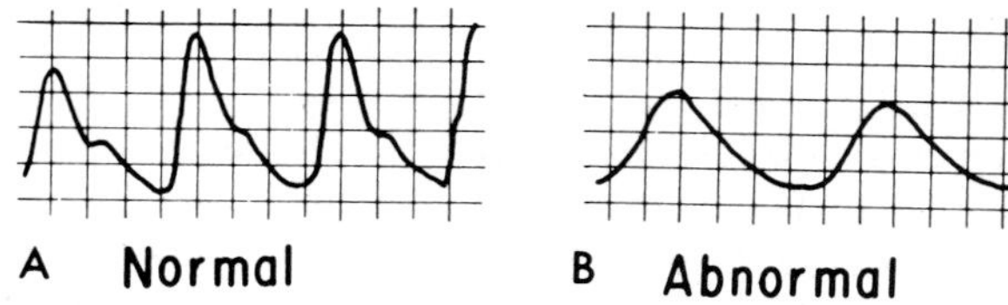

FIGURE 68–3. Photoplethysmographic digital artery waveforms objectively document arterial occlusive disease and diminish the need for angiography. *A*, A normal tracing. *B*, A tracing from a patient with obstructive Raynaud's syndrome.

Early in their experience, the authors used *hand arteriography* extensively in establishing the diagnosis of RS. Magnification hand arteriograms were obtained before and after ice water exposure and before and 24 hours after intra-arterial administration of reserpine. An example of a film sequence is shown in Figure 68–4. A typical pattern of total abolition of cold-induced vasospasm by adrenoreceptor blocking drugs was recognized and proved to be a reliable diagnostic test. The early arteriograms were of considerable importance in establishing the role of adrenoreceptor function in the pathophysiology of RS. Hand arteriography has been almost entirely replaced by vascular laboratory tests, especially the Nielsen test and digital plethysmography, in the diagnosis of RS.

The authors recommend upper extremity arteriography only in patients suspected of having large artery disease proximal to the palmar arch. This may be suspected by an absence of pulses on examination or unilateral development of digital ischemia.

Treatment

The goal of treatment in a patient with RS is palliation, because no curative treatment is available. It is important for the physician to understand the generally benign course of RS in most patients. The natural history is one of symptomatic periods interspersed with periods of improvement or even complete remission. Inexorable progression to severe finger ischemia or gangrene occurs rarely—only in the presence of an underlying obstructive arterial disease. The majority of patients with vasospastic RS have only mild to moderate symptoms and respond satisfactorily to avoidance of cold and tobacco. The use of oral contraceptives,[27] beta-adrenergic blockers,[31, 75] and ergotamine preparations[42, 48, 78, 83] is not recommended because each of these agents has been reported to exacerbate Raynaud's symptoms and equally effective alternative forms of therapy are generally available. Patients occasionally require pharmacologic intervention during the winter; such treatment is also indicated in patients with severe symptoms.

The objective evaluation of the efficacy of drug treatment of RS is impossible in the absence of any vascular laboratory test that accurately quantitates drug effect on the digital circulation. Until such a test is developed, the as-

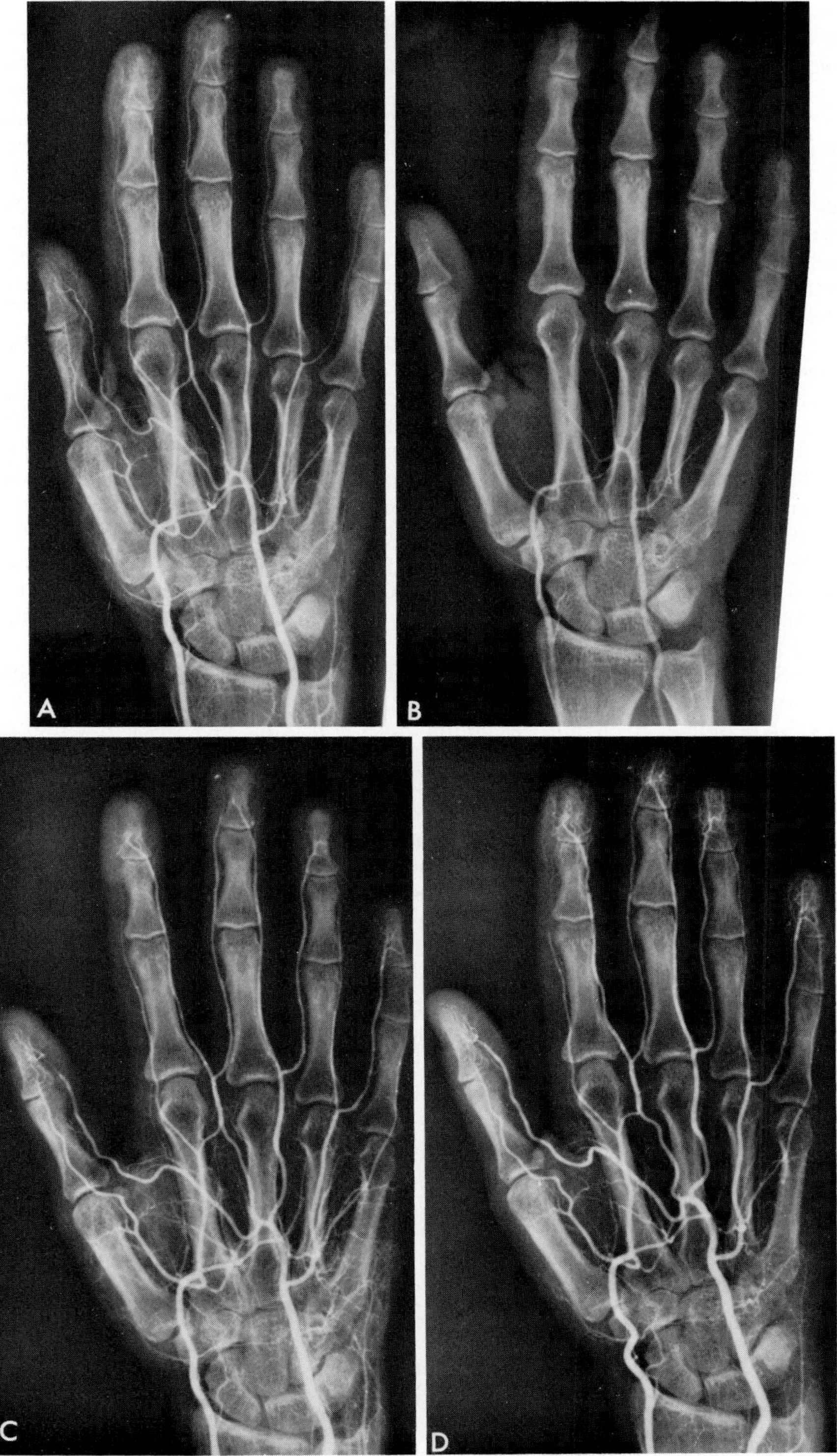

FIGURE 68–4. *A*, Hand arteriogram of a patient with Raynaud's syndrome before ice water exposure. *B*, After ice water exposure, prominent resting vasospasm and a marked vasospastic response to cold are present. *C* and *D*, Arteriograms obtained 48 hours after intra-arterial injection of reserpine and before and after ice water exposure. Resting vasospasm has been completely eliminated, and there is a marked decrease in the vasospastic response to cold.

sessment of drug response will be anecdotal and greatly hampered by such uncontrolled variables as environmental temperature, amount of environmental cold exposure, and the patient's emotional state. The efficacy assessments of all the drugs described in this section are anecdotal and are subject to all the inherent disadvantages of this method of drug evaluation.

Sympatholytic agents have been the mainstay of the pharmacologic therapy of RS.[1, 2, 18, 20, 77, 132, 138] Patients with vasospastic RS generally respond much more favorably to treatment than do those with obstructive RS. The effectiveness of medical treatment is limited not only by the presence of severe arterial obstructive disease but also by the presence of frequent side effects of drug treatment.[97]

Oral reserpine was one of the earliest drugs evaluated in the treatment of RS,[36, 87, 93] and daily doses of 0.25 mg to as high as 1.0 mg have been used clinically.[66] Other orally administered sympathetic blockers in clinical use that have been of modest benefit include guanethidine,[107] methyldopa,[133] isoxsuprine,[137] phenoxybenzamine,[107, 125] and prazosin.[135] The high dosages required when each of these agents is used as a single agent frequently lead to intolerable side effects. Low-dose combination regimens can sometimes reduce the frequency and severity of side effects; one such combination, consisting of guanethidine, 10 mg daily, and 1 to 2 mg of prazosin per day, has appeared beneficial in the treatment of RS in the authors' experience.[100] The authors have also used this drug combination in the treatment of patients with ischemic finger ulceration, but the results of drug therapy have been much less clear in this patient group.[125] There are few reported prospective, randomized, double-blind trials of any of these agents in the treatment of RS, and all reports of drug treatment of RS have relied on anecdotal end-points.

Sympathetic blockers have generally been replaced by calcium channel blockers in the treatment of symptomatic RS.[62] Nifedipine, given either as 30 mg orally at bedtime in a sustained-release formulation or as 10 mg orally three times a day, is the authors' current first-line drug.[84, 97] The sustained-release formulation appears to be tolerated better. Some patients who do not tolerate the standard formulation will be able to take the sustained-release formulation without having side effects. Controlled prospective trials have shown improvement in the vasospastic symptoms of patients with RS.[39, 110, 120] Diltiazem, another calcium channel blocker, may be equally effective. The addition of the alpha-adrenergic blocker prazosin may result in further improvement in patients who respond incompletely to a calcium channel blocker alone. Pentoxifylline, 400 mg three times per day, is a hemorrheologic agent that appears to be of benefit in some patients, but controlled trials are lacking.

The beneficial effect of intra-arterial reserpine in patients with RS was first reported by Abboud and associates in 1967.[1] Other investigators have confirmed the abilities of intra-arterial reserpine[2, 77, 102, 132] and tolazoline[104] to improve certain difficult cases, including those with digital ulcers. The effect is generally short-lived, however, lasting from a few hours to a few weeks. Additionally, repeated intra-arterial drug injections are hazardous and present a cumulative risk of arterial damage. An example of the effect of reserpine on cold-induced vasospasm is shown in Figure 68–4.

Bier-block reserpine, with injection of the medication intravenously into the "extravasated" extremity under tourniquet control, has been reported to be safe and appears to be at least as effective as the intra-arterial route of administration.[127] Unfortunately, parenteral reserpine is no longer available in the United States. Guanethidine administered by intravenous Bier block is currently under investigation.

The difficulty of treating patients with RS who have associated digital ulceration has prompted investigations of less conventional modalities. Infusion of prostaglandin E, and prostaglandin I_2, both of which are potent vasodilators and inhibitors of platelet aggregation,[123] has been studied by Clifford and associates[16, 17] and Pardy and associates,[92] with encouraging initial anecdotal results. Interestingly, a subsequent randomized, double-blind study of prostaglandin E, in patients with RS without digital ulceration showed no benefit.[82] Jarrett and coworkers used the fibrinolytic stimulating agent stanozolol in patients with RS, again with promising results.[60] This treatment, however, was selected on the basis of finding high fibrinogen levels in a number of patients. This abnormality has seldom been observed by the authors or by other investigators. Therefore, this experimental treatment is not expected to be generally applicable. Likewise, the technique of plasmapheresis has been used with satisfactory results in certain patients, supposedly on the basis of defibrination, although possibly involving lysis of established fibrin deposits, induced alterations of platelet function, or reduction of circulating immune complexes.[25, 91, 124] These treatments may be of great benefit to the individual patient in whom such unusual factors as abnormal serum proteins or viscosity may play a dominant role. However, they appear to be of little or no benefit in the majority of patients, who do not manifest these specific abnormalities.

Cervicothoracic sympathectomy has been performed frequently in past decades to treat both vasospastic RS and ischemic digital ulceration associated with small artery occlusive disease.[23, 65, 72] The reported rates of response to sympathectomy vary widely in different surgical series; generally, however, symptomatic recurrence has followed an initial period of improvement.[38, 43, 61] Whether this failure of long-term benefit is due to incomplete sympathectomy, regeneration of sympathetic nerves, or catecholamine hypersensitivity after denervation is uncertain. At present, the authors do not recommend or perform upper extremity sympathectomy in the treatment of patients with RS.

ASSOCIATED DISEASES

RS has been associated with a bewildering variety of clinical conditions, which at first glance appear to have little relationship to each other.[11] A list of conditions that have been associated with RS appears in Table 68–2. In the past, this array of disparate associated conditions significantly obscured the understanding of RS. It now appears clear that the associated conditions should be viewed from the perspective of being related to either vasospastic or obstructive RS. A majority of the conditions listed have distal upper extremity small artery obstruction as part of the disease process.

The type and severity of associated diseases that are encountered reflect, in significant part, local referral patterns. The authors found an associated autoimmune disease in 80 per cent of all patients with RS in the early years of their study[99] when only the more severely symptomatic patients from the community were referred. As awareness of their continued interest in this condition spread, patients with milder symptoms of shorter duration were also referred. Accordingly, the incidence of associated connective tissue disease in their patients dropped to 40 per cent and has been stable at this level in more recent years.

Table 68–2. Disorders Reported in Association With Raynaud's Syndrome

Autoimmune connective tissue diseases
- Dermatomyositis
- Henoch-Schönlein purpura
- Hepatitis B-antigen–induced vasculitis
- Mixed connective tissue disease
- Polyarteritis nodosa
- Polymyositis
- Reiter's syndrome
- Rheumatoid arthritis
- Scleroderma-CREST syndrome
- Sjögren's syndrome
- Systemic lupus erythematosus
- Undifferentiated connective tissue disease

Hypersensitivity angiitis (rapid-onset vascular occlusion)

Myeloproliferative disorders
- Leukemia
- Myeloid metaplasia
- Polycythemia rubra vera
- Thrombocytosis

Circulating globulins
- Cold agglutinins
- Cryoglobulinemia
- Malignancy
- Macroglobulinemia
- Multiple myeloma

Obstructive arterial diseases
- Atherosclerosis
- Buerger's disease

Peripheral embolization
- Atherosclerosis
- Thoracic outlet syndrome

Environmental conditions
- Repetitive trauma
- Vibration injury
- Cold injury

Drug-induced (without arteritis)
- Ergots
- Beta-blocking drugs
- Cytotoxic agents
- Oral contraceptives

Miscellaneous
- Chronic renal failure
- Drug-induced vasculitis
- Vinyl chloride disease
- Neurologic disorders
  - Central
  - Peripheral
    - Polyneuropathy
    - Neurofibromatosis
- Endocrine disorders
- Hematologic disorders
  - Disseminated intravascular coagulation

In the authors' experience, as well as that reported from other referral centers, approximately 40 per cent of patients with RS have the idiopathic variety caused by vasospasm alone, without evidence of an associated small artery obstructive disease.[96–99] Raynaud's syndrome, however, may be the first symptom of an otherwise silent systemic illness. Therefore, careful long-term follow-up is prudent in all such patients because the initial symptoms of Raynaud's attacks may precede the development of a detectable associated disease by months or even years.[97] The prognosis for vasospastic RS is benign; in most patients, it is a nuisance condition only, with no risk of subsequent tissue loss.

In 60 per cent of patients with RS, an underlying disorder associated with palmar and digital artery occlusive disease can be diagnosed using the evaluation plan outlined previously. The associated diseases found in the authors' most recently tabulated series of 631 patients with RS are shown in Table 68–3. In their experience and that of other referral centers,[96–99, 142] autoimmune connective tissue disorders are the most frequently diagnosed associated conditions, accounting for about 50 per cent of the associated diseases.

One third of patients with RS and connective tissue disease have scleroderma or a CREST variant; the remainder suffer from one or more of a variety of autoimmune diseases, including mixed connective tissue disease, rheumatoid arthritis, systemic lupus erythematosus, Sjögren's syndrome, or one of a number of other autoimmune conditions. A significant percentage of patients present with abnormal serologic study results and evidence of end-organ involvement but lack the pattern of a classically defined syndrome; they are classified as having undifferentiated connective tissue disease. Other patients have signs and

Table 68–3. Associated Disorders in 631 Patients With Raynaud's Syndrome (Oregon Health Sciences University Clinical Research Center, 1970–1987)

Disorder	Number of Cases (%)
Idiopathic (pure vasospasm with no associated disease)	236 (37.4)
CTDs	235 (37.2)
Scleroderma, CREST	85
Undifferentiated CTD	33
Mixed CTD	20
Rheumatoid arthritis	14
Systemic lupus erythematosus	13
Sjögren's syndrome	12
Polyarteritis nodosa	3
Reiter's syndrome	3
Suspected CTD	31
Overlap syndromes	8
Combined disorders (CTD + others)	5
Hypersensitivity angiitis (rapid-onset vascular occlusion)	22 (3.5)
Myeloproliferative disorders	1 (0.2)
Leukemia	1
Circulating globulins	13 (2)
Cryoglobulinemia	1
Gammopathy	3
Malignancy (solid)	9
Atherosclerosis obliterans	35 (5.5)
Buerger's disease	12 (1.9)
Frostbite	25 (4)
Trauma or vibration injury	10 (1.6)
Medication-induced disorder	10 (1.6)
Embolization	5 (0.8)
Other	9 (1.4)
Hypothyroidism	6
Chronic renal failure	3
Miscellaneous	18 (2.9)
Total patients	631 (100)

CTD, connective tissue disease.

Table 68–4. Risk of Patients With Raynaud's Syndrome Developing Connective Tissue Disease If They Present With No or 1⁺ Signs of Such a Disease

Authors, Date	Follow-Up (Years)	No Sign CTD		1⁺ Sign CTD	
		N	*(% Progression)*	*N*	*(% Progression)*
Blain et al, 1951[10]	5+	100	25	—	—
Gifford and Hines, 1957[37]	2+	280	4.6	—	—
Harper et al, 1982[46]	2	37	2.7	17	35.3
Gerbracht et al, 1985[35]	3.7	75	2.7	12	16.7
Sheiner and Small, 1987[116]	3.5	78	0	19	15.8
Priollet et al, 1987[105]	4.7	49	0	24	58.3
Fitzgerald et al, 1988[29]	2.7	33	9	25	32
Kallenberg et al, 1988[63]	6	29	3.4	35	25.7
Wollersheim et al, 1989[139]	3.5	51	7.8	20	65
Gentric et al, 1990[34]	4	16	6.3	9	11
Weiner et al, 1991[136]	4	40	0	23	17.4

CTD, connective tissue disease.

symptoms of more than one defined clinical syndrome and are categorized as having overlap syndromes.

The common pathophysiologic mechanism of RS in patients with connective tissue disorders is presumed to be patchy or transmural necrotizing vasculitis, possibly secondary to an antigen-antibody or autoantibody reaction.[11, 23] Subsequent inflammatory thrombosis results in areas of fibrous obliteration of multiple digital and palmar arteries. Once diffuse small artery obstruction is present, even a normal vasospastic response to cold will induce a Raynaud's attack. Thus, most patients with RS and autoimmune disease appear to have obstructive RS. Early in the course of autoimmune disease, however, patients may manifest spastic RS before the development of widespread small artery obstruction. It is estimated that RS is present in more than 80 per cent of patients with scleroderma or mixed connective tissue disease, in 25 per cent of patients with rheumatoid arthritis, and in 20 per cent of patients with systemic lupus erythematosus.[25, 96, 121] Interestingly, there is no current explanation for the predilection of autoimmune arteritis for the distal upper extremity arteries.

For a patient who presents for the evaluation of RS and does not have a connective tissue disease at the time of initial presentation, the risk of subsequently developing a connective tissue disorder appears to depend primarily on the presence or absence of other findings suggestive of connective tissue disease, such as a positive antinuclear antibody titer, sclerodactyly, or abnormal nailfold capillary microscopy findings. The published reports that the authors are aware of are listed in Table 68–4. Combining these results gives an average risk of developing connective tissue disease of 6 per cent at 3.3 years if there are no signs or symptoms at initial presentation and of 42 per cent at 4 years if there are one or more signs of a connective tissue disease at initial presentation.

Numerous other obstructive arterial diseases may be associated with RS, including atherosclerosis and Buerger's disease (thromboangiitis obliterans). Upper extremity involvement is frequently reported in Buerger's disease; between 20 and 50 per cent of these patients have associated obstructive RS.[5, 51, 53, 81] Distal embolization resulting in multiple palmar and digital arterial occlusions may result from a proximal innominate or subclavian artery lesion or, rarely, from arterial complications of thoracic outlet syndrome.[57, 101, 113] Various myeloproliferative disorders, including leukemia,[103, 112] myeloid metaplasia, thrombocytosis, and polycythemia rubra vera may be associated with digital artery obstruction and RS.[88] Pathologic increases in any of the formed elements of the blood may lead to hyperviscosity and cellular sludging, with subsequent small artery thrombosis.[41, 50] Hyperviscosity caused by circulating serum proteins has been described in numerous conditions and may result in digital ischemia in certain patients with multiple myeloma, cryoglobulinemia,[40] or an epithelial cell–derived malignancy.[47, 88, 126]

The occupational causes of RS are discussed in the section on epidemiology. Chronic vibration injury may cause digital artery obstruction after long exposure.[58] The cause of the syndrome in patients exposed to vibration for only a short period may reflect smooth muscle alteration induced by vibratory shear stresses.[8, 114] With longer exposure, arterial obstruction appears to predominate. A Raynaud-type syndrome with associated swelling and pain on cold exposure frequently follows frostbite injuries.[76]

Drug-induced RS appears primarily vasospastic, as exemplified by ergot and the beta-blockers.[31] The mechanism of action of the cytotoxic[130] and anovulatory[27] drugs in the production of RS is uncertain. The precise cause of RS in patients with one or more of the associated diseases listed under the miscellaneous category in Table 68–2 is unclear.

Of special interest has been a group of patients presenting with endocrine abnormalities[11] and RS. The associated endocrine conditions seen to date in the authors' patient group include hypothyroidism, Graves' disease, Addison's disease, Cushing's disease, and hypofunctioning pituitary tumors. The temporal association of these conditions with the onset of RS in certain patients has suggested a causal relationship, although to date there has been no explanation of any pathophysiologic mechanisms.

ISCHEMIC DIGITAL ULCERATION AND GANGRENE

Ischemic digital ulceration occurs infrequently. In the course of evaluating more than 900 patients with RS since

1970, the authors have encountered 100 patients with finger gangrene caused by small artery occlusive disease.[80, 94] The underlying diagnoses established in these patients are listed in Table 68–5. Digital ulceration never results from vasospasm alone; its occurrence invariably signals the presence of an underlying disease associated with digital artery obstruction. In the authors' experience, the four most commonly encountered associated diseases are connective tissue disorders, hypersensitivity angiitis, atherosclerosis, and Buerger's disease. More than half the patients with ischemic digital ulceration will have connective tissue disease, and one half of these patients will suffer from scleroderma or the CREST variant (chondrocalcinosis, RS, esophageal motility disturbance, sclerodactyly, and telangiectasias).

Hypersensitivity angiitis is an interesting condition characterized by the sudden onset of pain and digital cyanosis with rapid progression to ulceration and finger gangrene[9] in a previously asymptomatic patient. Twenty-seven patients in the authors' series presented in this manner. All had documented fixed digital artery obstruction as shown by plethysmography, angiography, or both, and in all patients, serologic test findings for autoimmune disease were initially negative. In 5 patients, serologic abnormalities developed during long-term follow-up and led to the diagnosis of an associated autoimmune condition. In 22 patients, however, all serologic test results remained consistently negative. Ischemic digital lesions healed with conservative treatment in all these patients, and no recurrences were noted with follow-up extending up to 15 years. This syndrome has been termed *hypersensitivity angiitis with rapid-onset vascular occlusion.* It is acknowledged that the authors' use of this term is speculative, and this condition does not manifest either the florid necrotizing panarteritis or systemic symptoms associated with the traditional hypersensitivity angiitides. The clinical picture of sudden-onset digital ischemia without systemic toxicity, with relatively rapid resolution, and with lack of recurrence is consistent with an immune vasculitis with distribution limited to the digital and palmar arteries, although specific antigens have yet to be identified.

All patients with digital ischemia undergo routine upper extremity three-cuff vascular laboratory evaluation, as well as recording of Doppler waveforms from the brachial, radial, ulnar, and digital arteries. As noted previously, hand arteriography is performed selectively. If a patient has normal pulses to the wrist, obstructive waveforms in all 10 fingers, and serologic abnormalities typical for autoimmune disease, arteriography is unlikely to show more than the palmar and digital artery obstructive disease documented by the noninvasive tests. The authors currently recommend arteriography only in patients with absent or diminished arm pulses, unilateral finger ischemia, or both. An example of hand arteriography showing marked arterial obstruction in a patient with finger ulceration is shown in Figure 68–5.

Table 68–5. Underlying Diagnosis Established in 100 Patients With Ischemic Finger Ulceration Secondary to Small Artery Occlusive Disease

Diagnosis	No. of Patients
Connective tissue disease	54
Hypersensitivity angiitis (ROVO)*	22
Thromboangiitis obliterans (Buerger's disease)	9
Atherosclerosis obliterans	9
Malignancy	4
Combined atherosclerosis and connective tissue disorder	2
Total number of patients	100

**ROVO, rapid-onset vascular occlusion.*

Treatment

Healing rates of 80 to 85 per cent for ischemic digital ulcers have been reported following a variety of unconventional therapies, including sympathectomy or vasodilator drug infusion.[23, 65, 72] In the authors' series of 100 consecutive patients with ischemic finger ulceration and gangrene associated with small artery disease, a conservative treatment regimen without sympathectomy was used.[80] This simple regimen consisted of gentle soap and water scrubs, débridement of necrotic tissue, fingernail removal to facilitate the drainage of underlying infection, administration of culture-specific antibiotics, and delayed length-conserving digital amputation débridement as required. With this approach, complete healing without recurrence was achieved in 88 per cent of patients. This outcome apparently reflects the natural history of the condition itself and is certainly not a specific response to this therapy. A representative photograph of a painful ischemic digital ulcer in a patient with digital artery obstruction is shown in Figure 68–6. Total healing was achieved in 4 weeks following conservative therapy. In the authors' experience, all recurrent digital ulcers have occurred in patients with connective tissue disease, most often scleroderma. The authors find no evidence that cervicothoracic sympathectomy or unconventional drug therapy is of any benefit and do not use them in the treatment of patients with ischemic finger ulceration.

Local digital artery sympathectomy performed by stripping the adventitia from distal digital arteries and dividing the terminal sympathetic nerve branches using microscopic assistance has been described in the treatment of finger ischemia.[30] These reports are anecdotal, and controlled clinical trials comparing this mode of therapy with other forms of treatment are lacking. In addition, distal microsurgical sympathectomy, like the proximal cervicothoracic procedure, does not address the underlying arterial obstructive disease present in patients with ischemic digital ulceration and has no effect on the fundamental local vascular fault in patients with spastic RS. Microsurgical arterial reconstruction of palmar and digital arteries has been reported in a few patients,[117] but the diffuse pattern of involvement in most patients limits the application of this technique to an insignificant minority.

SUMMARY

RS consists of episodic digital pallor or cyanosis with associated numbness induced by cold exposure or emo-

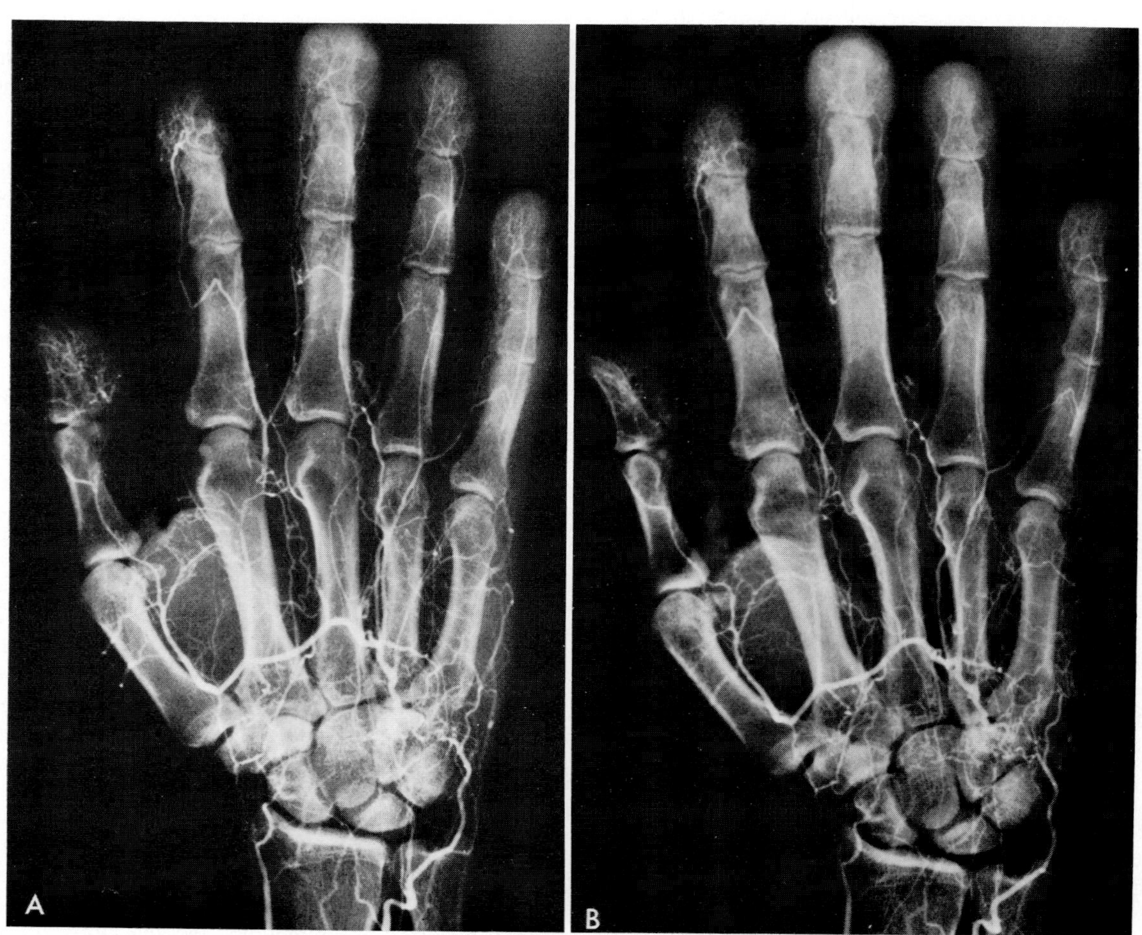

FIGURE 68–5. *A*, Hand arteriogram of a 41-year-old man with Buerger's disease, an ischemic digital ulcer, and Raynaud's syndrome. The widespread arterial obstruction is obvious. *B*, Same patient after ice exposure. This shows only minimal angiographic vasospasm and is typical of obstructive Raynaud's syndrome. Compare this pattern with the vasoconstrictive pattern after cold exposure in Figure 68–4*B*.

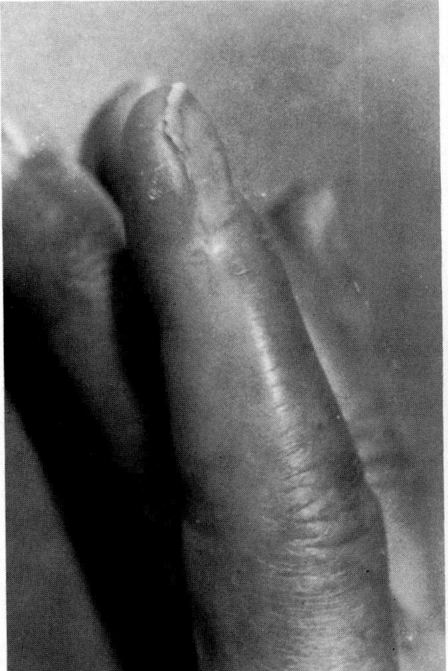
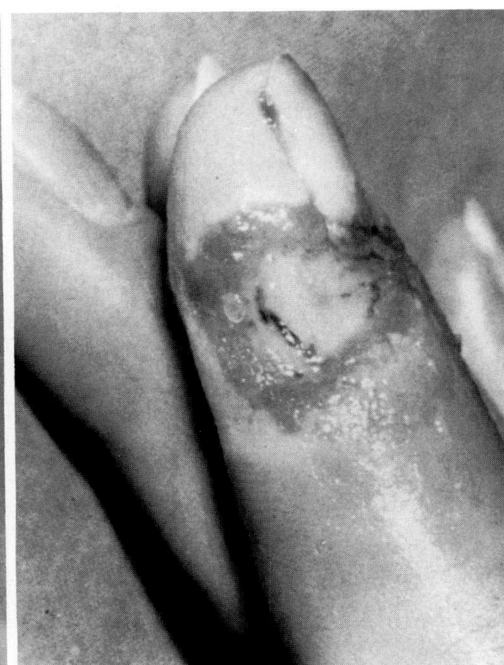

FIGURE 68–6. **Ischemic digital ulcer in a patient with scleroderma. Total healing was achieved using the conservative treatment regimen outlined.**

tional stimuli. The condition affects, to some degree, 20 to 30 per cent of patients in cool, damp climates, and a significant majority of affected patients are female. Available evidence suggests that Raynaud's attacks may be produced by two distinct pathophysiologic mechanisms. In certain patients, the digital arteries appear normal and episodic vasospasm is induced by an abnormally forceful muscular contraction of the digital artery. Other patients have significant palmar and digital artery obstructive disease with diminished arterial pressure in the fingers. In these patients, a presumably normal cold-induced arterial contraction is sufficient to induce an attack. The treatment of RS is entirely symptomatic because no curative therapy is available. Approximately 90 per cent of patients are adequately treated by cold and tobacco avoidance, and no drug therapy is necessary. For the remainder, the best results have been obtained with calcium channel blockers, specifically nifedipine, although drug treatment results in symptomatic improvement in only about 50 per cent of patients and is frequently associated with significant side effects. There is currently no evidence that regional surgical sympathectomy is of any long-term benefit in patients with RS.

A small number of patients develop severe finger ischemia, including ischemic finger ulceration with or without preceding RS. These patients all have severe palmar and digital artery obstructive disease caused by various associated disease processes. In the authors' experience, the most frequent have been the arteritis of autoimmune connective tissue disease, hypersensitivity arteritis, arteriosclerosis, and Buerger's disease. The treatment of these patients has been conservative, with local cleansing, antibiotics, and limited débridement as required. There is no convincing evidence that sympathectomy or vasodilator drug therapy is of benefit in the treatment of digital ischemia.

References

1. Abboud FM, Eckstein JW, Lawrence MS: Preliminary observations on the use of intra-arterial reserpine in Raynaud's phenomenon. Circulation 35:11, 1967.
2. Acevedo A, Reginato AJ, Schnell AM: Effect of intra-arterial reserpine in patients suffering from Raynaud's phenomenon. J Cardiovasc Surg 19:77, 1978.
3. Adams T, Smith RE: Effect of chronic cold exposure on finger temperature responses. J Appl Physiol 17:317, 1962.
4. Alexander S, Cummings C, Figg-Hoblyn L, et al: Usefulness of digital peaked pulse for diagnosis of Raynaud's syndrome. J Vasc Tech 12:71, 1988.
5. Allen EV, Brown GE: Thrombo-angiitis obliterans: A clinical study of 200 cases. Ann Intern Med 1:535, 1928.
6. Allen EV, Brown GE: Raynaud's disease: A critical review of minimal requisites for diagnosis. Am J Med Sci 1983:187, 1932.
7. Anderson CJ, Bardana EJ, Porter JM, et al: Anticentromere and antinuclear antibodies in Raynaud's syndrome. Clin Res 28:76A, 1980.
8. Azuma T, Onhashi T, Salsaguchi M: An approach to the pathogenesis of "white finger" induced by vibratory stimulation: Acute but sustained changes in vascular responsiveness of canine hindlimb to noradrenaline. Cardiovasc Res 14:725, 1980.
9. Baur GM, Porter JM, Bardana EJ, et al: Rapid onset of hand ischemia of unknown etiology: Clinical evaluation and follow-up of ten patients. Ann Surg 186:184, 1977.
10. Blain A III, Coller FA, Carver GB: Raynaud's disease: A study of criteria for prognosis. Surgery 29:387, 1951.
11. Blunt RJ, Porter JM: Raynaud's syndrome. Semin Arthritis Rheum 11:282, 1981.
12. Buchanan JL, Cranley JJ Jr, Linton RR: Observations on the direct effect of cold on blood vessels in the human extremity and its relation to peripheral vascular disease. Surgery 31:62, 1952.
13. Bunker CB, Terenghi G, Springall DR, et al: Deficiency of calcitonin gene-related peptide in Raynaud's phenomenon. Lancet 336:1530, 1990.
14. Chatterjee DS, Petrie A, Taylor W: Prevalence of vibration-induced white finger in fluorspar mines in Weardale. Br J Ind Med 35:208, 1978.
15. Chucker R, Fowler RC, Molomiza T, et al: Induced temperature

gradients in Raynaud's disease measured by thermography. Angiology 22:580, 1971.
16. Clifford PC, Martin MFR, Dieppe PA, et al: Prostaglandin E_1 infusion for small vessel arterial ischemia. J Cardiovasc Surg 24:503, 1983.
17. Clifford PC, Martin MFR, Sheddon EJ, et al: Treatment of vasospastic disease with prostaglandin E_1. Br Med J 2:1031, 1980.
18. Coffman JD: Effect of vasodilator drugs in vasoconstricted normal subjects. J Clin Pharmacol 8:302, 1968.
19. Coffman JD: Total and nutritional blood flow in the finger. Clin Sci 42:243, 1979.
20. Coffman JD: Vasodilator drugs in peripheral vascular disease. N Engl J Med 300:713, 1979.
21. Coffman JD, Cohen AS: Total and capillary fingertip blood flow in Raynaud's phenomenon. N Engl J Med 285:259, 1971.
22. Cupps TR, Fauci AS: The Vasculitides. Philadelphia, WB Saunders, 1981, pp 116–118.
23. Dale WA: Occlusive arterial lesions of the wrist and hand. J Tenn Med Assoc 57:402, 1964.
24. deTakats G, Fowler EF: Raynaud's phenomenon. JAMA 179:99, 1962.
25. Dodds AJ, O'Reilly MJG, Yates CJP, et al: Hemorrheological response to plasma exchange in Raynaud's syndrome. Br Med J 2:1186, 1979.
26. Downs AR, Gaskell P, Morrow I, et al: Assessment of arterial obstruction in vessels supplying the fingers by measurement of local blood pressures and the skin temperature response test—Correlation with angiographic evidence. Surgery 77:530, 1975.
27. Eastcott HHG: Raynaud's disease and the oral contraceptive pill. Br Med J 2:447, 1976.
28. Edwards JM, Phinney ES, Taylor LM Jr, et al: Alpha-2 adrenergic receptor levels in obstructive and spastic Raynaud's syndrome. J Vasc Surg 5:38, 1987.
29. Fitzgerald O, Hess EV, O'Connor GT, Spencer-Green G: Prospective study of the evolution of Raynaud's phenomenon. Am J Med 84:718, 1988.
30. Flatt AE: Digital artery sympathectomy. J Hand Surg 5:550, 1980.
31. Frolich ED, Tarayi RC, Dutson MP: Peripheral arterial insufficiency as a complication of beta-adrenergic blocking therapy. JAMA 208:2471, 1969.
32. Fyhrquist F, Saijonmaa O, Metsarinne K, et al: Raised plasma endothelin-1 concentration following cold pressor test. Biochem Biophys Res Commun 169:217, 1990.
33. Gates KN, Tyburczy JA, Zupan T, et al: The non-invasive quantification of digital vasospasm. Bruit 8:34, 1984.
34. Gentric A, Blaschek MA, Le Noach JF, et al: Serological arguments for classifying Raynaud's phenomenon as idiopathic. J Rheumatol 17:1177, 1990.
35. Gerbracht DD, Steen VD, Ziegler GL, et al: Evolution of primary Raynaud's phenomenon (Raynaud's disease) to connective tissue disease. Arthritis Rheum 28:87, 1985.
36. Gifford RW Jr: Reserpine and Raynaud's phenomenon [editorial]. N Engl J Med 285:290, 1971.
37. Gifford RW Jr, Hines EA Jr: Raynaud's disease among women and girls. Circulation 16:1012, 1957.
38. Gifford RW Jr, Hines EA Jr, Craig WM: Sympathectomy for Raynaud's phenomenon: Follow-up study of 70 women with Raynaud's disease and 54 women with secondary Raynaud's phenomenon. Circulation 17:5, 1958.
39. Gjorup T, Kelbaek H, Hartling OJ, et al: Controlled double blind trial of the clinical effect of nifedipine in the treatment of idiopathic Raynaud's phenomenon. Am Heart J 111:742, 1986.
40. Gorevic PD: Mixed cryoglobulinemia: Clinical aspects and long-term follow-up of 40 patients. Am J Med 69:287, 1980.
41. Goyle KG, Dormandy JA: Abnormal blood viscosity in Raynaud's phenomenon. Lancet 1:1317, 1976.
42. Graham MR: Methylsergide for prevention of headache: Experience in five hundred patients over three years. N Engl J Med 270:67, 1964.
43. Hall KV, Hillestad LK: Raynaud's phenomenon treated with sympathectomy: A follow-up study of 28 patients. Angiology 11:186, 1960.
44. Halperin JL, Coffman JD: Pathophysiology of Raynaud's disease. Arch Intern Med 139:89, 1979.
45. Halpern A, Kuhn PH, Shaftel HE, et al: Raynaud's phenomenon and serotonin. Angiology 11:151, 1960.
46. Harper FE, Maricq HR, Turner RE, et al: A prospective study of Raynaud phenomenon and early connective tissue disease: A five-year report. Am J Med 72:883, 1982.
47. Hawley PR, Johnston AW, Rankin JT: Association between digital ischemia and malignant disease. Br Med J 3:208, 1967.
48. Henry LG, Blockwood JS, Cowley JE, et al: Ergotism. Arch Surg 110:929, 1975.
49. Heslop J, Coggon D, Acheson ED: The prevalence of intermittent digital ischaemia (Raynaud's phenomenon) in a general practice. J R Coll Gen Pract [Occas Pap] 33:85, 1983.
50. Hild DH, Myers TJ: Hyperviscosity in chronic granulocytic leukemia. Cancer 46:1418, 1980.
51. Hill GL, Moelino J, Tumewee F, et al: The Buerger syndrome in Java: A description of the clinical syndrome and some aspects of the aetiology. Br J Surg 60:606, 1973.
52. Hirai M: Cold sensitivity of the hand in arterial occlusive disease. Surgery 85:140, 1979.
53. Hirai M, Shinoya S: Arterial obstruction of the upper limb in Buerger's disease: Its incidence and primary lesion. Br J Surg 60:124, 1979.
54. Holling HE: Digital ischemia. *In* Peripheral Vascular Disease: Diagnosis and Management. Philadelphia, JB Lippincott, 1972, p 137.
55. Holmgren K, Baur GM, Porter JM: The role of digital photoplethysmography in the evaluation of Raynaud's syndrome. Bruit 5:19, 1981.
56. Hutchinson J: Raynaud's phenomena. Med Press Circ 123:403, 1901.
57. James EC, Khun NT, Fedde CW: Upper limb ischemia resulting from arterial thromboembolism. Am J Surg 137:739, 1979.
58. James PB, Galloway RW: Arteriography of the hand in men exposed to vibration. *In* Taylor W, Pelmear PL (eds): Vibration White Finger in Industry. London, Academic Press, 1975, p 31.
59. Jamieson GG, Ludbrook J, Wilson A: Cold hypersensitivity in Raynaud's phenomenon. Circulation 44:254, 1971.
60. Jarrett PEM, Morland M, Browse NL: Treatment of Raynaud's phenomenon by fibrinolytic enhancement. Br Med J 2:523, 1978.
61. Johnston ENM, Summerly R, Birnstingly M: Prognosis in Raynaud's phenomenon after sympathectomy. Br Med J 1:962, 1965.
62. Kahan A, Weber S, Amor B, et al: Nifedipine and Raynaud's phenomenon [Letter]. Ann Intern Med 94:546, 1981.
63. Kallenberg CG, Wouda AA, Hoet MH, van Venrooij WJ: Development of connective tissue disease in patients presenting with Raynaud's phenomenon: A six-year follow-up with emphasis on the predictive value of antinuclear antibodies as detected by immunoblotting. Ann Rheum Dis 47:634, 1988.
64. Keenan EJ, Porter JM: Alpha-2 adrenergic receptors in platelets from patients with Raynaud's syndrome. Surgery 94:204, 1983.
65. Kirtley JA, Riddell DH, Stoney WS, et al: Cervicothoracic sympathectomy in neurovascular abnormalities of the upper extremities: Experience in 76 patients with 104 sympathectomies. Ann Surg 165:869, 1967.
66. Kontos HA, Wasserman AJ: Effect of reserpine in Raynaud's phenomenon. Circulation 39:259, 1969.
67. Krahenbuhl B, Nielsen SL, Lassen NA: Closure of digital arteries in high vascular tone states as demonstrated by measurement of systolic blood pressure in the finger. Scand J Clin Lab Invest 37:71, 1977.
68. Lafferty K, deTrafford JC, Roberts VC, et al: Raynaud's phenomenon and thermal entrainment: An objective test. Br Med J 286:290, 1983.
69. Leppert J, Aberg H, Ringqvist I, Sorensson S: Raynaud's phenomenon in a female population: Prevalence and association with other conditions. Angiology 38:871, 1987.
70. Lewis T: Experiments relating to the peripheral mechanism involved in spastic arrest of the circulation in the fingers, a variety of Raynaud's disease. Heart 15:7, 1929.
71. Lewis T, Pickering GW: Observations upon maladies in which the blood supply to digits ceases intermittently or permanently and upon bilateral gangrene of digits; Observations relevant to so-called Raynaud's disease. Clin Sci 1:327, 1933.
72. Machleder HI, Wheeler E, Barber WF: Treatment of upper extremity ischemia by cervico-dorsal sympathectomy. Vasc Surg 13:399, 1979.
73. Mackiewisz A, Piskorz A: Raynaud's phenomenon following long-

term repeated action of great differences of temperature. J Cardiovasc Surg 18:151, 1977.
74. Maricq HR, Weinrich MC, Keil JE, LeRoy EC: Prevalence of Raynaud phenomenon in the general population. J Chron Dis 39:423, 1986.
75. Marshall AJ, Roberts CJC, Barritt DW: Raynaud's phenomenon as a side effect of beta-blockers in hypertension. Br Med J 1:1498, 1976.
76. Martinez A, Golding M, Sawyer P: The specific arterial lesion in mild and severe frostbite: Effect of sympathectomy. J Cardiovasc Surg 35:495, 1965.
77. McFadyen IJ, Housley E, MacPherson AIS: Intra-arterial reserpine administration in Raynaud's syndrome. Arch Intern Med 132:526, 1973.
78. Merhoff CG, Porter JM: Ergot intoxication: Historical review and description of unusual clinical manifestations. Ann Surg 180:773, 1974.
79. Miller D, Waters DD, Warnica W, et al: Is variant angina the coronary manifestation of a generalized vasospastic disorder? N Engl J Med 304:763, 1981.
80. Mills JL, Friedman EI, Taylor LM Jr, et al: Upper extremity ischemia caused by small artery disease. Ann Surg 154:123, 1987.
81. Mills JL, Taylor LM Jr, Porter JM: Buerger's disease in the modern era. Am J Surg 154:123, 1987.
82. Mohrland JS, Porter JM, Smith EA, et al: A multiclinic, placebo-controlled, double-blind study of prostaglandin E_1 in Raynaud's syndrome. Ann Rheum Dis 44:754, 1985.
83. Miller-Schweinitzer E: Responsiveness of isolated canine cerebral and peripheral arteries to ergotamine. Arch Pharmacol 292:113, 1976.
84. Murdoch D, Brogden RN: Sustained release nifedipine formulations. Drugs 41:737, 1991.
85. Nerem RM: Vibration-induced arterial shear stress: The relationship to Raynaud's phenomenon of occupational origin. Arch Environ Health 26:105, 1973.
86. Nielsen SL, Lassen NA: Measurement of digital blood pressure after local cooling. J Appl Physiol 43:907, 1977.
87. Nobin BA, Nielsen SL, Eklov D, et al: Reserpine treatment of Raynaud's disease. Ann Surg 187:12, 1978.
88. O'Donnell JR, Keaveny TV, O'Connell LG: Digital arteritis as a presenting feature of malignant disease. Ir J Med Sci 149:326, 1980.
89. Okada A, Yamashita T, Nagano C, et al: Studies on the diagnosis and pathogenesis of Raynaud's phenomenon of occupational origin. Br J Ind Med 28:353, 1971.
90. Olsen N, Nielsen SL: Prevalence of primary Raynaud phenomena in young females. Scand J Clin Lab Invest 37:761, 1978.
91. O'Reilly MJG, Talops G, Robert VC, et al: Controlled trial of plasma exchange in treatment of Raynaud's syndrome. Br Med J 1:1113, 1979.
92. Pardy BJ, Lewis JD, Eastcott HHG: Preliminary experience with prostaglandins E_1 and I_2 in peripheral vascular disease. Surgery 88:826, 1980.
93. Peacock JH: The treatment of primary Raynaud's disease of the upper limb. Lancet 2:65, 1960.
94. Porter JM: Upper extremity digital gangrene caused by small artery occlusion. *In* Machleder HI (ed): Vascular Disorders of the Upper Extremity. Mt. Kisco, NY, Futura Publishing, 1983, p 107.
95. Porter JM: Raynaud's syndrome. *In* Sabiston DC Jr (ed): Textbook of Surgery. Philadelphia, WB Saunders, 1986, p 1925.
96. Porter JM, Bardana EJ Jr, Baur GM, et al: The clinical significance of Raynaud's syndrome. Surgery 80:756, 1976.
97. Porter JM, Friedman EI, Mills JL Jr: Raynaud's syndrome: Current concepts and treatment. Medical Tribune Therapaeia, 29:23, 1988.
98. Porter JM, Rivers SP, Anderson CJ, et al: Evaluation and management of patients with Raynaud's syndrome. Am J Surg 142:183, 1981.
99. Porter JM, Snider RL, Bardana EJ, et al: The diagnosis and treatment of Raynaud's phenomenon. Surgery 77:11, 1975.
100. Porter JM, Taylor LM Jr: Limb ischemia caused by small artery disease. World J Surg 7:326, 1983.
101. Porter JM, Taylor LM Jr, Friedman EI: Indications for cervical and first rib excisions. *In* Greenhalgh RM (ed): Indications in Vascular Surgery. Orlando, FL, Grune & Stratton, 1987, pp 101–118.
102. Porter JM, Wesche D, Rosch J, et al: Intra-arterial sympathetic blockade in the treatment of clinical frostbite. Am J Surg 132:625, 1976.
103. Powell KR: Raynaud's phenomenon preceding acute lymphocytic leukemia. J Pediatr 82:539, 1973.
104. Prandoni AG, Moser M: Clinical appraisal of intra-arterial Priscoline therapy in the management of peripheral arterial diseases. Circulation 9:73, 1954.
105. Priollet P, Vayssairat M, Housset E: How to classify Raynaud's phenomenon: Long-term follow-up study of 73 cases. Am J Med 83:494, 1987.
106. Raynaud M: On local asphyxia and symmetrical gangrene of the extremities. *In* Selected Monographs. London, New Sydenham Society, 1888.
107. Rivers SP, Porter JM: Clinical approach to Raynaud's syndrome. Vasc Diagn Ther 4:15, 1983.
108. Rivers SP, Porter JM: Management of Raynaud's syndrome. *In* Bergan JJ (ed): Clinical Surgery International. New York, Churchill Livingstone, 1984, p 185.
109. Rivers SP, Porter JM: Raynaud's syndrome and upper extremity small artery occlusive disease. *In* Wilson SE, Veith FJ, Hobson RW, et al (eds): Vascular Surgery: Principles and Practice. New York, McGraw-Hill, 1987, p 696.
110. Rodeheffer RJ, Rommer JA, Wigley F, et al: Controlled double-blind trial of nifedipine in the treatment of Raynaud's phenomenon. N Engl J Med 308:880, 1983.
111. Rosch J, Porter JM, Gralino BJ: Cryodynamic hand angiography in the diagnosis and management of Raynaud's syndrome. Circulation 55:807, 1977.
112. Rudolph RI: Vasculitis associated with hairy-cell leukemia. Arch Dermatol 116:1077, 1980.
113. Schmidt FE, Hewitt RL: Severe upper limb ischemia. Arch Surg 115:1188, 1980.
114. Schmid-Schonbein H: Critical closing pressure or yield shear stress as the cause of disturbed peripheral circulation? Acta Chir Scand 465(Suppl):10, 1976.
115. Shawket S, Dickerson C, Hazelman B, Brown MJ: Prolonged effect of CGRP in Raynaud's patients: A double-blind randomised comparison with prostacyclin. Br J Clin Pharmacol 32:209, 1991.
116. Sheiner NM, Small P: Isolated Raynaud's phenomenon—A benign disorder. Ann Allergy 58:114, 1987.
117. Silcott GR, Polich VL: Palmar arch arterial reconstruction for the salvage of ischemic fingers. Am J Surg 142:219, 1981.
118. Silman A, Holligan S, Brennan P, Maddison P: Prevalence of symptoms of Raynaud's phenomenon in general practice. Br Med J 301:590, 1990.
119. Singh S, de Trafford JC, Baskerville PA, Roberts VC: Digital artery calibre measurement—A new technique of assessing Raynaud's phenomenon. Eur J Vasc Surg 5:199, 1991.
120. Smith CD, McKendry RJR: Controlled trial of nifedipine in the treatment of Raynaud's phenomenon. Lancet 2:1299, 1982.
121. Strandness DE Jr: Episodic digital ischemia. *In* Peripheral Arterial Disease: A Physiologic Approach. Boston, Little, Brown, 1969, p 265.
122. Sumner DS, Strandness DE Jr: An abnormal finger pulse associated with cold sensitivity. Ann Surg 175:294, 1972.
123. Szczeklik A, Cryglewski RJ, Nizankowski R, et al: Prostacyclin therapy in peripheral arterial disease. Thromb Res 19:191, 1980.
124. Talpos G, White JM, Horrocks M, et al: Plasmapheresis in Raynaud's disease. Lancet 1:416, 1978.
125. Taylor LM Jr, Baur GM, Porter JM: Finger gangrene caused by small artery occlusive disease. Ann Surg 193:453, 1981.
126. Taylor LM Jr, Hauty MG, Edwards JM, et al: Digital ischemia as a manifestation of malignancy. Ann Surg 206:62, 1987.
127. Taylor LM Jr, Rivers SP, Keller F, et al: Treatment of digital ischemia with intravenous Bier block reserpine. Surg Gynecol Obstet 154:39, 1982.
128. Taylor W, Pelmear PL: Vibration White Finger in Industry. London, Academic Press, 1975.
129. Taylor W, Pelmear PL: Raynaud's phenomenon of occupational origin: An epidemiologic survey. Acta Chir Scand 465(Suppl):27, 1976.
130. Teutsch C, Lipton A, Harvey A: Raynaud's phenomenon as a side effect of chemotherapy with vinblastine and bleomycin for testicular carcinoma. Cancer Treat Rep 61:925, 1977.
131. Tietjen GW, Chien S, Leroy C, et al: Blood viscosity, plasma proteins, and Raynaud's syndrome. Arch Surg 110:1343, 1975.
132. Tindall JP, Whalen RE, Burton EE Jr: Medical uses of intra-arterial injections of reserpine: Treatment of Raynaud's syndrome and of

some vascular insufficiencies of the lower extremities. Arch Dermatol 110:233, 1974.
133. Varadi DP, Lawrence AM: Suppression of Raynaud's phenomenon by methyldopa. Arch Intern Med 124:13, 1969.
134. Velayos EE, Robinson H, Porciuncula FU, et al: Clinical correlation analysis of 137 patients with Raynaud's phenomenon. Am J Med Sci 262:347, 1971.
135. Waldo R: Prazosin relieves Raynaud's vasospasm. JAMA 241:1037, 1979.
136. Weiner ES, Hildebrandt S, Senecal JL, et al: Prognostic significance of anticentromere antibodies and anti-topoisomerase I antibodies in Raynaud's disease. A prospective study. Arthritis Rheum 34:68, 1991.
137. Wesseling H, denHeeten A, Wouda AA: Sublingual and oral isoxsuprine in patients with Raynaud's phenomenon. Eur J Clin Pharmacol 20:329, 1981.
138. Willerson JT, Thompson RH, Hookman P, et al: Reserpine in Raynaud's disease and phenomenon: Short-term responses to intra-arterial injection. Ann Intern Med 72:17, 1970.
139. Wollersheim H, Thien T, Hoet MH, Van Venrooy WJ: The diagnostic value of several immunological tests for anti-nuclear antibody in predicting the development of connective tissue disease in patients presenting with Raynaud's phenomenon. Eur J Clin Invest 19:535, 1989.
140. Yao JST, Gourmos C, Papathanasiou K, et al: A method for assessing ischemia of hands and fingers. Surg Gynecol Obstet 135:373, 1972.
141. Zamora MR, O'Brien RF, Rutherford RB, Weil JV: Serum endothelin-1 concentrations and cold provocation in primary Raynaud's phenomenon. Lancet 336:1144, 1990.
142. Zweifler AJ, Trinkaus P: Occlusive digital artery disease in patients with Raynaud's phenomenon. Am J Med 77:995, 1984.

69

Neurogenic Thoracic Outlet Syndrome

Ronald J. Stoney, M.D., and Stephen W. K. Cheng, M.S., F.R.C.S.

• • •

The term thoracic outlet syndrome (TOS) refers to a group of neurologic and vascular symptoms of the upper extremity caused by compression of the brachial plexus and the subclavian vessels by bony or soft tissue anomalies as they traverse the thoracic outlet region at the base of the neck. There are three major types. The *neurogenic* type of TOS consists mainly of pain, paresthesia, and often weakness of the upper limb, usually aggravated by the overhead posture. Autonomic disturbances are less common. These symptoms are caused by irritation of the brachial plexus along its course from the intervertebral foramina to the costoclavicular space. This is the predominant type, accounting for 90 to 95 per cent of all patients with TOS. Those affected are usually young adults in the 3rd to 5th decades of life, with a female:male ratio of 4:1. The *arterial* type of TOS is rare: it occurs in fewer than 5 per cent of cases. It is secondary to compression of the subclavian artery at the thoracic outlet, usually by bony abnormalities such as cervical ribs, rudimentary or anomalous first ribs, or old clavicle fractures. The affected artery may exhibit post-stenotic dilatation or frank aneurysm formation, and patients usually present with thromboembolic complications. The *venous* type of TOS, which is also uncommon, results from thrombosis of the axillary or subclavian vein, often associated with activity of the arm. This chapter deals with neurogenic TOS.

HISTORY

The clinical symptoms that constitute neurogenic TOS have been recognized for more than a century, but continuous controversy has surrounded its etiology and treatment. Some investigators have questioned its existence as a separate entity, partly because of the lack of specific objective diagnostic criteria and partly because the results of treatment are not always favorable.

Mechanical compression of the brachial plexus is considered to be the principal cause of neurologic complaints in symptomatic patients. Although there is no consensus about a treatment plan, conservative measures, which include exercise, physical therapy, and the administration of analgesics and muscle relaxants, are usually initiated first. Surgical decompression is generally reserved for patients in whom conservative treatment fails or for those whose conditions become disabling. The conflicting views of the pathophysiology proposed by different surgeons are reflected by the wide diversity of operative approaches currently used, including scalenotomy and scalenectomy, with or without excision of a cervical rib, the first rib, or both. The choice of operation depends on which anatomic structures are regarded by the surgeon to be the cause of compressive plexus symptoms. Four operative approaches are generally available: supraclavicular, transaxillary, infraclavicular, and parascapular. These approaches offer a variety of exposures of the brachial plexus and thoracic outlet structures and include comprehensive and limited access to this region.

Cooper first described the symptoms of vascular compression from a cervical rib in 1821.[1] In 1861, Coote was the first to excise a cervical rib for the treatment of TOS.[2] This was followed by the removal of a normal first rib by Murphy in 1910 to relieve neurologic symptoms that he termed brachial neuritis.[3] Later, Ochsner and colleagues[4] and Naffziger and Grant[5] reported on the role of the anterior scalene muscle in brachial plexus compression (the scalenus anticus [Naffziger] syndrome) and developed the technique of anterior scalenotomy. Various theories were subsequently introduced to explain the condition, including the theory of costoclavicular compression and the hyperabduction concept, which stressed the role of the pectoralis minor tendon. Peet and associates, in 1956, first used the term *thoracic outlet syndrome* to encompass the whole symptom complex.[6]

Concern with surgical procedures that were limited to the scalene muscle, particularly scalenotomy, led to anterior scalene resection. Persistent or recurrent symptoms appearing after scalenotomy suggested that a more extensive structural operation was necessary. The observation that cervical rib resection alleviated symptoms of brachial plexus irritation focused attention on the bony skeleton (first rib) as a key structure in the thoracic outlet. It was thought that first rib resection would remove the floor of this region, disconnect the anterior scalene muscle, and resect a portion of the middle scalene insertion, thus allowing the plexus to descend without restriction.

In the early 1960s, Clagett proposed first rib resection using the posterior thoracotomy approach for thoracic outlet decompression.[7] This was followed by the transaxillary approach to first rib resection described by Roos,[8] which has become the most popular operation for TOS since the early 1970s. Even second rib excision was performed by pioneers in this field. However, a significant proportion of these patients have symptomatic recurrences due to fibrotic encasement of the plexus trunks and reattachment of the anterior scalene muscle to the first rib bed. In these patients, supraclavicular reoperation and scalenectomy provided good results. Combined transaxillary first rib resection and supraclavicular radical scalenectomy was therefore introduced, followed later by supraclavicular scalenectomy and first rib resection alone. The rationale of routine first rib removal has since been questioned, and the tendency now is toward precise identification of the pathology followed by adequate decompression of the brachial plexus, often without resorting to any bony resection at all.

ETIOLOGY

Mechanical (Structural) Predisposition

The nerves and vessels in the region of the thoracic outlet traverse several narrow anatomic passages surrounded by osseous and soft tissue structures (Fig. 69–1). The *superior thoracic outlet* is bounded by the manubrium anteriorly, the spine posteriorly, and the first rib laterally. Within this rigid skeletal confine course the subclavian artery and vein and the five roots of the brachial plexus that emerge from the intervertebral foramina. The *interscalene space* is bounded by the anterior scalene muscle anteriorly, the middle scalene muscle posteriorly, and the first rib inferiorly. The subclavian artery and the three trunks of the brachial plexus traverse this intermuscular space. The *costoclavicular space* is formed by the clavicle and the subclavius muscle anteriorly, the anterolateral border of the first rib medially, and the scapula posteriorly. The subclavian vein also traverses this space.

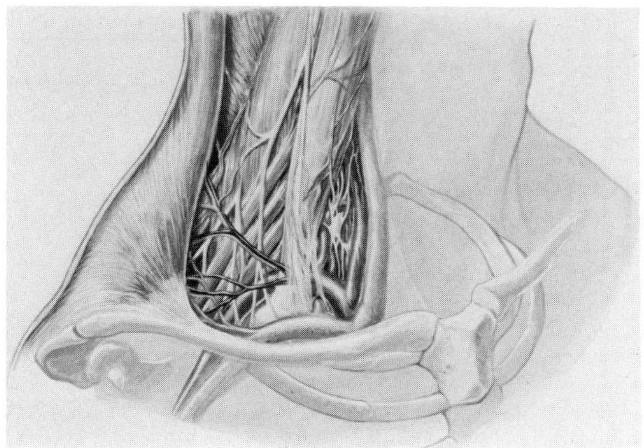

FIGURE 69–1. Anatomy of the thoracic outlet showing the relationship of the brachial plexus to the anterior and middle scalene muscles and the subclavian artery.

Anatomic anomalies or acquired pathology of the skeletal and soft tissue structures forming or bordering the three passages may cause mechanical compression or direct irritation of the brachial plexus and produce symptoms of neurogenic TOS (Table 69–1). These predisposing structures are discussed in the following sections.

Osseous Anomalies

The *cervical rib* was first reported by Cooper[1] and by Adson and Coffey.[9] The incidence of this anomaly in the normal population varies from 0.17 per cent to 0.74 per cent.[10, 11] Gruber classified cervical ribs into four types, from fibrous bands to a complete bony structure between the C7 vertebra and the first rib.[12] Jones postulated that in fetal life, the spinal nerves going to the limb buds block the growth of the cervical ribs, and an underdeveloped T1 nerve root results in development of a cervical rib.[13] When a cervical rib is present, the brachial plexus is displaced cranially, impinging on the apex of the scalene triangle. This is probably due to an anomalous middle scalene muscle that is displaced medially and superiorly and may have abnormal muscular insertions on the first rib, further compressing the nerves. Similarly, a *long transverse process of the C7 vertebra* can cause direct compression of the plexus or can indirectly compress it by serving as a base for the attachment of fibromuscular bands or an anomalous middle scalene muscle.

The *first rib* is located strategically: it is the only bony structure to border the three anatomic spaces through which the neurovascular bundle passes. It also serves as the osseous framework to which muscles and ligaments attach. Abnormal development or orientation of the first rib may lead to undue pressure on the lower trunks of the brachial plexus. Acquired pathology such as exostosis, tumors, abnormal callus formation, and fractures of the first rib or the clavicle can irritate the brachial plexus.

Table 69–1. Etiology of Thoracic Outlet Nerve Compression

Congenital	Acquired
Osseous	
Cervical rib	Fractured clavicle, callus, and pseudarthrosis
Long C7 transverse process	Fractured first rib
Abnormal or anomalous first rib	Exostosis or tumors
Soft Tissue	
Anomalous anterior scalene insertion	Scalene muscle injuries
Anomalous middle scalene insertion	Previous operations and scars
Scalene muscle interdigitations	Reattachment of the anterior scalene tendon
Scalene muscle hypertrophy	
Scalenus minimus	
Abnormal ligaments and fibrous bands	Soft tissue tumors
Brachial plexus anomalies	Brachial plexus schwannomas
Prefixed or postfixed brachial plexus	Direct brachial plexus injury
Posturing	
Sagging shoulders	
Heavy breasts	

Soft Tissue Anomalies

The role of the *anterior scalene muscle* was first recognized in the 1930s.[4, 5] The muscle normally inserts into the scalene tubercle on the first rib, anterior to the subclavian artery. However, variations are frequent.[14] Posterior displacement of the anterior scalene insertion narrows the interscalene space.[15] Likewise, anterior displacement of the *middle scalene* insertion[16] or an abnormally broad based insertion of the middle scalene will displace the brachial plexus anteriorly. Hypertrophy of one or both of the scalene muscles or anomalous interdigitations between the anterior and the middle scalene muscles are often encountered during operations for TOS. This muscle configuration can compress the nerve roots and trunks, especially if the latter are fixed or displaced by a cervical rib or ligament.

A *scalenus minimus* muscle is present in more than 50 per cent of the population.[17] It usually originates from the transverse process of the C7 vertebra, sometimes mixing with the anterior scalene muscle, and inserts on the first rib behind the scalene tubercle or on Sibson's fascia. In the majority of cases, the muscle crosses in front of the C8 and T1 nerve roots, and it may compress these roots against the inner border of the neck of the first rib (Fig. 69–2). Additional slips of the scalenus minimus may encase the subclavian artery. If atrophied, it represents a vertebrocostal ligament. Other muscular abnormalities, such as the pectoralis minor tendon,[18] were also thought to compress the trunks of the plexus, but this was never substantiated.

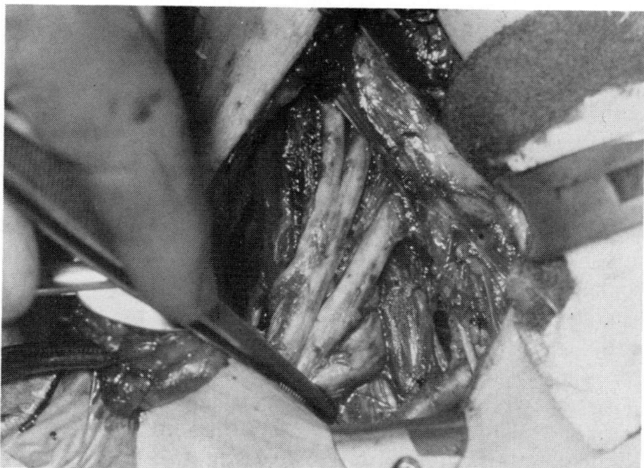

FIGURE 69–2. Operative photograph showing the right smallest scalene muscle crossing in front of the C8 and T1 nerve roots and compressing them against the middle scalene muscle and the first rib.

Congenital myofascial bands and ligaments are frequently identified during operative decompression of the thoracic outlet. Roos extensively classified a large number of these bands, which may or may not be associated with bony abnormalities.[19] These structures can arise from a cervical rib or the transverse process of the C7 vertebra, often course within the belly of the middle scalene muscle, and insert into the first rib or Sibson's fascia over the dome of the pleura. These fibromuscular structures can exert direct pressure on, or limit the mobility of, the lower cords of the brachial plexus.

The *brachial plexus* itself may be anomalous and predispose to compression. It can be *prefixed,* with a large contribution from the C4 root and displaced cranially, thus impinging on the apex formed by the scalene muscles, or *postfixed,* with contributions from the T2 root and displaced caudally, resulting in angulation by the first rib.

Acquired soft tissue pathology of the thoracic outlet includes post-traumatic fibrous scarring, postoperative reattachment of the anterior scalene tendon to the first rib bed, and inadequate first rib removal.

In some patients, TOS occurs in the absence of anatomic abnormalities or trauma. The relationship between the first rib and the clavicle is important to maintain the configuration of the costoclavicular passage. A narrow passage is believed to produce neurologic compression.[20] The normal costoclavicular angle is maintained by a balance of muscle tone. Newborns have a large costoclavicular space. Progressive bony growth leads to descent of the shoulders in infancy.[21] The trunks and cords of the brachial plexus are stretched over the first rib and may bring on neurologic symptoms in some patients.[22] The symptoms are often relieved by arm elevation. This is especially true in thin women with poor posturing and weak muscular support of the shoulder girdle. Drooping or sagging of the shoulders further increases acromioclavicular descent and induces additional compression of the nerves in the costoclavicular space. Pressure from tight brassiere straps in women with heavy breasts has also been postulated as a reason for depression of the clavicle.[23] Conversely, poor development of the rectus abdominis muscle results in an elevated sternum and first rib, leading to a narrow costoclavicular angle. Shoulder descent and weak rectus abdominis musculature are common in women and can explain the prevalence of this disorder in the female gender. Physical therapy directed toward strengthening the trapezius and rectus abdominis may improve the anatomic passage, minimize brachial plexus descent, prevent ascent of the first rib, and alleviate TOS symptoms.

Table 69–2. Classification of Thoracic Outlet Nerve Compression by Pathophysiology

Traumatic
Osseous
Fractures and callus
Soft tissue
Direct
Brachial plexus
Scalene muscles
Indirect
Work-related injuries
Cervical strain
Nontraumatic
Osseous
Cervical ribs and other bony anomalies
Soft tissue
Congenital muscular anomalies
Myofascial bands
Posture and shoulder descent

Trauma

The role of trauma of the scalene muscles in neurogenic TOS was first reported by Ochsner and colleagues.[4] They described three patients with symptoms after neck injury and theorized that fibrosis and spasm of the scalene muscles led to elevation of the first rib and impingement of the brachial plexus. Subsequent studies confirmed this relationship,[5] and scalenotomy was accepted as standard treatment at that time.

The association between a history of soft tissue injury of the neck and TOS has been increasingly recognized and has been found in up to 86 per cent of patients in some series.[24] Two groups of patients are evident. *Direct* trauma, either to the brachial plexus itself or to the muscles, is usually the result of whiplash flexion-extension injury to the neck after a rearend automobile accident. These patients often have a more abrupt onset of severe sensory symptoms but little, if any, motor disturbance. A second group, who suffer *indirect or work-related* repetitive microstress trauma, consists of patients whose jobs demand repeated elevation of the upper limb or heavy lifting, which places abnormal stress on the brachial plexus. Their symptoms are often worse with abduction of the arm. These patients' conditions tend to have a slow, progressive course over years, with a gradual evolution of disabling symptoms that are often aggravated by a minor event such as a cervical strain (Table 69–2).

The exact mechanism of how trauma precipitates TOS is still debated. Direct damage of the nerves of the brachial plexus or osseous fractures can explain some symptoms. In the majority of patients, these factors are absent and the role of the scalene muscles in symptom production becomes a focus of concern. Microscopic reports from other authors[25, 26] and the chapter authors' own studies have demonstrated histologic changes in the scalene muscles, the exact significance of which is still unknown. It is possible that the scalene muscles respond to trauma by inflammation and fibrosis, resulting in a chronically contracted, scarred muscular mass that will irritate the brachial nerves. An alternative, neurochemical theory suggests that an initial injury, whether gross or from repeated microtrauma, produces a local perineural inflammation in the soft tissues. In certain individuals, this can sensitize the local neural net to produce trophic and inflammatory factors (e.g., substance P), which in turn evoke an organizing extracellular response and scar formation. This perineural fibrosis and the consequent local vasoconstriction of the vasa nervorum produce local ischemia of the nerves. These same factors can stimulate tonic muscle growth and local hypertrophy. Ischemia, whether neurogenic in origin or from mechanical irritation, perpetuates the abnormal sensitivity of the perineural network and creates pathologic positive feedback, which eventually results in the neurologic symptoms of TOS.

In the past, experience of TOS decompression was gained from cervical rib operations. In the absence of a cervical rib, it was commonly believed that the first rib, because of its strategic position, played an active role in thoracic outlet nerve compression. This led to a large number of routine first rib resections in the 1960s and 1970s, particularly via the transaxillary route, whereas soft tissue abnormalities in the neck were not well identified. In fact, actual osseous anomalies account for only a small proportion of neurogenic TOS cases. The increasing identification of soft tissue pathology has led to the hypothesis that the syndrome of thoracic outlet nerve compression is probably a combination of a congenital *anatomic predisposition* to brachial plexus pressure and an inciting stimulus that evokes an inflammatory response to injury. The authors believe that the first rib probably has only a passive role in TOS: it provides a matrix to which myofascial elements adhere, and it is these elements that primarily cause nerve compression. This concept is further supported by the frequent observation of soft tissue anomalies and a normal first rib on supraclavicular explorations, consistent histopathologic abnormalities of the scalene muscles, and the authors' good results with thoracic outlet decompression with sparing of the first rib.

HISTOPATHOLOGY

There have been few histologic studies of actual scalene muscle pathology. Machleder and coworkers subjected frozen specimens of the anterior scalene muscle from pa-

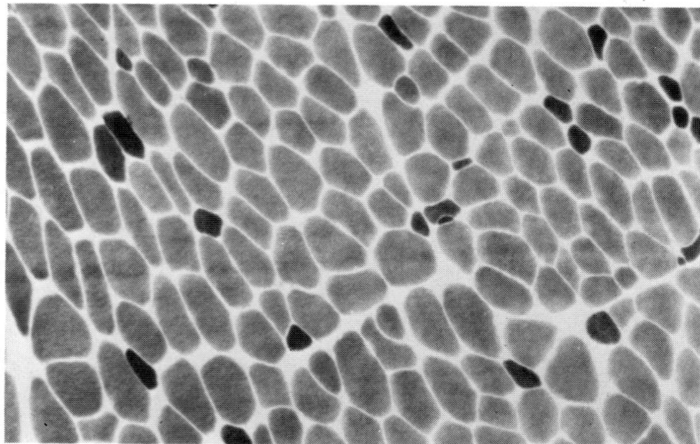

FIGURE 69–3. Photomicrograph of a section of the anterior scalene muscle in a patient with neurogenic thoracic outlet syndrome, stained for myofibrillar myosin adenosine triphosphatase at a pH of 9.4. Note the predominance of type I fibers (light stained) and the atrophy of type II fibers (dark stained).

tients with TOS to fiber typing.[25] Normal human skeletal muscles contain two main types of fibers with respect to fiber reactivity to histochemical staining. A slow-twitch (type I) fiber has a higher oxidative enzyme capacity and a lower glycolytic activity and is adapted to slow, tonic contractions. These fibers show increased reactivity to nicotinamide adenine dinucleotide hydrogenase–tetrazolium reductase (NADH-TR), a mitochondrial oxidative enzyme, and lower reactivity to myosin ATPase. A fast-twitch, quick-reacting (type II) fiber has low oxidative capacity with NADH-TR but increased reactivity with myosin ATPase. Normal skeletal muscles contain almost equal percentages of type I and type II fibers of about the same cross-sectional size, with individual variations determined by the pattern of contraction. Machleder and coworkers reported marked type I fiber predominance (85 per cent) and muscle hypertrophy in seven patients with TOS and muscle atrophy in four patients who had had prior tenotomy.

A more recent report by Sanders and associates, who used a computerized image analysis system for muscle fiber typing, confirmed a consistently abnormal pattern in the anterior and middle scalene muscles of patients with the traumatic type of TOS: an increase in the number of type I fibers and atrophy of type II fibers and a significant increase in connective tissue.[26] The chapter authors were able to demonstrate a similar predominance and hypertrophy of type I fibers, atrophy of type II fibers, and endomysial fibrosis in their series of more than 80 symptomatic TOS patients (Fig. 69–3). However, these pathologic studies have been hampered by the fact that it is difficult to obtain a good control group and many ''normal'' scalene muscles have similar findings.

These microscopic changes suggest that there is an abnormality in the anterior and middle scalene muscles that could play a role in brachial plexus compression. They also support the view that radical anterior and middle scalenectomy are necessary for complete decompression of the thoracic outlet. It may be assumed that repeated microtrauma or chronic stimulation of the muscle causes an adaptive transformation to slow-contracting fibers with increased tone and fibrosis. Prolonged tonic contraction of the muscles will reduce the interscalene space and displace or irritate the brachial plexus roots and trunks.

CLINICAL FEATURES

History and Symptoms

Patients with neurogenic TOS are usually women in their 3rd to 5th decades of life. They may have a previous history of cervicothoracic trauma due to either an accident or a work-related event. The onset is usually abrupt and related to a specific incident, although it may occasionally be insidious. Certain activities that involve stretching of the plexus or hyperabduction, such as typing, painting, and lifting heavy objects, predictably aggravate the condition.

Pain is the main symptom of neurogenic TOS. Depending on which nerve root is irritated, pain can be located along the side of the neck or in the lateral shoulder, the anterior chest, or the parascapular region, or it can radiate down the arm to the hand and fingers. Associated paresthesia and numbness in the distal extremity are also frequent. If the upper brachial nerve roots are principally affected, the pain is localized to the lateral aspect of the arm and shoulder areas. Ipsilateral headache, facial pain, or pain in the temporomandibular region may be present. The symptoms are often aggravated by elevation of the arm. Lower root involvement often produces pain in the inner aspect of the arm and forearm following an ulnar distribution. Frequently, however, all nerve roots are affected and it is difficult to differentiate the symptoms accurately into upper and lower plexus groups. Other, less constant complaints include a sense of clumsiness in the hands and fingers and episodic temperature changes or Raynaud's phenomenon in the digits.

Several musculoskeletal disorders in the cervical region mimic neurogenic TOS, and a list of differential diagnoses should always be kept in mind (Table 69–3). Nerve

Table 69–3. Differential Diagnosis of Thoracic Outlet Nerve Compression

- Nerve compression syndromes
  - Carpal tunnel syndrome
  - Ulnar nerve compression at the elbow
- Cervical spine pathology
  - Cervical spine injury
  - Cervical disc herniation
  - Spinal stenosis
- Neurologic diseases of the spine
  - Spinal cord tumor
  - Multiple sclerosis
- Shoulder disorders
  - Rotator cuff tendinitis or injury
  - Biceps tendinitis
  - Myositis of the shoulder muscles (trapezius, rhomboid, supra- or infraspinatus)
- Sympathetic disorders
  - Raynaud's disease
  - Reflex sympathetic dystrophy
- Other conditions
  - Angina
  - Migraine
  - Temporomandibular joint abnormalities

entrapment or compression syndromes, especially carpal tunnel syndrome or ulnar neuropathy at the elbow, shoulder pathology, and herniated cervical discs must be carefully excluded by physical examination and appropriate ancillary investigations before a diagnosis of thoracic outlet nerve compression is made. Sometimes, multiple levels of nerve compression exist. Upton and McComas introduced the term *double-crush syndrome* to describe the conditions of patients who have carpal tunnel syndrome or ulnar nerve entrapment and a second nerve compression at the cervical level.[27]

Physical Examination

A thorough physical examination should always be performed with the differential diagnosis in mind. The patient's posture and the presence of any deformities or scars in the cervicothoracic region are noted. The neck, shoulders, and upper limb should be examined in detail in order to recognize any bony prominence or spasm of the trapezius muscles. The hands are examined, with particular attention given to the color, temperature, muscle strength, and atrophy of the small muscles. Diagnostic tests for carpal tunnel syndrome or ulnar nerve entrapment (the Tinel and Phalen tests) must be carried out. The cervical spine and upper thoracic spine are examined for local tenderness and range of motion. The shoulder, elbow, and wrist joints are also examined for mobility and pathology. A most characteristic finding of TOS is the presence of supraclavicular tenderness. This can be elicited by palpating directly over the anterior scalene muscle or more posteriorly over the brachial plexus (Fig. 69–4). A positive response reproduces the symptoms of pain and paresthesia radiating from the neck down the arm. A complete neurologic examination of the sensory and motor functions of the upper limb is crucial to an accurate diagnosis. The examination concludes with a evaluation of the vascular system, with note taken of the presence or absence of bruits in the supraclavicular fossa and the character of the upper limb pulses. The blood pressures of both arms should be measured.

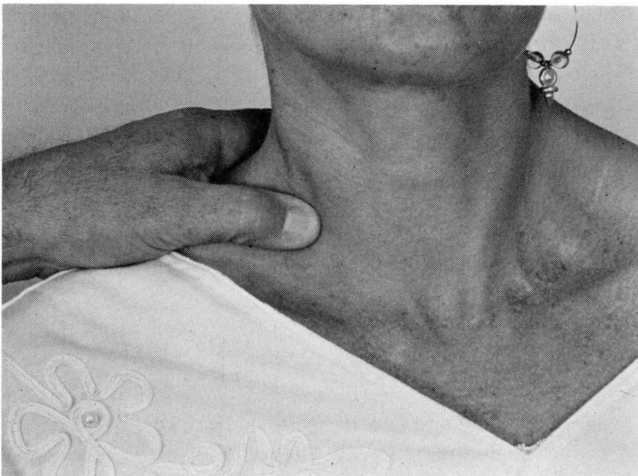

FIGURE 69–4. **Test for supraclavicular tenderness. The examiner palpates directly over the anterior scalene muscle with the thumb. A positive response would reproduce pain and paresthesia radiating from the neck down the arm.**

A number of postural maneuvers are often performed as part of the physical examination. Most of the tests are nonspecific and are not useful for diagnostic purposes. The *elevated arm stress test* maneuver introduced by Roos is, in the authors' experience, the most reliable. The patient is instructed to place both arms in 90 degrees of abduction and external rotation, with the shoulders braced posteriorly, and is then asked to open and close the hands slowly for 3 minutes. Test results are positive if the symptoms are reproduced. Most patients with neurogenic TOS are unable to complete this test.

The *Adson test*[9] is performed by asking the patient to elevate the chin and turn the head away from the affected side while taking a deep breath, with the arm abducted 90 degrees from the chest wall and the elbow flexed. A positive test response will produce paresthesia over the brachial plexus distribution and obliteration of the ipsilateral radial pulse. Once considered pathognomonic for TOS, this test has now been proved to be unreliable, producing negative results in many patients with TOS and often positive results in the asymptomatic normal population. A positive result indicates only pressure of the scalene muscle on the subclavian artery and is not related to associated brachial plexus compression unless neurogenic symptoms are reproduced. The *costoclavicular maneuver,* carried out by bracing the shoulders backward and downward in a "military" position, aims to demonstrate compression of the subclavian artery in the costoclavicular space.[20] Its value is also questionable.

The *upper limb or brachial plexus tension test,*[28, 29] first described by Elvey, is analogous to the straight leg raising test in the lower limb. It examines signs of adverse brachial plexus nerve tension in patients with upper limb pain by exerting an axial traction force on the peripheral nerve trunks and the cervical nerve roots. It involves the following steps: passive shoulder depression, shoulder abduction behind the coronal plane and external rotation of the arm, elbow extension and forearm supination, and wrist extension. The maneuvers are carried out in steps to the point of eliciting pain and paresthesia. This sequence of the procedure will exert progressively more stress on the nerve trunks (Fig. 69–5). Cadaver studies have confirmed actual strain and elongation of the C5 to T1 nerve roots during the procedure.[30] The effect of the test can be further augmented by adding lateral neck flexion away from the side being examined. Alternatively, the contralateral upper limb may be placed in a similar position to prestress the diseased side. This test has been shown to have a discriminative value in distinguishing between brachial plexus involvement and other causes of shoulder pain.

INVESTIGATIONS

The diagnosis of neurogenic TOS is usually made clinically based on the history and physical examination alone. A wide variety of diagnostic studies have been advocated by various investigators, but so far none have proved to be specific for thoracic outlet nerve compression. They serve only as ancillary tools for excluding other causes of upper

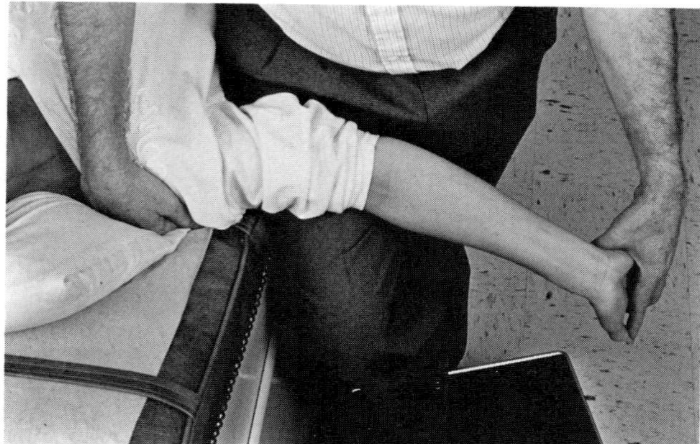

FIGURE 69–5. The upper limb (brachial plexus) tension test. The patient is positioned supine on the examination table, and the test is carried out in steps involving shoulder abduction behind the coronal plane with external rotation, elbow extension and forearm supination, and wrist extension. This test is analogous to the straight leg–raising test and places progressive increasing stress on the brachial plexus. Reproduction of symptoms implies nerve irritation at the cervical level.

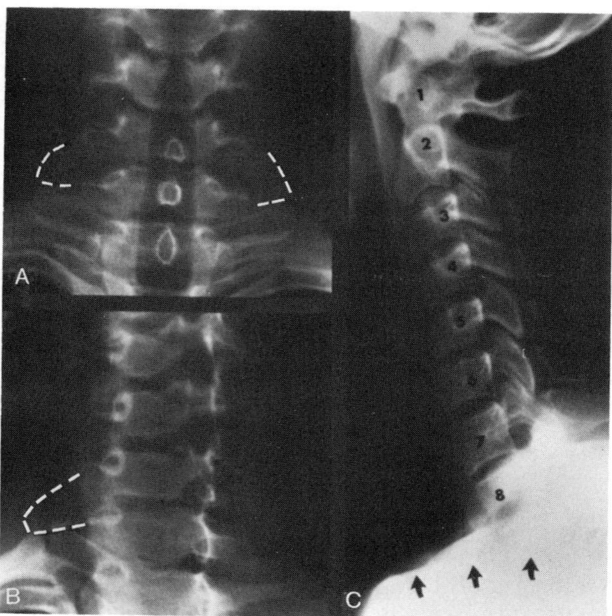

FIGURE 69–7. Anteroposterior and lateral radiographs of the cervical spine. *A* and *B*, Long transverse processes of the C7 vertebra *(dashed lines)*. *C*, Sagging of the shoulders suggests acromioclavicular descent and compression of the brachial nerves in the costoclavicular space.

limb pain. Excessive laboratory tests not only are unnecessary but also add expense and patient discomfort.

Radiologic Examination

Plain *cervical spine and chest x-ray studies* should be obtained for every patient. They provide valuable clues to the presence of cervical ribs, elongated C7 transverse processes, other bony aberrations of the first rib or spine, and clavicular fractures (Figs. 69–6 and 69–7). Signs of degenerative diseases of the cervical spine, such as narrowing of the intervertebral space and osteophytes, should be obvious. Additional information on the neural foramina can be obtained by an oblique projection. In patients with suspected cervical spine disease such as tumors, spinal stenosis, or a herniated disc, *computed tomography, myelography,* or *magnetic resonance imaging* may be employed. Sagittal magnetic resonance imaging in the plane of the brachial plexus is being investigated and in the future may provide an accurate means of assessing the point of actual compression of the nerves.

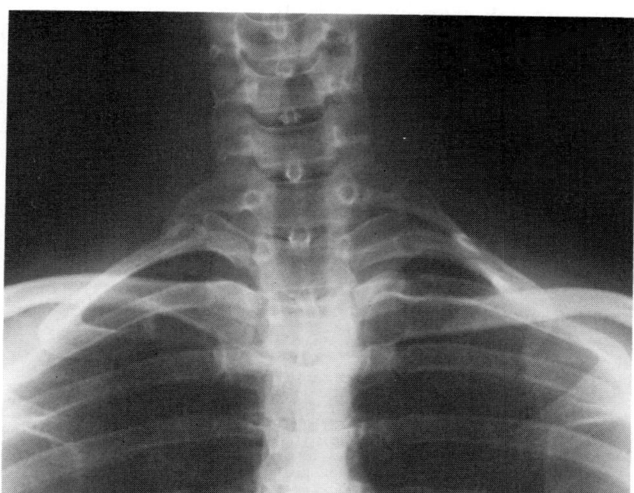

FIGURE 69–6. Anteroposterior radiograph of the cervical spine showing bilateral cervical ribs.

Arteriography is performed only when the patient is suspected of having a concomitant arterial complication of TOS, such as a supraclavicular bruit, a pulsatile mass, or vascular symptoms and signs of upper limb thromboembolism. Arteriography delineates the anatomy of the subclavian artery but is not useful for diagnosing neurogenic TOS. Many normal patients have abnormal subclavian arteriographic findings owing to artifacts introduced by posturing, whereas patients with nerve compression often have normal arteriographic findings. Moreover, the site of compression of the artery may not correspond to the site of nerve irritation. *Venography,* on the other hand, is diagnostic for subclavian vein thrombosis or stenosis at the level of the first rib.[31]

Electrophysiologic Studies

Many electrophysiologic studies have been proposed, but there is no standard objective diagnostic test for thoracic outlet nerve compression. The tests are beset with technical problems because the site of brachial plexus compression is often situated deep in the confines of the bony inlet and located proximally, at the level of the nerve roots near the intervertebral foramina. It is thus inaccessible to the application of an electrical stimulus. Many of these tests also have a wide range of normal values, which makes accurate interpretation of an abnormal result difficult. At best, a positive result indicates only a nonspecific disorder of nerve function. The authors do not find these studies helpful in establishing a diagnosis of TOS, and they are not carried out routinely.

The use of *ulnar nerve conduction velocities* in neurogenic TOS was popularized by Urschel and Razzuk.[32, 33] The technique involves placing electrodes at Erb's point at the base of the neck and on the hand and measuring the latency of an applied electrical impulse. Urschel and Razzuk reported a decrease in ulnar nerve conduction velocities in patients with TOS and a return to normal after surgical decompression. This observation has not been consistently reproduced,[34, 35] and the value of the test has been much disputed. *Electromyography* is a measure of muscle electrical activity and evaluates only motor neurons. Because the majority of patients with TOS have mainly sensory complaints, this test is helpful only in the few cases of TOS with muscular atrophy to exclude alternate diagnoses such as carpal tunnel syndrome, ulnar nerve entrapment, and cervical root disease. *F-wave responses* are likewise primarily motor and are therefore of limited value.[36] *Somatosensory evoked potentials* are obtained by recording the time required for a stimulus applied to the median or ulnar nerve to reach the brain. Early studies reported a good clinical correlation between TOS and abnormal somatosensory evoked potential results,[37] but the test is also nonspecific and its usefulness has not been demonstrated.

Noninvasive Vascular Laboratory Studies

Digital plethysmography, pulse volume recordings, and pressure measurements are of limited value in neurogenic TOS. They appear to be helpful only in patients with ischemic symptoms due to arterial TOS. Duplex scanning of the subclavian arteries and veins may show an aneurysm or venous thrombosis and may provide some anatomic information before angiography.

CONSERVATIVE TREATMENT

Once neurogenic thoracic outlet compression has been diagnosed, an initial period of supervised conservative treatment should be instituted before operative intervention is considered. Medications such as analgesics are used to control pain, and if muscular spasms are prominent, muscle relaxants can be prescribed. Patients are instructed to avoid placing the upper limb in positions that aggravate their symptoms, such as elevating the arm in work or during sleep. Occupational adjustments may be necessary to improve posture. Physical therapy consists of simple heat and cold application, massages, and application of ultrasound to the supraclavicular area. Shoulder girdle strengthening exercises are taught to women with poor muscular support. Stretching and joint mobilization maneuvers (e.g., the upper limb tension test) may be used to improve the range of shoulder motion. Active exercises may be assisted by passive transcutaneous nerve stimulation to the muscles.

Various local procedures, such as brachial plexus nerve blocks or anterior scalene muscle blocks by injection of local anesthetics, may grant temporary relief of symptoms. An improvement after injection is regarded by some authors as diagnostic of neurogenic TOS.[24]

Most patients, especially those with symptoms of recent onset, will experience some benefit with a few months of conservative therapy. Surgical decompression is indicated if conservative measures fail or result in worsening of the neurologic symptoms or if intractable pain leads to job loss or interferes with the activities of daily living. Muscle wasting or progressive loss of function of the upper limb also warrants surgical intervention. A concomitant cervical sympathectomy may be indicated if there is severe digital ischemia or reflex sympathetic dystrophy. The decision to operate should be made after a thorough discussion with the patient of the potential surgical complications, including nerve or vascular injury. The possibility of achieving only partial relief or of the recurrence of symptoms should be emphasized, particularly when the symptomatic period exceeds 2½ years.

OPERATIVE TREATMENT

The controversy surrounding neurogenic TOS is best exemplified by the diversity of surgical treatments available. Various combinations of scalenotomy, scalenectomy, first rib resection, and neurolysis of the brachial plexus may be carried out via one of four approaches: supraclavicular, transaxillary, infraclavicular, and parascapular.

Choice of Operation

The objectives of any surgical procedure aimed at relieving brachial plexus symptoms are to arrest the continued irritation of the brachial plexus roots and trunks and to restore an optimal environment for healing. Any abnormal osseous structure, such as a cervical rib, exostosis, an abnormal first rib, or fracture callus, should be removed. In the majority of patients, however, the skeletal framework of the thoracic outlet is normal, and it is in the treatment of this group of patients that surgical opinions differ.

Originally, the authors adopted the transaxillary approach popular in the 1960s and 1970s to remove the first thoracic rib rather than precisely exposing and decompressing the brachial plexus itself. Not surprisingly, a significant proportion of the patients had persistent or recurrent symptoms after transaxillary first rib resection alone. In these patients, supraclavicular reoperation disclosed reattachment of the anterior scalene muscle to the scarred bed of the first rib, as well as undisturbed myofascial anomalies and perineural scar. These patients' symptoms invariably improved after removal of the acquired scar and myofascial anomalies and radical scalenectomy. This experience prompted the authors to combine supraclavicular scalenectomy with transaxillary first rib resection.[38] The supraclavicular incision provided excellent exposure of the posterior two thirds of the first rib and the course of all four cervical nerve roots and the one thoracic nerve root making up the brachial plexus. The removal of the anterior scalene muscle after extraperiosteal mobilization and transaxillary excision of the first rib completed the procedure. The authors abandoned the transaxillary operation completely in 1983 and have achieved a 90 per cent success rate in relieving neurogenic symptoms with supraclavicular scalenectomy, brachial plexus neurolysis, excision of congenital and acquired compressive structures, and first rib resection.[39] With increasing experience with the supraclavicular procedure, they began to question the necessity of routine first rib resection. Since the late 1980s, the authors have performed supraclavicular radical scalenectomy, neurolysis, and excision of congenital and acquired factors while sparing the first rib. The rationale for this operation is based on the considerations discussed in the following sections.

Superior Exposure. Successful decompression of the brachial plexus requires full, unrestricted exposure of its entire course from the vertebral foramina to the clavicle. The supraclavicular approach provides a view unparalleled by the transaxillary or any other route. It allows direct visualization of the anatomic relationship between the bony and myofascial structures and of the course of the plexus through the scalene space in the thoracic outlet. This permits precise identification of the exact pathology of the offending structures, thus avoiding a blind first rib resection. Unlike with the transaxillary operation, simultaneous treatment of any anomalies of the scalene muscles is possible, so that every source of compression of the brachial plexus can be removed. The limitations in exposure of a transaxillary operation also pose additional hazards when a total neurolysis is attempted, particularly with long thoracic nerve and brachial plexus root and trunk injuries,[40] not to mention injuries of the related vascular structures.

Rationale of Radical Scalenectomy. In contrast to the conduct of previous supraclavicular operations, the authors believe that total removal of the scalene muscles is essential. After scalenotomy or transaxillary decompression, reattachment of the anterior scalene muscle to the rib bed is a frequent cause of operative failures. As the role of the scalene muscles in the pathogenesis of nerve compression and irritation has become clearer, a thorough mobilization and resection of the anterior scalene muscle from its origins at the transverse processes of the cervical vertebrae to its insertion at the first rib has been recognized as necessary. Removal of the middle scalene muscle from a level just caudal to and parallel to the course of the long thoracic nerve is also important because it affords access to the posterior aspect of the brachial plexus and frees the anterior surface of the first rib. This creates the potential space between the posterior aspect of the plexus and the first rib. Damage to the long thoracic nerve, which runs inside the muscle belly, is avoided with the extent of middle scalenectomy described.

Concept of Total Decompression. The authors advocate complete removal of all soft tissues, congenital and acquired, surrounding the brachial plexus to allow it to assume a free, unhindered course in the interscalene space. Some authors have attempted to divide neurogenic TOS symptoms into upper and lower plexus types and have proposed transaxillary first rib resection for lower plexus lesions, reserving the supraclavicular operation as a "staged" procedure in case of recurrences.[41] In the authors' experience, the symptoms produced in most patients are mixed, and diffuse plexus irritation requires total decompression. Subsequent scarring after an initial limited decompression of part of the plexus would make a second, staged operation difficult.

Rationale for Sparing the First Rib. The offending structures identified during supraclavicular decompression are usually soft tissue anomalies, particularly muscular interdigitation between the scalene muscles and myofascial bands and perineural scarring. The first rib is seldom in actual mechanical contact with the brachial plexus, except for the first thoracic root. After scalenectomy and a complete neurolysis, the brachial plexus runs an unobstructed course without impingement or displacement through the thoracic outlet. Resection of the first rib in these instances is unnecessary and poses additional problems of increased postoperative pain and shoulder immobility and a higher risk of pleural damage. Moreover, the bed of the resected first rib is often a site of excessive scarring, which contributes to late recurrences.

On the basis of the previously mentioned considerations, the authors have performed 45 consecutive supraclavicular thoracic outlet decompressions consisting of anterior and middle scalenectomy and neurolysis of the brachial plexus, without resection of the first rib. This operation has a lower morbidity and a shorter hospital stay, and the clinical results have been no different from those of the other operative approach the authors used, which was identical except that it also included resection of the first rib. A description of the technique follows.

Supraclavicular Scalenectomy

The operation is carried out under general anesthesia with endotracheal intubation. The patient is placed in a semi-recumbent (Fowler) position with the head turned away from the side of the operation. A curvilinear incision is made at the base of the neck, two fingerbreadths above the clavicle, beginning over the clavicular head of the sternocleidomastoid muscle and curving laterally and posteriorly for about 10 cm (Fig. 69–8). The platysma is incised, and subplatysmal flaps are raised superiorly to the level of the cricoid cartilage and inferiorly to the level of the clavicle. The sternocleidomastoid muscle is retracted medially, and its clavicular head is divided, if necessary. The use of a self-retaining miniframe retractor (Omni-Tract Surgical, Minnesota Scientific, St. Paul) produces multiple forces to displace and retain the soft tissues without the need for any hand-held retractors.

The lateral border of the internal jugular vein is identified, and mobilization of the scalene fat pad is begun at this point. The mobilization proceeds laterally onto the anterior surface of the anterior scalene muscle and inferiorly along the clavicle. The omohyoid muscle is resected. The phrenic nerve, which runs obliquely from lateral to medial

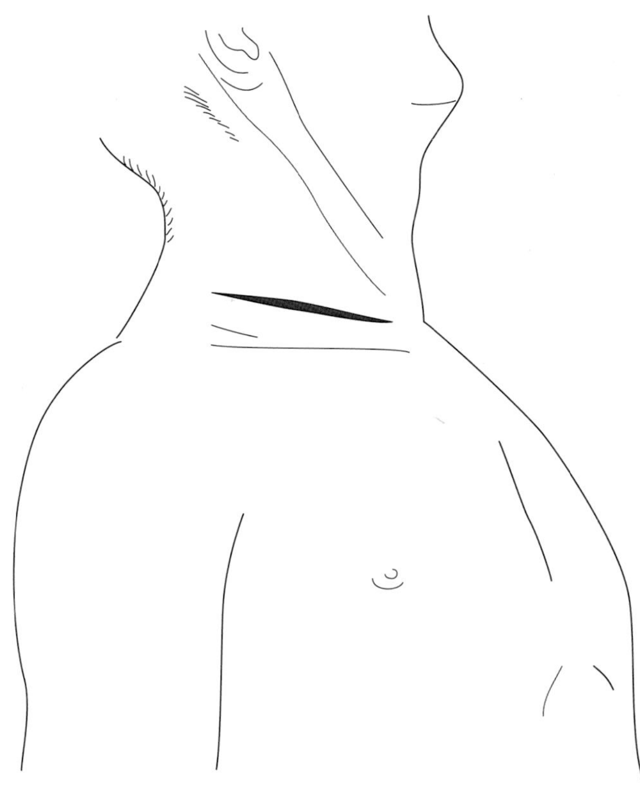

FIGURE 69–8. Supraclavicular incision used for anterior and middle scalenectomy. The incision is placed two fingerbreadths above the clavicle and curves laterally and posteriorly from the clavicular head of the sternocleidomastoid for about 10 cm.

across the anterior scalene muscle, is identified and gently dissected free. The scalene fat pad is reflected on a laterally based pedicle (Fig. 69–9*A*).

The phrenic nerve is retracted medially, and the anterior scalene muscle is mobilized down to its insertion to the first rib, with care taken to protect the subclavian artery and the trunks of the brachial plexus posteriorly (see Fig. 69–9*B*). Branches of the thyrocervical trunk may be encountered running across the anterior scalene muscle; they must be divided. The muscle insertion is detached flush with the first rib tubercle and is reflected superiorly. This allows optimal visualization of the anterior aspect of the plexus and the subclavian artery. Any muscle fibers that interdigitate with the middle scalene muscle between the trunks of the plexus or that encircle the subclavian artery are then divided. The dissection proceeds proximally until the origins of the anterior scalene muscle at the transverse processes of the upper cervical vertebrae are exposed and divided, and the anterior scalene muscle is removed as a single specimen.

Thorough mobilization of the roots and trunks of the brachial plexus is performed until gentle anterior displacement of these structures is possible. The dissection and neurolysis of the C8 and T1 roots of the plexus anteriorly may reveal a myofascial structure emerging between the C7 and C8 roots and crossing the proximal portion of C8 and T1 to attach to Sibson's fascia or the first rib (see Fig. 69–9*C*). When this appears as a well-developed muscle, it is termed the scalenus minimus. (Some investigators term it the scalenus pleuralis, the scalenus accessorius, or the scalenus anticus minor.) The authors have encountered this anomaly in nearly one third of their patients, always with associated compression of the lower roots against the neck of the first rib, as well as perineural scarring. Complete resection of these structures allows full dissection of the lower roots and trunks of the plexus from the neural foramina to the clavicle. Gentle displacement of the shoulder upward relaxes the roots of the plexus, allowing their mobilization and freeing any posterior attachments to the insertion of the middle scalene muscle on the first rib. This facilitates removal of the middle scalene muscle in a rib-sparing procedure that is described later.

The lateral border of the middle scalene muscle is explored until the point of emergence of the long thoracic nerve is determined. The middle scalene muscle is mobilized completely by gently displacing the trunks of the brachial plexus. Any interdigitating muscle fibers or anomalous bands passing between or compressing the nerve roots or trunks are removed. As this dissection progresses toward the posterior surface of the middle scalene muscle, the first rib will be easily felt behind the muscle. The middle scalene muscle is then transected on a line parallel and inferior to the course of the long thoracic nerve down to the anterior aspect of the neck of the first rib (see Fig. 69–9*D*). The muscle insertion, together with the periosteum, is removed entirely from the rib. This leaves a clean bony surface on the first rib, with no muscle adjacent to the brachial plexus. If a prominent transverse process of the C7 vertebra is encountered, it may be shortened with a rongeur or cut with a pair of heavy scissors.

First Rib Resection. Resection of the scalene muscles will allow access to the posterior part of the first rib. The intercostal muscles between the first and second ribs and

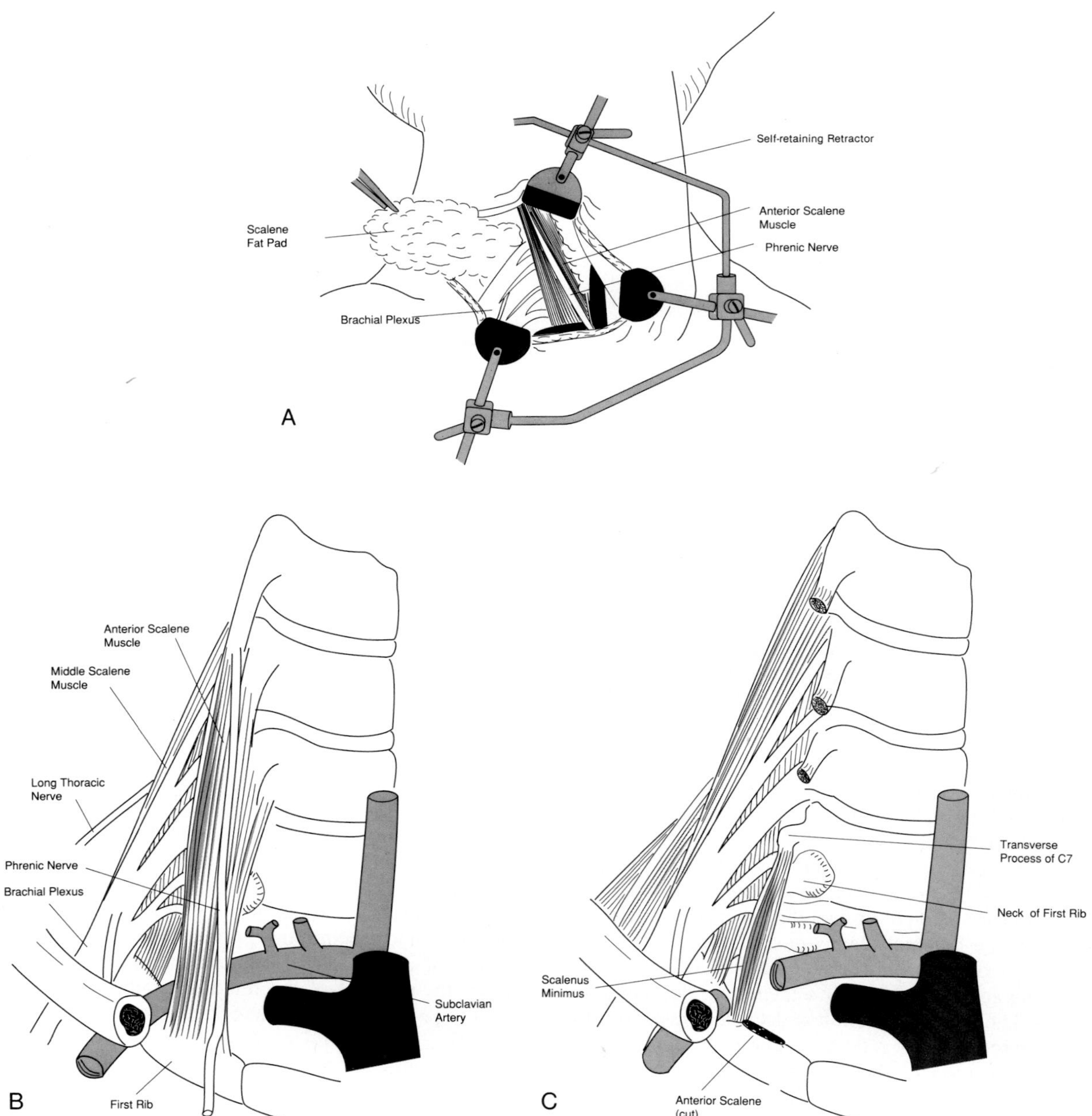

FIGURE 69–9. **Technique of supraclavicular scalenectomy. *A*, The exposure is facilitated by a self-retaining miniframe retractor. The scalene fat pad is mobilized and reflected on a laterally based pedicle. *B*, The anterior scalene muscle and the phrenic nerve, brachial plexus, and subclavian artery are dissected. The muscle is mobilized from its origin down to its insertion to the first rib and resected. *C*, After resection of the anterior scalene muscle, the brachial plexus can be visualized and any muscular interdigitations can be removed. The smallest scalene muscle is shown compressing the C8 and T1 nerve roots as it runs from the transverse process of the C7 vertebra and attaches to the first rib.**

Illustration continued on opposite page

the posterior scalene muscles are divided. Inferiorly, blunt finger dissection is used to separate and displace the pleura from the undersurface of the first rib. Medially, the lower trunks of the brachial plexus are gently dissected free, and total mobilization of the first rib is completed by retracting the clavicle anteriorly and the subclavian artery and brachial plexus laterally. The rib is then divided with a sagittal saw anterior to the scalene tubercle near the costochondral junction and posteriorly close to the spine and removed. If the proximal rib stump impinges on the T1 nerve root, a rongeur is used to remove additional offending bone.

First Rib Sparing. In the authors' experience, the first rib does not cause actual compression of the plexus and is not disturbed. If the medial neck of the first rib displaces the course of the T1 root of the plexus, a bone rongeur is used to remove a small rim of the medial border, allowing space for an unrestricted course of the root as it traverses the route from the intervertebral foramina to the junction with C8 to form the lower trunk (see Fig. 69–9*E*).

The brachial plexus is then carefully inspected, and each root and trunk is traced from the intervertebral foramina to the level of the clavicle. Any scar tissue and resid-

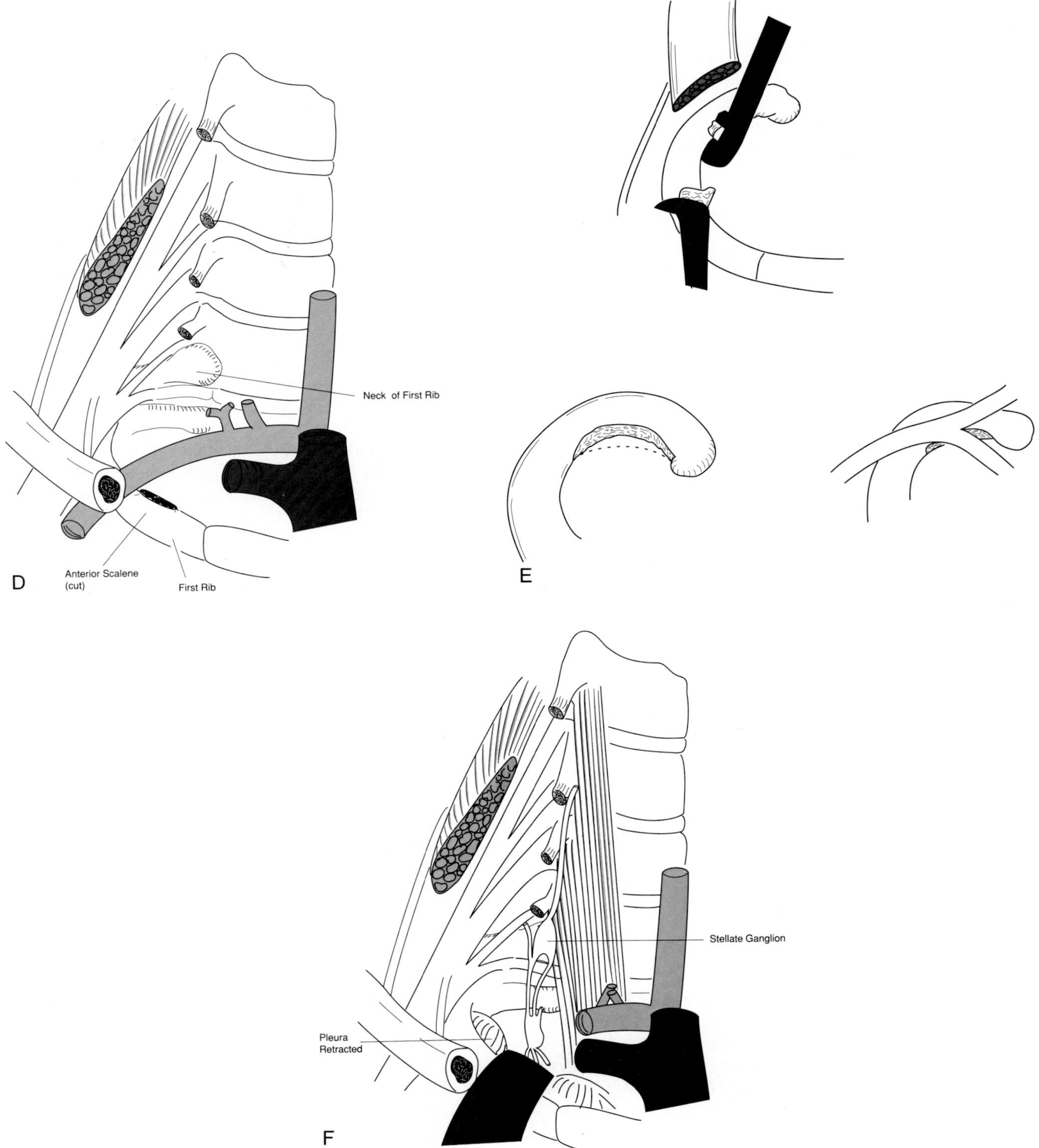

FIGURE 69–9. *Continued* *D*, The middle scalene muscle is transected on a line parallel and inferior to the long thoracic nerve, freeing the posterior aspect of the brachial plexus. *E*, Sagittal osteotomy of the medial border of the first rib using a bone rongeur, allowing the T1 root to course unrestricted to join the C8 root. *F*, Brachial plexus neurolysis is completed. The stellate ganglion lies close to the neck of the first rib, and a cervical sympathectomy may be accomplished by reflecting the dome of the pleura inferiorly.

ual muscle fibers are removed by a complete neurolysis until the nerves are skeletonized. For patients with prominent vasomotor symptoms, a *cervical sympathectomy* can be performed at the same time. The pleura is displaced laterally and inferiorly, and the stellate ganglion is identified at the medial side of the neck of the first rib (see Fig. 69–9*F*). The thoracic component (the lower half) of the ganglion is then divided from the inferior cervical sympathetic chain. The dissection is carried into the upper mediastinum, and the chain is removed together with the T2 and T3 sympathetic ganglia. Frozen section confirmation is obtained.

Hemostasis is secured, and the wound is inspected for any chylous or lymphatic leakage. The lung is inflated, and the pleura is examined for any disruption. If a pleural defect is detected, a small catheter is placed through the pleurotomy into the thoracic cavity and the air is evacuated by aspiration before closure. The catheter is later withdrawn from the closed wound. A smaller rent in the pleura can be closed directly with absorbable sutures. The mobilized prescalene fat pad is positioned loosely over the trunks of the brachial plexus to provide a soft insulating layer to help protect the nerves. The platysma is reapproximated, and the skin is closed with subcuticular sutures around a closed suction drain. An epidural catheter placed through a stab wound and positioned along the course of the proximal roots of the brachial plexus can be used for instillation of topical anesthetic agents for postoperative pain relief. Steroids may be administered via the same route to reduce scar tissue formation in reoperative cases.

Transaxillary First Rib Resection

This operation, although not used by the authors since the early 1980s, is still popular in the United States. It provides a superior cosmetic result and offers better access to the thoracic sympathetic trunk. In costoclavicular compression syndromes, it can provide adequate decompression. However, the transaxillary operation has the disadvantage of having a deep, limited exposure that allows inadequate identification of the offending pathology, especially when the nerve compression occurs at a more proximal level (the upper roots). Radical scalenectomy is not possible, and concomitant cervical rib or fibromuscular band excision is often difficult and hazardous. Removal of the posterior part of the first rib may be incomplete and carries the risk of long thoracic nerve damage. It has a higher rate of morbidity (particularly brachial plexus damage), a longer patient recovery time, and in the authors' prior experience, an unacceptably higher neurogenic recurrence rate.

The operation, as described by Roos,[8, 42] is performed with the patient placed in a lateral thoracotomy position. The ipsilateral arm is draped and is supported in an abducted and elevated position by an assistant during the entire operation. A transverse axillary incision, 10 to 15 cm long, is made over the second intercostal space just below the hairline. The incision is deepened between the pectoralis major and the latissimus dorsi muscles and is carried down to the chest wall. Care is taken to preserve the intercostobrachial nerve if possible. If the nerve is damaged or overstretched, pain and paresthesia in the region of the axilla and medial arm may be severe, and it is best to divide the nerve and accept a minor degree of postoperative anesthesia. A self-retaining retractor maintains the superficial exposure, and a tunnel is developed upward in the plane over the serratus anterior muscle and the rib cage toward the axilla. Small vessels that cross the axillary fat are divided. Blunt dissection is continued until the first rib is reached.

The first rib is mobilized by dissecting anteriorly up to the costochondral junction and posteriorly beyond the middle scalene muscle. The subclavian artery and vein and the lower trunks of the brachial plexus are carefully identified and preserved as they course above the rib. Exposure can be improved by having an assistant raise and stabilize the arm and shoulders and by the use of special deep Martinez retractors. Excessive traction on the brachial plexus should be avoided, and care should be taken to relax the arm periodically. Temporary traction injury to the T1 nerve root and subsequent causalgia are not uncommon postoperatively if these precautions are not observed. The long thoracic nerve should be protected as it runs posteriorly after exiting from the lateral edge of the middle scalene muscle.

Using sharp dissection and a periosteal elevator, the surgeon divides the intercostal muscles along the outer edge of the rib. The extraperiosteal plane is entered, and the pleura is gently separated from the inner side of the rib. The anterior scalene muscle is separated from the subclavian artery and is divided at its attachment to the scalene tubercle. The middle scalene muscle is likewise resected with scissors. The dissection plane should adhere to the rib to avoid injury to the long thoracic nerve. The rib is cleared of remaining soft tissue attachments and is divided with a rib cutter as posteriorly as possible, close to the transverse process of the vertebra, while the T1 root is retracted out of the way. Attention is then turned to the anterior aspect of the rib. With the subclavian vein protected, the rib is divided again medial to the anterior scalene tubercle or dislocated at the costochondral junction and removed. The stumps of the rib should be inspected and, if necessary, smoothened with a rongeur. Shortening the posterior stump is especially important to avoid undue pressure on the T1 root. The anterior scalene muscle is drawn downward and transected, with removal of as much of the distal half of the muscle as possible.

The brachial plexus is inspected, and any neurolysis is completed. The stellate ganglion and the thoracic sympathetic chain are easily visualized at the neck of the first rib, and a sympathectomy can be performed, although it is not commonly indicated. Hemostasis is secured, and pleural rents are repaired. The wound is closed over a small suction drain.

Combined Operation

The combined supraclavicular and transaxillary approach provides the best exposure to the upper and lower nerves of the brachial plexus. The transaxillary approach simplifies first rib resection, and supraclavicular exposure facilitates excision of soft tissue anomalies and scar. The supraclavicular scalenectomy is accomplished as described, and neurolysis is completed. Thereafter, transaxillary resection of the first rib is performed. This was the authors' preferred approach from 1980 to 1983, when the transaxillary route was abandoned because the supraclavicular route alone permitted identification and correction of all structures believed to be initiating the brachial plexus symptoms.

Parascapular Approach

First introduced by Clagett in 1962,[7] first rib excision via a posterior thoracotomy has the advantage of avoiding dense scarring in reoperations for TOS.[43] With the patient in a lateral decubitus position, a posterior thoracotomy incision is made. The incision is deepened through muscle, and the scapula is retracted upward. The serratus anterior and rhomboid muscles are divided, and the first rib is exposed by retracting the paraspinal muscles. The rib is mobilized and removed, and a neurolysis of the brachial plexus follows. A cervical sympathectomy can be performed extrapleurally by sectioning a small portion of the second rib. Despite the good results claimed by some surgeons,[44] this approach was never popular as a primary procedure and is not recommended because of the technical difficulties and the extensive muscle division.

Infraclavicular Approach

A 15-cm incision is made over the first rib, two fingerbreadths below and parallel to the clavicle, starting at the costochondral junction. The wound is deepened by splitting the sternal and clavicular fibers of the pectoralis major muscle, and retractors are inserted. The first rib is identified and dissected free by dividing the intercostal muscle at its inferior border and the anterior and middle scalene muscles superiorly. The pleura is gently separated from the inner surface of the rib, and the rib is divided with shears at the costochondral junction and retracted outward. The pleura is further swept away from the rib toward the spine. With a finger protecting the neurovascular bundle, the posterior end of the rib is transected as far backward as possible. With this approach, first described by Gol and associates,[45] good results have been reported.[46] This approach offers good exposure of the medial aspect of the first rib and its costoclavicular junction. It can be combined with a supraclavicular incision (paraclavicular approach) in cases in which extensive exposure of the entire first rib becomes necessary, particularly in association with surgical relief of effort thrombosis of the subclavian vein.[31] Alone, it does not allow adequate exposure of the posterior half of the rib or the roots of the plexus, and for this indication it is not recommended.

Intraoperative Monitoring

The adequacy of surgical decompression of the brachial plexus can be monitored intraoperatively by observing the pattern of thermal emission from the hand of the patient on the operated side. Previous experience in patients with cervical and lumbosacral radiculopathy has validated the usefulness of this technique.[47] The completeness of surgical decompression of the spinal nerve roots can be determined by observing the pattern of change in heat emission during the conduct of the operation. With an on-line infrared camera processed by a colorizer, the initial thermal image of the patient's hand is recorded preoperatively. This pattern is characterized by asymmetric cooling of the dorsum of the hand and involves multiple dermatomes, unlike disc disease, in which only one dermatome is affected. The same image is displayed on a small video terminal and is monitored continuously during the operation. A decrease in heat emission in the dermatome of the nerve root being manipulated is consistently observed. Conversely, an increase in heat emissivity is seen when myofascial anomalies or bony deformities are removed. A further rise in temperature is noted after successful neurolysis. This process is sensitive enough to direct further surgical exploration and decompression of affected nerve roots until a steady thermal state is achieved.

COMPLICATIONS

The thoracic outlet is the site of many vital neurovascular structures, and a thorough understanding of the anatomy is essential to the success of any operation. The surgeon should also bear in mind that diverse anatomic variations and anomalies exist in this region. The surgical complications include injuries to the nerves, vessels, and lymphatic structures in the neck (Table 69–4).

Nerve Injuries

Injuries to the nerves can be temporary, due to excessive manipulation or retraction, or permanent and cause significant disability or deformity. Injury to the *brachial plexus* is potentially serious because complete return of function is not universal. Most plexus injuries are a temporary neurapraxia, which is usually due to deep retraction. Permanent damage is rare, occurring in fewer than 1 per cent of cases, but paralysis of the arm has been reported.[40] It is more likely to occur after transaxillary operations because of the limited exposure and excessive retraction. During reoperations, the plexus may be encased by scar tissue

Table 69–4. Complications of Thoracic Outlet Operations

Intraoperative	Postoperative
Nerve injury Brachial plexus Long thoracic nerve Phrenic nerve Intercostobrachial nerve Vagus nerve and recurrent laryngeal nerve	Wound complications Wound infection Lymph collections
Vascular injury Subclavian vein Subclavian artery	Scar formation or accelerated healing
Thoracic duct injury Lymphatic fistula Lymphocele Chylothorax	
Pleural complications Pleural damage Pneumothorax Pleural effusion Hemothorax	

and can be damaged in the course of dissection. The T1 root lies close to the neck of the first rib and may be inadvertently severed by bone cutters during first rib resections. The resultant symptoms vary from severe causalgic pain to partial or total loss of sensation and paralysis of the limb. With supportive physical therapy, about 80 per cent of patients with brachial plexus neurapraxic injuries will have a complete recovery of function.

The *phrenic nerve,* which runs across the surface of the anterior scalene muscle from lateral to medial, is liable to injury in supraclavicular operations, usually as the result of retraction. Temporary paralysis of the nerve is occasionally revealed on the postoperative chest x-ray study, on which an elevation of the ipsilateral hemidiaphragm is observed. It can lead to a small basal pleural effusion or mild symptomatic respiratory embarrassment. Treatment is conservative, with chest physiotherapy.

The *long thoracic nerve* emerges on the lateral border of the middle scalene muscle. It serves as a landmark for the division of this muscle in supraclavicular operations. Injury can occur during careless middle scalenectomy because the nerve runs inside the belly of the muscle. In transaxillary rib resections, the nerve is not usually identified and can be injured as it runs along the serratus anterior or during division of the middle scalene muscle and the first rib posteriorly. Anatomic variations of the nerve are frequent; often, more than one root joins to form the main nerve inside the middle scalene muscle. Damage to the nerve or its branches will result in winging of the scapula.

The *vagus nerve or its recurrent branch* on the right side may be jeopardized as it courses in front of the subclavian artery. The *intercostobrachial nerve* can also be stretched during transaxillary exposure. The *cervical sympathetic chain* and the stellate ganglion lie close to the neck of the first rib. Damage to the ganglion during rib resection can produce Horner's syndrome.

Vascular Injuries

Injuries to the *subclavian artery* or its branches are rare. Occasionally, postoperative bleeding or a hemothorax occurs if a small branch is divided inadvertently and overlooked. Small tears in the vessel can be repaired easily. Under exceptional circumstances, a second infraclavicular incision may be necessary to gain proximal control of the subclavian vessels for bleeding. *Subclavian vein* damage more commonly follows transaxillary rib resections.

Lymphatic Injuries

In left supraclavicular approaches, the thoracic duct may be damaged during dissection as it turns laterally below the level of the transverse process of the C7 and runs in front of the subclavian artery to drain into the left innominate vein. The duct is seldom seen, but if it is injured, it should be ligated. A search is made for lymphatic leakage at the completion of the operation, and any small lymphatic leaks are sutured before the wound is closed. Small chylous collections in the postoperative period may be managed conservatively by aspiration and by avoiding regular meals to decrease chyle flow, but a gross lymphatic fistula or even a chylothorax usually requires re-exploration and ligation of the leaking duct.

Pleural Complications

Pleural damage was the most common complication in the authors' experience when first rib resection was routinely practiced: it occurred in about half of the cases. It is more frequent, and sometimes unavoidable, after extraperiosteal first rib resection. A small rent in the pleura can be adequately treated by direct suture repair or aspiration of the air with a small catheter before wound closure. A chest drain is necessary for a larger defect. Postoperative *pneumothorax* is rare and may be managed conservatively if it is small. *Pleural effusions* or *hemothorax* can develop as fluid and blood accumulate in the pleural cavity through a damaged pleura. Usually, observation or needle paracentesis offer adequate treatment.

Wound Complications

Wound infection is rare after TOS operations. A collection of serous fluid or lymph in the supraclavicular wound may pose an occasional problem. The swelling usually subsides with needle aspiration and administration of antibiotics. In rare instances, it becomes encapsulated, and operative removal is necessary together with ligation of any leaking lymphatic ducts.

POSTOPERATIVE MANAGEMENT

After the supraclavicular operation, the drains are usually removed within 48 hours, and the patient is discharged on the 3rd or occasionally on the 4th postoperative day. In difficult cases, usually reoperations, a wound catheter may be used for instillation of local anesthetic to alleviate pain and steroids to deter fibrosis. Passive arm movement is allowed immediately, and a physical therapy program is instituted. Patients should be warned that they may experience an initial period of worsening pain and limited range of motion for a few weeks, but the paresthesia and pain should start to decrease within a few days after surgery. Rehabilitation is usually gradual and may take months, and patients often have to make adjustments in the working environment until adequate function returns. The degree of recovery is usually dictated by the extent of nerve damage and the duration of symptoms before surgical treatment. Mild residual symptoms are not infrequent, especially in long-standing cases. Patients should be made aware of the fact that some deterioration over time may occur owing to scarring.

Healing and scar formation around the brachial plexus start early, and passive physical therapy should begin as soon as possible to achieve an optimal healing environment and prevent nerve immobility. Active mobilization and brachial plexus tension exercises of the arm and shoulder girdle are begun after discharge with the aim of recovering a full range of motion and preventing scar contraction that will encase and immobilize the nerves of the plexus.[28]

Abnormal healing and excessive scar formation around the brachial plexus can result in early recurrence of pain, tightness, muscle spasm, and limited motion. Vigorous physical therapy, steroid use, and interferon administration have been tried to alleviate these symptoms, without much success. Reoperation to remove the fibrous tissue may be necessary if the symptoms become unmanageable. Postoperative magnetic resonance imaging is a new means of assessing scar development. After a successful thoracic outlet decompression, some patients report burning pain and increased sympathetic tone in the upper extremity. There are often trigger zones in the supraclavicular area where palpation will aggravate the symptoms. Neuromas, nerve entrapment by scars, and reflex sympathetic dystrophy have been suggested as the cause. Stellate ganglion blocks, trigger point injections, and ultrasound can provide temporary relief.

Recurrences are noted in about 10 to 15 per cent of patients with neurogenic TOS, particularly with long follow-up (more than 2 years). The symptoms often recur or become worse, particularly after another episode of trauma or undue physical activity or microstress similar to that which led to the original irritation of the plexus. The symptoms are often protracted and the cause of significant disability. The results of reoperations are usually not as favorable, and the morbidity rate is high. Missed anomalies and scars from scalene muscle reattachment are still common findings at secondary operations after transaxillary rib resection. It is therefore the surgeon's responsibility to make an accurate initial diagnosis and identify and remove all offending structures at the initial operation so that the brachial plexus can be allowed to heal in the best possible environment.

References

1. Cooper A: On exostosis. *In* Cooper, Cooper, Travers (eds): Surgical Essays. 3rd ed. London, 1821, p 128.
2. Coote H: Exostosis of the left transverse process of the seventh cervical vertebra, surrounded by blood vessels and nerves; Successful removal. Lancet 1:360, 1861.
3. Murphy T: Brachial neuritis caused by pressure of first rib. Aust Med J 15:582, 1910.
4. Ochsner A, Gage M, Debakey M: Scalenus anticus (Naffziger) syndrome. Am J Surg 28:669, 1935.
5. Naffziger HC, Grant WT: Neuritis of the brachial plexus mechanical in origin: The scalenus syndrome. Surg Gynecol Obstet 67:722, 1938.
6. Peet RM, Hendriksen JD, Anderson TP, et al: Thoracic outlet syndrome: Evaluation of a therapeutic exercise program. Proc Mayo Clin 31:281, 1956.
7. Clagett OT: Presidential address: Research and prosearch. J Thorac Cardiovasc Surg 44:153, 1962.
8. Roos DB: Transaxillary approach for first rib resection to relieve thoracic outlet syndrome. Ann Surg 163:354, 1966.
9. Adson AW, Coffey JR: Cervical ribs: A method of anterior approach for relief of symptoms by division of the scalenus anticus. Ann Surg 85:839, 1927.
10. Etter LE: Osseous abnormalities of the thoracic cage seen in forty thousand consecutive chest photoroentgenograms. Am J Roentgenol 51:359, 1944.
11. Haven H: Neurocirculatory scalenus anticus syndrome in the presence of developmental defects of the first rib. Yale J Biol Med 11:443, 1939.
12. Gruber W: Über die Halsrippen des Menschen mit Vergleichend-Anatomischen Bemerkungen. St. Petersburg, 1869.
13. Jones FW: Discussion on cervical ribs: The anatomy of cervical ribs. Proc R Soc Med 6:95, 1913.
14. Kirgis HD, Reed AF: Significant anatomic relations in the syndrome of the scalene muscles. Ann Surg 127:1182, 1948.
15. Gage M, Parnell H: Scalenus anticus syndrome. Am J Surg 73:252, 1947.
16. Thomas GI, Jones TW, Stavney LS, et al: The middle scalene muscle and its contribution to the thoracic outlet syndrome. Am J Surg 145:589, 1983.
17. Lawson FL, McKenzie KG: The scalenus minimus muscle. Can Med Assoc J 65:358, 1951.
18. Lord JW Jr, Stone PW: Pectoralis minor tenotomy and anterior scalenotomy with special reference to the hyperabduction syndrome and "effort thrombosis" of the subclavian vein. Circulation 13:537, 1956.
19. Roos DB: New concepts of thoracic outlet syndrome that explain etiology, symptoms, diagnosis, and treatment. Vasc Surg 13:313, 1979.
20. Falconer MA, Weddell G: Costoclavicular compression of the subclavian artery and vein. Lancet 2:539, 1943.
21. Todd TW: The descent of the shoulder after birth: Its significance in the production of pressure-symptoms on the lowest brachial trunk. Anat Anz 41:385, 1912.
22. Swift TR, Nichols FT: The droopy shoulder syndrome. Neurology 34:212, 1984.
23. De Silva M: The costoclavicular syndrome: A "new cause." Ann Rheum Dis 45:916, 1986.
24. Sanders RJ, Pearce WH: The treatment of thoracic outlet syndrome: A comparison of different operations. J Vasc Surg 10:626, 1989.
25. Machleder HI, Moll F, Verity A: The anterior scalene muscle in thoracic outlet compression syndrome: Histochemical and morphometric studies. Arch Surg 121:1141, 1986.
26. Sanders RJ, Jackson CGR, Banchero N, et al: Scalene muscle abnormalities in traumatic thoracic outlet syndrome. Am J Surg 159:231, 1990.
27. Upton ARM, McComas AJ: The double crush in nerve-entrapment syndromes. Lancet 2:359, 1973.
28. Elvey RL: Brachial plexus tension tests and the pathoanatomical origin of arm pain. *In* Idczak RM (ed): Aspects of Manipulative Therapy. Melbourne, Lincoln Institute of Health Sciences, 1980, p 105.
29. Kenneally M, Rubenach H, Elvey R: The upper limb tension test: The SLR test of the arm. *In* Grant R (ed): Physical Therapy of the Cervical and Thoracic Spine. Churchill Livingstone, 1988, p 167.
30. Selvaratnam PJ, Glasgow EF, Matyas T: Differential strain produced by the brachial plexus tension test on C5 to T1 nerve roots. *In* Proceedings of the 6th Biennial Conference of Manipulative Therapists Association of Australia. 1989.
31. Thompson RW, Schneider PA, Nelken NA, et al: Circumferential venolysis and paraclavicular thoracic outlet decompression for "effort thrombosis" of the subclavian vein. J Vasc Surg 16:723, 1992.
32. Urschel HC, Razzuk MA: Management of the thoracic outlet syndrome. N Engl J Med 286:1140, 1972.
33. Urschel HC, Razzuk MA: The failed operation for thoracic outlet syndrome: The difficulty of diagnosis and management. Ann Thorac Surg 42:523, 1986.
34. Cherington M: Ulnar conduction velocity in thoracic-outlet syndrome. N Engl J Med 294:1185, 1976.
35. Wilbourn AJ: Evidence for conduction delay in thoracic outlet syndrome is challenged. N Engl J Med 310:1052, 1984.
36. Hongladarom T: "F"-wave conduction velocity in thoracic-outlet syndrome. N Engl J Med 295:1382, 1976.
37. Glover JL, Worth RM, Bendick PJ, et al: Evoked responses in the diagnosis of thoracic outlet syndrome. Surgery 89:86, 1981.
38. Qvarfordt PG, Ehrenfeld WK, Stoney RJ: Supraclavicular radical scalenectomy and transaxillary first rib resection for the thoracic outlet syndrome: A combined approach. Am J Surg 148:111, 1984.
39. Reilly LM, Stoney RJ: Supraclavicular approach for thoracic outlet decompression. J Vasc Surg 8:329, 1988.
40. Dale A: Thoracic outlet compression syndrome: Critique in 1982. Arch Surg 117:1437, 1982.
41. Sanders RJ, Haug CE, Pearce WH: Recurrent thoracic outlet syndrome. J Vasc Surg 12:390, 1990.
42. Roos DB: Experience with rib resection for thoracic outlet syndrome. Ann Surg 173:429, 1971.
43. Urschel HD Jr, Razzuk MA, Albers JE, et al: Reoperation for recurrent thoracic outlet syndrome. Ann Thorac Surg 21:19, 1976.

44. Johnson CR: Treatment of thoracic outlet syndrome by removal of first rib and related entrapments through posterolateral approach: A 22 year experience. J Thorac Cardiovasc Surg 68:536, 1974.
45. Gol A, Patrick DW, McNeel DP: Relief of costoclavicular syndrome by infraclavicular removal of first rib. J Neurosurg 28:81, 1968.
46. Nelson RM, Jenson CB: Anterior approach for excision of the first rib: Surgical technique. Ann Thorac Surg 9:30, 1970.
47. Hubbard J, Maultsby J, Wexler C: Lumbar and cervical thermography for nerve fiber impingement: A critical review. Clin J Pain 2:131, 1986.

Additional Reading

Sanders RJ, Haug CE: Thoracic outlet syndrome. A common sequela of neck injuries. Philadelphia, JB Lippincott, 1991.

70

Arterial Complications of Thoracic Outlet Compression

Edouard Kieffer, M.D., and Carlo Ruotolo, M.D.

• • •

Arterial complications of thoracic outlet compression have serious prognostic implications, although they are present in fewer than 5 per cent of operations performed for thoracic outlet syndrome (TOS). Long-standing compression of the subclavian artery (SA) may lead to major arterial lesions with thromboembolic complications that may in turn impair the function and even jeopardize the viability of the affected upper limb.[1–3] This chapter reviews the anatomic, clinical, and surgical aspects of these complications.

ANATOMIC LESIONS

Arterial complications of TOS are always secondary to significant, permanent, and long-standing compression—usually a congenital bony abnormality. There is usually a long delay before arterial lesions develop and symptoms appear. The mean age of patients having arterial complications is at least 10 years older than that of patients having neurologic or venous symptoms from TOS. Although the compression may involve any of the three consecutive narrowings of the thoracic outlet, it affects primarily the costoscalene passage and, less frequently, the costoclavicular passage. The SA compression occurs in the anteroposterior direction in the former case and cephalad to caudad in the latter. To the authors' knowledge, no case of arterial complication due to compression in the retropectoral passage has ever been reported. The following sections describe the causes of compression and the arterial pathology.

Elements of Compression

Congenital bony abnormalities are the most frequent causative factors. *Cervical ribs* are present in most patients with arterial complications of TOS. The arterial consequences of complete versus incomplete cervical ribs have been emphasized by several investigators.[4–6] Complete long cervical ribs are articulated or fused to a tubercle on the upper aspect of the first thoracic rib, just behind the distal insertion of the anterior scalene muscle. If a large, spatulated anterior end of the cervical rib is present, the resulting arterial compression may be accentuated. Incomplete short cervical ribs do not directly reach the first thoracic rib, although they are commonly associated with a fibrous band that follows the same trajectory as a complete cervical rib. Incomplete cervical ribs, when symptomatic, usually cause nerve compression, whereas complete cervical ribs appear as the main causative factor of arterial compression and complications. These complications may also develop as a result of an incomplete cervical rib or an elongated C7 transverse process, but this occurs much less frequently.[7, 8] In both situations, the bony abnormality is usually prolonged by a fibrous band inserted on the first thoracic rib just behind the tubercle of the anterior scalene muscle.

Congenital abnormalities of the *first thoracic rib* are less common than those of the cervical ribs; however, when present, they seem to be an even more frequent cause of arterial complications than are those of cervical ribs.[9] The most common abnormality is agenesis of the anterior part of the first rib. In these cases, the posterior part of the rib may be articulated with or fused to the second rib in the same manner that a complete cervical rib articulates with a normal first thoracic rib. In other cases, the anterior end of the partially agenetic first rib may be free and pulled upward by the anterior scalene muscle that inserts on it. Synostosis of the first two ribs,[6] bifidity,[10] or an abnormal tubercle of the first rib[11] are less frequently encountered.

Isolated *congenital bands,* as well as hypertrophic anterior scalene muscles, have been described in a small number of patients with arterial complications of TOS, although they are mainly responsible for neurologic symptoms.[11–14]

Acquired bony abnormalities affecting mainly the clavicle and, less frequently, the first thoracic rib are even less common.[15] Malunion of a fractured clavicle is more likely to cause arterial problems than is a hypertrophic callus. Anecdotal cases of hypertrophic callus or exostosis of the first thoracic rib, as well as cases of sequelae of osteomyelitis of the clavicle, have also been reported.

Whatever its cause, location, and mechanism, arterial compression is usually intermittent at its onset. Later, it becomes permanent as a result of various physiologic, pathologic, or traumatic factors. The most important of these factors is the physiologic drooping of the shoulder girdle, which usually takes place during the 3rd decade of life, especially in women.[5, 11] Whiplash cervical injuries may also precipitate arterial compression by causing trauma and subsequent fibrosis of the scalene muscles.

Arterial Lesions

The initial consequence of a tight, long-standing compression of the SA in the costoscalene or costoclavicular passage of the thoracic outlet is a localized stenosis. Even after many years, this lesion is probably entirely reversible by surgical decompression. However, with the passage of time and the mechanical trauma caused by shoulder motion, the arterial wall becomes thick and fibrotic, and inflammatory changes of the adventitia fix the artery to the surrounding structures. In most cases, a post-stenotic dilatation develops and is a characteristic complication of arterial compression in the thoracic outlet caused by the fragility of the SA in young persons. The most common mechanism of this dilatation, at least in compressions in the costoscalene passage, is post-stenotic turbulence,[5] which is secondary not only to the presence of a tight stenosis but also to an angulation in the frontal plane. Indeed, the bony abnormality usually pushes the artery upward in the lower cervical region, resulting in its acute angulation before it reaches the axillary region. The resulting vibrations and abnormal wall shear stress affect the fragile arterial wall, distending and rupturing components of the media and thus giving rise to a circumferential dilatation of the artery.[16, 17] Localized jet lesions may be present in very tight stenoses and account for the rare occurrence of saccular aneurysms. Similarly, repeated trauma from the moving clavicle may be responsible for a localized lesion of the upper aspect of the SA when compression takes place in the costoclavicular passage.

As described in Figure 70–1, these arterial lesions have several consequences, of which thromboembolic complications are the most common and potentially the most dangerous. An intimal lesion may occur either at the site of compression and stenosis of the SA (Fig. 70–2) or in the post-stenotic dilatation, often at the site of impact of the post-stenotic jet (Fig. 70–3). When distal pulses are normal, distal microembolization of platelet aggregates formed on this intimal lesion is now commonly considered to be the usual mechanism of Raynaud's syndrome and digital necrosis occurring as a complication of TOS. These microemboli are especially frequent in the thumb and index finger, probably as a result of the straightforward pathway through the radial artery as opposed to that through the ulnar artery. The formation of a mural thrombus is even more ominous.[18] Although mechanical factors are usually predominant, they may be accelerated by hematologic or hormonal disturbances, including the use of contraceptive pills.[1, 8] Ischemic consequences of the resulting macroembolization vary according to the site and extent of the distal occlusion. An isolated proximal embolus often has less serious consequences than a more distal one, owing to the greater possibilities of collateral circulation. If the SA abnormality is not corrected early, emboli will occur repeatedly, with progressive obliteration of the distal arterial bed and aggravation of the ischemia. In some cases, effective treatment may be impossible and major irreversible ischemia will follow. Thrombotic occlusion of the SA is rarely encountered, but when it does occur, occlusion usually remains initially limited to the subclavian and axillary arteries and a good collateral circulation develops. In these cases, distal ischemia is usually mild or even absent. When it occurs after many episodes of distal embolization, ischemia is usually severe and may even be irreversible because of difficulties in clearing the distal arterial bed. Retrograde embolization in the cerebral arteries, although rare, is a serious potential complication.[19, 20]

CLINICAL SYMPTOMS

Diagnosis is rarely made at an early stage, before the appearance of thromboembolic complications. Three different clinical situations may result in an early diagnosis: (1) a pulsatile supraclavicular mass revealing an asymptomatic subclavian aneurysm;[21] (2) isolated neurologic symptoms associated with a cervical rib or any bony abnormality of the thoracic outlet, a situation that, in the authors' opinion, warrants arteriography or an ultrasound study; and (3) an incidental finding in an arteriogram obtained for a symptomatic lesion of the opposite upper extremity.

In many cases, the disease remains undiagnosed until thromboembolic complications occur. The most frequent early symptoms are due to embolic occlusions of the digital arteries or palmar arch. Raynaud's syndrome or its equivalents, including episodic pallor, cyanosis, or both; paresthesiae; coldness; pain; and cold sensitivity of the hands and digits are commonly found at this stage of the disease. They must be recognized as vascular symptoms and their source properly managed before further showers of microemboli or a larger embolus results in ischemic lesions of the fingertips or even frank gangrene of part or all of one or more digits.[22] In the presence of such distal vascular findings, the following facts favor the diagnosis of arterioarterial embolism: (1) late age of onset; (2) predominant distribution in the radial artery of the hands and digits; (3) absence of other etiology, such as collagen vascular disease, occupational arterial trauma, or Buerger's disease; and (4) a strictly unilateral nature, clearly indicating their secondary origin.[6, 11] Although digital gangrene is diagnostic of arterial occlusion, Raynaud's syndrome or its equivalents may offer special clinical difficulties. Even if a TOS is recognized, these symptoms may have been wrongly attributed to sympathetic irritation because of nerve compression;[6] as a result, the arterial complications may be overlooked. Another diagnostic difficulty may arise from the coincidence of a

Arterial Compression

ARTERIAL STENOSIS

Poststenotic Dilatation

ANEURYSM

INTIMAL LESION

Thrombosis

Platelet Aggregates

Subclavian Artery Occlusion

Macroembolization

Microembolization

Distal

Retrograde

Distal

UPPER LIMB ISCHEMIA

Central Neurologic Complications (rare)

DISTAL ISCHEMIA RAYNAUD'S SYNDROME

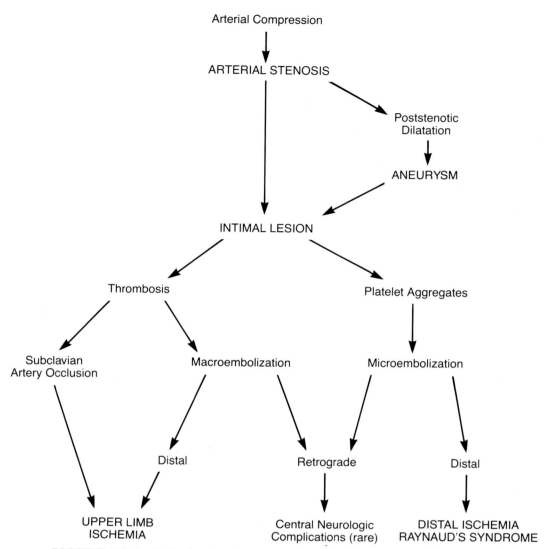

FIGURE 70–1. Pathophysiology of arterial complications of thoracic outlet syndrome.

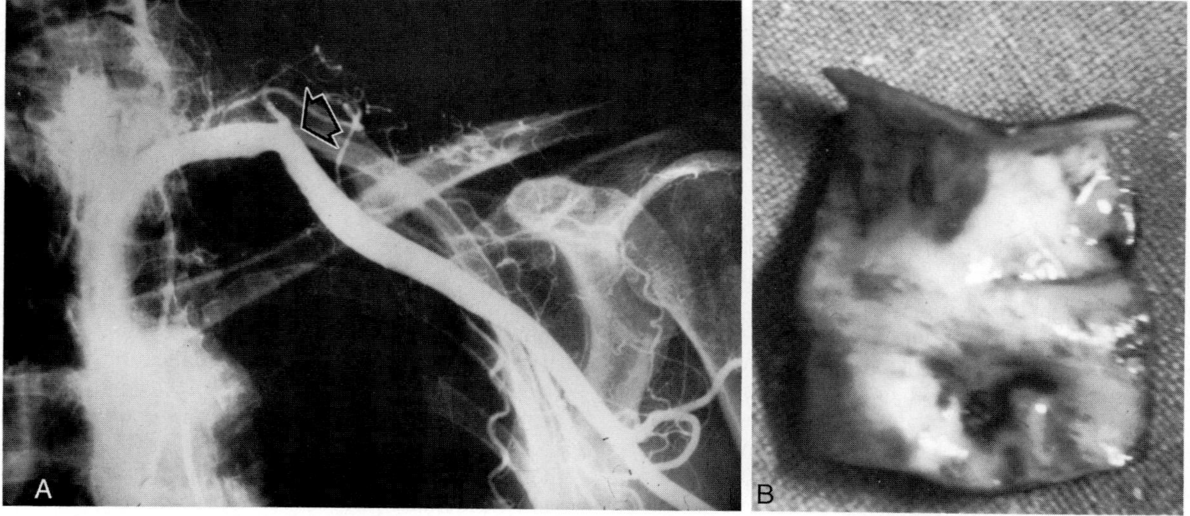

FIGURE 70–2. Preoperative arteriogram *(A)* and operative specimen *(B)* of a patient with unilateral Raynaud's syndrome and an ulcerated plaque at the point of compression of the subclavian artery by a cervical rib (*open arrow* in *A*).

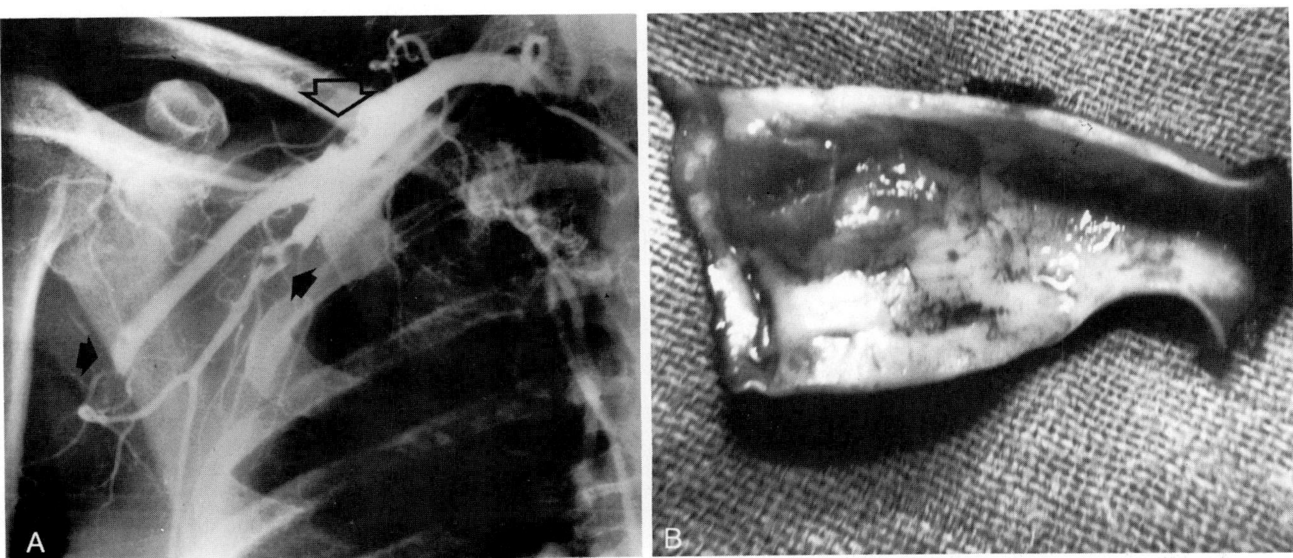

FIGURE 70–3. Preoperative arteriogram *(A)* and operative specimen *(B)* of a patient with acute embolic ischemia of the arm (*black arrows* in *A*) due to post-stenotic dilatation with mural thrombus of the subclavian-axillary artery (*open arrow* in *A*) secondary to an anomalous first thoracic rib.

cervical rib and Raynaud's syndrome from a different etiology, because both entities are sometimes encountered in a patient.

Microembolization may last months or even years before major embolic complications occur. Acute ischemia due to proximal embolism is the most frequent complication. A proximal arterial source accounts for 25 to 50 per cent of all upper extremity emboli,[23] and of these, complications of TOS are the most common. This source must be suspected in the presence of any proximal embolus in the upper extremity, especially if a cardiac source is not found. A major error would be to proceed to a standard isolated embolectomy only.[5, 13, 14, 24] This first episode of embolization usually has a favorable outcome, even if it is not surgically treated. The resulting ischemia may become subacute or chronic or even completely disappear owing to the development of collateral circulation; however, sooner or later, embolization will recur if its cause has not been eradicated through proper management. In these cases, ischemia becomes severe, it does not regress spontaneously, and surgical management becomes extremely difficult because of multiple emboli of different ages located at various levels in the limb. The outcome may be unfavorable in the more advanced cases, with major amputations becoming necessary. Subacute or chronic ischemia is usually produced by a proximal segmental occlusion with good collateral circulation. In a few cases, usually with isolated SA occlusion, ischemia does not develop, and it may be difficult to establish the differential diagnosis of chronic occlusions because of trauma, cardiogenic embolism, or even Takayasu's arteritis.

DIAGNOSTIC METHODS

Diagnosis is usually easy if the possibility of a TOS is considered when the clinician is faced with a patient who has an ischemic upper extremity. A clinical *history* of a fractured clavicle or first rib, with late complications of hypertrophic callus, malunion, or both, may suggest the diagnosis. More frequently, the presence of a cervical rib may have been known for some time from a previous chest roentgenogram. Symptoms secondary to associated nerve compression are present in only one third of cases.

The diagnosis may be established by *physical examination.* A pulsatile mass in the supraclavicular area is often palpable but does not usually correspond to the SA aneurysm itself. A more precise examination usually shows that the palpable abnormality is the bony abnormality pushing the artery upward; the arterial dilatation is slightly more distal, behind the clavicle. A bruit may be heard over the SA, occasionally only in extreme positions of the upper extremity. These positions may also diminish or even abolish the distal pulses. Although these findings have some value in these clinical circumstances, they are not specific because they are often present in normal persons.

Anteroposterior and oblique cervical spine and upper thoracic *roentgenograms* are most important because a bony abnormality is nearly always present. As previously mentioned, the most frequent is a cervical rib, usually long, complete, and fused or articulated to the first rib. Agenesis of the anterior part of the first thoracic rib is less commonly found; still rarer are other congenital abnormalities of the first rib or acquired abnormalities of the clavicle or first rib. The absence of a bony abnormality, however, should not rule out the diagnosis of arterial complications of TOS because a few cases have been described in which only muscular or fibrous elements of compression are present.

Noninvasive techniques have been used in the investigation of these patients. Doppler examination may be useful in describing and quantifying the postural changes in arterial circulation of the upper extremity. It may also localize the arterial occlusion and assess the collateral circulation. B-mode ultrasonography is useful in establishing the diag-

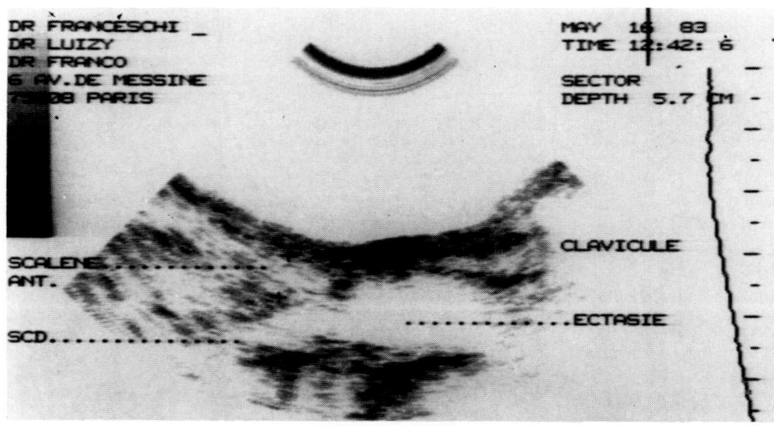

FIGURE 70–4. Ultrasonogram of a case of post-stenotic aneurysm of the subclavian artery.

nosis of post-stenotic dilatation (Fig. 70–4) and mural thrombus.

The *arteriogram* should visualize the entire upper extremity, from the aortic arch to the digital arteries. The usual technique is catheterization through the femoral artery and selective injection in the proximal SA.* Arteriographic diagnosis of arterial complications of TOS is not always easy.[24] Subtraction techniques are useful. A fusiform aneurysm is usually evident, especially if situated distal to a permanent arterial stenosis (Fig. 70–5). An irregular lining or filling defects strongly suggest the presence of mural thrombus (see Fig. 70–3). Arteriographic findings are seldom entirely normal, and some features may be difficult to recognize. Mural thrombus may obliterate part of the aneurysmal sac. In symptomatic patients, even the smallest post-stenotic dilatation is a strong clue to the diagnosis, and in these patients, mural thrombus will often be found at operation. The SA stenosis is not always evident on the anteroposterior view because compression in the costoscalene passage takes place in the same plane. Dynamic views will help define the exact site of compression. Arteriography is also helpful in demonstrating distal arterial occlusions and the development of the collateral circulation. In the presence of Raynaud's syndrome or distal gangrene due to occlusive disease of the digital arteries, magnification films, including those obtained after the intra-arterial injection of a vasodilator, may help in differentiating between local lesions and emboli.[25]

In a small number of patients with cervical ribs or other bony abnormalities and symptoms of thromboembolic disease of the upper extremity, the SA may appear grossly normal or only slightly dilated on the arteriogram (Fig. 70–6). In these rare situations, the authors strongly advocate *surgical exploration* as an integral part of the diagnostic work-up. Intraoperative arterial palpation is unreliable and may be dangerous because it entails the risk of mobilizing the thrombus, with further distal embolization. The authors believe that an exploratory longitudinal arteriotomy is best in these cases. This seemingly aggressive attitude is the only way to rule out with certainty a small intimal lesion, which must be treated if recurrent emboli are to be avoided.[7, 6, 10, 11] If the arterial intima appears normal, it is very simple to close the artery using a continuous suture, tailoring it to correct the post-stenotic dilatation.

*It should be remembered that if no lesion is visualized, this technique can miss a lesion near the origin of the SA.

SURGICAL MANAGEMENT

The treatment of arterial complications of TOS is surgical. Surgery must often be performed on an emergency or a semi-emergency basis, not only in the presence of acute or subacute ischemia of the upper extremity but also every time a mural thrombus has been recognized, because severe embolic complications are unpredictable and may rapidly become difficult to manage.[7] The three anatomic components of the disease process—arterial compression, subclavian-axillary arterial lesions, and less consistently, distal emboli—have to be treated simultaneously.

Surgical Approach

An ideal surgical approach should allow simultaneous thoracic outlet decompression, treatment of the subclavian-

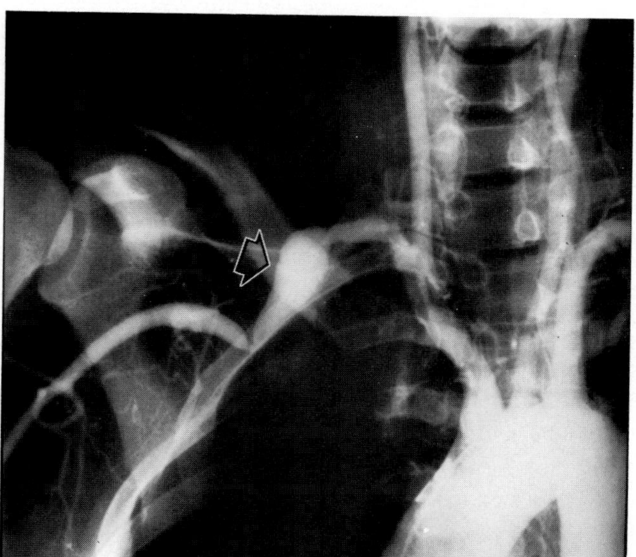

FIGURE 70–5. Post-stenotic aneurysm of the subclavian-axillary artery *(open arrow)* in an asymptomatic patient with a cervical rib.

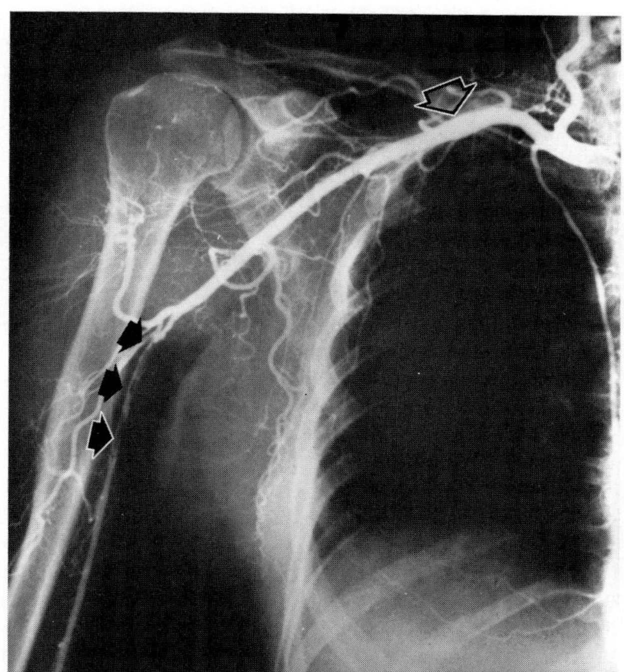

FIGURE 70–6. Minimal post-stenotic dilatation of the subclavian-axillary artery *(open arrow)* in a patient with brachial emboli *(black arrows)* and a cervical rib; mural thrombus of the subclavian-axillary artery was found at operation.

axillary arterial lesions, and upper dorsal sympathectomy if indicated. The whole upper extremity should be accessible to the surgeon to allow for distal embolectomy when necessary.

The *transaxillary approach* is largely used for isolated rib resection in the presence of neurologic symptoms. An associated upper dorsal sympathectomy may be easily added; however, this approach does not offer a satisfactory exposure of the subclavian-axillary artery and is therefore contraindicated in the management of arterial complications. The same objections apply to the *anterolateral thoracic approach.* In addition, a thoracic incision is an unwarranted surgical maneuver, even in young or middle-aged patients.

The *transclavicular approach* allows a wide exposure of the supraclavicular and axillary regions. One of two techniques may be used. Although temporary transection of the mid-part of the clavicle, followed by osteosynthesis, seems logical, it may lead to orthopedic complications such as malunion, hypertrophic callus of the clavicle, or both, with or without infection.[8] Resection of the mid-part or the medial two thirds of the clavicle is simpler and has a low incidence of cosmetic and functional impairment;[1, 11] however, because the same surgical procedures can be performed without dividing the clavicle using a supraclavicular approach, the only indications for clavicular resection are the rare cases of arterial complications from malunion or hypertrophic callus of the clavicle.

The *supraclavicular approach* offers complete exposure of the SA, a cervical rib, and muscular or fibrous bands.[11] With this approach, resection of the normal first rib is simple and safe, provided that the SA and the brachial plexus are entirely dissected and that the entire upper extremity is prepared and draped so that it may be raised when resection of the anterior part of the rib is undertaken. Complete resection of the posterior part of the first rib is easily achieved, and it is straightforward to detect and treat any type of associated muscular or fibrous abnormality. Difficulties may arise in the presence of arterial lesions extending to the axillary artery. In these cases, additional exposure is obtained through a deltopectoral or infraclavicular incision, leaving the clavicle undisturbed.[2, 3, 7]

Thoracic Outlet Decompression

Complete resection of a cervical rib or an abnormal first rib is obviously necessary. It seems logical to add routine resection of the normal first rib as is done in the more common neurologic forms of TOS. Clavicular resection should be performed in cases of malunion or hypertrophic callus complicating a fractured clavicle. In any case, resection of the bony abnormality must be accompanied by removal of any abnormal muscular or fibrous element. Scalenectomy seems definitely preferable to scalenotomy because the scalene muscles may reattach themselves to the bed of the resected cervical or first rib and be responsible for recurrent arterial or nerve compression.

Proximal Arterial Reconstruction

Arterial reconstruction is necessary in the presence of an arterial aneurysm or mural thrombosis, with or without distal thromboembolic complications. However, mild post-stenotic dilatation without clinical or radiologic evidence of mural thrombus deserves discussion. Many surgeons still consider this entity an indication for conservative management because of its anticipated regression after isolated arterial decompression.[4, 8, 21] The authors believe that it does not always represent a benign condition and dictates at least surgical exploration. The presence of intimal arterial disease or mural thrombus is difficult to rule out unless an exploratory arteriotomy is performed. Very few cases of actual regression of the dilatation after isolated arterial decompression have been reported. Severe arterial complications have been regularly reported after these conservative procedures.[10] Although the initial arterial lesions have not always been described precisely, these cases constitute a strong argument in favor of direct arterial reconstruction in the presence of a seemingly benign post-stenotic dilatation.

Surgical techniques have to be tailored to the arterial lesions. Resection is needed in the presence of a subclavian-axillary aneurysm. Excessive arterial length is usually obtained after resection of the cervical and first thoracic ribs; this allows for end-to-end anastomosis in most cases.[2, 3] In the presence of a lengthy arterial dilatation, a short segment of graft may have to be interposed to bridge the arterial defect. The preferred graft material is autogenous saphenous vein. When this material is unavailable, the authors favor the use of an arterial autograft[24] rather than a Dacron or polytetrafluoroethylene graft.

A mild fusiform post-stenotic dilatation should be opened longitudinally along its entire length and closed

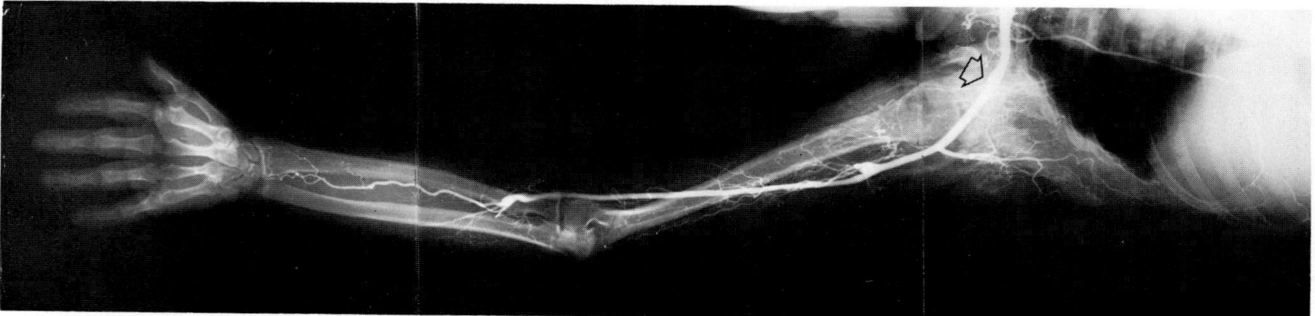

FIGURE 70–7. Postoperative arteriogram 4 years after bony decompression of thoracic outlet, resection and anastomosis of a subclavian aneurysm *(open arrow)*, embolectomy of the axillary and proximal brachial artery, upper dorsal sympathectomy, and brachial artery–interosseous artery saphenous vein bypass.

with a continuous tailoring suture after an intimal lesion has been ruled out or treated either by intimectomy or limited segmental resection. Although this technique appears easy and appealing, it may sometimes be difficult to perform. The use of an internal stent may be necessary for a suitable aneurysmorrhaphy. Proximal or distal transection of the artery may also be useful in dealing with arterial lesions extending behind the clavicle. This allows visualization of the entire diseased artery through the supra- or infraclavicular incision. After the aneurysmorrhaphy has been performed, the artery is placed in its normal position and an end-to-end anastomosis is performed. A limited arterial resection may be added if excessive arterial length is present.

In rare cases, an isolated intimal fibrous plaque without any associated arterial dilatation may be treated by intimectomy, with or without patch angioplasty closure of the artery.

Management of Distal Embolic Occlusions

Distal embolic occlusions often introduce major difficulties in the surgical treatment of these patients. They are usually multiple and diffuse, with emboli of different ages. Some occlusions are recent and easily cleared by thromboembolectomy; others are older, adherent to the arterial wall, and inaccessible to direct or indirect embolectomy. In such cases, unsuccessful surgical attempts at disobliteration may result in extensive thrombosis. In the presence of a seemingly old and well-compensated distal embolic occlusion, direct surgical treatment is to be avoided.[2, 3] In most of these cases, upper dorsal sympathectomy is probably all that is required.

If the distal arterial occlusion involves the large arteries, is apparently of recent onset, and results in severe distal ischemia, an attempt at direct revascularization is appropriate. It may be possible to perform an embolectomy by introducing a Fogarty balloon catheter through the distal SA at the site of proximal reconstruction. Distal passage of the catheter through the entire upper extremity is often difficult or impossible. Selective catheterization of the radial and ulnar arteries may also be difficult, and a separate approach to the brachial artery bifurcation is usually necessary. An intraoperative arteriogram is advisable in most cases. Persisting occlusion of the forearm or hand arteries requires a direct approach to the radial artery, the ulnar artery, or both, at the wrist. Selective embolectomy of the palmar arches is performed using a No. 2 Fogarty balloon catheter; closure of the arteriotomy is made under loupe magnification. In the presence of a chronic brachial occlusion, complicated by a proximal recent embolus, it may be sufficient to revascularize the deep brachial artery,[10] which plays the same physiologic collateral role in the upper extremity as does the deep femoral artery in the lower extremity, provided that the periarticular arterial network of the elbow is patent.

If embolectomy is impossible, ineffective, or incomplete, a distal bypass using autogenous vein may be performed in an attempt to revascularize one of the forearm arteries, usually the interosseous artery (Fig. 70–7).

Difficulty in clearing the distal arterial bed accounts for the incomplete revascularization of the forearm and hand in the most advanced cases. A large number of major amputations are still reported, often after multiple surgical attempts to revascularize the upper extremity.[1, 11, 24] Distal amputations are mentioned in most large series, and some patients, although they have a viable upper limb, will suffer disabling ischemic sequelae such as Raynaud's syndrome, Volkmann's contracture, claudication, or fatigability of the forearm. These results are in sharp contrast to those obtained in the absence of distal embolization, where clinical and anatomic results are consistently good if the initial surgical management has been appropriate.

References

1. Judy KL, Heymann RL: Vascular complications of thoracic outlet syndrome. Am J Surg 123:521, 1972.
2. Kieffer E, Jue-Denis P, Benhamou M, et al: Complications artérielles du syndrome de la traversée thoraco-brachiale: Traitement chirurgical de 38 cas. Chirurgie 109:714, 1983.
3. Cormier JM, Amrane M, Ward A, et al: Arterial complications of the thoracic outlet syndrome: Fifty-five operative cases. J Vasc Surg 9:778, 1989.
4. Blank RH, Connar RG: Arterial complications associated with thoracic outlet syndrome. Ann Thorac Surg 17:315, 1974.
5. Short DW: The subclavian artery in 16 patients with complete cervical ribs. J Cardiovasc Surg 16:135, 1975.
6. Swinton NW Jr, Hall RJ, Baugh JH, et al: Unilateral Raynaud's phenomenon caused by cervical–first rib anomalies. Am J Med 48:404, 1970.

7. Martin J, Gaspard DJ, Johnston PW, et al: Vascular manifestations of the thoracic outlet syndrome. A surgical urgency. Arch Surg 111:779, 1976.
8. Mercier C, Houel F, David G, et al: Les complications vasculaires des syndromes de la traversée thoraco-brachiale. Chirurgie 107:433, 1981.
9. Dumeige F, Andre J, Vargas R, et al: Les complications vasculaires des anomalies de la première côte. Chirurgie 112:584, 1986.
10. Banis JC Jr, Rich N, Whelan TJ Jr: Ischemia of the upper extremity due to noncardiac emboli. Am J Surg 134:131, 1977.
11. Bouhoutsos J, Morris T, Martin P: Unilateral Raynaud's phenomenon in the hand and its significance. Surgery 82:547, 1977.
12. Roos DB: Congenital anomalies associated with thoracic outlet syndrome. Am J Surg 132:771, 1976.
13. Dorazio RA, Ezzet F: Arterial complications of the thoracic outlet syndrome. Am J Surg 138:246, 1979.
14. Simon H, Gryska PF, Carlson DH: The thoracic outlet syndrome as a cause of aneurysm formation, thrombosis, and embolization. South Med J 70:282, 1977.
15. Melliere D, Escourrou J, Becquemin JP, et al: Ischémies aigues des membres: Complications tardives de cals hypertrophiques et de pseudarthroses. J Chir (Paris) 118:641, 1981.
16. Roach MR: Changes in arterial distensibility as a cause of poststenotic dilatation. Am J Cardiol 12:802, 1963.
17. Ojha M, Johnson KW, Cobbold RSC: Evidence of a possible link between poststenotic dilation and wall shear stress. J Vasc Surg 11:127, 1990.
18. Gunning AJ, Pickering GW, Robb-Smith AHT, et al: Mural thrombosis of the subclavian artery and subsequent embolism in cervical rib. Q J Med 129:133, 1964.
19. Al-Hassen HK, Sattar MA, Eklof B: Embolic brain infarction: A rare complication of thoracic outlet syndrome. A report of two cases. J Cardiovasc Surg 29:322, 1988.
20. De Villiers JC: A brachiocephalic vascular syndrome associated with cervical rib. Br Med J 2:140, 1966.
21. Pairolero PC, Walls JT, Payne WS, et al: Subclavian axillary artery aneurysms. Surgery 90:757, 1981.
22. Vayssairat M, Fiessinger JN, Housset E: Les nécroses digitales du membre supérieur: 86 cas. Nouv Presse Med 6:931, 1977.
23. Sachatello CR, Ernst CB, Griffen WO Jr: The acutely ischemic upper extremity: Selective management. Surgery 76:1002, 1974.
24. Etheredge S, Wilbur R, Stoney RJ: Thoracic outlet syndrome. Am J Surg 138:175, 1979.
25. Maiman MH, Bookstein JJ, Bernstein EF: Digital ischemia: Angiographic differentiation of embolism from primary arterial disease. Am J Roentgenol 137:1183, 1981.

71

Axillary-Subclavian Vein Thrombosis

Herbert I. Machleder, M.D.

• • •

In 1949, Hughes wrote, "The association of a more or less acute venous obstruction in the upper extremity of an otherwise perfectly healthy person constitutes a syndrome which, in the absence of accurate knowledge of the etiology and pathology, can be called the 'Paget-Schroetter syndrome,' after the first two to describe it as a clinical entity." He additionally credited Ranzi, of Pisa (1849), with being the first to suggest "effort" as the cause of the thrombosis.[1]

Since the time of Hughes' seminal review, it has been recognized that thrombosis of the axillary and subclavian veins occurs in a variety of clinical settings. It has become evident that the natural history and the development of symptoms are more often a consequence of the underlying pathologic anatomy than of the resulting thrombotic process even though the fundamental presenting abnormality may appear similar for primary and secondary subclavian vein occlusion. Significant disability (and pulmonary embolism), for example, is much more apt to follow thrombosis associated with thoracic outlet compression syndrome than thrombosis developing from central venous catheterization.[2–4]

There has been increasing use of the upper extremity veins for diagnostic venipuncture, intravenous infusion, central venous monitoring, long-term parenteral lines, indwelling cardiac pacemaker wires, and access for short- and long-term hemodialysis. One adverse consequence of the evolving importance of these veins for circulatory and cardiac access is the growing frequency of axillary-subclavian vein thrombosis. These contemporary iatrogenic problems have now been added to the traditionally recognized causes of venous thrombosis, which include spontaneous or effort thrombosis and systemic predisposing diseases such as neoplasm and myocardial failure.

PRIMARY THROMBOSIS: THE PAGET-SCHROETTER SYNDROME

Etiology and Pathogenesis

Primary thrombosis (also referred to as spontaneous or effort-related thrombosis) is a disorder of young, otherwise healthy individuals. Lowenstein studied the possible mechanical nature of what he suspected was venous compression and subsequent thrombosis. He noted that the subclavius tendon and the costocoracoid ligament, which follow the course of the clavicle, extend laterally from their insertion at the claviculosternal–first chondral junction. In some individuals (particularly those with subclavius muscle hypertrophy), during abduction of the arm, these structures cause compression of the vein against the underlying first rib and laterally against the scalenus anticus muscle (Fig. 71–1). Casts made of the vein often show a prominent ridge in this area.[5]

In addition, dissections have demonstrated a valve in the subclavian vein immediately adjacent to the lateral border of the first rib. At the time of surgical exploration or of follow-up venography after thrombolytic therapy, it has become evident that the subclavian vein is thickened, narrowed, and fibrotic at the border of the first rib. The valve often shows fibrosis and contraction of the leaflets. It has been suggested that the vein is progressively damaged during exercise by repetitive compression in the costoclavicular space, with consequent intimal roughening and thickening and subsequent thrombosis.[6, 7]

The possibility of an underlying coagulation abnormality has been suggested by several investigators. Blood hypercoagulability has not been substantiated as a common cause but may be of some significance in a select group of patients with either primary or secondary upper extremity venous thrombosis. Sundquist and coworkers studied the coagulation profiles of 60 consecutive patients with upper extremity venous thrombosis and noted that 16 per cent of the patients were taking conjugated estrogens for birth control.[8] Forty-nine per cent of these patients had defective

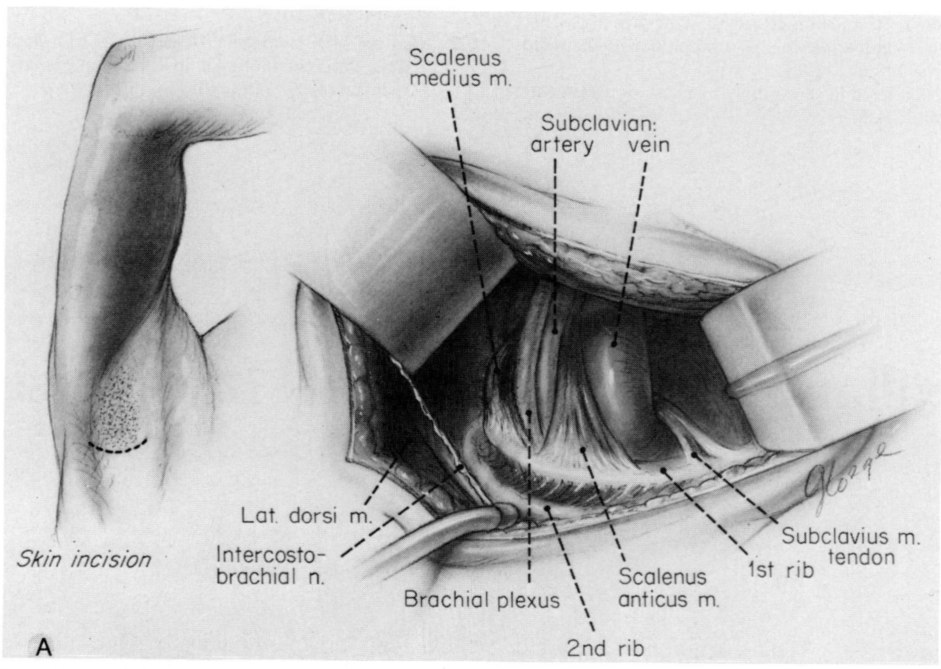

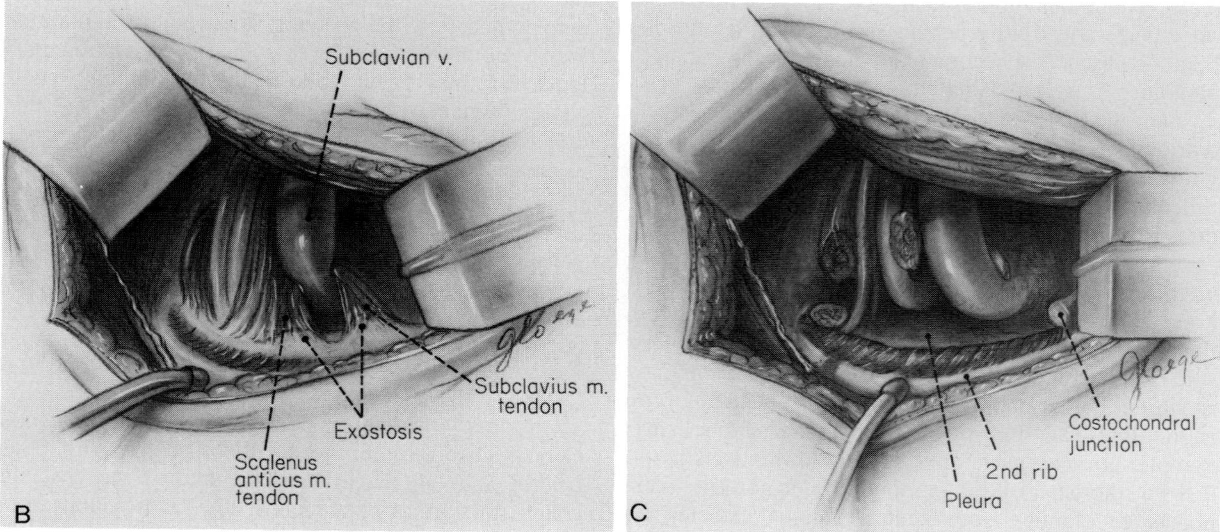

FIGURE 71–1. *A*, Anatomic relationship of structures of the thoracic outlet as seen from the transaxillary surgical approach. *B*, Compression of the axillary-subclavian vein seen in patients with the Paget-Schroetter variant of the thoracic outlet compression syndrome. *C*, Configuration of the thoracic outlet after removal of the first rib and lysis of the axillary-subclavian vein. (*A–C*, From Kunkel JM, Machleder HI: Treatment of Paget-Schroetter syndrome: A staged, multidisciplinary approach. Arch Surg 124:1153–1156, 1989. Copyright 1989, American Medical Association.)

fibrinolytic capacity, as measured in the circulation, or decreased fibrinolytic capacity of the venous endothelium, as measured in cephalic vein biopsy specimens from both the affected and contralateral arms. In contrast, patients with deep venous thrombosis of the lower extremity veins were found to have a 70 per cent incidence of impaired fibrinolytic defense mechanisms. It is unclear whether these changes represent a primary abnormality, a secondary abnormality, or a residual hematologic abnormality following an episode of thrombosis. Although coagulation and fibrinolytic changes may have significance in some female patients, upper extremity venous thrombosis of the Paget-Schroetter variety in men is almost certainly a direct consequence of structural compressive changes.

An accurate summary of the considerable literature on the subject indicates that acute thrombosis almost invariably arises in an area of chronic compression and stricture of the axillary-subclavian vein at the thoracic outlet. The vein is compressed between a hypertrophied scalene or subclavius tendon and the underlying first rib. A large exostosis is often found adjacent to the costosternal-clavicular junction at the insertion of the subclavius tendon (see Fig. 71–1).

Epidemiology

In all reported series, there is a male predominance, as well as a right upper extremity predominance. The thrombotic episode often follows upper extremity exertion, a factor recognized by the frequently used term *effort thrombosis* as well as by the association with thoracic outlet compression syndrome. In a University of California–Los Angeles study of 50 consecutive patients, 30 per cent were engaged in competitive sports, 36 per cent were laborers, and 34 per cent were sedentary workers. Seventy-six per cent of the patients had onset of the syndrome associated with vigorous use of the upper extremity.[9]

Although neurogenic thoracic outlet syndrome is far more common in women, the vascular complications are more common in men. Venous thrombosis is reported to occur in 1.5 to 12 per cent of patients presenting with thoracic outlet syndrome; conversely, the coincidence with thoracic outlet compression has been reported in 80 per cent of patients who present with Paget-Schroetter syndrome.[10, 11] In the University of California–Los Angeles series, vascular complications predominated in 15 per cent of the patients presenting with one of the thoracic outlet compression syndromes.

Clinical Features

There will almost invariably be complaints of swelling in the extremity, either arising rapidly or appearing slowly over a period of several weeks. Increased prominence of the veins in the hand and forearm, as well as a prominent venous pattern over the shoulder and hemithorax, is commonly noted and is often associated with a subtle cyanosis or mottling of the skin. Although severe pain is rarely reported, there are common complaints of heaviness and discomfort in the arm, which are exacerbated by activity and relieved by rest.

In the natural history of this disorder, resumption of normal activity after a period of recuperation following the episode of thrombosis frequently leads to symptoms related to upper extremity venous hypertension, which are exacerbated by using the arms in the overhead position. This position can be demonstrated venographically to occlude collateral vessels traversing the thoracic outlet. A number of patients also develop symptoms of neurogenic thoracic outlet syndrome, with radicular dysesthesias and muscle weakness such as a loss of grip strength and fine motor coordination.

Contrary to a frequently encountered opinion, repeated venography rarely shows recanalization following anticoagulant therapy alone, despite almost uniform clinical improvement and almost total absence of symptoms at rest after about 6 weeks of treatment. However, these patients are likely to have symptoms of venous hypertension during vigorous upper extremity activity and to remain at risk for recurrent thrombosis after early discontinuation of anticoagulation therapy.

The incidence of disabling symptoms related to the development of venous hypertension after an episode of axillary-subclavian vein thrombosis has been addressed by several authors. It ranges from a low of 25 per cent reported by Linblad and associates (Sweden)[13] to 40 per cent reported by Gloviczki and colleagues (Mayo Clinic),[2] 47 per cent reported by Donayre and associates (Los Angeles),[3] and 74 per cent reported by Tilney and coworkers (Boston).[12]

Although no episodes of pulmonary embolism were identified in the 320 pre-1949 cases reviewed by Hughes, a single case was reported in 1951 as part of a review of 300 cases.[14] In more recent publications, the incidence of pulmonary embolism has ranged between 10 and 30 per cent, depending on the diagnostic criteria and the tests used.[4] The increased incidence may be a function of better recognition with the use of more sophisticated techniques (e.g., arterial blood gas measurements, ventilation-perfusion scans, and pulmonary venography) rather than of a change in the epidemiology. Episodes of pulmonary embolism can occur during the acute thrombotic episode or subsequently, coincident with the recrudescence of arm symptoms that usually indicate recurrent thrombosis or extension of the original thrombotic process.

The incidence of symptoms seems to be lower in patients who have undergone at least 3 months of anticoagulation than in those treated by other conservative measures (72 per cent had good results vs 35 per cent).

The natural history of the disease reflects the development of venous hypertension due to chronic venous compression, with acute symptoms resulting from sudden thrombosis and obstruction of collateral veins. After resolution of acute thrombotic manifestations, patients may be relatively free of symptoms at rest, with edema resolving fairly promptly within 1 to 3 weeks.

Diagnosis

Despite the stereotypic presentation of this condition, the diagnosis is often missed initially.

Physical Examination

Characteristics noted in the physical examination vary with the interval from the onset of venous thrombosis to the time of evaluation. Nonpitting edema involving the forearm, the upper arm, and occasionally the hand and fingers usually resolves within 1 to 3 weeks, despite the possibility of considerable residual symptomatic exacerbation with arm use. Cyanosis, although commonly present initially, likewise resolves within several days to 3 weeks.

With resolution of the acute symptoms, increased collateral circulation is observed around the axilla and shoulder. However, other manifestations of elevated venous pressure are not readily evident during the clinical examination of these patients, and postphlebitic stigmata (characteristic of lower extremity venous thrombosis) are rarely encountered. In the early stages, tenderness to digital pressure over the axillary vein is usually found in the axilla. The vein may be firm and thrombotic or tense and distended, particularly when the arm is abducted. Despite its importance as a collateral venous pathway, the ipsilateral internal jugular vein is not unusually prominent; any enlargement should alert the examiner to the possibility of more central venous obstruction or a superior vena caval syndrome.[15]

Additional signs of neurovascular compression at the thoracic outlet are often evident. About 80 per cent of patients have stress test results positive for arterial compression, as assessed by pulse obliteration or axillary-subclavian artery bruit with Adson's test or with the costoclavicular maneuver. Forty-five per cent of patients will have evidence of brachial plexus compression when assessed by somatosensory evoked responses.[16, 17]

Laboratory Evaluation

Noninvasive Tests. Investigation of upper extremity venous thrombosis has included insonation of the axillary, subclavian, and brachial veins with continuous-wave Doppler assessment, duplex ultrasound scanning, magnetic resonance angiography, thermography, and impedance plethysmography.[18, 19] Computed tomography and magnetic resonance imaging have been helpful in specific cases; however, their overall usefulness in the author's experience is still quite limited. Although the diagnosis can be corroborated by these noninvasive tests, venography is the standard by which the diagnosis is established.[20]

Venography. Venography permits discrimination between stenosis, external compression, and thrombosis, and it identifies the site and extension of the occlusive process. However, proper performance and interpretation of *venography* are far more demanding than of upper extremity *arteriography.* Optimum visualization can be obtained by injection into the basilic vein, initially with the arm at the patient's side and then abducted to 90 degrees. Contrast injected into the cephalic vein may bypass axillary vein thrombus and is subject to increased dilution by collaterals, often failing to visualize the subclavian vein even in the absence of occlusion. Simultaneous bilateral upper extremity venography or transfemoral superior venacavography offers an even better opportunity to demonstrate the pathologic anatomy.

The typical venographic picture will demonstrate thrombosis from the jugular-subclavian junction extending peripherally to the axillary and often the brachial veins. Extension of the clot to involve the origin of the jugular vein, or more centrally, is rarely seen. Occasionally, the thrombus may undergo spontaneous lysis, revealing an irregular vein and a residual compressive abnormality at the costoclavicular space (Fig. 71–2).

The characteristic of high-grade stenosis with probable intermittent occlusion was suspected in 14 of Hughes' collected cases (those in which exploration of the vein failed to reveal any thrombus).[1] This phenomenon was analyzed later in more detail by McCleery and coworkers.[21] When the typical clinical picture is investigated angiographically, intermittent venous obstruction and thrombosis have been described.[22, 23]

When the contralateral vein is studied venographically, thrombosis or a compressive abnormality (or stricture) sufficient to result in collateral vein appearance will be found in about 65 per cent of patients, particularly when the arm is placed in an abducted position.[9, 24]

Venous pressures measured in conjunction with venography can enhance the value of the study, with normal resting values in the peripheral system measuring approximately 5 mmHg.[25] With abduction maneuvers, the occasional normal individual may show a maximum pressure increase of 7 to 9 mmHg, whereas patients with venous obstruction will demonstrate a rise of 12 to 30 mmHg.[11] Postexercise pressures are similarly elevated in affected individuals.[26]

In patients with intermittent subclavian vein compression, which may occasionally precede overt venous thrombosis, the abnormality can be more easily documented venographically in the sitting position than with the patient supine. All supine venography should be performed first with the arm at the side and again with the arm abducted to 90 degrees. The abnormality appears as a beak-like deformity of the subclavian vein at the thoracic outlet. Adams and associates described a group of patients with intermittent obstruction evaluated by venography and saline pressure manometry.[22] Venous pressures taken with the arm at the level of the right atrium, or in the supine neutral position, varied between 12 and 19 cm saline. With the shoulders braced backward and downward or hyperabducted, the asymptomatic side was 12 cm saline and the symptomatic side 37 cm saline.

Treatment

Paget treated his first case for 2 weeks with a "milk diet; six leeches every third night; and three grains of Mercury with chalk every night and morning." The patient "certainly improved, the arm decreasing, and its veins becoming less full. . . . He believed himself well at the end of May."[27] A host of physicians and surgeons (including this author) have attempted to better Paget's putative success.

From the first reported surgical thrombectomy in 1910 by Schepelmann to the present, aggressive surgical therapy has been repeatedly recommended to remove the occluding thrombus and relieve the compressive elements.[7, 28, 29] Nevertheless, primary surgical therapy has never enjoyed much

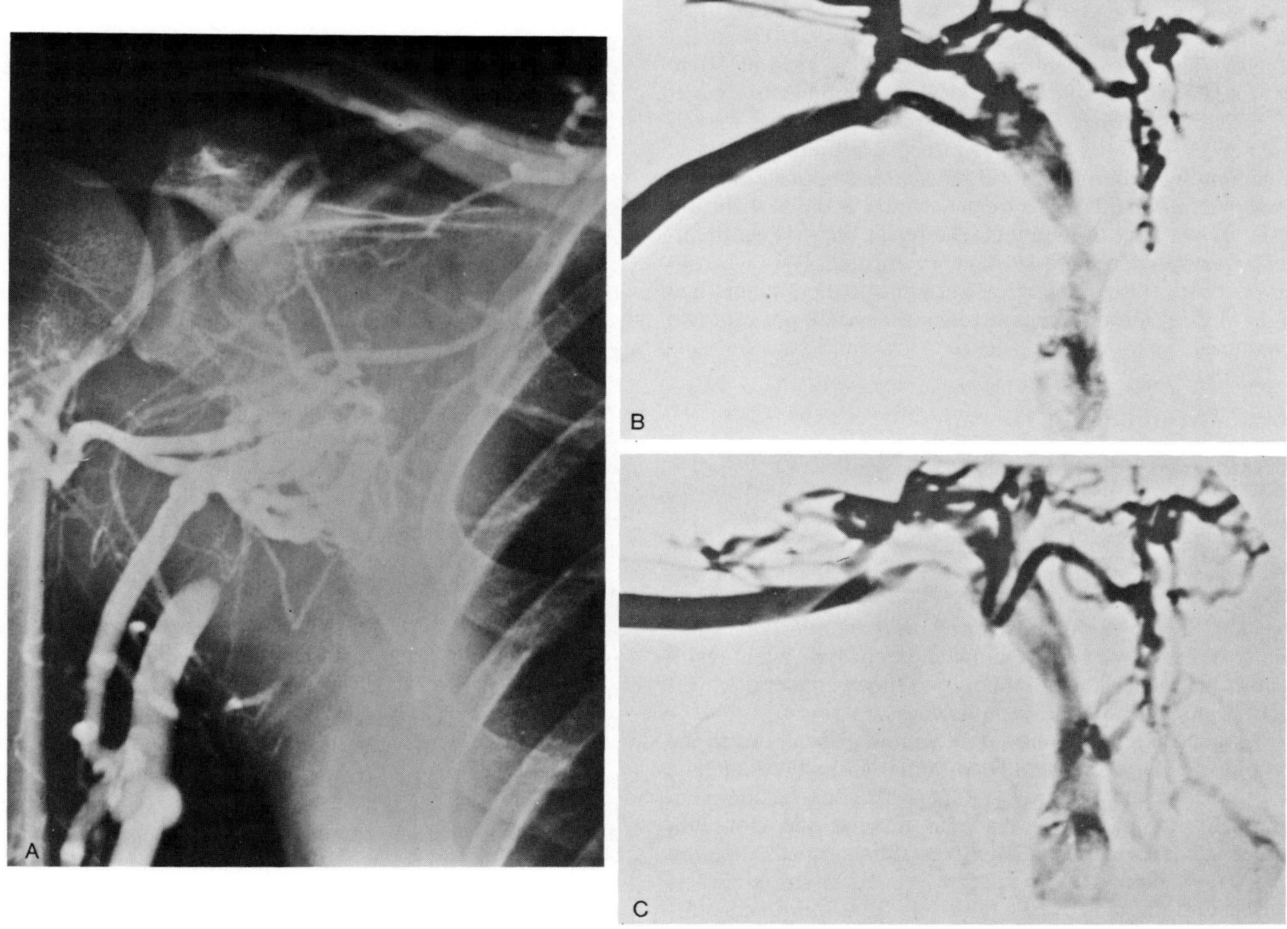

FIGURE 71–2. *A*, Right axillary-subclavian venogram in a 24-year-old woman with spontaneous edema and cyanosis of the right hand and arm. *B*, After clot lysis, a digital subtraction venogram (with the arm in neutral position, at the side) shows an area of venous compression at the thoracic outlet. Note the prominent collateral veins around the narrowed region. *C*, A venogram obtained with the arm in the outstretched position (abducted) shows high-grade compression at the thoracic outlet compared with compression shown with the arm in neutral position. (*A–C*, From Machleder HI: Upper extremity venous thrombosis. Semin Vasc Surg 3:221, 1990.)

success in the treatment of acute venous occlusion, and this experience is reflected in early results of axillary-subclavian thrombectomy.[28] The more favorable results in subsequent reports are difficult to assess in retrospect because follow-up venography was rarely used. Current understanding, based on pre- and posttreatment venographic findings, indicates that early improvement rarely coincides with reconstitution of direct subclavian vein patency. The development of venous collaterals is probably the most significant factor in the resolution of symptoms. Thrombectomy probably fails because of the intimal and structural vein damage that accompanies the thrombotic episode.

Recognition of these suboptimal results and the development of appropriate pharmacologic agents led to repeated attempts to use anticoagulant and thrombolytic therapy to treat the acute thrombus.[30]

Fibrinolytic Therapy

The first clinical trial of streptokinase, in 1959, studied the use of this fibrinolytic agent to dissolve upper extremity venous thrombi.[31] It seems appropriate, therefore, that thrombolytic therapy has reemerged as a primary treatment for the Paget-Schroetter syndrome. Unfortunately, the subsequent reports of the use of streptokinase describe varying results. Steed and associates used streptokinase in the treatment of subclavian vein thrombosis and achieved complete clot lysis in only one patient.[32] In a group of patients reported on by Machleder, 4 of 11 patients (36 per cent) treated with catheter-directed local streptokinase achieved complete clot lysis.[9]

More recently, there has been a shift to urokinase, which has a number of advantages despite its increased cost. It is relatively nonantigenic compared with streptokinase and is also direct acting (in converting plasminogen to the proteolytic enzyme plasmin) rather than having to form an activator complex with plasminogen, as does streptokinase. Both fibrinolytic agents can be used in either a *locally active* or a *systemically active* mode.

In a series of 18 cases reported from Germany in which the systemic thrombolytic approach was used, a loading dose of 150,000 to 250,000 IU of urokinase was followed by an infusion of 1000 to 2000 IU/kg/hr. The loading dose was given over 5 minutes, and all of these patients were given simultaneous heparin at 15 to 17 U/kg/hr. The fibrinogen concentration was kept at 50 to 100 mg/dl, and the activated partial thromboplastin time at 1.5 to 2 times normal. Coagulation parameters were reevaluated every 12 hours for a mean treatment time of 10 days. Treatment was continued for 3 days after demonstrable clot lysis. When patients were treated within 8 days of thrombosis, 82 per cent of the clots underwent lysis. When treatment was initiated after 10 days, no thrombolysis was observed. With this regimen, 39 per cent of the patients had slight bleeding from venopuncture sites and 28 per cent had hematuria.[33]

Local Thrombolytic Therapy

The superiority of local thrombolytic therapy over systemic infusion of fibrinolytic agents has been demonstrated, particularly for the treatment of axillary-subclavian vein thrombosis.[34, 35] This modality has been facilitated by the development of excellent catheter delivery systems and advances in endovascular techniques and equipment. In addition to allowing the avoidance of the systemic lytic state, locally directed and high regional doses of lytic agent result in considerably faster thrombolysis with a concomitant reduction in systemic lytic complications.[36]

After venography and visualization of thrombus in the brachial, axillary, or subclavian veins, a small catheter is positioned in the clot via the percutaneous basilic vein approach. An attempt is made to traverse the clot with either a guidewire or a catheter to establish a channel before infusion. A loading dose of 250,000 IU of urokinase is infused into the clot over 1 hour (4000 IU/min), and infusion is continued at this rate for an additional hour and then reduced to 1000 IU/min for up to 24 hours. Optimally, the catheter is kept within the visualized thrombus throughout the course of the infusion.[36]

Systemic heparinization is used to maintain the partial thromboplastin time at 1.5 times the control value if there is any evidence of thrombus formation in the segment of vein traversed by the catheter or if a prolonged thrombolytic infusion is anticipated after review of the initial response. After discontinuation of the fibrinolytic agent, full heparinization is maintained until anticoagulation with warfarin achieves a prothrombin time of 1.5 to 2 times control values. Warfarin anticoagulation is continued for 3 months to allow the phlebitic process and endothelial damage to resolve.[16, 36, 37]

Although follow-up venography after fibrinolytic therapy often reveals partial or complete clot lysis, there usually remains evidence of an underlying fixed anatomic compression with luminal irregularity at the level of the thoracic outlet. Paradoxically, resolution of symptoms seems to be independent of the post-thrombolytic venographic findings and is probably as much a consequence of collateral development and the prevention of clot propagation.

Surgical Therapy

With changes in concepts of pathophysiology (i.e., traumatic fibrosis of the axillary-subclavian vein with superimposed acute thrombosis), there have been renewed efforts to deal with the various mechanical factors surgically. However, Campbell and associates reported disappointing results after simple thrombectomy combined with vein patch angioplasty.[18]

When patients were treated relatively early in the postthrombotic period and the clot was well localized, Adams and DeWeese reported good results with acute thrombectomy and decompression of the costoclavicular space.[38] Aziz and coworkers reported similarly good results with clavicular resection, venous thrombectomy, and reconstruction, even 3 months after the initial thrombosis.[7] They suggested subtotal medial claviculectomy and lysis of the proximal subclavian vein by division of the constricting extravenous bands or costocoracoid ligament. Venotomy was performed at the site of the lesion, with thrombectomy and resection of the fibrotic valve or endovenous fibrous lesion. Vein patch venoplasty was performed in most patients to enlarge the usually fibrosed and narrowed vein. In two of the patients, a distal arteriovenous fistula was constructed.

Currier and colleagues reported using 6-mm polytetrafluoroethylene bypass grafts from the axillary to the internal jugular vein. These grafts were tunneled through the thoracic outlet, with three of the six grafts presumably remaining patent.[39] Avoidance of the undecompressed thoracic outlet (by removing the first rib or passing the graft over the clavicle) could be expected to improve the results of this type of bypass procedure. Although good results have been reported after resection of the first thoracic rib alone, it is difficult to establish whether these patients had symptoms as a consequence of continued peripheral venous hypertension or from the underlying neurogenic thoracic outlet compression syndrome.[40]

The Multi-Disciplinary Approach to Therapy

Surgical thrombectomy unfortunately has a very high incidence of failure because it is limited by the considerable thrombogenicity of the damaged vein segment and the difficulty of maintaining adequate anticoagulation in the early postoperative period. Additionally, although *thrombolytic* therapy can restore patency of the axillary-subclavian vein, when the underlying compressive abnormality remains or collateralization is inadequate, the patient continues to be at risk for rethrombosis or continues to experience symptoms of venous hypertension during exercise.

A more comprehensive, multi-disciplinary approach has been developed using pharmacologic and interventional radiologic techniques combined with corrective surgery to achieve excellent and consistent results that include relief of venous hypertension and prevention of rethrombosis.

In 1985, Taylor and associates reported the use of thrombolytic therapy to restore venous patency followed by first rib resection to decompress the thoracic outlet.[41] In 1986, Perler and Mitchell reported the results in a single patient in whom the underlying compressive stricture at the thoracic outlet was demonstrated and treated by transaxillary first rib resection. They used balloon angioplasty to

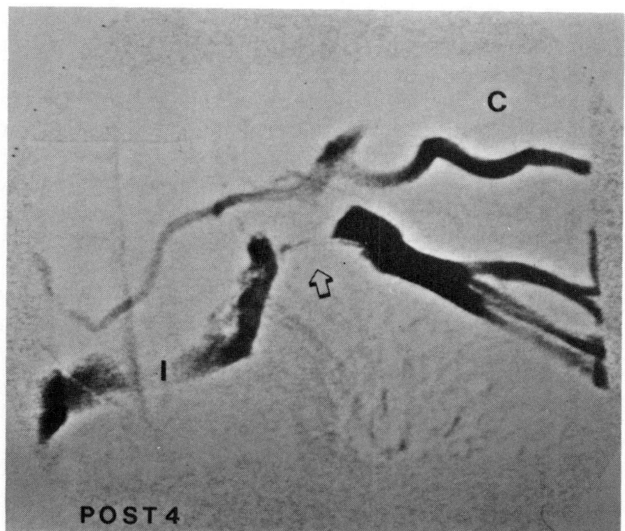

FIGURE 71–3. Residual area of compression *(arrow)* after successful thrombolytic therapy but before surgical correction. The area remains unchanged after four attempts at balloon dilatation. Balloon dilatation attempted before surgical decompression of the vein has a significant adverse effect on the ultimate outcome of venous patency. C, cephalic vein; I, innominate vein. (From Machleder HI: The role of thrombolytic agents for acute subclavian vein thrombosis. Semin Vasc Surg 5:86, 1992.)

correct a residual stricture found on follow-up venography.[42]

In 1989, Kunkel and Machleder reported the results of a new, staged, multi-disciplinary approach to therapy in a group of 25 patients. This therapeutic algorithm used catheter-directed thrombolytic therapy followed by anticoagulation, then thoracic outlet decompression, and finally transluminal balloon angioplasty to correct any residual stenosis[43] (Fig. 71–3). Studies have confirmed that the comprehensive, multi-disciplinary approach to therapy for this disorder is effective in restoring vein patency as well as reducing the risk of rethrombosis[9] (Fig. 71–4).

SECONDARY THROMBOSIS

Occlusion of either peripheral or central brachiocephalic veins is seen in a variety of clinical settings. Phlebitis

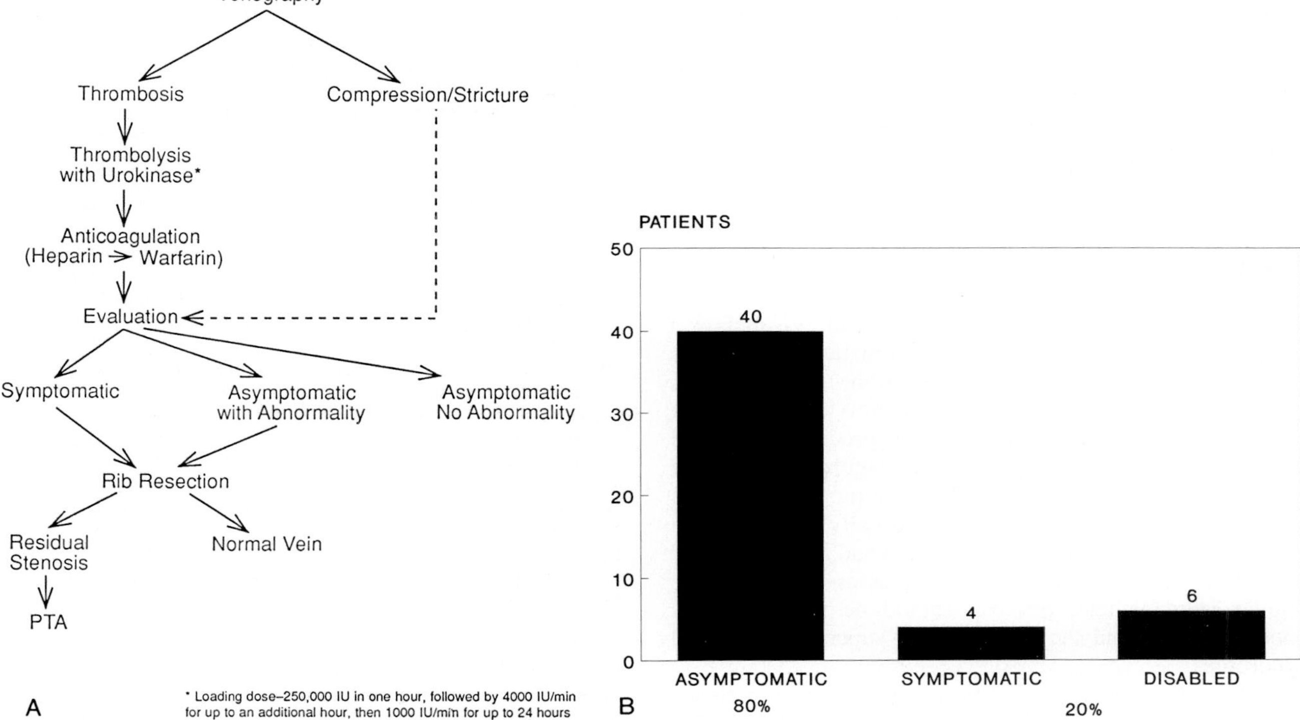

FIGURE 71–4. *A*, Staged multidisciplinary algorithm for the management of spontaneous "effort" thrombosis of the axillary-subclavian vein. PTA, percutaneous transluminal angioplasty. *B*, Final clinical result in 50 consecutive patients treated with this approach. (*A* and *B*, From Machleder HI: Evaluation of a new treatment strategy for Paget-Schroetter syndrome: Spontaneous thrombosis of the axillary-subclavian vein. J Vasc Surg 17:305, 1993.)

and localized thrombosis often occur during intravenous infusion, with the incidence being greater than 20 per cent when continuous infusions are longer than 24 hours in duration. The observation that intermittent infusions can reduce the incidence of thrombophlebitis has promoted the use of the heparin lock system of venous access.[44, 45] In the absence of a septic thrombophlebitis, these peripheral venous complications, although uncomfortable, rarely result in residual problems or extend to thrombosis of the axillary-subclavian segment.

Thrombosis of the subclavian vein often has an indolent course. With venous collateralization around the shoulder girdle being quite extensive, thrombosis of the axillary-subclavian vein arising from central venous catheters and diagnostic lines is often unrecognized and asymptomatic. Although these occlusions were formerly thought to be quite uncommon, an incidence of these clinically silent occlusions of between 20 and 30 per cent has been evident in several large prospective studies that used routine venographic follow-up examinations.[46–48]

Thrombosis can occur even in the absence of infusion, as has been documented in patients with permanent transvenous pacemaker wires evaluated by venography. In one such study, 35 per cent of patients had complete occlusion of the subclavian vein and an additional 35 per cent had developed a high-grade stenosis with signs or symptoms of venous obstruction. Temporary dialysis catheterization of the subclavian vein has likewise been implicated in causing subclavian stricture or stenosis. Commonly, the site of stenosis or occlusion is located at the thoracic outlet, in virtually the same position as the occlusion seen in spontaneously occurring effort thrombosis.[49]

Nineteen studies in the literature examined the incidence of *clinically diagnosed,* catheter-related thrombosis from 1973 to 1985. The incidence in 5970 cases was 5.3 per cent. In 9 studies comprising 539 patients studied *venographically,* the incidence was 28 per cent. In 10 reported studies from 1965 to 1987, the incidence of pulmonary embolism ranged from 9 to 25 per cent, with an average of 12.4 per cent.[50]

Treatment

Although generally asymptomatic, axillary-subclavian vein occlusions tend to become symptomatic when there is extension of the thrombotic process into the collateral veins or when there is a superimposed phlebitis of bacterial or fungal origin. In the absence of a septic process, the central line can often be salvaged by anticoagulation until the thrombotic process has stabilized. In the presence of septic thrombophlebitis, catheter removal is usually required, even with a rapid response to anticoagulation and antibacterial or antifungal agents. If thrombosis progresses to involve the jugular vein, catheter removal should be more urgently considered to avoid the possibility of superior vena caval syndrome.[15]

It has become apparent that many patients experience silent thrombosis of the axillary-subclavian vein with indwelling lines. This suggests a stable thrombus without obstruction of other major brachiocephalic veins. When thrombus is discovered incidentally, it has been the author's recommendation not to intervene with therapy or remove the catheter. With a large population of patients requiring long-term indwelling central venous lines, the author's philosophy has been to direct therapy toward preserving access rather than removing and reinserting lines via another site. When edema or rapidly enlarging collaterals suggest propagation of the thrombus to occlude collateral channels, this unstable thrombotic process requires therapy.

Thrombolytic Therapy

Peripheral venous infusion of a thrombolytic agent has been found to be ineffective even when infusion is into the ipsilateral extremity.[51] However, the central venous catheter can be partially withdrawn so that the urokinase infusion goes directly through the clot. The catheter can be exchanged over a guidewire when replacement is indicated. Alternatively, a second catheter can be placed, via the antecubital basilic vein, into or alongside the thrombus. A standard 3-day infusion of urokinase has been used, starting with 500 IU/kg for 10 minutes and followed by 500 IU/kg/hr. If there is no response, the dose can be increased to 2000 IU/kg/hr. After infusion, patients are anticoagulated with heparin while treatment with warfarin is initiated and maintained long-term.

References

1. Hughes ESR: Venous obstruction in the upper extremity (Paget-Schroetter's syndrome). A review of 320 cases. Int Abstr Surg 88:89, 1949.
2. Gloviczki P, Kazmier FJ, Hollier LH: Axillary-subclavian venous occlusion: The morbidity of a nonlethal disease. J Vasc Surg 4:333, 1986.
3. Donayre CE, White GH, Mehringer SM, Wilson SE: Pathogenesis determines late morbidity of axillosubclavian vein thrombosis. Am J Surg 152:179, 1986.
4. Harley DP, White RA, Nelson RJ, Mehringer CM: Pulmonary embolism secondary to venous thrombosis of the arm. Am J Surg 147:221, 1984.
5. Lowenstein PS: Thrombosis of the axillary vein. JAMA 82:854, 1927.
6. Gould EP, Patey DH: Primary thrombosis of the axillary vein: A study of eight cases. Br J Surg 16:208, 1937.
7. Aziz S, Straehley CJ, Whelan TJ: Effort related axillosubclavian vein thrombosis. Am J Surg 152:57, 1986.
8. Sundquist SB, Hedner U, Kullenberg HKE, Bergentz SE: Deep venous thrombosis of the arm: A study of coagulation and fibrinolysis. Br Med J 283:265, 1981.
9. Machleder HI: Evaluation of a new treatment strategy for Paget-Schroetter's syndrome: Spontaneous thrombosis of the axillary-subclavian vein. J Vasc Surg 17:305, 1993.
10. Roos DB: Thoracic outlet and carpal tunnel syndromes. *In* Rutherford RB (ed): Vascular Surgery. 2nd ed. Philadelphia, WB Saunders, 1984, pp 708–724.
11. Dunant JH: Effort thrombosis, a complication of thoracic outlet syndrome. Vasa 10:322, 1981.
12. Tilney NL, Griffiths HJG, Edwards EA: Natural history of major venous thrombosis of the upper extremity. Arch Surg 101:792, 1970.
13. Linblad B, Bornmyer S, Kullendorff B, Bergqvist D: Venous haemodynamics of the upper extremity after subclavian vein thrombosis. Vasa 19:218, 1990.
14. Barnett T, Levitt LM: Effort thrombosis of the axillary vein with pulmonary embolism. JAMA 146:1412, 1951.
15. Bean WB: Superior vena cava disorders. *In* Machleder HI (ed): Vascular Disorders of the Upper Extremity. 2nd ed. Mt. Kisco, NY, Futura, 1989, pp 297–301.
16. Kunkel JM, Machleder HI: Treatment of Paget-Schroetter syndrome: A staged, multidisciplinary approach. Arch Surg 124:1153, 1989.

17. Nuwer MR: Somatosensory evoked potentials in the assessment of upper extremity neurovascular compression. *In* Machleder HI (ed): Vascular Disorders of the Upper Extremity. 2nd ed. Mt. Kisco, NY, Futura, 1989, pp 189–203.
18. Campbell CB, Chandler JG, Tegtmeyer CJ, Bernstein EF: Axillary, subclavian, and brachiocephalic vein obstruction. Surgery 82:816, 1977.
19. Haire WD, Lynch TG, Lieberman RP, et al: Utility of duplex ultrasound in the diagnosis of asymptomatic catheter-induced subclavian vein thrombosis. J Ultrasound Med 10:493, 1991.
20. Haire WD, Lynch TG, Lund GB, et al: Limitations of magnetic resonance imaging and ultrasound-directed (duplex) scanning in the diagnosis of subclavian vein thrombosis. J Vasc Surg 13:391, 1991.
21. McCleery RS, Kesterson JE, Kirtley, Love RB: Subclavius and anterior scalene muscle compression as a cause of intermittent obstruction of the subclavian vein. Ann Surg 133:588, 1951.
22. Adams JT, DeWeese JA, Mahoney EB, Bob CG: Intermittent subclavian vein obstruction without thrombosis. Surgery 63:147, 1968.
23. Adams JT, McEvoy RK, DeWeese JA: Primary deep venous thrombosis of upper extremity. Arch Surg 91:29, 1965.
24. Stevenson IM, Parry EW: Radiological study of the etiological factors in venous obstruction of the upper limb. J Cardiovasc Surg 16:580, 1975.
25. Daskalakis E, Bouhoutsos J: Subclavian and axillary vein compression of musculoskeletal origin. Br J Surg 67:573, 1980.
26. Schubart PJ, Haeberlin JR, Porter JM: Intermittent subclavian venous obstruction: Utility of venous pressure gradients. Surgery 99:365, 1986.
27. Paget J: Clinical Lectures and Essays. London, Longmans, Green & Company, 1875.
28. Schepelmann E: Muench Med Wochenschr 57:2444, 1910. As cited in Hughes ESR: Venous obstruction in the upper extremity (Paget-Schroetter's syndrome). A review of 320 cases. Int Abstr Surg 88:89, 1949.
29. DeWeese JA, Adams JT, Gaiser DL: Subclavian venous thrombectomy. Circulation 42 (Suppl 2):159, 1970.
30. Molina JE: Thrombolytic therapy of axillary-subclavian venous thrombosis. Arch Surg 123:662, 1988.
31. Johnson AJ, McCarty WR: The lysis of artificially induced intravascular clots in man by intravenous infusions of streptokinase. J Clin Invest 38:1627, 1959.
32. Steed DL, Teodori MF, Peitzman AB, et al: Streptokinase in the treatment of subclavian vein thrombosis. J Vasc Surg 4:28, 1986.
33. Zimmerman R, Morl H, Harenberg J, et al: Urokinase therapy of subclavian-axillary vein thrombosis. Klin Wochenschr 59:851, 1981.
34. Becker GJ, Holden RW, Rabe FE, et al: Local thrombolytic therapy for subclavian and axillary vein thrombosis. Radiology 149:419, 1983.
35. Machleder HI: Venous disorders. *In* Machleder HI (ed): Vascular Disorders of the Upper Extremity. 2nd ed. Mt. Kisco, NY, Futura, 1989, pp 269–296.
36. Machleder HI: The role of thrombolytic agents for acute subclavian vein thrombosis. Semin Vasc Surg 5:82, 1992.
37. Smith-Behn J, Althar RE, Katz W: Primary thrombosis of the axillary/subclavian vein. South Med J 79:1176, 1986.
38. Adams JT, DeWeese JA: "Effort" thrombosis of the axillary and subclavian veins. J Trauma 11:923, 1971.
39. Currier CB Jr, Widder S, Ali A, et al: Surgical management of subclavian and axillary vein thrombosis in patients with a functioning arteriovenous fistula. Surgery 100:25, 1986.
40. Glass B: The relationship of axillary venous thrombosis to the thoracic outlet compression syndrome. Ann Thorac Surg 19:613, 1975.
41. Taylor LM, McAllister WR, Dennis DL, Porter JM: Thrombolytic therapy followed by first rib resection for spontaneous ("effort") subclavian vein thrombosis. Am J Surg 149:644, 1985.
42. Perler BA, Mitchell SE: Percutaneous transluminal angioplasty and transaxillary first rib resection; A multidisciplinary approach to the thoracic outlet compression syndrome. Am Surg 52:485, 1986.
43. Kunkel JM, Machleder HI: Treatment of Paget-Schroetter syndrome: A staged, multidisciplinary approach. Arch Surg 124:1153, 1989.
44. Weiss Y, Nissan S: A method for reducing the incidence of infusion phlebitis. Surg Gynecol Obstet 141:73, 1975.
45. Ferguson RL, Rosett W, Hodges GR, Barnes WG: Complications with heparin lock needles: A prospective evaluation. Ann Intern Med 85:583, 1976.
46. Axelsson CK, Efsen F: Phlebography in long-term catheterization of the subclavian vein: A retrospective study in patients with severe gastrointestinal disorders. Scand J Gastroenterol 13:933, 1978.
47. Smith VC, Hallett JW: Subclavian vein thrombosis during prolonged catheterization for parenteral nurtrition: Early management and long term followup. South Med J 76:603, 1983.
48. Feliciano DV, Mattox KL, Graham JM, et al: Major complications of percutaneous subclavian vein catheters. Am J Surg 138:869, 1979.
49. Davis D, Petersen J, Feldman R, et al: Subclavian venous stenosis: A complication of subclavian dialysis. JAMA 252:3404, 1984.
50. Horattas MC, Wright DJ, Fenton AH, et al: Changing concepts of deep venous thrombosis of the upper extremity: Report of a series and a review of the literature. Surgery 104:561, 1988.
51. Fraschini G, Jadeja J, Lawson M, et al: Local infusion of urokinase for the lysis of thrombosis associated with permanent central venous catheters in cancer patients. J Clin Oncol 5:672, 1987.

72

Upper Extremity Sympathectomy

John P. Harris, M.S., F.R.A.C.S., F.R.C.S., F.A.C.S., Paul M. Satchell, B.Sc.(Med.), F.R.A.C.P., Ph.D., M.B.A., and James May, M.S., F.R.A.C.S., F.A.C.S.

• • •

Upper extremity sympathectomy was once commonly performed for disorders as diverse as essential hypertension, bronchial asthma, angina pectoris, hyperthyroidism, and even the crises of tertiary syphilis.[59] In the absence of effective medical or surgical alternatives, the operation was one of the few options available to surgeons caring for patients with ischemic disorders of the upper extremity. Several advances have decreased the need for surgical sympathetic ablation. As a result of more effective medical therapy,[70] chemical sympathetic blockade,[37] and the development of percutaneous[82] and endoscopic surgical techniques[30, 42, 43] to disrupt the sympathetic nerve supply to the upper extremity, sympathectomy is now an infrequently performed operation with limited indications. Nevertheless, upper extremity sympathectomy retains a useful role, particularly in the treatment of severe hyperhidrosis and for selected upper extremity ischemic and post-traumatic pain syndromes.

The history of and past controversy over the exact anatomy, surgical approach, and indications for upper extremity sympathectomy have been reviewed by Welch and Geary.[78] Sympathetic control of the circulation was described by Bernard and Brown-Sequard in 1852. By 1889, Gaskell and Langley had mapped the anatomy of the autonomic nervous system. Alexander was the first surgeon to operate on the sympathetic nervous system when he performed a cervical sympathectomy for epilepsy in 1899.[79] Leriche, in 1913, described periarterial sympathectomy to increase blood flow to the extremities. Other surgeons, including Jonnesco, Brunning, Gask, and Royle, advocated more proximal upper extremity sympathetic interruption by excision of the stellate ganglion.[78]

Since then, the conflicting aims of achieving complete sympathectomy and avoiding the disability of Horner's syndrome, which occurs if the stellate ganglion is completely excised, have resulted in argument over the extent of sympathectomy, the amount of stellate ganglion to be resected, and the best way to do the procedure.[6, 12, 48, 65, 78] Many of these issues remain incompletely resolved.

SURGICAL ASPECTS OF UPPER EXTREMITY SYMPATHETIC NERVE SUPPLY

Preganglionic fibers supplying the upper limb are derived from cells in the intermediolateral column of the gray matter of the spinal cord between its second and ninth segments. Most vasoconstrictor fibers supplying the arteries of the upper extremity emerge from the spinal cord in the ventral roots of the second and third thoracic nerves. These arteries can be denervated by cutting the sympathetic trunk below the third thoracic ganglion and severing the rami communicantes of the second and third thoracic ganglia. The sympathetic nerve supply to the eccrine glands in the upper extremity may be similarly interrupted. It is necessary to divide the trunk below the fourth thoracic ganglion and divide its associated rami if the eccrine glands of the axilla are to be completely denervated. To produce sympathetic denervation of the upper extremity, it is unnecessary to excise any portion of the stellate ganglion or to divide the rami to the first thoracic ganglion.

Roos searches for and divides the nerve of Kuntz, an intrathoracic nerve passing from the second intercostal nerve to the T1 root.[61] Sympathetic fibers may pass from the spinal cord to the lower brachial plexus along this nerve, bypassing the sympathetic chain. However, in the authors' experience, inadequate excision of the T3 and T4 ganglia is more likely to result in incomplete sympathectomy than is failure to find the nerve of Kuntz.[46]

Sympathetic innervation of the digital arteries has been described by Morgan and colleagues.[50] Sympathetic nerve twigs pass from the digital nerves to the digital arteries. Sympathectomy can be performed in the hand by denervating the digital arteries using microsurgical techniques.[14, 23, 81]

INDICATIONS

The most common indications for upper extremity sympathectomy in modern vascular surgical practice are hyperhidrosis, ischemia, and to a lesser extent, post-traumatic pain syndromes.

The management of upper extremity ischemic disease and post-traumatic pain syndromes is dealt with elsewhere in this text. The results of sympathectomy for upper extremity ischemic[73] and post-traumatic pain syndromes[8, 55, 60, 75] are not as good as those achieved for hyperhidrosis. Although some investigators have abandoned the use of upper extremity sympathectomy for digital ischemia,[57, 73] the authors believe that upper extremity sympathectomy can help selected patients. The decision to proceed to surgical sympathectomy still depends on clinical judgment because a good response to temporary stellate ganglion blockade is only a limited guide to predicting the outcome of upper extremity sympathectomy.[76] In sharp contrast to the debate over the place of upper extremity sympathectomy in these conditions, there is general agreement that a predictably good outcome will follow upper extremity sympathectomy for hyperhidrosis.

Hyperhidrosis is sweating in excess of that required for normal thermoregulation. Sweating can be severe enough to warrant upper extremity sympathectomy. Primary, or essential, hyperhidrosis occurs in the absence of any known structural abnormality of the eccrine glands, sympathetic nerves, or ganglia. Hyperhidrosis is rarely secondary to systemic disorders, which include hyperthyroidism and pheochromocytoma. A good account of the differential diagnosis and nonoperative management of hyperhidrosis has been given by Fitzpatrick and coworkers.[13]

Most affected patients are young and otherwise healthy. The condition occurs in both sexes. Some authors have observed a familial tendency,[2] although this is disputed by others.[16] Sweating usually begins in childhood or adolescence. It is usually episodic and is precipitated by thermal, gustatory, or emotional stimuli specific to the individual. Although sweating may be exacerbated by hot weather, climate is not a major etiologic factor. The mechanism is unclear, but these stimuli result in hyperactivity of the sudomotor drive.[2] Sweating tends to be symmetric and is usually absent during sleep. In severe cases, sweat can drop from the hands, making handling paper impossible and shaking hands a social embarrassment. Moist skin can result in chronic dermatitis and fungal infections.

The clinical picture is usually so clear-cut that extensive investigation is not required.[2, 13] Patients who are mildly affected may get sufficient symptomatic relief with topical antiperspirant medication and atropine-like drugs.[13, 16] In severe hyperhidrosis, these measures are not effective enough, and surgical sympathectomy is indicated. However, it is desirable to allow patients with essential hyperhidrosis to try all conservative measures before reaching the conclusion that sympathectomy is the only cure. In rare instances, eccrine glands may be congenitally absent in some areas. These patients have compensatory localized sweating as their only form of cutaneous thermoregulation; sympathectomy is therefore inappropriate.[13]

Less common indications for upper extremity sympathectomy include cold injury,[12] rare forms of arteritis,[41, 77] vasospastic disease,[11] and unusual cardiac tachydysrhythmias.[51, 68]

SURGICAL APPROACHES

Several approaches to the sympathetic chain in the upper thoracic and lower cervical regions have been described. Smithwick popularized exposure of the sympathetic chain from behind after excision of a small section of the third rib together with the associated transverse process of the third thoracic vertebra.[71] This approach has been superseded by alternative techniques.

The anterior transthoracic exposure of the thoracodorsal sympathetic chain is achieved by a thoracotomy through the third intercostal space together with division of the costal cartilage of the third rib to increase the exposure.[53]

The axillary extrapleural approach[61] is performed after excision of the first rib. It has the following advantages: there is less postoperative pain because rib retraction is unnecessary, and the operating surgeon is able to determine beyond doubt the exact level of the sympathetic chain and identify and protect the T1 nerve root, which carries the motor fibers to the small muscles of the hand. Despite these advantages, the approach is technically demanding. In the authors' opinion, the supraclavicular[74] and axillary[4, 35] transthoracic approaches are safer options for surgeons who are unfamiliar with first rib resection for thoracic outlet syndrome.[56, 67]

Supraclavicular Approach

Supraclavicular sympathectomy is performed through a short incision above the medial one third of the clavicle, with the patient in the supine position.[74] The clavicular head of the sternomastoid is divided. The phrenic nerve runs down from the lateral to the medial border of the scalenus anterior muscle. The nerve is mobilized, and the scalenus anterior is divided. The subclavian artery is dissected to allow retraction without division of any of its branches. The scalenus pleuralis muscle is divided to allow the dome of the pleura to be displaced inferiorly. This muscle arises from the transverse process of the seventh cervical vertebra and attaches to the suprapleural membrane inferiorly. It always has a fibrous portion and may have a fleshy component as well. The pleura may be opened inadvertently if this muscle is not divided before the surgeon attempts to depress the apical pleura. Wood Jones stated that the scalenus pleuralis muscle is present in 35 per cent of cases.[84] In the authors' experience, it is present more frequently than this.

In the past, the authors removed the stellate ganglion to ensure facial symmetry after bilateral operations when the supraclavicular approach was used,[46] but Welch and Geary recommended that the T2 and T3 ganglia be excised and the stellate ganglion spared.[78] The authors now agree with this recommendation but find that the part of the sympathetic chain below the stellate ganglion can be more readily excised via the axillary transthoracic approach. Integrity of the pleural cavity should be checked by saline wound irrigation and postoperative chest x-ray studies.

An interesting but little known variation of anterior exposure for upper extremity sympathectomy is the anterior cervical approach.[38] A thyroid incision is made. The fascia on the medial border of the sternomastoid muscle is divided. The carotid sheath is retracted laterally, and the trachea and esophagus are retracted medially to expose the anterior surface of the vertebral bodies and the sympathetic chain on each side. The recurrent laryngeal nerve is at risk for injury, particularly on the right.

Axillary Transthoracic Approach

In 1949, Atkins described an approach to the upper extremity sympathetic chain through the axilla.[3] The technique was well described and illustrated by Little.[34] The patient is placed in the lateral position, and the arm is supported to prevent traction on the brachial plexus. Collapse and re-expansion of the lung can be controlled with a double-lumen endotracheal tube, but this is not essential because the lung can be retracted, provided that the patient is ventilated by hand by the anesthesiologist and is not on a ventilator.

A transverse incision is made beneath the hair-bearing area of the axilla. The intercostobrachial nerve should be identified and preserved. The thorax is entered through the second intercostal space. The long thoracic nerve, supplying the serratus anterior, is at risk while the intercostal opening is extended posteriorly. A small rib retractor is inserted and should be opened slowly and progressively to avoid rib fracture. Improved operative illumination can be provided in the manner described by McCaughan and May[40] (Fig. 72–1). This involves passing a malleable, cold light source through a stab incision in the fourth intercostal space in the mid-axillary line. This has the advantage of providing shadowless illumination of the sympathetic chain, relieving the assistants of the task of holding the light source still and, most importantly, removing a bulky object from the limited access between the retractor blades. The light source is easier to insert before the rib retractor is opened.

The sympathetic chain is identified, and the level is determined by counting down from the first rib at the apex of the thoracic cavity. The pleura overlying the sympathetic chain is incised. The sympathetic chain can then be encircled with a Silastic loop for gentle retraction so that the rami can be identified and divided. Care is taken to avoid excessive traction on the sympathetic chain, which might result in Horner's syndrome. The second to fourth thoracic ganglia are removed routinely. Immediate frozen section confirmation can be requested if there is doubt about the excised specimen.

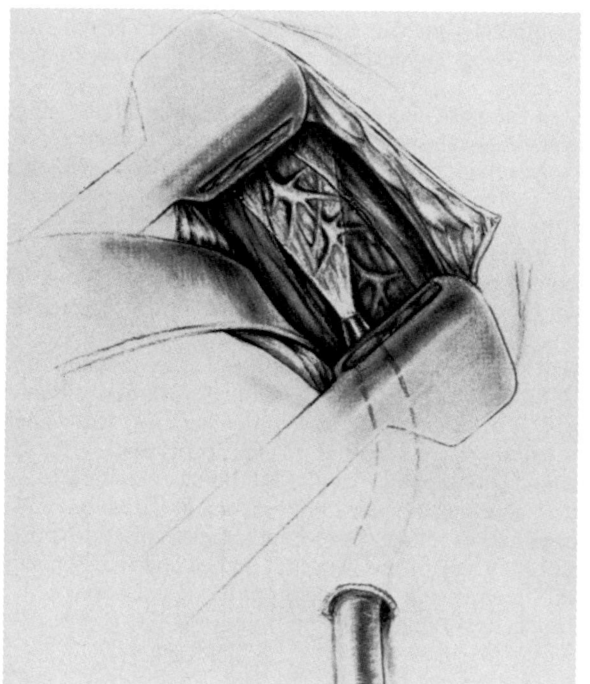

FIGURE 72–1. Axillary transthoracic exposure of the sympathetic chain. Shadowless illumination is obtained by passing a light source through the fourth intercostal space. A chest tube can be brought out through the same tract when the light source is withdrawn. (From McCaughan BC, May J: Illumination and access for transaxillary thoracic sympathectomy. Surg Gynecol Obstet 156:507, 1983. By permission of Surgery, Gynecology & Obstetrics.)

An underwater seal drain is conveniently brought out through the tract left in the fourth intercostal space after the light source has been removed. After reinflation of the lung is ensured, the chest is closed. The drain can usually be removed within 24 hours of surgery. Chest x-ray studies are taken to ensure that there is no intrathoracic collection or residual pneumothorax.

Campbell and associates consider it safe to perform bilateral axillary sympathectomy under the same anesthetic.[10] The authors prefer staged unilateral operations, particularly in older patients, in view of the adverse pulmonary function changes noted by Molho and coworkers.[47, 48]

Comparison of Supraclavicular and Axillary Sympathectomy

Most surgeons perform either supraclavicular[78] or axillary transthoracic[21] sympathectomy. The choice of operation is often based on personal preference or teaching. There have been attempts to provide information on the relative merits of the two procedures.[34, 46, 48]

The authors previously reported on a comparison of 28 supraclavicular and 34 axillary sympathectomies performed in 22 and 20 patients, respectively.[46] There was no significant difference in the length of hospital stay. Regardless of the technique used, significant complications occurred. Two supraclavicular sympathectomies for hyperhidrosis failed to produce a dry axilla. The most troublesome complication was post-sympathetic neuralgia, which occurred in 3 patients after supraclavicular sympathectomy. Most of the complications in the axillary group were respiratory and responded promptly to treatment. Although postoperative pain was more severe following axillary sympathectomy, this approach was recommended because of the superior exposure, easier access to the sympathetic chain for wide excision, avoidance of Horner's syndrome, and good cosmetic result.

Not all investigators agree with this recommendation. Molho and coworkers compared pulmonary function abnormalities in 12 patients who had supraclavicular sympathectomies with those in another 12 patients who underwent transaxillary sympathectomies.[48] Small airway resistance increased with both approaches. Because radiologic abnormalities and pulmonary function changes were more frequent after the axillary approach, they preferred supraclavicular sympathectomy. The functional changes were not great, however, and most function had returned to normal when reassessed 6 months after surgery.

OBJECTIVE ASSESSMENT OF THE RESULTS OF SYMPATHECTOMY

Methods for detecting sympathetic denervation are well established but have not found widespread clinical

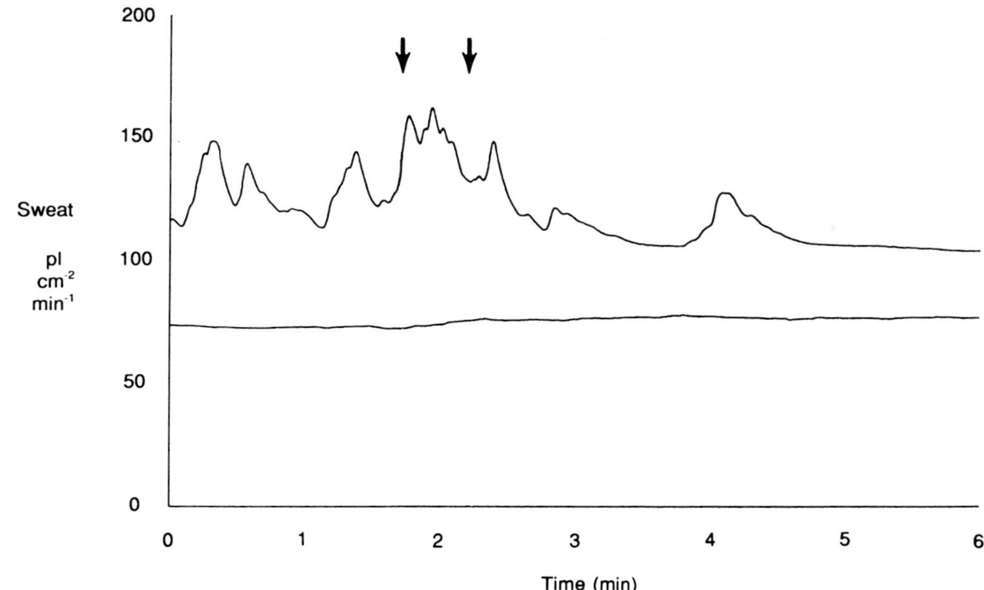

FIGURE 72–2. Finger sweat output before and after sympathectomy. The upper tracing shows fluctuations in left index finger sweating that occurred spontaneously and with altered arousal *(arrows)*, indicating intact sympathetic innervation. Complete sympathectomy is confirmed postoperatively (lower tracing), as there is no alteration in sweat output from the same finger, even with arousal and temperature change.

application because most are complex, relatively time consuming, and require powders,[62] electrodes, electrode paste, stimulators, or electrophoresis units.[25, 26, 39, 69] Furthermore, most are imprecise. The problems inherent with these tests are avoided with finger sudometry, which provides a sensitive measure of sudomotor drive to the fingers. Patients have only to insert a finger through a rubber diaphragm into a chamber.[66] Finger sudometry continuously measures the amount of sweat produced by a finger, thus allowing the effect of stimuli on sweat output to be quantified and the results of sympathectomy to be determined (Fig. 72–2). This technique and others are likely to have an increasing place in the surgical manipulation of the autonomic nervous system and be important adjuncts in the work-up of patients being considered for sympathectomy, particularly if reoperation is being considered.[29, 33]

Results of Sympathectomy for Hyperhidrosis

After upper extremity sympathectomy, relief of hyperhidrosis is usual. Patients undergoing this surgery are significantly younger than those having sympathectomy for other indications. Adar and colleagues failed to achieve a dry hand in only 7 of 198 sympathectomies in 100 patients suffering from hyperhidrosis.[2] They had no failures when frozen section histology was used to confirm excision of the sympathetic chain. Ninety-one patients who had a good initial result were followed up for an average of 18 months; 38 had completely dry hands, and 53 had some return of moisture, but in no case did the hyperhidrotic state recur. Greenhalgh and coworkers reported similarly good results in a smaller group of patients, some of whom were followed up for up to 10 years.[16] Mild gustatory sweating was common in the experience of Adar and colleagues, as was some form of compensatory perspiration.[2] Occasionally, patients have residual sweating in part of the axillae. This area can be delineated by starch-iodine testing and excised if symptoms are sufficiently troublesome.[16] In a study of 39 patients undergoing simultaneous bilateral supraclavicular sympathectomy for hyperhidrosis, Papa and colleagues concluded that there was no overt arrhythmogenic effect on the young, healthy heart after sympathectomy.[54] They also found that the beta-blocker–like effect persisted for at least 2 years. Extensive sympathetic denervation of the upper and lower extremities for hyperhidrosis should be avoided because orthostatic hypotension has been observed.[31]

Results of Endoscopic Sympathectomy for Hyperhidrosis

The results of endoscopic or percutaneous upper extremity sympathectomy are encouraging, and endoscopic sympathectomy is evolving as the preferred method for surgical control of hyperhidrosis.[24, 64]

Percutaneous sympathectomy has been performed as an outpatient procedure.[82] Kux reported complete relief of hand sweating in 63 patients after endoscopic sympathectomy, but 19 per cent still had some sweating in the axilla.[30] Malone and associates found that the technique could be readily learned and reported favorable results after 13 sympathectomies.[42, 43] With the adaptation of laparoscopic surgical techniques for thoracic applications, endoscopic sympathectomy is increasingly displacing open operation for hyperhidrosis as the low morbidity and good results of early reports[30, 42] are confirmed in further studies.[9, 32, 49] The patient benefits from early hospital discharge and avoids the morbidity associated with thoracotomy.[49] Patients are also more likely to accept bilateral procedures. In contrast, with open operation, about 20 per cent of patients who have had successful unilateral sympathectomy will not agree to have the other side operated on because of the pain experienced after the initial operation.[1, 72]

In an experimental study of endoscopic thoracic sympathectomy that compared techniques for sympathetic ablation, Massad and associates found that the excimer laser and the carbon dioxide laser produced discrete lesions with minimal damage to surrounding structures compared with radiofrequency-generated thermocoagulation and the neodymium: yttrium-aluminum-garnet laser.[44] In a review of the surgical management of primary hyperhidrosis, Moran and Brady summarized the results of endoscopic and surgical sympathectomy for hyperhidrosis.[49] Success was achieved in 90 per cent of 192 patients from three series who were treated endoscopically, compared with 97 per cent of 435 patients from six series who underwent cervical or transaxillary sympathectomy. Endoscopic sympathectomy was achieved by diathermy coagulation of the sympathetic chain, which may account for the lower success rate compared with that achieved with excision of the sympathetic chain.

As laparoscopic surgical instrumentation is modified and improved for thoracic endoscopic sympathectomy, results similar to those achieved with open operation may be obtained. The 10-mm laparoscope with a high-intensity light guide, a high-resolution video display, and the option for multiple operating ports facilitates precise dissection and excision of the thoracic sympathetic chain (Fig. 72–3).

Results of Sympathectomy for Hand and Digital Ischemia

Although the place of sympathectomy in upper extremity ischemic syndromes is controversial,[7, 27, 73] upper extremity sympathectomy can benefit selected patients with upper extremity ischemia, and several broad recommendations can be supported.

Only short-term benefit has followed upper extremity sympathectomy for Raynaud's syndrome not associated with digital artery occlusion.[5, 7, 15, 17, 19, 78] Symptoms usually recur within 2 to 3 years of surgery. Vasospastic changes in the hands may precede, by many years, clinical manifestations of collagen vascular disease.[11] Van de Wal and coworkers followed up 25 patients thought to have primary Raynaud's disease.[76] Collagen vascular disease was eventually discovered in 20 per cent. Upper extremity sympathectomy for the treatment of Raynaud's syndrome associated with collagen vascular disease, particularly scleroderma, does not retard the progression of hand ischemia.[22, 45]

Major upper extremity amputation for ischemia is rarely required,[80] although digital ischemia severe enough to warrant local amputation is relatively common. Detailed hand angiography can complement other investigations in detecting underlying reasons for upper extremity ischemia and determining whether arterial reconstruction is feasible.[18, 79, 84] Sympathectomy may be a useful adjunct to proximal arterial reconstruction, but this has not been firmly established. Most patients with digital ischemia will be helped by topical and systemic vasodilators and by stellate ganglion blockade.[73] Some surgeons have abandoned the use of upper extremity sympathectomy for digital ischemia;[56, 73] however, the authors have found that sympathectomy will relieve pain, improve digital perfusion, and decrease the need for amputation.[46] The best results are achieved in patients with digital arterial occlusion in the absence of Raynaud's syndrome.[76] Birnstingl found that the prognosis after sympathectomy for digital ischemia was better in males than in females.[7] These observations are supported in a long-term study by van de Wal and coworkers of 57 patients who had 72 thoracic sympathectomies for upper extremity ischemia.[76]

The authors continue to recommend upper extremity sympathectomy for patients with obliterative arterial disease threatening the viability of the hands or digits when the localization and extent of the arterial occlusions make reconstructive arterial surgery impossible. The ultimate prognosis depends on the underlying cause of the upper extremity ischemia.

Results of Sympathectomy for Post-Traumatic Pain Syndromes

Upper extremity sympathectomy can relieve post-traumatic pain syndrome; however, not all patients will benefit. The best results of sympathectomy for post-traumatic pain

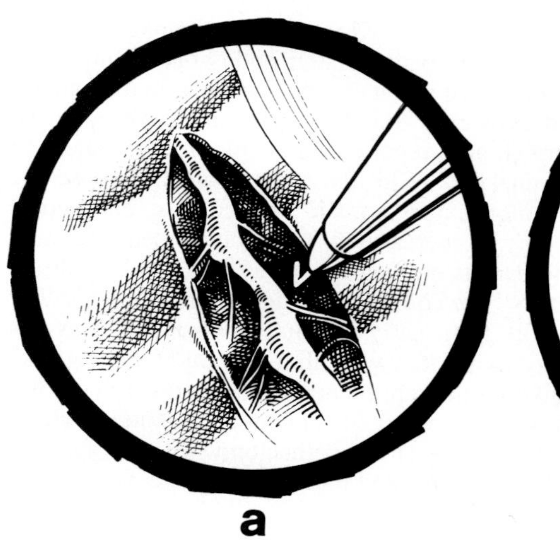

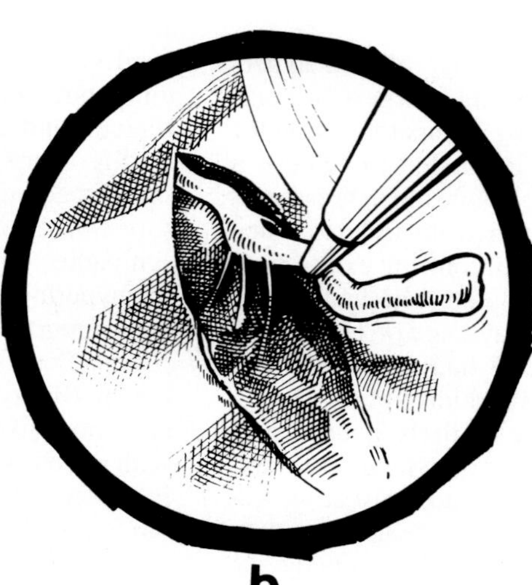

FIGURE 72–3. Endoscopic view of the thoracic sympathetic chain after the pleura has been incised *(a)*. Precise dissection of the sympathetic rami is facilitated by the magnified view *(b)*.

syndrome have been achieved when a diagnosis is made early, before physical changes occur.[52, 83, 85] Kleinert and colleagues reported on a large series of 506 patients with what they classified as post-traumatic sympathetic dystrophy.[28] Only 23 of these patients underwent axillary sympathectomy; 19 experienced permanent improvement, and there were four failures in patients with fixed pain patterns and established trophic changes. Thompson also stressed early recognition of the condition and treatment with physical therapy, analgesia, and repeated stellate ganglion blockade.[75] Buker and associates found that post-traumatic pain syndrome after high-velocity gunshot injury was more likely to require sympathectomy.[8]

Horowitz studied 11 patients in a civilian practice, all of whom were thought to have an iatrogenic basis for their symptoms.[20] Two of these patients had had prior surgery for thoracic outlet syndrome. Horowitz also stressed early recognition of the condition and reviewed the legal ramifications.

The authors would conclude that few patients with post-traumatic pain syndrome will require upper extremity sympathectomy. Most will get sufficient symptomatic relief from physical therapy, analgesia, and nerve blocks. Sympathectomy will be of most benefit when an accurate diagnosis has been made early, before trophic changes become established.

COMPLICATIONS

The complications the authors have encountered are listed in Table 72–1. At late follow-up, it is common to note numbness in the distribution of the intercostobrachial nerve after axillary sympathectomy and to a lesser extent in the distribution of the supraclavicular nerves following supraclavicular sympathectomy. These areas of sensory deficit are rarely commented on spontaneously by the patient.

Sweating on the contralateral side (compensatory hyperhidrosis) has been rare in the authors' experience, as have nasal congestion and visual disturbance associated with Horner's syndrome.

Severe postsympathetic neuralgia[36, 58] can be a devastating complication. Debilitating pain in the upper arm develops approximately 2 weeks after surgery. Three of the authors' patients were normal, stable individuals before the occurrence of this complication following supraclavicular sympathectomy. Major drug and alcohol dependence developed. Their symptoms, which lasted from 2 to 12 months, were eventually relieved with repeated brachial plexus nerve blocks and transcutaneous nerve stimulation.[46]

Lymphatic complications were observed only after supraclavicular sympathectomy, particularly on the left side, where the thoracic duct may be injured. Lymph fistulae can take several weeks to resolve.

The majority of complications observed after axillary transthoracic sympathectomy relate to the thoracotomy[63] and include incomplete expansion of the lung, pulmonary infection, and recurrent pneumothorax. The most serious complication encountered by the authors was an empyema, which required decortication (Fig. 72–4). Thoracotomy for decortication was required. Horner's syndrome is rare and is usually temporary if the sympathetic chain is divided below the stellate ganglion.

The complication of winged scapula is disfiguring, particularly in a young woman (Fig. 72–5). It is a preventable complication, and every effort should be made to identify and protect the long thoracic nerve to the serratus anterior. This nerve seems to be at greater risk with a thoracotomy through the short second intercostal space than with one through a lower interspace.

Temporary sweating of the palms may occur on the 3rd or 4th day after sympathectomy for hyperhidrosis. Greenhalgh and coworkers noted that temporary sweating was frequent following supraclavicular sympathectomy for hyperhidrosis.[16] It is important to be aware of this complication because the surgeon could be misled into believing that he or she has done an incomplete operation. This is important if metallic clips have been used for hemostasis, because clips indicating the upper limit of resection usually appear much lower than the superior border of the second rib on postoperative chest x-ray studies (Fig. 72–6). The authors have confirmed this observation by placing clips at

Table 72–1. Complications of 80 Upper Extremity Sympathectomies

Supraclavicular (n = 29)		Axillary (n = 51)	
Postsympathectomy neuralgia	3	Empyema	1
Pleural effusion	1	Winged scapula	2
Atelectasis	1	Pneumonia	2
Chylous fistula	2	Atelectasis	3
Lymphocele	1	Pneumothorax	2
Wound hematoma	1		
Totals	9		10

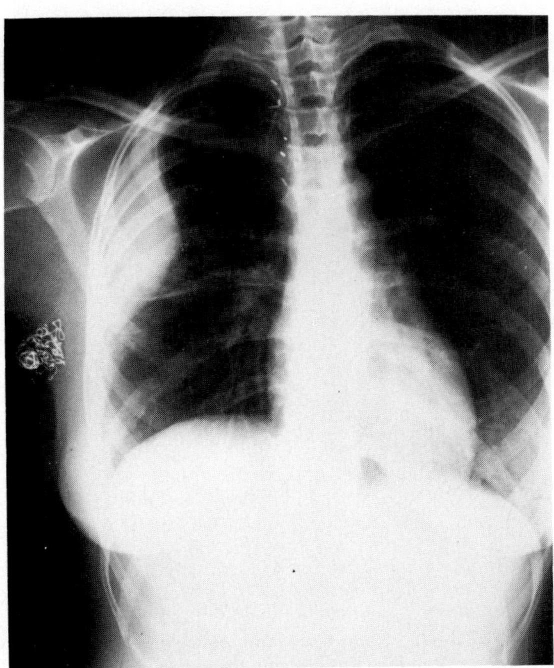

FIGURE 72–4. Empyema after axillary sympathectomy for hyperhidrosis.

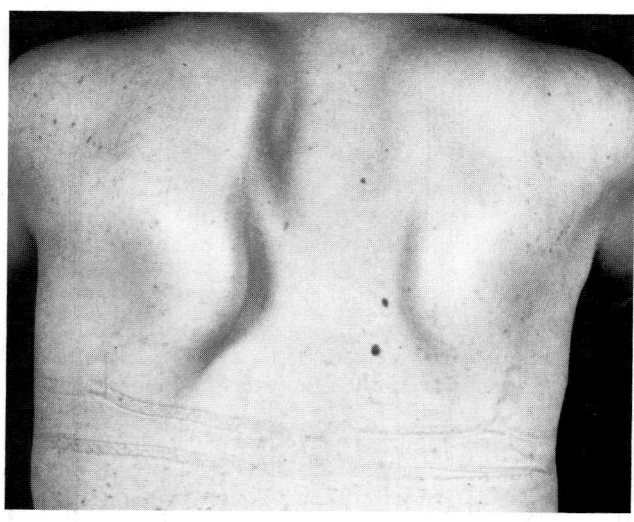

FIGURE 72–5. Winging of the scapula can result if the nerve supplying the serratus anterior is injured during axillary sympathectomy.

the superior border of the second rib just lateral to the sympathetic chain in patients undergoing thoracotomy for lung pathology through a large incision in which the second rib could be identified with complete confidence. In postoperative radiographs, clips consistently appeared to be below the second rib despite having been placed at its upper border.[46]

CONCLUSIONS

Upper extremity sympathectomy retains a useful place in modern vascular surgery to treat hyperhidrosis and selected ischemic and post-traumatic pain syndromes. Upper extremity sympathectomy can be achieved in different ways, including by endoscopic or percutaneous methods and by microsurgical sympathetic denervation of the fingers.

Endoscopic sympathectomy is replacing open operation as the method of choice for upper extremity sympathectomy, particularly for hyperhidrosis.

At least six surgical approaches have been described for upper extremity sympathectomy. The axillary transthoracic approach offers superior exposure, the capability of wider sympathetic excision, good cosmetic appearance, and avoidance of Horner's syndrome. In the absence of lung disease or the need to explore the root of the neck for vascular repair, this approach is recommended if open operation is required for upper extremity sympathectomy.

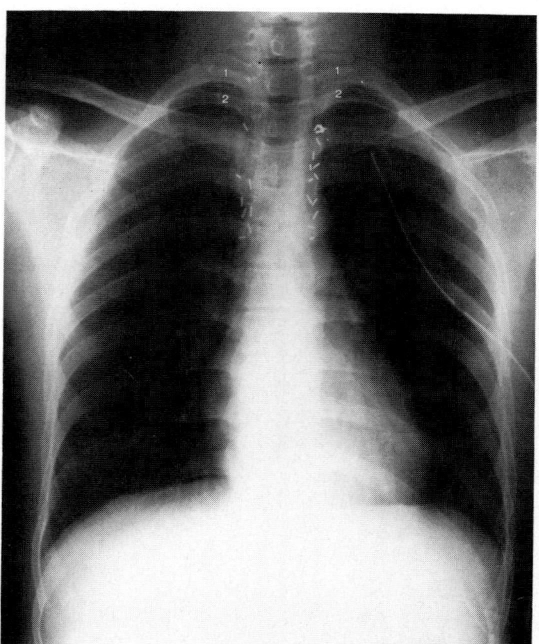

FIGURE 72–6. Chest x-ray study following bilateral axillary sympathectomy. Metallic clips indicate the excised portion of the sympathetic chain. The upper limit appears to be at the level of the third rib, despite a surgically higher level of resection and the development of dry hands clinically (see text).

References

1. Adams DCR, Poskitt KR: Surgical management of primary hyperhidrosis [Letter]. Br J Surg 78:1019, 1991.
2. Adar R, Kurchin A, Zweig A, et al: Palmar hyperhidrosis and its surgical treatment: A report of 100 cases. Ann Surg 186:34, 1977.
3. Atkins HJB: Peraxillary approach to the stellate and upper thoracic sympathetic ganglia. Lancet 2:1152, 1949.
4. Atkins HJB: Sympathectomy by the axillary approach. Lancet 1:538, 1954.
5. Baddeley RM: The place of upper dorsal sympathectomy in the treatment of primary Raynaud's disease. Br J Surg 52:426, 1965.
6. Berguer R, Smit R: Transaxillary sympathectomy (T_2 to T_4), for relief of vasospastic/sympathetic pain of upper extremities. Surgery 89:764, 1981.
7. Birnstingl M: Results of sympathectomy in digital artery disease. Br Med J 2:601, 1967.
8. Buker RH, Cox WA, Scully TJ, et al: Causalgia and transthoracic sympathectomy. Am J Surg 124:724, 1972.
9. Byrne J, Walsh TN, Hederman WP: Endoscopic transthoracic electrocautery of the sympathetic chain for palmar and axillary hyperhidrosis. Br J Surg 77:1046, 1990.
10. Campbell WB, Cooper MJ, Sponsel WE, et al: Transaxillary sympathectomy—Is a one-stage bilateral procedure safe? Br J Surg 69(Suppl):S29, 1982.
11. Coffman JD, Davies WT: Vasospastic disease: A review. Prog Cardiovasc Dis 18:123, 1975.
12. de Takats G: Sympathectomy revisited: Dodo or phoenix? Surgery 78:644, 1975.

13. Fitzpatrick TB, Eisen AZ, Wolff K (eds): Dermatology in General Medicine. 3rd ed. New York, McGraw-Hill, 1986.
14. Flatt AE: Digital artery sympathectomy. J Hand Surg 5:550, 1980.
15. Gifford RW, Hines EA, Craig W: Sympathectomy for Raynaud's phenomenon. Follow-up study of 70 women with Raynaud's disease and 54 women with secondary Raynaud's phenomenon. Circulation 19:5, 1958.
16. Greenhalgh RM, Rosengarten DS, Martin P: Role of sympathectomy for hyperhidrosis. Br Med J 1:332, 1971.
17. Hall KV, Hillestad LK: Raynaud's phenomenon treated with sympathectomy. Angiology 11:186, 1960.
18. Harris RW, Andros G, Dulawa LB, et al: Large-vessel arterial occlusive disease in symptomatic upper extremity. Arch Surg 119:1277, 1984.
19. Haxton H: The technique and results of upper limb sympathectomy. J Cardiovasc Surg 11:27, 1970.
20. Horowitz SH: Iatrogenic causalgia. Classification, clinical findings, and legal ramifications. Arch Neurol 41:821, 1984.
21. Jochimsen PR, Hartfall WG: Per axillary, upper extremity sympathectomy: Technique reviewed and clinical experience. Surgery 71:686, 1972.
22. Johnston ENM, Summerly R, Birnstingl M: Prognosis in Raynaud's phenomenon after sympathectomy. Br Med J 1:962, 1965.
23. Jones NF: Ischemia of the hand in systemic disease: The potential role of microsurgical revascularization and digital sympathectomy. Clin Plast Surg 16:547, 1989.
24. Kao M-C: Video endoscopic sympathectomy using a fiberoptic CO_2 laser to treat palmar hyperhidrosis. Neurosurgery 30:131, 1992.
25. Kennedy WR, Navarro MDX: Sympathetic sudomotor function in diabetic neuropathy. Arch Neurol 46:1182, 1989.
26. Kirno K, Kunimoto M, Lundin S, et al: Can galvanic skin response be used as a quantitative estimate of sympathetic nerve activity in regional anaesthesia? Anesth Analg 73:138, 1991.
27. Kirtley JA, Riddell DH, Stoney WS, et al: Cervicothoracic sympathectomy in neurovascular abnormalities of the upper extremities: Experiences in 76 patients with 104 sympathectomies. Ann Surg 6:869, 1967.
28. Kleinert HE, Cole NM, Wayne L, et al: Post-traumatic sympathetic dystrophy. Orthop Clin North Am 4:917, 1973.
29. Van Rhede van der Kloot EJH, Jörning PJG: Resympathectomy of the upper extremity. Br J Surg 77:1043, 1990.
30. Kux M: Thoracic endoscopic sympathectomy in palmar and axillary hyperhidrosis. Arch Surg 113:264, 1978.
31. Lieshout van JJ, Wieling W, Wesseling KH, et al: Orthostatic hypotension caused by sympathectomies performed for hyperhidrosis. Neth J Med 36:53, 1990.
32. Lin C: A new method of thoracoscopic sympathectomy in hyperhidrosis palmaris. Surg Endosc 4:224, 1990.
33. Lindquist C, Fedorcsak I, Steig P: Electrophysiological aid in high thoracic sympathectomy for palmar hyperhidrosis. Neurosurgery 24:449, 1989.
34. Little JM: Transaxillary transpleural thoracic sympathectomy. *In* Malt RA (ed): Surgical Techniques Illustrated. Boston, Little, Brown, 1977, vol. 2, p 15.
35. Little JM, May J: A comparison of the supraclavicular and axillary approaches to upper thoracic sympathectomy. Aust N Z J Surg 45:143, 1975.
36. Litwin MS: Postsympathectomy neuralgia. Arch Surg 84:591, 1962.
37. Loh L, Nathan PW: Painful peripheral states and sympathetic blocks. J Neurol Neurosurg Psychiatry 41:664, 1978.
38. Lougheed WM: A simple method for upper thoracic sympathectomy in patients requiring sympathectomy of the upper limb. Can J Surg 8:306, 1965.
39. Low PA, Caskey PE, Tuck RR, et al: Quantitative sudomotor axon reflex test in normal and neuropathic subjects. Ann Neurol 14:573, 1983.
40. McCaughan BC, May J: Illumination and access for transaxillary thoracic sympathectomy. Surg Gynecol Obstet 156:507, 1983.
41. MacLeod PM, Tyrrell CJ, Bliss B: Raynaud's phenomenon following cytotoxic chemotherapy successfully managed by dorsal sympathectomy. Eur J Surg Oncol 15:79, 1989.
42. Malone PS, Cameron AEP, Rennie JA: The surgical treatment of upper limb hyperhidrosis. Br J Dermatol 115:81, 1986.
43. Malone PS, Cameron AEP, Rennie JA: Endoscopic thoracic sympathectomy in the treatment of upper limb hyperhidrosis. Ann R Coll Surg Engl 68:93, 1986.
44. Massad M, LoCicero J, Matano J, et al: Endoscopic thoracic sympathectomy: Evaluation of pulsatile laser, non-pulsatile laser, and radiofrequency-generated thermocoagulation. Lasers Surg Med 11:18, 1991.
45. Mattassi R, Miele F, D'Angelo F: Thoracic sympathectomy: Review of indications, results and surgical techniques. J Cardiovasc Surg 22:336, 1981.
46. May J, Harris JP: Upper extremity sympathectomy: A comparison of the supraclavicular and axillary approaches. *In* Bergan JJ, Yao JST (eds): Evaluation and Treatment of Upper and Lower Extremity Circulatory Disorders. Orlando, FL, Grune & Stratton, 1984, p 159.
47. Molho M, Kurchin A, Ohry A, et al: Pulmonary functional abnormalities after upper dorsal sympathectomy. Am Rev Respir Dis 116:879, 1977.
48. Molho M, Shemesh E, Gordon D, et al: Pulmonary functional abnormalities after upper dorsal sympathectomy. A comparison between the supraclavicular and transaxillary approaches. Chest 77:651, 1980.
49. Moran KT, Brady MP: Surgical management of primary hyperhidrosis. Br J Surg 78:279, 1991.
50. Morgan R, Reisman NR, Wilgis EFS: Anatomic localization of sympathetic nerves in the hand. J Hand Surg 8:283, 1982.
51. Moss AJ, McDonald J: Unilateral cervicothoracic sympathetic ganglionectomy for the treatment of long QT interval syndrome. N Engl J Med 285:903, 1971.
52. Olcott C, Eltherington LG, Wilcosky BR, et al: Reflex sympathetic dystrophy—The surgeon's role in management. J Vasc Surg 14:488, 1991.
53. Palumbo LT: Anterior transthoracic approach for upper thoracic sympathectomy. Arch Surg 72:659, 1956.
54. Papa MZ, Schneiderman J, Tucker EBN, et al: Cardiovascular changes after bilateral upper dorsal sympathectomy: Short- and long-term effects. Ann Surg 204:715, 1986.
55. Patman RD, Thompson JE, Persson AV: Management of post-traumatic pain syndromes: Report of 113 cases. Ann Surg 177:780, 1973.
56. Pollak EW: Surgical anatomy of the thoracic outlet syndrome. Surg Gynecol Obstet 150:97, 1980.
57. Porter JM, Rivers SP, Anderson CJ, et al: Evaluation and management of patients with Raynaud's syndrome. Am J Surg 142:183, 1981.
58. Raskin NH, Levinson SA, Hoffman PM, et al: Postsympathectomy neuralgia amelioration with diphenylhydantoin and carbamazepine. Am J Surg 128:75, 1974.
59. Ravitch MM: A Century of Surgery. Philadelphia, JB Lippincott, 1982.
60. Roberts WJ: A hypothesis on the physiological basis for causalgia and related pains. Pain 24:297, 1986.
61. Roos DB: Transaxillary extrapleural thoracic sympathectomy. *In* Bergan JJ, Yao JST (eds): Operative Techniques in Vascular Surgery. New York, Grune & Stratton, 1980, p 115.
62. Rundles RW: Diabetic neuropathy: General review with report of 125 cases. Medicine 24:111, 1945.
63. Rutherford RB: Complications of sympathectomy. *In* Bernhard VM, Towne JB (eds): Complications in Vascular Surgery. 2nd ed. Orlando, FL, Grune & Stratton, 1985, p 69.
64. Salob SP, Atherton DJ, Kiely EM: Thoracic endoscopic sympathectomy for palmar hyperhidrosis in an adolescent female. J R Soc Med 84:114, 1991.
65. Sarkar SD: Assessment of sympathetic denervation following upper dorsal sympathectomy. Br J Clin Pract 22:59, 1968.
66. Satchell PM, Ware S, Barron J, Tuck R: Finger sudorometry and assessment of the sudomotor drive. J Neurosci Meth (In press).
67. Scher LA, Veith FJ, Samson RH, et al: Vascular complications of thoracic outlet syndrome. J Vasc Surg 3:565, 1986.
68. Schwartz PJ, Stone HL: Left stellectomy in the prevention of ventricular fibrillation caused by acute myocardial ischemia in conscious dogs with anterior myocardial infarction. Circulation 62:1256, 1980.
69. Shahani BT, Halperin JJ, Boulu P, Cohen J: Sympathetic skin response: A method of assessing unmyelinated axon dysfunction in peripheral neuropathies. J Neurol Neurosurg Psychiatry 47:536, 1984.
70. Smith CR, Rodeheffer RJ: Treatment of Raynaud's phenomenon with calcium channel blockers. Am J Med 78(Suppl 2B):39, 1985.
71. Smithwick RH: Modified dorsal sympathectomy for vascular spasm (Raynaud's disease) of the upper extremity. Ann Surg 104:339, 1936.

72. Sternberg A, Brickman S, Kott I, et al: Transaxillary thoracic sympathectomy for primary hyperhidrosis of the upper limbs. World J Surg 6:458, 1982.
73. Taylor LM, Baur GM, Porter JM: Finger gangrene caused by small artery occlusive disease. Ann Surg 193:453, 1981.
74. Telford ED: The technique of sympathectomy. Br J Surg 23:448, 1935.
75. Thompson JE: The diagnosis and management of post-traumatic pain syndromes (causalgia). Aust N Z J Surg 49:299, 1979.
76. van de Wal HJCM, Skotnicki SH, Wijn PFF, et al: Thoracic sympathectomy as a therapy for upper extremity ischemia. A long-term follow-up study. Thorac Cardiovasc Surg 33:181, 1985.
77. Vogelzang NJ, Bosl GJ, Johnson K, et al: Raynaud's phenomenon: A common toxicity after combination chemotherapy for testicular cancer. Ann Intern Med 95:288, 1981.
78. Welch E, Geary J: Current status of thoracic dorsal sympathectomy. J Vasc Surg 1:202, 1984.
79. White JC, Smithwick RH, Simeone FA: The Autonomic Nervous System: Anatomy, Physiology and Surgical Application. 3rd ed. New York, Macmillan, 1952.
80. Whitehouse WM, Zelenock GB, Wakefield TW, et al: Arterial bypass grafts for upper extremity ischemia. J Vasc Surg 3:569, 1986.
81. Wilgis EFS: Sympathectomy in the hand. *In* Bergan JJ, Yao JST (eds): Evaluation and Treatment of Upper Extremity and Lower Extremity Circulatory Disorders. Orlando, FL, Grune & Stratton, 1984, p 171.
82. Wilkinson HA: Radiofrequency percutaneous upper-thoracic sympathectomy technique and review of indications. N Engl J Med 311:34, 1984.
83. Wirth FP, Rutherford RB: A civilian experience with causalgia. Arch Surg 100:633, 1970.
84. Wood Jones F: Buchanan's Manual of Anatomy. London, Bailliere, Tindall & Cox, 1953, pp 962, 1152.
85. Zelenock GB, Cronenwett JL, Graham LM, et al: Brachiocephalic arterial occlusions and stenoses. Manifestations and management of complex lesions. Arch Surg 120:370, 1985.

73

Occupational Vascular Problems

James S. T. Yao, M.D., Ph.D.

• • •

Occupational injuries include those caused by work accidents and those caused by cumulative trauma due to the performance of repetitive motions. Injuries in the latter category result from small but additive amounts of tissue damage sustained through the performance of repetitive tasks; they are known collectively as cumulative trauma disorders. According to data released by the US Bureau of Labor Statistics, cumulative trauma disorders account for more than 50 per cent of all occupational illnesses in the United States today.[1] Although most of these injuries are musculoskeletal in origin, injuries to arteries and veins may also occur.[2] These injuries occur because of excessive or exaggerated physical activity induced in a working environment involving the shoulder or hands.

Arterial injuries in the form of occupational trauma include vibration-induced white finger, hypothenar hammer syndrome, electrical burns, acro-osteolysis, and athletic injuries.

VIBRATION-INDUCED WHITE FINGER

The term vibration-induced white finger was favored by the Industrial Injuries Advisory Council in 1970 to describe the occurrence of symptoms somewhat similar to those of Raynaud's disease but caused by exposure to vibration.[3] Other investigators have used the term Raynaud's phenomenon of occupational origin or traumatic vasospastic disease. Regardless of the terminology, the common and presenting symptoms are those of Raynaud's phenomenon owing to the prolonged use of vibrating mechanical tools.

In the very early stages of injury, vibration may cause slight tingling and numbness. Later, the tips of one or more fingers exposed to vibration suffer attacks of blanching, usually precipitated by cold. With continued exposure to vibration, the affected area increases in size and the blanching extends to those fingers exposed to vibration. Attacks of white finger typically last about 1 hour and are terminated with a reactive hyperemia (red flush) and often considerable pain. Prolonged exposure to vibration may induce a blue-black cyanotic appearance in the affected fingers. Only about 1 per cent of the cases progress to ulceration or gangrene.[4] It is well known that hand-held tools, such as pneumatic hammers and drills, grinders, and chain saws, are associated with vibration-induced white finger. The injury is not restricted to the use of a few types of tools but occurs in a variety of situations in which the hands of workers are subjected to significant vibration exposure.[3] Table 73–1 lists the types of tools that commonly cause vibration-induced white finger.

The first cases of this type of injury are usually considered to be those reported in Rome in 1911 by Loriga.[5] Blanching and numbness of the hands after using pneumatic drills was noted by Cottingham in 1918;[6] and subsequent reports by Taylor and Pelmear[7] and Ashe and associates[8] firmly established vibration-induced white finger as

Table 73–1. Tools Associated With Vibration-Induced White Finger

Pneumatic tools
Riveting
Caulking
Drilling
Clinching and flanging
Rotary burring tools
Pneumatic hammers
Chain saws
Grinders
Pedestal
Hand-held
Chipping hammers
Concrete vibrothickener
Concrete-leveling vibrotables

a distinct clinical entity in hand ischemia. According to Taylor and Pelmear,[7] the severity of the disease can be staged into five categories (Table 73–2); this classification has been accepted as a standard by workers in this field. This classification is of particular use in determining the level of compensation in labor disputes.

The exact mechanism of injury is unknown. Repetitive trauma from the vibration of the tool is obviously the main cause of the problem. Both the frequency of the vibration and the intensity of the trauma of the vibrating tool cause damage to the endothelium.[9] Local platelet adhesion appears to be an important factor in causing arterial occlusion. It has been shown that sympathetic hyperactivity in combination with local factors, such as vibration-induced hyperresponsiveness to cold of the digital vessels, may be responsible for finger blanching attacks.[10]

Diagnosis is made from a history of use of vibratory tools and the classic Raynaud's symptoms. For a vasospastic condition, the most promising single objective test is cold provocation with a recording of the recovery of digital temperature. Detection of digital artery occlusion is best achieved by recording the systolic pressure of the affected fingers with the transcutaneous Doppler ultrasound technique[11, 12] or, more recently, with the B-mode scanning technique.[13] In advanced stages of the disease, arteriographic examination is helpful. Barker and Hines first documented arterial occlusion by brachial arteriography in a group of workers with hand blanching and attacks of numbness.[14] Others have reported on the use of arteriography in investigating this injury, including Shatz,[15] Ashe and Williams,[16] and Wegelius.[17]

Arteriographic changes in vibration tool injury are largely confined to the hand. Multiple segmental occlusions of the digits are seen, and a corkscrew formation is sometimes observed.[17] The extent of digital artery occlusion depends on the duration of exposure to the vibratory tool. In advanced cases, occlusion of digital arteries is common. Of 80 workers (chippers) with vibration-induced white finger investigated at the Blood Flow Laboratory at Northwestern University, 25 (28 per cent) had a significant reduction in systolic pressure in one or more digits.[18] In 6 of the 25 workers, arteriography demonstrated occlusion of digital arteries (Fig. 73–1). Incompleteness of the palmar arch was seen not only in the symptomatic hand but also in the contralateral, asymptomatic hand (Fig. 73–2). Seventy-three of 80 workers (91 per cent) had symptoms of Raynaud's phenomenon. Forty-two (52 per cent) experienced bilateral symptoms, and 31 (37 per cent) had unilateral symptoms.

Treatment of vibration-induced white finger consists of symptomatic relief of Raynaud's symptoms. Surgical treatment is rarely indicated or needed. The most important step is to discontinue the use of the vibratory tool with job change or rotation. In most instances, prevention is more effective than cure. Factories should conform to acceptable standards as suggested by the American Conference of Governmental Industrial Hygienists in 1984[19] and perhaps develop automation to eliminate the human element in the working process. In advanced cases, a calcium channel blocker such as nifedipine (30 to 80 mg daily) may be useful. Calcium antagonists inhibit the response of arterial smooth muscle to noradrenalin and are reported to be effective.[20]

HYPOTHENAR HAMMER SYNDROME

The predisposing factor in the development of hypothenar hammer syndrome is the repetitive use of the palm

Table 73–2. Stages of Vibration-Induced White Finger

Stage	Condition of Digits	Work and Social Interference
0	Vibration exposed but no signs or symptoms	No complaints
0_T	Intermittent tingling	No interference with activities
0_N	Intermittent numbness	No interference with activities
1	Blanching of one or more fingertips with or without tingling and numbness	No interference with activities
2	Blanching of one or more fingers with numbness; usually confined to winter	Slight interference with home and social activities; no interference at work
3	Extensive blanching; frequent episodes in summer as well as winter	Definite interference at work, at home, and with social activities; restriction of hobbies
4	Same as 3: extensive blanching; most fingers; frequent episodes in summer and winter	Same as 3, but occupation changed to avoid further vibration exposures because of the severity of signs and symptoms

Updated from Taylor W, Pelmear PL (eds): Vibration White Finger in Industry. New York, Academic Press, 1975.

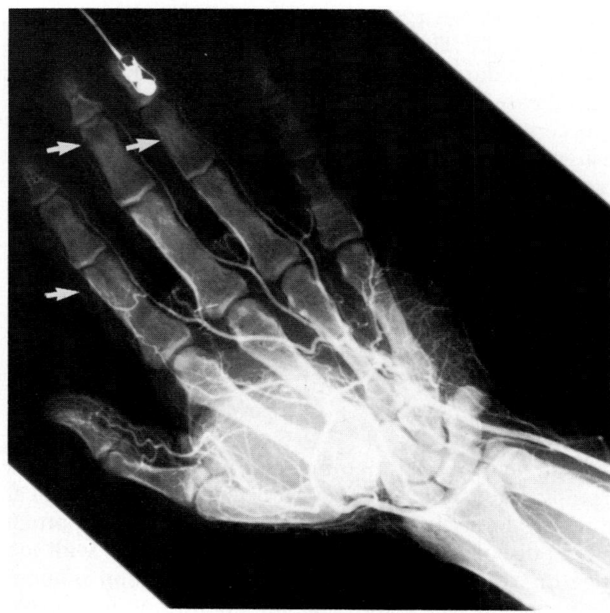

FIGURE 73–1. Arteriogram of the hand in a vibratory tool worker. There is occlusion of the digital arteries in the second, third, and fourth fingers *(arrows)*.

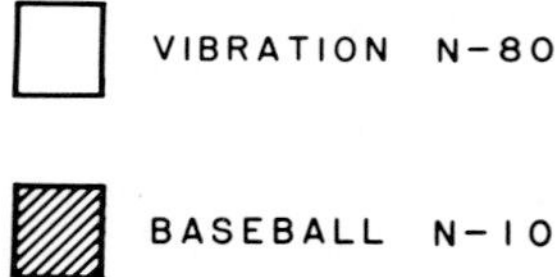

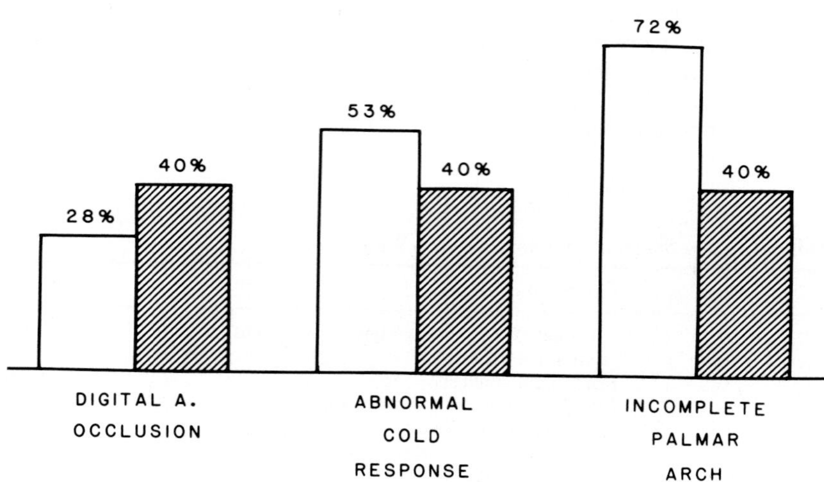

FIGURE 73–2. Incidence of abnormal cold response, digital artery occlusion, and incomplete palmar arch by Doppler examination in vibratory tool workers and baseball players. (From Bartel P, Blackburn D, Peterson L, et al: The value of non-invasive tests in occupational trauma of the hands and fingers. Bruit 8:15, 1984. Reproduced with permission.)

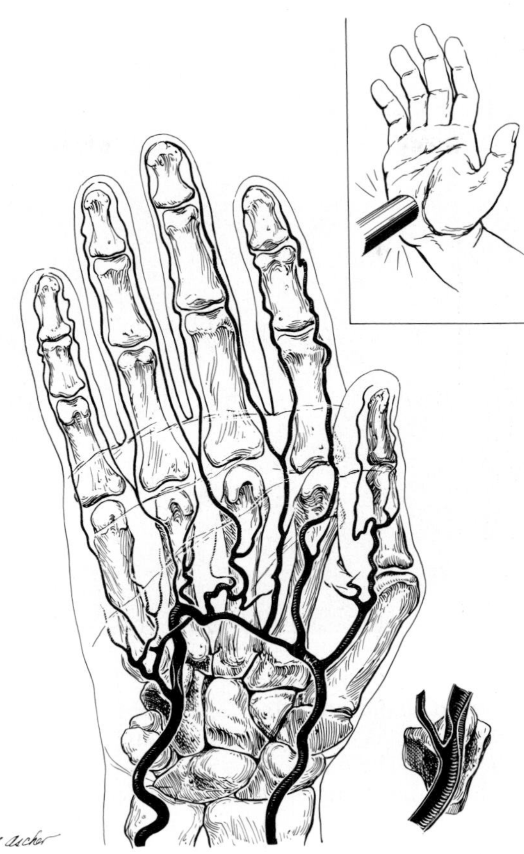

FIGURE 73–3. Mechanism of ulnar artery injury in a patient with hypothenar hammer syndrome. The terminal branch of the ulnar artery is vulnerable to injury because of its close proximity to the hamate bone *(inset)*.

of the hand in activity that involves pushing, pounding, or twisting. The anatomic location of the ulnar artery in the area of the hypothenar eminence places it in a vulnerable position. The terminal branches of the ulnar artery (deep palmar branch and superficial arch) arise in a groove called Guyon's tunnel, which is bounded medially by the pisiform and the hook of the hamate and dorsally by the transverse carpal ligament. Over a distance of 2 cm, the ulnar artery lies quite superficially in the palm, being covered only by skin, subcutaneous tissue, and the palmaris brevis muscle (Fig. 73–3). When this area is repeatedly traumatized, ulnar or digital arterial spasm, aneurysm formation, occlusion, or a combination of these lesions can result. Embolization from an aneurysm may cause multiple digital artery occlusions distally. The type of arterial abnormality observed will often depend on the nature of the damage to the vessel. Thus, intimal damage often results in thrombotic occlusion (Fig. 73–4), whereas injury to media causes palmar aneurysms (Fig. 73–5).[21, 22] This type of occupational injury has been called the hypothenar hammer syndrome.[23] In 1934, Von Rosen provided the first descriptive report of this condition,[24] and only recently has this condition been recognized as an occupational disease.[25] Table 73–3 lists the types of workers who developed this syndrome in reported series.[26] Of 79 workers who habitually used the hand as a hammer, Little and Ferguson found that 11 (14 per cent) showed evidence of ulnar artery occlusion in one or both hands.[27]

Clinically, the patient presents with symptoms of Raynaud's phenomenon, namely numbness, paresthesias, stiffness, coldness, and blanching of one or more digits of the dominant hand. In the series of patients described by Conn and colleagues, the ring finger was most commonly involved.[23] The traditional triphasic color (white-blue-red) changes and thumb involvement are uncommon.[26] Physical examination may disclose a prominent callus over the hypothenar eminence, coldness, or mottling of the involved fingertip, along with atrophic ulceration. A positive Allen

Table 73–3. Type of Employment in 33 Patients With Hypothenar Hammer Syndrome

Mechanic/auto repair	15
Lathe operator	3
Fitter and turner	2
Tire braider	2
Carpenter	2
Engineer	2
Machinist	2
Painter	1
Butcher	1
Gardener	1
Tool and die worker	1
Bus conductor	1

Modified from Pineda CJ, Weisman MH, Bookstein JJ, et al: Hypothenar hammer syndrome: Form of reversible Raynaud's phenomenon. Am J Med 79:561, 1985.

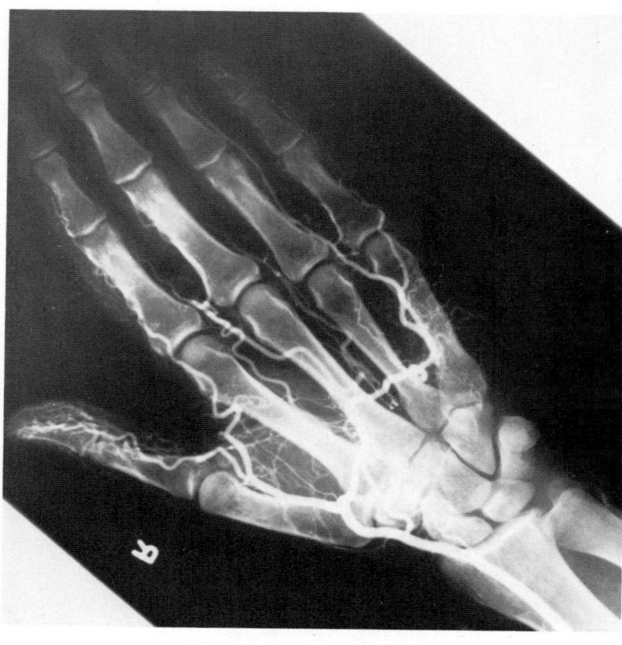

FIGURE 73–4. Occlusion of the ulnar artery in the palm of a patient with hypothenar hammer syndrome.

test result, indicating ulnar artery occlusion, is common. Occasionally, an aneurysm can be found as a pulsatile mass in the palm. The diagnosis is made by a history of trauma and presenting symptoms and can be confirmed by a noninvasive test. B-mode scanning is of particular value in detecting ulnar aneurysms. Arteriography is helpful both in the diagnosis of hypothenar hammer syndrome and in planning treatment. Arteriographic examination defines the type of vascular lesion (spasm, aneurysm, or occlusion), localizes its site and extent, and demonstrates the presence of significant collateral vessels. Not infrequently, an incomplete superficial palmar arch is seen in these patients, even in the asymptomatic hand.

Treatment of ulnar artery occlusion is often supportive,

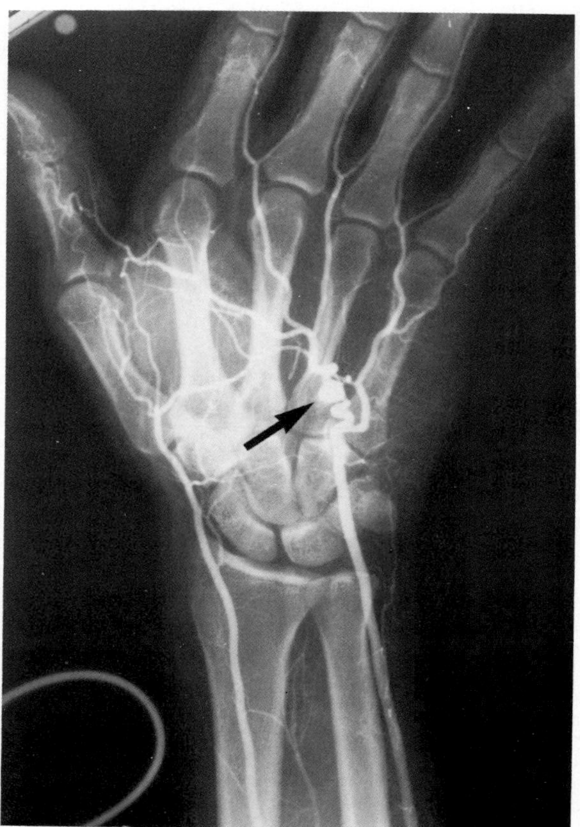

FIGURE 73–5. Arteriogram of the hand in a carpenter. Note the aneurysm of the ulnar artery *(arrow)* because of repetitive trauma from using the hand as a hammer.

and surgical intervention is seldom needed or possible. Aneurysm of the ulnar artery should be resected to eliminate the source of emboli and can be treated by resection of the aneurysm with end-to-end anastomosis of the artery or by an interposed vein graft. Satisfactory long-term results with this approach have been reported by Vayssairat and coworkers.[28]

OCCUPATIONAL ACRO-OSTEOLYSIS

Occupational acro-osteolysis was first described by Wilson and colleagues in workers exposed to polyvinylchloride.[29] Many of these people present with ischemic symptoms in the hand. Interestingly, they develop resorption of the distal phalangeal tufts similar to that seen with scleroderma. Once again, the dominant presenting symptoms are of Raynaud's phenomenon. Few reports of angiography in this syndrome have been published to document damage to the digital arteries.[30–32] The findings include multiple arterial stenoses and occlusions of the digital arteries, along with nonspecific hypervascularity adjacent to the areas of bony resorption. The reason for the hypervascularity is not clear, but it may be related to stasis of contrast in digital pulp arteries secondary to shortening and retraction of the fingers. Some of the digits in these patients were clubbed, a finding that has also been associated with hypervascularity in the fingertips.

ELECTRICAL BURNS

Electrical burns inflict their tissue destruction in relation to the voltage applied. Currents of less than 1000 volts cause injuries limited to the immediate underlying skin and soft tissues. High voltage (more than 1000 volts) usually causes extensive damage as it travels from the point of entrance to the point of exit. No tissue is immune to the devastating effects of high-voltage injury, and arterial injury may occur. The upper extremity, especially the hand because of its grasping function, is more commonly involved than other parts of the body. The arterial injury is often manifested by arterial necrosis with thrombus or bleeding, occasionally producing gangrenous digits. Bookstein described the angiographic changes in the upper extremity following electrical injury.[30] The findings include extensive occlusion of the ulnar and digital arteries and thrombosis of the radial artery. Arterial spasm may also be present. In late follow-up, damage of the media may cause aneurysm formation. Figure 73–6 shows a brachial artery aneurysm in a patient who had suffered electrical burns 9 months previously. Treatment depends on the associated soft tissue and bone injury. Major artery occlusion docu-

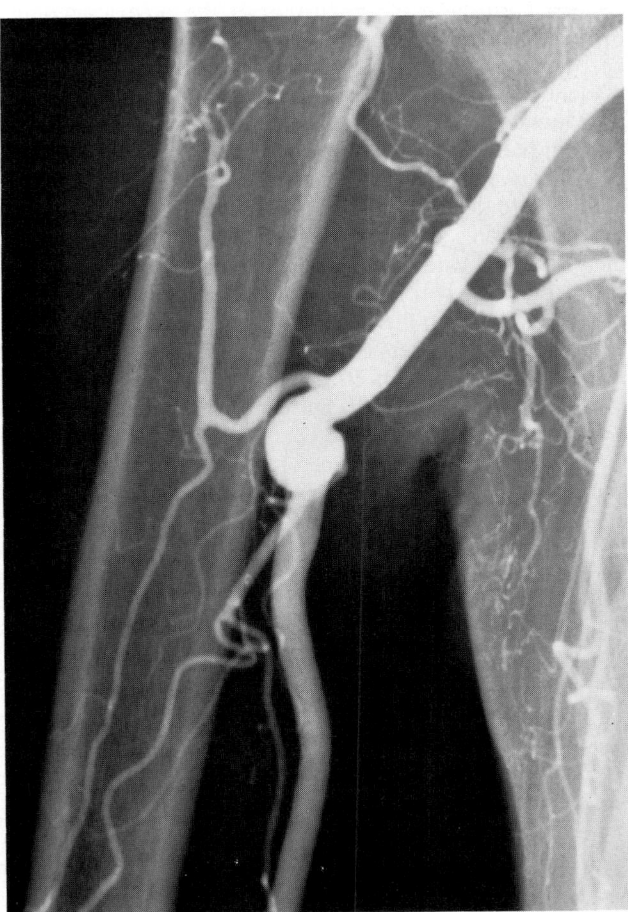

FIGURE 73–6. Aneurysm of the brachial artery in an electrician who had suffered a high-voltage electrical burn 9 months previously.

mented by arteriography requires bypass grafting, and good results have been reported.[33]

ATHLETIC INJURIES

Athletes, particularly professional players who engage in excessive or exaggerated hand or shoulder activity, may develop hand or upper extremity ischemia as a result of arterial injury. Hand ischemia is often manifested by Raynaud's phenomenon or symptoms of sudden arterial occlusion. Two types of arterial injuries are common: hand ischemia and thoracic outlet compression of the subclavian-axillary artery. The exact incidence is unknown; however, vascular injury has been reported in professional or competitive players engaged in athletic activities such as baseball, karate, volleyball, handball, Frisbee, lacrosse, weight-lifting, and butterfly swimming.[18, 26, 34–37]

Hand Ischemia

Repetitive trauma is the main cause of hand ischemia, and injuries to the digital arteries can occur in hypothenar hammer syndrome or with sudden occlusion of the radial or ulnar arteries. Nearly all hand activity involved in any sport may cause injury to the arteries because of blunt force. Hand ischemia, however, is more commonly seen in handball players, baseball catchers, and karate players. Figure 73–7 illustrates an occlusion of the palmar arch in a Frisbee player; sudden ischemia of all fingers occurred after he caught the Frisbee. It has been suggested that handball players with more than 200 hours of accumulated playing time are at greater risk for developing a symptomatic alteration in perfusion.[38, 39]

Professional baseball players, particularly the catchers, are likely to develop chronic hand ischemia. Many catchers have symptoms of Raynaud's phenomenon, especially in the off-season when they are engaged in outdoor activity in cool autumn or winter weather. Lowrey reported decreased digital perfusion to the index finger of the glove hand in 13 of 22 baseball catchers examined by Doppler flow detector and the Allen test.[40] Of 10 professional catchers studied in the author's laboratory, 40 per cent had evidence of digital artery occlusion (see Fig. 73–2).[18] Considering the speed of the baseball and the impact of the force exerted on the hands, perhaps arterial injury in professional baseball catchers occurs more frequently than expected.

Treatment of hand ischemia depends on the mode of presentation. In acute injury, a conservative approach using dextran 40 infusion and control of pain is the choice. Surgical intervention is rarely needed. Once again, prevention of injury is important and can be accomplished by the use of gloves with padding or other protective devices.[40]

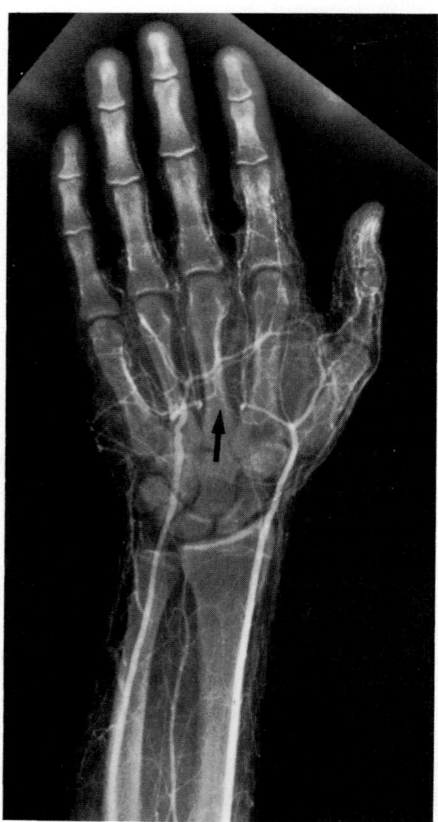

FIGURE 73–7. Occlusion of the palmar arch *(arrow)* in a Frisbee player. Because of the injury, there is poor filling of the contrast media in the second, third, fourth, and fifth fingers.

Thoracic Outlet Compression

Athletes who engage in overextended shoulder motion, such as baseball pitchers, butterfly swimmers, weight-lifters, and oarsmen, are potential candidates for thoracic outlet compression. Injuries to the subclavian artery or vein have been reported in these athletes. In professional baseball pitchers, the injury is most likely due to the violent throwing motion. The pitching mechanism consists of five phases: (1) wind-up, (2) cocking, (3) acceleration, (4) release and deceleration, and (5) follow-through. Most injuries occur during the acceleration and deceleration phases.[41] It has been estimated that the fast ball creates 600 inch-pounds of forward momentum at ball release; it is understandable that soft tissue injury may occur because of the force absorbed by the shoulder and the elbow.[42]

Symptoms are more common in pitchers whose throwing motion is overhand rather than sidearm. Symptoms are pain in the region of the elbow, with easy fatigue and loss of velocity after several innings of pitching. Raynaud's phenomenon has also been observed in these pitchers. Diagnosis is often difficult, and a complete evaluation by an orthopedic surgeon to rule out musculoskeletal abnormalities is mandatory. The use of duplex scanning and transcutaneous Doppler flow detection in pitching position helps to detect compression of the subclavian or axillary artery. Finally, definitive diagnosis is established by arteriography (Figs. 73–8 and 73–9).

Arterial injury in the pitching arm includes the subclavian artery,[35] the axillary artery,[34] and the posterior humeral circumflex artery.[43] Compression to the subclavian or axil-

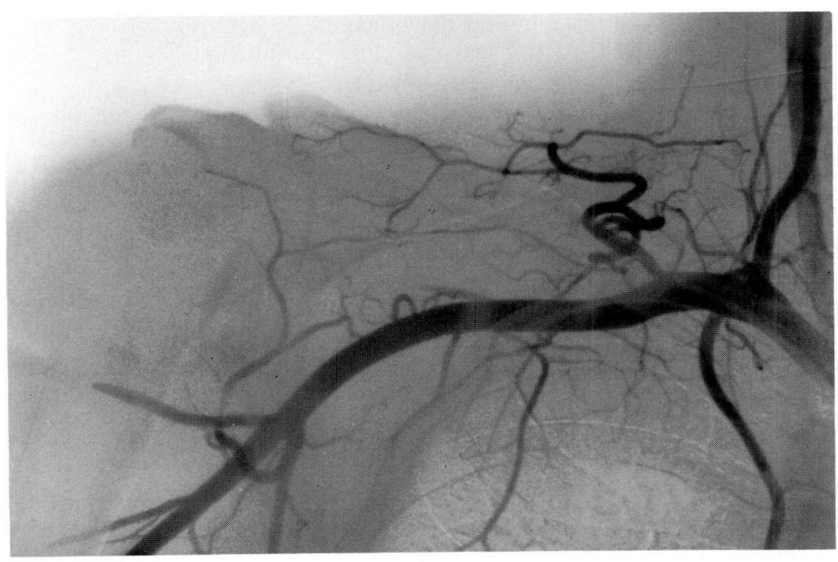

FIGURE 73–8. Arteriogram of the right subclavian artery in a professional baseball pitcher. No injury is seen when the arm is placed in neutral position.

lary artery is often due to hypertrophy of the anterior scalene muscle or the pectoralis minor muscle. In 1964, Cooley and colleagues were the first to report an axillary artery thrombus owing to pectoralis minor compression in a major league pitcher.[34] In 1978, Strukel and Garrick reported on three competitive baseball pitchers who suffered from thoracic outlet compression.[44] Until Fields' report on athletic injury in the thoracic outlet, the injury had received little attention.[45] The report by Fields and associates on a major league pitcher who suffered a catastrophic complication of stroke resulting from subclavian artery thrombosis is of great interest.[35]

Not only the main trunk of the subclavian-axillary artery is subjected to compression. Cahill and Palmer described the quadrilateral space syndrome; compression of the posterior humeral circumflex artery or nerve occurred in the quadrilateral space in 18 patients.[43] Additionally, aneurysm formation of the circumflex artery due to repetitive athletic activities has been reported.[46]

It has been recognized that the head of the humerus can cause compression to the axillary artery. As a result of repetitive compression, damage of the axillary artery causing a thromboembolic phenomenon has been reported in baseball pitchers.[47, 48]

In addition to arterial injury, thrombosis of the subclavian-axillary vein, the so-called effort thrombosis, has been reported in baseball pitchers,[49] weightlifters,[50] and competitive swimmers.[51]

Treatment depends on the extent of injury. Compression only is best treated by division of the offending muscle and tendon. Occlusion of a major artery requires bypass grafting together with decompression of the thoracic outlet. Venous thrombosis is best treated with heparin and standard anticoagulation therapy. Injury requires cessation of athletic

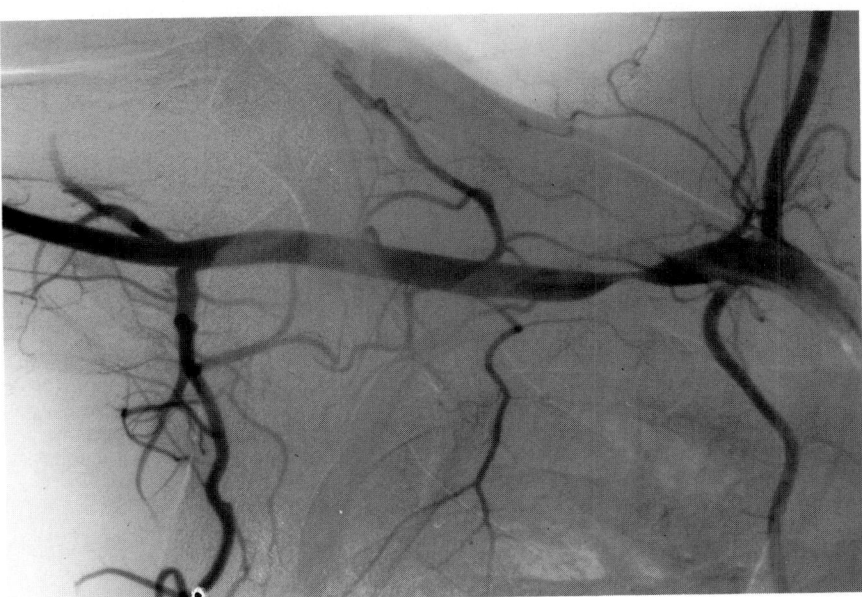

FIGURE 73–9. In the same patient shown in Figure 73–8, there is compression of the subclavian artery when the arm is placed in the pitching position (hyperabduction).

activity, with careful planning for rehabilitation. To return a professional athlete to full activity, close consultation with a trainer or sports medicine specialist is necessary.

References

1. Bureau of Labor Statistics Reports on Survey of Occupational Injuries and Illness in 1977–1989. Washington, DC, Bureau of Labor Statistics, US Department of Labor, 1990.
2. Rempel DM, Harrison RJ, Barnhart S: Work-related cumulative trauma disorders of the upper extremity. JAMA 267:838, 1992.
3. Griffin MJ: Vibration injuries of the hand and arm: Their occurrence and the evolution of standards and limits. London, Her Majesty's Stationery Office, 1980.
4. Yodaiken RE, Jones E, Kunicki R: The Raynaud phenomenon of occupational origin. *In* Altura BM, Davis E (eds): Advances in Microcirculation. Basel, Karger, 1985, vol. 12, pp 6–33.
5. Loriga G: Ill lavoro con i martelli pneumatic boll. Ispett Lavoro 2:35, 1911.
6. Cottingham CE: Effects of use of air hammer on hands of Indiana stone cutters [Bulletin]. US Bureau of Labor Statistics 19:125, 1918.
7. Taylor W, Pelmear PL (eds): Vibration White Finger in Industry. New York, Academic Press, 1975.
8. Ashe WF, Cook WT, Old JW: Raynaud's phenomenon of occupational origin. Arch Environ Health 5:63, 1962.
9. Newem RM: Vibration-induced arterial shear stress: The relationship to Raynaud's phenomenon of occupational origin. Arch Environ Health 26:105, 1973.
10. Bovenzi M: Some pathophysiological aspects of vibration-induced white finger. Eur J Appl Physiol 55:381, 1986.
11. Pearce WH, Yao JST, Bergan JJ: Noninvasive vascular diagnostic testing. *In* Ravitch MM (ed): Current Problems in Surgery. Chicago, Year Book Medical Publishers, 1983, vol. 20.
12. Sumner DS: Vascular laboratory diagnosis and assessment of upper extremity vascular disorders. *In* Machleder HI (ed): Vascular Disorders of the Upper Extremity. New York, Futura Publishing Company, 1983, pp 1–47.
13. Payne KM, Blackburn DR, Peterson LK, et al: B-mode imaging of the arteries of the hand and upper extremity. Bruit 10:168, 1986.
14. Barker NW, Hines EA Jr: Arterial occlusion in the hands and fingers associated with repeated occupational trauma. Mayo Clin Proc 19:345, 1944.
15. Shatz IJ: Occlusive arterial disease in the hand due to occupational trauma. N Engl J Med 268:281, 1963.
16. Ashe WF, Williams N: Occupational Raynaud's. II. Further studies of this disorder in uranium mine workers. Arch Environ Health 9:425, 1964.
17. Wegelius U: Angiography of the hand: Clinical and postmortem investigations. Acta Radiol [Diag] (Stockh) 315 (Suppl):1, 1972.
18. Bartel P, Blackburn D, Peterson L, et al: The value of noninvasive tests in occupational trauma of the hands and fingers. Bruit 8:15, 1984.
19. Threshold limit values approved by ACGIH for hand-arm vibration. Noise Regulation Reporter 11:3, 1984.
20. Kahan A, Amor B, Menkes CJ: Nifedipine and allied substances in the treatment of Raynaud's phenomenon. *In* Altura BM, Davis E (eds): Advances in Microcirculation. Basel, Karger, 1985, vol. 12, pp 95–104.
21. Kleinert HE, Burget GC, Morgan JA, et al: Aneurysms of the hand. Arch Surg 106:554, 1973.
22. Kleinert HE, Volianitis GJ: Thrombosis of the palmar arterial arch and its tributaries: Etiology and new concepts in treatment. J Trauma 5:447, 1965.
23. Conn J, Bergan JJ, Bell JL: Hypothenar hammer syndrome: Post-traumatic digital ischemia. Surgery 68:1122, 1970.
24. Von Rosen S: Ein Fall von Thrombose in der Arteria ulnaris nach Einwirkung von stumpfer Gewalt. Acta Chir Scand 73:500, 1934.
25. Short DW: Occupational aneurysm of the palmar arch. Lancet 2:217, 1948.
26. Pineda CJ, Weisman MH, Bookstein JJ, et al: Hypothenar hammer syndrome: Form of reversible Raynaud's phenomenon. Am J Med 79:561, 1985.
27. Little JM, Ferguson DA: The incidence of the hypothenar hammer syndrome. Arch Surg 105:684, 1972.
28. Vayssairat M, Debure C, Cormier J, et al: Hypothenar hammer syndrome: Seventeen cases with long-term follow-up. J Vasc Surg 5:838, 1987.
29. Wilson R, McCormick W, Tattum C, et al: Occupational acro-osteolysis. JAMA 201:577, 1967.
30. Bookstein JJ: Arteriography. *In* Poznanski AK (ed): The Hand in Radiologic Diagnosis With Gamuts and Pattern Profiles. 2nd ed. Philadelphia, WB Saunders, 1984, vol. 1, pp 97–112.
31. Veltman G: Raynaud's syndrome in vinylchloride disease. *In* Heidrich H (ed): Raynaud's Phenomenon. Berlin, TM-Verlag, 1979, pp 211–216.
32. Falappa P, Magnavita N, Bergamaschi A, et al: Angiographic study of digital arteries in workers exposed to vinyl chloride. Br J Ind Med 39:169, 1982.
33. Wang X, Roberts BB, Zapata-Sirvent RL, et al: Early vascular grafting to prevent upper extremity necrosis after electrical burns: Commentary on indications for surgery. Burns 11:359, 1985.
34. Tullos HS, Erwin WD, Woods GW, et al: Unusual lesions of the pitching arm. Clin Orthop 88:169, 1972.
35. Fields WS, Lemak NA, Ben-Menachem Y: Thoracic outlet syndrome: Review and reference to stroke in a major league pitcher. AJNR 7:73, 1986.
36. Green DP: True and false traumatic aneurysms in the hand: Report of two cases and review of the literature. J Bone Joint Surg 55A:120, 1973.
37. Ho PK, Dellon AL, Wilgis EFS: True aneurysms of the hand resulting from athletic injury: Report of two cases. Am J Sports Med 13:136, 1985.
38. Buckhout BC, Warner MA: Digital perfusion of handball players: Effects of repeated ball impact on structures of the hand. Am J Sports Med 8:206, 1980.
39. McCue FC III, Miller GA: Soft-tissue injuries to the hand. *In* Pettrone FA (ed): Upper Extremity Injuries in Athletes. St. Louis, CV Mosby, 1986, pp 85–94.
40. Lowrey CW: Digital vessel trauma from repetitive impacts in baseball catchers. J Hand Surg 1:236, 1976.
41. McLeod WD: The pitching mechanism. *In* Zarins B, Andrews JR, Carson WG Jr (eds): Injuries to the Throwing Arm. Philadelphia, WB Saunders, 1985, pp 22–29.
42. Sain J, Andrews JR: Proper pitching techniques. *In* Zarins B, Andrews JR, Carson WG Jr (eds): Injuries to the Throwing Arm. Philadelphia, WB Saunders, 1985, pp 34–36.
43. Cahill B, Palmer R: Quadrilateral space syndrome. J Hand Surg 8:65, 1983.
44. Strukel RJ, Garrick JG: Thoracic outlet compression in athletes: A report of four cases. Am J Sports Med 6:35, 1978.
45. Fields WS: Neurovascular syndromes of the neck and shoulders. Semin Neurol 1:301, 1981.
46. Nijhuis HHAM, Muller-Wiefel H: Occlusion of the brachial artery by thrombus dislodged from a traumatic aneurysm of the anterior humeral circumflex artery. J Vasc Surg 13:408, 1991.
47. McCarthy WJ, Yao JST, Schafer MF, et al: Upper extremity arterial injury in athletes. J Vasc Surg 9:317, 1989.
48. Rohrer MJ, Cardullo PA, Pappas AM, et al: Axillary artery compression and thrombosis in throwing athletes. J Vasc Surg 11:761, 1990.
49. Dale WA: Thoracic outlet compression syndrome. *In* Management of Vascular Surgical Problems. New York, McGraw-Hill, 1985, pp 562–587.
50. Baker CL, Thornberry R: Neurovascular syndromes. *In* Zarins B, Andrews JR, Carson WG Jr (eds): Injuries to the Throwing Arm. Philadelphia, WB Saunders, 1985, pp 176–188.
51. Vogel CM, Jensen JE: "Effort" thrombosis of the subclavian vein in a competitive swimmer. Am J Sports Med 13:269, 1985.

INDEX

Note: Page numbers in *italics* refer to illustrations; page numbers followed by t refer to tables.

ISBN 0-7216-3837-6

90038

9 780721 638379